*Tenth Edition* — *Volume II*

Davis — Christopher

# TEXTBOOK
# OF
# SURGERY

## THE BIOLOGICAL BASIS OF
## MODERN SURGICAL PRACTICE

*Edited by*

## DAVID C. SABISTON, Jr., M.D.

James B. Duke Professor and Chairman,
Department of Surgery,
Duke University Medical Center
Durham, North Carolina

W. B. SAUNDERS COMPANY PHILADELPHIA • LONDON • TORONTO

W. B. Saunders Company: West Washington Square
Philadelphia, Pa.   19105

12 Dyott Street
London, WC1A   1DB

833 Oxford Street
Toronto 18, Ontario

Listed here is the latest translated edition of this book together with the language of the translation and the publisher.
Portuguese (9th Edition) — Editora Guanabara Koogan, Rio de Janeiro, Brazil
Spanish (9th Edition) — Editorial Interamericana, Mexico

Davis-Christopher TEXTBOOK OF SURGERY

Vol. I  ISBN  0-7216-7866-1
Vol. II ISBN  0-7216-7867-x

Print No.:    9    8    7    6    5    4    3    2

# CONTENTS

## VOLUME I

# VOLUME II

## 57

## INDEX

# 33

# THE LIVER

*Marshall J. Orloff, M.D.*

## ANATOMY

### Embryology

The liver arises from the entoderm of the foregut and the mesoderm of the septum transversum (Fig. 1). In the 2.5 mm. embryo, approximately 4 weeks old, a diverticulum develops from the ventral floor of the foregut at the level of the future duodenum and extends into the septum transversum in close association with a capillary plexus that connects to the vitelline veins from the yolk sac. The caudal portion of the diverticulum develops into the cystic duct and gallbladder, and the cranial portion becomes the liver. In the early embryo, the two vitelline veins pass through the hepatic anlage to enter the sinus venosus of the heart in conjunction with the paired umbilical veins from the placenta. At a later stage, the vitelline veins form the portal vein and the hepatic veins, whereas the left umbilical vein becomes the ductus venosus which largely bypasses the liver and shunts oxygenated placental blood directly into the inferior vena cava. At birth, the ductus venosus closes and along with the remainder of the obliterated left umbilical vein becomes the ligamentum venosum and its continuation, the ligamentum teres hepatis, in the caudal free border of the falciform ligament, which connects the liver to the umbilicus and anterior body wall. In the adult, it is possible to catheterize the portal vein for diagnostic studies by surgically reopening the obliterated left umbilical vein through a small incision adjacent to the umbilicus. The other ligamentous attachments of the liver are derived from the two layers of the ventral mesentery between which the hepatic anlage develops. Table 1 shows the adult structures derived from the embryonic blood vessels and mesentery.

**TABLE 1** ADULT LIVER STRUCTURES DERIVED FROM EMBRYONIC BLOOD VESSELS AND MESENTERY

| Embryo | Adult |
|---|---|
| Right and left vitelline veins | Portal vein<br>Hepatic veins |
| Left umbilical vein, ductus venosus | Ligamentum venosum and ligamentum teres hepatis |
| Anterior portion of ventral mesentery | Falciform ligament<br>Right and left anterior coronary ligaments<br>Right and left triangular ligaments |
| Posterior portion of ventral mesentery | Gastrohepatic ligament<br>Hepatoduodenal ligament<br>Right and left posterior coronary ligaments<br>Right and left triangular ligaments |

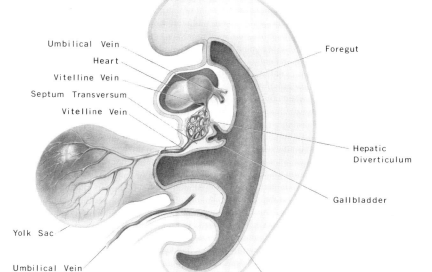

**Figure 1** Embryology of the liver shown in an embryo of approximately 4 mm.

Umbilical Vein
Heart
Vitelline Vein
Septum Transversum
Vitelline Vein
Yolk Sac
Umbilical Vein
Foregut
Hepatic Diverticulum
Gallbladder
Hindgut

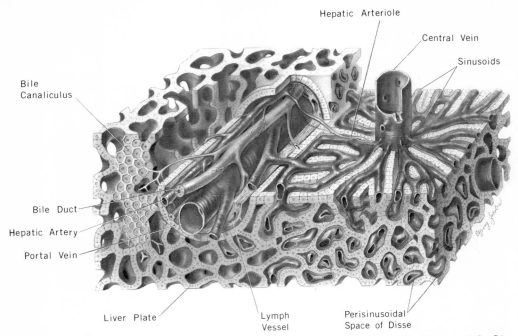

**Figure 2**   Three-dimensional model of liver. (After Elias, H., and Sherrick, J. C.: Morphology of the Liver. New York, Academic Press, 1969.)

## Microscopic Anatomy

The liver is covered by a thick capsule of collagen and elastic tissue, called Glisson's capsule, which extends into the parenchyma along the blood vessels and bile ducts. The capsule encases a spongelike mass of cells arranged in plates through which passes an intricate system of capillaries called sinusoids (Fig. 2). The sinusoids differ from ordinary capillaries in that their endothelial lining is made up of specialized phagocytic cells, the *Kupffer cells,* and they are more permeable to macromolecules than are systemic capillaries. The liver cell plates are one cell thick and have an intimate association with the sinusoids to facilitate maximal exchange of nutrients and products of metabolism. On microscopic examination the hepatic parenchyma appears to be distributed in poorly defined lobules (Fig. 3). At the center of each lobule is a central vein, a tributary of the hepatic venous outflow system that carries blood from the liver toward the heart. The central veins drain into progressively enlarging sublobular veins and intrahepatic veins until connections are made with the major hepatic veins that enter the inferior vena cava. At the periphery, between several lobules, is a collection of connective tissue called a portal tract or triad which contains branches of the portal vein, the hepatic artery, and the bile duct (Fig. 3). The branches of both the portal vein and hepatic artery empty directly into the sinusoids after a series of divisions and ramifications. In addition, the branches of the hepatic artery nourish the structures in the portal tracts. The bile duct system originates as fine bile canaliculi

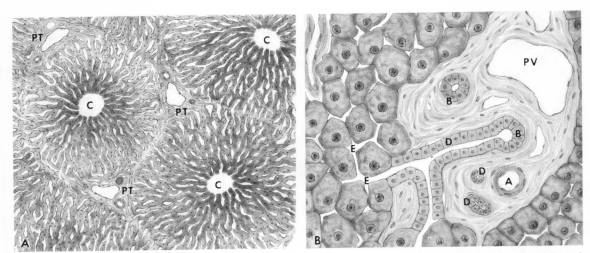

**Figure 3**   Microscopic appearance of normal liver, showing (*A*) lobular pattern and (*B*) components of portal triad. A, Hepatic artery; B, bile duct; C, central vein; D, bile ductule; E, bile canaliculi; PT, portal triad; PV, portal vein.

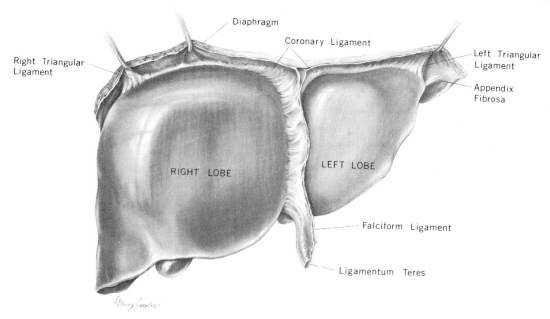

**Figure 4**  Ligaments of the liver.

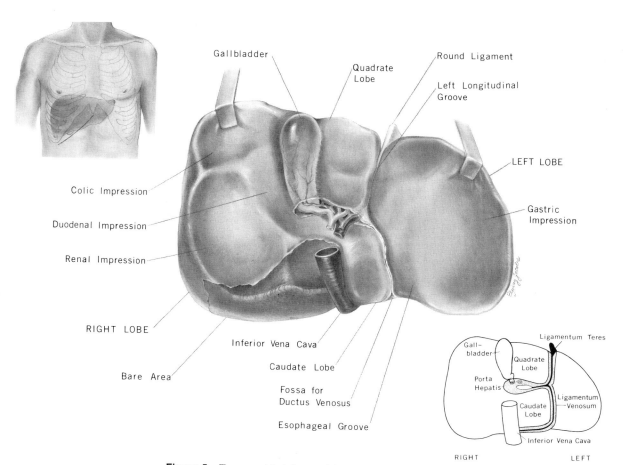

**Figure 5**  Topographic lobes and impressions of the liver.

located between the hepatic cells and forming a part of the cell membrane. Bile is secreted by the hepatocytes into the canaliculi. These bile capillaries drain into intralobular ductules and then into large bile ducts in the portal tracts.

### Gross Anatomy

**Topography.**    The liver is the largest organ in the body with a weight of from 1200 to 1600 gm. It occupies the right hypochondrium and much of the epigastrium and extends into the left hypochondrium. Its superior surface conforms to the under surface of the diaphragm and its inferior surface rests on the viscera in the upper abdomen. It is held in position mainly by intra-abdominal pressure. Except in the epigastrium, the organ is largely surrounded by the thoracic cage and in normal subjects usually cannot be palpated on physical examination. When the body is supine, the upper border of the liver is located between the levels of the fourth and fifth ribs anteriorly on the right, and at the level of the sixth rib anteriorly on the left. In the midaxillary line, the right lobe of the liver is covered by lung, pleura, and diaphragm down to the level of the eighth rib (dullness to percussion), and by the pleura and diaphragm alone between the eighth and tenth ribs (flatness to percussion).

The under surface of the liver is in contact with the duodenum, colon, kidney, and adrenal gland on the right, and with the esophagus and stomach on the left (see Fig. 5). The liver is covered by peritoneum except for an area on the posterior superior surface adjacent to the inferior vena cava which is in direct contact with the diaphragm and is called the bare area.

**Ligaments.**    The peritoneal reflections from the anterior abdominal wall, diaphragm, and abdominal viscera to the liver form 10 distinct ligaments (Fig. 4). These are:

1. The falciform ligament, which attaches the liver to the anterior abdominal wall between the diaphragm and umbilicus.

2. The ligamentum teres hepatis, which occupies the lower free border of the falciform ligament and represents the obliterated left umbilical vein.

3 and 4. The gastrohepatic ligament and hepatoduodenal ligament, which are the portions of the lesser omentum extending to the liver from the lesser curvature of the stomach and the proximal duodenum. These ligaments contain the hepatic artery, portal vein, and common bile duct. The hepatoduodenal ligament forms the anterior boundary of the epiploic foramen of Winslow.

5, 6, 7, and 8. The right and left anterior coronary ligaments and the right and left posterior coronary liga-

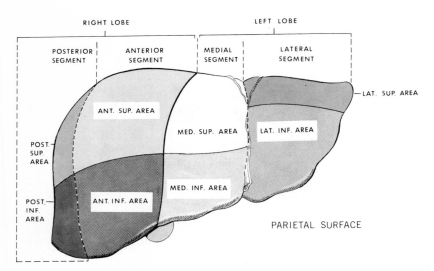

PARIETAL SURFACE

**Figure 6**  Anatomic lobes and segments of the liver.

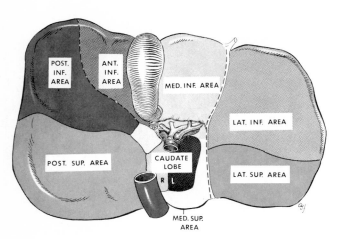

VISCERAL SURFACE

ments, which represent the peritoneal reflections from the diaphragm onto the liver.

9 and 10. The right and left triangular ligaments, which are produced by fusion of the anterior and posterior coronary ligaments at the right and left lateral borders of the liver.

**Lobes and Segments.** The falciform ligament divides the liver topographically, but not anatomically or functionally, into a large right lobe and a smaller left lobe. In addition, on the visceral surface several fissures and fossae arranged in the shape of an H demarcate two additional small lobes, the quadrate and caudate. The crossbar of the H is the porta hepatis in which are found the hepatic artery, portal vein, bile duct branches, lymphatics, nerves, and attachment of the lesser omentum (Fig. 5). Recent interest in and success with resection of portions of the liver have served to re-emphasize the fact that the classic topographic division of the liver into right and left lobes is not anatomically or functionally correct. The liver is similar to the lung in that it can be divided into anatomic segments on the basis of the pattern of branching of the hepatic artery, portal vein, and bile duct (Fig. 6). Accordingly, the true anatomic left lobe consists of a medial segment that lies to the right of

the falciform ligament and a lateral segment made up of the classic topographic left lobe. The topographic quadrate lobe is part of the anatomic left lobe. The true anatomic right lobe consists of anterior and posterior segments. The line of division between the anatomic right and left lobes is not marked on the surface but follows a line from the gallbladder fossa below to the inferior vena cava fossa above. The topographic caudate lobe is divided, according to its blood supply and bile duct drainage, between the anatomic right and left lobes. The hepatic veins have an interlobar distribution between the liver segments.

**Blood Supply, Lymphatics, and Nerves.** The liver is unique among the abdominal viscera in having a dual blood supply. The common hepatic artery arises from the celiac axis along with the left gastric artery and splenic artery, and courses to the liver in the lesser omentum to the left of the common bile duct and anterior to the portal vein (Fig. 7). It gives off three major branches, the gastroduodenal artery, supraduodenal artery, and right gastric artery, after which it divides into a right and left ramus. The right ramus passes behind the common hepatic duct and gives off the cystic artery before entering the liver. In over 40 per cent of subjects, variations from

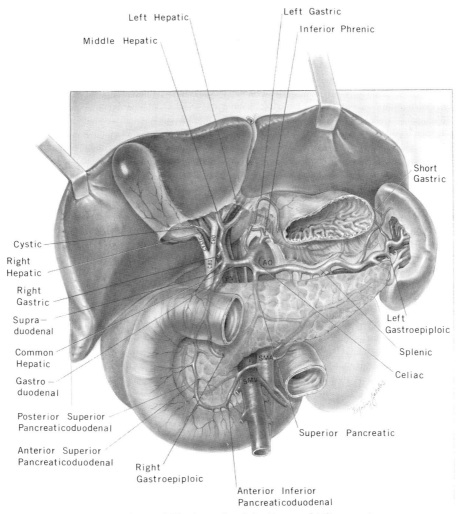

**Figure 7**    Arterial blood supply of the liver and biliary system.

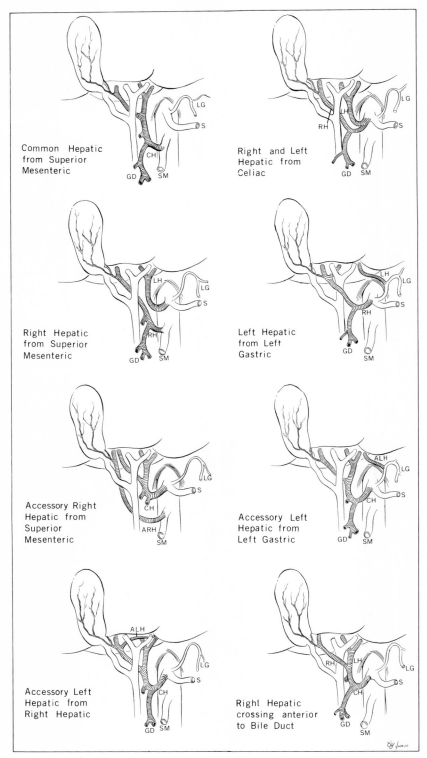

**Figure 8** Common variations in the anatomy of the hepatic artery. CH, Common hepatic artery; RH, right hepatic artery; LH, left hepatic artery; ARH, accessory right hepatic artery; ALH, accessory left hepatic artery; LG, left gastric artery; S, splenic artery; SM, superior mesenteric artery; GD, gastroduodenal artery.

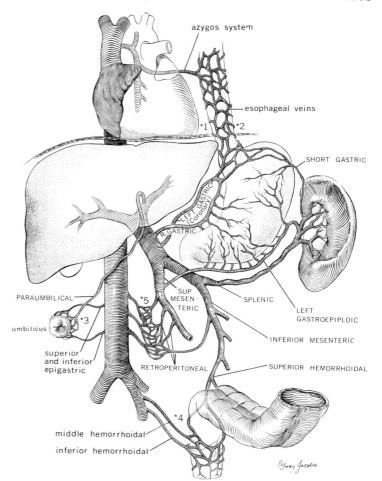

**Figure 9** The portal venous system, showing sites of portal-systemic anastomoses labeled 1 to 5. See text for description of these collateral communications.

the classic pattern occur (Fig. 8). The surgeon must be aware of these variations if he is to avoid serious operative accidents.

The valveless portal vein carries blood to the liver from the stomach, small intestine, large intestine, pancreas, and spleen. It is formed from the junction of the superior mesenteric vein and splenic vein behind the head of the pancreas, and passes posterior to the first part of the duodenum, through the hepatoduodenal ligament, to the porta hepatis where it divides into right and left branches. The hepatic artery and common bile duct lie anterior to it. The inferior mesenteric vein usually drains into the splenic vein. The tributaries of the portal vein connect with the systemic venous system in several areas (Fig. 9). In normal subjects these communications are of little importance, but in patients with portal hypertension they may assume great clinical significance. Portal-systemic anastomoses occur at the following sites:

1. The left gastric (coronary) vein, a tributary of the portal vein, connects with the esophageal plexus of veins and, in turn, with the azygos vein, hemiazygos vein, and other tributaries of the superior vena cava. Esophageal varices develop in the esophageal plexus as a result of portal hypertension.

2. The short gastric veins and left gastroepiploic vein, tributaries of the splenic vein, connect with the esophageal plexus.

3. The paraumbilical veins, tributaries of the portal

vein, and occasionally a persistent umbilical vein anastomose with the inferior and superior epigastric veins of the systemic system. These connections are the site of the caput medusae and the Cruveilhier-Baumgarten syndrome in patients with portal hypertension.

4. The superior hemorrhoidal vein, a tributary of the inferior mesenteric vein, communicates with the middle and inferior hemorrhoidal veins of the systemic circulation and may form large hemorrhoids in the presence of portal hypertension.

5. Retroperitoneal veins form communications between the portal vein, superior mesenteric vein, inferior mesenteric vein, pancreatic veins, and the tributaries of the inferior vena cava. In portal hypertension these communications produce striking "staining" of the peritoneum similar to a port-wine stain and familiar to surgeons, particularly because they cause troublesome bleeding during operations in patients with cirrhosis.

The venous outflow from the liver is carried by the valveless hepatic veins which enter the inferior vena cava just below the diaphragm (Fig. 10). Beginning with the central veins in the liver lobules, the venous effluent passes through progressively larger sublobular veins and collecting veins into the major right, middle, and left hepatic veins. The middle and left hepatic veins usually join and enter the vena cava as one vessel. Several smaller hepatic veins from the caudate lobe and other parts of the liver are consistently found. Because of their

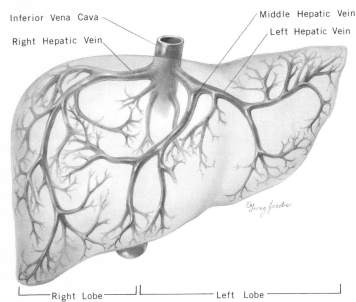

Inferior Vena Cava
Right Hepatic Vein
Middle Hepatic Vein
Left Hepatic Vein

Right Lobe ——————  Left Lobe ——————

**Figure 10**  The hepatic venous outflow system.

interlobar distribution the hepatic veins may be accidentally entered during resections of segments or lobes of the liver.

Recent interest in the role of the hepatic lymph in cirrhosis has focused attention on the lymphatic drainage of the liver. Between the liver cell plates and the sinusoids, tissue spaces called the perisinusoidal spaces of Disse are found, through which fluid exchange between the blood and the hepatocyte takes place. Fluid from these spaces drains into small lymphatic vessels in the portal tracts and then into major lymphatics which leave the liver in the porta hepatis and empty into the cisterna chyli from which the lymph drains into the thoracic duct. In addition, lymphatic vessels are found around the hepatic veins, in Glisson's capsule, and around the bile ducts. Many of these pass through the diaphragm and empty into the thoracic duct in the thorax. The lymph nodes to which the hepatic lymphatics connect are located in the porta hepatis, and these, in turn, connect with the celiac nodes and nodes around the termination of the inferior vena cava, along the left gastric artery, and near the pylorus.

The nerve supply to the liver consists of sympathetic fibers from the seventh to the tenth thoracic segments of the spinal cord and parasympathetic fibers carried in the right and left vagus nerves. The sympathetic nerves pass through the celiac ganglia. The nerves form an anterior and posterior hepatic plexus in the porta hepatis and are distributed throughout the liver along the blood vessels and bile ducts. The afferent innervation is carried in the sympathetic splanchnic nerves and in the right phrenic nerve. Hepatic pain is dull and is distributed over the area occupied by the liver, with occasional radiation to the right shoulder.

**Biliary System.**  The extrahepatic biliary system is described in detail in the next chapter. The intrahepatic biliary system originates in the tiny bile canaliculi located between the hepatic cells, into which bile is secreted. The canaliculi drain into progressively enlarging intralobular and segmental bile ducts which, in turn, drain into the main right and left hepatic ducts. In the porta hepatis, the right and left hepatic ducts unite to form the common hepatic duct which, in its descent toward the duodenum, is joined by the cystic duct to form the common bile duct.

## PHYSIOLOGY

### Functions of the Liver

Just as the heart is the focal organ in the circulatory system, and the brain is the hub of integrative activity, the liver is the center of metabolism in the body. The synthesis, modification, storage, breakdown, and excretion of many of the substances upon which life depends occur in the liver. The functions of the liver exceed those of all other organs in number and complexity. Although much remains to be learned about the many vital activities of the liver, the known functions can be divided into eight categories.

**Bile Formation and Excretion.**  Bile is composed of bilirubin, the salts of bile acids, cholesterol, phospholipids, inorganic salts, mucin, water, and a host of metabolites. It is secreted at the rate of 600 to 1000 ml. per day. The liver synthesizes bile acids from cholesterol, and bile represents the main route by which cholesterol is eliminated from the body. Substantial evidence indicates that the bile salts and organic ions in bile are secreted by an active process that involves independent transport mechanisms for the various components.

Bilirubin is formed mainly from the breakdown of hemoglobin in the reticuloendothelial system at various sites in the body, but particularly in the bone marrow and spleen. A small amount of bilirubin originates as a byproduct of hemoglobin synthesis in the bone marrow and from heme proteins other than hemoglobin, mechanisms that become significant only in certain rare diseases that produce "shunt hyperbilirubinemia." The first step in the process of hemoglobin breakdown involves the opening of the tetrapyrrole ring in the heme radical to form biliverdin-iron-globin. Next, the iron and globin components are separated to form biliverdin. Reduction of the biliverdin produces unconjugated bilirubin. This compound is largely insoluble in water and does not react with diazotized sulfanilic acid in the van den Bergh reaction unless it is first treated with alcohol to make it water-soluble. The unconjugated bilirubin is carried to the liver cell in the blood, bound mainly to albumin. In the liver, bilirubin is conjugated with glucuronic acid and to a much lesser extent with sulfate to form mainly bilirubin diglucuronide and a small amount of bilirubin sulfate. A microsomal enzyme, bilirubin UDP-glucuronyl transferase, catalyzes conjugation. The conjugated compounds are water-soluble and give the van den Bergh reaction without pretreatment with alcohol. In actuality, direct-reacting bilirubin may consist of two pigments, I and II, the major of which (II) is bilirubin diglucuronide and the other of which is believed to be the monoglucuronide or unconjugated bilirubin. Conjugated bilirubin is secreted into the bile canaliculi and is excreted via the bile ducts into the intestine, where it is reduced by bacteria to colorless compounds, mesobilirubinogen and stercobilinogen, collectively called urobilinogen. Much of the urobilinogen is excreted in the stool, where part of it is oxidized to the colored pigment urobilin. However, about one-third to one-half of the urobilinogen is reabsorbed from the intestine in what is called the enterohepatic circulation, and is carried to the liver, where it is again excreted or is transformed back to bilirubin. A small amount of the reabsorbed urobilinogen escapes processing by the liver and is excreted in the urine. Figure 11 summarizes the steps in the breakdown of hemoglobin.

**Carbohydrate Metabolism.** Hepatic synthesis, transformation, and breakdown of carbohydrates, fats, and proteins are so intimately related that the liver has been referred to as a metabolic pool.

The liver is capable of forming these major substances from each other so that separation of the metabolic processes is done mainly for discussion purposes. The liver converts pentoses and hexoses absorbed from the intestine to glycogen, the major form of carbohydrate storage in the body, by enzymatic mechanisms called glycogenesis. In reverse, the liver breaks down glycogen by glycogenolysis, and, thereby, serves as a primary source of glucose for the body. The liver converts glucose, via the hexose monophosphate shunt, to pentoses, which have several uses. They are metabolized to provide energy. They are used in the biosynthesis of nucleotides, nucleic acids, and adenosine triphosphate. They are used to produce 3-carbon compounds, such as pyruvic acid, which serve as precursors for active acetate, a compound that forms a link between carbohydrate, fat, and protein metabolism and plays a central role in the tricarboxylic acid cycle.

**Fat Metabolism.** The liver both synthesizes and catabolizes fatty acids and neutral fats. Fatty acids are transformed into 4-carbon compounds, the ketone bodies, and into 2-carbon compounds such as active acetate. Similarly, glycerol is broken down into active acetate. The liver is the predominant site of cholesterol synthesis and esterification, and it plays a major role in the synthesis and breakdown of phospholipids and lipoproteins.

**Protein Metabolism.** The liver synthesizes a large variety of proteins from amino acids. By deamination the liver forms sugars and fatty acids from amino acids, and by transamination it produces amino acids from non-nitrogenous compounds. The liver is the only organ that produces plasma albumin and alpha globulin, and it is the major site for the production of urea, the end prod-

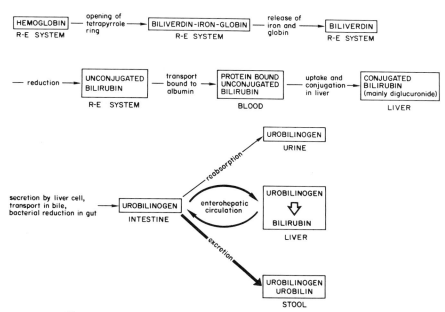

**Figure 11** Hemoglobin breakdown and bile pigment formation.

uct of protein metabolism. Beta globulin is also formed in the liver.

**Blood Coagulation.** The liver is the primary center for the synthesis of most of the proteins involved in blood coagulation. It manufactures fibrinogen, prothrombin, and factors V, VII, VIII, IX, XI, and XII. Vitamin K is required for the formation of prothrombin and factors VII, IX, and X.

**Vitamin Metabolism.** All the vitamins are stored in and utilized by the liver. It is the primary site for the storage of vitamins A, D, E, K, and $B_{12}$.

**Detoxification.** The liver is the detoxification center of the body. By oxidation, reduction, methylation, acetylation, esterification, and conjugation the liver degrades or modifies a great variety of endogenous substances such as the steroid hormones and exogenous drugs and chemicals.

**Phagocytosis and Immunity.** Through the Kupffer cells of its reticuloendothelial system, the liver serves as a large filter where bacteria, pigments, and other debris are removed from the blood by phagocytosis. Furthermore, the Kupffer cells are an important source of gamma globulin, which is involved in immune defense mechanisms.

### Hepatic Hemodynamics

Measurements of hepatic blood flow by indirect and direct methods have shown that the liver receives about one-fourth of the cardiac output. Liver blood flow in normal subjects averages 1500 ml. per minute (1000 ml. per minute per kilogram of liver), with a range of from 1000 to 1800 ml. per minute. The hepatic artery contributes about one-fourth of the blood flowing to the liver and the portal vein contributes about three-fourths (Fig. 12). The pressure in the portal vein ranges from approximately 7 to 10 mm. Hg (100 to 140 mm. saline), whereas the pressure in the hepatic artery is the same as the systemic arterial pressure. In the hepatic sinusoids, where the two systems join, the pressure is reduced to 4 to 8 mm. Hg. The pressure in the hepatic veins ranges from 3 to 6

mm. Hg and in the inferior vena cava at the level of the diaphragm it is about 2 to 5 mm. Hg. The consecutive pressure gradients assure movement of blood toward the heart. The oxygen content of portal vein blood is higher than that of systemic blood, averaging approximately 80 per cent saturation. The flow of blood to the liver is controlled by mechanical, neural, and humoral mechanisms. Rapid and striking changes in hepatic blood flow occur under various conditions such as exercise, fever, and shock. Thus, the liver is important in maintaining circulatory homeostasis.

### Effects of Hepatectomy

Studies in hepatectomized dogs have provided important information about liver function and have raised a number of questions not yet answered. Immediately following complete removal of the liver the animals awake from anesthesia and appear normal. After several hours, however, muscular weakness and depression of reflexes develop, followed in a short time by convulsions and death. These abnormalities are due to hypoglycemia and can be prevented by the administration of glucose. The animal treated with glucose survives in good health for up to 48 hours. However, despite the continued provision of sugar, restlessness, vomiting, and tachypnea ultimately develop, followed by ataxia, spasticity, coma, and death. The cause of death is unknown. A number of biochemical abnormalities have been observed, but none has been proved to be responsible for the terminal events. These include a mild increase in blood ammonia, a rise in the amino acid content of blood, cerebrospinal fluid, and brain, an elevation of blood uric acid, an increase in serum bilirubin and the appearance of bilirubin in the urine, a decrease in the proteins involved in blood coagulation, and a fall in blood urea.

### The Eck Fistula Dog

Performance of a portacaval shunt (Eck fistula) in normal animals results in a number of serious disturbances that suggest that sudden diversion of portal blood from the normal liver is incompatible with good hepatic function. In such animals a syndrome of central nervous system symptoms develops following the ingestion of meat which has come to be known as meat intoxication. In addition, animals with an Eck fistula have a decreased capacity to synthesize proteins, impaired bile formation, decreased hepatic storage of glycogen, a fall in serum cholesterol and fatty acids, a progressive rise in blood and urine uric acid, and a hypochromic anemia. The liver undergoes atrophy and accumulates fat, and polydipsia, polyuria, anorexia, weight loss, and lassitude develop. Unless care is meticulous, the animals do not survive for more than a few months. In dogs with experimental cirrhosis, construction of an Eck fistula does not produce the abnormalities observed in animals with an initially normal liver; this fact suggests that the liver can compensate for a gradual reduction in portal blood flow. Similarly, in

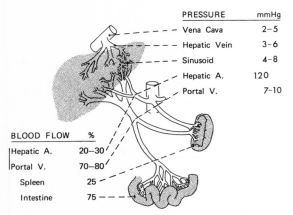

| PRESSURE | mmHg |
|---|---|
| Vena Cava | 2–5 |
| Hepatic Vein | 3–6 |
| Sinusoid | 4–8 |
| Hepatic A. | 120 |
| Portal V. | 7–10 |

| BLOOD FLOW | % |
|---|---|
| Hepatic A. | 20–30 |
| Portal V. | 70–80 |
| Spleen | 25 |
| Intestine | 75 |

**Figure 12** Pressures in the hepatic circulation and the percentage of contribution to hepatic blood flow made by the various components.

humans with extrahepatic obstruction of the portal vein due to thrombosis or atresia marked disturbances of hepatic function are not usually observed. One of the important unsettled issues regarding the therapeutic use of portacaval shunt in patients with cirrhosis is the question of whether or not diversion of portal blood away from a liver with an already reduced portal blood flow adversely affects liver function.

### Liver Regeneration

Liver regeneration is a phenomenon of fundamental biologic significance and of importance in the understanding and treatment of hepatic disease. The normal adult mammalian hepatocyte shows little turnover of nuclear DNA, rarely undergoes mitosis, and has a life span commensurate with the adult life of the organism, be it the rat or man. However, destruction or removal of part of the liver gives rise to mitotic activity and cell division of such intensity that the organ is reconstituted within days or weeks, depending upon the species. All of the mitotic activity involves mature cells, and there is no evidence of progenitor stem cells. Following removal of two-thirds of the liver, complete restoration requires 10 to 14 days in the rat, 6 to 8 weeks in the dog, and 4 to 6 months in man.

Extensive research has been directed at identifying the factors responsible for initiating and regulating the remarkable chain of events involved in liver regeneration. It has been suggested that liver injury or loss causes release of a humoral stimulant of hepatic origin, that partial hepatectomy removes an inhibitor of cell division that is normally present, and that total liver blood flow controls regeneration. None of these suggestions has received solid scientific support. Recently, however, it has been demonstrated that portal blood is essential for restoration of the liver, and convincing evidence indicates that there is a hepatotrophic portal blood factor (HPBF) that regulates hepatic regeneration. The nature and site of origin of the HPBF remain to be determined.

# DIAGNOSIS OF LIVER DISEASE

## HISTORY

Diseases of the liver produce a variety of symptoms depending on the etiology and nature of the underlying disturbance, and upon the rapidity with which liver damage occurs. Many of the symptoms are nonspecific. Nevertheless, certain symptoms occur with sufficient frequency in various hepatic diseases to alert the physician to the possibility that a liver disorder is the cause of the patient's illness (Table 2).

Jaundice is a common symptom of many liver diseases and is perhaps the complaint that most frequently leads the patient to seek medical attention. Jaundice is often accompanied by dark urine and sometimes by light stools. The investigation of a patient with jaundice should include a search

**TABLE 2**  COMMON SYMPTOMS AND SIGNS OF LIVER DISEASE

### Symptoms

Jaundice, dark urine, pruritus
Fatigue, malaise, myalgia, headache
Anorexia and nausea
Pain in right upper quadrant of abdomen
Fever
Hematemesis and melena
Pedal edema and abdominal enlargement (ascites)
Mental changes, forgetfulness, confusion
Weight loss
Purpura and epistaxis

### Signs

Jaundice
Hepatomegaly and liver tenderness
Splenomegaly
Fever
Ascites (with shifting dullness) and edema
Spider angiomas
Palmar erythema
Collateral veins in abdominal wall
Tremor, asterixis, mental confusion
Muscle wasting (shoulder girdles, extremities)
Xanthomas
Gynecomastia, testicular atrophy, loss of axillary and pubic hair
Hematemesis, melena, hematochezia
Purpura

for a history of transfusions of blood or blood products, injections, contact with jaundiced persons, occurrence of jaundice in the family, exposure to chemicals at work or in the home, and a record of travel. The possibility that jaundice is due to biliary obstruction requires questioning about fatty food intolerance, attacks of colic, bloating, and belching. Pruritus sometimes accompanies jaundice and may be the patient's predominant complaint.

Fatigue, malaise, headache, myalgia, arthralgia, and fever are frequent symptoms associated with acute hepatic inflammation and necrosis. Anorexia and nausea are striking manifestations of hepatitis, but are also found in chronic liver disease. Pain in the right hypochondrium may occur in most liver diseases as well as in disturbances of the biliary system. The distinction between continuous dull hepatic pain and biliary colic is of diagnostic importance.

Hematemesis and melena are complications of chronic liver disturbances, and particularly of cirrhosis. Liver disease must be considered, at least initially, in every patient with upper gastrointestinal bleeding. Similarly, ascites, dependent edema, weight loss, and a bleeding tendency are manifestations of severe and usually long-standing liver damage. Mental abnormalities such as forgetfulness, confusion, inability to concentrate, and personality changes are common symptoms of advanced cirrhosis. A history of alcohol intake and a dietary history are of great importance.

## PHYSICAL EXAMINATION

The findings on physical examination again depend on the type of liver disease and its chronicity. Jaundice, seen best in the sclerae, is an important sign. Hepatomegaly and liver tenderness are found frequently in both acute and chronic liver disease, whereas splenomegaly is a common finding in long-standing hepatic disorders. Fever occurs most often in acute inflammation and necrosis of the liver. Circulatory disturbances, such as spider angiomas seen usually on the face, neck, upper trunk, and arms, telangiectasis over the nose and cheeks, palmar erythema, and collateral veins beneath the skin of the abdomen are characteristic signs of chronic hepatic dysfunction. Similarly, ascites with shifting dullness, dependent edema, gynecomastia, testicular atrophy, loss of axillary and pubic hair, and muscle wasting are classic manifestations of cirrhosis. Neurologic disturbances such as tremor, asterixis, peripheral neuritis, and disorders of consciousness varying from confusion to coma are associated with severe destruction of the hepatic parenchyma. Xanthomas, which occur most often in the skin of the eyelids, extremities, and upper trunk, are found in liver diseases associated with chronic biliary obstruction. An interesting but uncommon sign of advanced liver disease is a sweet, musty odor of the breath called fetor hepaticus.

## LIVER FUNCTION TESTS

A large number of laboratory procedures are used to detect the presence of liver disease. Some of these measure functions of the liver, some measure activities that the liver shares with other organs and systems, and many measure biochemical changes that are associated with hepatic injury but have nothing to do with the known functions of the liver. Collectively, these studies are called liver function tests. Normal adult values for these tests are listed in Table 3.

### Bilirubin Metabolism

**Serum Bilirubin.** The liver conjugates and excretes bilirubin carried to it in the unconjugated form by the blood. Conjugated bilirubin is water-soluble and gives the prompt, direct red diazo reaction of van den Bergh. Unconjugated bilirubin is largely water-insoluble and must be pretreated with alcohol to give the van den Bergh reaction. The total concentration of bilirubin in normal serum is less than 1.2 mg. per 100 ml. and almost all of it is in the unconjugated form. A rise in unconjugated bilirubin in the blood occurs when there is an increased breakdown of hemoglobin and in certain liver disorders in which there is impaired uptake of bilirubin or a deficiency of the enzymes involved in bilirubin conjugation. Jaundice due mainly to an increase in conjugated bilirubin in the blood is found in intrahepatic and extrahepatic bile duct obstruction, in hepatocellular damage, and in certain rare diseases in

**TABLE 3**  NORMAL ADULT VALUES FOR LIVER FUNCTION TESTS

| | |
|---|---|
| Serum bilirubin, total | 0.3–1.2 mg./100 ml. |
| Serum bilirubin, direct | 0–0.25 mg./100 ml. |
| Serum bilirubin, indirect | 0.2–0.8 mg./100 ml. |
| Urine bilirubin | 0 |
| Urine urobilinogen | 0.2–3.3 mg./day |
| Fecal urobilinogen | 40–280 mg./day |
| Serum alkaline phosphatase | |
|   Bodansky | 1.5–4.0 units |
|   King-Armstrong | 3–13 units |
|   Bessey-Lowry | 0.8–3.0 units |
|   Shinowara-Jones-Reinhart | 2.8–8.6 units |
| SGOT | 8–40 units |
| SGPT | 5–35 units |
| Serum 5′-nucleotidase | 0.3–3.2 units |
| Serum leucine aminopeptidase (LAP) | 50–220 units |
| Serum lactic dehydrogenase (LDH) | 200–450 units |
| Prothrombin time | 80–100% of control |
| Fibrinogen | 200–400 mg./100 ml. |
| Bromsulphalein retention (45 min. after 5 mg./kg.) | 0–6% |
| Indocyanine green retention | 0–6 |
| Serum albumin | 4.7–5.7 gm./100 ml. |
| Serum globulins | 1.3–2.5 gm./100 ml. |
| Serum proteins, total | 6.5–7.9 gm./100 ml. |
| Serum alpha fetoprotein | 0 |
| Cephalin-cholesterol flocculation | 0 |
| Thymol turbidity | 0–4 units |
| Zinc sulfate turbidity | 0–4 units |
| Serum cholesterol | 140–280 mg./100 ml. |
| Serum cholesterol esters, fraction of total cholesterol | 66–72% |
| Arterial blood ammonia | 20–60 µg./100 ml. |

which the transport of bilirubin after conjugation is disturbed.

**Urine Bilirubin.** Normally, bilirubin is not present in the urine because the kidney is capable of excreting only the conjugated form of the pigment. Bilirubin appears in the urine in diseases in which there is an elevated level of conjugated bilirubin in the blood.

**Urine Urobilinogen.** The bilirubin excreted into the intestines is transformed into urobilinogen by intestinal bacteria. A substantial amount of the urobilinogen is reabsorbed, and a small portion of that which is reabsorbed is excreted in the urine (0.2 to 3.3 mg. per day). If renal function is normal, absence of urobilinogen in the urine occurs in obstruction to bile flow and when the intestines are sterilized with antibiotics. Increased urine urobilinogen is found in hepatocellular disease because the liver is unable to dispose of the reabsorbed pigment, and in conditions that produce an increase in hemoglobin breakdown. The pH of the urine influences renal excretion of urobilinogen.

**Fecal Urobilinogen.** Normally, fecal urobilinogen excretion ranges from 40 to 280 mg. per day. The excretion rate decreases markedly in biliary obstruction and increases in association with increased bilirubin production. Excretion rates in hepatocellular disease are variable.

## Serum Enzymes

**Alkaline Phosphatase.** These are a group of isoenzymes that hydrolyze phosphate esters in an alkaline medium. They occur in a number of tissues, including the liver, biliary system, bone, intestine, kidney, and placenta. Alkaline phosphatase in serum originates mainly from the bones (40 to 75 per cent), hepatobiliary system, and intestines. Recently, it has become possible to separate the isoenzymes of serum alkaline phosphatase according to their sites of origin, although the electrophoretic techniques are not yet available as routine laboratory procedures. Alkaline phosphatase is excreted from the body in bile. Elevations of serum alkaline phosphatase occur in a number of hepatobiliary disorders, as well as in osteoblastic diseases of bone, in pregnancy, and during normal growth. Among the hepatobiliary disorders, the most striking increases are observed in conditions that produce bile duct obstruction. In fact, the finding of a normal level of serum alkaline phosphatase is strong evidence against extrahepatic obstructive disease. Elevations of serum alkaline phosphatase occur also in metastatic neoplasms to the liver (in over 90 per cent of the cases with hepatomegaly), and in primary liver cancer, hepatic abscess, cholangitis, and diffuse liver damage. For many years, elevation of serum alkaline phosphatase was attributed solely to mechanical obstruction of the excretory pathway. Although biliary obstruction is clearly a major cause of regurgitation of the enzyme into the blood, recent evidence suggests that overproduction of alkaline phosphatase by the liver occurs in response to a variety of noxious stimuli, in the absence of impairment of bile flow.

**Glutamic Oxalacetic Transaminase (SGOT).** This enzyme facilitates the transfer of an amino group from glutamic acid to oxalacetic acid. It is found in skeletal muscle, kidney, brain, and pancreas but the highest levels occur in liver and heart. When tissues containing the enzyme are injured, it is released into the bloodstream. Neither the biliary system nor the kidney is an important route of GOT excretion. Normal serum contains up to 40 units of GOT. SGOT elevations are found in association with severe damage of cardiac and skeletal muscle, as well as in a variety of hepatic disorders. Marked elevations in excess of 300 units suggest the presence of acute hepatic inflammation or necrosis, and are most commonly observed in viral hepatitis.

**Glutamic Pyruvic Transaminase (SGPT).** This enzyme promotes the transfer of an amino group from glutamic acid to pyruvic acid. Its concentration in liver greatly exceeds that in other tissues or organs. Normal serum contains 35 units or less. Although it has been suggested that a rise in GPT is a more specific indicator of liver damage than an elevation of GOT, both enzymes increase similarly in various liver diseases.

**Other Enzymes.** Abnormal serum levels of lactic dehydrogenase (LDH), leucine aminopeptidase (LAP), isocitric dehydrogenase (ICD), cholinesterase, 5'-nucleotidase, and a number of other enzymes have been observed in various hepatic disorders as well as in diseases of other organs. While determinations of these enzymes may be of value, they have not displaced the other liver function tests and do not appear to significantly enhance the differential diagnosis of liver disease.

## Blood Coagulation Factors

The liver is the primary site for synthesis of most of the proteins involved in blood coagulation. Methods have been devised for measuring individual factors, such as fibrinogen, factor V, factor VII, and prothrombin, but they are seldom used. Rather, a composite test is employed that depends on the presence of all the factors in the prothrombin complex and is a useful indicator of liver disease. This test is called the prothrombin time, and the one-stage clotting method of Quick is most commonly used. The test is influenced by the levels of fibrinogen, prothrombin, and factors V, VII, and X. Normally, the prothrombin time is at least 80 per cent of the time obtained with control plasma. The prothrombin time is prolonged or, in other terms, the percentage of normal is decreased in hepatocellular disease because of depressed protein synthesis, and in obstructive jaundice because of impaired absorption of vitamin K, which is required for synthesis of the prothrombin complex. Normalization of the prothrombin test (30 per cent or greater increase within 24 hours) occurs in biliary obstruction following parenteral administration of vitamin K, but does not occur when the coagulation deficiency is due to liver damage. The prothrombin response to parenteral vitamin K is a useful method of distinguishing between hepatocellular and biliary disease.

## Dye Excretion

**Bromsulphalein Excretion (BSP).** Sodium phenoltetrabromphthalein disulfonate, or Bromsulphalein, is a synthetic dye that is removed from the blood mainly by the liver. Following intravenous injection, the dye is carried to the liver bound to albumin and alpha lipoprotein, is taken up by the hepatic cells by an active transport mechanism, is conjugated mainly with glutathione, and is excreted into the biliary canaliculi in both the free and conjugated forms by an active, carrier-mediated transport process. The dye is removed from the body in bile and is not reabsorbed from the intestines. In normal subjects, less than 6 per cent of an injected dose of 5 mg. per kilogram body weight is present in the blood 45 minutes after administration. The BSP test is a very sensitive measure of hepatic functional reserve, and retention of the dye is found consistently in patients with significant liver damage. It is the test that is most frequently abnormal in cirrhosis. Bilirubin competes with BSP for both the hepatic uptake and excretion transport mechanisms, and therefore the BSP test is not valid in the presence of a serum bilirubin greater than 5 mg. per 100 ml., or in obstruction of the bile ducts. Similarly, dyes used for radiographic visualization of the gallbladder compete with BSP for hepatic uptake, and the test should not be done for several days after biliary radiography. BSP retention regularly occurs in very obese patients, and occasionally occurs in the presence of significant fever. In shock, BSP may be retained because of impaired hepatic blood flow.

**Indocyanine Green Excretion (ICG).** Indocyanine green is a synthetic dye that is removed from the blood almost exclusively by the liver. It is excreted in the bile in an unconjugated form, and is not reabsorbed from the intestines. Evidence indicates that ICG and BSP utilize the same uptake and excretion transport mechanisms, and that agents that compete with BSP also compete with ICG. Experience with the ICG test suggests that it is similar to the BSP test in both sensitivity and limitations.

**Iodine-131-Rose Bengal Excretion.** Rose bengal is a synthetic phthalein dye that is removed from the blood almost entirely by the liver parenchymal cells and excreted in the bile. The dye can be labeled with $^{131}$I, and by positioning detectors over the head, liver, and abdomen, its disappearance from the blood, its hepatic uptake, and its excretion into the intestines can be determined. It has been suggested that the radioactive rose bengal test makes possible a differentiation between hepatocellular and obstructive jaundice, but the results have not been consistent. Rose bengal and Bromsulphalein are retained under similar circumstances.

### Protein Metabolism

**Serum Albumin.** The liver is the sole source of serum albumin. In normal subjects, the serum albumin concentration averages 5.2 gm. per 100 ml. by the commonly used salting out method, and 4.3 gm. per 100 ml. by the more accurate paper electrophoresis method. Serum albumin levels decline in hepatocellular damage and particularly when albumin is lost into the peritoneal cavity in ascites. Normal levels are not infrequently found in advanced liver disease, so that measurements of serum albumin do not serve as a sensitive test of liver function. Moreover, serum albumin changes are not specific for liver disease and are of little value in differential diagnosis.

**Serum Globulins.** Hyperglobulinemia occurs in acute and chronic liver disease, as well as in a number of nonhepatic illnesses. The elevations are due mainly to augmented gamma globulin production, although increases in alpha and beta globulins are sometimes found. Because gamma globulin is produced by the hepatic and extrahepatic reticuloendothelial system, it is not certain that the liver is completely responsible for a rise in gamma globulin. Changes in various serum protein fractions are detected by serum electrophoresis.

**Turbidity and Flocculation Tests.** There are a number of tests that do not measure liver function, but reflect qualitative and quantitative changes in serum proteins and are frequently positive in the presence of hepatocellular damage. The most frequently used studies in this category are the cephalin-cholesterol flocculation, the thymol turbidity, and the zinc sulfate turbidity. Flocculation of a cephalin-cholesterol suspension occurs upon the addition of serum containing decreased or altered albumin, increased or altered gamma globulin, altered alpha and beta globulins, or reduced alpha lipoproteins. Turbidity of a thymol-barbital buffer solution occurs upon exposure to serum containing increased gamma globulin, increased beta globulin, an increase of certain lipoproteins, or decreased or altered albumin. Turbidity of a zinc sulfate solution develops upon addition of serum containing an increase in gamma globulin. In all these tests, the degree of turbidity or flocculation is quantitated in terms of arbitrary units. None of the tests are abnormal in uncomplicated obstructive jaundice in the absence of liver injury. Unfortunately, the tests are often negative in the presence of advanced chronic hepatic disease, and are sometimes positive in disorders unrelated to the liver. Moreover, the tests do not indicate the severity of liver damage.

**Serum Alpha Fetoprotein.** Embryonic liver and yolk sac produce alpha fetoprotein, a globulin that is a normal constituent of fetal serum. Alpha fetoprotein is present in small quantities in serum at birth but it disappears early in life and is not normally present in adult human serum. The only adults in whom alpha fetoprotein has been found have been patients with primary hepatocellular carcinoma of the liver and with embryonic neoplasms of the ovary and testes. Serum alpha fetoprotein is becoming widely used as a test for primary liver cancer in areas where this disease is common. Its presence can be detected by a screening test that employs Ouchterlony immunodiffusion, or by a more precise quantitative immunoassay. A positive test has been obtained in from 46 to 82 per cent of patients with hepatoma, and no definite false-positive tests have been reported.

### Carbohydrate Metabolism

Although the liver plays a central role in carbohydrate metabolism, tests of this hepatic function are of limited value. The standard glucose tolerance test often produces a diabetic curve and glycosuria in patients with severe hepatocellular damage. The intravenous galactose tolerance test measures the specific capacity of the liver to convert galactose to glucose. Impaired clearance of galactose from the blood and its appearance in increased quantities in the urine indicate liver dysfunction.

### Lipid Metabolism

The liver is the major site of cholesterol synthesis and esterification, and the bile is the primary avenue of cholesterol elimination from the body. Serum cholesterol levels decrease, as does the esterified fraction, in severe liver damage. Intrahepatic or extrahepatic biliary obstruction, in the absence of severe hepatocellular injury, causes an increase in serum cholesterol. Cholesterol and cholesterol ester determinations are of limited value in the diagnosis of liver disease.

### Ammonia Metabolism

Ammonia is formed from nitrogenous substances in the intestines by the action of bacterial enzymes. Ammonia absorbed into portal blood is largely converted to urea by a highly efficient enzyme system in the liver, involving arginine, ornithine, and citrulline. In the presence of severe hepatic damage or portal-systemic venous connections, ammonia levels in peripheral arterial blood may rise above the normal concentration of less than 100 $\mu$g. per 100 ml. Although theoretically attractive, determinations of blood ammonia show no consistent correlation with the type or extent of hepatic damage and are of limited diagnostic value. The only circumstance in which measurement of blood ammonia is consistently helpful is in the patient with protein-related portal-systemic encephalopathy.

## LIVER BIOPSY

Biopsy of the liver is valuable in the diagnosis of liver disease as well as in the assessment of therapy. It is not a routine procedure, but is indicated in a variety of situations when there is doubt about the diagnosis or uncertainty about the activity of a pathologic process. If necessary, biopsy can be performed under direct vision through an abdominal incision or during peritoneoscopy. Usually, however, a percutaneous liver biopsy is possible, in which a cutting or aspirating needle is inserted through the right eighth or ninth intercostal space between the anterior and posterior axillary lines. When the liver is large, a subcostal approach may be used. Serious complications of the procedure have been reported to occur in only 0.3 to 0.4 per cent of the cases and consist mainly of bleeding and bile peritonitis. The mortality rate has been reported to be between 0.1 and 0.2 per cent. In patients with a prothrombin time less than 50 per cent, platelet count below 100,000, or with obstructive jaundice, the risk of needle biopsy is increased. Liver biopsy provides accurate information in patients with diffuse hepatic disease. Focal lesions in the liver may be missed.

## ROENTGENOGRAPHIC STUDIES

### Barium Contrast Upper Gastrointestinal Series

In our experience, the upper gastrointestinal series is a simple and accurate method of making the diagnosis of esophageal varices (Fig. 13). In a large series, this procedure provided accurate information in more than 90 per cent of the patients. Barium contrast x-rays of the esophagus, stomach, and duodenum have proved particularly helpful in the differential diagnosis of upper gastrointestinal hemorrhage because they demonstrate the presence or absence of lesions other than varices that may be responsible for bleeding, such as duodenal and gastric ulcers. This valuable diagnostic study can be performed safely at the time of bleeding in almost all patients.

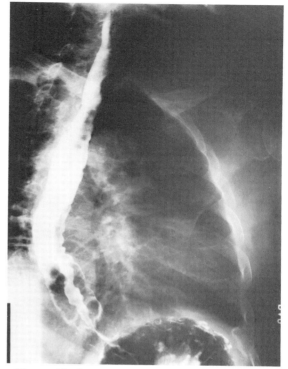

**Figure 13** Barium contrast upper gastrointestinal x-rays showing large esophageal varices.

### Portal Venography

Visualization of the portal venous system by the injection of contrast media is most valuable in the diagnosis and evaluation of portal hypertension, and occasionally may be helpful in the diagnosis of space-occupying lesions within the liver. Portal venography provides important information about the site of venous obstruction, the type and extent of portal-systemic collaterals, the size of the major components of the portal system, and, with appropriate timing, the rate of portal venous blood flow. Several methods are available for demonstrating the portal vasculature. The most frequently used technique is that of percutaneous splenoportography, which involves injection of a radiopaque dye into the spleen through a needle inserted through the left ninth or tenth intercostal space between the midaxillary and posterior axillary lines (Fig. 14). Bleeding from laceration of the spleen is an occasional serious complication of this procedure. Another technique is that of operative portal venography, in which a tributary of the portal vein is catheterized under direct vision at laparotomy. Catheterization of the umbilical vein through a small incision in the abdominal wall permits transumbilical portal venography, a technique that is particularly useful in splenectomized patients. Direct percutaneous needle puncture of the portal vein has been used to perform transhepatic portal venography. Finally, splenic arteriography performed by percutaneous catheterization of the splenic artery via the femoral artery permits

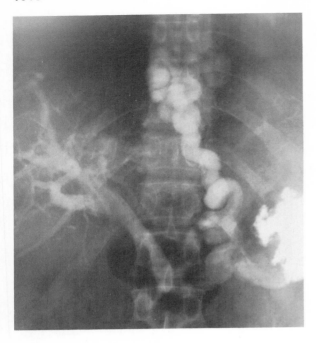

**Figure 14**   Splenoportogram in a patient with cirrhosis showing large gastroesophageal varices.

delayed visualization of the portal venous system by appropriately timed x-rays. None of these techniques are routine procedures that are required in all patients. All of them are associated with risks which must be weighed against the information to be obtained. However, usually they can be performed safely and often they are extremely useful.

### Hepatic Venography

Percutaneous catheterization of the hepatic veins via either the basilic vein in the arm or the femoral vein is a relatively simple procedure. Visualization of the inferior vena cava (vena cavography) may be combined with wedged hepatic venography. Injection of contrast medium into the hepatic veins may be used to determine retrograde blood flow in cirrhosis by showing filling of the portal vein, and to demonstrate hepatic vein occlusion in the Budd-Chiari syndrome and in veno-occlusive disease of the liver. Both hepatic venography and inferior vena cavography may be helpful in demonstrating space-occupying

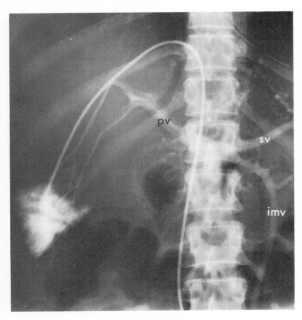

**Figure 15**   Hepatic venogram in a patient with cirrhosis showing retrograde filling of portal vein indicative of reversal of portal blood flow. pv, Portal vein; sv, splenic vein; imv, inferior mesenteric vein.

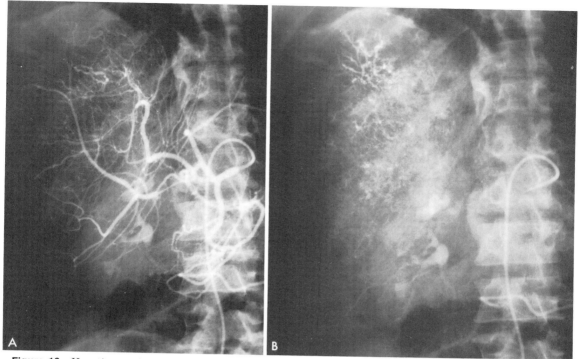

**Figure 16**   Hepatic arteriogram showing a large malignant neoplasm in the right lobe of the liver. *A*, Distortion of the arterial tree by the neoplasm. *B*, Extensive "tumor staining" during the venous phase of the study.

lesions situated in the posterior segments of the liver. Figure 15 shows a hepatic venogram.

### Hepatic, Celiac, and Superior Mesenteric Arteriography

Percutaneous selective catheterization of the hepatic, celiac, and superior mesenteric arteries for visualization of the splanchnic vasculature is a safe procedure that has become very valuable in the diagnosis of liver disease (Fig. 16). It is particularly useful for demonstrating space-occupying lesions, hepatic vascular lesions, the status of the arterial tree in cirrhosis, hemobilia, and injury to the liver associated with blunt trauma. With proper timing, superior mesenteric arteriography may be used to visualize the portal venous system and to demonstrate patency of portacaval shunts. We have found that selective injection of contrast medium into the left gastric artery is an excellent technique for delayed visualization of esophageal varices.

### Cholecystography and Cholangiography

Techniques for oral, intravenous, and direct percutaneous visualization of the biliary system are important in the diagnosis of biliary disease, and may be of help in the differential diagnosis of jaundice. They are discussed in detail in the next chapter.

## ESOPHAGOGASTROSCOPY

Many surgeons are of the opinion that esophagoscopy is the best means of determining the presence of esophageal varices and of demonstrating varix hemorrhage. In the face of massive bleeding, however, endoscopy may be difficult. The development of the flexible fiberoptic esophagogastroscope has made endoscopy a relatively simple bedside procedure that is usually well tolerated by patients. Esophagogastroscopy is not a substitute for barium contrast roentgenography in the diagnosis of upper gastrointestinal hemorrhage. Rather, the two procedures complement each other and together they improve diagnostic accuracy substantially. Esophagogastroscopy is the only reliable means of making the diagnosis of hemorrhagic gastritis.

## PORTAL PRESSURE MEASUREMENTS

### Wedged Hepatic Vein Pressure (WHVP)

Measurements of portal venous pressure are helpful in the diagnosis of portal hypertension and in the selection of appropriate surgical therapy. Under most circumstances the portal pressure can be determined indirectly by percutaneous hepatic vein catheterization via an arm vein or the femoral vein, and this procedure is used routinely in many clinics. The catheter tip is wedged in a hepatic venule and produces a static column of blood that extends back to the sinusoid. The pressures in the sinusoid, and in portal blood entering the sinusoid, are transmitted through the static blood to the catheter. The correlation between measurements of WHVP and portal pressure are extremely good under most conditions. When there is sinusoidal or postsinusoidal obstruction to portal blood flow, as occurs in the common forms of cirrhosis, portal pressure rises and WHVP increases correspondingly. In portal hypertension due to an extrahepatic block (presinusoidal), WHVP is normal and does not reflect portal pressure. During hepatic vein catheterization, the free hepatic vein and inferior vena cava pressures are always determined also, and the WHVP is usually expressed in terms of its difference from vena cava pressure.

### Splenic Pulp Pressure

The splenic pulp pressure reflects the pressure in the valveless portal venous system, and it can be measured by the same percutaneous technique as that used for splenoportography. Often the two procedures are combined. If necessary, splenic pulp pressure can be determined at the bedside.

### Umbilical Vein Catheterization

As described previously, the portal vein can be catheterized for direct pressure measurements through the umbilical vein, which is isolated through a small paraumbilical incision and forcefully reopened.

### Intraoperative Pressure Measurements

Direct pressure measurements are always made at operations for portal hypertension, both before and after a portacaval shunt is performed. These include the inferior vena cava pressure (IVCP), the free portal pressure (FPP), and the pressures on the hepatic and splanchnic sides of a clamp temporarily occluding the portal vein. The latter determinations are called the hepatic occluded portal pressure (HOPP) and the splanchnic occluded portal pressure (SOPP), respectively. When the liver is normal, HOPP is markedly lower than FPP. In cirrhosis with hepatic outflow obstruction, HOPP rises progressively and occasionally exceeds FPP, a finding that suggests that portal blood flow has reversed and the portal vein is serving as an outflow tract. Pressure measurements following construction of a portacaval shunt are essential,

and provide the only reliable means of determining that the anastomosis is functioning satisfactorily.

### Postoperative Pressure Measurements Following Portacaval Shunt

The patency of a portacaval shunt is readily determined by percutaneous catheterization via the femoral vein and performance of both angiography and measurements of portal and vena caval pressures.

## RADIOISOTOPE STUDIES

### Hepatic Blood Flow

Estimation of hepatic blood flow may be helpful in the assessment of portal hypertension and in the selection of appropriate therapy. Indirect methods for measuring liver blood flow involve the infusion of a tracer substance that is removed mainly, and preferably completely, by the liver. Bromsulphalein was the first tracer used for this purpose and the technique consisted of simultaneous measurements of concentrations in arterial and hepatic venous blood during a continuous intravenous infusion of the dye. Indocyanine green may be used instead of BSP. More recently, simple methods have been developed for measuring the blood disappearance rate of a radioactive tracer that is removed mainly by the liver. Either external monitoring or analysis of radioactivity in serial blood samples is used to measure removal of the injected tracer from the peripheral blood. Radioactive colloidal gold ($^{198}$Au), colloidal human serum albumin ($^{131}$I or $^{125}$I), colloidal technetium sulfide ($^{99m}$Tc), and colloidal chromic phosphate ($^{32}$P) have been used as tracers. All of the methods of estimating hepatic blood flow have several inherent sources of error which become magnified in the presence of liver disease. When liver damage is marked, hepatic uptake of the tracer is reduced regardless of changes in blood flow, and extrahepatic removal of the test substance increases, leading to unreliable results. A portacaval shunt further complicates the measurements.

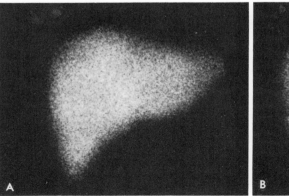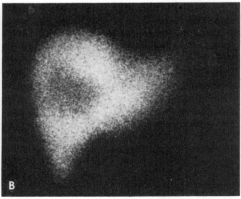

**Figure 17**  Scintillation scans following administration of colloidal technetium sulfide ($^{99m}$Tc), showing (A) normal liver and (B) large area of reduced radioactivity in right lobe of liver due to a metastasis from carcinoma of the colon.

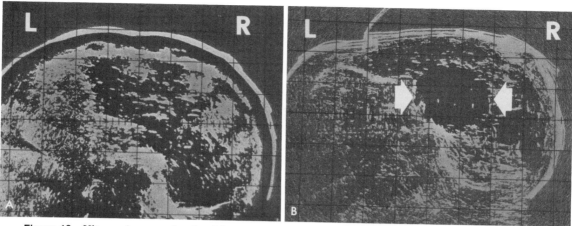

**Figure 18** Ultrasonic scans showing (*A*) normal liver and (*B*) large amebic abscess in right lobe of liver.

### Liver Scanning

Scintillation scanning following the administration of a radioisotope that selectively localizes in the liver is helpful in determining liver size and shape and in detecting lesions that occupy space within the hepatic parenchyma or compress the liver from without. Isotopically labeled colloidal gold ($^{198}$Au), colloidal human serum albumin ($^{131}$I or $^{125}$I), colloidal technetium sulfide ($^{99m}$Tc), rose bengal ($^{131}$I), and ammonium molybdate ($^{99}$Mo) are employed. Figure 17 shows typical scans.

## ULTRASONIC SCANNING

Ultrasonic scanning is a harmless, noninvasive procedure that has proved to be useful in the diagnosis of mass lesions in and around the liver. It involves the recording on an oscilloscope of the pattern of reflections or echoes that are produced by passing high-frequency ultrasonic waves into the body. Echoes are produced at interfaces between materials of different density. Normal liver parenchyma is homogeneous and produces no reflections (Fig. 18*A*). Tumors or abscesses within the liver produce abnormal echoes (Fig. 18*B*).

## HEMATOLOGIC STUDIES

Hematologic abnormalities are common in chronic liver disease. Gastrointestinal bleeding, of course, is a major complication of cirrhosis. In addition, chronic anemia is frequently found as a result of a decreased red blood cell survival time and poor nutrition. Hypersplenism, with a depression of any or all of the formed elements of the blood, is often associated with portal hypertension. Appropriate hematologic studies, including the usual complete blood count, platelet count, determinations of red cell indices, measurements of serum iron, and determinations of red blood cell survival time and splenic trapping of red cells, may

be important components of the diagnostic work-up.

## BALLOON TAMPONADE CONTROL OF BLEEDING

Control of upper gastrointestinal hemorrhage by esophageal or gastric balloon tamponade has been interpreted as evidence that the bleeding is coming from esophageal varices. This diagnostic procedure has been accurate in approximately 75 per cent of patients. It is infrequently indicated as a diagnostic procedure.

## JAUNDICE

Jaundice or icterus is a yellow discoloration of the tissues that results from staining with bilirubin. It is best observed in sites containing elastic tissue such as the sclerae and skin of the face and neck. Jaundice is easily recognizable when the conjugated bilirubin concentration in the serum reaches 2 to 3 mg. per 100 ml., or the unconjugated bilirubin level is 3 to 4 mg. per 100 ml. With experience jaundice can be detected at lower levels of serum bilirubin. Jaundice occurs in a substantial number of diseases and determination of the precise cause can be one of the more difficult problems in clinical medicine.

There is no satisfactory classification of jaundice that accounts for all conditions. The classic separation of jaundice into hemolytic, hepatocellular, and obstructive types is useful but does not explain all the pathophysiologic mechanisms that recent studies have clarified. Classification on the basis of the type of bilirubin, conjugated or unconjugated, that predominates in the blood is of limited clinical validity because of the frequent occurrence of mixed forms of hyperbilirubinemia. An understanding of bilirubin metabolism and of the stages at which it may be disturbed by disease provides the soundest approach to the differential diagnosis of icterus.

The metabolism and excretion of bilirubin in-

I. *Excessive bilirubin production usually due to hemolysis ("hemolytic jaundice")*
  A. Inherited hemolytic anemias
  B. Acquired hemolytic disorders
    1. Hemolytic anemias
    2. Sepsis
    3. Hemolysins (snake venom, mushrooms)
    4. Absorption of sequestered blood (hematomas, hemothorax, hemoperitoneum, infarcts)
    5. Burns
    6. Mismatched blood transfusions
    7. Massive blood transfusions
  C. Shunt hyperbilirubinemia
II. *Impaired transport of bilirubin to liver*
  Some types of Gilbert's syndrome
III. *Impaired hepatic conjugation of bilirubin*
  A. Inborn errors
    1. Crigler-Najjar syndrome
    2. Some types of Gilbert's syndrome
  B. Immaturity of enzyme systems
    1. Physiologic jaundice of newborn
    2. Jaundice of prematurity
IV. *Impaired hepatic transport and excretion of bilirubin after conjugation ("hepatocellular jaundice")*
  A. Acquired liver diseases (e.g., hepatitis, cirrhosis, neoplasms)
  B. Dubin-Johnson syndrome and Rotor syndrome
  C. Intrahepatic cholestasis (drug-induced, disease-related, and idiopathic)
V. *Mechanical bile duct obstruction ("obstructive jaundice")*
  A. Extrahepatic (stone, neoplasm, stricture, atresia, etc.)
  B. Intrahepatic

volve the formation of free bilirubin mainly from the breakdown of hemoglobin in the reticuloendothelial system; transport of the unconjugated bilirubin to the liver; uptake and conjugation of the bilirubin by the hepatic cell; excretion of the conjugated bilirubin by the hepatic cell into the bile; excretion of the bile along the biliary ducts into the intestines, where conjugated bilirubin is converted to urobilinogen. A classification of jaundice according to the stage at which bilirubin metabolism is disturbed is presented in Table 4 and Figure 19.

Increased production of bilirubin from hemolysis of red blood cells or during erythropoiesis, impaired transport of bilirubin to the liver, and impaired uptake and conjugation of bilirubin by the liver cell result in icterus due to unconjugated hyperbilirubinemia. The term "retention jaundice" has been used to describe this type, and it is not accompanied by impairment of bile flow. The jaundice in most of these disorders is mild, there is no bile in the urine, urine urobilinogen is not increased, and the liver function tests are usually normal.

Impaired transport and excretion of conjugated bilirubin by the hepatic cell produces jaundice with a substantial amount of conjugated bilirubin in the blood. The term "regurgitation jaundice" has been applied to this type. Most of the common liver diseases fall into this category. Because the damaged hepatic cells are unable to conjugate all

the bilirubin resulting from normal hemoglobin breakdown, an increase in unconjugated bilirubin develops along with the regurgitated conjugated pigment in the blood. Bile appears in the urine, urine urobilinogen levels rise, and liver function tests are usually abnormal. One group of disorders that produce impaired cellular excretion of conjugated bilirubin does not conform to the usual pattern of liver disease and presents problems in the differential diagnosis of obstructive jaundice. The term intrahepatic cholestasis has been used to describe these conditions. They are characterized by a clinical and biochemical picture similar to that of bile duct obstruction, normal or mildly abnormal liver function tests, and a histologic picture of bile stasis without mechanical obstruction. A growing number of drugs, including phenothiazine compounds, certain diuretics, testosterone derivatives, oral contraceptives, oral antidiabetes agents, and arsenicals, are known to injure the cellular excretion mechanism and cause intrahepatic cholestasis. A similar picture has been observed during pregnancy and, as a transient phenomenon, during viral hepatitis. In some instances, no etiologic agent can be identified.

Mechanical bile duct obstruction results in conjugated hyperbilirubinemia, along with an increase in unconjugated pigment in the blood. The mechanism is similar to that which occurs in primary liver disease, and the jaundice is of the regurgitation type. Bile appears in the urine but, if the obstruction is complete, urobilinogen is absent from the urine and stool, and the stools are light- or clay-colored. The serum alkaline phosphatase levels are significantly elevated, but the other liver function tests are usually normal early in the course of obstruction. However, repeated or long-standing obstruction or infection results in substantial liver damage and makes it difficult to distinguish the symptoms and findings from those of primary hepatic disease. Prolonged absence of bile from the intestine impairs the absorption of fat-soluble vitamin K and produces a decrease in prothrombin activity that can be corrected by parenteral administration of the vitamin. The prothrombin response to vitamin K is helpful in differentiating liver disease from biliary obstruction.

The first steps in the diagnostic approach to the patient with jaundice are the taking of a thorough history and the performance of a careful physical examination. These routine aspects of every work-up often provide crucial information that points to the diagnosis. Taking of the history should include pointed questions about rapidity of onset and course of the jaundice, color of the urine and stools, pruritus, weight loss, abdominal pain, digestive symptoms, malaise, anorexia, occupation, travel, jaundice in the family, contact with jaundiced persons, exposure to hepatotoxins, alcohol consumption, ingestion of drugs, transfusions, injections, and previous operations. The physical examination should include particularly careful palpation of the liver, gallbladder, and spleen, a search for the stigmata of cirrhosis, gross determination of stool color, and chemical exam-

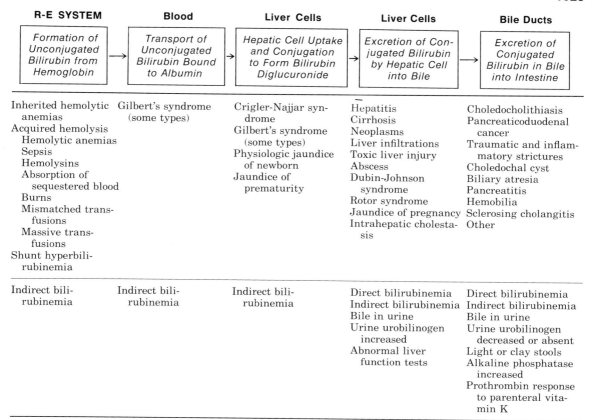

| R-E SYSTEM | Blood | Liver Cells | Liver Cells | Bile Ducts |
|---|---|---|---|---|
| Formation of Unconjugated Bilirubin from Hemoglobin | Transport of Unconjugated Bilirubin Bound to Albumin | Hepatic Cell Uptake and Conjugation to Form Bilirubin Diglucuronide | Excretion of Conjugated Bilirubin by Hepatic Cell into Bile | Excretion of Conjugated Bilirubin in Bile into Intestine |
| Inherited hemolytic anemias<br>Acquired hemolysis<br>  Hemolytic anemias<br>  Sepsis<br>  Hemolysins<br>  Absorption of<br>    sequestered blood<br>  Burns<br>  Mismatched trans-<br>    fusions<br>  Massive trans-<br>    fusions<br>Shunt hyperbili-<br>  rubinemia | Gilbert's syndrome<br>(some types) | Crigler-Najjar syn-<br>drome<br>Gilbert's syndrome<br>(some types)<br>Physiologic jaundice<br>of newborn<br>Jaundice of<br>prematurity | Hepatitis<br>Cirrhosis<br>Neoplasms<br>Liver infiltrations<br>Toxic liver injury<br>Abscess<br>Dubin-Johnson<br>syndrome<br>Rotor syndrome<br>Jaundice of pregnancy<br>Intrahepatic cholesta-<br>sis | Choledocholithiasis<br>Pancreaticoduodenal<br>cancer<br>Traumatic and inflam-<br>matory strictures<br>Choledochal cyst<br>Biliary atresia<br>Pancreatitis<br>Hemobilia<br>Sclerosing cholangitis<br>Other |
| Indirect bili-<br>rubinemia | Indirect bili-<br>rubinemia | Indirect bili-<br>rubinemia | Direct bilirubinemia<br>Indirect bilirubinemia<br>Bile in urine<br>Urine urobilinogen<br>increased<br>Abnormal liver<br>function tests | Direct bilirubinemia<br>Indirect bilirubinemia<br>Bile in urine<br>Urine urobilinogen<br>decreased or absent<br>Light or clay stools<br>Alkaline phosphatase<br>increased<br>Prothrombin response<br>to parenteral vita-<br>min K |

**Figure 19** Stages of bilirubin metabolism at which diseases produce jaundice, and the types of jaundice that result.

ination of the stool for blood. After the history and physical examination, the next steps involve determinations of the levels of direct-reacting and indirect-reacting bilirubin in the blood, and the amounts of bile and urobilinogen in the urine. Hyperbilirubinemia that is mainly of the unconjugated pigment, combined with the absence of bile in the urine, indicates that the icterus is of the retention type. In an adult patient, the odds are overwhelming that the cause is hemolysis of red blood cells. The liver function tests under these circumstances will be normal and appropriate hematologic studies, and other tests should be performed to identify the underlying disease.

If a substantial portion of the bilirubin in the blood is of the direct-reacting variety, as is commonly the case, and there is bile in the urine, the jaundice is of the regurgitation type and the problem is usually one of distinguishing between liver disease and bile duct obstruction. Liver function tests, stool color examination, and urobilinogen measurements should be performed. Normal liver function tests except for a depressed prothrombin activity and an elevated serum alkaline phosphatase, light- or clay-colored stools, absence of urobilinogen in the urine, a good prothrombin response to parenteral vitamin K, and a history and physical examination that are compatible indicate clearly that the jaundice is due to biliary obstruction that requires surgical relief. On the

other hand, abnormal liver function tests, a normal-colored stool, increased urobilinogen in the urine, a negative or incomplete prothrombin response to parenteral vitamin K, an enlarged liver, and the absence of symptoms of biliary tract disease such as abdominal colic and fatty food intolerance indicate that the jaundice should be treated by nonsurgical measures. Needless to say, the history and physical findings are of great importance in arriving at the correct diagnosis.

In a number of patients, perhaps 10 to 15 per cent, a diagnosis will not be possible on the basis of the initial work-up. Additional studies, repeated tests, and a period of observation will be required to determine the etiology of the jaundice. In some patients liver scan, liver biopsy, upper gastrointestinal x-rays, cholangiography, arteriography, peritoneoscopy, and duodenal drainage must be performed. Occasionally, laparotomy must be done for diagnostic as well as therapeutic purposes.

## PORTAL HYPERTENSION

Portal hypertension is a manifestation of various diseases of the liver and its circulation. It is the complication of hepatic disease that most frequently requires surgical treatment. Although the portal pressure in normal subjects varies considerably with activity, at rest it ranges from about 100 to 140 mm. saline (7 to 10 mm. Hg). In terms of pressure measurements, portal hypertension may be defined as a portal vein pressure of 250 mm. saline (18 mm. Hg) or greater in the presence of a normal pressure in the inferior vena cava. Stated in other terms, portal hypertension exists when the difference between portal and inferior vena cava pressure exceeds 150 mm. saline. More important, portal hypertension may be defined in terms of the pathologic disturbances it produces that compromise health and threaten life. Some of these disorders, such as bleeding esophageal varices and hypersplenism, are a direct reflection of the high pressure in the portal circulation and its collateral communications. Others, such as ascites, hepatic coma, peptic ulcers, and renal failure, are complicated manifestations of a number of factors including the portal hypertension, the underlying liver disease, and the required treatment.

## ETIOLOGY OF PORTAL HYPERTENSION

Table 5 lists the causes of portal hypertension. From both clinical and pathologic standpoints these may be divided into diseases within the liver and diseases of the blood vessels outside the liver. With the exception of the rare splanchnic arteriovenous fistulas, all the conditions cause portal hypertension by producing obstruction to portal blood flow.

Intrahepatic obstructive diseases account for more than 90 per cent of the patients with portal hypertension. Of these, portal cirrhosis associated with chronic alcoholism is by far the most common etiology in the United States. Postnecrotic cir-

**TABLE 5** ETIOLOGY OF PORTAL HYPERTENSION

I. *Intrahepatic obstructive disease*
  A. Portal cirrhosis (alcoholic, nutritional, Laennec's)
  B. Postnecrotic cirrhosis (posthepatitic idiopathic)
  C. Biliary cirrhosis
  D. Uncommon forms of cirrhosis and fibrosis (hemochromatosis, Wilson's disease)
  E. Alcoholic hepatitis
  F. Neoplasms and granulomas
  G. Schistosomiasis
  H. Veno-occlusive disease
  I. Congenital hepatic fibrosis
  J. Hepatoportal sclerosis
II. *Extrahepatic disease*
  A. Portal vein obstruction
    1. Congenital atresia or stenosis
    2. Thrombosis due to infection or trauma
    3. Cavernomatous transformation
    4. Extrinsic compression
  B. Hepatic vein (outflow) obstruction
    1. Budd-Chiari syndrome
    2. Constrictive pericarditis
  C. Excessive portal blood flow
    1. Arteriovenous fistula between hepatic artery and portal vein
    2. Arteriovenous fistula between splenic artery and vein

rhosis due to viral hepatitis is a fairly common cause of portal hypertension, whereas the incidence of biliary cirrhosis due to extrahepatic bile duct obstruction or primary intrahepatic disease is low. The other forms of intrahepatic obstruction are uncommon. Because cirrhosis is largely a disease of adulthood and, particularly in alcoholic cirrhosis, develops slowly over many years, patients with portal hypertension of the intrahepatic type are most often in the fifth or sixth decades of life. Moreover, they are usually in poor health because of the underlying liver disease, and the risk of operative treatment is significant.

Extrahepatic obstruction of the portal vein is most often due to thrombosis. Neonatal omphalitis is a relatively frequent cause, but often the etiology of the thrombosis cannot be determined. Cavernomatous transformation is most likely the end result of thrombosis and recanalization of the portal vein. Congenital atresia of the portal vein and extrinsic compression are rare causes of portal hypertension. Extrahepatic portal hypertension usually develops in childhood or early adult life. Furthermore, the patients usually do not have liver damage, are otherwise in good health, and usually tolerate both the complications of their circulatory disorder and the required surgical therapy quite well.

Extrahepatic obstruction of the hepatic venous outflow system occurs in a group of rare conditions called the Budd-Chiari syndrome. The obstruction is usually due to inflammatory or neoplastic thrombosis or fibrosis of the hepatic veins and, sometimes, of the adjacent inferior vena cava. The etiology of the process is often obscure, although some cases are associated with polycythemia vera and with neoplasms. Marked hepatomegaly and massive ascites are the most striking clinical findings. The condition has been relieved by construction of a side-to-side portacaval shunt.

## PORTAL HYPERTENSION DUE TO CIRRHOSIS

### PATHOPHYSIOLOGY

The widespread destruction of the hepatic parenchyma in cirrhosis leads to overgrowth of fibrous tissue and the formation of regenerative nodules in a pathologic rearrangement of liver architecture. As a result, the hepatic blood vessels are compressed and distorted. The branches of the hepatic vein, because of their low pressure and thin protective coat of connective tissue, are affected more than the other components of the vasculature, and hepatic venous outflow obstruction develops. This postsinusoidal obstruction is the fundamental hemodynamic lesion in the common forms of cirrhosis. Outflow obstruction leads to an increase in sinusoidal pressure which, in turn, is reflected in an elevation of portal pressure and a decrease in portal blood flow to the liver. In extreme stages of postsinusoidal obstruction, the valveless portal vein may become an outflow tract and conduct blood in a retrograde manner away from the liver, leaving the hepatic artery alone to nourish the parenchyma. An additional consequence of the disruption of hepatic integrity is the development of communications between the intrahepatic branches of the hepatic artery and portal vein, and between the tributaries of the portal vein and hepatic vein. The arteriovenous shunts contribute to the portal hypertension. Moreover, both types of shunts divert blood away from the hepatic parenchyma and compromise the nutrition of the liver cells. In an unsuccessful attempt to compensate for the reduction in portal flow to the liver, hepatic artery flow increases and the liver becomes dependent upon the hepatic artery for a major portion of its blood supply.

The elevated pressure in the portal vein leads to an enlargement of all the collateral venous connections between the portal and systemic circulations, and development of varicosities (see Fig. 9). In addition, splenomegaly develops. Blood flow through the collaterals is away from the liver, which further impairs hepatic nutrition. Despite their large size, the portal-systemic anastomoses are insufficient to accommodate the volume flow of portal blood and to overcome portal hypertension. Most prominent among the collaterals are those in the submucosa of the lower esophagus and upper stomach, and those around the umbilicus and anterior abdominal wall. Rupture of the esophageal varices often causes massive hemorrhage and is associated with a high mortality rate.

## NATURAL HISTORY OF CIRRHOSIS

Cirrhosis of the liver is a common and highly lethal disease. Currently in the United States it is the ninth leading cause of death, and in subjects older than 40 years it is the fourth ranking cause of mortality. Furthermore, during the past decade the death rate of cirrhosis increased more than that of any of the other common causes of death. Chronic alcoholism, the most frequent etiologic factor in cirrhosis, has been conservatively estimated to involve 6.5 million people in the United States. When the immediate families of patients are considered, chronic alcoholism affects the lives of some 20 million people in our country each year. During the past decade there has been an increase of 1.5 million chronic alcoholics. The social cost of cirrhosis in alcoholics has been estimated to exceed 2 billion dollars per year.

**TABLE 7** CAUSES OF DEATH IN 235 PATIENTS WITH CIRRHOSIS AND VARICES (Boston Inter-Hospital Liver Group, 1959–1961)[85]

|  | % of Deaths |
|---|---|
| Hemorrhage | 34 |
| Hepatic failure | 32 |
| Renal shutdown | 11 |
| Infection | 9 |
| Indeterminate and other | 14 |

The survival rates of patients admitted to general hospitals because of cirrhosis are shown in Table 6. In the classic study of Ratnoff and Patek, who examined in retrospect the histories of 386 patients admitted to five New York hospitals between 1916 and 1938, only one-third of the patients with ascites were alive after 1 year and only a few survived for 5 years. Survival rates for patients with jaundice and hematemesis were similar. In the more recent prospective study of the Boston Inter-Hospital Liver Group, 79 per cent of the patients who bled from esophageal varices were dead within 1 year of bleeding, and in the entire group of 467 patients, with and without bleeding, only 26 lived for 5 years. The results of these studies indicate that once a patient entered the hospital for treatment of cirrhosis, his chances of living for 1 year were similar to those of a patient with acute lymphocytic leukemia, and his chances of surviving 5 years were about the same as those observed in most untreated cancers.

The causes of death in patients with cirrhosis and varices were tabulated by the Boston Group (Table 7). Hemorrhage was responsible for one-third of the deaths, hepatic failure accounted for one-third, renal shutdown for 11 per cent, infection for 9 per cent, and miscellaneous causes for the remainder. These figures, which are similar to those obtained in other studies, clearly show that varix bleeding is a major cause of death in cirrhosis. This complication in particular has occupied the attention of surgeons and serves as the major indication for surgical therapy.

## BLEEDING ESOPHAGEAL VARICES

The most frequent cause of death from upper gastrointestinal bleeding is *rupture* of an esophageal varix with hemorrhage. Until recently, ap-

**TABLE 6** NATURAL HISTORY OF CIRRHOSIS

| Authors | Cases | Complications | Survival in % | | |
|---|---|---|---|---|---|
|  |  |  | 1 Year | 2 Years | 5 Years |
| Ratnoff and Patek (five New York Hospitals, 1916–1938) | 296 | Ascites | 32 | 17 | 7 |
|  | 245 | Jaundice | 26 | 23 | 5 |
|  | 106 | Hematemesis | 28 | 25 | 20 |
| Boston Inter-Hospital Liver Group (seven Boston Hospitals, 1959–1961) | 467 | Varices | 34 | 21 | 5.5 |
|  | 288 | Varices without bleeding | 43 | 25 | 8 |
|  | 179 | Varices with bleeding | 21 | 14 | 1.5 |

TABLE 8   MORTALITY OF FIRST VARICEAL HEMORRHAGE IN CIRRHOSIS

| Authors | Year Reported | Type of Hospital | Number of Patients | Mortality (%) |
|---|---|---|---|---|
| Ratnoff and Patek | 1942 | Five private-teaching | 106 | 40 |
| Higgins | 1947 | City indigent | 45 | 76 |
| Atik and Simeone | 1954 | City indigent | 59 | 83 |
| Nachlas, O'Neal, and Campbell | 1955 | City indigent | 102 | 59 |
| Cohn and Blaisdell | 1958 | City indigent | 456 | 74 |
| Taylor and Jontz | 1959 | Veterans | 102 | 45 |
| Merigan, Hollister, Gryska, Starkey, and Davidson | 1960 | City indigent | 74 | 76 |
| Orloff | 1962 | City indigent | 87 | 84 |
| | | Total | 1031 | Mean 73 |

proximately three out of four cirrhotic patients who entered the hospital with their first episode of bleeding varices failed to leave the hospital alive. Table 8, which shows the results of a number of studies conducted during the past 40 years, indicates that as of 1962 the immediate mortality rate of the first variceal hemorrhage averaged 73 per cent. From these statistics, it is apparent that the emergency treatment of bleeding esophageal varices is the single most important aspect of the therapy of portal hypertension.

The precipitating cause of rupture of esophageal varices is uncertain. It has been proposed that erosion of the mucosa by reflux acid-peptic esophagitis is involved. However, in a gross and microscopic study of the distal esophagus in 20 patients at the time of bleeding we found esophagitis in only one patient. Moreover, bleeding from esophageal varices has been reported in patients with proven gastric achlorhydria. The evidence strongly suggests that increased hydrostatic pressure is responsible for "blowout" rupture of esophageal varices.

### Emergency Diagnosis

In most patients who enter the hospital with upper gastrointestinal hemorrhage, the diagnosis of bleeding esophageal varices depends on affirmative answers to three questions. Does the patient have cirrhosis? Does the patient have portal hypertension and esophageal varices? Are the varices the site of the bleeding, rather than some other lesion such as duodenal or gastric ulcer, gastritis, or hiatus hernia? Information sufficient to answer these questions usually can be obtained within a few hours of the patient's admission to the hospital by means of an organized diagnostic plan that includes some, and if necessary all, of the following steps:

**1. History and Physical Examination.** A history of chronic alcoholism, hepatitis, jaundice, previous bleeding episodes, melena, abdominal swelling, edema, and mental abnormalities, and the absence of symptoms of peptic ulcer suggest the diagnosis of cirrhosis. The most important physical findings are hepatosplenomegaly, spider angiomas, palmar erythema, collateral abdominal veins, muscle wasting, jaundice, ascites, edema, and neu-

rologic signs such as tremor and asterixis. In many patients, not all these classic signs are present. Confirmation of gastrointestinal bleeding by aspiration of the stomach through a nasogastric tube and by gross and chemical examination of the stool is an essential early measure, and should really be considered part of the physical examination. A nasogastric tube is inserted in all patients.

**2. Blood Studies.** Blood samples for typing and crossmatching and for studies are drawn immediately on admission. The initial studies include a complete blood count, liver function tests (Bromsulphalein excretion, prothrombin, bilirubin, alkaline phosphatase, albumin, globulin, thymol turbidity, cephalin flocculation, glutamic oxalacetic transaminase, glutamic pyruvic transaminase), urea nitrogen, electrolytes, pH, and blood gases. The liver tests that are most consistently abnormal and of greatest value are the BSP excretion, if performed in the absence of marked jaundice and after hypovolemic shock has been corrected, and the prothrombin and serum bilirubin. It is not unusual for the other liver function tests to be normal in the presence of advanced cirrhosis.

**3. Esophagogastroscopy.** With the development of the flexible fiberoptic esophagogastroscope, endoscopy has become a well tolerated, relatively simple procedure that can be performed rapidly at the bedside in the emergency room. It is the best diagnostic measure for determining with certainty the presence or absence of gastritis and of the uncommon Mallory-Weiss syndrome, and, in combination with roentgenographic studies, it makes possible the diagnosis of esophageal varices with a high degree of confidence.

**4. Upper Gastrointestinal X-rays.** As soon as shock has been corrected and the patient's condition stabilized, a barium contrast upper gastrointestinal series is obtained. Parenteral fluid therapy and monitoring should continue throughout this procedure, and the physician in charge of treatment should accompany the patient to the radiology department and remain in constant attendance. When this is done, x-ray studies can be performed safely in almost all patients. It is to be emphasized that roentgenographic studies are directed at determining the presence or absence not only of esophageal varices, but also of other lesions such as a duodenal ulcer, gastric ulcer, or hiatus hernia. The literature contains many statements that suggest that esophageal varices are demonstrated in only 50 to 60 per cent of patients who have them. Our experience indicates that a skillful and interested radiologist can accurately demonstrate varices at the time of bleeding in more than 90 per cent of cirrhotic patients (see Fig. 13).

**5. Hepatic Vein Catheterization.** This relatively simple procedure has become a routine diagnostic measure in our institution. It is used to determine wedged hepatic vein pressure, free hepatic vein pressure, and inferior vena cava pressure. Hepatic venography is usually added to the studies, although it is not essential and does not yield information that is as important as that obtained from the pressure measurements. The main purpose of venography is to determine the direction of flow in the portal vein (see Fig. 15). WHVP accurately reflects portal pressure in the common forms of cirrhosis and establishes the diagnosis of portal hypertension with certainty.

*The emergency diagnosis of bleeding esophageal varices has been made accurately from information obtained in these first five steps in more than 95 per cent of our patients.* It has been regularly possible to complete these diagnostic measures within 6 hours of the patient's admission to the emergency room.

**6. Splenoportography and Splenic Manometry.** Visualization of the portal venous system is not regularly required for emergency diagnosis of varix hemorrhage in patients with cirrhosis. However, this procedure provides useful hemodynamic information about the pattern of collateral circulation and the volume of blood perfusing the liver, and it may ultimately provide a basis for selection of therapy. Consequently, we regularly perform splenoportography as part of the emergency work-up (see Fig. 14). In patients with normal liver function who are suspected of having extrahepatic portal obstruction, splenoportography provides crucial information about the site of obstruction and patency of the portal venous system, and it should be done routinely. Splenic manometry is usually combined with splenoportography and offers an alternative to hepatic vein catheterization. If desired, the splenic pulp pressure can be determined readily at the bedside by percutaneous puncture of the spleen under local anesthesia. Although this procedure does not determine the site of bleeding, it indicates the presence or absence of portal hypertension. Bleeding from esophageal varices infrequently occurs with a splenic pulp pressure below 300 mm. saline and rarely occurs with a pressure below 250 mm.

**7. Splenic, Hepatic, Celiac, Left Gastric, and Superior Mesenteric Arteriography.** Percutaneous selective catheterization and visualization of the splanchnic arteries provides interesting hemodynamic data about the status of the circulation in cirrhosis that some day may serve as the basis for

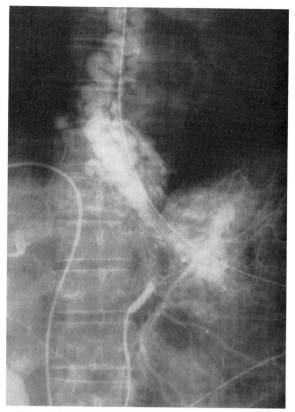

**Figure 20** Selective left gastric arteriogram with delayed visualization of large esophageal varices during the venous phase.

selecting patients for one or another form of treatment. However, selective arteriography is not at present an essential or routine emergency diagnostic procedure in cirrhotic patients with varix hemorrhage. With proper timing, injection of contrast media into the splenic artery or superior mesenteric artery provides delayed visualization of the portal vein and its collateral connections. Although this technique is not as consistent as splenoportography, it is particularly useful in patients whose spleen has been removed previously. We have found that selective injection of the left gastric artery frequently produces excellent delayed visualization of esophageal varices (Fig. 20).

**8. Radioisotope Hepatic Blood Flow.** While not a routine procedure or one that is necessary for making the diagnosis of bleeding esophageal varices, determination of liver blood flow is part of a hemodynamic investigation that may yield useful information for the future selection and evaluation of therapy. The most commonly used technique involves injection of a radionuclide and external monitoring of its disappearance rate from the blood. Radioactive colloidal technetium sulfide ($^{99m}$Tc), colloidal gold ($^{198}$Au), colloidal human serum albumin ($^{131}$I or $^{125}$I), and colloidal chromic phosphate ($^{32}$P) are used as tracers.

**9. Balloon Tamponade Control of Bleeding.** Control of bleeding by esophageal balloon tamponade

**TABLE 9**  DIAGNOSTIC FINDINGS IN 89 CONSECUTIVE CIRRHOTIC PATIENTS SUSPECTED OF
BLEEDING FROM ESOPHAGEAL VARICES*

| Final Diagnosis | Number of Cases | History Compatible with Cirrhosis | Physical Exam Compatible with Cirrhosis | Liver Function Tests Compatible with Cirrhosis | Varices on Upper GI X-ray | Other Lesion on Upper GI X-ray | Portal Hypertension on Splenic Manometry | Varices on Esophagoscopy |
|---|---|---|---|---|---|---|---|---|
| Bleeding varices | 74 | 74 | 74 | 74 | 70/74 | 4/74 | 2/2 | 2/2 |
| Peptic ulcer | 6 | 6 | 6 | 6 | 0/6 | 6/6 | – | 0/2 |
| Gastritis | 9 | 9 | 9 | 9 | 0/9 | 0/9 | 0/9 | 0/2 |

*From Emergency treatment of bleeding esophageal varices in cirrhosis, by Orloff, M. J. in Portal Hypertension, edited by Longmire, W. P., Jr., Current Problems in Surgery, edited by Ravitch, M. M., et al. Copyright © 1966, Year Book Medical Publishers. Used by permission.

is presumptive evidence that an esophageal varix is the site of bleeding. The balloon tamponade test is accurate in approximately three-fourths of patients. The development of new and better diagnostic measures has made this indirect diagnostic procedure almost obsolete.

Several years ago we evaluated the use of a vigorous emergency diagnostic approach in 89 consecutive adult patients in whom cirrhosis and varix hemorrhage were suspected on admission to our emergency room. In all of the patients a history was taken and physical examination, blood studies, and barium contrast upper gastrointestinal x-ray examinations were done. Splenic manometry and esophagoscopy with the rigid esophagoscope were performed only if the other measures failed to reveal the diagnosis. Table 9 summarizes the results of this diagnostic approach. Upper gastrointestinal x-rays correctly demonstrated the presence or absence of varices in 96 per cent of the patients. Roentgenography gave false-negative results in 4 per cent of the patients. Splenic manometry was performed in 11 patients in whom x-rays failed to show varices; in two patients, portal hypertension was found and bleeding varices were demonstrated subsequently at operation, whereas in nine patients the finding of a normal portal pressure corresponded to the absence of varices on x-ray. Esophagoscopy was performed in six patients in whom no varices were demonstrated by roentgenography; in two patients bleeding varices were observed and subsequently proved at operation, whereas in the other four patients the absence of varices was confirmed by endoscopy. In 97 per cent of the patients, the diagnostic work-up was completed within 6 hours of admission to the hospital. Fifty-nine of the 89 patients were subjected to emergency operations with the preoperative diagnosis of corrhosis and bleeding esophageal varices, and in each instance this diagnosis proved to be correct. Since this study was completed, we have added esophagoscopy with the flexible fiberoptic instrument and hepatic vein catheterization to the routine diagnostic work-up done in all patients. Our experience has shown that the diagnosis of varix hemorrhage in cir-

rhosis can be made rapidly and with a high degree of accuracy.

The differential diagnosis of upper gastrointestinal bleeding in 99 per cent of cirrhotic patients is confined to a consideration of six lesions in addition to ruptured varices. Three of these lesions, hemorrhagic gastritis, duodenal ulcer, and gastric ulcer, are common. The other three lesions, gastric cancer, hiatus hernia, and the Mallory-Weiss syndrome (a tear of the esophagogastric mucosa produced by forceful vomiting), are infrequent causes of bleeding. Each of these conditions produces characteristic symptoms, and each can be ruled in or out by the combination of esophagogastroscopy and barium contrast upper gastrointestinal x-rays. It is general experience that bleeding in cirrhotic patients originates from lesions other than esophageal varices in 20 to 25 per cent of cases. While this statistic should serve to alert the clinician to a spectrum of etiologic considerations, it should not be interpreted as an indication that the diagnosis of varix hemorrhage is particularly complicated or cannot be made with accuracy. In point of fact, once esophageal varices have been demonstrated, the chances that another lesion is responsible for the bleeding are less than 10 per cent. Furthermore, if instances of mild bleeding in cirrhotic patients with proven varices are eliminated, gastrointestinal hemorrhage will be found to arise from rupture of the varices in over 95 per cent of patients. Thus, demonstration of esophageal varices in a cirrhotic patient with significant upper gastrointestinal bleeding provides overwhelming odds that the varices are the source of the hemorrhage.

### Emergency Treatment

In view of the high mortality rate associated with varix hemorrhage in patients with cirrhosis, it is clear that the efforts of physicians must be concentrated on the prompt and definitive control of the first bleeding episode if the survival rate of these patients is to be improved. Emergency treatment of bleeding esophageal varices can be categorized into general measures of therapy, specific medical treatment aimed at stopping the bleeding, and specific surgical procedures for controlling the hemorrhage.

**General Measures of Emergency Therapy.** Cirrhosis of the liver is a severe, debilitating disease with remote manifestations, only one of which is bleeding from esophageal varices. Death after varix rupture is frequently due to hepatic decompensation, renal failure, or infection, rather than to exsanguination. Although control of bleeding is of primary importance, the effectiveness of therapy of the underlying liver disease often determines the outcome. Therefore, there are certain general principles of treatment that apply to all patients, regardless of the specific therapeutic measures used to stop the hemorrhage.

1. PROMPT RESTORATION OF THE BLOOD VOLUME. Vigorous replacement of blood loss with whole blood transfusions is essential. Large-bore intravenous catheters should be inserted in each arm at the start of therapy. Every effort is made to obtain fresh blood less than 12 hours old for administration because of the serious defects in coagulation associated with liver disease plus those superimposed by multiple transfusions. Bleeding cirrhotic patients usually have thrombocytopenia in addition to abnormalities of the protein blood clotting factors. In addition, recent evidence indicates that the red blood cells of cirrhotic patients are deficient in 2,3-diphosphoglyceric acid, a substance that mediates the dissociation of oxygen from hemoglobin. It has been proposed that this deficiency impairs the delivery of oxygen to the tissues. Since there is a progressive decline in 2,3-DPG levels in blood during storage, the use of fresh blood has been recommended to correct the abnormality in oxygen transport.

2. PREVENTION OF HEPATIC COMA. Although the nervous disorders associated with liver disease are diverse and poorly understood, the encephalopathy observed in patients with bleeding esophageal varices sometimes appears to be due to the absorption of large quantities of ammonia directly into the systemic circulation via portal-systemic collaterals. For this reason, measures directed at destroying ammonia-forming bacteria and eliminating all nitrogen from the gastrointestinal tract are initiated promptly. These include removal of blood from the stomach by lavage with iced saline through a nasogastric tube, instillation of cathartics (60 ml. magnesium sulfate) and neomycin (4 gm.) into the stomach, and thorough and repeated cleansing of the colon with enemas containing neomycin (4 gm. per liter of water). The fear that insertion of a nasogastric tube will perforate the varices is unfounded, and such a tube should be placed at the start of the diagnostic work-up. Although ammonia-binding agents, such as sodium glutamate and arginine, and ion exchange resins have been used, we have obtained no evidence that agents of this sort have been of value.

3. SUPPORT OF THE FAILING LIVER. Parenterally administered hypertonic glucose solutions containing therapeutic doses of vitamins K, B, and C are included in the initial treatment regimen. Appropriate amounts of electrolytes are added to the parenteral fluids. In general, administration of sodium is avoided because patients with advanced cirrhosis usually have an increase in total-body sodium and a tendency to retain salt and water.

4. CORRECTION OF HYPOKALEMIA AND METABOLIC ALKALOSIS. The vast majority of the many bleeding cirrhotic patients that we have studied have been found to have significant hypokalemia and a metabolic alkalosis preoperatively or immediately postoperatively. The deleterious effects of hypokalemia are well known. In addition, alkalosis has a number of harmful consequences that include: (1) interference with the release of oxygen to the tissues by shifting the oxyhemoglobin dissociation curve to the left; (2) in combination with hypokalemia, precipitation of cardiac arrhythmias, particularly in patients taking digitalis; (3) potentiation of ammonia toxicity by elevating the tissue concentration of ammonia, and increasing the passage of ammonia across the blood-brain barrier; and (4) production of tetany by lowering the level of ionized calcium in extracellular fluid. Correction of hypokalemia and metabolic alkalosis is undertaken soon after admission to the hospital and consists of parenteral administration of large quantities of potassium chloride supplemented, occasionally, by infusion of an acidifying agent such as ammonium chloride or arginine hydrochloride. Administration of potassium is usually required for several days in amounts occasionally as high as 400 mEq. per day.

5. FREQUENT MONITORING OF VITAL FUNCTIONS. The usual techniques are used to determine the magnitude of bleeding and adequacy of blood volume replacement. These include measurements of vital signs, of urine output by way of an indwelling catheter, of central venous pressure via a polyethylene catheter threaded through an arm cutdown into the superior vena cava, of hematocrit, and of rate of blood loss by continuous suction through a nasogastric tube. Serial measurements of arterial pH and blood gases are facilitated by insertion of an indwelling catheter into the radial artery, which also makes possible continuous recordings of blood pressure. Because of the systemic circulatory abnormalities and hyperdynamic state that frequently exist in bleeding cirrhotic patients, we have added serial determinations of cardiac output by the dye dilution technique, using indocyanine green, to our monitoring regimen, and often perform measurements of pulmonary artery wedge pressure by percutaneous insertion of a Swan-Ganz pulmonary artery catheter.

**Specific Emergency Medical Therapy.** Emergency medical treatment used specifically to stop varix bleeding includes esophageal balloon tamponade, intravenous posterior pituitary extract, and gastroesophageal hypothermia. Although each of these measures is capable of temporarily controlling bleeding esophageal varices, it has been our experience, as well as that reported by many other workers, that they have not significantly in-

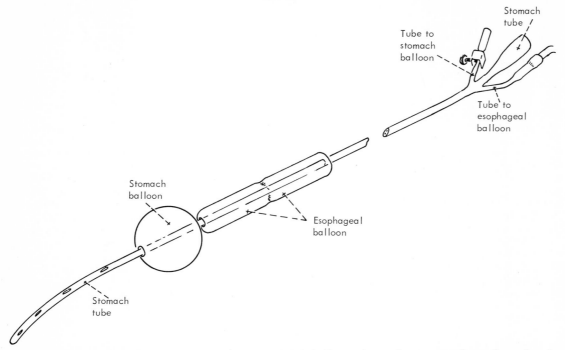

**Figure 21**  The Sengstaken-Blakemore triple-lumen, double-balloon tube used to tamponade esophageal varices. The gastric balloon is inflated first and pulled up against the cardia by continuous mild traction. The esophageal balloon directly compresses the varices in the lower esophagus. The third lumen is used for irrigation of the stomach and removal of blood and gastric contents.

fluenced the mortality rate of varix hemorrhage in cirrhotic patients.

1. ESOPHAGEAL BALLOON TAMPONADE. The most widely used nonoperative method of treatment has been esophageal balloon tamponade (Fig. 21). Since its introduction in 1930 by Westphal, and its popularization in 1950 by Sengstaken and Blakemore, balloon tamponade has been adopted by almost every hospital in the country as standard treatment for bleeding esophageal varices. As shown in Table 10, there is no doubt that this popular mode of therapy has initially stopped varix bleeding in many patients. The disheartening aspect of this form of management has been that

many of the patients have resumed bleeding when the balloons were deflated. Moreoever, we and others have observed frequent and sometimes lethal complications of balloon tamponade, which include perforation of the esophagus, asphyxiation from regurgitation of the balloon into the pharynx, and aspiration pneumonia. Most important, data from a number of institutions clearly indicate that balloon tamponade has failed to influence measurably the mortality rate of bleeding esophageal varices during a trial of 20 years. For these reasons, we have abandoned the use of balloon tamponade as a definitive form of treatment and use it only on infrequent occasions as a temporary measure

**TABLE 10**  RESULTS OF ESOPHAGEAL BALLOON TAMPONADE IN CIRRHOTIC PATIENTS WITH BLEEDING VARICES

| Authors | Year Reported | Number of Patients | Initial Control (%) | Ultimate Control (%) | Mortality (%) |
|---------|:---:|:---:|:---:|:---:|:---:|
| Reynolds, Freedman, and Winsor | 1952 | 32 | 66 | 50 | 47 |
| Hamilton | 1955 | 20 | 45 | — | 75 |
| Ludington | 1958 | 58 | 75 | 43 | — |
| Conn | 1958 | 50 | 70 | — | 82 |
| Read, Dawson, Kerr, Turner, and Sherlock | 1960 | 38 | 84 | 24 | 74 |
| Merigan, Hollister, Gryska, Starkey, and Davidson | 1960 | 68 | — | — | 80 |
| Orloff | 1962 | 45 | 56 | 20 | 82 |
| | | Total 311 | | | Mean 74 |

**TABLE 11**  RESULTS OF INTRAVENOUS POSTERIOR PITUITARY EXTRACT IN CIRRHOTIC PATIENTS WITH BLEEDING VARICES

| Authors | Number of Patients | Number of Trials | Initial Success (%) | Rebled (%) | Mortality (%) |
|---|---|---|---|---|---|
| Schwartz, Bales, Emerson, and Mahoney | 11 | 27 | 89 | Frequent | — |
| Merigan, Plotkin, and Davidson | 15 | 22 | 73 | Frequent | 93 |
| Shaldon and Sherlock | 8 | 25 | 100 | 63 | 75 |
| Orloff | 45 | 45 | 88 | Immediate operation | — |
| | 18 | 18 | 88 | 83 | — |

to prepare patients for operation when massive bleeding cannot be initially controlled by other means.

2. INTRAVENOUS POSTERIOR PITUITARY EXTRACT. It has been shown in both experimental animals and man that posterior pituitary extract reduces portal pressure and blood flow by constricting the splanchnic arterioles. The response is directly related to the dose and rapidity of injection, and in the usual clinical dosage range has a duration of 1 hour or less. However, as shown in Table 11, the transient reduction of portal pressure has been sufficient to stop varix hemorrhage temporarily in a large percentage of patients. Unfortunately, most of the patients have bled again unless operation was performed within 8 hours of treatment, and subsequent administration of the drug has been much less effective in stopping bleeding. It is apparent, therefore, that posterior pituitary extract alone is not a definitive form of treatment but may be of considerable immediate value while other measures are being readied or the patient is being prepared for operation. Every patient with bleeding esophageal varices is given posterior pituitary extract soon after admission to our institution. The agent is administered intravenously over a 15 to 20 minute period in a dose of 20 units diluted in 200 ml. of solution. We have not observed any cardiac abnormalities related to infusion of Pituitrin. This measure of therapy has largely replaced esophageal balloon tamponade as our means of obtaining immediate control of hemorrhage.

3. GASTROESOPHAGEAL HYPOTHERMIA. Use of gastroesophageal hypothermia to stop varix bleeding is based on the demonstration that lowering the temperature of the stomach to 10 to 14° C. abolishes the digestive activity of gastric juice and produces a significant reduction of blood flow in the stomach. Cooling is accomplished with balloons in the stomach and esophagus through which a cold alcohol-water solution is circulated. The rationale of gastroesophageal cooling in part hinges on the theory that rupture of esophageal varices is the result of reflux acid-peptic esophagitis. However, our recent studies have cast considerable doubt on the acid-peptic hypothesis. Experience with gastroesophageal hypothermia has been small but reports to date indicate that this technique, although often effective in temporarily stopping

bleeding, has failed to lower the mortality rate of varix hemorrhage and probably does not warrant serious consideration.

**Specific Emergency Surgical Therapy.** During the past quarter century, the widely accepted approach to the treatment of bleeding varices in patients with cirrhosis has involved the use of temporary nonsurgical emergency measures directed at stopping the hemorrhage so as to permit deliberate and methodical preparation of the patients for an elective portacaval shunt. This approach has been based on the belief that, on the one hand, it is often possible to stabilize and improve the underlying liver disease and, on the other hand, cirrhotic patients will not tolerate major operations performed under emergency circumstances in the face of hemorrhage. A wealth of evidence indicates that this approach has not substantially influenced survival of the bleeding cirrhotic population, since two-thirds to three-fourths of the patients have died during the initial bleeding episode and only 10 to 20 per cent have become eligible for elective therapy. Because of the failure of the "traditional" approach there has been considerable recent interest in emergency surgical management. Results obtained during the past 10 years have been encouraging and suggest that immediate operation is the treatment of choice in most patients. Experience is insufficient as yet to establish definite criteria for selection of patients for operation. Although it is clear that the risk of operation is great in patients with decompensated cirrhosis, it is also certain that such patients have little chance of surviving with nonoperative therapy. Currently, emergency operative treatment is largely confined to the use of two operations, transesophageal varix ligation and the emergency portacaval shunt. Both procedures stop varix bleeding in almost all patients, and the problem associated with them is mainly that of hepatic decompensation which may result when a critically ill patient with a severely damaged liver is subjected to anesthesia and major trauma, in addition to hemorrhage.

1. TRANSESOPHAGEAL VARIX LIGATION (Fig. 22). Since Boerema first described transesophageal ligation of esophageal varices in 1949, the reported experience with this procedure has not been large. Moreover, the cases have varied so greatly as to etiology, severity of the underlying disease, prior

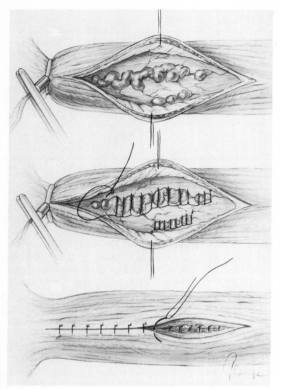

**Figure 22**  Technique of transesophageal varix ligation. (From Orloff, M. J.: Surgery, 52:103, 1962.)

treatment, and time lapse between onset of bleeding and ligation, that accurate assessment of the results is difficult. The mortality rate has ranged from 15 to 86 per cent. The largest reported series has involved 58 selected patients with an operative mortality rate of 45 per cent and a 1 year survival rate of 29 per cent. Because the value of this procedure was not clearly established, several years ago we undertook a prospective comparison of emergency transesophageal varix ligation and medical therapy. Every cirrhotic patient admitted to the hospital with varix bleeding was

included in the study with no attempt at selection. The diagnostic work-up was completed within 6 hours and, in the surgical group, operation was performed within 8 hours of admission to the hospital. The study was conducted in comparable groups of chronic alcoholics with moderate to advanced cirrhosis and massive varix hemorrhage. Approximately half the patients in each group had jaundice and ascites, and one-fourth had hepatic encephalopathy. When feasible, the patients who survived emergency surgical or medical therapy were prepared for and underwent an elective portacaval shunt at a later date.

The results of this study are included in the summary presented in Table 12. Emergency transesophageal varix ligation consistently controlled bleeding. The early survival rate was 54 per cent following operative ligation compared to 14 per cent in the medically treated patients. The 5 year survival rate was 21 per cent in the surgical group and 3 per cent in the medical group. Our experience showed that varix ligation is not a definitive procedure, but must be considered the first of two stages in treatment, the second stage of which is an elective portacaval shunt. The refusal of some patients to undergo an elective shunt was invariably associated with rebleeding and played a major role in the declining survival rate. Moreover, in evaluating the long-term results of both varix ligation and medical therapy, the mortality rate of the subsequent elective portacaval shunt must be considered.

A major reason for considering transesophageal varix ligation as emergency treatment for bleeding varices is the belief that it is an effective procedure of lesser magnitude than other emergency operations. Our experience has shown that such is not the case. The time required to perform the operation, the magnitude of the trauma, the metabolic response, and the effects on liver function are similar to those associated with emergency portacaval shunt. While varix ligation appears to have distinct advantages over medical therapy, it does not appear to be the best emergency surgical procedure available.

2. EMERGENCY PORTACAVAL SHUNT. Portalsystemic shunt is the only available definitive

**TABLE 12**  COMPARISON OF RESULTS OF EMERGENCY PORTACAVAL SHUNT, TRANSESOPHAGEAL VARIX LIGATION, AND MEDICAL TREATMENT IN PATIENTS WITH CIRRHOSIS AND BLEEDING VARICES

|  | Medical Treatment | Varix Ligation | Emergency Shunt |
|---|---|---|---|
| Number of patients | 59 | 28 | 40 |
| Jaundice | 25 (42%) | 16 (57%) | 23 (58%) |
| Ascites | 24 (41%) | 14 (50%) | 17 (43%) |
| Encephalopathy on admission | 15 (25%) | 7 (25%) | 8 (20%) |
| Mean liver index | 2.8 | 2.8 | 2.9 |
| Admission hemoglobin 11 gm./100 ml. or less | 41 (70%) | 20 (71%) | 28 (70%) |
| Varices demonstrated | 56 (95%) | 28 (100%) | 40 (100%) |
| Volume of blood transfused (mean) (liters) | 7.2 | 4.2 | 4.2 |
| Early survival (30 days and left hospital) | 10 (17%) | 15 (54%) | 21 (53%) |
| Five year survival | 2 (3%) | 6 (21%) | 17 (43%) |

## CUMULATIVE SURVIVAL

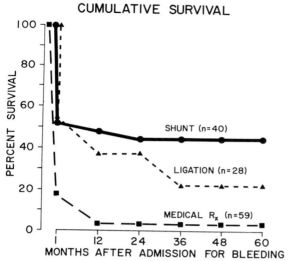

**Figure 23** Cumulative 5 year survival rates of patients with cirrhosis and varix hemorrhage following emergency portacaval shunt, transesophageal varix ligation, and medical treatment.

treatment for portal hypertension and esophageal varices. Numerous studies have shown that a technically satisfactory portacaval shunt will permanently solve the problem of bleeding varices in the vast majority of patients. The obvious potential advantage of performing this procedure under emergency circumstances is that, unlike other forms of treatment, it can be expected to provide both immediate and prolonged control of varix hemorrhage. The question is, can cirrhotic patients tolerate an operation of this magnitude when it is performed as an emergency in the face of bleeding? To answer this question, we have been conducting a prospective study of emergency portacaval shunt, similar to our comparative evaluation of varix ligation and medical therapy. The study has involved unselected alcoholic cirrhotics with advanced liver disease, and the diagnostic work-up and operation have been performed within 8 hours of admission to the emergency room. Our initial report in 1967 concerned 40 patients, the survivors among which have now been followed for at least 5 years. The results in this group are shown in the comparative summary in

Table 12 and Figure 23. The early survival rate was 53 per cent, compared to 54 per cent for varix ligation and 17 per cent for medical therapy. The 5 year survival rate was 43 per cent, compared to 21 per cent for varix ligation and 3 per cent for medical treatment. Since our initial report, we have performed emergency portacaval shunt in an additional 65 unselected patients. The operative survival rate for the total group of 105 patients was 47 per cent, and the long-term survival rate to date (1 to 9 years) is 40 per cent (Table 13). The experience of others with emergency portacaval shunt is shown in Table 14. All but one of these studies were retrospective in nature, and all involved selected patients; therefore, they cannot be compared with our experience in an unselected population.

The results of these studies indicate that emergency portacaval shunt has produced a significant improvement in immediate and long-term survival of cirrhotic patients with bleeding esophageal varices. As is true of survival statistics for cancer and other lethal disorders, the absolute survival rate is of limited meaning unless it is viewed in the context of the natural history of the disease. The 5 year survival rate in our experience to date is 14 times greater than that associated with emergency medical therapy followed by elective portacaval shunt in the few patients who survive. Undoubtedly, some patients with advanced cirrhosis will not survive with any form of therapy currently available. The problem is that criteria for identifying such patients are not yet known. The development of sound criteria for selection of patients for various forms of treatment unquestionably will improve the results of operative management. Until such guidelines are developed by well controlled, prospective studies it would appear that emergency portacaval shunt is the therapy of choice for most cirrhotic patients who bleed from esophageal varices.

3. OTHER EMERGENCY OPERATIONS. A host of other operative procedures have been used as emergency treatment of bleeding esophageal varices. Included among these are gastric or esophageal transection, sometimes combined with extensive ligation of the veins around the distal esophagus and upper stomach; esophagogastrectomy with or without interposition of a segment of colon or jejunum; splenectomy alone or with

**TABLE 13** RESULTS OF A PROSPECTIVE STUDY OF EMERGENCY PORTACAVAL SHUNT IN 105 UNSELECTED PATIENTS WITH ALCOHOLIC CIRRHOSIS AND BLEEDING ESOPHAGEAL VARICES

| | % of 105 | | % of 105 |
|---|---|---|---|
| Jaundice on admission | 50 | Operative survival | 47 |
| Ascites on admission | 53 | Long-term survival (1–9 years) | 40 |
| Encephalopathy on admission | 24 | Control of bleeding | 97 |
| Previous history of encephalopathy | 18 | Encephalopathy postoperatively – all types | 24 |
| Varices demonstrated by x-ray | 100 | Chronic postoperative encephalopathy – | |
| Alcoholic cirrhosis on biopsy | 100 | protein-related | 4 |
| Alkalosis and hypokalemia, preoperative | | Abstinence from alcohol post- | |
| and postoperative | 81 | operatively | 73 |

**TABLE 14**  OVERALL IMMEDIATE RESULTS OF EMERGENCY PORTACAVAL SHUNT IN THE
THERAPY OF BLEEDING ESOPHAGEAL VARICES IN CIRRHOTIC PATIENTS

| Authors | Year | Number of Patients | Type of Evaluation | Operative Survival (%) |
|---|---|---|---|---|
| Orloff | 1971 | 105 | Prospective — Unselected patients | 47 |
| VA Cooperative Study | 1971 | 50 | Prospective — Selected patients | 52 |
| Mikkelsen | 1962 | 37 | Retrospective — Selected patients | 65 |
| Wantz and Payne | 1961 | 34 | Retrospective — Selected patients | 59 |
| Ekman and Sandblom | 1964 | 30 | Retrospective — Selected patients | 83 |
| Balasegaram and Damodaran | 1970 | 30 | Retrospective — Selected patients | 70 |
| Megevand | 1970 | 30 | Retrospective — Selected patients | 70 |
| Adson | 1967 | 30 | Retrospective — Selected patients | 73 |
| Weinberger | 1965 | 29 | Retrospective — Selected patients | 72 |
| Preston and Trippel | 1965 | 25 | Retrospective — Selected patients | 56 |
| Hoffman, Jepson, and Harris | 1969 | 20 | Retrospective — Selected patients | 55 |

coronary vein ligation; combination of splenectomy, resection of the proximal two-thirds of the greater curvature of the stomach, ligation of gastric and esophageal varices, ligation of the left gastric artery, and, sometimes, vagotomy and pyloroplasty; ligation of the hepatic, left gastric, and splenic arteries; external drainage of the thoracic duct; and an extracorporeal or subcutaneous shunt between the umbilical and saphenous veins. Although some success has been obtained with each of these procedures, often in a small number of cases, general experience with them has not been good for a variety of reasons, and they do not warrant serious consideration.

**Postoperative Care Following Emergency Portacaval Shunt.**  Cirrhotic patients who bleed from esophageal varices are among the most seriously ill patients in any hospital, regardless of the specific therapy used to control the bleeding. In those who undergo emergency portacaval shunt, the expertness of the postoperative care is a major factor in determining survival. All such patients should be admitted to an intensive care unit with equipment and personnel geared to managing the complicated problems associated with this disease. Specific prophylactic and therapeutic aspects of postoperative care are as follows:

1. MONITORING. Careful monitoring of vital signs, central venous pressure, urine output, arterial pH, arterial and alveolar gases, fluid balance, body weight, and abdominal girth are essential. Serial electrocardiograms and determinations of cardiac output, peripheral resistance, and pulmonary artery wedge pressure with a Swan-Ganz catheter often are very helpful. Serial measurements of liver function, of the formed elements in the blood, including platelets, of blood coagulation, of serum electrolytes, and of renal function must be done.

2. PARENTERAL FLUID THERAPY. Patients with cirrhosis are often water-logged even before the onset of bleeding from varices, and they have a markedly impaired capacity to excrete water loads. The bleeding episode and the operation intensify renal sodium and water retention and exaggerate the already existing fluid intolerance. Parenteral

fluid therapy should be calculated to maintain such patients on the dry side. Fluid losses are replaced by a solution of 10 per cent dextrose in water containing vitamins B, C, and K. The total volume usually amounts to 1500 to 2000 ml. per day, based on daily losses of 500 ml. of nasogastric aspirate, 500 to 1000 ml. of urine, 800 to 1000 ml. of insensible water, and a *gain* of 250 to 500 ml. from endogenous water formation. Sodium is given only to replace nasogastric losses, which rarely exceed 30 to 40 mEq. per day. Parenteral potassium therapy is started as soon as the urine output is adequate, and is given in whatever amounts are necessary to maintain the serum potassium concentration between 4 and 5 mEq. per liter. Usually, the requirement is 150 to 200 mEq. per day, but doses as high as 400 mEq. per day may be necessary. If a metabolic alkalosis develops that is unresponsive to potassium replacement, parenteral ammonium chloride or arginine hydrochloride is given slowly so as to lower the arterial blood pH below 7.50. In addition to crystalloid fluid therapy, it is often necessary to add colloid therapy to replace continuing losses of blood and plasma. Transfusions of fresh blood are given for blood loss or a hematocrit below 30 per cent. Type-specific, single-donor plasma, fresh-frozen plasma, or salt-poor concentrated albumin is given for losses of fluid into the operation site and peritoneal cavity (acute ascites), as determined by the combined measurements of abdominal girth, central venous pressure, urine output, body weight, and a hematocrit showing hemoconcentration.

A major shortcoming of current parenteral fluid therapy is its caloric deficiency. It is estimated that a patient who has undergone an emergency portacaval shunt for varix hemorrhage has a metabolic response that consumes 4000 to 5000 calories per day for the first few postoperative days. Two liters of 10 per cent dextrose in water provides a total of only 800 calories. There is reason to believe that the postoperative cirrhotic patient may benefit from early nutritional therapy. For this reason, recently we have initiated an investigation of parenteral hyperalimentation with a concentrated glucose-amino acid solution starting on the first day postoperatively.

3. PULMONARY THERAPY. Pulmonary complications, particularly infection and wet lung, are a major cause of morbidity and mortality in patients with cirrhosis and bleeding varices. Often it is necessary to maintain the patient on a respirator for several days postoperatively. In most cases, mechanical ventilatory support can be provided through an endotracheal tube that may be left indwelling for 48 to 72 hours. Occasionally it is necessary to perform a tracheostomy for ventilation and tracheobronchial toilet, but it should be recognized that complications of tracheostomy, particularly bleeding, are more frequent in cirrhotic patients. Portable chest x-rays are obtained daily in patients on respirators or those having pulmonary problems. The decision to taper off and then discontinue mechanical ventilatory support is based on measurements of arterial blood and alveolar gases, ventilatory volumes, chest x-rays, and physical findings.

All patients not on a respirator are given continuous oxygen therapy by nasal catheter, nasal prongs, or mask for 5 to 7 days postoperatively because of the frequent cardiovascular abnormalities and arteriovenous shunting that exist in cirrhosis. From the start, all patients receive intensive respiratory therapy that consists of intermittent tracheobronchial aspiration, postural drainage, chest physiotherapy, intermittent positive-pressure respiration, frequent turning, encouragement to cough and breathe deeply, and the use of blow bottles and a humidifier. Diuretics may be of value in the treatment of pulmonary edema due to left heart failure or infection.

4. HYPERDYNAMIC CIRCULATION. Numerous studies have shown that patients with cirrhosis and portal hypertension frequently have a hyperdynamic state that consists of a decrease in vascular tone and peripheral resistance, an increase in cardiac index, an increase in venous oxygen saturation with widespread peripheral arteriovenous shunting, and marked pulmonary arteriovenous admixture. These abnormalities are sometimes intensified by bleeding from esophageal varices or performance of a portacaval shunt, and high-output cardiac failure may develop, particularly in older patients and those with far advanced liver disease. Patients with a hyperdynamic state are digitalized immediately postoperatively, before there are any signs of cardiac failure. Vigorous correction of hypovolemia is undertaken simultaneously. Once blood volume is restored, fluids are restricted to avoid circulatory overload, and diuretics are used if there are any signs of overhydration. Positive inotropic drugs are used when appropriate.

5. DELIRIUM TREMENS. Alcoholic cirrhotic patients frequently have delirium tremens following hemorrhage alone or in combination with a portacaval shunt or other operation. There is not a close temporal correlation between alcohol withdrawal and the development of this serious disorder; we have observed postoperative delirium tremens

weeks and months after ingestion of alcohol was stopped. Delirium tremens by itself, in the absence of bleeding or an operation, is associated with a mortality rate of 20 to 35 per cent. When added to the stress of hemorrhage or major surgery, the mortality rate climbs to 50 to 60 per cent. Initial treatment consists of administration of a central nervous system depressant. We prefer intramuscular magnesium sulfate in doses of 5 gm. every 2 to 4 hours. If magnesium sulfate therapy is not rapidly effective, chlordiazepoxide hydrochloride (Librium) is added in a dose of 25 to 50 mg. intramuscularly every 4 hours. Supportive treatment in the form of adequate parenteral fluids containing concentrated glucose and vitamins, antipyretic agents, and pulmonary therapy is important. This hyperactive, hypermetabolic disorder must not be confused with hepatic encephalopathy, since the use of a central nervous system depressant in hepatic encephalopathy may be lethal. Intravenous alcohol is a severe hepatotoxin, and there is no basis for its use in cirrhotic patients with postoperative delirium tremens. Parenteral paraldehyde has no advantages over other hypnotic drugs and, in the author's opinion, should not be used because of the frequent soft tissue abscesses and noxious odor it produces.

6. HEPATIC FAILURE. The majority of patients appear to be in surprisingly good condition immediately following an emergency portacaval shunt. However, by the second or third postoperative day there is evidence of some deterioration of liver function in almost all patients. In many patients the liver dysfunction stabilizes and then improves, but in some it progresses to hepatic coma and the full syndrome of hepatic failure, with jaundice, severe abnormalities of blood coagulation, ascites, and renal insufficiency. Liver failure is the most frequent cause of death in cirrhotic patients who bleed from esophageal varices, whether or not they have had a portacaval shunt.

The subject of hepatic coma is discussed in detail later in this chapter. It should be emphasized that the hepatic coma that occurs during the immediate postoperative period is due to liver cell failure, and is *not* related to ammonia intoxication or systemic shunting of nitrogenous substances absorbed from the intestines. Unfortunately, there is no specific therapy for hepatic failure, and all that can be done is to provide parenteral nutritional support and symptomatic therapy of the individual abnormalities that arise. There is no evidence that exchange transfusion, hemodialysis, or extracorporal perfusion of the blood through a pig, baboon, or human liver is of value in this situation. Spontaneous recovery sometimes occurs.

Because it is rarely possible to remove all of the blood from the gastrointestinal tract preoperatively, neomycin therapy (1 gm. every 6 hours via the nasogastric tube), cathartics (60 ml. magnesium sulfate per day via the nasogastric tube), and a daily neomycin enema (4 gm. in 1 quart of water) are continued for 3 days postoperatively. If continued beyond 3 days, troublesome diarrhea usually follows. With this regimen, significantly elevated blood ammonia levels or signs of nitrogen-related encephalopathy rarely occur within the first postoperative week.

7. GASTRIC ACID HYPERSECRETION. The subjects of gastric acid hypersecretion and peptic ulcer following portacaval shunt are discussed in detail later in this chapter. To protect against this complication, nasogastric suction is continued for 3 or 4 days postoperatively. As soon as the nasogastric tube is removed, the patient is started on hourly antacid therapy until his oral dietary intake is good, and then the antacid schedule is changed to between meals and at bedtime. An antacid that does not contain sodium is used. Antacid therapy and avoidance of ulcerogenic foods are continued for life.

8. RENAL FAILURE. The subject of renal failure is discussed in detail later in this chapter. There are two common forms of renal dysfunction following varix hemorrhage and portacaval shunt. The first is acute tubular necrosis which results from a period of hypotension and consequent renal ischemia. It is manifested by oliguria, azotemia, hyperkalemia, a low fixed urine specific gravity and osmolality, substantial quantities of sodium in the urine, and a urine sediment containing casts and red blood cells. Treatment consists of stringent fluid restriction, measures to reduce serum potassium, and, if necessary, hemodialysis. The second renal disorder is spontaneous renal failure associated with hepatic decompensation, the so-called "hepatorenal syndrome." It is more insidious in onset than acute tubular necrosis and is manifested initially by progressive azotemia without striking oliguria. In contrast to acute tubular necrosis, the urine specific gravity is variable and ranges up to 1.020, there is almost no sodium in the urine, the osmolality of the urine is high, and the urine sediment is normal. There is no specific treatment for spontaneous renal failure, and therapy is directed at reversing the hepatic decompensation, minimizing dilutional hyponatremia, and correcting problems as they appear. There is no indication for the use of diuretics and, in fact, they may intensify the renal abnormality. Numerous vasoactive agents have been used for the purpose of improving renal blood flow, but none have influenced the outcome significantly. Hemodialysis has created more problems than it has solved. The mortality rate of the combined syndrome of hepatic and renal decompensation is very high.

9. INFECTION. Substantial evidence indicates that patients with cirrhosis have a high incidence of infection, perhaps because of their debilitated general condition. Surprisingly, wound and intraperitoneal infections following emergency portacaval shunt have been uncommon in our experience. However, pulmonary infections have been common and urinary tract infections not infrequent. The value of prophylactic antibiotic therapy in this condition has not been established. Appropriate antibiotics are given for proven infections, always on the basis of bacterial cultures and antibiotic sensitivity tests. We routinely obtain cultures of tracheal aspirates and urine during the early postoperative period to avoid delays in therapy should infection develop.

10. NUTRITION. Nutritional therapy is very important in liver disease. Oral diet is started as soon as the patient tolerates removal of the nasogastric tube for 24 hours, usually on the fifth or sixth postoperative day. Initially, a 200 mg. sodium, 4000 calorie, high carbohydrate, regular fat, 20 gm. protein, bland diet is introduced. There is no basis for restricting fat, and doing so only serves to make the diet unpalatable. The protein content of the diet is increased in 20 gm. increments every 3 to 4 days up to 80 gm., and the patient is carefully observed for signs of encephalopathy. If the patient tolerates 80 gm. of protein per day, he is discharged on a 60 gm. protein diet after having received a diet list and specific instructions from a dietician. Rigorous sodium restriction is continued for several months and, even after a year has elapsed, sodium intake is not allowed to advance above 2.5 gm. per day. Daily therapeutic doses of vitamins B and C are added to the diet.

11. ALCOHOLISM. Perhaps the major factor that determines long-term survival following portacaval shunt is abstinence or failure to abstain from alcohol (Table 15). It is vitally important that a frank discussion be held with the patient regarding the extremely serious dangers of further ingestion of alcohol. The help of psychiatrists and social workers should be obtained while the patient is in the hospital and continued after discharge. It is incumbent upon the surgeon to exploit his special relationship with the patient in a long-term effort to cure the underlying cause of the patient's liver disease.

12. FOLLOW-UP. A lifelong program of follow-up evaluation and treatment is a crucial part of the care of cirrhotic patients who have undergone portacaval shunt. The liver disease cannot be cured, but it can be stabilized to the point of permitting a long and productive life in reasonable comfort. After discharge from the hospital, out-

**TABLE 15** INFLUENCE OF RESUMPTION OF ALCOHOLISM FOLLOWING EMERGENCY PORTACAVAL SHUNT ON SURVIVAL

| Survivors of Portacaval Shunt | Length of Follow-up (Years) | Resumption of Alcohol | | | Abstinence from Alcohol | | |
|---|---|---|---|---|---|---|---|
| | | No. | % | Mortality (%) | No. | % | Mortality (%) |
| 21 | 5-8 | 13 | 26 | 46 | 36 | 74 | 3 |
| 49 | 1-8 | 6 | 29 | 50 | 15 | 71 | 7 |

patient visits are scheduled weekly for the first 8 weeks, monthly for the remainder of the first postoperative year, and every 3 months thereafter for the remainder of the patient's life.

### Elective Treatment

In patients who have not undergone an emergency portacaval shunt and have recovered from an episode of bleeding esophageal varices, there is general agreement that elective surgical treatment directed at overcoming portal hypertension is indicated, provided there is a reasonable likelihood that the patient will survive the elective operation. Our studies of 27 patients who recovered from their first bleeding episode and qualified for surgical therapy but were not operated upon showed that 93 per cent bled again, 74 per cent died from the subsequent hemorrhage, and all were dead within 5 years. The only consistently effective treatment for portal hypertension is the portal-systemic shunt which, when performed properly, will protect more than 90 per cent of patients against subsequent varix hemorrhage. Therefore, one episode of varix bleeding is an indication for elective shunt therapy in all cirrhotic patients, unless they have hepatic decompensation. Unfortunately, only 10 to 20 per cent of bleeding cirrhotic patients survive nonsurgical emergency therapy and recover sufficient hepatic function to become eligible for elective shunt.

What criteria can be used to predict the likelihood of a patient surviving an elective shunt procedure without serious sequelae? The answer to this question is not known with any degree of certainty, and is particularly difficult because the decision not to operate is tantamount to accepting a lethal outcome. The criteria for selection of patients for operation have been undergoing progressive change as knowledge regarding the underlying liver disease and its management has accumulated. The results of liver function tests such as the level of serum albumin, the amount of BSP retention, or the magnitude of prothrombin deficiency do not correlate well with the response to shunt except at the extremes. In the final analysis, the decision concerning operation is based on a composite of many features of a patient's disease, determined during a period of intensive medical treatment in the hospital. Certain features are ominous; thus, the presence of substantial jaundice, of ascites that cannot be stabilized, of repeated bouts of encephalopathy, of advanced muscle wasting, and of a poor appetite indicate that operation should not be undertaken. Studies of hepatic blood flow may prove in the future to be of additional help in selecting patients for operation. If these general criteria have been followed, the operative mortality rate has been in the acceptable range of 10 per cent. It should be emphasized that, whenever possible, patients are prepared for an elective operation during a 3 to 6 week period in the hospital with a regimen directed at improving nutrition, slowly restoring blood volume and red cell mass, correcting electrolyte and acid-base abnormalities, and unloading excess fluid.

There are several untoward sequelae of the portal-systemic anastomosis. The most important of these is postshunt encephalopathy which presumably is due to shunting of ammonia, or some nitrogenous substance absorbed from the intestine, directly into the systemic circulation. The reported incidence of this disturbing complication has varied considerably, but has been in the range of 5 to 15 per cent of patients. Because ammonia is formed by the action of bacteria on nitrogenous substances in the terminal ileum and colon, encephalopathy often can be controlled by limiting the protein content of the diet and by the use of intestinal antibiotics such as neomycin. If these measures fail, operative exclusion of the colon by ileostomy or ileosigmoidostomy may be effective. The central nervous system disorders associated with liver disease are discussed in greater detail later in this chapter.

The development of peptic ulcer is another potential complication of portal-systemic shunt. Hepatic bypass of a potent intestinal hormone that stimulates gastric acid hypersecretion is a regular consequence of a portacaval anastomosis. This

**TABLE 16** RESULTS OF ELECTIVE PORTAL-SYSTEMIC SHUNT IN PATIENTS WITH CIRRHOSIS

| Authors | No. of Patients | Type of Shunt | Operative Mortality (%) | Varix Rebleeding (%) | 5 Year Survival (%) |
|---|---|---|---|---|---|
| McDermott, Palazzi, Nardi, and Mondet | 237 | 166 splenorenal 71 portacaval | 23 | 15 | 54 |
| Barnes et al. | 173 | 103 portacaval 70 splenorenal | 13 | 14 | 39 |
| Mikkelsen, Turrill, and Pattison | 173 | All portacaval | 12 | 7 | 44 |
| Linton, Ellis, and Geary | 169 | 129 splenorenal 47 portacaval | 12 | 19 | 50 |
| Wantz and Payne | 97 | All portacaval | 11 | 5 | 68 (4 year) |
| Walker | 50 | All portacaval | 6 | 12 | 70 |
| Child | 56 | All portacaval | 12 | 0 | — |
| Orloff | 54 | All portacaval | 4 | 2 | 59 |

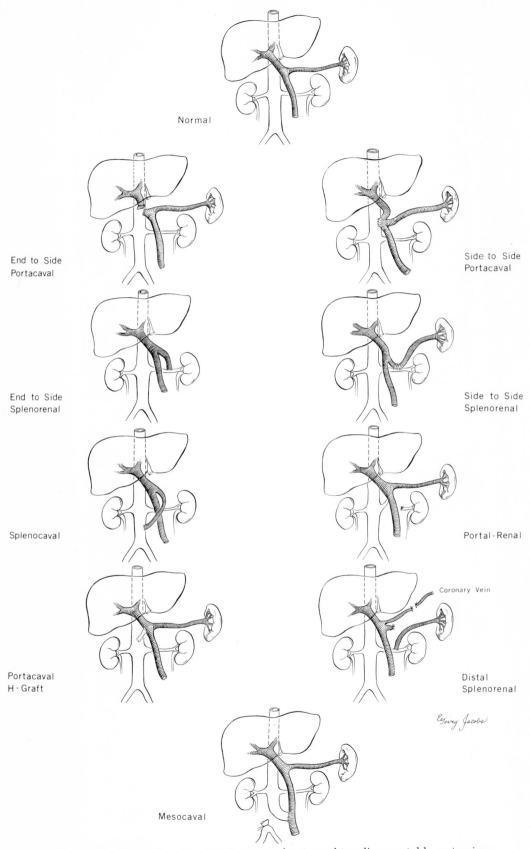

Normal

End to Side
Portacaval

Side to Side
Portacaval

End to Side
Splenorenal

Side to Side
Splenorenal

Splenocaval

Portal-Renal

Portacaval
H-Graft

Coronary Vein

Distal
Splenorenal

Mesocaval

**Figure 24** Types of portal-systemic venous shunts used to relieve portal hypertension.

phenomenon is discussed in detail later in this chapter. It would seem prudent to institute ant-acid therapy and a dietary ulcer regimen following shunt operations.

Venous shunt therapy, of course, represents treatment of the complications of cirrhosis and has no direct beneficial effect on the liver disease itself. In contrast to the effects of portacaval shunt in experimental animals with normal livers, the influence of the operation on liver function in humans with cirrhosis and portal hypertension is variable. In our studies, hepatic function did not change or improved moderately in the majority of patients following operation. Deterioration of hepatic function has been related more closely to whether or not the patient resumed the ingestion of alcohol than to any other factor. Beyond any doubt, the portal-systemic shunt prevents subsequent varix bleeding in the vast majority of patients. Moreover, 39 to 70 per cent of the patients subjected to elective treatment have survived 5 years (Table 16). The crucial question of whether a comparable, selected group of patients who were treated medically rather than surgically would survive as long has not yet been answered. Two prospective studies of this important matter are currently in progress and should soon provide valuable information. On the basis of our current knowledge, and until adequate information to the contrary is available, the elective portacaval shunt is indicated in patients who have bled one or more times from esophageal varices.

**Choice of Portal-Systemic Shunt.** Because the portal venous system contains no valves, it is possible to decompress it at various points, provided the anastomosis with the low-pressure systemic venous system is of sufficient size to accommodate a large flow of blood. Several types of portal-systemic shunts are available for relief of portal hypertension (Fig. 24). The most commonly used procedures are the end-to-side and side-to-side anastomoses between the portal vein and inferior vena cava, and the end-to-side splenorenal shunt. The end-to-side portacaval shunt accomplishes splanchnic decompression by shunting all splanchnic venous blood into the inferior vena cava and, at the same time, it decompresses the liver sinusoid by eliminating the contribution of portal venous blood to hepatic inflow and pressure. However, it rarely lowers hepatic sinusoidal pressure to normal and sinusoidal hypertension often persists because hepatic arterial blood continues to encounter difficulty in leaving the liver through the obstructed hepatic venous outflow system. The side-to-side portacaval shunt produces splanchnic decompression equivalent to the end-to-side anastomosis, but it accomplishes significantly greater hepatic decompression by allowing egress of liver blood in a retrograde direction through the portal vein into the low-pressure vena cava. The side-to-side shunt converts the portal vein into an outflow tract, and portal blood does not continue to perfuse the liver. An important question about the side-to-side anastomosis concerns the theoretical possibility that it creates an intrahepatic

arteriovenous fistula in which hepatic arterial blood leaves the liver via the portal vein without having made contact with the hepatic cells and having contributed to hepatic nutrition and metabolism. Studies in experimental animals suggest that arteriovenous shunting occurs to some degree but is compensated for by an increase in afferent hepatic arterial blood flow so that hepatic nutrition is not compromised.

Although the two types of direct portacaval shunt produce similar splanchnic decompression and are equally effective in relieving and preventing varix hemorrhage, the overall hemodynamic effects of the two procedures are distinctly different. Hence, there has been a continuing controversy regarding the comparative advantages and disadvantages of the end-to-side and side-to-side anastomoses. In a series of studies, we have compared the effects of the two types of shunt on hepatic blood flow, liver function, liver morphology, and ammonia tolerance in dogs with experimental cirrhosis, and on hepatic function, ammonia tolerance, the 5 year incidence of hepatic coma and encephalopathy, and the 5 year survival rate in cirrhotic humans who were operated on for bleeding esophageal varices. The results are shown in Table 17. There were no significant differences between end-to-side and side-to-side portacaval shunt in any of the parameters that were evaluated. We have concluded that there is no advantage of one type of direct portacaval shunt over the other except under one circumstance, namely, when there is spontaneous reversal of portal flow as suggested by a pressure on the hepatic side of a clamp occluding the portal vein (HOPP) that is higher than the free portal pressure (FPP). In this circumstance the side-to-side portacaval shunt is clearly the procedure of choice since the end-to-side anastomosis obliterates the already existing portal venous outflow tract and, thereby, increases sinusoidal hypertension to the point of causing intractable ascites that may be lethal.

The splenorenal anastomosis is a variant of the side-to-side, in-continuity shunt. It utilizes tributaries of the portal vein and vena cava which, obviously, are of smaller size than the parent vessels. It is followed by a lower incidence of protein-related portal-systemic encephalopathy than the direct portacaval anastomosis because it shunts a small volume of nitrogen-containing portal blood to the systemic circulation. At the same time, it does not decompress the portal bed as effectively as the direct portacaval shunt, is associated with a significant incidence of varix rebleeding, and has a high incidence of thrombosis. In the author's opinion it is the procedure of choice only in rare instances when severe and intractable hypersplenism complicates portal hypertension and requires splenectomy. The most commonly used type of splenorenal shunt involves removal of the spleen and anastomosis of the end of the splenic vein to the side of the left renal vein. However, a central side-to-side splenorenal shunt can be done in continuity, without splenectomy. It has been proposed that the latter operation permits

TABLE 17  COMPARISON OF END-TO-SIDE AND SIDE-TO-SIDE PORTACAVAL SHUNT IN DOGS
WITH EXPERIMENTAL CIRRHOSIS AND IN CIRRHOTIC HUMANS WHO WERE
TREATED FOR BLEEDING ESOPHAGEAL VARICES

|  | End-to-Side Shunt | Side-to-Side Shunt |
|---|---|---|
| *Cirrhotic Dogs* | | |
| Hepatic blood flow | 17% mean decrease | 18% mean decrease |
| Ammonia tolerance — mean peak blood $NH_3$ | 881 μg./100 ml. | 884 μg./100 ml. |
| Effects on liver function | Same | |
| Effect on liver morphology | Same | |
| *Cirrhotic Humans* | | |
| Number of patients | 25 | 35 |
| Ammonia tolerance — mean peak blood $NH_3$ | 543 μg./100 ml. | 532 μg./100 ml. |
| Liver function index | 1.6 | 1.7 |
| Hepatic coma and encephalopathy (all causes) | 25% | 23% |
| Five year survival | 48% | 57% |

continued portal venous perfusion of the liver, but it is doubtful that such is the case since the principles that govern the hemodynamics of a valveless system dictate that flow is in the direction of the area of lowest pressure, i.e., the splenorenal anastomosis.

The mesocaval shunt is an anastomosis between the upper end of the divided inferior vena cava and the side of the superior mesenteric vein. In principle, it is hemodynamically similar to the side-to-side portacaval shunt. In patients with extrahepatic portal hypertension due to occlusion of the portal vein, this type of shunt is very effective. However, in adult cirrhotic patients it is doubtful that this procedure represents a first choice. Cirrhotic patients have a tendency to retain salt and water, and division of the inferior vena cava may lead to intractable edema of the lower extremities.

The use of H grafts between the intact portal vein and inferior vena cava has been attempted sporadically during the past 20 years. Synthetic prostheses and autogenous veins have been employed for this purpose. In general, the use of grafts in the venous system has had a long history of failure, so that there is justifiable skepticism about the possibility of consistent long-term patency of the H graft. However, success has been reported in a small number of cases. We have not yet encountered a case in which use of an H graft has been necessary or indicated.

An unsettled issue of great importance regarding the use of portacaval shunt concerns its effects both on liver cell function (presumably related to liver blood flow) and on portal-systemic encephalopathy (presumably related to hepatic bypass of nitrogenous substances absorbed from the intestines). When portal blood is completely shunted away from the liver, further liver damage might be anticipated unless there is a compensatory increase in hepatic arterial blood flow. The adequacy of the hepatic arterial compensation has not been precisely determined. It has been proposed that a worsening of liver function or outright hepatic failure following portacaval shunt is due to sudden diversion of needed blood away from the liver. The familiar hepatic dysfunction that follows creation of a portacaval shunt (Eck fistula) in the dog with a normal liver is cited as evidence for this proposal. The fact that patients with extrahepatic occlusion of the portal vein do not usually have significant hepatic dysfunction, either before or after portal-systemic anastomosis, has been interpreted as resulting from the combination of a long period of adaptation to diminished portal flow and an initially normal hepatic parenchyma. On the basis of data obtained from a small group of subjects, Warren and his associates concluded that cirrhotic patients with normal or near-normal hepatic blood flow, who often appear to be the best-risk patients with the least severe liver disease, are intolerant of sudden shunting of portal blood, and often die of progressive hepatic failure. On the other hand, Warren et al. proposed that patients with moderately reduced hepatic blood flow tolerated a portacaval shunt well, since the bypass produced little further reduction in the blood supply to the liver. In contradiction to these proposals, Price and his colleagues concluded from intraoperative hemodynamic studies in 24 patients that neither hepatic blood flow before or after portacaval shunt, nor the amount of reduction of flow caused by the shunt, correlated with survival or other long-term effects of the operation. In order to settle this issue, it is vitally important that these hemodynamic studies be extended to a large number of patients.

On the presumption that portacaval shunt injures the liver and increases portal-systemic encephalopathy in patients with a large hepatopetal portal flow, Warren and his associates have recently advocated a modified shunting procedure that is believed to selectively decompress esophageal varices while, at the same time, preserving blood flow to the liver and avoiding systemic shunting of intestinal blood. The operation consists of a distal splenorenal shunt in which the splenic side of the divided splenic vein is anastomosed to the intact left renal vein, and gastrosplenic isolation aimed at diverting the gastroesophageal venous flow through the shunt.

Gastrosplenic isolation is accomplished by ligation of the coronary vein, the right gastric vein, and the right gastroepiploic vein and division of the gastrohepatic, gastrocolic, and splenocolic ligaments. The most recent report of Warren et al. indicates that the operation has been attempted electively in 28 selected patients with various forms of mild to moderate liver disease, good liver function, and excellent liver blood flow. The operative mortality rate was 32 per cent. Ascites and intraperitoneal bleeding were frequent postoperative problems. Although several patients died of liver failure, none of the survivors developed portal-systemic encephalopathy during observation periods of from 2 months to 4 years. While theoretically attractive, the value of this procedure remains to be established by long-term studies of survival, incidence of shunt thrombosis, frequency of rebleeding, and incidence of liver failure and encephalopathy.

In the hope of improving liver blood flow after end-to-side portacaval shunt, Maillard, Benhamou, and Rueff recently reported a procedure for arterializing the hepatic stump of the portal vein and its use in 10 patients. The value of this operation remains to be determined.

**Prophylactic Portacaval Shunt.** Because of the very high mortality rate associated with varix bleeding, some workers have advocated prophylactic performance of portacaval shunt in patients with demonstrable varices who have never bled. Although once a patient has bled from esophageal varices he is almost certain to bleed again, there is nothing to suggest that the mere demonstration of varices in a patient with no history of bleeding permits a prediction regarding the likelihood of varix rupture. In fact, recent statistics indicate that only one-fourth to one-third of patients with esophageal varices who have no history of bleeding will subsequently have varix hemorrhage. Thus, two-thirds to three-fourths of the patients subjected to prophylactic portacaval shunt would undergo an operation to prevent a complication that would not have developed had they not received surgical therapy. Herein lies the fallacy of prophylactic shunt.

Recently, prophylactic portacaval shunt was compared with medical therapy in three prospective studies that were performed in selected cirrhotic patients with esophageal varices that had not bled. All three studies showed that prophylactic shunt, while protecting the patients against bleeding, had no influence on survival of selected patients. Interestingly, it appears that the criteria for selection of patients may have influenced the outcome, because in a fourth and most recent prospective study by Conn and Lindenmuth, prophylactic portacaval shunt in cirrhotic patients with both varices and ascites has significantly prolonged survival. During a 40 month observation period, 91 per cent of the shunted patients have survived, while only 56 per cent of the medically treated patients have lived. Until further data are available, however, there is little to recommend the prophylactic operation.

## ASCITES

Ascites is a serious complication of cirrhosis. In many patients, it develops suddenly in association with severe hepatocellular damage and is a manifestation of hepatic decompensation. In others, it develops gradually and persists as a chronic disturbance that leads to progressive discomfort, nutritional depletion, and debilitation.

The pathogenesis of ascites is best explained by Starling's hypothesis, which states that the exchange of fluid across capillary membranes is a result of the hydrostatic pressure and osmotic pressure on each side of the membrane. Although several factors may be involved in the pathogenesis of ascites, including the serum albumin concentration, the sodium ion, and hormones such as aldosterone, results of recent studies indicate that increased pressure within the liver plays a major role in ascites formation and is the primary mechanism responsible for transudation of ascitic fluid. Moreover, substantial evidence suggests that the intrahepatic hypertension in cirrhosis is a result of hepatic venous outflow obstruction.

Experimentally, ascites is produced by any procedure that obstructs hepatic venous outflow, but does not result from obstruction of portal venous or hepatic arterial inflow. Furthermore, in experimental ascites the fluid leaks into the peritoneal cavity from the surface and hilum of the liver, a finding that suggests that it originates from some intrahepatic disturbance. Under experimental circumstances, therefore, hepatic outflow obstruction is the sine qua non for ascites formation. In man, a similar striking difference is seen in the ascites-producing effects of outflow and inflow obstruction. In the Budd-Chiari syndrome, a condition resulting from occlusion of the hepatic veins, massive ascites is an invariable complication. In contrast, ascites rarely accompanies extrahepatic obstruction of the portal vein. Comparative observations such as these, both experimental and clinical, plus substantial supporting evidence obtained from hemodynamic and histopathologic studies in man, have led to the conclusion that hepatic outflow block is involved in the pathogenesis of ascites in cirrhosis.

A number of studies have demonstrated a marked increase in the flow of lymph in the hepatic hilar lymphatics and thoracic duct in association with experimental ascites, hepatic outflow obstruction, or experimental cirrhosis. A similar increase in lymph flow in the thoracic duct has been observed in humans with cirrhosis and with congestive heart failure, and the marked enlargement of the lymphatics in the hilum of the cirrhotic liver, so familiar to surgeons who have performed operations for portal hypertension, has been documented by careful histopathologic studies. The bulk of evidence indicates that the augmented production of hepatic lymph is in large part a mechanical phenomenon resulting from obstruction to the outflow of blood from the liver sinusoids and the consequent spillover of the plasma portion of the blood into the perisinusoidal spaces

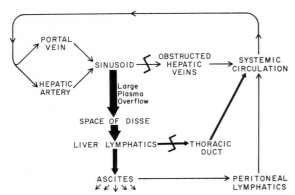

**Figure 25** The chain of events in ascites formation. Hepatic venous outflow obstruction and the resultant intrahepatic hypertension play a primary role in causing transudation of ascitic fluid. (From Orloff, M. J., et al.: Arch. Surg., 93:119, 1966.)

and lymphatics. Ascites, in turn, has been attributed to the inability of the lymphatic system to accommodate the excessive formation of lymph, with resultant leakage of fluid into the peritoneal cavity from the overburdened hepatic lymphatics. This chain of events in ascites formation is depicted in Figure 25.

Humans with cirrhosis and ascites present a characteristic picture of marked salt and water retention, secondary hyperaldosteronism, hypervolemia, and dilutional hyponatremia. It is generally believed, although not proved by scientific data, that ascites precedes the hyperaldosteronism and sodium retention, and that a decrease in nonsplanchnic or "effective blood volume" is the stimulus to aldosterone hypersecretion. However, recent studies by Lieberman and his colleagues indicate that sodium retention antedates ascites formation and probably plays a role in its pathogenesis. Furthermore, studies in our laboratory have uncovered an aldosterone-regulating mechanism in the liver which is activated by increased intrahepatic pressure, and have shown that aldosterone hypersecretion and renal sodium retention precede the appearance of experimental ascites. Thus, it appears possible that increased intrahepatic pressure sets in motion a sequence of events that includes leakage of fluid, increased secretion of aldosterone, and retention of sodium by the kidney, all of which contribute to the formation and persistence of ascites.

In the vast majority of cirrhotic patients, ascites disappears in response to a regimen consisting of abstinence from alcohol, a nourishing diet, salt restriction, and one or more of a variety of diuretic

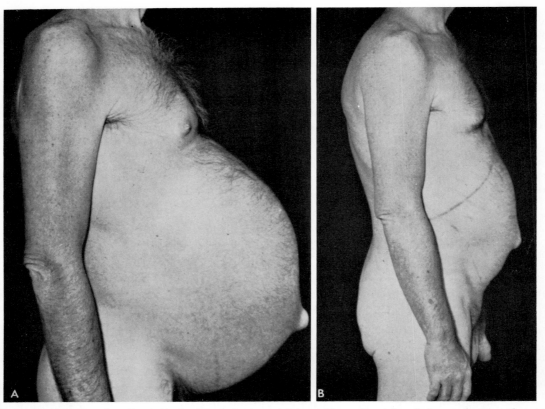

**Figure 26** Photographs of a patient with cirrhosis and intractable ascites taken before and after side-to-side portacaval shunt. *A*, Preoperatively, when ascites was massive. *B*, Six weeks after side-to-side portacaval shunt. (From Orloff, M. J.: Amer. J. Surg., 112:287, 1966.)

and antialdosterone drugs. Nevertheless, in a small but disturbing group of patients, ascites is refractory to these measures. It is for this group that the surgeon has attempted to devise operative measures of relief. If it is assumed, on the basis of substantial evidence, that increased hydrostatic pressure within the liver is important in the pathogenesis of ascites, it should be possible to relieve ascites by reducing the intrahepatic pressure. Theoretically, decompression of the obstructed hepatic vascular bed may be accomplished, to a greater or lesser degree, by reducing the inflow of blood to the liver or by improving the outflow of blood from the liver. Inflow-reducing procedures include ligation of the hepatic artery and the end-to-side portacaval shunt, both of which have been used in the treatment of cirrhotic ascites. Hepatic artery ligation no longer merits serious consideration, because it is an unpredictable operation that is associated with a high mortality rate. Improving the outflow of blood from the liver by a direct attack on the hepatic veins is not possible. However, numerous studies have demonstrated that the valveless portal vein is capable of serving as an

outflow tract and that the objective of hepatic decompression is realized by a side-to-side portacaval shunt.

In a series of experiments, we evaluated the effects of portacaval shunts on ascites. These studies showed that the side-to-side portacaval shunt was effective in relieving ascites, overcoming intrahepatic hypertension, eliminating the hypersecretion of aldosterone that follows hepatic outflow occlusion, and reducing the markedly augmented thoracic duct lymph flow to normal. The end-to-side portacaval anastomosis was much less effective than the lateral anastomosis in relieving the sequelae of increased pressure in the liver.

On the basis of these experimental observations, we have performed side-to-side portacaval shunt in 13 selected patients with alcoholic cirrhosis and truly intractable ascites. All of our patients failed to respond to prolonged and intensive medical treatment for ascites before operation was considered. Twelve of the 13 patients (92 per cent) survived the operation, and all the survivors have been relieved of ascites, salt retention, and hyperaldosteronism for periods ranging from 3 to 8

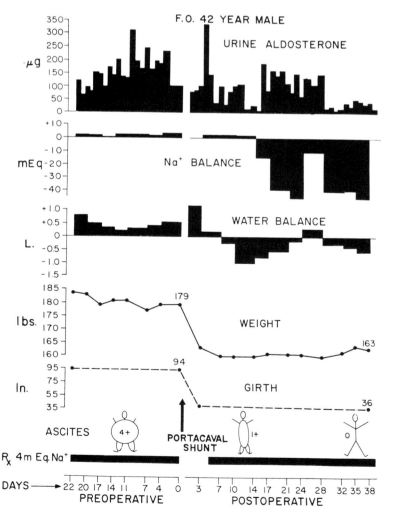

**Figure 27** Results of a metabolic balance study of the patient shown in Figure 26, conducted before and after treatment of intractable ascites by side-to-side shunt. (From Orloff, M. J.: Amer. J. Surg., *112*:287, 1966.)

years (Fig. 26). The most notable feature of the response to operation, other than relief of ascites, has been a striking improvement in nutrition and vigor accompanied by substantial gains in lean tissue mass and body fat. Figure 27 shows the effects of the shunt on water and electrolyte balance and on aldosterone excretion in one of our patients. Our small but consistent experience has led to the conclusion that side-to-side portacaval shunt is of lasting benefit when used in carefully selected cirrhotic patients with truly intractable ascites who have failed to respond to vigorous and expert medical management. It must be emphasized that the number of such patients is small.

## HEPATIC COMA

The central nervous system disorders associated with hepatic cell failure and portal-systemic shunting are included under the umbrella of the term "hepatic coma" and represent the most common terminal event in cirrhosis. The etiology and pathogenesis of most of these disturbances are unknown. In a small percentage of patients, hepatic coma appears to be due to ammonia intoxication resulting from hepatic bypass through spontaneous or surgical portacaval shunts of ammonia absorbed from the intestines, or to the inability of the damaged liver to transform ammonia to urea. The symptoms are related to the amount of nitrogen in the intestine and to the level of blood ammonia, and are described by the terms "portal-systemic encephalopathy" and "exogenous hepatic coma." Ammonia is believed to produce central nervous system depression by interfering with aerobic glycolysis in the brain. In most patients with hepatic coma, the neurologic abnormalities are unrelated to intestinal ammonia absorption but appear to be a mysterious manifestation of hepatic failure.

Hepatic coma occurs under a variety of circumstances in patients with advanced liver damage. Often, it is an aspect of progressive clinical deterioration. Not infrequently it occurs following an episode of varix bleeding or after major operations of any type in cirrhotic patients. It may be precipitated by infection, disorders of fluid and electrolyte balance, certain diuretics such as chlorothiazide, sedatives and analgesics, a bout of alcohol ingestion, or paracentesis.

The incidence of portal-systemic encephalopathy due to shunting of ammonia absorbed from the intestine in patients with a portacaval shunt is not known. Hepatic coma has been reported to occur in from 5 to 30 per cent of shunted patients but, unfortunately, most reports combine all neurologic sequelae under the term encephalopathy, including instances of central nervous system disturbance due to liver cell failure as well as the chronic or recurring disorders due to systemic shunting of nitrogenous substances. In our experience with 218 portacaval shunts, the incidence of protein-related portal-systemic encephalopathy was 7 per cent.

The symptoms and signs of hepatic coma from any cause are nonspecific and run the gamut of alterations of consciousness. In the early stage, called "hepatic precoma," a variety of personality changes occur, including euphoria, untidiness, inability to concentrate, insomnia, and mild confusion. Later, depression and disorientation progressing to stupor and unconsciousness develop. Occasionally, convulsions occur. Asterixis or "liver flap" is a characteristic sign which consists of a flapping, rough tremor best demonstrated by having the patient dorsiflex the hands and spread the fingers. The electroencephalogram shows paroxysms of bilaterally synchronous, high-voltage, slow waves. Fluctuations of the symptoms and level of consciousness are usual.

The treatment of hepatic coma is generally supportive and nonspecific. In the most common form, which is related to liver cell failure, there is no correlation between the level of blood ammonia and the severity of symptoms, and measures directed at lowering blood ammonia are of little benefit. In patients with portal-systemic encephalopathy related to intestinal ammonia absorption, elimination of protein from the diet, removal of nitrogen from the gastrointestinal tract by cathartics and enemas, and administration of intestinal antibiotics such as neomycin may be helpful. In chronic intractable encephalopathy, bypass of the colon by ileostomy or ileosigmoidostomy may be indicated if other measures have failed. The use of ammonia-binding agents, such as glutamic acid and arginine, and of ion exchange resins has met with little success. Similarly, the use of oral lactulose, a nonabsorbable synthetic disaccharide composed of galactose and fructose that is believed to diminish ammonia absorption by lowering colonic pH and inducing mild diarrhea, has been associated with inconsistent results. Treatment of abnormalities known to precipitate hepatic coma and support of liver failure with parenteral glucose and vitamins are of value. Spontaneous recovery from hepatic coma occurs with sufficient frequency to make evaluation of the efficacy of therapy difficult.

In recent years, numerous attempts have been made to treat hepatic coma associated with liver failure by exchange transfusion, hemodialysis, peritoneal dialysis, cross circulation with a human or baboon donor, and extracorporal perfusion of the patient's blood through an isolated liver obtained from a pig, baboon, or human cadaver. Although several of these techniques have produced dramatic improvement in consciousness for brief periods, they have not influenced the mortality rate of the disease. Exchange transfusion is the simplest of these procedures and it has been used most widely. However, the results have not been significantly different from those obtained with noninvasive measures of therapy.

## GASTRIC ACID HYPERSECRETION AND PEPTIC ULCER

The association of peptic ulcer and cirrhosis of the liver has been the subject of numerous studies.

The diagnosis of the two diseases has been based on clinical information in some investigations, and on autopsy findings in others. All of the studies have been retrospective in nature, and all of them have suffered from a lack of suitable controls. The reported incidence of peptic ulcer in patients with cirrhosis has ranged from 2.6 to 24 per cent. Depending upon the references cited, it is possible to conclude that ulcer disease is either more frequent or less frequent in cirrhotic patients than in a comparable noncirrhotic population. Neither conclusion is valid, and the facts remain to be determined by a careful prospective clinical evaluation.

Studies in humans concerning the influence of cirrhosis on gastric acid secretion have almost all demonstrated a depression of basal and histamine-stimulated acid production or no change from the normal. Our studies of the intestinal phase of gastric secretion in cirrhotic patients showed a secretory response within the normal range. Thus, there is no evidence that liver disease per se stimulates the gastric parietal cells.

In contrast to the studies in cirrhosis, it has been observed repeatedly in experimental animals that

portacaval shunt produces profound gastric acid hypersecretion. The nature and cause of this excessive acid production associated with portacaval shunt has been determined only recently. Studies in our laboratory have demonstrated conclusively that it is due to unmasking of the intestinal phase of gastric secretion by hepatic bypass of an intestinal hormone that is normally almost totally degraded by the liver (Fig. 28). The hormone has been shown to originate from the jejunum in both dogs and humans and to be released by the entry of any type of food into the intestine or by intestinal distention. The hormone has been extracted in crude form from hog intestinal mucosa and has been found to be a peptide of low molecular weight. The acid hypersecretion is confined to the intestinal phase of gastric secretion and does not involve the cephalic or gastric phases.

The relationship of the exaggerated intestinal phase of gastric secretion to the development of peptic ulcer in patients with a portacaval shunt is uncertain. It is generally believed that there is an abnormally high incidence of peptic ulcer in shunted cirrhotic patients, and that ulcer disease runs an unusually virulent course in these patients. At least 15 studies of this matter, all retrospective and without suitable controls, have been performed. The frequency of peptic ulcer has ranged from 1.7 to 16 per cent, and the results have been equally divided between those suggesting a causal relationship between shunt and ulcer, and those showing only a coincidental association between the two diseases. In a prospective study in progress, we have observed a 6 per cent chronic ulcer incidence in a group of 34 shunted patients followed for 5 or more years. The true relationship of portacaval shunt to peptic ulcer remains to be determined by prospective studies involving a large number of patients. In view of the invariable gastric acid hypersecretion following shunt operations, it would seem prudent to institute antacid therapy and a dietary ulcer regimen postoperatively.

### RENAL FAILURE

Between 10 and 15 per cent of patients who die from advanced liver disease have renal failure. In some instances the renal disorder can be attributed to a specific kidney injury such as acute tubular necrosis resulting from shock associated with bleeding esophageal varices, or nephropathy secondary to sodium or potassium depletion produced by excessive use of diuretics in the treatment of ascites. In many cases, however, azotemia and oliguric renal failure develop spontaneously from no discernible cause. Such cases are commonly referred to as the "hepatorenal syndrome," although some workers object to the use of this term because the exact relationship of the liver disease to the associated renal dysfunction has not been identified.

There is no specific kidney lesion in the spontaneous renal failure associated with hepatic decompensation and, in fact, microscopic examination of

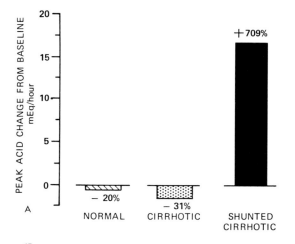

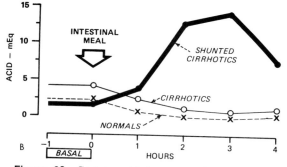

**Figure 28** Gastric acid hypersecretion in humans with portacaval shunts due to hepatic bypass of an intestinal hormone. *A* shows mean peak gastric acid response and *B* shows mean 4 hour gastric acid response to an intestinal meal in normal, cirrhotic, and shunted cirrhotic humans. (From Orloff, M. J., et al.: Ann. Surg., *170*:515, 1969.)

the kidney usually reveals normal architecture or only trivial abnormalities. A cadaver kidney allograft obtained from a cirrhotic donor who died of renal failure has been reported to have functioned promptly and normally when transplanted into a living recipient. The evidence indicates that the renal dysfunction is caused by a disturbance in the blood flow to the kidney resulting from an underlying systemic circulatory abnormality. A number of studies have shown a decrease in renal plasma flow and glomerular filtration rate, an increase in renal vascular resistance, and a redistribution of flow within the kidney such that a disproportionate amount of blood is routed to the medulla. Since these changes frequently occur in the presence of an increased cardiac output, it is apparent that some systemic mechanism produces a diversion of blood flow from the kidneys to other parts of the body. There is reason to believe that the disturbance in renal blood flow is a manifestation of the hyperdynamic circulatory abnormality found in advanced liver disease in which there is a loss of peripheral vascular tone and widespread arteriovenous shunting.

Spontaneous renal failure is most commonly observed in patients with advanced cirrhosis whose hepatic function is deteriorating. Many of the patients have ascites that is progressively refractory to treatment. During the early stages oliguria is not striking and the physician usually first becomes aware of the renal disorder when he finds elevated levels of urea and creatinine in the blood which increase progressively. Unlike acute tubular necrosis due to hypotension and renal ischemia, the urine in spontaneous renal failure is moderately concentrated (1.016 to 1.020), contains almost no sodium, has substantial quantities of potassium, has an osmolality that often exceeds that of plasma, and is free of protein, casts, and red blood cells. As the renal disorder progresses, dilutional hyponatremia and water retention become marked, and oliguria develops. Toward the end, hyperkalemia may become prominent. In most instances, there should be no difficulty in distinguishing this syndrome from acute tubular necrosis, since the latter is usually characterized by early oliguria, a fixed urine specific gravity around 1.010, an increase in sodium and decrease in potassium in the urine, a low urine osmolality, and a highly abnormal urine sediment. Terminally, patients with spontaneous renal failure often show the combined effects of loss of liver and kidney function such as hepatic coma, severe azotemia, hypotension, ascites, edema, and defects in blood coagulation.

The mortality rate of spontaneous renal failure associated with decompensated cirrhosis exceeds 70 per cent, and in some reports has approached 100 per cent. There is no specific treatment for the condition, and therapy is focused on improving liver function. A search should be made for specific causes of renal dysfunction, since they may be amenable to treatment. Because of the marked sodium and water retention and the consequent dilutional hyponatremia and waterlogging, intakes of sodium and fluids are restricted. Diuretic therapy is of no value in this disorder, and may be harmful. Attempts have been made to improve renal blood flow by the use of mannitol, colloid infusions, norepinephrine, metaraminol, aminophylline, dopamine, and other vasoactive substances but there is no solid evidence that these agents have significantly influenced the course of the renal disease or survival. Hemodialysis has been unsuccessful in the treatment of spontaneous renal failure and, because of the multisystem abnormalities that occur in decompensated cirrhosis, has been associated with serious complications.

## PORTAL HYPERTENSION DUE TO EXTRAHEPATIC PORTAL OBSTRUCTION

Portal hypertension due to extrahepatic portal obstruction is a strikingly different condition from intrahepatic portal hypertension. The patients are usually much younger and most often are children. They do not have liver disease and, consequently, have a much greater tolerance for bleeding and for operations. Except in infancy, they rarely have ascites, and hepatic coma due to liver cell failure does not develop. Because the portal vein is usually obliterated, a direct portal vein to vena cava anastomosis cannot be performed for portal decompression. Finally, age and the related technical matter of adequate vessel size influence treatment. Patients with extrahepatic portal obstruction come to the attention of the surgeon usually because of bleeding from esophageal varices or splenomegaly. Although hematemesis is the most common symptom, the bleeding sometimes presents as melena. Exsanguinating hemorrhage does not occur nearly as often as in cirrhosis. On physical examination, splenomegaly is almost always found but the liver is not palpable. Dilated collateral veins in the abdominal wall may be striking. The liver function tests usually are normal, but hematologic studies often reveal peripheral cytopenia that reflects hypersplenism. The hypersplenism is infrequently severe. Upper gastrointestinal x-rays and esophagogastroscopy demonstrate varices. Because the obstruction is presinusoidal, hepatic vein catheterization shows a normal wedged hepatic vein pressure. Splenic manometry and splenoportography are crucial diagnostic procedures and regularly demonstrate the presence of portal hypertension, the site of the portal obstruction, and the size of the vessels available for portal decompression.

The definitive treatment of extrahepatic portal obstruction is the portal-systemic venous shunt. However, for technical reasons related to the size of the vessels required for the shunt, temporizing hemostatic measures may have to be used in infants and young children until they have grown to the point where an adequate anastomosis is feasible. The mesocaval shunt usually should not be performed before the age of 4, and splenorenal shunt is often not feasible before the age of 7 or 8. Consequently, the emergency treatment of varix bleeding in infants and young children consists of blood transfusions and, when necessary, medical measures such as esophageal balloon tamponade and intravenous Pituitrin. Failure to control bleeding is an indication for transesophageal varix ligation. Rebleeding following these temporizing measures is the rule, but it is usually well tolerated and controllable until the child reaches a suitable age.

The types of portal-systemic anastomoses used in patients with an obliterated portal vein are the superior mesenteric vein–inferior vena cava shunt and the splenorenal shunt. The mesocaval shunt has been followed by a lower incidence of rebleeding and appears to be the procedure of choice. Both operations have been associated with operative mortality rates below 5 per cent. Other operative procedures, such as esophagogastrectomy with intestinal interposition, are associated with a high mortality rate and incidence of failure, and are indicated only when a portal-systemic shunt is impossible.

## LIVER TRAUMA

Because of its size, the liver is the solid viscus most frequently injured by perforating wounds of the abdomen; it is involved in approximately 20 to 25 per cent of patients who have received perforating trauma. In blunt injuries to the abdomen, liver damage occurs in 5 to 10 per cent of the patients. As a result of the marked increase in automobile accidents, blunt liver trauma has become a common clinical entity.

Liver wounds vary greatly in direct relationship to the type and magnitude of the trauma. Stab wounds often cause relatively simple lacerations, while gunshot injuries frequently traverse the full depth of the liver and may produce widespread destruction of hepatic tissue. Blunt injuries range from simple subcapsular hematomas to complicated stellate fractures and, occasionally, central rupture of the liver parenchyma. Direct damage to the hilar structures and avulsion of hepatic veins may occur with both perforating and blunt injuries, and present complicated problems that are often lethal.

Because the liver is highly vascular, tolerates anoxia poorly, and is an unpaired organ upon which life depends, hepatic injuries generally are more difficult to treat than other forms of abdominal trauma. Moreover, as a result of its location, injuries to certain parts of the liver are not easily accessible to rapid surgical repair. Consequently, liver trauma carries a higher mortality rate than injury to any other abdominal viscus. Furthermore, liver wounds are often associated with injuries to other organs and systems which complicate treatment and significantly increase the mortality rate. It is common for a patient with liver trauma to have concomitant extra-abdominal injuries of the head, thorax, or long bones, as well as intra-abdominal wounds of the spleen, pancreas, kidney, duodenum, or colon. Table 18 shows the

**TABLE 18**   RELATIONSHIP OF NUMBER OF ORGANS INJURED TO MORTALITY RATE IN 134 CASES OF LIVER TRAUMA

| Number of Organs Injured | Cases | Deaths | Mortality (%) |
|---|---|---|---|
| *Gunshot Wounds* | | | |
| Liver alone | 9 | 1 | 11 |
| Liver + 1 | 15 | 2 | 13 |
| Liver + 2 | 10 | 3 | 30 |
| *Blunt Trauma* | | | |
| Liver alone | 6 | 0 | 0 |
| Liver + 1 | 60 | 8 | 13 |
| Liver + 2 | 20 | 7 | 35 |
| Liver + 3 or more | 14 | 9 | 64 |

direct relationship of the mortality rate of liver trauma to the number of other organs injured.

### Diagnosis

Since it is general policy to perform exploratory laparotomy in all gunshot wounds of the abdomen, the diagnosis of liver injury under such circumstances is made by direct inspection at operation and does not present any diagnostic difficulties. However, in stab wounds and blunt trauma to the abdomen, the decision regarding whether or not to operate is based on obtaining diagnostic evidence of intraperitoneal organ damage. As a result of its rich blood supply, hemorrhage and shock dominate the clinical picture of liver trauma in many patients. In addition, the patient with a liver injury usually complains of pain in the right upper quadrant of the abdomen and on physical examination there are distinct signs of peritoneal irritation such as tenderness and rigidity in the right hypochondrium and hypoactive or absent bowel sounds. Occasionally, pain in the right shoulder from diaphragmatic irritation is a prominent feature. Laboratory studies reveal an elevated white blood cell count and a fall in the hematocrit and hemoglobin concentration, although early in the course hematocrit and hemoglobin determinations may be of no value. Liver function tests rarely provide useful information during the initial 12 hours following injury, when the diagnosis must be made. Abdominal and chest x-rays are of limited value, but may demonstrate signs of blood in the peritoneal cavity, an elevated right hemidiaphragm, and telltale fractures of the right lower ribs. Sometimes, evidence on abdominal x-rays of injury to other organs such as the spleen, duodenum, or colon, an abnormal intravenous pyelogram, or an elevated serum amylase from pancreatic injury provides the indications for performing a laparotomy at which liver damage is discovered.

The most helpful diagnostic procedures in our experience are the abdominal tap and hepatic arteriography. Although a negative tap does not rule out serious intra-abdominal organ damage, a tap productive of free blood is obtained in over 80 per cent of patients with liver injury. Several tech-

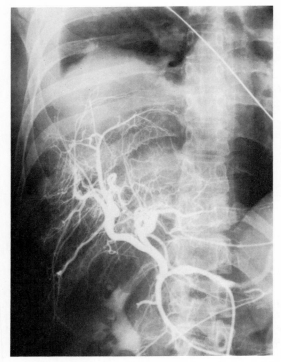

**Figure 29**   Hepatic arteriogram in a patient with blunt abdominal trauma showing distortion of the vasculature due to herniation of the liver into the thorax through a ruptured right diaphragm.

niques of abdominal paracentesis are used, including aspiration from an 18 gauge spinal needle inserted into each of the four abdominal quadrants, aspiration from a plastic catheter inserted into the peritoneal cavity through a needle, and aspiration from a plastic catheter following irrigation of the peritoneal cavity with 1 or 2 liters of saline. Selective hepatic, splenic, and superior mesenteric arteriography is a safe and extremely valuable procedure in the diagnosis of abdominal injury. Hepatic arteriography is used in our clinic whenever there is a question about the diagnosis of liver trauma, and it has proved to be highly accurate and very helpful (Fig. 29). Finally, the radioisotope liver scan is sometimes of value in the diagnosis of liver wounds, although it infrequently yields information not provided by other diagnostic measures.

### Treatment

**Preoperative Preparation.**   Liver trauma requires emergency surgical therapy. In some hepatic injuries, hemorrhage is so massive that operative control of bleeding is the only possible means of resuscitation, and operation should be undertaken promptly without preoperative preparation. In most liver wounds, however, several hours of preoperative treatment facilitates the operation and improves the chances of survival. Usually preoperative therapy is undertaken simultaneously with the diagnostic work-up. The following are im-

portant preoperative preparatory measures used in all but minor liver wounds:

1.  Shock is corrected by restoration of the blood volume with whole blood transfusions administered through two large-bore plastic catheters inserted via a cutdown in each arm. Because of the potential coagulation defects associated with liver damage, liver resection, and multiple transfusions of stored blood, correction of hypovolemia involves as much fresh blood (less than 12 hours old) as can be obtained.

2.  Assurance of adequate ventilation is a matter of first priority along with the treatment of shock. This involves the administration of oxygen, and may require insertion of a thoracostomy catheter to evacuate blood or air, insertion of an endotracheal tube, and mechanical ventilatory support.

3.  Vital functions are monitored by insertion of a central venous pressure catheter through an arm cutdown into the superior vena cava, a radial artery catheter for arterial pressure recordings, an indwelling bladder catheter for hourly measurements of urine output, and a rectal or esophageal probe for temperature recordings. The patient is connected by body surface leads to an electrocardiograph for continuous recordings of the electrocardiogram. Arterial pH and blood gases, blood urea nitrogen, and serum electrolytes are determined.

4.  Both the chest and the abdomen are shaved and prepared with antiseptic soap for operation.

5.  A hypothermia blanket is placed on the operating table so that total-body cooling can be initiated as soon as anesthesia is induced.

6.  Equipment for intraoperative cholangiography and visceral angiography is brought to the operating room, if not already present, and appropriate scout x-rays are taken before induction of anesthesia. The surgeon should not find himself in the position of needing these studies and discovering after the abdomen has been entered that he has failed to provide for the necessary equipment.

**Operative Treatment.**   The operative treatment of liver wounds is based on three important principles: (1) excision of devitalized liver tissue; (2) securing liver hemostasis; and (3) drainage of the peritoneal cavity to prevent bile collections. Excision of devitalized liver tissue is essential to prevent the often lethal sequelae of delayed necrosis, infection, and late hemorrhage. Unroofing of deep missile tracts, segmental liver resection, or hepatic lobectomy in extensive injuries may be necessary to accomplish this important objective. Securing liver hemostasis is accomplished by direct suture, but the use of hemostatic agents or resection of the liver may be required. Through-and-through perforating injuries with bleeding in the depths of the liver should never be treated by simply suturing closed the surface openings of the wound, since such a maneuver often leads to an expanding intrahepatic hematoma with serious consequences. Instead, the wound should be laid open throughout its length and the bleeding points should be controlled by direct suture. Drainage of the peritoneal cavity is necessary to remove the bile that invariably leaks from the hepatic wound. If the bile is not evacuated, infected bile collections or bile peritonitis may develop. Drainage is accomplished by the combined use of Penrose drains and sump drains that are placed on suction. In addition, in recent years some workers have advocated deliberate T tube drainage of the common bile duct or cholecystostomy on the assumption that controlled extrahepatic biliary drainage will prevent bile leakage from the liver wound. While theoretically attractive, there is no solid evidence to indicate that controlled drainage of the common bile duct accomplishes the objective for which it was proposed. To the contrary, Lucas et al. have demonstrated in extensive experimental and clinical studies that drainage of the common bile duct does not reduce intrahepatic biliary pressure, does not diminish bile drainage from the liver wound, and is associated with increased morbidity, mortality, and stress ulceration in patients with liver trauma. Furthermore, Lucas et al. have emphasized that insertion of a T tube into a small common bile duct may damage the duct. For these reasons, we do not advocate the routine use of controlled extrahepatic biliary drainage in liver trauma.

In extensive liver injury, there are certain technical maneuvers of which the surgeon must be aware if he is to control bleeding. Reflection of the duodenum by a Kocher maneuver so as to gain fingertip control of the afferent blood supply to the liver is a simple first step in the approach to serious hepatic injuries. Occlusion of the hepatic artery and portal vein by cross-clamping the porta hepatis with a vascular clamp (Pringle maneuver) is helpful in controlling and repairing extensive liver wounds, and in performing hepatic resections. Vascular inflow occlusion is tolerated for 20 minutes when body temperature is normal, and for 60 minutes under hypothermia of 30° C. The time period can be extended by releasing the occluding vascular clamp for several minutes at appropriate intervals so as to produce intermittent vascular occlusion. Division of the falciform, coronary, and triangular ligaments provides access to all parts of the liver except the bare area and major hepatic veins, and should be done early in operations for wounds of the posterior and superior segments.

Liver wounds that involve the major hepatic veins are the most difficult to repair and have the highest mortality rate because of their inaccessibility and the danger of both exsanguination and air embolism. Such injuries must be recognized promptly and approached rapidly by extending the usual midline abdominal incision into the thorax through the seventh or eighth right intercostal space. The diaphragm is divided down to the orifice of the inferior vena cava. In addition to occlusion of hepatic vascular inflow, occlusion of the inferior vena cava below the liver and above the liver in the pericardial cavity is used to isolate and repair the injured hepatic veins. Clamping of the inferior vena cava for more than 15 to 20 minutes produces severe hypotension, so the use

**TABLE 19** METHODS OF OPERATIVE TREATMENT USED IN 204 CASES OF PERFORATING AND BLUNT LIVER TRAUMA

| | Number of Cases |
|---|---|
| Suture of liver | 104 |
| Suture and hemostatic agents | 43 |
| Resection of liver | 24 |
| Laparotomy alone | 22 |
| Died without operation | 7 |

of intermittent occlusion may be required. Additional techniques for isolating the large hepatic veins involve combined occlusion of the inferior vena cava and aorta above the celiac axis so as to avoid hypotension from pooling of blood in the lower half of the body, unroofing of the inferior vena cava within the liver from a posterior approach, and insertion of an internal shunt into the vena cava through the right atrium.

The methods of operative treatment used in 204 cases of perforating and blunt liver trauma are listed in Table 19.

**Postoperative Complications.** Table 20 shows the postoperative complications in 100 cases of blunt liver trauma. Infection is the most frequent problem following liver injury. Subphrenic, subhepatic, and intrahepatic abscesses, peritonitis, wound infection, and wound dehiscence occur with disturbing frequency. The importance of thoroughly irrigating the peritoneal cavity and wound with antibiotic solutions at the time of operation, and of closing the abdominal incision with retention sutures, cannot be overemphasized.

Respiratory complications such as pneumonia, atelectasis, pulmonary edema, and "shock lung" are common in all types of major trauma. The use of mechanical ventilatory assistance delivered through an endotracheal tube or tracheostomy, an intensive program of tracheobronchial toilet, and careful monitoring of arterial pH and blood gases, pulmonary function, and radiographic changes in the lungs are essential aspects of postoperative care.

Secondary hemorrhage from necrosis and infection of hepatic tissue is a major cause of delayed death following liver trauma. Moreover, it is not uncommon for serious coagulopathies to de-

**TABLE 20** POSTOPERATIVE COMPLICATIONS IN 100 CASES OF BLUNT LIVER TRAUMA

| | Incidence (%) |
|---|---|
| Infection—intra-abdominal and wound | 22 |
| Respiratory problems | 19 |
| Hemorrhage | 14 |
| Renal failure | 9 |
| Stress ulcer | 6 |
| Pancreatitis | 5 |
| Other | 14 |

**TABLE 21**  CAUSES OF 151 DEATHS FROM
LIVER TRAUMA FROM 1960 TO 1970

|  | Per Cent of Deaths |
|---|---|
| Liver hemorrhage—intraoperative and postoperative | 53 |
| Respiratory failure | 14 |
| Infection—intra-abdominal and wound | 12 |
| Pancreatitis | 8 |
| Stress ulcer bleeding | 6 |
| Other | 7 |

**TABLE 23**  MORTALITY RATE OF BLUNT
LIVER TRAUMA

| Authors and Year Reported | Cases | Mortality (%) |
|---|---|---|
| Edler, 1887 | 96 | 78 |
| O'Neill, 1940 | 100 | 81 |
| Mikesky et al., 1956 | 24 | 71 |
| Crosthwait et al., 1962 | 43 | 30 |
| Shafton et al., 1963 | 38 | 55 |
| McClelland and Shires, 1965 | 31 | 26 |
| Orloff et al., 1967 | 100 | 24 |
| Lucas and Walt, 1970 | 65 | 28 |

velop in patients with liver injuries as a result of the combination of hepatic dysfunction and replacement of the blood volume with banked blood. To the extent possible, fresh blood transfusions should be used to restore platelets, replenish the protein blood clotting factors, and provide 2,3-DPG for delivery of oxygen to the tissues.

Renal failure associated with hepatic trauma is almost always due to acute tubular necrosis resulting from a period of hypotension and renal ischemia. Although this complication cannot be prevented in all cases, it can be minimized by a vigorous program of resuscitation starting when the patient first enters the emergency room. The development of stress ulceration with gastrointestinal hemorrhage is not uncommon in patients with massive trauma of any type. Prophylaxis against this complication includes continuous nasogastric suction during the first several days postoperatively, followed by hourly oral antacid therapy beginning immediately upon removal of the nasogastric tube. Finally, liver failure rarely develops as a direct result of an uncomplicated hepatic injury or from resection of the hepatic tissue, but frequently occurs when other complications, such as sepsis or pulmonary failure, are added to the liver trauma. There is no specific treatment for hepatic failure, but the use of parenteral hyperalimentation may be helpful and has become a regularly used measure in our management of serious liver wounds.

**Traumatic Hemobilia.**  An unusual but interesting complication of liver trauma is hemobilia. This disorder usually follows central rupture of the liver, or suture of lacerations on the liver surface without obliteration of dead space in the depths of the hepatic substance. The communication between the vasculature and the biliary tract de-

velops as a result of necrosis of a portion of liver parenchyma within a closed space. Symptoms may occur at any time, but commonly they appear 3 to 4 weeks after injury and consist of episodes of biliary colic due to passage of blood clots down the bile ducts, mild jaundice, and gastrointestinal bleeding that presents as melena or, less often, hematemesis. Elevations of the serum alkaline phosphatase and bilirubin usually accompany the attacks, and sometimes the SGOT is increased. Hepatic arteriography is particularly useful in establishing the diagnosis, and splenoportography, cholangiography, and radioisotope liver scanning may be helpful. Although many different operations have been used, definitive treatment consists of either resection of the lesion or ligation of the ends of the contributing blood vessels. Intraoperative angiography and cholangiography are helpful in localizing the involved part of the liver.

### Mortality

A significant number of patients with liver trauma die before reaching the hospital. Moreover, hepatic injury is often associated with trauma to other organs and systems, and death is sometimes due to associated injuries. Patients who die as a direct result of the liver wound usually succumb from hepatic hemorrhage, respiratory complications, or infection in the peritoneal cavity or wound (Table 21).

The mortality rate of perforating liver injuries has been reduced from more than 60 per cent prior to 1940 to approximately 10 per cent at present (Table 22). Stab wounds of the liver are associated with a mortality rate of only 2 to 3 per cent, while

**TABLE 22**  MORTALITY RATE OF PERFORATING LIVER TRAUMA

| Author and Year Reported | Cases | Mortality (%) | Stab Wounds No. | Mortality (%) | Gunshot Wounds No. | Mortality (%) |
|---|---|---|---|---|---|---|
| Sparkman and Fogelman, 1954 | 92 | 11 | 34 | 3 | 58 | 16 |
| Amerson and Blair, 1959 | 167 | 13 | 68 | 0 | 99 | 21 |
| Crosthwait et al., 1962 | 297 | 12 | — | — | — | — |
| Shafton et al., 1963 | 73 | 12 | 61 | 8 | 12 | 33 |
| McClelland and Shires, 1965 | 228 | 9 | — | — | — | — |
| Lucas and Walt, 1970 | 539 | 10 | 290 | 2 | 249 | 18 |

gunshot injuries are more often lethal because of the magnitude of liver damage and the frequent involvement of other organs. The mortality rate of blunt trauma to the liver has been reduced significantly to about 30 per cent during the past decade as a result of better organized emergency care and more effective operative treatment (Table 23). Nevertheless, blunt liver injury remains the most lethal form of trauma to the abdominal viscera.

## PYOGENIC LIVER ABSCESS

Although pyogenic liver abscess was fairly common prior to the antibiotic era, it is found infrequently now. Invasion of the liver by bacteria occurs along the following routes:

1. Ascending biliary infection from cholangitis due to calculi in the common bile duct or to an obstructing pancreaticoduodenal cancer is the most frequent cause of hepatic abscess.

2. Hematogenous invasion of the liver via the portal vein from intraperitoneal infections such as suppurative appendicitis, diverticulitis, or omphalitis is another relatively common route. Occasionally, such conditions are associated with a suppurative thrombophlebitis of the portal vein, called pyelophlebitis, which gives rise to multiple liver abscesses.

3. Hematogenous spread by way of the hepatic artery occurs in systemic infections such as bacterial endocarditis.

4. Direct extension of infection into the liver from peritonitis or a diseased gallbladder is an unusual mechanism for hepatic abscess formation.

5. Finally, implantation of microorganisms during liver trauma is responsible for some cases of abscess.

The clinical symptoms of pyogenic liver abscess consist of fever often accompanied by chills, pain in the right upper abdomen, anorexia, and weight loss. In one-half to two-thirds of the patients, the liver is enlarged and tender. Jaundice and a right-sided pleural effusion occur in one-fourth of the patients. Leukocytosis is almost invariable and anemia is common. The liver function tests often show abnormalities similar to those found in viral hepatitis. These include enzyme elevations, Bromsulphalein retention, positive turbidity and flocculation tests, hyperbilirubinemia, and, particularly, an elevation of serum alkaline phosphatase. A positive blood culture is found in one-third to one-half of the cases. X-rays of the abdomen and chest and fluoroscopy show elevation and fixation of the right hemidiaphragm. Occasionally, a diagnostic air-fluid level below the right diaphragm and a pleural effusion above are seen. The liver scan is an important diagnostic procedure, and hepatic arteriography may be helpful. A serious complication of pyogenic liver abscess is rupture into the pleural cavity.

The treatment of pyogenic liver abscess consists of antibiotics and surgical drainage. Selection of the appropriate antibiotics depends on the causative organism; *Escherichia coli* and *Staphylococcus aureus* are the bacteria most frequently found, but many different organisms have been cultured from liver abscesses. Surgical drainage may be performed by an extraserous transthoracic approach or by a transabdominal approach, depending upon the location of the lesion. Fear of the transabdominal approach, based on the high mortality rate observed in the preantibiotic era, is no longer justified. In fact, under most circumstances entry into the peritoneal cavity is preferable because of the high incidence of multiple hepatic and extrahepatic abscesses and the likelihood that these will be missed by an extraserous approach. The overall mortality rate of liver abscess in recent reports has ranged from 11 to 26 per cent.

## AMEBIC LIVER ABSCESS

It has been estimated that infection with *Entamoeba histolytica* involves from 5 to 20 per cent of the population in the United States. The reported incidence of amebic liver abscess in patients with intestinal amebiasis has varied from 1 to 25 per cent. Hepatic complications of amebic infection are usually found in middle-aged males. Liver abscess is always due to spread of intestinal amebiasis via the portal vein. However, cysts or trophozoites are found in the stool in less than one-fourth of the patients with hepatic infection. The liver abscess is most often solitary and in the right lobe, and its contents have a characteristic appearance of anchovy paste on exposure to air.

The clinical symptoms of amebic liver abscess consist of pain in the right hypochondrium or lower chest sometimes with radiation to the right shoulder, fever, chills, sweating, anorexia, and weight loss. Diarrhea is an inconstant feature of the present or past history. Hepatomegaly and liver tenderness are the most important physical findings. The infrequent abscess of the left lobe of the liver may present as a tender mass in the epigastrium or left hypochondrium. Pulmonary abnormalities occur in one-fourth of the patients. Jaundice is unusual.

Laboratory studies show a leukocytosis and often an anemia. Elevation of the serum alkaline phosphatase and Bromsulphalein retention are frequently but inconsistently found, and the serum albumin concentration is almost invariably decreased. The liver function tests are usually normal. Sigmoidoscopy shows active colitis in only a small percentage of patients with liver abscess. Parasites are found in the stool and in specimens obtained by sigmoidoscopy in about 20 per cent of patients. The radiographic and liver scan findings are similar to those observed in pyogenic liver abscess, and are of great importance in making the diagnosis. Recently, ultrasonic scanning of the liver has proved to be of equal value to the radio-isotope scintillation scan in diagnosing hepatic abscess and following its progress (see Fig. 18B).

A number of serologic tests are used to detect amebic infection. The indirect hemagglutination test, the gel diffusion precipitin test, and the latex agglutination test are positive in nearly 100 per cent of patients with amebic liver abscess. The first two of these procedures require up to 48 hours to perform, while the latex agglutination test can be done in a few minutes. All patients suspected of having amebiasis should undergo serologic testing. The diagnosis of amebic liver abscess is made at present on the basis of a compatible history and physical examination, an abnormal radioisotope or ultrasonic liver scan, positive serologic tests, and a prompt response to amebicidal drug therapy.

The complications of amebic liver abscess consist of secondary pyogenic infection, which is usually accompanied by a sudden increase in toxic signs and symptoms, and of rupture of the abscess into the lung, pleural cavity, peritoneal cavity, pericardium, or bowel. The development of pulmonary signs and symptoms should suggest the possibility of rupture. In contrast to the era prior to 1960, complications of amebic liver abscess are now infrequent in the United States.

The primary treatment of amebic liver abscess is drug therapy. Although some workers continue to perform needle aspiration of the abscess for diagnosis and initial treatment, most authorities have abandoned the routine use of aspiration. Metronidazole is a safe and very effective agent against both extraintestinal and intestinal amebic infection, and it is rapidly becoming the therapeutic agent of choice. It has been reported to cure most hepatic abscesses in early trials. Prior to the use of metronidazole, treatment involved the use of an extraintestinal amebicide, such as emetine or chloroquine, followed by therapy with an intestinal amebicide such as diiodohydroxyquin (Diodoquin) or chiniofon. The response to treatment is determined by disappearance of clinical symptoms and signs, and progressive shrinkage of the hepatic defect on serial liver scans. Persistence of the abscess after drug therapy is an indication for needle aspiration. The indications for surgical treatment of amebic liver abscess are few, and they arise infrequently. Failure of an abscess to respond to either drug therapy or aspiration, and secondary bacterial infection of an abscess call for surgical drainage by either an extraserous or transperitoneal approach. Rupture of a liver abscess into adjacent viscera usually requires operative treatment.

The mortality rate of amebic liver abscess that is diagnosed during life and has not been neglected is now less than 5 per cent.

## ECHINOCOCCUS CYST

Hydatid disease is common in many parts of the world, but it is a rare condition in the United States and is found mainly in immigrants who bring the disease to this country. Two forms of the echinococcus tapeworm produce disease in man,

*Echinococcus granulosus* and *Echinococcus multilocularis.* The adult tapeworm lives in the intestine of the dog, from which ova are passed in the stool. The ova are ingested by an intermediate host, usually sheep, cattle, and pigs but occasionally man, and hatch into embryos in the duodenum. The embryos pass into the portal venous system and are filtered out by the liver, although occasionally they escape to the lung or other organs. In the liver, the embryos reproduce asexually and form multiloculated cysts. The cyst in the liver usually has a well defined wall with an inner germinative layer and a thick outer laminated layer which often calcifies. The cyst fluid contains numerous embryonal scolices called "hydatid sand." The cycle is completed when a dog feeds on the infected tissues of an intermediate host, and the scolices develop into mature tapeworms in the dog's intestines.

Hydatid cysts frequently are present for many years without producing symptoms. Often, the discovery of a liver mass on physical examination or the pathognomonic finding of a calcified, round mass in the liver on x-ray leads to the diagnosis (Fig. 30). Liver scans and hepatic arteriography may be helpful in defining the lesion. Eosinophilia occurs in one-fourth of the cases. A complement fixation test and the response to intradermal injection of cyst fluid (Casoni test) are positive in the vast majority of patients. Several serologic tests that indicate hydatid infection are also available.

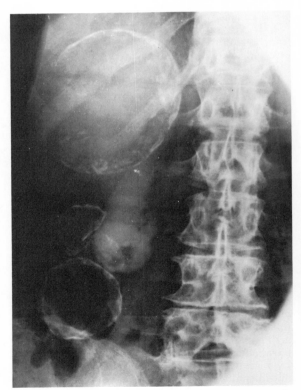

**Figure 30**  Calcified masses in the right upper quadrant indicative of echinococcus cysts in the liver, discovered during an oral cholecystogram performed for right upper quadrant abdominal pain.

The major cause of morbidity and mortality associated with echinococcus cyst of the liver is rupture of the cyst. Rupture into the bile ducts produces a syndrome of biliary colic, jaundice, urticaria, and fever. Rupture into the peritoneal cavity results in abdominal pain, urticaria, anaphylactic shock, and the development of multiple intra-abdominal cysts. Rupture into the pleural cavity causes pain, cough, fever, and the development of empyema. Rarely, hydatid cysts rupture into the gastrointestinal tract. Secondary infection of liver cysts with pyogenic bacteria occurs sometimes and produces the signs and symptoms of pyogenic liver abscess.

The treatment of hydatid cyst is surgical removal. Usually the cyst can be removed by shelling out, but occasionally hepatic resection is required. In order to prevent seeding of the cyst contents, preliminary aspiration and instillation of hydrogen peroxide, absolute alcohol, or formalin are done. Care must be taken to avoid spilling viable scolices into the peritoneal cavity. The defect in the liver that remains after removal of the cyst should be closed or marsupialized. The mortality rate for treatment of uncomplicated cysts is less than 5 per cent.

## BENIGN NEOPLASMS AND CYSTS

Usually, benign neoplasms of the liver are of clinical significance only in that they pose problems in differential diagnosis from more serious lesions. The most common benign tumor is the hemangioma, a lesion of blood vessels that presents the microscopic appearance of endothelium-lined cystic spaces filled with blood. The liver is the parenchymatous organ in which hemangiomas are most frequently found. The tumors vary greatly in size. They are usually asymptomatic, although they may grow so large as to compress adjacent viscera. When clinically significant, they present as an abdominal mass and produce x-ray, angiographic, and liver scan abnormalities. The most serious complication of the hepatic hemangioma is rupture with massive intraperitoneal hemorrhage, an event that has been reported with some frequency. Treatment is required when the tumors become clinically significant and consists of excision or hepatic lobectomy. Radiation therapy may be effective and is indicated in inoperable lesions.

Hepatic adenomas are rare tumors of liver cells or bile duct epithelium. They are usually asymptomatic and when discovered at laparotomy may be mistaken for primary or metastatic cancers. They require excision only when large.

Hamartomas are congenital collections of normal hepatic cell plates, bile ducts, blood vessels, and fibrous tissue in an abnormal arrangement. They are developmental disturbances and are not true neoplasms. They may be single or multiple and vary greatly in size. Some are quite large and are palpable on physical examination. Usually, they are asymptomatic. No treatment is necessary unless they are very large. Hamartomas are of clinical significance mainly because of the difficulty in distinguishing them from malignant tumors on gross examination.

Cysts of the liver are uncommon. Most of the solitary cysts are congenital lesions caused by arrest in the development of the bile ducts. Some single cysts originate from trauma, and in rare instances true neoplastic cystadenomas are found. Multiple cysts of the liver, or polycystic disease, represent congenital bile duct anomalies; associated polycystic disease of the kidneys is found in half of the patients and accompanying cystic disease of other organs has been reported. Other congenital anomalies are often found in patients with polycystic disease. Both solitary cysts and polycystic disease are usually not discovered until adulthood.

Cysts of the liver are usually asymptomatic and come to the attention of a physician because of the finding of an enlarged liver or a mass in the abdomen. Liver function is normal. X-rays of the abdomen, liver scans, and hepatic arteriography are helpful in demonstrating the presence of a liver mass. Treatment consists of excision of the cyst, hepatic resection, or external drainage with packing. Polycystic disease requires no treatment and is compatible with long life if serious associated anomalies are absent.

## MALIGNANT NEOPLASMS

### Primary Cancer

Primary cancer of the liver is uncommon in the United States, but in Africa and Asia it is one of the most frequent malignant neoplasms. Only the Caucasian race is relatively free of liver cancer. The disease occurs in infants, and in parts of Africa and Asia it is common in children and young adults, but in North America it predominates in the fifth and sixth decades of life. Two-thirds to three-fourths of hepatic cancers in the United States develop in patients with cirrhosis, particularly cirrhosis of the postnecrotic type. The incidence of liver cancer among cirrhotic patients is approximately 5 per cent. Patients with hemochromatosis also have a high incidence of hepatic carcinoma. In Africa and Asia, a number of carcinogenic substances in food and infestation of the liver with certain parasites have been implicated in the etiology of liver cancer. In particular, there is suggestive evidence that aflatoxin, a potent hepatocarcinogen from the plant *Aspergillus flavus* that is contained in food, plays an etiologic role in the frequent occurrence of cancer of the liver.

There are two major forms of liver cancer. These are liver cell carcinoma (hepatocellular carcinoma, hepatoma) and bile duct carcinoma (cholangiocarcinoma). A third type that represents a mixture of the other two and is called hepatobiliary carcinoma or cholangiohepatoma is infrequent compared to the two major malignant neoplasms. An uncommon variant of liver cell carcinoma seen most often in infants, hepatoblastoma, is the most amenable of the hepatic malignant tumors to cure by resection. Liver cell carcinomas outnumber bile duct cancers five to one. Other primary liver cancers are rare. Carcinoma of the liver metastasizes widely, but the most frequent sites are the lungs and regional lymph nodes.

The clinical features of liver carcinoma in the United States most often consist of a rapid increase of signs and symptoms in a patient with cirrhosis and include the appearance of ascites, edema, jaundice, anemia, weakness, and weight loss. Occasionally, hepatic carcinoma is responsible for the first episode of bleeding varices. In noncirrhotic patients, the common symptoms are weakness, weight loss, dull pain in the hypochondrium, abdominal swelling, edema, and fever. The usual signs are nodular hepatomegaly and ascites. Jaundice is found in about one-third of the patients when first seen. Hemorrhage into the peritoneal cavity is an occasional terminal event.

All the liver function tests may be abnormal, but elevation of the serum alkaline phosphatase and SGOT and Bromsulphalein retention are the most consistent biochemical abnormalities. The appearance of alpha fetoprotein in the serum shows a high correlation with the presence of liver cell carcinoma and strongly suggests the diagnosis. Hepatic arteriography, radioisotope liver scanning, ultrasonic liver scanning, splenoportography, and needle liver biopsy alone or under direct vision during peritoneoscopy may provide the diagnosis.

The treatment of primary carcinoma of the liver is hepatic resection when the lesion is solitary and there are no regional or distant metastases. Unfortunately, these circumstances rarely occur and cure of the disease by resection, while possible and definitely worth considering, is infrequent. Orthotopic liver allotransplantation has been attempted in a number of cases of hepatic cancer but, to date, has not resulted in cure of the disease. Radiation therapy is of no value. Infusion of chemotherapeutic agents, such as methotrexate and 5-fluorouracil, into the hepatic artery has provided brief palliation in occasional patients. Duration of life after discovery of hepatic cancer averages only 3 to 4 months.

## Metastatic Cancer

Because of its rich and unique blood supply, the liver is the most common organ to be involved by metastatic cancer. One-half to two-thirds of the patients who die of cancer of the gastrointestinal tract, pancreas, breast, and ovary, and one-third of the patients who die of lung and kidney cancers, have liver metastases. Neoplasms spread to the liver by way of the portal vein, hepatic artery, and lymphatics and by direct extension. Right upper quadrant abdominal pain, anorexia, weight loss, nodular hepatomegaly, and ascites are the most common clinical features. Jaundice occurs in one-fourth of the cases. Bromsulphalein retention and elevation of serum alkaline phosphatase are consistent findings, and SGOT is frequently increased. Hepatic arteriography, liver scans, portography, and needle liver biopsy help to make the diagnosis. The yield of liver biopsy is increased by perform-

ing the procedure under direct vision during peritoneoscopy. Although rare cases of metastatic carcinoma have been cured by hepatic resections performed after control of the primary neoplasm, the vast majority of hepatic metastases are incurable. Chemotherapy by hepatic arterial infusion has resulted in palliation in occasional cases. Duration of life following discovery of liver metastases varies according to the nature of the primary neoplasms, but it rarely exceeds 1 year.

## REFERENCES

*General*

 1. Popper, H., and Schaffner, F.: Liver: Structure and Function. New York, McGraw-Hill Book Company, 1957.
 2. Popper, H., and Schaffner, F.: Progress in Liver Diseases. Volume 3. New York, Grune & Stratton, 1970.
 3. Schiff, L.: Diseases of the Liver. 3rd ed. Philadelphia, J. B. Lippincott Company, 1969.
 4. Schwartz, S. I.: Surgical Diseases of the Liver. New York, McGraw-Hill Book Company, 1964.
 5. Sherlock, S.: Diseases of the Liver and Biliary System. 4th ed. Oxford, Blackwell Scientific Publications, 1968.

*Anatomy*

 6. Douglass, B. E., Baggenstoss, A. H., and Hollenshead, W. H.: The anatomy of the portal vein and its tributaries. Surg. Gynec. Obstet., *91*:562, 1950.
 7. Elias, H., and Sherrick, J. C.: Morphology of the Liver. New York, Academic Press, 1969.
 8. Gilfillan, R. S.: Anatomic study of the portal vein and its main branches. Arch. Surg., *61*:449, 1950.
 9. Michels, N.: The hepatic, cystic and retroduodenal arteries and their relations to the biliary ducts. Ann. Surg., *133*:503, 1951.

*Physiology*

*Bile Formation*

10. Brauer, R. W.: Hepatic blood supply and the secretion of bile. In: Taylor, W., ed.: The Biliary System. Oxford, Blackwell Scientific Publications, 1965, pp. 41-67.

*Bilirubin Metabolism*

11. Arias, I. M.: The excretion of conjugated bilirubin by the liver cell. Medicine, *45*:513, 1966.
12. Gregory, C. H.: Studies of conjugated bilirubin. III. Pigment I, a complex of conjugated and free bilirubin. J. Lab. Clin. Med., *61*:917, 1963.
13. Klatskin, G.: Bile pigment metabolism. Ann. Rev. Med., *12*:211, 1961.
14. Lester, R., and Schmid, R.: Bilirubin metabolism. New Eng. J. Med., *270*:779, 1964.

*Protein Metabolism*

15. Miller, L. L., and Bale, W. F.: Synthesis of all plasma protein fractions except gamma globulin by the liver. J. Exp. Med., *99*:125, 1954.

*Blood Coagulation*

16. Spector, I., and Corn, M.: Laboratory tests of hemostasis. The relation to hemorrhage in liver disease. Arch. Intern. Med., *119*:577, 1967.
17. Walls, W. D., and Losowsky, M. S.: The hemostatic defect of liver disease. Gastroenterology, *60*:108, 1971.

*Hepatic Hemodynamics*

18. Brauer, R. W.: Liver circulation and function. Physiol. Rev., *43*:115, 1963.
19. Grayson, J., and Mendel, D.: Physiology of the Splanchnic Circulation. Monographs of the Physiological Society. Arnold, London, 1965.
20. Greenway, C. V., and Stark, R. D.: Hepatic vascular bed. Physiol. Rev., *51*:23, 1971.
21. Reynolds, T. B., and Redeker, A. G.: Hepatic hemodynamics and portal hypertension. In: Popper, H., and Schaffner, F., eds.: Progress in Liver Diseases. Volume 2. New York, Grune & Stratton, 1965.

22. Shoemaker, W. C., and Elwyn, D. H.: Liver: Functional interactions within the intact animal. Ann. Rev. Physiol., *31*:227, 1969.

*Hepatectomy*

23. Bollman, J. L., and Mann, F. C.: Studies on the physiology of the liver. XVIII: The effect of removal of the liver on the formation of ammonia. Amer. J. Physiol., *92*:92, 1930.
24. Bollman, J. L., Mann, F. C., and Magath, T. B.: Studies on the physiology of the liver. Effect of total removal of the liver on formation of urea. Amer. J. Physiol., *69*:371, 1924.
25. Bollman, J. L., Mann, F. C., and Magath, T. B.: Studies on the physiology of the liver. The effect of total removal of the liver on deaminization. Amer. J. Physiol., *78*:258, 1926.
26. Mann, F. C.: Studies in the physiology of the liver. I. Technic and general effects of removal. Amer. J. Physiol., *55*:285, 1921.
27. Mann, F. C.: The effects of complete and partial removal of the liver. Medicine, *6*:419, 1927.

*Eck Fistula*

28. Harper, H. A., Gardner, R. E., Johansen, R., Galante, M., and McCorkle, H. J.: Amino acid tolerance in experimental portacaval anastomosis. Surgery, *29*:210, 1951.
29. McDermott, W. V., Jr., and Adams, R. D.: Episodic stupor associated with an Eck fistula in the human with particular reference to the metabolism of ammonia. J. Clin. Invest., *33*:1, 1954.
30. Silen, W., Mawdsley, D. L., Weirich, W. L., and Harper, H. A.: Studies of hepatic function in dogs with Eck fistula or portacaval transposition. Arch. Surg., *74*:964, 1957.
31. Whipple, G. H., Robscheit-Robbins, F. S., and Hawkins, W. B.: Eck fistula liver subnormal in producing hemoglobin and plasma proteins on diets rich in liver and iron. J. Exp. Med., *81*:171, 1945.

*Liver Regeneration*

32. Becker, F. F.: The normal hepatocyte in division: Regeneration of the mammalian liver. In Popper, H., and Schaffner, F., eds.: Progress in Liver Disease. Volume 3. New York, Grune & Stratton, 1970, p. 60.
33. Bucher, N. L. R.: Experimental aspects of hepatic regeneration. New Eng. J. Med., *277*:686, 738, 1967.
34. Chandler, J. G., Lee, S., Krubel, R., Rosen, H., and Orloff, M. J.: The roles of inter-liver competition and portal blood in regeneration of auxiliary liver transplants. Surg. Forum, *22*:341, 1971.
35. Fisher, B., Szuch, P., and Fisher, E. R.: Evaluation of a humoral factor in liver regeneration utilizing liver transplants. Cancer Res., *31*:322, 1971.
36. Lee, S., Edgington, T. S., and Orloff, M. J.: The role of afferent blood supply in regeneration of liver isografts in rats. Surg. Forum, *19*:360, 1968.
37. Lee, S., Keiter, J. E., Rosen, H., Chandler, J. G., and Orloff, M. J.: Influence of blood supply on regeneration of liver transplants. Surg. Forum, *20*:369, 1969.
38. Moolten, F. L., and Bucher, N. L. R.: Regeneration of rat liver: Transfer of humoral agent by cross circulation. Science, *158*:272, 1967.

**Diagnosis of Liver Disease**

*Liver Function Tests*

39. Clermont, R. J., and Chalmers, T. C.: The transaminase tests in liver disease. Medicine, *46*:197, 1967.
40. Combes, B.: The importance of conjugation with glutathione for sulfobromophthalein sodium (BSP) transfer from blood to bile. J. Clin. Invest., *44*:1214, 1965.
41. Combes, B., Wheeler, H. O., Childs, R. W., and Bradley, S. E.: The mechanisms of Bromsulphalein removal from the blood. Trans. Ass. Amer. Physicians, *69*:276, 1956.
42. Goresky, C. A.: Initial distribution and rate of uptake of sulfobromophthalein in the liver. Amer. J. Physiol., *207*:13, 1964.
43. Leevy, C. M., Smith, F., Longueville, J., Paumgartner, G., and Howard, M. M.: Indocyanine green clearance as a test for hepatic function. J.A.M.A., *200*:236, 1967.

44. Müting, D., and Reikowski, H.: Protein metabolism in liver disease. In: Popper, H., and Schaffner, F., eds.: Progress in Liver Diseases. Volume 2. New York, Grune & Stratton, 1965, p. 84.
45. Newton, M. A.: The clinical application of alkaline phosphatase electrophoresis. Quart. J. Med., *36*:17, 1967.
46. Owen, J. A., and Robertson, R. F.: Paper electrophoresis of serum proteins in hepatobiliary disease. Lancet, 2: 1125, 1956.
47. Posen, S.: Alkaline phosphatase. Ann. Intern. Med., *67*:183, 1967.
48. Quick, A. J.: Hemorrhagic Diseases and Thrombosis. 2nd ed., Philadelphia, Lea & Febiger, 1966, p. 391.
49. Rappaport, S. F., Ames, S. B., Mikkelsen, S., and Goodman, J. R.: Plasma clotting factors in chronic hepatocellular disease. New Eng. J. Med., *263*:278, 1960.
50. Ratnoff, O. D.: Hemostatic mechanisms in liver disease. Med. Clin. N. Amer., *47*:721, 1963.
51. Reinhold, J. G.: Flocculation tests and their application to the study of liver disease. In: Sobotka, H., and Stewart, C. P., eds.: Advances in Clinical Chemistry. Volume 3. New York, Academic Press, 1960, p. 83.
52. Watson, C. J.: The importance of the fractional serum bilirubin determination in clinical medicine. Ann. Intern. Med., *45*:351, 1956.
53. Wheeler, H. O., Meltzer, J. I., and Bradler, S. E.: Biliary transport and hepatic storage of sulfobromophthalein sodium in unanaesthetized dog, in normal man, and in patients with hepatic disease. J. Clin. Invest., *39*:1131, 1960.
54. Zieve, L., Hill, E., Hanson, M., Falcone, A. B., and Watson, C. J.: Normal and abnormal variations and clinical significance of the one-minute and total serum bilirubin determinations. J. Lab. Clin. Med., *38*:446, 1951.
55. Zimmerman, H. J., and West, M.: Serum enzyme levels in the diagnosis of hepatic disease. Amer. J. Gastroent., *40*:387, 1963.

*Liver Biopsy*

56. Linder, H.: Limitations and dangers in percutaneous liver biopsies with the Menghini needle. Proceedings of the Third World Congress of Gastroenterology, *3*:373, 1966.
57. Menghini, G.: One-second needle biopsy of the liver. Gastroenterology, *35*:190, 1958.
58. Nelson, R. S.: The development and function of a liver biopsy program: training of personnel, description of a modified Vim-Silverman needle and clinical value of 500 biopsies. Amer. J. Med. Sci., *227*:152, 1951.
59. Zamcheck, N., and Klausenstock, O.: Needle biopsy of the liver. II. The risk of needle biopsy. New Eng. J. Med., *249*:1062, 1953.
60. Zamcheck, N., and Sideman, R. L.: Needle biopsy of the liver. I. Its use in clinical and investigative medicine. New Eng. J. Med., *249*:1020, 1953.

*Roentgenography*

61. Boijsen, E., Eckman, C. A., and Olin, T.: Coeliac and superior mesenteric angiography in portal hypertension. Acta Chir. Scand., *126*:315, 1963.
62. Kahn, P. C., and Alexander, F. K.: Total hepatic angiography and vascular dynamics in liver disease. Amer. J. Gastroent., *52*:317, 1969.
63. Kirsh, I. E., Blackwell, C. C., and Bennett, H. D.: Roentgen diagnosis of esophageal varices: comparison of roentgen and esophagoscopic findings in 502 cases. Amer. J. Roentgen., *74*:477, 1955.
64. Kreel, L., Jones, E. A., and Tavill, A. S.: A comparative study of arteriography and scintillation scanning in space-occupying lesions of the liver. Brit. J. Radiol., *41*:401, 1968.
65. Lavoie, P., Jacob, M., Leduc, J., Legare, A., and Viallet, A.: The umbilicoportal approach for the study of splanchnic circulation: technical, radiological and hemodynamic considerations. Canad. J. Surg., *9*:338, 1968.
66. Leger, L. H.: Splenoportography: Diagnostic Phlebography of the Portal Venous System. Springfield, Ill., Charles C Thomas, 1966.
67. Viamonte, M., Jr., Warren, W. D., and Foman, J. J.: Liver panangiography in the assessment of portal hyperten-

sion in liver cirrhosis. Radiol. Clin. N. Amer., 8:147, 1970.

*Esophagogastroscopy*

68. Conn, H. O., Binder, H., and Brodoff, M.: Fiberoptic and conventional esophagoscopy in the diagnosis of esophageal varices. Gastroenterology, 52:810, 1967.
69. Conn, H. O., Smith, H. W., and Brodoff, M.: Observer variation in the endoscopic diagnosis of esophageal varices. New Eng. J. Med., 272:830, 1965.

*Portal Pressure Measurements*

70. Leevy, C. M., and Gliedman, M. L.: Practical and research value of hepatic vein catheterization. New Eng. J. Med., 258:738, 1958.
71. Reynolds, T. B., Ito, S., and Iwatsuki, S.: Measurement of portal pressure and its clinical application. Amer. J. Med., 49:649, 1970.
72. Viallet, A., Legare, A., and Lavoie, P.: Hepatic and umbilico-portal catheterization in portal hypertension. Ann. N. Y. Acad. Sci., 170:177, 1970.
73. Warren, W. D., and Muller, W. H.: Clarification of some hemodynamic changes in cirrhosis and their surgical significance. Ann. Surg., 150:413, 1959.

*Radioisotope Liver Blood Flow*

74. Restrepo, J. E., Warren, W. D., Nalon, S., and Muller, W. H., Jr.: Radioactive gold technique for the estimation of liver blood flow: Normal values and technical considerations. Surgery, 48:748, 1960.
75. Shaldon, S., Chiandussi, L., Guevara, I., Caesar, J., and Sherlock, S.: The estimation of hepatic blood flow and intrahepatic shunted blood flow by colloidal heat-denatured human serum albumin labeled with I¹³¹. J. Clin. Invest., 40:1346, 1961.
76. Warren, W. D., Fomon, J. J., Viamonte, M., and Zeppa, R.: Preoperative assessment of portal hypertension. Ann. Surg., 165:999, 1967.

*Radioisotope Liver Scanning*

77. McAfee, J. G., Ause, R. G., and Wagner, H. N., Jr.: Diagnostic value of scintillation scanning of the liver. Arch. Intern. Med., 116:95, 1965.

*Ultrasonic Scanning*

78. Lehman, J. S.: Ultrasound in the diagnosis of hepatobiliary disease. Radiol. Clin. N. Amer., 4:605, 1966.

**Jaundice**

79. Hanger, F. M.: Diagnostic problems of jaundice. Arch. Intern. Med., 86:169, 1950.
80. Hoffman, H. N., II, Whitcomb, F. F., Jr., Butt, H. R., and Bollman, J. L.: Bile pigments of jaundice. J. Clin. Invest., 39:132, 1960.
81. Ingelfinger, F.: Differential diagnosis of jaundice. Disease-a-Month, Nov., 1958.
82. Schenker, S., Balent, J., and Schiff, L.: Differential diagnosis of jaundice: A report of a prospective study of 61 proved cases. Amer. J. Dig. Dis., 7:449, 1962.
83. Schiff, L.: The differential diagnosis of jaundice. Postgrad. Med., 41:39, 1967.
84. With, T. K.: Bile Pigments: Chemical, Biological and Clinical Aspects. New York, Academic Press, 1968.

**Natural History of Cirrhosis**

85. Garceau, A. J., and the Boston Inter-Hospital Liver Group: The natural history of cirrhosis. I. Survival with esophageal varices. New Eng. J. Med., 268:469, 1963.
86. Popper, H., Davidson, C. S., Leevy, C. M., and Schaffner, F.: The social impact of liver disease. New Eng. J. Med., 281:1455, 1969.
87. Powell, W. J., Jr., and Klatskin, G.: Duration of survival in patients with Laennec's cirrhosis: influence of alcohol withdrawal, and possible effects of recent changes in general management of the disease. Amer. J. Med., 44:406, 1968.
88. Ratnoff, O. D., and Patek, A. J., Jr.: Natural history of Laennec's cirrhosis of the liver: analysis of 386 cases. Medicine, 21:207, 1942.

**Bleeding Esophageal Varices**

*Natural History*

89. Atik, M., and Simeone, F.: Massive gastrointestinal bleeding: a study of 296 patients at City Hospital of Cleveland. Arch. Surg., 69:355, 1954.
90. Baker, L. A., Smith, C., and Lieberman, G.: The natural history of esophageal varices. Amer. J. Med., 26:228, 1959.
91. Cohn, R., and Blaisdell, F. W.: The natural history of the patient with cirrhosis of the liver with esophageal varices following the first massive hemorrhage. Surg. Gynec. Obstet., 106:699, 1958.
92. Higgins, W. H., Jr.: The esophageal varix: A report of one hundred and fifteen cases. Amer. J. Med. Sci., 214:436, 1947.
93. Liebowitz, H. R.: Pathogenesis of esophageal varix rupture. J.A.M.A., 175:874, 1961.
94. Merigan, T. C., Jr., Hollister, R. M., Gryska, P. F., Starkey, G. W. G., and Davidson, C. S.: Gastrointestinal bleeding with cirrhosis: study of 172 episodes in 158 patients. New Eng. J. Med., 263:579, 1960.
95. Nachlas, M. M., O'Neil, J. E., and Campbell, A. J. A.: The life history of patients with cirrhosis of the liver and bleeding esophageal varices. Ann. Surg., 141:10, 1955.
96. Orloff, M. J., and Thomas, H. S.: Pathogenesis of esophageal varix rupture: A study based on gross and microscopic examination of the esophagus at the time of bleeding. Arch. Surg., 87:301, 1963.
97. Taylor, F. W., and Jontz, J. G.: Cirrhosis with hemorrhage. Arch. Surg., 78:786, 1959.

*Emergency Diagnosis*

98. Orloff, M. J.: Emergency treatment of bleeding esophageal varices in cirrhosis. In: Longmire, W. P., Jr., ed.: Portal hypertension. Curr. Probl. Surg., July, 1966.
99. Viamonte, M., Jr., Warren, W. D., Fomon, J. J., and Martinez, L. O.: Angiographic investigations in portal hypertension. Surg. Gynec. Obstet., 130:37, 1970.

*Emergency Medical Therapy*

100. Conn, H. O.: Hazards attending the use of esophageal tamponade. New Eng. J. Med., 259:701, 1958.
101. Conn, H. O., and Simpson, J. A.: Excessive mortality associated with balloon tamponade of bleeding varices. J.A.M.A., 202:587, 1967.
102. Hamilton, J. E.: Management of bleeding esophageal varices associated with cirrhosis of liver. Ann. Surg., 141:637, 1955.
103. Ludington, A. G.: A study of 158 cases of esophageal varices. Surg. Gynec. Obstet., 106:519, 1958.
104. Merigan, T. C., Plotkin, G. R., and Davidson, C. S.: Effect of intravenously administered posterior pituitary extract on hemorrhage from bleeding varices. New Eng. J. Med., 266:134, 1962.
105. Orloff, M. J., Halasz, N. A., Lipman, C., Schwabe, A. D., Thompson, J. C., and Weidner, W. A.: The complications of cirrhosis of the liver. Ann. Intern. Med., 66:165, 1967.
106. Read, A. E., Dawson, A. M., Kerr, D. N. S., Turner, M. D., and Sherlock, S.: Bleeding oesophageal varices treated by oesophageal compression tube. Brit. Med. J., 1:227, 1960.
107. Reynolds, T. B., Freedman, T., and Winsor, W.: Results of the treatment of bleeding esophageal varices with balloon tamponade. Amer. J. Med. Sci., 224:500, 1952.
108. Schwartz, S. I., Bales, H. W., Emerson, G. L., and Mahoney, E. B.: Use of intravenous pituitrin in treatment of bleeding esophageal varices. Surgery, 45:72, 1959.
109. Shaldon, S., and Sherlock, S.: The use of vasopressin (Pitressin) in the control of bleeding from oesophageal varices. Lancet, 2:222, 1960.
110. Wangensteen, S. L., and Smith, R. S., III: Intragastric cooling for upper gastrointestinal bleeding. Ann. N.Y. Acad. Sci., 115:328, 1964.

*Emergency Transesophageal Varix Ligation*

111. Orloff, M. J.: A comparative study of emergency transesophageal ligation and nonsurgical treatment of bleeding esophageal varices in unselected patients with cirrhosis. Surgery, 52:103, 1962.

112. Rothwell-Jackson, R. L., and Hunt, A. H.: The results obtained with emergency surgery in the treatment of persistent haemorrhage from gastro-oesophageal varices in the cirrhotic patient. Brit. J. Surg., 58:205, 1971.

*Emergency Portacaval Shunt*

113. Adson, M. A.: Emergency portal-systemic shunts. Surg. Clin. N. Amer., 47:887, 1967.
114. Balasegaram, M., and Damodaran, A.: Emergency shunt surgery for bleeding oesophagogastric varices. Aust. New Zeal. J. Surg., 40:152, 1970.
115. Edmonson, H. T., Jackson, F. C., Juler, G. L., Siegel, B., and Perrin, E. B.: Clinical investigation of the portacaval shunt. IV. A report of early survival from the emergency operation. Ann. Surg., 173:372, 1971.
116. Ekman, C. A., and Sandblom, P.: Shunt operation in acute bleeding from esophageal varices. Ann. Surg., 160:531, 1964.
117. Hoffman, D. C., Jepson, R. P., and Harris, J. D.: Experiences with emergency porta-caval shunt. Aust. Ann. Med., 18:238, 1969.
118. Mikkelsen, W. P.: Emergency portacaval shunt. Rev. Surg., 19:141, 1962.
119. Orloff, M. J.: Emergency portacaval shunt: a comparative study of shunt, varix ligation and nonsurgical treatment of bleeding esophageal varices in unselected patients with cirrhosis. Ann. Surg., 166:456, 1967.
120. Orloff, M. J.: Emergency treatment of bleeding esophageal varices. In: Markoff, N. G., ed.: The Therapy of Portal Hypertension. Stuttgart, Georg Thieme Verlag, 1968, p. 211.
121. Orloff, M. J.: Emergency treatment of bleeding esophageal varices in alcoholic cirrhosis. In: Sardesai, V. M., ed.: Biochemical and Clinical Aspects of Alcohol Metabolism. Springfield, Ill., Charles C Thomas, 1969, p. 288.
122. Peskin, G. W., Crichlow, R. W., Berggren, R. B., and Miller, L. D.: Portacaval shunt in the emergency treatment of variceal bleeding. Surgery, 56:800, 1964.
123. Preston, F. W., and Trippel, O. H.: Emergency portacaval shunt. Arch. Surg., 90:770, 1965.
124. Rousselot, L. M., Gilbertson, F. E., and Panke, W. F.: Severe hemorrhage from esophagogastric varices. Its emergency management with particular reference to portacaval anastomosis. New Eng. J. Med., 262:269, 1960.
125. Wantz, G. E., and Payne, M. A.: Experience with portacaval shunt for portal hypertension. New Eng. J. Med., 265:721, 1961.
126. Weinberger, H. A.: Emergency portacaval shunt for esophagogastric hemorrhage. Arch. Surg., 91:333, 1965.

*Postoperative Care Following Emergency Portacaval Shunt*

127. Del Guercio, L. R. M., Coommaraswamy, R. P., Feins, N. R., Woolman, S. B., and State, D.: Pulmonary arteriovenous admixture and the hyperdynamic cardiovascular state in surgery for portal hypertension. Surgery, 56:74, 1964.
128. Gabuzda, G. J.: Nutrition and liver disease. Practical considerations. Med. Clin. N. Amer., 54:1455, 1970.
129. Glickman, L., and Herbsman, H.: Delirium tremens in surgical patients. Surgery, 64:882, 1968.
130. Isbell, H., Fraser, H. F., Wikler, A., Belleville, R. E., and Eisenman, A. J.: An experimental study of the etiology of "rum fits" and delirium tremens. Quart. J. Stud. Alcohol, 16:1, 1955.
131. Nielson, J.: An intensive one year study of delirium tremens in Copenhagen. Acta Psychiat. Scand., Supp. 187, 41:32, 1965.
132. Siegel, J. H., Greenspan, M., Cohn, J. D., and Del Guercio, L. R. M.: The prognostic implications of altered physiology in operations for portal hypertension. Surg. Gynec. Obstet., 126:249, 1968.
133. Siegel, J. H., and Williams, J. B.: A computer based index for the prediction of operative survival in patients with cirrhosis and portal hypertension. Ann. Surg., 169:191, 1969.
134. Sloop, R. D., and Orloff, M. J.: An important syndrome of metabolic alkalosis in patients with cirrhosis, bleeding varices, and portacaval shunt. Surg. Forum, 17:37, 1966.

*Elective Portacaval Shunt*

135. Barnes, B. A., Ackroyd, F. W., Battit, G. E., Kantrowitz, P. A., Schapiro, R. H., Strole, W. E., Jr., Todd, D. P., and McDermott, W. V.: Elective portosystemic shunts: morbidity and survival data. Ann. Surg., 174:76, 1971.
136. Child, C. G., III: The Shattuck Lecture: The portal circulation. New Eng. J. Med., 262:837, 1955.
137. Eckman, C. A.: Portal hypertension. Acta Chir. Scand., 113:1, 1957.
138. Grace, N. D., Muench, H., and Chalmers, T. C.: The present status of shunts for portal hypertension in cirrhosis. Gastroenterology, 50:684, 1966.
139. Hallenbeck, G. A., Wollaeger, E. E., Adson, M. A., and Gage, R. P.: Results after portal-systemic shunts in 120 patients with cirrhosis of liver. Surg. Gynec. & Obstet., 116:435, 1963.
140. Linton, R. R., Ellis, D. S., and Geary, J. E.: Critical comparative analysis of early and late results of splenorenal and direct portacaval shunts performed in 169 patients with portal cirrhosis. Ann. Surg., 154:446, 1961.
141. McDermott, W. V., Palazzi, H., Nardi, G. L., and Mondet, A.: Elective portal systemic shunt. New Eng. J. Med., 264:419, 1961.
142. Mikkelson, W. P., Turrill, F. R., and Pattison, A. C.: Portacaval shunt in cirrhosis of the liver. Clinical and hemodynamic aspects. Amer. J. Surg., 104:204, 1962.
143. Rousselot, L. M., Panke, W. F., Bono, R. F., and Moreno, A. H.: Experiences with portacaval anastomosis: analysis of 104 elective end-to-side shunts for prevention of recurrent hemorrhage from esophagogastric varices (1952 through 1961). Amer. J. Med., 34:297, 1963.
144. Schapiro, R. H., Strole, W. E., Jr., Todd, D. P., and McDermott, W. V., Jr.: Elective portosystemic shunts: morbidity and survival data. Ann. Surg., 174:76, 1971.
145. Sedgwick, C. E., Poulantzas, J. K., and Miller, W. H.: Portasystemic shunts in 102 patients with portal hypertension. New Eng. J. Med., 274:1290, 1966.
146. Walker, R. M., Shaldon, C., and Vowles, K. D.: Late results of portacaval anastomosis. Lancet, 2:727, 1961.

*Choice of Portal-Systemic Shunt*

147. Bernstein, J. E., Nutting, R. O., and Orloff, M. J.: Comparison of the effects of end-to-side and side-to-side portacaval shunts on liver function, liver blood flow, and ammonia metabolism in dogs and man. S. Forum, 19:328, 1968.
148. Britton, R. C., and Voorhees, A. B., Jr.: Selective portal decompression. Surgery, 67:104, 1970.
149. Britton, R. C., Voorhees, A. B., Jr., and Price, J. B., Jr.: Perfusion of the liver following a side-to-side portacaval shunt. Surgery, 62:181, 1967.
150. Maillard, J. N., Benhamou, J. P., and Rueff, B.: Arterialization of the liver with portacaval shunt in the treatment of portal hypertension due to intrahepatic block. Surgery, 67:883, 1970.
151. Panke, W. F., Rousselot, L. M., and Burchell, A. R.: A sixteen-year experience with end-to-side portacaval shunt for variceal hemorrhage: analysis of data and comparison with other types of portasystemic anastomoses. Ann. Surg., 168:957, 1968.
152. Price, J. B., Jr., Britton, R. C., and Voorhees, A. B., Jr.: The significance and limitations of operative hemodynamics in portal hypertension. Arch. Surg., 95:843, 1967.
153. Reynolds, T. B., Hudson, N. M., Mikkelsen, W. P., Turrill, F. L., and Redeker, A. G.: Clinical comparison of end-to-side and side-to-side portacaval shunt. New Eng. J. Med., 274:706, 1966.
154. Salam, A. A., Warren, W. D., LePage, J. R., Viamonte, M. R., Hutson, D., and Zeppa, R.: Hemodynamic contrasts between selective and total portal-systemic decompression. Ann. Surg., 173:827, 1971.
155. Tamaki, A., Golby, M., and Orloff, M. J.: Effects of side-to-side portacaval shunt on hepatic hemodynamics and metabolism. Surg. Forum, 19:324, 1968.
156. Turcotte, J. G., Wallin, V. W., Jr., Child, C. G., II: End-to-side versus side-to-side portacaval shunts in patients with hepatic cirrhosis. Amer. J. Surg., 117:108, 1969.
157. Warren, W. D., and Muller, W. H., Jr.: Clarification of some

hemodynamic changes in cirrhosis and their surgical significance. Ann. Surg., *150*:413, 1959.

158. Warren, W. D., Zeppa, R., and Fomon, J. J.: Selective transsplenic decompression of gastroesophageal varices by distal splenorenal shunt. Ann. Surg., *166*:437, 1967.

*Prophylactic Portacaval Shunt*

159. Conn, H. O.: Prophylactic portacaval shunts. Ann. Intern. Med., *70*:859, 1969.
160. Conn, H. O., and Lindenmuth, W. W.: Prophylactic portacaval anastomosis in cirrhotic patients with esophageal varices. Interim results with suggestions for subsequent investigations. New Eng. J. Med., *279*:725, 1968.
161. Conn, H. O., and Lindenmuth, W. W.: Prophylactic portacaval anastomosis in cirrhotic patients with esophageal varices and ascites. Amer. J. Surg., *117*:656, 1969.
162. Jackson, F. C., Perrin, E. B., Smith, A. G., Dagradi, A. E., and Nadal, H. M.: A clinical investigation of the portacaval shunt. II. Survival analysis of the prophylactic operation. Amer. J. Surg., *115*:22, 1967.
163. Resnick, R. H., Chalmers, T. C., Ishihara, A. M., Garceau, A. J., Callow, A. D., Schimmel, E. M., O'Hara, E. T., and the Boston Inter-Hospital Liver Group: A controlled study of the prophylactic portacaval shunt. A final report. Ann. Intern. Med., *70*:675, 1969.

**Cirrhotic Ascites**

164. Hyatt, R. E., and Smith, J. R.: The mechanism of ascites. Amer. J. Med., *16*:434, 1954.
165. Lieberman, F. L., Denison, E. K., and Reynolds, T. B.: The relationship of plasma volume, portal hypertension, ascites, and renal sodium retention in cirrhosis. The overflow theory of ascites formation. Ann. N.Y. Acad. Sci., *170*:202, 1970.
166. Madden, J. L., Lore, J. M., Jr., Gerold, F. P., and Ravid, J. M.: The pathogenesis of ascites and a consideration of its treatment. Surg. Gynec. Obstet., *99*:385, 1954.
167. Orloff, M. J.: Surgical treatment of intractable cirrhotic ascites. In: Longmire, W. P., Jr., ed.: Portal Hypertension. Curr. Probl. Surg., July, 1966, p. 28.
168. Orloff, M. J.: Effect of side-to-side portacaval shunt on intractable ascites, sodium excretion, and aldosterone metabolism in man. Amer. J. Surg., *112*:297, 1966.
169. Orloff, M. J.: Pathogenesis and surgical treatment of intractable ascites associated with alcoholic cirrhosis. Ann. N.Y. Acad. Sci., *170*:273, 1970.
170. Orloff, M. J., Ross, T. H., Baddeley, R. M., Nutting, R. O., Spitz, B. R., Sloop, R. D., Neesby, T., and Halasz, N. A.: Experimental ascites. VI. The effects of hepatic venous outflow obstruction and ascites on aldosterone secretion. Surgery, *56*:83, 1964.
171. Orloff, M. J., Spitz, B. R., Wall, M. H., Thomas, H. S., and Halasz, N. A.: Experimental ascites. IV. A comparison of the effects of end-to-side and side-to-side portacaval shunts on intractable ascites. Surgery, *56*:784, 1964.
172. Orloff, M. J., Wright, P. W., DeBenedetti, M. J., Halasz, N. A., Annetts, D. L., Musicant, M. E., and Goodhead, B.: Experimental ascites. VII. The effects of external drainage of the thoracic duct on ascites and hepatic hemodynamics. Arch. Surg., *93*:119, 1966.
173. Parker, R. G. F.: Occlusion of the hepatic veins in man. Medicine, *38*:369, 1959.
174. Sherlock, S., and Shaldon, S.: The aetiology and management of ascites in patients with hepatic cirrhosis. A review. Gut, *4*:95, 1963.
175. Welch, C. S., Welch, H. F., and Carter, J. H.: The treatment of ascites by side-to-side portacaval shunt. Ann. Surg., *150*:428, 1959.

**Hepatic Coma**

176. Brown, H., Trey, C., and McDermott, W. V., Jr.: Lactulose treatment of hepatic encephalopathy in outpatients. Arch. Surg., *102*:25, 1971.
177. Gabuzda, G. J.: Hepatic coma: Clinical considerations, pathogenesis, and management. Advances Intern. Med., *11*:11, 1962.
178. McDermott, W. V., Jr.: Metabolism and toxicity of ammonia. New Eng. J. Med., *257*:1076, 1957.
179. McDermott, W. V., Jr., Barnes, B. A., Nardi, G. L., and Ackroyd, F. W.: Postshunt encephalopathy. Surg. Gynec. Obstet., *126*:585, 1968.

180. Orloff, M. J., Wall, M. H., Hickman, E. B., and Neesby, T.: The influence of the stomal size of portacaval shunts on peripheral blood ammonia levels. Ann. Surg., *158*:172, 1963.
181. Read, A. E.: The medical treatment of hepatic coma. In: Read, A. E., ed.: The Liver. Colston Papers, Volume 19. London, Butterworths, 1967, p. 191.
182. Resnick, R. H., Ishihara, A., Shimmel, A., and Chalmers, T. C.: A controlled trial of colon by-pass in chronic hepatic encephalopathy. Gastroenterology, *54*:1057, 1968.
183. Trey, C., and Davidson, C. S.: The management of fulminant hepatic failure. In: Popper, H., and Schaffner, F., eds.: Progress in Liver Diseases. Volume 3. New York, Grune & Stratton, 1970, p. 282.
184. Zieve, L.: Pathogenesis of hepatic coma. Arch. Intern. Med., *118*:211, 1966.

**Gastric Acid Hypersecretion and Peptic Ulcer**
**Associated with Liver Disease and Portacaval Shunt**

185. Clarke, J. S., Ozeran, R. S., Hart, J. C., Cruze, K., and Crevling, V.: Peptic ulcer following portacaval shunt. Ann. Surg., *148*:551, 1958.
186. Orloff, M. J., Abbott, A. G., and Rosen. H.: Nature of the humoral agent responsible for portacaval shunt-related gastric hypersecretion in man. Amer. J. Surg., *120*:237, 1970.
187. Orloff, M. J., Chandler, J. G., Alderman, S. J., Keiter, J. E., and Rosen, H.: Gastric secretion and peptic ulcer following portacaval shunt in man. Ann. Surg., *170*:515, 1969.
188. Orloff, M. J., Villar-Valdes, H., Abbott, A. G., Williams, R. J., and Rosen, H.: Site of origin of the hormone responsible for gastric hypersecretion associated with portacaval shunt. Surgery, *68*:202, 1970.
189. Orloff, M. J., Villar-Valdes, H., Rosen, H., Thompson, A. G., and Chandler, J. G.: Humoral mediation of the intestinal phase of gastric secretion and of acid hypersecretion associated with portacaval shunts. Surgery, *66*:118, 1969.
190. Ostrow, J. D., Timmerman, R. J., and Gray, S. J.: Gastric secretion in human hepatic cirrhosis. Gastroenterology, *38*:303, 1960.
191. Thompson, J. C.: Alterations in gastric secretion after portacaval shunting. Amer. J. Surg., *117*:854, 1969.

**Renal Failure Associated with Liver Disease**

192. Baldus, W. P., and Summerskill, W. H. J.: The kidney in hepatic disease. In: Foulk, W. T., ed.: Diseases of the Liver. New York, McGraw-Hill Book Company, 1968, p. 107.
193. Goresky, C. A., and Kummer, G.: Renal failure in cirrhosis of the liver. Canad. Med. Ass. J., *90*:353, 1964.
194. Papper, S.: The role of the kidney in Laennec's cirrhosis of the liver. Medicine, *37*:299, 1958.
195. Papper, S.: The kidney in liver disease. In: Strauss, M. B., and Welt, L. G., eds.: Diseases of the Kidney. Boston, Little, Brown & Company, 1963, p. 841.
196. Shear, L., Hall, P. W., III, and Gabuzda, G. J.: Renal failure in patients with cirrhosis of the liver. II. Factors influencing maximal urinary flow rate. Amer. J. Med., *39*:199, 1965.
197. Shear, L., Kleinerman, J., and Gabuzda, G. J.: Renal failure in patients with cirrhosis of the liver. I. Clinical and pathologic characteristics. Amer. J. Med., *39*:184, 1965.

**Portal Hypertension Due to**
**Extrahepatic Portal Obstruction**

198. Clatworthy, H. W., Jr., and Boles, E. T., Jr.: Extrahepatic portal bed block in children: pathogenesis and treatment. Ann. Surg., *150*:371, 1959.
199. Clatworthy, H. W., Jr., and DeLorimer, A. A.: Portal decompression procedures in children. Amer. J. Surg., *107*:447, 1964.
200. Mikkelsen, W. P.: Extrahepatic portal hypertension in children. Amer. J. Surg., *111*:333, 1966.
201. Vorhees, A. B., Jr., Harris, R. C., Britton, R. C., Price, J. B., and Santulli, T. V.: Portal hypertension in children: 98 cases. Surgery, *58*:540, 1965.

202. Walker, R. M.: Treatment of portal hypertension in children. Proc. Roy. Soc. Med., 55:770, 1962.

## Liver Trauma

203. Amerson, J. R., and Blair, R. D.: Traumatic liver injuries. Amer. J. Surg., 25:648, 1959.
204. Crosthwait, R. W., Allen, J. E., Murga, F., Beall, A. C., Jr., and DeBakey, M. E.: The surgical management of 640 consecutive liver injuries in civilian practice. Surg. Gynec. Obstet., 144:650, 1962.
205. Donovan, A. J., Turrill, F. L., and Facey, F. L.: Hepatic trauma. Surg. Clin. N. Amer., 48:1313, 1968.
206. Kindling, P. H., Wilson, R. F., and Walt, A. J.: Hepatic trauma with particular reference to blunt injury. J. Trauma, 9:17, 1969.
207. Lucas, C. E., and Walt, A. J.: Critical decisions in liver trauma. Arch. Surg., 101:277, 1970.
208. Madding, G. F., and Kennedy, P. A.: Trauma to the Liver. 2nd ed. Philadelphia, W. B. Saunders Company, 1971.
209. McClelland, R. N., and Shires, T.: Management of liver trauma in 259 consecutive patients. Ann. Surg., 161:248, 1965.
210. Shafton, G. W., Gliedman, M. L., and Capelletti, R. R.: Injuries of the liver. A review of 111 cases. J. Trauma, 3:63, 1963.
211. Sparkman, R. S., and Fogelman, M. J.: Wounds of the liver. Ann. Surg., 139:690, 1954.
212. Whelan, T. J., and Gillespie, J. T.: Treatment of traumatic hemobilia. Ann. Surg., 162:920, 1965.
213. Wright, P. N., and Orloff, M. J.: Traumatic hemobilia. Ann. Surg., 160:42, 1964.

## Pyogenic Liver Abscess

214. Altemeier, W. A., Schowengerdt, C. G., and Whiteley, D. H.: Abscesses of the liver: Surgical considerations. Arch. Surg., 101:258, 1970.
215. Butler, T. J., and McCarthy, C. F.: Pyogenic liver abscess. Gut, 10:389, 1969.
216. Gaisford, W. D., and Mark, J. B. D.: Surgical management of hepatic abscess. Amer. J. Surg., 118:317, 1969.
217. Halasz, N. A.: Subphrenic abscess: Myths and facts. J.A.M.A., 214:724, 1970.
218. Joseph, W. L., Kahn, A. M., and Longmire, W. P., Jr.: Pyogenic liver abscess. Changing patterns in approach. Amer. J. Surg., 115:63, 1968.
219. Ostermiller, W., Jr., and Carter, R.: Hepatic abscess: current concepts in diagnosis and management. Arch. Surg., 94:353, 1967.
220. Warren, K. W., and Hardy, K. S.: Pyogenic hepatic abscess. Arch. Surg., 97:40, 1968.

## Amebic Liver Abscess

221. Abbruzzese, A. A.: Hepatic amebiasis. Amer. J. Gastroent., 54:464, 1970.
222. Adi, F. C.: Clinical features of hepatic amoebiasis. W. Afr. Med. J., 14:181, 1965.
223. Elsdon-Dew, R.: The epidemiology of amoebiasis. Advances Parasit., 6:1, 1968.
224. Grigsby, W. P.: Surgical treatment of amebiasis. Surg. Gynec. Obstet., 128:609, 1969.
225. Lamont, N. M., and Pooler, N. R.: Hepatic amebiasis: a study of 250 cases. Quart. J. Med., 27:389, 1958.

226. Powell, S. J.: Drug therapy of amoebiasis. Bull. W.H.O., 40:953, 1969.

## Echinococcus Cyst

227. Hankins, J. R.: Management of complicated hepatic hydatid cysts. Ann. Surg., 158:1020, 1963.
228. Katz, A. M., and Pan, C.: Echinococcus disease in the United States. Amer. J. Med., 25:759, 1958.
229. West, J. T., Hillman, F. J., and Rausch, R. L.: Alveolar hydatid disease of the liver: Rationale and techniques of surgical treatment. Ann. Surg., 157:548, 1963.

## Primary Liver Cancer

230. Curutchet, H. P., Terz, J. J., Kay, S., and Lawrence, W.: Primary liver cancer. Surgery, 70:467, 1971.
231. Edmondson, H. A., and Steiner, P. E.: Primary carcinoma of the liver. A study of 100 cases among 48,900 necropsies. Cancer, 7:462, 1954.
232. El-Domeiri, A. A., Huvos, A. G., Goldsmith, H. S., and Foote, F. W.: Primary malignant tumors of the liver. Cancer, 27:7, 1971.
233. Ishak, K. G., and Glunz, P. R.: Hepatoblastoma and Hepatocarcinoma in infancy and childhood. Cancer, 20:396, 1967.
234. Lin, T. Y.: Primary cancer of the liver. Scand. J. Gastroent., Supp. 6, 5:223, 1970.
235. Nikaidoh, H., Boggs, J., and Swenson, O.: Liver tumors in infants and children. Arch. Surg., 101:245, 1970.
236. Pack, G. T., and Islami, A. H.: Surgical treatment of tumors of the liver. In: Pack, G. T., and Ariel, I. M., eds.: Treatment of Cancer and Allied Diseases. Volume 5. 2nd ed. New York, Hoeber Medical Division, Harper & Row, 1962.
237. Purves, L. R., Bersohn, F., and Geddes, E. W.: Serum alpha-feto-protein and primary cancer of the liver in man. Cancer, 25:1261, 1970.
238. Reuter, S. R., Redman, H., and Sickers, D. B.: The spectrum of angiographic findings in hepatoma. Radiology, 94:89, 1970.

## Metastatic Liver Cancer

239. Bengmark, S., Domellöf, L., and Hafström, L.: The natural history of primary and secondary malignant tumors of the liver. Digestion, 3:56, 1970.
240. Fenster, L. F., and Klatskin, G.: Manifestations of metastatic tumors of the liver; a study of 81 patients subjected to needle biopsy. Amer. J. Med., 31:238, 1961.
241. Flanagan, L., Jr., and Foster, J. H.: Hepatic resection for metastatic cancer. Amer. J. Surg., 113:551, 1967.
242. Jaffe, B. M., Donegan, W. L., Watson, F., and Spratt, J. S., Jr.: Factors influencing survival in patients with untreated hepatic metastases. Surg. Gynec. Obstet., 127:1, 1968.
243. Mansfield, C. M., Kramer, S., Southard, M. E., and Mandell, G.: Prognosis in patients with metastatic liver disease diagnosed by liver scan. Radiology, 93:77, 1969.
244. Pack, G. T., and Brasfield, R. D.: Metastatic cancer of the liver: The clinical problem and its management. Amer. J. Surg., 90:704, 1955.
245. Schaefer, J., and Schiff, L.: Liver function tests in metastatic tumor of the liver. Gastroenterology, 49:360, 1965.

# 34

# THE

# BILIARY SYSTEM

*Marshall J. Orloff, M.D.*

## ANATOMY

The biliary system and liver develop together from a diverticulum that arises in the embryo from the ventral floor of the foregut and extends into the septum transversum. The caudal portion of this diverticulum becomes the gallbladder, cystic duct, and common bile duct, whereas the cranial portion develops into the liver and hepatic bile ducts.

The gallbladder is a thin-walled, pear-shaped organ covered by peritoneum and attached to the inferior surfaces of the right and quadrate lobes of the liver. Normally, it is 7 to 10 cm. long and 3 to 5 cm. in diameter and has a capacity of 30 to 60 ml. Anatomically, it is divided into a fundus or tip, which protrudes from the anterior edge of the liver, a corpus or body, an infundibulum called Hartmann's pouch, and a narrow neck that leads into the cystic duct (Fig. 1). Topographically, the

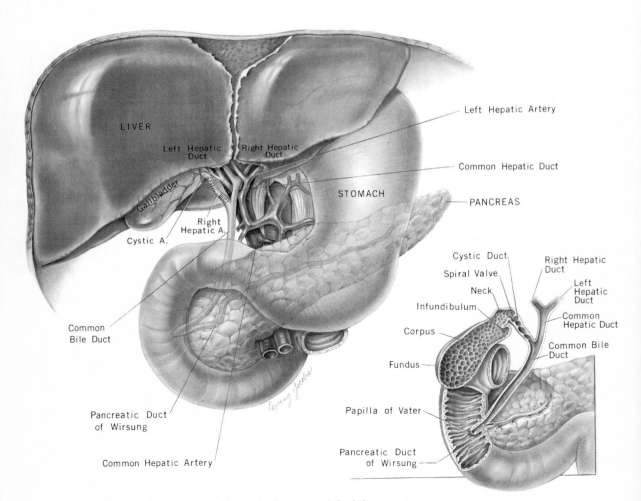

**Figure 1**  Anatomy of the biliary system.

fundus of the gallbladder is located behind the ninth right costal cartilage at the junction of the costal margin with the right border of the rectus abdominis muscle.

The cystic duct from the gallbladder is about 2 to 4 cm. long and contains prominent mucosal folds called spiral folds or valves of Heister. It is questionable whether these folds have any valvular function in regulating bile flow. The cystic duct joins the right lateral aspect of the common hepatic duct to form the common bile duct (Fig. 1).

The extrahepatic bile duct system originates from the liver as the right and left hepatic ducts, each of which is 1 to 2 cm. long and drains the respective lobe of the liver. The two ducts join to form the common hepatic duct, a 2 to 4 cm. long structure in the porta hepatis. The union of the common hepatic duct with the cystic duct gives rise to the common bile duct, which is 8 to 15 cm. long and 5 to 10 mm. in outside diameter. The common bile duct descends in the hepatoduodenal ligament to the right of the hepatic artery and anterior to the portal vein, passes behind the first part of the duodenum and through the pancreas, and enters the descending duodenum on its posteromedial aspect about 10 cm. distal to the pylorus at the papilla of Vater. The choledochoduodenal junction is an oblique passageway through the duodenal wall occupied by the common bile duct and the main pancreatic duct of Wirsung.

These two ducts usually join in a common channel, the ampulla of Vater, which opens into the duodenum at the papilla of Vater; however, the two ducts may join before entering the duodenal wall or may empty into the duodenum through separate openings. The muscle of the choledochoduodenal junction, called the sphincter of Oddi, regulates the flow of bile and consists of several components. The two major components are the sphincter ductus choledochi, which surrounds the common bile duct within the duodenal wall proximal to its junction with the pancreatic duct, and the sphincter ampullae, which surrounds the common ampulla of Vater (Fig. 2).

The arterial blood supply to the common bile duct comes mainly from the retroduodenal artery, a branch of the gastroduodenal artery. The gallbladder is nourished by the cystic artery, which originates from the right hepatic artery, to the right of and behind the common hepatic duct, and divides into anterior and posterior branches. During cholecystectomy, the cystic artery is usually found in the cystic triangle of Calot, a space bounded by the liver, the common hepatic duct, and the cystic duct. The triangle contains the right hepatic artery with its cystic artery branch, a large lymph node, and, in its depths, the right branch of the portal vein. Venous drainage from the extrahepatic biliary system is into the portal vein. Lymphatic vessels from the gallbladder join

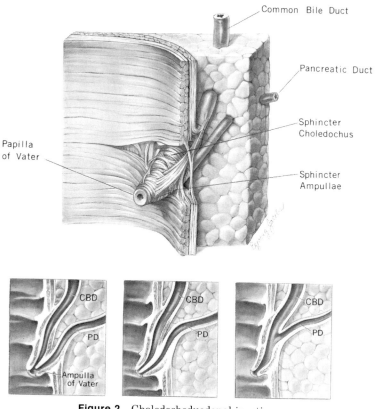

Common Bile Duct

Pancreatic Duct

Sphincter Choledochus

Sphincter Ampullae

Papilla of Vater

CBD  PD  Ampulla of Vater

CBD  PD

CBD  PD

**Figure 2**  Choledochoduodenal junction.

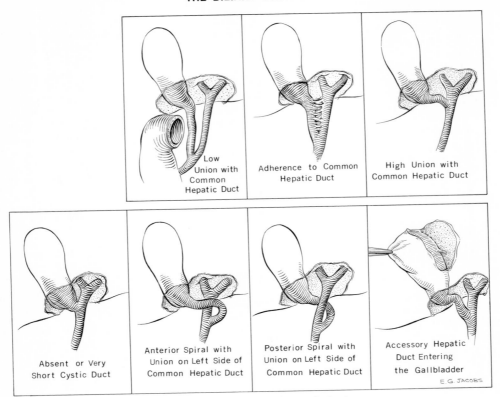

**Figure 3**  Anomalies of the cystic duct.

those from the liver to empty into the cisterna chyli and thoracic duct. Lymph nodes at the neck of the gallbladder, at the junction of the cystic duct and hepatic ducts, and at the end of the common duct play a prominent role in the lymphatic drainage and are regularly enlarged in cholecystitis. The innervation of the biliary system is similar to that of the liver. Vagal stimulation causes contraction of the gallbladder, whereas sympathetic stimulation produces the reverse actions. The effect of vagal stimulation on the sphincter of Oddi is variable.

Histologically, the gallbladder consists of a mucosa of columnar epithelium, a muscularis, a subserosa, and a serosa. Mucous glands are found only in the neck. Gallbladder inflammation characteristically produces invaginations of the mucosa into the muscularis called Rokitansky-Aschoff sinuses. The bile ducts are lined by columnar epithelium and contain mucous glands.

A most striking and, for the surgeon, dangerous feature of the anatomy of the extrahepatic biliary system is its *variability.* Variations in the bile ducts, cystic artery, and hepatic artery are very common. For this reason, biliary operations require extremely careful technique. Anomalies of the gallbladder are rare and include congenital absence, duplications, left-sided gallbladder with the cystic duct entering the left side of the common bile duct or left hepatic duct, and location of the gallbladder partially or completely within the

liver. "Floating gallbladder," in which the vesicle is suspended from the liver by a peritoneal mesentery, is the most common anomaly and occasionally results in acute torsion of the organ.

Anomalies of the cystic duct are shown in Figure 3. Some of these variations are common and the surgeon must be aware of them in performing cholecystectomy. Variations in the other extrahepatic bile ducts are of less surgical significance, although they occur in one of 10 humans. The most important common anomaly of the bile ducts consists of one or more accessory hepatic ducts, which enter the gallbladder directly from the liver. If such ducts are overlooked during excision of the gallbladder, persistent leakage of bile into the peritoneal cavity may result. This possibility constitutes one reason for draining the gallbladder bed following cholecystectomy.

Anomalies of the hepatic arteries were discussed in the previous chapter, and those of the cystic artery are shown in Figure 4. Variations in the origin and location of the arterial blood supply to the gallbladder are very common.

Injuries to the bile ducts during cholecystectomy usually result from failure to recognize anatomic variations in the biliary tree and its blood supply. The consequences of such injuries are often very serious, and they underscore the importance to surgeons of a thorough knowledge of anatomy. The mechanisms whereby some of these injuries occur are illustrated in Figure 5.

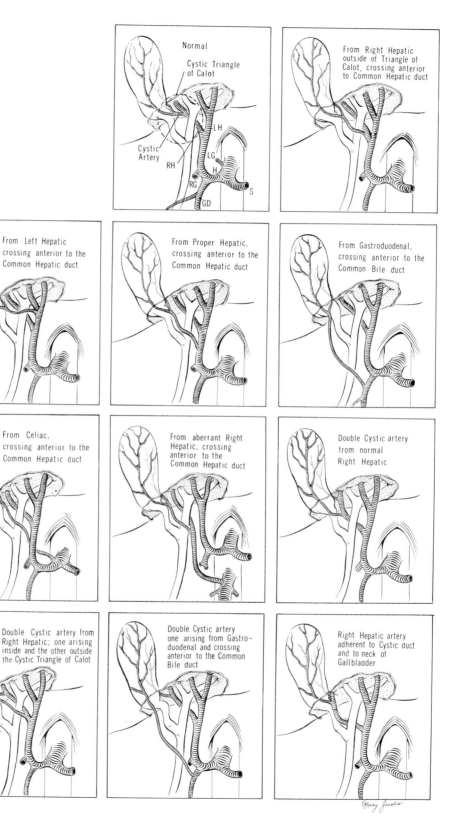

**Figure 4** Anomalies of the cystic artery.

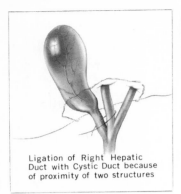

Ligation of Right Hepatic
Duct with Cystic Duct because
of proximity of two structures

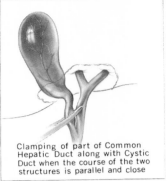

Clamping of part of Common
Hepatic Duct along with Cystic
Duct when the course of the two
structures is parallel and close

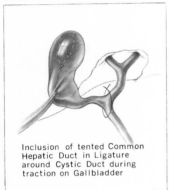

Inclusion of tented Common
Hepatic Duct in Ligature
around Cystic Duct during
traction on Gallbladder

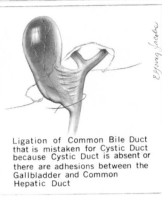

Ligation of Common Bile Duct
that is mistaken for Cystic Duct
because Cystic Duct is absent or
there are adhesions between the
Gallbladder and Common
Hepatic Duct

**Figure 5** Mechanisms whereby injuries to the bile ducts may occur during cholecystectomy.

## PHYSIOLOGY

Bile secreted by the liver into the biliary canaliculi is a solution of bile salts, bile pigments, electrolytes, cholesterol, lecithin, fatty acids, proteins, and a large number and variety of products of hepatic metabolism. The bile salts are glycine and taurine conjugates of cholic and chenodeoxycholic acid, which are formed in the liver from cholesterol. Added to these two primary bile acids are two derivatives, deoxycholic acid and lithocholic acid, which are formed in the intestine by bacterial enzymes and are absorbed in the enterohepatic circulation of bile salts. The bile acids behave as anions and are balanced by the cations sodium and potassium to form salts. The bile pigments are mainly bilirubin diglucuronide and a small amount of urobilinogen. Electrolytes are present in concentrations similar to those found in plasma and consist mainly of sodium, potassium, calcium, chloride, and bicarbonate. The pH of bile normally ranges from 6.0 to 8.8.

Bile has a number of important functions. It plays a role in the hydrolysis and absorption of lipids through a complex mechanism of emulsification. It is involved in the absorption of minerals such as calcium, iron, and copper, of cholesterol, and of the fat-soluble vitamins, A, D, K, and E. It activates and stimulates secretion of certain digestive enzymes, such as pancreatic lipase. It provides alkali for the neutralization of gastric acid in the duodenum. Finally, bile serves as a vehicle for the excretion of numerous compounds metabolized by the liver.

The functions of the extrahepatic biliary system consist of the transport of bile secreted by the liver to the intestines, the regulation of bile flow, and the storage and concentration of bile. The liver secretes 600 to 1000 ml. of bile per day. Liver bile has a specific gravity of 1.011, and 97 per cent of its content is water. The gallbladder concentrates the bile at least 5 to 10 times by absorbing water and electrolytes, and excretes a product with a specific gravity of 1.040. The absorptive capacity of the gallbladder mucosa is greater than that of the small intestine per unit of surface. Normally, the gallbladder does not absorb bile pigments, bile salts, proteins, or lipids. In addition to its absorptive function, the mucosa secretes a thick mucus, and it is this substance that constitutes the so-called white bile in hydrops of the gallbladder associated with cystic duct obstruction.

In the absence of food in the intestine, bile secreted continuously by the liver is retained within the bile ducts as a result of steady contraction of the sphincter of Oddi. As the biliary pressure rises, the bile refluxes into the gallbladder where it is concentrated and stored. Entrance of food into the duodenum causes the release of *cholecystokinin*, an intestinal hormone that produces contraction of the gallbladder, relaxation of the sphincter of Oddi and duodenum, and free flow of bile into the intestine. Cholecystokinin was isolated and purified in 1968 by

Jorpes and Mutt. It has been found to be identical to pancreozymin, a substance that stimulates the pancreas to secrete an enzyme-rich fluid, and the two agents are believed to be a single hormone, sometimes called CCK-PZ. Cholecystokinin is a peptide hormone that consists of 33 amino acid residues and has a molecular weight of approximately 4300. Of great interest, the C-terminal pentapeptide amide, in which the physiologic activity is concentrated, is identical to that of the hormone gastrin. It is believed that nervous stimuli, mediated by the vagus nerves, participate in the process of gallbladder emptying, although motor function is normal after vagotomy and hormonal stimulation appears to be the most important mechanism that regulates the flow of bile into the duodenum. Fats and proteins are strong stimuli to gallbladder contraction, whereas carbohydrates have little effect on motor activity. Following cholecystectomy, regulation of bile flow is dependent entirely on the sphincter of Oddi.

The bile secretory pressure of the liver varies throughout the day but averages 300 mm. saline. At rest, the pressure within the gallbladder averages only 100 mm., so that with the sphincter of Oddi contracted bile is directed into the gallbladder for storage and concentration, and the gallbladder dilates. When the gallbladder contracts in response to a meal, the pressure rises to from 200 to 300 mm., and this hydrostatic force plus inhibition of the sphincter of Oddi by cholecystokinin and nervous impulses causes the sphincter to open completely and bile to flow into the duodenum. Pressures in the bile ducts greater than 350 mm. cause suppression of hepatic bile secretion.

*Pain* from the gallbladder and bile ducts is produced by stretching or distention of the biliary tree, or by abnormal tension of the biliary musculature (spasm). It is often accompanied by nausea and vomiting. Such pain is transmitted by visceral sensory fibers in the splanchnic nerves connected to the seventh to tenth thoracic segments, and is perceived in the epigastrium. As a result of the motor activity in the biliary system and the related changes in pressure, biliary pain often has an intermittent component. Inflammation of the gallbladder causes referral of the visceral sensory impulses to somatic segments, giving rise to pain in the right hypochondrium, infrascapular area, substernal area, and, occasionally, as a result of connections with the phrenic nerve, the right shoulder tip. If inflammation of the gallbladder spreads to the adjacent parietal peritoneum, such as occurs in acute cholecystitis, well localized somatic sensory pain develops. Most of the common analgesics used to relieve biliary tract pain, such as morphine and meperidine, unfortunately produce spasm of the sphincter of Oddi and duodenum and actually increase the pressure in the biliary tree. Distention of the gallbladder or bile ducts may cause a reflex decrease in coronary blood flow and cardiac arrhythmias, and is believed to explain the association of biliary tract disease and cardiac abnormalities.

## DIAGNOSIS

### History and Physical Examination

The history and physical examination play important roles in the diagnosis of biliary diseases. Biliary symptoms fall into three major categories, namely, pain, jaundice, and digestive disturbances sometimes called dyspepsia. Several varieties of pain are produced by diseases of the biliary system, but the most common type is colic in the right upper quadrant of the abdomen with radiation to the back or tip of the scapula. Biliary colic is, in fact, a continuous pain that waxes and wanes in intensity. Jaundice has been discussed at length in the previous chapter. The jaundice associated with extrahepatic biliary obstruction is of the *regurgitation* type, with light or clay-colored stools, dark urine, mixed bilirubinemia with a predominance of the conjugated, direct-reacting fraction, bilirubin in the urine, and, sometimes, pruritus. Jaundice due to a stone in the common bile duct often is intermittent, while jaundice caused by neoplastic obstruction of the biliary tree is usually relentless and progressive. The term "dyspepsia" refers to a number of vague and nonspecific symptoms that are commonly associated with biliary disease. It includes excessive belching, flatulence, bloating, nausea, constipation, and intolerance for fried and fatty foods, onions, cabbage, and tomatoes.

Physical findings produced by biliary diseases include jaundice, light or clay-colored stools, and tenderness in the right upper quadrant and epi-

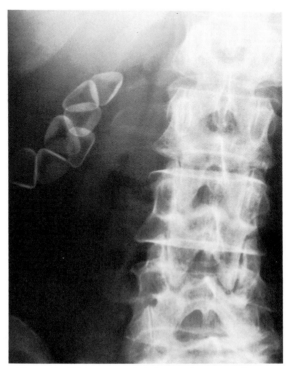

**Figure 6**  Plain x-ray of abdomen showing radiopaque calculi in gallbladder.

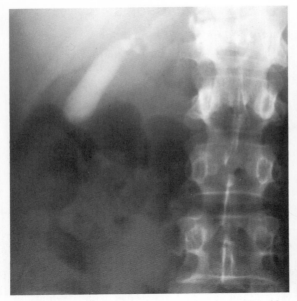

**Figure 7**  Plain x-ray of abdomen showing gallbladder opacified by "milk of calcium" bile.

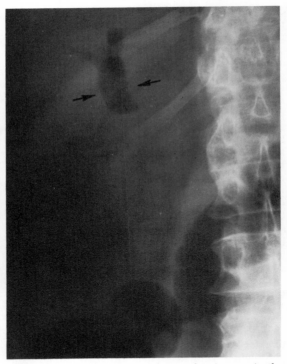

**Figure 8**  Plain x-ray of abdomen showing gas in the biliary tree from a biliary-enteric fistula.

gastrium of the abdomen. When the gallbladder is acutely inflamed, signs of parietal peritoneal irritation such as muscle guarding or rigidity appear, fever develops as a systemic manifestation of the inflammation, and the gallbladder sometimes can be palpated as a tender mass in the upper abdomen. In obstructive jaundice due to a periampullary neoplasm, a distended, nontender gallbladder can be palpated in about one-fourth of the cases.

### Roentgenographic Studies

The diagnosis of biliary tract disease is in large part dependent on roentgenographic studies.

**Plain X-rays of the Abdomen.**  Plain x-rays of the abdomen may be helpful in directing attention to or making the diagnosis of biliary disease. Between 10 and 15 per cent of gallstones contain sufficient calcium to be seen on plain abdominal films (Fig. 6). An uncommon condition called "milk of calcium" bile, which consists of a collection of calcified debris, may cause opacification of the dependent portion of the gallbladder or of the entire organ (Fig. 7). This sediment of calcium carbonate is associated with obstruction of the cystic duct and chronic gallbladder inflammation. Gas in the bile ducts is a diagnostic sign of an abnormal communication between the biliary system and gastrointestinal tract (Fig. 8). Emphysematous cholecystitis is an unusual inflammation of the gallbladder due to gas-producing bacteria that results in gas in the wall and lumen of the gallbladder (Fig. 9). Intestinal obstruction due to a gallstone that has eroded through the biliary tree and into the intestine, called gallstone ileus, is a well known complication of cholecystitis and produces the characteristic roentgenographic signs of

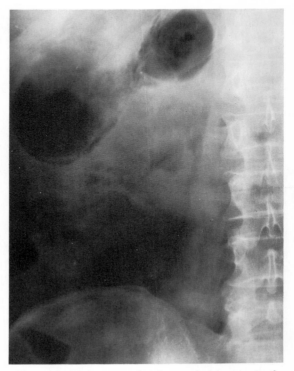

**Figure 9**  Plain x-ray of abdomen showing gas in the lumen and wall of the gallbladder due to emphysematous cholecystitis.

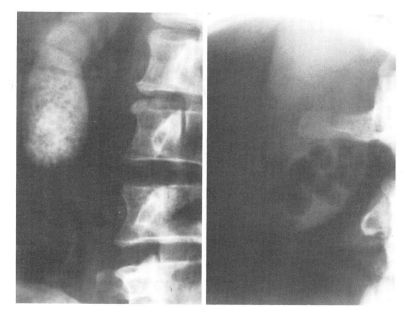

**Figure 10** Radiolucent calculi demonstrated by oral cholecystography in two patients with symptoms of chronic cholecystitis.

dilatation of the bowel. Finally, a dilated loop of small intestine adjacent to an inflamed gallbladder, the so-called sentinel loop, represents a localized ileus and may be of diagnostic significance.

**Oral Cholecystography.** In 1924, Graham and Cole produced radiographic opacification of the gallbladder by the oral administration of an organic iodide-containing dye and initiated a new era in x-ray diagnosis. A wide variety of iodinated organic agents that are absorbed from the intestine, excreted by the liver in the bile, and concentrated in the gallbladder are now available for

visualization of the biliary system. Failure of visualization of the gallbladder usually indicates obstruction of the bile ducts or inability of the gallbladder to concentrate the dye. However, other causes of failure must be ruled out and include inadequate dose of dye, failure of intestinal absorption, inadequate hepatic excretion due to liver disease, and, rarely, a full gallbladder or improper radiographic technique. Administration of a double dose of dye or administration of dye daily for 4 days sometimes demonstrates a gallbladder that could not be visualized with the standard technique. Visualization of the gallbladder rarely

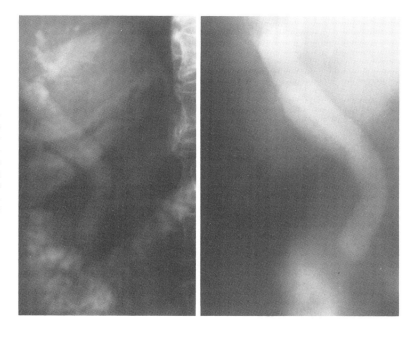

**Figure 11** Intravenous cholangiogram from patient with acute cholecystitis showing good visualization of the bile ducts, but nonvisualization of the gallbladder. As is usual, at operation a stone was found blocking the cystic duct. The x-ray on the right is a tomogram, which is used to show the common bile duct in greater detail.

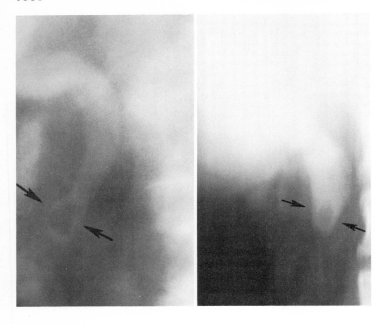

Figure 12 Intravenous cholangiograms showing calculi in the common bile ducts of two patients who had had cholecystectomy several years previously.

occurs when the serum bilirubin is above 4 mg. per 100 ml., and does not usually occur when the serum bilirubin exceeds 3 mg. per 100 ml.

The two most important diagnostic findings of oral cholecystography are radiolucent shadows in the opaque dye and failure of visualization of the gallbladder. The radiolucent shadows are almost always due to gallstones and are diagnostic of disease (Fig. 10). Failure of visualization, however, should be interpreted cautiously and requires a careful consideration of the patient's history, physical findings, and results of other studies. Approximately 5 per cent of nonvisualized gallbladders prove to be normal and no cause for nonvisualization can be identified.

**Intravenous Cholecystography and Cholangiography.** The development of dyes such as sodium iodipamide that do not require concentration in the gallbladder for visualization of the biliary system is the basis for intravenous cholangiography. Although this procedure was originally aimed at demonstrating the extrahepatic bile ducts, it can be employed to visualize the gallbladder. Intravenous cholangiography and cholecystography are used in patients who cannot take the dye orally, in patients who have had a cholecystectomy, and when demonstration of the extrahepatic bile ducts is desired. The procedure is of particular value in patients suspected of having acute cholecystitis, which is usually associated with obstruction of the cystic duct (Fig. 11). Such patients have nausea and vomiting and cannot tolerate oral administration of dye. Visualization of the gallbladder by intravenous cholecystography eliminates the diagnosis of acute cholecystitis. Dilatation or stricture of the bile ducts, choledocholithiasis, choledochal cysts, and cystic duct remnants may be demonstrated by intravenous cholangiography (Fig. 12). A successful study is unusual in the presence of a serum bilirubin greater than 4 mg. per 100 ml. Intravenous cholangiography should not be performed without clear indications because rare hypersensitivity reactions to the dye resulting in circulatory collapse and death have been reported.

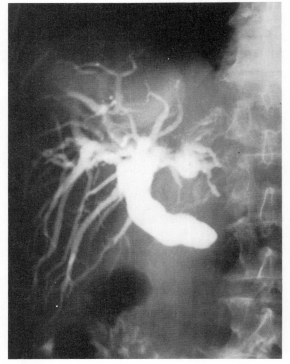

Figure 13 Percutaneous transhepatic cholangiogram from a patient with obstruction of the common bile duct due to carcinoma of the head of the pancreas.

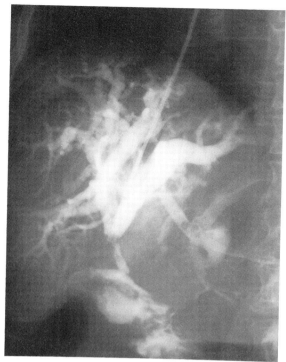

**Figure 14**   Transjugular cholangiogram from a patient with a stricture of the common bile duct produced by injury during cholecystectomy.

**Percutaneous Transhepatic Cholangiography.**   Instillation of opaque media into the biliary system by percutaneous needle puncture of a bile duct has been used primarily in jaundiced patients to determine whether biliary obstruction is extrahepatic or intrahepatic (Fig. 13). Leakage of bile, bleeding, and accidental perforation of other viscera are significant hazards of this technique, and it is generally performed when determination of the site of obstruction may make possible a lifesaving operation. When surgical therapy is indicated, operation is usually undertaken immediately after the cholangiographic study. Failure to visualize the biliary tree after repeated attempts usually means that the obstruction is intrahepatic

and that the extrahepatic biliary system is small in caliber. In carefully selected cases, transhepatic cholangiography may provide valuable information about the nature and site of biliary obstruction, and may make it possible to avoid unnecessary operations.

**Transjugular Cholangiography.**   Another direct percutaneous method of visualizing the biliary system in selected jaundiced patients involves catheterization of a hepatic vein via the internal jugular vein in the neck, and entry into a bile duct by puncture across the wall of the hepatic vein (Fig. 14). The method has been successful in visualizing the bile ducts in about three-fourths of the trials. Because the peritoneal cavity is not entered and the liver capsule is not punctured, the transjugular technique has the advantages over transhepatic cholangiography of avoiding the dangers of bile peritonitis and bleeding and, therefore, of not requiring an immediate operation when extrahepatic biliary obstruction is found. However, transjugular cholangiography has been associated with a disturbing incidence of septicemia and fever due to entry of infected bile directly into the venous outflow from the liver.

**Duodenoscopy and Transduodenal Cholangiography.**   The recent development of flexible fiberoptic endoscopes has made it possible to perform duodenoscopy consistently. Often it is possible to catheterize the common bile duct through the papilla of Vater, and to obtain a cholangiogram following the injection of dye (Fig. 15). With some frequency the pancreatic duct is also visualized. This technique may be of value in jaundiced patients for differentiating between intrahepatic and extrahepatic jaundice, and for distinguishing between stones and neoplasms obstructing the common bile duct.

**Operative and Postoperative Direct Cholangiography.**   Visualization of the extrahepatic bile ducts by instillation of dye via a catheter in the cystic duct or common bile duct during operations on the biliary system has become an important method for identifying stones and other abnormalities. During cholecystectomy, many surgeons perform operative cholangiography via the cystic duct routinely to help decide whether or

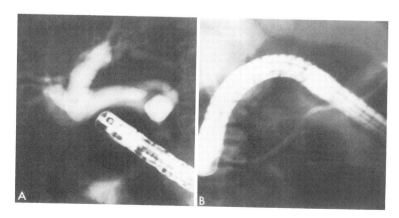

**Figure 15**   Transduodenal cholangiograms showing (A) dilatation of the common bile duct caused by stenosis of the sphincter of Oddi, and (B) a normal pancreatic duct.

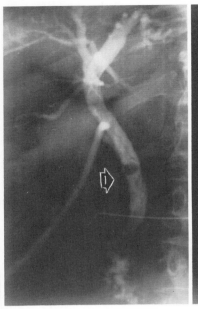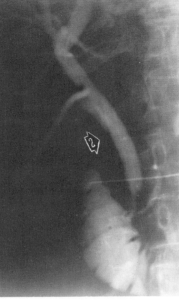

**Figure 16** Intraoperative T tube cholangiograms taken after exploration of the common bile duct showing (1) a calculus that had been overlooked, and (2) appearance on a repeat cholangiogram following removal of the stone.

not to explore the common bile duct for stones. Following exploration of the common bile duct, almost all surgeons obtain a tube cholangiogram before terminating the operation to be certain that stones or strictures have not been overlooked (Fig. 16). For similar reasons, tube cholangiograms are regularly obtained postoperatively before biliary drainage is discontinued.

**Barium Contrast Upper Gastrointestinal X-rays.** The upper gastrointestinal series is an important study in the investigation of patients suspected of having biliary disease. Because the symptoms of gastrointestinal diseases such as peptic ulcer and hiatus hernia often mimic those of biliary disorders, it is important to establish the presence or absence of extrabiliary disturbances that may account for symptoms. The upper gastrointestinal x-rays may be helpful in the differential diagnosis of obstructive jaundice, and particularly in distinguishing between neoplastic and calculus obstruction. Widening of the duodenal sweep, the "reverse 3" sign of Frostberg, distortion of the duodenal mucosa, and displacement of the stomach are important radiographic signs of carcinoma of the head of the pancreas.

A valuable adjunct to the routine upper gastrointestinal series is *hypotonic duodenography.* The technique involves relaxation of the duodenum by the intramuscular administration of a blocking agent such as propantheline during the instillation of barium and air into the duodenum by mouth or via a properly positioned tube. The method is particularly useful in demonstrating pancreaticoduodenal neoplasms in patients with obstructive jaundice (Fig. 17).

**Splanchnic Arteriography.** Splanchnic arteriography is of value mainly in the differential diagnosis of jaundice. As described in the previous

chapter, hepatic arteriography is useful in demonstrating various liver diseases that produce jaundice. Furthermore, celiac arteriography is becoming increasingly accurate in demonstrating pancreatic disease, particularly cancer of the head of the pancreas.

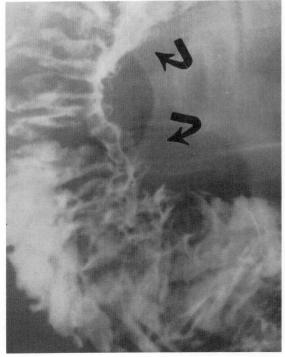

**Figure 17** Hypotonic duodenography with barium in a patient with carcinoma of the head of the pancreas.

## Biochemical Studies

The use of liver function tests in the differential diagnosis of jaundice is discussed in detail in the preceding chapter. The hallmarks of extrahepatic bile duct obstruction are an elevation of serum bilirubin, with a preponderance of the direct-reacting, conjugated fraction, and a parallel rise in serum alkaline phosphatase. A rise in the serum 5'-nucleotidase level, similar to that of alkaline phosphatase, also occurs. Depression of prothrombin activity that can be corrected by parenteral administration of vitamin K is characteristic of prolonged obstructive jaundice. Appearance of bilirubin in the urine and, if obstruction is complete, disappearance of urobilinogen from the urine and stool are regular biochemical abnormalities produced by biliary obstruction. In uncomplicated obstructive jaundice of short duration, the other liver function tests are usually normal. However, in long-standing bile duct obstruction, or in biliary infection such as cholangitis, abnormalities of all of the common liver function tests and particularly of the enzyme levels may develop.

Because of the intimate association of diseases of the biliary system and pancreas, determinations of serum amylase and lipase and of urinary diastase are frequently indicated. Elevations of these enzymes are often found in patients with acute biliary inflammations in the absence of gross disease of the pancreas. The frequent occurrence of biliary disorders in patients with diabetes requires determinations of blood and urine sugar.

## Liver Biopsy

The role of percutaneous needle biopsy of the liver in the diagnosis of jaundice is discussed in the previous chapter. It may be of help in distinguishing between jaundice due to liver disease and extrahepatic obstructive jaundice.

## Duodenal Drainage

Aspiration of bile from a tube inserted via the nose or mouth into the duodenum may provide valuable information in the diagnosis of biliary disease and in the differential diagnosis of jaundice. Instillation of magnesium sulfate or olive oil into the duodenum causes contraction of the gallbladder and permits collection of bile emanating from the gallbladder. By proper timing of specimens, bile from the extrahepatic ducts and fresh liver bile may be obtained. The finding of cholesterol and calcium bilirubinate crystals on microscopic examination of the duodenal aspirate strongly suggests the presence of gallstones. Cytologic studies for cancer cells may provide evidence of carcinoma of the biliary ducts or duodenum. Duodenal drainage is indicated when other diagnostic studies fail to yield positive results in patients with symptoms suggestive of biliary disease.

## Peritoneoscopy

Peritoneoscopy or laparoscopy is occasionally of value in the differential diagnosis of jaundice. Direct visualization of the peritoneal cavity may reveal the dilated normal gallbladder associated with malignant biliary obstruction, peritoneal and hepatic metastases from a pancreaticoduodenal cancer, the shrunken, diseased gallbladder of chronic cholecystitis, or the "pearls" of fat necrosis associated with acute pancreatitis. Needle biopsy of suspicious lesions in the liver can be done under direct vision during peritoneoscopy.

## GALLSTONES

The vast majority of diseases of the extrahepatic biliary system are associated with gallstones. Approximately 15 million people in the United States have cholelithiasis, and about 350,000 gallbladders are removed surgically each year because of calculi. Gallstone disease occurs in approximately 10 per cent of the adult population of our country and in about 20 per cent of persons over the age of 40, and so this condition is one of the most common disorders of adult life. The incidence of cholelithiasis increases progressively with age; approximately one-third of persons in their eighth decade of life have calculi. At the same time, the occurrence of gallstones in children associated with hemolytic anemias is by no means rare, and the finding of cholelithiasis in young adults, particularly pregnant women, is not unusual. Biliary calculi develop about four times more frequently in women than in men, although with age the incidence among males progressively approaches that among females.

Gallstones are formed from the constituents of bile. The three major components are cholesterol monohydrate, calcium carbonate, and calcium bilirubinate. Other inorganic salts of calcium and small quantities of a variety of organic and inorganic substances may be found in some stones. In the United States, the vast majority of calculi are "mixed" stones that contain cholesterol as the predominant component. "Pure" cholesterol stones and "pure" pigment calculi are uncommon. The latter are formed only in disorders causing increased bilirubin production (Fig. 18).

The pathogenesis of gallstones is not completely understood, and undoubtedly several mechanisms are involved. For more than a century, three major factors have been considered to be of etiologic importance: (1) a primary physicochemical disorder of bile, (2) stasis of bile, and (3) infection or inflammation of the biliary system. In recent years, substantial evidence has been obtained to suggest that a primary abnormality in the physicochemical composition of bile plays an important role in gallstone formation.

More than 90 per cent of the dry weight of bile is made up of three constituents: bile salt (cholate, chenodeoxycholate, and deoxycholate), phospholipid (90 per cent of which is lecithin), and cholesterol. Lecithin is insoluble in aqueous systems, but it takes up water to form liquid crystals. Cholesterol is completely insoluble in aqueous solutions, but it is incorporated into the lecithin

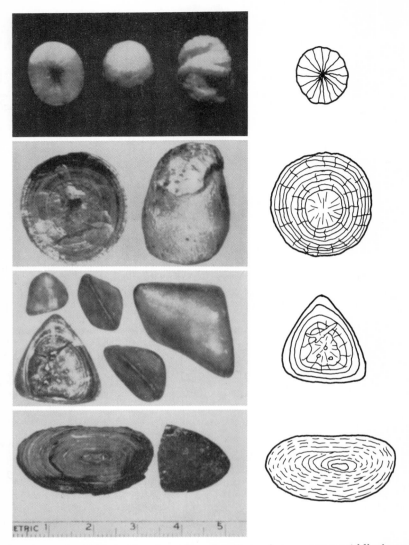

**Figure 18**  Various types of gallstones. *Top* shows "pure" cholesterol stone; *upper middle* shows laminated mixed stone; *lower middle* shows faceted mixed stone; *bottom* shows pigment stone. (From Juniper, K., Jr. In: Paulson, M., ed.: Gastroenterologic Medicine. Philadelphia, Lea & Febiger, 1969; upper middle photo from Juniper, K., Jr.: Mod. Treatm., 5:480, 1968.)

liquid crystals. Bile salts are water-soluble, and they have the unique capacity to form highly charged polymolecular aggregates called micelles. The bile salts solubilize the lecithin liquid crystals with the incorporated cholesterol by forming mixed micelles. The capacity of these mixed micelles to keep cholesterol in solution is related to the relative concentrations of lecithin and bile salts. This important relationship can be expressed on triangular coordinates in a phase diagram devised by Admirand and Small (Fig. 19). The limits of cholesterol solubility at various relative concentrations of bile salt, lecithin, and cholesterol in solutions of various dilutions are defined by such a diagram. The line ABC in Figure 19 represents the maximal solubility of cholesterol in varying mixtures of bile salt and lecithin. Mix-

tures falling below the ABC line are in a single liquid phase and are not completely saturated with cholesterol (i.e., cholesterol is completely solubilized), while those above the ABC line are oversaturated with cholesterol and, therefore, contain insoluble cholesterol crystals. Substantial evidence suggests that the formation of bile containing more cholesterol than can be dissolved in the bile salt-lecithin micelle is responsible for the initiation of gallstone formation. Admirand and Small concluded from studies in humans that bile from normal subjects fell entirely within the micellar zone and was unsaturated with cholesterol, while bile from patients with cholelithiasis was saturated or supersaturated with cholesterol.

The source of the abnormal lithogenic bile is uncertain. It could be formed in the liver, or it

**Figure 19** Admirand and Small's phase diagram in which three major components of bile are plotted on triangular coordinates. Line ABC represents the maximal solubility of cholesterol in varying mixtures of bile salt and lecithin. Any combination of bile salt, lecithin, and cholesterol may be expressed as a single point within the triangle. For example, a mixture having 80 moles of bile salt, 15 moles of lecithin, and 5 moles of cholesterol would be plotted at point P, well within the micellar zone where cholesterol is completely dissolved.

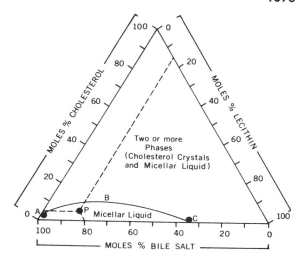

could result from alterations that occur in the gallbladder and bile ducts. It has been shown that gallstones produced in the hamster by a fat-free, high-glucose diet are associated with the production of abnormal bile by the liver. Furthermore, hepatic bile obtained from American Indians of the Southwest who have a very high incidence of gallstones has been found to be abnormal. In addition, it has been reported that patients with cholesterol cholelithiasis have a markedly reduced bile acid pool size; this results in a decrease in secretion of both bile acids and lecithin, and a reduced capacity of bile to solubilize cholesterol. Thus, gallstones may be due to decreased hepatic bile salt production rather than increased cholesterol secretion.

Certain evidence suggests that alteration of normal hepatic bile by the gallbladder may play a role in stone formation. While the normal gallbladder reabsorbs only water and electrolytes, it has been known for many years that the inflamed gallbladder can reabsorb bile salts and thereby change the physicochemical composition of bile. Moreover, recent studies in mice fed a cholesterogenic diet indicate that reabsorption of bile salts by a damaged gallbladder mucosa is responsible for gallstone formation in these animals. The formation of calcium bilirubinate stones, so common in the Orient in association with *Ascaris lumbricoides* or *Escherichia coli* infection, is believed to be due to hydrolysis of soluble bilirubin diglucuronide in bile by β-glucuronidase produced by the infectious organisms, and the subsequent precipitation of the free bilirubin with calcium.

The recent progress in identifying the physicochemical abnormalities in gallstone formation has led to attempts to dissolve gallstones in vivo. Some years ago it was shown that human gallstones dissolved when placed in the gallbladder of dogs, pigs, sheep, and goats. Recent studies have demonstrated that human cholesterol calculi can be dissolved in vitro by an appropriate lecithinbile salt mixture. Finally, Danzinger et al. in 1972 reported the disappearance or reduction in size of gallstones in four of seven patients given chenodeoxycholic acid orally for periods of 6 to 22 months. While the feasibility of medical therapy of cholelithiasis is far from established, the results of these preliminary studies present an exciting possibility.

The role of infection in the pathogenesis of cholelithiasis is uncertain. Although bacteria are commonly found in inflamed gallbladders and in stones, substantial evidence indicates that normal bile is usually sterile. The inflamed gallbladder mucosa has a markedly altered permeability, which permits the absorption of bile acids and the movement of inorganic salts into the gallbladder lumen. It is possible that these changes alter the distribution of the constituents of bile and cause precipitation of cholesterol. Equally important may be the role of excessive cellular debris and increased protein secretion, which occur in response to inflammation and may form a nidus for gallstones. Finally, the effects of bacterial enzymes on the constituents of bile may alter solubility conditions and lead to precipitation of cholesterol or bilirubin.

Stasis has been proposed as a factor in gallstone formation, in part on the basis of experimental studies regarding the production of calculi. Chronic spasm of the sphincter of Oddi is believed to be a cause of stasis. It is postulated that stasis leads to excessive reabsorption of water by the gallbladder and an increased concentration of bilirubin and cholesterol in bile. The resultant physiochemical imbalance may cause precipitation of the organic constituents and the development of calculi.

Symptomatic chronic cholecystitis is almost always associated with cholelithiasis. At the same time, a substantial number of patients with calculi have silent stones that do not produce symptoms. Estimates of the percentage of calculi that are asymptomatic have ranged from 10 per cent to as high as 50 per cent.

# INFLAMMATORY DISEASES OF THE BILIARY SYSTEM

## CHRONIC CHOLECYSTITIS

### Pathogenesis

Chronic cholecystitis is a disease distinguished by the pathologic findings of chronic inflammation and by a clinical course in which the systemic manifestations of inflammation are not prominent. Approximately 95 per cent of the cases are associated with gallstones. The pathogenesis of this condition is not clear despite the attention it has received. It is not a usual bacterial inflammation, although bacteria may play a primary or secondary role. The theories regarding etiology are several. Prominent among these is the proposal that chronic cholecystitis is caused by mechanical or chemical irritation. According to this proposal, gallstones form before inflammation occurs. The calculi then cause inflammation by pressure on the mucosa and lead to the formation of mucosal ulcers. The inflammation is promoted by the irritating effect of constituents of bile, particularly when there is bile stasis. These chemicals may cause inflammation in the absence of stones. Bacterial invasion may occur as a secondary event.

A second theory proposes that bacterial infection is the primary cause of chronic cholecystitis. Bacteria are believed to gain access to the gallbladder along the bile ducts, via the lymphatics, and by way of the arterial and venous circulations. Undoubtedly, some cases of cholecystitis, particularly those associated with systemic infections, have a bacterial etiology. However, the absence of bacteria in normal bile and the frequent failure to culture organisms in diseased gallbladders cast some doubt on the suggestion that bacteria commonly cause cholecystitis.

### Diagnosis

The diagnosis of chronic cholecystitis is based mainly on the history, physical examination, and x-ray studies. The symptoms fall into two categories: vague digestive complaints, sometimes called dyspepsia, and attacks of biliary colic. The digestive disturbances include postprandial belching, nausea, bloating, flatulence, and constipation and are often related to the ingestion of fried or fatty foods or such items as cabbage and onions. These symptoms are due to reflex disorders of gastrointestinal motility and by themselves are nonspecific.

Attacks of biliary colic are quite distinctive. They are due to distention of the biliary tree as a result of a calculus transiently obstructing the cystic duct or common bile duct or as a consequence of spasm of the sphincter of Oddi. They often begin after a heavy meal or at night and last for several hours to several days. The pain is severe and, unlike other forms of colic, is continuous, with waves of increasing intensity. The pain begins in the epigastrium and, as it pro-

gresses, radiates to the right costal margin, to the back below the tip of the scapula, and sometimes to the right shoulder. Radiation to the substernal area and left hypochondrium is occasionally observed. Deep respiration intensifies the pain, but movement does not. At the height of the pain, nausea and vomiting frequently occur. As the pain subsides, the patient is left with residual soreness.

The physical findings are not striking. Mild to moderate tenderness and guarding in the epigastrium and right hypochondrium are the only significant signs. The gallbladder is usually not palpable except in hydrops of the gallbladder, a condition in which the cystic duct is obliterated and the gallbladder becomes distended with mucus. Fever is usually absent or low-grade. Transient bilirubinemia is not uncommon.

Roentgenographic studies represent the best means of confirming the suspicion that a patient has chronic cholecystitis. The demonstration of gallstones by cholecystography or, occasionally, by plain abdominal x-rays provides the only certain evidence of the disease. Failure of visualization of the gallbladder, particularly on repeated studies, strongly suggests chronic cholecystitis if added to a history of typical symptoms. Duodenal drainage may provide important information and is indicated if the diagnosis is in doubt.

Severe attacks of biliary colic may be confused with a large number of diseases, including peptic ulcer, pancreatitis, hiatus hernia, diverticulitis, mesenteric thrombosis, myocardial infarction, and pleurisy. The importance of ruling out these conditions by appropriate studies, particularly when gallstones are not demonstrable, should be apparent.

### Management

The treatment of symptomatic chronic cholecystitis is surgical removal of the gallbladder. The operative mortality of this procedure is less than 1 per cent. The treatment of a patient with clear-cut symptoms by any means other than cholecystectomy is almost always associated with recurrence of symptoms and often with the development of serious complications.

The treatment of a patient whose gallbladder fails to be visualized by cholecystography is a matter of judgment. Under such circumstances, operation should be performed only in the presence of strongly suggestive symptoms and after repeated x-ray studies. Moreover, the absence of other diseases that might account for the symptoms should be demonstrated.

The treatment of patients with silent stones discovered incidentally is controversial. The probability that such calculi will become symptomatic is considerable, and the possibility exists that serious complications such as acute cholecystitis, obstructive jaundice, cholangitis, and biliary fistula will develop. Long-term follow-up studies of patients with asymptomatic calculi have shown that symptoms developed in approximately 50 per cent, and complications such as acute cholecystitis and common duct obstruction developed in 25 per cent, usually within 5 years of discovery of the stones. The low mortality rate and morbidity of elective cholecystectomy add support to the argument for surgical treatment. Nevertheless, the decision regarding therapy must take into account the health of the patient, risk of operation, and the life expectancy. In general, operation is advisable in patients less than 60 years of age who are in good health.

Symptomatic gallstones have been shown to play a potentiating role in pancreatitis and in coronary insufficiency. Removal of the gallbladder often has a beneficial effect on these diseases and is recommended.

## ACUTE CHOLECYSTITIS

### Etiology and Pathology

Acute cholecystitis is characterized clinically by the presence of systemic and local signs of inflammation, and pathologically by the presence of an acute inflammatory process in the gallbladder. In more than 90 per cent of the patients it is associated with gallstones. The failure to find bacteria in more than half the cases suggests that it is not usually caused by a bacterial infection. It is currently believed that acute cholecystitis is a chemical inflammation, sometimes with secondary bacterial enhancement.

Acute cholecystitis is initiated by calculus obstruction of the cystic duct. The subsequent overconcentration of the bile trapped in the gallbladder is believed to produce inflammation of the mucosa and an outpouring of fluid, which causes marked distention of the gallbladder and the development of a high intraluminal pressure. If the obstruction is not relieved spontaneously or surgically, the blood supply to the gallbladder may be compromised, and necrosis and perforation may result. Bacterial invasion produces an empyema of the gallbladder and facilitates necrosis. Gangrene and perforation occur in 10 to 15 per cent of the patients with acute cholecystitis. The perforation is usually walled off by omentum and surrounding organs; this produces a pericholecystic abscess, subphrenic abscess, or biliary-enteric fistula. Free perforation with bile peritonitis occurs in only 1 per cent of the cases.

### Diagnosis

The most prominent symptom of acute cholecystitis is severe abdominal pain. Initially, it may be characteristic of biliary colic, but soon it becomes a continuous pain in the right hypochondrium intensified by movement and respiration. One or two episodes of vomiting accompany the pain. Fever (101 or 102° F.) regularly occurs and may be accompanied by chills. A history of previous symptoms of chronic cholecystitis is often obtained.

The physical findings consist of marked tenderness and rigidity in the right upper quadrant and epigastrium. A mass representing the gallbladder and adherent omentum is palpable in about one-fourth of the cases. Mild jaundice is common and is usually due to associated inflammation of the bile ducts and liver rather than to biliary obstruction.

Laboratory studies show a polymorphonuclear leukocytosis and often a mild elevation of serum bilirubin and alkaline phosphatase. The serum amylase level is commonly increased. Plain x-rays of the abdomen infrequently show a calculus. Oral cholecystography is often not possible because of the patient's nausea and vomiting. On intravenous cholangiography, the common bile duct is seen but the gallbladder is not visualized, a finding of diagnostic value. Visualization of the gallbladder by cholangiography rules out the diagnosis of acute cholecystitis.

The differential diagnosis of acute cholecystitis involves a consideration of most acute abdominal diseases and some extra-abdominal disorders. These include pancreatitis, perforated peptic ulcer, appendicitis, strangulation obstruction of the intestines, mesenteric occlusion, pyelonephritis, salpingitis, acute hepatitis, myocardial infarction, acute congestive heart failure, and right lower lobe pneumonia. In elderly patients, symptoms and signs may not be well developed, and diagnosis may be difficult.

### Treatment

The therapy of acute cholecystitis is not uniform. In the past, medical treatment of acute cholecystitis was the rule, and a number of physicians continue to employ this approach. Approximately 75 to 90 per cent of patients respond to a medical regimen consisting of nasogastric suction, parenteral fluids, and antibiotics, and are well within 2 to 14 days of the onset of the acute attack. Such patients are subjected to an elective cholecystectomy 2 or 3 months later. Failure to respond to medical treatment is an indication for an emergency operation and, because the patient is often seriously ill, simple drainage of the gallbladder occasionally may be the only safe procedure possible. A second operation for removal of the gallbladder must be done at a later time. Advocates of medical therapy argue that the vast majority of patients respond, that there are advantages in making certain of the diagnosis and preparing the patient for operation over a period of time, and that early operation may be difficult because of inflammation and edema and may not permit exploration of the common bile duct when indicated.

Contrary to this point of view, in the United States there has been a progressive shift toward early surgical treatment, within 24 to 72 hours of the onset of the attack. The failure of medical therapy in some patients, the frequent necessity of a compromise operation in patients who do not respond, the requirement for two periods of hospitalization, the danger of perforation, and the fact that all patients must eventually undergo cholecystectomy form the basis for advocating early surgical therapy in most patients. Moreover, the mortality rate associated with early operation has been only slightly greater than that of elective cholecystectomy. It has been general experience that removal of the acutely inflamed gallbladder and, if necessary, exploration of the common bile duct are quite safe and almost always possible when performed early, and may be less difficult than a dissection through scar tissue performed 2 to 3 months after the acute attack. It should be emphasized that simple drainage of the gallbladder by cholecystostomy is the treatment of choice in an occasional patient in whom technical difficulties are encountered. In elderly patients and diabetics, difficulty in judging the progress of the disease makes early surgical treatment imperative.

### Emphysematous Cholecystitis

This is an unusual form of acute cholecystitis in which gas accumulates in the lumen and wall of the gallbladder as a result of infection with a variety of gas-forming enteric bacteria. Gangrene of the gallbladder frequently results. The condition has been reported in males more than in females, and about one-third of the reported patients have had diabetes mellitus. The roentgenographic picture is striking and provides the diagnosis (see Fig. 9). Treatment consists of intensive antibiotic therapy and early operative removal or drainage of the gallbladder. Although the risk of gallbladder perforation is significant, some patients have recovered with medical therapy alone.

## CHOLEDOCHOLITHIASIS

Calculi in the extrahepatic bile ducts usually originate in the gallbladder, although they may form in the biliary ducts. Choledocholithiasis develops in 10 to 20 per cent of patients with gallbladder stones. Although stones in the bile ducts may be silent, they usually produce biliary obstruction, which is often incomplete and intermittent. In addition, they may be associated with bile duct infection and, if present for long periods, may be responsible for significant liver damage and occasionally for secondary biliary cirrhosis.

### Diagnosis

Choledocholithiasis in its classic form produces a syndrome of jaundice, biliary colic, and fever. However, in a substantial number of patients one or more symptoms of this triad are absent. Jaundice occurs in about 80 per cent of the patients and is characteristically fluctuating in nature. Progressive, relentless jaundice is unusual and suggests the presence of neoplastic obstruction rather than stones. The jaundice is accompanied by dark urine and light stools, but clay-colored stools lasting for a significant length of time do not usually occur. Biliary colic due to distention of the bile ducts is a common early symptom of choledocholithiasis. The pain is similar in nature and location to gallbladder colic and is often accompanied by restlessness, nausea, and vomiting. Fever and chills occur in only one-third of the patients with

bile duct stones. A past history of the dyspeptic symptoms of chronic cholecystitis is common.

Physical findings include tenderness and rigidity in the epigastrium and right hypochondrium in proportion to the existence and severity of infection. The liver is often palpable and tender if cholangitis is present. The gallbladder usually is not palpable, even in the presence of severe biliary obstruction. According to the autopsy studies of Courvoisier in the late nineteenth century, the gallbladder was normal and usually distended in obstructive jaundice due to neoplasm, but was seldom distended in obstructive jaundice due to calculi because of pre-existing cholecystitis and fibrosis. These observations have become known as *Courvoisier's law.*

The diagnosis of choledocholithiasis usually, although by no means invariably, involves the differential diagnosis of jaundice. The hyperbilirubinemia shows a predominance of conjugated bilirubin, there is bilirubin in the urine, and, if the obstruction is complete, urine and stool urobilinogen are decreased. Serum alkaline phosphatase is consistently elevated, even in the absence of jaundice. The enzyme, turbidity, and flocculation liver function tests are usually normal except in long-standing obstruction or when cholangitis is present. Intravenous cholangiography may show calculi, or dilatation of the common bile duct greater than 15 mm. if performed in the absence of marked jaundice. The finding of crystals in the duodenal aspirate is suggestive of biliary stones.

In patients with jaundice, the most important diagnostic considerations include obstructive jaundice due to neoplasm, intrahepatic cholestasis, and regurgitation jaundice due to primary liver disease. Neoplastic obstruction of the bile ducts is usually complete and relentless, and occurs in a patient with debilitating manifestations of cancer and no history of dyspeptic symptoms; stone obstruction is usually incomplete and fluctuating. Intrahepatic cholestasis usually does not produce pain, a history of ingestion of one of the causative agents may be obtained, and a history of dyspeptic symptoms is usually absent. Jaundice due to hepatic cell damage is regularly associated with typical liver function test abnormalities and the absence of colicky pain. Occasionally, cholangiography by the percutaneous transhepatic, transjugular, or transduodenal technique may be required to differentiate these three forms of jaundice.

Other diagnostic possibilities, particularly in patients without jaundice, include renal or intestinal colic, acute congestive heart failure, acute hepatitis, and the numerous diseases that may produce acute abdominal pain.

### Treatment

The treatment of choledocholithiasis involves surgical exploration of the common bile duct and removal of the calculi after preparation of the patient for operation, which may require parenteral vitamin K therapy. Usually, this is combined with treatment of the associated gallbladder disease by cholecystectomy. Occasionally, choledochotomy is required for newly formed or overlooked calculi in patients who have previously undergone cholecystectomy.

In every operation on the gallbladder, the surgeon must decide whether or not to explore the common bile duct. Such explorations are not performed routinely because of the increased morbidity and slightly increased mortality associated with them. The indications for exploring the common bile duct as a supplement to cholecystectomy are: (1) palpable stone or mass in the common bile duct; (2) dilatation of the common bile duct greater than 12 mm.; (3) jaundice at the time of operation or in the patient's recent history; (4) evidence of stones on operative cholangiogram; (5) small stones in the gallbladder that are smaller in diameter than the diameter of the cystic duct; and (6) a single faceted stone in the gallbladder.

In some instances, duodenotomy and division or partial resection of the sphincter of Oddi must be added to choledochotomy in order to remove stones impacted in the ampulla of Vater and relieve biliary obstruction. Following choledochotomy, most surgeons drain the common bile duct with a T tube and perform direct cholangiography before terminating the operation and again 7 to 10 days postoperatively, before removing the T tube, in order to be certain that biliary calculi have not been overlooked.

Retained or recurrent bile duct calculi are a serious problem. In approximately 5 per cent of patients who have had a cholecystectomy, stones in the bile duct are discovered at a later date. The incidence is higher in patients who have undergone common bile duct exploration initially than in patients who have had an initial cholecystectomy without choledochotomy (Fig. 20). Although many of these represent calculi that were overlooked at the initial operation, there is no question that in some instances they are new stones formed in the bile ducts. Primary bile duct stones are characteristically ovoid, nonfaceted, and soft. The treatment of retained or recurrent choledocholithiasis is reoperation and surgical removal unless there are strong contraindications related to increased operative risk. When there is concomitant stenosis of the papilla of Vater, when the stones have the characteristics of primary ductal calculi, or when the stones are impacted in the small intrahepatic ducts and cannot be extracted, a choledochoduodenostomy (or choledochojejunostomy) or partial excision of the sphincter of Oddi (sphincteroplasty) should be added to the operation to assure free passage of remaining or yet-to-be-formed calculi into the duodenum. In the case of intrahepatic stones, it is sometimes possible to remove them by surgically exposing the bile ducts through the liver.

## ACUTE SUPPURATIVE CHOLANGITIS

Infection in the bile ducts, or cholangitis, is common in patients with choledocholithiasis. In most instances, it responds to intensive antibiotic therapy and the patient can be operated on electively for treatment of the underlying calculous disease. Should it not respond promptly to medical treatment, an emergency operation is necessary to remove the obstructing stones and decompress the biliary tree. Thus, cholangitis varies considerably in severity, but it is usually a readily controllable condition.

In recent years, an acute, fulminating form of cholangitis has been clearly recognized in which

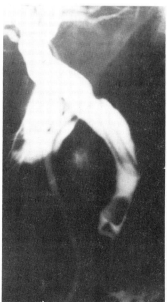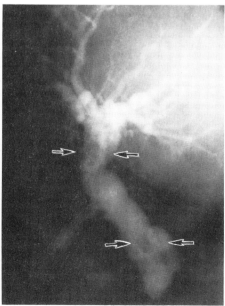

**Figure 20** Retained stones in the common bile duct demonstrated by postoperative T tube cholangiograms in two patients who had undergone cholecystectomy and choledochotomy.

the bile ducts contain frank pus under high pressure. This entity is called acute suppurative cholangitis, and it is the most serious complication of calculous biliary tract disease. The suppurative inflammation of the bile ducts usually results from the combination of duct obstruction and infection, most often with gram-negative organisms. The obstruction is almost always due to gallstones, although noninflammatory strictures and, rarely, neoplastic obstruction may be responsible. The clinical picture is characterized by jaundice, high fever, chills, right upper quadrant pain, hepatomegaly, liver tenderness, and marked leukocytosis. Marked systemic toxicity culminating in shock and prostration may develop. In addition to conjugated hyperbilirubinemia and increased serum alkaline phosphatase, elevations of the glutamic oxaloacetic transaminase and glutamic pyruvic transaminase may be pronounced. Thrombocytopenia is a frequent finding. Positive blood cultures are often obtained.

Acute suppurative cholangitis is uniformly fatal unless the obstruction is relieved. Multiple liver abscesses invariably develop if the biliary tree is not decompressed. Therefore, the treatment consists of emergency surgical drainage of the common bile duct combined with intensive chemotherapy. If the patient's condition permits, cholecystectomy and removal of calculi in the bile ducts may be done at the time of the emergency operation, but biliary drainage is the sine qua non of therapy. Even with surgical treatment, mortality rates have averaged 30 per cent.

A common form of cholangitis in the Orient, but one that is rare in the United States, is recurrent pyogenic cholangitis or oriental cholangiohepatitis. It is seen most commonly in Chinese in association with a combination of parasitic and bacterial infection of the biliary tract. The parasites most often involved are Ascaris and the liver fluke *Clonorchis sinensis*. Calculi are regularly found in the common bile duct. The disease produces widespread inflammation and scarring throughout the biliary system, and often results in liver abscesses and extensive destruction of hepatic tissue. Definitive treatment consists of removal of the stones combined with wide drainage of the common bile duct through a choledochoduodenostomy or sphincteroplasty. Appropriate chemotherapy, of course, is added.

## PRIMARY SCLEROSING CHOLANGITIS

Primary sclerosing cholangitis, known also as "stenosing cholangitis," "fibrosing cholangitis," and "obliterative cholangitis," is a rare, diffuse, chronic inflammation of unknown etiology that involves the extrahepatic bile ducts. It occurs at least three times more commonly in males than in females, and has been reported in patients ranging in age from 20 to 67 years. It is characterized by marked thickening of the common bile duct and sometimes the hepatic ducts, with extreme narrowing of the lumen due to inflammation and edema of the submucosa and subserosa. Adjacent lymph nodes are often enlarged, but the gallbladder is usually normal and free of calculi. There is no specific microscopic lesion. Involvement of the liver invariably occurs as a result of the chronic extrahepatic biliary obstruction, and may progress to the development of secondary biliary cirrhosis and portal hypertension.

### Etiology

The cause of this unusual disorder is unknown. Bacterial, viral, and autoimmune etiologies have been proposed, but there is no objective evidence to support any of these factors. Cultures of the bile and biliary tissue are often sterile. The condition has been found in association with a number of other diseases, including chronic ulcerative colitis, Riedel's struma, scleroderma, regional enteritis, thrombocytopenic purpura, orbital pseudotumor, and fibrous retroperitonitis and mediastinitis. Of these, chronic ulcerative colitis is by far the most common associated disorder, and involvement of the intrahepatic bile ducts as well as the extrahepatic biliary system in these cases is not uncommon. Several authors have proposed that the term primary sclerosing cholangitis be reserved for cases in which there are no associated diseases, and that all other cases be classified as "secondary sclerosing cholangitis." A number of patients originally thought to have primary sclerosing colangitis have proved on follow-up to have sclerosing bile duct carcinoma, and this neoplasm must always be considered in the differential diagnosis. As experience with primary sclerosing cholangitis has increased, the following criteria have been established for the diagnosis: (1) absence of gallstones; (2) absence of previous biliary surgery; (3) absence of biliary tract malignant disease on long-term follow-up; (4) absence of primary biliary cirrhosis on biopsy; (5) absence of associated diseases such as ulcerative colitis or retroperitoneal fibrosis; (6) generalized thickening and stenosis of the extrahepatic bile ducts; and (7) progressive obstructive jaundice. With application of these criteria, fewer than 50 cases have been reported in the literature.

### Diagnosis

The clinical manifestations of primary sclerosing cholangitis are variable, but obstructive jaundice is the key feature of the picture. The jaundice may be intermittent initially, but ultimately it becomes continuous and progressive and may be accompanied by pruritus. Intermittent low-grade fever, chills, malaise, weakness, weight loss, nausea and vomiting, and dull abdominal pain in the right upper quadrant and epigastrium are frequent symptoms. The liver is often palpable and tender on physical examination, and the usual stigmata of portal hypertension may be present. Liver function studies show hyperbilirubinemia, with a preponderance of the direct-reacting pigment, and an elevation of the serum alkaline phosphatase. Other abnormalities of liver function are variable, depending on the stage of the disease. Oral and intravenous cholangiography are seldom possible because of the jaundice, and attempts at percutaneous transhepatic cholangiography usually fail because the lumen of the bile ducts is so tiny. Transjugular cholangiography may be informative, although no cases in which this technique was used have been reported. Operative cholangiograms are characteristic and show a common bile duct irregularly narrowed to threadlike size, with beading of the intrahepatic ducts and a "pruned-tree" appearance. The diagnosis can be made only by surgical exploration of the biliary tract.

### Treatment

Prolonged T tube drainage of the common bile duct and long-term adrenal steroid therapy are the essential elements of treatment. Forceful dilatation of the common duct may be required for insertion of the T tube. Although beneficial effects of biliary decompression have been documented, the mechanism by which this procedure influences the disease is not clear. The T tube should be left in place until cholangiograms show satisfactory dilatation of the biliary tree and free flow of dye into the duodenum. The undiseased gallbladder should not be removed at the time of the initial exploration because, in cases in which the disease is confined to the common bile duct, it may be used at a later time for biliary decompression via a cholecystoduodenostomy. Biopsies of the liver and bile ducts should always be obtained at the time of operation. Antibiotic therapy is indicated when positive cultures of bile are obtained, and attempts to decrease the viscosity of bile by the administration of bile salt cholegogues may have some limited value. On the presumption that the disease has an autoimmune etiology, treatment with the immunosuppressive agent azathioprine has been attempted, but experience is insufficient to judge the merits of such therapy. In the secondary form of the disease associated with chronic ulcerative colitis, total colectomy may be of benefit.

The mortality rate of primary sclerosing cholangitis is uncertain. Until the past decade, almost all of the patients died, usually of liver damage or the complications of portal hypertension. However, with proper therapy, a number of patients have recovered and remained asymptomatic for prolonged periods of time. The specter of bile duct carcinoma dictates a guarded prognosis at least for 5 years after the onset of symptoms.

## STENOSIS OF THE SPHINCTER OF ODDI AND STENOSING PAPILLITIS

Stenosis of the sphincter of Oddi, from spasm or fibrosis, and inflammatory stenosis of the papilla of Vater are conditions that may cause the clinical manifestations of common bile duct obstruction and pancreatitis. However, their clinical importance is uncertain and a matter of controversy.

The vast majority of cases are associated with calculi in the common bile duct or gallbladder and are believed to result from the inflammatory response to the choledocholithiasis and cholecystitis. A small number of primary cases without biliary calculi have been reported, and the etiology of these is unknown.

Stenosis of the sphincter or the papilla is believed to be responsible for some cases of persistence of symptoms following cholecystectomy, the *postcholecystectomy syndrome,* for some forms of recurrent pancreatitis, and for some cases of obstructive jaundice in the absence of choledocholithiasis or other demonstrable etiologic processes. The most frequent clinical manifestation is pain, usually in the form of attacks of biliary colic. Some patients have intermittent clinical or subclinical jaundice, with increased serum bilirubin and alkaline phosphatase, and attacks of pancreatitis with elevations of serum amylase and lipase. Cholangiographic demonstration of dilatation of the common bile duct above 1.5 cm., unusual narrowing of the terminal portion of the duct, and delay in emptying of the contrast medium into the duodenum are helpful in making the diagnosis preoperatively.

Operations for stenosis of the sphincter or the papilla in the absence of gallstones should be undertaken only after other causes of the symptoms have been excluded by a thorough diagnostic investigation. At operation, the stenosis should be demonstrated by inability to pass a 3 mm. probe into the duodenum through a choledochotomy, by operative cholangiography, or by radiomanometry. The latter technique involves pressure and flow measurements in the common bile duct and is used frequently in Europe but not in the United States. The operation of choice is transduodenal sphincteroplasty in which part of the sphincter of Oddi is excised. Some surgeons have reported comparable benefits from choledochoduodenostomy. In all initial explorations of the common bile duct during operations for calculus disease, calibration of the sphincter of Oddi with a probe or dilator is an integral part of the surgical procedure. A number of surgeons have advocated the performance of a sphincteroplasty whenever evidence of terminal duct stenosis is obtained during a routine exploration. However, the added potential morbidity and mortality of this procedure must be weighed against its potential benefits in routine initial choledochotomies.

## BILIARY FISTULAS AND GALLSTONE ILEUS

Internal biliary fistulas may result from external trauma, operative injuries, penetration of duodenal ulcers, invasion of cancers from adjacent viscera, infections in the liver and right upper quadrant of the abdomen, and unsuccessful reconstructive or bypass operations in the bile ducts. However, the vast majority of fistulas arise spontaneously in patients with advanced calculous cholecystitis, and result from adherence of the inflamed gallbladder or common bile duct to an adjacent viscus and erosion of a gallstone into the adherent organ. Gallstones have been known to erode into every major segment of the gastrointestinal tract, as well as into the liver, kidney, urinary bladder, uterus, vagina, portal vein, inferior vena cava, pleural cavity, pericardial sac, and bronchus. Three-fourths of the spontaneous fistulas are between the gallbladder and duodenum. Next in declining frequency are abnormal communications between the gallbladder and common bile duct, the gallbladder and colon, and the common duct and duodenum. The symptoms of biliary fistulas are those of the underlying calculous cholecystitis to which are often added episodes of biliary infection. Choledocholithiasis is found in a high percentage of cases. In addition to the usual signs of cholecystitis in diagnostic studies, gas in the biliary tree and reflux of contrast medium into the bile ducts or gallbladder are often seen on x-rays following a barium meal or barium enema. The treatment of biliary fistulas consists of operative separation and repair of the adherent viscus and the usual surgical treatment of the biliary disease. Because of the frequency of choledocholithiasis, common bile duct exploration is often necessary.

Most gallstones that enter the gastrointestinal tract are either passed in the stool or vomited, but in 10 to 15 per cent of spontaneous internal biliary fistulas, a gallstone obstructs the intestinal tract to produce the condition known as gallstone ileus. This disorder accounts for 1 to 3 per cent of all cases of intestinal obstruction, and for about 20 per cent of nonstrangulating intestinal obstructions in patients over the age of 65. The obstructing gallstone is usually larger than 2.5 cm. in diameter, and a stone as large as 17.5 cm. in greatest diameter has been recovered from a patient with gallstone ileus. It is likely that some of the stones enlarge while in the intestine. In a collective review, the site of the obstruction was found to be in the terminal ileum in 59 per cent, in the mid-ileum in 24 per cent, in the jejunum in 9 per cent, and in the duodenum, colon, and rectum in the remaining 8 per cent of the cases.

### Diagnosis of Gallstone Ileus

The diagnosis of gallstone intestinal obstruction is being made with increasing frequency as physicians are becoming more aware of this condition. Typically, gallstone ileus occurs in elderly women with advanced calculous cholecystitis who present with the usual picture of simple mechanical intestinal obstruction, i.e., cramping abdominal pain, vomiting, obstipation, distention, and obstructive peristalsis. The presenting symptoms infrequently reflect an acute inflammatory episode coincident with the formation of the fistula, although a history consistent with biliary disease can be obtained from many of the patients. Frequently, the patient gives a recent past history suggestive of repeated episodes of intermittent intestinal obstruction associated with passage of

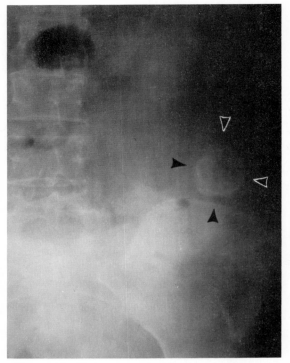

**Figure 21**  Plain x-ray of abdomen of patient with intestinal obstruction due to gallstone ileus, showing calculus in an ectopic location.

the gallstone down the intestinal tract. This phenomenon, called "tumbling" obstruction, is highly suggestive of gallstone ileus. Clinical jaundice from stones in the common bile duct is seen in 10 to 20 per cent of the patients.

Abdominal x-rays are the key to the diagnosis. In addition to the usual picture of mechanical intestinal obstruction, gas in the biliary tree can be seen in a high percentage of cases. This diagnostic roentgenographic sign is overlooked too often. In some cases, the obstructing gallstone in an ectopic location can be identified (Fig. 21). Contrast x-rays often demonstrate the fistula, but they are rarely indicated in the presence of intestinal obstruction.

### Treatment of Gallstone Ileus

The treatment of gallstone ileus is surgical correction of the intestinal obstruction after preparation of the patient with parenteral fluid therapy and nasointestinal intubation. The obstructing stone is removed through an enterotomy. Careful palpation of the entire intestinal tract, with removal of any other stones that are found, is an essential part of the operation. Recurrence of gallstone ileus due to overlooked calculi in the intestine has been reported in 5 to 10 per cent of the cases.

Treatment of the biliary disease and the biliary-enteric fistula depends on the condition of the patient. The gallbladder is usually involved in an inflammatory mass with the attached intestine. If the patient is in good condition, division of the fistula, cholecystectomy, and, if indicated, exploration of the common bile duct may be done at the initial operation. However, if the patient is in poor condition, as is frequently the case, treatment of the underlying disease is best reserved for a second operation.

Spontaneous closure of a biliary fistula sometimes occurs after the gallbladder empties its contents into the intestine, particularly if there is no obstruction in the common bile duct. However, if the biliary disease is not treated, the majority of patients have significant symptoms, and serious complications such as obstructive jaundice, cholangitis, and carcinoma of the gallbladder develop in many. Therefore, subsequent elective surgical treatment of the biliary disease is generally recommended. Needless to say, the general condition of the patient will influence the decision regarding a second operation.

Until recently, gallstone ileus was associated with a high mortality rate because of the advanced age and poor condition of many of the patients and because of frequent delays in diagnosis and treatment. In the past decade, the mortality rate has been reduced to 10 to 15 per cent.

## HYPERPLASTIC CHOLECYSTOSES

The hyperplastic cholecystoses are a group of benign, degenerative lesions in which there is excessive proliferation of gallbladder tissue. Unlike true papillomas of the gallbladder, they are not neoplasms. According to Jutras et al., included among these uncommon conditions are cholesterolosis, adenomyomatosis, neuromatosis, lipomatosis, fibromatosis, and hyalinocalcinosis (calcified gallbladder). In cholecystograms, they often appear as filling defects in an otherwise normal gallbladder. Most of these lesions are discovered at operations or in roentgenograms in patients who do not have symptoms of biliary disease. However, occasionally they are associated with symptoms similar to those of chronic calculous cholecystitis. Cholecystectomy is recommended only for patients with well documented symptoms that cannot be accounted for by other diseases after a thorough investigation. Relief of symptoms following removal of the gallbladder has been reported.

## ACALCULOUS CHOLECYSTITIS

In approximately 5 per cent of cases of acute and chronic cholecystitis, no calculi are demonstrable in the biliary system. Some of these cases are attributable to specific causes such as bacterial infections, congenital anomalies, pancreatitis, obstruction of the cystic duct by neoplasm, fibrosis, or kinking, thrombosis of the blood supply to the gallbladder, and stenosis of the sphincter of Oddi or papilla of Vater. However, in a substantial number of cases, the etiology is unclear. The clinical manifestations are identical to those of acute or chronic calculous cholecystitis, and it is not until operation that the absence of gallstones is dis-

covered. Cholecystectomy is followed by relief of symptoms in only two-thirds to three-fourths of the cases. While excision of a grossly diseased gallbladder is indicated whether or not calculi are demonstrated, removal of a normal-appearing gallbladder is unwarranted even though the operation was undertaken because of definite symptoms.

## SYMPTOMS AFTER CHOLECYSTECTOMY

Ninety to ninety-five per cent of patients subjected to cholecystectomy for chronic cholecystitis are relieved of symptoms. However, in a small number of patients, symptoms continue or new complaints develop after operation. The causes of these disturbances are several, and they have been lumped together under the term "postcholecystectomy syndrome." The conditions responsible for symptoms after cholecystectomy may be categorized as follows:

1. *Diseases of other systems.* Included in this category are functional disorders and conditions such as peptic ulcer, pancreatitis, hiatus hernia, and coronary insufficiency. The discovery of these diseases does not necessarily indicate an error in initial diagnosis, although this is often the case. This group represents the most frequent cause of the postcholecystectomy syndrome.

2. *Organic biliary tract disease.* This category includes overlooked cholelithiasis, a large cystic duct stump in which calculi may develop, stenosis of the sphincter of Oddi, and injuries to the biliary ducts. These disorders require surgical correction.

3. *Biliary dyskinesia.* This is presumed to be a functional disorder of the bile ducts that causes abnormal elevations of pressure and disturbances of bile flow in the biliary system. The existence of this condition as a demonstrable clinical entity has been questioned.

A significant reduction in the incidence of symptoms after cholecystectomy will occur if every patient is evaluated thoroughly before biliary surgery is undertaken.

## INJURIES TO THE EXTRAHEPATIC BILIARY SYSTEM

### EXTERNAL TRAUMA

Because of the protected location of the extrahepatic biliary system, injuries to the gallbladder and bile ducts from external trauma are uncommon. Moreover, biliary wounds are usually associated with injuries to adjacent viscera, particularly the liver, colon, small intestine, and pancreas, and the symptoms and signs of the associated organ damage frequently dominate the clinical picture. Perforating trauma due to gunshot wounds, stab wounds, and needle lacerations during liver biopsy and percutaneous cholangiography make up the bulk of biliary injuries. Wounds caused by blunt trauma are rare, and are usually the result of automobile accidents.

The clinical manifestations of biliary wounds are initially caused by leakage of bile and bleeding. Although bile in the peritoneal cavity of experimental animals has been found to cause a severe peritonitis and a high mortality rate, human bile is usually sterile and produces only a mild inflammatory reaction. However, if bile leakage continues for several days, large fluid losses, loculated collections, and secondary infection are common sequelae. Pain in the right upper abdomen, abdominal tenderness and rigidity, absence of bowel sounds, fever, and leukocytosis are the usual clinical findings. If the blood vessels to the biliary tract or liver are damaged, shock from bleeding may occur. A positive abdominal tap productive of bile or blood is often obtained. Since isolated biliary injuries are rare, the clinical manifestations are frequently those of associated wounds of the liver or intestinal tract.

The treatment of biliary tract injuries consists of prompt operation and surgical repair of the damage. In the case of gallbladder wounds, cholecystectomy is usually necessary. Wounds of the bile ducts are repaired by direct reconstruction when possible, or by a bypass anastomosis between the biliary system (bile duct or gallbladder) and intestine (duodenum or jejunum). Catheter drainage of the biliary tree is an essential adjunct. In cases involving common bile duct injury or retroperitoneal hematomas in the right upper quadrant of the abdomen, it is important to examine thoroughly the retroduodenal portion of the common duct by reflecting the duodenum medially by means of a Kocher maneuver. The mortality rate of biliary wounds is almost entirely related to associated injuries of other viscera.

## ACQUIRED STRICTURES DUE TO OPERATIVE INJURY

### Etiology

Almost all of the acquired strictures of the bile ducts are due to accidental injury during operations, and this condition is one of several very serious complications of biliary surgery. In the large experience of the Lahey Clinic with the treatment of 958 patients with bile duct strictures, 97 per cent of the strictures were due to surgical trauma. While a few cases were associated with gastroduodenal and pancreatic operations, 96 per cent of the injuries occurred during the course of operations on the biliary tract. In 3 per cent of the cases, the strictures were due to nonsurgical causes such as erosion by gallstones, inflammatory conditions, and blunt external trauma. The mechanism of surgical injury was identifiable in only one-third of the cases and consisted of recognized direct damage to the bile duct, ligation of the bile duct, massive bleeding managed by blind clamping of the blood vessels, and difficulties in dissection due to adhesions and inflammation. There is no doubt that almost all surgical injuries to the bile ducts can be avoided if the surgeon has a thorough knowledge of the frequent anatomic variations in the porta hepatis, performs a careful dissection of the hepatic artery, cystic artery, and junction of the cystic duct with the common hepatic duct, is familiar with the principles that govern the management of bleeding in the right upper quadrant, and is aware of the occasional necessity of identifying and intubating the common bile duct during difficult operations for penetrating duodenal ulcer.

As might be expected from the age and sex incidence of calculous cholecystitis, biliary strictures occur most commonly in middle-aged women. The site of the stricture is usually around the level of the junction between the cystic duct and common hepatic duct. In the Lahey Clinic series, 40 per cent of the strictures were confined to the common hepatic duct, 28 per cent involved both the common hepatic and common bile ducts, and 23 per cent occurred in the common bile duct alone. Fortunately, only 10 per cent of the injuries occurred at a level above the common hepatic duct.

### Diagnosis

When injuries to the bile ducts are recognized at the time of their occurrence during cholecystectomy, substantial morbidity and mortality can be prevented. Immediate repair by plastic reconstruction, end-to-end duct anastomosis, or biliary-intestinal anastomosis provides an excellent chance of normal biliary function. Unfortunately, the initial damage is frequently overlooked. The most common clinical manifestations of bile duct injury are the onset of obstructive jaundice within 48 hours after operation and the appearance of bile in sizable quantities from an external drain site or from the wound during the first postoperative week. These two telltale signs may be accompanied by fever and chills and light or clay-colored stools. Laboratory studies show hyperbilirubinemia, with substantial conjugated pigment, and an elevated serum alkaline phosphatase. If a drain is in place, x-rays following instillation of a contrast medium may demonstrate the fistula.

In some patients, the early manifestations abate, go unheeded, or do not occur. In such cases, the patient may present weeks, months, and occasionally years after operation with a history of intermittent jaundice and attacks of cholangitis consisting of fever, chills, clay-colored stools, and continuous dull pain in the right hypochondrium. Tender hepatomegaly and sometimes splenomegaly are found on examination, and laboratory studies show leukocytosis, hyperbilirubinemia, elevated serum alkaline phosphatase, and, depending on the timing in relation to infection, elevations of SGOT and SGPT. Prothrombin activity may be depressed. In time, liver damage may progress to biliary cirrhosis. Portal hypertension and hypersplenism develop in 15 to 20 per cent of patients because of liver disease resulting from continuing biliary obstruction and infection. Hepatic failure, bleeding from esophageal varices, and systemic infection are common complications.

In most cases, the diagnosis is clear-cut. However, in some instances, radiographic visualization of the bile duct stricture by transhepatic or transjugular cholangiography may be necessary for diagnosis.

### Treatment

Biliary strictures are fatal if uncorrected. Therefore, attempts at surgical correction are indicated, even if repeated operations are required. However, the greatest chances for success, other than those associated with immediate repair at the time of injury, are provided by the first reconstructive operation. It should be planned carefully and undertaken by a surgeon with experience in such procedures. The patient should be prepared for operation, if indicated, with antibiotics to control infection, parenteral nutritional therapy, and parenteral vitamin K. If the patient has portal hypertension and hypersplenism and has bled from esophageal varices, a splenorenal shunt should be performed prior to the biliary reconstruction. Dissection of the porta hepatis may be associated with significant bleeding in the presence of portal hypertension.

The most important determinants of the out-

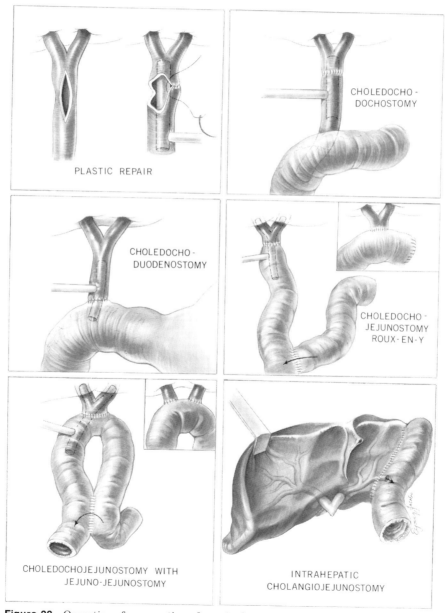

**Figure 22** Operations for correction of acquired traumatic strictures of the bile ducts.

come of biliary reconstruction are the site of the stricture and the condition of the proximal bile duct. Other factors that bear on the outcome are the amount of inflammation and scarring, the number of previous attempts at correction, and the extent of liver damage. An important initial step in operations for biliary strictures is identification of the proximal duct by needle aspiration and assessment of the biliary tree by operative cholangiography through a needle or a catheter inserted in the duct.

The operations used for correction of biliary strictures are illustrated in Figure 22. Plastic repair by vertical excision of the stricture and horizontal closure of the duct can be used in minor strictures of the common bile duct but is infrequently possible. End-to-end anastomosis of the bile duct after excision of the stricture is the procedure of choice, provided there is an adequate length of vascularized distal duct, and the anastomosis can be performed *without tension*. It is important to resist the temptation to perform a duct-to-duct anastomosis under any tension, since such repairs invariably fail. Anastomoses of the bile duct to the duodenum, a loop of jejunum combined with a jejunojejunostomy, or a defunctionalized segment of jejunum by the Roux-en-Y technique give comparable results. Again, it is important to avoid tension at the anastomosis, and this consideration sometimes limits the use of duodenum. The jejunal segment or loop should be at least 16 inches removed from the stream of intestinal contents to minimize reflux into the biliary tree, although substantial evidence indicates that such reflux is harmless in the absence of obstruction. Finally, resection of the left lobe of the liver and anastomosis of an intrahepatic bile duct to the jejunum may be attempted if no other procedure is feasible. Use of this procedure is predicated on the demonstration that the selected duct communicates freely with the ductal system in the right lobe of the liver, so that it is essential to obtain a cholangiogram through the duct to be used for the anastomosis before proceeding with the definitive operation. The success of intrahepatic cholangiojejunostomy has been limited.

There is controversy regarding the use of rubber stents across the anastomosis, and no controlled studies of this matter have been done. At one time, internal stents were regularly inserted and allowed to pass spontaneously or were removed at a second operation, but these are rarely used today. At present, it is general practice to insert a T tube or Y tube stent that exits to the outside and can be easily removed at a later time. The external limb of the stent must always be brought out through a site at a distance from the biliary anastomosis (proximal or distal bile duct, or intestine), since bringing it out through the anastomosis results in a high incidence of recurrence of stricture. Many surgeons leave the stent in place for months and even years. However, when these long-indwelling tubes are removed, they are invariably plugged and covered with biliary sludge and debris; this finding suggests that they have stimulated a reaction within the duct and have been an impediment to biliary drainage. Experimental evidence indicates that a rubber tube in the common bile duct stimulates a foreign body inflammation that increases with time. There is reason to doubt that a stent will prevent formation of scar tissue, and it is possible that the foreign body may increase fibrosis. Cole et al. reported 29 successful operations without the use of internal drainage. It is our practice to use rubber stents in biliary reconstructions, but to remove them after obtaining a cholangiogram within a few weeks of operation.

Some results of reconstructive operations for biliary stricture are shown in Table 1. An operative mortality rate of 5 to 10 per cent and an overall mortality rate of 15 to 20 per cent have been observed in patients treated by experienced surgeons. With long-term follow-up it is likely that the mortality increases to 25 or 30 per cent. Hepatic failure, hemorrhage from esophageal varices or during operation, and infection are the most frequent causes of death. Operations for biliary stricture are associated with significant morbidity in about one-fourth of the cases. Common complications include wound infections, intraperitoneal abscesses, biliary fistula, a variety of bleeding problems, and various degrees of hepatic insufficiency.

Two-thirds to three-fourths of patients are cured of their biliary stricture by present surgical techniques. The severity of pre-existing liver damage influences the overall results and provides an impetus for early diagnosis and prompt surgical treatment.

**TABLE 1** RESULTS OF OPERATIONS FOR ACQUIRED BILIARY STRICTURE

| Authors | No. Patients | No. Operations | Excellent | Results (%) Good | Poor | Died | Lost |
|---|---|---|---|---|---|---|---|
| Warren, Mountain, and Midell (1971) | 987 | 1553 | 52 | 26 | 4 | 13 | 4 |
| Waters, Nixon, and Hodgins (1959) | 191 survivors | 217 | 30 | 31 | 39 | ? | |
| Cole, Ireneus, and Reynolds (1955) | 122 | 188 | 76 | | 7 | 16 | |

# EXTRAHEPATIC BILIARY CARCINOMA

## CARCINOMA OF THE GALLBLADDER

Carcinoma of the gallbladder is not a common neoplasm. It makes up about 1 per cent of all cancers and 3 per cent of cancers of the digestive system. It has been estimated to develop in 1 to 2 per cent of patients with cholelithiasis. It occurs in women three or four times more commonly than in men, and its incidence increases with age. Three-fourths of the patients are over the age of 60. Histologically, 85 to 90 per cent of malignant lesions of the gallbladder are adenocarcinomas, and the remainder are mainly undifferentiated carcinomas and squamous cell cancers. Other malignant tumors are rare. The neoplasm spreads most often by direct extension to the liver, bile ducts, and adjacent viscera, by the lymphatics to the regional lymph nodes, and by intraperitoneal seeding. Metastases outside of the peritoneal cavity are infrequent.

From 80 to 90 per cent of patients with carcinoma of the gallbladder have gallstones. Although postulated, a cause-and-effect relationship between cholelithiasis and cancer has not been established. Attempts to demonstrate a specific carcinogenic effect of gallstones in experimental animals have not been successful. However, in hamsters with cholesterol pellets in the gallbladder a significant increase in gallbladder carcinoma occurred following oral administration of the carcinogen dimethylnitrosamine, and this finding led to the conclusion that the cholesterol "stone" produced nonspecific irritation of the gallbladder mucosa that enhanced the development of cancer. Although there are several valid reasons for advocating cholecystectomy in patients with silent gallstones, a significantly increased risk of gallbladder cancer is not one of them. Long-term studies of patients with asymptomatic calculi have shown an incidence of carcinoma below 1 per cent, and the overall incidence of gallbladder cancer in all patients with cholelithiasis is less than 2 per cent.

The early symptoms of carcinoma of the gallbladder are those of the associated calculous cholecystitis. During this stage, the cancer may be discovered incidentally in a gallbladder removed because of inflammation. Such circumstances provide the best chance of cure, although it is by no means very good. Later, the symptoms include persistent right upper quadrant pain, weight loss, anorexia, nausea, and vomiting. Obstructive jaundice due to invasion of the bile ducts occurs in 50 to 60 per cent of patients, and is accompanied by the usual laboratory findings. In about half the patients, a mass is palpable in the right subcostal area, and hepatomegaly is common. Serum alkaline phosphatase is elevated in many patients, including those without jaundice. Cholecystography in nonicteric patients almost always reveals nonvisualization of the gallbladder. Radioisotope liver scans often demonstrate hepatic defects, and he-

patic arteriograms may provide evidence of malignant disease in both the gallbladder and the liver.

The prognosis of carcinoma of the gallbladder is very poor. Of the few patients who are cured, most are those in whom the lesion is removed incidentally by a simple cholecystectomy for calculous cholecystitis. Even in this fortuitous situation, the cure rate is less than 5 per cent. In approximately three-fourths of the patients, surgical resection of the tumor is not possible because it has spread to adjacent vital organs or distantly. When the neoplasm is localized, radical cholecystectomy with excision of liver tissue surrounding the gallbladder bed and removal of regional lymph nodes has been advocated. Under unusual circumstances, right hepatic lobectomy has been performed. These radical cancer operations have been associated with a 15 to 20 per cent operative mortality rate and have only occasionally cured the disease. The overall 5 year survival rate of patients with carcinoma of the gallbladder is between 1 and 2 per cent. The mean survival time after discovery of gallbladder cancer is less than 6 months, and 80 per cent of the patients die within one year.

## CARCINOMA OF THE BILE DUCTS

Carcinoma of the extrahepatic bile ducts, like gallbladder cancer, is a highly lethal neoplasm, but it is about one-third as common. Less than 1 per cent of biliary operations are performed for this tumor. Carcinoma of the ampulla of Vater, or more accurately, the papilla of Vater, is believed to arise from the duodenal mucosa and is not included in the group of bile duct cancers. In contrast to gallbladder cancer, carcinoma of the bile ducts occurs more frequently in men than in women, the ratio being between 3 to 2 and 2 to 1. The peak incidence is in the sixth and seventh decades of life. Gallstones are found in about one-fourth to one-third of the cases, and are usually confined to the gallbladder.

Almost all of the bile duct tumors are adenocarcinomas. Approximately one-third of them develop in the distal common bile duct, one-third in the middle of the extrahepatic duct system, one-fourth around the junction of the hepatic ducts, and the remainder throughout the biliary tree. The tumor regularly extends submucosally up and down the bile ducts for a considerable distance, and so complete extirpation is usually difficult. In addition, it frequently invades the liver and adjacent viscera, spreads to the regional lymph nodes, and seeds elsewhere in the peritoneal cavity. At the time of operation, more than three-fourths of the lesions have been found on gross examination to have extended beyond the bile duct.

The clinical manifestations of bile duct carcinoma are jaundice, aching pain in the right hypochondrium, weight loss, anorexia, and pruritus. The jaundice is usually relentless, but it sometimes fluctuates, and in some patients it does not occur. In a few patients cholangitis with fever and chills develops. On physical examination, in addition to jaundice, most patients have hepatomegaly and about one-third have a palpable gallbladder. The serum alkaline phosphatase is elevated in almost all patients, even in the absence of hyper-bilirubinemia. Barium contrast upper gastrointestinal x-rays show distortion of the duodenum in a substantial number of patients. Transjugular or transhepatic cholangiography demonstrates the obstructing lesion but is usually unnecessary.

The prognosis of bile duct carcinoma is among the poorest of all cancers. A 3 year survival rate of 4 per cent has been reported for 173 patients treated at the Lahey Clinics, and a 5 year survival rate of 1.6 per cent has been observed in 78 patients treated at the Mayo Clinic. More than 80 per cent of the patients have died within 1 year of the discovery of the disease, and the mean survival time generally has been less than 6 months. With rare exceptions, only those lesions occurring in the distal common bile duct have been amenable to radical resection with hope of cure. Such tumors have been treated by pancreaticoduodenectomy (Whipple operation). Of 27 patients so treated at the Lahey Clinic, 22 per cent were alive and free of disease 4 years after operation. A large number of palliative operations have been employed in the treatment of bile duct carcinoma, but they have been associated with a high mortality rate and only limited success. It is doubtful that extensive efforts to obtain biliary diversion are often worthwhile.

An uncommon and unique bile duct cancer that has received recent attention is the *sclerosing carcinoma* of the intrahepatic hilar bile ducts. This well differentiated adenocarcinoma usually develops in the major hepatic ducts at their junction, and presents a problem in differential diagnosis from sclerosing cholangitis. It often has an insidious onset and runs a slow course characterized by obstructive jaundice, weight loss, and intermittent episodes of fever due to sepsis. Death is often due to hepatic failure or infection. At operation, the bile ducts are markedly thickened and their lumen is greatly narrowed. Treatment consists of forceful dilatation and T tube external drainage of the involved ducts or, when possible, a proximal biliary-intestinal anastomosis such as an intrahepatic cholangiojejunostomy. Survival for several years following palliative decompression has been observed. However, cure of this neoplasm has not been reported to date.

# CONGENITAL ANOMALIES OF THE BILE DUCTS

## CHOLEDOCHAL CYST

Cystic dilatation of the common bile duct is an uncommon congenital lesion that may produce symptoms in infancy but more often is discovered at some time during the first two decades of life. More than 500 cases have been reported in the literature, 83 per cent of which have been diagnosed in patients below the age of 30. Female patients have outnumbered males 3 or 4 to 1. The lesion is usually characterized by a well circumscribed dilatation of the common duct. The terminal bile duct distal to the lesion may be narrowed or, rarely, obliterated, but the intrahepatic biliary tree is usually normal. The etiology of the condition is unknown, although many theories have been proposed. Among these is the theory that the cyst is a congenital malformation that results from an abnormality of epithelial cell pro-

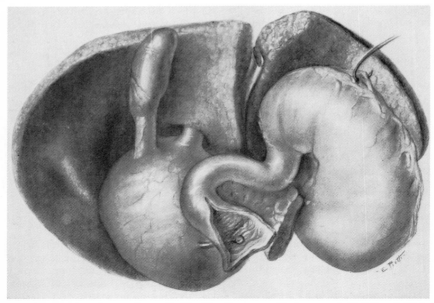

**Figure 23**  Choledochal cyst. (From Gross, R. E.: The Surgery of Infancy and Childhood. Philadelphia, W. B. Saunders Company, 1953.)

liferation during development of the bile ducts, and the proposal that the cyst results from the combination of a congenital weakness in the bile duct wall and distal duct obstruction.

### Pathology

Choledochal cysts have been classified into three anatomic categories. Type I is an aneurysmal dilatation of the common bile duct, and it is by far the most frequent form (Fig. 23). Type II is a diverticulum that arises laterally from the wall of the common bile duct. Only 13 cases of this type have been reported. Type III, of which only nine cases have been reported, arises in the terminal intra-duodenal portion of the common bile duct, involves the entrance of the pancreatic duct, and is lined by duodenal mucosa inside and out. It has been called a choledochocele, and it may represent an entero-genous cyst rather than a true choledochal cyst. To these three types, Longmire et al. have added a rare fourth type in which the common and hepatic ducts have multiple diverticula. This condition has been called polycystic formation or diverticulosis of the bile ducts.

Choledochal cysts have been found to vary in size from 3 to 25 cm. in diameter. The cyst wall is composed of fibrous tissue with interspersed elastic and smooth muscle fibers. The internal lining consists of columnar epithelium, but it is often destroyed by inflammation and the pressure of the distending fluid. Surprisingly, gallstones are only occasionally found in the biliary system or in the cyst. Carcinoma in the cyst or the adjacent bile ducts has been reported in 14 cases, an unusually high incidence.

### Diagnosis

The clinical manifestations of choledochal cyst are often intermittent and are due to filling of the cyst with fluid and resultant compression of the biliary tree. A triad of abdominal pain, jaundice, and a palpable abdominal mass in the right hypo-chondrium has been classically associated with this condition. The pain in the right hypochon-drium is usually colicky and most severe during episodes of jaundice, but it may be dull and con-stant. Jaundice with dark urine and light stools is characteristically intermittent, but, particularly in infants, it may be continuous and raise the possibility of biliary atresia. Laboratory studies confirm the obstructive nature of the jaundice. The abdominal mass is typically cystic and nontender on palpation. In at least one-third of the patients, all of the elements of the clinical triad are not present. Additional symptoms in some cases in-clude fever and chills (cholangitis), nausea, vomit-ing, and anorexia. If untreated, choledochal cyst produces liver damage, which progresses to biliary cirrhosis and portal hypertension with all of its sequelae. In some instances, the portal hyperten-sion results from compression of the portal vein by the cyst. Rupture of the cyst with bile peritonitis has been reported a number of times.

In addition to the usual laboratory tests used in the diagnosis of jaundice, barium contrast upper gastrointestinal x-rays and hypotonic duodenog-raphy may be of value in showing displacement and distortion of the duodenum. Intravenous chol-angiography in the patient without jaundice, and percutaneous transhepatic or transjugular chol-angiography may demonstrate the cystic dilata-tion of the common bile duct. Ultrasonic scanning has been successful in demonstrating the abdomi-nal mass in several instances. In all cases, the precise relationship of the cyst to the biliary tree should be demonstrated by cholangiography at operation.

### Treatment

Once a choledochal cyst has produced symptoms, it is almost invariably fatal unless it is treated surgically. Treatment of the rare type II diverticu-lum consists of simple excision, while the rare type III choledochocele is treated by transduo-denal excision of the cyst wall so as to create a wide opening into the duodenum. The common type I fusiform cyst is currently treated either by excision combined with a biliary-intestinal anas-tomosis or by anastomosis of the cyst to the in-testinal tract. Excision of the cyst may be difficult and has seldom been practiced in the United States, although it is popular in Japan. Anastomo-sis of the cyst to the intestinal tract may take the form of cystoduodenostomy, cystojejunostomy using a loop of intestine, and cystojejunostomy by the Roux-en-Y technique. The Roux-en-Y anas-tomosis has been associated with somewhat better results than the other two techniques, and there would appear to be some advantage in avoiding reflux of intestinal contents into the cyst by using a defunctionalized limb of intestine. Incidental cholecystectomy should be performed because of the significant postoperative incidence of chole-cystitis and gallstones. The current mortality rate of choledochal cyst treated by surgical decompres-sion is 5 to 10 per cent. The long-term results of operative therapy are quite good, although second-ary operations to correct stenosis at the biliary-intestinal anastomosis are sometimes necessary.

## ATRESIA OF THE BILE DUCTS

During early embryonic life the gallbladder and bile ducts are represented by solid cords. Failure of the cords to canalize leads to atresia of part or all of the biliary system. In the majority of instances, the atresia involves the extrahepatic ducts or the intrahepatic ducts and is not amenable to surgical therapy. However, in 10 to 15 per cent of the patients, only the distal common bile duct is atretic and correction may be accomplished by connecting the gallbladder or proximal common bile duct to the duodenum or jejunum. Some types of biliary atresia are shown in Figure 24. Other variations have been observed.

### Diagnosis

The onset of jaundice in patients with biliary atresia is classically described as occurring during the middle or end of the first week of life, because

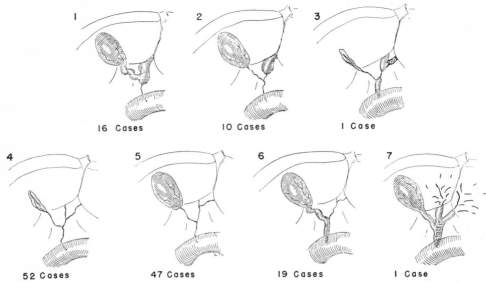

**Figure 24**  Types of biliary atresia encountered by Gross in 146 patients. The conditions in the upper row are surgically correctable; those in the lower row are inoperable. (From Gross, R. E.: The Surgery of Infancy and Childhood. Philadelphia, W. B. Saunders Company, 1953.)

of clearing of bilirubin in utero across the mother's placenta. However, a significant number of patients are observed to have jaundice at birth, and some patients have been described who did not become icteric until several weeks after birth. The influence of observer error in determining the time of onset of jaundice is difficult to assess. Onset of jaundice after the first month of life is rarely due to biliary atresia. The jaundice is progressive, although there are often small fluctuations, until a high plateau is reached after several weeks. Dark urine and light or clay-colored stools accompany the icterus. Small amounts of pigment may appear in the feces from time to time as a result of desquamation of intestinal epithelial cells and secretion of intestinal mucus stained with bilirubin. During the first month after birth, the infant usually grows normally, has a good appetite, and is alert and active. Subsequently, anorexia develops and the baby becomes irritable. As the disease progresses, the abdomen enlarges owing to hepatomegaly and often splenomegaly and ascites. Ultimately, biliary cirrhosis and portal hypertension develop, with all of the usual manifestations of these conditions. Death is usually due to liver failure, malnutrition, or bleeding from esophageal varices or a coagulopathy. Associated congenital anomalies, particularly of the cardiovascular system, occur in 15 to 30 per cent of cases.

Laboratory studies show a high serum bilirubin with substantial quantities of conjugated pigment, bilirubin in the urine, absence of urobilinogen in the urine and stool, elevated serum alkaline phosphatase, depressed prothrombin, and variable abnormalities of hepatic enzyme and turbidity tests. Rising or sustained high levels of serum bilirubin with a significant direct-reacting fraction on weekly determinations over a period of several weeks are helpful in making the diagnosis early in the course of the disease.

The diagnosis of biliary atresia may be very difficult. The differential diagnosis of neonatal jaundice includes the neonatal hepatitis syndrome, choledochal cyst, inspissated bile syndrome (the existence of which, as a discrete entity, is now doubtful), physiologic jaundice of the newborn or of prematurity, sepsis, hemolytic diseases, galactosemia, cytomegalic inclusion disease, syphilis, the Crigler-Najjar syndrome, and toxoplasmosis. Most of these conditions can be ruled out by appropriate laboratory studies and observations of the course of the disease over a brief period of time. However, differentiation of biliary atresia from the neonatal hepatitis syndrome presents a major problem and may not be possible. The time of onset, progression of jaundice, obstructive pattern, and results of laboratory studies may be identical in the two conditions. The incidence of neonatal hepatitis is similar to that of biliary atresia. On liver biopsy, both conditions may show giant cell transformation of the parenchymal cells, disorganization of the hepatic architecture, bile duct proliferation, and bile stasis, and there is substantial overlapping of the microscopic findings in the two diseases. In a study of diagnostic accuracy, Hays and his associates observed that the differentiation of biliary atresia and the neonatal hepatitis syndrome was erroneous or indeterminate in 40 per cent of needle liver biopsies, 38 per cent of open liver biopsies, and 20 per cent of operative cholangiograms. Herein lies the dilemma in the management of biliary atresia.

## Treatment

Biliary atresia is invariably fatal if not relieved by surgery. Survival ranges from 3 to 90 months, with a mean of 19 months. The majority of patients die within 2 years of birth. Approximately 10 to 15 per cent of the patients have potentially correctable anomalies, and 5 to 6 per cent have been actually cured by surgical therapy. It is essential that all patients with biliary atresia undergo laparotomy for determination of the feasibility of surgical correction and for appropriate treatment. However, because of the difficulties in preoperative diagnosis and the hazards of operation in jaundiced infants who do not have biliary atresia, there is considerable controversy about the timing of exploratory laparotomy. Many clinicians advocate operation during the first month of life on the basis that delay causes irreparable liver damage that may be fatal even if the obstruction is relieved. Others argue that waiting for 2 or 3 months will help to sort out the patients whose jaundice is due to conditions other than biliary atresia, and who may recover spontaneously unless they are subjected to the trauma of operation. It is important to point out that operations in patients with the neonatal hepatitis syndrome not only are risky because of the general adverse effects of trauma in the presence of liver disease, but also are associated with the hazard of damaging the tiny biliary tree during the exploratory dissection of the porta hepatis. It would seem that delaying operation until approximately 3 months of age has merit.

The operative approach initially is directed at making the diagnosis. A liver biopsy with frozen section examination is obtained for histologic information which may be of value. If the gallbladder can be identified, it is aspirated to determine the presence of bilirubin-stained bile as an indicator of intact cystic and hepatic ducts. Operative cholangiography, if necessary with occlusion of the hepatoduodenal ligament to direct dye into the intrahepatic bile ducts, is then performed via the gallbladder. If the cholangiogram shows an intact biliary tree, the diagnosis is not biliary atresia and nothing further is done. If the cholangiogram demonstrates a correctable anomaly, or nonvisualization of the bile ducts, or if no gallbladder can be identified, an extremely careful and meticulous dissection of the hepatoduodenal ligament and porta hepatis is undertaken in the hope of finding an intact proximal ductal system. Cholangiography via intact-appearing ducts may be helpful in assessing the situation. Anastomosis of the gallbladder or proximal common bile or hepatic duct to the duodenum or jejunum by the loop or Roux-en-Y technique is performed in the fortunate circumstance of finding a reparable lesion. Although a variety of palliative operations have been attempted in patients with uncorrectable anomalies, none of these have influenced longevity and they do not appear worthwhile. Moreover, an occasional patient believed to have irreparable biliary atresia has recovered spontaneously following laparotomy, undoubtedly because of an error in diagnosis such as that which might be associated with the rare hypoplasia (rather than atresia) of the biliary system.

Transplantation of the liver is currently the most promising new therapeutic modality in the treatment of biliary atresia. Several patients are now living and well between 2 and 3 years after orthotopic liver transplantation for otherwise fatal atresia of the bile ducts.

## REFERENCES

### General

1. Glenn, F.: Atlas of Biliary Tract Surgery. New York, Macmillan Company, 1963.
2. Hess, W.: Surgery of the Biliary Passages and the Pancreas. Princeton, N.J., D. Van Nostrand Company, 1965.
3. Smith, R., and Sherlock, S.: Surgery of the Gallbladder and Bile Ducts. London, Butterworth & Company, 1964.

### Anatomy

4. Boyden, E. A.: The anatomy of the choledochoduodenal junction in man. Surg. Gynec. Obstet., 104:641, 1957.
5. Daseler, E. H., Anson, B. J., Hambley, W. C., and Reimann, A. F.: Cystic artery and constituents of the hepatic pedicle. Surg. Gynec. & Obstet., 85:47, 1947.
6. Flanney, M. G., and Caster, M. P.: Congenital anomalies of the gallbladder. Surg. Gynec. Obstet., 103:439, 1956.
7. Kune, G. A.: The influence of structure and function in the surgery of the biliary tract. Ann. Roy. Coll. Surg., 47:78, 1970.
8. Michels, N. A.: Blood Supply and Anatomy of the Upper Abdominal Organs. Philadelphia, J. B. Lippincott Company, 1955.

### Physiology

9. Ivy, A. C., and Goldman, L.: Physiology of biliary tract. J.A.M.A., 113:2413, 1939.
10. Johnson, L. R., and Grossman, M. I.: Intestinal hormones as inhibitors of gastric secretion. Gastroenterology, 60:120, 1971.
11. Jorpes, J. E.: The isolation and chemistry of secretin and cholecystokinin. Gastroenterology, 55:157, 1968.

### Roentgenographic Studies in Diagnosis

12. Baker, H. L., Jr., and Hodgson, J. R.: Further studies on the accuracy of oral cholecystography. Radiology, 74:239, 1960.
13. Eaton, S. B., Benedict, K. T., Jr., Ferrucci, J. T., Jr., and Fleischli, D. J.: Hypotonic duodenography. Radiol. Clin. N. Amer., 8:125, 1970.
14. Kittredge, R. D., and Finby, M.: Percutaneous transhepatic cholangiography. Amer. J. Roentgen., 101:592, 1967.
15. Seldinger, S. I.: Percutaneous transhepatic cholangiography. Acta Radiol., Supp. 253, 1966.
16. Shehadi, W. H.: Clinical Radiology of the Biliary Tract. New York, McGraw-Hill Book Company, 1963.
17. Weiner, M., and Hanafee, W. N.: A review of transjugular cholangiography. Radiol. Clin. N. Amer., 8:53, 1970.

### Gallstones

18. Admirand, W. H., and Small, D. M.: The physicochemical basis of cholesterol gallstone formation in man. J. Clin. Invest., 47:1043, 1967.
19. Bouchier, I. A. D., and Freston, J. W.: The aetiology of gallstones. Lancet, 1:340, 1968.
20. Dam, H.: Determinants of cholesterol cholelithiasis in man and animals. Amer. J. Med., 51:596, 1971.
21. Danzinger, R. G., Hofmann, A. F., Schoenfield, L. J., and Thistle, J. L.: Dissolution of cholesterol gallstones by chenodeoxycholic acid. New Eng. J. Med., 286:1, 1972.
22. Isselbacher, K. J.: A medical treatment for gallstones? New Eng. J. Med., 286:40, 1972.
23. Juniper, K.: Physicochemical characteristics of bile and their relation to gallstone formation. Amer. J. Med., 39:98, 1965.

24. Juniper, K.: Cause of gallstone disease. Mod. Treatm., *5*:480, 1968.

25. Rains, A. J. H.: Gallstones: Causes and Treatment. Springfield, Ill., Charles C Thomas, 1964.

26. Sampliner, R., and Bennett, P. H.: Gallbladder disease in Pima Indians demonstrative of high prevalence and early onset by cholecystography. New Eng. J. Med., *283*:1358, 1970.

27. Small, D. M.: Gallstones. New Eng. J. Med., *279*:588, 1968.

28. Small, D. M.: The formation of gallstones. Advances Intern. Med., *16*:243, 1970.

29. Vlahcevic, Z. R., Bell, C. C., Jr., Buhac, I., Farrar, J. T., and Swell, L.: Diminished bile acid pool size in patients with gallstones. Gastroenterology, *59*:165, 1970.

**Chronic Cholecystitis**

30. Colcock, B. P., Killen, R. B., and Leach, N. G.: The asymptomatic patient with gallstones. Amer. J. Surg., *113*: 44, 1967.

31. Colcock, B. P., and Perez, B.: The treatment of cholelithiasis. Surg. Gynec. Obstet., *117*:529, 1963.

32. Comfort, M. W., Gray, H. K., and Wilson, J. M.: The silent gallstone: A ten to twenty year follow-up study of 112 cases. Ann. Surg., *128*:931, 1948.

33. Lund, J.: Surgical indications in cholelithiasis: Prophylactic cholecystectomy elucidated on the basis of long-term follow-up on 526 nonoperated cases. Ann. Surg., *151*: 153, 1960.

34. McSherry, C. K., and Glenn, F.: Surgical aspects of biliary tract disease. Amer. J. Med., *51*:651, 1971.

35. Method, H. L., Mehn, W. H., and Frable, W. J.: "Silent" gallstones. Arch. Surg., 85:338, 1962.

36. Ravdin, I. S., Fitz-Hugh, T., Jr., Wolferth, C. C., Barbieri, E. A., and Ravdin, R. G.: Relation of gallstone disease to angina pectoris. Arch. Surg., 70:333, 1955.

37. Wenckert, A., and Robertson, B.: The natural course of gallstone disease. Eleven year review of 781 nonoperated cases. Gastroenterology, 50:376, 1966.

**Acute Cholecystitis**

38. Bartlett, M. K., Quinbey, W. C., and Donaldson, G. A.: Surgery of the biliary tract. II. Treatment of acute cholecystitis. New Eng. J. Med., *254*:200, 1956.

39. Becker, W. F., Powell, J. I., and Turner, R. J.: A clinical study of 1,060 patients with acute cholecystitis. Surg. Gynec. Obstet., *104*:491, 1957.

40. Branch, C. D., and Zollinger, R. M.: Acute cholecystitis: A study of conservative treatment. New Eng. J. Med., *214*:1173, 1936.

41. Glenn, F., and Thorbjarnarson, B.: The surgical treatment of acute cholecystitis. Surg. Gynec. Obstet., *116*:61, 1963.

42. Marshall, J. F., and Hartzog, D. C.: Acute emphysematous cholecystitis. Ann. Surg., *159*:1011, 1964.

43. Massie, J. R., Coxe, J. W., III, Parker, C., and Dietrick, R.: Gallbladder perforations in acute cholecystitis. Ann. Surg., *145*:825, 1957.

44. Pines, B., and Rabinovitch, J.: Perforation of the gallbladder in acute cholecystitis. Ann. Surg., *140*:170, 1959.

45. Rosoff, L., and Meyers, H.: Acute emphysematous cholecystitis. Amer. J. Surg., *111*:410, 1966.

46. Strohl, E. R., Diffenbaugh, W. G., Baker, J. H., and Cheema, M. H.: Gangrene and perforation of the gallbladder. Surg. Gynec. Obstet., *114*:1, 1962.

47. Welch, C. E.: Cholecystectomy for acute cholecystitis. Surgery, *49*:284, 1961.

**Choledocholithiasis**

48. Bartlett, M. K., and Dreyfuss, J. R.: Residual common duct stones. Surgery, *47*:202, 1960.

49. Bartlett, M. K., and Waddell, W. R.: Indications for common duct exploration. New Eng. J. Med., *258*:164, 1958.

50. Colcock, B. P., and Liddle, H. V.: Common-bile-duct stones. New Eng. J. Med., *258*:264, 1958.

51. Longmire, W. P., Jr., and Rangel, D. M.: Difficult problems encountered in the management of biliary obstruction due to stones and other benign conditions. Advances Surg., *4*:105, 1970.

52. Madden, J. L., Chien, J. Y., Kondaloft, S., and Parekh, M.: Choledochoduodenostomy, an unjustly maligned surgical procedure? Amer. J. Surg., *119*:45, 1970.

53. Madden, J. L., Vanderheyden, L., and Kondaloft, S.: The nature and surgical significance of common duct stones. Surg. Gynec. Obstet., *126*:3, 1968.

54. Smith, R. B., III, Conklin, E. F., and Porter, M. R.: A five year study of choledocholithiasis. Surg. Gynec. Obstet., *116*:731, 1963.

**Acute Suppurative Cholangitis**

55. Dow, R. W.: Acute obstructive suppurative cholangitis. Ann. Surg., *169*:272, 1969.

56. Glenn, F., and Moody, F. G.: Acute obstructive suppurative cholangitis. Surg. Gynec. Obstet., *113*:265, 1961.

57. Hinchey, E. J.: Acute obstructive suppurative cholangitis. Amer. J. Surg., *117*:62, 1969.

58. Mage, S.: Surgical experience with cholangiohepatitis (Hong Kong disease) in Canton Chinese. Ann. Surg., *162*:187, 1965.

59. Reynolds, B. M.: Acute obstructive cholangitis: a distinct clinical syndrome. Ann. Surg., *150*:299, 1959.

60. Stock, F. E.: Oriental cholangiohepatitis. Proc. Roy. Soc. Med., *61*:223, 1968.

**Primary Sclerosing Cholangitis**

61. Cutler, B., and Donaldson, G. A.: Primary sclerosing cholangitis and obliterative cholangitis. Amer. J. Surg., *117*:502, 1969.

62. Glenn, F., and Whitsell, J. C., II: Primary sclerosing cholangitis. Surg. Gynec. Obstet., *123*:1037, 1966.

63. Krieger, J., Seaman, W. B., and Porter, M. R.: The roentgenologic appearance of sclerosing cholangitis. Radiology, 95:369, 1970.

64. Longmire, W. P., Joseph, W. L., Levin, P. M., and Mellinkoff, S. M.: Diagnosis and treatment of cholangiolitic hepatitis (primary biliary cirrhosis). Ann. Surg., *162*:356, 1965.

65. Myers, R. N., Cooper, J. H., and Padis, N.: Primary sclerosing cholangitis. Complete gross and histologic reversal after long-term steroid therapy. Amer. J. Gastroent., *53*:527, 1970.

66. Perry, A. W., Djang, E., Katrouni, G., and Ludington, L. G.: Primary sclerosing cholangitis. Amer. J. Surg., *121*: 743, 1971.

67. Sherlock, S.: Chronic cholangitides: Aetiology, diagnosis, and treatment. Brit. Med. J., *3*:515, 1968.

68. Thorpe, M. E. C., Scheuer, P. J., and Sherlock, S.: Primary sclerosing cholangitis, the biliary tree, and ulcerative colitis. Gut, 8:435, 1967.

69. Warren, K. W., Athanassiades, S., and Mange, J. J.: Primary sclerosing cholangitis. Amer. J. Surg., *111*:23, 1966.

**Stenosis of the Sphincter of Oddi and Stenosing Papillitis**

70. Bartlett, M. K.: Might gallstones and recurrent pancreatitis have a common cause? Arch. Surg., 95:887, 1967.

71. Cattell, R. B., and Colcock, B. P.: Fibrosis of the sphincter of Oddi. Ann. Surg., *137*:797, 1953.

72. Grage, T. B., Lober, P. H., Imamoglu, K., and Wangensteen, O. H.: Stenosis of the sphincter of Oddi. Surgery, 48: 304, 1960.

73. Jones, S. A., Smith, L. L., and Gregory, G.: Sphincteroplasty for recurrent pancreatitis. Ann. Surg., *147*:180, 1958.

74. Nardi, G. L., and Acosta, J. M.: Papillitis as a cause of pancreatitis and abdominal pain. Ann. Surg., *164*:611, 1966.

**Biliary Fistulas, Gallstone Ileus**

75. Cooperman, A. M., Dickson, E. R., and ReMine, W. H.: Changing concepts in the surgical treatment of gallstone ileus: A review of 15 cases with emphasis on diagnosis and treatment. Ann. Surg., *167*:377, 1968.

76. Fjermeros, H.: Gall-stone ileus. Case reports and review of 178 cases from Scandinavia and Finland. Acta Chir. Scand., *128*:186, 1964.

77. Glenn, F., and Mannix, H., Jr.: Biliary enteric fistula. Surg. Gynec. Obstet., *105*:693, 1957.

78. Hudspeth, A. S., and McGuirt, W. F.: Gallstone ileus. A continuing surgical problem. Arch. Surg., *100*:668, 1970.

79. Raiford, T. S.: Intestinal obstruction caused by gallstones. Amer. J. Surg., *104*:383, 1962.

80. Thomas, H. S., Cherry, J. K., and Averbook, B. D.: Gallstone ileus. J.A.M.A., *179*:625, 1962.

81. Warshaw, A. L., and Bartlett, M. K.: Choice of operation for gallstone intestinal obstruction. Ann. Surg., *164*: 1051, 1966.

**Hyperplastic Cholecystoses**

82. Jutras, J. A., Longtin, J. M., and Levesque, H. P.: Hyperplastic cholecystoses. Amer. J. Roentgen., *83*:795, 1960.

**Acalculous Cholecystitis**

83. Glenn, F., and Mannix, H.: The acalculous gallbladder. Ann. Surg., *114*:670, 1956.

84. Hoerr, S. O., and Hazard, J. B.: Acute cholecystitis without gallbladder stones. Amer. J. Surg., *111*:47, 1966.

85. Munster, A. M., and Brown, J. R.: Acalculous cholecystitis: Amer. J. Surg., *113*:730, 1967.

**Symptoms after Cholecystectomy**

86. Colcock, B. P., and McManus, J. E.: Experience with 1,356 cases of cholecystitis and cholelithiasis. Surg. Gynec. Obstet., *101*:161, 1955.

87. Glenn, F.: A 26 year experience in the surgical treatment of 5,037 patients with nonmalignant biliary tract disease. Surg. Gynec. Obstet., *109*:591, 1959.

88. Womack, N. A., and Crider, R. L.: Persistence of symptoms following cholecystectomy. Ann. Surg., *126*:31, 1947.

**Injuries to the Extrahepatic Biliary System**

89. Diethrich, E. B., Beall, A. C., Jr., Jordon, G. L., Jr., and DeBakey, M. E.: Traumatic injuries to the extrahepatic biliary tract. Amer. J. Surg., *112*:756, 1966.

90. Cattell, R. B., and Braasch, J. W.: Primary repair of benign strictures of the bile duct. Surg. Gynec. Obstet., *109*: 531, 1959.

91. Cole, W. H.: Strictures of the common duct. Surgery, *43*:320, 1958.

92. Lary, B. G., and Scheibe, J. R.: Effect of rubber tubing on healing of common duct anastomoses. Surgery, *32*:789, 1952.

93. Longmire, W. P., Jr.: Early management of injury to the extrahepatic biliary tract. J.A.M.A., *195*:111, 1966.

94. Longmire, W. P., Jr., and Lippman, H. N.: Intrahepatic cholangiojejunostomy. An operation for biliary obstruction. Surg. Clin. N. Amer., *36*:849, 1956.

95. Manlove, C. A., Quattlebaum, F. W., and Ambrus, L.: Nonpenetrating trauma to the biliary tract. Amer. J. Surg., *97*:113, 1959.

96. Penn, I.: Injuries of the gall-bladder. Brit. J. Surg., *49*:636, 1961–62.

97. ReMine, W. H., and Ferris, D. O.: Surgery for biliary strictures. Surg. Clin. N. Amer., *47*:877, 1967.

98. Walters, W., Nixon, J. W., Jr., Hodgins, T. E., and Ramsdell, J. A.: Strictures of the common and hepatic bile ducts. Arch. Surg., *78*:908, 1959.

99. Warren, K. W., and McDonald, W. M.: Facts and fiction regarding strictures of the extrahepatic bile ducts. Ann. Surg., *159*:996, 1964.

100. Warren, K. W., Mountain, J. C., and Midell, A. I.: Management of strictures of the biliary tract. Surg. Clin. N. Amer., *51*:711, 1971.

**Extrahepatic Biliary Carcinoma**

101. Altemeier, W. A., Gall, E. A., Culbertson, W. R., and Inge, W. W.: Sclerosing carcinoma of the intrahepatic (hilar) bile ducts. Surgery, *60*:191, 1966.

102. Appleman, R. M., Morlock, C. G., Dahlin, D. C., and Adson, M. A.: Long-term survival in carcinoma of the gallbladder. Surg. Gynec. Obstet., *117*:459, 1963.

103. Braasch, J. W., Warren, K. W., and Kune, G. A.: Malignant neoplasms of the bile ducts. Surg. Clin. N. Amer., *47*:627, 1967.

104. Cattell, R. B., Braasch, J. W., and Kahn, F.: Polypoid epithelial tumours of the bile ducts. New Eng. J. Med., *266*:57, 1962.

105. Fahim, R. B., McDonald, J. R., Richards, J. C., and Ferris,

D. O.: Carcinoma of the gallbladder; a study of its mode of spread. Ann. Surg., *156*:144, 1962.

106. Gerst, P. H.: Primary carcinoma of the gallbladder, a thirty-year summary. Surgery, *153*:369, 1961.

107. Glenn, F., and Hays, D. M.: The scope of radical surgery in treatment of malignant tumors of the extrahepatic biliary tract. Surg. Gynec. Obstet., *99*:529, 1954.

108. Hamm, J. M., and Mackenzie, D. C.: Primary carcinoma of the extrahepatic bile ducts. Surg. Gynec. Obstet., *118*:977, 1964.

109. Hardy, M. A., and Volk, H.: Primary carcinoma of the gallbladder. A ten year review. Amer. J. Surg., *120*:800, 1970.

110. Kowalewski, K., and Todd, E. F.: Carcinoma of the gallbladder induced in hamsters by insertion of cholesterol pellets and feeding dimethylnitrosamine. Proc. Soc. Exp. Biol. Med., *136*:482, 1971.

111. Kuwayti, K., Baggenstoss, A. H., Stauffer, M. H., and Priestly, J. T.: Carcinoma of the major intrahepatic and the extrahepatic bile ducts exclusive of the papilla of Vater. Surg. Gynec. Obstet., *104*:357, 1957.

112. Quattlebaum, J. K., and Quattlebaum, J. K., Jr.: Malignant obstruction of the major hepatic ducts. Ann. Surg., *161*:876, 1965.

113. Sako, K., Seitzinger, G. L., and Garside, E.: Carcinoma of the extrahepatic bile ducts: Review of the literature and report of six cases. Surgery, *41*:416, 1957.

114. Solan, M. J., and Jackson, B. T.: Carcinoma of the gallbladder. A clinical appraisal and review of 57 cases. Brit. J. Surg., *58*:593, 1971.

115. Strauch, G. O.: Primary carcinoma of the gallbladder, presentation of 70 cases from the Rhode Island Hospital and a cumulative review of the last 10 years of the American literature. Surgery, *47*:368, 1960.

116. Tanga, M. R., and Ewing, J. B.: Primary malignant tumors of the gallbladder: Report of 43 cases. Surgery, *67*:418, 1970.

117. Van Heerden, J. A., Judd, E. S., and Dockerty, M. B.: Carcinoma of the extrahepatic bile ducts. Amer. J. Surg., *113*:49, 1967.

**Choledochal Cyst**

118. Alonso-Lej, F., Rever, W. B., Jr., and Pessagno, D. J.: Congenital choledochal cyst, with a report of 2, and an analysis of 94 cases. Surg. Gynec. Obstet., *108*:1, 1959.

119. Kasai, M., Asakura, Y., and Taira, Y.: Surgical treatment of choledochal cyst. Ann. Surg., *172*:844, 1970.

120. Lee, S. S., Min, P. C., Kim, G. S., and Hong, P. W.: Choledochal cyst. A report of nine cases and review of the literature. Arch. Surg., *99*:19, 1969.

121. Trout, H. H., and Longmire, W. P., Jr.: Long-term follow-up study of patients with congenital cystic dilation of the common bile duct. Amer. J. Surg., *121*:68, 1971.

122. Tsardakas, E. N., and Robnett, A. H.: Congenital cystic dilatation of common bile duct; report of 3 cases, analysis of 57 cases, and review of literature. Arch. Surg., *72*:311, 1956.

**Atresia of the Bile Ducts**

123. Bennett, D. E.: Problems in neonatal obstructive jaundice. Pediatrics, *33*:735, 1964.

124. Hays, D. M., and Snyder, W. H.: Life-span in untreated biliary atresia. Surgery, *54*:373, 1963.

125. Hays, D. M., Wooley, M. M., Snyder, W. H., Reed, G. B., Bwinn, J. L., and Landing, B. H.: Diagnosis of biliary atresia: relative accuracy of percutaneous liver biopsy, open liver biopsy, and operative cholangiography. J. Pediat., *71*:598, 1967.

126. Holder, T. M.: Atresia of the extrahepatic bile duct. Amer. J. Surg., *107*:458, 1964.

127. Krovetz, L. T.: Congenital biliary atresia: I. Analysis of thirty cases with particular reference to diagnosis. Surgery, *47*:453, 1960.

128. Krovetz, L. T.: Congenital biliary atresia: II. Analysis of the therapeutic problem. Surgery, *47*:468, 1960.

129. Longmire, W. P., Jr.: Congenital biliary hypoplasia. Ann. Surg., *159*:335, 1964.

130. Stowens, D.: Congenital biliary atresia. Ann. N. Y. Acad. Sci., *111*:337, 1963.

# 35

# THE PANCREAS

*W. Dean Warren, M.D., and Robert Zeppa, M.D.*

## ANATOMY

A thorough understanding of the anatomy of the pancreas will facilitate a clear understanding of the disorders requiring surgical intervention and the various techniques employed in their treatment. Because of the importance in clinical management of an understanding of these features of pancreatic anatomy, the salient anatomic characteristics will be emphasized and are clearly illustrated in Figure 1.

### Fixed Retroperitoneal Position Crossing the Upper Abdomen behind the Lesser Omental Bursa

The pancreas lies transversely in the upper abdomen, extending from the duodenal curve on the right to the hilus of the spleen on the left. It generally lies in a retrogastric position and crosses the vertebral column just below the celiac axis. Because of this relatively *fixed* position and its close association with the vertebral column, the pancreas is prone to injury by blunt trauma. The classic syndrome is the steering wheel injury in which the thrust of impact is delivered to the epigastrium with splitting or transection of the pancreas at its anatomic neck, or that portion overlying the vertebral column. The pancreas crosses behind the lesser omental bursa and, thus, much of it is hidden from view by the stomach, transverse colon, and gastrohepatic and gastrocolic ligaments. Consequently, injuries or tumors of the neck, body, and tail of the gland may easily be overlooked. Pseudocysts of the pancreas are the result of duct disruption and leakage of pancreatic juice. As the peritoneal coverage of the anterior pancreatic surface is quite thin, the fluid disrupts this membrane, thereby entering the

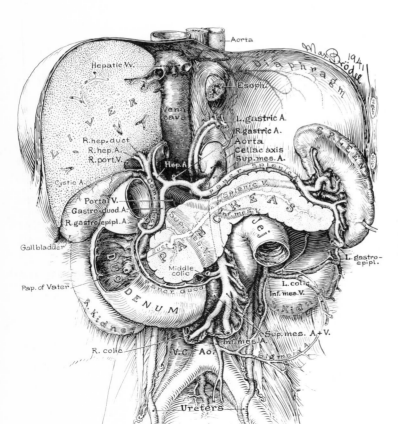

**Figure 1** Relationships of the pancreas to other structures in the upper abdomen. (From Trimble, I. R., Parsons, J. W., and Sherman, C. P.: Surg. Gynec. Obstet., *73*:711, 1941.)

lesser omental bursa; thus, pseudocysts of the pancreas are typically confined to this area.

The lack of a mesentery partially explains the low rate of resectability and curability of cancer of the pancreas. This is due not only to the early direct invasion of the posterior abdominal wall but also to the anatomy of pancreatic lymph drainage. Several groups of nodes, including celiac, suprapancreatic, subpyloric, subhepatic, superior mesenteric, aortic, and splenic nodes, drain the pancreas and their excision is accomplished only with a "node picking" type of procedure rather than an en bloc resection with wide surgical margins.

### Joint Blood Supply for the Duodenum and Head of the Pancreas

One of the important limitations in pancreatic surgery is the inability to perform safely a simple total pancreatectomy. This is largely due to the joint blood supply of the head of the pancreas and the second portion of the duodenum; the superior and inferior pancreaticoduodenal arteries course within the pancreatic substance and would be sacrificed during total pancreatectomy, thus impairing markedly the duodenal blood supply and incurring the risk of ischemic necrosis. The common bile duct also traverses the head of the pancreas immediately before it enters the duodenal wall and this poses an additional hazard in simple total pancreatectomy. The Whipple operation was designed to overcome the dangers of simple total pancreatectomy and also to achieve a wider margin of resection for malignancy. In this procedure the head and varying portions of the body and tail of the pancreas are resected along with the duo-

denum, the terminal end of the common bile duct, and a portion of the stomach. Reconstruction involves anastomosis of the jejunum to the residual pancreas, the common bile duct, and the stomach proximally and distally, to minimize the danger of jejunal ulceration.

Recently, the so-called radical distal pancreatectomy (or 95 per cent pancreatectomy) has been designed to resect all of the pancreas except the small crescent necessary to protect the pancreaticoduodenal arteries. Child and his associates have employed this operation with great success in the treatment of benign pancreatic diseases.[19]

The remainder of the blood supply of the pancreas comes primarily from branches of the splenic and superior mesenteric arteries. The venous drainage of the pancreas in general follows that of the arterial system. Of clinical significance is the fact that the body and tail of the pancreas are drained by small venous tributaries into the splenic vein. These vessels are fragile and easily torn during dissection; for this reason resection of the body and tail of the pancreas is frequently combined with splenectomy to minimize dissection and simplify the procedure.

### Intimate Association with Vital Vascular Structures

The pancreas in its transverse course passes immediately anterior to the inferior vena cava, the aorta, and the superior mesenteric artery and vein and lies anterior or slightly inferior to the splenic artery and vein. One of the great dangers in both penetrating and nonpenetrating injuries of the pancreas is the possibility of injury to one of these

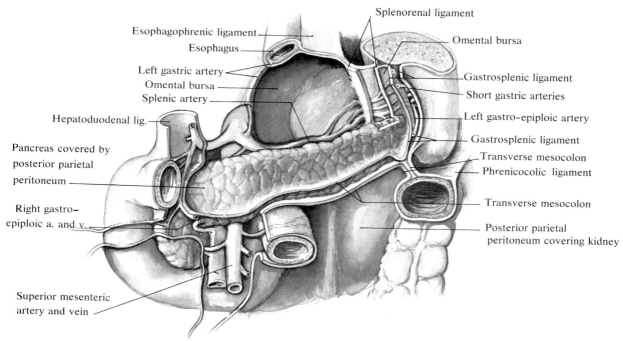

**Figure 2** Vascular structures near the pancreas. (From Healey, J. E., Jr.: A Synopsis of Clinical Anatomy. Philadelphia, W. B. Saunders Company, 1969.)

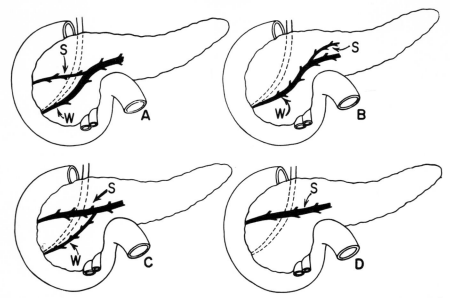

**Figure 3** Diagrammatic illustration of several variations in the size and connections of the main duct of Wirsung (W) and the accessory duct of Santorini (S). *A,* The arrangement reported in the majority of dissections. *B,* Santorini's duct draining the midportion of the gland and connecting directly into the duct of Wirsung. *C* and *D,* The duct of Santorini as the major pancreatic duct. *D,* Although relatively rare, obliteration of the duct of Wirsung gives the surgeon great difficulty when attempting to catheterize the pancreatic duct preliminary to pancreatogram following sphincterotomy. (From Ellison, E. H., and Carey, L. C. In: Davis, L., ed.: Christopher's Textbook of Surgery. 9th ed. Philadelphia, W. B. Saunders Company, 1968.)

large vessels. The pancreas may obscure the site of hemorrhage, and extensive mobilization or even transection of the pancreas may be necessary to control the bleeding vessel. Massive hemorrhage remains the principal cause of death in injuries involving the pancreas. A related problem is the dangerous hemorrhage sometimes seen with necrotizing pancreatitis and pseudocysts of the pancreas; the splenic or superior mesenteric vessels are usually the source of such bleeding (Fig. 2).

### Relationship of the Pancreatic Duct and Common Bile Duct at the Ampulla of Vater

There are numerous variations in the anatomic relationships between the common bile duct and the pancreatic duct. At one extreme each duct terminates in duodenum through an entirely separate papilla and at the other end of the spectrum the two ducts jointly share a conduit, a centimeter or more in length, which terminates at the papilla of Vater. It has been well demonstrated, however, that in most patients with chronic pancreatitis there is some degree of a "common channel" between the two ducts. This has been shown both at operation and at autopsy by injection into the common bile duct with reflux into the pancreatic ductal system. From the available data it appears that this relationship is far more common in patients with pancreatitis than in the normal population. This anatomic association is important to help explain the role of biliary tract disease in the development of pancreatitis through obstruction at the ampulla of Vater, induced either by

spasm or stones. In addition, papillitis with fibrosis and stenosis is seen in other types of pancreatitis. Sphincteroplasty in many instances can decompress both the biliary and pancreatic ductal systems (Fig. 3).

### The Fleshy Characteristic of Normal Pancreas

The normal pancreas is a soft, friable organ that holds sutures very poorly. If there is a large, dilated pancreatic duct, this problem is simplified, as a direct duct to intestine anastomosis can be carried out. Frequently, however, the open face of the pancreatic remnant must be inserted into a loop of jejunum. Following a Whipple procedure for carcinoma, one of the most serious complications and frequent causes of death is leakage at the pancreaticojejunostomy.

### Innervation of the Pancreas

Pancreatic secretion is controlled to some extent through its vagal innervation. This has led to proposed treatment of acute pancreatitis with vagolytic drugs and chronic pancreatitis with bilateral vagotomy combined with gastrojejunostomy. Although these therapeutic concepts are still controversial, the influence of the vagus on the pancreas is unquestioned. Of greater surgical importance is the splanchnic innervation of the pancreas which mediates the sensation of pain. Procedures to block the splanchnic nerves temporarily or to divide them have been utilized in the treatment of pancreatic disorders that are accompanied by severe pain, namely carcinoma of the pancreas and chronic pancreatitis. The left splanchnic nerve innervates the great majority of the pancreas but failure to control pain in a significant number of cases has led to bilateral splanchnicectomy when a maximal effort at pain control is needed. Although performed relatively infrequently, splanchnicectomy and splanchnic blocks are important tools in the management of the severe pain of pancreatic cancer and chronic pancreatitis.

## MICROSCOPIC ANATOMY

The pancreas is a complex structure composed of two strikingly different types of tissue having widely disparate functions. The exocrine or digestive portion of the organ is composed of a compound acinar gland divided into lobules clearly demarcated by loose connective tissue septa. In turn, the septa are traversed by nutrient blood vessels, nerves, and lymphatics. The acini are composed of a single row of pyramidal epithelial cells converging toward a central lumen and resting at the opposite pole on a well demarcated basal lamina (Fig. 4).

The basilar portion of the acinus cells contains the tubular and cisternal elements of the rough endoplasmic reticulum as well as mitochondria appearing in the shape of long rods with well developed cristae and matrix granules. The Golgi complex is also located in this region of the cell. The free surfaces of the acinar cells forming the interface with the lumen of the acinus contain few short and irregular microvilli. The apical cytoplasm in this area is usually loaded with zymogen droplets and in some preparations these droplets may be seen discharging into the lumen of the acinus (Fig. 5). The lumen of each acinus is continuous with the lumen of the terminal duct, which is bounded by centroacinar cells. These cells have been so named because they are surrounded by and appear to extend toward the center of the lumen of the acinus. These are cuboidal to low columnar cells which are pale-staining with hematoxylin and eosin. This terminal portion of the duct system drains proximally into the intralobular or intercalated ducts. The latter are lined by cells that are similar in appearance to the centroacinar cells and are low columnar in variety. In turn, the intercalated ducts are involved in the secretion of water and electrolytes.

Intimately associated with the acinar structure of the exocrine pancreas are small masses of endocrine cells composing the islets of Langerhans. These are scattered throughout the pancreas and are frequently found to number in excess of one

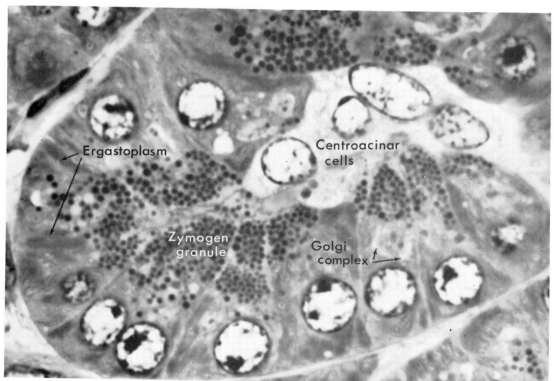

**Figure 4**   Photomicrograph of human pancreas, showing an acinus and its centroacinar cells. The ergastoplasm, Golgi complex, and zymogen granules of the acinar cells are clearly identifiable. The fixation of the nuclei is less than ideal, but adequate preservation of this organ from postmortem material is difficult. Formalin, osmium fixation, Epon section, stained with toluidine blue, × 3200. (Courtesy of S. Ito; from Bloom, W., and Fawcett, D. W.: A Textbook of Histology. 9th ed. Philadelphia, W. B. Saunders Company, 1968.)

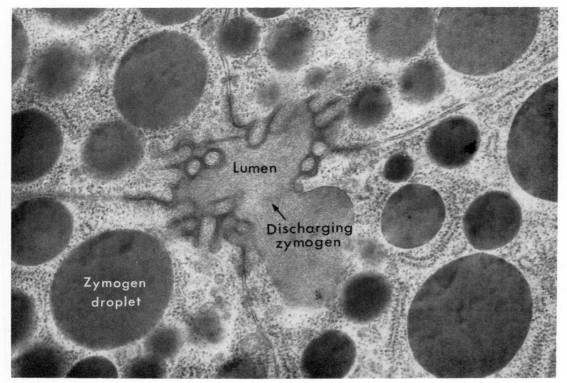

**Figure 5**   Electron micrograph of the lumen of an acinus and the apical portions of four acinar cells. Large dense zymogen droplets or granules are found in the cell apex. The limiting membrane of one of these has fused with the cell membrane and its zymogen is being discharged into the lumen. The free surface of the acinar cells bears short microvilli. × 38,000. (From Bloom, W., and Fawcett, D. W.: A Textbook of Histology. 9th ed. Philadelphia, W. B. Saunders Company, 1968.)

million per gland. The islets are clearly demarcated by a thin layer of reticular fibers. Occasionally, the endocrine cells may be found isolated or in smaller groups scattered among the acinar cells. They may be identified by differential staining since secretory granules cannot be identified within the endocrine cells on routine hematoxylin and eosin staining. However, special techniques have revealed that there are at least three types of endocrine cells which in fact do contain distinctive granules. The alpha cell contains granules that are insoluble in alcohol, while the granules of the other most common type, the beta cell, are soluble in alcohol. Morphologically intermediate between the alpha and beta cells is the delta cell which contains granules that are usually somewhat larger but less dense than the granules in the alpha cell. The physiologic significance of the delta cells in the islets is not clear, whereas the alpha cells have been associated with the production of the hormone glucagon and the beta cells with insulin (Fig. 6).

## EMBRYOLOGY

An endodermal pouch on the dorsal wall of the duodenum may be seen in the 3 mm. human

embryo and identified as the first appearance of the pancreas. Somewhat later, an additional pouch, sometimes two, appears on the inferior portion of an angle formed by the duodenum and the developing hepatic buds. This latter pouch (or pouches) constitutes the ventral pancreas. The dorsal pancreas grows more rapidly than the ventral and rotation of the duodenum and common bile duct carries the ventral pancreas to the right. Subsequently, fusion occurs between dorsal and ventral pancreas and the latter is situated caudally, forming most of the head.

Lobular arrangement within the pancreas becomes evident at about the fourth month of fetal existence, and the lobules are usually small and well separated by connective tissue. Acinus formation may be seen approximately 1 month earlier, the acini appearing as small groups of cells along the lateral walls and distal ends of the ducts. Continued proliferation of the ducts is associated with formation of new acini and these tend to bulge outward, developing small lumina that appear clustered around the ends of the ducts. The duct cells that are surrounded by acinar cells then become known as the centroacinar cells (see earlier).

Before the acini begin to develop, islets of Langerhans may be discovered in association with the ducts. The first group to be identified undergoes primary degeneration and a second genera-

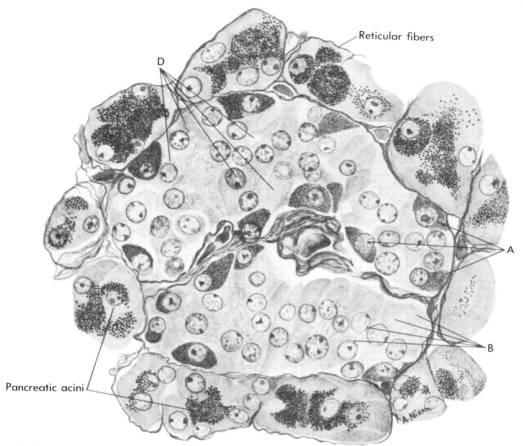

D

Reticular fibers

A

B

Pancreatic acini

**Figure 6** Section of human pancreas. The central part of the figure is an islet of Langerhans with granular cells of types alpha, beta, and delta. Mallory-azan stain, × 960. (After Bloom, 1931; from Bloom, W., and Fawcett, D. W.: A Textbook of Histology. 9th ed. Philadelphia, W. B. Saunders Company, 1968.)

tion appears sometime during the fourth month of gestation.

## CONGENITAL ANOMALIES

*Annular pancreas* is a relatively rare congenital malformation which occasionally first causes symptoms during adult life. The symptoms may result from obstruction to the duodenum at the site of the annulus or from chronic pancreatitis and peptic ulcer. The initial symptom may be jaundice, and evaluation of the biliary tract may reveal a dilated common duct with or without stones. While the precise etiology of this abnormality is not clear, two major theories consider the condition to be due to either (1) the failure of the ventral anlage of the pancreas to rotate with the duodenum or (2) hypertrophy of both the ventral and dorsal pouches. On examination, the annular pancreas contains normal acinar and islet tissue. When the symptoms are primarily those of obstruction, a bypass operation is clearly the procedure of choice, usually a duodenojejunostomy. Resection

or division of the annulus is considered inadvisable because of the risk of fistula formation and duodenal leakage since the pancreatic tissue may be dispersed throughout the duodenal wall.

Pancreatic heterotopia is a more common congenital malformation.[8] The ectopic pancreas may be found almost anywhere along the gastrointestinal tract. However, in descending order of frequency, it is found in the duodenum, stomach, and jejunum (Fig. 7). There is lesser involvement of Meckel's diverticulum and the wall of the ileum. Interestingly, about one-fourth of all the reported gastrointestinal diverticula of embryonic origin are found to have ectopic pancreatic tissue within them. The clinical significance of these aberrant foci of pancreatic tissue depends upon the complications they provoke. These complications include ulceration, hemorrhage, and obstruction either because of the size of the pancreatic mass per se or because it serves as the focal point for the development of an intussusception. The differentiation of ectopic pancreas from a primary neoplasm of the organ affected is sometimes difficult and resolved only by excision.

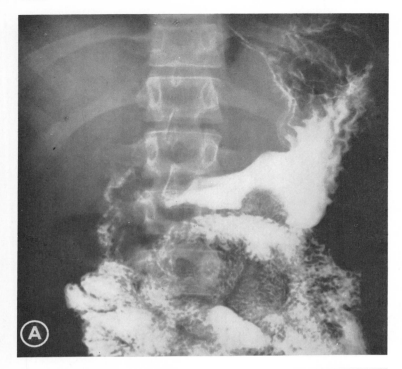

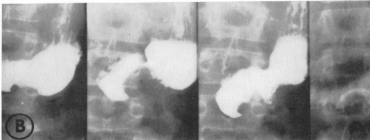

Figure 7 A, Typical round, smooth filling defect of an aberrant pancreas occurring on the greater curvature of the stomach. B, Fluoroscopy and spot films of the antrum demonstrate an umbilication at the site of a central duct. (From Ellison, E. H., and Carey, L. C. In: Davis, L., ed.: Christopher's Textbook of Surgery. 9th ed. Philadelphia, W. B. Saunders Company, 1968.)

## FUNCTION

### EXOCRINE

The first demonstration of the effect of vagal stimulation on pancreatic secretion was recorded by Heidenhain in 1875.[42] This was confirmed and further defined by Pavlov and his brilliant group of co-workers who also demonstrated the presence of inhibitory fibers in the vagus nerves.[65] Pavlov's student Babkin was the first to demonstrate that all the secretory nerves to the pancreas are cholinergic even when derived from the sympathetic nervous system.[4]

At the turn of the century, Bayliss and Starling demonstrated the existence of a substance in duodenal mucosa that stimulated pancreatic secretion, to which they gave the name *secretin*.[9] They demonstrated that the greatest concentration of the hormone was in the duodenum and that it could be found for variable distances in the mucosa farther down the intestinal tract. These contributions were initial milestones in the endeavor to understand pancreatic function, and their validity remains unchallenged today.

Despite the accumulation of a wealth of information since the observations of Heidenhain, a clearly defined schema of an integrated exocrine function of the pancreatic gland is not yet clear. Examination of the digestive function of the gland clearly defines two separate components. The first, water and electrolyte secretion, is thought to be located in the centroacinar and intercalated duct cells. The stimulated flow rate in man may reach more than 4.5 ml. per minute; however, tonicity is independent of flow rate. The osmotic pressure of the juice is isotonic with and responds to changes in plasma osmolality. The sum of the concentrations of sodium and potassium is approximately equal to that found in the plasma and remains independent of the rate of flow of pancreatic secretion. The pH of the juice varies from 7 to 8.7 and the specific gravity from 1.007 to 1.042. The most important anion in pancreatic juice is bicarbonate which appears in a concentration range of 25 to 170 mEq. per liter. The concentration of bicarbonate varies directly with the rate of flow, increasing at high flow rates and vice versa. Chloride ion varies inversely with bicarbonate and the sum of bicarbonate and chloride concentrations falls between 154 and 175 mEq. per liter. Bicarbonate in the juice is not simply a reflection of the metabolic activity of the gland since injected radioactive carbon dioxide appears promptly in the juice with a specific activity measured to be five times greater than that in plasma.

Secretin, which was defined by Jorpes as a linear polypeptide containing 27 amino acids, stimulates the flow of pancreatic juice at high rates and contains large amounts of bicarbonate. The hormone is released from the duodenal mucosa in the presence of hydrochloric acid, proteolytic byproducts, fatty acid soaps, and amino acids such as glutamic acid. Conversely, the flow of pancreatic juice and the concentration of bicarbonate are reduced by the action of antidiuretic hormone.

The mechanism of secretion of large volumes of bicarbonate-rich juice is not clear. Two hypotheses are most prevalent. The first, proposed by Janowitz, describes the primary secretion of isotonic bicarbonate with alteration in the final concentrations being due to an exchange for chloride in the collecting system. This scheme favors an increase in the exchange at low flow rates. The alternative hypothesis favors the unicellular concept which describes the secretion of both bicarbonate and chloride at variable rates. At present there are insufficient data to establish the absolute supremacy of either concept although many of the experimental findings support the exchange hypothesis.

The other component of exocrine function consists of the elaboration and secretion of small volumes of fluid rich in enzymatic activity. This is protein-rich fluid of high specific gravity containing the active and inactive forms of the enzymes trypsin, chymotrypsins A and B, carboxypeptidases A and B, ribonuclease, and deoxyribonuclease in addition to amylase and lipase. Extensive studies on protein synthesis in the acinar cells revealed that secretory proteins are formed on the ribosomes and then transferred across the membranes of the rough endoplasmic reticulum which appear as cisterns in electron micrographs. Smooth buds develop from the rough cisterns in the region of the Golgi apparatus which then form into small vesicles containing newly synthesized secretory protein. These vesicles coalesce, perhaps receiving some membrane from the Golgi to form immature zymogen granules partially filled with protein. Maturation of these granules occurs during their movement from the basilar portion of the cell toward the free surface and probably involves either the extrusion of water or the internal transport of additional protein (Fig. 8).

Pancreatic enzyme production is adaptive, depending upon the composition of the diet. The ingestion of a carbohydrate-rich diet has been shown to lead to an increase in the synthesis of amylase and decrease in chymotrypsinogen. The rapid turnover of protein in the pancreas associated with enzyme synthesis requires the presence of me-

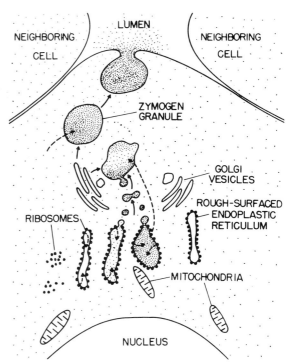

**Figure 8** Scheme of intracellular protein transport in the pancreas. After the secretory proteins are formed on the ribosomes they are transferred across the membranes of the rough-surfaced cisternae, where they accumulate. Smooth membranes bud from the ends of the rough-surfaced cisternae in the centrosphere (Golgi) region and form small vesicles containing newly synthesized secretory proteins. Small vesicles coalesce, possibly receiving additional membrane from the Golgi vesicles to form immature zymogen granules, partly filled with secretory protein. Mature zymogen granules are formed by extrusion of water or by transport of additional protein across the membrane of the zymogen vacuoles (or both). *Solid arrows* depict migration of membrane. *Dashed arrows* depict transmembrane transport of protein. Dots depict secretory protein. (From Hokin, L. E. In: American Physiological Society: Handbook of Physiology. Section 6, Alimentary Canal; Volume II, Secretion. Edited by C. F. Code. Baltimore, Williams & Wilkins, 1968; adapted from Palade, G. E., et al. In: de Reuck, A. V. S., and Cameron, M. P., eds.: Ciba Foundation Symposium, Exocrine Pancreas. London, J. & A. Churchill, 1962, pp. 23–55.)

thionine. The administration of ethionine, an analog of the essential amino acid, leads to a reduction in the synthesis of enzymes and also to structural damage to the gland with the loss of acinar cells and fibrosis.

In common with secretory function elsewhere in the gastrointestinal tract, the regulation of pancreatic exocrine secretion is bimodal. There are neural cholinergic effects as well as potent hormonal stimuli. The results of early studies indicate that a substantial portion of the secretory innervation to the pancreas enters the gland in the region of the choledochoduodenal junction. The vagus nerves provide secretory fibers to both acinus and islet cells and, in addition, distribute motor fibers to the smooth muscle of the major ducts. Both trunks of the vagus nerves appear to be involved. Stimulation of the vagus nerves provokes a secretory response that is characterized by the appearance of pancreatic juice of high specific gravity rich in enzyme activities, with only a modest increase in volume. This response may be mimicked by cholinergic drugs and blocked by atropine. Further, stimulation of the vagus nerves potentiates the actions of both hormones pancreozymin and secretin. Both of the hormones are released from the duodenal mucosa in response to similar stimuli. Pancreozymin does not significantly alter the flow of water or electrolytes from the pancreas but it profoundly stimulates the output of enzymes, whereas secretin, as previously mentioned, provokes the secretion of a thin watery pancreatic juice rich in bicarbonate ions. While this information suggests that the integrated control of pancreatic secretion may be viewed as the action of the two duodenal hormones operating against a background of vagal activity, there is as yet no clear-cut evidence that vagotomy in man has any effect upon the response of the pancreas to secretin stimulation.

In addition to the stimulatory effects of the intestinal hormones secretin and pancreozymin, there is evidence that suggests that a gastric phase of pancreatic secretion may exist. Pancreatic secretion may be provoked by injecting pure gastrin or by stimulating the antral release of endogenous gastrin by distention or manipulation of intraluminal pH. Conversely, the pancreatic response to a meal may be reduced considerably following partial gastrectomy. The pancreatic response to administered gastrin involves secretion of both bicarbonate and protein.

The stimulatory action of secretin forms the basis of the clinically useful test in which the duodenum is intubated, secretin administered, and pancreatic juice aspirated through an indwelling tube. While the normal range of responses must be established for each laboratory, the minimal volume to be expected approximates 100 ml. per hour, with the secretion of 15 to 20 mEq. of bicarbonate ion and 700 units of amylase.[6, 16, 24, 41, 43, 46, 52]

## ENDOCRINE

The relationship between the pancreas and diabetes mellitus was established by von Mering and Minkowski in 1889 who described diabetes in a dog following removal of the pancreas.[79] The thesis describing the internal secretion of the pancreas was established by their observations. The knowledge that glycosuria was an important factor in the disease had been recognized since ancient times. It was during the seventeenth and eighteenth centuries that diagnosis of the disease earned the diagnosticians the vulgar appellation of "piss prophets," obviously reflecting a certain association with the observation of Willis that the urine of the diabetic patient was "wonderfully sweet as if imbued with honey or sugar." By 1922 Banting and Best had obtained potent pancreatic extracts that were active against hyperglycemia and by 1926 Abel had crystallized insulin and found it had a molecular weight of 6000 and was clearly defined as two polypeptide chains linked by a disulfide bridge.

Insulin is the product of the beta cell within the islands of Langerhans, and the beta granules of these cells represent the storage form of the hormone. The release of insulin by the beta cell is stimulated by alterations in the concentration of blood sugar. In isolated, perfused pancreas preparations, an increase in the concentration of glucose was found to be followed by an increase in insulin release, and reduction in the concentration of the sugar was attended by the reciprocal event. Further, after chronic continuous intravenous administration of glucose to animals an increased amount of islet tissue may be found in the pancreas and during this interval body weight of the animal slowly decreases. The amino acid leucine and some sulfonyl urea compounds are known to cause the release of insulin from beta cell granules. In addition, evidence has been obtained from man that has shown that the hormone secretin causes the release of insulin, which may be measured in the portal venous blood within minutes following intravenous administration of the hormone. These studies have clearly defined the mechanism involving digestive function in the homeostasis of blood sugar. In animals, secretin also causes an increase in pancreatic blood flow and oxygen consumption associated with insulin release. This action of secretin may explain the discrepancy between the findings that vagotomy appears to have no effect upon glucose metabolism and, conversely, that stimulation of the vagus nerve has been shown to cause insulin release. Presumably, this action is the result of the effect of vagal stimulation upon acid secretion and, in turn, the stimulation of secretin release by acid in the duodenum.

Glucagon is the other internal secretion of the pancreas and is a polypeptide composed of 29 amino acid residues with a molecular weight of 3482. Glucagon is a hyperglycemic stimulating hormone that acts through the induction of the breakdown of liver glycogen with consequent release of glucose into the circulation. This effect upon blood sugar may be the most important mechanism whereby glucagon provides the release of insulin. The hormone also has exocrine effects which have been noted following administration of exogenous glucagon. Infusion at a dose of 40 $\mu$g. per kilogram has resulted in striking reduction in the volume of pancreatic juice secreted through a fistula in man. Other effects of glucagon include (1) inhibition of gastric acid secretion, (2) inhibition of gastric and intestinal motility, (3) stimulation of the flow of bile, and (4) stimulation of Brunner's glands and intestinal secretion.

A physiologic role for delta cells is unknown; however, it is possible that they are involved in the development of gastrin-secreting tumors of the pancreas,[7, 12] since gastrin has been demonstrated in the pancreas by immunoassay and immuno-fluorescence.

## ACUTE PANCREATITIS

The morbid process of pancreatic distress identified as acute pancreatitis includes a broad spectrum of visible alterations ranging from minimal edema to autolysis. The attack rate of the disease is unknown; however, it constitutes a relatively common cause of emergency admission to hospitals. An example of the experience at a university medical center with this problem is reflected in the fact that 98 patients suffering from acute pancreatitis were admitted to the University of Miami Affiliated Hospitals during a 1 year period (1970). Twelve of these patients died (12.2 per cent), usually exhibiting refractory shock and acute pulmonary insufficiency.

Just as the gross and microscopic manifestations of pancreatitis are variable, so are the concepts concerning the etiology of the disease. Attempts to discover a single precise etiologic factor have occupied medical investigators for more than 100 years. At present, there is general agreement that some combination of ductal obstruction, with or without reflux of duodenal or biliary contents and vascular insufficiency, imposed upon the stimulated exocrine pancreas is responsible for initiating the process of acute pancreatitis.

### Obstruction and Reflux

Simple obstruction of the major pancreatic ducts, complete or partial, has been considered by some to be the basic cause of this disease. The incidence of ductal obstruction in the postmortem examination in fatal pancreatitis does not support this thesis. Autopsies in 100 consecutive patients dying of pancreatitis in the Los Angeles County General Hospital revealed duct obstruction in only three of the cadavers. Further, deliberate ligation of the major pancreatic duct in treatment of chronic relapsing pancreatitis has not caused the acute disease. These anecdotal data do not preclude the possibility of pancreatitis developing as a result of duct obstruction when powerful stimulatory factors affect exocrine function simultaneously. In experiments involving laboratory animals, obstruction of the pancreatic duct is followed by acinar atrophy (the experiments of Banting and Best). However, when experimental duct obstruction is imposed in association with stimulation to pancreatic secretion, pancreatitis will be induced in the majority of the subjects.

The role of bile or duodenal reflux into the pancreatic ducts in the etiology of human pancreatitis is equally obscure. Opie (1901) first proposed that bile reflux into pancreatic ducts was a cause of acute hemorrhagic pancreatitis. The "common channel theory" that he postulated was based on the discovery of a biliary stone lodged in the ampulla of Vater with the terminal bile and pancreatic ducts in free communication in a patient who died of acute pancreatitis. The theory provided an attractive and easily digestible

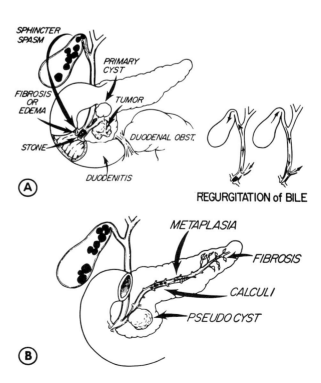

**Figure 9** *A*, Conditions associated with and thought to contribute to acute pancreatitis: occlusion of the sphincter of Oddi results in obstruction of the pancreatic duct and permits regurgitation of bile through a common channel; it can result from reflex spasm, stone, fibrosis, or edema. Duodenal obstruction distal to the sphincter may cause reflux of duodenal contents. An enlarging tumor or cyst may result in intrapancreatic obstruction. *B*, Recurrent pancreatitis with fibrosis and metaplasia of the ductal epithelium, calculus formation, or the development of a pancreatic pseudocyst may lead to secondary obstruction of the pancreatic ducts, thus fostering further attacks. (From Ellison, E. H., and Carey, L. C. In: Davis, L., ed.: Christopher's Textbook of Surgery. 9th ed. Philadelphia, W. B. Saunders Company, 1968.)

explanation for the well recognized association of biliary stones and pancreatitis. Unfortunately, the anatomic features required to support a common channel hypothesis appear to exist in only one-third of all subjects. Further, bidirectional reflux, that is, bile into pancreatic ducts and pancreatic juice into bile ducts, has been observed in humans without pancreatitis and, in addition, the pressure in the pancreatic duct exceeds bile duct pressure under normal conditions. Investigative efforts using animal models have not answered all of the inquiries concerning reflux. For example, Claude Bernard (1855) was unsuccessful in an attempt to create the lesion by injecting bile and sweet oil into the pancreatic ducts of dogs. The active perfusion of the pancreatic ducts with normal bile at normal pressures apparently does not cause pancreatitis. Treatment of the bile by incubation with pancreatic juice, trypsin, or bacteria and then injection of this material into the pancreatic ducts at increased pressures (sufficient to injure the finer radicals) is usually effective in provoking acute hemorrhagic pancreatitis.

Acute pancreatitis has also been attributed to the reflux of duodenal contents into the pancreatic duct. Such duodenopancreatic reflux has been demonstrated to occur in humans, and this concept has the added attraction of describing a mechanism which per se includes activation of proteolytic ferments. Despite this, it has been shown that continuous perfusion of the pancreatic duct with either duodenal or biliary secretions does not cause pancreatitis in experimental animal models even though intraductal activation of pancreatic enzymes occurs. This is true so long as forceful injection retrograde through the duct is not the mechanism for the introduction of the materials into the pancreatic ductal system. On the other hand, the experimental construction of closed-loop duodenal obstruction with biliary exclusion (Pfeffer preparation) is followed by a most virulent form of acute pancreatitis. The severity of the lesion may be modified by the administration of antibiotics or by pancreatic duct ligation. At present, the clinical significance of these laboratory observations is difficult to assess except to say that the obstructed duodenum may elaborate a factor or factors which may provoke pancreatic inflammation (Fig. 9).

### Vascular Factors

Interference with the arterial blood supply to the pancreas has been shown to cause pancreatic lesions. The magnitude of the pancreatic injury appears to correlate well with the degree of occlusion of the terminal vascular radicals (Figs. 10 to 14). Panum (1862) provoked focal hemorrhagic infarcts by injecting wax particles into the pancreatic arteries of animals. It has been shown recently that gradations in the severity of pancreatic inflammation may be obtained by the injection of microspheres of various sizes into the pancreaticoduodenal arteries of animals. The smallest spheres (8 to 20 $\mu$) provoked the most severe forms of acute pancreatitis, suggesting that these smaller par-

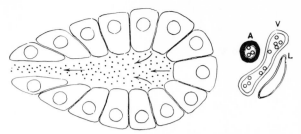

**Figure 10** Normal pancreas. Schematic representation of acinar cell grouping in normal pancreas. Arrows indicate direction of flow of enzymes (stippling) into duct. A, V, and L signify arterial, venous, and lymphatic vessels, respectively, in the interstitial area. (From Anderson, M. C., et al.: Surg. Clin. N. Amer., 47:127, 1967.)

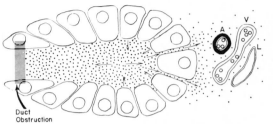

**Figure 11** Early pancreatitis: Enzymes enter interstitial area. (From Anderson, M. C., et al.: Surg. Clin. N. Amer., 47:127, 1967.)

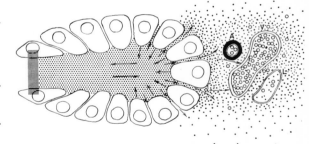

**Figure 12** Pancreatitis: Enzymes increase vascular permeability. (From Anderson, M. C., et al.: Surg. Clin. N. Amer., 47:127, 1967.)

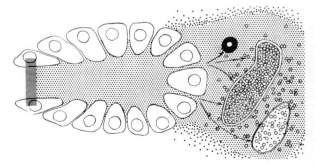

**Figure 13** Pancreatitis: (1) Massive interlobular extravasation, (2) venous dilatation and stasis, (3) red blood cells enter lymphatic circulation, (4) reduced circulating blood volume leading to splanchnic arterial constriction. (From Anderson, M. C., et al.: Surg. Clin. N. Amer., 47:127, 1967.)

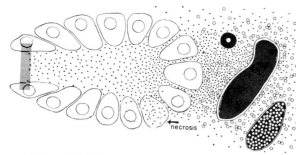

**Figure 14** Necrotizing pancreatitis: Arterial spasm, venous thrombosis, lymphatics obstructed with red blood cells, progressing to vascular insufficiency and finally cell death. (From Anderson, M. C., et al.: Surg. Clin. N. Amer., *47*:127, 1967.)

ticles occlude the terminal arterial supply, thus precluding the possibility of collateral arterialization which might maintain the viability of the acinar structures.

The importance of a vascular factor in determining the severity of the inflammatory process in the pancreas is suggested by the studies of Popper. He produced edematous pancreatitis in rats by ligation of the pancreatic ducts in conjunction with the administration of secretin. Subsequent and temporary occlusion of the gastroduodenal artery in this model was followed by the development of full-blown hemorrhagic pancreatitis.

### Clinical Disease

Despite the extensive literature describing experimental pancreatitis, the etiology of the human disease is unknown. Evidence in favor of ductal obstruction or reflux is meager and seems to apply to a disappointingly small number of patients. In the United States, the majority of persons who present with pancreatitis are chronic alcoholics. Many studies have sought to expose a direct toxic effect of alcohol on the pancreatic acini of experimental animals, but to date these efforts have been singularly unsuccessful. The most prevalent hypothesis concerning the role of alcohol in the production of the disease considers (1) the stimulated production of excessive amounts of highly alkaline juice, leading to alkalinization of the gland which results in instability of the zymogen membranes, *in combination with* (2) spasm of the sphincter of Oddi due to duodenal irritation as a local effect of alcohol. This hypothesis has the sanctity of conforming to experimental models that describe pancreatitis resulting from duct obstruction and stimulated secretion. The accuracy of the tenet remains to be proved. It has also been suggested that ethanol may interfere with the pancreatic production of naturally occurring trypsin inhibitor. However, at this time no data are available to support this concept.

Other significant factors that may have an etiologic role in clinical pancreatitis include biliary tract disease (10 to 20 per cent of patients) and operation (the "postoperative" group, 10 to 15 per cent of patients); about 10 to 15 per cent of pa-

tients acquire the disease in the absence of recognized contributory factors (idiopathic group). In addition, a multitude of infrequently cited causes include drug therapy such as corticosteroids and chlorothiazide, hyperparathyroidism, pregnancy, carcinoid disease, hyperlipemia, periarteritis nodosa, and trauma.

## DIAGNOSIS

The signs and symptoms of acute pancreatitis are variable in severity and dependent upon the structural alterations within the gland. In the milder edematous form of the disease, the patient usually complains of penetrating upper abdominal pain, often radiating to the flanks, shoulders, and back. On physical examination there is epigastric tenderness and a low-grade fever. In severe hemorrhagic pancreatitis, the patient may present with a rigid abdomen and signs of shock including sweating, tachycardia, and hypotension. Nausea, vomiting, and abdominal distention are common and jaundice may be detected in 20 to 25 per cent of patients. Rarely, discoloration of the skin may be visible in the flanks (Gray-Turner sign) or about the umbilicus (Cullen's sign) (Fig. 15).

In patients with the milder form of the disease, the differential diagnosis must consider biliary tract disease, peptic ulcer, appendicitis, and intestinal obstruction. Hemorrhagic pancreatitis must be differentiated from other catastrophic abdominal illness including strangulation obstruction, perforated peptic ulcer, and mesenteric vascular and intra-abdominal vascular crises which include ruptured abdominal aortic or dissecting aneurysms.

The association of high serum amylase activity in pancreatitis was first reported by Elman (1929) with the recommendation for its use as a diag-

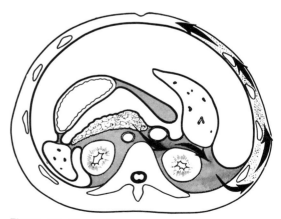

**Figure 15** Hemorrhage through the retroperitoneal space into the subcutaneous fat leads to ecchymosis and discoloration in one or both flanks (Gray-Turner sign). A deposit of iron salts may lead to permanent discoloration. (From Ellison, E. H., and Carey, L. C. In: Davis, L., ed.: Christopher's Textbook of Surgery. 9th ed. Philadelphia, W. B. Saunders Company, 1968.)

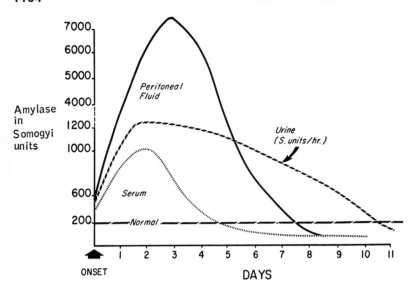

**Figure 16** Knowledge of the relative amylase values in the serum, urine, and peritoneal fluid is helpful when subsiding pancreatitis is suspected. (From Ellison, E. H., and Carey, L. C. In: Davis, L., ed.: Christopher's Textbook of Surgery. 9th ed. Philadelphia, W. B. Saunders Company, 1968.)

nostic test. Prior to this observation, the recognition of pancreatitis was confined to the operating or autopsy rooms. Usually the serum amylase is elevated within 2 to 12 hours of the onset of symptoms and returns to normal within 3 or 4 days. Pseudocyst formation may be associated with prolonged hyperamylasemia. At present it is impossible to predict either the certainty of pancreatitis or the severity of the process from the blood level of amylase activity. In general it may be stated that the higher this activity the greater the probability of acute pancreatitis. Hyperamylasemia may be found in patients with biliary tract disease, alcoholism in the absence of pancreatitis, perforated peptic ulcer, intestinal obstruction, mesenteric thrombosis, ectopic pregnancy, and, often, after the use of drugs such as meperidine (Demerol) or morphine.

The rate of urinary amylase excretion has been found to reflect the amount of amylase released from the pancreas into the blood. The use of the urinary amylase test in addition to serum amylase determination will magnify the precision of the diagnosis of acute pancreatitis by a factor of 2. The urinary excretion of amylase in excess of 1000 units per hour is found almost exclusively in patients with acute pancreatitis, whereas lesser rates of amylase excretion are more frequently associated with other diseases (Fig. 16).

Elevation in the serum and urinary lipase activities is associated with acute pancreatitis. Interpretations of the results of the lipase tests are subject to the same constraints as applied to the amylase determinations since hyperlipasemia has been recorded in patients with nonpancreatic gastrointestinal disease.

In some patients, thoracentesis or paracentesis may be indicated to aid in establishing an accurate diagnosis. Examination of the fluid obtained for both lipase and amylase activity may be helpful since the enzyme levels may be increased in these fluids for prolonged periods of time. A smear and culture of the fluid are important to rule out the presence of bowel contents and infection.

X-ray examinations of the chest and abdomen may be useful in establishing the diagnosis of pancreatitis. Roentgenograms of the abdomen may reveal pancreatic or biliary calcifications that suggest the pancreas as the site of origin for the patient's symptoms. The identification of a single dilated loop of small bowel, usually in the left upper quadrant, provides contributory evidence for the diagnosis. When the patient's condition permits, roentgenographic examination of the upper gastrointestinal tract with barium may be helpful. The C loop described by the course of the duodenum may be enlarged as a result of swelling of the head of the pancreas, and the contrast pattern of the duodenal mucosa may be coarse owing to the swelling imposed by lymphatic and venous obstruction. On lateral films the stomach may be displaced anteriorly because of extensive retroperitoneal edema surrounding the pancreas which resembles an extensive phlegmon. This abnormality may herald the accumulation of fluid in the lesser sac either derived from the pancreatic juice or due to abscess formation (Fig. 17).

Other laboratory studies have less value as aids in the confirmation of the diagnosis of acute pancreatitis yet may be of singular importance in guiding the therapy. The hematocrit must be followed serially as a guide to the repletion of plasma volume. An elevation in hematocrit is a common finding in patients first seen with severe pancreatitis. Hypocalcemia is a common accompaniment to severe necrotizing pancreatitis, and serum levels below 9 mg. per 100 ml. are common. Hypocalcemia may persist for many days, even after serum amylase activity has returned to normal. Electrocardiographic abnormalities that may attend this electrolyte disturbance include variable prolongation of the Q-T segment, suppression of the S-T segment, and flattening of the T waves. These findings may be seen in hypokalemia as

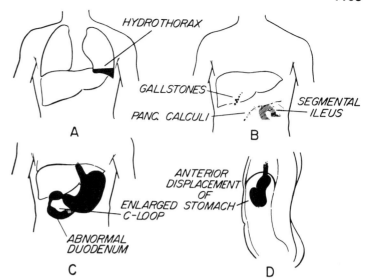

**Figure 17** Some of the more common roentgenographic findings in acute pancreatitis. (From Ellison, E. H., and Carey, L. C. In: Davis, L., ed.: Christopher's Textbook of Surgery, 9th ed. Philadelphia, W. B. Saunders Company, 1968.)

well, and this abnormality may exist in combination with hypocalcemia.

Many patients with pancreatitis present with tachypnea and about one-third of the fatalities due to pancreatitis are associated with respiratory failure. When rapid and shallow respirations are observed, blood gas analysis is indicated, including determination of $pO_2$, $pCO_2$, and pH. The finding of abnormal gas exchange should be regarded as an ominous sign indicating the need for respiratory assistance.

### THERAPY

Shock complicating the course of acute pancreatitis requires prompt and aggressive therapy. This potentially lethal complication is due to a critical reduction in plasma volume. Hemodynamic studies of such patients have revealed reductions in mean arterial blood pressure and cardiac output associated with an increase in peripheral resistance. Rapid expansion of the constricted plasma volume will reverse these hemodynamic changes and result in increased urine output and correction of the accompanying metabolic acidosis. Control of the rates of administration of the large volumes of colloid and crystalloid solutions required for resuscitation may be achieved most successfully by serial monitoring of central venous pressure, hematocrit, urine output, $pO_2$, pH, and $pCO_2$. Additional therapy is aimed at the suppression of pancreatic secretion, relief of pain, correction of specific electrolyte disorders, and prevention of abscess formation.

Continuous nasogastric suction is used to inhibit hydrogen ion-stimulated release of secretin and pancreozymin-cholecystokinin. In addition, swallowed air is aspirated, to prevent increase in the distention that may be present when the patient is first seen. Anticholinergic agents such as propantheline bromide may be administered in the attempt to suppress pancreatic secretion. These agents should be avoided if clinical shock is evident and in patients with glaucoma.

Relief of severe pain which usually accompanies acute pancreatitis may be difficult. The most effective drugs, morphine and meperidine, both cause spasm of the sphincter of Oddi, resulting in increased intrabiliary pressures. The requirement for large doses of these drugs in the therapy of such pain may be avoided if splanchnic nerve block is successful.

As indicated previously, hypokalemia or hypocalcemia or both may occur and precipitate disturbances in cardiac function. Repletion with intravenous potassium salts must be accompanied by electrocardiographic monitoring, and they must be administered cautiously when any degree of oliguria is present. The intravenous injection of calcium salts is reserved for the therapy of tetany as signaled by the appearance of positive Chvostek or Trousseau signs.

The use of antienzyme preparations in the therapy of acute pancreatitis is prevalent in Europe. Theoretically, inhibition of proteolytic activity might affect the course of pancreatitis. The release of trypsin from the afflicted gland is capable, in turn, of activating pancreatic kallikrein, another proteolytic ferment which splits the vasoactive decapeptide, kallidin, from an $\alpha_2$ globulin. This peptide is a potent vasodilator and hypotensive agent. An antitryptic-antikallikrein polypeptide (Trasylol) has been extracted from bovine parotid glands. This agent has been shown to inhibit trypsin, chymotrypsin, kallikrein, and plasmin. Despite the demonstration of potent in vitro antiproteolytic activity, the efficacy of Trasylol in modifying experimental pancreatitis is still unclear. It is probable that the drug is not effective in preventing or modifying acute severe hemorrhagic pancreatitis but it may reduce the mortality that attends experimental duct obstruction. The clinical data concerning the use of Trasylol are even more controversial owing primarily to the anecdotal quality of the recorded experience. One prospective study has failed to demonstrate significant therapeutic benefit following the use of the agent.

Antibiotics are usually given to patients with severe acute pancreatitis. The rationale for this therapy has been based on experimental data showing an improvement with antibiotic therapy in the survival of animals suffering pancreatitis provoked by duodenal obstruction. The clinical efficacy of antibiotic therapy is not known although the institution of such therapy is clearly indicated if sepsis complicates the course of pancreatitis. Occasionally, abscess of the lesser sac occurs during the course of this illness and antimicrobial therapy in addition to surgical drainage is mandatory. The appearance of retroperitoneal or lesser sac sepsis is usually signaled by the appearance of high fever, chills, and prostration and the rapid development of a retrogastric mass. Occasionally, all of these signs may be mimicked by acute massive pancreatic necrosis with the rapid release of large amounts of ferments. Should an exploratory celiotomy uncover massive necrosis without abscess formation, the patient may be helped by removal of necrotic tissue or drainage of the peripancreatic fluid. In general, the therapy of acute pancreatitis is considered to be nonoperative; however, a more aggressive approach should be strongly considered when massive necrosis or infection is in evidence.[1-3, 14, 21, 28, 29, 35, 40, 54, 55, 57, 59, 60-64, 66, 68, 70, 72, 75, 77, 78, 85-89, 93]

## TRAUMA

The majority of pancreatic injuries seen in large urban centers come from penetrating wounds of the abdomen. The surgical management of isolated pancreatic injuries has been greatly improved in the last decade and should but rarely cause death. As the pancreas is closely approximated by several other organs, its involvement in multiple organ injuries is rather common. In addition, the aorta, inferior vena cava, superior mesenteric artery and vein, and splenic vessels pass along the posterior surface of the pancreas. Thus, while multiple organ injury will increase the mortality, by far the major cause of death in wounds involving the pancreas is an associated blood vessel injury with massive hemorrhage.

The fixed retroperitoneal position of the pancreas, especially as it crosses the vertebral column, makes the pancreas extremely vulnerable to injury in nonpenetrating upper abdominal trauma, with the head and neck of the gland being most susceptible. A not uncommon finding is laceration of the neck of the gland, which lies anterior to the vertebral column; occasionally there is complete disruption with exposure of the superior mesenteric vessels. Failure to visualize the pancreas during abdominal exploration for trauma has led

to many complications and even death. This mistake is usually made when there is an obvious injury to another organ, such as deep liver laceration, which seemingly accounts for the patient's clinical findings.

## DIAGNOSIS

Of primary concern in the early management of abdominal trauma is whether or not operation is necessary. Until recently this was not a problem with penetrating injuries, as the accepted practice was to explore all patients. However, there are now an increasing number of surgeons who believe that exploration is not indicated in a large percentage of abdominal stab wounds, and in some centers even some bullet wounds of the abdomen may be followed expectantly. This practice requires careful assessment at frequent intervals of the patient's general condition and abdominal findings. Thus, in some penetrating as well as nonpenetrating injuries, the accumulation and interpretation of data regarding the possibility of serious intra-abdominal injury are of great importance.

Instigation for abdominal exploration comes primarily from signs of peritonitis or serious intra-abdominal hemorrhage. In some patients severe injury is first evidenced by signs of abdominal distention, tenderness, or rigidity. In other instances changes in vital signs, a decrease in hematocrit, and a falling urinary output may be seen with normal abdominal findings. In doubtful circumstances a four-quadrant paracentesis may facilitate early exploration by demonstrating intra-abdominal bleeding or fluid accumulation with a high amylase content.

An isolated injury to the pancreas may produce little early evidence of severe intra-abdominal injury. By far the most frequent cause for immediate operation is evidence of intra-abdominal bleeding. When this is not present the abdominal findings may be minimal for 2 to 3 days, after which time tenderness and distention usually occur. An elevated serum amylase is most helpful in minimizing the delay in diagnosis, although there is not total agreement that hyperamylasemia, of itself, is an indication for abdominal exploration. With nonpenetrating trauma a patient actually may be asymptomatic for weeks or months, until a pseudocyst develops or distal pancreatitis occurs secondary to a ductal stricture.

## SURGICAL TREATMENT

There are a variety of surgical techniques that are useful in the management of different types of pancreatic injury. The most useful procedures include the following:

### External Drainage of the Injured Tissue

This is a fundamental method and is used in the majority of patients. When there is contusion or laceration, with no evidence of major duct disruption, external drainage is usually the treatment of choice. It should be emphasized that "sump-type" drainage should be employed, as this technique has been shown to be superior to simple drainage. Although there will be a significant occurrence of fistulas and pseudocysts, the safety of the procedure warrants its frequent utilization.

### Re-establishment of Pancreatic Duct Drainage

The need for these procedures is greatest in transection injuries due to blunt trauma. One approach is to anastomose the two severed ends of the duct but the fact that these ducts are frequently quite small poses a considerable technical problem. A technique of increasing popularity is Roux-en-Y drainage of the disrupted pancreas. The anastomosis is usually performed to the severed end of the distal remnant of pancreas with simple closure of the opened surface of the proximal segment. However, if there is reason to suspect possible ductal obstruction in the head, then each pancreatic segment can be drained into the Roux-en-Y loop (Fig. 18). These procedures have the advantage of maximal preservation of pancreatic tissue and are most clearly indicated for localized transecting injuries of the head and neck. Although simple closure of both ends of the transected pancreas has been advocated, in our experience this has led to death from traumatic pancreatitis of the distal (obstructed) remnant and should be used rarely.

### Excision

There is rarely an indication for total pancreatectomy for trauma but both distal and proximal subtotal pancreatectomy are being utilized with increasing frequency. An edematous, lacerated, hemorrhagic tail of the pancreas is frequently handled more safely by excision than by the more conservative methods of external or internal drainage. These are instances in which the

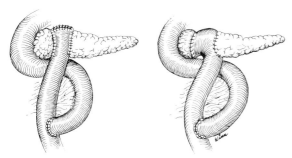

**Figure 18**   Diagrammatic illustration of a Roux-en-Y pancreaticojejunostomy. In this instance both proximal and distal pancreas were anastomosed to the loop following a transection injury to the neck of the pancreas. Note the isoperistaltic character of the drainage limb, which protects against reflux of intestinal contents. The Roux-en-Y technique is widely used in drainage procedures for chronic pancreatitis and pancreatic cysts. *Left,* redrawn (from Jones, R. C., and Shires, G. T.: Arch. Surg., *90*:502, 1965.)

experience and judgment of the surgeon are of great importance. The Whipple operation for resection of the head of the pancreas is a procedure of considerably greater magnitude than simple distal pancreatectomy. However, when there is extensive disruption of the duodenum and the head of the pancreas, a Whipple procedure may be the safest method of management. An increasing number of these operations have been done in recent years and with an apparently lowered mortality in these extremely serious injuries. The postoperative morbidity is not as great as that seen following operation for malignant disease, and near-normal nutritional and metabolic status is usually attained.[31, 50, 51, 80]

## CHRONIC PANCREATITIS

The term *chronic pancreatitis* (or chronic relapsing pancreatitis) implies continuing anatomic changes of pancreatitis even during long asymptomatic periods. Such chronicity can be difficult to establish as several bouts of acute pancreatitis may occur with return to an essentially normal status. Also, most patients with early chronic pancreatitis have asymptomatic periods. The concept is useful, nevertheless, in that it designates a stage of pancreatitis characterized by essentially irreversible change.

The etiology of chronic pancreatitis presumably is as varied as that of acute pancreatitis. There are well established relationships with such conditions as biliary tract disease, chronic alcoholism, mumps, hyperparathyroidism, and a genetic disorder characterized by excessive urinary excretion of certain amino acids, especially cystine and lysine. However, the actual pathogenesis of chronic pancreatitis remains unknown. Although there is a direct effect of alcohol on the pancreas, a primary "cirrhosis" type of reaction has not been confirmed. Many believe that obstruction at the ampulla of Vater is a factor common to biliary tract disease and alcoholism. Spasm and edema of the sphincter of Oddi with biliary tract disease is generally accepted, while alcohol presumably causes edema and inflammation of the papilla of Vater by its local effects. Neither of these concepts has been proved, nor, in fact, has the concept of ampullary obstruction been totally accepted. However, intrapancreatic duct obstruction at one or more places can be demonstrated in most instances of advanced chronic pancreatitis.

### DIAGNOSIS

#### Clinical Manifestations

Diagnosis can be a difficult task and a considerable number of patients with "idiopathic" chronic pancreatitis are treated for psychiatric problems before the true nature of their disease is established. Nevertheless, the syndrome is now well known and a high index of suspicion should lead to the correct diagnosis in most instances. The "typical" patient is a heavy drinker who begins to experience attacks of abdominal pain. The pain is usually epigastric in location and frequently radiates to the left hypochondrium and into the back. With an elevation in serum amylase, serum lipase, or urinary amylase during an acute exacerbation, the diagnosis is strengthened (see diagnosis of acute pancreatitis).

From a practical standpoint the basic tool of diagnosis is documentation of attacks of acute pancreatitis with less severe but continuing symptoms between periods of exacerbation. The confirmation of permanent pathologic changes is sometimes difficult but if the classic triad of *weight loss, diabetes,* and *steatorrhea* has developed, severe pancreatic disease can be assumed to be present.

### Laboratory Aids

In addition to the conventional laboratory tests for acute pancreatitis, the diagnosis of chronic pancreatitis relies heavily upon demonstrating changes in the exocrine functions or endocrine functions (or both) of the pancreas. One simple approach is to examine the stool chemically or microscopically for an increase in fat, and steatorrhea is demonstrated in many patients with grossly normal stools. With improved methods for duodenal aspiration, the measurement of pancreatic enzymes following a meal or secretin stimulation has added greatly to accuracy in detecting relatively early changes in exocrine function. In similar fashion, a glucose tolerance test will frequently be abnormal in spite of a normal fasting blood sugar. Obstructive jaundice can occur with chronic pancreatitis and when it is present the differential diagnosis from tumor can be difficult.

### Radiographic Aids to Diagnosis

Pancreatic calcification in combination with the clinical history just presented is presumptive evidence of chronic pancreatitis. Such calcifications may be intraductal or diffusely scattered within the parenchyma. Cholecystography is an important adjunct to diagnosis, and primary biliary tract disease is frequently the key to the diagnosis of associated chronic pancreatitis. An upper gastro-intestinal series is occasionally helpful and hypotonic duodenography has increased the accuracy of diagnosis by elucidating more subtle changes in pancreatic-duodenal anatomy. Improvements in pancreatic scanning have given hope that this technique will become increasingly helpful in diagnosis. Selective angiography is generally nonspecific and does not warrant routine utilization.

### Indications for Operative Intervention

The one virtually unassailable indication for operative intervention is the diagnosis of primary biliary tract disease as evidenced by gallstones or nonvisualization of the gallbladder on repeated examinations. However, it should be emphasized that a "normal" gallbladder may not be visualized

for several days after an attack of acute pancreatitis. Apart from this group of patients, the indications for operation are often controversial. This reflects the inability to ascertain the point at which the disease is unresponsive to medical therapy, the fear of mortality and morbidity from an operation, and the uncertainty of obtaining relief of symptoms by the surgical procedure. Theoretically, it would seem advisable to institute surgical therapy before pancreatic function is seriously impaired, but the patient usually seen in the surgical service has had multiple attacks of pancreatitis requiring either admission to the hospital or treatment in the emergency room, and is found to have far-advanced chronic pancreatitis.

## SURGICAL TREATMENT

The multiplicity of procedures recommended for the surgical treatment of chronic pancreatitis is indicative of the failure of any one operation to satisfy the needs of all patients. One of the problems in assessment of surgical therapeutics has been the tendency of a surgeon to apply one or two operations to virtually all patients with the disease. Each patient must be individually studied and the nature and extent of the disease carefully documented in order to facilitate rational choice of a surgical procedure. The fundamental principles of surgical therapy are as follows:

**Correction of Primary Biliary Tract Disease.** As the available evidence overwhelmingly supports the concept that primary biliary tract disease can initiate pancreatitis, it is logical that correction of the biliary tract disease should be a major aim of surgical therapy.

**Relief of Ductal Obstruction.** Improvement in pancreatic function is one of the aims of pancreatic ductal decompression. In patients seen fairly soon after onset of the disease, the relief of obstruction is thought to diminish the likelihood of recurrent episodes of acute pancreatitis and thus stop, or at least delay, further pancreatic fibrosis. However, in most cases the pancreatic changes are quite diffuse and significant improvement is hard to document; that further deterioration can occur was documented by DuVal and Enquist. From an empiric viewpoint the major achievement of successful relief of ductal obstruction has been the control of pain.

**Relief of Pain.** It is widely believed that the pain of chronic pancreatitis is caused by ductal distention secondary to incomplete ductal obstruction. This concept has been tested by procedures designed to decompress the pancreatic ducts, and successful control of pain has been confirmed by several reliable investigators. Other approaches to control of pain include extirpation of all or a major portion of the pancreas and interruption of the splanchnic nerves, the mediators of visceral pain.

### Surgical Procedures and Indications for Their Use

**Operations on the Biliary Tract.** The one unquestioned indication for operation in chronic pan-

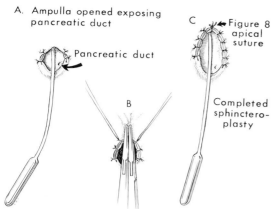

A. Ampulla opened exposing pancreatic duct

Pancreatic duct

C — Figure 8 apical suture

B

Completed sphincteroplasty

**Figure 19** Diagrammatic illustration of a sphincteroplasty. When performed in this manner, and as contrasted to simple sphincterotomy, obstruction rarely recurs. (Courtesy of S. Austin Jones and Louis L. Smith, Loma Linda University and University of California, Irvine.)

creatitis is associated primary biliary tract disease. Simple removal of a chronically diseased gallbladder, with or without common duct stones, has successfully controlled the pancreatitis in about 80 per cent of such patients. As these are relatively safe procedures, without significant metabolic sequelae, there is universal agreement as to their usefulness in the therapy of pancreatitis. However, simple nonvisualization of the gallbladder, as occurs frequently during acute exacerbation of pancreatitis, should not be misconstrued as primary biliary tract disease. Cholecystectomy frequently has been augmented by sphincteroplasty when there are multiple common duct stones or when symptoms recur after operation upon the biliary tract.

**Sphincteroplasty.** It has been shown that a simple sphincterotomy will generally close within a few weeks' time with restoration of preoperative common bile duct pressure. However, a properly performed sphincteroplasty has been shown to remain widely patent and to alleviate completely common bile duct obstruction at the ampulla (Fig. 19). The use of sphincteroplasty in the management of chronic pancreatitis is based upon the theory that ampullary obstruction is a basic mechanism causing pancreatitis in some patients and that a "common channel" is found in the great majority of patients with chronic pancreatitis. If the bile duct is widely opened, this should, therefore, decompress the pancreatic duct also (Fig. 20). That sphincteroplasty can have significant success in the control of the symptoms of pancreatitis is indicated by the studies of Jones et al.[48] and Nardi and Acosta.[60] However, correct utilization of this procedure demands that intrapancreatic ductal obstruction must be ruled out, usually by operative pancreatography. If intrapancreatic obstruction is found, other procedures must be substituted for, or combined with, sphincteroplasty if a successful result is to be anticipated. In the absence of intrapancreatic ductal obstruction or dilatation, 75 to 90 per cent of patients undergoing sphincteroplasty should have a good to excellent result. The lower figure is for alcoholic pancreatitis and the better results are obtained in biliary and "idiopathic" pancreatitis.

**Direct Pancreatic Ductal Drainage.** The general indications for the use of direct duct decompression procedures are intrapancreatic duct strictures (which invalidate sphincteroplasty) and the desire to preserve endocrine function sufficient to avoid insulin dependency. The initial concept of retrograde drainage of the pancreas by anastomosis of the major pancreatic duct to a loop of jejunum was that of DuVal.[25] Subsequent modifications have

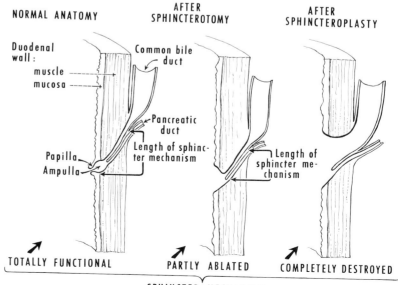

**Figure 20** Diagrammatic demonstration of the differences between sphincteroplasty and sphincterotomy. Physiologic studies have confirmed the loss of sphincteric function following a sphincteroplasty. (Courtesy of S. Austin Jones and Louis L. Smith, Loma Linda University and University of California, Irvine.)

NORMAL ANATOMY

AFTER SPHINCTEROTOMY

AFTER SPHINCTEROPLASTY

Duodenal wall:
muscle
mucosa

Common bile duct

Pancreatic duct

Length of sphincter mechanism

Papilla

Ampulla

Length of sphincter mechanism

TOTALLY FUNCTIONAL

PARTLY ABLATED

COMPLETELY DESTROYED

SPHINCTER MECHANISM

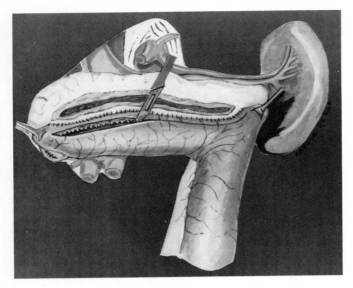

**Figure 21** Diagrammatic illustration of a longitudinal pancreaticojejunostomy. Note the opening of a dilated pancreatic duct throughout most of its length. A Roux-en-Y loop of jejunum is being opened following placement of the inferior row of sutures. (Courtesy of C. B. Puestow, Veterans Administration Hospital, Hines, Ill.)

been developed to increase the efficacy of this operation, the most basic alteration being recommended by Puestow and Gillesby.[69] In the Puestow procedure a long, longitudinal incision is made throughout the length of the duct until all strictures have been opened (Fig. 21). A Roux-en-Y loop of jejunum is then anastomosed over this widely opened ductal system, thus affording free drainage to areas obstructed between ductal strictures (Fig. 22). Such procedures have in general been successful in controlling pain in 80 per cent or more of patients but there is rarely evidence of significant improvement of pancreatic endocrine function. Of great importance is preservation of the islet cell mass, as few patients are immediately converted to insulin-dependent diabetics. This remains the greatest advantage of such procedures over the use of major pancreatic resections.

**Extirpative Procedures.** Total and near-total

pancreatectomies have been accomplished by a number of investigators and excellent relief of pain has been achieved, whereas less extensive resections (50 to 75 per cent) are followed by a significant failure rate. An important addition to the therapy of severe chronic pancreatitis has been the work of Child and his associates[19] in the development of the 95 per cent distal pancreatectomy (Fig. 23). This procedure, which leaves the stomach and duodenum in their normal anatomic position, has been quite successful in the relief of pain and is superior to the Whipple procedure and total pancreatectomy in that exocrine replacement and nutritional restoration are more readily accomplished. In addition, the mortality has been surprisingly low, especially in the University of Michigan series. However, the great deterrent to routine use of these procedures is the conversion of the patient from a non-insulin-dependent status to that of an insulin-dependent diabetic. The possi-

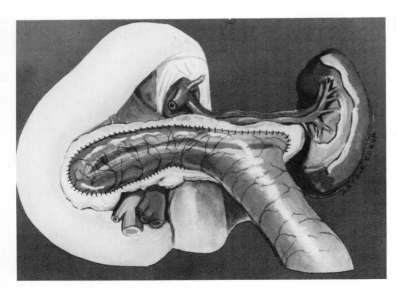

**Figure 22** The completed longitudinal pancreaticojejunostomy. Note the preservation of the entire pancreas. (Courtesy of C. B. Puestow, Veterans Administration Hospital, Hines, Ill.)

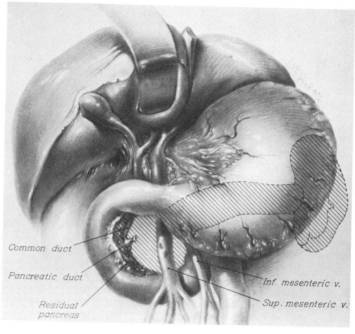

**Figure 23** General anatomic relationships of the pancreas demonstrated in a diagrammatic illustration of a 95 per cent pancreatectomy. This operation is of great value in the treatment of chronic pancreatitis. Note the small crescent of residual pancreas preserved for the protection of the pancreaticoduodenal arteries and the common bile duct. The superior mesenteric artery is not shown. (From Child, C. G., III, et al.: Surg. Gynec. Obstet., *129*:49, 1969.)

Common duct

Pancreatic duct

Residual pancreas

Inf. mesenteric v.

Sup. mesenteric v.

ble long-range complications are significant for any patient but in the alcoholic there is the added danger of diabetic acidosis or overdosage of insulin during periods of inebriation. The postpancreatectomy diabetic is frequently quite "brittle," requiring meticulous management of diet and insulin dosage. Deaths from diabetic complications are well documented in the literature and in the authors' series at least two patients have died within a few months after operation from failure to follow their prescribed regimen. However, these procedures, especially the 95 per cent pancreatectomy, have provided relief of pain and rehabilitation of patients who have not been helped by one or more of the drainage procedures. In nonalcoholic patients with advanced pancreatitis and alcoholic patients already insulin-dependent preoperatively, serious consideration should be given to such a procedure as the initial operation.

**Splanchnicectomy.** This procedure has been used by a number of investigators in the treatment of pancreatitis but the greatest experience has been in European clinics.[25] There is good documentation of initial control of pain in more than half the patients, although the duration of pain control need not necessarily be permanent. In the authors' experience, this operation has been particularly helpful when there has been failure of other operations to control the severe pain of pancreatitis and the patient is not considered a good social or medical candidate for pancreatectomy.[13, 15, 19, 23, 25, 26, 34, 36, 48, 49, 53, 69, 76, 83, 92]

## PANCREATIC CYSTS

A simple classification of cystic lesions of the pancreas is outlined in Table 1. Other than

cystadenomas, cystadenocarcinoma, and pseudocysts, pancreatic cysts are either quite rare in this country or usually diagnosed as an incidental finding at operation or autopsy. The so-called "retention cysts," which accounted for a significant proportion of the large series reported by Warren et al.,[8] are really obstructed pancreatic ducts and are managed coincidentally with the tumor or chronic pancreatitis.

Cystadenomas are benign lesions that are considered premalignant and may be difficult to differentiate from cystadenocarcinoma. Characteristically, both of these tumors develop slowly and unless obstruction of the common bile duct occurs, there are few early symptoms other than vague upper abdominal distress. A palpable mass is frequently discernible and barium studies, angiography, and pancreatic scan will usually give additional evidence of a pancreatic lesion. In the absence of pre-existing pancreatitis or pancreatic trauma, suggesting pseudocyst, a neoplastic cyst should be suspected when a large pancreatic mass can be clearly delineated preoperatively.

**TABLE 1** PANCREATIC CYSTS

A. True cysts
    congenital
    retention
    parasitic
    dermoid
B. Pseudocysts
C. Cystic tumors
    adenomatous
    carcinomatous

Whenever feasible, excision of neoplastic cysts should be accomplished. Five year survival following resection of a cystadenocarcinoma is not rare and the premalignant nature of the cystadenoma makes excision desirable. If extirpation is not possible, internal drainage of the cyst is indicated; external drainage may be followed by persistent fistula or growth of cancer to the abdominal wall.

## PANCREATIC PSEUDOCYSTS

Pseudocysts of the pancreas are thought to develop secondary to rupture of a pancreatic duct with escape of pancreatic juice into the surrounding tissues or spaces. The fluid becomes loculated and a fibrous wall results from the secondary inflammatory reaction. There is no epithelial lining to such a cyst wall, and this differentiates it from the various types of true cysts. Characteristically, the lesser omental bursa is the site of cyst formation and the cyst wall evolves from and is densely adherent to adjacent organs, i.e., duodenum, stomach, liver, and colon. There are numerous anatomic variations; mediastinal cysts, for instance, are well recognized. Occasionally the pancreatic fluid will reach the greater peritoneal cavity via a patent foramen of Winslow or leakage from a pseudocyst and *pancreatic ascites* may develop (see later).

### CLINICAL MANIFESTATIONS

A pseudocyst of the pancreas should be suspected in any patient with a history of pancreatitis or pancreatic trauma and a large retrogastric mass. Although some patients are essentially asymptomatic, in most instances there is upper abdominal pain or discomfort, loss of appetite, and weight loss. A mass is frequently palpable but is more clearly characterized by radiographic examination of the upper gastrointestinal tract. Figure 24 demonstrates the general type of radiographic findings but many variations are seen, dictated by the size and location of the cyst. With demonstration of such a large retrogastric mass, a persistently high serum amylase is strong confirmatory evidence of a pseudocyst; however, a significant proportion of pancreatic pseudocysts are seen in patients with a normal serum amylase. Other evidence of chronic pancreatitis such as pancreatic calcification, diabetes, or steatorrhea is also helpful. Generally, the typical history and radiographic findings readily establish the presumptive diagnosis.

It should be noted that a radiographically demonstrable retrogastric mass is frequently present 7 to 14 days after an episode of severe (necrotizing) pancreatitis. In these circumstances the mass may be composed of massively edematous

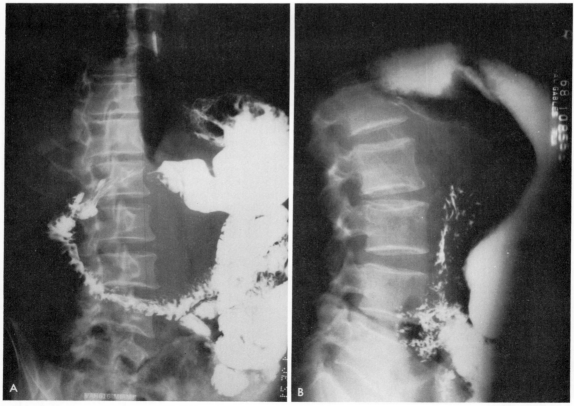

**Figure 24**   Radiographic findings "typical" of pancreatic pseudocysts. *A,* Markedly widened, smoothly contoured duodenal loop. *B,* Marked anterior displacement of the stomach indicative of a large retrogastric mass.

pancreas and retroperitoneal tissues without actual pseudocyst formation. Unless operation is imperative because of abscess, bleeding, or worsening of the patient's clinical status, a mass of this type will frequently resolve spontaneously. There is still considerable controversy as to how these early "cysts" should be handled. In the absence of sepsis, with normal vital signs and general clinical improvement, it is the authors' opinion that operative intervention should be withheld.

## Treatment

Nonoperative management of pseudocysts has been recommended but there do not appear to be enough data to substantiate this position. Some confusion in this regard exists because of differences in terminology. Thus, an acute lesser sac fluid accumulation, pancreatic abscess, and "chronic" pseudocyst can all be included under a definition of pseudocyst of the pancreas. The acute collections usually resolve spontaneously and an expectant regimen is generally justified. On the other hand, pancreatic abscess demands surgical intervention and external drainage is clearly the treatment of choice for most patients. In such situations a sump type of drain is more effective in fluid removal as bits of solid debris are usually present and seriously interfere with simple external drainage. However, the point at which an "acute" fluid accumulation becomes a "chronic" pseudocyst is a moot question. This is important because it implies both failure of spontaneous resolution and "maturity" of the cyst wall. The latter characteristic has been found to occur in an experimental model at about 4 weeks, while in the human 6 weeks might be more appropriate. In both the experimental animal and retrospective patient studies, the mature, or solidly formed, cyst wall lessened the complications of internal drainage procedures. There is general agreement that the chronic pseudocyst deserves surgical management to control symptoms and, presumably, lessen the incidence of the serious complications of bleeding, sepsis, or rupture of the cyst.

In the surgical management of pseudocyst (the term utilized here to denote chronicity) there are three primary methods: excision, external drainage, and internal drainage.

### Excision

Although it has several theoretical advantages, excision should be reserved for small cysts of the body or tail of the pancreas with minimal attachments to adjacent organs. Failure to observe this has resulted in an unacceptably high mortality.

### External Drainage

This was the treatment of choice for most surgeons until the relatively recent past. This judgment was predicated upon the belief that external drainage carried a lower mortality than internal drainage procedures. While it was readily demon-

strated that the morbidity of persistent fistula and recurrence of the cyst were greater with external drainage, it was not realized that the mortality (generally due to bleeding or sepsis) was as high as that following internal drainage procedures. However, external drainage is still the preferred technique for infected cysts, pancreatic abscesses, and cysts requiring drainage during the 4 to 6 week period required for maturation of the cyst wall.

### Internal Drainage

The choice of operation and surgical technique employed must be founded upon the following fundamental principles: (1) a suture anastomosis to the fibrous cyst wall cannot be relied upon to prevent leakage; (2) reflux of gastrointestinal contents into the cyst cavity should be prevented; and (3) dependent drainage is highly desirable. Of the several methods of internal drainage, by far the most useful are transgastric cystgastrostomy and cystojejunostomy to a Roux-en-Y loop of jejunum.

The transgastric cystgastrostomy has advantages of speed and ease of performance. As the cyst wall is densely adherent to the posterior wall of the stomach, suture anastomosis is unnecessary, and, therefore, leakage into the peritoneal cavity can be obviated. The cystgastrostomy is performed by opening the anterior wall of the stomach and then incising through the posterior gastric wall into the cavity of the cyst. In order to minimize reflux of gastric contents into the cyst cavity, the cystgastrostomy incision should be short (generally 4 cm. or less) and if a biopsy of the cyst is desirable it should be obtained at a site other than through the gastrostomy. Careful hemostasis should be obtained as gastrointestinal bleeding is one of the major complications of cystgastrostomy as well as of the other types of drainage of pancreatic pseudocysts. Another potential disadvantage of cystgastrostomy is the lack of dependency of the drainage orifice when there is a very large cyst with depression of the transverse colon and mesocolon. Postoperatively cystgastrostomy patients should be maintained on gastric decompression with parenteral alimentation for at least several days. The gastric decompression can be accomplished effectively by a gastrostomy tube to which a small Penrose drain is sutured at its tip. The drain is passed through the cystgastrostomy site and helps prevent premature closure of the drainage orifice while suction on the gastrostomy catheter maintains gastric decompression.

A cystojejunostomy with a Roux-en-Y loop is an excellent procedure with the advantage that truly dependent drainage usually can be achieved with this operation. The Roux-en-Y loop, if sufficiently long (at least 30 cm.), protects against reflux of intestinal contents and a large drainage orifice is both possible and desirable. This allows for biopsy of the cyst wall and at the same time helps to prevent premature closure of the anastomotic site. In a number of instances the cystojejunostomy anastomosis has broken down and the usual sequence of events has been successful treatment of the recurrent pseudocyst at a second operation with the same loop of jejunum. Although the cystojejunostomy is a somewhat more demanding surgical procedure, it is certainly well within the capability of a well trained surgeon and is probably the choice for very large pancreatic pseudocysts.

The mortality inherent in any type of drainage procedure, whether external or internal, is closely related to the two major complications of bleeding or inadequate drainage and sepsis. The bleeding may come from the area of anastomosis, from the cyst wall, or from erosion of one of the large vessels adjacent to the cyst wall, frequently the splenic artery. Aggressive treatment of hemorrhage will frequently allow a successful outcome and reoperation should not be delayed unnecessarily.[11, 18, 20, 32, 38, 67, 81, 84]

## PANCREATIC ASCITES

An entity related to pseudocyst of the pancreas that is being recognized with increasing frequency is pancreatic ascites. This condition has been associated with leaking pseudocysts of the pancreas in the majority of cases thus far reported, and there has been evidence of communication of the pancreatic ductal system with the free peritoneal cavity in most instances. The usual clinical finding is a relatively small pseudocyst that has leaked into the peritoneal cavity and has a direct connection with the pancreatic ductal system. The diagnosis usually can be established readily by demonstrating a high amylase content in the ascitic fluid. Surgical therapy consists of drainage of the abdomen with appropriate drainage of the cystic lesion of the pancreas or duct. The results thus far have indicated an excellent response with little tendency to reaccumulation of ascites. It is of great importance to have a high index of suspicion of this condition in alcoholics with ascites, since confusion with cirrhotic ascites might easily occur. As medical therapy of pancreatic ascites is frequently unsuccessful and the surgical procedure for resistant cirrhotic ascites (side-to-side portacaval shunt) would be inappropriate and perhaps severely damaging, the necessity for establishing the type of ascites is obvious.[17, 74]

## TUMORS OF THE PANCREAS

Tumors of the pancreas most commonly originate from the two major histologic components of the organ, and thus may be classified appropriately into neoplasms of (1) exocrine origin and (2) endocrine origin.

### NEOPLASMS OF THE EXOCRINE GLANDS

The most common tumor of the pancreas is carcinoma of the exocrine glands. It is a disease of the aged with a peak incidence in the eighth decade; two-thirds of its victims are over 60 years of age. During those intervals of time when longevity was increasing with discernible rates, the incidence of pancreatic cancer increased as well, resulting in a trend toward increasing mortality from this disease.

### Symptoms

The symptoms of pancreatic cancer depend upon the location of the tumor. Regardless of the anatomic site, pain is the most common initial complaint. Characteristically, the pain is vague in quality but located in the epigastrium with radiation to the back. In tumors of the body and tail, the pain may be described in the left upper quadrant and back. Characteristically, the pain may be less severe in the erect position, and back pain may be eased by bending forward and flexing the left thigh. Rapid weight loss has been reported as the second most frequent complaint. The exact reason for this is not clear, but may be related to anorexia due to the abdominal pain and anxiety associated with undiagnosed illness. Frequently the abdominal pain due to cancer of the body or tail of the pancreas is not diagnosed until the disease is far advanced. Findings on routine gastrointestinal x-rays are usually negative early in the course of the disease.

Jaundice is an early sign in carcinoma of the head of the pancreas, particularly when the tumor is located in the periampullary area. For this reason, tumors of the head are likely to be less advanced than tumors of the body or tail at the time of surgical exploration.

### Diagnosis

The early diagnosis of carcinoma of the body of the pancreas requires a high index of suspicion, leading to early laparotomy. Frequently, patients arrive at near-terminal status during lengthy and often unproductive evaluation in the attempt to find the origin of vague abdominal pain. When jaundice is present, contributing to the triad composed of jaundice, weight loss, and pain, surgical exploration is usually carried out much sooner after the patient's initial complaints. Some of these patients will present with a palpable gallbladder in addition to jaundice (Courvoisier's law.) Conventional wisdom describes distention of the gallbladder when the common bile duct is obstructed by cancer, but not when the duct is obstructed by a stone. The reason given is that the gallbladder containing stones is fibrotic and incapable of distention. Clinical experience should tell us that this is not true, since the discovery of stones in a gallbladder distended as a result of carcinoma of the pancreas is not a rare event. The probable cause of distention of the gallbladder associated with obstruction of the common bile duct relates to the completeness of the occlusion. Obstruction due to stones is most often partial in extent, whereas obstruction by carcinoma is frequently complete, even at the onset.

Abnormalities of clinical chemical findings may

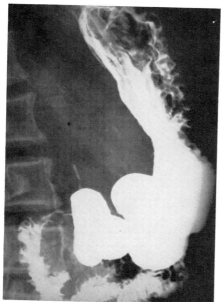

**Figure 25**  The "inverted 3" sign in a patient with an advanced adenocarcinoma of the head of the pancreas. Note the associated smoothing of the duodenal mucosal pattern. (From Ellison, E. H., and Carey, L. C. In: Davis, L., ed.: Christopher's Textbook of Surgery. 9th ed. Philadelphia, W. B. Saunders Company, 1968.)

be minimal or absent in this disease. In jaundiced patients with cancer of the head of the pancreas, laboratory tests reveal only those data which are indicative of the extrahepatic biliary obstruction, i.e., elevation of serum alkaline phosphatase ac-

tivity and high serum bilirubin concentration. This relative lack of utility of chemical studies in helping to establish the diagnosis of carcinoma of the pancreas has served as a stimulus for the study of other diagnostic techniques, primarily physical in nature. Examination of the upper intestinal tract with barium may be helpful in almost one-third of the patients with cancer of the head of the pancreas in demonstrating widening of the duodenal C loop, the "inverted three" sign, and evidence of external pressure on or invasion of the duodenum (Fig. 25). Percutaneous transhepatic cholangiography has been helpful when a tapered obstruction of the common bile duct is discovered. Radioisotopic scanning of the pancreas has been useful in some cases; however, there is no unanimity of opinion concerning the accuracy of this method. Selected visceral angiography has received attention as a potentially useful technique. The identification of a "tumor blush" in the distribution of the pancreatic blood supply may be diagnostic. Obviously, the degree of vascularization of the neoplasm is the most important factor influencing the accuracy of angiographic diagnosis, and this may vary considerably. Some tumors contain a rich microvascular network, whereas in others the vascularity is poor. Another technique that has recently received modest attention involves the use of ultrasound for the diagnosis of mass lesions within the abdominal cavity. Although echographic diagnosis of pancreatic lesions has been attempted, the resolution of the method is not yet established.

At present, it is fair to conclude that graphic visualization of the pancreas has not been accomplished satisfactorily and there is no technique

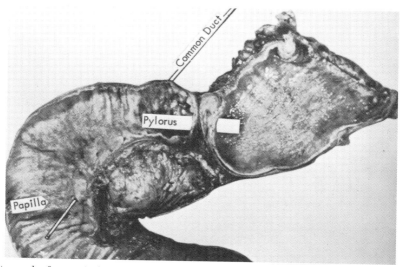

**Figure 26**  Photograph of a surgical specimen of carcinoma of the head of the pancreas. This 60 year old man gave a history of anorexia and mild abdominal distention for 8 weeks. Four weeks before admission he became jaundiced and thereafter lost 36 pounds in weight. At operation a tumor approximately the "size of a golf ball" was found in the head of the pancreas. Pancreaticoduodenectomy was performed. The patient died 48 hours postoperatively; at autopsy no residual tumor was found in the pancreas and no metastases were found in the lymph nodes or liver. (From Franz, V. K.: Atlas of Tumor Pathology, Section VII, Fascicles 27 and 28, Tumors of the Pancreas. Washington, D.C., Armed Forces Institute of Pathology, 1959.)

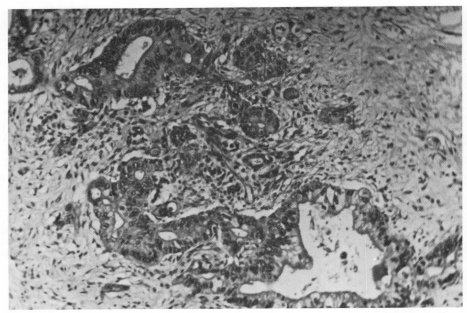

**Figure 27** Photomicrograph of this well differentiated adenocarcinoma showing tall columnar cells, some of them goblet cells, forming ducts. (From Franz, V. K.: Atlas of Tumor Pathology, Section VII, Fascicles 27 and 28, Tumors of the Pancreas. Washington, D.C., Armed Forces Institute of Pathology, 1959.)

available that has sufficient precision or reproducibility of results to be of important diagnostic value. The most precise diagnostic technique remains exploratory celiotomy in the hands of an experienced surgeon.

### Therapy

Pancreaticoduodenectomy is the only therapy with proven efficacy for the cure of cancer of the head of the pancreas. Unfortunately, the rate of success is modest, being approximately 10 per cent of patients who have had such resections. More frequently the exploration reveals a neoplasm that is incurable because of (1) metastases to other organs or lymph nodes or (2) invasion of vascular structures such as the portal vein and superior mesenteric vessels. Recently, the operative mortality associated with this procedure has

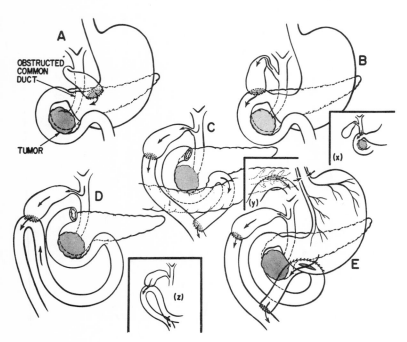

**Figure 28** Palliative procedures for nonresectable tumors of the head of the pancreas. *A,* Cholecystogastrostomy. *B,* Cholecystoduodenostomy and (x), choledochoduodenostomy. *C, D,* and (z), Several modifications of a cholecystojejunostomy. (y), Drainage of an obstructed pancreatic duct into the jejunum. *E,* Gastroenterostomy included to prevent duodenal obstruction. Vagotomy is added as a precaution against peptic ulceration, since the alkaline juices of the biliary tract have been routed away from the gastrojejunostomy. (From Ellison, E. H., and Carey, L. C. In: Davis, L., ed.: Christopher's Textbook of Surgery. 9th ed. Philadelphia, W. B. Saunders Company, 1968.)

been reduced to below 10 per cent, and studies involving as many as 40 patients have reported no deaths.

The operative procedure involves resection of the distal stomach, duodenum, and either part or all of the pancreas (Figs. 26 and 27). Total pancreatectomy has the advantage of precluding the appearance of local recurrence of the tumor in the pancreatic remnant. The major disadvantage rests in the fact that this procedure results in permanent diabetes mellitus and the continuing requirement for insulin therapy. Reconstruction of the gastrointestinal tract requires anastomosis between the biliary system (usually the common bile duct) and the jejunum, gastrojejunostomy, pancreaticojejunostomy, and establishment of intestinal continuity between the Roux-en-Y jejunal limb via a jejunojejunostomy. Vagotomy is advocated by some as an ancillary measure to inhibit gastric acid secretion and, in turn, the potential for gastrojejunal ulceration. In addition, the reconstruction requires that the inflow of alkaline bile and pancreatic juice be diverted proximal to the gastrojejunostomy to further protect against marginal ulceration.

If pancreaticoduodenectomy is not indicated because of the operative findings of incurability, then biliary diversion to relieve jaundice should be performed (Fig. 28). Cholecystoenterostomy is simple and effective. The possibility of impending duodenal obstruction must be considered and evaluated, and gastrojejunostomy should be a frequent accompaniment to biliary decompression. Surgical palliation may be improved by the addition of chemotherapy. The drug of choice is 5-fluorouracil, usually given intravenously.[10,30,33,39,44,56,71,73,82,91]

## Neoplasms of the Endocrine Glands

Recognition of hypoglycemia caused by pancreatic tumors of islet origin is a recent development dating to 1927. The first surgical cure of hyperinsulinism was reported in 1929, following the removal of an islet cell tumor.

### Symptoms

Symptoms of insulin-producing tumors are those of spontaneous hypoglycemia. The complaint may be of "fits" or "spells" which may represent a wide range of nervous system manifestations. Usually the attack of symptoms has a uniformity of psychophysical presentation, as well as time sequence in any given patient. The attacks occur in the fasting state, with blood sugar concentrations of less than 50 mg. per 100 ml., and are relieved promptly by the administration of sugar (Whipple's triad).

### Diagnosis

The simplest test for establishing the diagnosis of insulin-producing tumor was described by Whipple. It consists of withholding food from the patient and confirming Whipple's triad. This should be performed only in the hospital environ-

ment under continuous observation. It is not without risk, since convulsions, coma, and death may be precipitated by the hypoglycemia. Other useful tests include measurement of the serum insulin levels, which should be the most precise determinant in making the diagnosis and has the virtue of being risk-free. The tolbutamide infusion test may be helpful, but carries the risk of induced hypoglycemia. Tolbutamide is administered intravenously and provokes the release of insulin from the tumor. This results in a precipitous fall in blood sugar with delayed return to fasting levels.

### Therapy

Surgical therapy for insulin-producing tumors has been complicated by the fact that these neoplasms are usually small and difficult to find. Further, multiple tumors have an appearance frequency of 10 to 15 per cent and heterotopic location of an adenoma is not uncommon. Such complexity associated with the precise anatomic localization of the offending tissue has resulted in the requirement for subtotal pancreatectomy or pancreaticoduodenectomy for some of these patients.

Recently a new drug, diazoxide, has been introduced into the therapeutic armamentarium available for the treatment of hypoglycemia. This agent suppresses the release of insulin from both normal pancreatic islet tissue and adenomas, and its use has promised a future of nonoperative therapy for this difficult problem. While the magnitude of the effect of the blood sugar is only partially explained by the inhibition of insulin release, nonetheless the clinical efficacy of the agent has been striking.[37,45,58,90]

### Zollinger-Ellison Syndrome

Since the original report by Zollinger and Ellison in 1955, suggesting that non-beta cell tumors of the pancreatic islets might have causal relationship to severe, atypical peptic ulcer disease, this supposition has been confirmed handsomely. Furthermore, the tumors have been found to synthesize the polypeptide gastrin, and abnormally high concentrations of this substance have been detected in the circulating blood of these patients.

The diagnosis is suggested by the severity and resistance to therapy of the ulcer disease. Frequently, the peptic ulceration is discovered in atypical sites, such as distal duodenum or proximal jejunum. These patients have a marked elevation in basal acid secretion, presumably due to the perpetual and near-maximal stimulation of the parietal cell mass by the abnormal levels of circulating gastrin. Additional exogenous stimulation in the form of a monamine oxidase test with histamine or Histalog provokes little increase over the basal acid secretion. The diagnosis is confirmed by finding the serum gastrin concentrations to be elevated (greater than 1200 picograms per milliliter).

As in insulinomas, the surgical therapy of this condition is complicated by an inability to obtain

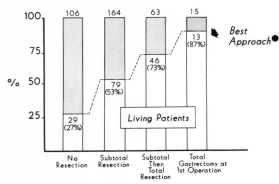

**Figure 29** Total gastrectomy at the initial surgical procedure has resulted in the greatest survival. Death in those patients undergoing total gastric resection after previous gastric surgery has been related to the need for emergency operations in poor-risk patients. (From Wilson, S. D., and Ellison, E. H.: Amer. J. Surg., *111*:787, 1966.)

precise anatomic localization of the offending tissue. First, more than 60 per cent of these tumors are malignant and many have metastasized by the time of discovery. Second, the benign lesions are often multiple. Experience has demonstrated clearly that total gastrectomy is the procedure of choice for this disease. The greatest percentage survival has been shown for patients who have undergone this operative procedure when compared to comparable patients subjected to operations of lesser magnitude[27, 94] (Fig. 29).

## SELECTED REFERENCES

Anderson, G., and Johnson, S. R.: Treatment of acute necrotizing pancreatitis. Acta Chir. Scand., *134*:311, 1968.
*This paper emphasizes the potential benefit of early and aggressive surgical therapy in acute necrosis of the pancreas. It reaffirms the concept of early surgery for selected patients proposed earlier by Lord Moynihan.*

Anderson, M. C.: Review of pancreatic disease. Surgery, *66*:434, 1969.
*This is a well written and succinct review of diseases of the pancreas.*

Banks, P. A., and Janowitz, H. D.: Some metabolic aspects of exocrine pancreatic disease. Gastroenterology, *56*:601, 1969.
*This is a well documented review article from a clinic with extensive experience in the study of normal and abnormal pancreatic function in man and animals. It is concise and well written.*

Banting, F. G., and Best, C. H. J.: The internal secretion of the pancreas. J. Lab. Clin. Med., *7*:251, 1922.
*This paper is a milestone in the efforts of investigators to obtain insulin from pancreatic extracts. Banting and Best induced acinar atrophy by ligation of the pancreatic ducts and subsequently obtained potent hypoglycemic extracts from the residual viable islet tissue.*

Barbosa, J. J. de C., Docherty, M. B., and Waugh, J. M.: Pancreatic heterotopia. Review of the literature and report of 41 authenticated surgical uses of which 25 were clinically significant. Surg. Gynec. Obstet., *82*:527, 1946.
*This paper is a valuable reference work, serving as a catalog of pancreatic heterotopia.*

Bayliss, W. M., and Starling, E. H.: The mechanism of pancreatic secretion. J. Physiol., *28*:325, 1902.
*This is a classic paper, containing the first description of the humoral control of pancreatic secretion by secretin.*

Cameron, J. L., Brawley, R. K., Bender, H. W., and Zuidema, G. D.: The treatment of pancreatic ascites. Ann. Surg., *170*:668, 1969.
*The authors make an excellent presentation of a large personal experience with chronic pancreatic ascites. Diagnostic methodology is clearly presented; confusion with cirrhotic ascites should be guarded against, as a substantial percentage of cases of both types of ascites occur in alcoholic patients. Operative radiographic examinations clearly establish duct disruption as a primary causative mechanism. Surgical therapy usually requires drainage of a pseudocyst of the pancreas or direct drainage of the leaking pancreatic duct.*

Child, C. G., Frey, C. F., and Fry, W. J.: A reappraisal of removal of ninety-five per cent of the distal portion of the pancreas. Surg. Gynec. Obstet., *129*:49, 1969.

Fry, W. J., and Child, C. G.: Ninety-five per cent distal pancreatectomy for chronic pancreatitis. Ann. Surg., *162*:543, 1965.
*These papers announce and confirm the importance of a major new tool for the treatment of chronic pancreatitis, the 95 per cent pancreatectomy. While not performed routinely, this procedure has greatly enhanced the surgical armamentarium with which to combat this difficult disease. In the authors' hands the mortality and morbidity have been surprisingly low and relief of symptoms excellent. The long-term results are influenced chiefly by the continued use of alcohol and drugs and the complications of diabetes.*

Cope, O., Culver, P. J., Mixture, C. G., Jr., and Nardi, G. L.: Pancreatitis, diagnostic clue to hyperparathyroidism. Ann. Surg., *145*:857, 1957.
*This important contribution calls attention to the relationship between pancreatitis and hyperparathyroidism.*

Dreiling, D. A., Druckerman, L. J., and Hollander, F.: The effect of complete vagisection and vagal stimulation on pancreatic secretion in man. Gastroenterology, *20*:578, 1952.
*An important set of observations concerning the quantitative aspects of vagal control of pancreatic secretion in man. The authors demonstrated a lack of effect by vagotomy on secretin-stimulated pancreatic secretion.*

Elman, R., Arneson, N., and Graham, E. A.: Value of blood amylase estimations in diagnosis of pancreatic disease: Clinical study. Arch. Surg., *19*:943, 1929.
*Although he is not often credited, Dr. Elman was the first to demonstrate the elevation of serum amylase in patients with pancreatitis.*

Folk, F. A., and Freeark, R. J.: Reoperations for pancreatic pseudocysts. Arch. Surg., *100*:430, 1970.
*The authors have had extensive experience in pancreatic surgery and utilize case presentations to highlight the various pitfalls incumbent on the treatment of pancreatic pseudocysts. An analysis of some of the causes of postoperative complications is pertinent and the general success achieved by reoperation is properly emphasized. However, sepsis, one of the major problems in the treatment of pseudocysts, was not encountered in this series.*

Halsted, W. S.: Retrojection of bile into the pancreas, a cause of acute hemorrhagic pancreatitis. Bull. Johns Hopkins Hosp., *12*:179, 1901.

Opie, E. L.: Etiology of acute pancreatitis. Bull. Johns Hopkins Hosp., *12*:182, 1901.
*These two papers laid the foundation for the "common channel theory" as an etiologic factor in the development of acute pancreatitis. Professor Opie described such an anatomic arrangement from postmortem studies and Professor Halsted demonstrated that the probable cause was the invasion of the pancreatic ducts by bile.*

Jones, R. C., and Shires, G. T.: The management of pancreatic injuries. Arch. Surg., *90*:502, 1965.
*This paper from one of the leading centers for the study of trauma is concise yet presents clearly the problems of pancreatic injury. The use of several surgical procedures is outlined and the resulting morbidity and mortality carefully analyzed. Aggressive treatment of pancreatic ductal injuries and resection of extensively traumatized pancreatic tissue has progressively lowered the mortality specifically due to the pancreas. Associated injuries continue to be the major cause of death.*

Jones, S. A., Steedman, R. A., Kellen, T. B., and Smith, L. L.:

Transduodenal sphincteroplasty (not sphincterotomy) for biliary and pancreatic disease. Amer. J. Surg., *118*:292, 1969.

*This paper, from the originators of the sphincteroplasty technique, is a most illuminating critique of the usefulness and limitations of this operation. The technical details necessary for a successful procedure are clearly outlined and the physiologic differences between sphincteroplasty and sphincterotomy documented. The careful analysis of mortality and immediate morbidity is impressive, as is the study of the long-term results of the operation. This report substantiates the usefulness of the procedure when correctly utilized and confirms the superior results with patients with primary biliary tract disease and other types of nonalcoholic pancreatitis as compared to those with alcoholic pancreatitis.*

Kalser, M. H., Leite, C. A., and Warren, W. D.: Fat assimilation after massive distal pancreatectomy. New Eng. J. Med., *279*:570, 1968.

*Careful documentation of the exocrine metabolic effects of 95 per cent pancreatectomy is presented. The surprisingly great residual function and ease of clinical management are in contrast to those seen after total pancreatectomy, which requires duodenal resection. When 20 to 25 per cent of normal pancreas was preserved, there were no clinical problems with either endocrine or exocrine function.*

Panum, P. L.: Experimentalle Beitrage zur Libre von der Embolie. Virchow's Arch. Path. Anat., *25*:308, 1862.

*This paper records for the first time the importance of the pancreatic circulation in the pathogenesis of pancreatitis. Professor Panum occluded small pancreatic arteries with paraffin emboli and described the changes of pancreatic inflammation.*

Pavlov, I. P.: The Works of the Digestive Glands. Translated by W. H. Thompson. London, Charles Griffin Company, 1910.

*This classic description of the neural influence on pancreatic secretion gives clear demonstration that the vagus is the secretory nerve of the pancreas and describes the first successful chronic pancreatic fistula preparation.*

Von Mering, J., and Minkowki, O.: Diabetes mellitus nach Pankreasexstirpation. Arch. Exp. Path. Pharmakol. 26:371, 1889.

*The authors were the first to establish the relationship between diabetes and the pancreas. They observed diabetes in a dog following removal of the pancreas.*

Warren, K. W., Braasch, J. H., and Thum, C. W.: Diagnosis and surgical treatment of carcinoma of the pancreas. Curr. Probl. Surg., June, 1968.

*This is an up-to-date and comprehensive treatise on the therapy of pancreatic cancer, and is an excellent reference source.*

Warren, W. D., Marsh, W. H., and Sandusky, W. R.: An appraisal of surgical procedures for pancreatic pseudocyst. Ann. Surg., *147*:903, 1958.

*This study, using an experimental model plus an extensive clinical survey, considers the fundamental principles of treating pancreatic pseudocysts. An understanding of the usefulness of a variety of procedures facilitates the correct choice of operation for a condition in which individual differences are of great importance.*

Webster, P. D., and Zieve, L.: Alterations in serum content of pancreatic enzymes. New Eng. J. Med., *267*:604, 1962.

Webster, P. D., and Zieve, L.: Alterations in serum content of pancreatic enzymes. New Eng. J. Med., *267*:654, 1962.

*These two manuscripts together are parts of a review of the significance of changes in pancreatic serum enzymes. The papers contain many helpful references and much important information.*

Whipple, A. O., and Frantz, V. K.: Adenoma of islet-cells with hyperinsulinism. A review. Ann. Surg., *101*:1299, 1935.

*This paper records the relationship between islet adenoma and hyperinsulinism. This is one of Dr. Allen Whipple's many firsts.*

Whipple, A. O., Parsons, W. W., and Mullins, C. R.: Treatment of carcinoma of the ampulla of Vater. Ann. Surg., *102*:763, 1935.

*This is the classic description of pancreaticoduodenectomy, or Whipple's procedure. This operation continues to be the surgical therapy of choice for carcinoma of the head of the pancreas or tumors of the ampulla of Vater.*

Zollinger, R. M., and Ellison, E. H.: Primary peptic ulcerations of the jejunum associated with islet-cell tumors of the pancreas. Ann. Surg., *142*:709, 1955.

## REFERENCES

1. Anderson, G., and Johnson, S. R.: Treatment of acute necrotizing pancreatitis. Acta Chir. Scand., *134*:311, 1968.
2. Anderson, M. C.: Review of pancreatic disease. Surgery, *66*:434, 1969.
3. Anderson, M. C., Schoenfeld, F. B., Iams, W. B., and Suwa, M.: Circulatory changes in acute pancreatitis. Surg. Clin. N. Amer., *47*:127, 1967.
4. Babkin, B. P.: Secretory Mechanisms of the Digestive Glands. 2nd ed. New York, Hoeber Medical Division, Harper & Row, 1950.
5. Balfour, J. F.: Pancreatic pseudocysts: Complications and their relation to the timing of treatment. Surg. Clin. N. Amer., *50*:395, 1970.
6. Banks, P. A., and Janowitz, H. D.: Some metabolic aspects of exocrine pancreatic disease. Gastroenterology, *56*:601, 1969.
7. Banting, F. G., and Best, C. H. J.: The internal secretion of the pancreas. J. Lab. Clin. Med., 7:251, 1922.
8. Barbosa, J. J. de C., Docherty, M. B., and Waugh, J. M.: Pancreatic heterotopia. Review of the literature and report of 41 authenticated surgical uses of which 25 were clinically significant. Surg. Gynec. Obstet., *82*:527, 1946.
9. Bayliss, W. M., and Starling, E. H.: The mechanism of pancreatic secretion. J. Physiol., *28*:325, 1902.
10. Beall, M. S., Dyer, G. A., and Stephenson, H. E., Jr.: Disappointments in the management of patients with malignancies of pancreas, duodenum and common bile duct. Arch. Surg., *101*:461, 1970.
11. Becker, W. F., Pratt, H. S., and Ganji, H.: Pseudocysts of the pancreas. Surg. Gynec. Obstet., *127*:744, 1968.
12. Behrens, O. K., and Bromer, W. W.: Glucagon, Vitamins and Hormones. Volume 16. New York, Academic Press, 1958.
13. Berk, J. E., and Guth, P. H.: Chronic pancreatitis. Med. Clin. N. Amer., *54*:479, 1970.
14. Bolooki, H., Minkowitz, S., Giammona, S. T., and Jude, J. R.: Respiratory failure in acute pancreatitis. J. Surg. Oncol., *3*:31, 1971.
15. Brom, B., and Kalser, M. H.: Diagnosis of pancreatic disease. J. Florida Med. Ass., *58*:29, 1971.
16. Brooks, F. P., and Manfredo, H.: The control of pancreatic secretion and its clinical significance. Amer. J. Gastroent., *42*:42, 1964.
17. Cameron, J. L., Brawley, R. K., Bender, H. W., and Zuidema, G. D.: The treatment of pancreatic ascites. Ann. Surg., *170*:668, 1969.
18. Cerilli, J., and Faris, T. D.: Pancreatic pseudocysts: delayed versus immediate treatment. Surgery, *61*:541, 1971.
19. Child, C. G., Frey, C. F., and Fry, W. J.: A reappraisal of removal of ninety-five percent of the distal portion of the pancreas. Surg. Gynec. Obstet., *129*:49, 1969.
20. Coghill, C. L.: Hemorrhage in pancreatic pseudocysts. Ann. Surg., *167*:112, 1968.
21. Cope, O., Culver, P. J., Mixter, C. G., Jr., and Nardi, G. L.: Pancreatitis, diagnostic clue to hyperparathyroidism. Ann. Surg., *145*:857, 1957.
22. Doubilet, H., and Mulholland, J. H.: Recurrent acute pancreatitis: Observations on etiology and surgical treatment. Ann. Surg., *128*:609, 1948.
23. Doubilet, H., and Mulholland, J. H.: Eight-year study of pancreatitis and sphincterotomy. J.A.M.A., *160*:521, 1956.
24. Dreiling, D. A., Druckerman, L. J., and Hollander, F.: The effect of complete vagisection and vagal stimulation on pancreatic secretion in man. Gastroenterology, *20*:578, 1952.
25. DuVal, M. K., Jr.: Caudal pancreaticojejunostomy for chronic relapsing pancreatitis. Ann. Surg., *140*:775, 1954.

26. DuVal, M. K., Jr., and Enquist, I. F.: Surgical treatment of chronic pancreatitis by pancreaticojejunostomy. An eight-year reappraisal. Surgery, 50:965, 1961.

27. Ellison, E. H., and Wilson, S. D.: The Zollinger-Ellison syndrome: reappraisal and evaluation of 260 registered cases. Ann. Surg., 160:512, 1964.

28. Elman, R., Arneson, N., and Graham, E. A.: Value of blood amylase estimations in diagnosis of pancreatic disease: Clinical study. Arch. Surg., 19:943, 1929.

29. Facey, F. L., Weil, M. H., and Rosoff, L.: Mechanism and treatment of shock associated with acute pancreatitis. Amer. J. Surg., 111:374, 1966.

30. Filly, R. A., and Freimanis, A. K.: Echographic diagnosis of pancreatic lesions. Radiology, 96:575, 1970.

31. Foley, W. J., Gaines, R. D., and Fry, W. J.: Pancreaticoduodenectomy for severe trauma to the head of the pancreas and associated structures. Ann. Surg., 170:759, 1969.

32. Folk, F. A., and Freeark, R. J.: Reoperations for pancreatic pseudocysts. Arch. Surg., 100:430, 1970.

33. Frantz, V. K.: Tumors of the Pancreas. In: Atlas of Tumor Pathology. Section VII. Washington, D.C., Armed Forces Institute of Pathology, 1959.

34. Fry, W. J., and Child, C. G.: Ninety-five per cent distal pancreatectomy for chronic pancreatitis. Ann. Surg., 162:543, 1965.

35. Gambill, E. E., and Mason, H. L.: One hour value for urinary amylase in 96 patients with pancreatitis. J.A.M.A., 186:130, 1963.

36. Gillesby, W. J., II, and Puestow, C. B.: Pancreaticojejunostomy for chronic relapsing pancreatitis: An evaluation. Surgery, 50:859, 1961.

37. Gray, R. K., Rösch, J., and Grothman, J. H., Jr.: Arteriography in the diagnosis of islet-cell tumors. Radiology, 97:39, 1970.

38. Greenstein, A., De Maio, E. F., and Nabseth, D. C.: Acute hemorrhage associated with pancreatic pseudocysts. Surgery, 69:58, 1971.

39. Grosfield, J. L., Clatworthy, H. W., Jr., and Hamondi, A. B.: Pancreatic malignancy in children. Arch. Surg., 101:370, 1970.

40. Halsted, W. S.: Retrojection of bile into the pancreas, a cause of acute hemorrhagic pancreatitis. Bull. Johns Hopkins Hosp., 12:179, 1901.

41. Harper, A. A.: Physiologic factors regulating pancreatic secretion. Gastroenterology, 36:386, 1959.

42. Heidenhain, R.: Beiträge zur Kenntnis des Pankreas. Arch. Ges. Physiol., 10:557, 1875.

43. Hokin, L. E.: Metabolic aspects and energetics of pancreatic secretion. In: American Physiological Society: Handbook of Physiology. Section 6, Alimentary Canal, Volume II, Secretion, ed. C. F. Code. Baltimore, Williams & Wilkins, 1967.

44. Howard, J. M.: Pancreatico-duodenectomy: Forty-one consecutive Whipple resections without an operative mortality. Ann. Surg., 168:629, 1968.

45. Howard, J. M., Moss, N. H., and Rhoads, J. E.: Hyperinsulinism and islet-cell tumors of the pancreas with 398 recorded tumors. Surg. Gynec. Obstet., 90:417, 1950.

46. Janowitz, H. D., and Dreiling, D. A.: The Pancreatic Secretion of Fluid and Electrolytes. Ciba Foundation Symposium on the Exocrine Pancreas, Normal and Abnormal Function. London, J. & A. Churchill, 1962.

47. Jones, R. C., and Shires, G. T.: The management of pancreatic injuries. Arch. Surg., 90:502, 1965.

48. Jones, S. A., Steedman, R. A., Kellen, T. B., and Smith, L. L.: Transduodenal sphincteroplasty (not sphincterotomy) for biliary and pancreatic disease. Amer. J. Surg., 118:292, 1969.

49. Jordan, G., and Grossman, M. I.: Pancreaticoduodenectomy in the management of chronic relapsing pancreatitis. Surgery, 41:871, 1957.

50. Jordan, G. L.: Pancreatic fistula. Amer. J. Surg., 119:200, 1970.

51. Jordan, G. L., Overton, R. T., and Werschky, L. R.: Traumatic transections of the pancreas. Southern Med. J., 62:90, 1969.

52. Jorpes, J. E., and Mutt, V.: The gastrointestinal hormones, secretin and cholecystokinin-pancreozymin. Ann. Intern. Med., 55:395, 1961.

53. Kalser, M. H., Leite, C. A., and Warren, W. D.: Fat assimila-

tion after massive distal pancreatectomy. New Eng. J. Med., 279:570, 1968.

54. Krongrad, E., and Feldman, F.: Acute hemorrhagic pancreatitis, electrolyte and electrocardiographic changes. Amer. J. Dis. Child., 119:143, 1970.

55. Lefer, A. M., Glenn, T. M., O'Neill, T. J., Lovett, W. L., Gersinger, W. T., and Wangensteen, S. L.: Inotropic influence of endogenous peptides in experimental hemorrhagic pancreatitis. Surgery, 69:220, 1971.

56. Liewendahl, K., and Kvist, G.: Evaluation of pancreatic scanning. Acta Med. Scand., 188:75, 1970.

57. McHardy, G., Craighead, C. C., Balart, L., Cradie, H., and LaGrange, C.: Pancreatitis—intrapancreatic proteolytic trypsin activity. J.A.M.A., 183:527, 1963.

58. Meyer, E. M.: Diazoxide and the treatment of hypoglycemia. Ann. N.Y. Acad. Sci., 150:191, 1968.

59. Montgomery, W. H., and Miller, F. C.: Pancreatitis and pregnancy. Obstet. and Gynec., 35:658, 1970.

60. Nardi, G. L., and Acosta, J. M.: Papillitis as a cause of pancreatitis and abdominal pain: role of evocative test, operative pancreatography and histologic evaluation. Ann. Surg., 164:611, 1966.

61. Nelp, W. B.: Pancreatitis induced by steroid therapy. Arch. Intern. Med., 108:702, 1961.

62. Opie, E. L.: Etiology of acute pancreatitis. Bull. Johns Hopkins Hosp., 12:182, 1901.

63. Panebianco, A. C., Scott, S. M., Dart, C. H., Jr., Takaro, T., and Schegaray, H. M.: Acute pancreatitis following extracorporeal circulation. Ann. Thorac. Surg., 9:562, 1970.

64. Panum, P. L.: Experimentelle Beitrage zur Libre von der Embolie. Virchow's Arch. Path. Anat., 25:308, 1862.

65. Pavlov, I. P.: The Work of the Digestive Glands. Translated by W. H. Thompson. London, Charles Griffin Company, 1910.

66. Pfeffer, R. B., Lazzarini-Robertson, A., Jr., Safadi, D., Mixter, G., Jr., Secoy, C. F., and Hinton, J. W.: Gradations of pancreatitis, edematous through hemorrhagic, experimentally produced by controlled injection of microspheres into blood vessels in dogs. Surgery, 51:764, 1962.

67. Polk, H. C., Jr., Zeppa, R., and Warren, W. D.: Surgical significance of differentiation between acute and chronic pancreatic collections. Ann. Surg., 169:444, 1969.

68. Popper, H. L., Necheles, H., and Russell, K. C.: Transition of pancreatic edema into pancreatic necrosis. Surg. Gynec. Obstet., 87:79, 1948.

69. Puestow, C. B., and Gillesby, W. J.: Retrograde surgical drainage of the pancreas for chronic relapsing pancreatitis. Arch. Surg., 76:898, 1958.

70. Rich, A. R., and Duff, G. L.: Experimental and pathological studies on pathogenesis of acute hemorrhagic pancreatitis. Bull. Johns Hopkins Hosp., 58:212, 1936.

71. Robertson, G. C., and Eeles, G. H.: Syndrome associated with pancreatic acinar cell carcinoma. Brit. Med. J., 2:708, 1970.

72. Robinson, T. M., and Dunphy, J. E.: Continuous perfusion of bile protease activators through the pancreas. J.A.M.A., 183:530, 1963.

73. Ross, D. E.: Cancer of the pancreas. A plea for total pancreatectomy. Amer. J. Surg., 87:20, 1954.

74. Schindler, S. C., Schaefer, J. W., Hull, D., and Griffin, W. O.: Chronic pancreatic ascites. Gastroenterology, 59:453, 1970.

75. Shader, A. E., and Paxton, J. R.: Fatal pancreatitis. Amer. J. Surg., 111:369, 1966.

76. Silen, W., Baldwin, J., and Goldman, L.: Treatment of chronic pancreatitis by longitudinal pancreaticojejunostomy. Amer. J. Surg., 106:243, 1963.

77. Tilney, N. L., Collins, J. J., Jr., and Wilson, R. D.: Hemorrhagic pancreatitis. A fatal complication of renal transplantation. New Eng. J. Med., 274:1051, 1966.

78. Trapnell, J. E., and Anderson, M. C.: Role of early laparotomy in acute pancreatitis. Ann. Surg., 165:49, 1967.

79. Von Mering, J., and Minkowski, O.: Diabetes mellitus nach Pankreasexstirpation. Arch. Exp. Path. Pharmakol., 26:371, 1889.

80. Walters, R. L., Gaspard, D. J., and Germann, T. D.: Traumatic pancreatitis. Amer. J. Surg., 111:364, 1966.

81. Warren, K. W., Athanassiades, S., Frederick, P., and Kune,

G. A.: Surgical treatment of pancreatic pseudocysts: review of 183 cases. Ann. Surg., *163*:886, 1966.

82. Warren, K. W., Braasch, J. H., and Thum, C. W.: Diagnosis and surgical treatment of carcinoma of the pancreas. Curr. Probl. Surg., June, 1968.

83. Warren, W. D., Leite, C. A., Baumeister, F., Poucher, R. L., and Kalser, M. H.: Clinical and metabolic response to radical distal pancreatectomy for chronic pancreatitis. Amer. J. Surg., *113*:77, 1967.

84. Warren, W. D., Marsh, W. H., and Sandusky, W. R.: An appraisal of surgical procedures for pancreatic pseudocyst. Ann. Surg., *147*:903, 1958.

85. Waterman, N. G., Walsky, R., Kasdan, M. L., and Abrams, B. L.: The treatment of acute hemorrhagic pancreatitis by sump drainage. Surg. Gynec. Obstet., *126*:963, 1968.

86. Watts, G. T.: Total pancreatectomy for fulminant pancreatitis. Lancet, *2*:384, 1963.

87. Webster, P. D., and Zieve, L.: Alterations in serum content of pancreatic enzymes. New Eng. J. Med., *267*:604, 1962.

88. Webster, P. D., and Zieve, L.: Alterations in serum content of pancreatic enzymes. New Eng. J. Med., *267*:654, 1962.

89. Weiner, S., Gramatica, L., Voegle, L. D., Hauman, R. L., and Anderson, M. C.: Role of the lymphatic system in the pathogenesis of inflammatory disease in the biliary tract and pancreas. Amer. J. Surg., *119*:55, 1970.

90. Whipple, A. O., and Frantz, V. K.: Adenoma of islet-cells with hyperinsulinism. A review. Ann. Surg., *101*:1299, 1935.

91. Whipple, A. O., Parsons, W. W., and Mullins, C. R.: Treatment of carcinoma of the ampulla of Vater. Ann. Surg., *102*:763, 1935.

92. White, T. T., Lawinski, M., Stacher, G., Pangtay Tea, J., Michoulier, J., Murat, J., and Mallet-Guy, P.: The treatment of pancreatitis by left splanchnicectomy and coeliac ganglionectomy. An analysis of 146 cases. Amer. J. Surg., *112*:195, 1966.

93. White, T. T., Morgan, A., and Hopton, D.: Postoperative pancreatitis. A study of 70 cases. Amer. J. Surg., *120*:132, 1970.

94. Zollinger, R. M., and Ellison, E. H.: Primary peptic ulcerations of the jejunum associated with islet-cell tumors of the pancreas. Ann. Surg., *142*:709, 1955.

# 36

# THE SPLEEN

*Gordon W. Philpott, M.D., and Walter F. Ballinger, M.D.*

Knowledge of splenic function and splenic disorders has become of increasing importance to the surgeon. Many diseases of the spleen, both primary and secondary, will respond to splenectomy. The operative techniques are seldom a problem for most well trained surgeons. All too frequently, however, important preoperative and postoperative decisions depend entirely upon the wisdom and judgment of the hematologist. For optimal patient management, the surgeon must evaluate the advisability and proper timing of splenectomy with a clear understanding of the disease process and the risks attendant upon surgical intervention.

## HISTORICAL ASPECTS

The spleen has been of interest to many scientific and nonscientific authors for over 2000 years. Galen regarded it as an organ full of mystery, and interesting and imaginative functions such as mirth, anger, and speed in running have been ascribed to the spleen.

A more realistic role of the spleen as a filtering mechanism was suggested by physicians and philosophers such as Plato and Aretaeus, who believed that the spleen "strained black blood or black bile" and helped keep the liver "bright and pure." Aretaeus of Cappadocia (c. A.D. 150) recognized splenic enlargement, which he thought was due to a derangement in this hypothetically important "black bile."

Marcello Malpighi (1659) first described some of the microscopic anatomy of the spleen, including the malpighian corpuscles. He also conclusively demonstrated that the spleen was an organ of the vascular system, located in the splanchnic bed.

Matthis, Barbette, Clark, and Morgagni published some of the earliest studies on the effects of splenectomy in the dog. Each of these investigators clearly showed that the spleen was not necessary for a healthy life, just as Aristotle had suggested centuries before.

Although post-traumatic splenectomies may have been performed by military surgeons earlier, splenectomy for nontraumatic disorders was first performed in the modern era by Quittenbaum (1826) and Wells (1876). Survival, however, was not achieved until 1887, when Spencer Wells removed the spleen of a patient with hereditary spherocytosis. Plagued by problems with hemorrhage and infection, surgeons for the next 35 years seldom performed the operation, except for trauma,

twisted splenic pedicle, or massive tumors. Splenectomy in leukemia was particularly disastrous and the lack of any survivors caused physicians and surgeons to abandon the operation in all patients with leukemia. Only recently has this ban been lifted in carefully selected patients with hypersplenism from leukemic infiltration.[23-25]

As techniques have improved, splenectomy for the cure or alleviation of hematologic disease once again has become accepted. Since Moynihan (1921) wrote exhaustive reviews on splenectomy, little has been added to the techniques of splenectomy.[18] Important advances have occurred in understanding splenic function and dysfunction and in new methods of diagnosis of hematologic disease. Some of these investigations will be mentioned in the appropriate sections.

## ANATOMY

During early embryonic life, the spleen develops from the coalescence of several small subperitoneal swellings. These mesodermal masses arise in the left side of the dorsal mesogastrium, and by 3 months of gestation, they have merged into the adult form of a spleen, occasionally maintaining persistent fetal lobulations. The dorsal mesogastrium becomes the gastrosplenic ligament containing the short gastric vessels. The peritoneal reflections from the splenic capsule to adjacent organs form the surgically important suspensory ligaments of the spleen. These are the splenophrenic, splenorenal, and splenocolic, as well as the gastrosplenic (Fig. 1).

Accessory spleens occur in 14 to 30 per cent of those requiring splenectomy for hematologic diseases. These probably arise from the failure of complete coalescence of normal primordial spleen buds or the formation of spleen buds in unusually distant locations. Another possible explanation is that some splenic tissue becomes pinched off the main mass during development. The most common locations for accessory spleens are in the hilus, in the various suspensory ligaments of the spleen, particularly the gastrosplenic and splenocolic ligaments, and in the greater omentum. Accessory splenic tissue also rarely occurs in the mesentery of the gastrointestinal tract, or in the pelvis (Fig. 2).

The spleen is a highly vascular organ composed of a specialized capillary bed between the splenic artery and portal venous system. The normal adult

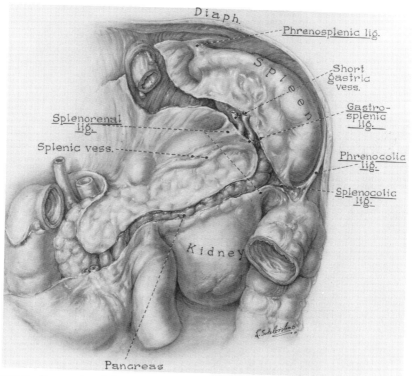

**Figure 1** Suspensory ligaments of the spleen. (From Splenectomy, by Ballinger, W. F., and Erslev, A. J., in Current Problems in Surgery, edited by Ravitch, M. M., et al. Copyright © 1965, Year Book Medical Publishers. Used by permission.)

spleen weighs approximately 100 to 225 gm., and is usually not palpable. It is bordered superiorly and laterally by the diaphragm and lower rib cage, inferiorly by the colon, medially by the stomach, and posteriorly by the kidney. The tail of the pancreas extends into the hilus and often is quite close to the spleen. Peritoneal attachments from the surrounding structures to the splenic capsule are of surgical importance. The splenophrenic, splenorenal, and splenocolic ligaments are usually relatively avascular and can be easily transected to bring the spleen and hilus medially and anteriorly into the level of the wound. All of the suspensory ligaments of the spleen, however, contain collaterals, which can be quite large with impairment of the splenic venous or arterial blood flow. The gastrosplenic ligament, containing the short gastric vessels, extends from the greater curvature of the fundus and body of the stomach to the spleen. This ligament is often extremely short in the superior portion and transection must be done carefully. The splenic pedicle, located in the most medial portion of the splenorenal ligament, contains the splenic artery, vein, and lymphatics, and often the tail of the pancreas. The splenic artery arises from the celiac plexus and follows an irregular course along the superior border of the pancreas. The splenic vein, which is just inferior to the artery, courses posterior to the pancreas before joining the hepatic portal system.

The vessels enter the hilus and branch out along

the trabeculae, which form the connective tissue framework, dividing the spleen into smaller and smaller interconnected compartments. Branches of the trabecular arteries pass into both the white pulp and red pulp, proceeding peripherally to communicate through capillaries and sinuses with the venous channels, located in the marginal areas (Fig. 3). The complex microcirculation through the splenic substance is incompletely understood, but the distribution of blood flow is at least partially controlled by an opening and closing of the smaller central arteries and arterioles leading into the splenic sinuses.

The white pulp is composed of lymphatic tissue and lymphoid follicles, or malpighian bodies, that surround the central arteries. They contain predominantly lymphocytes, plasma cells, and macrophages distributed throughout a reticular network.

The marginal zone between the red and white pulp is an ill defined vascular space that varies in size, depending upon its contents. Sometimes it contains only plasma and, at other times, a variety of cellular elements. Foreign materials are preferentially sequestered in this zone, as well as in the red pulp.

The red pulp is composed of interconnected cords of reticular cells, which form an irregular honeycomb throughout the red pulp. The sinuses lie between the cords and provide meandering channels from the arterial to the venous circula-

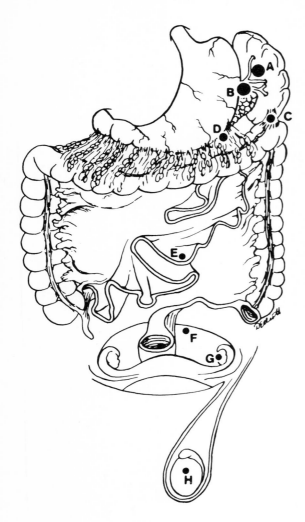

**Figure 2** Location of accessory spleens. *A*, Splenic hilus. *B*, Adjacent to splenic vessels and tail of pancreas. *C*, Splenocolic ligament. *D*, Greater omentum. *E*, Mesentry, *F*, Presacral region. *G*, Adnexal region. *H*, Peritesticular. (From Splenectomy for hematological disorders, by Schwartz, S., et al., in Current Problems in Surgery, edited by Ravitch, M. M., et al. Copyright © 1971, Year Book Medical Publishers. Used by permission.)

**Figure 3** Microcirculation of the spleen. (From Weiss, L. In: Greep, R. O., ed.: Histology. Copyright 1966, McGraw-Hill Book Company. Used with permission of McGraw-Hill Book Company.)

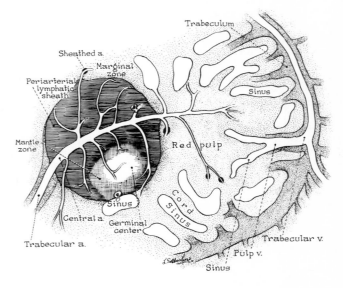

tions. There is considerable variation in the size and type of connections between the central arterioles, after they leave the white pulp, and the cords and sinuses. Some end as terminal vessels in the cords. Others empty into the sinuses by tiny openings. Phagocytes line some of the capillaries directly beneath the endothelial membrane, accounting for much of the filtering of foreign material by the spleen. Although the splenic sinuses are 35 to 40 $\mu$ in diameter, they have frequent gaps of 2 to 3 $\mu$ in their lining membrane, which constrict and impede erythrocytes as they move between the cords and sinuses.

Blood flows through the spleen by a number of these different routes. Normal healthy blood elements pass rapidly through the normal spleen by any number of the various routes. Abnormal or aged elements, on the other hand, are often retarded and entrapped in the normal splenic substance. When the spleen is enlarged, even normal blood elements can be impeded and engulfed, giving rise to a hypersplenic state.

## PHYSIOLOGY AND PATHOPHYSIOLOGY

The human spleen has a number of well known functions including the filtering of blood elements and foreign material, hematopoiesis, and, in some situations, the production of lymphocytes and antibodies. It may also have an endocrinologic role as a partial regulator of bone marrow function, but available data are inconclusive. The fact that normal health is possible without a spleen indicates that other tissues in the body can assume these duties when the spleen is absent.

Approximately 350 liters of blood flows through a normal spleen daily. Normal blood elements usually pass rapidly through the spleen, while defective and aged cells and foreign material are removed. The mechanisms by which abnormal cells are filtered are not completely defined. The slit-like gaps and narrow channels in the cords and sinuses are undoubtedly one way that the spleen can retain odd-shaped cells, such as spherocytes and elliptocytes. The methods of filtering normal-shaped cells, with either abnormal particles or

membrane coating, are not known. Chromium ($^{51}$Cr) tagging experiments have shown that normally few cells are filtered in one passage through the spleen, attesting to the efficiency by which the bone marrow produces cells of standard size and shape. The normal bone marrow, however, does make a significant number of cells with abnormal particles, which usually appear in the circulation after splenectomy. These include Howell-Jolly bodies, siderocytes, Pappenheimer bodies, and Heinz bodies (Fig. 4). The spleen can clean out bits of cellular "debris," such as these fragments of nuclear and cytoplasmic material, without necessarily removing the cells. Sequestration of these cells not only allows the spleen to cleanse and filter abnormal cells and particles, but permits a weakening and "aging" of the erythrocytes. Although this process is not well understood, crowding in the pulp probably leads to glucose deprivation, reduction in high-energy phosphates, and deterioration of the sodium pump. With each incident of congestion, this metabolic damage increases, until the aged cell is phagocytized by the reticuloendothelial system. In a normal person, this amounts to 20 ml. of red cells daily. The spleen may also participate in the maturation of erythrocytes, by somehow altering the volume-surface ratio. Target cells (Fig. 4) temporarily appear after splenectomy, suggesting a disproportionate shrinkage in red cell volume, until other tissue in the body takes over the functions of the spleen. After splenectomy in patients without hematologic diseases, anemia and polycythemia do not occur, and red cell survival remains unchanged. These facts suggest that the filtering function of the spleen is quickly assumed by remaining reticuloendothelial tissue and that red cell production must decrease, since a significant vascular component is removed by splenectomy, without ensuing polycythemia.

Normal leukocytes are removed from the circulation by the reticuloendothelial system including the spleen. When the spleen is removed, a temporary leukocytosis occurs, predominantly a lymphocytosis. This is of no known consequence, except that it can confuse the postoperative picture. In the rare disorder splenic neutropenia,

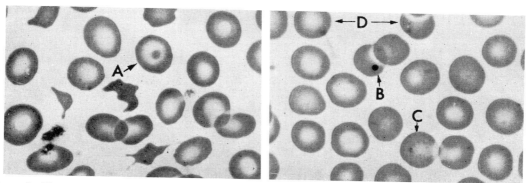

**Figure 4** Photomicrograph of blood smears of patients splenectomized because of idiopathic thrombocytopenic purpura. Note the target cell (*A*), the Howell-Jolly body (*B*), the stippling (*C*), and the barely perceptible Pappenheimer bodies (*D*). (From Wintrobe, M. M.: Clinical Hematology. 6th ed. Philadelphia, Lea & Febiger, 1967.)

leukocytes are preferentially removed by the spleen.

Platelets are also filtered out of the circulation by the spleen. When coated with antibodies, platelets are removed at a much greater rate, giving rise to thrombocytopenia. Following splenectomy, the circulating levels of both the coated and normal platelets rise, sometimes to over 1 million per cubic millimeter. The cause of this thrombocytosis has never been adequately determined. One hypothesis is that it is simply a matter of decreasing sequestration and destruction of platelets. Another hypothesis is that the splenectomy also removes a suppressant of bone marrow platelet production or release; and still another hypothesis is that the bone marrow is geared to regulate the overall platelet mass at a certain size, and when a compartment normally containing a significant portion of the platelet pool is removed, the overall platelet concentration rises.

The reticuloendothelial cells in the adult spleen are involved in the normal production of monocytes, lymphocytes, and plasma cells. Hematopoiesis of the other blood elements occurs in the fetal spleen, but normally stops between the sixth and eighth months of gestation. Hematopoietic stem cells then remain in the spleen in a dormant state, but can be reactivated after a prolonged and intense demand for blood cell formation. This extramedullary hematopoiesis apparently is performed in a less favorable environment than in the bone marrow, because there is often cell death in situ and premature release of early erythroid and myeloid cells. The mature cells are characterized by a great deal of anisocytosis and poikilocytosis. Megakaryocyte fragments and giant platelets are often observed. However, it is possible that this dyshematopoiesis is related to the underlying disease process, rather than to the extramedullary hematopoiesis per se. Thus, for example, in myeloid metaplasia, the abnormal proliferation of the primitive mesenchymal precursors from which the hematopoietic system takes origin leads to overgrowth of connective tissue in the bone marrow and reactivation of marrow stem cells in the spleen and liver, and might explain the close association of polycythemia vera, myeloid metaplasia, and myelogenous leukemia.

Antibodies are normally produced by cells within the spleen. Splenectomy can lead to a slight temporary reduction in antibody formation. In acquired hemolytic anemia, splenic neutropenia, and idiopathic thrombocytopenic purpura, antibodies to specific cellular elements are produced. Splenectomy then not only will remove an organ designed to sequester antibody-coated cells, but also will reduce antibody production, at least temporarily.

## HYPERSPLENISM

Hypersplenism is the inappropriate sequestration and destruction of blood elements with reduction in circulating red blood cells, white blood cells, or platelets.

**TABLE 1**  CLASSIFICATION OF POTENTIAL HYPERSPLENIC DISORDERS

*Primary hypersplenism*
　Congenital hemolytic anemia
　　Hereditary spherocytosis
　　Hereditary elliptocytosis
　　Pyruvate kinase deficiency
　　Hemoglobinopathies (sickle cell anemia, etc.)
　　Thalassemia
　　Porphyria hematopoietica
　Acquired hemolytic anemia: "autoimmune"
　Idiopathic thrombocytopenic purpura
　Thrombotic thrombocytopenic purpura
　Primary splenic neutropenia
　Primary splenic pancytopenia
*Secondary hypersplenism*
　Inflammation
　　Acute: typhoid fever, rubella, chickenpox, etc.
　　Bacterial subacute endocarditis
　　Chronic
　　　Tuberculosis
　　　Syphilis
　　　Boeck's sarcoid
　　　Beryllium disease
　　　Rheumatoid arthritis (Felty's syndrome)
　　　Disseminated lupus erythematosus
　　　Malaria
　　　Trypanosomiasis
　　　Schistosomiasis
　　　Leishmaniasis
　　　Echinococcosis
　　　Histoplasmosis
　　　Cryptococcosis
　Congestion
　　Cirrhosis of liver
　　Portal vein obstruction
　　Splenic vein obstruction
　　Congestive heart failure
　Ingestion
　　Gaucher's disease
　　Neimann-Pick disease
　　Amyloidosis
　　Hyperlipemia
　Infiltration
　　"Benign": infectious mononucleosis
　　"Neoplastic"
　　　Hodgkin's disease
　　　Lymphoma
　　　Leukemia
　　　Agnogenic myeloid metaplasia
　　　Histiocytosis (Hand-Schüller-Christian; Letterer-Siwe)
　　　Polycythemia vera

*Primary hypersplenism* includes a group of diseases in which the spleen becomes hypertrophic in response to a sustained and heavy workload (Table 1). In these conditions, the abnormal cells or platelets are removed so efficiently that the resulting cytopenia becomes of greater concern than the presence of the abnormal cells.

*Secondary hypersplenism* includes a group of diseases (Table 1) in which an enlarged spleen leads to increased destruction of normal or abnormal blood cells or platelets. Secondary hypersplenism can thus be caused by primary hypersplenism, by inflammation, by congestion, by ingestion of macromolecular colloids, or by infiltration of normal or abnormal cells. It must be emphasized that splenomegaly is not necessarily associated with hypersplenism (e.g., splenic cysts or some cases of infectious mononucleosis), and conversely, pancytopenia may be associated with splenomegaly without being caused by it (e.g., bone marrow failure with secondary extramedullary hematopoiesis). Many diseases involve both bone marrow and spleen and it is of importance in patients with cytopenia and splenomegaly to establish a diagnosis of hypersplenism and adequately evaluate bone marrow function before splenectomy is considered.

### Diagnostic Evaluation of Hypersplenism

The decision to perform a therapeutic splenectomy depends upon an accurate assessment both of the size of the spleen and of the degree of hypersplenism. An enlarged spleen usually can be demonstrated by careful physical examination, roentgenographic examination, or radioisotopic scanning. The spleen normally cannot be palpated or percussed. Splenomegaly can result in significant dullness to percussion at or above the left ninth intercostal space. Bimanual examination, with the left side of the patient tilted upward, will often help in the differentiation between an enlarged spleen (with its typical notch) and the left lobe of the liver, a pancreatic cyst, a large left kidney, or a colonic tumor.

A normal spleen usually can be outlined on a supine x-ray of the abdomen. An enlarged spleen displaces the stomach medially and inferiorly and the splenic flexure of the colon posteriorly and inferiorly. The outline of the spleen can be accentuated by introducing air or contrast material into the stomach or colon. Tomograms may also be of assistance in outlining an atypical spleen, but are seldom necessary.

Two methods for radioisotopic scanning are cur-

rently in use. In the first method, autogenous erythrocytes are heated to 50° C. for 1 hour and tagged with $^{51}$Cr. The heated red blood cells become spheroid and are trapped and destroyed by the spleen, which is then selectively visualized by scintillation scanning. A less selective method, but one giving as good or better results, employs a sulfur colloid linked to indium-113m or to technetium-99m, which is picked up by the reticuloendothelial system, predominantly in the liver and the spleen (Fig. 5). A third method uses labeled Rh-positive cells, coated with anti-Rh antibodies, but is seldom used today in the determination of splenic size.

The functional abnormalities in hypersplenism may be revealed in the peripheral blood by anemia, leukopenia, or thrombocytopenia. However, the circulating red cells, white cells, or platelets can remain at normal levels indefinitely, because the bone marrow can increase its rate of hematopoiesis by a factor of 6 to 10 times, as long as the metabolic requirements are met. The peripheral blood smear may show characteristic abnormalities such as spherocytes, elliptocytes, target cells, leukoblasts, and megakaryocyte fragments.

The increased destruction of red cells that occurs in hemolytic anemia usually results in a compensatory rise in the rate of erythrocyte production, as evidenced by increases in the reticulocyte count, the erythroid-myeloid ratio in the bone marrow, and the turnover of iron. There are frequently elevations of the serum bilirubin and fecal urobilinogen, and gallstones are common. In acquired hemolytic anemia, the Coombs test is often positive, indicating abnormal protein coating of the red cells that may or may not be due to true "autoantibodies."

Splenic sequestration and destruction of red blood cells can be evaluated indirectly by measuring the rate of cellular destruction or the degree

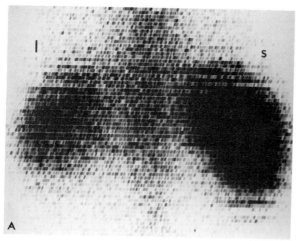 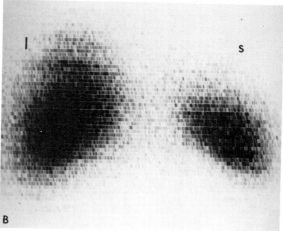

**Figure 5**   Two technetium-sulfur colloid spleen and liver scans, showing in (A) an enlarged spleen (s) on the right side of the scan, and in (B) a normal-sized spleen (s). Both scintiscans were taken from the posterior, so that the spleen (s) in each is outlined on the right-hand side and the liver (l) on the left. The scan in (A) is from a patient with splenomegaly due to portal hypertension. (Courtesy of Dr. E. J. Potchen, Department of Radiology, Washington University, St. Louis, Missouri.)

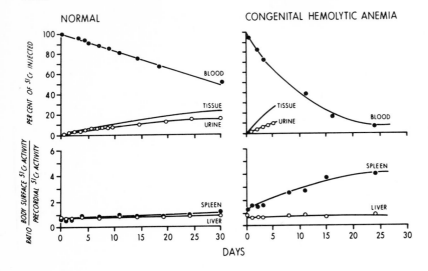

**Figure 6** Chromium-51-labeled erythrocyte determinations in normal and hemolytic anemia. In hemolytic anemia, radioactivity disappears from the circulation and accumulates in the tissue much more rapidly than normal with the spleen taking up more [51]Cr than does the liver. (From Splenectomy for hematological disorders, by Schwartz, S., et al., in Current Problems in Surgery, edited by Ravitch, M. M., et al. Copyright © 1971, Year Book Medical Publishers. Used by permission. After Jandl, J., et al., J. Clin. Invest., *35*:842, 1956.)

of compensatory production, and directly by measuring splenic sequestration of labeled cells. Transfusion requirements will give a rough, but useful, estimate of the rate of red cell destruction. Since the adult human loses approximately 20 ml. of red cells per day, under normal conditions, in 10 days he will have lost approximately 200 ml. of erythrocytes (blood volume × hematocrit × $\frac{1}{RBC\ life\ span}$ or, in a 70 kg. man, 5000 × 48/100 × 1/120 = 20 ml.). Thus, if the transfusion requirements are in excess of one unit of blood every 10 days, it can be assumed that the patient has a shortened red cell life span with accelerated destruction.

A more sophisticated measurement of the rate of disappearance of red cells from the circulation and the sequestration of these cells in the spleen utilizes [51]Cr-tagged autologous erythrocytes. A measured half-life of less than 20 to 25 days is considered an accelerated rate of red cell destruction. The relative role of the spleen in this destruction of erythrocytes can be further assessed by daily scanning over the spleen, liver, and precordium (Fig. 6). A selective rise in the ratio of radioactivity in the spleen as compared to the liver or precordium suggests significant splenic sequestration. With this technique, a satisfactory result from splenectomy may be predicted with a degree of accuracy approaching 90 per cent in situations in which the half-life of [51]Cr-labeled erythrocytes is below 50 per cent of normal (less than 15 days) and the spleen-liver ratio is greater than two.

The normal half-life of circulating granulocytes is so short (6 to 12 days) that attempts to assess a decreased longevity of leukocytes have not been clinically helpful. Also, there is no satisfactory clinical method of correlating metabolic effects of increased destruction of leukocytes and the relative importance of the spleen in this destruction.

Determination of platelet life span, using [51]Cr tagging, has been of some clinical usefulness in evaluating increased destruction of thrombo-

cytes.[3, 25] The normal life span of 7 to 10 days can be significantly reduced in patients with splenomegaly and in many cases of idiopathic thrombocytopenic purpura. When thrombocytopenia is due to increased destruction, the bone marrow will often show a compensatory increase in immature megakaryocytes. Evaluation of the use of surface scanning after injection of [51]Cr-labeled platelets is still incomplete. This technique may eventually prove to be a helpful diagnostic test in predicting the value of splenectomy.

## POTENTIAL HYPERSPLENIC DISORDERS AMENABLE TO SPLENECTOMY

Table 1 lists a classification of disorders in which splenectomy may be therapeutic. "Primary hypersplenism," as used in this classification, includes the hematologic disorders in which hypersplenism occurs in association with a spleen that is not afflicted with another disease. "Secondary hypersplenism" includes diseases in which hyperactivity results from splenomegaly due secondarily to a variety of other hematologic and nonhematologic disorders. Although this classification is useful in consideration of hypersplenic disorders, it is somewhat arbitrary. A number of authors prefer to limit the term "primary hypersplenism" to primary splenic neutropenia and to primary splenic pancytopenia.[23, 25]

### CONGENITAL HEMOLYTIC ANEMIAS

#### Hereditary Spherocytosis

Spherocytic anemia is also called familial hemolytic anemia, chronic hereditary hemolytic jaundice, and chronic acholuric jaundice. Since Minkowski (1900) first described the familial associations, this disease is now known to be transmitted as an autosomal dominant trait, causing a defect in the red cell membrane. It is

**TABLE 2** AUTOHEMOLYSIS TEST—PER CENT HEMOLYSIS, 37° C., 48 HOURS*

| Red Cells | Without Glucose | With Glucose | With Adenosine Triphosphate |
|---|---|---|---|
| Normal | 2–6% | <1% | <1% |
| Hereditary spherocytosis | 10–20% | 2–3% | 2–3% |
| Pyruvate-kinase deficiency | 10–20% | 10–20% | 2–3% |
| Glucose-6-phosphate dehydrogenase deficiency | 2–6% | 2–3% | 2–3% |

*From Splenectomy by Ballinger, W. F., and Erslev, A. J., in Current Problems in Surgery, edited by Ravitch, M. M., et al. Copyright © 1965. Year Book Medical Publishers. Used by permission.

characterized by small, dense spheroid erythrocytes that have increased osmotic fragility, as first demonstrated by Chaufford in 1907. As the spherocytes pass into the splenic pulp, they are impeded by the normal gaps and channels, resulting in glucose and ATP deprivation, membrane fragmentation, and cell disruption.

Besides the familial history, the common clinical manifestations are anemia, jaundice, and splenomegaly. The anemia is usually not severe, with hemoglobin determinations ranging between 9 and 12 gm. per 100 ml. Anemic "crises" with fever, chills, abdominal pain, vomiting, tachycardia, and dyspnea are not uncommon. They are accompanied by jaundice and increased reticulocytosis and occasionally are severe enough to be fatal. Cholelithiasis occurs in 30 to 60 per cent of these patients, but is uncommon before 10 years of age.[3, 23]

Spherocytes can be identified from peripheral blood smears and osmotic fragility tests. Also, spontaneous autohemolysis tests demonstrate an increased lysis of erythrocytes, which is partially corrected by the addition of glucose or adenosine triphosphate (Table 2).

Splenectomy is the treatment of choice and should be performed as soon as the diagnosis is established, even with compensated hemolytic anemia. If gallstones are present, concomitant cholecystectomy should also be performed. In very young patients, it is probably advisable to delay splenectomy until the third or fourth year. Although there is a difference of opinion among writers, splenectomy before the age of 4 years may predispose to an increased risk of infection.

### Hereditary Elliptocytosis

This is a familial disease which is usually of little clinical significance. It is characterized by oval and rod-shaped erythrocytes which constitute 50 to 90 per cent of the red cells on peripheral blood smears. Reticulocytosis and hyperbilirubinemia respond well to splenectomy in the few patients who do have anemia.[3, 23, 25]

### Pyruvate-Kinase (P-K) Deficiency

This disorder is one of the nonspherocytic hereditary hemolytic anemias first described by Baty in 1930. It is caused by an autosomal recessive defect in the enzymatic synthesis of high-energy phosphates (ATP) from glucose utilization. Homozygous patients have a high infant mortality. Those who survive develop poorly and have a severe macrocytic hemolytic anemia with splenomegaly. Studies with $^{51}$Cr-tagged erythrocytes show that the spleen is a major site for hemolysis. Splenectomy can help these patients by reducing the transfusion requirements and improving the anemia.[3, 23] It is important to distinguish between P-K deficiency and the numerous other forms of hereditary nonspherocytic hemolytic anemias caused by glucose-6-phosphate dehydrogenase (G-6-PD) deficiencies. The multiple genetic variants that give rise to G-6-PD-deficient red cells seldom cause splenomegaly and do not require splenectomy. The autohemolysis test will distinguish between these enzyme-deficient patients. The proportion of hemolyzed red cells after incubation at 37° C. for 48 hours, without glucose, is greater than normal with P-K deficiency, but not with G-6-PD deficiency (Table 2). Furthermore, the addition of glucose to the media will not reduce the autohemolysis with P-K deficiency as it does with normal cells, with spherocytes, and to some extent with G-6-PD-deficient cells. The addition of ATP reduces the hemolysis in all the hereditary hemolytic anemias as it does with normal erythrocytes.

### Sickle Cell Anemia

This disorder, first described by Herrick in 1910, is the most important disease of the group of hereditary hemoglobinopathies. An abnormality in the beta chain of hemoglobin produces the characteristic crescent-shaped, or sickled, red cells, under appropriate conditions of low oxygen tension. As a disease peculiar to Negroes, it is clinically manifested by episodes of acute abdominal pain, jaundice, bone and joint pains, hematuria, priapism, leg ulcers, and a variety of neurologic symptoms. In a few patients, splenic engorgement with hypersplenism and hemolytic crisis occurs early in the course of the disease. Splenectomy is helpful in these patients, to reduce transfusion requirements and to hasten the natural process of "autosplenectomy" that occurs in most patients by multiple painful splenic infarctions over a period of years.[3, 23, 25]

### Thalassemia Major

This disorder, known also as Cooley's anemia, Mediterranean anemia, target cell anemia, and erythroblastic anemia, was first described by Cooley and Lee in 1925. Transmitted as a dominant genetic trait, it is characterized by an ineffective production of abnormal erythrocytes owing to defects in the hemoglobin peptide chains. Clinical manifestations include a muddy yellow skin color, retarded growth with a large head and facial bones, cardiac dilatation, leg ulcers, inter-current infections, and hepatosplenomegaly. The hyphochromic, microcytic anemia may be severe and the peripheral blood smear shows character-istic target cells with decreased osmotic fragility, fragmented forms, stippled cells, and multiple nucleated red blood cells. Reticulocyte and leuko-cyte counts are high, whereas platelet counts are usually normal. Serum bilirubin is usually only slightly elevated and serum iron is high, with a saturated iron-binding protein. Gallstones occur in about a quarter of the patients. Splenectomy can be palliative to decrease transfusion require-ments and to eliminate an enlarged uncom-fortable spleen.[3, 23, 25]

### Porphyria Hematopoietica

This is an extremely rare disorder caused by an intrinsic defect in porphyrin synthesis of red cells, leading to hemolysis and accelerated red cell production. The porphyrins cause excessive photo-sensitivity and debilitating bullous dermatitis. The hypersplenic condition can be greatly bene-fited by splenectomy.[3, 23, 25]

## ACQUIRED HEMOLYTIC ANEMIA

Nonhereditary hemolytic anemias can be acquired during life by exposure to a variety of chemicals, drugs, bacteria, and physical agents. These can usually be alleviated by removal of the offending agent and temporary support with corti-costeroids and transfusions.[3, 25] There is also a type of hemolytic anemia that is of unknown eti-ology and that is believed to be due to an auto-immune mechanism. This type of acquired hemo-lytic anemia was first described by Chauffard and Troisier in 1908 and is more common in women over 50 years of age. Clinically, it may be mani-fested as a chronic and rather mild anemia or as an acute fulminant crisis with chills, fever, back-ache, jaundice, hemoglobinuria, and uremia. Splenomegaly occurs in over half of the cases, and gallstones are not uncommon. The patient's red cells are coated with abnormal proteins and the serum of these patients contains gamma globulins that agglutinate their own as well as normal erythrocytes. The coated and agglutinated red cells are trapped by the entire reticuloendothelial system, including the spleen. The positive direct and indirect Coombs tests in these patients indi-cate abnormal protein coating of erythrocytes and antibodies in the serum. They do not prove the presence of a true "autoantibody" to red cells, however, since the tests could be positive because of nonspecific adsorption of various previously formed antigen-antibody complexes.[3, 23, 25]

Corticosteroids and transfusions are relatively successful therapy, with 55 to 90 per cent of the patients showing remission. Only about 25 per cent maintain it, however, and then long-term steroid therapy or splenectomy is needed. Trans-fusion matching may be extremely difficult and

carefully washed red cells and potent saline-active antisera are often needed to obtain a successful crossmatch. Splenectomy is indicated when cortico-steroids cannot be given, or are ineffective after 4 to 6 weeks. The demonstration of splenic seques-tration of $^{51}$Cr-tagged red cells, with a spleen to liver ratio greater than 2:1 indicates a favorable response to splenectomy. Immediate response occurs in about 50 per cent of unselected cases and in 80 per cent of cases with significant splenic sequestration. Relapses are frequent with all forms of therapy, but tend to be less frequent after a good response to splenectomy.[3, 23, 25]

## IDIOPATHIC THROMBOCYTOPENIC PURPURA

This disease, which is also known as purpura hemorrhagica and "immunologic" thrombocyto-penic purpura, was first described as a clinical entity by Werlhof in 1735, and was first shown to be due to thrombocytopenia by Brohm in 1883. It is a syndrome characterized by decreased numbers of circulating platelets, abundant megakaryocytes in the bone marrow, and a shortened platelet life span; it probably has an immunologic pathogene-sis. Much confusion has resulted from the inclu-sion of a number of disorders with purpura second-ary to drug or toxic reactions, viral and bacterial infections, lymphoproliferative diseases, and dis-seminated lupus erythematosus in the category of idiopathic thrombocytopenic purpura (ITP). As the name implies, the etiology is unknown, and at present the term should be reserved for cases in which the well known causes of secondary throm-bocytopenia cannot be identified. The acute cases of ITP, which occur mostly in children, may rep-resent responses to inapparent viral infections, but are still included in this syndrome. Chronic cases can occur at any age, but are most common in 15 to 35 year old women.

A large majority of patients, particularly those with chronic ITP, have platelet-agglutinating and complement-fixing antibodies. A circulating anti-platelet factor, with the characteristics of an anti-body, has been demonstrated in a large proportion of these patients and normal transfused platelets are rapidly destroyed until splenectomy is per-formed.[14]

The spleen plays an important role in this dis-ease for two, and perhaps three, reasons. First, the spleen contributes to the production of the anti-platelet "antibodies." Whether these are true "autoantibodies" or antibodies directed against foreign antigens with adsorption of the antigen-antibody complex to the platelets is not known. In any case, slight temporary reduction in titers fol-lows splenectomy. Platelet-agglutinating anti-bodies can be demonstrated in the circulation for some time after splenectomy, even in patients in clinical remission.[3, 23, 25] This attests to the sec-ond, and probably the most important, role of the spleen in this disease, namely the sequestration and removal of coated platelets. Harrington and associates demonstrated that blood from ITP patients, transfused into normal matched recipients, could cause rapid thrombocytopenia and that "sensitized" platelets are selectively sequestered in the spleen.[10, 14] The infusion of [51]Cr-tagged platelets causes a rise of radioactivity, predominantly in the spleen. The site of platelet removal may depend upon the severity of the disease, with the spleen filtering out "lightly" sensitized platelets and the liver removing the more "heavily" coated ones. Besides these two major roles, the spleen may have some suppressive effect on maturation or release, or both, of platelets from the bone marrow.[8] This, however, is still a controversial theory.

The clinical manifestations of ITP include petechiae, ecchymosis, epistaxis, bleeding gums, vaginal bleeding, gastrointestinal hemorrhage, hematuria, and central nervous system bleeding. The course is sometimes cyclic, with exacerbations occurring during menses. Palpable splenomegaly occurs in 2 to 3 per cent of patients. Laboratory findings include very low platelet counts, often 50,000 or less, prolonged bleeding times, normal clotting times, and increased capillary fragility. Platelet life spans are reduced and the bone marrow contains normal or increased numbers of megakaryocytes. Erythrocyte and leukocyte counts are usually normal.

The treatment of ITP depends upon the age of the patient, the severity of the disease, and the duration of thrombocytopenia. Acute ITP in children under the age of 16 years has an excellent prognosis, with approximately 80 per cent of patients having a complete and permanent spontaneous remission within 3 to 6 months.[23] Corticosteroids may be of use in the acute period to increase platelet levels and avert the danger of severe hemorrhage. The use of steroids, however, has not improved the overall prognosis for recovery, nor has it reduced the incidence of chronic ITP, which occurs in 10 to 20 per cent of these patients.

The proper treatment of chronic ITP and acute ITP in older patients is somewhat more controversial. Both corticosteroids and splenectomy are useful and effective therapy. Corticosteroids will increase circulating platelet levels in as high as 90 per cent of acute cases and in 60 per cent of chronic cases.[8] In most series, however, sustained clinical remissions are much less frequent with corticosteroids (Table 3), ranging from 14 to 38 per cent, depending upon the chronicity of the disease.[4, 5, 7, 10, 19] Furthermore, complications of prolonged administration of corticosteroids, such as nervousness, hyperglycemia, azotemia, and hypertension, are not uncommon.

Splenectomy, which was first advocated for this disease by Kaznelson in 1916, has proved to be a more effective therapy in chronic ITP (Table 3). An increase in platelets is almost always noted within 2 to 3 days of removal of all the splenic tissue, with circulating levels sometimes exceeding 1 to 2 million thrombocytes. Sustained remission occurs in 57 to 90 per cent of patients in reported series, with most "permanent" success rates more than 80 per cent (Table 3). As with corticosteroids, success rates are somewhat better with acute ITP than with the chronic disease. In most series, splenectomy has also proved effective following therapeutic failure with steroids (Table 3). Operative mortality is relatively low (1 to 3 per cent) with most surgical deaths occurring in emergency splenectomies done for uncontrolled hemorrhage.[23] Postoperative complications occur in about 10 to 15 per cent of patients and are usually correctable. Postoperative thrombocytosis, even as high as 1 to 2 million, is seldom a problem and rarely is prophylactic anticoagulation indicated.

Although some investigators routinely advocate almost immediate splenectomy, most clinicians prefer first to give corticosteroids. With ITP of short duration, it is reasonable to give a trial on steroids for several weeks to a few months. If sustained remission results upon withdrawal of the drug, no further therapy is needed. If a reasonable dosage of corticosteroids does not result in a satisfactory increase in circulating platelets, or if relapse occurs, splenectomy is indicated. In patients with chronic ITP, steroids should be given to effect an increase in circulating platelets, if possible, and splenectomy performed without further delay.

Relapse of ITP following splenectomy, which occurs in 20 to 40 per cent of cases, is seldom due to a "missed" accessory spleen. However, this possibility should be evaluated in these cases by careful isotopic scanning and selective arteriography. Only those patients with positive findings of re-

**TABLE 3** SUSTAINED REMISSIONS WITH CORTICOSTEROIDS AND SPLENECTOMY IN PATIENTS WITH IDIOPATHIC THROMBOCYTOPENIC PURPURA

| Authors | No. of Patients | Sustained Remissions (%) | | |
|---|---|---|---|---|
| | | Steroids | Splenectomy | Splenectomy after Steroid Failure |
| Carpenter et al., 1959 | 50 | 38 | 81 | 73 |
| Doan et al., 1960 | 167 | 16 | 85 | 78.5 |
| Bunting et al., 1961 | 134 | 14 | 57 | — |
| Myers, 1961 | 71 | 14 | 83 | — |
| Block et al., 1966 | 67 | — | 90 | 100 |
| Washington University Hospitals (unpublished) | 148 | — | 75 | 75 |

tained splenic tissue merit re-exploration. Some patients with relapse of ITP after splenectomy have been successfully treated with immunosuppressive drugs such as azathioprine or cyclophosphamide.[25]

## THROMBOTIC THROMBOCYTOPENIC PURPURA

In 1925, Moschcowitz described a syndrome of purpura, fever, hemolytic anemia, varied neurologic symptoms, and renal abnormalities. Since then, some 300 cases of thrombotic thrombocytopenic purpura (TTP) have been reported. Some patients with this disease have benefited from splenectomy, which was first successfully performed for TTP in 1951. The syndrome is caused by hyaline thrombosis of terminal arterioles and capillaries, which may be due to an immune mechanism. The course is usually a rapid one, with progression until death. Less than 30 reported patients have had sustained remissions. Adrenocorticosteroids or splenectomy alone seems to give few remissions. The combination of prednisone and splenectomy seems to be more rewarding. It is sometimes advantageous to utilize both modalities, so that steroid dosages can be reduced to acceptable levels.[9, 23, 25]

## SPLENIC NEUTROPENIA AND SPLENIC PANCYTOPENIA

These two rather rare conditions of unknown etiology were first described by Doan and associates. Some authors prefer to limit the term "primary hypersplenism" to cases classified as splenic neutropenia or splenic pancytopenia.[23, 25] These diseases are characterized by splenomegaly, a normal or hyperplastic bone marrow, and leukopenia, or by varying degrees of pancytopenia. Clinical manifestations may include fever, recurrent infections, purpura, pallor, and pain in the left upper quadrant. Lymph nodes are not enlarged, in spite of the relative lymphoproliferation seen in peripheral blood, which is sometimes marked enough to suggest "premalignant lymphoma." Corticosteroids are occasionally of limited, temporary benefit in these diseases. When the diagnosis is made, splenectomy is indicated and usually curative. In some series, a few patients with initial improvement have been reclassified later as having lymphoma.

## SECONDARY HYPERSPLENISM

There are a wide variety of diseases that give rise to splenomegaly and secondary splenic hyperfunction (see Table 1). Inflammation, congestion, ingestion, and infiltration are the major underlying disease processes.

### Inflammation

Acute infections can be associated with hemolysis of circulating erythrocytes, as well as with decreased production. This rare state occurs when reticuloendothelial overreactivity leads to splenomegaly. The "acute splenic tumor" can lead to a decrease in other circulating cells as well. Adequate therapy of the acute infection relieves the secondary hypersplenism.

Chronic infections and inflammatory states (see Table 1) may be associated with reticuloendothelial hyperplasia, splenomegaly, and secondary hypersplenism. Worldwide, malaria is probably the most common cause of splenomegaly, which may reach huge proportions and may cause enough symptoms to require splenectomy.[3, 23, 25] In leishmaniasis, Boeck's sarcoid, tuberculosis, and so forth, splenectomy is indicated when clinical manifestations of hyperfunction are significant, or the splenomegaly results in pain and impairment of respiration. Enlarged spleens rupture more easily with minor trauma and prophylactic removal is sometimes advisable.

Rheumatoid arthritis, after several years' duration, may become associated with splenomegaly and neutropenia (Felty's syndrome). Corticosteroids may be of minimal benefit in correcting the neutropenia, but often this is temporary. Splenectomy can be of lasting benefit, not only in correcting the leukopenia, but sometimes in ameliorating the arthritis as well.[22]

Secondary hypersplenism develops in about 5 per cent of patients with sarcoidosis, with thrombocytopenic purpura, hemolytic anemia, leukopenia, or spontaneous splenic rupture. Splenectomy should be considered in these people, since the hematologic deficiencies are usually corrected after removal.

### Congestion

Congestive splenomegaly with pancytopenia (Banti's syndrome) can occur with portal hypertension. The spleen is no longer believed to be the primary source of this disorder, but rather it is secondarily involved as a result of increased blood pressure within the splenic or hepatic portal veins.[3, 23, 25] Splenic congestion with sequestration and destruction of circulating blood elements results. Splenectomy will usually correct the cytopenias, but a portal-systemic venous shunt usually is necessary to lower the portal hypertension. Removal of a large spleen can reduce portal hypertension by decreasing the influx of blood into the congested portal system by as much as 40 per cent. However, reduction is usually temporary and a portacaval or splenorenal shunt is preferable to prevent recurrent variceal bleeding. Shunting procedures are seldom indicated for isolated congestive hypersplenism without other symptoms, predominantly variceal bleeding. Successful portal-systemic decompression usually corrects the secondary hypersplenism over a period of several months, although occasionally persistent hypersplenism has required later splenectomy.

### Ingestion

In diseases such as Gaucher's disease and Niemann-Pick's disease, the reticuloendothelial system ingests "foreign" macromolecules and undergoes hyperplasia, with splenomegaly and sequestration of blood elements. This eventually results in secondary hypersplenism, which can be corrected by splenectomy. Splenectomy may also be indicated to relieve symptoms, such as respiratory distress or abdominal discomfort, caused by a massively enlarged spleen.

### Infiltration

In a number of diseases, abnormal cells infiltrate the splenic parenchyma, which can result in splenomegaly and secondary hypersplenism. For the surgeon, myeloid metaplasia, the lymphomas, and the leukemias are the most important diseases in this category, since splenectomy may become necessary.

**Myeloid Metaplasia.** This disease is also called agnogenic myeloid metaplasia and chronic non-leukemic myelosis and currently is considered to be a myeloproliferative disorder in which there is an excessive proliferation of primitive mesenchymal elements. Connective tissue proliferates in the bone marrow, spleen, liver, and lymph nodes, with a concomitant proliferation of hematopoietic stem cells in the spleen, liver, and long bones. Overgrowth of fibroblasts eventually obliterates the bone marrow, resulting in myelofibrosis. Although the same fibrotic process can eventually occur in the spleen or liver, the predominant process in these organs is extramedullary hematopoiesis. This current theory of the pathogenesis of the myeloproliferative disorders is more acceptable than the previously held belief that myelofibrosis caused a compensatory extramedullary hematopoiesis. The close association between myeloid metaplasia, polycythemia vera, and myelogenous leukemia is more compatible with the current theory of pathogenesis and even suggests that the mesenchymal stem cells may be altered by a malignant process. Confirmation of these theories, however, is still lacking, even though it is now quite clear that removal of a spleen involved with myeloid metaplasia does not necessarily result in decreased formation of cellular blood elements.[12, 23, 25]

Most patients with myeloid metaplasia are middle-aged to older, and present with anemia, weight loss, and pressure symptoms from splenomegaly. Dyspnea, pallor, edema, bleeding, infections, pruritus, and bone pain are not uncommon during the course of the disease, which ranges from 1 to 20 years. Hematologic findings include anemia, with anisocytosis and poikilocytosis. The white blood count is usually reduced, but can exceed 50,000, with a leukocyte alkaline phosphatase that is usually high. Modest thrombocytopenia is seen in about one-third to one-half of the patients; normal platelet counts are found in about one-fourth of the patients; and thrombocytosis is seen in 5 to 25 per cent of patients with this disease. Splenic scans and erythrocyte survival times are important diagnostic tests to indicate possible benefit from splenectomy. Corticosteroids, testosterone, alkylating agents, and radiotherapy are of some use in myeloid metaplasia. Deterioration in spite of medical therapy is an indication for splenectomy. Even though removal of the spleen does not alter the general course of the disease, it is often palliative by decreasing transfusion requirements, by relieving symptoms of splenomegaly, and by halting bleeding episodes.[12, 23, 25]

**Hodgkin's Disease, Lymphosarcomas, and Leukemia.** The spleen can be infiltrated by malignant cells during the various stages of these diseases. This may lead to secondary hypersplenism, or to absolutely no clinically detectable abnormality. Splenectomy may be indicated in both of these situations, either as palliative treatment or as a part of a diagnostic staging laparotomy.[1–3, 13–15, 17, 20, 23–25] Palliative therapy can be useful when chemotherapy and radiotherapy fail to prevent splenic infiltration and splenomegaly. This can result in troublesome symptoms from the size or from the hypersplenism.

These diseases can, of course, also affect the marrow, altering the hematologic picture. In deciding on the potential efficacy of splenectomy, it is essential to establish that the bone marrow is normal, or hypercellular, and that splenomegaly and hypersplenism exist. Red cell survival, transfusion requirements, and splenic scans are helpful. The use of scanning techniques, however, has not been a completely reliable indicator in these situations, because scans show sequestration in only about half of the patients with lymphomas who eventually improve with splenectomy. There is still controversy about the efficacy of splenectomy for palliation in Hodgkin's disease, with some authors favoring it and others much less enthusiastic.[20, 23] Palliative splenectomy for lymphosarcoma and for lymphocytic leukemia has been more uniformly accepted. In chronic myelogenous leukemia, splenectomy is seldom indicated, although some authors feel it can be helpful in permitting further chemotherapy. In reticulum cell sarcoma, results seem to be favorable, but quite short-lived, since operation is usually performed late in the course of the disease. In all of these diseases, it may be better to perform splenectomy when hypersplenism first becomes evident and not to wait until the terminal stages.

Recently, splenectomy has been advocated as part of a diagnostic laparotomy for staging patients with Hodgkin's disease.[1, 2, 13, 15, 17] Precise staging is useful in selecting the proper therapy, as well as in predicting patient survival. Exploratory laparotomy with splenectomy, liver biopsy, and para-aortic lymph node biopsy has markedly improved the staging of Hodgkin's disease, causing an alteration in preoperative evaluation in a fourth to a half of the patients in reported series (Table 4). Clinical evaluation of splenic involvement has proved to be incorrect more often than evaluation of liver and abdominal lymph node involvement. Preoperative determination of splenic involvement, including the use of isotopic scans, has proved inaccurate in about 35 per cent of patients with Hodgkin's disease who have been selected for diagnostic laparotomy. Clinical evaluation of liver involvement was incorrect in 10 to 25

**TABLE 4**  COMPARISON OF CLINICAL AND HISTOLOGIC STAGING FOR HODGKIN'S DISEASE. TOTAL OF 205 PATIENTS*

| Preoperative Clinical Status | Histol.+ Cases No. Examined | Per Cent Clinically Incorrect |
|---|---|---|
| 1. Spleen | | |
|   a) Clin. involved | 33/53 | 37.7 |
|   b) Clin. uninvolved | 49/150 | 32.7 |
|      Total | — | 34.0 |
| 2. Liver | | |
|   a) Clin. involved | 8/42 | 81.0 |
|   b) Clin. uninvolved | 12/163 | 7.4 |
|      Total | — | 22.4 |
| 3. Para-aortic Lymph Nodes | | |
|   a) Clin. involved | 45/64 | 29.7 |
|   b) Clin. uninvolved | 13/99 | 13.1 |
|   c) Clin. equivocal | 6/34 | — |
|      Total | — | 19.6 |

*Data from Kadin et al., 1971; Allen et al., 1969; Lowenbraun et al., 1970; and Presant et al., unreported series at Washington University Hospitals.

per cent of the reported cases, and abdominal lymphatic evaluation was incorrect in 15 to 25 per cent of the patients. Liver involvement does not seem to occur without splenic involvement. It is important to emphasize that the reported series in which diagnostic laparotomies have been utilized comprise selected patients. As the indications for staging operation are extended to asymptomatic patients with clinically more localized disease, fewer restaged cases will probably result.

Many authors believe splenectomy is also helpful in Hodgkin's disease because it makes subsequent radiotherapy easier. The radiotherapy port in the left upper quadrant can be limited to the splenic hilus (marked at laparotomy with metal clips), thus reducing the amount of radiation to the left kidney and lung. Laparotomy also allows bilateral oophoropexy in young women to move the ovaries out of the direct field of radiation. Although this is not completely effective in protecting the ovaries from radiation damage, ovarian function persists after radiotherapy in about half of the patients with oophoropexies. Although laparotomy has clearly improved the precise staging of patients with Hodgkin's disease and thus has altered treatment in a significant number, it is not yet possible to show improvement in survival rates because the follow-up period is still too short. No mortality from a staging operation has been reported (with the possible exception of one case), but this undoubtedly will occur as use of the procedure increases in popularity.[13] The reported complication rate is low, but it may be more significant than previously believed.

In the Washington University Hospitals series of 35 patients, the total complication rate was 31 per cent, with most of these being minor complications, such as atelectasis, pneumonitis, urinary tract infections, and minor wound infections.

Major complications due to the operation developed in only two patients — in both cases, subphrenic abscess. It must be emphasized that the eventual worth of subjecting patients to diagnostic laparotomy has not been established. However, at the present time, it does not seem justified to recommend this procedure as a routine approach to staging all unstaged patients. Until more data are available, diagnostic laparotomy, with splenectomy, should probably be limited to selected patients in whom there is a relatively high possibility of altering the subsequent therapy.

## RUPTURE OF THE SPLEEN

Splenic rupture is not uncommon, in spite of the fact that the spleen seems well protected by the ribs and muscular parieties.[6, 16] The spleen is a rather friable, vascular organ, suspended by ligaments that are attached to an adherent capsule, and even relatively minor trauma can result in avulsion of the splenic substance, or tearing of vessels in the suspensory ligaments, causing profuse bleeding. No injury to the spleen should be considered trivial, since delay in diagnosis and institution of the proper therapy can result in serious consequences. The reported mortality of approximately 10 per cent in isolated splenic rupture can be reduced by rapid diagnosis and therapy. Concomitant injuries to other organs are frequent with major trauma and account for a higher mortality and morbidity (15 to 25 per cent) of splenic injury.

The classification of splenic rupture, based on the etiology and the interval between onset and obvious manifestations, is a clinically useful one (Table 5).

**Penetrating Trauma.**  Most penetrating wounds that involve the spleen are obvious and warrant little discussion. Injury from high-speed missiles occasionally can be a diagnostic problem for the unwary physician, particularly if the missile follows an erratic course after entering the skin. Missiles such as bullets quite frequently do not follow a straight trajectory after entering the body, and injury to any organ, including the spleen, should be considered in all such patients. Hemopneumothorax in association with splenic injury indicates penetration of the lung, pleura, and diaphragm and a transthoracic approach for splenectomy is often preferable to remove clot and repair the damaged thoracic structures. If such an approach is used, careful consideration should be

**TABLE 5**  CLASSIFICATION OF SPLENIC RUPTURE

1. Penetrating trauma
  a) transabdominal
  b) transthoracic
2. Nonpenetrating trauma
  a) immediate rupture
  b) delayed rupture
3. Operative trauma
4. Spontaneous rupture

given to abdominal exploration, which usually requires a separate abdominal or a thoracoabdominal incision.

**Nonpenetrating Trauma.** Automobile accidents are the most common causes of blunt trauma to the spleen, even in children (in whom sledding and bicycle accidents are often the cause of splenic rupture). The spleen can be avulsed from its pedicle, fractured through the capsule and parenchyma, or ruptured beneath an intact capsule to give rise to a subcapsular hematoma. Bleeding is usually profuse with the first two, although a completely avulsed splenic artery can temporarily close with spasm, particularly in children. Delayed exsanguinating hemorrhage can occur when spasm ceases and the thrombus is pushed out. Delayed rupture, which occurs in 15 per cent of nonpenetrating splenic injuries, usually results from a subcapsular hematoma, which becomes manifest anytime from a day to several weeks after an injury. Approximately 75 per cent of delayed ruptures are diagnosed within 2 weeks of injury. Delayed rupture not infrequently is heralded by sudden, profuse bleeding and shock, after an episode of minor trauma is forgotten. Delay in diagnosis leads to relatively high mortality rates.

Spontaneous rupture is rare in a normal spleen; it is more often associated with diseased spleens. Rupture with minimal trauma, or spontaneous rupture, has been reported in malaria, mononucleosis (usually in the second to fourth weeks of the disease), sarcoidosis, acute and chronic leukemia, congestive splenomegaly, polycythemia vera, and acquired hemolytic anemia. Rapid, early splenectomy gives an excellent prognosis of survival.

Operative trauma to the spleen necessitating "incidental" splenectomy occurs in a significant number of operations in the left upper quadrant. Such injury is most common in operations involving the stomach and splenic flexure of the colon. Even small tears in the capsule almost always require splenectomy because of the real danger of hemorrhage.

### Clinical Manifestations of Ruptured Spleen

Although some patients, on admission, may be moribund in severe hemorrhagic shock or, at the other extreme, totally asymptomatic, the condition of most patients falls between these two extremes.[6, 16] There is usually some evidence of hypovolemia, particularly tachycardia and orthostatic hypotension. Most patients have varying degrees of generalized abdominal pain, often accompanied by nausea. In only about a third of the patients with splenic rupture and no other abdominal injuries is the pain localized to the upper quadrant. Pain radiating into the left shoulder (Kehr's sign) is relatively frequent (15 to 75 per cent of patients, depending upon the series), and can often be elicited by placing the patient in the Trendelenburg position. There is usually tenderness in the left upper quadrant and often it can be elicited as rebound tenderness.

Occasionally, there is a fixed mass or fixed area of dullness (Ballance's sign) in the left upper quadrant, due to subcapsular or extracapsular hematoma surrounded by omentum. Shifting dullness and a "doughy" feel to the abdomen are uncommon signs of extensive intraperitoneal bleeding. If clinical and laboratory evaluation does not demonstrate the splenic injury, repeated examinations often do. The importance of continued clinical evaluation in suspected splenic injury cannot be overemphasized.

Certain laboratory and radiologic tests can be of help. The white blood cell count often is increased to levels of 15,000 to 20,000. An initial hematocrit is often misleading, but serial determinations usually show a fall. Radiologic examinations are often not conclusive, but occasionally will show an enlarged spleen, without sharp outlines, that compresses the stomach medially and the transverse colon inferiorly. The left kidney and psoas shadows may be indistinct, and sometimes the left diaphragm is elevated. The presence of rib fractures can be helpful in the diagnosis of a splenic rupture, since they are present in about 20 per cent of splenic injuries. Hematuria in association with left rib fractures usually means a damaged spleen as well. An uncommon, but helpful radiographic finding occurs when blood dissects into the gastrosplenic ligament, causing a serrated appearance of the greater curvature of the stomach. Arteriograms of the splenic artery can be diagnostic in difficult cases (Fig. 7), but are seldom needed. Splenic scanning can also be helpful (Fig. 8), and is a procedure that can be done in most institutions.[21]

Paracentesis with an 18 or 20 gauge needle, or a small polyethylene catheter, can be helpful in difficult diagnostic situations. The presence of blood from a four-quadrant tap does much to confirm the diagnosis, and may be expected in as many as 50 per cent of cases with splenic rupture. The procedure, however, is not without some danger, particularly when there are dense peritoneal adhesions or abdominal distention, and a negative tap does not exclude injury to any of the abdominal

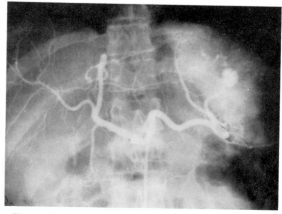

**Figure 7** A selective splenic arteriogram showing a subcapsular hematoma following blunt trauma to the abdomen.

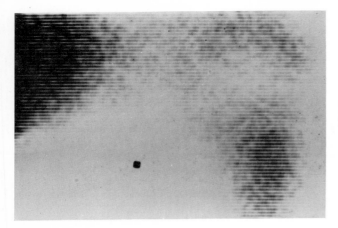

**Figure 8**  A technetium-sulfur colloid scan done 1 week after minor abdominal trauma. A large subcapsular hematoma can be seen in the mid-portion of the spleen, which is outlined to the right. A portion of the left lobe of the liver can be seen to the left of the umbilical marker (black square). (Courtesy of Dr. E. J. Potchen.)

organs. In the authors' viewpoint, there is little justification for *routine* four-quadrant taps in *all* cases of abdominal trauma, but rather the procedure should be limited to situations with *questionable* indications for abdominal exploration.

Once the diagnosis is made, or even highly suspected, laparotomy is indicated. Correction of hypovolemia with whole blood, or lactated Ringer's solution, or plasma expanders until blood is available, should proceed during the evaluation and while transporting the patient to the operating room. Delay for unnecessary diagnostic procedures or "to get the patient in better shape" for operation can be catastrophic. With trauma, a midline incision is preferable, since it allows rapid splenectomy and a complete exploration for injury to other organs, which occurs in about a third of patients with ruptured spleens. Hemorrhage from the spleen can be quickly controlled by clamping the pedicle between two fingers, dividing the lateral attachments, and delivering the spleen into the wound, where careful removal can be easily accomplished. A complete abdominal exploration must then be performed. Isolated splenic rupture treated in this way has a favorable prognosis, with a mortality of 1 per cent or less. The higher reported mortality rates (10 to 25 per cent) are due in large part to associated fatal injuries.[3, 6, 16, 23]

It seems clear that some injuries to the spleen do correct themselves. The occurrence of pseudocysts and old, well organized hematomas and the fact that splenic puncture usually does not lead to hemorrhage attest to this fact. The likelihood, however, that traumatic or spontaneous rupture of the spleen will correct itself is exceedingly small and should, under no circumstances, encourage delay in operation.

Splenosis may also be a late manifestation of previous splenic injury, although the etiology of this condition is still in some doubt. These small bits of splenic tissue scattered throughout the peritoneal cavity probably arise from fragmentation and autotransplantation, and are probably not true accessory spleens. They become of clinical significance if they cause intestinal obstruction, or if they are mistaken for peritoneal nodules due to other causes, such as carcinomatosis.

## LESS COMMON SPLENIC DISEASES

**Splenic Cysts.**  Parasitic and nonparasitic cysts rarely occur in the spleen. Echinococcus is the only parasitic infection reported to cause splenic cysts, which occur in less than 2 per cent of people with echinococcal infection. Nonparasitic cysts are either true cysts lined by epithelium or pseudocysts. Pseudocysts probably arise from old hematomas or splenic infarcts. True cysts are exceedingly rare. In the last 25 years, only one of the eight splenic cysts removed at Barnes Hospital has been lined with epithelium (Fig. 9). Splenectomy, and not aspiration, is the treatment of choice for all cysts.

**Neoplasms.**  Primary tumors of the spleen are also rare. Benign tumors include hamartomas, angiomas, and endotheliomas. Malignant primary tumors are all sarcomas, which grow and spread rapidly before clinical manifestations of a left quadrant mass, cachexia, and ascites occur. Cure is infrequent, but palliation can be achieved with splenectomy. Although metastases to the spleen (other than lymphomas) are felt to be rare, they are not uncommon in autopsy series of advanced lung and breast carcinomas.[3]

**Abscesses.**  Septicemia can rarely result in splenic abscess. Trauma or infarcts in sickle cell disease are the usual antecedent lesions. Splenic scans can be a valuable diagnostic aid. Splenectomy is preferable treatment, but drainage can help if removal is not possible.

**Ectopic Spleen.**  In rare instances, a lengthened splenic pedicle allows for a "wandering spleen" which may present as a mobile mass. It is of clinical significance only in that it can be mistaken for a tumor or a cyst, such as an ovarian cyst, or it can twist on its pedicle. Torsion of the spleen demands emergency splenectomy.

**Splenic Artery Aneurysms.**  Although these are quite rare, they are clinically important because of occasional rupture. They occur in women more

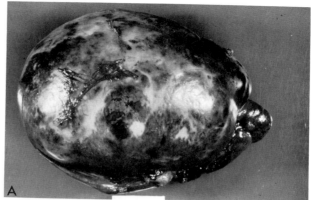

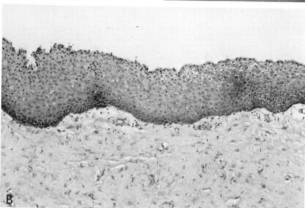

**Figure 9**   *A*, Anterior view of a spleen containing a large congenital cyst, lined with squamous epithelium (*B*).

than men, are usually asymptomatic, and may be seen on plain roentgenographs as a thin calcified rim. Excision seems advisable, unless there are complicating factors.

## SPLENECTOMY

**Preoperative Preparation.** Since emergency splenectomy is seldom necessary except for rupture, careful preparation prior to operation is usually possible. With splenic rupture, whole blood should be administered, but operation should not be delayed in the face of continuing hemorrhage. In patients with coagulation disorders that require preoperative transfusions, fresh blood obtained in plastic or siliconized containers is preferable, to preserve platelets as much as possible. Patients with severe thrombocytopenia usually benefit from platelet packs, but it is seldom worthwhile to give them before the splenic pedicle is clamped, since infused platelets are rapidly destroyed by the spleen.[25] In some patients with hematologic disorders, such as acquired hemolytic anemia and lymphomas, the blood bank should be given sufficient warning, since satisfactory matching is often difficult. Patients who have been receiving corticosteroids need adequate coverage during the operative period. Doubling the maintenance dose on the evening prior to operation, and again on the

day of operation, is usually satisfactory. Postoperatively, the dose can be slowly tapered back to maintenance levels and, it is hoped, then eventually discontinued. General anesthesia is preferable for splenectomy, with ether a good choice of agent, since it produces a significant decrease in the size of the spleen.

**Operative Technique.** After the induction of anesthesia, a nasogastric tube should be passed to decompress the stomach. Left subcostal, upper midline, and left paramedian skin incisions all give adequate exposure. The choice of skin incision is dictated by the indications for operation and the individual preference of the surgeon. For splenectomy alone, a left subcostal incision gives excellent exposure and allows removal of even a massively enlarged spleen if the incision is extended into the flank and across the midline (Fig. 10). Midline and left paramedian incisions are preferable for ruptured spleens, and are often more desirable for severe coagulation disorders, for massively enlarged spleens, and for "staging" operations. Thoracoabdominal incisions are seldom necessary, unless there is an associated pulmonary or diaphragmatic injury (Fig. 11).

The spleen is mobilized by dividing the lateral peritoneal attachments from the colon, left kidney, and diaphragm. These ligaments are usually avascular, but may contain large vessels, especially in portal hypertension or myeloid metaplasia.

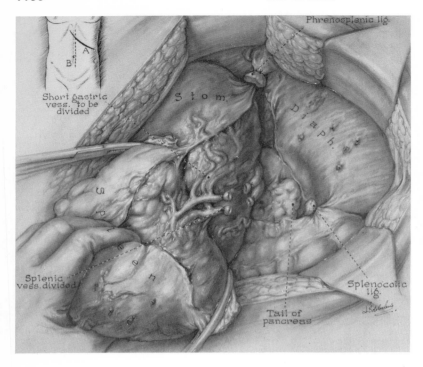

**Figure 10** The spleen just before removal with only a few short gastric vessels still intact. Abdominal incisions for splenectomy are depicted in the upper left. (From Splenectomy, by Ballinger, W. F., and Erslev, A. J., in Current Problems in Surgery, edited by Ravitch, M. M., et al. Copyright © 1965, Year Book Medical Publishers. Used by permission.)

Adhesions to the diaphragm must be divided and can sometimes cause troublesome hemorrhage. Electrocoagulation can be helpful. The spleen and hilus then can be rotated forward and medially, and a pack placed in the fossa to help control oozing and to keep the spleen in the wound. The short gastric vessels are divided, with care not to damage the greater curvature of the stomach. After identification of the tail of the pancreas, which extends into the hilus, the splenic artery and vein are ligated and transected. This can often be best accomplished by approaching the hilus posteriorly. Some surgeons prefer to identify and ligate the splenic artery through the gastro-

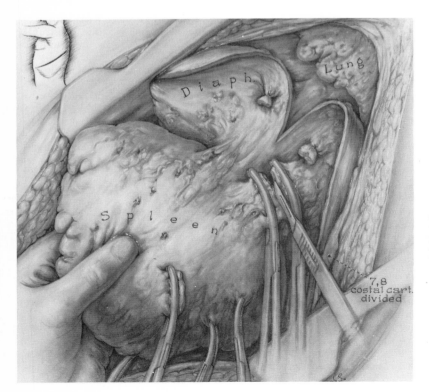

**Figure 11** Thoracoabdominal incision with good exposure of dense splenophrenic adhesions. (From Splenectomy, by Ballinger, W. F., and Erslev, A. J., in Current Problems in Surgery, edited by Ravitch, M. M., et al. Copyright © 1965, Year Book Medical Publishers. Used by permission.)

splenic and gastrocolic ligaments before mobilizing the spleen. "Early" ligation of the splenic artery is sometimes difficult with enlarged lymph nodes or with a massively enlarged spleen, but can facilitate dissection by decreasing the size of the spleen and lessening troublesome hemorrhage.

After the spleen is removed, meticulous hemostasis is accomplished; the pancreas and stomach are carefully examined for injury and the splenic fossa is irrigated with saline. Drainage is usually not necessary, unless there has been extensive tissue damage and bleeding from dissection or from injury, or unless the pancreas has been damaged. Sump drains are preferable when the pancreas is injured. Since infection can spread retrograde down a drain from the exterior, attachment of a splenic drain to sterile drainage is preferable.

Accessory spleens, which are often present (14 to 30 per cent of patients), should be found and removed, particularly when the patient has a hematologic disorder. These occur, in the order of decreasing frequency, in the hilus and along the splenic vessels, the gastrosplenic and splenocolic ligaments, the gastrocolic ligament, the splenorenal ligament, the greater omentum, the mesentery of the intestine, and the pelvis (see Fig. 2). When "staging" for lymphoma, the splenic hilus and areas of lymph node biopsy should be tagged with metal clips. The periaortic lymph nodes in the upper abdomen, as well as along the lower aorta, should be examined and biopsied. The liver is also biopsied, preferably in both lobes.

**Postoperative Management.** Persistent hemorrhage can occur in the immediate postoperative period. If continued transfusions are required, and the abdominal girth is increasing, re-exploration is mandatory. Often in such situations, intraperitoneal blood and clot are found, but no specific bleeding site is identified. Evacuation of the clot, irrigation with saline, and packing for several minutes will usually control any oozing.

The most common complication of splenectomy is left lower lobe atelectasis. Helpful preventive measures include vigorous deep breathing and coughing, blow bottles, intermittent positive-pressure exercises, and endotracheal suctioning. Rarely bronchoscopy is needed. Pneumonia and pleural effusion can occur. A left pleural effusion may also be due to a left subphrenic abscess. Fluid collections under the left diaphragm may become infected, develop into a subphrenic abscess, and require drainage. Injury to the pancreas or stomach is not common, but does occur. Gastric injury usually results in subphrenic abscess and gastrocutaneous fistula. Pancreatitis, with or without subsequent fistula or pseudocyst, occurs somewhat more frequently.

The danger of postoperative thrombosis from excessively high platelet counts has been overemphasized. Thrombocytosis with counts as high as 1 to 2 million is not a routine indication for prophylactic anticoagulants. The only exception to this might be in myeloid metaplasia, where thrombosis is more common.[25] Counts of over 1 to 2 million with myeloid metaplasia should be treated with anticoagulants, or with thrombocytophoresis. Patients with thrombosis, of course, should be treated with anticoagulants, bed rest, and leg wraps. Thrombophlebitis and pulmonary emboli are not common and often do not correlate with the platelet count.

The risk of infections in children after splenectomy may be higher than in adults,[11] but this remains controversial. This possibility has caused some authors to advocate prophylactic antibiotics after splenectomy in patients under 2 years of age. Actually, this increased risk seems to correlate more with the type of disease process than with the *age* of the patient. Thalassemia, myeloid metaplasia, Wiskott-Aldrich syndrome, and lipoidosis all carry increased risks of infection, regardless of age.

## SELECTED REFERENCES

Glatstein, E., Guernsey, J. M., Rosenberg, S. A., and Kaplan, H. S.: The value of laparotomy and splenectomy in the staging of Hodgkin's disease. Cancer, 24:709, 1969.
*An important current reference presenting a series of patients that forms the basis for the expanding use of exploratory laparotomy and splenectomy in "staging" patients with Hodgkin's disease. This approach is well supported by early data, but, as the authors emphasize, further investigation is needed to define and confirm its eventual clinical usefulness.*

Schwartz, S. I., Adams, J. T., and Bauman, A. W.: Splenectomy for Hematologic Disorders. Curr. Probl. Surg., May, 1971.
*This monograph is an excellent current review of this increasingly important area. The surgically important hematologic disorders are described in detail with a concise presentation of pathophysiology, important diagnostic procedures, therapy, and results. The authors combine an extensive personal experience with a thorough review of the literature to provide a useful reference.*

Wintrobe, M. M.: Clinical Hematology. 6th ed. Philadelphia, Lea & Febiger, 1967.
*This outstanding text remains the standard hematology reference.*

## REFERENCES

1. Aisenberg, A. C., Goldman, J. M., Raker, J. W., and Wang, C. C.: Spleen involvement at the onset of Hodgkin's disease. Ann. Intern. Med., 74:544, 1971.
2. Allen, L. W., Ultmann, J. E., Ferguson, D. J., and Rappaport, H.: Laparotomy and splenectomy in the staging of Hodgkin's disease. J. Lab. Clin. Med., 74:845, 1969.
3. Ballinger, W. F., II, and Erslev, A. J.: Splenectomy. Curr. Probl. Surg., February, 1965.
4. Block, G. E., Evans, R., and Zajtchun, R.: Splenectomy for idiopathic thrombocytopenic purpura. Arch. Surg., 92:484, 1966.
5. Bunting, W. L., Kiely, J. M., and Campbell, D. C.: Idiopathic thrombocytopenic purpura. Arch. Intern. Med., 108:733, 1961.
6. Calamel, P. M., Cleveland, H. C., and Waddell, W. R.: Ruptured spleen. Surg. Clin. N. Amer., 43:445, 1963.
7. Carpenter, A. F., Wintrobe, M. M., Fuller, E. A., Haut, A., and Cartwright, G. E.: Treatment of idiopathic thrombocytopenic purpura. J.A.M.A., 171:1911, 1959.
8. Dameshek, W.: Controversy in idiopathic thrombocytopenic purpura. J.A.M.A., 173:1025, 1960.
9. Distenfeld, A., and Oppenheim, E.: The treatment of acute thrombotic thrombocytopenic purpura with corticosteroids and splenectomy. Arch. Intern. Med., 65:245, 1966.
10. Doan, C. A., Bouroncle, B. A., and Wiseman, B. K.: Idiopathic and secondary thrombocytopenic purpura. Clinical study and evaluation of 381 cases over a period of 28 years. Ann. Intern. Med., 53:861, 1960.

11. Eraklis, A. J., Kevy, S. V., Diamond, L. K., and Gross, R. E.: Hazard of overwhelming infection after splenectomy in childhood. New Eng. J. Med., 276:1225, 1967.

12. Fishman, N., and Ballinger, W. F., II: Splenectomy for agnogenic myeloid metaplasia and myelofibrosis. Arch. Surg., 90:240, 1965.

13. Glatstein, E., Guernsey, J. M., Rosenberg, S. A., and Kaplan, H. S.: The value of laparotomy and splenectomy in the staging of Hodgkin's disease. Cancer, 24:709, 1969.

14. Harrington, W. J., Minnick, M., Hollingsworth, J., and Moore, C. V.: Demonstration of a thrombocytopenic factor in the blood of patients with thrombocytopenic purpura. J. Lab. Clin. Med., 38:1, 1951.

15. Kadin, M. E., Glatstein, E., and Dorfman, R. F.: Clinico-pathologic studies of 117 untreated patients subjected to laparotomy for the staging of Hodgkin's disease. Cancer, 27:1277, 1971.

16. Lieberman, R. C., and Welch, C. S.: A study of 248 instances of traumatic rupture of the spleen. Surg. Gynec. Obstet., 127:961, 1968.

17. Lowenbraun, S., Ramsey, H., Sutherland, J., and Serpick, A. A.: Diagnostic laparotomy and splenectomy for staging Hodgkin's disease. Ann. Intern. Med., 72:655, 1970.

18. Moynihan, B. G. A.: The spleen and some of its diseases. The Bradshaw Lecture of 1920 (The Royal College of Surgeons of England). Philadelphia, W. B. Saunders Company, 1921.

19. Myers, M. C.: Results of treatment in 71 patients with idiopathic thrombocytopenic purpura. Amer. J. Med. Sci., 242:295, 1961.

20. O'Brien, P. H., Hartz, W. H., Derlacki, D., and Graulich, K.: Splenectomy for hypersplenism in malignant lymphoma. Arch. Surg., 101:348, 1970.

21. O'Mara, R. E., Hall, R. C., and Dombroski, D. L.: Scinti-scanning in the diagnosis of rupture of the spleen. Surg. Gynec. Obstet., 131:1077, 1970.

22. O'Neill, J. A., Jr., Scott, H. W., Jr., Billings, F. T., and Foster, J. H.: The role of splenectomy in Felty's syndrome. Ann. Surg., 167:81, 1968.

23. Schwartz, S. I., Adams, J. T., and Bauman, A. W.: Splenectomy for hematologic disorders. Curr. Probl. Surg., May, 1971.

24. Strumia, M. M., Strumia, P. V., and Bassert, D.: Splenectomy in leukemia; hematologic and clinical effects of 34 patients and review of 299 published cases. Cancer Res., 26:519, 1966.

25. Wintrobe, M. M.: Clinical Hematology. 6th ed. Philadelphia, Lea & Febiger, 1967.

# 37

# HERNIAS

*Lloyd M. Nyhus, M.D., and C. Thomas Bombeck, M.D.*

## HISTORICAL ASPECTS

The early history of interest in the problem of hernia is that of the discipline of surgery. The names associated so intimately with the subject of hernia are familiar because of the pioneering thrust these men gave to surgery in general, e.g., Celsus, Henri de Mondeville, Guy de Chauliac, and Ambroïse Paré.[72]

The Egyptian papyri do not contain reference to the operative treatment of hernia, but the Papyrus Ebers (1552 B.C.) recommended diet and externally applied pressure (truss?) for its treatment. The word *barbaric* is frequently used in terms of surgery during the middle ages, and no less so for the treatment of hernia (Fig. 1). Major development in the knowledge of hernial anatomy and treatment occurred during the eighteenth century. Percival Pott (1714–1788) of London refuted many of the old theories concerning the etiology of hernia and methods of treatment based on these theories.[57] He was probably the first to suggest the congenital origin of hernias.

### The Modern Era of Hernial Surgery: Nineteenth and Twentieth Centuries

Early in the nineteenth century, four men contributed significant descriptions of inguinal anatomy: Camper,[12] Cooper,[17] Hesselbach,[33, 34] and Scarpa.[63] In 1801, Pieter Camper published the description of the fascia that bears his name. The skilled anatomist Sir Astley Cooper (1768–1841) published his two-volume work, *The Anatomy and Surgical Treatment of Abdominal Hernia*, in 1804 and 1807. First descriptions credited to Cooper include: transversalis fascia, internal ring, inguinal canal, correct formation of femoral sheath by the transversalis fascia, and the complete description of Camper's fascia. He paid little attention to the "ligament of the pubis," now called Cooper's ligament, and he certainly had no idea of how important this structure would become in the modern treatment of hernia. Franz Kaspar Hesselbach (1759–1816) described the triangle that bears his name in 1814 while he was prosector in the anatomic theater of Würzburg. Finally, in this quartet of anatomists must be included Antonio Scarpa (1747–1832) for whom a superficial layer of fascia is named. He is also credited with being the first to describe a sliding hernia (1821).

The nineteenth century brought anesthesia, hemostasis, and antisepsis, which made modern surgery possible. As in every area of surgery, these advances allowed rapid development of the science of hernial surgery. Wide acceptance soon was attained in Europe and America for the operation consisting of ligature and excision of the sac at the external ring and suturing of the pillars around the cord to reduce the size of the ring. This procedure was described in 1877 by Vincenz Czerny (1842–1916).[18] It is to Henry O. Marcy (1837–1924) of Boston that the modern era of hernial surgery is credited.[47, 48] His understanding of the importance of the transversalis fascia and of the anatomic contribution of fascial repair of the internal ring was reported in 1871. Parenthetically, this was 12 years before Bassini did his first operation for hernia, and 16 years before Bassini published his first paper on the subject.

Marcy's writings, however, did not stimulate the imagination of his contemporary surgeons, and further refinements in technique were suggested by Sir William Macewen (1886),[46] Lucas-Championnière (1892),[44] and Alexander H. Ferguson (1899).[23]

It remained for Edoardo Bassini (1844–1924) (Fig. 2) to present a reconstruction technique of the inguinal floor with transposition of the cord.[8] His operation (1884) included high ligation of the sac and reinforcement of the floor of the canal by suturing the conjoined tendon to the inguinal ligament beneath the cord, thus placing the cord under the external oblique aponeurosis. Bassini at this time held the chair of clinical surgery at the University of Padua. Independently and almost simultaneously, William S. Halsted (1852–1922), Professor of Surgery at Johns Hopkins, developed an operation similar to that of Bassini. The Halsted operation (Halsted I) transposed the cord above the external oblique aponeurosis.[30] This procedure was first mentioned in 1889. The Halsted II operation (1893) did not transpose the cord but added imbrication of the aponeurosis of the external oblique muscle in performing the closure. The first mention of imbrication

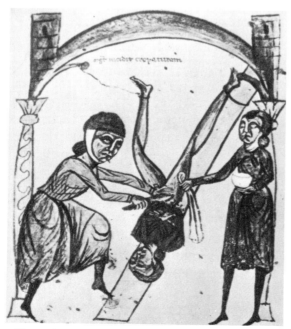

**Figure 1** Hernia operation in Trendelenburg position. From a thirteenth century manuscript. (Courtesy of L. M. Zimmerman.)

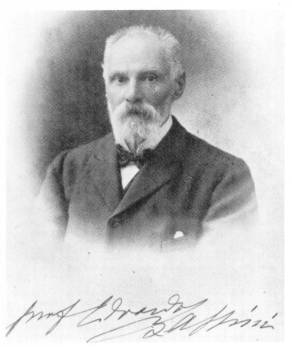

**Figure 2**   Edoardo Bassini (1844–1924). (Courtesy of L. M. Zimmerman.)

is credited to E. Wyllys Andrews (1856–1927)[4] of Chicago. The ludicrous overuse of eponyms in this field can be appreciated when we learn that the Halsted II procedure is also known as the Ferguson-Andrews operation since Ferguson left the cord in its normal anatomic position and Andrews stressed the imbrication of the external oblique aponeurosis.

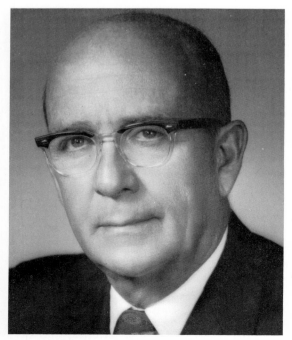

**Figure 3**   Chester B. McVay (b. 1911).

The use of the iliopectineal ligament (Cooper's ligament), or *ligamentum pubicum superius*, B.N.A., to anchor the medial parietal wall in the repair is credited to Georg Lotheissen (1868–1935)[42] of Vienna. The use of this structure as an integral part of hernial repair has been popularized by Chester B. McVay (b. 1911)[51] (Fig. 3) of South Dakota and the operation is known throughout the United States as the McVay repair.

The importance of the posterior inguinal wall in the etiology as well as repair of hernias was recognized relatively late. One of the strongest advocates of the transversalis fascia layer repair was P. W. Harrison (1883–1962).[32] A thickening in the transversalis fascia layer, the iliopubic tract, has received minimal attention from anatomists and surgeons alike. Depicted by Hesselbach (1814), it was described in detail in 1836 by Thomson.[67] In the past several decades, use of this structure has been recommended by a small number of surgeons interested in the anatomy of the groin (Clark and Hashimoto, 1946;[14] Donald, 1948;[19] Griffith, 1959;[28] and Nyhus, 1964.[54]).

After such a long period of interest in this anatomic area, controversy still abounds. The last chapter on the history of groin anatomy and operative repair of hernia defects has not been written.

## GROIN HERNIA

### ANATOMY OF INGUINAL AND FEMORAL CANALS

As in all areas of the abdomen, the abdominal wall in the groin is composed of multilaminar arrangements of muscle, their aponeuroses, fascia, fat, and either skin or peritoneum. The abdominal wall at the level of the groin may be divided into two groups of laminae, an outer and an inner. These two groups are mirror images of each other and are divided by the inguinal canal and spermatic cord (Table 1; Fig. 4).

Since by definition any hernia is a protrusion of normal cavity contents through the fascial and muscular layers designed to contain them, it is obvious that groin hernias are due to failure of the inner lamina of the abdominal wall, not of the outer.

#### External Oblique Aponeurosis

The external oblique muscle arises from the lower eight ribs posteriorly and sweeps downward

**TABLE 1**  LAYERS OF THE ABDOMINAL WALL

| | |
|---|---|
| Skin | |
| Fat (abdominal panniculus) | |
| Fascia (Scarpa's) | |
| Aponeurosis and muscle (external oblique) | Superficial stratum |
| Inguinal canal, muscle (internal oblique) and spermatic cord | |
| | |
| Aponeurosis and muscle (transversus abdominis) | |
| Fascia (transversalis) | Deep stratum |
| Fat (preperitoneal fat) | |
| Peritoneum | |

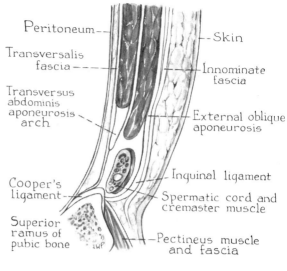

**Figure 4** A parasagittal schematic representation of the musculoaponeurotic relationships in the middle of the right inguinal canal, viewed from the lateral aspect of the section. The closer approximation, via their common insertion into the pectineal line of the pubis, of the superficial (external oblique, inguinal ligament) layer to the deep (transversus abdominis, transversalis fascia) musculoaponeurotic layer in the medial portion of the groin is demonstrated. (From Condon, R. E. In: Nyhus, L. M., and Harkins, H. N.: Hernia. Philadelphia, J. B. Lippincott Company, 1964.)

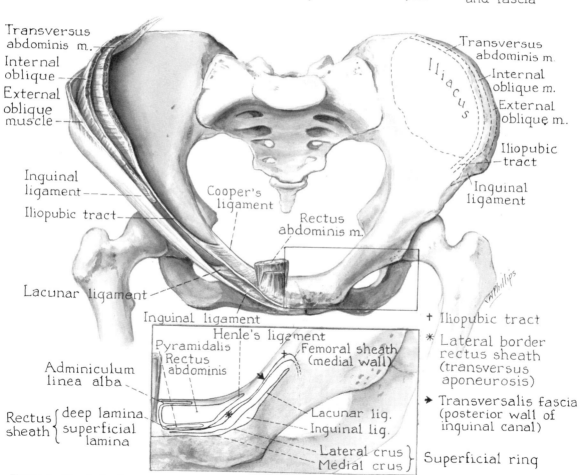

**Figure 5** The skeletal origins of the three flat muscles are indicated in the main figure. The origins of the internal oblique and transversus abdominis muscles are not only from the crest of the ilium but also partly from iliacus fascia and the iliopectineal arch (not shown). The complex insertions of the muscle layers of the groin into the body and superior ramus of the pubis are depicted in the inset (left side). The inferior portions of each of the three muscles of the groin have been preserved in this dissection to illustrate the relationships between these layers. The drawing shows well the relationship between the femoral sheath and canal (removed) and the insertions of the iliopubic tract and lacunar ligament. The internal oblique muscle arches above the spermatic cord and across the groin to insert into the deep lamina of the rectus sheath, usually somewhat superior to the line of transection depicted here. (From Condon, R. E. In: Nyhus, L. M., and Harkins, H. N.: Hernia. Philadelphia, J. B. Lippincott Company, 1964.)

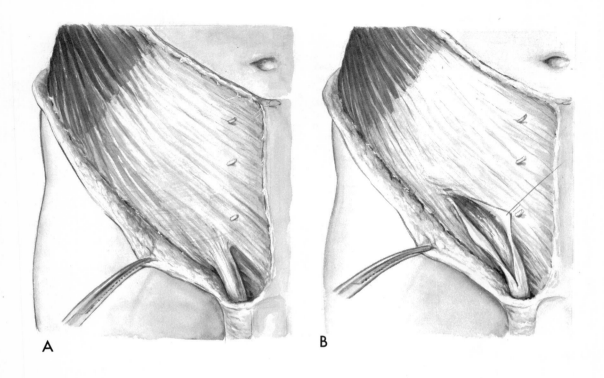

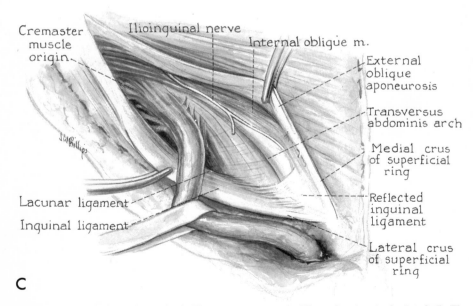

**Figure 6**   Dissection of the inguinal canal. *A,* The intact external oblique lamina is depicted. *B,* The external spermatic fascia and innominate fascia have been incised through the superficial inguinal ring. *C,* The external oblique aponeurosis has been opened widely and the spermatic cord mobilized by transecting many of its areolar (cremasteric fascia) attachments to the walls of the inguinal canal. (From Condon, R. E. In: Nyhus, L. M., and Harkins, H. N.: Hernia. Philadelphia, J. B. Lippincott Company, 1964.)

and around the trunk as a broad, flat muscle. The muscle fibers give way to their flat tendon of insertion, the external oblique aponeurosis, at the linea semilunaris, located in approximately the midclavicular line. The aponeurosis is attached to the iliac crest and the anterior superior iliac spine laterally (Fig. 5), and inserts rather broadly into the linea alba medially. It makes up a portion of the rectus sheath only very medially and does not attach to the lateral edge of the sheath, that structure being composed of deeper layers. Inferiorly, the aponeurosis is slightly thickened and folded back upon itself to form the inguinal ligament. As such, this structure is not a true ligament, since its function is not to stabilize bone. The lower edge of the inguinal ligament is loosely bound to the fascia lata by the innominate fascia. This fascia also serves to bind together the collagenous fibers of both the aponeurosis and the inguinal ligament. Medially the inguinal ligament inserts on the pubic tubercle, and fans downward onto the superior pubic ramus as the lacunar ligament. The medial attachment of the inguinal ligament is continuous with the insertion of the aponeurosis into the linea alba.

### External Inguinal Ring (Fig. 6)

Just above the inguinal ligament and lateral to its insertion onto the pubic tubercle, the fibers of the external oblique aponeurosis split to form a triangular opening, the external or superficial inguinal ring. The ring serves as the point of egress for the spermatic cord in the male and the round ligament in the female. It has no role in

diagnosis, prevention, or treatment of inguinal hernia.

### Internal Oblique Muscle

The internal oblique muscle is the central and most muscular layer of the abdominal wall. It originates from the lateral half of the inguinal ligament and the iliac fascia, from the anterior two-thirds of the middle lip of iliac crest, and from the lower portion of the lumbar aponeurosis near the crest. The aponeurosis of this muscle proceeds medially to fuse with the aponeurosis of the transversus abdominis muscle to form the anterior and, in the upper abdomen, posterior rectus sheaths. The fused aponeuroses then proceed medially to insert into the linea alba as the rectus sheath. The lowermost portion of the internal oblique, below the semilunar line of Douglas, contributes only to the anterior rectus sheath. In that area, it fuses with the transversus abdominis aponeurosis to form the sheath, but in only 5 per cent of persons does it fuse laterally to the sheath to form a "conjoined tendon." That anatomic structure is more a rarity than a constant finding, and its description should be deleted from the hernia literature.

Inferiorly and laterally the internal oblique originates from the inguinal ligament and the iliac crest and from deeper structures derived from the transversalis fascia. The medial margin of this insertion forms an arch over the internal inguinal ring. From this point fibers of the muscle arch downward and envelop the spermatic cord as it issues from the internal ring (Fig. 7). These fibers form the cremaster muscle. This muscle is impor-

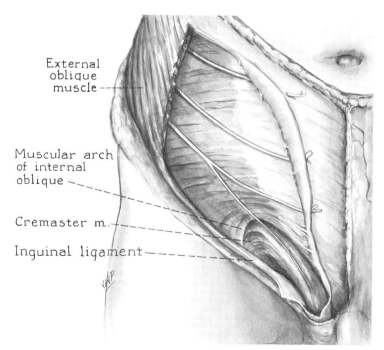

**Figure 7** Deeper dissection of the groin (right side) to show the internal oblique muscle layer. The spermatic cord has been left in situ. (From Condon, R. E. In: Nyhus, L. M., and Harkins, H. N.: Hernia. Philadelphia, J. B. Lippincott Company, 1964.)

External oblique muscle

Muscular arch of internal oblique

Cremaster m.

Inguinal ligament

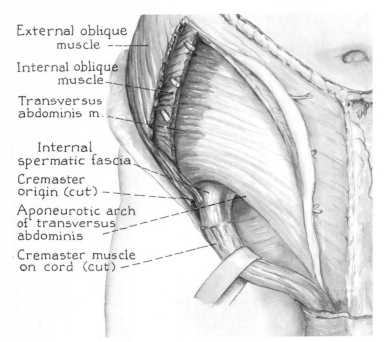

External oblique
   muscle

Internal oblique
   muscle

Transversus
abdominis m.

Internal
spermatic fascia

Cremaster
origin (cut)

Aponeurotic arch
of transversus
abdominis

Cremaster muscle
on cord (cut)

**Figure 8**   Dissection to show the deepest of the three muscle layers of the groin. The spermatic cord has been mobilized to show the arching muscular and aponeurotic lower margin of the transversus abdominis (the transversus abdominis arch). Inferior to this arch, the posterior wall of the inguinal canal is formed by transversalis fascia. (From Condon, R. E. In: Nyhus, L. M., and Harkins, H. N.: Hernia. Philadelphia, J. B. Lippincott Company, 1964.)

tant in hernia repair only in that it should be completely removed to expose the internal ring.

### Transversus Abdominis

This is the most internal of the three flat muscles of the abdominal wall. It rises by fleshy fibers from the lateral portion of the iliopubic tract, from the inner lip of the iliac crest, the lumbodorsal fascia, and from the inner surfaces of the cartilages of the lower six ribs. It passes medially in a transverse fashion around the lateral aspect of the abdomen onto the anterior abdominal wall. At a point lateral to the rectus sheath, its muscular fibers are replaced by a tendinous aponeurosis, which fuses with the internal oblique aponeurosis to form the rectus sheath. The lower free margin of this muscle arches with the internal oblique from the lateral origin of that muscle over the internal inguinal ring to form a free edge over the ring and above the floor of the inguinal canal medial to the ring (Fig. 8). This arch, called the transversus abdominis aponeurotic arch, occasionally fuses with the arch of the internal oblique aponeurosis to form a "conjoined tendon" or falx inguinalis, but in only 5 per cent of cases. The common finding is that the transversus aponeurosis joins the internal oblique at the rectus sheath. The arch forms the upper margin of the area through which inguinal hernias of all types protrude. The arch itself forms a basic component of the anatomic repair of all inguinal hernias.

### Endoabdominal Fascia

The endoabdominal or transversalis fascia is the most important layer in the prevention of groin and other abdominal wall hernias. This fascial layer forms a bag that holds the abdominal viscera within, and separates them from, the muscular and bony layers of the abdomen without. Various portions of the bag are known by different names, depending on the external structure at that point. Thus, the endoabdominal fascia underlying the transversus abdominis muscle and its aponeurosis is known as the transversalis fascia (Fig. 9).

### Hesselbach's Triangle

This classic anatomic designation is given to the area bounded superiorly by the falx inguinalis, laterally by the inferior epigastric vessels, and inferiorly by the inguinal ligament. As is already clear, the designation is confusing, since none of the three borders of the triangle is in the same layer of the abdominal wall. The inguinal ligament is superficial to the falx inguinalis (when one exists), and both layers are superficial to the inferior epigastric vessels. Use of this term in the description of hernia repair should be abandoned. More correctly, the boundaries of the floor of the inguinal canal, which is what Hesselbach intended to describe, should be limited to structures within that floor. These comprise the transversalis fascia and its analogs. For a complete understanding of these structures, the most important of the groin structures in hernia surgery, the reader is referred to classic works by Condon[16] and by Anson, Morgan, and McVay.[6] A full understanding of the anatomy and physiology of this layer is basic to a successful treatment of groin hernia.

### Transversalis Fascia Analogs

In several locations in the endoabdominal fascial sac, there exist thickenings or condensations of the

**Figure 9** Posterior (internal) view of the right groin following removal of the peritoneum, preperitoneal fat and lymphatics, and the iliacus fascia. The spermatic cord has been transected just internal to the deep inguinal ring. The structures of the transversus abdominis lamina are well shown. The inferior epigastric vein is more frequently a double channel where it lies upon the rectus abdominis, and its junction with the external iliac vein is often a little more proximal.

This drawing is also a good illustration of the difficulties of medical illustration in the groin region, problems similar to those faced by the cartographer in attempting to depict a curved surface on a flat plane. In order to present a drawing with no discontinuities, increasing distortion and exaggeration must be introduced as one proceeds from the central focus to the margins of the picture. The geographic exaggerations of a world map drawn on Mercator's projection are analogous to those of this figure. (From Condon, R. E. In: Nyhus, L. M., and Harkins, H. N.: Hernia. Philadelphia, J. B. Lippincott Company, 1964.)

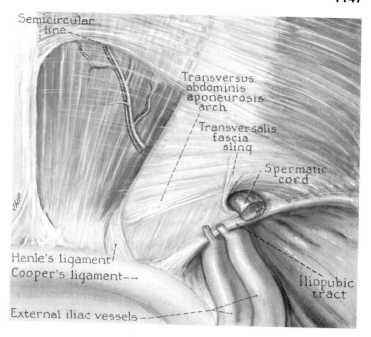

fascia, which are continuous with and integral to the sac itself (Fig. 10). These condensations, termed transversalis fascial analogs, usually are formed at points of insertion of various muscle groups, or at points of attachment of other fascial or aponeurotic structures into the fascial sac itself. Four important fascial analogs are: the transversalis fascial sling, the transversus abdominis aponeurotic arch, the iliopubic tract, and the iliopectineal ligament (Cooper's ligament).

**Transversalis Fascial Sling.** The transversalis fascial sling reinforces the medial margin of the internal inguinal ring. The internal ring itself is the site of exitus of the spermatic cord from the abdominal cavity. It is located midway between the anterior superior iliac spine and the pubic tubercle, and is 2 cm. above the inguinal ligament. As the cord structures exit through the ring, they turn medially and inferiorly to traverse the inguinal canal. As they perforate the transversalis fascia at the internal ring, they carry a prolongation of the transversalis fascia with them, the internal spermatic fascia. Because of the abrupt inferomedial turn that the cord structures take, this tubular projection of fascia is bent inferomedially, forming a fold at its lower medial margin. This fold has been likened to a monk's hood. The fold itself forms a slinglike thickened condensation in the transversalis fascia at the medial and inferior margin of the ring.

**Transversus Abdominis Aponeurotic Arch.** The transversus abdominis aponeurotic arch has already been mentioned. It forms the superior border of the floor of the inguinal canal and consists of the fused aponeurosis of the transversus abdominis with the transversalis fascia.

**Iliopubic Tract.** The iliopubic tract is another fascial condensation wholly integral to the endoabdominal fascial sac (Fig. 11). It arises from the iliopectineal arch, which is a fibrous condensation of endoabdominal fascia, spanning the iliopsoas muscles as they exit from the pelvis. Via this arch, the tract gains insertion on the anterior superior iliac spine and inner lip of the wing of the ilium. From its insertion it extends inferomedially above and slightly behind the inguinal ligament. Immediately after its origin, it arches over the femoral vessels forming the anterior portion of the femoral sheath. It then fans out to insert along the superior border of the pubic ramus and the pubic tubercle, and into the body of the pubis. Its lateral, recurved portion, that is, the portion that curves down to the pubic ramus immediately after the ligament passes over the femoral vessels, forms the medial boundary of the femoral canal. It is this fanlike recurved portion that ordinarily closes the femoral canal, and not the lacunar ligament, which is external to it.

**Cooper's Ligament.** On the posterior aspect of the superior ramus of the pubis and extending posterolaterally from it along the rim of the true pelvis is the iliopectineal line. Periosteum of the pelvis along the line is intimately fused with another condensation of the transversalis fascia and iliopubic tract to form Cooper's ligament. It is anatomically constant and always strong in character.

### Preperitoneal Space and Preperitoneal Fat

Between the transversalis fascia and peritoneum is the preperitoneal space, which is loosely filled with fat and fibrous tissue and is the internal analog of the abdominal panniculus without. It varies in thickness and density with the body

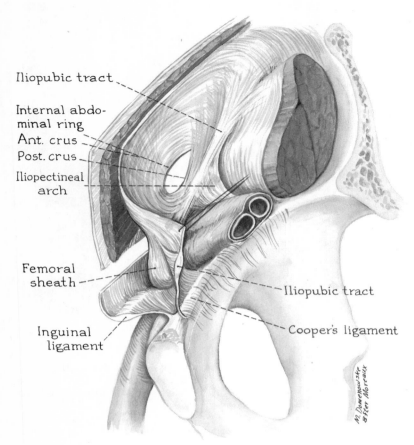

Iliopubic tract

Internal abdominal ring

Ant. crus

Post. crus

Iliopectineal arch

Femoral sheath

Inguinal ligament

Iliopubic tract

Cooper's ligament

**Figure 10** Fasciomusculoaponeurotic components of the lower abdominal wall. Right posterior oblique view. Note relationship of the transversalis fascia to the structures in the posterior inguinal wall. Spermatic cord has been removed and the iliopubic tract is reflected to demonstrate fascial continuity with the femoral sheath. The posterior inguinal wall (transversus abdominis–transversalis fascia lamina) is firmly "rooted" to the thigh at this point. The crura of the internal abdominal ring also are well shown. (From Nyhus, L. M.: Surg. Clin. N. Amer., *44*:1305, 1964.)

**Figure 11** Relation of the iliopubic tract to the femoral vessels and to Gimbernat's ligament. Medial cross section of right lower abdominal wall, viewed medial to lateral. (From Nyhus, L. M.: Surg. Clin. N. Amer., *44*:1305, 1964.)

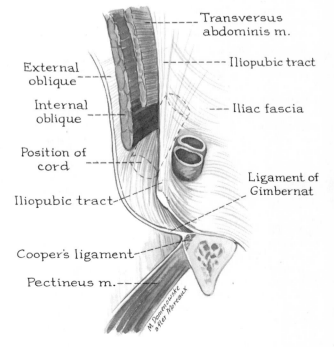

Transversus abdominis m.

External oblique

Iliopubic tract

Internal oblique

Iliac fascia

Position of cord

Iliopubic tract

Ligament of Gimbernat

Cooper's ligament

Pectineus m.

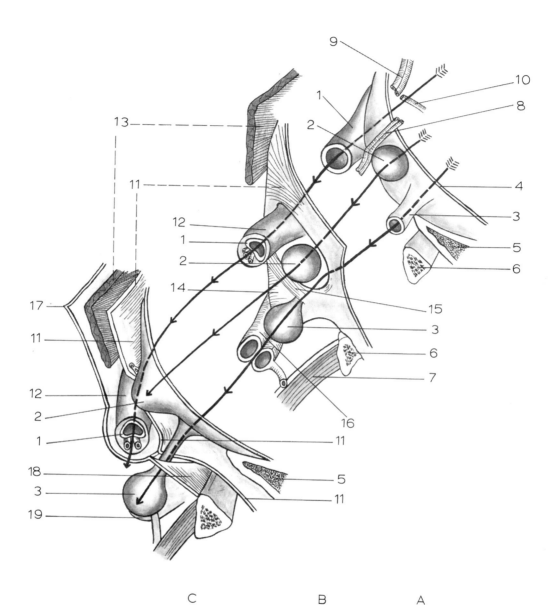

**Figure 12** Formation of hernias of the groin.
*A,* Peritoneal protrusions:
  1. Indirect inguinal hernial sac
  2. Direct inguinal hernial sac
  3. Femoral hernial sac
  4. Peritoneum
  5. Bladder
  6. Pubic bone
  7. Pectineus muscle
  8. Inferior epigastric vessels
  9. Spermatic vessels
  10. Vas deferens
(From Gaster, J.: Hernia: One Day Repair. New York,
Hafner Publishing Company, 1970.)

*B,* Transversus musculoaponeurotic fascial lamina:
  11. Transversalis aponeurosis and fascia
  12. Internal spermatic fascia
  13. Internal oblique muscle
  14. Femoral sheath
  15. Iliopubic tract
  16. Femoral vessels
*C,* Diagrammatic arrangement of groin:
  17. External oblique aponeurosis
  18. Gimbernat's ligament
  19. Fossa ovalis

habitus of the individual and may in the extremely thin person represent only a potential space.

### Peritoneum

Deep to the preperitoneal space and forming its innermost boundary is the peritoneum. In the groin, as elsewhere, the peritoneum is a thin elastic membrane, which serves only to provide a lubricating surface for its contained viscera. Because of the elastic character of the peritoneum, it does not act in the prevention of hernia.

### Spermatic Cord

The spermatic cord is formed at the internal ring by the confluence of the vas deferens from the testis with the spermatic artery and veins, which are descending into the ring to the testis. In the normal male these structures are also joined by a slip of fibrous tissue, the ligamentum vaginale, which is the remnant of the processus vaginalis of the peritoneum. At the ring the testicular vein is formed by the confluence of the pampiniform plexus of veins, which provide venous drainage of the spermatic cord and testis. As these structures exit through the deeper layers of the abdominal wall, they pursue an oblique downward course for 5 to 7 cm. into the scrotum, through the inguinal canal.

As the cord structures pass through the internal ring, transversalis fascia is reflected onto the cord as the internal spermatic fascia. The internal oblique muscle then contributes muscular fibers, which invest the cord as the cremaster muscle. The cremaster-covered cord then proceeds downward toward the pubic tubercle and the external inguinal ring. As it passes through the external ring, the investing fascia of the external oblique aponeurosis, Gallaudet's fascia,[24] is reflected onto the cord, covering the remaining slips of the cremaster muscle as the external spermatic fascia. The cord then enters the scrotum.

### Femoral Canal

This space, the femoral canal, is ordinarily closed by the reflected fibers of the iliopubic tract as they swing around the external iliac vein to attach to Cooper's ligament. It is a common misconception that the medial boundary of this canal is formed by the recurved fibers of the inguinal ligament. Those fibers and indeed that entire fascial layer is within the superficial stratum of the abdominal wall. The next most superficial layer is the inguinal ligament and its recurrent portion, the lacunar ligament. Thus the hernia sac protrudes through the internal femoral ring lateral to the recurved portion of the iliopubic tract, across Cooper's ligament, which is posterior to the sac, and beneath the inguinal ligament. It protrudes through the fossa ovalis, which is the defect in the fascia lata left for entrance of the greater saphenous vein. The fossa ovalis is loosely closed with the cribriform fascia, which is a prolongation of the innominate fascia from the abdominal wall (Fig. 12).

## PHYSIOLOGY OF INGUINAL CANAL STRUCTURES

In the normal person, two mechanisms act to preserve the integrity of the inguinal canal and to prevent protrusion of abdominal contents through the internal ring. The first of these is the sphincter action of the transversus abdominis and internal oblique muscles at the internal ring. The ring is attached to the transversus abdominis muscle via the transversalis fascial sling which reinforces the medial and inferior margin of the ring. When the transversus abdominis contracts it pulls the transversalis fascial sling superiorly and laterally. This serves both to close the internal ring around the cord structures and to pull the internal ring superiorly and laterally, under the buttress formed by the internal oblique. For this action to be effected, the transversalis fascia and its structures must be movable beneath the internal and external obliques. Any operative procedure that fixes the transversalis fascia or internal ring to a more superficial fixed structure, such as the inguinal ligament, destroys the sphincter action of the transversus abdominis.

The second mechanism closing the inguinal canal is the shutter action of the transversus abdominis aponeurotic arch, which normally is upwardly convex at rest, and is straightened and flattened when the transversus abdominis and internal oblique muscles are tensed (Fig. 13). Any tensing action brings the arch in apposition to the inguinal ligament, thereby covering the cord and buttressing the floor of the inguinal canal. It has been postulated that the occurrence of direct inguinal hernia is due primarily to a higher than normal position of this tranversus aponeurotic arch, so that when the abdominal musculature is stimulated and the arch brought down, it does not reach the inguinal ligament and iliopubic tract, thereby leaving a weakened area in the floor of the inguinal canal, which is defended only by the transversalis fascia. The incidence of recurrent

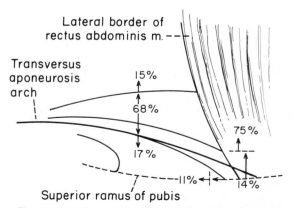

**Figure 13** The relationships of the insertion of the transversus abdominis arch to the lateral border of the rectus abdominis and to the superior ramus of the pubis as found in a group of 135 dissections of the groin. (From Condon, R. E. In: Nyhus, L. M., and Harkins, H. N.: Hernia. Philadelphia, J. B. Lippincott Company, 1964.)

hernia following various repairs and, indeed, all direct hernias have been attributed to this "congenital" malformation.

## DIAGNOSIS, INCIDENCE, AND PROGNOSIS

### Diagnosis

Diagnosis of hernia is made usually on the basis of physical examination rather than history. In children, however, the mother's insistence upon having observed a lump in the groin should alert the examiner to the presence of a groin hernia even if the first examination is negative. Similarly, chronic use of a truss may cause such a degree of scarring that the hernial sac does not readily fill with bowel. A negative examination in this setting should be followed after several days by success if the patient leaves the truss off in the interim. Dragging sensations or pain in the groin suggests the presence of a hernia. Modest pain is common at the outset, but as time progresses, sensations in the area become those of only vague discomfort.

Examination of the groin is best accomplished with the examiner seated on a low chair before the standing patient. The examination consists of the following: (1) observation of the groin area for evidence of a bulge or swelling while the patient coughs or tenses the abdominal musculature, preferably while holding a deep breath; (2) repetition of the preceding step with the index finger invaginated into the external ring for palpation of bulges or significant pressure impulses against the examining finger (note that an enlarged external ring without a palpable mass or impulse does *not* connote the presence of a hernia); and (3) repetition of steps 1 and 2 while the patient is lying down. At one time it was considered important to differentiate preoperatively between direct and indirect hernias during examination, but this seems less important now when surgeons are able to make an accurate diagnosis and perform an appropriate technical procedure at the operating table. Femoral hernias must be differentiated from inguinal hernias during the examination because their presence often means that a different operative approach is indicated. The common error is to miss a femoral hernia. If, on accurate palpation, the swelling protrudes below the inguinal ligament it is femoral; if above, it is inguinal. A number of other "lumps and bumps" appear in the groin which must be differentiated from hernial swellings. These include: (1) inguinal adenitis; (2) ectopic testis; (3) hydrocele of the cord; (4) psoas abscess; (5) femoral adenitis; and (6) saphenous varix.

### Incidence

Accurate figures for the incidence are difficult to obtain. Statistics available are those from the 1960 survey of the U.S. Department of Health, Education, and Welfare,[69] which found that hernia occurred in approximately 15 per 1000 of the population interviewed, i.e., 3 million Americans. The same government agency found that 40 mil-

lion days of restricted activity per year could be attributed to this problem. Each person with a hernia averaged almost 16 days of restricted activity as a result of the condition. More important, the total amount of work loss by the populace with hernias was 10 million days, a figure that reflects the prevalence of hernias in the male population. The economic aspects of the hernial problem are further revealed by the National Health Survey of 1960. In one year, 1957–1958, 450,000 hernia repairs were performed. This represented 7 per cent of all nonobstetrical surgery performed during that year. Tonsillectomy was the only operative procedure performed with greater frequency.

Approximately 50 per cent of all hernias are indirect inguinal and one-quarter are direct inguinal. Incisional and ventral abdominal hernias represent about 10 per cent, followed by femoral, 6 per cent; umbilical, 3 per cent; esophageal hiatus, 1 per cent; and miscellaneous rarer types, 2 per cent. The total balance tips in favor of the groin hernias, roughly 75 per cent of all. Parenthetically, it should be noted that 86 per cent of all groin hernias occur in males, yet 84 per cent of all femoral hernias occur in females. It must be emphasized, however, that the most common groin hernia found in the female is the indirect inguinal, and the incidence of femoral hernia in females is so high only because of the relatively rare incidence of femoral hernia in males.

### Prognosis after Treatment

In this modern era of surgery, *recurrence* of the hernia after operative treatment remains a real problem. The poorer results are related to many factors, including: (1) failure of the operating room surgeon to understand the fine nuances of the surgical anatomy within the groin; (2) failure to use meticulous operative technique for the *common* hernia repair; and (3) failure to follow all patients operated upon so that each surgeon is aware of his technical shortcomings.[29] Until this subject is taken seriously, 100,000 patients per year will continue to be disappointed upon the recurrence of what was thought to be a simple problem.

## THE DANGER OF HERNIA

### Mortality

Morbidity and economic factors have been discussed. Unfortunately, death rates from this potentially curable entity remain high. A 1964 survey of the Department of Health, Education and Welfare showed that 2030 persons died from intestinal obstruction due to hernia. A similar report in 1967 listed hernia associated with intestinal obstruction as one of the 10 leading causes of death in the United States.[26]

### Incarceration, Strangulation, and Intestinal Obstruction

The sine qua non of danger is protrusion of a hollow viscus outside its normal environment through a ring of variable size. If the viscus becomes caught by the ring and cannot be replaced, it has become incarcerated. If in addition blood flow to or from the protruding viscus is compromised, the process of strangulation begins, with ultimate necrosis of the bowel if left unattended. Incarcerated hernias are difficult to differentiate from those in which the strangulating process has begun and therefore are considered to be surgical emergencies.

Incarcerated hernias may or may not cause intestinal obstruction, but essentially all hernias involving bowel that reach the stage of vascular compromise do cause the signs and symptoms of intestinal obstruction. There are two exceptions, namely, Richter's hernia, i.e., one side of the bowel wall is involved, and Littre's hernia, i.e., the incarceration and strangulation of a Meckel's diverticulum. In all patients with signs and symptoms of intestinal obstruction all potential hernia sites must be visualized and palpated, and contrariwise all patients with incarcerated or strangulated hernia should be carefully reviewed for the presence of intestinal obstruction. Femoral, indirect inguinal, and umbilical hernias are more likely to cause strangulation of bowel because these sacs have smaller necks that tend to be surrounded by rings of rigid tissue. Direct inguinal hernias usually have a broad neck and incarceration with attendant complications is infrequent.

Recognition of impending or actual strangulation is extremely important since emergency measures (operation) are indicated. Pain in the region of the hernial swelling and particularly tenderness to palpation are ominous signs. Sudden change from a state of hernial reducibility to irreducibility and discoloration of the tissues over the swelling are additional signs of strangulation.

Without signs of strangulation, an incarcerated hernia of short duration may be carefully reduced by gentle but firm pressure upon the swelling. It is possible to reduce the bowel content from its extracavitary position but not release the bowel from the peritoneal sac, i.e., reduction en masse. Thus, patients must be observed for a period following reduction to assure restoration of normal bowel activity.

## INGUINAL HERNIA IN CHILDHOOD

Infants and children with *inguinal* hernias nearly always have the *indirect* type. The hernias are related to abnormal descent of the testis and failure of normal obliteration of the processus vaginalis. Direct hernias in childhood are quite rare.

### Diagnosis

Difficulties may arise in determining the presence of an inguinal hernia in infants; usually the older child presents no problem. A fat pad in infants may obscure the bulge, but careful inspection and palpation will usually suffice to establish the diagnosis. Palpation of the spermatic cord at its entrance into the scrotum may create, when rolling the fingers from side to side, a sensation of silk rubbing on silk if a hernia is present. In female infants, the lack of the spermatic cord may create further difficulties, but again the sensation of gliding silk ("silk glove" test) may be helpful. A definite history from the mother of a lump in the groin plus these suggestive findings is sufficient indication for operative exploration.

### Treatment

There is general agreement that once the diagnosis of inguinal hernia is established, elective surgical repair should be performed. In general it is rare to find an infant or child of such poor risk that an operation cannot be done. Further, it is fallacious to believe that hernias in this age group heal spontaneously or that the application of a truss will obliterate the funicular process.

Since the cause of hernia here is failure of the processus vaginalis to become obliterated, and no muscular weakness is present, surgical treatment should include only obliteration of the hernial sac (by high ligation and transection, with or without excision of the distal sac). Thus, operative techniques that reinforce the abdominal wall ordinarily should not be used and the wound is reconstituted but not reconstructed.

## INGUINAL HERNIAS IN ADULTS

Hernias may be classified as either funicular or diffuse. The former type protrudes through a tight fibrous ring of some sort, almost always at the site of exitus of some structure from the endoabdominal fascial sac. Indirect inguinal hernias, femoral hernias, and umbilical hernias are all funicular. These hernias tend to incarceration, obstruction, and even strangulation, because of the tight ring through which the herniating viscera protrude. In addition to causing the usual symptoms of dragging discomfort at the site of herniation, these hernias are always potentially disastrous and must be repaired whenever found.

Diffuse hernias, on the other hand, lack the tight constricting ring at the site of exitus from the endoabdominal fascial sac. Most ventral hernias, direct inguinal hernias, and lumbar hernias fit this classification.

In the indirect inguinal hernia the protruding viscus exits from the endoabdominal fascial sac through the internal inguinal ring. The herniating viscus, therefore, always has the same coverings as the investments of the spermatic cord, and does not actually protrude through any layer of the abdominal wall. By its nature, it always requires a preformed or at least a potential sac, which in this instance is the patent processus vaginalis. It is therefore a true congenital defect. Depending on the length of the patent processus vaginalis, the indirect inguinal hernia may protrude into the inguinal canal or through the external ring, or extend into the scrotum.

### Indirect Hernia

The processus vaginalis testis is the peritoneal tube through which the fetal testis reaches the scrotum from its intraperitoneal origin in the seventh to eighth month. Normally it obliterates completely to form a fibrous cord, the ligamentum vaginale, which extends from a dimple on the parietal peritoneum deep to the internal ring down through the inguinal canal into the scrotum to the tunica vaginalis and testis. It may only partially obliterate anywhere along the course of its descent. The various anomalies of processus obliteration are frequently associated. An undescended testicle or a testicle in the inguinal canal is always associated with an indirect inguinal hernia. The high association of either testicular or cord hydroceles with inguinal hernias is well known.

Indirect inguinal hernias may be further subdivided with regard to the extent of dilatation of the internal inguinal ring. An infantile or childhood hernia may have a normal or only slightly enlarged internal inguinal ring, with the major defect being only protrusion of bowel into a patent processus vaginalis. It should be emphasized that a simple patent processus vaginalis is not a hernia, but that it possesses a high potential of becoming one.

If the hernia has been present for some time, the internal ring may be enlarged. Such a hernia is frequently found in the young adult. If the ring enlarges sufficiently to begin to push the inferior epigastric vessels medially, a simple adult hernia is present. If the enlargement impinges on the floor of the inguinal canal, a combined indirect-direct hernia, is present. Occasionally the ring is dilated sufficiently without displacement of the inferior epigastric vessel to impinge on the floor of the inguinal canal. This condition results in an outpouching of peritoneum around the inferior epigastric vessels, so that both direct and indirect hernial sacs exist, straddling those vessels. This is the pantaloon hernia.

### Direct Hernia

In a direct hernia the protruding viscus does not herniate through a preformed ring. The transversalis fascia weakens and bulges outward in front of the hernial mass. In the case of the direct inguinal hernia, the weakness in the wall of the sac is in the floor of the inguinal canal medial to the internal inguinal ring and medial to the inferior epigastric vessels. In the past, the location of the inferior epigastric vessels lateral to the hernia has been considered important. In our experience, these vessels may be anywhere with regard to the location of the direct hernia, and may even be a part of the wall of the hernial sac.

Most recurrent hernias are direct, resulting after the repair of indirect inguinal hernia. A few recurrent hernias will be indirect. In every instance, a recurrent indirect hernia is due to failure of the initial operating surgeon to remove the patent processus vaginalis (hernial sac) from the cord at the internal ring. As long as a peritoneal outpouching is left through the internal ring, hernia is a threat. The sac may be left in the cord if the sac is divided at the internal ring.

## INGUINAL HERNIA REPAIR

Currently, controversy exists regarding the proper layers of the abdominal wall to be used for repair of inguinal hernia. On this basis the types of repair have been divided into the posterior (transversalis fascia lamina) and anterior (external-internal oblique lamina). Proponents of the posterior repair insist that the reconstruction of the inguinal canal and of the internal inguinal ring should be accomplished with preservation of deep groin anatomy. Transversalis fascial structures should be sutured to transversalis fascial structures. Layers normally found superficial to the inguinal canal and its content should not be used to reinforce the posterior wall of the inguinal canal. This approach is based on the concept that the basic hernial defect lies within the deep structures of the abdominal wall, that is, those deep to the internal oblique, and therefore the repair should reside within those layers.

On the other hand, proponents of the anterior type of repair do not make the distinction between superficial and deep layers of the abdominal wall, and consequently use superficial structures such as the external oblique aponeurosis and inguinal ligament as either anchoring points or artificial buttresses for repair of the internal ring and floor of the inguinal canal. Surgeons who use the anterior lamina ignore the fact that the superficial stratum of the abdominal wall musculature is movable upon the deep stratum and vice versa. Artificial attachment of the deep layer to the superficial layer results in strain at the suture line or attachment, and this may be the reason for the high incidence of recurrence with this type of hernia repair. Nonetheless, a large fund of experience has been reported with repairs described by Halsted, Bassini, Andrews, and Ferguson. Rarely, the anatomic layers of the deep stratum of the abdominal wall may be insufficient to permit repair strictly within that layer, and the more superficial procedures may be required.

A single operative technique is not appropriate in all patients. The approach must be designed at the operating table to properly handle the following variations: (1) small indirect inguinal; (2) medium indirect inguinal; (3) large indirect and direct inguinal; and (4) femoral hernias.[31]

### Small Indirect Inguinal Hernia

The basic pathologic feature here is a patent processus vaginalis with minimal dilatation of the internal abdominal ring. After removal of the hernial sac and high ligation of the neck of the sac, restoration of the transversalis fascia surrounding the spermatic cord at the internal ring will suffice. Since the hernial sac tends to enlarge the ring medially, the sutures are placed medial to the

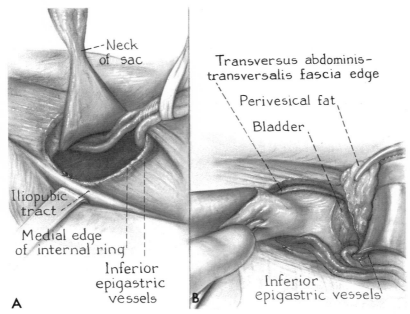

**Figure 14**   Repair of small indirect inguinal hernia. Identification of the internal ring. *A,* The vas and vessels have been separated from the peritoneum posteriorly. The vas turns medially while the vessels continue upward. Note how the neck of the sac is freed and pulled beyond the internal ring for ligation well above the neck. The medial boundary of the internal ring is now well defined after removal of the internal spermatic fascia. The iliopubic tract is exposed by downward retraction of the inguinal ligament. The iliopubic tract blends with that fascia adjacent to the ligated external spermatic artery. *B,* The retractor inserted into the internal ring pulls the medial edge of the internal ring and inferior epigastric vessels medially. The sac has been opened, and a finger inserted into the sac pulls the peritoneum out. The perivesical fat has been dissected from the peritoneum to expose bladder muscle. This dissection affords high ligation of the sac medially. (From Griffith, C. A.: Surg. Clin. N. Amer., *39:*531, 1959.)

cord structures. Although this is the simplest of all hernial defects to correct, it is also the most common and a meticulous anatomic dissection and repair here gives great satisfaction. Griffith[28] in 1959 described a technique for this repair (Figs. 14 to 16), an anterior approach to the posterior inguinal wall.

### Medium Indirect Inguinal Hernia and Attenuated Posterior Inguinal Floor

Occasionally, the internal ring has expanded (enlarged) further medially, and the posterior inguinal wall appears attenuated. In this instance the sutures are "walked" from the internal ring

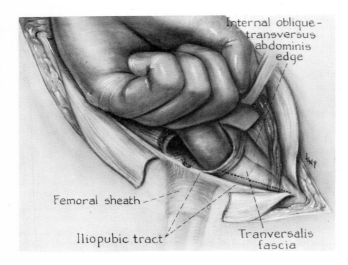

**Figure 15**   Repair of small indirect inguinal hernia. The hole in transversalis fascia. The sac has been ligated and removed. A finger inserted through the internal ring, behind the transversalis fascia preperitoneally down to the pubic spine, palpates the inguinal floor. A section of inguinal ligament has been diagrammatically removed to show the transversalis fascia comprising the inguinal floor. This diagram demonstrates that the iliopubic tract continues with that fascia adjacent to the ligated external spermatic artery. This fascia is also continuous with the femoral sheath. The stump of the external spermatic artery is therefore a landmark for the fascia comprising the inferior edge of the internal ring. Superiorly, the transversalis fascia continues beneath transversus abdominis aponeurosis. (From Griffith, C. A.: Surg. Clin. N. Amer., *39:*531, 1959.)

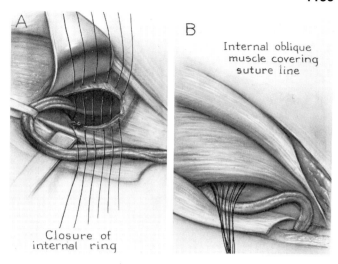

**Figure 16** Repair of small indirect inguinal hernia. Repair of the internal ring. *A*, Sutures are placed through transversalis fascia and only transversalis fascia. The cord structures are displaced laterally. The reconstructed ring admits only the tip of a hemostat. The repair has been made possible by removal of cremaster muscle and retraction as illustrated. *B*, Retractors have been removed to allow the inguinal ligament and the internal oblique and transversus abdominis muscles to assume their normal positions at rest. The internal ring is buttressed by overlying muscle. (From Griffith, C. A.: Surg. Clin. N. Amer., *39*:531, 1959.)

closure medially between the aponeurotic arch of transversus abdominis and iliopubic tract until the pecten of the pubis is reached. Thus, in addition to the plastic closure of the internal ring, the posterior inguinal floor has been strengthened. Small direct hernias are handled in the same manner except that dissection of the internal ring is unnecessary.

### Large Indirect and Direct Inguinal Hernia

These are the most difficult problems. As the indirect hernia enlarges, it breaks down the posterior inguinal wall medial to the internal ring, so that in essence the surgeon must reconstruct the entire posterior inguinal wall and form a new internal inguinal ring. McVay has popularized the Cooper's ligament repair for this problem and has reported a 3.6 per cent overall recurrence rate; this result is unexcelled by any other author in the world literature.[31] Because of the importance of this contribution we quote from his description of the technique (Fig. 17).

In addition to the presence of the congenital hernial sac, *a large indirect inguinal hernia*, because of the greatly enlarged abdominal inguinal ring, has destroyed the posterior wall of the inguinal canal. In accomplishing the repair of this type of hernia, one must not only remove the hernial sac and make a snug abdominal inguinal ring, but also reconstruct a new posterior inguinal wall [Fig. 17].

Through the years, innumerable devices have been used to obtain muscular, aponeurotic and fascial material to replace the posterior inguinal wall. Some of them have merit while others are based on false anatomic premises. Any hernioplasty which fastens the new posterior inguinal wall to the inguinal ligament is anatomically unsound. It should be the object of every hernia operation to return the region to the normal anatomic state.

When the posterior inguinal wall is destroyed in part or in toto by a large indirect inguinal hernia, aponeuroticofascial tissue must be borrowed somewhere to close the defect. The simplest device is to use the aponeurosis and fused fasciae of the transversus abdominis immediately above and medial to the defect [Fig. 17]. This aponeuroticofascial plate also contains the lowest aponeurotic fibers of the internal oblique muscle. Where

it lies over the rectus abdominis muscle, it is known as the rectus sheath. This layer is the ideal material because it is primarily aponeurotic. The fasciae, of which the innermost layer is the transversalis fascia, serve to bind the aponeurotic fibers together into a firm and intact layer. Fascia or muscle does not meet the requirements for a satisfactory layer to close a hernial defect.

Another sound surgical principle is that layers should be approximated without tension. If one sutures the strong edge of the transversus abdominis aponeurosis to Cooper's ligament, there is considerable tension on the suture line. The same difficulty is encountered in the classic herniorrhaphies which use the inguinal ligament as the anchoring structure. To obviate tension, the relaxing incision [Fig. 17] should be used in every instance in which the posterior inguinal wall is reconstructed. A modification of the relaxing incision is the turning downward of a triangular flap of the rectus sheath. The slide of the rectus sheath made possible by the relaxing incision seems more physiologic than the flap method because the normal direction of musculoaponeurotic pull is maintained. . . .

Before the new posterior inguinal wall can be transferred into position, all of the attenuated old posterior inguinal wall and hypertrophied cord fasciae must be excised [Fig. 17]. The peritoneal hernial sac must be dissected out and the neck of the sac ligated as for any indirect inguinal hernia. For an accurate repair of this hernia, one must have an evenly cut margin of transversus abdominis aponeurosis above, from abdominal inguinal ring to Cooper's ligament. Below, the glistening margin of Cooper's ligament must be seen medially and the edge of the anterior femoral sheath laterally. When these margins have been carefully dissected and the peritoneal sac excised, one is then ready to repair the hernia [Fig. 17c].

After making the relaxing incision [Fig. 17a and b], the strong cut edge of the transversus abdominis aponeurosis is sutured to Cooper's ligament from the pubic tubercle to within a few millimeters of the external iliac vein [Fig. 17d]. This maneuver not only reconstructs the posterior inguinal wall, but also re-establishes a normally broad insertion into Cooper's ligament and thus obviates the possibility of the development of a femoral hernia. It should be noted that the relaxing incision [Fig. 17d] is now a considerable defect in the rectus sheath, protected behind by the rectus and pyramidalis muscles and their fasciae.

The next suture is the transition suture which approxi-

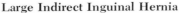

Large Indirect Inguinal Hernia          Direct Inguinal Hernia

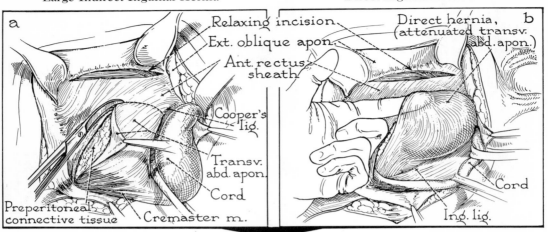

## RECONSTRUCTION OF THE POSTERIOR INGUINAL WALL

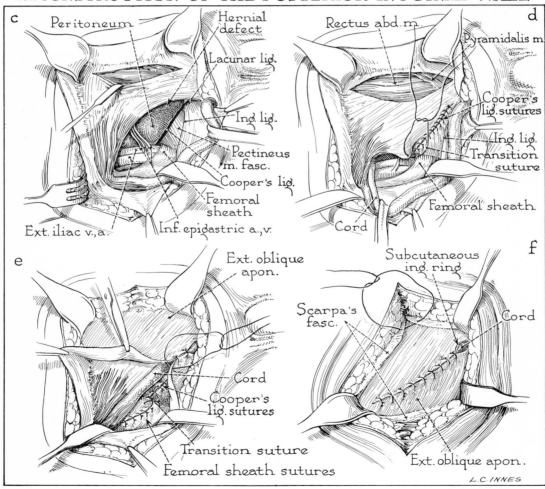

**Figure 17**  Hernioplasty for large indirect and direct inguinal hernias. *a,* Cutting out the attenuated portion of the posterior inguinal wall in a large indirect inguinal hernia. *b,* Attenuated posterior inguinal wall that is to be removed in a direct inguinal hernia. *c, d, e,* and *f,* Successive steps in the reconstruction of the posterior inguinal wall. Hernioplasty for both large indirect and direct inguinal hernias. (From McVay, C. B. In: Davis, L.: Christopher's Textbook of Surgery. 9th ed., Philadelphia, W. B. Saunders Company, 1968.)

mates the edge of the transversus abdominis aponeurosis to the medial wall of the femoral sheath and pectineus muscle fascia. This suture is necessary to close the angle and permit the line of closure to come up from the level of Cooper's ligament to the more superficial level of the anterior femoral sheath. This distance is represented by the diameter of the external iliac vein.

The remaining defect is closed by suturing the transversus abdominis aponeurosis, or in case the layer is muscular at this point, the transversalis fascia, to the anterior layer of the femoral sheath. This re-establishes the normal continuity of transversalis fascia into the anterior femoral sheath. This line of sutures is continued laterally until a snug abdominal inguinal ring is made just as it is done for the repair of the small- to medium-sized indirect inguinal hernia. The spermatic cord is dropped in against the new posterior inguinal wall and the external oblique aponeurosis closed over it [Fig. 17*e* and *f*], thus re-establishing the obliquity of the inguinal canal. The subcutaneous inguinal ring is snugly closed.[52]

Repair of a large direct hernia is performed in a similar manner to replace the destroyed posterior inguinal wall. The only difference in the technique is the management of the peritoneal sac. High ligation of the peritoneal sac is mandatory in the operation for indirect inguinal hernia, but the broad neck of the direct inguinal hernia precludes the necessity of even opening the peritoneum.

### Femoral Hernia

By popular usage, femoral hernia has been separated from indirect and direct inguinal hernias because of its exit beneath the inguinal ligament. We believe as others[31] that it should be considered a third variety of inguinal hernia. Its anatomic boundaries are familiar to us after study of the posterior inguinal wall: (1) superior—iliopubic tract (anterior femoral sheath); (2) inferior—Cooper's ligament; (3) lateral—femoral vein; and (4) medial—insertion of iliopubic tract into Cooper's ligament (previously said to be lacunar ligament).

The McVay Cooper's ligament repair is very satisfactory for repair of femoral hernia. Other techniques include the "low approach"[45] and the inguinal approach (Annandale,[5] Moschcowitz,[53] Ruggi[61]). Resurgence of interest in the preperitoneal approach, particularly for femoral hernia, has occurred during the past decade.[54] For safety, for visualization of anatomic structures, and for ease of performance of ancillary procedures, the posterior or preperitoneal approach to the repair of femoral hernia is recommended. It is unquestionably superior to the direct anterior and subinguinal approaches.

**Posterior (Preperitoneal) Approach to Femoral Hernia.** The skin incision for the preperitoneal approach is different from that employed for the anterior approach (Fig. 18). It is oriented horizontally and is placed approximately three fingerbreadths above the pubic tubercle. One-third extends over the rectus muscle and two-thirds lateral to it. The edges of the skin incision are retracted and dissection is carried to the preperitoneal space. With blunt dissection the preperitoneal fat is dissected away from the lower abdominal wall.

The hernial sac can readily be seen protruding into the femoral canal medial to the external iliac vein and just lateral to the reflected fibers of the iliopubic tract, and anterior to Cooper's ligament (Fig. 19). The femoral canal is closed by apposition of the iliopubic tract to Cooper's ligament (Fig. 20).

A direct hernia may be repaired through this approach with excellent results.[41, 55, 59] However, since some authors[25, 49] report high recurrence rates following the preperitoneal approach and repair we do not recommend it for general use at this time. A Cooper's ligament repair may be carried out from the same approach. Cooper's ligament is readily identifiable at the inferomedial aspect of the wound as it proceeds posteriorly from the pubic tubercle along the iliopectineal line. As with the anterior approach, sutures are placed through the transversus abdominis

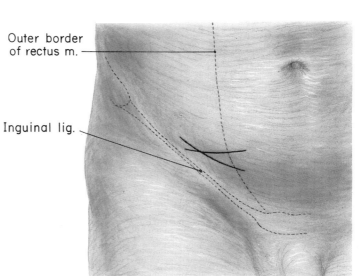

**Figure 18**   Incisions used in the anterior and preperitoneal approaches. The preperitoneal area is approached through the short, horizontal incision. The direct anterior approach is achieved through the longer incision in the lines of skin tension. (From Nyhus, L. M., and Bombeck, C. T.: GP, *33*:115, 1966.)

Outer border of rectus m.

Inguinal lig.

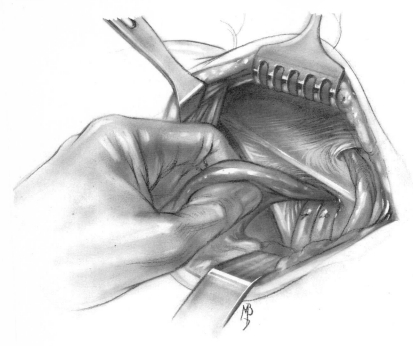

**Figure 19** Femoral hernia. The peritoneal sac of the femoral hernia is reduced by traction and blunt dissection. (From Nyhus, L. M. In: Nyhus, L. M., and Harkins, H. N.: Hernia. Philadelphia, J. B. Lippincott Company, 1964.)

aponeurotic arch and Cooper's ligament in the medial aspect of the repair, a transition suture is placed between the transversus arch, iliopubic tract, and Cooper's ligament, and finally the lateral portion of the repair is completed with sutures through the transversus arch and the iliopubic tract.

When Cooper's ligament repair is performed

through the posterior approach, the transversus abdominis aponeurosis is seen to be apposed to Cooper's ligament with a deceptive lack of tension. This lack of tension is due to the incision in the transversus abdominis, which was used to enter the preperitoneal space. When the operative wound in the transversus abdominis is closed at the end of the procedure, tension again is placed

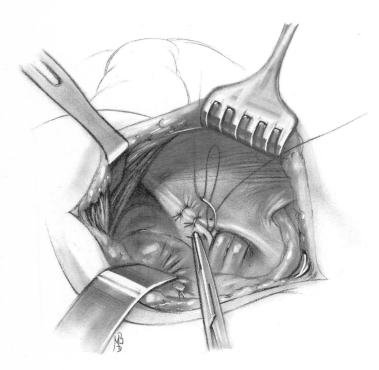

**Figure 20** Femoral hernia. The femoral canal is narrowed by sutures placed between the iliopubic tract above and Cooper's ligament below. (From Nyhus, L. M.: In: Nyhus, L. M., and Harkins, H. N.: Hernia. Philadelphia, J. B. Lippincott Company, 1964.)

on this aponeurosis and therefore upon the suture line. Consequently, a relaxing incision must be placed as before.

**Anterior Inguinal Wall Repairs.** The classic Bassini operation consists of suturing the transversus abdominis aponeurotic arch to the lacunar and inguinal ligaments beneath the cord. The various modifications of Halsted,[30] Lucas-Championnière,[44] Andrews,[4] and Ferguson[23] are well known. Literally millions of hernia patients have been cured by these techniques. These latter techniques have been used throughout the world much more frequently than the repair of the posterior inguinal wall presented in detail here. On the other hand, an inordinate rate of recurrence persists (5 to 20 per cent) following the anterior wall repair. Whether this is due to a basic failure of the anatomic repair, failure of the surgeon to take the necessary time to do a good repair, or the presence of a basic defect in the collagen synthesis of hernia patients[56] is not known.

## SPECIAL PROBLEMS, HERNIAS, AND MISCELLANEA

### Appendectomy

In the past it was debatable whether the appendix should be removed during repair of a right inguinal hernia. A good rule for the experienced surgeon is to do so if the appendix is adequately exposed and the patient can tolerate the procedure. It is unlikely that any harm will result from removal of the appendix in an otherwise uncomplicated hernia repair,[21] although most surgeons generally do not perform the procedures simultaneously.

### Cooper's Hernia

The sac follows the femoral canal but additional tracts pass into the scrotum, toward the labium majus, and toward the obturator foramen.[2]

### Division of the Spermatic Cord

Surgical castration, with removal of the testicle on the involved side, division of the spermatic cord at the internal ring, and complete closure of the ring, has been used as a method of treatment of inguinal hernia particularly in aged men and after multiple recurrent hernias. Prior written permission must be obtained if this is contemplated.

If cord division is planned without removal of the testicle, great care must be exercised in dissection of the cord to prevent embarrassment of the collateral blood supply of the testicle (Fig. 21).

### Exploration of the Opposite Side in Children

Controversy continues whether the opposite groin should be explored in the infant undergoing repair of unilateral inguinal hernia. The incidence of a second hernia appearing on the contralateral

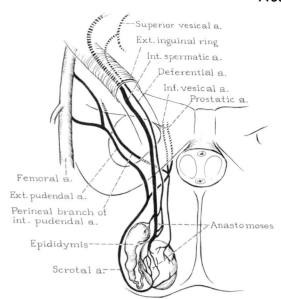

**Figure 21** Schematic drawing of both primary and collateral circulation of the testis. (From Nyhus, L. M. In: Artz, C. P., and Hardy, J. D., eds.: Complications in Surgery and Their Management. 2nd ed. Philadelphia, W. B. Saunders Company, 1967.)

side following repair of a clinically unilateral hernia has been reported to be between 3 and 31 per cent. There is an apparent discrepancy between this observation in a series of patients following their first herniorrhaphy, and the findings of other surgeons who report a much higher incidence of patent processus vaginalis on the other side when contralateral exploration is performed at the time of original operation. This has been used as justification for always exploring the contralateral side should conditions permit. Santulli[62] has compared two groups of pediatric patients presenting with unilateral inguinal hernia. In one group the hernia was repaired and nothing further was done; in the second group, the hernia was repaired and contralateral exploration carried out. A 14 year follow-up was conducted on the first group and in 12 per cent a contralateral hernia subsequently developed. In the second group, with contralateral exploration, a patent processus vaginalis was found on the opposite side in 56 per cent. On the basis of this finding, we do not recommend contralateral exploration. Cavanagh and Schnug[13] have stated what appear to be adequate criteria for contralateral exploration.

Given a surgeon familiar with pediatric surgery, an experienced anesthesiologist, an otherwise healthy baby, and an operation that is proceeding rapidly and smoothly, there appears to be little risk associated with bilateral exploration; however, if the baby is premature or has any associated illness, or should the surgeon have any difficulty with his initial repair, or if anesthesia is not being well tolerated, contralateral exploration should not be done. If the baby is being operated on for incarceration, contralateral exploration should not be done.

In short, exploration of the opposite side depends to a large extent on the condition of the patient and the experience of the surgeon.

### Hesselbach's Hernia (External Femoral Hernia)

This hernial sac passes into the pelvis lateral to the femoral vessels but below the inguinal ligament and iliopubic tract. It is usually associated with an indirect hernia on the same side.

### Incarcerated and Strangulated Hernias

An incarcerated hernia is, by definition, simply an irreducible one. Incarceration of itself would not be a particularly emergent condition were it not for the possible supervention of strangulation of the incarcerated viscus. Strangulation of a hernia is a true surgical emergency and must be treated as soon as the diagnosis is made. The most commonly strangulated groin hernia is the femoral, but because it is a rare hernia compared with the inguinal hernia, there are fewer strangulated femoral hernias than there are strangulated inguinal hernias.

The usual vigorous efforts of the surgeon to reduce an incarcerated hernia must be tempered with the awareness of two possible complications. The first of these is "reduction en masse," wherein the hernia, with sac, is reduced within the endoabdominal fascia, so that even though the external bulge is reduced, the hernia remains incarcerated within the sac. Therefore, following reduction of any incarcerated hernia the patient must be carefully observed for signs of continuing intestinal obstruction.

The second possibility is the potentially catastrophic event of reduction of a strangulated, nonviable piece of bowel within the abdominal cavity. At the first sign of strangulation of a hernia all attempts at reduction must be abandoned and the patient operated upon immediately.

### Inguinal Hernia in the Female

Indirect inguinal hernia does occur in the female, in which case the sac is adherent to the round ligament since there is no spermatic cord. Because the round ligament serves no useful function, it can be divided at its exit from the internal ring and, following excision of the sac, the entire internal ring can be closed tightly. Inasmuch as no compromise is required to preserve a spermatic cord, recurrent hernia is almost unknown in the female.

### Interparietal and Interstitial Hernias

These hernias represent a subgroup of inguinal hernia. The sac or sacs, in addition to the normal course, burrow within the abdominal wall, i.e., preperitoneally, where the sac lies between the peritoneum and the transversalis fascia; in the abdominal wall, where the sac lies between the transversalis fascia and the transversus abdominis, internal oblique, and external oblique muscles; or superficially, where the sac lies between the external oblique aponeurosis and the skin.[40, 43]

### Lacunar Ligament Hernia (Laugier's Hernia or Velpeau's Hernia)

These hernias pass through Gimbernat's ligament. Incision of the ligament may be necessary for reduction of the incarcerated mass.[58]

### Lipoma of the Cord

Lobulated preperitoneal fat may project down the cord at the internal ring. Since this fat pad presents as a mass, it may be mistaken for an indirect inguinal hernia. Whenever a lipoma of the cord is identified (usually found at the lateral margin of the cord), it should be excised to prevent confusion as to diagnosis at a later date.

### Obturator Hernia

This hernia passes through the obturator foramen or canal in the os innominatum. It is a "hidden" hernia, and diagnosis is difficult. The diagnosis is suggested by a pain that passes down the inner side of the thigh to the knee (Howship-Romberg sign). If the hernial sac content is incarcerated or strangulated, a mass may be felt on rectal examination. These hernias are five times more commonly seen in females than in males. Most of the patients who have this type of hernia are elderly, weak, and often emaciated. Because of the rigid walls of the orifice, strangulation frequently occurs.

The defect may be approached by the abdominal, preperitoneal, inguinal, or obturator routes.[71] Tissue surrounding the defect is of poor quality and it is often necessary to patch the defect with prosthetic material such as Teflon or Marlex.[60]

### Pectineal Hernia (Cloquet's Hernia)

This hernia enters the femoral canal and then perforates the aponeurosis of the pectineus muscle. Thus it does not present at the fossa ovalis. This hernia was first described by Callisen[11] and later in more detail by Cloquet.[15]

### Perineal Hernia

Defects occur in the muscle floor of the pelvis through which peritoneal sacs project. Fortunately these hernias are usually reducible, and strangulation seldom occurs. There are three types: (1) anterior—protrudes anterior to the transverse perinei muscles and starts as a defect in the levator ani; these hernias usually contain bladder and are found most frequently in females; (2) posterior—similar to anterior but protrudes posteriorly in the levator ani or between this muscle and the coccyx; these sacs contain ileum and are also most commonly found in women; and (3) complete rectal prolapse. These hernias may be approached by the abdominal and perineal route or by synchronous use of both.[9, 27, 39]

### Prevascular Hernia

This is a hernia found within the femoral sheath but anterior to the femoral vessels. It is rare, and it may be treated by either the Cooper's ligament or iliopubic tract repair.[10, 68]

## Prosthetic Materials

Many artificial aids to hernia repair have been used in past years. These include fascial sutures, fascia lata grafts taken from the thigh, ox fascia, dermal grafts, and all of the various prosthetic meshes such as stainless steel, nylon, tantalum, and finally Marlex or polypropylene.[1, 3, 37, 38, 65, 70] With the currently available methods of repair, these ancillary measures should rarely be required. Nonetheless, should the autogenous tissues be so deficient as to make it impossible to close the defect of a direct inguinal hernia, the newer plastic meshes such as Marlex or polypropylene can be employed.

## Retrovascular Hernia (Serafini's Hernia)

This is a hernia that passes within the femoral sheath but exits posterior to the femoral vessels.[64]

## Sciatic Hernia

The rarest of all hernias, it makes its exit through the greater or lesser sacrosciatic foramen. The mass presents below the fold in the buttock. It may be approached by the abdominal or sciatic route, but occasionally a synchronous technique is advantageous.[66]

## Sliding Inguinal Hernias

Occasionally the cecum on the right or the sigmoid colon on the left makes up a portion of the sac wall in an indirect inguinal hernia. In that instance, special care must be exercised to avoid opening the bowel or devascularizing it when dealing with the sac. For this reason, since it is difficult to determine whether a sliding hernia is present until the hernial sac is opened, the sac of an indirect hernia is always opened on its anterior medial aspect. The hernia itself is due to failure of fusion of the two leaves of peritoneum as they cover the colon; these leaves are allowed to evert around the colon as it protrudes into a hernial sac. Once the sac has been inverted the repair is carried out as for any other indirect inguinal hernia. In the female, especially the infant and child, the sliding hernia may also contain portions of the female genital tract, but these are dealt with in the same fashion as the colon, with imbrication of the peritoneal sac behind the protruding structure.

## Supravesical Hernia

This is another rare hernia first described by Sir Astley Cooper. Keynes[35] has cataloged the types and treatment extensively.

# ABDOMINAL WALL HERNIA

Abdominal wall hernia may be defined as any protrusion of the abdominal viscera through the endoabdominal fascial sac. Examples are umbilical, epigastric, lumbar (both superior and inferior), spigelian, and ventral incisional hernia.

## Umbilical Hernia

Umbilical hernia is a true congenital defect, occurring through the patent umbilical ring following obliteration of the umbilical vessels after delivery. It is considerably more common in Negro infants than in Caucasian, but the reason for this difference is not clear. True umbilical hernia is to be distinguished from omphalocele, which is due to failure of abdominal wall closure in the midline about the umbilicus, in early intrauterine life.

The hernia is present in 10 per cent of Caucasian infants and in 40 to 90 per cent of Negro infants. In almost all of these, the patent umbilical ring closes spontaneously by the age of 2 years. Opinion is currently divided regarding whether any umbilical hernia in a child ever requires operation except for urgent indication. Some surgeons advise nothing but observation of the hernia until the child is 2 years old, and then surgical correction should a defect greater than 1 cm. persist. Other authors, on the basis of a large series of patients observed for many years, recommend no operation at all on the assumption that all umbilical hernias eventually close.[36]

Incarceration and strangulation of umbilical hernias, although rare, do occur. Rupture of an umbilical hernia may also occur, especially in cases of blunt abdominal trauma. In these instances, the hernia is dealt with in the same way as any strangulated hernia or any external rupture of the abdominal viscera.

In distinction to infantile umbilical hernia, umbilical hernia in the adult must always be treated with the same dispatch used for the treatment of an inguinal hernia, for it is known to be liable to incarceration or strangulation or both. Spontaneous or traumatic rupture of umbilical hernia in pregnancy or in cirrhosis with ascites is not uncommon. Baron[7] has indicated that surgical repair of an umbilical hernia in the cirrhotic patient may precipitate variceal hemorrhage. He attributes this to interruption of collateral venous channels that moderate portal venous pressure.

**The Repair.** The classic repair for umbilical hernia is that proposed by Mayo[50] in 1907, the "pants-over-vest" method. Farris[22] has proposed that the Mayo repair for umbilical hernia may not be necessary. On the basis of both experimental and human operative experience, he has advocated a simple transverse closure of the defect with good results.

The poor results with umbilical hernia repair prior to the use of the Mayo operation were most likely due to the poor surgical technique and unsuitable suture material that characterized the period. With advances in surgical technique, better suture material, and better anesthesia, simple closure of the defect, whether in the transverse or vertical plane, has become the treatment of choice.

Recurrence of an umbilical hernia is rare, and only isolated reports have appeared in the literature. Should hernia recurrence become a problem in any individual patient, owing to the size of the umbilical hernia, a prosthetic mesh repair may be required.

## Epigastric Hernia

All hernias occurring in the midline of the abdomen, with the exception of those of the umbilicus, are collectively referred to as hernias of the linea alba. These hernias are far more common above the umbilicus than below and are termed epigastric hernias. They are much more common than generally realized, occurring in approximately 5 per cent of the general population at autopsy. Most are small and asymptomatic and therefore undiagnosed.

It may be difficult to diagnose a small epigastric hernia consisting only of a tag of omentum herniated through the linea alba. The presence of unexplained upper abdominal symptoms, especially in the obese patient, which are aggravated when the patient reclines on his back, should lead one to suspect this diagnosis. This latter finding, pain on reclining, is thought to be due to traction on the incarcerated tissue.

Pain in the linea alba is also a common presenting finding in other upper abdominal diseases. Therefore, a thorough survey for intra-abdominal disease must be carried out before epigastric hernia is incriminated. The diagnosis is easily made by palpation of a small subcutaneous mass in the linea alba.

Current accepted treatment of epigastric hernia is simple closure of the defect. These hernias are frequently multiple, and a wide exposure of the linea alba through a vertical midline skin incision is indicated.

## Ventral (Incisional) Hernia

Incisional hernia is the one true iatrogenic hernia. Principles of treatment of incisional hernia should therefore begin with principles of prevention, that is, principles of proper wound closure. The most common cause of incisional hernia is wound infection, and this should be borne in mind during closure of possibly contaminated wounds. Proper principles of wound closure are dealt with elsewhere in this volume.

Transverse incisions are associated with a significantly lower incidence of wound disruption and incisional hernia than are vertical incisions. Nonetheless, vertical incisions continue to be used for operations on the alimentary tract when transverse incisions would suffice. The anatomic reason for the superiority of transverse incisions is simple. All strata of the abdominal wall, save the rectus abdominis muscle, are collections of fibers, either muscular or fascial, that are oriented in a horizontal direction. The tension exerted by the muscular layers of the abdominal wall is directed horizontally. Vertical incisions are therefore always placed across the lines of force exerted by the abdominal musculature and are always closed under tension. In transverse incisions, tension exerted by the abdominal musculature tends more to appose the edges of the incision than to disrupt them.

More than with any other hernia of the abdominal wall, obesity plays a role in recurrence after ventral hernia repair. Extreme obesity may be regarded as a contraindication to the repair of any incisional hernia, except in the emergent situation.

Incisional hernias, if small, are subject to the same complications as funicular hernias in any other area of the body. They are usually large and diffuse, however. Because of the trauma that has occurred at the operative site, incarceration is relatively common in these hernias, but since they are diffuse, strangulation is rare. One dreaded complication is spontaneous rupture of an incisional hernia with evisceration. Because of the relative fragility of the overlying scar in the superficial layer covering the hernia, this complication is relatively more common with this type of hernia than it is with others.

The treatment of incisional hernia is simple closure of the defect, but this may require a complicated procedure. An incisional hernia is always due to separation of the suture line originally used to close the operative wound. Frequently, the same factors that caused the suture line separation and herniation in the first place will still be operable when a second suture line is placed at the same site. Furthermore, each time a wound disrupts the defect grows larger and more difficult to close. This is especially true of hernias that have occurred through vertical incisions. The surgeon is frequently faced with an ovoid, ever widening defect that is oriented vertically and must be closed under tension.

As might be expected because of the difficult nature of the defect, the absence of suitable contiguous tissues to be used in the repair, and the consequent high recurrence rate, the number of operative procedures proposed for the correction of incisional hernia is high. Prosthetic meshes, autogenous or heterologous fascia, and special suture techniques were first devised for repair of these hernias.

Preoperative treatment of the patient includes correction of any nutritional or metabolic deficits that may be present to contribute to recurrence of the hernia, reduction of weight if the patient is obese, and finally treatment of ancillary systemic conditions which, through augmentation of intra-abdominal pressure, may contribute to recurrence. Some measures to increase intra-abdominal volume may also be necessary in patients with chronic pulmonary dysfunction. Reinsertion of abdominal content that has been within the hernial sac for an indeterminate length of time may severely limit diaphragmatic excursion in these patients, and possibly result in severe embarrassment of pulmonary function. Very large incisional hernias may even contribute to pulmonary dysfunction by compromise of the efficiency of the cough mechanism in patients with chronic bronchitis and emphysema. Under these circumstances, repair of the hernia is indicated because of respiratory disease, not despite it.

Incisional hernias are treated by three types of operation, varying as to their complexity. In the first, simple closure, nothing is necessary save simple reapproximation of the edges of the fascial defect at the transversalis fascial level and above. This repair is probably sufficient for hernias occurring through transverse incisions and for other small incisional hernias. Special attention must be paid to the ends of the wound created, for it is here that recurrent herniation is most likely to occur.

For larger incisional hernias and those with gaping fascial defects, two relatively complicated types of operation are used, those using autogenous tissues and those using prosthetic devices.

### Spigelian Hernia

Spigelian hernia, or spontaneous lateral ventral hernia as it is sometimes called, may be defined as a protrusion through the spigelian fascia. The spigelian fascia is that area of the transversus abdominis aponeurosis lateral to the edge of the rectus sheath, but medial to the spigelian line. The spigelian line is the point of transition of the transversus abdominis muscle to its aponeurotic tendon. The fascia begins at about the level of the eighth or ninth costal cartilage and extends downward to the pubic tubercle. It is widest at a point just below the umbilicus in the region of the semilunar line of Douglas. Most spigelian hernias occur at the widest and therefore weakest area of the spigelian fascia, but they have been reported at the lowermost extent of this fascia, wherein they are easily confused with direct inguinal hernia. The distinction is easily made, since a lower spigelian hernia always protrudes through the transversus abdominis aponeurotic arch, while a direct hernia protrudes below it. Spigelian hernias, being small, are of the funicular type and have a high incidence of incarceration and strangulation.

The treatment is straightforward. A transverse skin incision is made over the defect and carried down through the external oblique aponeurosis, which is opened in the direction of its fibers. The hernial sac is identified, isolated, opened, ligated, and closed in the usual fashion. The transversus abdominis aponeurotic defect can usually be closed with a few interrupted nonabsorbable sutures. Wound closure is carried out in the usual fashion. Cases reported in the literature are too few for assessment of recurrences to be possible.

### Lumbar Hernia (Petit's Triangle Hernia and Grynfeltt's Hernia)

These are also relatively rare hernias, only 250 to 300 cases having been reported in the literature. The more common of the two is superior lumbar hernia, or Grynfeltt's. Probably superseding both of these, however, are incisional hernias resulting from nephrectomy or traumatic hernias of the lumbar region.

The inferior lumbar triangle is an anatomic area of weakness, bounded posteriorly by the latissimus dorsi, anteriorly by the external oblique, and inferiorly by the iliac crest. Its floor is formed by the internal oblique and transversus abdominis muscles. The superior triangle or triangle of Grynfeltt-Lesshaft is situated above and anterior to Petit's triangle and is normally covered by the latissimus

dorsi and serratus posterior inferior muscle. The boundaries of the triangle are the twelfth rib above, which forms the base, and the anterior border of the internal oblique anteriorly. The floor is ordinarily the quadratus lumborum muscle mass. It is more constant and larger than Petit's triangle, which accounts for the higher incidence of hernia through it. Etiologically, hernias through these triangles are either spontaneous or traumatic. Congenital hernias have also been described in this region. The incidence of strangulation is approximately 10 per cent.

Because of the anatomy of these hernias, treatment is difficult. Until the advent of satisfactory mesh repairs, the basic principle of treatment of Petit's triangle hernia was that advocated by Dowd[20] in 1907, which involved closure of the defect by a pedicle flap of tensor fascia lata and gluteus maximus from below the iliac crest, with side-to-side apposition of the external oblique and latissimus dorsi. Repair of the upper triangle is essentially the same, depending on the development of flaps from adjacent structures. The basic principle of repair of all lumbar hernias is initial closure of the transversalis fascial defect.

With the increasing use of mesh prostheses, it seems likely that the treatment of choice is the employment of one of these aids. If the hernia is small, operative repair by suture of the external oblique to the latissimus dorsi, with or without fascia lata reinforcement, has been successful.

In addition to the aforementioned two varieties of lumbar hernia, there have been isolated reports of hernias occurring through congenital defects or eventrations of other portions of the posterior abdominal wall. Most of these are treated by simple closure of the defect, or by pedicle flap or prosthetic closure should the defect be large. The most common posterior hernia is the postnephrectomy incisional hernia. Its repair is essentially the same as that for incisional hernia in any location.

## SELECTED REFERENCES

Anson, B. J., and McVay, C. B.: Surgical Anatomy. 5th ed. Philadelphia, W. B. Saunders Company, 1971.
*This two-volume monograph includes the finest review of hernial anatomy available today. The section on the abdominal wall represents a distillate of over 30 years of active study, both in the anatomy laboratory and at the operating room table.*

Condon, R. E.: Surgical anatomy of the transversus abdominis and transversalis fascia. Ann. Surg., 173:1, 1971.
*By reproducing in color a photograph of the posterior inguinal wall, Condon has helped "clear the air" of many anatomic misconceptions of groin anatomy. This report gives a succinct but exceptionally clear description of the posterior inguinal wall.*

Fruchaud, H.: Traitement chirurgical des hernies de l'aine chez l'adulte. Paris, G. Doin & Cie, 1956.

Fruchaud, H.: Anatomie chirurgical des hernies de l'aine. Paris, G. Doin & Cie, 1956.
*These two monographs are beautifully illustrated. All interested in this subject should review these fine works.*

Glassow, F.: Recurrent inguinal and femoral hernia. Brit. Med. J., 1:215, 1970.
*The Shouldice Hospital in Thornhill, Ontario, is unique because the only operations performed there are related to the*

*problem of hernia. Between 1945 and 1967, 50,000 primary hernial repairs were performed with a recurrence rate of 0.7 per cent. The technique used in this astounding mass of hernia operations was multiple-layer closure — beginning with imbrication of the attenuated posterior inguinal wall — with continuous stainless steel wire sutures.*

Griffith, C. A.: Inguinal hernia: an anatomic-surgical correlation. Surg. Clin. N. Amer., *39*:531, 1959.
*Crediting H. O. Marcy for original work relating to plastic closure of the internal ring, Griffith shows in this article a fine technique for repair of the small indirect hernia in the adult.*

Halvorson, K., and McVay, C. B.: Inguinal and femoral hernioplasty — a 22 year study of the authors' methods. Arch. Surg., *101*:127, 1970.
*What is the true recurrence rate after hernial repair? Unfortunately most glowing reports in the world literature fail to assure sufficient follow-up time. These authors after diligent study have suggested a formula by which a more accurate recurrence rate can be assured. The following table represents their method of predicting recurrence up to 25 years after the operation.*

| All Patients Followed | Multiply Rate |
|---|---|
| One year | 5.0 |
| Two years | 2.5 |
| Five years | 1.5 |
| Ten years | 1.2 |

*When these rates were applied to their own series, an impressive accuracy was noted. Any author reporting results of hernial surgery with follow-up of less than 10 years would be well advised to calculate the 25 year potential for recurrence in his series.*

Lytle, W. J.: The deep inguinal ring, development, function and repair. Brit. J. Surg., *57*:531, 1970.
*The closing mechanism of the internal ring is well described in this short paper. The student of hernial repair should read carefully all the works of Lytle.*

McVay, C. B., Read, R. C., and Ravitch, M. M.: Inguinal hernia. Curr. Probl. Surg., Oct. 1967.
*This monograph gives a tripartite summary of hernial repair today. McVay presents the complete repair of the posterior inguinal wall which he has popularized so successfully. Read reviews the preperitoneal approach and Ravitch clearly presents the classic Halsted-Ferguson procedure.*

Nyhus, L. M., and Harkins, H. N.: Hernia. Philadelphia, J. B. Lippincott Company, 1964.
*Details of all facets of hernial problems are presented. A multiauthor text, it contains diverse views as to the appropriate approach to groin hernias. It also includes sections on diaphragmatic hernia, industrial hernia, muscle hernia, and medicolegal problems related to hernia surgery.*

Usher, F. C.: The repair of incisional and inguinal hernia. Surg. Gynec. Obstet., *131*:525, 1970.
*The use of prosthetic material in hernial repair has found a place in the surgical armamentarium largely as a result of the work of Usher. This paper updates the subject and it also includes reference for further reading.*

Zimmerman, L. M., and Anson, B. J.: The Anatomy and Surgery of Hernia. 2nd ed. Baltimore. Williams & Wilkins, 1967.
*The anatomic genius of Anson is combined here with the fine surgical knowledge of Zimmerman to produce a beautifully illustrated and overall fine text.*

## REFERENCES

1. Abel, A. L., and Hunt, A. H.: Stainless steel wire for closing abdominal incisions and for the repair of herniae. Brit. Med. J., 2:379, 1948.
2. Aird, I.: A Companion in Surgical Studies. 2nd ed. Baltimore, Williams & Wilkins, 1957.
3. Ali, M.: Cutis strip and patch repair of large inguinal hernias. New Eng. J. Med., 251:932, 1954.
4. Andrews, E. W.: Imbrication of lap joint method: A plastic operation for hernia. Chicago Med. Rec., 9:67, 1895.
5. Annandale, T.: Case in which a reducible oblique and direct inguinal and femoral hernia existed on the same side and were treated by operation. Edinburgh Med. J., 21:1087, 1876.
6. Anson, B. J., Morgan, E. H., and McVay, C. B.: Surgical anatomy of the inguinal region based upon a study of 500 body-halves. Surg. Gynec. Obstet., 111:707, 1960.
7. Baron, H. C.: Umbilical hernia secondary to cirrhosis of the liver — complications of surgical correction. New Eng. J. Med., 263:824, 1960.
8. Bassini, E.: Nuovo metodo per la cura radicale dell'ernia. Atti Cong. Ass. Med. Ital. (1887), 2:179, 1889.
9. Blair, C. R., Nay, H. R., and Rucher, C. M.: Surgical repair of rectal prolapse. Surgery, 53:625, 1963.
10. Burton, C. C.: Inguinopectineal hernias — a classification and correlation. Int. Abstr. Surg., 97:419, 1953.
11. Callisen, H.: Herniorum rariorum luga acta societatis medicae hafniae. Hanniae, 2:321, 1777.
12. Camper, P.: Icones herniarum. Francofurti ad Moenum, Varrentrapp and Wenner, 1801.
13. Cavanagh, C. R., and Schnug, G. E.: Inguinal hernias in infants and children. Northwest Med., 61:598, 1962.
14. Clark, J. H., and Hashimoto, E. I.: Utilization of Henle's ligament, iliopubic tract, aponeurosis transversus abdominis and Cooper's ligament in inguinal herniorrhaphy. Surg. Gynec. Obstet., 82:480, 1946.
15. Cloquet J.: Recherches anatomiques sur les hernies de l'abdomen. Thèse. Paris, 1817.
16. Condon, R. E.: The anatomy of the inguinal region. In: Nyhus, L. M., and Harkins, H. N.: Hernia. Philadelphia, J. B. Lippincott Company, 1964.
17. Cooper, A. P.: The Anatomy and Surgical Treatment of Abdominal Hernia. 2 volumes. London, Longman & Co., 1804–1807.
18. Czerny, V.: Studien zur Radikulbehandlung der Hernien. Wein. Med. Wschr., 27:497, 1877.
19. Donald, D. C.: The value derived from utilizing the component parts of the transversalis fascia and Cooper's ligament in the repair of large indirect and direct inguinal hernias. Surgery, 24:662, 1948.
20. Dowd, C. N.: Congenital lumbar hernia at the triangle of Petit. Ann. Surg., 45:245, 1907.
21. Eiseman, B., Robinson, R. M., and Brown, J. H.: Simultaneous appendectomy and herniorrhaphy without prophylactic antibiotic therapy. Surgery, 51:578, 1962.
22. Farris, J. M.: Umbilical hernia. In: Nyhus, L. M., and Harkins, H. N.: Hernia. Philadelphia, J. B. Lippincott Company, 1964.
23. Ferguson, A. H.: The Technique of Modern Operations for Hernia. Chicago, Cleveland Press, 1907.
24. Gallaudet, B. B.: A Description of the Planes of Fascia of the Human Body. New York, Columbia University Press, 1931.
25. Gaspar, M. R., and Casberg, M. A.: An appraisal of preperitoneal repair of inguinal hernia. Surg. Gynec. Obstet., 132:207, 1971.
26. Gaster, J.: Hernia — One Day Repair. Darien, Conn., Hafner Publishing Co., 1970.
27. Goligher, J. C.: Prolapse of the rectum. In: Nyhus, L. M., and Harkins, H. N.: Hernia. Philadelphia, J. B. Lippincott Company, 1964.
28. Griffith, C. A.: Inguinal hernia: an anatomic-surgical correlation. Surg. Clin. N. Amer., 39:531, 1959.
29. Guy, C. C., Werelius, C. Y., and Bell, L. B., Jr.: Five years' experience with tantalum mesh in hernia repair. Surg. Clin. N. Amer., 35:175, 1955.
30. Halsted, W. S.: The radical cure of hernia. Bull. Johns Hopkins Hosp., 1:12, 1889.
31. Halverson, K., and McVay, C. B.: Inguinal and femoral hernioplasty. Arch. Surg., 101:127, 1970.
32. Harrison, P. W.: Inguinal hernia: A study of the principles involved in the surgical treatment. Arch. Surg., 4:680, 1922.
33. Hesselbach, F. K.: Anatomisch-chirurgische Abhandlung über den Ursprung der Leistenbrücke. Wurzburg, Baumgärten, 1806.
34. Hesselbach, F. K.: Nueste anatomisch-pathologische Untersuchungen uber den Ursprung und das Fortschreiten der

Leisten- und Schnekel-bruche. Wurzburg, Baumgartner, 1814.

35. Keynes, W. M.: Supravesical hernia. In: Nyhus, L. M., and Harkins, H. N.: Hernia. Philadelphia, J. B. Lippincott Company, 1964.

36. Kiesewetter, W. B.: Hernias—inguinal and umbilical. Amer. J. Surg., *101*:656, 1961.

37. Koontz, A. R.: Dead (preserved) fascia grafts for hernia repair: clinical results. J.A.M.A., *89*:1230, 1927.

38. Koontz, A. R.: The use of tantalum mesh in inguinal hernia repair. Surg. Gynec. Obstet., *92*:101, 1951.

39. Koontz, A. R.: Perineal hernia. In: Nyhus, L. M., and Harkins, H. N.: Hernia. Philadelphia, J. B. Lippincott Company, 1964.

40. Koontz, A. R., and Stafford, E. S.: Unusual types of interparietal hernia. Arch. Surg., *71*:723, 1955.

41. Lindholm, A., Nilsson, O., and Tholin, B.: Inguinal and femoral hernias. Arch. Surg., *98*:19, 1969.

42. Lotheissen, G.: Zur Radikaloperation der Schenkelhernien. Zbl. Chir., *25*:548, 1898.

43. Lower, W. E., and Hicken, N. F.: Interparietal hernias. Ann. Surg., *94*:1070, 1931.

44. Lucas-Championnière, J.: Cure radicale des hernies; avec une étude statistique de deux cents soizante-quinze opérations et cinquante figures intercalées dans le texte. Paris, Rueff et Cie, 1892.

45. Lytle, W. J.: Femoral hernia. Ann. Roy. Coll. Surg. Eng., *21*:244, 1957.

46. Macewen, W.: On the radical cure of oblique inguinal hernia by internal abdominal peritoneal pad, and the restoration of the valved form of the inguinal canal. Ann. Surg., *4*:89, 1886.

47. Marcy, H. O.: A new use of carbolized catgut ligatures. Boston Med. Surg. J., *85*:315, 1871.

48. Marcy, H. O.: The radical cure of hernia by the antiseptic use of the carbolized catgut ligature. Trans. A.M.A., *29*:295, 1878.

49. Margoles, J. S., and Braun, R. A.: Preperitoneal versus classical hernioplasty. Amer. J. Surg., *121*:641, 1971.

50. Mayo, W. J.: Radical cure of umbilical hernia. J.A.M.A., *48*:1842, 1907.

51. McVay, C. B.: Inguinal and femoral hernioplasty: anatomic repair. Arch. Surg., *57*:524, 1948.

52. McVay, C. B.: The hernias. In: Davis, L., ed.: Christopher's Textbook of Surgery. 9th ed. Philadelphia, W. B. Saunders Company, 1968.

53. Moschcowitz, A. V.: Femoral hernia: a new operation for the radical cure. New York J. Med., 7:396, 1907.

54. Nyhus, L. M.: An anatomic reappraisal of the posterior inguinal wall. Special consideration of the iliopubic tract and its relation to groin hernias. Surg. Clin. N. Amer., *44*:1305, 1964.

55. Nyhus, L. M.: The preperitoneal approach and iliopubic tract repair of all groin hernias. In: Nyhus, L. M., and Harkins, H. N.: Hernia. Philadelphia, J. B. Lippincott Company, 1964.

56. Peacock, E. E., Jr.: Personal communication, 1971.

57. Pott, P. A.: A Treatise on Ruptures. London, C. Hitch and L. Hawes, 1756.

58. Priesching, A.: Laugerische Hernia. Arch. Klin. Chir., *281*:411, 1956.

59. Read, R. C.: Preperitoneal exposure of inguinal herniation. Amer. J. Surg., *116*:653, 1968.

60. Rogers, F. A.: Strangulated obturator hernia. In: Nyhus, L. M., and Harkins, H. N.: Hernia. Philadelphia, J. B. Lippincott Company, 1964.

61. Ruggi, G.: Metodo operative nuovo per la cura radicale dell'ernia crurale. Bull. Sci. Med. Bologna Sev., 7:223, 1892.

62. Santulli, T. V., and Shaw, A.: Inguinal hernia: Infancy and childhood. J.A.M.A., *176*:110, 1961.

63. Scarpa, A.: Sull'ernia del revineo. Pavia, P. Bizzoni, 1821.

64. Serafini, G.: Sulle varieta dell'ernia crurale e particolarmente sull'ernia crurale retrovascolare intravaginale e sull'ernia pettina. Policlinico (Chir.), *24*:230, 1917.

65. Smith, R. S.: Adjuncts in hernial repair: a consideration of basic principles. Arch. Surg., *78*:868, 1959.

66. Thomas, G. I.: Sciatic hernia. In: Nyhus, L. M., and Harkins, H. N.: Hernia. Philadelphia, J. B. Lippincott Company, 1964.

67. Thomson, A.: Cause anatomique de la hernie inguinale externe. J. Conn. Méd. Prat., *4*:137, 1836.

68. Turner, D. P. B.: Prevascular femoral hernia. Brit. J. Surg., *41*:77, 1953.

69. U.S. Department of Health, Education and Welfare: National Health Survey on Hernias. Series B, No. 25, Dec. 1960.

70. Usher, F. C.: The repair of incisional and inguinal hernias. Surg. Gynec. Obstet., *131*:525, 1970.

71. Wakeley, C. P. G.: Obturator hernia. Brit. J. Surg., *26*:515, 1939.

72. Zimmerman, L. M., and Anson, B. J.: Anatomy and Surgery of Hernia. 2nd ed. Baltimore, Williams & Wilkins, 1967.

# 38

# PEDIATRIC SURGERY

*Thomas M. Holder, M.D., and Lucian L. Leape, M.D.*

Pediatric surgery is that branch of surgery devoted to surgical care and management of infants and children. It bears the same relation to surgery that pediatrics does to internal medicine. The conditions treated surgically in the pediatric age group are usually congenital malformations, neoplasms, or the result of trauma. Most are amenable to definitive treatment and thus offer the deep satisfaction of lifelong cure.

Since the infant's response to disease is quite different from the adult's, it is necessary to be aware of these differences when caring for him.[20] Perhaps the single most important difference is the much greater lability of babies. Because of a higher metabolic rate the young infant has a more rapid turnover of water and metabolites and a higher oxygen consumption. His body weight usually doubles in the first 6 months. This increased caloric requirement results in an increase in fluid requirement as well. For example, a 5 kg. infant requires about 500 cc. of intravenous fluids per day (100 cc. per kilogram body weight at this size) to meet his metabolic requirement. An equivalent amount for a 70 kg. adult would be 7000 cc. per day, far more than usual needs.

Because of the greater surface area as compared to body mass, the small infant loses heat much more rapidly than an adult. Accordingly, he is much more susceptible to changes in ambient temperature. Temperature control mechanisms are poorly developed in the small infant, especially the premature. If his body temperature is significantly above or below normal, there is a marked increase in oxygen consumption as well. Particularly in the operating room, measures must be taken to conserve body heat or core temperature will drop significantly.

Respiratory problems are common in young infants after operation. There are several reasons for this. First, the neonate is an obligatory nose breather. Accordingly, nasogastric intubation decreases the airway by obstructing one naris. Second, the ribs are soft and horizontal so that intercostal action contributes much less to ventilation than the diaphragm. Third, the infant airway is much more easily compromised by a small amount of edema (such as that caused by an endotracheal tube). One millimeter of edema of the mucosa of a 6 mm. trachea quadruples the airway resistance. Finally, infants mobilize secretions poorly because of inadequate cough reflexes. Assiduous respiratory care is mandatory if these patients are to survive.

Since the diagnostic approach to a patient is usually determined by the predominant symptom or sign, diseases will be grouped by major clinical symptoms. No attempt is made to provide encyclopedic coverage. Rather, major conditions encountered in infancy and childhood requiring surgical treatment are described as part of the differential diagnosis of the major presenting symptom. For more details, the reader is referred to several excellent textbooks of pediatric surgery or to monographs on specific subjects.

## RESPIRATORY DISTRESS

Respiratory distress in the newborn is commonly life-threatening, often progressive, and frequently caused by an entity amenable to surgical cure. Whether manifested merely by an increase in respiratory rate, or attended by stridor, retractions, cyanosis, and other signs of oxygen deficiency, the exact cause must be rapidly identified and appropriate treatment instituted. In broad terms the causes of respiratory distress are abnormalities of ventilation, impaired oxygen diffusion, and the shunting of blood from venous to arterial circuits without oxygenation.

Most of the surgically treated problems produce abnormalities of ventilation. These may result from airway obstruction (as in vascular ring compressing the trachea), poorly functioning muscles of respiration (as in phrenic paralysis or central nervous system disorders), or decrease in lung volume (such as from pneumothorax or a diaphragmatic hernia).

Poor oxygen diffusion may result from pneumonia, atelectasis, hyaline membrane disease, or pulmonary congestion and edema due to congestive heart failure. Most of the entities in this category are treated by nonoperative means. Shunting may occur either in the heart or in the lungs. The intrapulmonary shunt is usually the result of blood perfusing unoxygenated alveoli, as in atelectasis. Intracardiac shunting results from septal defects. At times it may be difficult to differentiate pulmonary from cardiac causes of distress. In general, cyanosis due to pulmonary causes improves with oxygen administration, while that due to an intracardiac shunt does not.

In the infant or child with respiratory distress, either with or without cyanosis and retraction, a posteroanterior and lateral chest x-ray film is the most helpful single diagnostic study and should be obtained promptly in any patient with these symptoms. No infant is too sick for a chest x-ray. The cause of the respiratory difficulty is usually apparent. Additional studies may be necessary to further delineate the cause of the symptoms, but at least a provisional diagnosis usually can be made from the chest x-ray.

Further diagnostic studies, if needed, should demonstrate the cause of the respiratory distress with the least risk to the patient. Some patients, particularly neonates or the critically ill, will not tolerate extensive diagnostic evaluation. The choice of specific procedures should be based on the most likely diagnosis in view of the clinical picture; one should not employ all procedures available to exclude every diagnostic possibility. If there is stridor and retraction, upper airway obstruction is likely. Cyanosis and tachypnea without stridor are more suggestive of a pulmonary or cardiac problem. Physical examination may reveal the cause of obstruction, for example, a large cervical mass, cystic hygroma with laryngeal or tongue involvement, or micrognathia. Since the infant is primarily a diaphragmatic breather, marked abdominal distention from any cause will interfere with ventilation.

If there is no obviously visible cause, a reasonable stepwise approach to a patient with respiratory distress is: (1) obtain a chest x-ray; (2) pass a tube through each naris (to detect choanal atresia); (3) obtain an esophagogram (to detect vascular ring or other structure compromising the esophagus and the trachea); (4) look at the larynx and pharynx (to detect a mass, a web, or compression); (5) perform tracheobronchoscopy and obtain a tracheogram to detect subglottic or other narrowing not seen on previous roentgenographic studies. Laryngoscopy should be done first if the patient has severe airway obstruction, and an endotracheal tube is introduced if necessary to relieve the obstruction and perhaps localize the area of narrowing.

## DIAPHRAGMATIC HERNIA

The Bochdalek diaphragmatic hernia is one of the surgical emergencies of the newborn. While not all infants with the posterolateral diaphragmatic defect have symptoms as newborns, most do, and the risk to these infants is high.

**Anatomy and Embryology.** The septum transversum forms caudal to the heart at about the eighth week of fetal life and grows posteriorly to meet the dorsal mesentery of the foregut to form the central portion of the diaphragm. Pleuroperitoneal folds develop on each side and progress posteriorly and laterally, dividing the thoracic from the abdominal cavity. Arrest of the process at this time results in a posterolateral diaphragmatic defect—the persistent pleuroperitoneal canal of Bochdalek. Muscle fibers grow between these folds to form the true diaphragm by about the end of the ninth week. The process is usually complete on the right before the left, partially explaining the 90 per cent predominance of the defect on the left. About this same time the gut returns to the abdomen from the base of the umbilical cord. If the pleuroperitoneal canal is still open, the gut returning to the abdominal cavity will pass through the defect into the chest and not complete the normal process of intestinal rotation. The abdominal viscera in the chest compress the ipsilateral lung and prevent its development to the normal size. The abdominal cavity likewise does not develop to its normal size.

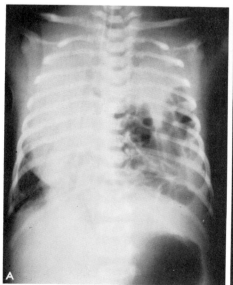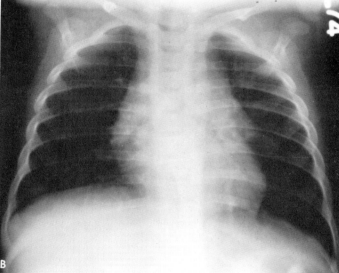

**Figure 1** *A*, X-ray appearance of a 12 hour old male with a Bochdalek diaphragmatic hernia showing air-filled loops of intestine in the left chest with marked mediastinal shift and compression of the right lung. *B*, Same patient at age 10 months showing complete expansion of both lungs.

**Pathophysiology.** With the first breath an infant begins to swallow air, which promptly passes to the small bowel. As the air enters the intestine the volume occupied by the intestine increases. Since the gut is in the chest, and the thoracic volume is relatively fixed, the increase in volume of the intestine occurs at the expense of the most easily compressed of the thoracic contents, the lungs. As pressure increases, there is a shift of the mediastinum with compression of the contralateral lung. The increased intrathoracic pressure and mediastinal shift impede venous return.

The result of this expanding mass is severe hypoxia and respiratory acidosis. These factors have an effect on the labile pulmonary vasculature of the neonate, producing an increase in pulmonary vascular resistance.

**Symptoms and Signs.** Symptoms and signs vary from severe respiratory difficulty from the time of delivery to no respiratory symptoms at all. Most of these infants do reasonably well initially but have progressive difficulty as the gut fills with air and are in severe respiratory distress within a few hours. On physical examination most patients have a scaphoid abdomen, a barrel-shaped chest, and some degree of cyanosis and respiratory distress. On listening to the chest, the most striking finding is that the heart is best heard well over toward the right anterior axillary line (in the 90 per cent of patients whose defect is on the left). Breath sounds are decreased or absent on the involved side. To the disappointment of the physical diagnosis enthusiast, bowel sounds are seldom heard in the chest.

Some patients have few or no respiratory symptoms but have intermittent or partial intestinal obstruction. These symptoms usually occur after the neonatal period.

**Diagnosis.** Diagnosis is by chest x-ray. There are loops of air-filled bowel in the chest. Those patients who are in respiratory distress usually show a marked mediastinal shift away from the hernia (Fig. 1).

**Treatment.** Treatment is prompt reduction and repair of the hernia. The hypoxia and acidosis cannot be corrected until the lung can be expanded. The acidosis can, however, be improved by intravenous sodium bicarbonate, and this should be given empirically. The anesthetic should not be given by mask as more air will be forced into the intestine. An endotracheal tube is passed in the awake infant, who is then lightly anesthetized.

The operative approach is through the abdomen (Fig. 2). The advantages of the abdominal approach as opposed to the thoracic are: (1) the diaphragmatic defect is not repaired under the difficult

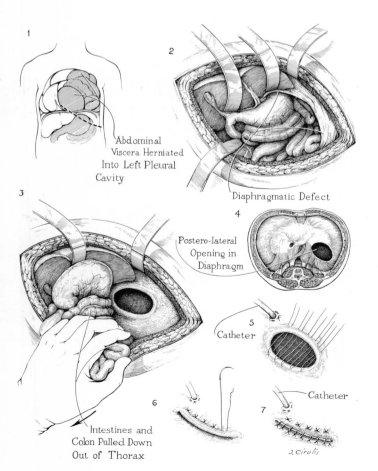

1

Abdominal Viscera Herniated Into Left Pleural Cavity

2

Diaphragmatic Defect

3

4

Postero-lateral Opening in Diaphragm

5
Catheter

6

7
Catheter

Intestines and Colon Pulled Down Out of Thorax

J. Cirulis

**Figure 2** Technique of repair of Bochdalek diaphragmatic defect. An abdominal approach has a decided advantage. A catheter can either be placed through the diaphragm and brought out through a stab wound in the abdomen or brought directly out through the chest wall. In either case it is connected to an underwater seal. Gastrostomy is helpful in preventing postoperative intestinal distention. (From Gross, R. E.: An Atlas of Children's Surgery, Philadelphia, W. B. Saunders Company, 1970.)

conditions of trying to push the viscera back into the too-small abdominal cavity (hence a more secure closure can be obtained); (2) if there are peritoneal bands obstructing the duodenum or other manifestations of incomplete rotation, they can be readily corrected; and (3) a gastrostomy is easily performed. The viscera are removed from the thorax and the defect in the diaphragm is closed. In the rare instance when there is insufficient diaphragm for a primary closure, it may be closed with a synthetic prosthesis or rotated flap of abdominal wall musculature. A gastrostomy is performed to decompress the stomach and intestinal tract postoperatively. Since the abdominal cavity is small, return of all the viscera that were in the chest to the abdominal cavity may cause a marked increase in intra-abdominal pressure with decreased diaphragmatic excursion and ventilation. Venous return is also impaired. If there is moderate tension in closing the abdomen, a ventral hernia should be left either by closing only the skin or by closing the abdominal wall with a temporary prosthesis, similar to the therapy of omphalocele.[16] If a prosthesis is used, abdominal wall closure can be accomplished 7 to 10 days later without undue tension. A chest tube is left in the pleural space and connected to underwater drainage.

The postoperative care in these infants is critical. Arterial pH, $pO_2$, and $pCO_2$ should be closely monitored via an arterial catheter. If these show even moderate acidosis, hypoxia, or hypercarbia, the patient should be given ventilatory assistance.

In patients who survive, the mediastinum shifts back toward the midline, and the ipsilateral lung gradually expands over the next 5 to 10 days to occupy the hemithorax. The lung has the capacity to grow alveoli after birth. On long-term follow-up the lungs are found to be normal by clinical evaluation and x-ray examination.

**Results.** Survival rate is about 50 per cent for those infants who are in respiratory difficulty during the first 24 hours of life. Many of these babies have a severely hypoplastic lung. The patient who does not have symptoms until after 24 hours of life has a much better outlook, with a mortality of less than 5 per cent. Presumably the lungs in these latter infants are less severely affected.

## PNEUMOTHORAX

Pneumothorax is not rare in the neonate. It may occur spontaneously as a result of birth trauma or from a ruptured bleb or cyst. In infants and, less often, children who have elements of bronchiolar obstruction or infection, air may leak back along the bronchi into the mediastinum with subsequent rupture into the pleural space producing a pneumothorax.

In most cases pneumothorax in infants is small, causes no symptoms, and needs no therapy other than observation to see that the air is decreasing rather than increasing in amount. If a tension pneumothorax develops, respiratory distress may be severe. Physical examination reveals a rapid respiratory rate, cyanosis, and retraction. There are no breath sounds on the involved side. Diagnosis is made by chest x-ray. Treatment is by insertion of an intercostal catheter connected to an underwater seal. This is safer than aspiration since it provides a vent in case of continued or recurrent leak. The tube should remain in place until the air leak is well sealed, usually a matter of 3 to 5 days. Premature removal of the tube is apt to be followed by recurrence of the pneumothorax.

Pneumomediastinum may cause caval obstruction. It is more difficult to treat since there is not a single space that can be easily evacuated. Therapy is usually not necessary, but if the patient is in distress, aspiration of the mediastinum may remove enough air to tide the patient over until the air is absorbed.

## INFANTILE LOBAR EMPHYSEMA

Marked overdistention of a single lobe (or segment) of lung may be the cause of respiratory distress in the infant. This condition was first described by Nelson in 1932 and first successfully treated by Gross in 1945.

**Pathophysiology.** Lobar emphysema may result from partial bronchial obstruction or, less commonly, primary alveolar fibrosis. External bronchial compression may result from an abnormal vessel or lymph node. Intrinsic obstruction can result from bronchomalacia, bronchostenosis, or redundant mucosal fold. In about half the patients, no cause can be found. As the lobe becomes overinflated, the remaining lobes of the ipsilateral lung are compressed and the diaphragm is depressed. As distention progresses, herniation of the distended lobe across the flexible anterior mediastinum may occur, causing compression of the contralateral lung. The emphysematous lobe acts as any large intrathoracic mass, compressing the normal intrathoracic structures and interfering with ventilation. In addition, the increased intrathoracic pressure produces a shift of the mediastinum and may impede venous return to the heart.[15]

**Symptoms and Signs.** The patient is usually in respiratory distress with tachypnea, dyspnea, and cyanosis. On auscultation, the breath sounds are decreased on the involved side. Hyperinflation and decreased expansions of the affected side may be noted. In some patients symptoms appear shortly after birth and are rapidly progressive. In about half, the onset of symptoms is during the first month of life, and in most of the others, during the first 4 months of age. Rarely the disorder is seen in an older child with congenital heart disease (10 to 15 per cent).

**Diagnosis.** Diagnosis is by chest x-ray (Fig. 3). The classic findings are (1) radiolucency of the lung field with bronchovascular markings present; (2) wedge-shaped densities adjacent to the affected lobe representing the atelectatic other lobes; (3)

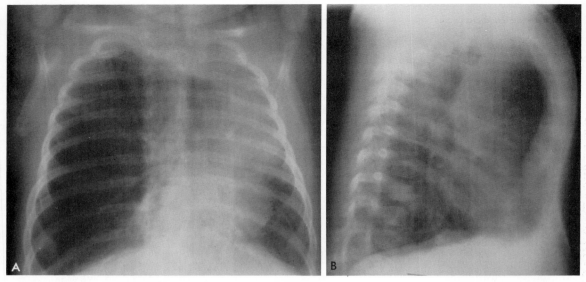

**Figure 3**   *A*, X-ray appearance of infantile lobar emphysema of the middle lobe. The mediastinum is displaced to the left with herniation of the middle lobe across the midline. The right lower lobe is compressed along the right heart border and the right hemidiaphragm depressed. *B*, The lateral projection shows a large radiolucent area in the upper anterior mediastinum where the middle lobe has expanded across the mediastinum.

depression of the ipsilateral half of the diaphragm; (4) mediastinal shift to the opposite side; and (5) retrosternal radiolucency indicating herniation across the mediastinum. Bronchograms are occasionally necessary to demonstrate obstruction in atypical cases.

**Treatment.**   Surgical resection of the diseased lobe is curative and often life-saving.

**Results.**   Operative mortality is low. In rare cases a second lobe will become involved. Long-term follow-up studies have occasionally demonstrated decrease in vital capacity beyond that expected from the volume of the lung removed. This indicates that there may be other residual lung disease.

## CYSTIC MALFORMATIONS OF THE LUNG

Congenital cystic disease of the lung is uncommon. Cysts are the result of faulty embryogenesis, are lined by cuboidal or columnar ciliated epithelium, and usually communicate with the tracheobronchial tree. One variety in this spectrum of disease, cystic adenomatoid malformation, consists primarily of the glandular components of the lung and presents as a predominantly solid tumor of the lung in the neonate.

**Pathophysiology.**   The cysts may be single or multiple and are usually segmental or lobar in distribution. Occasionally an entire lung may be involved. In the neonate the cysts are usually large and cause symptoms because of their size. Bronchial communication often permits air to enter more easily than to escape, resulting in a progressive enlargement of the cyst. In older infants and children infection in the cyst is common.

**Symptoms.**   Symptoms are those of an intrathoracic mass or superimposed infection—dyspnea, tachypnea, wheezing, cyanosis, cough, and fever.

**Diagnosis.**   Diagnosis is made by chest x-ray, which shows one or more air-filled cysts varying in size, at times causing a mediastinal shift. Air-fluid levels are more common in infected cysts than in those that are not. Cystic adenomatoid malformation presents as a large, rather homogeneous solid pulmonary mass. Differential diagnosis includes pneumothorax, infantile lobar emphysema, diaphragmatic hernia, acquired cystic disease of the lung secondary to staphylococcal pneumonia, and pulmonary manifestations of cystic fibrosis.

**Treatment.**   Treatment is resection of the involved lobe or lobes. It is not wise to aspirate the cyst except in extreme emergency because of the risk of tension pneumothorax. If necessary as a life-saving measure, aspiration should be followed by immediate thoracotomy and resection of the cyst. The results are good. Infants tolerate pulmonary resection well.

## STAPHYLOCOCCAL PNEUMONIA

Staphylococcal pneumonia occurs in persons of all ages, but is most often seen in infants and young children. Peribronchial abscesses occur, with escape of air into the lung parenchyma and development of pneumatoceles. If the abscess is subpleural in location, rupture into the pleural space results in a pneumothorax or empyema or both. Staphylococcal pneumonia in the early phases may be a rapidly progressive, fulminating disease. Close x-ray surveillance is necessary

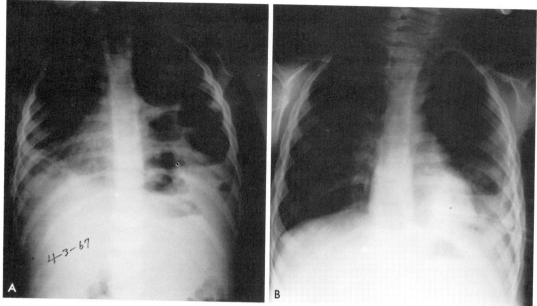

**Figure 4** *A,* Staphylococcal pneumonia with pneumatoceles on the left, mediastinal shift to the right, and right empyema which has been drained by an intercostal catheter. *B,* Four weeks later the right empyema and pleural thickening have subsided. On the left all but one of the pneumatoceles have subsided. A left empyema developed which is being drained by a tube. Over the next 2 months complete resolution occurred.

during this phase of the disease to keep abreast of the progression of the disease process. The patients are febrile and have rapid respirations and dyspnea.

**Diagnosis.** Diagnosis is by chest x-ray showing pneumatoceles and frequently empyema and pneumothorax (Fig. 4). Culture of the Staphylococcus from the nose or throat is suggestive; from a tracheal aspirate or the pleural space it is confirmatory.

**Treatment.** Treatment of the pneumonia is by antibiotics, usually methicillin or cephalothin. Therapy of the complications is surgical. The pneumatoceles rarely become large enough to cause respiratory distress. If they do, tube drainage is safer than aspiration. Pneumothorax, pleural effusion, and empyema are frequent complications and require tube drainage of the pleural space. Drainage early in the course of empyema is much more efficient than drainage after loculation has occurred.

Once the infection has been controlled by antibiotics, progression of the process ceases. Antibiotics are usually required for several weeks to control the infection. Therapy should be continued until the patient has been afebrile for 10 to 14 days and the white and differential blood counts have returned to the normal range for a similar period of time. The pneumatoceles will regress over a period of weeks or months. If there has been an empyema, there may be marked pleural thickening that restricts ventilation. In spite of the alarming x-ray appearance, the thick pleura will almost always resolve, though it may take several months. Decortication is seldom required.[10]

## VASCULAR RING

Vascular rings cause symptoms similar to those of other conditions discussed here and should be considered in the differential diagnosis. The symptoms may be caused by compression of the trachea or compression of the esophagus with resulting aspiration of formula. Diagnosis can usually be made by barium swallow and tracheogram. Treatment is division of the appropriate vessel.

## ESOPHAGEAL ATRESIA AND TRACHEOESOPHAGEAL FISTULA

Esophageal atresia and tracheoesophageal fistula (TEF) may occur as separate entities but usually occur in combination. First described in 1697 by Thomas Gibbon, esophageal atresia was not successfully treated until 1939 when Ladd in Boston and Leven in St. Paul obtained the first survivors. These two infants were treated by multiple operations which required months of hospitalization. Two years later Cameron Haight performed the first successful primary repair.

**Embryology.** Tracheoesophageal fistula is presumably the result of failure of complete midline fusion of the tracheoesophageal septum. Esophageal atresia probably results from epithelial overgrowth in the esophageal lumen along the course of the lateral esophageal grooves.

**Classification.** The important factors in the pathophysiology, symptoms, and therapy are whether both esophageal atresia and tracheoesophageal fistula are present, and if so, their

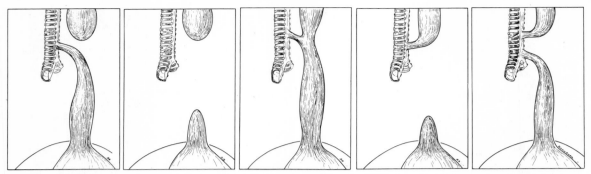

**Figure 5** Types of esophageal atresia and tracheoesophageal fistula (TEF) in order of decreasing frequency from left to right: esophageal atresia with distal TEF; esophageal atresia (without TEF); tracheoesophageal fistula (without esophageal atresia); esophageal atresia with proximal TEF; esophageal atresia with proximal and distal TEF.

anatomic relation; i.e., is the fistula proximal or distal to the atresia? The following classification shows the different anomalies (Fig. 5) with their relative frequency (based on 1058 patients, from the survey of the Surgical Section of the American Academy of Pediatrics).

| | |
|---|---|
| Esophageal atresia with distal TEF | 86.5 per cent |
| Esophageal atresia (without TEF) | 7.7 per cent |
| Isolated TEF (without esophageal atresia) | 4.2 per cent |
| Esophageal atresia with proximal TEF | 0.8 per cent |
| Esophageal atresia with proximal and distal TEF | 0.7 per cent |

### Esophageal Atresia with Distal Tracheoesophageal Fistula

**Anatomy.** In this most common form of the anomaly the esophagus ends as a dilated, blind pouch in the upper chest at or above the level of the carina. The distal esophagus originates from a small fistulous communication with the membranous portion of the distal trachea.

**Pathophysiology and Symptoms.** Since esophageal atresia prevents the passage of oral contents to the stomach, the proximal pouch fills with saliva and the infant *drools excessively.* If offered water or formula, he is likely to aspirate it into the trachea, *cough,* and become *cyanotic.*

Crying or coughing increases intratracheal pressure which in the presence of a tracheoesophageal fistula causes air to pass through the fistula into the esophagus. If there is a distal fistula the stomach and small bowel become distended, causing elevation of the diaphragms. Periodically, the stomach is decompressed back through the fistula, flooding the tracheobronchial tree with gastric secretions, leading to chemical tracheobronchitis, pneumonitis, and atelectasis, which is followed by bacterial pneumonia.

**Diagnosis.** Since untreated esophageal atresia is a uniformly fatal disease, it is imperative that the diagnosis be confirmed or excluded in any patient in whom it is suspected. The earlier the diagnosis is made, the fewer the pulmonary complications and the better the chance of survival. It is a simple matter to place a small catheter into the upper esophagus, inject 0.5 to 1 ml. of contrast medium, and obtain posteroanterior and lateral x-rays of the chest. If the esophagus ends as a blind pouch, atresia is confirmed. The presence of air in the stomach in this instance indicates a communication of the distal esophagus with the trachea (Fig. 6). The absence of gas in the abdomen usually indicates esophageal atresia without tracheoesophageal fistula. (Occasionally, in the presence of a tracheoesophageal fistula that is very narrow, no gas will have reached the abdomen.)

Esophageal atresia can also be detected by the inability to pass a rather stiff (14 to 16 French) Robinson catheter more than a short distance into the esophagus. Unfortunately, a tube of the size passed through the nose of a neonate can easily coil in the upper esophageal pouch, leading the examiner to the false conclusion that it has been passed into the stomach. The presence of the tube in the stomach must be confirmed by x-ray to exclude esophageal atresia. On this same film the pulmonary status or other causes of respiratory distress can be detected.

**Treatment.** The principal cause of death in these infants is pulmonary complications. Prior to operation therapy must be directed first toward clearing the pneumonia that is almost always present. Prompt decompressive gastrostomy will prevent reflux of gastric contents into the trachea, and sump catheter decompression of the proximal esophageal pouch will prevent further aspiration. Appropriate antibiotics, high humidity, and frequently endotracheal suction are also indicated. With intravenous fluids the patient can be safely cared for for several days until the lungs clear sufficiently to permit safe thoracotomy.

Surgical correction consists of division of the tracheoesophageal fistula with closure of the tracheal side of the fistula and anastomosis of the small distal esophageal segment to the dilated proximal pouch. Discrepancy in the size of the segments and tension due to a gap between the two ends lead to a significant number of leaks. A retropleural approach minimizes this hazard

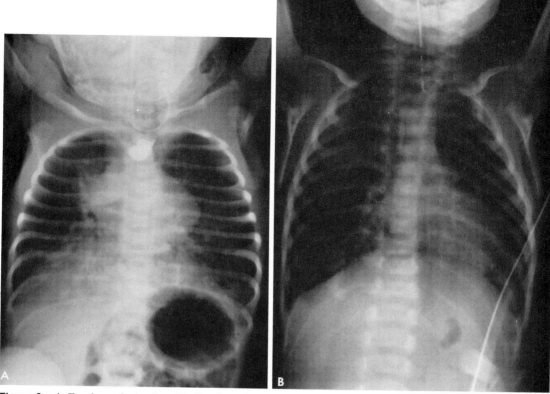

**Figure 6**  *A,* Esophageal atresia with distal tracheoesophageal fistula is demonstrated in this x-ray by contrast medium in the blind upper esophageal pouch and air in the stomach. Note right upper and lower lung field infiltrates. A gastrostomy was performed shortly after this film. *B,* Same patient 48 hours later showing effect of gastrostomy. The lungs are clear, and the diaphragm is no longer elevated by distended gut. The patient is in a much better condition to tolerate a thoracotomy.

since it results in a localized infection rather than empyema should a leak occur.

Immediate postoperative management is primarily concerned with pulmonary care. High humidity, antibiotics, pharyngeal suction, and often endotracheal suction are necessary.

**Results.** Two factors that greatly influence survival rate are associated anomalies (present in about half these infants) and the size of the patient (about one-third are premature by weight). In the infant over 6 pounds without associated anomalies, the survival rate is over 90 per cent, while in the infant weighing less than 4 pounds with associated anomalies, it is less than 20 per cent. Pneumonia, atelectasis, and retained secretions are the major causes of death.[11]

Some small premature infants or infants with associated anomalies benefit from a staged operative approach in which gastrostomy is done immediately and division of the fistula is carried out a day or two later. The infant is then fed by gastrostomy and the upper pouch is decompressed. After increase in size to 4½ to 5 pounds, or treatment of the associated anomaly, the definitive esophageal anastomosis is performed.

An anastomotic leak is a major complication. If the procedure has been done retropleurally and the space is well drained, a small leak is likely to close spontaneously. Recurrent tracheoesophageal fistula is the result of an anastomotic leak and requires division. The most frequent late complication is anastomotic stricture, which usually responds to esophageal dilatation.

### Esophageal Atresia without Tracheoesophageal Fistula

Esophageal atresia without tracheoesophageal fistula presents a somewhat different therapeutic problem since the distal esophageal segment is short and there is a long gap between the two esophageal pouches. Howard has advocated stretching the proximal esophageal pouch with a 12 F mercury-loaded bougie twice daily to make a primary anastomosis possible. This approach has yielded varied results. The other approach is to perform a gastrostomy for feeding and cervical esophagostomy for proximal pouch drainage. Later a colon interposition is employed to connect the proximal esophagus and the stomach. Small bowel segments or a gastric tube can also be used for this purpose.

### Tracheoesophageal Fistula without Esophageal Atresia

Tracheoesophageal fistula without esophageal atresia often presents a difficult diagnostic problem. These patients have recurrent bouts of pneumonia, they often cough when taking liquids, and they have increased intestinal gas with abdominal distention (from air passing through the fistula). Cine-esophagogram may or may not demonstrate a communication between the esophagus and trachea. It often shows poor peristalsis in the distal esophagus. The fistula is best visualized from the tracheal side in the infant by means of an infant fiberoptic Foroblique cystoscope. Another method is to perform esophagoscopy while dye is placed through an endotracheal tube and the patient is forcefully ventilated by the anesthesiologist. This forces air and dye through the fistula, demonstrating the abnormal communication.

Once a fistula has been demonstrated by any means, it should be divided. Most of the fistulas occur at or above the level of the second thoracic vertebra and can be repaired through a cervical approach.

## ESOPHAGEAL STENOSIS

Congenital stenosis of the esophagus is not common. Patients with esophageal stenosis, however, may present with respiratory difficulty secondary to aspiration of formula, recurrent pneumonia, or dysphagia. Diagnosis is by barium swallow and esophagoscopy. Short stenotic segments usually respond to esophageal dilation. A rare one is resistant to dilation and will require resection and esophagoesophagostomy.

## VOMITING

Although occasional regurgitation of formula is quite common in infants, persistent vomiting, the vomiting of bile-stained material, or forceful vomiting is abnormal, and its cause should be investigated. In the neonate bile-stained vomitus is almost always indicative of intestinal obstruction. Nonobstructive causes of vomiting must also be considered, such as increased intracranial pressure (subdural hematoma, hydrocephalus), electrolyte imbalance (adrenogenital syndrome), and, particularly, sepsis.

Abdominal distention is a prominent feature of distal small bowel and colonic obstruction but is absent with obstruction above the proximal jejunum. Most normal infants will pass a meconium stool during the first 24 hours of life. Interestingly, many neonates with small bowel obstruction will pass one or two meconium stools. They simply evacuate the colon of meconium distal to the obstruction. The fact that an infant has passed a stool or does not have abdominal distention therefore does not exclude intestinal obstruction.

After a thorough physical examination to detect extra-abdominal causes of vomiting and evaluation of the abdomen for signs of intra-abdominal sepsis or an abdominal mass, recumbent and upright roentgenograms of the abdomen are of primary diagnostic importance. On plain x-ray of the abdomen it is not possible in the neonate to differentiate colon from small bowel. This distinction must be made by barium enema if the correct diagnosis is to be made and proper therapy instituted. If the vomitus does not contain bile, the pathologic lesion is proximal to the ampulla of Vater and will be best delineated by barium swallow.

Pulmonary complications of vomiting (aspiration and aspiration pneumonia) are a major cause of death for neonates with intestinal obstruction. To avoid this complication the stomach should be promptly aspirated in any infant suspected of having intestinal obstruction.

An important part of operative correction of neonatal obstruction is a gastrostomy to reduce the chance of postoperative vomiting with the hazard of aspiration. The advantages of a gastrostomy over a nasogastric tube are (1) the larger tube employed does a more efficient job of decompressing the stomach; (2) a tube through the nose and pharynx interferes with the infant's moving pharyngeal and tracheal secretions, whereas gastrostomy does not; and (3) a gastrostomy can be used for feeding purposes once intestinal peristalsis has returned to normal in the premature or ill neonate. It is a helpful and safe procedure in pediatric surgery.[12]

Another consideration in neonates with intestinal obstruction is the use of parenteral feeding (intravenous hyperalimentation). In many patients it takes a long time for proper gastrointestinal function to be established. It is probably wise to place a central venous catheter early in the postoperative period and start parenteral feeding. If the intestinal tract promptly begins to function satisfactorily, the catheter can be removed. If not, the patient has not reached a state of malnutrition and severe negative nitrogen balance before this valuable form of therapy is instituted.

## DUODENAL OBSTRUCTION

Duodenal obstruction in the neonate is the result of duodenal atresia or stenosis, annular pancreas (with associated atresia or stenosis), or peritoneal bands secondary to incomplete intestinal rotation.

**Embryology.** The duodenum is the one portion of the gastrointestinal tract in which a solid phase is known to exist in early fetal life. Lack of recanalization results in atresia or stenosis. Annular pancreas is thought to be the result of failure of the tip of the ventral pancreatic anlage to rotate with the duodenum. As a consequence, it becomes wrapped around the second portion of the duodenum.

**Clinical Findings.** The principal symptom is vomiting of bile-stained material. On rare occasions the obstruction is proximal to the ampulla of Vater and the vomitus is not green. With atresia the vomiting usually starts the first day of life. If there has been an asymptomatic period of a few days prior to onset of symptoms, malrotation is more likely. Stenosis causes less severe symptoms, and the patient may have little difficulty until solids are added to the diet. Abdominal distention is not a prominent feature though there may be fullness in the epigastrium if the stomach is distended. The state of hydration depends on how soon after birth the diagnosis is made. About one-fourth of patients with duodenal atresia also have Down's syndrome (mongolism).

**Diagnosis.** Diagnosis of duodenal obstruction is made by upright x-ray of the abdomen, which shows the typical "double bubble" of stomach and dilated duodenum with no other small bowel gas (Fig. 7). The presence of air distal to the duodenum indicates partial obstruction—stenosis or malrotation.

**Therapy.** Extensive preoperative preparation is not required if the diagnosis has been promptly made. The stomach should be emptied by a nasogastric tube. If the patient is dehydrated, intravenous fluids are given. Since the obstruction is high and the gut proximal to it can be easily decompressed, perforation is not a danger. If operation must be delayed and there is any question of malrotation with midgut volvulus, a barium enema should be obtained to exclude this possibility.

A right upper transverse incision gives excellent exposure of the duodenum. If there is an intrinsic atresia or stenosis, the duodenum is mobilized by an extensive Kocher maneuver to allow a generous duodenoduodenostomy without tension. The area of the common bile duct and ampulla of Vater is avoided. No attempt is made to resect the obstruction; it is simply bypassed. If annular pancreas is present or there is a long atretic segment, the proximal dilated duodenum segment is connected in a retrocolic fashion to the proximal jejunum by a side-to-side anastomosis.

Postoperatively the stomach is decompressed by gastrostomy and the patient is maintained on intravenous fluids (with or without parenteral feeding) until oral feedings can be tolerated. Complications are pneumonia, sepsis, and postoperative intestinal obstruction.

**Results.** About two-thirds of patients with duodenal obstruction survive. Associated anomalies and prematurity significantly influence the mortality rate and are responsible for half the deaths. Respiratory and anastomotic complications cause most of the remaining deaths and are preventable.[8]

Some parents of infants with duodenal atresia and mongolism prefer not to have the infants operated upon. If the diagnosis of mongolism is not definite, the stomach can be safely decompressed by a nasogastric tube for the 48 to 72 hours required to obtain a confirmatory chromosome analysis.

## JEJUNOILEAL ATRESIA

In the neonate distal small bowel and colonic obstructions present much the same clinical picture and may be due to atresia or stenosis of the jejunum, ileum (most common), or colon (rare), meconium ileus, malrotation, or Hirschsprung's disease (Fig. 8).

**Etiology.** Current thinking holds that the etiology of atresia of the small bowel is usually, if not always, the result of an in utero vascular accident. Similar lesions can be produced experimentally by ligation of the mesenteric vessels of the fetal dog. Microscopic examination of resected gut distal to an atretic area shows squamous epithelial cells in the lumen, indicating that the gut was patent at some previous time. The gut is often shorter than normal in these infants. Associated intra-abdominal adhesions and calcifications also implicate a previous catastrophic event. The mechanism of the vascular accident is unknown, but it could result from volvulus, thrombosis, embolus, or intussusception.

**Clinical Findings.** The most prominent symptom is vomiting of bile-stained material from the first day or two of life. The abdomen is distended and may have been so from birth. The infant may be dehydrated both from vomiting and from fluid loss into the dilated loops of intestine.

**Diagnosis.** X-ray of the abdomen shows dilated loops of gut usually with air-fluid levels. Barium enema shows a normally rotated, small, unused colon (Fig. 9). (This "microcolon" is actually normal but because of proximal obstruction contains little or no material. It will function normally.)

**Treatment.** Preoperative preparation consists

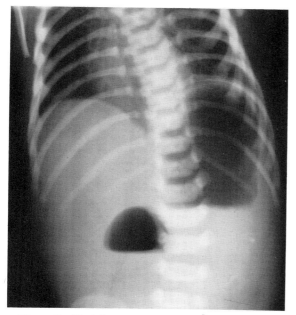

**Figure 7** Upright roentgenogram of a neonate with duodenal atresia showing the classic "double bubble" of stomach and dilated duodenum. There is no distal gas.

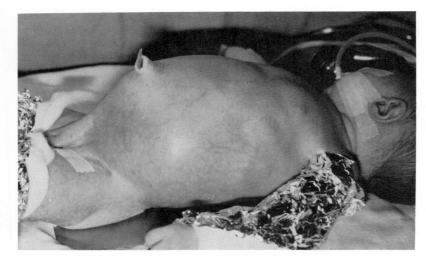

**Figure 8** Abdominal distention of this degree in a newborn with symptoms of intestinal obstruction is indicative of distal small bowel or colonic obstruction.

of gastric decompression, vitamin K administration, and, if the patient's condition warrants, intravenous fluids and plasma. This should not take more than 4 hours. If preoperative chest x-ray shows aspiration pneumonia, antibiotics, usually penicillin and kanamycin, are given.

Operation is through either a transverse incision just above the umbilicus or an upper abdominal midline incision. It is important that the markedly dilated segment of intestine just proximal to the atretic segment be resected (Fig. 10). Even if the gut is shortened and an appropriate effort to conserve intestine is being made, this grossly dilated pouch must be removed. It will not

function properly and will result in chronic functional obstruction.[8] Intestinal continuity is established by an end-to-end anastomosis. Because of the small caliber of the distal gut the anastomosis must be done with great care. We prefer a single-layer anastomosis using inverting horizontal mattress sutures of 5–0 vascular silk placed from within the lumen. A Stamm gastrostomy provides postoperative gastric decompression.

Since some of these infants have difficulty in the postoperative period with mechanical obstruction or short intestine, parenteral feeding is of value. If there is less than 12 inches of small intestine, the outlook for survival is bleak.

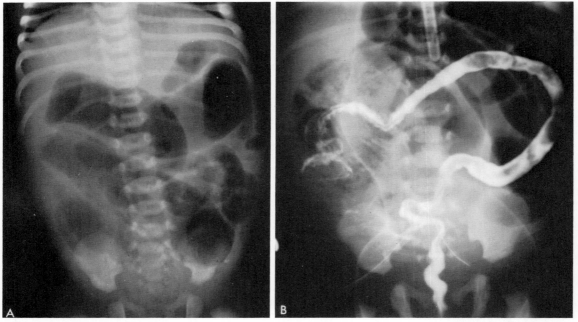

**Figure 9** *A,* Typical x-ray of a newborn with distal small bowel or colonic obstruction. It is not possible on a plain film of the abdomen to distinguish large from small bowel gas in patients of this age. *B,* Barium enema in a patient with small bowel obstruction shows a small unused colon.

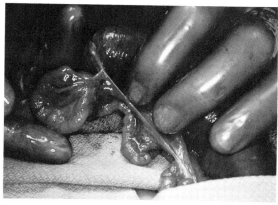

**Figure 10** Operative photograph of ileal atresia, showing the proximal bowel to end blindly, a V-shaped mesenteric defect, and the decompressed tiny distal intestine.

**Results.** Louw in South Africa has reported a 90 per cent survival rate in infants with small bowel atresia. The overall survival rate is closer to 65 per cent. Prematurity and associated anomalies are not nearly as frequent as with duodenal atresia. Anastomotic and pulmonary complications account for most of the deaths.

## MECONIUM ILEUS

Meconium ileus is the earliest manifestation of cystic fibrosis and is present in approximately 10 to 15 per cent of patients with this disease.

**Etiology and Pathology.** Cystic fibrosis is a hereditary disease transmitted as an autosomal recessive trait. For a family with one affected child there is a 25 per cent chance that each subsequent child will have the disease. Cystic fibrosis involves the lungs, pancreas, liver, and skin as well as the gut. The meconium contains an abnormal mucoprotein. There is also a decrease or absence of pancreatic exocrine function.

The terminal ileum is filled with firm, small, gray concretions and is of small caliber. Just proximal to this, the ileum is markedly dilated and filled with a thick, very viscid, and exceedingly sticky meconium which intestinal peristalsis is incapable of propelling. The proximal ileum is less dilated and the meconium is liquid (Fig. 11).

Some patients with meconium ileus have associated atresia, presumably the result of a prenatal volvulus of a segment of the dilated intestine. This may be associated with intra-abdominal calcification.

**Diagnosis.** Clinical findings are similar to those in patients with intestinal atresia—bilious vomiting and abdominal distention. Dilated meconium-filled loops of ileum may be palpable. A family history of cystic fibrosis provides strong support for a diagnosis of meconium ileus.

X-rays of the abdomen reveal findings similar to those in other forms of neonatal distal intestinal obstruction. There may, however, be fewer fluid levels, a greater variety in the size of intestinal loops, and a granular appearance in some of the dilated loops of gut. The loops may be arranged in concentric circles and change little with upright positioning. Barium enema shows a small, unused, normally positioned colon. If there is reflux of barium into the terminal ileum, the small concretions typical of meconium ileus may be seen. A sweat chloride level over 60 mEq. per liter is diagnostic.

**Treatment.** Preoperative preparation is similar to that for neonates with other forms of intestinal obstruction. Because of the particular susceptibility of these patients to pulmonary infections, every effort should be made to avoid sources of contamination. High-humidity environment may help prevent pulmonary secretions from becoming so tenacious that they plug bronchi.

Operative therapy consists of resection of the segment of markedly dilated ileum containing the very sticky meconium. The terminal ileum is irrigated with the mucolytic agent N-acetylcysteine in a 2 per cent concentration. (More concentrated solutions are irritating.) Either the proximal or distal end of the remaining ileum is brought out as a vent with anastomosis of the other end to the side of the vented segment just below the abdominal wall.[4] Alternatively, the ends of the intestine are brought out as a "double-barrel" Mikulicz ileostomy.

Occasionally at operation a relatively short segment of ileum is involved and can be evacuated by enterostomy and irrigation with 2 per cent N-acetylcysteine, so that resection is avoided. Whether resection is required or not, a gastrostomy is performed for gastric decompression.

A few patients have a mild form of the disease and may respond to nonoperative forms of treatment. One is administration of acetylcysteine by mouth and by enema. Another is use of Gastrografin enemas in which the hypertonic contrast medium loosens concretions by causing a shift of

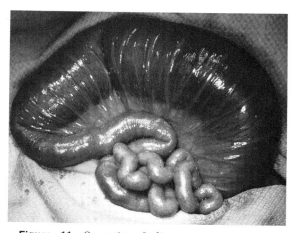

**Figure 11** Operative findings in a patient with meconium ileus. The terminal ileum is small and contains small, firm concretions. The portion just proximal to this is dilated and contains exceedingly sticky meconium.

fluid into the gut. There is a concomitant decrease in blood volume. It is dangerous to persist in either of these forms of treatment if prompt relief is not obtained.

Postoperative care is similar to that in jejuno-ileal atresia. Special care is taken to avoid pneumonia. If an ileostomy vent has been used, it is closed later extraperitoneally under local anesthesia to avoid a second general anesthesia. Pancreatic enzyme supplementation must be added to the formula.

**Results.**   While 75 to 80 per cent survive the intestinal obstruction, these patients are still faced with all the pulmonary and nutritional problems of cystic fibrosis. Only about 50 per cent survive the first 6 months.

After the neonatal period obstruction can occur in patients with cystic fibrosis because of inspissated intestinal contents. This is likely to occur if pancreatic supplementation has been deleted from the diet. This condition has been termed meconium ileus equivalent. Nonoperative management by long-tube intestinal decompression plus administration of pancreatic enzymes or N-acetylcysteine through the tube and by enema is usually successful. The inspissated intestinal contents in the cecum or terminal ileum may act as a lead point for an intussusception in the older infant or child. This often requires operative reduction.

## MALROTATION OF THE INTESTINE

Malrotation may produce duodenal or distal small bowel obstruction in the neonate as well as in the older child. High obstruction is due to compression of the duodenum by Ladd's bands, and distal obstruction to compression by midgut volvulus. In addition, malrotation may produce chronic malabsorption (celiac-like syndrome).

**Embryology.**   Malrotation or, more accurately, incomplete rotation, results from arrest of the normal rotation of the midgut (that portion of the intestine supplied by the superior mesenteric artery — from the duodenum to the midcolon). About the tenth week of fetal life the midgut returns to the abdominal cavity from the coelomic extension in the base of the umbilical cord. As the gut returns, it rotates in a counterclockwise direction. Pivoting around the superior mesenteric artery, the duodenum passes inferiorly to the vessels while the ileocecal area passes superior to the vessels and ultimately rests in the right lower quadrant. If the rotational process is arrested when the cecum is in the epigastrium or right upper quadrant, there is no posterior peritoneal attachment of the small bowel mesentery from the ligament of Treitz to the right lower quadrant, nor does the ascending colon have its posterior peritoneal attachments to the right posterior abdomen. Peritoneal bands, presumably those normally attaching the right colon to the posterior peritoneum, connect the cecum and proximal colon to the right upper quadrant. In so doing they cross

and often obstruct the duodenum. If the duodenum has not rotated inferior to the superior mesenteric vessels, the distal duodenum and jejunum remain on the right side of the spine and there is no ligament of Treitz.[21]

**Clinical Findings.**   Symptoms in the neonate are those of duodenal or low intestinal obstruction. Bile-stained vomitus is present. Abdominal distention may or may not be present. Symptoms may be present from the first day of life. Sometimes there is an asymptomatic period followed by a sudden onset of symptoms due to midgut volvulus. The infant may deteriorate rapidly. Bloody stools can be a prominent feature. This is a catastrophic event and requires prompt treatment.

In the somewhat older infant or child chronic symptoms are likely to result from partial duodenal obstruction. There is recurrent vomiting and poor weight gain. Chronic diarrhea, malnutrition, and abdominal distention may occasionally result from malrotation. The cause of this symptom complex is not clear. It is thought to be the result of partial midgut torsion with venous obstruction, mucosal edema, and malabsorption.

**Diagnosis.**   Diagnosis is by x-ray. Plain films of the abdomen show either duodenal or distal obstruction. Duodenal obstruction is less apt to be as complete as, or to be accompanied by as much duodenal dilatation as, duodenal atresia. With volvulus there are dilated loops of small bowel with air-fluid levels. On occasion when volvulus is associated with a high degree of duodenal obstruction, almost no small bowel gas is present.

Barium enema shows the cecum in the right upper quadrant or epigastrium. With midgut volvulus the proximal colon is wrapped around the root of the small bowel mesentery, and barium enema may not fill the proximal colon. Barium swallow done in patients with symptoms of chronic high intestinal obstruction shows a "corkscrew" duodenum with the duodenum passing down the right side of the spine into the proximal portion of jejunum, which is also on the right.

**Treatment.**   Because of the risk of vascular occlusion volvulus requires prompt operation. A very short time of preoperative preparation may be required to restore the blood volume if the patient is in shock. On opening the abdomen, the surgeon notes that the colon is not in the right gutter but is wrapped around the root of the small bowel mesentery. The entire small bowel should be delivered onto the abdominal wall and rotated in a counterclockwise direction until the volvulus has been reduced. Nonviable gut must be resected. Unfortunately, that is sometimes the entire midgut. If this extensive resection is required, the wisest course may be to exteriorize only that portion of the gut which is definitely not viable and return any questionable areas to the abdomen. Laparotomy the following day may reveal that some of the remaining intestine is still viable. If not, the patient's chance for survival is nil. Parenteral feeding is not indicated since it merely delays the inevitable outcome.

The duodenal obstruction is relieved by division

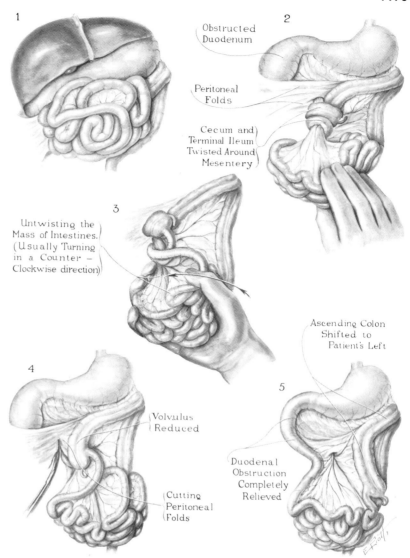

1

2
Obstructed
Duodenum

Peritoneal
Folds

Cecum and
Terminal Ileum
Twisted Around
Mesentery

3
Untwisting the
Mass of Intestines.
(Usually Turning
in a Counter –
Clockwise direction)

Ascending Colon
Shifted to
Patient's Left

4

5

Volvulus
Reduced

Duodenal
Obstruction
Completely
Relieved

Cutting
Peritoneal
Folds

**Figure 12** Operative treatment of malrotation with midgut volvulus and duodenal obstruction. (From Gross, R. E.: An Atlas of Children's Surgery. Philadelphia, W. B. Saunders Company, 1970.)

of the peritoneal bands crossing the duodenum. Occasionally intrinsic obstruction of the duodenum is associated with malrotation, and it should be looked for. The proximal colon is returned to the left side of the abdomen. Intestinal fixation procedures are unnecessary (Fig. 12). Postoperative care usually presents no particular problems unless an extensive resection is required.

**Results.** Survival exceeds 95 per cent if resection is not required and there is no significant associated anomaly.

## AGANGLIONIC MEGACOLON (HIRSCHSPRUNG'S DISEASE)

Hirschsprung, the noted Danish pediatrician, presented his classic description of "Constipation in Newborns Due to Dilatation and Hypertrophy of the Colon" before the Berlin Congress of Children's Disease in 1886. The paper was published in 1888. The Dutch surgeon Ruysch is generally credited with the first recorded description 200 years earlier. A true understanding of the nature of the pathology did not come until 60 years later when Swenson and Bill in 1948 described an operative procedure to excise the entire aganglionic segment by an abdominoperineal pull-through technique.

**Pathology.** The basic defect in Hirschsprung's disease is absence of ganglionic cells of the myenteric plexuses of Auerbach in the involved segment of colon. This absence of ganglion cells extends from the anus proximally for various distances, usually to involve the rectum and a portion of the sigmoid colon. Aganglionosis may, however, on unusual occasions involve the entire colon and, rarely, the entire small bowel as well.

Even more rarely, skip areas with intervening normal bowel have been reported. The rectum, however, is not skipped.

**Physiology.** The absence of parasympathetic innervation leads to lack of peristalsis in the involved portion of colon. Histochemical studies also indicate sympathetic overactivity in the aganglionic segment leading to increased muscle tone. The result is a functional obstruction. The colon just proximal to this area dilates and the musculature becomes hypertrophied as it works to propel the fecal stream through the distal obstruction.

If pressures are measured in the colonic lumen in patients with Hirschsprung's disease, there is no evidence of peristaltic activity in the aganglionic segment. Persistaltic pressures in the proximal colon are higher than normal.

**Clinical Findings.** Almost all patients with Hirschsprung's disease have some difficulty during the neonatal period. In some the clinical picture is the same as that in other forms of neonatal intestinal obstruction, with green vomitus and abdominal distention. In others the symptoms are less impressive. It is, however, usually possible to obtain a history that the infant was constipated in the neonatal period. Constipation persists and frequent enemas, suppositories, and laxatives are given for relief, even in the infant.

This chronic obstruction leads to enterocolitis in some infants. They may become quite ill with diarrhea, dehydration, and sepsis. The colitis may proceed to perforation. Enterocolitis is the most dangerous complication of Hirschsprung's disease and carries a high mortality.

The child with Hirschsprung's disease has passed from a constipated infancy into a constipated childhood and must be distinguished from the much larger number of children who are constipated from other causes. The child with Hirschsprung's disease has had symptoms from birth. He seldom soils his underclothing, and on rectal examination the stool is at least 2 to 3 cm. above the sphincter. Stool may be passed after the digital examination. Some of these children go for 2 to 3 weeks without passing stools. In constipation from other causes the onset of symptoms occurs after the neonatal period, the child usually soils his underpants frequently, and rectal examination reveals a large quantity of stool just at the sphincter.

**Diagnosis.** Diagnosis can usually be made with ease by barium enema in the older infant or child (Fig. 13). There is a relatively normal-sized rectum and rectosigmoid with considerable dilatation of the colon just proximal to this. The colon empties poorly. In the neonate, plain x-rays of the abdomen may be indistinguishable from those in distal small bowel obstruction. Barium enema, however, will show a relatively normal-appearing colon. The disparity in size has not yet developed. The colon empties poorly, however, and considerable barium will be present in the colon 24 hours later. This retention is highly suggestive of Hirschsprung's disease. A feathered appearance of the colonic mucosa is suggestive of superficial ulceration and is an indication of enterocolitis.

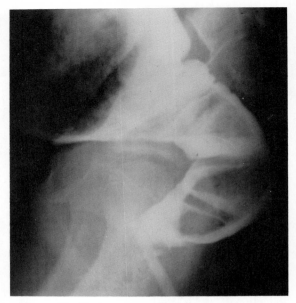

**Figure 13**  Barium enema in this older boy shows a normal-sized rectum with marked dilatation of the rectosigmoid, which is typical of Hirschsprung's disease.

The diagnosis is proved by rectal biopsy though this is not usually necessary with older infants and children. A full-thickness biopsy of the lateral rectal wall about 2 cm. above the mucocutaneous junction will reveal absence of myenteric ganglion cells if the patient has Hirschsprung's disease. Experienced radiologists and pathologists are most helpful in making the diagnosis of Hirschsprung's disease. Lack of familiarity on their part leads to much confusion in this diagnosis.

**Treatment.** The treatment of Hirschsprung's disease, as indicated by Swenson, is resection of the entire aganglionic segment with anastomosis at the anus.[23] This is an extensive procedure and is not well tolerated by the sick infant. Preliminary colostomy above the aganglionic segment permits delay of the corrective procedure until the patient can better tolerate it. It should be determined by frozen section that there are ganglion cells present at the colostomy site. Definitive resection is done when the patient is 6 months to a year old. Older patients usually do not require a preliminary colostomy unless the dilated segment is huge and decompression would facilitate anastomosis.

In addition to the Swenson pull-through operation, two modifications of that procedure have gained favor in recent years. In the Duhamel operation the ganglionic proximal colon is brought down posterior to the aganglionic rectum, which is not resected. They are connected by a side-to-side anastomosis. This procedure has particular merit for the patient who has aganglionosis of the entire colon. The small bowel can be connected to a long segment of rectum and sigmoid to provide adequate absorptive surface (colon) while providing a peristaltic segment (small bowel) down to the anus.

In the Soave procedure, the surgeon leaves the aganglionic rectal musculature in place, removes the rectal mucosa, and brings the normal peristaltic ganglionic segment down through the rectal muscular cuff. The advantage of this procedure is that it requires no pelvic dissection outside the rectum.

For patients with a very short aganglionic segment, resection of a strip of the rectal musculature posteriorly (in essence, a myotomy of the aganglionic segment) can be accomplished from inside the anus.

**Results.** The mortality for the older infant and child is 2 to 3 per cent. For the infant with enterocolitis the mortality is as high as 50 per cent. The functional results are quite good in 95 per cent of patients.

## IMPERFORATE ANUS

Imperforate anus is perhaps not the most accurate description of the anorectal malformations under discussion but is the one accepted by general usage. The anatomy in this group of anomalies is complicated. To give some idea of how complicated it is, a classification in outline form recently proposed by an international group of experts requires 30 lines.

**Embryology.** In the 4 mm. embryo the allantois connects with the hindgut in a terminal cavity, the cloaca. The urorectal septum divides the ventral urogenital portion from the dorsal rectal portion of the 5 mm. embryo down to the pubococcygeal line. Lateral ingrowth of mesenchyma completes the division below this level.

Alterations of this division result in a rectourinary fistula. In the female, müllerian ducts are interposed between the dorsal and ventral portions, so rectourinary fistulas do not occur (except cloacal anomalies). The distal vagina develops from sinovaginal buds which originate from the epithelium of the dorsal wall of the urogenital sinus. (Rectovaginal fistulas are the result of maldevelopment in this area.)

The terminal hindgut forms the upper portion of the anal canal. The lower portion is formed from the proctodeum. The anal sphincter is formed from still another source—mesoderm—and is almost always present.

**Pathology.** Anatomic conditions that are important in therapy are:

1. The height of the rectal pouch—is it above the pubococcygeal line (high pouch) and hence has not descended through the puborectalis sling?

2. Is there a fistula, and if so, to what? In the male fistulas may connect the rectum to the perineum, urethra, or bladder, and, in the female, to the vulva, vestibule, vagina, or perineum. The large majority of patients do have a fistula to one of these locations.

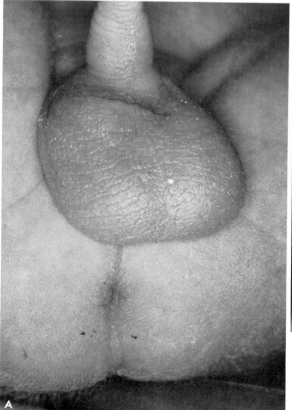

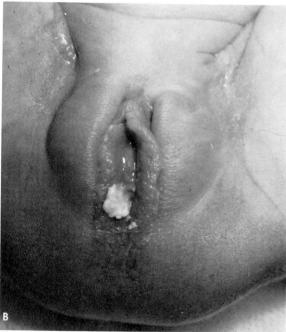

**Figure 14** *A,* Imperforate anus in a boy. *B,* Imperforate anus in a girl with rectal fistula to the fourchette.

A description of the anomaly should be anatomic and include this information. For example, "low imperforate anus with rectovaginal fistula" is more useful than a complicated system of letters and numbers.

Usually grouped with imperforate anus are rectal atresia (in which there is a normal anus distal to the atretic rectal area), anal stenosis, and anal membrane.

**Symptoms.** If there is a perineal or vaginal fistula that is large enough to decompress the colon, there may be no symptoms in the neonatal period. In these patients constipation usually develops later as stools become formed. If there is no external fistula or the fistula is small, typical symptoms of low intestinal obstruction appear.

**Diagnosis.** The diagnosis of imperforate anus is made by inspection of the perineum (Fig. 14). The height of the rectal pouch is determined by lateral x-rays in the upside-down position taken after swallowed air has had ample time to reach the rectum (24 hours of age). An opaque marker is placed on the anus, and the center of the x-ray beam is directed at the greater trochanter. This technique has the limitation that meconium in the pouch may prevent air from reaching the distal end of the pouch, giving a false impression of a high atresia. Conversely, if the baby is crying at the time the film is exposed, the increased intra-abdominal pressure may push the pouch down, giving the false impression of a low pouch. In general, the high pouch that has not descended through the puborectalis sling is more than 1.5 cm. above the anus on x-ray and appears above a line drawn from pubis to coccyx. A low pouch is below these points.

The physical findings are more important. If there is a perineal fistula (including ectopic anteriorly displaced anus and fistula opening along the median scrotal raphe) or fistula to the vaginal fourchette or low vagina, the operative approach is from the perineum. A retrograde urethrogram in the male may demonstrate a fistulous communication between the rectum and the posterior urethra or the base of the bladder. These patients, as well as those with no fistula, need a combined abdomin-operineal operation.

Imperforate anus is associated with other congenital anaomalies about half the time. Some of these are life-threatening, and their recognition is important to the immediate care of the patient. Esophageal atresia is present in about 5 per cent of patients and should be looked for prior to operation in all patients. Urologic anomalies are frequent. A cystourethrogram and intravenous pyelogram should be done to detect these associated anomalies. Congenital heart disease is common. Sacral anomalies are frequent with high imperforate anus.

**Treatment.** In almost all girls, and in those boys with perineal fistulas, the condition can be corrected by a perineal anoplasty. In these patients the rectum is normally positioned through the puborectalis sling. The fistulous opening is dissected back to the rectal pouch, which is freed to allow it to be sutured without tension to the anal skin in the normal position. In patients with anteriorly displaced anus this can usually be accomplished by a simple incision posteriorly and suture of the mucous membranes of the perineal skin. This procedure can be safely done in the neonatal period.

For the boy with a high pouch or urinary tract fistula and the girl with cloacal anomalies, the best functional results are obtained by definitive operation when the child is older. The initial therapy therefore is creation of a colostomy. With a divided colostomy that completely diverts the fecal stream there are fewer complications, and there is less chance of urinary tract infection in patients with urinary tract fistulas. Either sigmoid or transverse colostomy can be used.

The most important feature of the definitive repair is the accurate placement of the rectum through the puborectalis sling of the levator ani complex just behind the urethra. Stephens advocates a posterior approach just below the sacrum with removal of the coccyx for better visualization of the levator musculature.[22] The colon is mobilized by an abdominal approach, passed through the previously identified puborectalis and external sphincters, and sutured to the anal skin. Some surgeons feel the posterior approach does not appreciably aid in the identification of the puborectalis and identify this muscle from above. The urinary fistula is divided in the course of the mobilization of the distal rectal pouch and the urethral end is sewn over the catgut.

**Results.** Mortality is appreciably influenced by associated anomalies. Except for these, operative mortality is about 2 per cent.

Functional results are good for those with a low pouch that can be corrected by a perineal approach. Ninety to ninety-five per cent of these patients have essentially normal bowel control. Patients with a high pouch have a poorer result. Only about one-half have good functional control, though most can acquire socially acceptable control with diet, laxatives, and enemas.

## GASTROESOPHAGEAL REFLUX

After the first month of life gastroesophageal reflux is not normal. In 1947 Neuhauser and Berenberg coined the term "chalasia" to apply to the condition of an infant who has free gastroesophageal reflux without a demonstrable hiatal hernia. The term implies that the basic pathologic lesion is one of excessive relaxation of the distal esophagus.

Chalasia is seen during the first few months of life. Symptoms are those of vomiting or spitting up of formula, usually shortly after feedings, and often when the baby has been returned to the crib and placed in a horizontal position. Chalasia is a self-limiting process and is best treated by keeping the patient propped upright in an infant seat for 4 to 6 weeks.

Hiatal hernia is discussed in detail elsewhere.

In infants it is often overlooked. Some patients originally diagnosed as having chalasia are subsequently shown to have reflux secondary to a hiatal hernia. Symptoms are similar to those of chalasia. In addition, the vomiting may be forceful. On occasion patients may aspirate gastric contents, and may have resulting recurrent pneumonitis. They even may have frank airway obstruction with apnea. Some fail to gain weight. In the older child symptoms may be the result of esophageal stricture caused by a prolonged esophagitis from gastric reflux. Anemia may also be the result of esophagitis.

**Diagnosis.** Diagnosis of gastroesophageal reflux is made roentgenographically by barium swallow. If a portion of the cardia is demonstrated above the diaphragm, a true hiatal hernia exists. Esophagitis is detected by esophagoscopy. Strictures may be demonstrated by both these diagnostic approaches.

**Treatment.** For uncomplicated hiatal hernia and gastroesophageal reflux without esophagitis, the infant is treated by being propped in an upright (60 degrees) position 24 hours a day. About two-thirds of patients will respond to this therapy. If, however, the patient fails to gain weight or has episodes of aspiration with this treatment, he will benefit from an antireflux operation. Patients with esophagitis should be followed closely to see that it subsides. Older children will benefit from antacids. If esophagitis persists, operation is indicated. If stricture is present, repair of the hiatal hernia alone may not be sufficient. Esophageal resection with colon or small bowel interposition may be required.

## CONGENITAL HYPERTROPHIC PYLORIC STENOSIS

Hypertrophic pyloric stenosis is the most common condition requiring an operation in infancy. The operation is the Fredet-Ramstedt procedure. In 1907 Fredet suggested that the circular muscles at the pylorus be divided, with the mucosa left intact. The muscular layer was then closed transversely. In 1912 Ramstedt showed that the muscular closure was not necessary.

**Etiology.** The cause of pyloric stenosis is obscure. There is a hereditary factor involved. Boys are affected four times as often as girls. Relatives of female patients with pyloric stenosis are, however, more likely to have the disease than relatives of affected males. It seems likely that there is some autonomic nervous imbalance, perhaps due to immature ganglion cells, which leads to muscular hypertrophy.

**Pathology.** There is marked hypertrophy of the circular musculature at the pylorus. The enlarged musculature encroaches on the pyloric lumen, and there is often edema of the pyloric mucosa. There is disagreement as to whether the ganglion cells of the pylorus are normal or not.

**Symptoms.** Symptoms are the result of the par-

tial gastric outlet obstruction. Vomiting usually starts at about 1 week of age. Some authorities think this initial asymptomatic period occurs because it takes time for mucosal edema to develop. The edema further narrows the already compromised pyloric canal. Vomiting becomes progressively more frequent and forceful (projectile). Bile is not present in the vomitus, which does occasionally contain coffee-ground material. There is a decrease in the number and volume of stools. The baby is hungry and takes his feedings with vigor. After regaining birth weight and perhaps some additional weight, he begins to lose weight. The loss of hydrogen, chloride, and potassium ions leads to a metabolic alkalosis.

**Physical Findings.** Physical examination usually reveals a hungry baby of 2 to 6 weeks of age with signs of dehydration. Prominent peristaltic waves may be seen traversing the upper abdomen from left to right as the gastric contractions work against the obstructed pylorus. Although several attempts may be required, it is almost always possible to palpate the hypertrophied pyloric "tumor" characteristically described as an "olive." The "tumor" is best palpated when the stomach is empty—either just after the infant has vomited or after the stomach has been aspirated. Good abdominal relaxation is necessary. With the thighs flexed on the abdomen and the baby pacified with a sugar nipple, deep palpation of the epigastrium usually reveals the typical, firm, transverse mass which can be rolled under the examining fingers.

**Diagnosis.** Diagnosis is made by palpating the pyloric mass. If the mass is not palpable, roentgenographic visualization of the stomach and duodenum should be done. This will detect pyloric stenosis when present or perhaps other causes of vomiting when it is not present. If pyloric stenosis is demonstrated, the surgeon should persist in his attempt to palpate the tumor before operating because pylorospasm may present a similar x-ray appearance.

**Treatment.** Preoperative preparation consists of correction of dehydration and alkalosis. If this is not severe, oral electrolyte solutions will usually suffice. If there is moderate electrolyte imbalance or dehydration, or if the patient cannot retain clear liquids by mouth, intravenous replacement is required. In most cases this is not necessary. In many infants diagnosis is made early in the course of the symptoms and only oral fluids overnight are required preoperatively. Because of the pyloric obstruction there is marked delay in gastric emptying. The stomach should therefore be aspirated before induction of anesthesia to avoid the hazard of vomiting and aspiration.

Operative correction is that described by Ramstedt. A longitudinal incision is made on the anterior superior avascular portion of the pylorus through the entire length of the pyloric canal and the friable muscle fibers are split with a blunt instrument. The mucosa bulges into the incision, increasing the size of the pyloric lumen (Fig. 15).

Manometric studies after pyloromyotomy have shown that gastric peristalsis does not return for

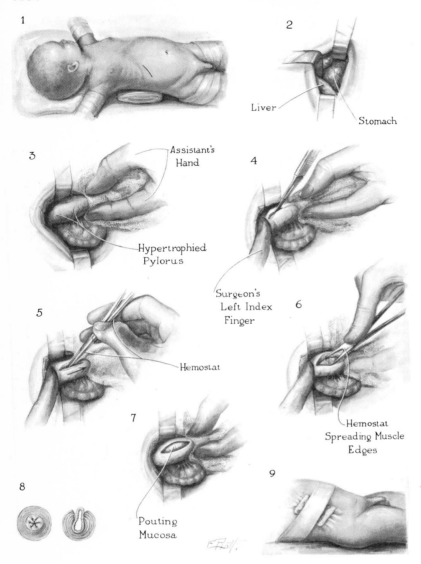

1

2

Liver

Stomach

3

Assistant's Hand

4

Hypertrophied Pylorus

5

Surgeon's Left Index Finger

6

Hemostat

7

Hemostat Spreading Muscle Edges

8

Pouting Mucosa

9

**Figure 15** Operative technique for Fredet-Ramstedt pyloromyotomy. An alternate incision that gives excellent exposure in a 3 to 4 cm. transverse skin incision midway between the xiphoid and the umbilicus with longitudinal midline incision through the linea alba. (From Gross, R. E.: An Atlas of Children's Surgery. Philadelphia, W. B. Saunders Company, 1970.)

12 to 18 hours. Clear liquid feedings are started after that time. Feedings are then advanced to full formula over the next 2 to 3 days, when the patient can be discharged.

**Results.** Results of operation are excellent. Mortality is currently less than 0.5 per cent. Complications are rare. Inadequate pyloromyotomy is rarely seen if the operation is performed by a competent surgeon. Duodenal perforation at the time of myotomy is not common. If recognized and closed, it carries little risk.[3]

Medical treatment of pyloric stenosis is based on the fact that if the infant can be kept alive the symptoms will usually subside. Antispasmodics, frequent small feedings with refeeding after vomiting, good nursing care, and several weeks of hospitalization are usually required. This form of therapy is not recommended.

## GASTROINTESTINAL BLEEDING

Massive gastrointestinal bleeding in the pediatric age group is not common. Small quantities of blood in the stool are. Some of the entities discussed in this section will at times present with symptoms other than bleeding but are discussed here because bleeding is often a prominent feature.

In the diagnostic approach to any patient with bleeding from the gastrointestinal tract it is important to know the color and quantity of blood, whether it is passed in vomitus or by rectum, if there is any evidence of a generalized bleeding disorder, if there are associated symptoms, and if, indeed, the material is blood. When passed in the stool, chocolate, tomato-based foods, red Jello, and some medications may look like blood to both parent and physician. Check it chemically to be sure.

Swallowed blood may be vomited. In the neonate, this may be blood swallowed during delivery. Fetal hemoglobin can be easily distinguished from adult hemoglobin and thus the source of the blood differentiated. In older patients, swallowed blood is usually from a nosebleed.

Vomiting of blood means the bleeding source is proximal to the ligament of Treitz. Tarry stools imply upper gastrointestinal bleeding, while a bright red color implies bleeding in the left colon or below. Blood from the upper gastrointestinal tract will be passed as red if the transit time is reduced or bleeding is brisk. Blood in the stool is only very rarely the result of malignant disease in the pediatric age group and hence does not cause the same concern as it does in the adult.

Bleeding disorders can usually be detected by a history of easy bruising or excessive bleeding after small cuts. Children have enough incidental trauma that they are repeatedly challenged. A peripheral smear, platelet count, prothrombin time, and partial thromboblastin time will detect most generalized bleeding disorders.

Diagnosis is usually made by upper or lower gastrointestinal x-rays, esophagoscopy, sigmoidoscopy, or, rarely, celiac arteriography. There are, however, a number of children in whom physical examination and all diagnostic studies are negative, and the diagnosis and therapeutic approach have to be made entirely on clinical grounds. When faced with this problem in a patient bleeding per rectum, it is probably worthwhile to proceed with laparotomy after one massive bleed requiring transfusion. The cause of bleeding will be found and can be corrected in about half these patients. If there is chronic loss of small quantities of blood, the chance of finding and correcting the cause of bleeding is not good. If transfusion has been required on several occasions to maintain hemoglobin, laparotomy is warranted. In upper gastrointestinal bleeding, uncontrolled hemorrhage is the indication for laparotomy.

The neonate is an exception to these guidelines. He should have a laparotomy only as a last resort when blood volume cannot be maintained by transfusion. Only rarely is a surgically correctable lesion present. The usual cause is some form of hemorrhagic disease of the newborn even though the prothrombin time may be normal. These infants should be treated with vitamin K and transfusion.

Massive upper gastrointestinal bleeding in the child, as in the adult, is most likely the result of bleeding from esophageal varices or ulceration in the stomach or duodenum. Both are discussed in detail elsewhere. It is well to remember that the etiology of these entities in the pediatric patient usually differs from that in the adult. Portal hypertension is most likely the result of an extrahepatic block, usually secondary to portal vein thrombosis. There may have been an omphalitis or umbilical vein catheterization in the neonatal period. Since these children have a relatively normal liver, the prognosis is much better than it is for those whose obstruction is the result of liver disease. Intrahepatic block in children is due to postnecrotic cirrhosis, congenital hepatic fibrosis, hepatic changes secondary to cystic fibrosis, Wilson's disease, and congenital cystic disease of the liver (and kidneys).

Ulcers are usually associated with other diseases—burns, central nervous system disease, generalized infection, or steroid therapy. Few in the small child are the result of the usual acid-pepsin disease.

## MECKEL'S DIVERTICULUM

Meckel's diverticulum is the most common cause of massive rectal bleeding in the pediatric age group.

**Embryology and Pathology.** Meckel's diverticulum is the persistence of the communication of the yolk sac with the intestine—a remnant of the vitelline duct. The diverticulum arises on the antimesenteric border of the ileum at about the junction of its middle and distal thirds. Infrequently it is attached to the umbilicus by a fibrous cord and rarely it contains a patent communication with the umbilicus. Ectopic gastric mucosa is often present. Bleeding is usually the result of ulceration of the normal ileal mucosa (of the diverticulum or adjacent ileum) by acid secretion of the ectopic gastric mucosa. Boys are affected three times as frequently as girls.

**Symptoms.** Meckel's diverticula are present in 1 to 2 per cent of the population. Most are asymptomatic. Those that do cause symptoms usually do so early in life, but symptoms may occur at any age. In the pediatric age symptoms are present in half the cases during the first 2 years of life. Massive rectal bleeding, which is either painless or associated with mild, vague abdominal discomfort, is the most frequent symptom. The blood at first is dark but usually becomes bright. Chronic loss of small quantities of blood is not likely to be caused by Meckel's diverticulum. Since it is almost impossible to demonstrate a Meckel's diverticulum by x-ray, the diagnosis is made on clinical grounds alone.

While bleeding is the most common symptom, Meckel's diverticulum may also produce other symptoms. Cramping abdominal pain and vomiting may result from intussusception when the diverticulum acts as a lead point, or obstruction may be secondary to a fibrous band extending to the umbilicus. Pain may also result from perforation of an ulcer or volvulus of the diverticulum with infarction. Symptoms and physical examination may be suggestive of appendicitis.[7]

**Treatment.** Treatment of Meckel's diverticulum is treatment of its complications. For those who bleed, transfusion is usually necessary prior to operative removal of the diverticulum. This may require resection of the adjacent ileum.

In patients who are operated upon with a tentative diagnosis of appendicitis and do not have an inflamed appendix, the ileum should be explored to detect an inflamed or perforated diverticulum. Patients with intestinal obstruction due to a fibrous band or small bowel intussusception require operation for relief of the obstruction and removal of the diverticulum.

## POLYPS

### Colonic Polyps

Colonic polyps in children may be solitary, multiple, or diffuse. The juvenile polyp is not a premalignant lesion and is often self-limited. Diffuse polyposis of the colon is often familial and premalignant. Bleeding from polyps is not massive. It is often associated with an urge to defecate, and there may be an excess of mucus in the stool. Blood is usually mixed with the stool. Diagnosis is by digital examination, sigmoidoscopy, and barium enema. X-ray visualization requires a well prepared colon devoid of feces. Air contrast studies may be helpful.

**Treatment.** Approximately 70 per cent of polyps are within the reach of the sigmoidoscope and should be removed. For juvenile polyps beyond the reach of the sigmoidoscope, no therapy is necessary unless symptoms persist. Barium enema a year later will often show that the polyp is no longer present. Diffuse familial polyposis requires a subtotal colectomy with ileoproctostomy. Subsequent periodic sigmoidoscopic visualization and fulguration of any recurring polyps in the rectum are required.

Rectal bleeding in children is almost never the result of malignant disease. While carcinoma of the colon does occur in children, it is rare. Barium enema shows a sessile or napkin-ring lesion. Treatment is similar to that in the adult.

### Small Bowel Polyps

Small bowel polyps may cause bleeding but are more likely to cause symptoms by acting as a lead point for an intussusception. They may be associated with brown pigmented spots around the lips and on the buccal membrane — the Peutz-Jeghers syndrome. There is frequently a family history of intestinal polyps and there are often other polyps in the colon or stomach.

**Symptoms.** The most frequent symptom is cramping abdominal pain secondary to intussusception (which may spontaneously reduce). Chronic blood loss with anemia is also frequent. Diagnosis is usually on clinical grounds — cramping abdominal pain, palpable abdominal mass, pigmented spots around the lips, and a positive family history. Visualization of small bowel polyps by roentgenography is often difficult. Associated colonic and gastric polyps are demonstrated by upper and lower gastrointestinal roentgenograms, sigmoidoscopy, or gastroscopy.

**Treatment.** Small bowel intussusception may require resection. If not, the intussusception is reduced with resection of the polyp or polyps. All palpable polyps should be removed with resection of as little intestine as possible. Although some small bowel polyps have a histologic appearance suggesting malignancy, they do not behave as malignant lesions.

## ANAL FISSURE

Anal fissure is the most common cause of blood in the stool in the pediatric age group. Fissures are acute and superficial, are frequently encountered during the first 2 or 3 years of life, and may be single or multiple. They may be located at any part of the anus. They occur at the mucocutaneous junction and are the result of trauma from a hard, bulky, constipated stool or diarrhea. The cardinal symptom is pain on defecation. Blood in the stool is usually scant and streaked on the surface.

Almost all fissures-in-ano in infants will heal with nonoperative treatment. In fact, some will have healed by the time the patient is seen by the physician. Therapy is warm sitz baths, relief of constipation by diet control and laxatives, anesthetic ointment, and rectal dilations. Rarely a chronic fissure will develop which will require operative excision. If pain on defecation persists, it will lead to chronic constipation, which can be a much more difficult problem than the original fissure.

## ULCERATIVE COLITIS

Any discussion about gastrointestinal bleeding in the pediatric age group would be incomplete without mention of ulcerative colitis. It is discussed in detail elsewhere. It can occur in infancy but is seen much more frequently in the prepubertal and adolescent child. It should be considered in the differential diagnosis in any child with lower gastrointestinal bleeding.

## ABDOMINAL WALL ABNORMALITIES

The most common defect in the abdominal wall in infants and children is indirect inguinal hernia. Umbilical hernias are also common, particularly in Negroes. Both are discussed in detail elsewhere, but a short comment here is warranted.

## INGUINAL HERNIA

The diagnosis of inguinal hernia is usually made when the parent notes a groin or scrotal mass (90 per cent are in boys) that is intermittently present, particularly when the patient cries or strains. Incarceration is common, especially in the first year of life. Elective repair should therefore be undertaken when the diagnosis is made. Since the defect in the indirect inguinal hernia of childhood is a persistent patency of the processus vaginalis, treatment consists of high ligation of the sac.

Incarceration, should it occur, can usually be reduced and the hernia repaired as an elective procedure a day or two later when the edema has subsided. There is a higher rate of recurrence in infants who are operated on when the hernia is incarcerated than in those in whom repair is carried out as an elective procedure (less than 1 per cent). If the incarceration cannot be reduced, the patient must, of course, be operated on promptly.

The most common sliding hernia in infancy occurs in the little girl with an indirect inguinal hernia containing a tube and ovary as the sliding component. Hydroceles in infant boys are common and are associated with about 15 per cent of inguinal hernias. Those not associated with hernias will usually regress eventually and hence do not require operation during infancy. Aspiration is ineffective and therefore contraindicated.

Umbilical hernias in pediatric patients, unlike inguinal hernias in the same age group or umbilical hernias in the adult, seldom become incarcerated and tend spontaneously to close the fascial defect. Umbilical hernias, therefore, need not be repaired during infancy. Those that persist into childhood should be repaired because of the danger of incarceration in later life.

## Omphalocele and Gastroschisis

Omphalocele and gastroschisis are uncommon abdominal wall defects of the newborn. Omphalocele is the herniation of abdominal contents into the base of the umbilical cord. The peritoneal sac is not covered by skin, as in an umbilical hernia, but by Wharton's jelly and amniotic membrane, i.e., the components of the umbilical cord. Gastroschisis is a full-thickness abdominal wall defect lateral to the umbilical cord without any sac or covering for the eviscerated intestines.

**Embryology.** From the sixth to the tenth week of fetal life the coelomic cavity is too small to accommodate the developing viscera. During this time a portion of the intestine normally occupies a coelomic extension into the base of the umbilical cord. Increase in size of the coelomic cavity is accompanied by return and rotation of the intestine. If this process is arrested, an omphalocele and associated malrotation of the intestine result.

If one side of the lateral somatic fold fails to develop, *gastroschisis* results, with a normally developed cord arising in the midline. Lack of development of the cephalic portion of the somatic fold results in ectopia cordia and pericardial defects, while failure of caudal somatic development results in exstrophy of the bladder — both of which may be associated with omphalocele.

**Clinical Findings.** Omphalocele varies in size from very small, containing only a knuckle of small bowel, to very large, containing liver, spleen, and most of the gastrointestinal tract. The sac may be quite thin and in danger of rupture or may be rather thick and tough. Rupture of the sac can occur prenatally, during delivery, or after birth. Over half the patients have other congenital anomalies.

In gastroschisis there is no sac. The matted, dusky, edematous gut (usually stomach, small bowel, and a portion of colon) makes an exit from the abdominal wall through a smooth, fibrous defect adjacent to the intact cord. There may be a strip of skin between the cord and defect. The defect is almost always at the right of the cord and usually 3 to 4 cm. in diameter. Frequently the gut is short. Peritonitis is always present.

**Treatment.** Initial therapy is to protect the intact sac or the intestines if they are exposed. A sterile, moist towel or gauze sponge wrapped around the abdomen is satisfactory. If the intestine is exposed, antibiotics should be given and particular efforts must be taken to combat heat loss. The stomach is decompressed with a nasogastric tube to prevent vomiting and distention of gut, which will hamper subsequent closure.

For the small intact omphalocele the sac is simply excised, the abdominal cavity explored, and the defect closed primarily. If there is a problem from malrotation or other anomalies, it is corrected. The medium-sized omphalocele can be treated in the same fashion if, on manual reduction of its contents, there is no compromise in ventilation in the unanesthetized patient. A gastrostomy should be added to the procedure to insure gastric decompression in the postoperative period.

In the patient with a large omphalocele it is not possible to return the viscera to the small abdominal cavity and close the fascial defect without markedly elevating the intra-abdominal pressure. The result is an elevation of the diaphragm beyond the point where adequate ventilation is possible, as well as compression of the vena cava, impeding venous return to the heart. These infants are best treated by suturing a plastic (Silon) prosthesis to the fascial defect over the intact sac without closure of the skin. The result is a prosthetic cylinder containing the sac and viscera (Fig. 16). The viscera are progressively forced back into the abdominal cavity as the cylinder is shortened daily by placing a row of sutures proximal to the cylinder end. Usually in 7 to 10 days the prosthesis can be removed and a fascial closure obtained. During this time the stomach is decompressed by gastrostomy, and the patient is given parenteral feeding and antibiotics. Infection is a hazard.[1]

Nonoperative therapy of omphalocele with intact sac consists of protecting the sac from rupture and allowing it to scar down and become epithelialized. The sac is painted with Mercurochrome or Zephiran. In time a remarkable reduction in the size of the defect occurs. There is probably a place for this approach in the very small premature infant with a large omphalocele or with severe extra-abdominal associated anomalies. Prolonged hospitalization is required.

In the patient with gastroschisis or ruptured omphalocele, the problem is more difficult. If pri-

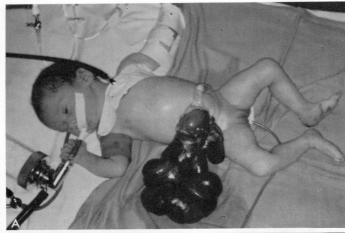

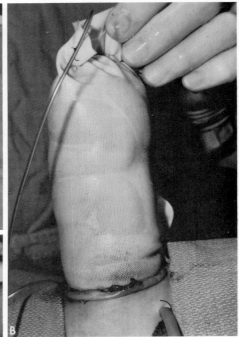

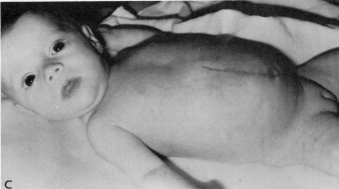

**Figure 16** *A,* Gastroschisis with evis-ceration of stomach, small bowel, and colon just to the right of the umbilical cord. The gut is thickened, matted and dusky. *B,* A prosthetic cylinder covering the intestine is sutured to the fascia of the defect. The cyl-inder will be progressively shortened over the next 7 to 10 days, so that the intestine is forced back into the abdominal cavity. *C,* Same patient after removal of prosthesis and closure of defect.

mary closure can be accomplished, this should be done. Direct closure, however, is usually impossi-ble for patients with gastroschisis. These patients are treated in the same manner as those with a large omphalocele except that the prosthesis is in direct contact with the intestine since there is no sac. Gastrostomy, parenteral feeding, and anti-biotics are essential supportive measures. Because peritonitis is present before repair, sepsis is a significant hazard.

**Results.** For the patient with a small omphalo-cele without associated anomalies, the risk is quite small. For the patient with a large omphalocele, overall mortality is 40 to 50 per cent, and for pa-tients with gastroschisis or ruptured omphalocele the mortality is 50 to 75 per cent. Many of these deaths are related to associated anomalies.

## JAUNDICE

Jaundice is common in pediatric patients, but it is not often due to obstruction. In the first few months of life biliary atresia may cause obstruc-tive jaundice. In the older child, choledochal cysts may cause obstruction. Common duct stones and

carcinoma of the head of the pancreas, the com-mon causes of obstructive jaundice in the adult, are rare in children but have been reported.

## BILIARY ATRESIA

Biliary atresia is an interesting but poorly understood entity. All or some of the intrahepatic and extrahepatic biliary ducts consist of fibrous cords with little or no lumen. The etiology is not clear. One possibility is faulty embryogenesis. A more likely explanation is that fibrosis of previ-ously normal ducts occurs in fetal life or in the early postnatal period. There is progressive de-velopment of biliary cirrhosis, portal hypertension, ascites, and liver failure. Life expectancy is about 18 months though some children live for several years.[17]

**Clinical Findings.** The onset of jaundice is usu-ally during the first week of life but may not be noted until 6 to 8 weeks of age. The stools become acholic and the urine dark. Intermittently the stools may be brown or yellow, presumably be-cause of desquamation of jaundiced mucosal cells. For some time the patient's general condition appears to be good. Then, as liver failure develops, there is a progressive deterioration. The liver is usually enlarged and firm, as is the spleen. Ascites and hemorrhoids may be present later in the course of the disease. Jaundice is unremitting, with total bilirubin in the 10 to 20 mg. per 100 ml. range.

**Differential Diagnosis.** There are many other causes of jaundice in the neonatal period which must be differentiated from biliary atresia. The most common cause of neonatal jaundice is so-called physiologic jaundice of the newborn, which is a result of an immature glucuronyl transferase enzyme system. Jaundice from this cause is usually cleared by 2 weeks of age. Jaundice beyond that period is pathologic, and therefore its cause should be investigated. Other causes of jaundice include bacterial sepsis, syphilis, cytomegalic inclusion disease, toxoplasmosis, erythroblastosis fetalis or other hemolytic disease, familial nonhemolytic icterus, "enclosed" hemorrhage, pancreatitis, cystic fibrosis, galactosemia, and some drugs. These entities can usually be detected by history or appropriate laboratory tests.

Inspissated bile syndrome and neonatal hepatitis also cause jaundice at this age and usually cannot be differentiated from biliary atresia by the usual liver function tests. While serum transaminase tends to be high with hepatitis and alkaline phosphatase high with obstruction, these findings are not consistent. The iodine-131 rose bengal test is probably the most helpful test in making a distinction between obstruction and hepatocellular disease in the neonate. Unfortunately, it cannot always be relied upon to give a clear-cut distinction.

**Treatment.** For those patients in whom biliary atresia cannot be excluded, a limited laparotomy with liver biopsy and operative cholangiogram will provide the diagnosis. This should be carried out by 8 weeks of age, before irreparable liver damage has occurred in patients who otherwise have a surgically correctable lesion. If the extrahepatic ductal system is patent, the procedure is terminated since the patient does not have extrahepatic biliary atresia. Liver biopsy will probably differentiate between intrahepatic atresia and neonatal hepatitis.

If cholangiogram reveals atresia of the common bile duct, the duct is anastomosed to the intestine. A Roux-en-Y connection to the jejunum is less likely to result in cholangitis than a direct connection of the duct to the duodenum.

If only a small gallbladder is visualized by cholangiography, and none of the ductal system is demonstrated, the proximal extrahepatic biliary tree should be thoroughly explored in search for any patent extrahepatic ducts. If one is present, it is connected to the intestine as with atresia of the common bile duct.

**Results.** A survey of the members of the Surgical Section of the American Academy of Pediatrics revealed that only 12 per cent of 843 patients with biliary atresia had a surgically correctable lesion, i.e., a patent biliary duct outside the liver

that could be connected to the gut. Of this correctable group, half subsequently died of cirrhosis, portal hypertension, or cholangitis, usually related to advanced disease at the time of correction. Half were long-term survivors.

Since in such a large proportion of patients biliary atresia is not amenable to current operative procedures, a number of other drainage procedures have been attempted. These include insertion of tubes into the liver for drainage into the gut and the placement of the cut surface of the left lobe of the liver into the intestine. Neither of these has been successful. Indeed it is likely that any drainage procedure not based on a mucosa-to-mucosa anastomosis will fibrose and obliterate any communication which may have been established. Anastomosis of the thoracic duct to the esophagus has resulted in a transient fall in bilirubin but does not alter the progression of liver failure.

Liver transplantation for biliary atresia has proved technically feasible. Because of rejection there are at present no long-term survivors, but transplantation does appear to be the brightest light on the horizon for these unfortunate infants.

## CHOLEDOCHAL CYST

Choledochal cyst or idiopathic dilatation of the common bile duct is of two types. Most commonly there is a diffuse dilatation of the extraduodenal common duct with a relatively narrow neck. Obstruction usually results from dilatation of the cyst with kinking of the distal duct. Choledochal cysts are rare lesions.

**Clinical Findings.** The onset of jaundice is usually during childhood but infrequently occurs during the neonatal period. There may be associated epigastric or right upper quadrant discomfort. A cystic mass is usually palpable in the right upper abdomen. Symptoms characteristically are intermittent and chronic. Most children have been treated for hepatitis before the diagnosis is made. Girls are affected three times more often than boys.

**Diagnosis.** Liver function tests indicate obstruction and are often quite helpful in making the distinction from hepatitis. Upper gastrointestinal series may demonstrate an extrinsic mass displacing the duodenum.

**Treatment.** Operative cholangiogram may be helpful in determining the anatomy of the cyst, i.e., whether it is a diffuse or diverticular type. The latter can be excised with T tube drainage of the common bile duct. The diffuse lesions are best treated by Roux-en-Y drainage to the jejunum.

**Results.** Mortality is about 10 per cent. The long-term outlook is governed by postoperative cholangitis, reported to occur in 15 to 25 per cent of patients.

## ABDOMINAL MASSES

The presence of a palpable abdominal mass in an infant or child is a cause for alarm and always requires a complete investigation. The outlook for the newborn with an abdominal mass is better than that for the older child. More than half of abdominal masses found in newborns are renal in origin. Multicystic dysplastic kidney is the most common, although hydronephrosis (from a variety of causes) is also common. Intestinal duplications, hydrometrocolpos, and neuroblastoma follow in that order.[6] In the child, neoplasms, particularly Wilms' tumor and neuroblastoma, are more common.

### Diagnosis

Physical examination is frequently helpful in determining the etiology of the mass. The location, mobility, and consistency (whether cystic or solid) are important clues. If there are signs or symptoms of intestinal obstruction, duplication, meconium ileus, or malrotation must be considered. Extraintestinal masses rarely cause intestinal obstruction. The presence of other conditions may suggest the diagnosis. Absence of abdominal muscles ("prune belly" syndrome) is usually associated with severe hydronephrosis and hydroureter. Dehydration or sepsis may suggest renal vein thrombosis.

Plain roentgenograms of the abdomen are always indicated and usually helpful. The intravenous pyelogram, however, is most likely to give significant information since the majority of newborn masses are renal in origin. Total-body opacification is frequently helpful in identifying avascular lesions such as cysts, hematomas, and infarcted organs, abscess cavities, and so forth. This entails use of early films during the vascular mixing phase of the intravenous pyelogram to show absence of opacification. The presence of calcium suggests intrauterine intestinal perforation, neuroblastoma, or teratoma.

If the diagnosis is not clear from these studies,

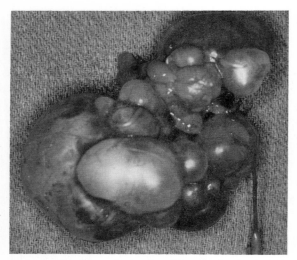

**Figure 17** The unilateral multicystic dysplastic kidney is the most common cause of abdominal mass in the newborn. It is often associated with atresia of the upper ureter, as in this specimen.

additional radiologic investigation is indicated. Cystogram or sinogram in the case of abnormal external genitalia may be helpful in further delineating the nature of a pelvic or low abdominal mass, as well as defining the presence of massive vesicoureteral reflux which may cause hydronephrosis or hydroureter. The recent introduction of ultrasonic scanning ("sonography") enables the physician to further refine the differentiation between cystic and solid tissue masses. This is particularly helpful in the renal region where the differentiation between hydronephrosis and tumor is of some significance. In the case of a large mass that appears clinically to be malignant, the use of venography or arteriography may be of assistance not only in determining the nature of the mass but also in planning its removal. Radioisotope scanning of the liver and kidneys may provide additional information. In almost all cases surgical exploration is indicated both to establish the diagnosis and for treatment.

## MULTICYSTIC KIDNEY

The most common abdominal mass in the neonate, multicystic dysplastic kidney, is also the easiest to treat (Fig. 17). Unlike polycystic kidneys, this lesion is unilateral, nonfamilial, and almost always discovered early in life. There is no associated cystic disease of other organs. Since the opposite kidney is almost always normal, the lesion is no threat to life. These dysplastic kidneys vary greatly in appearance, with multiple cysts of different sizes, some as large as 10 to 20 cm., and usually little in the way of recognizable renal parenchyma. Intravenous urography reveals absence of excretory function of the affected kidney, but usually shows a normal pyelogram on the opposite side. Treatment is removal, and the prognosis is excellent.

## HYDRONEPHROSIS

Hydronephrosis in the newborn often carries a poor prognosis since renal function may be severely compromised by the time of diagnosis. Especially if there is bilateral hydronephrosis, the mortality may be quite high. In most instances the kidney will not be opacified on intravenous urography. Total-body opacification or sonography will reveal the mass to be cystic. Cystography will reveal viscoureteral reflux in a large proportion of patients and will thus outline the extent of the pathologic process. If there is severe bilateral involvement, and especially if there is chemical evidence of renal failure, extensive reconstruction is unwise. These patients can be greatly improved by temporary tubeless urinary diversion, with creation of a cutaneous stoma between the urinary tract and the skin high in the ureter or at the pelvis of the kidney. This provides effective drainage without the hazard of infection and stone formation attendant upon the use of a catheter. Renal failure is often dramatically reversed in a matter of a few days. Urinary reconstruction can be carried out months or years later when there has been maximal return of renal function. The decrease in size of the dilated portions of the urinary tract is usually striking. With prompt tubeless diversion the mortality can be greatly reduced.

## URETEROPELVIC OBSTRUCTION

Obstruction at the junction between the kidney pelvis and the ureter may be caused by stenosis or atresia (Fig. 18). Frequently there is an aberrant vessel which may or may not be related to the hypoplastic segment. Adequate drainage is obtained either by a Y-V-plasty to the ureteropelvic junction or by excision of the stenotic segment with anastomosis of the ureter to the kidney pelvis. Part of the dilated redundant pelvis should be excised to facilitate urine propulsion. Temporary catheter drainage is essential. In some cases, when the condition is unilateral and when the renal parenchyma is exceedingly thin and unlikely ever to regain significant function, nephrectomy is indicated. In most patients, however, the kidney is well worth saving, and a reconstructive procedure should be performed.

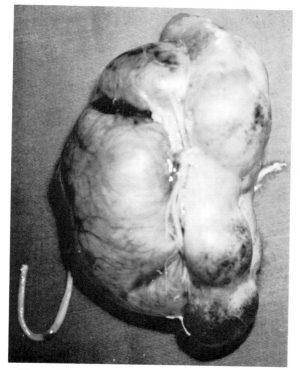

**Figure 18**　Massive hydronephrosis with destruction of renal parenchyma due to long-standing ureteropelvic obstruction.

## VESICOURETERAL REFLUX

Reflux in the newborn is sometimes the result of an abnormality of the vesicoureteral junction but usually occurs as a consequence of distal obstruction, as from posterior urethral valves or bladder neck obstruction or from a neurogenic bladder. It is also commonly seen in association with massive hydronephrosis and hydroureter in the "prune belly" syndrome with or without urethral obstruction. Most of these patients will profit from a period of tubeless diversion prior to reconstructive efforts. In the patient with isolated vesicoureteral reflux, reimplantation of the ureters usually produces excellent results (see discussion under Urinary Tract Infection later in this chapter). If there is an obstruction (such as posterior urethral valves) this must be relieved by endoscopic or transvesical resection, which can be done at the time of reimplantation of the ureters. The temporary diversion stoma can also be closed at that time. In patients with a neurogenic bladder, and in most with the "prune belly" syndrome, successful reconstruction cannot be done, so a permanent form of urinary diversion must ultimately be provided. At present the ileal conduit is the most satisfactory method of long-term urinary diversion. This can be done when the patient is 1 to 3 years of age when social considerations make it necessary to provide dry and odorless urinary control.

## DUPLICATIONS OF THE ALIMENTARY TRACT

Although they may present at any age, many duplications are first noted in the newborn period. Duplications may occur at any level of the intestinal tract from the mouth to the anus. Absence of an adequate communication between the second lumen and the primary enteric canal leads to accumulation of mucous secretions and cystic dilatation, thus the original term of "enterogenous cysts."

**Pathology.**　Duplications may be cystic or tubular. They are located on the mesenteric side of the involved gut and usually have a common muscular wall with at least a portion of the adjacent intestine. Some connect with the adjacent gut lumen, and some do not. Tubular duplications have a common muscular wall with a long segment of intestine. Others may be separate from the adjacent bowel and on occasion traverse the diaphragm to reside in the posterior mediastinum. The mucosa may be that of the adjacent gut or of any other part of the alimentary tract, including the stomach.[19]

**Clinical Findings.**　Symptoms are *obstruction* due to encroachment of the distended cyst on the adjacent intestine, *pain* from the distention of the cyst wall, or *bleeding*, which may be massive if it is caused by ulceration secondary to ectopic gastric mucosa. Intestinal obstruction and the presence of a mobile *mass* strongly suggest a duplication. Volvulus may also occur, or the patient may be asymptomatic and the mass discovered during a physical examination. This is especially likely to be true with gastric duplications. Pyloric duplications are commonly mistaken for congenital hypertrophic pyloric stenosis because of the symptoms of repeated projectile vomiting of non-bile-stained material. Rectal duplications may cause rectal prolapse. Thoracic duplications may cause dysphagia or tracheal compression.

**Diagnosis.** Upper gastrointestinal series may show a filling defect in esophageal, gastric, and duodenal duplications. Barium enema is of value in revealing a colonic duplication. Thoracic duplications are usually visible on chest x-ray. The presence of hemivertebrae and a mass suggests a duplication.

**Treatment.** Since duplication cysts are located on the mesenteric side of the intestinal lumen and have a common wall with the normal channel, simple excision is difficult. With duplications located in the small bowel, segmental excision and end-to-end anastomosis is the procedure of choice. If the duplication is quite long, or is located in an area where resection is not possible, division of the common wall or "windowing" may produce adequate decompression so that the cyst no longer fills. Long tubular duplications that would require an extensive resection are best treated by resection of the mucosa through multiple incisions, with the muscularis of the duplication left in situ.

**Results.** Although these may be complicated anomalies and, in the case of lower colon and rectal duplications, may be associated with urinary tract anomalies as well, surgical correction is usually possible and a good result is to be expected. Mortality is about 5 per cent overall.

## HYDROMETROCOLPOS

Hydrometrocolpos, or fluid accumulation in the vagina and uterus, occurs as the result of prenatal obstruction to the outlet of the vagina with excessive secretion due to circulating maternal estrogens. The most common cause is imperforate hymen, the result of failure of degeneration of the epithelial plate of the müllerian tubercle. Vaginal atresia may result if there is persistence of the solid cord stage of fused müllerian ducts.

Patients present with a suprapubic mass which usually extends up to the umbilicus or higher. It may be mistaken for a distended bladder and the true nature not suspected until the bladder is emptied. Since this condition may assume truly massive proportions, there may be rectal and urinary obstruction. Diagnosis is established by physical examination. When a bulging imperforate hymen is noted, hymenotomy relieves the obstruction as well as any secondary pressure on the urinary or intestinal tracts.

If there is vaginal atresia, a combined abdominoperineal approach is indicated. After drainage of fluid from above, the atretic end of the vagina is pressed into the perineum where it can be safely incised and drained. In these patients a catheter must be left in the vagina for an extended period of time so that an epithelium-lined tract will be established. Intravenous pyelogram is indicated to assess the extent of damage to the upper urinary tract.

Leakage of fluid from the fallopian tubes, especially if there is a communication between the bladder and the vagina (urogenital sinus) may lead to peritonitis and death. Adequate drainage of both the vagina and the bladder (cutaneous vesicostomy) is required. Many of these patients have a septate vagina and bladder. Imperforate anus is also commonly seen as an associated anomaly. These patients may present very difficult problems in diagnosis and therapy and should not be surgically approached by the inexperienced.

## CYSTS

Cystic abdominal masses are typically soft, ballotable, and quite mobile. They are not readily distinguished from duplications except that they seldom, if ever, cause intestinal obstruction. Mesenteric cysts are the most common but omental cysts, lymphangiomatous cysts (cystic hygroma), and ovarian cysts are also found. Cysts may be small or large, single or multiloculated, and lobulated or smooth, and may contain serous, chylous, or hemorrhagic fluid. True cysts are thin-walled and thus are easily distinguished from duplications, which have a thick wall equal to that of the normal intestine.

**Clinical Findings.** Most cysts are asymptomatic unless exceedingly large, when they may present as abdominal distention or, rarely, with respiratory distress due to elevation of the diaphragm. In older children abdominal pain may be the presenting symptom, resulting from mesenteric traction in the upright position produced by the weight of the cyst. Physical examination usually reveals a rounded, soft mass which is markedly mobile. X-ray of the abdomen shows an area of absent intestinal gas shadows. Barium studies may help localize the cyst, and excretory urogram occasionally shows ureteral displacement or obstruction. Ultrasonic scanning is of value in differentiating cysts from solid tumors.

**Treatment.** Since these structures are benign and usually do not involve the wall of the intestine or other vital structures, they usually can be "shelled out." On occasion local intestinal resection may also be necessary. In the treatment of ovarian cysts, an attempt should be made to preserve normal tissue if possible. Lymphangiomatous cysts are typically retroperitoneal. Resection is usually possible since vital structures are not actually invaded.

**Results.** The outlook is excellent.

## NEUROBLASTOMA

In addition to being the most common solid tumor of childhood, neuroblastoma is among the most interesting because of its occasional capacity for spontaneous regression. Indeed, of *documented* cases of spontaneous disappearance of cancer, approximately one-fourth were neuroblastomas. It is, however, a highly malignant tumor that often carries a dim outlook. Recognition of neuroblastoma as a distinct entity occurred during that great age of descriptive pathology, the late nineteenth century. The term "neuroblastoma" was coined by Wright in 1910.

**Pathology.** Neuroblastoma is the result of malignant proliferation of the primitive precursors of sympathetic ganglion cells and, as such, arises from the areas where these cells are found: the adrenal glands and the sympathetic ganglionic chain. Grossly these tumors are frequently hemorrhagic and multilobulated, and may or may not have a capsule. Soft areas, often the result of necrotic degeneration, alternate with areas of firm nodularity. Histologically the "pure" neuroblastoma is highly cellular, often appearing somewhat lymphoid. Rosettes of dark cell nuclei are frequently seen interspersed with bands of pale fibrillar tissue. With the more differentiated form of the tumor (ganglioneuroma) only ganglion cells and stroma are present and the ganglion cells are mature. In most tumors, both mature and immature cells are present.

Neuroblastoma accounts for 10 to 20 per cent of solid malignant lesions in childhood. Fifty to eighty per cent of neuroblastomas arise within the abdomen, most from the adrenal medulla, but some from paravertebral ganglion cells. Although the mean age is 2½ years at the time of diagnosis, as many as 40 per cent appear within the first year of life.

**Clinical Findings.** The presence of an abdominal mass is the usual initial finding. Typically the mass is "fixed," irregular in contour, and frequently quite large. It is much less regular and smooth than a Wilms' tumor and tends to be more medially located. Abdominal pain, distention, vomiting, and diarrhea are found, in order of decreasing frequency. Weight loss and weakness are present in approximately 25 per cent of patients. Despite the fact that these tumors arise from sympathetic ganglion precursors and many patients excrete catecholamines and their metabolites in excessive amounts, very few patients have hypertension. An occasional patient presents with neurologic symptoms due to extension of tumor into the spinal canal.

X-rays show calcification in more than 50 per cent of the tumors. Metastases are evident in 60 to 90 per cent of patients at the time of diagnosis. In addition to regional lymph nodes, liver, bones, lungs, subcutaneous tissue, and brain are most commonly affected. Bone marrow biopsy often reveals neuroblastoma cells. The presence of bony metastases carries a particularly poor prognosis. Liver metastases, on the other hand, are quite common in neonates and small infants, and do not necessarily carry an ominous prognosis.

**Diagnosis.** In addition to plain films of the abdomen, which should show the mass and often calcification, excretory urogram is always indicated.

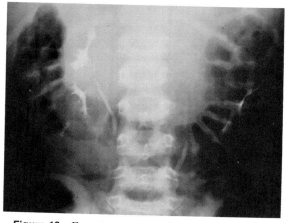

**Figure 19**   Excretory urogram in a 4 year old girl with neuroblastoma. There is an upper abdominal midline mass which displaces the left kidney down and laterally without distortion of the collecting system.

cated. Unlike Wilms' tumor, neuroblastoma seldom causes evidence of intrarenal distortion, although significant displacement and deformity of the kidney may be seen (Fig. 19). Hydronephrosis occasionally is seen as a result of compression of the ureter or the kidney pelvis. As with Wilms' tumor, the use of inferior vena cavograms may be of value in planning operative extirpation. Bone marrow aspiration is always indicated to determine the extent of metastatic dissemination.

Catecholamines and their breakdown products, including vanillylmandelic acid (VMA), homovanillic acid (HVA), epinephrine, and norepinephrine, can be found in the urine of most patients. The normal values vary with the size and age of the patient. Hence adult values are not applicable to the pediatric patient.[24]

**Treatment.** Although spontaneous regression does occur, it is rare and should never be considered in planning therapy. Total surgical excision offers the best chance for cure. The use of "triple therapy" further improves survival. Because of the propensity of this tumor to invade adjacent structures, total surgical excision may be impossible. If radical total excision offers a significant risk to the patient's life or to vital structures, an incomplete excision is preferred since many cures have been obtained in spite of the retention of significant amounts of tumor. Even the removal of large quantities of necrotic debris appears to be of some benefit, so this should be undertaken in the massive tumors.[13] Alternatively, biopsy followed by radiation therapy and later resection may be employed. Although neuroblastoma is moderately radiosensitive, radiation therapy as a sole form of treatment gives poor results and should not be relied upon. Even in the presence of proven bony metastases, removal of the primary tumor should be attempted since occasional cures have been reported.

CHEMOTHERAPY. The use of cyclophosphamide (Cytoxan) and vincristine has improved cure rates after surgical therapy. Used alone, these drugs seldom effect cures. As with other uses of chemotherapy, their value is considerably enhanced if the bulk of tumor tissue can be removed surgically so that cancerocidal action is concentrated on a smaller number of cells. Repeat doses over long periods of time appear to give the best results. Metastases may completely disappear with the use of chemotherapy.

RADIATION THERAPY. Radiation to the tumor bed, as well as to the liver if it is involved, should be part of the "triple therapy" employed routinely in the treatment of neuroblastoma. In young children 1000 to 1500 rads is given in 6 to 10 days. This dose is usually adequate because of the high radiosensitivity of this lesion. In older children doses of 2400 to 4500 rads are used. Results from radiation therapy are also significantly enhanced by surgical removal of the bulk of the tumor when possible. Bony recurrences may be treated effectively with radiation therapy.

Follow-up at frequent intervals is necessary for several years after diagnosis and initial treatment. Repeat chest and bone x-rays, as well as intravenous pyelogram, are indicated during this followup. If preoperative urinary assay demonstrated elevated catecholamine levels, then measurement of these in the follow-up period is a useful and reliable way of detecting recurrences (Fig. 20).

**Results.** Although neuroblastomas in extra-abdominal locations such as the chest or cervical region carry a reasonably good prognosis, with cure rates of 50 to 90 per cent, those arising in the abdomen have a much poorer outlook. The average survival from six large series is 19 per cent. Survival for infants less than 1 year of age is two to three times this great. Surprisingly, the presence of metastatic disease to the liver in the *infant* does not seem to significantly alter the prognosis in neuroblastoma. Many of these patients survive. Histologic evidence of maturation correlates well with prognosis. If the majority of cells are of the ganglioneuroma type, long-term

cure rates are high. Conversely, if no "mature" cells are seen, few patients survive.

## WILMS' TUMOR

The development of effective treatment for Wilms' tumor is one of the important "success stories" in cancer therapy. Above all else, it offers convincing evidence of the value of an aggressive approach to tumors even when metastases have occurred. As the result of combination therapy, employing surgical resection, radiation treatment, and chemotherapy, 80 per cent of affected children are now cured.

Although the classic description of the embryoma of the kidney by Max Wilms, a German surgeon, was published in 1899, the tumor had been described many times before, and, specifically, the characteristic occurrence of embryonic tubal and connective tissue as the distinguishing characteristic was described by Birch-Hirschfeld in 1898. Because these tumors are found at an early age, and because of their peculiar histologic characteristics, it is generally accepted that they are related to embryologic errors and originate from fetal tissue. The histologic appearance varies from patient to patient, and in different parts of a tumor from a single patient. Abortive tubules or glomeruli may be seen surrounded by hyperchromatic round cells or a mixture of smooth and striated muscle or myxomatous tissue.

Wilms' tumors constitute 15 to 40 per cent of solid tumors of childhood, but undoubtedly carry the best prognosis of any intra-abdominal neoplasm.

**Clinical Findings.** The average age at time of diagnosis is 3 years, although these tumors may be found at any age from the newborn period to adulthood. The presenting symptom is usually an abdominal mass, noted by either the parent or the examining physician, frequently on a "rou-

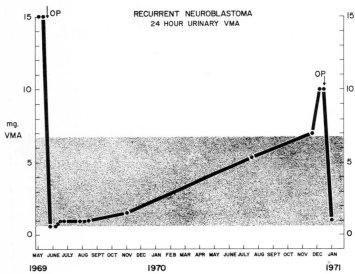

RECURRENT NEUROBLASTOMA
24 HOUR URINARY VMA

**Figure 20** VMA excretion in a 3 year old with neuroblastoma. He had no symptoms or evidence of mass after the first resection. The second operation was undertaken solely because of the elevated VMA. The shaded area represents normal values for an adult. The value of 5 mg. in July, 1970, was clearly abnormal for a child of this size and should have prompted exploration at that time.

tine" examination or evaluation for unrelated symptoms. Abdominal pain is present in about 20 per cent of patients; fever and hematuria are found in 15 to 20 per cent. Other symptoms such as malaise, nausea, vomiting, constipation, or diarrhea are occasionally present but sufficiently nonspecific to be of little value in diagnosis. Hypertension may be found in half or more of patients. Secondary infection of the urinary tract is also occasionally seen. Ninety per cent of patients will have a palpable mass in the flank on physical examination. If the mass is large, differentiation from neuroblastoma or other tumors may be exceedingly difficult. The major differential diagnostic problem, however, is hydronephrosis.

**Diagnosis.** Abdominal x-rays will usually show a mass, occasionally (10 per cent) with calcification. Excretory urogram in most patients will show the characteristic findings of Wilms' tumor: distortion of the pelvis and calices as they are stretched out over the tumor, rather than displacement or obstruction from an extrarenal mass (Fig. 21). If there is nonfunction of the kidney on excretory urogram, hydronephrosis is much more likely than Wilms' tumor. This distinction should be made by retrograde pyelogram. Renal scan and the use of ultrasonic scanning may also be of value. Arteriography is seldom indicated but may be of value in confusing situations.

Chest x-ray must be obtained to determine if pulmonary metastases are present since these are noted at the time of diagnosis in 20 to 50 per cent of patients. In contrast with neuroblastoma, bony metastases are rare. If the tumor is large or pulmonary metastases are already present, inferior

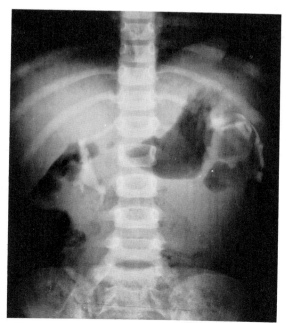

**Figure 21** Intravenous pyelogram in a 3 year old girl with a left Wilms' tumor demonstrating caliceal distortion and lateral displacement. The right kidney is normal.

vena cavogram is indicated to assess preoperatively the extent of venous involvement. The excretory urogram of the opposite kidney must be carefully inspected since approximately 6 per cent of patients with Wilms' tumor have involvement of both kidneys.

**Treatment.** The history of treatment of Wilms' tumor is one of increasing success as additional modalities were employed. In the 1930s Ladd and Gross demonstrated that the cure rate in Wilms' tumor could be improved by early ligation of the renal pedicle, decreasing metastases secondary to operative manipulation. Postoperative irradiation was added in the 1940s, and cure rates doubled. The addition of actinomycin D at the time of surgery and subsequently has further substantially increased survivals. There is no longer any significant doubt that "triple therapy" gives the best results in the treatment of this tumor.[5]

OPERATIVE TREATMENT. In patients with hematuria or a nonfunctioning kidney, cystoscopy should be performed prior to operation to rule out the presence of distant implants in the bladder. If found, these should be excised and radiation therapy given to the bladder as well as the tumor bed postoperatively.

Radical surgical excision is the most important feature of treatment of Wilms' tumor, and few patients have been cured without removal of the tumor. A long transperitoneal incision is used with a thoracoabdominal extension if additional exposure is desired. Incision of the peritoneum laterally permits reflection of the colon medially so that the renal vessels may be exposed and ligated prior to further tumor manipulation. The entire tumor mass must be removed together with the renal and periaortic lymph nodes. If there is caval invasion, resection may be performed. In massive tumors with extension beyond the capsule, resection of parts of adjacent organs such as the intestine, diaphragm, or liver may also be indicated. Such invasion does not constitute a hopeless situation, and every attempt must be made at complete removal, consistent with safety to the patient. On rare occasions, in truly huge tumors with multiple organ involvement, preoperative irradiation may be of value to shrink the tumor to more manageable proportions. If this approach is chosen, however, a biopsy must be obtained first to establish the nature of the mass.

In all cases the opposite kidney must be explored both by palpation and by careful examination because of the high incidence of bilateral disease. When bilateral involvement is present, partial nephrectomy or "shelling out" of the tumor is indicated. In some cases preoperative radiation to both kidneys designed to shrink the tumor is advisable. The "shelling out" operation may then be carried out, leaving a functioning kidney on both sides. At least one patient has been reported in whom bilateral nephrectomy and renal homotransplantation was carried out with long-term survival. Obviously a period of hemodialysis is indicated in such patients to make sure that they will not succumb to metastatic disease.

CHEMOTHERAPY AND RADIATION. There is now ample evidence from well controlled studies that the addition of actinomycin D substantially improves survival. Seventy-five micrograms per kilogram is given over a 5 day period starting at the time of operation. Repeat courses are administered every 6 to 12 weeks. Supravoltage radiation therapy, 3000 rads to the tumor bed in a 3 week period, is given to children in the 2 to 5 year age group, with appropriately lower or higher doses for those younger or older. Metastatic disease, commonly in the lungs, is treated with irradiation and chemotherapy. If the tumor is well localized, surgical resection carries an equally high cure rate. There are many patients reported who are long-term survivors after treatment of pulmonary metastases.

Although the period of maximal risk of recurrence is the first 2 years after resection, and the great majority of recurrences appear within 6 months, recurrences as late as 29 years later have been reported. Frequent follow-up with chest x-ray and, less frequently, intravenous pyelogram is necessary. As already indicated, lung metastases, if they occur, should be treated with the same aggressiveness as the original primary.

Congenital renal tumors discovered in the newborn period are almost always both clinically and histologically benign, showing profuse mesenchymal proliferation. Some authors have referred to these as hamartomas or mesoblastic nephromas. Since they are not true Wilms' tumors, surgical excision is sufficient for cure. Indeed, there is ample evidence that chemotherapy and radiation therapy in this age group carry a higher risk than their omission.

**Results.** Cure rates of better than 90 per cent can be expected in children in whom there is no evidence of metastatic disease at the time of operation. Even in those with metastases, long-term cure rates of 40 to 50 per cent are to be expected.

## TERATOMA

Teratoma may present as an abdominal mass. Most often these tumors occur in the sacrococcygeal area but they may also be located in the gonads, anterior mediastinum, neck, or nasopharynx.

**Pathology.** Teratomas are true congenital neoplasms which contain tissue of at least two embryologic germ layers. The origin of these tumors is not clear, but they are thought to arise from pluripotent or totipotent cells that do not respond in the usual way to normal differentiation in the developing embryo. They may be predominantly cystic or solid, often contain calcium, and may contain malignant components. In general, the solid tumors are more likely to be malignant.

**Clinical Findings.** Most teratomas are detected because a mass is noted. Symptoms usually are the result of encroachment of the tumor on some other adjacent structure. Sacrococcygeal teratomas with a presacral component or presacral teratomas may cause partial bladder and rectal obstruction. Cervical, nasopharyngeal, and mediastinal teratomas may cause airway obstruction. These tumors are usually smooth, round, and often quite large.

Teratomas of the sacrococcygeal, retroperitoneal, cervical, and nasopharyngeal areas tend to be detected in the first few months of life. Indeed, most are noted in the neonatal period. Those arising in the anterior mediastinum and gonads are most often detected in children or young adults.

**Diagnosis.** Diagnosis is suspected when a mass is noted in a location where teratomas occur, particularly if it contains calcium (Fig. 22). The calcium is often rather coarse or dense. Not all teratomas contain calcium, however, and for these the diagnosis is more difficult.

**Treatment.** Treatment is excision. Teratomas of the sacrococcygeal region may be quite vascular. The blood supply is from the middle sacral artery, and this should be divided early in the course of the dissection. If there is a presacral extension up to the sacral promontory, a combined abdominosacral approach will be required.

**Results.** Most teratomas are benign and carry a good prognosis. About 10 per cent of teratomas are malignant. The frequency of malignancy varies with location. In the sacrococcygeal region the outlook is much better for patients who have the teratoma removed in the neonatal period than for those operated on later—7 per cent malignancy during the first 4 months of life compared to 42

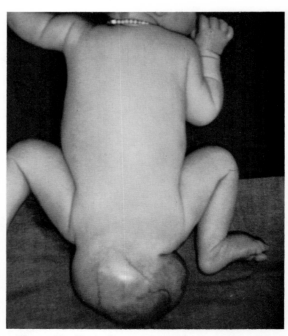

**Figure 22** Typical sacrococcygeal teratoma in a newborn infant. Despite its grotesque appearance, this tumor seldom involves vital structures, and complete excision may be accomplished.

per cent malignancy in patients 4 months to 15 years of age.[25]

# ABDOMINAL PAIN

Abdominal pain is a frequent complaint in childhood. The causes are innumerable. Of children whose main symptom is abdominal pain when they see a physician, less than 10 per cent will have a surgical disease. Within this group, however, are most who have a serious, life-threatening illness.

Symptoms of fever, irritability, vomiting, and abdominal pain in children are nonspecific and may be present with most kinds of infection or febrile episodes. They are also the symptoms of appendicitis.

The surgical conditions causing abdominal pain are most often detected by a thorough examination of the abdomen. For this reason it is mandatory that an adequate examination be obtained. Unfortunately, even with almost infinite patience, it is sometimes impossible to gain the cooperation of some ill infants and children. In this circumstance, a satisfactory examination can be obtained by sedating the patient to the point of sleep. (An opiate should not be used since it relieves pain.) Chloral hydrate or a short-acting barbiturate by rectum will produce sleep without masking tenderness. A thorough physical examination is essential to detect the extra-abdominal causes of abdominal pain.

## APPENDICITIS

Appendicitis is the most common cause of a surgical abdomen in children. The high incidence of ruptured appendicitis in pediatric patients (18 to 45 per cent in reported series) is related to (1) parental delay in seeking medical aid and (2) physician delay in making the diagnosis. Improvement in the former will result only from widespread public education. The latter will improve with the acceptance (1) that abdominal pain should not be treated over the telephone, (2) that in spite of the time consumed, a thorough abdominal examination is essential, and (3) that if it is not possible to make the diagnosis at the time of the original examination the patient should be examined again in 2 to 4 hours.

The other important factor in childhood appendicitis is the recognition and proper preoperative preparation of the very ill child. Almost all deaths and most of the complications from appendicitis occur in patients whose appendix has ruptured. Preoperative preparation of the patient with ruptured appendix and peritonitis should be prompt but adequate and includes expansion of blood volume, hydration, correction of acidosis, treatment of infection with antibiotics, and reduction of fever. Rough guidelines to indicate that the patient is sufficiently prepared for operation include a pulse below 120, rectal temperature below 39° C., and an adequate output of ketone-free urine.

Appendicitis is discussed in detail elsewhere.

## INTUSSUSCEPTION

Intussusception is the telescoping of one portion of the bowel into the segment just distal to it. Some intussusceptions reduce spontaneously. Many, however, progress to produce intestinal obstruction and impairment of blood supply with gangrene and perforation.

**Etiology.** Intussusception may result when a lead point, such as a polyp or Meckel's diverticulum, is carried along downstream by the intestinal peristalsis, taking its attachment with it. While a lead point is common in adults, it is uncommon in pediatric patients. Gross reported that only 6 per cent of his 702 pediatric patients with intussusception had a lead point.[7]

The idiopathic variety is probably the result of a disturbance in intestinal motility in which there is segmental spasticity and atony. When a peristaltic wave hits a spastic segment just proximal to an atonic segment, the former may be intussuscepted into the latter. Adenovirus, which is known to cause enteric symptoms, has been recovered from the stool in 46 per cent of patients with idiopathic intussusception at a time when 3.6 per cent of the general population harbored the virus. Resulting lymphoid hyperplasia in the bowel wall may act as a lead point. Idiopathic intussusception is decreasing in frequency. Intussusception may also occur a few days after abdominal operation when intestinal peristalsis is returning.

The usual idiopathic intussusception is ileocolic (ileum intussuscepts into colon). Small bowel intussusception is likely to have a lead point and tends to occur in older children.

**Clinical Findings.** Eighty-five per cent of pediatric intussusceptions occur in patients between 2 months and 2 years of age. The infant has usually been healthy. He exhibits a sudden onset of cramping abdominal pain and crying, often pulls his legs up onto his abdomen with the pains, and frequently vomits. Between episodes, which usually occur at 15 to 30 minute intervals, he is usually completely asymptomatic. Frequently the patient passes bloody mucous (currant jelly) stools. Rectal bleeding may be a prominent feature. If seen between episodes of pain during the asymptomatic period (which may be as long as 2 or 3 hours), the infant looks deceptively healthy. After a number of hours he becomes quite ill.

On physical examination a "sausage-shaped" mass is palpable in 90 per cent of patients, usually in the right upper quadrant. The mass, however, may be difficult to palpate. It is moderately soft, not particularly tender, and somewhat mobile. Sedation of the patient may be necessary for an adequate examination. The stool is usually guaiac-positive, even if not grossly bloody.

**Diagnosis.** Diagnosis may be made on clinical grounds. Plain x-ray of the abdomen is likely to show more than the usual amount of small bowel gas. The right lower quadrant may be empty of cecal gas and a mass may be seen. Intussusception into the colon can be diagnosed by barium enema.

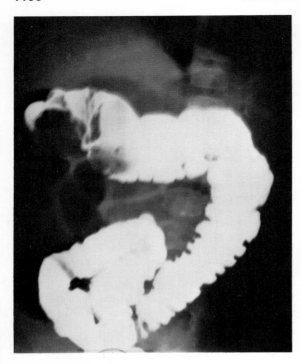

**Figure 23** Roentgenogram taken at the time of barium enema reduction of an intussusception. The intussusceptum can be seen at the hepatic flexure.

**Figure 24** Technique of operative reduction of intussusception. (From Gross, R. E.: An Atlas of Children's Surgery. Philadelphia, W. B. Saunders Company, 1970.)

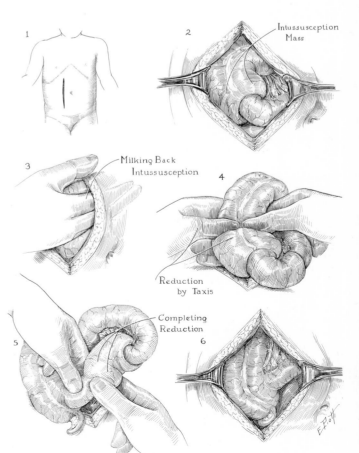

Any infant or child suspected of having an intussusception should have a prompt barium enema — day or night (Fig. 23). Unfortunately, barium enema is of no value in the diagnosis of small bowel intussusception.

**Treatment.** Reduction may be accomplished by hydrostatic pressure (first advocated by Hirschsprung) or operatively. If the intussusception is irreducible, resection is required. Hydrostatic reduction by barium enema under fluoroscopic control is a safe form of therapy if the following criteria are observed: (1) the surgeon should see the patient and the usual preoperative preparations should be carried out before any attempt is made at reduction; (2) the hydrostatic pressure is not to exceed $3^1/_2$ feet; (3) no manipulation of the abdomen is attempted (this further increases the intracolonic pressure and risk of bowel rupture); (4) reduction is not considered successful unless there is free reflux of barium into the ileum (if the ileum does not fill freely, operation is required at once); (5) the patient is admitted to the hospital for 24 hours of observation, and if symptoms persist, operation is mandatory; and (6) reduction by barium enema is not attempted in the infant with x-ray evidence of marked intestinal obstruction with acute toxicity or with clinical signs of strangulated bowel.[18]

Barium enema reduction has the limitations that it is of no value in the patient with small bowel intussusception and usually does not detect any lead point as the cause of the intussusception. The major dangers of barium enema reduction stem from the very factors that make it an appealing form of therapy — its ease and simplicity. The perforations and deaths that have occurred with its use have been in the hands of enthusiasts who have extended the indications or ignored the precautions just listed.

For patients with intussusception who are not candidates for hydrostatic reduction, or in whom it is unsuccessful, operation is performed as soon as adequate preparation has been carried out. Some surgeons consider this the safest form of therapy in all patients.

Operative reduction is illustrated in Figure 24. A lead point, if present, should be resected. If the reduction is unsuccessful, if the intestine is not viable, or if the patient is quite sick and toxic, the involved intestine should be resected. In some situations exteriorization is safer than primary anastomosis.

**Results.** Gross reports no deaths in patients with symptoms of less than 24 hours. With symptoms of over 24 hours' duration, the reported mortality is as high as 40 per cent. The importance of early diagnosis is obvious.

# URINARY TRACT INFECTION

Infections of the urinary tract are surprisingly common in preschool and school-age children, even in the absence of symptoms. Unlike respiratory infections, infections of the urinary tract frequently indicate an underlying organic lesion. It is important that the diagnosis be established by culture of properly obtained clean-voided urine and not by urinalysis. Studies have shown that pyuria is grossly unreliable as an indicator of urinary tract infection. If an infection is diagnosed by culture, not only must it be treated, but the underlying cause must be sought.[2]

Appropriate evaluation consists of a voiding cystourethrogram, excretory urogram, cystoscopy and urethral calibration, and assessment of renal function by creatinine clearance. Occasionally the use of renal scans, retrograde pyelography, and cystometrograms are of value. Most of the time the latter are not necessary, however, and simple x-ray studies and cystoscopy will delineate the disorder. An aggressive diagnostic approach is indicated, for not only is the yield great (approximately 50 per cent) but the chance of permanent cure by surgical methods is quite high.

# URETHRAL STENOSIS

A significant percentage of girls with recurring urinary tract infections are found to have marked narrowing of the urethra when it is calibrated at the time of cystoscopy. This narrowing may be present at the meatus or at the midurethral level (Lyon's ring) and is presumably a congenital malformation. The possibility that such narrowing is the result of chronic urethritis (bacterial or otherwise) cannot be excluded.

**Diagnosis.** In most cases the patient will give few if any symptoms to indicate difficulty in voiding that suggests the degree of obstruction that is found. In girls, the urinary stream is seldom observed by the mother, so this information is usually not available. X-rays also are unreliable and may show a proximal dilatation when no obstruction exists. Urethral calibration with bougies à boule, done with the patient anesthetized at the time of cystoscopy, is the only way of establishing the presence of significant stenosis. Urethral stenosis is sometimes seen in association with vesicoureteral reflux and may be the underlying obstructing mechanism.

**Treatment.** The treatment of urethral stenosis is urethrotomy. This is easily accomplished with an Otis urethrotome or with a surgical scalpel. Urethrotomy must be carried out to a diameter two to three times the original size to be effective (settings 24 to 34 F). Temporary incontinence frequently results but rapidly resolves as the healing process takes place. Urethrotomy is to be preferred to urethral dilations, since the latter usually need to be repeated periodically for sustained effect. If urethral stenosis is the only lesion discovered, the chances of cure of the recurring urinary tract infections by urethrotomy are excellent.

# VESICOURETERAL REFLUX

Undoubtedly one of the most controversial subjects of the past decade, vesicoureteral reflux is seen with considerable frequency among girls who are evaluated for recurring urinary tract infections.

**Etiology.** Reflux occurs when there is a breakdown of the normal one-way valve action of the vesicoureteral junction. These are several causes:

1. Obstruction. The most common form of obstruction in young girls is urethral stenosis (see the preceding section), and relief of this obstruction may bring about disappearance of the reflux. In boys, posterior urethral valves are the most common cause of lower urinary tract obstruction.

2. Neurogenic bladder. Patients with neurogenic bladder from any cause (myelomeningocele is the most common in the pediatric age group) may have vesicoureteral reflux caused by the inadequacy of the bladder wall itself. In these patients reflux cannot be corrected by the standard methods of reimplantation, and in most some form of urinary diversion will ultimately be necessary.

3. Chronic urinary tract infection. Some have felt that *all* vesicoureteral reflux is a result of changes of the vesicoureteral junction secondary to recurring infections. Although this mechanism undoubtedly accounts for some, many infections are the *result* of the reflux and will not respond to antibacterial treatment until the reflux is corrected. In about one-fourth of patients the reflux is the result of recurring urinary tract infections alone.

4. Congenital malformation of the vesicoureteral junction. The most common cause of reflux appears to be a malformation of the insertion of the ureter into the bladder. Some of these patients, especially males, may not have any history or evidence of urinary infection, although most do. It is in these patients that the best results of reimplantation surgery are to be expected.

**Pathophysiology.** The significance of vesicoureteral reflux is that it may produce renal damage if allowed to persist. Reflux permits a bladder infection to ascend to the kidneys and cause pyelonephritis. There is some evidence that reflux is frequently present when pyelonephritis occurs in the pediatric age group. Even in the absence of infection, reflux can cause significant damage to the kidney since it exposes this low-pressure system to the high intravesical voiding pressure every time the patient micturates.

**Diagnosis.** The presence and the extent of reflux can be determined only by instillation of radiopaque contrast medium into the bladder. Although reflux can sometimes be demonstrated in the anesthetized patient, it is its presence during the normal act of voiding that is of significance. For this reason, a voiding cystourethrogram in the awake patient is recommended. The presence of prominent or dilated ureteral orifices at cystoscopy is suggestive, but not diagnostic, of reflux, and may be misleading. Many patients with severe reflux have surprisingly normal-appearing ureteral orifices.

**Treatment.** In the evaluation of vesicoureteral reflux it is essential that patients with neurogenic bladder be identified since they will not benefit from a reimplantation operation. Further, it is mandatory that any form of a distal obstruction be corrected prior to (and often instead of) reconstructive reflux surgery. If the patient has no evidence of upper urinary tract damage (hydronephrosis or hydroureter), and if lower urinary obstruction has been ruled out, a trial of antibacterial therapy with one of the usual agents such as sulfisoxazole (Gantrisin), nalidixic acid (NegGram), or nitrofurantoin (Furadantin) is indicated. Six months' antibacterial therapy with frequent urine culture checks to make sure the urine is, in fact, being kept sterile will correct the reflux in those patients in whom infection is the sole etiologic basis. If at the end of 6 months the reflux persists, further medicinal therapy is unlikely to be successful, and reconstructive surgery is indicated.

Although many surgical techniques have been suggested, the Leadbetter-Politano method of reimplantation of the ureter, which creates a submucosal tunnel, has received widest acceptance. Properly performed, the operation can be expected to be 95 per cent successful in preventing reflux. Failures are usually in patients with dilated ureters in whom a ureteral-tailoring procedure is indicated. Either obstruction or persistent reflux can occur. Their detection requires periodic follow-up x-ray studies. On the whole, however, the operation has proved eminently satisfactory, and the great majority of patients are cured both of the reflux and of recurring urinary tract infections.[9]

## POSTERIOR URETHRAL VALVES

Urinary infection in a newborn male is almost always secondary to urinary tract obstruction or a neurogenic bladder. In this age group urinary obstruction may be due to posterior urethral valves (Fig. 25). Marked degrees of hydronephrosis and hydroureter can result from this obstruction which clearly is present long before birth. Ureters may be so dilated that they resemble the sigmoid colon, and when filled with radiocontrast material suggest a barium enema study. Severe renal destruction can occur, and may be irremediable. Especially in patients with severe hydronephrosis, the use of temporary tubeless drainage high in the ureter or at the renal pelvis is indicated (Fig. 26). This will permit maximal return of renal function as well as shrinkage of the ureters to normal size so that reconstruction can be carried out at a later date under optimal circumstances. The valves themselves may be resected endoscopically, through a perineal urethrotomy, or transvesically, depending on whether other reconstructive measures must be carried out. Vesicoureteral reflux is almost always present and requires reimplantation of the ureters. Delay of such reconstructive surgery until the patient is 1 or 2 years of age greatly facilitates the procedure, and is another reason for temporary tubeless diversion.[14]

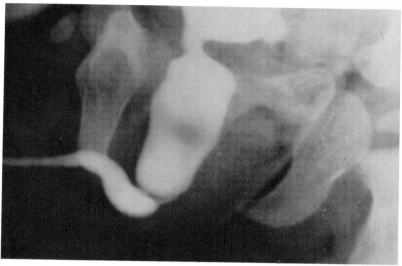

**Figure 25**   Voiding cystourethrogram in patient with posterior urethral valves. Note massive dilatation of posterior urethra and false impression of bladder neck contracture.

**Figure 26**   Method of performing in-continuity loop ureterostomies in child with massive hydronephrosis and hydroureter. Kinking of the ureter must be relieved so that the segment brought to the skin readily conducts urine out from the kidney.

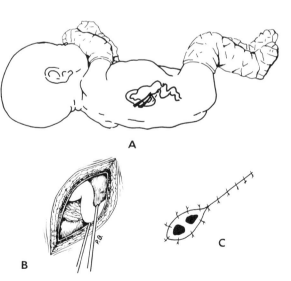

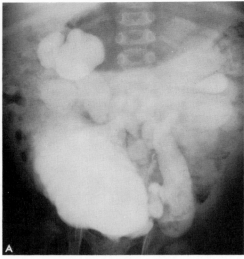
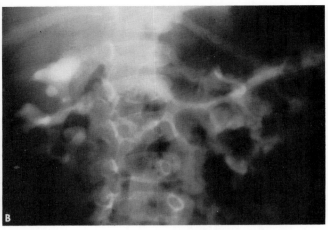

**Figure 27**  *A,* A cystogram of an 8 month old child with myelomeningocele, showing bilateral reflux and two massively dilated ureters and kidneys. Note large irregular-shaped bladder. *B,* Intravenous pyelogram of same patient 6 months after bilateral cutaneous ureterostomies. Note marked decrease in hydronephrosis and excellent urine-concentrating ability.

## NEUROGENIC BLADDER

Neurogenic bladder is a relatively common condition of infancy, being secondary to myelomeningocele in most patients. At the present time little can be done in the way of reconstructive surgery to permit adequate bladder function. It is essential that these patients receive urinary diversion early enough so that they do not suffer progressive renal damage both from inadequate drainage and from chronic infection (Fig. 27). This may require ileal conduit in the first year or two of life. For more detailed discussion of problems of diagnosis and management of neurogenic bladder, the reader is referred to the section in the chapter on the urinary system.

## MISCELLANEOUS CAUSES OF URINARY TRACT INFECTION

There are numerous other urinary tract anomalies that are first brought to the surgeon's attention because of recurring urinary tract infections: ureterocele, ectopic ureters, duplicated collecting systems, vesicoureteral obstruction, and so forth. In general, the diagnosis of these entities is made in the same fashion as that of those that have already been discussed: use of contrast radiography and cystoscopy. Treatment consists of correction of the defect and restoration of a normal urinary tract, which is usually possible. There remain a number of patients, perhaps as many as 40 to 50 per cent, in whom no organic underlying cause for recurring urinary tract infections can be found. These patients are particularly frustrating for the physician and bear witness to the inadequacy of current diagnostic methods. Neverthe-

less, in the absence of evidence of damage to the upper urinary tract the long-term prognosis for these patients is good. Many will respond to a prolonged course of antibacterial therapy. The important principle is that they be carefully followed and monitored by periodic cultures so that recurring infections may be promptly detected and treated.

## SELECTED REFERENCES

Gross, R. E.: The Surgery of Infancy and Childhood. Philadelphia, W. B. Saunders Company, 1953.
*This text is a classic. It is easy to read and contains a vast amount of material based, for the most part, on Dr. Gross' own experience at the Boston Children's Hospital. Despite being published in 1953, it still contains some of the most informative reading in pediatric surgery. The mortality statistics and some forms of therapy are not current.*

Gross, R. E.: An Atlas of Children's Surgery. Philadelphia, W. B. Saunders Company, 1970.
*This atlas with excellent illustrations by Janis Cirulis and Etta Piotti covers many of the operations in pediatric surgery. A short discussion of operative technique is included. The drawings and text are clear and concise.*

Mustard, W. T., Ravitch, M. M., Snyder, W. H., Jr., Welch, K. J., and Benson, C. D.: Pediatric Surgery. 2nd ed. Chicago, Year Book Medical Publishers, 1970.
*This two-volume text is the standard reference work in pediatric surgery and provides a comprehensive coverage of virtually all aspects. It is a multiauthor book with 80 contributors, many of them leading authorities on their subjects. Recently revised, it is up-to-date with current references and excellent illustrations.*

Swenson, O.: Pediatric Surgery. 3rd ed. New York, Appleton-Century-Crofts, 1969.
*This two-volume text written by Dr. Swenson and 24 of his colleagues at the Chicago Children's Memorial Hospital and Northwestern University Medical School is unusually well organized for a work with so many authors. The discussion of Hirschsprung's disease, particularly, is outstanding. Most other topics are also very well covered. This is a good and complete text.*

Rickham, P. P., and Johnston, J. H.: Neonatal Surgery. New York, Appleton-Century-Crofts, 1970.

*The major surgical diseases of the newborn are presented in this compendium which represents the experience of the Alder Hey Children's Hospital. Although various specialists of the staff have contributed to it, the bulk of the book is written by the senior authors and reflects their vast experience in this field. A large segment is devoted to organizational and nonoperative care aspects of neonatal surgery, duly emphasizing the importance these aspects have in determining the overall outcome. Although primarily of interest to the specialist, who will find in here virtually all he needs, it is also a valuable reference for the student seeking more detailed information than is available in the standard texts.*

## REFERENCES

1. Allen, R. G., and Wrenn, E. L., Jr.: Silon as a sac in the treatment of omphalocele and gastroschisis. J. Pediat. Surg., 4:3, 1969.
2. Allen, T. D.: Pathogenesis of urinary tract infection in children. New Eng. J. Med., 273:1421, 1965.
3. Benson, C. D., and Loyd, J. R.: Infantile pyloric stenosis. Amer. J. Surg., 107:429, 1964.
4. Bishop, H. C., and Koop, C. E.: Management of meconium ileus: Resection, Roux-en-Y anastomosis and ileostomy irrigation with pancreatic enzymes. Ann. Surg., 145:410, 1957.
5. Farber, S.: Chemotherapy in the treatment of leukemia and Wilms' tumor. J.A.M.A., 198:154, 1966.
6. Griscom, T.: The roentgenology of neonatal abdominal masses. Amer. J. Roentgen., 93:447, 1965.
7. Gross, R. E.: The Surgery of Infancy and Childhood. Philadelphia, W. B. Saunders Company, 1953.
8. Hays, D. M.: Intestinal atresia and stenosis. Curr. Probl. Surg., Oct. 1969.
9. Hendren, W. H.: Ureteral reimplantation in children. J. Pediat. Surg., 3:649, 1968.
10. Hendren, W. H., and Haggerty, R. J.: Staphylococcic pneumonia in infancy and childhood. J.A.M.A., 168:6, 1958.
11. Holder, T. M., and Ashcraft, K. W.: Esophageal atresia and tracheoesophageal fistula. Curr. Probl. Surg., Aug. 1966.
12. Holder, T. M., Leape, L. L., and Ashcraft, K. W.: Gastrostomy: Its use and dangers in pediatric patients. New Eng. J. Med., In press.
13. Koop, C. E., and Hernandez, J. R.: Neuroblastoma. Experience with 100 cases in children. Surgery, 56:726, 1964.
14. Leape, L. L., and Holder, T. M.: Temporary tubeless urinary diversion in children. J. Pediat. Surg., 5:288, 1970.
15. Leape, L. L., and Longino, L. A.: Infantile lobar emphysema. Pediatrics, 34:246, 1964.
16. Meeker, I. A., and Kincannon, W. H.: The role of ventral hernia in the correction of diaphragmatic defects in the newborn. Arch. Dis. Child., 40:146, 1965.
17. Pickett, L. K.: Obstructive jaundice. In: Mustard, W. T., et al., eds.: Pediatric Surgery. 2nd ed. Chicago, Year Book Medical Publishers, 1969, p. 732.
18. Ravitch, M. M.: Intussusception in Infants and Children. Springfield, Ill., Charles C Thomas, 1959.
19. Ravitch, M. M.: Duplications of the alimentary canal. In: Mustard, W. T., et al., eds.: Pediatric Surgery. 2nd ed. Chicago, Year Book Medical Publishers, 1969, p. 831.
20. Rickham, P. P.: Neonatal physiology and its effect on pre- and postoperative management. In: Rickham, P. P., and Johnston, J. H., eds.: Neonatal Surgery. New York, Appleton-Century-Crofts, 1969, p. 33.
21. Snyder, W. H., Jr., and Chaffen, L.: Malrotation of the intestine. In: Mustard, W. T., et al., eds.: Pediatric Surgery. 2nd ed. Chicago, Year Book Medical Publishers, 1969, p. 808.
22. Stephens, F. D.: Congenital Malformations of the Rectum, Anus and Genitourinary Tract. Edinburgh, E. and S. Livingstone, 1963.
23. Swenson, O.: Pediatric Surgery. 3rd ed. New York, Appleton-Century-Crofts, 1969, p. 734.
24. Voorhess, M. L.: Urinary catecholamine excretion by healthy children. Pediatrics, 39:252, 1967.
25. Waldhausen, J. A., Kilman, J. W., Vellios, F., and Battersby, J. S.: Sacrococcygeal teratoma. Surgery, 54:933, 1963.

# 39

# SURGICAL DISORDERS OF THE EARS, NOSE, PARANASAL SINUSES, PHARYNX, AND LARYNX

*James B. Snow, Jr., M.D.*

## THE EARS

Progress in surgery of the ear began in 1853 when Sir William Wilde of Dublin, father of Oscar Wilde, advocated a postauricular incision for the drainage of subperiosteal abscesses in acute mastoiditis. The next major advance occurred with Hermann Schwartze's introduction in 1873 of the complete mastoidectomy. This operation gained great popularity because of its effectiveness in resolving acute mastoiditis. Emanuel Zaufal recognized that this operation did not solve the problem in the presence of a cholesteatoma and in 1890 described the radical mastoidectomy, in which the disease process in the middle ear, antrum, and mastoid cell area is exteriorized by removal of the posterior and superior portion of the bony canal wall. Bondy observed that removal of the tympanic membrane remnants and auditory ossicles was not always necessary to exteriorize cholesteatomas and in 1910 introduced the modified radical mastoidectomy in which a cholesteatoma lateral to the ossicles could be exteriorized and the hearing preserved. In the 1930s Lempert popularized endaural incisions. The development of the binocular surgical microscope by Holmgren and improved illumination set the stage for the introduction of tympanoplasty by Wullstein and Zöllner in the early 1950s.[25] The next major advance occurred in 1952 when Rosen mobilized the stapes in a patient with otosclerosis.[19] Shea introduced stapedectomy in 1958 and brought a century of surgery for the middle ear to a dramatic climax.[22] More recently, House's endolymphatic sac surgery and translabyrinthine and middle cranial fossa approaches for the internal auditory meatus bring into view new horizons.[9, 10]

## ANATOMY OF THE EAR

The external auditory canal makes a slightly S-shaped curve. The outer one-third has a cartilaginous skeleton, and the inner two-thirds has a bony skeleton. Sebaceous glands and hair are borne in the outer one-third. The plane of the tympanic membrane makes an angle of 55 degrees with the long axis of the external auditory canal. The tympanic membrane is divided into the pars tensa

and the pars flaccida. The pars tensa is composed of three layers: the outer stratified squamous epithelium, which is continuous with the skin of the canal; the fibrous layer; and the inner mucous membrane, which is continuous with the rest of the mucous membrane of the middle ear. The fibrous layer thickens toward the periphery of the tympanic membrane to form the annulus tympanicus, which rests in the sulcus tympanicus, a groove in the most medial aspect of the canal. The fibrous layer ends at the anterior and posterior malleolar folds. The pars flaccida has only two layers, the stratified squamous epithelium laterally and the mucous membrane medially (Fig. 1). The long process of the malleus is embedded in the fibrous layer of the tympanic membrane, and the short process projects laterally. The head of the malleus articulates with the body of the incus. The lenticular process of the incus articulates with the head of the stapes. The footplate of the stapes articulates with the oval window (Fig. 2).

The middle ear space is irregular and compressed laterally. The part superior to the level of the tympanic membrane is the epitympanum or attic. The mesotympanum lies directly medial to the tympanic membrane. The hypotympanum is inferior to the level of the tympanic membrane. The basal turn of the cochlea makes an impression of the medial wall of the middle ear called the promontory. The roof or tegmen of the tympanum is opposite the middle cranial fossa. The tegmen tympani

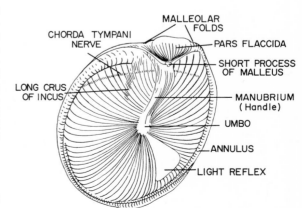

**Figure 1**   Landmarks of the right tympanic membrane. (From Saunders, W. H. In: Prior, J. H., and Silberstein, J. S.: Physical Diagnosis, The History and Examination of the Patient. St. Louis, C. V. Mosby Company, 1963.)

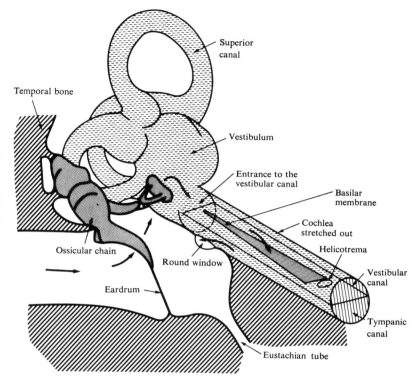

**Figure 2** Functional diagram of the external, middle, and inner ear with the cochlea unrolled. (From von Békésy, G. In: Theoretical and Mathematical Biology, edited by Talbot H. Waterman and Harold J. Morowitz. © 1965, Xerox.)

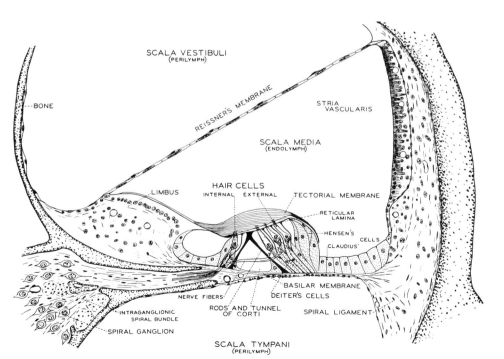

**Figure 3** Cross section of a turn of the cochlea. (From Davis, H., et al.: J. Acoust. Soc. Amer., *25*:1180, 1953.)

extends posteriorly to become the tegmen of the antrum and mastoid process. The middle ear communicates with the mastoid process through the antrum. All mastoid air cells communicate one through another with the antrum. Pneumatic cells also extend into the petrous pyramid from the antrum, attic, and hypotympanum. The floor of the middle ear is the roof of the jugular fossa.[2]

The cochlea makes two and three-quarters turns in the human. A cross section through the modiolus or central bony framework shows in each turn the scala vestibuli, the scala media, and the scala tympani (Fig. 3). The scala vestibuli is separated from the scala media by Reissner's membrane. The scala media is separated from the scala tympani by the basilar membrane. The organ of Corti with its hair cells and their supporting cells rests on the basilar membrane. The hairs of the hair cells are in contact with the tectorial membrane. Dendrites of the first-order neurons, whose cell bodies are in the spiral canal of Rosenthal in the modiolus, arborize about the base of the hair cells.

The axons terminate in the dorsal and ventral cochlea nuclei in the medulla. The pathway to the auditory cortex consists of at least four orders of neurons and includes the superior olivary complexes, the lateral lemnisci, the inferior colliculi, and the medial geniculate bodies. Crossing of the midline occurs at the level of the brain stem nuclei and the inferior colliculi. In man the auditory cortex lies in the posterior portion of the superior temporal gyrus in the sylvian fissure, which is called Heschl's gyrus.

The saccule is spherical and is connected with the scala media through the canalis reuniens of Hensen (Fig. 4). The saccular duct joins the utricular duct to form the endolymphatic duct. The utricle is larger than the saccule and is ovoid. The utricle has five openings for the three ampullated ends of the semicircular canals, the crus simplex of the horizontal semicircular canal, and the crus commune of the superior and posterior semicircular canals. The endolymphatic duct extends through the vestibular aqueduct to the endolymphatic sac, which is located between sheaves of dura on the posterior surface of the petrous pyramid.

The membranous labyrinth contains endolymph. The space between the bony labyrinth and the membranous labyrinth is filled with perilymph. The perilymphatic space communicates with the subarachnoid space through the cochlear aqueduct which enters the scala tympani. The endolymph is chemically similar to intra-cellular fluid with a high $K^+$ concentration and a low $Na^+$ concentration, whereas the perilymph resembles extracellular fluid with a low $K^+$ and a high $Na^+$. There is a resting direct current potential difference of 80 millivolts between the endolymph in the scala media and the perilymph, and the endolymph is positively charged relative to the perilymph.

## PHYSIOLOGY OF THE EAR

The external auditory canal maintains the temperature and humidity of the external environment of the tympanic membrane, and this environment varies very little regardless of the ambient temperature or humidity. The canal is self-cleansing. Debris is carried by the migration of a sheet of desquamated epithelial cells from the center of the tympanic membrane to its periphery and from the medial portion of the canal to its lateral extent.[13]

### Auditory Function

Sound waves impinging upon the tympanic membrane set the tympanic membrane in motion. Movement of the tympanic membrane in turn causes movement of the malleus, incus, and stapes. Movement of the stapes results in pressure changes in the fluid in the inner ear. These pressure changes result in deformation of the basilar membrane. A traveling wave is propagated in the basilar membrane from the base to the apex of the cochlea. Along the length of the basilar membrane, a point of maximal displacement occurs with each traveling wave. The location of the point of maximal displacement depends upon the frequency of the stimulating tone. High-frequency tones cause maximal displacement near the base of the cochlea. As the frequency of the stimulating tone is decreased, the point of maximal displacement moves from the base to the apex.

Displacement of the basilar membrane causes movement of the organ of Corti and deformation of the hairs of the hair cells. As the hairs of the hair cells are bent away from the modiolus, a depolarization occurs within the hair cell. An alternating current potential known as the cochlear potential or cochlear microphonic occurs in response to stimulation of the hair cells. The cochlear potential faithfully reproduces the frequency and intensity of the acoustic stimulation through a wide intensity range. A chemical transmitter is released in the region of the end-boutons of the afferent eighth nerve fibers. This chemical transmitter initiates a depolarization of the dendritic terminals of the afferent nerve.

## TRAUMA AND FOREIGN BODIES

Blunt trauma to the pinna results in a subperichondrial hematoma. When bleeding occurs between the cartilage and the perichondrium, the pinna becomes a reddish purple, shapeless mass. Since the perichondrium carries the blood supply to the cartilage, the cartilage undergoes avascular

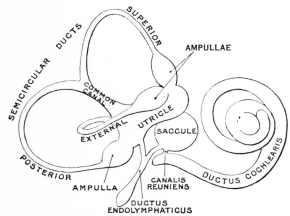

**Figure 4** Membranous labyrinth. (After Goss, C. N., ed.: Gray's Anatomy of the Human Body. 27th ed. Philadelphia, Lea & Febiger, 1959.)

necrosis if the hematoma is present on both sides of the cartilage, and with time the pinna becomes shriveled. A hematoma may become organized and calcify, resulting in the cauliflower ear characteristic of wrestlers and boxers. Treatment consists of incision for aspiration of the clot, and packing of the skin and perichondrium tightly onto the cartilage by means of a molded splint of cotton soaked in benzoin and a pressure dressing to approximate the cartilage and its blood supply.

Lacerations of the pinna extending through skin, cartilage, and skin are repaired by suturing of the skin margins of the wound, external splinting of the cartilage of the pinna with molded cotton impregnated with benzoin, and protective dressing. Sutures are not placed in the cartilage.

Perichondritis of the pinna results in the accumulation of pus between the perichondrium and the cartilage and leads to avascular and septic necrosis of the cartilage. The infection persists for long periods. The treatment for perichondritis is wide incision for drainage followed by application of a pressure dressing to approximate the cartilage and its blood supply. Systemic antibiotic therapy is indicated. Often, perichondritis results from a gram-negative rod infection, and culture and sensitivities are of considerable importance. Incisions in the skin of the pinna on its lateral surface for drainage of hematomas and perichondritis should be made just anterior to the antihelix so that the scar will not be visible on the lateral view of the ear.

Incision of superficial infections of the pinna is to be avoided for fear of initiating perichondritis.

Foreign bodies of the external auditory canal are a common problem. Beads, erasers, beans, and other objects may be inserted by children and their siblings into their ears. An insect may find its way into the ear canal and is particularly annoying to the patient until it is killed or removed. Foreign bodies are removed by passing a blunt

hook deep to the foreign body and raking it out (Fig. 5). A forceps is likely to push smooth foreign bodies ahead of it. If the foreign body is far medial, it is difficult to remove without injuring the tympanic membrane and ossicular chain. If a child is uncooperative or the mechanical problem is difficult, a general anesthetic is used for the removal of a foreign body. Metal and glass beads may be removed by irrigation, but care is used to be certain that the foreign body is not hygroscopic like a bean, because swelling with the addition of water will complicate its removal. An insect is killed to give the patient immediate relief and facilitate its removal by filling the ear canal with mineral oil. The dead insect is removed with a forceps.

The force of blows to the mandible may be transmitted to the anterior wall of the external auditory canal, which is the posterior wall of the glenoid fossa. In fractures of the anterior wall of the canal fragments may be displaced to such a degree that stenosis of the canal results. The displaced fragments are excised under general anesthesia.

The tympanic membrane may be perforated with twigs of a tree, cotton applicators, and other objects placed in the ear canal, missiles such as hot slag in welding, and a sudden overpressure in an explosion (acoustic trauma). Perforations of the tympanic membrane may be associated with dislocations of the ossicular chain. Most perforations of the tympanic membrane heal spontaneously in 6 weeks. It is important to avoid infection during the healing period. Instrumentation and topical applications carry with them the risk of introducing microorganisms. Prophylactic antibiotic therapy in the form of oral penicillin for the first 7 days is recommended. If the perforation fails to heal or if there is a persisting conductive hearing loss suggesting discontinuity of the ossicular chain, the middle ear is explored and repaired.

## Fractures of the Temporal Bone

Basal skull fractures result from blunt trauma to the head, particularly to the occipital area. Basal skull fractures are in essence fractures of the temporal bone, and they are a frequent cause of profound sensorineural hearing loss. Bleeding from the ear following an injury to the skull is pathognomonic of a fracture of the temporal bone whether the bleeding is medial to an intact tympanic membrane, from the middle ear through a rupture of the tympanic membrane, or from a fracture line in the ear canal. Hemotympanum gives the tympanic membrane a blue-black color. Usually, there is a communication with the subarachnoid space through the fracture line. Often there is cerebrospinal fluid otorrhea. Cleaning of the ear canal should be avoided for fear of introducing microorganisms. The immediate danger to the patient is the development of meningitis. Therefore, prophylactic antibiotic therapy is initiated and continued for 7 to 10 days. More fractures of the temporal bone are longitudinal (80 per cent) than transverse (20 per cent) to the long axis of the petrous pyramid. Longitudinal fractures extend

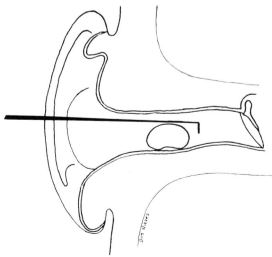

**Figure 5** Technique for the removal of foreign bodies of the ear canal. The foreign body is raked out with a blunt Day hook.

through the middle ear into the ear canal and cause rupture of the tympanic membrane. Transverse fractures extend across the cochlea and fallopian canal to produce a profound, permanent sensorineural hearing loss and a facial paralysis.[7] Approximately 35 per cent of longitudinal fractures produce a sensorineural hearing loss, and approximately 15 per cent produce facial paralysis. The fracture extending through the middle ear may result in a dislocation of the ossicular chain that requires subsequent repair. Persistence of a facial paralysis requires decompression of the facial nerve under certain circumstances.

## INFECTIOUS DISEASES

### External Otitis

Infection of the ear canal occurs in a diffuse form involving the entire canal, called external otitis generalisata, and a localized form due to furunculosis, called external otitis circumscripta. The diffuse form may be caused by a gram-negative rod such as *Escherichia coli, Pseudomonas aeruginosa,* or Proteus or by *Staphylococcus aureus.* Rarely a fungus may play a pathogenic role. Furunculosis is usually due to *Staphylococcus aureus.*

Patients with diffuse external otitis complain of itching, pain, foul-smelling discharge, and loss of hearing if the canal becomes swollen or filled with purulent debris. Tenderness on traction of the pinna and on pressure over the tragus tends to distinguish it from otitis media. The skin of the external auditory canal appears red, swollen, and littered with moist purulent debris.

Treatment with topical antibiotics and corticosteroids is efficacious. Systemic therapy is rarely necessary unless there is a spreading cellulitis about the ear. Furuncles of the canal should be allowed to resolve because incision may lead to a spreading perichondritis of the pinna.

### Acute Otitis Media

Acute otitis media is an infectious inflammatory process in the middle ear usually secondary to an upper respiratory tract infection. It is the most common localized infection in children. Most children between 1 and 5 years of age have two or three episodes of acute otitis media each winter. Acute otitis media may be viral or bacterial. Viral otitis media may resolve, or the middle ear may be secondarily invaded by bacteria. Acute suppurative otitis media is caused by group A beta hemolytic streptococcus, *Diplococcus pneumoniae, Staphylococcus aureus,* and *Haemophilus influenzae. H. influenzae* occurs in the age group under 5. In older children and adults, streptococcal infections are most common, followed by pneumococcal and staphylococcal infections. In children under 5 years of age the same relative frequencies occur, but *Haemophilus influenzae* may predominate or take any place in the ranking. Rarely *Escherichia coli, Klebsiella pneumoniae,* and Bacteroides may produce acute otitis media.

Penicillin is the drug of choice for acute otitis

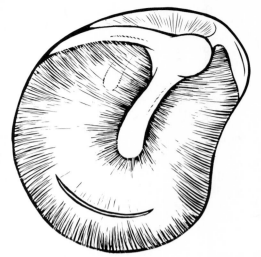

**Figure 6**  Myringotomy incision that occupies one-fourth of the circumference of the tympanic membrane midway between the umbo and the annulus tympanicus. (From Donaldson, J. A. In: Davis, L., ed.: Christopher's Textbook of Surgery. 8th ed. Philadelphia, W. B. Saunders Company, 1964.)

media in patients over 5 years of age. In those under 5 years of age, ampicillin is preferred because of the frequency of *Haemophilus influenzae* infections. The treatment is continued for 12 days to insure resolution and prevention of the sequelae of streptococcal infections.

A myringotomy is indicated if the tympanic membrane is bulging or if the systemic symptoms and signs such as pain, fever, vomiting, and diarrhea are severe. A large curvilinear incision is made parallel to the annulus in the inferior quadrants midway between the umbo and the canal wall (Fig. 6). The appearance and movement of the tympanic membrane and the patient's hearing are followed until there is complete resolution. The management of incomplete resolution is discussed under serous and secretory otitis media.

The infectious complications of acute otitis media are acute mastoiditis, petrositis, labyrinthitis, facial paralysis, conductive and sensorineural hearing loss, epidural abscess, meningitis, brain abscess, lateral sinus thrombosis, subdural empyema, and otitic hydrocephalus. The most common intracranial complication of acute otitis media is meningitis.

### Acute Mastoiditis

In acute otitis media, the infection almost invariably extends through the mastoid antrum into the mastoid cells. However, the term acute mastoiditis is not used clinically until destruction of the bony partitions between the mastoid air cells has occurred. Progression of the acute infectious process in the mastoid process is so regularly aborted by antibiotic therapy that clinically apparent acute mastoiditis has become a rare condition. The responsible bacteria are the same as those for acute otitis media.

Acute mastoiditis becomes clinically apparent 14 days or more after the onset of acute otitis media as one of the cortices of the mastoid process is destroyed. Usually associated with this destruction of the mastoid cortex is an exacerbation of the aural pain, fever, and otorrhea. The pain tends to be persistent and throbbing, and the discharge is usually creamy and profuse. Increasing hearing loss is characteristic of acute mastoiditis.

The lateral mastoid cortex is most frequently the first to be destroyed and a postauricular subperiosteal abscess develops. The first signs are thickening of the postauricular tissue, reduced mobility of the skin over the mastoid cortex, and blunting of the postauricular crease. As pus exudes from the mastoid cortex deep to the periosteum, an erythematous, hot, tender, fluctuant postauricular mass develops which displaces the pinna laterally and inferiorly.

In acute otitis media, there is increased radiographic density of the mastoid air cells owing to swollen mucous membrane and purulent fluid in the air cells. In coalescent mastoiditis the air cell partitions become indistinct, and the degree of radiopacity decreases. The individual septa can no longer be seen as one air cell coalesces with another. The resulting radiographic picture suggests the appearance of shattered ice on which hot water has been poured.

In early cases of acute mastoiditis in which there are the postauricular signs of tenderness and edema but no fluctuant subperiosteal abscess, antibiotic therapy may result in complete resolution with spontaneous healing of the tympanic membrane, reventilation of the middle ear, and return of the hearing to the preinfection level.

In the presence of a subperiosteal abscess, complete exenteration of the mastoid air cells (Schwartze operation) should be performed. The operation should include inspection of a small area of the middle and posterior fossa dura to exclude an epidural abscess. The objective of the complete mastoidectomy is to drain the abscess in the mastoid air cells and antrum (Fig. 7). Through-and-through drainage of the middle ear is provided by the myringotomy or perforation anteriorly and through the antrum posteriorly. The goals of this surgery are resolution of the infection, prevention of intracranial infectious complications, spontaneous healing of the perforation of the tympanic membrane, reventilation of the middle ear, and return of the hearing to the preinfection level.

### Serous and Secretory Otitis Media

Serous and secretory otitis media are manifested as sterile effusions in the middle ear. Such effusions result from incomplete resolution of acute otitis media or from eustachian tube obstruction due to inflammatory processes in the nasopharynx, allergic manifestations, hypertrophic adenoids, or benign or malignant nasopharyngeal neoplasms. Normally the middle ear is ventilated three to four times per minute as the eustachian tube opens during swallowing. If the patency of the eustachian tube is compromised, oxygen in the middle ear is absorbed by the blood in the vessels of the mucous membrane of the middle ear, and a relative negative pressure develops. At first there is mild retraction of the tympanic membrane. Soon a transudate of fluid occurs from the blood in the vessels in the mucous membrane of the middle ear. The presence of fluid in the middle ear may be recognized by an amber or dark gray color of the tympanic membrane, immobility of the tympanic membrane, and conductive hearing loss. Rarely an air-fluid level or bubbles of air may be seen through the tympanic membrane.

Treatment is directed toward correcting the underlying condition in the nasopharynx. Myrin-

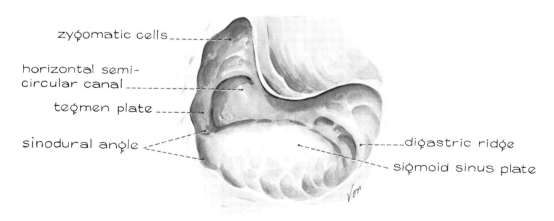

zygomatic cells

horizontal semi-circular canal

tegmen plate

sinodural angle

digastric ridge

sigmoid sinus plate

Completed mastoidectomy,
moderate pneumatization

**Figure 7**  Complete mastoidectomy (Schwartze operation) for acute mastoiditis. All pneumatic cells in the mastoid process are removed, and the antrum is drained. The posterior and superior bony canal wall is left in place. (From Shambaugh, G. E., Jr.: Surgery of the Ear. 2nd ed. Philadelphia, W. B. Saunders Company, 1967.)

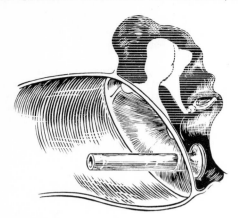

**Figure 8** Tympanostomy tube placed through a myringotomy incision for ventilation of the middle ear in serous and secretory otitis media. (From Donaldson, J. A. In: Davis, L., ed.: Christopher's Textbook of Surgery. 8th ed. Philadelphia, W. B. Saunders Company, 1964.)

gotomy for aspiration of the fluid and insertion of a tympanostomy tube for ventilation of the middle ear ameliorate the problem of eustachian tube obstruction regardless of the cause (Fig. 8). In children thorough adenoidectomy is frequently a necessary part of the treatment. Allergic evaluation and management with either elimination of the allergen from the patient's environment or desensitization therapy is helpful if there is an underlying allergic manifestation. Antibiotic therapy for bacterial rhinitis and sinusitis is similar to that outlined for acute otitis media. Immunologic investigation is occasionally helpful. The Valsalva maneuver and politzerization are employed in the absence of tympanostomy tubes.

### Chronic Otitis Media

Chronic otitis media means a permanent perforation of the tympanic membrane. Such perforations result from acute otitis media, mechanical trauma, thermal and chemical burns, and blast injuries. Chronic otitis media can be divided into two major categories depending upon the type of perforation present. There is a benign tubotympanic type, with a central perforation of the tympanic membrane, and a dangerous type, with a pars flaccida or marginal perforation.

A central perforation is one in which there is some substance of the tympanic membrane between the rim of the perforation and the bony sulcus tympanicus. These perforations result most commonly from acute otitis media produced by relatively virulent microorganisms. Exacerbations of the chronic otitis media result in painless, purulent otorrhea which may be foul-smelling and occur secondary to upper respiratory infections and when water gains access to the middle ear in bathing and swimming.

The middle ear can generally be repaired in chronic otitis media with a central perforation. A tympanoplasty provides sound protection for the round window and restores sound-pressure transformation to the oval window.[25] Wullstein categorized tympanoplastic procedures into five types

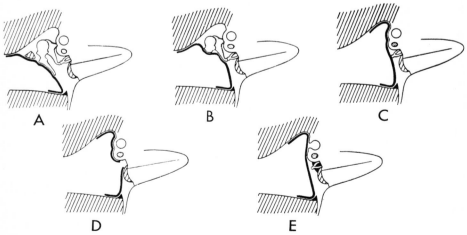

**Figure 9** Five types of tympanoplasty: *A,* Type I: Perforation of the tympanic membrane repaired with soft tissue graft to the tympanic membrane remnants. *B,* Type II: Perforation of the tympanic membrane and discontinuity of the ossicular chain repaired by soft tissue graft to the tympanic membrane remnants and by rearrangement of the ossicles, bony graft, or prosthesis. *C,* Type III: Perforation of the tympanic membrane and destruction of the incus and malleus repaired by applying to the tympanic membrane remnants a soft tissue graft which is placed in contact with the head of the stapes (columellar effect). *D,* Type IV: Perforation of the tympanic membrane with destruction of the superstructure (head, neck, and crura) of the stapes repaired by creating an air-filled space between the round window and the eustachian tube to provide sound protection for the round window. *E,* Type V: Perforation of the tympanic membrane with destruction of the stapedial superstructure and fixation of its footplate repaired by protecting the round window from sound and fenestrating the horizontal semicircular canal. (From Shambaugh, G. E., Jr.: Surgery of the Ear. 2nd ed. Philadelphia, W. B. Saunders Company, 1967.)

(Fig. 9). The Type I tympanoplasty is applicable to the patient with a perforation of the tympanic membrane in which the ossicular chain is intact and mobile. The Type I tympanoplasty, sometimes called a myringoplasty, restores the tympanic membrane by the use of a graft of soft tissue such as temporalis muscle fascia. A Type II tympanoplasty is required if there has been greater damage to the middle ear. Disruption of the ossicular chain, which often occurs as a result of necrosis of the long process of the incus, must be repaired in addition to grafting of the tympanic membrane.[8] Often the remnant of the incus can be repositioned to re-establish the continuity of the ossicular chain. A Type III tympanoplasty is required for a still more severely damaged middle ear in which the malleus and incus are not usable and only the stapes remains. Under these circumstances, the graft is placed in contact with the head of the stapes to produce a columellar effect similar to the single middle ear ossicle or columella found in birds. Tympanoplasty Types I, II, and III include sound protection for the round window as well as sound-pressure transformation for the oval window. In more severe degrees of damage to the middle ear in which the superstructure of the stapes has been destroyed, only sound protection of the round window can be achieved by grafting from the promontory to the inferior remnant of the tympanic membrane. This Type IV tympanoplasty creates a small closed space that communicates with the eustachian tube and provides an air-filled cushion over the round window. A Type V tympanoplasty is utilized when the footplate of the stapes is fixed. It provides sound protection for the round window as in a Type IV tympanoplasty and fenestration of the horizontal semicircular canal for the admission of acoustic energy into the inner ear. This type of tympanoplasty is rarely used.

The dangerous type of chronic otitis media occurs with pars flaccida and marginal perforations. Pars flaccida perforations lead into the epitympanum and are called attic perforations. Marginal perforations usually occur in the posterior-superior portion of the pars tensa. There is no substance of tympanic membrane between the periphery of the perforation and the bony sulcus tympanicus. The annulus tympanicus has been destroyed.

Theories of the pathogenesis of perforations of the pars flaccida include progressive retraction of the pars flaccida secondary to eustachian tube obstruction, rupture during acute otitis media, and hyperactivity of the basal layer of the epidermis of the pars flaccida due to long-standing inflammation in the middle ear. Each of these mechanisms may result in an invasive cholesteatoma.[20]

A cholesteatoma occurs when the middle ear is lined with stratified squamous epithelium. The stratified squamous epithelium desquamates in this closed space. The desquamated epithelial debris cannot be cleared and accumulates in ever enlarging concentric layers. This debris serves as a culture medium for microorganisms. Cholesteatomas have the ability to destroy bone, including the tympanic ossicles, probably because of the elaboration of collagenase.

Pars flaccida and marginal perforations are very frequently associated with cholesteatomas. Those cholesteatomas arising in association with pars flaccida perforations are classified as primary acquired cholesteatomas and may develop as an integral part of the development of the perforation or from the migration of stratified squamous epithelium once the perforation has occurred.

Marginal perforations are produced by acute otitis media with an especially virulent bacterium, particularly a group A beta hemolytic streptococcus, or in association with other infectious diseases such as diphtheria, chickenpox, or measles. This necrotizing otitis media destroys large areas of the tympanic membrane, including the annulus tympanicus and the middle ear mucous membrane, as well as the ossicles and their vascular and ligamentous support. During the healing process, the remaining epithelium of the mucous membrane of the middle ear migrates to cover the denuded areas. Likewise, the stratified squamous epithelium of the ear canal migrates into the middle ear to re-epithelialize the denuded areas. Once the stratified squamous epithelium is established in the middle ear, it begins to desquamate and a cholesteatoma results. Cholesteatomas developing by this mechanism are classified as secondary acquired cholesteatomas.

The presence of a cholesteatoma greatly increases the probability of the development of a serious complication such as a purulent labyrinthitis, facial paralysis, or intracranial suppurations. The propensity of cholesteatomas to produce these complications stems from their ability to destroy bone and the persistence of infection in the area bearing cholesteatoma.

Cholesteatomas are usually recognized by the small bits of white, amorphous debris in the middle ear and by the destruction of the external auditory canal bone superior to the pars flaccida or marginal perforation. Cholesteatomas are often associated with aural polyps which may conceal the epithelial debris and bone destruction. Radiography of the temporal bone occasionally demonstrates destruction of bone due to an otherwise unsuspected cholesteatoma. A radiolucency in the area of the antrum measuring greater than 1 cm. in diameter should be considered suspicious of cholesteatoma.

Cholesteatomas require surgical treatment. The objective of the surgery is to exteriorize the cholesteatoma and if possible remove it. In a radical mastoidectomy, the middle ear including the attic, the antrum, and the mastoid air cell area are converted into one cavity that communicates with the exterior through the ear canal (Fig. 10). If the cholesteatoma lies superficial to the remnants of the tympanic membrane and ossicles, a modified radical mastoidectomy can be performed (Fig. 11). The modified radical mastoidectomy spares the tympanic membrane remnants and ossicles and preserves the remaining hearing. Under unusually favorable circumstances, the

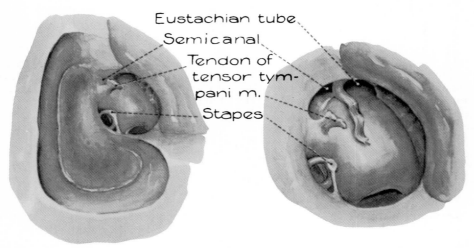

**Figure 10**   Radical mastoidectomy for cholesteatoma. The cholesteatoma-bearing area is exteriorized by converting the pneumatic cell area, antrum, and middle ear into one cavity that is accessible through the external auditory canal. (From Shambaugh, G. E., Jr.: Surgery of the Ear. 2nd ed. Philadelphia, W. B. Saunders Company, 1967.)

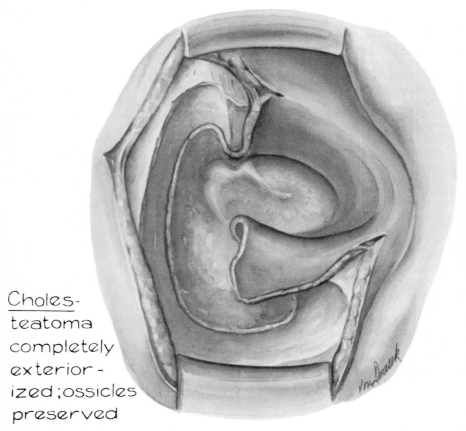

**Figure 11**   Modified radical mastoidectomy for exteriorizing cholesteatoma that is superficial to the remnants of the tympanic membrane and ossicles. The remnants of the tympanic membrane and ossicles are preserved. (From Shambaugh, G. E., Jr.: Surgery of the Ear. 2nd ed. Philadelphia, W. B. Saunders Company, 1967.)

cholesteatoma can be completely removed, and the middle ear reconstructed. Exteriorization or removal of the cholesteatoma greatly reduces the chance of intracranial complications. The primary goal of surgery for cholesteatoma is to make the ear safe, and the secondary goal is to maintain and improve the hearing.

## CONGENITAL MALFORMATIONS

The auricle may stand out too far from the skull and be termed an outstanding ear, lop ear, or protruding ear. The basic deformity is a lack of development of the antihelix. This deformity can be corrected surgically by weakening the spring of the cartilage of the pinna so that an antihelical fold can be created. This deformity is ideally corrected at age 5 to 6 years.

Preauricular cysts and sinuses are fairly common and may be unilateral or bilateral. They are usually asymptomatic but may become infected and require incision and drainage and later excision. Complete excision is difficult because of the ramification of these sinuses in close proximity to the branches of the facial nerve. Excision is recommended only if recurrent infection has become a problem.

Severe congenital deformities of the ear are spoken of as microtia and are frequently associated with urinary tract malformations. There may be major developmental defects in the pinna resulting in relatively small and misshaped external ears. With absence of a major portion of the auricular cartilage, surgical reconstruction rarely produces a satisfactory cosmetic result. An artistic prosthesis is the best solution to this cosmetic problem. Microtia is often associated with stenosis or atresia of the external auditory canal. These deformities are often associated with developmental abnormalities in the middle ear resulting in profound conductive hearing losses. The course of the facial nerve in the temporal bone may also be abnormal, and surgical repair of the sound-pressure transformation apparatus of the middle ear is hazardous. In unilateral defects with normal hearing in the other ear, middle ear reconstruction is not recommended because of the danger of facial nerve injury. However, if there is a bilateral profound hearing loss, attempts at reconstruction should be made. A bone conduction hearing aid will contribute to the habilitation if surgical reconstruction is not feasible. Congenital malformations of the inner ear resulting in profound sensorineural hearing losses may or may not be associated with abnormalities of the external and middle ear. The evaluation of congenital malformation of the ear is facilitated by radiography of the temporal bone.

## IDIOPATHIC DISEASES

### Otosclerosis

Otosclerosis is the most common cause of a progressive conductive hearing loss in the adult with a normal ear drum. Otosclerosis is a disease of the bone of the otic capsule with predilection for the anterior part of the oval window. Histologically, foci of otosclerosis show irregularly arranged, immature bone interspersed with numerous vascular channels. As the focus of the otosclerotic bone enlarges, it causes ankylosis of the footplate of the stapes and produces a conductive hearing loss. A second site of predilection is the posterior part to the oval window.

Otosclerosis tends to run in families. It is more common in women than in men. Approximately 10 per cent of the adult white population have foci of otosclerosis. Only one in 10 of these, or approximately 1 per cent of the white population, has clinical otosclerosis as evidenced by conductive hearing loss. Otosclerosis is rare in blacks, American Indians, and Japanese. It is common in Asiatic Indians. Otosclerosis also produces a sensorineural hearing loss if the focus is adjacent to the scala media. The conductive hearing loss becomes clinically evident in the late teenage and early adult years. The fixation of the stapes may progress rapidly during pregnancy. The conductive hearing loss can be corrected surgically in the vast majority of instances. With microsurgical techniques, the stapes is removed and replaced by a prosthesis. The most widely used prosthesis is one composed of stainless steel wire and cellulose sponge. The wire, which is shaped like a shepherd's crook, is crimped around the long process of the incus, and the sponge is placed in the oval window (Fig. 12). A membrane forms across the oval window which embeds the stainless steel wire in it. The sound conduction characteristics of this arrangement are excellent. The complication of a profound sensorineural hearing loss occurs in 2 to 4 per cent of patients. If a good initial hearing result is obtained, ordinarily a good result is maintained.

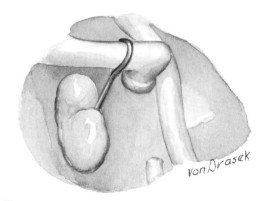

**Figure 12** Stapedectomy with replacement of the stapes with a stainless steel wire and cellulose sponge prosthesis. The wire is crimped around the long process of the incus, and the cellulose sponge is in the oval window. (From Shambaugh, G. E., Jr.: Surgery of the Ear. 2nd ed. Philadelphia, W. B. Saunders Company, 1967.)

### Meniere's Disease

Meniere's disease is characterized by hearing loss, tinnitus, and recurrent prostrating vertigo. The pathologic change in the inner ear is generalized dilatation of the membranous labyrinth, or endolymphatic hydrops. Only one ear is involved in 85 per cent of the patients with Meniere's disease. The sensorineural hearing loss is initially more severe in the lower frequencies than in the higher frequencies. The hearing tends to fluctuate. It is depressed after an attack of vertigo. The tinnitus has a low-pitched, roaring quality and is worse just before, during, and after an attack of vertigo. The attacks of vertigo occur suddenly, last from a few to 24 hours, and subside gradually. The attacks are associated with nausea and vomiting. The patient often has a full feeling or a pressure sensation in the affected ear. Over the course of many years, the hearing becomes progressively worse.

Neither medical nor surgical therapy has been demonstrated to be effective in Meniere's disease. A number of operations have been advocated for the treatment of the patient who is disabled by the frequency of the recurrent attacks of vertigo. Von Fick introduced the sacculotomy in which the saccule is ruptured with a pick placed through the footplate of the stapes. Cody has advocated the placement of a stainless steel tack through the footplate of the stapes so that a sacculotomy is performed each time the membranous labyrinth begins to distend. House has advocated the production of an artificial communication between the membranous labyrinth and subarachnoid space.[9] A labyrinthectomy can be performed if the vertigo is sufficiently disabling and the hearing has degenerated to a useless level.

### Bell's Palsy

Bell's palsy is an idiopathic unilateral facial paralysis that develops suddenly and is accompanied by pain in the postauricular area. All divisions of the nerve are paralyzed; this distinguishes the disease from a supranuclear lesion. The lesion is in the vertical portion of the intratemporal course of the nerve. The initial pathologic changes are hyperemia and edema. The edema compresses the blood supply to the nerve because of the bony confines of the fallopian canal. A conduction block develops without death or degeneration of the axons. Release of the pressure on the nerve results in rapid recovery of function. This type of paralysis is spoken of as neurapraxia. It should be differentiated from axonotmesis in which the pressure on the nerve is sufficiently severe to result in death of the axons distal to the compression within a period of several days. Neurotmesis designates complete transection of the facial nerve. In neurapraxia the flow of axoplasm has been interrupted; with resumption of the flow of axoplasm, the function of the distal axon recovers.

Nerve excitability testing is performed to determine whether neurapraxia or axonotmesis or neurotmesis exists. As long as muscular contraction can be induced at approximately the same direct current stimulus intensity on the affected side as on the normal side, the paralysis is probably a neurapraxia, and complete recovery may be anticipated. Loss of nerve excitability is an indication for decompression of the facial nerve by removing the bone of the fallopian canal through a mastoidectomy approach. Approximately 85 per cent of all patients with idiopathic facial nerve paralysis recover spontaneously. If recovery has not begun at 3 weeks after the onset of the facial paralysis, the chance of spontaneous recovery is greatly reduced. Ordinarily, facial nerve decompression is performed 3 weeks after the onset if there has been no recovery, or at any time when the nerve excitability deteriorates.

## NEOPLASMS

Squamous cell and basal cell carcinomas frequently develop on the pinna of those who are exposed to the sun. Early lesions can be successfully treated with irradiation or cautery and curettage. Surgical excision of a V-shaped wedge or larger amounts of the pinna is required in more advanced lesions. Invasion of cartilage usually dictates against radiation therapy and makes surgery the treatment of choice. Squamous cell and basal cell carcinomas also arise in the external auditory canal and under these circumstances require extensive resection in order to offer the best chance of cure. En bloc resection of the external auditory canal with sparing of the facial nerve is performed for lesions that are limited to the ear canal and have not invaded the middle ear.[5] Squamous cell carcinoma may arise in the middle ear. Persistent otorrhea of chronic otitis media predisposes to squamous cell carcinomas arising in the middle ear and the external auditory canal. Squamous cell carcinoma involving the middle ear requires resection of the temporal bone to obtain an adequate margin around the tumor.

Ceruminomas arise in the outer one-third of the external auditory canal. Although these tumors appear to be benign histologically, they behave in a malignant manner and should be widely excised.

Chemodectomas arise in the middle ear. These nonchromaffin paragangliomas are called glomus jugulare or glomus tympanicus tumors depending on their site of origin. The glomus tympanicus tumor arises from the area of Jacobson's nerve in the tympanic plexus on the promontory of the middle ear. The glomus jugulare tumor arises from the glomus jugulare body in the jugular bulb. Both tumors consist of rich networks of vascular spaces surrounded by epithelioid cells. Usually the tumors grow slowly, and symptoms may not be evident until the tumor is quite large. Pulsatile tinnitus, facial nerve paralysis, otorrhea, hemorrhage, vertigo, and paralysis of cranial nerves IX, X, XI, and XII are often the presenting symptoms and signs. Characteristically, a red mass that pulsates and blanches with compression with a pneumatic otoscope can be seen in the ear canal or middle ear.

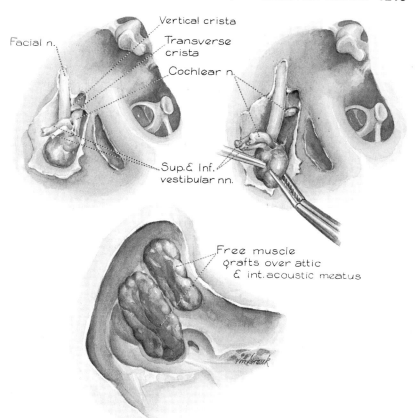

**Figure 13** Translabyrinthine approach to the internal auditory canal for acoustic neurinomas. (From Shambaugh, G. E., Jr.: Surgery of the Ear. 2nd ed. Philadelphia, W. B. Saunders Company, 1967.)

There may be x-ray evidence of bone erosion in the mastoid process, middle ear, or petrous pyramid. Treatment consists of excision of the smaller tumors with or without a radical mastoidectomy. With large lesions, radiation therapy is the treatment of choice.

Acoustic neurinomas account for approximately 7 per cent of all intracranial tumors. They arise twice as often from the vestibular division of the eighth nerve as from the auditory division. These tumors are derived from Schwann cells. Initially, they produce tinnitus and a neural hearing loss. The patient complains of unsteadiness or imbalance. True vertigo is not a common complaint. The hearing loss is predominantly a high-tone loss with greater impairment of the speech discrimination than would be expected with a cochlear lesion producing the same amount of pure-tone hearing loss. Békésy audiometry is Type III or IV.[11] Loudness recruitment is absent. Tone decay is present. The short increment sensitivity index is low.[12] Hallpike caloric testing usually shows canal paresis on the involved side.[4] Initially, the tumor is confined to the internal auditory meatus. As it increases in size, it projects into the cerebellopontine angle and begins to compress the cerebellum and brain stem. With the passage of time, the fifth and ultimately the seventh cranial nerves become involved. Papilledema is a late sign of acoustic neurinomas. Early diagnosis is based on auditory findings suggesting a neural loss of hearing, hypoactivity on caloric stimulation, laminagraphy and polytomography of the internal auditory meatus, and myelography of the posterior fossa. Large acoustic neurinomas are removed through an occipital craniotomy. For the removal of small tumors microsurgical approaches have been developed that utilize a translabyrinthine route if no useful hearing remains and a middle cranial fossa route for the preservation of the remaining hearing (Fig. 13). Both routes allow preservation of the facial nerve. For very large tumors, the combined occipital and translabyrinthine approach offers the best chance of complete removal.[10]

## THE NOSE AND THE PARANASAL SINUSES

In ancient India, adultery was punished by amputation of the nose. Suśruta circa A.D. 1000 described the reconstruction of the nose with a pedicle flap from the cheek. Another ancient Indian method described the forehead flap. Tagliacozzi in Renaissance Italy developed the arm-to-nose pedicle graft. Sir William Ferguson in 1845 introduced an approach for tumors of the nose and paranasal sinuses. It included splitting the lip in the midline as well as a horizontal incision along the inferior orbital rim to reflect the soft tissues of the face laterally. Ingals introduced nasal septal surgery by partial excision of the nasal septum for deviation of the septum in 1882. This operation was later improved by Krieg in 1899 and by Freer in 1902.

In 1903, Killian was the first to operate for an infection in the frontal sinus; and in 1904, he refined the submucous resection of the nasal septum. Joseph, at the turn of the century in Berlin, developed techniques and principles upon which the modern rhinoplasty is based.

## ANATOMY OF THE NOSE AND PARANASAL SINUSES

The skeleton of the nose consists of the nasal bones, the ascending processes of the maxilla, the upper lateral cartilages, the lower lateral cartilages, and the septal cartilage. The nasal septum makes up the medial wall of each nasal cavity. The lateral wall of each nasal cavity provides the attachment for the three turbinates. The inferior turbinate is the largest of the three. It extends from far anterior in the nasal cavity to the choana. The middle turbinate is somewhat smaller. Although it extends to the choana, its anterior tip is 2 cm. posterior to the anterior tip of the inferior turbinate. Its attachment to the lateral wall of the nasal cavity is oblique from superior anteriorly to inferior posteriorly. The superior turbinate arises from the far posterior-superior portion of the lateral wall of the nasal cavity. Inferior to the inferior turbinate is the inferior meatus. The nasolacrimal duct opens into the inferior meatus. The middle meatus lies between the middle turbinate and the inferior turbinate. The ostia of the maxillary and anterior ethmoid cells and the nasofrontal duct are in the middle meatus. The superior meatus lies between the superior turbinate and the middle turbinate. The ostia of the posterior ethmoid cells are in the superior meatus. The ostium of the sphenoid sinus is in the posterior part of the superior meatus, the sphenoethmoid recess.

## TRAUMA AND FOREIGN BODIES

### Nasal Fracture

The nose is a vulnerable leading part. Fractures of the nasal bones are the most common fractures of the facial bones. Fractures of the nose may involve the ascending processes of the maxillas and the nasal processes of the frontal bones as well as the nasal bones. A fracture of the nose is nearly always an open fracture. The skin of the dorsum of the nose may be lacerated, and the mucous membrane in the nasal cavity is nearly always torn. The most common deformity is a deviation of the nasal bones to the right with depression of the nasal bones on the left, characteristically occurring with a right hook. Fractures of the nose may be associated with septal fractures and hematomas.

Fractures of the nasal bones are almost always associated with bleeding from the nose due to the tear of the mucous membrane. A fracture should be suspected if blunt injury causes bleeding from the nose. Soft tissue swelling occurs fairly promptly and may tend to obscure the underlying bony

deformity. Ecchymosis may spread into the upper and lower eyelids. The diagnosis can ordinarily be established by gentle palpation of the dorsum of the nose. Any deformity suggests a fracture. At times instability and crepitus may be demonstrated as well as point tenderness. X-rays of the nasal bones will tend to confirm the diagnosis. Linear radiolucencies parallel to the long axis of the nasal bones are usually nutrient vessels. Radiolucencies transverse to the long axis of the nasal bones are usually fractures. Displacement of the bony fragments may be demonstrated; however, the degree of displacement is more readily determined by physical examination.

Fractures of the nasal complex are often associated with fractures of other facial bones, and x-rays of the paranasal sinuses are obtained if there is suspicion of fracture of the other facial bones. Trauma to the facial bones is often associated with a cerebrospinal fluid rhinorrhea. After injury to the central portion of the face, the patient is specifically examined for cerebrospinal fluid rhinorrhea by having him tip his head forward and collecting any drainage from the nose. Any watery fluid is examined for glucose content to differentiate cerebrospinal fluid from nasal mucus. Cerebrospinal rhinorrhea requires prophylactic antibiotic therapy to prevent meningitis. The patient is instructed to avoid blowing the nose. In most cases cerebrospinal fluid rhinorrhea ceases spontaneously. If the rhinorrhea does not cease within 14 to 21 days, the dural leak is repaired through a frontal craniotomy.

Nasal fractures in adults may be reduced under local anesthesia. General anesthesia is necessary for the reduction of nasal fractures in children. The local anesthesia required is similar to that used for a rhinoplasty. Thorough anesthesia is the key to a satisfactory reduction of the nasal bones. The fracture is manipulated into a good position by internal traction on the fracture fragments with a blunt periosteal elevator in association with external traction with the fingers. The need for internal and external splinting depends on the postreduction stability of the fracture.

If blunt trauma to the nose is neglected, it results in permanent deformity which ultimately requires septal surgery to improve the airway and rhinoplasty to improve the appearance of the nose.

Fractures of the nasal septum may be reduced at the same time as the reduction of the fracture of the nasal bone. Often these fractures are difficult to maintain in a position of good alignment and require a subsequent submucous resection of the nasal septum.

Septal hematomas lie between the quadrilateral cartilage and the perichondrium. If the perichondrium has been elevated from both sides of the septal cartilage, the cartilage will undergo avascular necrosis. Septal hematomas frequently become infected, and abscess formation produces avascular and septic necrosis of the septal cartilage which results in a saddle deformity of the nose. Septal hematomas are incised and drained as soon as the diagnosis is made. An incision in the mucoperichondrium over the anterior part of the hematoma allows access for aspiration. The perichondrium is placed in contact with the septal cartilage by packing the nasal cavity with petrolatum gauze.

Septal abscesses are located between the cartilage and the perichondrium. They may involve both sides of the cartilage. Septal abscesses are incised and drained under general anesthesia as soon as the diagnosis is established. Incisions are made bilaterally if there is pus on both sides of the septum. A small rubber drain is sutured to a lip of the wound until the drainage subsides. Vigorous systemic antibiotic therapy is employed.

### Deviations of the Nasal Septum

Deviations of the nasal septum may be caused by trauma or occur as developmental abnormalities, particularly in persons with highly arched palates. The nasal bones and septum are frequently fractured at the time of birth. This injury is of the greenstick type, and often it will correct itself. However, correction is usually simply accomplished by moving the nose digitally back toward the midline. Slight anterior traction is applied to the tip of the nose during this maneuver. No internal or external splinting is required.

Deviations of the nasal septum produce varying degrees of nasal obstruction and predispose the patient to sinusitis, particularly if the deviation tends to obstruct one of the ostia of the paranasal sinuses during acute inflammatory processes, and to epistaxis as a result of drying air currents over the deflected septum. The caudal edge of the nasal septum may be dislocated and produce an external deformity at the columella.

Deviations of the septum are corrected by submucous resection of the nasal septum. In this procedure, the mucoperichondrium is elevated from both sides of the septum. The deviated cartilage and bone are resected or remodeled to straighten the septum.

Perforations of the nasal septum may be secondary to nasal surgery or repeated trauma, as in picking the nose. In the past, perforations due to syphilis and tuberculosis were common. Perforations of the septum produce crusting about their margins and repeated epistaxis. Small perforations whistle. Septal perforations are closed by the development of opposing mucoperichondrial flaps over free grafts of fascia.[6]

Rhinoplasty is performed for physiologic as well as cosmetic purposes. A deformed nose is usually associated with airway obstruction. The aims of rhinoplasty are to eliminate the airway obstruction and to correct the external deformity of the nose. Usually rhinoplasty is performed under local anesthesia. The surgical procedure is directed toward the cartilaginous and bony framework of the nose. The soft tissue of the nose conforms postoperatively to the modification of the bony and cartilaginous framework. As a general rule, modification of each element of the nasal skeleton is necessary in order to achieve aesthetically pleasing results. Saddle deformities of the nose may be corrected by augmentation with autogenous bone or silicone rubber implants.

### Foreign Bodies

Children put all manner of objects in their noses. Erasers, beans, buttons, pebbles, wool nap, paper, and sponge rubber are common foreign bodies. A foreign body in the nasal cavity produces a severe inflammatory reaction and causes a foul-smelling, bloody, unilateral discharge. Removal of the foreign body is facilitated by producing vasoconstriction anterior to it with a topical sympathomimetic amine such as phenylephrine. The foreign body is removed by placing a blunt hook posterior to it and raking it anteriorly. Attempts at grasping smooth, firm foreign bodies with forceps tend to push them farther posteriorly. General anesthesia is used if good cooperation from a child cannot be obtained by gentle reassurance.

If a foreign body dwells long in the nose, mineral salts are deposited on it and produce a rhinolith. The rhinolith tends to conform to the contour of the nasal cavity, and its removal is usually difficult.

## SINUSITIS

Acute rhinitis is the usual manifestation of a common cold. Acute sinusitis is usually initiated by an acute respiratory tract infection of viral etiology. Nearly all cases of acute sinusitis and most cases of chronic sinusitis respond well to antibiotic therapy. The complications of acute and chronic sinusitis often require surgery, as does unresponsive chronic sinusitis. Complications of maxillary sinusitis are rare. Ethmoid sinusitis is frequently complicated in children by orbital cellulitis and abscess. Eighty per cent of all cases of orbital cellulitis are secondary to ethmoid sinusitis. In the patient who presents with erythema and swelling of the eyelids, proptosis, and displacement of the globe laterally and inferiorly, the source of the infection is sought by inspection of the nose for mucopus in the middle meatus and radiography of the paranasal sinuses for ethmoid sinusitis. Ethmoid sinusitis and its orbital cellulitis respond well to systemic antibiotic therapy. If the proptosis fails to subside or progresses, incision and drainage of the abscess, which is between the lamina papyracea and the orbital periosteum, is performed through a Killian incision that extends from the lateral aspect of the nose to the eyebrow. The orbital periosteum is elevated from the medial wall of the orbit so that the abscess cavity can be reached. The optic nerve tolerates 11 to 14 mm. of proptosis. The point at which extraocular motion is lost is also the limit of stretch of the optic nerve. Therefore, incision and drainage of an orbital abscess is performed prior to complete loss of extraocular motion to prevent permanent blindness.

Frontal sinusitis may cause intracranial complications such as meningitis, epidural abscess, subdural empyema, and brain abscess. In severe acute frontal sinusitis that fails to respond promptly to systemic antibiotic therapy, the anterior wall of the frontal sinus is trephined through an incision in the medial part of the eyebrow. An opening of approximately 7 to 8 mm. is made, and a catheter is placed in the sinus to maintain drainage. Trephination is performed in an attempt to prevent the intracranial complications of frontal sinusitis.

Fractures of the frontal sinus lead to the development of mucoceles. Mucoceles result from duplication of the mucous membrane. They gradually enlarge and destroy the floor of the frontal sinus; and as they expand into the orbital cavity, they produce proptosis and inferior and lateral displacement of the eye. Mucoceles and other other forms of chronic frontal sinusitis that do not respond to medical management can be managed surgically by an osteoplastic flap approach for obliteration of the frontal sinus (Fig. 14). The incision in the bone is made at the periphery of the frontal sinus, and the anterior wall is rotated inferiorly on the hinge of periosteum at the floor of the sinus. Infected mucous membrane is removed with a motor-driven burr, and the cavity of the frontal sinus is obliterated by the implantation of fat taken from the abdominal wall.

Approximately 25 per cent of cases of chronic maxillary sinusitis are secondary to a dental infection. In chronic maxillary sinusitis, radiographs of the apices of the teeth should be obtained to exclude the possibility of a periapical abscess.

Chronic maxillary sinusitis that does not respond to medical management may be controlled with the Caldwell-Luc operation, which is a maxillary sinusotomy performed through an incision in the canine fossa. The bone of the anterior wall of the maxillary sinus is resected to permit access to the interior of the sinus for removal of infected mucous membrane, cysts, and epithelial debris. Drainage of the maxillary sinus is improved by creating a nasoantral window in the inferior meatus.

Chronic ethmoid sinusitis is usually associated with allergic rhinitis and the formation of nasal polyps. In those persons in whom the formation of nasal polyps and the symptoms of ethmoid sinusitis cannot be controlled adequately by intranasal polypectomy and medical management including desensitization, an ethmoidectomy is indicated. Ethmoidectomy is performed intranasally and through an external approach utilizing a Killian incision. In the external ethmoidectomy, the orbital periosteum is elevated, and the lamina papyracea is removed to give access to the ethmoid air cells. Infected mucous membrane, polypoid tissue, and epithelial debris are removed. The anterior one-half of the middle turbinate is excised to create a large opening between the ethmoid air cells and the nasal cavity. In essence, an ethmoid-

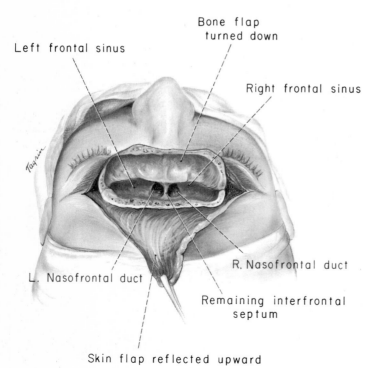

Bone flap
turned down

Left frontal sinus

Right frontal sinus

R. Nasofrontal duct

L. Nasofrontal duct

Remaining interfrontal septum

Skin flap reflected upward

**Figure 14** Approach to the frontal sinuses by the use of an osteoplastic flap for obliteration of the sinuses. (From Goodale, R. L., and Montgomery, W. W.: Arch. Otolaryng., 79:522, 1964.)

VIEW FROM HEAD OF THE TABLE

ectomy incorporates the ethmoid air cell area into the nasal cavity.

Chronic sphenoid sinusitis that does not respond to medical management may be controlled by an operation in which the sphenoid sinus is approached through an external ethmoidectomy. After an external ethmoidectomy has been accomplished, the anterior wall of the sphenoid sinus is resected to remove infected mucous membrane, polypoid tissue, and epithelial debris. The anterior and inferior walls of the sphenoid sinus are removed. In this way, the interior of the sphenoid sinus is incorporated in the posterior part of the nasal cavity and the nasopharynx, and in essence, the sphenoid sinus is eliminated as a separate entity.

## EPISTAXIS

Bleeding from the nose is a common clinical problem. Ninety per cent of the time epistaxis is from a plexus of vessels in the anterior-inferior part of the septum. In the other 10 per cent of cases nasal bleeding occurs from the posterior part of the nose, particularly from far posterior in the inferior meatus at the junction of the inferior meatus and the nasopharynx. It is from this area that persons with arteriosclerosis and hypertension are likely to bleed. This type of bleeding may be difficult to control and is associated with a 4 to 5 per cent mortality. Mild epistaxis from the anterior part of the nasal septum is usually effectively controlled by steady pressure applied by squeezing the mobile portion of the nose between the index finger and thumb for 5 to 10 minutes. Treatment for epistaxis that is not controlled by this simple measure requires visualization of the bleeding point. The bleeding point can be controlled temporarily and anesthesia achieved with pressure applied over a cotton pledget impregnated with a vasoconstrictor and a topically active local anesthetic such as tetracaine (Pontocaine). The bleeding point can be cauterized chemically or with electrocautery. Silver nitrate is preferred as the

cauterizing agent since it produces satisfactory intravascular coagulation without a severe burn of the mucous membrane. If the bleeding cannot be easily controlled with cautery or if the bleeding point cannot be visualized, strips of 1/2 inch petrolatum gauze are used to apply pressure to the bleeding point. Pressure is applied as atraumatically as possible. This method is preferred in a bleeding tendency since the periphery of a cauterized area may begin to bleed.

In order to pack the posterior part of the nasal cavity, the choana is obstructed with a postnasal pack (Fig. 15). The postnasal pack is made by folding and rolling 4 × 4 inch gauze squares into a tight pack and tying the pack with two strands of No. 2 black silk. The ends of one tie are oriented inferiorly, and the ends of the other tie are oriented superiorly. After topical anesthesia of the nose, nasopharynx, and pharynx has been induced, a catheter is introduced through the nasal cavity on the side of the bleeding and brought out through the mouth. The superiorly oriented ends of the tie are tied to the catheter, and the catheter is withdrawn from the nose as the pack is placed posterior to the soft palate into the nasopharynx. The inferiorly oriented ends of the tie are trimmed below the level of the soft palate so that they can be utilized in removing the pack. The superiorly oriented strands are held taut while the nasal cavity is firmly packed with petrolatum gauze. If the bleeding point is in the inferior meatus, this area is packed tightly. The superiorly oriented strands are tied over a roll of a 4 × 4 inch gauze square. The packing is left in place for 4 days. Prophylactic antibiotic therapy is indicated to prevent sinusitis and otitis media. Patients requiring postnasal packing generally have serious systemic vascular diseases. They have a low arterial pO2 while the packing is in place and should remain in an oxygen-enriched atmosphere. Severe epistaxis is often associated with preexisting liver disease. Large amounts of blood may have been swallowed prior to the nasal packing. Blood is eliminated from the gastrointestinal

**Figure 15** Packing of the nose for epistaxis with a postnasal pack and an anterior nasal pack. (From Boies, L. R., et al.: Fundamentals of Otolaryngology, A Textbook of Ear, Nose and Throat Diseases. 4th ed. Philadelphia, W. B. Saunders Company, 1964.)

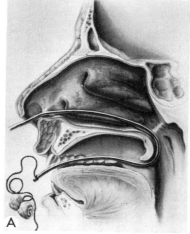
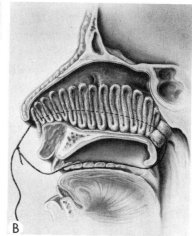

A

B

tract as promptly as possible by the use of cathartics and enemas. Sterilization of the gastrointestinal tract to prevent the breakdown of blood by microorganisms and the absorption of ammonia is indicated in the presence of liver disease. Replacement of blood that has been lost as a result of the epistaxis is carried out as indicated by the hemoglobin and hematocrit determinations as well as by the patient's vital signs.

A particularly debilitating form of epistaxis occurs in hereditary hemorrhagic telangiectasia (Rendu-Osler-Weber disease). Patients with this disease have frequent bleeding from the nose and gastrointestinal tract. Often the bleeding from the nose is sufficient to cause a chronic anemia that cannot be overcome by iron supplementation. A septal dermoplasty, in which the mucous membrane of the anterior portions of the nasal cavity is replaced with a split-thickness skin graft, is very effective in reducing the severity and frequency of the epistaxis so that the hemoglobin concentration may be brought to the normal level.[21]

## CONGENITAL MALFORMATIONS

### Choanal Atresia

Choanal atresia is a malformation in which the opening of the nasal cavity into the nasopharynx is obstructed by a partition of mucous membrane and bone. The malformation may occur unilaterally or bilaterally. If it occurs bilaterally, it produces respiratory distress in the neonate. Newborn infants are obligatory nasal breathers. If there is obstruction to the nasal airway, asphyxia will occur. The newborn presses his tongue against the roof of his mouth during the inspiratory effort. Fortunately, crying with its attendant mouth breathing often allows some ventilatory exchange. This diagnosis should be made in the delivery room. Choanal atresia should be considered in the infant who makes respiratory effort but fails to accomplish ventilatory exchange. The immediate

solution to the problem is the insertion of an oral airway. The nursing care of the oral airway during the next 2 to 3 weeks must be extremely meticulous. After 2 to 3 weeks the newborn learns to breathe through his mouth, and the danger abates. Some advocate perforation of the atretic area in the neonatal period for the insertion of polyethylene tubes. This operation often fails to provide permanent improvement, and a better repair can be performed when the child is 4 to 5 years of age through a transpalatal approach (Fig. 16). With careful nursing supervision of the oral airway, a tracheotomy can be avoided in the neonatal period. The diagnosis is made by attempting without success to pass a catheter through the nose into the pharynx. The diagnosis is confirmed by instilling radiopaque dye into the nasal cavity and taking a lateral x-ray of the nasopharynx in the supine position. If choanal atresia is present, the dye pools in the posterior part of the nasal cavity.

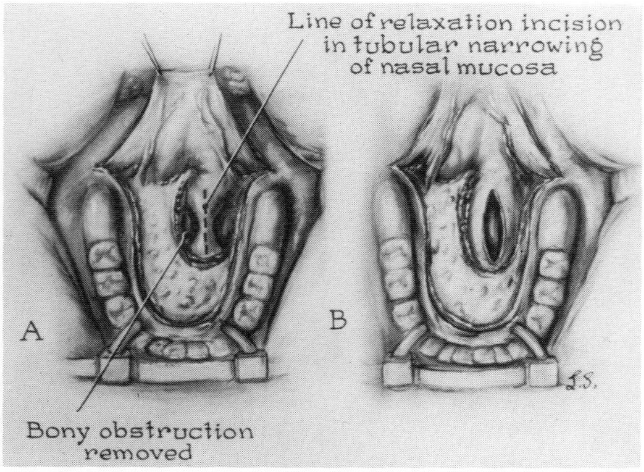

### Nasal Gliomas, Encephaloceles, and Meningoceles

Nasal glioma may present as a malformation of the dorsum of the nose evident at birth or as a mass in the nasal cavity. Nasal gliomas often have intracranial connections. To avoid the development of cerebrospinal fluid rhinorrhea, a frontal craniotomy is performed to exclude the possibility of an intracranial extension prior to the removal of the nasal glioma.[24] Encephaloceles and meningoceles may present in the nasal cavity through defects in the cribriform plate. Clinically they have an appearance similar to that of a nasal polyp. Nasal polyps ordinarily arise from the middle meatus. If what appears to be a nasal polyp does not arise from the middle meatus, thorough investigation to exclude an encephalocele or meningocele is carried out prior to operative intervention. Laminagraphy of the cribriform plate may demonstrate the associated defect in the floor of the anterior cranial fossa.

## NEOPLASMS

### Benign Tumors of the Nose and Paranasal Sinuses

Squamous cell papillomas occur in the nasal cavity and are thought to be caused by papovaviruses. Exophytic papillomas occasionally recur after excision but have a benign course. Inverted papillomas are invasive and behave in a locally malignant manner. They destroy soft tissue and bone and tend to recur following excision. They require removal with a large margin of normal tissue. Fibromas, hemangiomas, and neurofibromas occur occasionally in the nasal cavity. Fibromas, neurolemmomas, and ossifying fibromas occur in the paranasal sinuses.[1]

### Malignant Tumors of the Nose and Paranasal Sinuses

The most common malignant tumor occurring in the nose and paranasal sinuses is the squamous

**Figure 16**  Transpalatal approach for repair of choanal atresia. (From Cherry, J., and Bordley, J. E.: Ann. Otol., 75:911, 1966.)

cell carcinoma. Adenoid cystic carcinomas, adeno-carcinomas (particularly in the ethmoid sinuses), mucoepidermoid carcinomas, malignant mixed tumors, lymphomas, fibrosarcomas, osteosarcomas, chondrosarcomas, and melanomas also occur in the nose and paranasal sinuses.[1] Metastatic tumors may involve the paranasal sinuses, and the most common tumor to metastasize to the paranasal sinuses is the hypernephroma.

Early squamous cell and basal cell carcinomas of the skin of the nose are treated with radiation therapy or cauterization and curettage. Larger carcinomas involving cartilage require excision. Nasal septal carcinomas often require sacrifice of the columella as well as adjacent structures.

A combination of radiation therapy in a tumoricidal dose and radical resection gives the best survival rates in carcinomas and sarcomas of the nasal cavities and paranasal sinuses. Malignant tumors of the lateral wall of the nose require lateral rhinotomy. Malignant tumors of the maxillary sinus require partial or radical maxillectomy.[14] A radical maxillectomy includes exenteration of the orbit. Malignant tumors of the ethmoid sinus require radical resection of the ethmoid complex including exenteration of the orbit and partial maxillectomy. Malignant tumors of the frontal sinus and the sphenoid sinus are not satisfactorily resected and are usually treated with radiation therapy. Lymphomas limited to the nasal cavities or paranasal sinuses are treated with radiation therapy. Disseminated lymphomas require chemotherapy. Melanomas arising in mucous membrane are treated with surgery and radiation therapy, with only rare success.

## THE PHARYNX

Celsus is generally recognized as the first to describe tonsillectomy in his first century *De medicina*. However, the Asiatic Indians frequently performed the operation 1000 years earlier.

### ANATOMY OF THE PHARYNX

For descriptive purposes the pharynx can be divided into the nasopharynx, oropharynx, and hypopharynx. However, from a functional point of view, the pharynx remains united by the constrictors of the pharynx. They have a common insertion in the median pharyngeal raphe and form a musculomembranous tubular passage from the base of the skull to the opening of the esophagus. The lymphoid structures of the pharynx include the pharyngeal tonsil or adenoid, the palatine tonsils, the lateral bands, and the lingual tonsils.

### FOREIGN BODIES

Foreign bodies of the pharynx are likely to be found in four locations: the palatine tonsils, the lingual tonsils, the valleculae, and the pyriform sinuses. Sharp foreign bodies such as fish bones are particularly likely to lodge in the palatine tonsils and the lingual tonsils. Smooth, small, oval

foreign bodies such as capsules are likely to come to rest in the valleculae. Irregular sharp foreign bodies are likely to be retained in the pyriform sinuses. Rarely foreign bodies are coughed into the nasopharynx and become trapped there. Radiopaque foreign bodies may be located in a lateral neck x-ray. Foreign bodies in the palatine tonsil are removed by grasping the foreign body with a hemostat. Foreign bodies in the nasopharynx require general anesthesia for their removal. Foreign bodies of the hypopharynx are removed at direct laryngoscopy under local anesthesia.

## NASOPHARYNX

### The Adenoids

Adenoid hyperplasia in childhood often leads to obstruction of the eustachian tubes and the choanae. This lymphoid hyperplasia may be physiologic or secondary to infectious and allergic manifestations. Obstruction of the eustachian tubes leads to serous or secretory otitis media, recurrent acute otitis media, and exacerbations of chronic otitis media. Obstruction of the choanae produces mouth breathing, a hyponasal voice, and rhinorrhea.

Serous or secretory otitis media is the most common indication for the removal of the adenoid tissue. A sterile effusion in the middle ear in a child lasting 6 weeks or longer, occurring de novo or following acute otitis media, that does not respond to medical management responds regularly but not invariably to adenoidectomy. The use of myringotomies with the insertion of tympanostomy tubes increases the chance of success.

Chronic otitis media in children is another common indication for adenoidectomy. The procedure reduces the severity and frequency of exacerbations of chronic otitis media. It prepares the patient for subsequent mastoidectomy and tympanoplasty. Recurrent acute otitis media is a fairly frequent indication for these procedures. Many children between the ages of 1 and 6 years have two or three episodes of acute otitis media per year which completely resolve with antibiotic therapy. On the other hand, the child who is on antibiotic therapy for otitis media half of the time should be considered for this procedure. The duration of the pain, the presence of spontaneous perforation, the regularity with which myringotomy is required, and the associated systemic symptoms deserve consideration. Febrile convulsions with acute otitis media weigh heavily in favor of adenoidectomy since antibiotic therapy ordinarily is not initiated prior to the convulsion.

Persistent nasal obstruction due to adenoid hyperplasia is a problem in which the age of the patient is considered as well as the severity since lymphoid tissue reaches a relative and absolute maximum at puberty. Persistent and recurrent purulent rhinorrhea in spite of adequate antibiotic therapy is occasionally encountered in association with adenoidal hyperplasia and chronic adenoiditis. Chronic sinusitis in children without an underlying immunologic or other defense mechanism defect such as agammaglobulinemia or hypogammaglobulinemia, pancreatic fibrosis, and Kartagener's syndrome is relatively rare but is rather regularly improved or eliminated by adenoidectomy.

An adenoidectomy is performed under general anesthesia. The adenoid tissue is sheared from the posterior nasopharyngeal wall with a guillotine-type adenotome placed posterior to the soft palate. The lymphoid tissue is removed superficial to the fascia of the superior constrictor of the pharynx without damaging the fascia or the underlying musculature.

### Tornwaldt's Cyst

Cysts frequently form in the region of the medial recess of the nasopharynx. These cysts become symptomatic when they become infected. There may be persistent purulent drainage which has a foul taste and odor. Symptoms of eustachian tube obstruction and sore throat may be prominent. Excision or marsupialization of the cyst with an adenotome is the treatment of choice.

### Benign Neoplasms of the Nasopharynx

Juvenile angiofibromas are very vascular tumors that occur in pubescent males. They develop in the vault of the nasopharynx from the area of the basisphenoid and grow to large size. Angiofibromas may extend into and obstruct the nasal cavity, and their extensions may develop parasitic attachments distant to their site of origin. They may encroach upon the paranasal sinuses and the orbit. Histologically, these tumors are composed of fibrous tissue and numerous thin-walled vessels without contractile elements. Angiofibromas tend to involute at maturity.

Epistaxis is the major problem with angiofibromas, and the magnitude of the bleeding can be very great. The tumors are red and quite firm. Those portions of the tumor that project into the airway often become ulcerated during upper respiratory tract infections and bleed from the ulcerated surface. Their surgical removal is necessitated by recurrent massive bleeding. The extent of the tumor can be determined radiographically. The pterygomaxillary fissure is often widened on the lateral view of the nasopharynx by the extension of the tumor into the infratemporal fossa. These tumors give a characteristic vascular pattern on angiography. Usually, they are removed through a transpalatal approach. Often a lateral rhinotomy offers significant advantages. The blood loss during excision is often very great, and rapid blood replacement is required. These tumors are moderately responsive to radiation therapy. It is often the treatment of choice for the tumor that has invaded the paranasal sinuses and the orbit.

### Malignant Neoplasms of the Nasopharynx

Malignant tumors of the nasopharynx include squamous cell carcinomas, adenocarcinomas, adenoid cystic carcinomas, mucoepidermoid carci-nomas, malignant mixed tumors, melanomas, chordomas, sarcomas including fibrosarcoma, rhabdomyosarcoma, liposarcoma, and myxosarcoma, plasmacytomas, and lymphomas. Among children, the lymphomas and lymphosarcomas are the most common malignant tumors arising from and secondarily involving the nasopharynx. Among the carcinomas, lymphoepithelioma or squamous cell carcinoma is the most common type.

Carcinoma of the nasopharynx occurs at relatively young ages, and there is an unusually high incidence among the Chinese.[15] The majority of patients with carcinoma of the nasopharynx present with nasal or eustachian tube obstruction. Obstruction of the eustachian tube may result in a middle ear effusion. The nasal obstruction may be associated with purulent, bloody rhinorrhea and frank epistaxis. The more dramatic symptoms resulting from cranial nerve paralysis and cervical lymph node metastasis are unfortunately common presenting complaints. Metastasis tends to be limited to the neck until the late stages of the disease. A granular mass or ulcer may be seen in the nasopharynx. The palate may be deformed by the bulk of the nasopharyngeal mass, or its mobility may be limited by paralysis of the levator veli palatini. Not infrequently the tumor extends deep to the mucous membrane, appears only as a slight fullness, and produces no abnormality of the mucous membrane. It is this feature of carcinoma of the nasopharynx that makes biopsy through apparently normal mucous membrane occasionally fruitful.

The diagnosis is made by biopsy of the primary tumor. Adequate access to the nasopharynx ordinarily requires general anesthesia. General anesthesia also allows the opportunity to judge the extent of the primary lesion by palpation. Biopsy of the metastasis in the neck should be avoided until the nasopharynx has been inspected and palpated, and any suspicious lesion has been biopsied. Biopsy of the cervical metastasis violates the integrity of the block of tissue that is removed in a radical neck dissection. It may result in implantation of the tumor in the skin and subcutaneous tissue. The necessity for demonstrating the tumor in the nasopharynx prior to treatment remains even if a histologic diagnosis is obtained from biopsy of the cervical metastasis.

The treatment of choice for carcinoma of the nasopharynx is irradiation with a supervoltage source. The radiation should be delivered to the primary tumor-bearing area of the nasopharynx and to both sides of the neck whether there is clinically demonstrated metastasis or not. Surgery plays no role in the initial therapy of carcinoma of the nasopharynx. Those cervical metastases that remain clinically palpable following radiation therapy or that subsequently become apparent should be eradicated by radical neck dissection. As a general rule, control of the metastatic lesions should be attempted only after there is evidence that the primary lesion has been controlled. Occasionally, the primary lesion in the nasopharynx persists after radiation therapy without evidence of local or distant metastasis. Under these circumstances, cryosurgery may be applied to the persisting tumor in the nasopharynx. The overall 5 year survival for carcinoma of the nasopharynx is approximately 35 per cent.

## OROPHARYNX

### Peritonsillar Abscess

Peritonsillar cellulitis and abscess are complications of acute tonsillitis in which the infection has spread deep to the tonsillar capsule. Pus forms between the tonsillar capsule and the superior constrictor of the pharynx, and the tonsil is displaced medially. The uvula becomes tremendously edematous and is displaced to the opposite side. The soft palate is very red and displaced forward. There is marked trismus due to irritation of the pterygoid muscles, and the head is held tilted toward the side of the abscess. It is painful for the patient to talk and to swallow. Swallowing is so painful that the patient drools. The breath is foul-smelling. The temperature is usually 38 to 40° C. Peritonsillar cellulitis or abscess does not occur in children under the age of 10 to 12 years and is usually caused by a group A beta hemolytic streptococcus. If a cellulitis without pus formation exists, it will respond in a matter of 24 to 48 hours to penicillin therapy. If pus is present, it may resolve or require incision and drainage. The pus may be difficult to locate. Incision is performed as the mucous membrane takes on a pale yellow color overlying the pus. The patient is placed in the sitting position to avoid aspiration of the pus. Under topical anesthesia, the incision is made in the anterior pillar parallel to its free edge. The incision need only split the mucous membrane, and the pus is obtained by spreading gently with a hemostat. No drain is required because the abscess cavity is emptied by each swallow.

These abscesses tend to recur and are an indication for tonsillectomy which is performed 6 weeks after the acute infection. At the time of tonsillectomy, 1 to 2 ml. of pus is usually encountered between the capsule and the tonsillar fossa. This persistent abscess is the apparent reason for the recurrence of these abscesses.

### Parapharyngeal Abscess

Parapharyngeal abscess may occur in infants and young children as well as in adults secondary to streptococcal pharyngitis or tonsillitis. Pus forms in the parapharyngeal space secondarily from the breakdown of lymphadenitis. The pus is located lateral to the superior constrictor of the pharynx and adjacent to the carotid sheath. The tonsil and soft palate may be displaced medially, but there may be no inflammatory reaction in the pharynx. There is marked swelling in the anterior cervical triangle. Penicillin is the antibiotic of choice. Once it becomes fluctuant, the abscess is incised and drained. The abscess is not drained through the lateral pharyngeal wall because of the proximity of the internal carotid artery and the internal jugular vein. An incision is made in a skin fold over the anterior border of the sternocleidomastoid muscle. The anterior border of the muscle is identified, and blunt dissection is carried toward the carotid sheath where the pus is encountered. A drain is sewn in place until the drainage subsides.

### Retropharyngeal Abscess

Retropharyngeal abscess occurs in infants and young children and is rare after the age of 10 years. These infections are located between the constrictors of the pharynx and the prevertebral fascia. They are secondary to pharyngitis and due to the breakdown of retropharyngeal lymphadenitis. Infants with retropharyngeal abscesses usually present with stridor and hyperextension of the neck. A lumbar puncture is the appropriate diagnostic procedure in a febrile infant who presents in opisthotonos. If the cerebrospinal fluid is normal, the possibility of a retropharyngeal abscess must be excluded. The diagnosis is made by palpating the posterior pharyngeal wall. The infant is held in the prone position for the examination so that if the abscess is ruptured during the examination, the pus will flow out of the infant's mouth and not be aspirated. The abscess has a boggy fluctuant texture, and the bodies of the cervical vertebrae are not palpable. Inspection of the pharynx may not demonstrate the abscess because the whole posterior pharyngeal wall may be displaced forward and there may be no inflammatory reaction in the mucous membrane. In order to maintain the airway the child should be allowed to hyperextend the neck. A tracheotomy is rarely necessary. In addition to penicillin therapy, the posterior pharyngeal wall should be incised under general endotracheal anesthesia with the patient in the Rose position. The mucous membrane at the posterior wall of the pharynx is incised vertically. The incision need only split the mucous membrane. The pus is obtained by gently spreading a hemostat in the wound toward the retropharyngeal space. No drain is necessary because the abscess cavity tends to be emptied on swallowing.

### Tonsillectomy

Recurrent acute bacterial tonsillitis due to a group A beta hemolytic streptococcus occurring three to four times during the year in children from 2 to 7 years of age can be adequately managed with penicillin or other appropriate antibiotics if given for 12 days. The rationale for this length of treatment is that a shorter period may not eliminate a streptococcal infection. In addition to inappropriate selection of antibiotics and inadequate duration of therapy, passage of the streptococcus among family members is a cause of failure in the medical management of tonsillitis. This situation requires simultaneous cultures of the whole family and simultaneous treatment of all carriers. In spite of these precautions, in some patients tonsillitis repeatedly develops within a few days after the completion of adequate treatment. When this pattern cannot be altered by medical management, tonsillectomy is indicated.

Chronic tonsillitis with persistent sore throat, either briefly relieved or not at all relieved by antibiotic therapy, constitutes another indication for tonsillectomy. One peritonsillar abscess is an indication for tonsillectomy.

In adults, tonsillectomy is performed under local or general anesthesia. In children, general anesthesia is required. The technique involves an incision in the free edge of the tonsillar pillars. The dissection of the tonsil from the tonsillar fossa is carried out in the plane between the tonsillar capsule and the superior constrictor muscle of the pharynx and is completed by closing a snare placed inferior to the lower pole of the tonsil. The objective is to remove the tonsil and its capsule intact and spare the musculature of the tonsillar fossa.

### Carcinoma of the Tonsil

Carcinoma of the tonsil accounts for 1.5 to 3 per cent of all cancers and is second in frequency only to carcinoma of the larynx among malignant tumors of the upper respiratory tract. It is predominantly a disease of males. Squamous cell carcinoma is the predominant histologic type. These carcinomas may be exophytic with superficial ulceration or deeply invasive. At times they present as lobulated submucosal masses. The tumor frequently extends into the base of the tongue. Carcinoma of the tonsil usually remains asymptomatic until it has reached considerable size. Sore throat is the most common presenting complaint, and pain often radiates to the ear on the same side. Not infrequently the patients present with a metastatic mass in the neck as the first symptom. The diagnosis is established by biopsy of the primary lesion. A promising method of treatment consists of radiation therapy and surgery. A tumoricidal dose of radiation is delivered to the tonsillar fossa and to the same side of the neck. Radical resection of the tonsillar fossa, hemimandibulectomy with disarticulation of the temporomandibular joint, and radical neck dissection are carried out 6 weeks after completion of radiation therapy. The 5 year survival for carcinoma of the tonsil treated by irradiation is approximately 25 per cent.

### HYPOPHARYNX

### Diverticulum of the Hypopharynx

Diverticula of the hypopharynx result from herniation of the mucous membrane of the hypopharynx through weak points in the inferior constrictor muscle; they occur in the older age group. These pulsion diverticula almost always occur on the left side. The sac lies between the prevertebral fascia and the left posterolateral wall of the esophagus. While the origin of the diverticulum is the hypopharynx, the esophagus is compressed by the diverticulum. During deglutition, the diverticulum fills with food and fluid. When the patient lies down, the diverticulum empties into the pharynx, and aspiration of food and fluid into the lower respiratory tract may occur and result in recurrent and debilitating pneumonitis. The diverticulum is demonstrated with a barium swallow. Diverticula are managed surgically by excision through a cervical incision or by endoscopic cautery of the party wall between the cervical esophagus and the diverticulum.

## LARYNX

Caelius Aurelianus credits Asclepiades with having first employed tracheotomy in cynanche (probably diphtheria) in the century before the birth of Christ. In 1778, the French surgeon Pelletan performed a successful laryngofissure for the removal of a bolus of meat that had become entrapped between the vocal cords. In 1854, Manuel Garcia, a Spanish singing teacher, succeeded in observing his own larynx with two mirrors and the sun as a light source. In 1856, Türck and Czermak independently developed the laryngoscope in Vienna. Following the development of the laryngoscope peroral endolaryngeal surgery flourished in many centers. In the 1870s Bergman performed laryngotomies for removal of parts of the larynx involved with carcinoma. Billroth in 1873 performed the first successful laryngectomy.

### ANATOMY OF THE LARYNX

The skeleton of the larynx consists of the thyroid cartilage, the cricoid cartilage, the arytenoid cartilages with the corniculate and cuneiform cartilages, and the epiglottis. Phylogenetically the arytenoid cartilages are the oldest elements of the laryngeal skeleton. This fact emphasizes the primeval role of the larynx as a sphincter rather than a conduit for air. The cricoid cartilage completely encircles the airway and maintains its patency. The arytenoid cartilages articulate with the cricoid cartilage. The true vocal cords are attached to the vocal processes of the arytenoid cartilages and to the isthmus of the thyroid cartilage. The superior surfaces of the true vocal cords are flat, and the inferior surfaces are concave. The inferior surfaces of the false vocal cords are flat, and the superior surfaces of the false vocal cords are convex. The true vocal cords and the false vocal cords make a double-layered sphincter. The configuration of the true vocal cords makes them a good barrier to the ingress of air and a poor barrier to the egress of air. The configuration of the false vocal cords makes them a poor barrier to the ingress of air and a good barrier to the egress of air. The true vocal cords can be thought of as an inlet valve, and the false vocal cords as an outlet valve.

### PHYSIOLOGY OF THE LARYNX

The primary function of the larynx is that of a sphincter. During deglutition both the true vocal cord sphincter and false vocal cord sphincter are closed, and the epiglottis is drawn posterior over the closed sphincters and serves as a watershed deflecting food and fluid into the pyriform sinuses. The larynx also serves as a sphincter during parturition, coughing, and defecation. At these times, it serves primarily as an outlet valve.

During the lifting of heavy objects and climbing hand over hand as in climbing a tree, the pull of the shoulder girdles on the thorax tends to expand the thoracic cage. The larynx limits the ingress of air as an inlet valve and thereby stabilizes the thorax.

The larynx serves as the sounding source for speech. A fundamental tone is produced by the movement of the vocal cords which is brought about by the flow of exhaled air past lightly approximated vocal cords. The fundamental tone and its overtones are modified into meaningful symbols or speech by articulators such as the pharynx, palate, tongue, teeth, and lips. Synchrony of the vibration of the two vocal cords exists normally at any given instant, but aperiodicity over time also occurs. The fundamental tone varies with the sex and age of the individual. Adult males produce a fundamental tone of 125 Hz., and adult females produce a fundamental tone of 250 Hz. In the healthy voice, the overtones of these fundamental tones are whole-number multiples of the fundamental tone. The predominance of harmonic overtones gives the voice a musical quality. The distribution of the harmonics gives the voice a timbre which is characteristic of that individual. In the healthy voice there are frequent changes in the frequency of the fundamental tone which provide it with a melodious quality. The normal speaker uses changes in frequency rather than changes in intensity for emphasis.

## PATHOPHYSIOLOGY OF THE LARYNX

Various pathologic changes in the vocal cords result in the prominence of nonharmonic noise components in the voice. In contrast to the healthy musical voice, overtones that are not whole-number multiples of the fundamental tone produce a noisy voice or hoarseness. Structural changes in the vocal cords result in greater aperiodicity and asynchrony of the vibration of the vocal cords. Aperiodicity and asynchrony disrupt the harmonic relationships of the voice by limiting the possibility of the occurrence of overtones that are whole-number multiples of the fundamental tone. Characteristically, the abnormal voice is monotonous. A monotone may occur because of loss of flexibility in the frequency range of the larynx due to a disease process or it may be acquired as a habit, particularly in speakers who tend to use increases in intensity for emphasis rather than changes in frequency. Structural changes in the vocal cords often interfere with their approximation and result in air wastage which gives the voice a breathy quality.

## STRUCTURAL CHANGES IN THE TRUE VOCAL CORDS SECONDARY TO MISUSE AND ABUSE OF THE VOICE

Abuse and misuse of the voice can result in structural changes in the true vocal cords. Using the voice too loudly and too long produces acute and chronic changes in the true vocal cords. Prolonged use of intensity rather than frequency for emphasis, the employment of a monotone, the affectation of a frequency that is too low, and a very abrupt onset of high intensities (sharp glottal attack) produce structural changes in the true vocal cords.

### Polyps of the Vocal Cords

Polyps of the true vocal cords develop in response to using the voice too loudly and too long, as in the person who must speak over a great deal of background noise in a factory or who demonstrates wares in a department store or barks at a circus or carnival. Chronic subepithelial edema develops in the lamina propria of the true vocal cords. Similar pathologic changes result from chronic allergic reactions and the chronic inhalation of irritants such as tobacco smoke and industrial fumes. Such polypoid swellings of the free edge of the true vocal cord interfere with the approximation of the true vocal cords and with the maintenance of periodicity and synchrony of the vibration of the vocal cords. They produce hoarseness and give a breathy quality to the voice. To restore the voice, polyps are removed with biting forceps at direct laryngoscopy under local or general anesthesia.

### Vocal Nodules

Vocal nodules are caused by using a fundamental frequency that is unnaturally low and using the voice too loudly and too long. Vocal nodules occur in children as well as adults, and are likely to occur in robust, athletic boys 8 to 12 years of age who yell a great deal. Men affect an unnaturally low pitch to give an air of authority; women do it to give an impression of sexiness; and

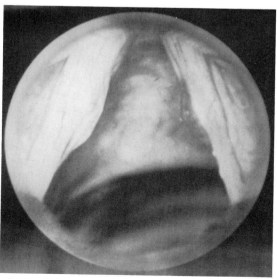

**Figure 17** Direct laryngoscopic view of vocal nodules during inspiration. (From the Jacques Holinger Memorial Fund Collection, courtesy of Dr. Paul H. Holinger.)

young boys probably do it to identify with older males in the family or community. Vocal nodules are condensations of hyaline connective tissue in the lamina propria at the junction of the anterior one-third and the posterior two-thirds of the true vocal cord (Fig. 17). These nodules produce hoarseness and give the voice a breathy quality. In adults, these lesions are removed at direct laryngoscopy to restore the voice. However, it is necessary to begin voice therapy prior to the surgery, because if the underlying misuse of the voice is not corrected, the nodules will recur. In children, surgical removal is not usually necessary because the vocal nodules will regress with voice therapy, which consists of voice rest, reduction in intensity and duration of voice production, and elevation of the pitch.

### Contact Ulcers

Contact ulcers of the larynx are thought to result from misuse and abuse of the voice, particularly in the form of a sharp glottal attack. They occur unilaterally or bilaterally over the vocal process of the arytenoid. The presence of these lesions causes mild pain on phonation and swallowing and varying degrees of hoarseness. The ulcers have a shaggy or granular base. They are biopsied at direct laryngoscopy to exclude the possibility of carcinoma. Voice therapy is important to correct the underlying misuse of the voice. However, prolonged voice rest is required for contact ulcers to heal.

## TRAUMA

Trauma has replaced infectious diseases such as diphtheria, streptococcal croup, syphilis, tuberculosis, rhinoscleroma, and typhoid fever as the most common cause of laryngeal stenosis. Automobile accidents in which the patient is thrown forward and the larynx is crushed between the cervical vertebrae and the object against which he decelerates are the single most important cause of laryngeal stenosis. Children may fracture the larynx by falling against the handlebars of a bicycle or riding a horse or bicycle under a taut line. Another cause of laryngeal stenosis is the high tracheotomy in which a perichondritis of the cricoid cartilage results from the pressure of the tube on the cartilage. Prolonged endotracheal intubation frequently results in subglottic stenosis, as do infectious processes.

Fractures of the thyroid cartilage may result in supraglottic, glottic, or transglottic stenosis. Persons with long slender necks are more likely to sustain supraglottic injuries in which the hyoid bone is also fractured. The suprahyoid muscles are disrupted, and the thyrohyoid membrane is ruptured. Fracture of the cricoid cartilage results in subglottic stenosis. Fractures of the cricoid cartilage are more likely to occur in males with short, thick necks and are relatively rare in females. Often a blow to the neck spares the larynx but transects the trachea.

Patients with crush injuries of the larynx complain of pain on swallowing. Hoarseness may progress to aphonia. Hemoptysis is usually present. Progressive dyspnea due to upper respiratory obstruction is to be anticipated. Subcutaneous emphysema is usually present in fractures of the larynx or trachea. The laryngeal cartilages cannot be distinctly palpated, nor can the trachea, owing to soft tissue swelling. On indirect laryngoscopy, the laryngeal lumen appears disrupted or obliterated, and there may be exposed cartilage and lacerated mucous membrane. Vocal cord paralysis may be noted. X-rays of the lateral neck and laminagrams of the larynx may indicate the type and degree of injury. Lateral neck x-rays may demonstrate associated fractures or dislocations of the cervical vertebrae.

In the initial management of the patient with a laryngeal fracture, a tracheotomy is performed and followed by direct laryngoscopy and tracheoscopy. Often, patients with multiple injuries are treated with a tracheotomy because of the upper airway obstruction, and the reason for the need for the tracheotomy is forgotten during the management of the thoracic and abdominal or perhaps intracranial injuries. The laryngeal trauma is rediscovered 10 or so days later when it appears that it would be appropriate to remove the tracheostomy tube. Evaluation of the larynx should be performed early to be certain that there has not been a fracture of the laryngeal cartilages that requires early repair.

The repair of the fracture is carried out through a transverse incision in the neck. In order to gain access to the interior of the larynx, a laryngofissure is performed by dividing the thyroid cartilage at its isthmus, or the fracture in the thyroid and cricoid cartilage is utilized. Mucous membrane lacerations are repaired, and the cartilages are returned to their normal alignment. Internal splinting is maintained with a solid-core mold for 6 weeks. Failure to reduce a dislocated or fractured cartilage leads to laryngeal stenosis. Late repair of laryngeal stenosis can sometimes be accomplished by an arytenoidectomy. At other times a supraglottic partial laryngectomy is required to restore the airway and the functional integrity of the laryngeal sphincter.[18] A keel is often employed to repair the angle of the anterior commissure. Subglottic stenosis is repaired by excision of the stenotic area and internal splinting for a period of 6 weeks or more. Tracheal stenosis may be managed by dilations, excision of the stenotic area with end-to-end anastomosis of the trachea if the defect is not greater than 2 cm. in length, or excision of the stenotic area with internal splinting for 6 weeks or more.

## FOREIGN BODIES OF THE LARYNX, TRACHEOBRONCHIAL TREE, AND ESOPHAGUS

Foreign bodies are retained in the larynx as a general rule because they are sharp and stick into the mucous membrane or are irregular and soft and are caught between the two vocal cords in laryngospasm. A frequently fatal laryngeal foreign body is a bolus of meat. The resulting laryngospasm completely occludes the larynx, and death takes place rapidly unless a Pelletan is present and establishes an alternate airway by performance of a prompt tracheotomy. This "café coronary" may be distinguished from a myocardial infarct by the respiratory effort without exchange and the marked suprasternal, intercostal, and subxiphoid retraction. Foreign bodies of the larynx induce a degree of laryngospasm that makes their removal difficult without general anesthesia. Even with a nonobstructing foreign body, a tracheotomy is often the first step in its removal, particularly with subglottic foreign bodies such as sand or grass burrs. The site of the foreign body is exposed with a laryngoscope, and the foreign body is grasped, disengaged, and removed with alligator or other appropriate forceps.

Smooth objects such as nuts, kernels of corn, watermelon seeds, beans, peas, and plastic toys pass through the larynx into the tracheobronchial tree. At the onset, there is severe spasmodic coughing which continues for approximately 30 minutes. During this period of time, the foreign body migrates from one portion of the tracheobronchial tree to another. It more frequently comes to rest in the right bronchus because the right bronchus is larger than the left and makes less of an angle with the long axis of the trachea, and the carina is to the left of the midline of the tracheal lumen. As it finally comes to rest, the coughing subsides, and a latent period begins during which the patient is free of symptoms. The mistaken inference is often made by the family and the physician in attendance that the foreign body has been coughed out. However, careful auscultation of the chest may demonstrate an expiratory wheeze and the signs of obstructive emphysema. The most common mechanism of the bronchial obstruction due to a foreign body is a one-way valve through which air may enter the bronchus distal to the foreign body during inspiration but its egress is limited on expiration. This type of obstruction produces emphysema distal to the foreign body. The obstructive emphysema may become apparent radiographically only on expiration (Fig. 18). The mediastinum shifts away from the obstructed lung, and the obstructed portion of the lung becomes radiolucent compared to the normal lung. This type of partial obstruction of the bronchus is likely to occur with the aspiration of nuts. In the evaluation of a patient with a suspected nonradiopaque foreign body of the bronchus, comparison of inspiratory and expiratory chest x-rays and fluoroscopy of the chest may demonstrate obstructive emphysema that would not be apparent on inspiration x-rays.

A foreign body that completely obstructs the bronchus causes the rapid development of a more serious pathophysiologic state. Complete atelectasis of the obstructed lung occurs as a result of absorption of the remaining air in the lung. The mediastinum shifts toward the atelectatic lung, and the remaining lung undergoes compensatory emphysema (Fig. 19). The atelectatic lung is useless as far as ventilatory exchange is concerned, and the efficiency of the emphysematous lung is greatly reduced. Rapid cardiorespiratory failure occurs unless the foreign body is removed. This type of complete bronchial obstruction is likely to occur with smooth hygroscopic foreign bodies like beans that swell in the bronchus.

Vegetable foreign bodies are very poorly tolerated. Metallic and plastic foreign bodies that cause partial obstruction of the bronchus may be tolerated for long periods. Nuts, particularly peanuts, produce a very severe tracheobronchitis. After the latent period of 24 hours, the patient develops a cough productive of purulent sputum, and a febrile course begins. A long-indwelling foreign body of the bronchus may produce bronchiectasis, recurrent pneumonitis, lung abscess, and em-

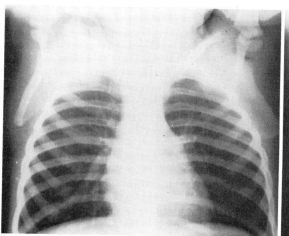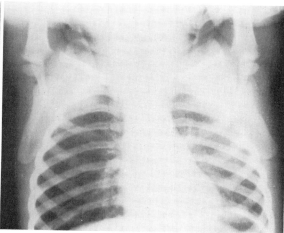

**Figure 18** Posterior-anterior radiographs of the chest on inspiration (left) and expiration (right) from a child with a peanut in the right bronchus. The inspiratory film appears normal. On expiration, the obstructive emphysema becomes evident with radiolucency of the right lung compared to the left and shift of the mediastinum to the left.

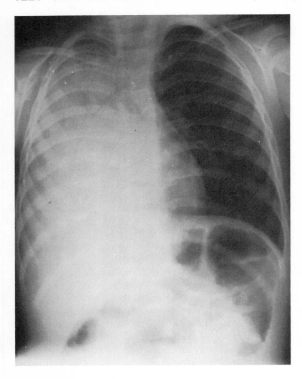

**Figure 19**  Posterior-anterior radiograph of the chest of a child with a pinto bean in the right bronchus. There is atelectasis of the right lung and compensatory emphysema of the left lung.

pyema. Tracheobronchial foreign bodies are removed under general anesthesia through bronchoscopes with forceps designed specifically for each type of foreign body.

Foreign bodies of the esophagus are likely to lodge just below the cricopharyngeus muscle. Ninety-five per cent of esophageal foreign bodies are found in this location. Other locations are the gastroesophageal junction and the indentations of the esophagus caused by the left bronchus and the arch of the aorta. The constrictors of the pharynx are very strong and can propel almost any irregular object through the cricopharyngeus muscle (Fig. 20). Once the foreign body has passed the cricopharyngeus, the muscular activity is very weak, and progress occurs mainly by gravity. Therefore, irregular objects are brought to a very abrupt stop just below the cricopharyngeus muscle.

The symptoms of a foreign body of the esophagus are dysphagia and pain in the suprasternal area on swallowing. Bulky foreign bodies in the cervical esophagus may produce upper airway ob-

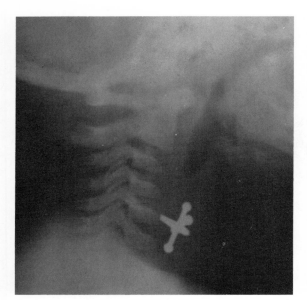

**Figure 20**  Lateral radiographic view of the neck demonstrating a jack in the cervical esophagus of a child.

struction by extrinsic pressure through the membranous posterior wall of the trachea. Foreign bodies can be identified on a lateral neck x-ray if they are radiopaque (Fig. 20). If they are radiolucent, evidence of a foreign body may still be obtained since the foreign body tends to hold the esophageal walls apart and air may be seen in the cervical esophagus. If the foreign body cannot be located on a lateral neck x-ray, PA and lateral chest x-rays are taken. If the foreign body cannot be located in this manner, an esophagogram may demonstrate it. A small pledget of cotton saturated with a solution of barium sulfate may hang on a sharp foreign body. A foreign body of the esophagus is removed under general anesthesia through an esophagoscope. The foreign body is grasped, disengaged, and removed as a trailing foreign body or through the esophagoscope with a foreign body forceps appropriate to the object. The longer a foreign body remains in the esophagus, the greater the risk of perforation of the esophagus. Perforation of the esophagus results in air and soft tissue swelling in the paraesophageal tissue, which may be demonstrated on physical examination and radiographically.

## INFECTIOUS DISEASES

### Croup

There are two forms of croup, epiglottitis and laryngotracheobronchitis. Croup occurs primarily in children over 1 year and under 5 years of age. It may be viral or bacterial. Parainfluenza Type I is the most frequently isolated agent in viral croup. *Haemophilus influenzae*, Staphylococcus, and Streptococcus also cause croup. Both epiglottitis and laryngotracheobronchitis may produce the rapid onset of upper respiratory obstruction with inspiratory stridor and suprasternal, supraclavicular, intercostal, and subxiphoid retractions. The voice may be hoarse, and the cough has a brassy quality with subglottic edema. With firm depression of the tongue, the epiglottis in epiglottitis appears as a rounded, red mass like a cherry on the base of the tongue. In laryngotracheobronchitis, the major problem is subglottic edema. The treatment for both conditions is a humidified atmosphere. The airway obstruction results in part from edema, but there are also tenacious mucoid secretions. Humidification of the inspired atmosphere liquefies this material, and the patient may cough it out to reduce the degree of airway obstruction. Antibiotic therapy is initiated at the onset of the disease, and ampicillin is the drug of choice since the infection is frequently caused by *Haemophilus influenzae*. Corticosteroid therapy is also initiated in an attempt to reduce the inflammatory swelling. A tracheotomy is far more likely to be required in epiglottitis than in laryngotracheobronchitis. The decision regarding a tracheotomy depends on the evaluation of the amount of ventilatory exchange that is taking place, the degree of fatigue of the patient, and the respiratory and pulse rates. Development of cyanosis is a late sign, and the decision to perform a tracheotomy should be made prior to the advent of this ominous sign. Blood gas determinations are not of great value in this particular situation because the clinical situation may change so rapidly. If it appears that the ventilatory exchange is inadequate, the necessary ventilatory effort cannot be maintained, or there is a progressive increase in the pulse rate above 140 per minute, a tracheotomy is performed. The airway emergency is converted to an elective tracheotomy by inserting an endotracheal tube or a bronchoscope. General anesthesia is induced, and the tracheotomy is performed in a relaxed patient under unhurried and ideal circumstances. This approach reduces the incidence of the complications such as pneumothorax.

### Tracheotomy

The indications for tracheotomy fall into three broad categories: upper respiratory obstruction, inability to handle upper respiratory secretions, and inability to handle lower respiratory secretions. Among those causes of upper respiratory obstruction that frequently require tracheotomy are congenital malformations of the upper respiratory tract, croup, diphtheria, foreign bodies, bilateral vocal cord paralyses, neoplasms of the larynx, postintubation edema, allergic reactions, and maxillofacial and laryngeal trauma. The importance of a tracheotomy in patients who are having difficulty handling upper respiratory secretions became well recognized during the polio epidemics. Neurologic problems other than infections, such as intracranial trauma and neoplasms, also lead to difficulty in handling upper respiratory secretions. Patients with ineffective respiratory effort on a neurologic or mechanical basis, chronic obstructive pulmonary disease, and parenchymal infections may have difficulty handling lower respiratory secretions.

A tracheotomy has several advantages and disadvantages. It relieves upper respiratory obstruction. It allows more effective access to the lower respiratory tract for suctioning the tracheobronchial tree. It decreases the dead space and reduces the work required for effective ventilation. A tracheotomy can readily be used as a route for the delivery of respiratory assistance. It eliminates the normal warming and humidification of the inspired air by bypassing the upper respiratory tract. A very serious disadvantage of the tracheotomy is the loss of an effective cough. It opens the lower respiratory tract to environmental pathogens and increases the vulnerability to Pseudomonas infections.

### Juvenile Papillomas of the Larynx

Papillomas of the larynx are thought to be of viral etiology. Although these lesions may occur as early as 1 year of age, they more commonly make their appearance in the second and third year of life. Papillomas may recur promptly after excision. Exuberant growth from multiple sites in the larynx makes maintenance of an adequate airway difficult. Eventually, most children with laryngeal papillomas require a tracheotomy. The papillomas are periodically removed gingerly at direct laryngoscopy under general anesthesia to maintain the voice so that the child can recite in class and to maintain the airway.

## CONGENITAL MALFORMATIONS

Congenital malformations of the larynx may produce varying degrees of airway obstruction. Among the well recognized causes of laryngeal obstruction encountered in the immediate neonatal period are bilateral vocal cord paralyses and subluxation of the arytenoids secondary to traumatic delivery, laryngomalacia or the exaggerated infantile larynx, stenosis and atresia of the larynx, cysts, and subglottic hemangioma.[23] Tracheal obstruction may be due to intrinsic tracheal lesions such as tracheomalacia, absence of tracheal rings, and tracheal stenosis, and to extrinsic tracheal compression from tumors of the thyroid, thymus, esophagus and mediastinum, and the vascular rings. Tetany of the newborn with laryngospasm is usually recognized by other characteristics of this condition. Newborns with tracheoesophageal fistulas certainly have respiratory distress due to aspiration, but usually no true airway obstruction.

In the delivery room, exposure of the vocal cords with a laryngoscope will relieve the obstruction of an exaggerated infantile larynx, in which the flexible epiglottis and arytenoids prolapse into the glottis with inspiration. Inserting a laryngoscope will not relieve obstruction from bilateral vocal cord paralyses, stenosis, or subglottic hemangiomas. Insertion of a 3.5 mm. bronchoscope will improve ventilation in these laryngeal lesions but will not relieve tracheal obstruction until the bronchoscope is passed beyond it. These maneuvers are of the utmost risk to a newborn and should not be undertaken unless the infant's exchange is inadequate for survival. In general, if the exchange is adequate, the infant should be managed expectantly in the neonatal period. Most forms of congenital stridor improve with time. Inappropriate instrumentation may convert a tolerable degree of airway obstruction into one requiring a tracheotomy. A tracheotomy in a newborn is hazardous and difficult to manage.

## LARYNGOCELES

Laryngoceles are epithelium-lined diverticula of the laryngeal ventricle and may be located internal or external to the laryngeal skeleton. An internal laryngocele may displace and enlarge the false vocal cord and may result in hoarseness and airway obstruction. External laryngoceles pass through the thyrohyoid membrane and present as a mass in the neck over the thyrohyoid membrane. The mass rises with the larynx on swallowing. Internal and external laryngoceles may coexist. Laryngoceles are more common in glassblowers,

wind instrument musicians, and others who develop high intraluminal pressures. Initially, laryngoceles are filled with air and expand and collapse with changes in the intraluminal pressure. They are expanded during the Valsalva maneuver. They appear as a smooth, ovoid, radiolucent mass on x-rays of the neck. Laryngoceles may fill with mucoid fluid and may become infected, under which circumstance the term laryngopyocele is appropriate. External laryngoceles are excised through a transverse cervical incision. The sac is dissected from surrounding tissue to its point of penetration of the thyrohyoid membrane. The sac is transected, and the mucous membrane of the ventricle is repaired. Internal laryngoceles are managed by the same approach but require extension of the dissection into the larynx through a thyrotomy.

## NEOPLASMS

Benign neoplasms including papillomas, fibromas, myxomas, chondromas, neurofibromas, hemangiomas, and so forth, may involve any part of the larynx including the true vocal cords. Such lesions can ordinarily be removed at direct laryngoscopy with restoration of the voice, the airway, and the functional integrity of the laryngeal sphincter.

### Malignant Neoplasms of the Larynx

The vast majority of malignant neoplasms of the larynx are squamous cell carcinomas. Squamous cell carcinoma of the larynx accounts for approximately 2 per cent of all cancer deaths. It is a disease mainly of males, with a sex ratio of eight to one. The peak incidence of carcinoma of the larynx is in the fifth and sixth decades of life. Laryngeal carcinoma occurs more commonly in persons with a large ethanolic intake. It rarely develops in a person who does not smoke. Leukoplakia results from the inhalation of irritants such as tobacco smoke that contain known potent carcinogens including 3,4-benzpyrene and other polycyclic aromatic hydrocarbons. It is a premalignant condition from which carcinoma may develop after a period of months or years.

Carcinoma may arise from the mucous membrane of any part of the larynx; however, there is a predilection for the true vocal cords, particularly the anterior portions of the true vocal cords. The epiglottis, pyriform sinus, and postcricoid area also are common points of origin of carcinoma. For purposes of clinical staging and end result reporting, carcinomas of the larynx can be divided into supraglottic, glottic, transglottic, and hypopharyngeal lesions. Supraglottic lesions involve the epiglottis, aryepiglottic fold, and false vocal cords. Glottic lesions are limited to the area of the true vocal cords. Transglottic lesions include the glottic area and extend into the supraglottic and subglottic areas. Hypopharyngeal lesions may be divided into lesions of the pyriform sinus, postcricoid area, and posterior pharyngeal wall.

The natural history of the carcinoma varies considerably from one location to another. The early symptom of carcinoma of the true vocal cords is hoarseness. In any patient with hoarseness lasting 2 weeks indirect laryngoscopy should be done. Any discrete lesions of the mucous membrane of the larynx should be biopsied. Carcinomas of the true vocal cord limited to the middle one-third of the true vocal cord and not impairing the mobility of the cord are treated with radiation therapy or cordectomy with an overall 5 year survival rate of 85 to 95 per cent. Since cordectomy results in permanent hoarseness and irradiation usually results in a return of the voice to normal, radiation therapy is the treatment of choice. Cordectomy is reserved for the 5 to 15 per cent who have persistent carcinoma following radiation therapy. The likelihood of metastasis in early carcinoma of the true vocal cord is very slight.

The mobility of the vocal cord becomes impaired in more advanced carcinomas as a result of invasion of the intrinsic musculature and cartilage. With invasion of the intrinsic musculature, the rate of metastasis increases. With invasion of the thyroid cartilage, the rate of 5 year survival with radiation therapy decreases precipitously. Surgery becomes the treatment of choice for lesions that involve the anterior commissure where cartilage is very early invaded and for larger glottic lesions in which the mobility of the true vocal cord is impaired. Often a partial vertical hemilaryngectomy can be performed and will preserve the phonatory and sphincteric functions of the larynx.[16] In more advanced cases, total laryngectomy is required, and the laryngectomy may be combined with a radical neck dissection if palpable metastases are present. In view of the fact that only 15 to 20 per cent of patients with glottic carcinomas have nonpalpable metastasis present at the time of initial treatment, a radical neck dissection is not performed electively.

Supraglottic carcinomas tend to be asymptomatic until they reach considerable size. They may produce hoarseness by secondary involvement of the vocal cords, or they may produce pain on swallowing as the first symptom. Often the pain radiates to the ears. Not infrequently, a patient with a supraglottic carcinoma presents with the chief complaint of a swelling in the neck which represents a metastasis. The chance of nonpalpable metastasis being present is 35 per cent. In many patients with supraglottic carcinomas, the tumor can be completely removed by performing a supraglottic partial laryngectomy with preservation of the phonatory and sphincteric function of the larynx.[17] If the glottis is involved, a total laryngectomy is required. These procedures are usually combined with a radical neck dissection on the same side as the tumor.

Transglottic lesions represent more advanced glottic carcinomas in which the tumor has secondarily invaded the subglottic area as well as the supraglottic area. Metastasis to the same side is present in 50 per cent of patients. Subglottic extension of the carcinoma requires a total laryngectomy and radical neck dissection on the same side.

The overall 5 year survival rate for patients with supraglottic, glottic, or transglottic carcinomas treated with total laryngectomy for all stages approximates 65 per cent.

Pyriform sinus carcinomas tend to remain asymptomatic for long periods of time. Often the patient presents with dysphagia and pain on swallowing which may radiate to the ear on the same side. Often the presenting complaint is a mass in the neck which represents a metastasis. Depending on the location of the lesion in the pyriform sinus, a partial laryngectomy can sometimes be accomplished with preservation of the phonatory and sphincteric functions of the larynx. More often, a total laryngectomy is required. Either of these procedures is combined with a radical neck dissection on the same side. The 5 year survival rate for all stages is 30 per cent.

Postcricoid carcinoma has a female predominance of 10 to 1. Women with the Plummer-Vinson syndrome have a predilection for the development of postcricoid carcinoma. The presenting complaint is usually pain on swallowing and dysphagia. Metastasis to both sides of the neck is common. The treatment required is total laryngectomy and radical neck dissection on one side followed by radical neck dissection on the other side in approximately 6 weeks. The 5 year survival rate for all stages is 25 per cent.

The use of preoperative radiation therapy in conjunction with surgery for advanced carcinoma of the larynx is being studied in numerous centers to determine the effectiveness of combined therapy as compared with that of surgery alone.[3]

A total laryngectomy requires the formation of a permanent tracheostomy in which the trachea is transected and anastomosed to the skin of the lower part of the neck. Rehabilitation of the postlaryngectomy patient requires the development of alaryngeal or esophageal speech. In this technique, the patient draws air into the esophagus during inspiration and gradually eructs the air through the cricopharyngeus muscle. The opening of the esophagus vibrates and serves as the sounding source. The sound is articulated by the pharynx, palate, tongue, teeth, and lips into speech. For those persons who, because of age or other physical or emotional reasons, cannot develop alaryngeal speech, an electrolarynx can serve as the sounding source for modification by the articulators. The oscillator of the electrolarynx is placed in the submandibular area, and the sound is articulated into speech. Most persons who require a laryngectomy may return to their former occupation. With proper guidance in their rehabilitation, the laryngectomee may resume all his activities except swimming.

## SELECTED REFERENCES

Glorig, A.: Audiometry: Principles and Practices. Baltimore, Williams and Wilkins, 1965.
*This text in audiology is an authoritative introduction to the measurement of hearing.*

Jackson, C., and Jackson, C. L.: Broncheosophagology. Philadelphia, W. B. Saunders Company, 1950.

*This text is the most comprehensive discussion of peroral endoscopy available.*

Maloney, W. H.: Otolaryngology. New York, Harper & Row, 1969.
*This is a comprehensive encyclopedia of otology, maxillofacial surgery, bronchoesophagology, and head and neck oncology by many authorities.*

Prior, J. A., and Silberstein, J. S.: Physical Diagnosis, The History and Examination of the Patient. St. Louis, C. V. Mosby Company, 1963.
*The section on physical diagnosis of the ears and upper respiratory tract by William H. Saunders is superb.*

Shambaugh, G. E., Jr.: Surgery of the Ear. 2nd ed. Philadelphia, W. B. Saunders Company, 1967.
*This textbook is a comprehensive source of information in operative otology. It is authoritative and well written.*

## REFERENCES

1. Ash, J. E., and Raum, M.: An Atlas of Otolaryngic Pathology. Washington, D.C., Armed Forces Institute of Pathology, 1949.
2. Bast, T. H., and Anson, B. J.: The Temporal Bone and the Ear, Springfield, Ill., Charles C Thomas, 1949.
3. Biller, H. F., Ogura, J. H., Davis, W. H., and Powers, W. E.: Planned preoperative irradiation for carcinoma of the larynx and laryngopharynx treated by total and partial laryngectomy. Laryngoscope, 79:1387, 1969.
4. Cawthorne, T., Dix, W. R., Hallpike, C. S., and Hood, J. D.: The investigation of vestibular function. Brit. Med. Bull., 12:131, 1956.
5. Conley, J. J., and Novack, A. J.: The surgical treatment of malignant tumors of the ear and temporal bone. Arch. Otol., 71:635, 1960.
6. Fairbanks, D. N. F.: Closure of large nasal septum perforations. Arch. Otol., 91:403, 1970.
7. Fredrickson, J. M., Griffith, A. W., and Lindsay, J. R.: Transverse fracture of the temporal bone, a clinical and histopathologic study. Arch. Otol., 78:770, 1963.
8. Hough, J. V. D.: Tympanoplasty with the interior fascial graft technique and ossicular reconstruction. Laryngoscope, 80:1385, 1970.
9. House, W. F.: Subarachnoid shunt for drainage of hydrops. Arch. Otol., 79:328, 1964.
10. House, W. F.: Transtemporal bone microsurgical removal of acoustic neuromas. Arch. Otol., 80:601, 1964.
11. Jerger, J.: Békésy audiometry in analyses of auditory disorders. J. Speech Hearing Res., 3:275, 1960.
12. Jerger, J., Shedd, J. L., and Harford, E.: On detection of extremely small changes in sound intensity. Arch. Otol., 69:200, 1959.
13. Litton, W. B.: Epithelial migration over tympanic membrane and external canal. Arch. Otol., 77:254, 1963.
14. Martin, H.: Surgery of Head and Neck Tumors. New York, Harper & Row, 1957.
15. Muir, C. S., and Shanmugaratnam, L.: Cancer of the Nasopharynx. Flushing, N.Y., Medical Examination Publishing Co., 1967.
16. Ogura, J. H., and Biller, H. F.: Glottic reconstruction following extended frontolateral hemilaryngectomy. Laryngoscope, 75:2181, 1965.
17. Ogura, J. H., and Dedo, H. H.: Glottic reconstruction following subtotal glottic-supraglottic laryngectomy. Laryngoscope, 75:865, 1965.
18. Ogura, J. H., and Powers, W. E.: Functional restitution of traumatic stenosis of the larynx and pharynx. Laryngoscope, 74:1081, 1964.
19. Rosen, S.: Mobilization of the stapes to restore hearing in otosclerosis. New York J. Med., 53:2650, 1953.
20. Ruedi, L.: Pathogenesis and treatment of cholesteatoma in chronic suppuration of the temporal bone. Ann. Otol., 66:283, 1957.
21. Saunders, W. H.: Hereditary hemorrhagic telangiectasis. Its familial pattern, clinical characteristics and surgical treatment. Arch. Otol., 76:245, 1962.
22. Shea, J. J., Jr.: Fenestration of the oval window. Ann. Otol., 67:932, 1958.
23. Snow, J. B.: Clinical evaluation of noisy respiration in infancy. J. Lancet, 85:504, 1965.
24. Walker, E. A., and Resler, D. R.: Nasal gliomas. Laryngoscope, 73:93, 1963.
25. Wullstein, H.: The restoration of function of the middle ear in chronic otitis media. Ann. Otol., 65:1020, 1956.

# 40

# THE MOUTH, TONGUE, JAWS, AND SALIVARY GLANDS

*Milton T. Edgerton, M.D.,
and Gaylord S. Williams, M.D.*

## HISTORICAL ASPECTS

There is evidence to indicate that surgery was performed in and about the mouth as early as 3000 B.C.[24] On a wall of the tomb of Hesi-re at Saqqara in Egypt, near the ruins of ancient Memphis, was found a picture of a seated dentist with instruments in his left hand.[34] A Babylonian cuneiform inscription, dating from about 2000 B.C., and now preserved in the British Museum, exorcises the toothworm (believed to be the cause of dental decay until the eighteenth century A.D.) The Edwin Smith Surgical Papyrus, now in the New York Academy of Medicine Library, and dating from the Egypt of 1700 B.C., presents 27 head injury cases with descriptions of fractures and dislocations of the jaw and injuries to the lips and chin, generally with diagnosis, treatment, and prognosis given. From about the sixth century B.C. through the second century of the Christian era, the Greeks developed a system of medicine that was the basis of treatment in Europe until near the end of the fifteenth century A.D. Hippocrates (born about 460 B.C.) is credited with having described a method for reduction of fractures of the lower jaw by binding together the firm teeth on each side of the break with linen thread or gold wire and supporting loose teeth by similar ligatures.[24] Cor-

nelius Celsus, a Roman of the first century A.D., in his multivolume work, *De medicina*, described ulcers of the mouth, which the Greeks called aphthae; small tumors of the gingiva, called parulides by the Greeks; a method for extracting teeth with forceps; treatment for toothache; incision and drainage for abscesses; and reduction of fractures of the jaw very similar to methods of the Egyptians. Galen (A.D. 131–201) wrote voluminously explaining all disease in the light of pure, dogmatic theory substituting a strict system of medical philosophy for the plain notation and interpretation of facts as taught by Hippocrates. His work was so well accepted as authoritative that "European medicine remained at a dead level for nearly fourteen centuries."[19]

From the death of the Prophet in A.D. 632, the religion of Mohammed spread east to Persia and west along both shores of the Mediterranean to Spain and north through central Europe. Parchments from libraries of overrun provinces traveled by ship and by camel to the various capitals, including Samarkand and Cairo, where they were translated into Arabic. Thus, Islamic and Arabic medicine fell under the influence of Galenic dogma.[24] Medicine in this period of the Dark Ages in Europe and the Mediterranean basin was, for the most part, nonsurgical, because of religious proscriptions against cut-

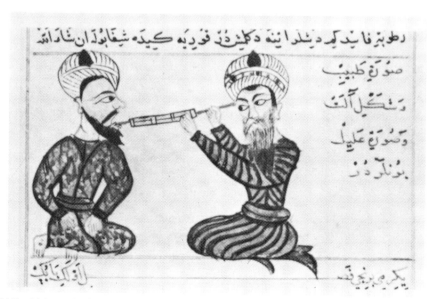

**Figure 1** Old Turkish method (c. A.D. 1465) of treating pyorrheic gingivitis by cauterizing the affected area with a hot cautery iron thrust down through a protective sleeve or tube to prevent injury to the surrounding tissues from the heat of the burning iron.

ting human flesh. Most treatment consisted of experiments in chemistry and pharmacology. Cautery became extremely popular (Fig. 1). In the twelfth century, with the dawning of the Renaissance, medicine again began to move forward. Theodoric, Bishop of Cervia (1205–1298), advocated that wounds should heal by primary intention. William, in his *Praxeox totius medicinae*, in 1275, first described intermaxillary fixation. He advised not only the binding together of firm teeth adjacent to a fracture in the mandible, but also binding of them into contact with the corresponding teeth in the maxilla. Fallopius (1528–1562) adopted the term "hard" and "soft" palate and described the fifth, seventh, and ninth cranial nerves. Eustachius (1520–1574) published in 1563 *Libellus de dentibus*, the first treatise ever written on the anatomy of the teeth and containing the first description of the periodontal membrane.

The celebrated French surgeon, Ambroïse Paré (1510–1590) described methods of transplanting and reimplanting teeth; he used obturators to close cleft or perforated palates; extracted teeth, drained dental abscesses, and set fractured jaws.[24]

In the seventeenth century, the specialties of dentistry and oral surgery began to develop. More than 100 works were published on dentistry.[9] Wilhelm Fabry (1556–1634) reported more than 600 cases, many of which dealt with oral surgical problems running the gamut from toothache to tumor. Anselme Louis Bernard Jourdain-Berchillet (1734–1816) was trained in surgery but specialized in dentistry and oral surgery. In 1778, he published his major work, *Treatise on the Diseases and Essentially Surgical Operations of the Mouth.* In this, he described the treatment of abscesses, caries, and necrosis of the jaws, diseases of salivary glands and ducts, ranuli, calculi, various tumors, hemorrhages, and maxillary sinus problems. He felt that general surgeons needed more special dental knowledge, and that dentists "lacked a sufficiently broad surgical view."

The effect of the elevator and depressor muscles on fragments in mandibular fractures was described by F. Chopart and P. J. Desault in 1779.[24]

In the nineteenth and twentieth centuries, because of advances in technology, all forms of surgery advanced exponentially. The rapid developments of asepsis, x-ray diagnosis, blood transfusions, antibiotics, and endotracheal anesthesia made possible what we now know as modern surgical management of lesions about the mouth.

Aseptic technique has been practiced rigorously and generally only in the twentieth century. Understanding of the germ theory of disease and its pragmatic application began in the latter half of the nineteenth century, notably with Lister (1827–1912) and his antiseptic technique. Principal advocates of the aseptic system were Sir William Macewen (1848–1924), a pupil of Lister, and Ernst von Bergmann (1836–1907), a Berliner, who introduced steam sterilization. Clean, white surgical gowns replaced the handy old frock coat at the operating table only in the 1880s, and rubber gloves were introduced by Halsted in 1890. Infection was so feared that a casual glance through any text on facial fractures antedating World War II reveals that open surgical reductions of mandibular fractures were avoided because of high risk. Antibiotics and chemotherapeutic agents have changed this.

The modern attempt to treat cancer of the head and neck by surgical excision probably began with Billroth's resection of the cervical esophagus and larynx on December 31, 1873.[15] Sir Henry T. Butlin, surgeon to St. Bartholomew's Hospital in London, 1885, published a monograph entitled *Diseases of the Tongue.* Without any of the advantages of modern surgery, Butlin courageously and repeatedly attempted by operation to control cancer of the tongue. He even excised the mandible and portions of the soft tissues and lymphatics of the upper cervical region. He reported more than 100 cases of cancer of the tongue that he had treated personally, performing total glossectomy on many. He noted that in the early nineteenth century, in England alone, more than 750 persons died of cancer of the tongue per year. At a time when American surgeons were making very little effort to cure this type of cancer, Butlin pointed out that "even the smallest, earliest, and most insignificant epithelioma of the tongue could produce cervical lymph node metastases," and, therefore, he concluded, "the surgeon would still be needed for the treatment of the regional metastases even if other methods for controlling the primary lesion should appear."

Röntgen, in 1895, and the Curies, in 1898, introduced the use of the roentgen ray and radium in the treatment of cancer. As is so often true with a new modality, overtreatment and enthusiasm led to discouraging results. Quinby, Janeway, and others contributed importantly to studies in the use of radiation.

In 1906, Crile presented a paper on "Excision of Cancer of the Head and Neck," in which he stated: "The operative treatment is hampered by tradition and conventionality, and the tragic ending of so large a proportion of these cases has held back lay and even professional confidence." He pointed out that less than 1 per cent of patients with head and neck cancer died from metastases to distant tissues, and he became convinced of the necessity of performing wider local excision and radical block dissection of the lymphatics of the neck. Crile was the first to describe staged, bilateral neck dissection. He was able to demonstrate in a personal series that the patient receiving such an en bloc neck dissection had a 25 per cent better chance of living for 3 years without disease than one treated for the primary lesion only.

In 1923, Brewer of New York presented statistics from several New York hospitals that indicated that the results of surgical treatment of cancer of the lip were far superior to those obtained with radium treatment. He felt that the treatment of cancer of the cheek by radium offered more promise. About that time, Sir Harold Gillies in England and Staige Davis and Vilray Blair in this country were pointing out the problems of deformity resulting from the treatment of head and neck cancer and developing techniques for the reconstruction of the face and jaws of these patients once the cancer had been controlled. Reluctance to perform adequate surgical resections led to a disappointing number of cancer recurrences and caused physicians to look again toward radiation therapy. Radium was tried in the form of plaques and molds in the early 1920s and, shortly thereafter, Evans and Cade in Great Britain reported the use of interstitial radium therapy for tongue cancer.

When the 200 kV roentgen ray machine was developed, the therapeutic use of external radium became less popular. Coutard (1937) made an outstanding contribution to head and neck cancer by showing the value of fractionation of x-radiation over a period of approximately 3 weeks, thus greatly reducing damage to overlying normal structures and skin. During the early 1930s, irradiation treatment for oral cancer was very common in America, but gradually physicians began to see increasing numbers of cases of irradiation necrosis and of radioresistant tumors.

Later came the recognition of sarcomas that were indeed *caused* by the irradiation that had been used in the treatment of the primary cancer. Just as surgeons had learned that some tumors appeared to be inoperable, radiotherapists began to appreciate that some of these tumors were not responsive to irradiation. Surgeons such as Hayes Martin, William MacFee, Grant Ward, J. B.

Brown, and Louis Byars were obtaining the salvage of many patients previously deemed incurable. Discriminating radiotherapists began to realize that patients with thyroid cancer, salivary gland cancer, and cancers within the jaw or facial bones were *usually not candidates for irradiation treatment*. It was recognized that many squamous cell cancers responded poorly, if at all, to irradiation.[15]

During World War II, striking improvements were made through the use of endotracheal anesthesia, more adequate transfusion with major surgery, and the advent of antibiotics. These changes, and the surgical skills learned by many physicians in dealing with the war wounded, contributed to a marked reduction in the operative mortality in operations on the head and neck. It became increasingly clear that even wider local excisions of oral cavity cancer could be accomplished with low mortality. Many surgeons treating head and neck cancer were trained in the use of modern reconstructive techniques and thus were emboldened to enlarge the reasonable limits of resection. The concept of "excision in continuity" as previously advocated by Halsted in the treatment of cancer of the breast, and by Miles in abdominoperineal resection was regularly applied to oral and laryngeal cancer. As a larger number of patients were cured of their cancers, of necessity more attention was focused on the resulting deformities. Plastic surgeons began to realize that they could contribute much to the rehabilitation of patients with head and neck cancer.[15]

In 1949, Baclesse advocated extending the total treatment time of fractionated external irradiation from 3 to 8 or 10 weeks. In this way, he reduced some of the severe acute irradiation reactions and allowed greater doses to be applied to the tumor. Paterson and Parker had already published, in 1938, their work on the use of low-intensity radium needles. Shortly afterward, the supervoltage machine was developed as a possible improvement in the method of administration. The radiologists of this period began to stress the importance of "knowing the exact site of origin of a tumor rather than the amount of anatomic involvement." Nonetheless, the results with the radiation therapy in almost all clinics in America continued to be disappointing and, after 1945, physicians returned again to modern types of surgery for primary treatment. In 1942, Wookey reported combined therapy by surgery and irradiation for the treatment of intraoral cancer, and Fletcher followed a similar program. Ward and Edgerton and others emphasized the value of preoperative irradiation in reducing exfoliation in many types of oral cavity cancer. Smith and Gehan (1959) at the National Clinical Center, in extensive wound-washing studies, demonstrated that preoperative irradiation does indeed reduce cell viability.

The use of modern methods of reconstructive surgery employed both at the time of tumor resection and shortly afterward has greatly reduced deformity and shortened hospital stay for many patients in recent years. Inevitably, new and complex methods of irradiation are being continuously developed but each will require some years for adequate evaluation of late effects. Chemotherapy to date has been disappointing in its effect on head and neck cancer and is not sufficiently successful for clinical use, except in conjunction with surgery and irradiation.[15]

Modern treatment of lesions about the mouth, tongue, jaws, and salivary glands demands the attentions of numerous medical, surgical, and paramedical disciplines in order to deliver optimal health care benefits to the patient. General practitioners, dentists, pedodontists, orthodontists, oral surgeons, plastic surgeons, general surgeons, ear, nose, and throat surgeons, radiotherapists, chemotherapists, prosthetists, prosthodontists, speech therapists, social workers, and even cosmeticians may all have a role to play in the diagnosis, operation, reconstruction, and ultimate rehabilitation of patients undergoing treatment for lesions or disease in this area. Because of this, there is a growing tendency in major medical centers for the utilization of a combined cooperative multidisciplinary team approach to the management of complex lesions in the head and neck region.

# LIPS

## CONGENITAL MALFORMATIONS AND DEVELOPMENTAL ANOMALIES

### Clefts

The incidence of cleft lip with or without cleft palate is variously reported as between 1 in 800 and 1 in 1300 live births. This is related to the racial and ethnic composition of the particular community. Cleft lip is eight times as frequent in Caucasians as in Negroes. The usual cleft lip runs vertically upward from the vermilion to the floor of the nose. These clefts may be complete or incomplete and may be unilateral or bilateral. They are caused by a lack of fusion of a single central prolabium with one or both of two lateral mesodermal masses. These units normally come together in the central face of the embryo and fuse between the fourth and seventh weeks of embryonic life. Failure of normal fusion of this tripartite junction of mesodermal masses results in any of the aforementioned types of cleft. Aplasia or hypoplasia of the median mesodermal mass results in the rare central facial cleft of the upper lip.[40] This is the true midline "harelip" seen in rodents. Median clefts of the lower lip are extremely rare but do occur. These represent a failure of the union of the mandibular arch at the ventral midline. They are frequently associated with a cleft in the midline of the mandible in the region of the symphysis and with a bifid tongue. Rare lateral or transverse facial clefts may extend into the cheeks from the commissures of the mouth. These may be unilateral or bilateral and vary in degree. They seldom extend beyond the anterior border of the masseter muscle. Rare oblique facial clefts (meloschisis) extend through the upper lip and toward the eye along an oblique line, passing lateral to both the philtrum and nostril.

The usual type of cleft lip is associated with a cleft palate, and occurs three times as frequently as cleft palate alone. Cleft lip alone is seen predominantly (2:1) with the male sex; cleft palate alone is twice as common in the female. Cleft lip with associated cleft palate occurs with equal frequency in males and females.

**Classification.** The usual type of vertical paramedian clefts are divided into two main categories: (1) clefts of the primary palate, and (2) clefts of the secondary palate. The primary palate comprises the lip and alveolar ridge and is demarcated posteriorly by the incisive foramen (just behind the upper alveolar ridge). Posterior to the incisive foramen, the hard and soft palates compose the

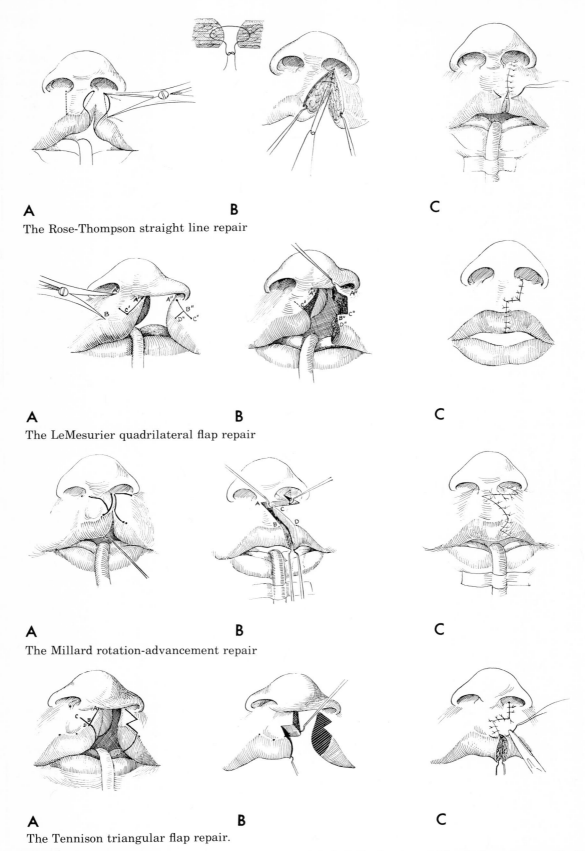

| A | B | C |
|---|---|---|

The Rose-Thompson straight line repair

| A | B | C |
|---|---|---|

The LeMesurier quadrilateral flap repair

| A | B | C |
|---|---|---|

The Millard rotation-advancement repair

| A | B | C |
|---|---|---|

The Tennison triangular flap repair.

**Figure 2** *A*, Markings; *B*, incisions; *C*, closure. (From Stark, R. B. In: Converse, J. M., ed.: Reconstructive Plastic Surgery. Volume III. Philadelphia, W. B. Saunders Company, 1964.)

secondary palate. Clefts of the primary palate (lip or alveolus or both) may vary from an incomplete cleft, with only slight notching of the lip, to a complete cleft extending into the floor of the nose. Clefts of the primary palate may be unilateral or bilateral and may or may not be associated with clefts in the secondary palate. Clefts of the secondary palate (the hard and the soft palate behind the incisive foramen) may also be incomplete or complete and may be unilateral or bilateral in the region of the hard palate.[22]

**Treatment.** Clefts of the lip (primary palate) are usually closed surgically during the first 3 months of life. Some surgeons prefer to close the lip deformity within the first few days after birth in order to take advantage of passively transferred maternal immunity and allow the parents to take home a nearly normal child. Most prefer to delay operation until the child is 2 to 3 months of age, when structures are larger, and anesthesia is safer. Some surgeons apply the Rule of Tens— that is, they delay closure of the lip until the child has reached a weight of 10 pounds and has a hemoglobin of 10 gm. or greater. This usually occurs when the child is 10 weeks of age or older.

To avoid future deformity, the closure of a cleft lip must be performed with meticulous accuracy, with a fine-layered plastic closure. The defect in a cleft lip deformity involves not only a transverse gap in the soft tissues but also a loss of vertical length of the lip. These two aspects of the deformity must be simultaneously corrected as the defect is surgically closed. In general, lateral lip tissue is brought in by some modification of the Z-plasty principle and used to add tissue to the cleft area, thus increasing the vertical length of the lip on the cleft side to restore symmetry. This is done by one of four basic methods. The first, the straight-line (Rose-Thompson) technique, is occasionally satisfactory for minimal incomplete clefts and notching of the lip.[38, 46] In larger clefts, this procedure sacrifices too much normal tissue and may destroy the shape of the cupid's bow. Straight-line closures tend to contract, producing a notching deformity in the vermilion.[9] If this repair is used, vertical height is gained by curving the lateral borders of the wound with the concavities of the incision toward the cleft after excising the deformed philtrum.

Three modern techniques that are commonly employed all utilize the principle of the Z-plasty. These methods include the quadrilateral flap of Mirault and LeMesurier,[26] the rotation-advancement technique of Millard,[31] and the triangular flap technique first described by Tennison[44] (Fig. 2). All of these may be considered variations of the Z-plasty with the adjacent sides of the cleft as the central limb of the Z-plasty. The techniques vary only in the positioning and lengths of the lateral limbs of the Z-plasty. Vertical height of the repaired side of the lip is provided by transverse incisions across both the lateral and medial lip elements and rotation of the created flap; these transverse incisions correspond to the lateral

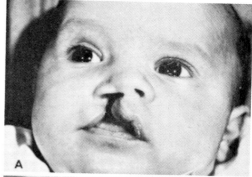

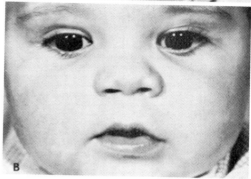

**Figure 3** *A,* Complete cleft lip with some nostril distortion. *B,* Seven months after rectangular flap repair (LeMesurier). (From Stark, R. B. In: Converse, J. M., ed.: Reconstructive Plastic Surgery. Volume III. Philadelphia, W. B. Saunders Company, 1964.)

limbs of the Z-plasty. Rotation or transposition of the flaps lengthens the central limbs at the expense of lip width. Geometrically, the amount of height that is gained depends upon the angle and distance of the transverse incisions. Practically speaking, the height that can be gained also depends upon the extent to which the tissue can be mobilized toward the midline (Fig. 3).

Bilateral clefts of the lip (primary palate) present an even more strikingly grotesque congenital deformity. The problems of surgical repair are frequently compounded by an elevated, protruding prolabium and premaxilla, which usually appears to be suspended from the dome of the nose by a very short columella. The timing of surgical repair for bilateral clefts is essentially the same as for unilateral clefts. As in unilateral cleft repairs, very little or no tissue is discarded or excised in the repair. All of these children suffer from a deficiency of tissue in the region of the upper lips, and great care must be taken to preserve every possible landmark of the normal lip elements. Occasionally, bilateral clefts must be repaired in stages in order to allow muscular action of the repaired side of the lip to mold the premaxilla inward toward the dental arch and thus facilitate closure of the opposite side of the lip. Surgical osteotomy and setback of the premaxilla may on occasion be necessary (Fig. 4).

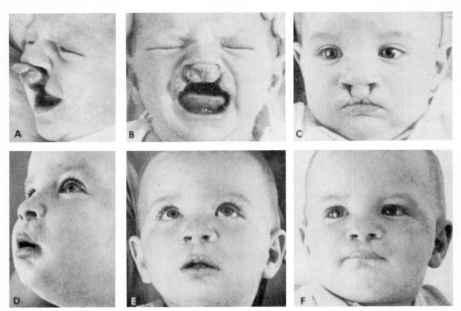

**Figure 4**  A and B, Bilateral complete cleft of lip with protruding premaxilla, absence of columella, wide nostril flare, and small prolabium. C, The premaxilla has been put back into the alveolar arch and lateral vermilion flaps have been attached to the prolabium for blood supply and cupid's bow. D, E, and F, Forked flap from prolabium has produced primary columella lengthening. Medial advancement of lateral triangular flaps has narrowed alar flares and incorporated the prolabium as a philtrum. (From Millard, D. R.: Transactions of the International Society of Plastic Surgeons, Second Congress. Edinburgh, E. & S. Livingstone, 1959.)

### Congenital Sinuses (Mucous Pits)

These usually appear as a symmetrically placed pair of dimples on the vermilion border of the lower lip, one on each side of the midline. These slitlike pits are the external orifices of blind sinuses, which extend downward through the orbicularis oris muscle, to end blindly just beneath the mucosal surface of the lower lip or gingiva. They are lined with squamous cell epithelium and numerous mucous glands empty into the lumen of the pits near their blind end. They are usually asymptomatic but cause vermilion deformity and are usually associated with cleft lip or palate. Heredity is the most important factor in their etiology[47] (Fig. 5). The most effective treatment is precise surgical excision of the entire sinus tract after staining of the lumen by filling it with aqueous methylene blue dye. All attached mucous glands whose ducts drain into the sinus must be removed with the tract. Failure to do so may result in the formation of a mucoid cyst.

### Retention Cysts

Small retention cysts may involve the mucous glands of the lips. These are mucoceles, due to plugging of the ducts of the mucous glands. They appear as small, nontender masses which appear to be filled with fluid. They are usually asymptomatic except for their annoying bulk. Treatment consists of surgical extirpation. The defect thereby created can be closed by simple sutures or left to heal by secondary intention.

### Microstomia

Children born with extremely small mouths occasionally present problems in feeding. Micro-

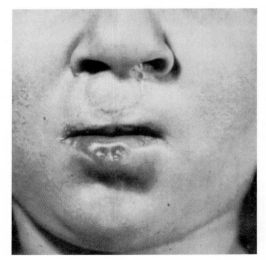

**Figure 5**  Congenital lip sinuses. The illustration shows bilateral, symmetrically situated sinus openings at the apices of a pair of nipple-like protrusions of the lower lip. Note the associated bilateral cleft lip, shown postoperatively. (From Wang, M. K. H., Macomber, W. B., Converse, J. M., and Wood-Smith, D. In: Converse, J. M., ed.: Reconstructive Plastic Surgery. Volume II. Philadelphia, W. B. Saunders Company, 1964.)

stomia is usually associated with a small, retruded jaw (micrognathia). The small mouth opening rarely requires surgical intervention and is best left to enlarge by normal growth and development.

### Double Lip

Congenital double lip occurs most frequently in the upper lip. The deformity is not obvious when the mouth is closed; however, with the mouth open a double vermilion is exhibited with a transverse furrow of varying depth between the reduplicated lips. The buccal portion of the double vermilion is rather loose and redundant. Treatment consists of transverse excision of the buccal redundancy with primary closure.[47]

### Peutz-Jeghers Syndrome

Melanin-like spots of pigmentation on the lips may be associated with multiple intestinal polyposis. This syndrome was first described by Peutz in 1921 and expounded on by Jeghers and associates in 1949. The syndrome is congenital and inherited. The lip (and occasionally buccal) lesions are benign and are significant in calling attention to the possible presence of intestinal polyposis.[33]

## INJURIES DUE TO TRAUMA

### Lacerations

Lacerations of the lip frequently involve both the mucosal and skin surfaces with division of the intervening musculature. Because of the circular and radial distribution of the perioral musculature, full-thickness lacerations tend to open widely when the muscle is divided. Because of this, inexperienced clinicians may be led to suspect tissue loss when the problem is largely tissue retraction. In closing lacerations of the lip, it is most important to reconstitute accurately the vermilion-cutaneous junction. Even a slight disparity in reconstituting this line will produce an obvious deformity. Therefore, it is most important to repair lip lacerations with good lighting, good assistance, and good anesthesia. It is quite helpful to tattoo temporarily the vermilion-cutaneous junction on either side of a laceration with a 25 gauge needle dipped in aqueous methylene blue, penetrating the skin along the vermilion edge on either side of the laceration prior to the infiltration of local anesthetic. The first skin suture is usually placed at the vermilion-cutaneous junction (Fig. 6). Local anesthetics and vasoconstrictors tend to blanch out the color differentiation between the vermilion and facial skin and, once injected, make the junction line difficult to appreciate. A few needle pricks with methylene blue prior to local anesthetic injection can greatly simplify accurate alignment of the vermilion-cutaneous junction.

Through-and-through lacerations should be closed in layers with absorbable suture material in the muscle and subcutaneous tissues. Copious irrigation and complete hemostasis are essential.

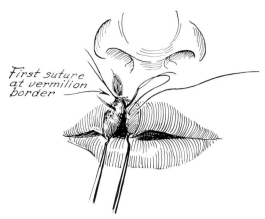

**Figure 6** Repair of vertical lacerations of the vermilion-cutaneous margin. The first skin suture should be used for approximation of the vermilion-cutaneous border. Accurate approximation of this line will avoid conspicuous irregularity of the lip after healing takes place. (From Dingman, R. O. In: Converse, J. M., ed.: Reconstructive Plastic Surgery. Volume II. Philadelphia, W. B. Saunders Company, 1964.)

The skin can be closed with 5-0 or 6-0 silk or nylon. The mucosa is loosely closed with similar-sized silk, polyglycolic acid, or chromic gut.

The lips and most of the face are blessed with an excellent blood supply. Because of this, stellate lacerations with multiple tiny flaps of tissue will usually heal quite well if accurately repaired. Very fine sutures and use of very few buried sutures should be the rule for repairing this type of laceration.

Because of Vincent's spirochetes, fusiform bacilli, and numerous pathogenic anaerobes in the human mouth, it is advisable to give penicillin in therapeutic doses by mouth for several days following closure of lip lacerations involving the oral surface.[33] This is especially true if the tissues have been crushed by the injury.

### Burns

Thermal burns of the lips generally involve the exposed skin and mucosal surfaces. They are treated in much the same way as cutaneous burns elsewhere on the body, depending on the depth of burn injury. Topical antibiotic ointment therapy may be applied with care about the mouth and will greatly relieve burn pain. It should be emphasized that the presence of a thermal burn about the mouth or nares should *not* be taken as an absolute indication for a tracheotomy. Certainly, burns in this area should alert the surgeon to the *possible* need for a tracheotomy, but it is becoming increasingly evident that routine tracheotomy for all patients with perioral burns is not only unnecessary but indeed *contra*indicated, unless there are definite signs of upper airway obstruction.[32] Elevation of the head of the patient's bed, croup tent, short courses of anti-inflammatory steroids, and wider use of prolonged endotracheal intubation will serve to further decrease the need for tracheotomy.

Burns of the inner surfaces of the lips, from the accidental ingestion of very hot liquids, are almost never deeper than second-degree. These are usually adequately managed by giving the patient a mild, orally administered analgesic. Alcoholic mouthwashes may be painful and irritating, and topical opiates are unnecessary.

One of the most frequently seen chemical burns of the lips is that due to lye in attempted suicides. This strong alkali penetrates the tissues of the lip, saponifies the fat, and reacts with the proteins to form soluble alkaline proteinates. The combination of lye with fats to form soaps is an exothermic reaction generating sufficient additional heat to damage surrounding tissue. The hygroscopic nature of lye produces cellular dehydration and cell death. The soluble alkaline proteinates formed tend to penetrate deeply into the tissues where they cause delayed further injury and increase in the depth of the burn wound.

The treatment of lye burns of the mouth should consist of early, copious, and prolonged irrigation with cold tap water. Water dilutes the injurious lye, washes away the noxious agent, and decreases the mass action and exothermic effect of the chemical reaction, thereby diminishing the inflammatory reaction. This is best done with a small rubber hose attached to a water faucet, so that large volumes of fresh, clean water can be used to irrigate the mouth continuously for at least 12 hours. Systemic steroids also are helpful in diminishing the inflammatory reaction, and penicillin should be given as with any other burn. Attempts at chemical neutralization of the lye are fraught with many hazards and have proved to be inferior to simple water irrigation.[49]

Electrical burns of the lips are most frequently seen in small children who are apt to chew on electrical cords or place the ends of extension cords in their mouths. Saliva creates a short circuit across the terminals within the plug, causing an electrical burn. Tissue destruction with electrical burns is sudden and extensive. Extensive, deep coagulation necrosis is instantaneously produced by the extreme temperatures of the electrical arc. If the child is well grounded, the current flow through his body may cause cardiac arrest.

The initial treatment of electrical burns of the lips should be conservative and not unlike the treatment of any other form of burn. Antibiotics should be administered for 5 days. Debridement should be limited to the excision of obviously dead and necrotic tissue, should be done without anesthesia, and should produce no bleeding. The wound should generally be allowed to heal spontaneously, and reconstructive efforts should be reserved until well after healing has occurred, and the scars have softened and matured. Delayed bleeding from the coronary labial arteries of the lips is frequently seen following electrical burns. This is easily controlled with a hemostat and a simple catgut ligature.

## INFECTIONS REQUIRING SURGERY

### Labial Abscess or Cellulitis

The skin of the lips is well endowed with hair follicles, sweat glands, and sebaceous glands. Minor infections due to blockage of these openings in the skin, producing pustules or small abscesses, are not infrequent. Warm soaks and appropriate surgical drainage are usually adequate therapy. Numerous persistent or recurrent infections should be treated with the appropriate antibiotics following culture. The usual offending organism is the Staphylococcus. Larger abscesses can be drained through the buccal surface of the lips and cheeks to lessen the production of visible external scars. When this is done, a small drain should be sutured in the intraoral wound at two points and left in place for 3 days. Cellulitis of the lips almost always indicates a streptococcal infection and is usually treated with penicillin.

### Herpetic Stomatitis

Herpetic stomatitis is a herpes simplex virus infection that presents as yellowish papulovesicular lesions which may be discrete or occur in groups. First, a small vesicle appears and ruptures early. A small ulceration then occurs. Symptoms consist of pain and burning in the region of the ulcer, particularly when the ulcer is touched. After a 10 to 12 day course, the lesion usually clears spontaneously.[3] Topical steroids such as triamcinolone and Orabase may speed symptomatic recovery. Early herpetic lesions may respond to topical 5-fluorouracil cream, but this has no efficacy once an ulcer has developed. Locally recurrent herpetic lesions may respond to subcutaneous injection of small amounts of triamcinolone at the site of recurrence. Chronic cases respond to viral vaccines.

### Canker Sores

Canker sores occurring on the buccal surface of the lips are characteristically small, superficial ulcerations, which are exquisitely tender and irritated by acid foods. The are usually surrounded by an inflammatory halo of erythema. These lesions are usually associated with gastrointestinal upsets, dehydration, or nutritional disturbances. They respond well to a bland diet, oral fluids, avoidance of acid foods and juices, and vitamin supplementation. Symptomatic relief may be obtained by holding promethazine (Phenergan) syrup in the mouth in the region of the lesion for 5 to 10 minutes before swallowing. One teaspoon of the syrup every 2 hours during waking hours is sufficient for most adults. The Phenergan acts locally as a topical anesthetic and when swallowed has a systemic sedative effect. Tetracycline syrup, held in the mouth for its topical action and then swallowed, may shorten the course of these lesions.

### Noma

Noma is a rapidly progressive gangrenous stomatitis that is rarely seen in well nourished persons. It occurs in patients with general debility

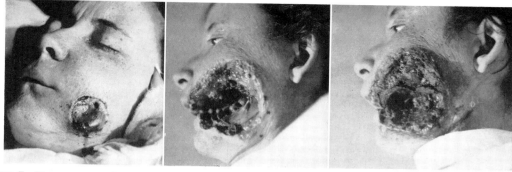

**Figure 7**  Noma; progressive gangrenous loss of entire cheek. (From Brown, J. B., and Fryer, M. P. In: Davis, L., ed.: Christopher's Textbook of Surgery. 9th ed. Philadelphia, W. B. Saunders Company, 1968.)

and metabolic dyscrasias (Fig. 7). These lesions rapidly invade and destroy soft tissues about the mouth, may involve bone, and frequently have a fatal termination. They are more common in children and occur after measles and other contagious diseases. They are initiated by anaerobic bacteria, among which are found fusospirochetal organisms.[21]

### Moniliasis

Moniliasis (thrush) is the most common fungus disease involving the oral cavity. Its incidence is increased in patients on antibiotic therapy. The acute form produces multiple, white, adherent, curdlike patches, irregularly distributed over the mucosal surfaces. Inflammation and fissuring of the labial commissures and encrustations on the lip frequently accompany the intraoral lesions. The specific treatment agent is nystatin (Mycostatin).[3]

### Syphilis

Syphilis, in its primary form, may produce a chancre on the lips. This is a foul, discharging, dirty ulcer without the surrounding characteristic hardness of carcinoma. Treatment is by systemic antisyphilitic therapy.

Other, infrequently encountered infections involving the lips include actinomycosis, histoplasmosis, molluscum contagiosum, and lymphogranuloma venereum.

## BENIGN TUMORS OF THE LIPS

Benign tumors may arise from any of the tissues forming the lips. The epithelium, dermis, fibrous tissue, fat, muscle, blood vessels, lymphatics, nerves, or specialized glands may occasionally produce benign tumors. Treatment of these lesions is usually surgical excision and microscopic examination for confirmation of the diagnosis and identification of the margins of the specimen. Larger lesions will require special reconstructive procedures and are best treated by plastic surgery techniques at the time of the initial excision.

### Nevi

Nevi may be subdivided microscopically into three groups, based on the depth of penetration of nevus cells across the dermal-epidermal junction: (1) Intradermal nevi have most of the nevus cells within the dermis. They are frequently raised above the skin surface, may contain hair, and show varying degrees of pigmentation. (2) Junctional nevi show the nevus cells to be concentrated at the junction between the dermis and epidermis. They are usually flat, do not contain hair, and may vary in depth of pigmentation. (3) Compound nevi show nevus cells distributed through both the dermis and junctional zones. They may be elevated or sessile and may or may not contain hair. It is generally agreed that intradermal nevi never become malignant and that junctional nevi may become malignant. Compounded nevi have been reported to become malignant, by a few authors. Any nevus of the lip (or elsewhere) that shows change in either size or pigmentation, or in any way appears to be undergoing change, by itching or bleeding for example, should be surgically excised. Similarly, any pigmented nevus that is chronically irritated should be excised.

### Papillomas

These are commonly referred to as "skin tags." They are frequently seen about the face and neck and are usually multiple. Microscopically, they appear to be primarily epithelial hyperplasias. The matrix of the skin tag shows a pattern of randomly arranged, delicate fibers that resemble the pattern of normal dermis. They vary in size but are usually less than 1 cm. in diameter. They are usually soft and pedicled on a stalk of soft skin. Surgical excision is the treatment of choice.

### Fibromas

These benign tumors arise in the deeper layers of the skin and contain mesodermal or epithelial elements. They may be classified as fibrolipoma, myofibroma, angiofibroma, or neurofibroma. Those with a gelatinous stroma are referred to as fibromyxomas. These tumors are rare but may occur in the lip. Treatment is by local surgical excision.

### Lipomas and Myomas

Lipomas and myomas may rarely occur on the lips. These benign tumors are excised surgically for diagnosis and cure.

### Hemangiomas

Benign vascular malformations or hamartomas, hyperplasias, and vascular ectasias may occur in the lips. Classification is based on the clinical characteristics and the histology of these angiomas. In general, they can be grouped into three categories: (1) capillary angiomas; (2) cavernous angiomas; and (3) telangiectases.

**Capillary Angiomas.** Capillary angioma, often called strawberry nevus, is usually present at, or appears shortly after, birth. It tends to be polypoid, raised, and bright red to purple in color, occasionally is bosselated, and involves the dermis and subcutis. Lesions that are superficial are bright red, but those with deep components tend to be darker in color. They may grow rapidly and are occasionally complicated by ulceration and infection. Spontaneous involution usually begins by the age of 2 or 3 years and is first noted by the appearance of patchy, pale areas, usually near the center of the lesion. Gradually, the tumor shrinks and involutes, losing its vascular color. When involution is complete, the site may appear normal or may show loose, wrinkled skin with slight atrophy and occasionally a few telangiectatic vessels.[35]

Treatment of capillary hemangiomas in the past has consisted of cryotherapy, injection of sclerosing agents, surgical excision, and x-ray or radium therapy. Most of these methods have produced cosmetic results that are definitely inferior to those after natural involution. Uncomplicated capillary hemangiomas that are not disturbing function or causing troublesome frequent bleeding are best followed conservatively. Most will undergo natural involution with supe-

rior final results. If the hemangioma continues to enlarge alarmingly, the involution can frequently be dramatically stimulated and hastened by the oral administration of prednisolone, given in high doses (40 mg. every 2 days for 10 days), to otherwise healthy babies in whom there is no contraindication to this form of therapy.[50]

X-ray therapy, either as superficial irradiation or in the form of radium implantation, is, unfortunately, still frequently advocated as a method for "inducing regression" of these lesions. This treatment of benign disease is mentioned here only to criticize it. The late sequelae of radiation damage include atrophy, dermatitis, and scarring in surrounding normal tissue, cessation of underlying bony growth and development, radionecrosis, and even late development of malignant neoplastic changes. These complications present problems of much greater magnitude than the original lesion.

**Cavernous Angiomas.** These are tumor-like aggregates of larger dilated vessels or sinusoidal blood spaces in a fibrous stroma. They are usually not present at birth, but appear during early childhood. They extend into the subcutaneous tissue with poorly defined borders. Histologically, the vessels appear more mature and lack the angioblastic qualities of the capillary hemangioma. Also, unlike capillary hemangiomas, they show no tendency for involution and, indeed, usually show insidious, progressive enlargement. Irradiation is contraindicated and has no more effect on the cavernous hemangioma than on the surrounding normal tissues. Interruption of feeding vessels, by ligation or by injection embolization, has been used with variable success. Usually, surgical resection and reconstruction will give the best results[35] (Fig. 8).

**Telangiectases.** *Nevus flammeus* (port-wine stain) is a macular, pink to purple vascular malformation that is frequently distributed along the course of peripheral nerves. Most of these nevi are

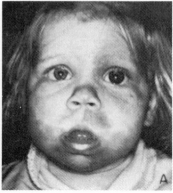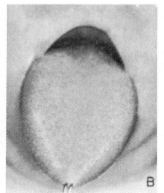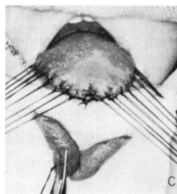

**Figure 8**    This child was born with a massive facial hemangioma of mixed type. In *A*, the external port-wine stain component is obvious, and her open bite secondary to macroglossia is also apparent. The grossly and diffusely enlarged tongue *(B)* was adequately reduced in size by wedge excision of the tip and lateral margins *(C)*. The child can now close her mouth and her dentition has been freed from the distorting forces of a large tongue. (From Edgerton, M. T., and DeVito, R. T. In: Converse, J. M., ed.: Reconstructive Plastic Surgery. Volume III. Philadelphia, W. B. Saunders Company, 1964.)

present at birth and do not tend to grow or involute. They do not respond to irradiation, freezing, or surgical abrasion. Many are managed by the application of cosmetics to hide the discoloration, but this does not relieve the "sense of deformity" and plastic surgeons are now using more "color-matched" skin grafts from the neck or scalp to replace these lesions on the lips and face.

*Venous varix* (senile hemangioma, venous lake) may appear as a solitary, deep blue nodule on the lips. It resembles a blood blister, but is not tense. It empties easily with pressure. These lesions tend to persist unless excised for cosmetic purposes.[35]

*Osler-Rendu-Weber syndrome* (hereditary hemorrhagic telangiectasia) is characterized by discrete, red, small, superficial punctate telangiectatic lesions on the skin and oral mucous membranes. They may be flat or slightly raised and are seldom more than a few millimeters in diameter. They are frequently accompanied by lesions on the fingers, face, and nasal mucous membranes. These lesions are prone to ulceration and hemorrhage and are frequently associated with arteriovenous fistulas in the lungs and vascular malformations of the liver. When seen on the lips, they should arouse suspicion of the other facets of the syndrome. The lip lesions can be controlled by cautery or excision.[35]

### Lymphangiomas

These are growths of thin-walled, vascular spaces that contain lymph. They may involve the lips and cheeks, producing visible deformity. They show no tendency toward spontaneous involution. They are not radiosensitive. Treatment, if indicated, is surgical, and if incomplete the lesions are likely to recur.[35]

### Pyogenic Granulomas

These are localized, superficial polypoid masses of new capillaries within an edematous matrix. They are devoid of epithelium and grossly resemble polyps of granulation tissue. In spite of their name, an infectious etiology for these lesions is not firmly established. These lesions may occur at any age and symptoms of pain or tenderness are variable. They tend to bleed easily when traumatized. Treatment should be by surgical excision with microscopic confirmation of the diagnosis to rule out the presence of other lesions that may mimic pyogenic granuloma, i.e., Kaposi's disease and metastatic renal cell carcinoma.[35]

### Epidermal Inclusion Cysts (Sebaceous Cysts)

These occur commonly on the skin of the lips. They are more common in people with thick, oily skin. They result from occlusion of the drainage pores of the sebaceous glands, and are usually firm and discrete. Palpation of the cyst and moving it about beneath the skin will frequently demonstrate traction umbilication of the skin at the site of the occluded pore. These cysts are best treated by excising a small, elliptical sliver of skin containing the punctum along with the underlying cyst.

### Keratoacanthomas

These common benign cutaneous tumors may arise from the hair follicles on the lips. Their rapid growth and histologic appearance may lead the surgeon, and occasionally the pathologist, to make a diagnosis of squamous carcinoma. Keratoacanthoma is, however, a benign tumor that runs a self-limited course. If untreated, it may produce a cicatricial deformity of the lips. This tumor is limited to the white races, and has its highest incidence in persons between the ages of 50 and 70. The etiology of keratoacanthoma is unclear. Actinic rays, chemical carcinogens, trauma, genetic factors, and viral factors may all play a role in its etiology. Clinically, the tumors may appear as dome-shaped buds with a pink to reddish hue. Later in the evolution of the tumor, the epithelium over the center of the dome breaks down to reveal a central keratin plug. Ultimately the keratin plug detaches, leaving a crater-shaped lesion. Finally, the lesion becomes ulcerated and then regresses completely, healing by scar formation. Treatment is by surgical excision with primary closure. The specimen must be submitted to the pathologist for accurate histopathologic diagnosis. Other methods of treatment such as curettage, cautery, diathermy, or x-ray therapy will usually prove curative for keratoacanthoma, but will make accurate pathologic diagnosis difficult or impossible. The excision of large keratoacanthomas may make it advisable for the surgeon to use pedicle flaps or grafts or both to reconstruct the lips.[20]

### Keratoses

These rough, scaly, slightly raised lesions occur at the vermilion-cutaneous junction, usually on the lips of elderly patients with fair skin who are chronically exposed to solar radiation. They may give rise to squamous cell carcinomas of the lips. Chronic labial keratoses are best excised by a "lip shave" procedure with mucosal advancement (Fig. 9). The full thickness of the skin should be excised and the tissue should be examined microscopically.[15, 42]

### Leukoplakia

This condition commonly presents with slightly elevated, white patches on the buccal mucosa, tongue, palate, or lip vermilion. Treatment should initially consist of the removal of any possible mouth irritants such as tobacco or snuff. General mouth cleanliness and hygiene should be encouraged and any caries or rough teeth should receive prompt dental care. Daily abrasion with a stiff-bristle toothbrush will clear up the superficial varieties. After these conservative measures have been tried, persistent lesions should be excised and examined microscopically as this condition is definitely precancerous.[4]

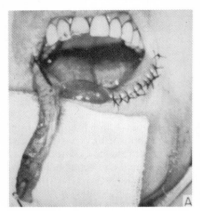
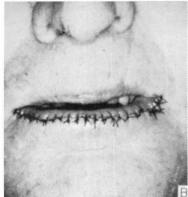
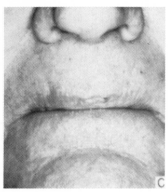

**Figure 9** Resection of the vermilion border with mucosal advancement ("lip shave") done for leukoplakia or chronic keratoses of the vermilion is shown in progress *(A)*, at completion *(B)*, and in the late postoperative period *(C)*. (From Edgerton, M. T., and DeVito, R. T. In: Converse, J. M., ed.: Reconstructive Plastic Surgery. Volume III. Philadelphia. W. B. Saunders Company, 1964.)

## Squamous Cancer of the Lips

Almost all "lip cancer" arises at the skin-vermilion junction. Basal cell cancers and melanomas arising in the skin of the lips are considered elsewhere in this book.

Lip carcinoma accounts for approximately 15 per cent of all malignant diseases of the head and neck and roughly 1 per cent of all cancers. They almost always occur on the lower lip, and 87 per cent occur in males.[1] They are rarely seen in persons below the age of 40 and there is an increasing incidence with advancing age. Persons with light-colored skin, blue eyes, and light-colored hair who tend to freckle (rather than tanning) when exposed to sunlight appear to be highly susceptible. Carcinoma of the lip is rarely seen in blacks. There is a definite correlation between lip cancer and exposure to sunlight.[1] The incidence of these cancers gradually increases in susceptible persons as the equator is approached from the extreme northern or southern latitudes. Persons spending most of their lives out of doors, in higher elevations, where the effects of actinic irradiation are stronger, also are more susceptible to the development of lip cancer. Other factors that frequently turn up in the histories of patients with lip cancer, and that are believed to have some etiologic significance, include syphilis, prior gamma irradiation, excessive use of tobacco (particularly smoking of pipes with clay stems), and the heavy drinking of alcohol.

Diagnostic work-up with a suspected lip cancer should include biopsy of the lesion. Biopsies are 100 per cent accurate if positive.[5] If negative, they should be repeated. Bidigital examination of the floor of the mouth and the submental and submaxillary triangles for metastatic disease should be carried out. Both sides of the entire neck should be carefully palpated for enlarged lymph nodes. A chest x-ray may reveal metastases.

**Classification.** Clinically, lip cancer presents as one of two major types: (1) exophytic lesions in which superficial proliferation predominates, or (2) endophytic lesions in which invasion, ulceration, and early involvement of muscle, bone, and skin predominate (Fig. 10). Histologically, epidermoid carcinoma accounts for 99 per cent of all lip cancers.[5] These are usually well differentiated. Basal cell carcinoma occasionally appears on the lips but this can, more often than not, be demonstrated to be associated with basal cell carcinoma arising in the skin surrounding the lips. Melanoma is occasionally seen as a primary lip cancer.

The metastatic behavior of lip cancer is characterized by relatively late spread to regional lymph nodes except in the undifferentiated lesions. The metastatic route is to the facial and submental lymph nodes and the nodes along the anterior portion of the submaxillary gland, and then to the jugular chain. Invasion of the mandible is usually late and occurs via direct soft tissue extension, usually entering the mental foramen to reach the marrow cavity. Distant metastasis to the

lungs and liver occurs late and is rare. When
death occurs it is usually due to uncontrolled
tumor in the neck.

**Principles of Treatment.**  The management of carcinoma of the lip must be individualized in every
case. Factors that enter into the decision include:

1. The age of the patient. Younger patients are
more likely to have early metastases than older
ones.[7]

2. The reliability of the patient and the logistical
practicality for close follow-up of the patient. Patients in whom the potential for close follow-up
seems dubious are better served by a diagnostic
dissection of the regional lymph nodes at the time
of the initial resection of the lip primary. Experience has shown that large recurrences may appear
rapidly in the neck, and they are most difficult to
treat.

3. The nature of the lesion. The endophytic,
invasive type carcinoma tends to metastasize
much earlier than the exophytic type.[7]

4. The size of the lesion. Lesions less than 1 cm.
in size only rarely will have metastasized to the
neck, and these smaller lesions can usually be
managed by local lip resection. Lesions larger
than 1 cm. in size are much more likely to have
spread to the regional nodes. The size of the lesion
is usually correlated with its duration on the lip.
The longer a lesion has been present, the more
likely that metastasis will have occurred to the
nodes in the neck.[7]

5. The histologic gradation of the cell malignancy. High-grade or undifferentiated carcinoma
is more likely to develop early metastasis than
low-grade, well differentiated tumors.

6. Staging. The presence of palpable enlarged
or indurated nodes in the submental area or neck
is a definite indication for radical neck dissection
to remove regional nodes.

7. Recurrent or persistent lesions. In those lesions which have previously been treated inadequately wide re-resection of the lip with in-continuity cervical node dissections should be done.

8. The experience and ability of the surgeon.
Those who undertake to treat lip carcinoma
should be thoroughly familiar with the techniques
of neck dissection, and should be competent in the

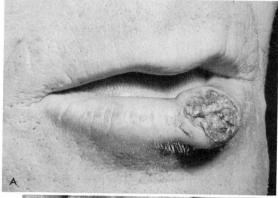
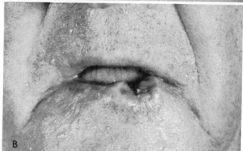

**Figure 10**  *A*, Exophytic carcinoma of lower lip with
central ulceration and raised, rolled borders. *B*, Ulcerating carcinoma of lower lip with diffuse infiltration. (From
Ackerman, L. V., and del Regato, J. A.: Cancer: Diagnosis, Treatment, and Prognosis. 4th ed. St. Louis, The
C. V. Mosby Company, 1970.)

planning, elevation, mobilization, and transportation of local flap tissue for immediate reconstruction.

Small primary lip cancers of the well differentiated type are adequately treated by local
resection. The "V-excision" is a popular method
that facilitates the closure (Fig. 11). Surgical
treatment of larger lip lesions, in which adequate
resection makes necessary the excision of more
than one-half of the lip, demands a thorough
knowledge of many ingenious local and distant

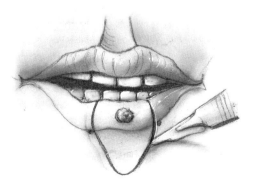
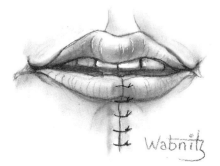

**Figure 11**  Small squamous carcinoma of lower lip treated by V-excision with direct closure. (From Loré, J. M., Jr.:
An Atlas of Head and Neck Surgery. Philadelphia, W. B. Saunders Company, 1962.)

flap techniques that have been designed for lip reconstruction. For the larger lesions, invasive lesions, those with a highly malignant histologic pattern, recurrent lesions, or lip cancers in patients in whom adequate follow-up is doubtful, a "diagnostic" bilateral supraomohyoid neck dissection is recommended at the time of resection of the lip lesion. Depending on microscopic findings, the neck dissection may be extended to include a full neck dissection on one or both sides of the neck (if there is frozen section evidence of nodal metastases on either side).

Radiotherapy still has many advocates as a primary modality in the treatment of lip cancer. A typical course of radiation therapy lasts several weeks with daily treatments five times a week, which is followed by breakdown of the tumor with ulceration and slow healing. In favorable lesions, the cure rate for radiation therapy is 80 to 90 per cent and approaches that of surgery.[18] However, radiation therapy produces considerable morbidity, does not provide pathologic check on the margins of treatment, and usually does not encompass the regional nodes. When cervical nodes are involved, radiation therapy is much less effective than surgical neck dissection. Prior radiotherapy usually increases the problems with wound healing if recurrence develops and surgery is then required.

Melanomas of the lip require wide, radical, surgical resection with incontinuity dissection of the nodal drainage areas in the neck. Radiotherapy is not effective. Chemotherapy for this lesion has thus far been disappointing.

# ORAL CAVITY

## CONGENITAL MALFORMATIONS AND DEVELOPMENTAL ANOMALIES

### Cleft Palate

Clefts of the secondary palate, from the incisive foramen posteriorly to the tip of the uvula, develop during the seventh to twelfth weeks of embryonic life.[40] Normally, two lateral mesodermal shelves develop and fuse in the midline during this time, separating the oral and nasal cavities. Prior to fusion these shelves hang downward alongside the tongue. During the seventh week, as the tongue descends into the oral cavity, they begin to fuse from anterior to posterior. The soft palate is formed by the ninth week; the uvula is completed by the twelfth week. Insults to the developing embryo during this time may produce arrest in this development process, resulting in clefts of the secondary palate.[39] The defect may vary from total, complete, bilateral cleft of the hard and soft palate, with wide communication between the oral and nasal cavities, to a cleft manifested by only slight notching of the tip of the uvula (Fig. 12).

Occult submucosal clefts of the palate occur with an intact mucous membrane, but lack of fusion of the muscle masses in the midline. These are usually associated with a notching of the posterior edge of the bony hard palate and a midline cleft of the uvula. Submucosal clefts quite often cause the

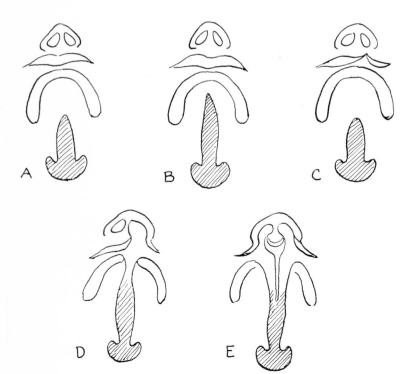

**Figure 12** Classification of cleft palate (after Kernahan and Stark, 1958). The division between primary palate (prolabium, premaxilla, and anterior septum) and secondary palate is the incisive foramen. *A*, Incomplete cleft of the secondary palate. *B*, Complete cleft of the secondary palate (extending as far as the incisive foramen). *C*, Incomplete cleft of the primary and secondary palate. *D*, Unilateral complete cleft of the primary and secondary palate. *E*, Bilateral complete cleft of the primary and secondary palate. (From Converse, J. M. In: Converse, J. M., ed.: Reconstructive Plastic Surgery. Volume III. Philadelphia, W. B. Saunders Company, 1964.)

child to have rhinolalia aperta or typical "cleft palate speech."

**Treatment.** Clefts of the palate are repaired surgically when the child is between 1 and 2 years old. This operation requires the use of general endotracheal anesthesia, which is much easier and safer when the child has reached this age. It is desirable to have the palate repair completed by the time the child begins meaningful attempts at speech. If the repair is unduly delayed, the child will develop faulty speech habits which will be difficult, if not impossible, to correct with later speech therapy.[9]

The operations utilized to repair a palatal cleft vary, but most are designed to close the medial cleft with the aid of bilateral relaxing incisions to release the soft tissues of the hard and soft palates. Recent operations also stress lengthening or retrodisplacement of the soft palate by local soft tissue flaps. Elevation and mobilization of mucoperiosteal flaps from the oral surface of the hard palate will allow pushback and lengthening of the soft tissues. Pushback procedures create open defects in the mucous membrane of the floor of the nose, which, if left to heal by cicatrization and epithelialization, will contract and cause postoperative shortening of the palate — partially negating the pushback procedure. Operations incorporating island flaps or the Z-plasty principle have now

been designed to close these defects on the nasal surface of the repaired palates.

Flaps of mucosa and muscle may be elevated from the posterior pharyngeal wall and attached to the posterior aspect of the soft palate to form a bridge of tissue that will reduce the velopharyngeal opening and provide a posterior point of fixation for the pushed-back palate. This procedure is known as "a posterior pharyngeal flap." More intricate muscle-plasty operations may be used to selectively reposition the levator veli palatini muscles more posteriorly within the soft palate in order to obtain a better mechanical advantage for elevation of the important dome of the soft palate.[14]

Cleft palate surgery is exacting and demanding. Each patient's repair should be individualized. It should never be attempted by the "occasional palate surgeon."

### Pierre Robin Syndrome

This congenital anomaly is characterized by a small mandible, retrodisplacement of the chin, and consequent posterior displacement and ptosis of the tongue into the hypopharynx, producing upper airway obstruction (Fig. 13). It was described in 1923 by the French stomatologist Pierre Robin, who emphasized its frequent fatal termination.[37] Clefts of the secondary palate are found in 40 per cent of the children with this syndrome. The exact

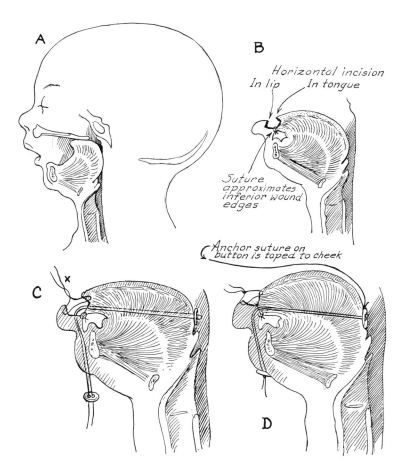

**Figure 13** A, Cross-section drawing of an infant with micrognathia, glossoptosis, and upper airway obstruction. With the mentum in retroposition the genioglossus muscle is unable to hold the tongue forward. When a cleft palate is also present, the tip of the tongue may be displaced into the nasopharynx. B, Cross section showing the horizontal incisions in the tip of the tongue and the labial mucosa with a suture approximating the inferior wound margins. C, A heavy tension suture connects a button beneath the chin to one on the posterior surface of the tongue by way of the lip and tongue incisions. A retrieving suture is tied to the tongue button and brought out through the mouth. A suture is placed on either side of the tension suture to approximate the muscle layer of the lip and tongue. D, The superior wound margins are approximated. (From Randall, P. In: Converse, J. M., ed.: Reconstructive Plastic Surgery. Volume III. Philadelphia, W. B. Saunders Company, 1964.)

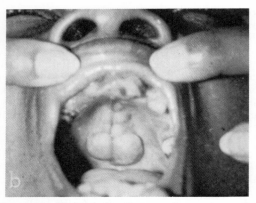

**Figure 14**   Multilobulated torus palatinus in an adult. (From Ochsner, A. In: Ochsner, A., and DeBakey, M. E., eds.: Christopher's Minor Surgery. 8th ed. Philadelphia, W. B. Saunders Company, 1959.)

etiology is unknown. Many believe the retrognathia is due to intrauterine pressure against the chin caused by sharp flexion of the head downward and forward, delaying forward development of the mandible. The degree of airway obstruction may vary from minimal to quite severe. Infants with greater degrees of airway obstruction expend all of their energy in breathing and cannot eat without choking. Without treatment they rapidly die from exhaustion or sudden respiratory obstruction. Only the very mildest forms should be treated by positioning (the child is kept on his side or in a prone position and is fed with his head held in a vertical, upright position). If the child has an episode of cyanosis, surgical intervention becomes urgent. Several operations have been described that relieve the obstruction by fixing the tongue forward to the lip or hypoplastic mandible by sutures or strips of fascia.[12, 27] The ultimate growth potential of these hypoplastic mandibles is unpredictable. Most develop to approximately normal size; others may require later secondary corrective surgery.

### Torus Palatinus

This relatively common and usually insignificant lesion is an exostosis in the midline of the hard palate (Fig. 14). It is occasionally seen in newborns, but is more common after adolescence. Its major significance is that it is occasionally mistaken for a neoplasm. The bone is usually symmetrically distributed on both sides of the midline and is covered with normal mucosa. Excision should be advised if there is chronic irritation of the overlying mucosa or if a full upper denture is to be worn.

### Ranula

A ranula is a thin-walled, bluish retention cyst located beneath the tongue in the anterior floor of the oral cavity. It is due to obstruction of a mucous gland or one of the sublingual salivary glands. Ranulas are filled with a thick, crystal-clear, mucoid fluid. They are soft and fluctuant, but not

painful. They are usually unilateral and form slowly. They occasionally rupture spontaneously, but usually recur. Treatment consists of marsupialization of the cyst by excision of the anterior, superior wall and suturing of the remaining posterior cyst wall to the mucous membrane of the floor of the surrounding oral cavity. Because of the thinness of the walls of these cysts, excision by enucleation is virtually impossible, and the attempt may result in obstruction of the ipsilateral Wharton's duct.

## INJURIES

### Burns (Thermal Trauma)

Thermal and electrical burns are rarely seen within the oral cavity beyond the lips and tongue tip. Chemical burns of the oral, palatal, or lingual mucosa due to the accidental or suicidal ingestion of caustics or acids are occasionally seen. These should be immediately treated with copious and prolonged water irrigation, systemic steroids, elevation of the patient's head, nothing by mouth and parenteral alimentation, and penicillin. Rapidly developing edema may necessitate a tracheotomy. Surgery is reserved for late sequelae and contractures. The oral mucous membrane demonstrates a remarkable capacity for rapid healing.

### Lacerations

Because of the extreme vascularity of the cheeks, tongue, and mouth, bleeding from lacerations is usually profuse. Hemorrhage is best controlled initially by digital pressure and packing. The application of multiple hemostats in deep lacerations of the cheeks and floor of the mouth to control bleeding in an emergency room is unnecessary and may frequently result in damage to branches of the facial, trigeminal, lingual, or hypoglossal nerve, or to one of the major salivary ducts. Local anesthetic agents containing vasoconstrictor drugs (epinephrine 1:100,000) are recommended for use within the mouth. Adequate lighting, good assistance and anesthesia, and proper instruments are indispensable for efficient repair of intraoral lacerations. After hemostasis is obtained, the membranes are loosely approximated with a proper suture material. Plain catgut sutures will rupture after a few days in the mouth and should not be used. Chromic catgut or polyglycolic acid sutures will last for several weeks, and they do not require later removal. Silk sutures are excellent for repair of intraoral lacerations, but most will require subsequent removal. Monofilament nylon and wire sutures are stiff, bristly, and uncomfortable and should not be used within the mouth.

### Dislodged Teeth

Recently dislodged permanent teeth should not be discarded. They can be replaced in an intact alveolar bone socket and wired in place with a high percentage of tooth survival. If the root canal of the tooth is treated and filled prior to replacement or shortly thereafter, the percentage of tooth survival approaches 95 per cent. These free dental grafts are exposed to a traumatized, contaminated oral cavity and should be protected with prophylactic penicillin therapy.

### Chronic Trauma

Chronic trauma to the lining tissues of the oral cavity may induce reactive hyperkeratosis or leukoplakia. If prolonged, this may lead to dyskeratosis with dissolution of the epithelial basement membrane and cancer. Irritants such as smoke, snuff, chewing tobacco, strong condiments, alcohol, oral trauma from various dental sources, hot spicy foods, allergy, galvanism, and lesions secondary to avitaminosis A have all been incriminated in the development of oral leukoplakia. Reactive patches appear as grayish white plaques on the epithelial membrane. Initial treatment should consist of identification and elimination of all irritant factors. If the lesion does not disappear within 2 weeks, it should be surgically excised and the defect closed or grafted. Long periods of "watchful waiting" are definitely contraindicated, and may allow the development of invasive carcinoma.

## INFECTIONS REQUIRING SURGERY

The greatest number of infections within the oral cavity are odontogenic in origin. Lacerations of the soft tissues or fractures of the maxilla or mandible account for a small percentage of infections. Extension of infection from an obstructed salivary gland or blood-borne septic emboli from infection elsewhere in the body are unusual. Most oral cavity infections arise from periapical or periodontal infection. They may be associated with cysts, root fragments, or pericoronal pockets.

The bacteria found in infections of the oral cavity are characteristically mixtures of the same organisms that make up the oral flora—unless the flora has been altered by previous antibiotic therapy. Virtually all are penicillin-sensi-

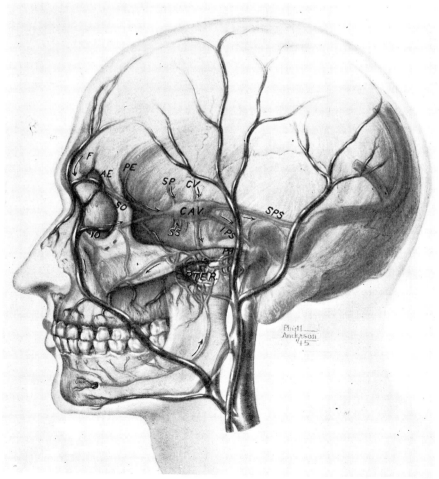

**Figure 15**   The venous tributaries of the cavernous sinus, including those from the teeth. The arrows (indicate the direction of blood flow. (From Archer, W. H.: Oral Surgery. 4th ed. Philadelphia, W. B. Saunders Company, 1966.)

tive. Fungal infections (i.e., actinomycosis) are slow in development and progression and are difficult to diagnose. Biopsies and special culture techniques may be required.

Anatomically, bacterial infections of the oral cavity may extend into the sublingual area, the mental and submental areas, the buccal space, the submandibular or submaxillary areas, the pterygomandibular space, the parapharyngeal space, the zygomaticotemporal space, or the fascial planes of the neck. Massive infections may threaten the airway and necessitate a tracheotomy.

A much feared complication of maxillary or mandibular infection is cavernous sinus thrombophlebitis. Veins of the upper jaw drain via the anterior facial vein or pterygoid plexus into the ophthalmic veins and thence to the cavernous sinus.

Septic phlebitis in the lower jaw may spread along the inferior dental vein into the pterygoid plexus and thence by way of the ophthalmic veins or the vein of Vesalius to the cavernous sinus (Fig. 15). Surprisingly, fatal cavernous sinus thrombosis arising from infections in the *lower* jaw has been reported with twice the frequency of that arising from infections in the *upper* jaw.[4] Treatment is by massive intravenous doses of antibiotics and by anticoagulants. The causative abscess should, of course, be drained.

In general, the treatment of bacterial oral cavity infection should consist initially of large doses of antibiotics. A high circulating antibiotic blood level is desirable prior to manipulation or drainage of the abscess. Relatively small collections such as gumboil or pericoronal abscess may be drained into the mouth. Larger abscess extensions require external incisions through a line of election beneath the mandible in a dependent position. Drainage is maintained by a rubber or gauze drain left in the wound for several days.

## BENIGN TUMORS OF THE MOUTH

Nonmalignant tumors or abnormal growths within the soft tissues of the oral cavity arise most frequently from the gingival tissues or the mucoperiosteal membrane of the alveolar processes of the maxilla or mandible. These include fibromas, hyperplasias, pyogenic granulomas, hemangiomas, gingival hyperplasia caused by diphenylhydantoin sodium, peripheral giant cell tumors, and neuromas. Second in frequency are the hyperplasias of the lining mucosa of the cheeks and lips from chronic trauma. Third in frequency are benign tumors found on or beneath the mucosa of the cheek. These include fibromas, fibropapillomas, lipomas, hemangiomas, mixed tumors, and traumatic neuromas. Fourth in the order of frequency are benign growths on the palate, including fibromas, fibropapillomas, acute inflammatory papillary hyperplasia, and mixed tumors. The least common site in the oral cavity for the occurrence of nonmalignant tumors is the floor of the mouth. Here may be found mixed tumors, myxofibromas, and dermoid cysts.

Most benign tumors of the oral cavity are readily diagnosed by observation, palpation, and radiographic studies. When the diagnosis is not readily made by these means, biopsy is indicated. Once diagnosed, all benign oral cavity tumors should be treated by simple, total, surgical excision. Radiotherapy has no role in their treatment. Excised surgical specimens should always be examined microscopically by a competent pathologist to confirm the diagnosis.

## MALIGNANT NEOPLASMS OF THE SOFT TISSUES OF THE ORAL CAVITY

### Sarcoma

This rare neoplasm of the lips and cheeks may mimic a benign tumor. It usually appears as a solid, firm growth with an intact mucosal covering. It is frequently seen many years after radiotherapy to the area. Biopsy is usually diagnostic. Treatment is by wide surgical excision. Most sarcomas are resistant to irradiation.

### Adenocarcinoma

Adenocarcinomas occur in the mouth more frequently than sarcomas. They arise in minor salivary glands in the soft tissues of the oral cavity, and they often pursue a more malignant course than their counterparts arising from the major salivary glands. Because of their submucosal origin, they exfoliate few cells and cytologic studies are of little help in diagnosis. Adenocystic carcinoma, sometimes referred to as cylindroma, shows a marked invasive tendency and characteristically spreads widely along nerve sheaths.

### Epidermoid Carcinoma

By far the most frequent malignant neoplasm of the oral cavity is squamous cell carcinoma. It constitutes 95 to 97 per cent of all malignant lesions in this area. In 1968, carcinoma of the buccal cavity and pharynx accounted for 2 per cent of the mortality from all forms of cancer in the United States. Carcinoma of the oral cavity is best considered anatomically by region.

**Floor of the Mouth.** Fifteen per cent of oral cavity cancers arise in the crescent-shaped area bounded anteriorly by the inferior dental arch and posteriorly by the inferior surface of the tongue.[1] Squamous cell carcinoma accounts for nearly all lesions. The average age for development of floor of the mouth carcinoma is around 60 years. Ninety-seven per cent of carcinomas in this area occur in males.[5] Carcinoma in this area usually presents as an infiltrative lesion with a fissure-like ulceration. Spread is rapid to involve the contralateral side and the mandible. The tongue may be involved and this may make exact origin of the tumor difficult to determine. Assessment of the extent and staging of the tumor are best done by bimanual palpation. Biopsy is easily accomplished and is always indicated. X-rays of the mandible are indicated to determine bony involvement.

Carcinoma of the floor of the mouth frequently presents with metastases in the submaxillary nodes. These are the primary drainage sites,[1] but subsequent spread to the deep cervical nodes is frequent.

Treatment of carcinoma of the floor of the mouth must be varied according to the size and staging of the primary tumor. Smaller primaries away from the mandible are well controlled with either radiation therapy or surgical excision. Larger primaries that encroach upon or involve the mandible require a composite resection of the floor of the mouth, partial mandibulectomy, and en bloc neck dissection (Fig. 16). Regardless of the treatment of the primary lesion, a neck dissection should be performed on the ipsilateral side of the lesion. If the tumor encroaches on the midline, or if positive nodes are found on the ipsilateral side, the neck dissection should be complemented by at least a supraomohyoid dissection of the contralateral side. Studies and experience have shown that in 50 per cent of all patients with carcinoma of the floor of the mouth nodal metastases in the neck will develop within the first year.[29] Thus, a neck dissection is advisable, *even in the absence*

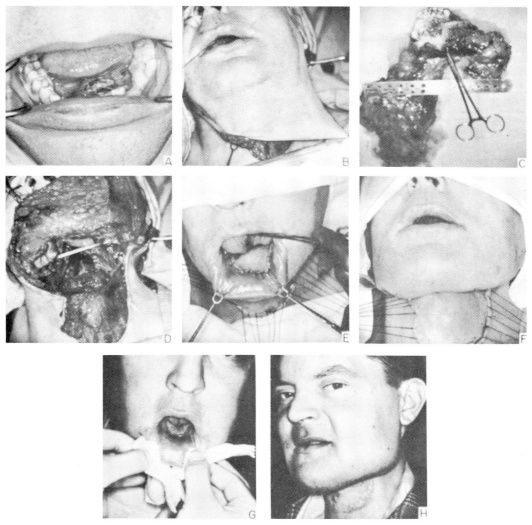

**Figure 16**  Photographs demonstrating resection of a floor of the mouth carcinoma with a composite resection of the mandible in continuity with a radical neck dissection and repair by an apron flap technique. The lesion is demonstrated preoperatively in *A*. The superiorly based apron flap is shown elevated in *B*. The resected specimen is seen in *C*. The mandibular arch is shown reconstituted with an internal metallic splint in *D*. The apron flap is shown wrapped around the metallic splint and sutured to the labial mucosa in *E*. A split-thickness skin graft covers the flap donor site on the anterior neck in *F*. The final result is shown in *G* and *H*. This technique obviates the need for using tongue tissue to close the defect and also permits immediate restoration of mandibular contour. (From Edgerton, M. T., and DeVito, R. T. In: Converse, J. M., ed.: Reconstructive Plastic Surgery. Volume III. Philadelphia, W. B. Saunders Company, 1964.)

*of clinically suspicious nodes.* The prognosis for 5 year survival is 60 per cent in the absence of palpable nodes in the neck. The presence of clinically positive nodes reduces this figure to 30 per cent.

**Buccal Mucosa.** The lining of the cheeks extending from the upper to the lower gingivobuccal gutters and from the oral commissures posteriorly to the ascending ramus of the mandible gives rise to 10 per cent of oral cavity cancer. Cancer in this area is more frequent in the older age groups. It is nine times as frequent in males as in females.[5] Certain chronic irritants such as chewing tobacco and betel nut have been shown to be causative.[1] Carcinoma in this area is preceded by leukoplakia more frequently than carcinoma in any other part of the oral cavity.[5] Squamous cancer in the buccal mucosa tends to be better differentiated and slower-growing and to have a lower rate of nodal metastasis than cancer of the floor of the mouth or tongue. Nodal metastases usually occur first in the submaxillary and upper cervical nodes. The primary lesions are usually painless exophytic growths or ulcerations of the mucosa in areas of leukoplakia or hyperkeratosis. Diagnosis is by direct inspection, bimanual palpation, and biopsy. Treatment for early lesions is surgical excision and reconstruction. Radiation therapy yields a somewhat lower cure rate. The exophytic, verrucous lesions offer a much more favorable prognosis

than the ulcerating endophytic type. Adequate surgical resection will almost invariably require excision of the overlying skin of the cheek, so that a through-and-through cheek defect is produced. Immediate flap reconstruction should be performed and will greatly reduce the functional impairment and cosmetic deformity (Fig. 17). The determinate 5 year survival (all methods of treatment) is about 43 per cent.[1]

**Gingivae and Hard Palate.** Squamous carcinoma is rare in the hard palate, infrequent in the upper gingiva, and fairly common in the lower gingiva, where it accounts for 12 per cent of oral cavity cancer.[5] There is no detectable difference in the incidence between the sexes. The average age of patients with gingival carcinomas is about 60. Characteristically, the tumor is usually a well differentiated carcinoma in the molar area. Nodal metastases develop in 40 to 65 per cent of these patients.[51] Patients usually complain of difficulty in wearing dentures, pain on mastication, or blood-streaked saliva. Biopsy and mandibular and maxillary x-rays are indispensable diagnostic procedures.

Surgery is the preferred method of treatment for gingival and palatal carcinoma. Since all but the earliest lesions involve bone, which has relatively little resistance to irradiation, this form of therapy is not desirable.[15] Some surgeons precede

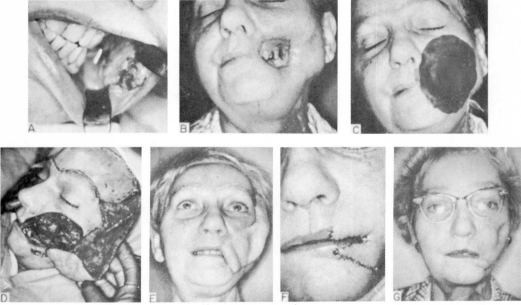

**Figure 17** Middle-aged woman with a massive carcinoma of the buccal mucosa (A). Wide excision with in-continuity lymphatic dissection was performed and a clean oral fistula obtained by suturing skin edges to mucosa (B). Convalescence was facilitated by the use of a rubber-dam "patch" held on the cheek with dermatome cement (C), so that the patient could talk and eat with surprising ease and comfort. Early repair was undertaken using a total forehead flap, pedicled on the side of the defect, with the donor site covered by a split-thickness graft from the infraclavicular area (D). Note that if the original neck dissection had not been done so as to spare the external carotid artery, reconstruction would have been much more complicated. The distal end of the forehead flap was folded upon itself to provide buccal lining, and the flap sutured into place (D and E). Subsequent division of the pedicle and construction of a commissure (F) produced a very satisfactory functional and cosmetic result (G). (From Edgerton, M. T., and DeVito, R. T. In: Converse, J. M., ed.: Reconstructive Plastic Surgery. Volume III. Philadelphia, W. B. Saunders Company, 1964.)

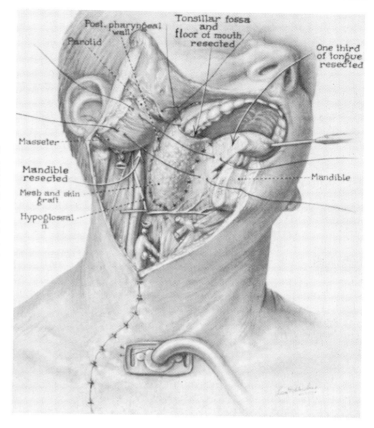

**Figure 18**   Drawing demonstrating the technique used for large posterior defects. The split-thickness skin graft is mounted on a framework of tantalum mesh and sutured into place. A vascular bed for the graft is provided by adjacent tissue such as a cervical flap or masseter muscle. A tie-on dressing is applied intraorally so that firm contact is maintained between the graft and its bed. (From Edgerton, M. T., and DeVito, R. T. In: Converse, J. M., ed.: Reconstructive Plastic Surgery. Volume III. Philadelphia, W. B. Saunders Company, 1964.)

operation for gingival carcinoma with a course of preoperative irradiation, feeling that this reduces the incidence of exfoliation metastasis.[28] Palatal carcinoma is usually of salivary gland origin and is relatively radioresistant. Since adequate excision of lower gingival carcinoma involves at least a partial mandibulectomy with opening of the tissue planes of the upper portion of the neck, a radical neck dissection should be performed on the ipsilateral side at the time of resection of the primary tumor. In palatal and upper gingival carcinoma, if there are no clinically palpable nodes in the neck, an expectant, careful follow-up without neck dissection is justified. Five year survival is 25 to 35 per cent.

**Oropharynx.** This region includes the soft palate, pharyngeal walls, tonsil, lingual tonsil, and posterior one-third of the tongue. Carcinoma here occurs predominantly in males with a peak incidence in those about 60 years old. The tonsil is the most common primary site, and carcinoma of the tonsil accounts for 10 per cent of all head and neck cancers.[5] Pain on swallowing, frequently referred to the ear, is a common presenting complaint. An enlarging upper cervical mass beneath the angle of the mandible is frequently noted. In addition to palpation, direct and indirect laryngoscopy is a useful diagnostic tool. Histologically, carcinoma in this region is usually a more undifferentiated variety of squamous cell carcinoma than

that found elsewhere in the oral cavity.[1] Lymphosarcoma also is frequently seen in this lymphoid-rich area of Waldeyer's ring.

The treatment of oropharyngeal carcinoma is by radical surgical extirpation, with a composite resection including a partial mandibulectomy and en bloc dissection of the neck with flap reconstruction (Fig. 18), or by radiation therapy alone, or by combinations of these modalities. Oropharyngeal carcinomas frequently cross the midline in the soft palate and base of the tongue, making operation less feasible or necessitating bilateral neck dissections to remove the nodal drainage areas. The 5 year survival for patients with carcinoma of the oropharynx, presenting—as they usually do—with stage 3 or stage 4 disease, treated by any form of therapy, is distressingly low and averages approximately 15 to 25 per cent overall.[1]

# TONGUE

## CONGENITAL MALFORMATIONS AND DEVELOPMENTAL ANOMALIES

### Thyroglossal Duct Cysts

The pyramidal lobe of the thyroid gland arises from a median pharyngeal diverticulum during embryogenesis. The tongue, which develops later, surrounds the opening of this diverticulum at the foramen cecum. Normally, the diverticulum becomes obliterated and all but the lower portion is resorbed. Failure of obliteration of the diverticulum at any point along its course from the base of the tongue to the thyroid gland may result in the formation of a thyroglossal duct cyst. This situation is very similar to the development of a hydrocele at any level of the spermatic cord and testicle. The hyoid bone develops after the diverticulum is formed and may pass behind, in front of, or around the diverticulum. Clinically, patients present with a midline cystic mass in the neck. The mass may steadily enlarge or fluctuate in size. These cysts usually appear before adulthood, and one-third of the cases are seen in children under 10 years of age. The cysts are usually freely movable beneath the strap muscles and are nontender. If spontaneous perforation or previous surgical drainage of the cyst has occurred, a thyroglossal duct fistula may be present. Treatment is by total excision of the cyst and the entire thyroglossal duct tract. If infection is present, the cyst should first be drained and several weeks later excised. Complete excision of the tract is essential and this requires resection of the central portion of the hyoid bone. The tract must then be completely removed up through the base of the tongue.

### Lingual Thyroid

Failure of descent of the midline pharyngeal diverticulum and the two lateral diverticula from the fourth pharyngeal pouches may result in all of the thyroid tissue remaining in the base of the tongue. This is mentioned only to caution against resection of a mass of reddish brown thyroid tissue from the base of the tongue without first checking to be sure that thyroid is present in its normal position beneath the strap muscles.

### Ankyloglossia

Ankyloglossia and "tongue-tie" are terms applied to a short lingual frenulum. If severe, this condition may cause an infant to have difficulty in nursing and may subsequently result in some speech impediment. The condition is readily treated by transverse incision and longitudinal closure of the frenulum, preferably with a Z-plasty, under local anesthesia.

### Median Rhomboid Glossitis

This condition, sometimes called grooved tongue, results from embryologic failure of the lateral halves of the tongue to fuse before the tuberculum impar becomes interposed between them, just anterior to the circumvallate papillae. This results in a rhomboid plaque of tissue in the midline of the tongue immediately anterior to the circumvallate papillae. It produces no symptoms and should be recognized to avoid confusion with neoplastic lesions. This condition requires no treatment.

### Bifid Tongue

This is an extremely rare congenital anomaly resulting from total lack of fusion of the two halves of the tongue in embryogenesis. This condition should be repaired surgically before the child begins meaningful speech.

## INJURIES DUE TO TRAUMA

Lacerations of the tongue bleed freely and may be difficult to expose for repair. Exposure may be facilitated by injection of local anesthetic into the tip of the tongue and passing a suture through the tip to be used for retraction. Lidocaine or procaine, with 1:100,000 epinephrine, gives good anesthesia of adequate duration and hemostasis. Larger bleeding vessels should be carefully grasped with hemostats and ligated with absorbable ligatures. The tongue mucosa should then be carefully approximated with silk or absorbable sutures. If catgut is used, the sutures may be placed in an inverted fashion with the knots buried so that they will have less tendency to untie with the constant motion of the tongue against the palate. The patient should be kept on a liquid diet for several days and advised in the use of a mouthwash. Penicillin should be administered daily for 3 to 4 days.

## INJURIES DUE TO INFECTION

### Syphilis

Syphilis in the oral cavity is quite likely to involve the tongue and may present as a primary chancre or as a secondary gumma. Syphilitic glossitis is always associated with a positive serologic test for syphilis.[33] Because of numerous varieties of spirochetes normally in the mouth, dark-field examination may be misleading. Syphilitic ulcers of the tongue are frequent in the midline and near the base or tip of the tongue. They should always be biopsied to rule out a malignant neoplasm. Treatment consists of a complete course of antisyphilitic medication.

### Lichen Planus

This chronic disease may affect the skin and oral mucous membranes. It characteristically produces hyperkeratotic nodules with associated inflammatory changes. The lesions may appear white or bluish white, and be confused with leukoplakia. The bluish color of these white, often lacelike lesions is helpful in differentiating them from leukoplakia. Lichen planus has not definitely been associated with the development of malignant change. Spontaneous remissions may occur. Vitamin A therapy has been reported to be of value in treatment.

## BENIGN TUMORS OF THE TONGUE

### Granular Cell Myoblastoma

The myoblastoma is a benign, firm, usually small, spherical mass which may occur in the tongue. While its designation implies origin in muscle tissue, it is not invariably found in relation to striated muscle and is probably not histogenetically derived from muscle cells. Myoblastomas probably arise from perineural fibroblasts; however, their origin remains in debate. They have no malignant potential and are readily cured by local surgical excision. When they occur submucosally, the overlying epithelium may undergo striking hyperplasia, sometimes simulating the development of carcinoma (pseudoepitheliomatous hyperplasia).[36]

### Lymphangioma and Cavernous Lymphangioma

These are tumors of the lymph vessels. Many are present at birth as congenital collections of proliferating lymph vessels, quite like cavernous hemangiomas. They have tiny white and red tufts on the surface that are pathognomonic. They may cause great enlargement of the tongue (macroglossia). Surgical excision and debulking of the tumor may be required to establish and maintain an airway, but some tongue should be left, even if it contains residual lymphangioma.

### Amyloidosis

This condition may present in the tongue and associated structures of the oral mucosa as submucosal, chiefly perivascular deposits or as solitary multiple nodules. Macroglossia, often to a severe degree, may develop. With enlargement of the tongue, indentations of the teeth along the border become very prominent and impaired

mobility may be observed. The upper airway may become obstructed. Ulcerations of the mucosa may also develop. Biopsy will establish the diagnosis. Surgical reduction of the huge tongue may greatly relieve some patients.

## MALIGNANT NEOPLASMS OF THE TONGUE

Malignant neoplasms of the tongue usually arise from the mucosa and are mostly epidermoid carcinomas. Those of the posterior one-third of the tongue behave like oropharyngeal lesions. Tongue carcinoma accounts for approximately 15 per cent of all cases of malignant disease of the head and neck. Eighty per cent of cases of tongue cancer occur in males.[14] Tongue carcinoma is unusual in persons below age 40 and has a peak incidence in those around age 60. Chronic alcoholism, heavy use of tobacco, poor oral hygiene, syphilis, and the Plummer-Vinson syndrome have all been incriminated as etiologic factors. Premalignant changes of leukoplakia and erythroplasia frequently precede the development of tongue cancer. Clinically, carcinoma of the tongue usually presents as a chronic, nonhealing, painless ulcer. Early involvement of submaxillary and digastric nodes is frequently seen. Biopsy, cultures of the lesion, and x-rays of the mandible and chest are essential diagnostic aides. Ninety-five per cent of all malignant neoplasms of the tongue are epidermoid carcinoma.[1,5] Adenocarcinoma is occasionally seen. Sarcoma and metastatic car-

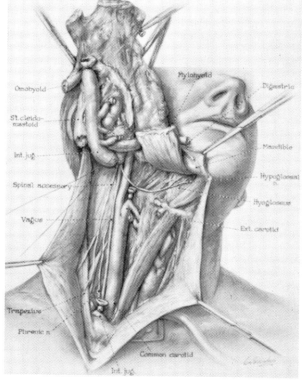

Figure 19  Drawing showing the extent of the usual radical neck dissection. The specimen is retracted superiorly. As is shown, resection of the posterior belly of the digastric muscle permits high ligation of the internal jugular vein and also facilitates dissection around the hypoglossal nerve. (From Edgerton, M. T., and DeVito, R. T. In: Converse, J. M., ed.: Reconstructive Plastic Surgery. Volume III. Philadelphia, W. B. Saunders Company, 1964.)

cinoma to the tongue from a distant primary are rare.

In the treatment of carcinoma of the oral tongue, it should be remembered that in half of all patients with nonpalpable nodes in the neck metastasis to these nodes will already have occurred *at the time of diagnosis, regardless of the size of the primary.*[15] Therefore, resection of a tongue carcinoma should always include an en bloc neck dissection at least on the side of the lesion (Fig. 19). For larger primaries or lesions approaching or encroaching upon the midline, a staged, bilateral neck dissection is always indicated. If the mandible is eroded by tumor or adherent to the primary, a composite resection including hemiglossectomy, partial mandibulectomy, and neck dissection is indicated. The treatment of lymph node metastasis in the neck is surgical. The primary reason for surgical failure is too timid a resection of the tongue and failure to adequately clear the nodal drainage areas. The overall 5 year survival rate for carcinoma of the oral tongue is approximately 40 per cent and has improved in recent years with bolder resections of the tongue.

## JAWS

The bony upper and lower jaws in the human are sometimes referred to as the upper maxilla and lower maxilla. Thus, when the two jaws are wired together after injury, the method is called "intermaxillary fixation." More commonly the lower maxilla is known as the mandible. The upper jaw or "maxilla" comprises several membrane bones fused together to form a single functioning unit. This includes two maxillary bones, two palatine bones, and, laterally, the two zygomas which form the bony prominence of each cheek. The upper jaw is thus fixed to the base of the skull and the orbit. The external nose is attached to its anterior surface, the upper teeth emerge from its alveolar process, and the two antral cavities lie within this bony complex on either side of the nasal cavity.

The mandible is composed of heavy cortical bone arising from Meckel's cartilaginous anlage. It articulates with the base of the skull at each glenoid fossa to form the temporomandibular joints. These joints are located just anterior to each bony ear canal. Movements of the mandible are controlled by powerful muscles of mastication and its rigid arch plays a vital role as a base for movements of the tongue and for elevation of the larynx in swallowing and speech. An intact arch of the mandible is critical to maintenance of an adequate air passage into the trachea. Severe deformity of the mandible and chin occasions great psychologic damage to the patient.

Surgical conditions involving the jaws may be conveniently divided on the basis of the etiology of the deformity. Deformities may be thought of as congenital or developmental, traumatic, metabolic, infectious, or neoplastic.

## CONGENITAL MALFORMATIONS AND DEVELOPMENTAL ANOMALIES

### MAXILLA

More than 100 syndromes involving abnormal development of the jaw have been described. Most may be greatly improved by surgical methods.

#### Hypoplastic Conditions

These include "dishface" deformities associated with recession of the maxilla, lateral constrictions of the upper arch, and craniofacial dysostoses such as Crouzon's disease or Apert's syndrome (Fig. 20). Maxillary hypoplasias usually result from premature fusion of bony epiphyses and incomplete descent of the midface beneath the skull. There is often associated brachycephaly of the cranial bones and exorbitism, producing a frog-faced appearance of the patient.

Surgical correction is best accomplished by extensive osteotomies of the maxilla to bring the midface and nose forward and re-establish occlusion of the teeth. These techniques are performed in increasingly younger children in order to improve eye function and overcome deformity before school age. Bone grafting to supplement depressed areas is often required.

#### Hyperplasias of the Maxilla

Symmetric or asymmetric overgrowths of the upper jaw may occur, producing giantism or hypertrophy of the middle face. This giantism may result from congenital arteriovenous fistulas within the bone or from the presence of plexiform neurofibromatosis associated with von Recklinghausen's syndrome. When the hyperplasia is symmetric and midline, it may be associated with ocular or orbital hypertelorism (Fig. 21). Most of these children have normal intelligence and surgical correction is effected by geometric osteotomies in association with intracranial exposure in order to protect the brain. This permits resection of excessive bone and translocation of the orbits, upper jaw, and nose, as required.[16,45]

Enlargement of the peripheral nerve to the affected part is often seen with cases of giantism associated with neurofibromatosis. These patients should receive surgery at an early age, and total resection of the neurofibroma is both unnecessary and undesirable.

#### Bony Clefts of the Maxilla

In addition to the common clefts of the upper lip and palate, patients may be seen with lateral facial clefts. These usually occupy an oblique position, running from the mouth in a cephalic direction. They may open into the floor of the nose or they may pass lateral to the nose to the midpoint of the floor of the bony orbit. The antrum may be totally absent on one or both sides and little bone is present beneath the eye to provide support. Rarely, one will encounter patients with midline

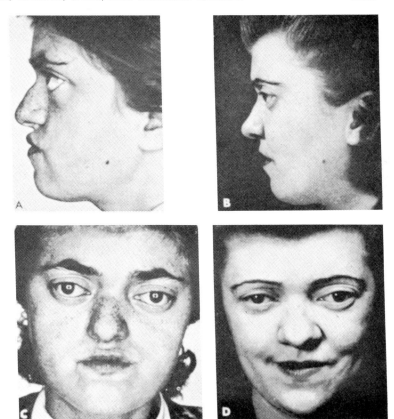

**Figure 20** Surgical correction of Crouzon's disease by maxillary osteotomy and forward traction procedures. *A*, Before operation. *B*, After operation. *C*, Before operation. *D*, After operation. (From Gillies, H., and Harrison, S. H.: Brit. J. Plast. Surg., *3*:123, 1950.)

clefts of the upper or lower jaw. Some children are born with complete mandibular agnathia or absence of the premaxillary bony segment. Such patients require complex surgical correction involving bone grafting and, at times, pedicle flap migration.

### Other Congenital Syndromes Involving the Maxilla

These include the Byzantine arch of the hard palate with its extremely narrow and high vault producing obstruction of the nasal airway. The

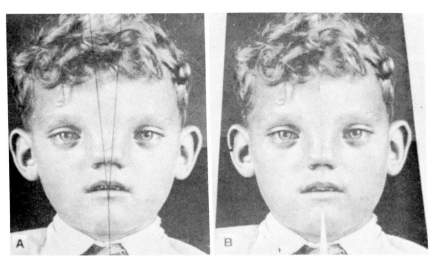

**Figure 21** *A*, Hypertelorism and excessive width of the upper portion of the face. *B*, Same photograph as *A* with central wedge removed as marked, showing more normal head and face contour. (From Webster, J. P., and Deming, E. G.: Plast. Reconstr. Surg., *6*:1, 1950.)

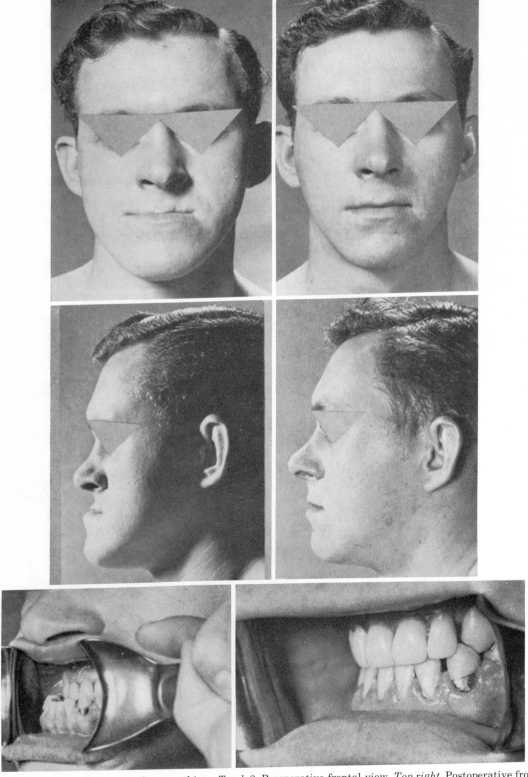

**Figure 22**   Surgically corrected prognathism. *Top left*, Preoperative frontal view. *Top right*, Postoperative frontal view. *Middle left*, Preoperative lateral view. *Middle right*, Postoperative lateral view. *Bottom left*, Preoperative malocclusion. *Bottom right*, Postoperative balanced occlusion. (From Archer, W. H.: Oral Surgery. 4th ed. Philadelphia, W. B. Saunders Company, 1966.)

airway may be opened by surgical division of the bony palate, rapid orthodontic expansion of the upper jaw, and insertion of a stabilizing bone graft.

Children with one of the oro-facial-digital syndromes (OFD I or II) often have constricting mucosal adhesions producing notches in the upper and lower alveolar processes. They also have lobulated tongues, small mandibles, cleft palates, and associated underdevelopment of the maxilla. Multiple reconstructive procedures on tongue, lips, and palate are quite helpful to such children.

## THE MANDIBLE

### Hypoplasia of the Mandible (Micrognathia)

Micrognathia is probably most commonly seen with the Pierre Robin syndrome consisting of symmetric underdevelopment of the chin with breathing problems (see Fig. 13) and associated clefts of the soft palate (present in 45 per cent of the patients). Other hypoplasias include asymmetric underdevelopment of one side of the bony face and narrow lower arches with a "pointed chin," owing to lack of development of the symphysis. Lack of development of the mandibular condyles, bilaterally or unilaterally, may produce

ankylosis. Very rarely, total absence (agnathia) of the lower jaw has been encountered. All these conditions may be helped by appropriate reconstructive techniques.

### Hyperplasia (Prognathism)

Mandibular overgrowth is most commonly symmetric and results in the condition known as prognathism. This deformity usually does not become evident until late childhood or adolescence. With growth of the mandibular body and ramus, the chin and lip are carried forward to produce deformity and associated malocclusion of the teeth. Failure to correct may result in a severe sense of deformity and premature loss of dentition. Correction usually involves appropriate bilateral osteotomies of the ramus or body of the mandible with appropriate retropositioning of the chin to improve both appearance and occlusion (Fig. 22). The condition may be unilateral and, if so, the surgical correction is modified appropriately.

### Developmental Anomalies of the Second Branchial Arch

These produce characteristic deformities involving the middle and external ear, the mandible, and at times the facial nerve (Fig. 23). Unlike the

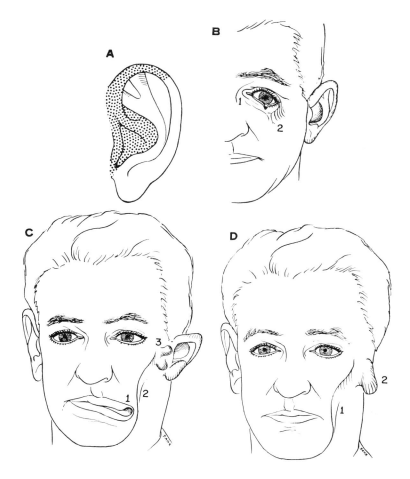

**Figure 23** *A*, Representation of contributions by branchial arches 1 (dotted area) and 2 (white area) to normal adult ear. The second branchial arch is represented by antihelix and lower helical crus. *B*, Treacher Collins syndrome (deficient maxillary process). Abnormal palpebral obliquity, coloboma, absence of cilia on medial two-thirds of lower lid, lack of malar development, abnormal hair above ear. Deformities are restricted to structures developing from the maxillary process. *C*, First branchial syndrome (mandibular arch). Macrostomia, hemignathia, and abnormalities of the helical crus and tragus (usually associated with preauricular tabs). Deformities are restricted to the first branchial arch derivatives. *D*, First and second branchial arch syndrome. Hemignathia and abnormalities of the entire auricle. Deformities are restricted to derivatives of dorsal part of branchial arches 1 and 2. These two arches normally combine in this area to form auricle, ramus of mandible, and temporomandibular joint. (From Stark, R. B., and Saunders, D. E.: Plast. Reconstr. Surg., *29*:229, 1962.)

case in Pierre Robin syndrome, the relative growth rate of the mandible may not be expected to improve with development. Instead, the deformity becomes progressively more severe with increasing age. Such children often require serial augmentation of the affected mandible with bone grafts in order to increase both length and height of the jaw. Many require associated building up of the soft tissues in the overlying parotid region. If reconstruction is performed at an early age, improved dental health and occlusion will be maintained. The associated ear deformities require separate staged reconstructive techniques.

## INJURIES

Most injuries to the jaw are secondary to mechanical trauma associated with falls, fights, or automobile accidents. The membranous bone comprising the support to the upper jaw has great capacity to absorb force with deceleration injuries. This property of energy absorption has saved many lives by protecting the brain from lethal injury when the facial bones crumple from a severe blow.[43]

The muscles attached to the upper jaw are small and lack the strength and leverage of those inserting on the mandible. Consequently, reduction of maxillary fractures does not require strong or prolonged fixation. The fractures usually occur in well defined patterns located at weak points in the bone.[25] In contrast, fractures of the mandible are often accompanied by severe displacement as a result of the pull of the strong muscles of mastication. Methods of mandibular fixation must thus be more secure and maintained for longer periods than in the case of fractures of the upper jaw.[11]

### Mandibular Fractures

Diagnosis of fracture of the mandible is best made by simple physical examination. Point tenderness will usually be found along the lower border of the mandible at the location of the fracture line. Crepitus and movement at this point are usually identified (Fig. 24). The patient will usually complain of some "abnormal" position of his teeth when he attempts to close his mouth. Numbness of the lower lip will be seen if the inferior alveolar nerve has been damaged. Fractures of the body of the mandible are often compounded into the oral cavity.

Treatment of mandibular fractures is most often accomplished by simple intermaxillary wiring or elastic band fixation of the remaining healthy teeth. Soft metallic bars are applied to the remaining teeth in each fracture fragment of the

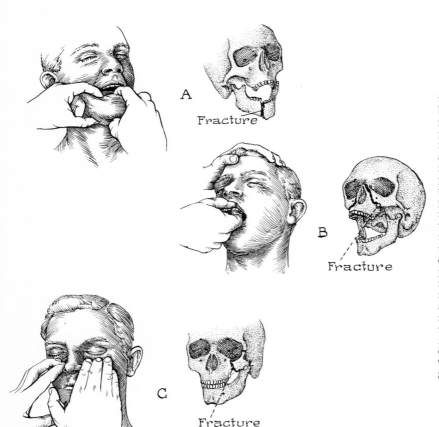

Figure 24   Manual examination for diagnosis of fractured bones of the face and jaws; careful examination with bimanual palpation will reveal the vast majority of facial fractures. In *A*, a gentle rocking motion of the fingers will reveal movement or pain at the site of fractures of the mandibular body or symphysis. In *B*, the top of the head is fixed and an attempt is made to move the hard palate by grasping the upper central incisor teeth. Midface fractures will often reveal slight movement or pain. In *C*, the examiner feels for symmetry of the infraorbital rim, or for a step or "notch" along the normal smooth lateral rim of the orbit. (From Edgerton, M. T. In: Ballinger, W. F., II, Rutherford, R. B., and Zuidema, G. D., eds.: The Management of Trauma. Philadelphia, W. B. Saunders Company, 1968.)

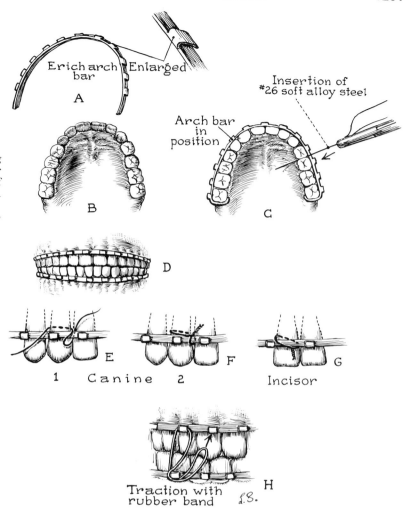

**Figure 25** Method of applying soft metallic arch bars to upper or lower jaw in preparation for use of intermaxillary elastic band fixation of a fractured maxilla or mandible: The soft metal Erich bar is bent to fit against the dental arch and allowed to curve about the most posterior tooth. Soft steel wires are then passed about the necks of the molar teeth and about the bar to make the latter secure. *E, F,* and *G* illustrate the variations in applying the wire when it is necessary to use a canine tooth as one point of fixation. This method prevents the tendency of such forces to slowly extract the anchored tooth. Once the arch bars are properly attached, elastic bands may be applied to the metal hooks, as shown in *H,* to bring the jaw fragments and teeth into satisfactory occlusion. (From Edgerton, M. T. In: Ballinger, W. F., II, Rutherford, R. B., and Zuidema, G. D., eds.: The Management of Trauma. Philadelphia, W. B. Saunders Company, 1968.)

upper and lower jaws, and small elastic bands are used to draw these arch bars and fragments into position so that the teeth will mesh in normal occlusal relationship (Fig. 25). When inadequate teeth remain for this type of stabilization, open reduction may be required. Open reduction may be accomplished through either the intraoral or extraoral route, and a steel wire fixation of the bone in the reduced position is accomplished. This type fixation is also desirable in patients with displaced fractures when one or more of the fragments do not contain teeth, in children with only deciduous dentition, and in patients with disruption of both maxillary and mandibular arches.

In recent years plastic surgeons have used open reduction increasingly to reduce morbidity with jaw fractures. Such fixation reduces the period of required intermaxillary fixation. If the patient with a jaw fracture has missing teeth that are unaccounted for at the time of initial examination, a chest x-ray should be obtained to be certain that the tooth has not been aspirated. Formerly surgeons recommended the extraction of *all*

*teeth lying within the fracture line of the jaw,* but it is now recognized that many of these teeth may be saved if the fracture is handled conservatively.

Some patients with fractures may be edentulous but may still have an intact denture. This may be used to help align the fragments of the lower jaw by attaching it by circumferential wires to splint the fractured mandible. Circumferential wiring without the aid of a denture as a splint may be used to secure bone fragments with oblique fracture lines. The formerly popular external skeletal pin fixation appliances proved to be cumbersome and unnecessary. They are rarely used for mandibular fractures today. An exception to this is seen in the case of compound injuries such as gunshot wounds of the lower jaw where large segments of bone may be missing and *external* fixation techniques must bridge the bony defect.

### Fractures of the Mandibular Condyle

Most condylar neck fractures should be treated conservatively by restoring dental occlusion with simple intermaxillary elastic band fixation for a

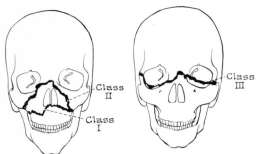

**Figure 26** Diagram showing the usual lines of fracture in LeFort's Class I, II, and III fractures. (From Edgerton, M. T. In: Ballinger, W. F., II, Rutherford, R. B., and Zuidema, G. D., eds.: The Management of Trauma. Philadelphia, W. B. Saunders Company, 1968.)

3 week period. If the head of the condyle has been badly displaced in a young child, open reduction is probably desirable to reduce the likelihood of progressive unilateral growth arrest of the jaw. With condyle fractures, the external auditory canal should be examined carefully as it may be fractured by the backward force of the condylar head against the bony ear canal.

Dislocations of the temporomandibular joint usually occur when the head of the condyle comes forward through a tear in the anterior joint capsule. The jaw may be locked in an open-bite position with considerable pain and muscle spasm. Local injection of lidocaine (Xylocaine) and downward traction on the molar teeth will often reduce the dislocation. At times, general anesthesia is required. A history of recurrent dislocation is indication for a reconstruction of the joint capsule by plastic techniques.

### Fractures of the Upper Jaw

Middle face fractures usually involve the two maxillas and the paired palatine bones. In 1900 Rene LeFort[25] classified these fractures as follows (Fig. 26).

1. LeFort I fractures (transverse maxillary fractures of Guerin). The fractured segment contains the upper teeth, the palate, lower portions of the pterygoid processes, and a portion of the wall of each maxillary sinus.

2. LeFort II fractures (pyramidal fractures). These fractures also contain the nasal bones and the frontal processes of the maxilla. The malar bones are usually not displaced with this fracture. Significant widening of the inner canthi of the eyes and bridge of the nose usually results with this fracture and there is often destruction of the ethmoid sinus cells.

3. LeFort III fractures (craniofacial disjunction). The maxillas, nasal bones, and zygomatic compound are separated as a unit from the cranial attachments (Fig. 26). Failure to recognize and reduce this type of fracture may result in severe elongation deformity of the central face. Unless it is corrected at the time of primary injury, late repair may be extremely difficult.

Diagnostic features of upper jaw fractures include malocclusion, open-bite deformity, and mobility of the upper jaw and hard palate (when upper teeth are grasped between the examiner's thumb and index finger). Stereoscopic roentgenograms in the Waters position (Fig. 27) provide an excellent x-ray view to visualize midface fractures. If the cribriform plate has been fractured,

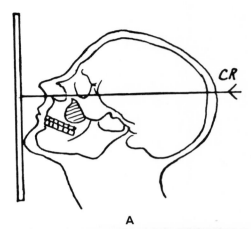

**A**

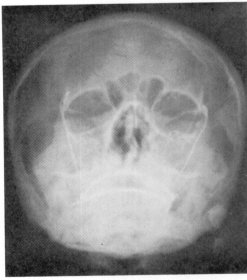

**B**

**Figure 27** Waters position. Posterior-anterior view for maxillary sinuses, maxilla, orbits, and zygomatic arches. This projection also may be helpful in demonstration of fractures of the nasal bones and nasal processes of the maxilla. In this view the petrous ridges are projected just below the floors of the maxillary sinuses. A, Position of the patient in relation to the film in the central ray. B, Waters view showing internal wire suspension for fixation in fractures of the middle third of the face. (From Dingman, R. O. In: Converse, J. M., ed.: Reconstructive Plastic Surgery. Volume II. Philadelphia, W. B. Saunders Company, 1964. A modified from Zizmor, J. In: Kazanjian, V. H., and Converse, J. M.: The Surgical Treatment of Facial Injuries. 2nd ed. Baltimore, Williams & Wilkins Company, 1959.)

watery cerebrospinal fluid may issue from the nostrils. To the patient this fluid has a salty taste. Treatment of these fractures is best carried out by direct surgical exposure with replacement and wiring together of the pieces of the bony puzzle. A suspension wire sling may be required to draw the maxilla into firm position against the base of the skull. The ends of the wires are allowed to emerge in the space behind the upper lip where they may be fixed to the arch bar, or attached to an upper tooth.

### Associated Fractures of the Zygomatic Compound

The malar bone is extremely dense, forming the prominence of each cheek. This bone is commonly fractured with injuries to the upper jaw. Such fractures may or may not involve displacement of the upper teeth or maxillas. The zygoma is often driven into the antrum and beneath the orbit. There are six common types of zygomatic fracture, based on the displacement of the bone and the required method of reduction (Fig. 28). These fractures tear the lining of the maxillary sinus and cause hematoma within the sinus cavity. The floor of the orbit may be displaced, causing injury to the globe or subsequent diplopia. The cheek bone is flattened, the lateral palpebral ligament may be displaced downward. One-half

of the upper lip is often numb. Irregularity of the bone may be felt by the examining finger when the rim of the orbit is palpated.

Treatment involves closed (Fig. 29) or open reduction to replace the bony parts and fix them with appropriate transosseous wiring. When possible, it is desirable to avoid packing the antral cavity. Existing lacerations or physiologic incisions within the "lines of skin relaxation" are used for exposure. In the case of zygomatic arch fractures, an incision may be made in the temple to allow an elevator to be passed beneath the arch and force the bone laterally into normal position (Gillies maneuver). Head caps with external wire fixation should be avoided whenever possible and are rarely necessary in the reduction of these fractures. If double vision is persistent after healing, it may be corrected by secondary repositioning of the orbit in approximately 80 per cent of the patients.

In approximately 7 per cent of all patients with major fractures in the upper and lower jaws, injuries to the cervical vertebrae may be found. Careful examination and x-rays of the neck are thus indicated in all such patients. It is imperative, on initial examination, to establish the presence of an adequate airway in all patients, and in many cases of displaced fracture of the mandible a tracheotomy is required.

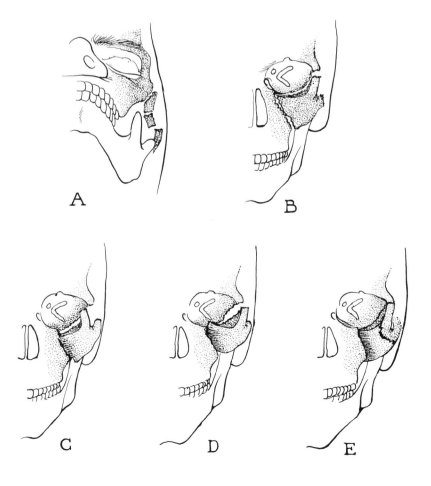

**Figure 28**  Simple classification of displaced fractures of the zygomatic compound: One in 20 fractures of the malar compound shows no significant displacement, and treatment is not required. One-tenth involve the arch only *(A)*, one-third show inward or downward displacement without rotation *(B)*, one-tenth show medial rotation of the upper part of the zygoma toward the midline *(C)*, one-fifth are rotated laterally *(D)*, and one-fifth are complicated by additional fractures of the central heavy portion of the malar bone *(E)*. These various types of fracture may be readily determined on examination and x-ray, and their recognition is of considerable help in planning operative reductions. (From Edgerton, M. T. In: Ballinger, W. F., II, Rutherford, R. B., and Zuidema, G. D., eds.: The Management of Trauma. Philadelphia, W. B. Saunders Company, 1968.)

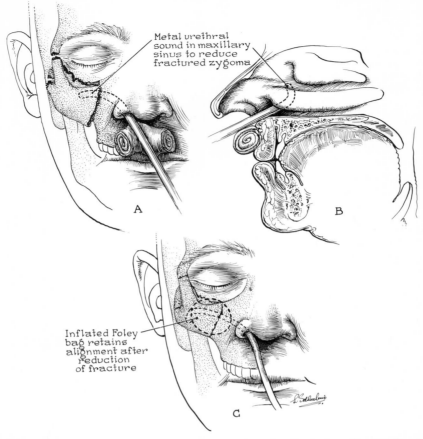

**Figure 29**   Early nonrotated fractures of the zygoma may at times be effectively reduced by the simple insertion of a metal urethral sound through the thin medial wall of the antrum by means of the nasal cavity. The tip of the sound may then be directed up beneath the solid central portion of the malar bone and a leverage action brought to bear against the bone from within. The roll of gauze acts as a fulcrum to protect the upper lip, and strong outward force can then be brought to bear on the zygoma. At times the bone will actually be heard to "click" back into place. If the zygoma does not remain stable in the reduced position, a Foley bag catheter can be inserted by the same route and the bag inflated until the bone receives adequate support. (From Edgerton, M. T. In: Ballinger, W. F., II, Rutherford, R. B., and Zuidema, G. D., eds.: The Management of Trauma. Philadelphia, W. B. Saunders Company, 1968.)

## INFECTIOUS DEFORMITY OF THE JAWS

The most common problem associated with infection in jaw bone results from diseased teeth with root abscesses and secondary osteomyelitis. This may result in chronic draining sinuses with pain, sequestration, and loss of bone. If infection is severe, nonunion of the mandible may result. Treatment usually requires surgical debridement, removal of sequestra, adequate soft tissue closure with drainage, and appropriate antibiotic therapy. If the upper jaw is involved, the infection may enter the antrum and require the surgeon to open and drain the sinus.

Chronic infections such as tuberculosis and actinomycosis must be recognized in patients with low-grade chronic drainage. They may be diagnosed by appropriate stains, cultures, and biopsies of tissue. Syphilis of the jawbone is now quite rare, but should be considered if associated defects in the bone and cartilaginous support of the nose and hard palate are seen.

In recent years, increasing numbers of patients with radio-osteonecrosis of the jaw have been seen following the treatment of cancer. This is sometimes an inevitable complication of adequate treatment of malignant disease; however, a characteristic of this type of bone infection is the severe pain that accompanies it, *even in the absence of significant change on x-ray examination of the bone.* Treatment usually requires wide removal of the damaged bone as spontaneous recovery is almost always prolonged and unpleasant. Spontaneous sequestration of dead bone is so delayed in such patients that surgical intervention at an early date is indicated.

## DEFICIENCY STATES AND METABOLIC DERANGEMENTS INVOLVING THE JAWS

Surgical treatment is of considerable value in many patients with metabolic disorders of bone. This includes young patients with fibrous dysplasia involving, commonly, the maxilla or mandible. Such patients may have associated disorders involving the long bones of the extremities and some will have a sensorineural hearing loss. The extensive facial deformities may be corrected by surgical sculpturing of the involved bones. X-ray therapy should be avoided for such conditions.

Other patients may suffer from ossifying fibromas with localized enlargement of the upper or lower jaw, or they may experience a cyst formation associated with parathyroid adenomas, producing giant cell tumors within the bones. In the mandible, such a condition may result in pathologic fractures. Bone grafting and cyst removal may be required.

## BENIGN TUMORS OF THE JAWS

Most benign tumors of the upper and lower jaw may be readily excised surgically once the diagnosis is established. Radiolucent lesions on x-ray often prove to be dental or root cysts. Radicular dentigerous cysts may cause considerable expansion of the alveolar cortex. Radiopaque benign tumors such as cementomas, osteomas, odontomas, and torus palatinus tumors are also quite common.

Fibromas and osteofibromas are frequently encountered. Most of these benign lesions may be removed by straightforward intraoral surgical techniques. If the resulting cavities are large and the mandibular bone has been weakened, the cavity may be filled with iliac crest bone chips to accelerate healing and provide strength.

## MALIGNANT TUMORS OF THE JAWS

### Adamantinoma (Ameloblastoma)

This interesting tumor appears to arise from the embryonic enamel organ of teeth and may be found in either the upper or the lower jaw. It is a slow-growing, low-grade malignant tumor that is known to metastasize to the bones or lungs at times. The histologic appearance is characteristic on biopsy, but local removal by curettement is commonly followed by recurrence. Wide excision of the lesion with bone grafting is the treatment of choice with larger lesions. Smaller lesions may be excised without grafting. The x-ray picture of these lesions shows a characteristic radiolucent "soap bubble" appearance.

### Osteogenic Sarcoma

Osteogenic sarcoma may involve either the mandible or the upper jaw. The condition carries a very grave prognosis, but may occasionally be cured by extremely wide resection. Reconstruction of the jaw should be deferred for a reasonable period because of the high incidence of early local recurrence. Postoperative radiation therapy should be used if the surgical margins are in doubt after resection.

### Osteochondrosarcoma

This type of cancer may be seen to develop after a history of repeated removal of bony tumors diagnosed as osteochondromas. With each successive recurrence, there may be change in the histologic appearance of the tumor. Wide removal of this lesion at the first opportunity may prevent this progressive and ominous change in clinical character. This tumor is sometimes encountered in children.

### Metastatic Carcinoma

The mandible, and less commonly the upper jaw, may be the seat of occasional metastatic tumors. Most commonly, these arise from the breast, thyroid, or prostate. In some instances, the metastasis to the mandible may produce the first symptoms of the patient's disease. Biopsy usually provides the diagnosis.

### Bone Grafting for Jaw Reconstruction

Bone grafting to the jaw is most commonly required to reconstruct the mandibular arch. Autogenous bone taken from the patient's iliac crest or rib cage provides the most suitable donor material (Fig. 30). Studies using radioactive material to label the cells of the bone graft would suggest that some of these cells remain viable after transplantation to the jaw region. If bony union is established with the recipient bone, creeping replacement of the cells within the bone graft appears to occur. A period of demineralization of the bone graft develops and reaches its peak about 6 months after surgery. After this, the healthy bone graft develops increased density and strength, manifested by greater density on radiologic examination. It would appear that normal mechanical stresses must be placed on the grafted bone if optimal strength and mineralization are to develop. The transplantation of bone that contains a growing epiphysis to the jaw in children has been followed by only very limited and clinically insignificant growth. Such bone grafts, utilizing a metatarsal bone, the head of the fibula, or a rib with contained epiphysis, have not produced growth sufficient to match the growth of the normal mandible on the opposite side of the child's face.

Successful bone grafting is correlated with the richness of vascularity of the soft tissue pocket into which the bone is placed, with the degree of bone contact against adequately bleeding recipient bone, with the absence of dead space and hematoma about the graft in the immediate postoperative period, and with the adequacy of fixation of the bone to its recipient site in the immediate weeks following transplantation. Within these guidelines of good technical bone grafting, reconstruction of the upper or lower jaw has proved to be quite successful.

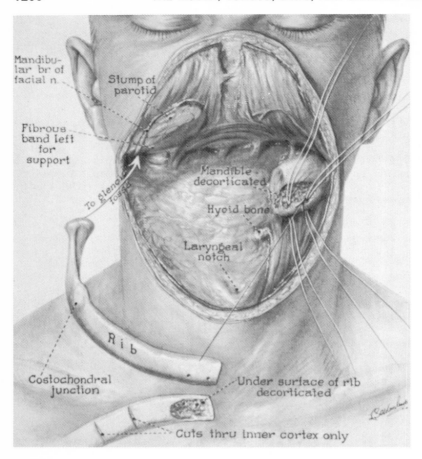

**Figure 30** Diagram showing late repair of a mandibular defect after hemimandibulectomy. The osteochondral graft of rib is taken from the opposite side of the chest so that the natural curve of the rib will match that of the mandibular angle. Small cuts through the inner cortex permit further shaping of the rib at the time of implantation. (From Edgerton, M. T., and DeVito, R. T. In: Converse, J. M., ed.: Reconstructive Plastic Surgery. Volume III. Philadelphia, W. B. Saunders Company, 1964.)

## SALIVARY GLANDS

The salivary glands are tubuloacinar glands arising from ectodermal and entodermal invaginations. They may be described as major and minor glands. There are six major salivary glands consisting of three pairs, namely, the parotid, submaxillary, and sublingual glands. Just beneath the mucosa of the oral cavity and pharynx, there are numerous minor salivary glands. All of these minor glands give mucous or mixed secretions except for von Ebner's posterior lingual gland. This produces a pure serous secretion.

Samuel White of Hudson, New York, is credited with the first successful surgical removal of the parotid gland, in 1808. Since that time, surgery has been increasingly useful in treating problems of the salivary glands.

### TRAUMA

Mechanical injury to the face may result in the division of parotid glandular tissue or Stensen's duct. When the duct is divided, the two ends should be carefully identified and, after appropriate wound debridement, repaired over a small plastic catheter that is allowed to emerge into the oral cavity (Fig. 31). Closure of the skin over the injured glandular tissue will usually be followed by satisfactory healing. Late complications of injury to the parotid may include the development of salivary-cutaneous fistulas or obstruction to the duct with resulting acute enlargement of the gland. Chronic salivary fistulas that persist for more than 3 months may require reconstruction; a pedicled strip of facial skin is used to redirect the secretions into the oral cavity. Acute obstruction or ligation of the duct may result in atrophy of the entire parotid gland on that side of the face. Contour reconstruction of the face by dermal grafts or synthetic implant may be required after such an event.

Children suffering from cerebral palsy or patients with damage to the tongue and lips following surgical procedures for cancer may be troubled by chronic drooling (ptyalism). Considerable help can be provided for such patients by transplantation of Stensen's ducts so that they enter the pharynx posteriorly. Further help for drooling may be provided by excision of the submaxillary glands to reduce salivary production.[8, 48]

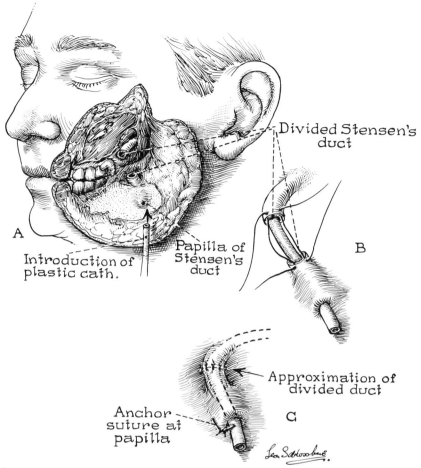

**Figure 31** Explosion injury to the cheek resulted in multiple fractures with division of the parotid duct approximately 1½ inches before its entrance into the oral cavity. The proximal end of the duct was found at operation and identified by the slow discharge of serous parotid secretion. The distal cut end was found by a retrograde threading of a polyethylene catheter from the duct papilla on the oral mucosa. Six-zero silk sutures were then placed in the submucosa of the duct to carry out fine closure of the divided duct with interrupted sutures. The catheter is anchored to the oral mucosa to prevent its slipping out in the postoperative period and is removed 2 weeks later. (From Edgerton, M. T. In: Ballinger, W. F., II, Rutherford, R. B., and Zuidema, G. D., eds.: The Management of Trauma. Philadelphia, W. B. Saunders Company, 1968.)

## INFECTIONS OF SALIVARY GLANDS (SIALADENITIS)

Isolated abscesses in the salivary glands are uncommon but may require incision and drainage if they develop. Low-grade infection is probably the most common cause of obstruction within the major salivary ducts and may be associated with the production of calculi.

Acute suppurative sialadenitis (parotid or submaxillary) may develop as a postoperative complication in patients who receive poor mouth care or when secretions are below the normal level. This condition causes severe sepsis and high fever and is dangerous to life. Such patients respond poorly to antibiotics and often require radical surgical excision of the necrotic gland. The condition is also seen postoperatively in children, but the prognosis is better in this group.

Recurrent acute sialadenitis may develop in some patients with reduced secretions. It is believed that these infections often ascend from the oral cavity by means of the major ducts. Ligation of the duct produces relief of symptoms and good results in about 65 per cent of the patients. Those who do not respond to this method may require parotidectomy or removal of the submaxillary gland.[10]

## METABOLIC DISORDERS

Calculi may form in the sublingual, submaxillary, or parotid ducts. Most commonly they are found near the duct orifice. They are thought to result from improper diet and abnormal salivary pH within the oral cavity, but prevention of further stone formation in such patients is difficult. Infection is present with many calculi, but in some instances may be secondary to the obstruction itself. Diagnosis is readily made by palpating the stone with the aid of a small lacrimal duct probe and the use of an intraoral radiograph of the duct in question. Once located, stones may usually be removed by incising the duct directly over the stone by the intraoral route. In some instances, residual infection of the gland after stone removal may make it necessary to carry out total sialoadenectomy.

Sialosis with chronic enlargement of the salivary glands may result from a variety of conditions. These include chronic states of malnutrition such as beriberi, sarcoidosis, and Mikulicz's syndrome. Elderly patients will frequently show a reduction in salivary gland secretion with paradoxical secondary gland enlargement and symptoms of xerostomia (dryness of the mouth). These conditions usually do not require surgical intervention but may be relieved by the use of lemon juice to stimulate secretions and by the administration of a sialogenous agent such as pilocarpine (1 mg. twice a day). In certain collagen disorders such as Sjögren's syndrome, the lack of tear formation by the lacrimal glands may be relieved by transplantation of the distal ends of the parotid ducts into the conjunctival sacs.

## SALIVARY TUMORS

Neoplasms of the salivary glands constitute approximately 5 per cent of all head and neck tumors. They provide the major cause for salivary gland surgery. Approximately 70 per cent of salivary gland tumors occur in the parotid gland and approximately 70 per cent of this group are benign. Roughly 60 per cent of submaxillary gland tumors are malignant.[17] The following classification of salivary tumors is useful:
A. Benign Tumors
   1. Mixed tumors (pleomorphic adenomas)
   2. Warthin's tumors (papillary cystadenoma lymphomatosum)
   3. Lymphoepithelial tumors (Mikulicz's disease and Sjögren's syndrome)
   4. Hemangiomas (capillary, cavernous, arteriovenous fistulas)
   5. Lymphangiomas (including hygroma)
   6. Oncocytic adenomas
   7. Miscellaneous benign conditions (including epidermoid cysts, lipomas, and branchial cleft cysts)
B. Malignant Tumors
   1. Mucoepidermoids (low-grade and high-grade types)
   2. Adenocarcinomas
      a. Adenoid-cystic (cylindromatous) type
      b. Acinic cell type
   3. Malignant mixed tumors
   4. Squamous cell carcinomas
   5. Undifferentiated carcinomas
   6. Salivary sarcomas
   7. Melanomas
   8. Metastatic cancers to the salivary gland or contained lymph nodes

### Diagnosis of Parotid Tumors

Most parotid tumors arise as slow-growing, firm, nodular masses that are sometimes mistaken for lymph nodes in the upper neck. They are usually painless and less than 30 per cent of those that are malignant will have produced paralysis of one or more branches of the facial nerve. Sialography with duct injection and x-ray is of interest but only rarely aids with treatment planning. X-ray of the chest and examination of the cervical lymph nodes may give evidence of metastatic spread. *Biopsy is required before final commitment to a surgical plan is made.*

Although needle biopsy has been popular in recent years, Ackerman and others have demonstrated that withdrawal of the needles will drag viable tumor cells outward into the skin. These microscopic nests of cells will implant and grow along the tract and thus complicate later treatment or lead to recurrence (Fig. 32). If the skin overlying the tumor is adherent or ulcerated, it will obviously be sacrificed at operation, and a direct biopsy may be taken directly through this skin at the initial examination. If the skin is uninvolved, it should be reflected from the surface of the tumor as the initial step at operation. The surgeon may then take a direct scalpel biopsy of the most prominent portion of the tumor, and send it to the pathology laboratory for frozen section. The modern cryostat now makes it possible for a competent pathologist to give a reliable frozen section diagnosis of most salivary tumors. The surgeon may then determine accurately whether the facial nerve should be saved or sacrificed in the ensuing dissection. By this approach, he avoids the danger of doing a simple lobectomy for an unsuspected parotid cancer.

Some surgeons prefer to perform a superficial lobectomy of the parotid gland if they suspect the lesion to be a mixed tumor. This approach is troublesome when the frozen section reveals a cancer of a histologically aggressive type.

In all benign parotid tumors and, indeed, with many of the smaller malignant tumors, great care should be taken to preserve the branches of the facial nerve. The patient's lips and eyelids should be left exposed during the operation so that any stimulation of the nerve can be detected (Fig. 33). We do not recommend the use of faradic current nerve stimulators as the method is less localizing than simple mechanical stimulation and may fatigue the nerve more readily. Most surgeons prefer to find the facial nerve by first exposing the proximal part of the nerve at the stylomastoid foramen. The tumor and parotid gland are rolled forward as the branches of the nerve are exposed. Some surgeons inject the parotid duct with methylene blue at the beginning of the operation to help outline the nerve branches and ducts. Others find the resultant staining of the gland undesirable. The operation is tedious and should be undertaken only by those very familiar with the anatomy of the region. Even with great gentleness transient paralysis of the face will sometimes be present after removal of a benign tumor. The

A

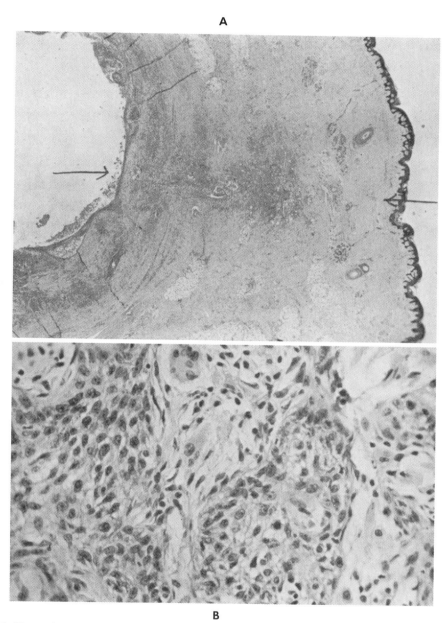

B

**Figure 32**  *A*, Photomicrograph of excised skin and portion of a node. The arrows point to a needle tract made 16 days previously. *B*, Undifferentiated squamous carcinoma in the needle tract, demonstrated in *A*. (From Ackerman, L. V., and Wheat, M. W., Jr.: Surgery, *37*:342, 1955.)

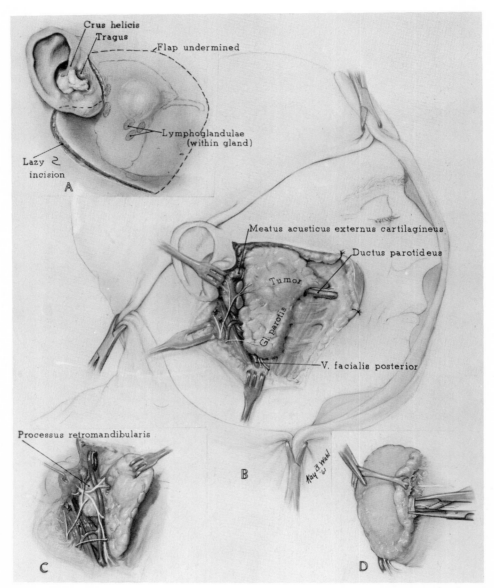

**Figure 33**  *A*, The incision is made long enough to facilitate complete exposure of the gland. The lower segment often need not extend quite so far posteriorly. *B*, The field exposed with the elevated flap sutured to the cheek. Note the common facial vein and marginal mandibular nerve at the lower pole of the parotid gland. *C*, Posterior approach to the facial nerve with the superficial lobe partly dissected from the nerve, and the retromandibular lobe still partly attached. This is the best approach for tumors located anteriorly. Note the greater auricular nerve with a small severed branch to the parotid capsule. *D*, Anterior approach, dissecting the anterior margin and elevating the gland from the facial nerve branches. Stensen's duct can be used as a tractor. This is the best approach for tumors located posteriorly or in the deep lobe. (From Robinson, D. W., and Masters, F. W. In: Converse, J. M., ed.: Reconstructive Plastic Surgery. Volume III. Philadelphia, W. B. Saunders Company, 1964.)

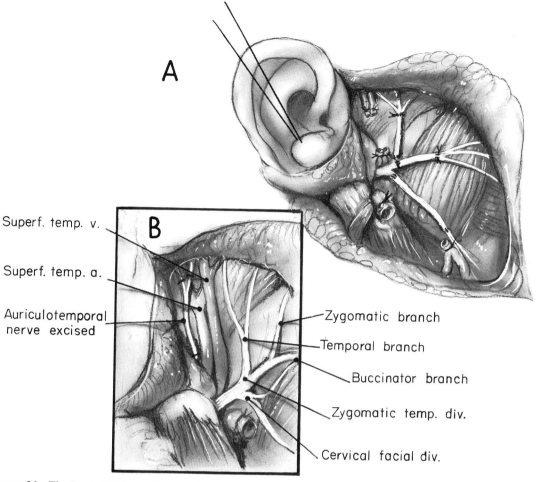

Superf. temp. v.

Superf. temp. a.

Auriculotemporal
nerve excised

Zygomatic branch

Temporal branch

Buccinator branch

Zygomatic temp. div.

Cervical facial div.

**Figure 34**  The inset *(B)* shows the usual anatomy of the facial nerve with its branches. *A* demonstrates repair of multiple branches of the facial nerve by free nerve grafts from the greater auricular nerve. (From Loré, J. M., Jr.: An Atlas of Head and Neck Surgery. Philadelphia, W. B. Saunders Company, 1962.)

patient should be warned of this possibility in advance and told that several months may be required for recovery of facial movements. Any surgical injury to a major branch of the facial nerve should be repaired immediately by suture or nerve grafting (Fig. 34). Following parotid resection with preservation of the facial nerve, about 50 per cent of the patients will have abnormal sweating of the skin overlying the parotid region in response to eating and other stimulation. This condition is known as gustatory sweating or Frey's syndrome. It is believed to be due to injury of the branches of the auriculotemporal nerve with subsequent crossed regeneration of fibers following surgery. It usually appears within 3 to 9 months after operation. Many such patients will find that these symptoms spontaneously improve. Frey's syndrome is rarely, if ever, seen in patients who have had *total* resection of the facial nerve along with the removal of malignant parotid tumors.

The mixed tumor of the parotid will recur in progressively more malignant forms if any attempt is made to remove it by simple "enucleation" techniques. The tiny nests of tumor cells may be seen extending through and beyond the gross capsule of these tumors. *An abundant layer of normal parotid tissue must be removed around the margins of mixed tumors in order to produce a consistent cure.*

### Surgical Treatment of Malignant Salivary Tumors

Malignant parotid tumors may require, because of their size or location, removal of portions of the facial nerve, overlying adherent skin, portions of the mandible, or segments of the external auditory canal, or in-continuity removal of the lymph nodes of the neck. In some instances, the deep surface of the tumor may involve the wall of the internal carotid artery, requiring its resection and the use of a vein graft to re-establish carotid circulation to the brain. Cranial nerves such as the vagus or hypoglossal may be involved, and if the patient has a history of pain in the face, the auriculotemporal nerve should be traced to the gasserian ganglion and resected with biopsy at that point.

Radical neck dissection of the regional cervical lymph nodes should be reserved for salivary tumors that are accompanied by enlarged and palpable nodes, for large or rapidly growing primary tumors, and for tumors diagnosed histologically as squamous carcinoma, malignant mixed tumor, adenoid-cystic carcinoma, or the high-grade variety of mucoepidermoid carcinoma. Lymph node metastasis to the neck is distinctly less common in the other types of malignant parotid and submaxillary tumors.

### Use of Immediate Reconstructive Techniques at the Time of Tumor Removal

Surgery continues to offer the best chance of cure with salivary gland tumors. Approximately 50 per cent of the patients receiving parotid resection remain free of disease. Approximately 800 deaths per year from salivary gland cancer are recorded in the United States. The most dramatic improvement in the treatment of salivary gland cancer in the past decade has been the increased use of immediate reconstructive techniques that make radical excisional surgery more acceptable to the patient.[23] These techniques include immediate transfer of the masseter muscle to the paralyzed corner of the mouth when the facial nerve must be removed; use of dermal ligaments and modified tarsorrhaphy to support paralyzed eyelids;[13] primary nerve grafts to the facial nerve (when distal and proximal nerve segments remain available);[30] free skin grafts and rotation flaps from neck or forehead to replace cutaneous defects; and occasionally primary bone grafting to replace the mandible. It is now inexcusable to leave any patient with an uncorrected facial nerve paralysis whose prognosis for remaining life exceeds even 1 or 2 years.

### Submaxillary Gland Tumors

Because of the deep location of the submaxillary gland and the high incidence of malignancy, lymph node dissection should be performed more often than in parotid cancer. Often the mylohyoid muscle and portions of the mandible must be resected to give adequate local tumor margins. At times, tumors of the submaxillary gland will also require removal of the lingual and hypoglossal nerves to provide adequate margins.

### Minor Salivary Gland Tumors

The most frequent tumors of the minor salivary glands occur in the palate and the majority of these are mixed tumors. When mixed tumors lie over the bony hard palate, it is sometimes wise to remove this bone en bloc with the tumor and immediately apply a split-thickness skin graft to the subjacent mucosa of the nasal floor. *Almost 75 per cent of the salivary gland tumors in the palate prove to be malignant.* Patients with such tumors require full-thickness resections of portions of the hard and the soft palate. Although hard palate defects may be managed by the use of a dental prosthesis, defects involving the posterior border of the soft palate are often best managed by an immediate reconstruction, using a flap of mucosa and muscle from the posterior pharynx (Fig. 35). When a prosthesis is to be used, a preoperative dental impression of the palate and upper jaw should be made. Many patients who remain well after resection of a malignant tumor of the palate will benefit from a subsequent pedicle flap reconstruction of the palate. Once the palate is reconstructed, they will not have to rely on a dental prosthesis for the remainder of their lives.

### Use of Radiation Therapy for Salivary Gland Tumors

Surgical excision offers the best method for cure of most salivary tumors other than lymphomas or metastatic tumors. However, in certain circumstances postoperative radiation therapy appears to improve the cure rate. Such treatment is indicated if the surgeon feels that there is residual cancer after radical resection, or if the pathologist reports "cancer extending to the margins of the resection." In such instances, postoperative cobalt therapy

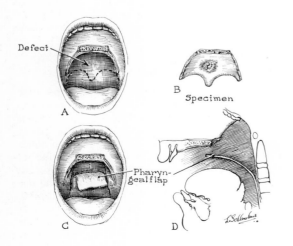

**Figure 35** Drawings showing the defect *(A)* is produced with adequate excision of soft palate tumors *(B)*. To restore velopharyngeal competency, a large posterior pharyngeal flap is elevated at the time of resection *(C and D)* and sutured into place. (From Edgerton, M. T., and DeVito, R. T. In: Converse, J. M., ed.: Reconstructive Plastic Surgery. Volume III. Philadelphia, W. B. Saunders Company, 1964.)

should be initiated as soon as satisfactory wound healing has been obtained. Other advanced parotid cancers that are clearly nonresectable may be controlled for many months by appropriate x-ray therapy.[6, 41]

### Chemotherapy for Salivary Tumors

In occasional circumstances, methotrexate or 5-fluorouracil therapy may produce limited regression of malignant neoplasms of the parotid or submaxillary gland. Such treatment, however, is often disappointing and serves primarily as late palliation rather than for improved cure rate. Infusion of the advanced parotid tumor with cyclophosphamide (Cytoxan) administered by retrograde catheter in the superficial temporal artery has produced marked regression in a few special tumors.

## SELECTED REFERENCES

Bardwil, J. M., Luna, M. A., and Healey, J. E.: Salivary glands. In: MacComb, W. S., and Fletcher, G. H.: Cancer of the Head and Neck. Baltimore, Williams & Wilkins Company, 1967, p. 357.
  *A concise review of anatomy and more recent pathologic classification of parotid tumors. The results reported with postoperative radiotherapy in selected cases are of interest.*

Converse, J. M., ed.: Reconstructive Plastic Surgery. Philadelphia, W. B. Saunders Company, 1964, Volume III, Chapters 34–39.
  *A very thorough treatise covering the basic aspects of cleft lip and palate surgery. It is well illustrated and referenced and provides a lucid introduction to this subject in full.*

Foote, F. W., Jr., and Frazelle, E. L.: Tumors of the major salivary glands. In: Atlas of Tumor Pathology. Section IV, Fascicle II. Washington, D.C., Armed Forces Institute of Pathology, 1954.
  *A classic paper on the classification, histology, and prognosis of salivary gland tumors.*

Hanna, D. C. Salivary gland tumors. In: Gaisford, J. C., ed.: Symposium on Cancer of the Head and Neck. Volume 2. St. Louis, C. V. Mosby Company, 1969, p. 352.
  *A sound review of the practical surgical management of parotid tumors with emphasis on reconstructive techniques.*

## REFERENCES

 1. Ackerman, L. V., and del Regato, J. A.: Cancer: Diagnosis, Treatment and Prognosis. 4th ed. St. Louis, C. V. Mosby Company, 1970, pp. 183–254 and 276–296.
 2. Ackerman, L. V., and Wheat, M. W., Jr.: The implantation of cancer—an avoidable surgical risk? Surgery, 37:341, 1955.
 3. Archard, H. O.: Biology of the human oral integument. In: Fitzgerald, T. B., et al., eds.: Dermatology in General Medicine. New York, McGraw-Hill Book Company, 1971, pp. 804–808.
 4. Archer, W. H.: Oral Surgery. 4th ed. Philadelphia, W. B. Saunders Company, 1966, pp. 384–388 and 563–566.
 5. Bales, H. W.: Head and neck tumors. In: Clinical Oncology for Medical Students and Physicians, A Multidisciplinary Approach. 3rd ed. New York, American Cancer Society, 1970–1971, pp. 228–261.
 6. Bardwil, J. M., Luna, M. A., and Healey, J. E.: Salivary glands. In: MacComb, W. S., and Fletcher, G. H.: Cancer of the Head and Neck. Baltimore, Williams & Wilkins Company, 1967, p. 357.
 7. Brown, J. B., and Fryer, M. P.: The Mouth, Tongue, Jaws and Salivary Glands. In: Davis, L., ed.: Christopher's Textbook of Surgery. 9th ed. Philadelphia, W. B. Saunders Company, 1968, pp. 323–357.
 8. Cohen, I. K., Holmes, E. C., and Edgerton, M. T.: Parotid duct transplantation for correction of drooling in patients with cancer of the head and neck. Surg. Gynec. Obstet., 133:663, 1971.
 9. Converse, J. M., ed.: Reconstructive Plastic Surgery. Philadelphia, W. B. Saunders Company, 1964, Volume III, Chapters 34–39.
10. Diamant, H., and Salen, B.: Akut varig parotid opusc. Med. (Stockholm), 9:56, 1964.
11. Dingman, R. O., and Natvig, P.: Surgery of Facial Fractures. Philadelphia, W. B. Saunders Company, 1964.
12. Douglas, B.: The treatment of micrognathia associated with obstruction by a plastic procedure. Plast. Reconstr. Surg., 1:300, 1946.
13. Edgerton, M. T.: Surgical correction of facial paralysis—a plea for better reconstruction. Trans. Southern Surg. Ass., 1966, p. 341.
14. Edgerton, M. T., and Dellon, A. L.: Surgical retrodisplacement of the levator veli palatini muscle. Plast. Reconstr. Surg., 47:154, 1971.
15. Edgerton, M. T., and DeVito, R. T.: Reconstructive surgery in treatment of oral, pharyngeal and mandibular tumors. In: Converse, J. M., ed.: Reconstructive Plastic Surgery. Philadelphia, W. B. Saunders Company, 1964, pp. 963–1037.
16. Edgerton, M. T., Udvarhelyi, G. B., and Knox, D. L.: The surgical correction of ocular hypertelorism. Ann. Surg., 172:473, 1970.
17. Foote, F. W., Jr., and Frazelle, E. L.: Tumors of the major salivary glands. In: Atlas of Tumor Pathology. Section IV, Fascicle II. Washington, D.C., Armed Forces Institute of Pathology, 1954.
18. Freund, R. H.: Principles of Head and Neck Surgery. New York, Appleton-Century-Crofts, 1967, p. 291.
19. Garrison, F. H.: An Introduction to the History of Medicine. 4th ed. Philadelphia, W. B. Saunders Company, 1929.
20. Ghadially, F. N.: Keratoacanthoma. In: Fitzgerald, T. B., et al., eds.: Dermatology in General Medicine. New York, McGraw-Hill Book Company, 1971, pp. 425–435.
21. Glickman, I.: The oral cavity. In: Robbins, S. L.: Pathology. 3rd ed. Philadelphia, W. B. Saunders Company, 1967, pp. 770–817.
22. Grabb, W. C., Rosenstein, S. W., and Bzoach, K. R.: Cleft Lip and Palate. Boston, Little, Brown and Company, 1971.
23. Hanna, D. C.: Salivary gland tumors. In: Gaisford, J. C., ed.: Symposium of Cancer of the Head and Neck. Volume 2. St. Louis, C. V. Mosby Company, 1969, p. 352.
24. Leake, D.: History of oral surgery. In: Guralnick, W. C., ed.: Textbook of Oral Surgery. Boston, Little, Brown and Company, 1968, pp. 1–8.
25. LeFort, R.: Fractures de la machoire supérieure. Cong. internat. de med., Paris, 1900, sect. de chir. gén., pp. 275–278.
26. LeMesurier, A. B.: The quadrilateral Mirault flap operation for harelip. Plast. Reconstr. Surg., 33:26, 1964.
27. Lewis, S. R., Lynch, J. B., and Blocker, T. G., Jr.: The use of facial slings for tongue stabilization in the Pierre Robin syndrome. Plast. Reconstr. Surg., 42:237, 1968.
28. MacComb, W. S., Fletcher, G. H., and Healey, J. E., Jr.: Intra-oral cavity. In: MacComb, W. S., and Fletcher, G. H.: Cancer of the Head and Neck. Baltimore, Williams & Wilkins Company, 1967, pp. 89–151.
29. MacFee, W. F.: Carcinoma of the floor of the mouth; clinical observations and surgical treatment. Ann. Surg., 149:172, 1959.
30. Miehlke, A.: Nerve grafting for restoration of lost facial expression. In: Conley, J.: Cancer of the Head and Neck. Washington, Butterworths, 1967, p. 550.
31. Millard, D. R.: Refinements in rotation-advancement cleft lip technique. Plast. Reconstr. Surg., 33:26, 1964.
32. Moncrief, J. A.: Burns. In: Schwartz, S. I., et al., eds.: Principles of Surgery. New York, McGraw-Hill, 1969, pp. 211–212.
33. Ochsner, A.: Diseases of the mouth. In: Ochsner, A., and DeBakey, M. E., eds.: Christopher's Minor Surgery. 8th ed. Philadelphia, W. B. Saunders Company, 1959, pp. 270–283.
34. Proskauer, C., and Witt, F. H.: Bildgeschichte der Zahnheilkunde. Colonge, Dumont, 1962.

35. Reed, R. J., and O'Quinn, S. E.: Vascular neoplasms. In: Fitzgerald, T. B., et al., eds.: Dermatology in General Medicine. New York, McGraw-Hill Book Company, 1971, pp. 533–547.

36. Robbins, S. L.: Textbook of Pathology. 3rd ed. Philadelphia, W. B. Saunders Company, 1967, pp. 1313–1367.

37. Robin, P.: Backward lowering of the root of the tongue causing respiratory disturbances. Bull. Acad. Nat. Med., 89:37, 1923.

38. Rose, W.: Harelip and Cleft Palate. London, H. K. Lewis and Company, 1891.

39. Stark, R. B.: Pathogenesis of harelip and cleft palate. Plast. Reconstr. Surg., 13:20, 1954.

40. Stark, R. B.: Embryology of cleft lip and palate. In: Converse, J. M., ed.: Reconstructive Plastic Surgery. Philadelphia, W. B. Saunders Company, 1964, pp. 1355–1358.

41. Stewart, J. B., Jackson, A. W., and Chew, M. K.: The role of radiotherapy in the management of malignant tumors of the salivary glands. Amer. J. Roentgen., 102:100, 1968.

42. Stoll, H. L.: Squamous cell carcinoma. In: Fitzgerald, T. B., et al., eds.: Dermatology in General Medicine. New York, McGraw-Hill Book Company, 1971, pp. 407–422.

43. Swearingen, J. J.: Tolerances of the Human Face to Crash Impact. Report from the Office of Aviation Medicine. Washington, D.C., Federal Aviation Agency, July, 1965.

44. Tennison, C. W.: The repair of unilateral cleft lip by the stencil method. Plast. Reconstr. Surg., 9:115, 1952.

45. Tessier, P., Guiot, G., Rougerie, J., Delbet, P., and Pastoriza, J. Ostéotomies cranio-naso-orbito-faciales. Hypertélorisme. Ann. Chir. Plast., 12:103, 1967.

46. Thompson, J. E.: An artistic and mathematically accurate method of repairing the defect in cases of harelip. Surg. Gynec. Obstet., 14:498, 1912.

47. Wang, M. K. H., and Macomber, W. B.: Deformities of the lips and cheeks. In: Converse, J. M., ed.: Reconstructive Plastic Surgery. Philadelphia, W. B. Saunders Company, 1964, pp. 829–833.

48. Wilkie, T. F.: Surgical treatment of drooling. Follow-up report of five years experience. Plast. Reconstr. Surg., 45:549, 1970.

49. Wolfort, F. G., DeMeester, F., Knorr, N., and Edgerton, M. T.: Surgical management of cutaneous lye burns. Surg. Gynec. Obstet., 131:873, 1970.

50. Zarem, H. A., and Edgerton, M. T.: Induced resolution of cavernous hemangiomas following prednisolone therapy. J. Plast. Reconstr. Surg., 39:76, 1967.

# 41

# NEUROSURGERY

## Guy L. Odom, M.D., and Associates

## HISTORICAL ASPECTS

### Robert H. Wilkins, M.D.

The American student who is interested in the history of neurosurgery has a unique advantage. This specialty is of relatively recent origin and has been developed mainly in the English-speaking countries. For this reason, classic works in neurosurgery are usually obtainable and understandable.[3,8] In addition, there are several excellent reviews of neurosurgical history that are written in English.[2,5,7]

These reviews all point out the fact that although the great majority of neurosurgical procedures have been developed recently, the history of trepanation dates back to the Neolithic Period. In widely separated geographic locations, archeologists have discovered human skulls containing crainectomy defects. Furthermore, in many of these skulls there are evidences of healing along the bony edges, indicating that the "patient" survived the operation. The rationale for these procedures is not known, since there are no written records from this era, but it is conceivable that seizures, headaches, or mental changes might have been the symptoms that led to this drastic form of treatment.

The oldest known writing dealing with surgical topics, the Edwin Smith Papyrus, is of special interest to the neurosurgeon. This treatise dates back to the seventeenth century B.C. and contains the first descriptions of the cranial sutures, the meninges, the external surface of the brain, the cerebrospinal fluid, and the intracranial pulsations. Brain injuries are related to changes in the function of other parts of the body, and hemiplegic contractures are well described. In addition, quadriplegia, urinary incontinence, and priapism are noted to occur in association with cervical vertebral dislocation. The Egyptian physicians of that period had a surprising knowledge of rudimentary neuroanatomy and neurophysiology, but their treatment of injuries of the central nervous system was only supportive. Significantly, trepanation is not mentioned in the Edwin Smith Papyrus.

The writings of Hippocrates contain the first recorded descriptions of trepanation, and his instruments and methods were very similar to their modern counterparts. In addition, Hippocrates dealt with other subjects of neurosurgical interest. He discussed epilepsy, the co-existence of spinal deformity with pulmonary tubercles, and the functional effects of compression of the spinal cord. He devised a method for reducing vertebral dislocations, and described permanent and transient facial paralyses, sciatica, and the complex of headache, visual disturbance, and vomiting. The ability of Hippocrates as an observer is well demonstrated by his descriptions of aphasia, unconsciousness, respiratory and cardiac irregularity, carphologia, pupillary inequality, and ophthalmoplegia associated with cerebral disease. He realized that a blow on one side of the head occasionally is followed by convusions or paralysis of the contralateral side of the body, and he recognized the poor prognosis of the patient with a head injury complicated by a dural laceration. These and other observations made the works of Hippocrates a beacon to surgeons for over 2000 years, until the development of anesthesia, asepsis, and cerebral localization in the nineteenth century established the foundation of modern neurosurgery.

The introduction of anesthesia and asepsis vastly increased the scope of surgery in general and made brain surgery feasible. Such operations were not performed often, however, because there was no way to locate lesions that did not involve the skull. The problem was solved when it was discovered by Jean Bouillaud, Paul Broca, Gustav Fritsch, Eduard Hitzig, David Ferrier, and others that there is focal representation of bodily function in the brain. This third fundamental concept—cerebral localization—became an important part of the foundation upon which modern neurosurgery was built.

Another vital advancement made during the late nineteenth century was the development of the technique of osteoplastic craniotomy by Wilhelm Wagner, which was later facilitated by the use of Leonardo Gigli's wire saw. The introduction of this technique permitted the exploration of relatively large areas of the cortex, and in so doing significantly extended the limits of brain surgery.

British surgeons were among the first to take advantage of these new developments, and they guided neurosurgery through its infancy in the last two decades of the nineteenth century. William Macewen, professor of surgery at the University of Glasgow, and a powerful figure in international surgical circles, was a pioneer in surgery of the central nervous system. Macewen was a pupil of Joseph Lister, and he strongly believed in Lister's principles of antisepsis. His phenomenal success in treating intracranial abscesses rarely has been equaled since that time, despite the subsequent introduction of antibiotics.

Rickman Godlee also applied Lister's principles of antisepsis to neurosurgery in 1884, when he became the first surgeon to attack an intracranial tumor that had been localized solely by neurologic means. William Bennett was another of these pioneering British surgeons. In 1888 he introduced the operation of posterior rhizotomy for the relief of pain.

The most outstanding surgeon in this field at that time, however, was Victor Horsley of London. He devoted the majority of his efforts to clinical and experimental neurosurgery, with exceptional results. Although he made myriad contributions, Horsley is best remembered today as the first surgeon to remove a neoplasm from the spinal canal (1887), and the first to attempt retrogasserian neurotomy for tic douloureux (1890). He also introduced bone wax (1892), and described a stereotactic apparatus for intracranial procedures in 1908, with Clarke.

During the early development of neurosurgery, it was common for neurologists to diagnose the disease, devise the operation, and direct the surgeon in its performance. For example, Hughes Bennett localized the brain tumor that was removed in 1884 by Rickman Godlee, and William Gowers diagnosed the spinal cord tumor that was removed by Victor Horsley in 1887. In the United States, similar situations were encountered frequently. William Spiller, at the University of Pennsylvania, directed Charles Frazier in the performance of a successful retrogasserian neurotomy in 1901, and 10 years later directed Edward Martin in the performance of the first cordotomy. Similarly, Charles Dana at the Cornell University Medical College proposed posterior rhizotomy as performed a short time later by William Bennett in London and Robert Abbe in New York. Two outstanding neurologists of a later generation, Otfrid Foerster in Germany and Clovis Vincent in France, actually became neurosurgeons to facilitate the procedures they devised. Foerster, for example, independently devised the operation of cordotomy and performed classic studies of cortical function and peripheral sensory innervation.

A host of general surgeons tried their hands at neurosurgery during its formative years at the turn of the century. Most were soon discouraged by the innumerable difficulties accompanying this type of surgery. Between 1886 and 1896, for example, more than 500 different general surgeons reported brain operations they had performed, but between 1896 and 1906 the number fell below 80.

Fortunately, during this time a young surgeon at Johns Hopkins University took an interest in neurosurgery and decided to devote his full attention to it. With little help, Harvey Cushing advanced neurosurgery from its infancy through its childhood.[1] He standardized operating technique, and by applying the rigid principles of William Halsted to neurosurgical procedures, Cushing was able to make major reductions in operative morbidity and mortality. Before Cushing's time hemorrhage had presented an almost insurmountable problem during brain surgery. In his typically thorough manner, Cushing mastered the techniques of others for compressing the scalp, waxing the diploë, and so forth, and then he introduced the silver clips and electrocautery that have become virtually indispensable for the control of intracranial and intraspinal bleeding.

Brain tumors also attracted Cushing's attention, and during the course of his career more than 2000 patients with brain tumors were seen in his clinic. With the aid of several brilliant assistants, such as Percival Bailey, Louise Eisenhardt, and Paul Bucy, Dr. Cushing classified these tumors morphologically, described their biologic behavior, and formulated their surgical treatment. The standardization of technique and the classification of brain tumors were only two of Harvey Cushing's many contributions. There are few areas of modern neurosurgical interest that are not based to some extent on the important investigations of this one man.

Another such giant was Walter Dandy. Dandy worked with Cushing for a short time at the Johns Hopkins Hospital before Cushing moved on to the Peter Bent Brigham Hospital. Dandy stayed at Johns Hopkins, and before he had finished his residency in surgery, he made two very important discoveries. In association with Kenneth Blackfan, he established the modern concept of hydrocephalus and developed the operations of choroid plexectomy and third ventriculostomy for the relief of communicating and obstructive hydrocephalus. A few years later, in 1918 and 1919, he introduced pneumoventriculography and pneumoencephalography, which have proved to be of inestimable diagnostic value to neurosurgeons since that time. As was true of Cushing, Dandy's contributions to neurosurgery were legion and his many pupils have influenced profoundly the subsequent course of modern neurosurgery.

A third such contributor was the Portuguese neurologist, Antonio Caetano de Abreu Freire Egas Moniz. Moniz was unusually talented in a number of fields other than medicine, but he still found time to produce more than 300 medical publications. With neurosurgeon Pedro Manuel de Almeida Lima, he introduced the diagnostic technique of carotid arteriography in 1927 and initiated prefrontal lobotomy for psychiatric illnesses in 1936. For the latter work, Egas Moniz received a Nobel Prize in 1949.

Despite the outstanding work of Cushing, Dandy, and Moniz, most advancements in neurosurgery have been made slowly by the patient efforts of many pioneers. The subsequent developments in the various areas of neurosurgery are outlined in the remainder of this chapter.

## SELECTED REFERENCES

Walker, A. E.: History of Neurological Surgery. Baltimore, Williams & Wilkins Company, 1951.
*This book is the standard history of neurosurgery, with 18 chapters on various aspects of the specialty by 12 contributors. It also contains 14 biographic sketches of pioneering neurosurgeons, and a bibliography containing 2371 references.*

Wilkins, R. H.: Neurosurgical Classics. New York, Johnson Reprint Corp., 1965.
*This is a collection of 52 of the most outstanding written contributions in the field of neurologic surgery. These have been compiled into 38 groups, each of which is accompanied by a commentary and a list of related references. The 15 works originally printed in other languages have been translated into English.*

## REFERENCES

1. Fulton, J. F.: Harvey Cushing. A Biography. Springfield, Ill., Charles C Thomas, 1946.
2. Horrax, G.: Neurosurgery: An Historical Sketch. Springfield, Ill., Charles C Thomas, 1952.
3. Morton, L. T.: A Medical Bibliography (Garrison and Morton): An Annotated Check-list of Texts Illustrating the History of Medicine. 3rd ed. Philadelphia, J. B. Lippincott Company, 1970.

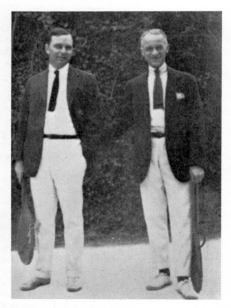

**Figure 1** Walter Dandy (left) and Harvey Cushing (right) after a game of tennis in 1921. (From Fulton, J. F.: Harvey Cushing. A Biography. 1946. Courtesy of Charles C Thomas, Publisher, Springfield, Ill.)

4. Penfield, W.: Neurosurgery, yesterday, today and tomorrow. J. Neurosurg., 6:6, 1949.
5. Sachs, E.: History and Development of Neurological Surgery. New York, P. B. Hoeber, 1952.
6. Scarff, J. E.: Fifty years of neurosurgery, 1905–1955. Int. Abstr. Surg., 101:417, 1955.
7. Walker, A. E.: History of Neurological Surgery. Baltimore, Williams & Wilkins Company, 1951.
8. Wilkins, R. H.: Neurosurgical Classics. New York, Johnson Reprint Corp., 1965.

# DIAGNOSTIC STUDIES

*M. Stephen Mahaley, Jr., M.D.*

## Skull X-rays

Plain film roentgenographic examination of the neurosurgical patient remains an extremely valuable though often underemphasized aid in diagnosis.[16] In instances of cranial trauma, skull films are used in outlining linear, comminuted, or depressed skull fractures; foreign bodies such as missile or bone fragments; pneumocephalus; and air-fluid levels in the sphenoid sinus. With intracranial mass lesions, a shift of the calcified pineal gland may indicate the side of a lesion. Separation of the cranial suture lines and presence of a "hammered silver" appearance of the calvarium characterize chronically increased intracranial pressure in children. Pathologic calcification may be visible in lesions such as tumors, toxoplasmosis, tuberous sclerosis, and vascular structures. Certain congenital abnormalities such as hydrocephalus, platybasia, craniosynostosis, encephalocele, and microcephaly often require skull x-rays for accurate evaluation. In postoperative cases, skull films may be quite helpful in evaluating obliteration of the subdural space when tantalum dust and silver clips have been used as markers,[18] in determining tumor recurrence when such markers have been placed in the tumor bed at the time of original surgery, and in searching for retained foreign bodies following trauma surgery. It is recommended that a routine chest x-ray be obtained for all neurosurgical patients suspected of having an intracranial or intraspinal mass lesion. It is not uncommon for a patient with signs and symptoms of a nervous system mass to harbor an asymptomatic pulmonary lesion such as a carcinoma.

## Spine X-rays

Plain spine x-rays are secured whenever a pathologic process is suspected in the cervical, dorsal, or lumbosacral area.[16] In instances of trauma, fractures and dislocations may be apparent, and subsequent films become essential as one attempts reduction and realignment. Congenital spine problems, such as spondylolisthesis, kyphoscoliosis, spina bifida, and diastematomyelia, can be evaluated. Views of the interspace area may reveal degenerative disc disease or infection while changes (lytic or blastic) in the bony structure may suggest a neoplastic process. Erosion of the bony pedicles often indicates the site of an expanding mass within the spinal canal.

## Lumbar Puncture

The diagnostic lumbar puncture is essential to the establishment of the diagnosis of meningitis or subarachnoid hemorrhage and is valuable in other diagnoses. However, particularly as regards the neurosurgical patient, one must be aware of the possible rapid neurologic deterioration of a patient with a focal mass lesion such as a brain abscess, tumor, or hematoma when cerebrospinal fluid is removed from the spinal route. As part of the route of a lumbar puncture, cerebrospinal fluid pressure should be noted, with the patient as relaxed as possible and without any compressive force upon the neck or abdominal areas. The cerebrospinal fluid should be compared with water, as a control, for color and clarity. Cerebrospinal fluid should be examined for protein and sugar content, cells, reactivity with syphilis, and colloidal gold. Protein electrophoretic patterns, when available, are used instead of colloidal gold reactions, and Millipore cerebrospinal fluid cytology may be an added diagnostic aid.[8, 19] Several special techniques are *not* part of a routine diagnostic lumbar puncture: the Queckenstedt maneuver to determine the patency of the spinal canal,[13] the Tobey-Ayer maneuver for testing the patency of the transverse venous sinuses,[17] and isotope cisternography, in which radioactive materials are injected intrathecally in an attempt to clarify diagnostic problems such as cerebrospinal fluid rhinorrhea,[3] hydrocephalus, including normal-pressure hydrocephalus,[6, 12] and shunt tube patency.

## Subdural Tap

Diagnostic tapping of the subdural space represents a technique useful primarily in children with nonfused cranial sutures.[11] A lumbar puncture or special subdural tap needle containing a solid stylus is passed through the scalp at an angle and then perpendicularly through the coronal suture line just lateral to the anterior fontanelle. The stylus is withdrawn after the needle tip passes through the dura, and any fluid issuing forth is collected. This technique serves not only to establish the diagnosis of the subdural hematoma or effusion but also may effectively treat such lesions. The volume and color of the fluid should always be noted and the fluid cultured when indicated.

## Myelography

Myelography is a radiographic means of outlining the contents of the spinal canal, utilizing positive (Pantopaque) or negative (air) contrast media. As regards Pantopaque myelography, this technique has been adequately described[14] and has proved invaluable as a diagnostic aid with disorders such as ruptured discs, osteoarthritic ridges and spurs, spinal tumors, angiomatous malformations on the surface of the cord, and spinal extradural hematomas. When the Queckenstedt maneuver is positive (sluggish or nonreactive) indicating probable block in the continuity of the cerebrospinal fluid pathway, a small amount of intrathecal Pantopaque usually suffices to delineate the location and configuration of the lesion. Air myelography[7, 15] is the procedure of choice in outlining lesions of the upper cervical cord and foramen magnum: meningiomas, neurinomas, Arnold-Chiari malformations, syringomyelia,[1] and hydromyelia.

## Pneumoencephalography

Pneumoencephalography is used less frequently now to localize brain tumors because of its possible deleterious effect on intracranial hydrodynamics in the presence of a mass lesion. However, it remains the definitive diagnostic procedure for cortical atrophy, hydrocephalus, porencephaly, focal cicatrix, and seizure disorders not accompanied by localizing signs of increased intracranial pressure.[16] Fractional pneumoencephalography permits the identification of cerebellar tonsillar location early in the study, gives exquisite detail of posterior fossa structures without confusing overlying supratentorial air, and allows control of the movement of air during the study.

## Ventriculography

Ventriculography with oxygen or air is utilized in cases of hydrocephalus either in the newborn or in older patients with evidence of increased intracranial pressure, when an air study from the spinal route might be complicated by tissue herniation at the tentorial notch or foramen magnum. The transcoronal suture approach can be used in children, and in adults a twist drill opening in the skull or a burr hole is used to permit passage of the ventricular needle. Positive contrast materials such as Pantopaque may be needed to outline small acoustic neurinomas and anatomic structures in the posterior third ventricle and aqueduct areas.[10]

## Angiography

Cerebral angiography is possible by several approaches—carotid, brachial, or femoral artery catheterization—depending largely upon the disease suspected. Angiography has to a great degree supplanted air study as the definitive diagnostic study for supratentorial tumors (neoplasms, abscesses, and hematomas) and, of course, is the definitive study in the diagnosis of aneurysms, arteriovenous malformations, and arterial occlusive disease.

## Electroencephalography

Electroencephalography is most useful in the diagnosis of seizure disorders, metabolic disturbances, and certain encephalitides.[4] It is used as an indicator of brain death. The brain surface corticogram is used extensively in surgery for epileptic disorders. It should be remembered, however, that the neurologic examination, brain scan, or angiography may provide a more definitive localization of intracranial pathologic change than the electroencephalogram, which may be completely normal in extracerebral lesions, such as meningiomas.

## Brain Scanning

Isotopic brain scanning has gained enormous popularity in recent years, and both technique and accuracy have shown continuous improvement.[2, 5] It has proved useful in neoplasms, abscesses, subdural hematomas, and cerebral infarctions, and as a study of relative cerebral blood flow. It is being used to follow brain tumor patients postoperatively for evidence of recurrence.

## Electromyography

Electromyography, combined with nerve conduction studies, has proved valuable in the initial evaluation and subsequent following of peripheral nerve injuries.[9] When neurologic signs and myelography are not conclusive, the electromyogram may aid in localization of spinal root lesions.

## REFERENCES

1. Conway, W. L.: Hydrodynamic studies in syringomyelia. J. Neurosurg., 27:501, 1967.
2. Davis, C. H., Jr., Alexander, E. J., Witcofski, R. L., and Maynard, C. D.: Brain scanning with 99m technetium. J. Neurosurg., 24:987, 1966.
3. DiChiro, G., Ommaya, A. K., Ashburn, W. L., and Briner, W. H.: Isotope cisternography in the diagnosis and follow-up of cerebrospinal fluid rhinorrhea. J. Neurosurg., 28:522, 1968.
4. Gibbs, F. A., and Gibbs, E. L.: Atlas of Electroencephalography. 2nd ed. Reading, Mass., Addison-Wesley Publishing Company, Volumes I, II, III, 1950, 1952, 1964.
5. Gilson, A. J., and Smoak, W. M., III: Central Nervous System Investigation with Radionuclides. Springfield, Ill., Charles C Thomas, 1971.
6. Heinz, E. R., Davis, D. O., and Karp, H. R.: Abnormal isotope cisternography in symptomatic occult hydrocephalus. A correlative isotopic-neuroradiological study in 130 subjects. Radiology, 95:109, 1970.
7. Jirout, J.: Pneumomyelography. Springfield, Ill., Charles C Thomas, 1969.
8. Koss, L. G.: Diagnostic Cytology and Its Histopathologic Basis. 2nd ed. Philadelphia, J. B. Lippincott Company, 1968.
9. Krusen, F. H., ed.: Handbook of Physical Medicine and Rehabilitation. 2nd ed. Philadelphia, W. B. Saunders Company, 1971.
10. Lang, E. K., and Russell, J. R.: Pantopaque ventriculography: demonstration and assessment of lesions of the third ventricle and posterior fossa. J. Neurosurg., 32:5, 1970.
11. Matson, D. D.: Neurosurgery of Infancy and Childhood. 2nd ed. Springfield, Ill., Charles C Thomas, 1969.
12. Ojemann, R. G., Fisher, C. M., Adams, R. D., Sweat, W. H., and New, P. F. J.: Further experience with the syndrome of "normal" pressure hydrocephalus. J. Neurosurg., 31:279, 1969.
13. Queckenstedt, M. E.: Zur Diagnose der rückenmarks Kompression. Deutsch. Z. Nervenheilk., 55:316, 1916.
14. Shapiro, R.: Myelography. Chicago, Year Book Medical Publishers, 1962.
15. Southworth, L. E., Jimenez, J. P., and Goree, J. A.: A practical approach to cervical air myelography. Amer. J. Roentgen., 107:486, 1969.
16. Taveras, J. M., and Wood, E. H.: Diagnostic Neuroradiology. Baltimore, Williams & Wilkins Company, 1964.
17. Tobey, G. L., Jr., and Ayer, J. B.: Dynamic studies of cerebrospinal fluid in differential diagnosis of lateral sinus thrombosis. Arch. Otolaryng., 2:50, 1925.
18. Veith, R. G., Tindall, G. T., and Odom, G. L.: The use of tantalum dust as an adjunct in the postoperative management of subdural hematomas. J. Neurosurg., 24:514, 1966.
19. Wilkins, R. H., and Odom, G. L.: Cytological changes in cerebrospinal fluid associated with resections of intracranial neoplasms. J. Neurosurg., 25:24, 1966.

# INTRACRANIAL TUMORS

*M. Stephen Mahaley, Jr., M.D.*

The brain may host malignant or nonmalignant neoplasms, and brain tumors have been recognized to possess several rather unique features: a broad spectrum of cell types participating in neoplasms of different histologic patterns and a variety of growth characteristics; the rarity of metastasis of malignant gliomas despite rapid local growth and invasiveness; a peculiar vascular proliferation as part of the neoplastic process in many malignant gliomas;[8] and a difference in predominant tumor type and tumor location between children and adults. Brain tumors are usually classified according to tissue of origin and cell type. Table 1 lists the incidence of various intracranial neoplasms operated upon at Duke University Medical Center over a span of approximately 10 years. The biologic behavior of intracranial tumors varies as much as the methods of classification. In any evaluation of the treatment of intracranial tumors, the exact neuropathologic classification of each case represents the foundation upon which other statistical studies must be based.

**TABLE 1** 705 INTRACRANIAL NEOPLASMS —DUKE SERIES*

| Neoplasm | No. | % |
|---|---|---|
| Glioblastoma multiforme | 150 | 21.3 |
| Ependymoblastoma | 23 | 3.3 |
| Ependymal spongioblastoma | 11 | 1.6 |
| Astroblastoma | 6 | .9 |
| Medulloblastoma | 23 | 3.3 |
| Mixed glioma | 19 | 2.7 |
| Neuroblastoma | 3 | .4 |
| Astrocytoma | 96 | 13.6 |
| Oligodendroglioma | 17 | 2.4 |
| Ependymoma | 40 | 5.7 |
| Spongioblastoma | 11 | 1.6 |
| Ganglioneuroma | 6 | .9 |
| Pinealoma | 5 | .7 |
| Microglioma | 1 | .1 |
| Neuroepithelioma | 1 | .1 |
| Acoustic neurinoma | 39 | 5.5 |
| Neurinoma, V | 2 | .3 |
| Neurofibroma | 2 | .3 |
| Meningioma | 89 | 12.6 |
| Hemangioblastoma | 9 | 1.3 |
| Hemangioma | 3 | .4 |
| Hemangiopericytoma | 1 | .1 |
| Osteoma | 2 | .3 |
| Chondroma | 1 | .1 |
| Pituitary tumor | 28 | 4.0 |
| Craniopharyngioma | 17 | 2.4 |
| Cholesteatoma | 8 | 1.1 |
| Metastases | 90 | 12.8 |
| Teratoma | 2 | .3 |

*Data compiled by Information Science Division, Community Health Sciences Department, Duke University Medical Center.

The most common brain tumors are the gliomas, and in adults the most frequent glioma is unfortunately the most malignant—the glioblastoma multiforme, characterized histologically by pleomorphism of cell types, invasiveness, mitotic figures, hemorrhage, necrosis, and vascular wall proliferation.[2,9] Other gliomas (astrocytomas, oligodendrogliomas, spongioblastomas, and ependymomas) show lesser degrees of malignancy or are totally benign in growth characteristics. Extracerebral neoplasms include such tumors as the pituitary adenoma, meningioma, acoustic neurinoma, and cholesteatoma. In children, the most common brain tumor is the medulloblastoma, a malignant neoplasm of the cerebellar vermis.[6] Other posterior fossa neoplasms (ependymoma, cerebellar astrocytoma, and pontine glioma) make up the majority of the childhood tumors.

### Symptoms and Signs

Symptoms that may arise from a brain tumor include headache, nausea and vomiting due to increased intracranial pressure, and seizures and focal neurologic deficits due to the local effects of tumor growth. A seizure without obvious cause commencing in adult life should be considered a symptom of brain tumor until proved otherwise; childhood seizures, on the other hand, less often indicate the presence of an intracranial neoplasm. Tumors of the pituitary gland often present with endocrine disturbances, the first symptom frequently being loss of menses in women and impotence in men; later, visual field defects characteristic of optic nerve or chiasmal compression may occur as the tumor enlarges above the sella turcica. Tumors of the eighth cranial nerve usually present with tinnitus and unilateral hearing loss.

On examination, signs of increased intracranial pressure may be evidenced as papilledema or an alteration in the state of consciousness. A focal neurologic deficit, such as weakness, sensory loss, or visual field defect, may be seen with supratentorial tumors, as brain tissue is compressed or infiltrated by tumor. Acoustic neurinomas usually cause neurosensory hearing loss and absence of caloric responses on the side of the tumor. Posterior fossa tumors may cause dystaxia due to the local tumor effect and generalized increased intracranial pressure signs due to blockage of the fourth ventricle and resulting noncommunicating hydrocephalus. A pontine glioma should be suspected whenever a child presents with bilateral sixth nerve palsies or progressive cranial nerve palsies or both and long tract signs, usually without hydrocephalus. A child with a cerebellar astrocytoma frequently has a rather insidious onset of ipsilateral dystaxia and may show a head tilt toward the side of the tumor. Optic nerve gliomas, also occurring most frequently in children, usually cause visual loss with optic atrophy; large tumors of the chiasm cause signs of increased intracranial pressure from blockage of the third ventricle.

**TABLE 2** INTRACRANIAL NEOPLASMS—DUKE SERIES*

| Neoplasm | Scan† | Skull | CAG | BAG | PEG | Key: +/cases % + Vent. | EEG |
|---|---|---|---|---|---|---|---|
| Astrocytomas Grades I & II | 3/3 100% | 2/3 67% | 1/1 100% | | | | 1/1 100% |
| Astrocytomas Grades III & IV | 24/26 92% | 7/15 47% | 16/17 94% | 2/4 50% | 2/3 67% | 1/1 100% | 16/19 84% |
| Ependymomas Grades I & II | 0/1 0% | 0/1 0% | | | 1/1 100% | | 0/1 0% |
| Ependymomas Grades III & IV | 2/2 100% | 0/2 0% | 1/1 100% | 1/1 100% | | | |
| Medulloblastomas | 2/2 100% | 0/2 0% | | 1/1 100% | 2/2 100% | 1/1 100% | 0/1 0% |
| Undifferentiated gliomas | 1/2 50% | 1/2 50% | 2/2 100% | 0/1 0% | 1/1 100% | | 1/2 50% |
| Meningiomas | 16/16 100% | 8/15 53% | 10/11 91% | 2/2 100% | 1/1 100% | | 7/13 54% |
| Metastases | 35/41 85% | 3/21 14% | 14/17 82% | 2/7 29% | 5/6 83% | 3/4 75% | 17/24 71% |
| Acoustic neurinoma | 1/1 100% | 1/1 100% | | | | | 0/1 0% |
| Pituitary tumors | 3/6 50% | 5/6 83% | 1/2 50% | | 3/3 100% | | 2/3 67% |
| Craniopharyngiomas | 1/3 33% | 3/3 100% | 1/2 50% | | 2/2 100% | | |
| Other neoplasms | 4/9 44% | 3/5 60% | 3/4 75% | | 4/4 100% | 2/2 100% | 1/3 33% |

*From Gilson, S. J., and Smoak, W. M., III, Central Nervous System Investigation with Radionuclides. 1971. Courtesy of Charles C Thomas, Publisher, Springfield, Illinois.

†Technetium-99m

## Diagnosis

Studies such as brain scanning, electroencephalography, arteriography, and pneumoencephalography are used in tumor diagnosis and localization. Most tumor suspects are screened first with plain skull x-rays, electroencephalogram, and brain scan (Table 2). Ependymomas, oligodendrogliomas, and meningiomas most frequently cause pathologic intracranial calcification visible on plain skull x-rays. Meningiomas may cause hyperostosis or erosion of the adjacent calvarium near their dural attachments. A pineal shift may be the only clue on plain skull x-rays as to the side of the tumor. If a focal area of abnormality is seen on these studies, angiography is generally the next study performed. The neoplasm may show up as an avascular area with displacement of normal vessels or as a "tumor stain" with radiographic filling of vessels within the tumor or its capsule (Fig. 2). Even though less often used for brain tumor diagnosis than other studies, now pneumoencephalography still offers the surest screen of the entire intracranial cavity for tumor and is the diagnostic tool most likely to reveal small neoplasms, whether they be within the brain parenchyma or in the subarachnoid or cisternal spaces.

## Treatment

Whether benign or malignant, any enlarging intracranial mass ultimately threatens survival. Whenever possible, surgical resection of the tumor remains the therapy of choice. However, it is well recognized that it is almost never possible to surgically cure a patient of a glioblastoma multiforme.[3] Sometimes the tumor, though histologically benign, is in a vital area such as the motor strip or speech region, so that total surgical extirpation is precluded. A benign meningioma may present in a "malignant" location, such as the clivus or the tuberculum sellae, so that complete removal without sacrifice of essential central nervous system structures is very difficult. In cases of tumors of the third ventricle, hypothalamus, or pineal region, where noncommunicating hydrocephalus plays an important role in the illness, a palliative shunt procedure for rerouting of the cerebrospinal fluid may produce dramatic relief of many of the symptoms and signs secondary to the tumor, although the lesion itself may not be surgically resectable. High-voltage radiation therapy is utilized in many cases when surgical resection seems unwise or when incomplete resection is necessary.[7] Tumors such as medulloblastomas and ependymomas in children, and perhaps craniopharyngiomas,[4] have shown radiosensitivity. In adults, the chromophobe adenoma of the pituitary gland and some gliomas appear radiosensitive. Cooperative studies are currently under way to determine more precisely the effectiveness of radiation therapy (cobalt-60) for gliomas and the potential usefulness of chemotherapy in the management of malignant gliomas.[1]

Investigational studies have indicated an anti-

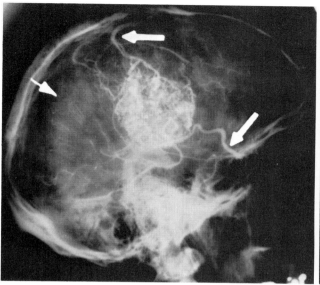
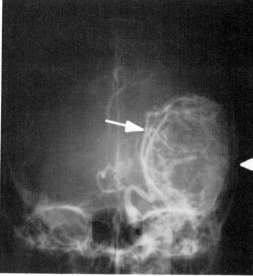

**Figure 2** Angiograms, showing vascular stain of a malignant glioma (*left,* lateral view) and a benign meningioma (*right,* anteroposterior view). *Left,* The characteristic early venous filling (broad arrows) due to neoplastic arteriovenous shunting seen in malignant gliomas during the capillary phase (thin arrow) of the brain circulation. *Right,* The lateral meningeal attachment and origin (broad arrow) of the meningioma, with medial displacement of the middle cerebral artery (thin arrow).

genic potential for cerebral neoplasms,[5, 10] and current studies are being directed toward screening the general and specific immune competence of brain tumor patients in an effort to control more effectively those cases that defy surgical cure.

Surgery for metastatic tumors merits special consideration, pertaining to one's philosophy regarding management of these often difficult cases, particularly when a primary lesion is known to exist elsewhere in the body. The lung represents the most common primary site in the male, and the breast in the female. Unfortunately, surgery for the most common metastases to the brain offers little as regards prolongation of survival time,[11] although the prognosis following intracranial surgery for metastases from other primary sites such as the gastrointestinal and genitourinary tract is sometimes quite good. Since the period of *useful* survival may be lengthened by removal of an intracranial metastasis, it is our general practice to consider surgical resection of a likely intracranial metastasis when it represents the only intracranial lesion as judged by all diagnostic criteria, when the general medical condition of the patient permits surgery, when the tumor is surgically approachable, and when the patient or his family realize the uniqueness of the situation. It is occasionally discovered that a tumor stain seen by angiography in a patient known to have had a previous malignant disease elsewhere in the body is, in fact, a meningioma and not a metastasis at all. In such instances, surgery may be the only way to establish the true diagnosis and may rescue what otherwise might be considered a hopeless case.

## REFERENCES

1. Brain Tumor Study Group, National Cancer Institute, National Institutes of Health, Bethesda, Md.
2. Frankel, S. A., and Serman, W. J.: Glioblastoma multiforme. J. Neurosurg., *15*:489, 1958.
3. Jelsma, R., and Bucy, P. C.: Glioblastoma multiforme. Its treatment and some factors affecting survival. Arch. Neurol., *20*:161, 1969.
4. Kramer, S., McKissock, W., and Cancannon, J. P.: Craniopharyngiomas. Treatment by combined surgery and radiation therapy. J. Neurosurg., *18*:217, 1961.
5. Mahaley, M. S., Jr.: Immunological considerations and the malignant glioma problem. Clin. Neurosurg., *15*:175, 1968.
6. Matson, D. D.: Neurosurgery of Infancy and Childhood. 2nd ed. Springfield, Ill., Charles C Thomas, 1969.
7. Moss, W. T.: Therapeutic Radiology. St. Louis, C. V. Mosby Company, 1959.
8. Nystrom, S.: Pathological changes in blood vessels of human glioblastoma multiforme. Acta Path. Microbiol. Scand., *49*:1, 1960.
9. Roth, J. G., and Elvidge, A. R.: Glioblastoma multiforme: a clinical survey. J. Neurosurg., *17*:736, 1960.
10. Trouillas, P., and Lapras, C.: Immunothérapie active des tumeurs cérébrales. Neurochirurgie, *16*:143, 1970.
11. Veith, R. G., and Odom, G. L.: Intracranial metastases and their neurosurgical treatment. J. Neurosurg., *23*:375, 1965.

## SPONTANEOUS INTRACRANIAL HEMORRHAGE

*Robert H. Wilkins, M.D.*

When intracranial bleeding occurs in the absence of head trauma, it usually happens within the subarachnoid space or within the substance of the brain.

## Spontaneous Subarachnoid Hemorrhage and Intracranial Aneurysms[7, 8, 12, 14, 16]

### Subarachnoid Hemorrhage

Characteristically, this type of bleeding has an explosive onset, causing severe headache, nausea, vomiting, and perhaps loss of consciousness, with or without a concomitant seizure. These symptoms are most likely due to the sudden increase in intracranial pressure caused by a jet of arterial blood at a mean pressure of perhaps 100 to 150 mm. Hg squirting into a space filled with cerebrospinal fluid having a pressure of about 10 to 15 mm. Hg. Fortunately, the bleeding ceases after about 10 to 20 ml. or so of blood has escaped, perhaps as a result of a transient muscular spasm in the walls of the arteries adjacent to the site of bleeding. Then, as the blood induces a sterile meningitis over the ensuing hours, stiff neck, minor fever, and photophobia develop. Occasionally, headaches may precede the dramatic onset of subarachnoid hemorrhage, and there may be one or two "small leaks," but these events usually go unrecognized.

The ictal event itself may be precipitated by physical stress, but more than a third of patients sustain the subarachnoid hemorrhage during sleep. An unusually high number of patients who have experienced a subarachnoid hemorrhage are noted to be hypertensive when they are brought to the hospital. However, in many instances this systemic arterial hypertension simply reflects a physiologic response (the Cushing reflex) to increased intracranial pressure. It has not been possible to obtain accurate information on a large group of these patients as to their previous blood pressure, especially during the hours just preceding the ictus.

Retinal hemorrhages may develop, because the blood in the subarachnoid spaces about each optic nerve compresses the central retinal vein at its exit from the nerve, thus causing retrograde venous distention back to the eye itself. Changes in the electrocardiogram, primarily involving altered and delayed ventricular repolarization, may also occur in association with subarachnoid hemorrhage, but the etiology of these electrocardiographic changes is obscure.

Roughly 10 per cent of the patients will die within 24 hours of their first major subarachnoid hemorrhage, largely as a result of the damage done to the brain by concomitant intracerebral hemorrhage, by herniation of the uncus of one or both temporal lobes over the tentorial edge against the midbrain, or by infarcts and hemorrhages within the midbrain and pons that are secondary to downward displacement of the brain stem by the acute increase in the supratentorial pressure just described.

The survivors frequently recover within a few days with little or no neurologic deficit, only to face two more serious threats: cerebral arterial spasm and recurrent subarachnoid hemorrhage.

**Cerebral Arterial Spasm.** Cerebral arterial spasm is demonstrated in cerebral arteriograms as a narrowing of previously normal arteries.[17] This phenomenon is encountered in the arteriograms of about 40 per cent of patients with subarachnoid hemorrhage. It characteristically does not appear until a few days after the bleeding episode, and then it lasts for a few weeks. In a large proportion of these patients, cerebral arterial spasm appears to be simply an epiphenomenon, but in some it is associated with decreased blood flow through the involved arteries, and cerebral ischemia and infarction in the area they supply. Therefore, under the latter circumstances, such arterial spasm can increase both the morbidity and mortality associated with subarachnoid hemorrhage.

After the first bleeding episode, the patient's subsequent course depends a great deal on whether an aneurysm, arteriovenous malformation, or some other detectable lesion was responsible. In an extensive cooperative study involving 19 medical centers, the causes of spontaneous (i.e., non-traumatic) subarachnoid hemorrhage in 5834 cases were found to be intracranial aneurysm in 51 per cent, cerebral angiomatous malformation in 6 per cent, and both in 0.7 per cent.[14] A small number of additional patients had hypertensive intracerebral hemorrhages, primary or metastatic brain tumors, cerebral emboli, blood dyscrasias, anticoagulant therapy, eclampsia, intracranial infections, spinal angiomatous malformations, and so forth. In the remainder, the etiology of the hemorrhage was never satisfactorily explained.

**Recurrent Bleeding.** The patients in whom arteriography of both carotid and both vertebral circulations is normal seldom have any recurrence of bleeding, and their prognosis is very good. On the other hand, an untreated aneurysm is likely to rupture again within 2 weeks, and the second rupture has a higher morbidity and mortality than the first. Often the original blood in the subarachnoid spaces about the aneurysm will organize into an imperfect barrier of fibrous tissue. It is usually not adequate to prevent a recurrent rupture of the aneurysm, but may be dense enough to deflect the recurrent bleeding into the cerebral substance, with devastating results. This points up the necessity for early cerebral arteriography in these patients in order to detect those with treatable lesions.

Occasionally, an aneurysm will compress adjacent structures, such as the third cranial nerve, as it enlarges.[10] Under these circumstances, the aneurysm may be detected before it ruptures. It is extremely important that these cases be identified promptly, since the treatment of an unruptured aneurysm is not complicated by intracranial hemorrhage or cerebral arterial spasm and therefore it has a much better prognosis.

Similarly, a small percentage of the aneurysms of the internal carotid artery occur within the cavernous sinus. Such an aneurysm may compress the adjacent ipsilateral third, fourth, fifth, and sixth cranial nerves as it enlarges, but if it ruptures it will cause a carotid-cavernous fistula rather than a subarachnoid hemorrhage.[10] Though this does not involve a serious threat to the patient's life, it may cause a series of disabling complications from an annoying bruit to bilateral blindness. Here again, it is important to recognize and treat this type of aneurysm before it ruptures.

### Cerebral Aneurysms

As stated earlier, congenital cerebral arterial aneurysms (called berry aneurysms because of their resemblance to berries) account for slightly more than half of all cases of spontaneous subarachnoid hemorrhage. These typically develop at vessel forks, and may be etiologically related to congenital deficiencies in the muscular arterial media that occur at these locations. As the aneurysm enlarges, its internal elastic lamina frays apart, and its dome consists primarily of the remaining adventitial connective tissue. The turbulent and irregular flow of the blood entering the aneurysm through its relatively narrow neck contributes to its enlargement, and also to the laminations of thrombus that are frequently laid down within its sac. These thrombi may be looked upon as the body's attempts to obliterate the aneurysm. As such, they are usually inadequate to prevent rupture of the aneurysm, especially after it becomes larger than 1 cm. in diameter. However, this process may be aided by certain therapeutic measures to be described, with the result of successful obliteration of the aneurysm.

Although they seem to be due to a congenital weakness of the arterial wall, cerebral aneurysms seldom rupture or otherwise make their presence known during childhood. Instead, they are one of the causes of "stroke" or "cerebrovascular accident in the adult. Atherosclerosis, inflammation, and other pathologic processes may also involve the walls of a congenital aneurysm. Furthermore, several other types of aneurysms may occur on the

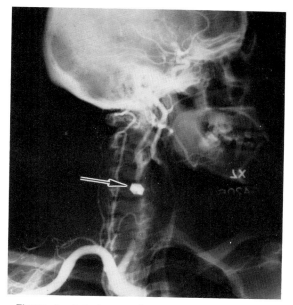

**Figure 4**  Arteriogram from same case as shown in Figure 3, after gradual occlusion of the right common carotid artery with a metal clamp (arrow). The arteries distal to the clamp fill via collaterals. The aneurysm is no longer visualized, and is presumably filled with an organizing thrombus.

larger cerebral arteries, and may be demonstrated angiographically. These include: (1) fusiform atherosclerotic aneurysms or ectasias involving mainly the proximal internal carotid arteries or the vertebrobasilar complex; (2) mycotic aneurysms, usually involving the distal branches of

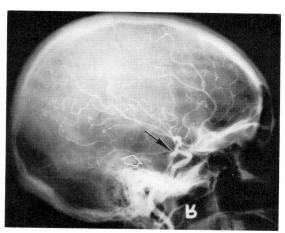

**Figure 3**  Arteriographic demonstration of an aneurysm (dark arrow) on the right internal carotid artery at the origin of the posterior communicating artery (just below tip of dark arrow). The white arrow points to the posterior cerebral artery.

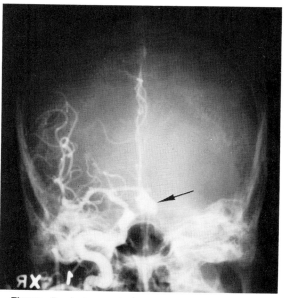

**Figure 5**  Anteroposterior view of a right carotid arteriogram, demonstrating an aneurysm (arrow) originating from the junction of the right anterior cerebral and anterior communicating arteries.

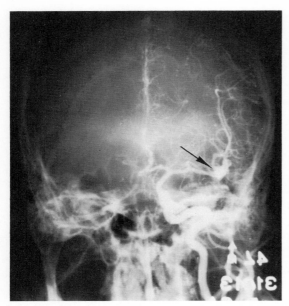

**Figure 6** Anteroposterior view of a left carotid arteriogram, showing an aneurysm (arrow) of the left middle cerebral artery.

the middle cerebral arteries; (3) dissecting aneurysms; (4) traumatic aneurysms; and (5) luetic aneurysms. But these are unusual or rare forms of intracranial aneurysm, and a discussion of their pathogenesis and treatment is beyond the scope of this chapter.

Congenital berry aneurysms occur almost any-

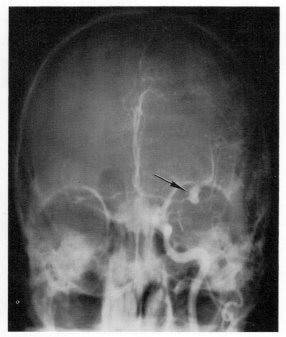

**Figure 7** Arteriogram from a case similar to that shown in Figure 6, but also demonstrating marked spasm of the intracranial arteries.

where along the components and larger branches of the arterial circle of Willis, but especially at a few specific locations. Most of these aneurysms are located at the junction of the posterior communicating artery with the internal carotid artery (Figs. 3 and 4), at the junction of the anterior communicating artery with one of the anterior cerebral arteries (Fig. 5), or at the first major branching of the middle cerebral artery (Figs. 6 and 7). Another, less common site is the terminal bifurcation of the basilar artery. Approximately 20 per cent of patients with intracranial aneurysms have more than one, and this of course complicates their management.

### Management of Subarachnoid Hemorrhage

In a patient with a spontaneous subarachnoid hemorrhage the diagnosis should be verified by lumbar puncture at the first opportunity. A few milliliters of the bloody cerebrospinal fluid should be centrifuged, and the appearance of the supernatant fluid noted. Oxyhemoglobin will appear in the cerebrospinal fluid a few hours after the hemorrhage and then bilirubin will appear and will persist for 2 to 3 weeks.[1, 15] Therefore, during the first few days after the hemorrhage, the presence of xanthochromia in the supernatant will establish that bleeding has occurred and that the bloody cerebrospinal fluid is not the result of a traumatic lumbar puncture. Similarly, when cerebrospinal fluid is obtained 1 to 3 weeks after hemorrhage, the red blood cells are usually not present and xanthochromia may be the only proof that bleeding did occur. There may also be an abnormally low cerebrospinal fluid sugar value, probably because of the obstruction by the blood of routes of entry of sugar from the bloodstream into the cerebrospinal fluid.

The patient should then be transferred as soon as possible to a neurosurgical center equipped to treat intracranial aneurysms. He is maintained at strict bed rest in peaceful surroundings to minimize the danger of rebleeding, and bilateral carotid arteriography is performed within 24 hours to visualize the anterior cerebral circulation. If no abnormalities are found, a left retrograde brachial arteriogram is performed on the following day to visualize the vertebrobasilar circulation. If this is likewise normal, the patient is kept at bed rest for 1 month from the time of his hemorrhage and is then allowed to resume all of his previous activities. It has also been our policy to repeat the bilateral carotid arteriography 1 week after the first set, just to be sure that a small aneurysm was not overlooked because of faulty radiographic technique or some other reason. For the doctor, it is intellectually unsatisfying that the source of the subarachnoid hemorrhage cannot be demonstrated in such patients. But it is far better for the patient, since he seldom has either a residual neurologic deficit or a recurrence of this problem.

### Surgical Treatment of Aneurysm

If an aneurysm is demonstrated arteriographically, the neurosurgeon must then decide whether, when, and how to treat it. The location and size of the aneurysm play an important role. A small percentage of aneurysms can be considered inoperable from the start, and others, such as those originating at the basilar bifurcation, carry a prohibitive operative mortality except in the hands of a few neurosurgeons who have become especially skilled in their treatment.

Another important factor is the condition of the patient. If he is alert and neurologically normal, the surgeon may wish to operate immediately, taking the risk that cerebral arterial spasm may then develop in its usual delayed fashion and complicate the patient's postoperative course. On the other hand, if the patient is comatose and hemiplegic, surgery is ordinarily delayed unless there is arteriographic evidence of a significant intracerebral hematoma. In that unusual situation, the immediate evacuation of the hematoma via craniotomy is sometimes worthwhile.

Usually, though, the patient is somewhere between these extremes, and the surgeon decides to delay surgical treatment. By the judicious use of bed rest, controlled hypotension to reduce the blood pressure within the aneurysm, and antifibrinolytic agents to try to retard the rate of lysis of blood clots on both sides of the aneurysmal wall, the surgeon is often able to delay operating on an intracranial aneurysm until the initial intracranial hypertension and the delayed cerebral arterial spasm have subsided, and conditions are more favorable for a good result. This regimen exposes the patient to the risk of a devastating recurrent hemorrhage, but at present this is the lesser of two evils.

Surgical therapy of intracranial aneurysms is aimed at the prevention of rebleeding by encouraging the development of clotting within the aneurysm, by strengthening its walls, or by removing it entirely from the cerebral circulation (Table 3). A variety of agents and techniques have been used for many years, and new ones are being developed constantly. Their very number attests to their deficits.

Theoretically, an aneurysm is best treated by removing it from the cerebral circulation, while keeping the arteries from which it arises intact. If the aneurysm is accessible surgically and has a narrow neck that involves only a short segment of its parent artery, this goal can be accomplished by placing a metal clip or ligature about its neck. Though it leads to the best theoretical result, such a procedure is attended by various hazards, such as the possible rupture of the aneurysm while it is being exposed. Even in experienced hands, with use of the most modern equipment such as the operating microscope, the operative mortality may approach 25 to 30 per cent.

These same hazards also apply to the reinforcement of the aneurysm by wrapping it with strips of muscle, fascia, cloth, or other material or by coating it with plastic. But, unlike the cases in which just the neck of the aneurysm must be exposed to accept a clip or ligature, in these cases the entire aneurysm, including its previous point of rupture,

**TABLE 3** SURGICAL TREATMENT OF ANEURYSMS

1. Exclusion of the aneurysm from the circulation
   a. With maintenance of flow through the parent artery—clip or suture ligation of the neck of the aneurysm
   b. Sacrificing the parent artery—clip or suture ligation of the parent artery on each side of the aneurysm ("trap" ligation)
2. Reinforcement of the aneurysm wall
   a. Muscle, fascia, or other biologic materials
   b. Muslin, or other types of cloth
   c. Acrylic resins, or other types of plastic
3. Reduction of blood pressure and flow within the aneurysm, and promotion of intra-aneurysmal thrombosis
   a. Systemic hypotension
   b. Systemic administration of antifibrinolytic agents
   c. Carotid ligation—common vs. internal carotid, rapid vs. gradual ligation
   d. Carotid ligation combined with ligation of the proximal portions of the contralateral anterior cerebral artery
   e. Ligation of the parent artery proximal to the aneurysm
   f. Electric thrombosis of the aneurysm, or the injection or insertion of foreign materials, such as hairs or iron particles, into the aneurysm, either stereotactically or after operative exposure of the aneurysm

must be dissected free of the surrounding tissue before it can be adequately reinforced.

The last technique, involving the reduction of pressure and promotion of thrombosis within the aneurysm, carries with it the danger of distal cerebral ischemia and infarction, especially if such treatment is complicated by cerebral arterial spasm. Gradual occlusion of the common carotid artery over 7 to 10 days has been found to be safer than rapid occlusion of the common or internal carotid artery or than gradual occlusion of the internal carotid artery, since it allows for the development of collateral circulation through the external carotid system. Such carotid ligation, usually performed with a specially designed metal clamp, will result in significant long-term reduction in the pressure within the proximal components of the circle of Willis, but it has less effect on more distal pressures.

Despite the dangers implicit in the surgical treatment of intracranial aneurysms, most neurosurgeons proceed anyway because of the poor prognosis of most untreated aneurysms. Each case must be individualized for treatment, but some generalizations may be made. Aneurysms of the internal carotid artery may be treated by common carotid ligation, or may be clipped intracranially if they are accessible and have a small neck. Aneurysms of the anterior communicating–anterior cerebral complex may be clipped intracranially, but there are sizable technical difficulties associated with this procedure. Carotid ligation is of value when the aneurysm is supplied by only one carotid tree, i.e., when the proximal portion of the contralateral anterior cerebral artery is developmentally hypoplastic or has been purposely ligated via a craniotomy. Aneurysms of the middle cerebral artery seldom have a narrow neck that can be easily ligated, and they may be too far distal to be helped by carotid ligation. Many are therefore treated by reinforcement. Aneurysms of the vertebral and basilar arteries either are considered inoperable or are attacked directly. Proximal ligation of the vertebral artery is very hazardous and has not been shown to be of any value.

Blood within the subarachnoid space from any cause will obliterate the arachnoidal villi and other arachnoidal channels that are important in the normal absorption of cerebrospinal fluid. This frequently results in mild hydrocephalus for a few days or weeks until the blood has been absorbed. However, in some cases the communicating hydrocephalus will persist, and some type of shunt operation (e.g., ventriculoatrial or lumbar-peritoneal) may then be required.

## SPONTANEOUS INTRACEREBRAL HEMORRHAGE, CEREBRAL MICROANEURYSMS, AND ANGIOMATOUS MALFORMATIONS

Whereas congenital berry aneurysms bleed primarily into the subarachnoid space, and only at times bleed into the cerebral substance, the intracranial bleeding associated with hypertension and with angiomatous malformations is just the reverse. It occurs mainly within the substance of the brain, and extends into the subarachnoid space or ventricular system in only a portion of the patients.

### Hypertensive Hemorrhage

By hypertensive intracerebral hemorrhage, we mean the spontaneous development in the previously hypertensive patient of bleeding within the basal ganglia on one side (most common site), or within the pons, cerebellum, or other sites.

A century ago, Charcot and Bouchard grossly dissected the brains of persons dying of intracerebral hemorrhages and found objects a few millimeters in size that they assumed to be intracerebral microaneurysms. Later investigators raised the possibility that Charcot and Bouchard had actually seen small blood clots rather than tiny aneurysms.[2] More recent studies, using postmortem arterial injections and special histologic techniques, have established the presence of miliary microaneurysms measuring 300 to 900 $\mu$ in diameter, especially along the lenticulostriate arterial branches in elderly hypertensive subjects.[13] It is assumed that these are the weak points from which intracerebral hemorrhages arise in hypertensive patients.

If the hemorrhage occurs in the pons, the patient usually loses consciousness quickly. The pupils are characteristically small and there are bilateral pyramidal signs and various abnormalities of conjugate eye movements. Ordinarily this type of hemorrhage is fatal.[5]

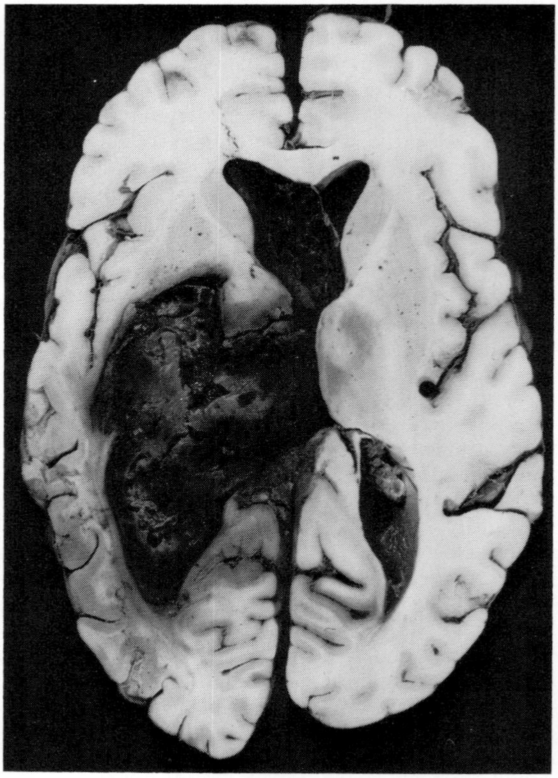

**Figure 8** Horizontal section of the brain from a hypertensive patient who died of a spontaneous intracerebral hemorrhage. The bleeding originated in the region of the left basal ganglia and ruptured into the left lateral ventricle.

If the hemorrhage originates in the cerebellar hemisphere, its prompt recognition on clinical grounds is imperative to permit evacuation of the clot before the condition ends fatally. The typical picture consists of progressive neurologic deterioration from intracranial bleeding in the presence of hypertension, with vomiting, early inability to walk, vertigo, headache, paresis of conjugate lateral gaze, and so forth, combined with the lack of hemiparesis, sensory deficit, homonymous field defect, or aphasia.[6] Since the clot is quite tenacious, it cannot be simply evacuated through a burr hole with a needle and syringe. A suboccipital craniectomy and surgical evacuation of the hematoma with suction are required.

Similarly, a craniotomy is required if a hematoma is to be evacuated from the region of the basal ganglia. This operation is not performed often, however, because of the devastating effects of the hemorrhage. The patient typically experiences a headache and then, over minutes to hours, develops hemiplegia, aphasia (if the hemorrhage is in the dominant hemisphere), and loss of consciousness.[5] The hemorrhage is frequently extensive, and it may break into the ventricular system. It is associated with a high mortality rate, even when the clot is evacuated soon after onset, and the few survivors usually retain their severe neurologic deficit. Therefore, most neurosurgeons simply verify the diagnosis by lumbar puncture (often bloody cerebrospinal fluid) and carotid arteriography (an avascular mass in the region of the basal ganglia on one side, with no evidence of aneurysm, angiomatous malformation, or other cause), and give the patient supportive care. If he survives, a rehabilitation program is then of value.

### Angiomatous Malformations[8, 11, 12, 14]

The exact classification of intracranial angiomatous malformations is still a debated subject, but for this discussion, three varieties are important. Telangiectasias (capillary angiomas) and cavernous angiomas are typically solitary developmental malformations within the brain substance that are too small to be visualized by angiography. They may serve as the site of origin of a large spontaneous intracerebral or intracerebellar hemorrhage, with the lesion itself being destroyed by the hemorrhage. This type of hematoma is frequently accessible surgically, and the diagnosis can at times be verified by microscopic examination of a biopsy from the walls of the hematoma. The prognosis of the treated case depends on the exact location and extent of the hemorrhage, but in general it is good.

Arteriovenous malformations are usually much larger, and most often can be visualized angiographically in the distribution of the middle cerebral artery. The superficial portions of the malformation may cover part of the cerebral surface, but the lesion frequently extends like a cone down to the ventricular surface. Therefore, the intracerebral hemorrhage that may occur from these lesions may spill into the subarachnoid space or ventricular system.

Besides bleeding, arteriovenous malformations may "steal" blood from the surrounding brain, and may cause a significant increase in cardiac output.

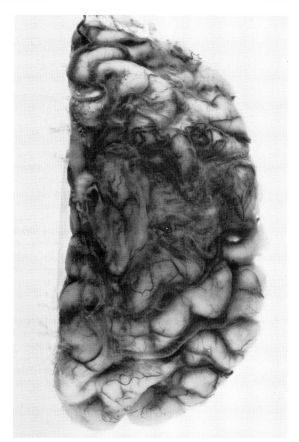

**Figure 10** Superior aspect of the right cerebral hemisphere, showing a large arteriovenous malformation that had caused headaches and seizures during life.

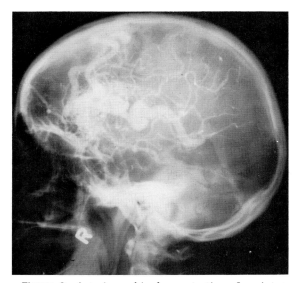

**Figure 9** Arteriographic demonstration of an intracranial arteriovenous malformation.

Likewise, patients with large arteriovenous malformations may have a variety of symptoms and signs aside from those directly related to bleeding, such as headaches, cranial bruits, convulsive seizures, mental deterioration, or a hemispheric neurologic deficit. Therefore, in contrast to intracranial aneurysms, arteriovenous malformations may frequently be diagnosed by angiography before they bleed. On the other hand, arteriovenous malformations tend to bleed earlier in life than aneurysms, with the peak incidence in persons between 15 and 20 years.

Surgical treatment by ligation of the ipsilateral carotid arteries or of the arterial branches directly feeding the arteriovenous malformation does not have lasting value since collateral feeders quickly enlarge and the malformation persists. Repeated embolization of these malformations with plastic spheres of graded sizes or with other materials introduced via the internal carotid artery in the neck to promote intravascular thrombosis has proved to be a satisfactory alternative in some cases. But adequate control in many instances requires surgical excision of the entire malformation if its location and size will permit such a procedure. It may also be necessary to perform a craniot-

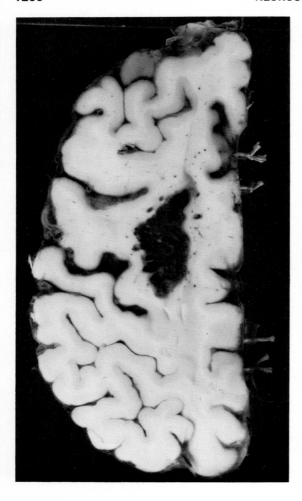

**Figure 11**   A horizontal section of the right cerebral hemisphere from the same case as shown in Figure 9. The arteriovenous malformation extended like an inverted pyramid from a broad base on the cerebral cortex to a small tip abutting against the lateral ventricle.

omy to evacuate an intracerebral hematoma even if the malformation cannot be resected.

The symptoms of untreated arteriovenous malformations tend to increase with time, and recurrent episodes of bleeding are common. The prognosis of lesions treated surgically depends on the size and location of the malformation, and the extent of cerebral destruction from intracerebral hemorrhage, direct surgical trauma, and cerebral infarction due to arterial interruption. As a general rule, about 60 per cent of patients from whom it is possible to excise an arteriovenous malformation will be free of symptoms or have only minimal symptoms, and another 20 per cent will be partly disabled but still able to work.

## SPONTANEOUS INTRASPINAL HEMORRHAGE

### Angiomatous Malformations[3, 4, 9, 18]

The various types of angiomatous malformation encountered intracranially are also encountered within the spinal canal, but it is the location of the lesion in respect to the cord rather than the pathologic type that usually determines the clinical syndrome that results. A lesion that is partially or totally intramedullary will usually cause thrombotic infarction of or hemorrhage into the adjacent spinal cord (hematomyelia), with a resultant myelopathy, whereas a lesion that is primarily extramedullary but intradural will often cause subarachnoid hemorrhage or will compress the adjacent cord by its bulk. Typically, in both types patients will experience a progressive loss of spinal cord function, punctuated by sudden and often painful increases in their neurologic deficits with each episode of hemorrhage.

Myelography will often reveal the abnormal vessels as serpentine defects in the oil column. Often they may also be studied in better detail by selective arteriography, frequently via transfemoral catheterization of the intercostal artery or arteries that feed the malformation.[3, 4]

Despite the relative ease with which these lesions may be diagnosed, the results of treatment have been quite disappointing. Even with careful removal of the accessible malformations by means of microneurosurgical techniques, the damage that has already been done to the cord remains, and the surgical interruption of feeding arteries may cause further ischemia and infarction of the cord adjacent to the malformation.

### Neoplasms

Neoplasms of various sorts account for a significant percentage of the cases of spontaneous spinal subarachnoid hemorrhage, so they must be considered in the differential diagnosis of these cases along with angiomatous malformations.

### Spinal Epidural Hemorrhage

Patients suffering from a spinal epidural hemorrhage typically experience severe back pain at the level of the hemorrhage, associated with a rapidly progressive paraparesis or quadriparesis. The bleeding usually originates from some point in the extensive epidural venous plexus within the spinal canal, and it may be initiated by minor trauma, such as stretching or sneezing. Also, a number of these patients are receiving anticoagulant medication at the time of onset of their hemorrhage.

It is extremely important that diagnosis be made early, by history, physical examination, and myelography, so the clot can be evacuated surgically as soon as possible. With early diagnosis and operation, it may be possible to completely restore or significantly improve neurologic function. This is even more important in view of the fact that few of these patients ever have another such hemorrhage.

### SELECTED REFERENCES

Krayenbühl, H., Maspes, P. E., and Sweet, W. H.: Progress in Neurological Surgery. Volume 3. Chicago, Year Book Medical Publishers, 1969.
*In this book are 12 comprehensive papers by various experts dealing with virtually all aspects of the treatment of spontaneous intracranial hemorrhages due to aneurysms, arteriovenous malformations, microangiomas, and hypertension.*

Pool, J. L., and Potts, D. G.: Aneurysms and Arteriovenous Anomalies of the Brain. New York, Hoeber Medical Division, Harper & Row, 1965.
*This is an excellent recent study of the experience with intracranial aneurysms and arteriovenous malformations gained at the Neurological Institute of New York.*

Sahs, A. L., Perret, G. E., Locksley, H. B., and Nishioka, H.: Intracranial Aneurysms and Subarachnoid Hemorrhage. A Cooperative Study. Philadelphia, J. B. Lippincott Company, 1969.
*This 296 page volume constitutes a detailed analysis of 6368 cases of intracranial aneurysms and subarachnoid hemorrhage that were contributed to a cooperative study from 18 medical centers in the United States and one in England between 1958 and 1965. It represents the largest and best analyzed series of such cases.*

### REFERENCES

1. Barrows, L. J., Hunter, F. T., and Banker, B. Q.: The nature and significance of pigments in the cerebrospinal fluid. Brain, 78:59, 1955.
2. Cole, F. M., and Yates, P.: Intracerebral microaneurysms and small cerebrovascular lesions. Brain, 90:759, 1967.
3. Djindjian, R., Houdard, R., and Hurth, M.: Les angiomes da la moelle. Paris, Sandoz Editions, 1969.
4. Doppman, J. L., DiChiro, G., and Ommaya, A. K.: Selected Arteriography of the Spinal Cord. St. Louis, Warren H. Green, 1969.
5. Fisher, C. M.: Clinical syndromes in cerebral hemorrhage. In: Fields, W. S., ed.: Pathogenesis and Treatment of Cerebrovascular Disease. Springfield, Ill., Charles C Thomas, 1961, pp. 318–338.
6. Fisher, C. M., Picard, E. H., Polak, A., Dalal, P., and Ojemann, R. G.: Acute hypertensive cerebellar hemorrhage: Diagnosis and surgical treatment. J. Nerv. Ment. Dis., 140:38, 1965.
7. Hamby, W. B.: Intracranial Aneurysms. Springfield, Ill., Charles C Thomas, 1952.
8. Krayenbühl, H., Maspes, P. E., and Sweet, W. H.: Progress in Neurological Surgery. Volume 3. Chicago, Year Book Medical Publishers, 1969.
9. Odom, G. L.: Vascular lesions of the spinal cord: Malformations, spinal subarachnoid and extradural hemorrhage. Clin. Neurosurg., 8:196, 1962.
10. Odom, G. L.: Ophthalmic involvement in neurological vascular lesions. In: Smith, J. L., ed.: Neuro-Ophthalmology. Springfield, Ill., Charles C Thomas, 1964, pp. 1–96.
11. Olivecrona, H., and Ladenheim, J.: Congenital Arteriovenous Aneurysms of the Carotid and Vertebral Arterial Systems. Berlin, Springer-Verlag, 1957.
12. Pool, J. L., and Potts, D. G.: Aneurysms and Arteriovenous Anomalies of the Brain. New York, Hoeber Medical Division, Harper & Row, 1965.
13. Russell, R. W. R.: Observations on intracerebral aneurysms. Brain, 86:425, 1963.
14. Sahs, A. L., Perret, G. E., Locksley, H. B., and Nishioka, H.: Intracranial Aneurysms and Subarachnoid Hemorrhage. A Cooperative Study. Philadelphia, J. B. Lippincott Company, 1969.
15. Tourtellotte, W. W., Metz, L. N., Bryan, E. R., and De Jong, R. N.: Spontaneous subarachnoid hemorrhage. Factors affecting the rate of clearing of the cerebrospinal fluid. Neurology, 14:301, 1964.
16. Walton, J. N.: Subarachnoid Hemorrhage. Edinburgh, E. & S. Livingstone, 1956.
17. Wilkins, R. H., Alexander, J. A., and Odom, G. L.: Intracranial arterial spasm: A clinical analysis. J. Neurosurg., 29:121, 1968.
18. Wyburn-Mason, R.: The Vascular Abnormalities and Tumours of the Spinal Cord and Its Membranes. London, Henry Kimpton, 1943.

# CRANIOCEREBRAL INJURIES

## *Guy L. Odom, M.D.*

Accidental injury has become the fourth leading cause of death in the United States with the increase in the number of motor vehicles, and the leading cause in the age group of 1 to 44 years. Approximately 50,000 deaths a year result from automobile accidents in this country. It is estimated that injuries to the head occur in 72 per cent of persons involved in automobile accidents and 1 of every 10 such injuries is dangerous or fatal.

### Classification of Craniocerebral Injuries

Scalp
    Laceration
    Subgaleal hematoma
Skull
    Fracture, simple vs. compound
        Linear
        Depressed
Cerebrum
    Concussion
    Contusion
    Laceration
Hemorrhage
    Extradural
    Subdural

Subarachnoid
Intracerebral
Penetrating wounds

Although this classification may be helpful, most patients have a combination of these injuries, not a single one. In severe accidents, Braunstein reports that 44 per cent of the patients with head injuries sustain injuries to other parts of the body.

### Initial Examination

It is frequently difficult to make a definite diagnosis or to evaluate a patient completely from a neurologic standpoint immediately after an injury. In this complex situation one must determine whether the patient is in *shock*, whether *multiple injuries* have occurred, whether there is *evidence of increasing intracranial pressure,* and whether there is *evidence of spinal cord involvement.*

### The Question of Shock and Airway

The presence of vascular *shock* and the adequacy of the *airway* are the two most important clinical determinations to be made when the patient is first examined, and these two problems are given priority over all other aspects of the examination and immediate therapy. The presence of shock usually indicates that the patient has sustained multiple injuries and the examiner's attention should be directed to other organs of the body, even though the patient may be unconscious.

A severe head injury alone seldom results in shock unless there has been extensive scalp laceration with profuse bleeding that has been unattended.

The most common causes of shock associated with head injuries are rupture of an abdominal organ, intrathoracic bleeding, and fracture of the femur or pelvis. The treatment of shock demands priority over everything else, *unless* it is obvious that the patient has an *extradural hematoma.* It is essential that the patient *not be moved* for x-rays or other procedures until the usual methods are carried out to combat shock. No attempt is made to repair scalp lacerations during the initial phase of observation. The wound should be covered with a sterile dressing and a tight elastic bandage applied. If large arterial bleeders are present, the vessels may be clamped or ligated, and repair or further examination of the wound is deferred until the patient's condition has stabilized.

The maintenance of an adequate airway is as essential as treating shock. The air passage may become obstructed by blood, mucus, and vomitus. This may be avoided by the use of suction and positioning with someone in constant attendance. In extensive faciomaxillary injuries or in the unconscious patient with respiratory difficulty, tracheotomy may be a lifesaving procedure.

### Associated Spinal Injuries

The early recognition of a spinal injury is of extreme importance in order to prevent further damage to the spinal cord. This is seldom a problem in the conscious patient, but it may be difficult to determine in the unconscious person. In the comatose patient, the absence of deep reflexes in the lower extremities, diaphragmatic respirations, and the failure of painful stimulation to produce reflex movement in the lower portion of the body while it does so over the arms or shoulders indicates involvement of the spinal cord.

### Observation and Treatment

At the time of the initial clinical evaluation, if the patient has a closed head injury, it may be necessary to observe the patient for a period of time to determine whether the problem will require surgical or nonsurgical treatment. This decision may depend upon whether signs of increasing intracranial pressure due to intracranial hematomas or cerebral edema develop. The parameters to be monitored include level of consciousness, blood pressure, pulse, respiration, pupils, eye movements, motor responses to command or pain, and electrolytes.

If personnel and facilities are not available for surgery, the patient should be immediately transferred, if not in shock, to a neurosurgical center.

One of the first changes to occur with rising intracranial pressure may be a *decrease in level of consciousness.* The patient becomes restless, confused, and lethargic. If intracranial pressure continues to rise, the patient becomes stuporous and finally comatose.

Blood pressure, pulse, and respiration should be recorded every 15 minutes for 1 to 2 hours, then every 30 minutes, and finally every hour depending on the individual case. *Rising blood pressure and slowing of pulse rate* and *irregular respirations* are indications of acute increased intracranial pressure.

The pupils should be checked each time the vital signs are recorded. Unilateral dilatation of the pupil followed by fixation to light is indicative of third nerve compression from herniation of the medial aspect of the temporal lobe over the edge of the tentorium.[9, 17] Bilateral constriction and fixation of pupils suggest pontine involvement and poor prognosis. The spinociliary reflex is useful in determining brain stem involvement. A normal reflex results in ipsilateral pupillary dilatation in response to pinching of the skin of the neck and is lost in progressive brain stem dysfunction.

Rising intracranial pressure may produce *changes in motor function* such as increasing hemiparesis, increasing spasticity on one or both sides with increased muscle tone, increased deep tendon reflexes, ankle clonus, and Babinski sign. The development of decorticate posturing (lower extremities extended and rigid with upper extremities flexed at the elbows) and decerebrate posturing (upper and lower extremities extended and rigid) is indicative of progressive midbrain involvement.[8]

Electrolytes should be checked every 2 to 3 days. Electrolyte imbalance, which has been found to occur following cerebral injury, may produce confusion, drowsiness, coma, and convulsions.[12] This syndrome may be difficult to differentiate from expanding intracranial lesions.

### Scalp Laceration

A scalp wound, whether single or multiple, may involve the underlying skull and should always be considered a potentially serious problem. The scalp should be shaved widely about the laceration and thoroughly cleansed. The wound is then palpated with a sterile glove in an attempt to determine whether there is involvement of the underlying skull. The scalp edges are debrided and closed in layers without tension. When there is a scalp defect that cannot be closed primarily, a local pedicle scalp flap may be needed to close the defect and cover the underlying exposed bone or dura.[10] If this is done, it is necessary to outline the flap to maintain maximal blood supply and venous drainage. If the secondary defect cannot be closed without tension, a skin graft is used.

### Linear Skull Fracture

Linear skull fractures seldom present a problem unless they extend into air spaces (otorrhea and rhinorrhea), cross middle meningeal channels, become widely separated (tear of underlying dura), or are compounded. In the latter instance, the fracture line is thoroughly inspected for trapped particles of hair or other foreign material between the bone edges of the fracture line. With a blow to the head it is not unusual for the edges of the linear fracture to spring open several millimeters and immediately close, retaining foreign debris in the fracture line. When this occurs, it is necessary to debride the bone edges by placing a trephine opening adjacent to the fracture line and removing a narrow strip of bone from both sides of the fracture with rongeurs.

One of the most serious complications of linear skull fractures is cerebrospinal fluid rhinorrhea. Fractures involving the cribriform plate or the posterior wall of the frontal sinus are the most frequent causes of this complication which opens a pathway for infection into the subarachnoid space. If there is not an associated compound depressed fracture, the patient can be followed for 7 to 10 days to determine if the drainage will stop. During this period of time, the head of the bed is elevated, antibiotics are given, and the patient is advised not to blow his nose. If the leak does not cease spontaneously, the dural tear is closed by exploring the anterior fossa by means of a bilateral frontal craniotomy.[10]

Cerebrospinal fluid otorrhea is a leak of subarachnoid fluid from the external auditory meatus and is caused by fractures extending into the petrous ridge. These patients are treated conservatively and seldom require surgery to close the dural tear.

In cases of linear fractures with separation of the bone edges, there may be laceration of the underlying dura with herniation of cerebral tissue. This complication occurs more frequently in children and may result in a leptomeningeal cyst which may progressively increase in size.[14, 15]

### Depressed Fracture

In simple depressed fractures there are two instances when the fracture may be treated conservatively: first, if the inner table is depressed several millimeters and there is no associated focal neurologic deficit; and, second, if the depressed fragment overlies the sagittal or transverse sinus. In the latter situation, the underlying venous sinus may have been lacerated by the sharp edge of the depressed bone and elevation of the fragment may necessitate ligation of the sinus to control hemorrhage.

Simple depressed or simple comminuted depressed fractures are treated by outlining a suitable scalp flap which will extend several centimeters beyond the margins of the involved bone. After the scalp has been reflected from the depressed fragments, the periosteum is incised and separated between the fragments and the intact skull. A burr hole is then placed in the skull adjacent to the depression with a piecemeal elevation of the fragments. Care must be taken to separate the dura from the inner surface of each individual fragment. If the dura is torn, there may be contusion, laceration, or hemorrhage into the underlying cortex. If the dura is intact but bluish in color it should be opened and underlying hemorrhage or contused cortex removed. After careful hemostasis, the dura is closed and bone fragments replaced.

The seriousness of the compound depressed fracture depends upon associated laceration of the underlying dura and cortex or subdural or intracerebral hemorrhage. These wounds are frequently contaminated by foreign material and must be cleansed thoroughly and debrided. The comminuted depressed bone fragments are removed and occasionally edges of the intact skull must be debrided with rongeurs. If the dura is discolored it should be opened to be certain that there is not an associated subdural hematoma or contusion or hemorrhage in the underlying cortex. The devitalized brain is removed and the dura is closed. If the edges of the dura cannot be approximated, a small fascial graft is inserted. The scalp is closed with through-and-through steel sutures. Drains should not be used.

Carrington, Taren, and Kahn report that in compound comminuted depressed fractures in children, the bone fragments may be replaced without danger of infection after they are thoroughly cleansed. In 76 cases treated by means of this technique, infection occurred in only two cases and in these there was no spread of infection intracranially.

### Extradural Hemorrhage

Extradural hemorrhage most commonly occurs from a tear of the middle meningeal artery and accompanying veins secondary to a linear fracture in the temporal bone, and initially is seldom associated with cerebral involvement (Fig. 12).

The typical history of an extradural hemorrhage is that of a minor head injury with a short period of

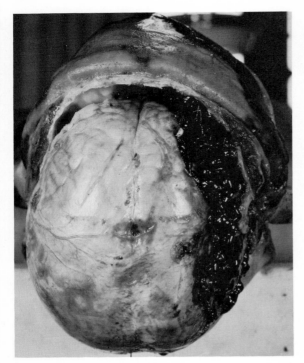

**Figure 12**  Autopsy specimen revealing an extradural hematoma on the right.

unconsciousness.[7] There is then an interval during which the patient is alert and has no neurologic involvement. In a short time, however, progressive severe headache, nausea, and vomiting may develop. These symptoms are followed by impairment in state of consciousness, which at first may be very gradual and later abruptly change to coma. During the period of lethargy, there may be decrease in voluntary movements on one side of the body. As the intracranial pressure increases, the blood pressure becomes elevated, with slowing of the pulse rate. The accumulation of blood displaces the medial aspect of the temporal lobe over the edge of the tentorium, with compression of the oculomotor nerve which produces dilatation of the pupil.[8, 15] Bilateral rigidity and extension of the extremities may occur. The hematoma must be evacuated at this time without additional diagnostic studies. If surgery is delayed, further herniation of the hippocampal gyrus occurs with compression of the posterior cerebral artery at the edge of the tentorium and infarction of the occipital lobe. This further increases intracranial pressure and results in midbrain hemorrhage and death.

If an extradural hemorrhage is suspected, a trephine hole should be placed in the temporal bone immediately, instead of awaiting further developments. The evacuation of an extradural hemorrhage is carried out by means of a subtemporal craniectomy. Endotracheal anesthesia is used to provide an adequate airway. The entire side of the head is prepared and draped. An incision is made in the temporal region, 2 to 3 cm. anterior to the ear with the lower end of the incision extending

down to the zygomatic arch. A trephine opening is placed in the bone and rapidly enlarged with rongeurs. The clot is removed by suction and if the site of bleeding is not obvious, the middle meningeal artery should be followed down into the middle fossa and the foramen spinosum packed with a small piece of cotton and bone wax. If a third nerve palsy was present before operation, the dura should be opened and the middle fossa explored for a hippocampal herniation. If a molded herniation is encountered, it should be removed by suction or the edge of the tentorium should be sectioned. During the closure the dura is sutured to the periosteum to prevent reaccumulation of blood in the epidural space and displacement of the dura and brain.

### Subdural Hematoma

Subdural hematomas are divided into acute, subacute, and chronic types. This division is a rather arbitrary one depending upon the time between injury and surgical intervention. Acute subdural hematomas are considered to be those that deteriorate and require surgery during the first 24 hours, subacute those requiring surgery 2 to 14 days after the injury, and chronic those requiring surgery after 14 days.

The symptoms of an acute subdural hematoma occur immediately after the injury and are difficult to differentiate from those of an extradural hematoma. The patient with acute subdural hematoma usually sustains a severe head injury with contusion of the cerebrum as well as bleeding into the subdural space. The type of operation indicated depends upon the consistency of the clot. If the clot is liquid, it can be evacuated by multiple trephinations and a small temporal craniectomy. A temporoparietal skull flap is required if a solid clot is encountered. The wound should be drained. Acute subdural hematomas may occur bilaterally; therefore, if such a lesion is encountered on one side, an exploratory trephination should be done on the opposite side as well. The operative mortality of acute subdural hematomas during the first 24 hours is 82 per cent.[1]

**Chronic Subdural Hematoma.**  The injury responsible for a chronic subdural hematoma may be rather trivial and in a number of cases may not be recalled as part of the history. Headache is the most common complaint and may be progressive from the time of the accident. Progressive focal neurologic signs and lethargy may occur, with papilledema and pupillary inequality; however, it is not infrequent for patients to be free of headache and focal neurologic signs.[2] To complicate the diagnostic problem, cerebrospinal fluid pressure may be normal in spite of the presence of a large chronic subdural hematoma.

X-rays of the skull may or may not reveal a fracture. Poppen reported fractures in only 8 of 119 patients.[13] The pineal gland may be displaced away from the side of a unilateral lesion, but may remain in the midline in bilateral subdural hematomas (Fig. 13). Poppen reported displacement of

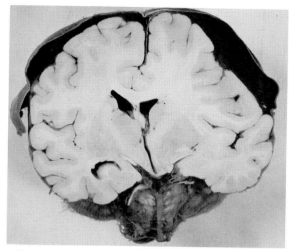

**Figure 13**   Autopsy specimen revealing bilateral subdural hematomas.

the pineal gland in 40 of 119 patients,[13] and Brock in 22 of 114 cases.[1]

The brain scan is helpful in screening patients for intracranial mass lesions and may reveal subdural hematomas that were unsuspected from a clinical standpoint. Approximately 80 per cent of patients with chronic subdural hematoma have a positive brain scan.[4, 18] Contusion of the scalp and subgaleal hematoma may be confused with subdural hematoma on brain scans.

Pneumoencephalography or arteriography[16] may be necessary to establish the diagnosis of a chronic subdural hematoma. Arteriography is usually the procedure of choice, since it does not change intracranial dynamics. The arteriographic pattern of chronic subdural hematoma (Fig. 14) is very typical, with the convexity of the displaced vessels toward the midline and displacement of the anterior cerebral artery toward the opposite side. If there is inward displacement of cortical vessels and no shift of the anterior cerebral artery, a bilateral subdural hematoma should be suspected and looked for by angiography or burr holes.

The chronic subdural hematoma can usually be evacuated by a small subtemporal craniectomy with frontal and parietal trephination. The temporal incision should be placed as part of the anterior limb of a temporoparietal skull flap. This is done in case there is solid clot that cannot be removed by through-and-through irrigation or in case postoperative recurrence of the hematoma necessitates a flap as a second procedure. The outer membrane is removed in the exposed area and the inner membrane is incised in a stellate fashion after it is gently separated from the arachnoid. The dura is left open beneath the temporal muscle to permit the escape of fluid from the subdural space.

## SELECTED REFERENCES

Browder, J.: A résumé of the principal diagnostic features of subdural hematoma. Bull. N. Y. Acad. Med., *19*:168, 1943.
   *This is an excellent review of the symptoms and signs in 289 cases of subdural hematoma.*

Jefferson, G.: Tentorial pressure cone. Arch. Neurol. Psychiat., *40*:857, 1938.
   *This article contains a very good review of the literature and an excellent discussion of the pathophysiology of the tentorial pressure cone.*

Kahn, E. A., Crosby, E. C., Schneider, R. C., and Taren, J. A.: Correlative Neurosurgery. Springfield, Ill., Charles C Thomas, 1969.
   *This text contains an excellent chapter devoted to closure of various types of scalp defects with pedicle scalp flaps and grafts.*

## REFERENCES

1. Brock, S.: Injuries of the Brain and Spinal Cord and Their Coverings. New York, Springer Publishing Company, 1960.
2. Browder, J.: A résumé of the principal diagnostic features of subdural hematoma. Bull. N. Y. Acad. Med., *19*:168, 1943.
3. Carrington, K. W., Taren, J. A., and Kahn, E. A.: Primary repair of compound skull fractures in children. Surg. Gynec. Obstet., *110*:203, 1960.
4. Cowan, R. J., Maynard, C. S., and Laster, K. R.: Technetium-99m pertechnetate brain scans in the detection of subdural hematomas: A study of the age of the lesion as related to the development of a positive scan. J. Neurosurg., *32*:30, 1970.
5. Echlin, F.: Traumatic subdural hematoma—acute, subacute and chronic; analysis of 70 operated cases. J. Neurosurg., *6*:294, 1949.
6. Echlin, R. A., Sordillo, S. V. R., and Garvey, T. Q., Jr.: Acute, subacute and chronic subdural hematoma. J.A.M.A., *16*:1345, 1956.
7. Gurdjian, E. S., and Webster, J. E.: Extradural hemorrhage. Int. Abstr. Surg., *75*:206, 1942.
8. Jefferson, G.: Bilateral rigidity in middle meningeal hemorrhage. Brit. Med. J., *2*:683, 1921.
9. Jefferson, G.: Tentorial pressure cone. Arch. Neurol. Psychiat., *40*:857, 1938.

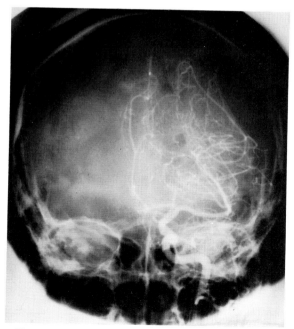

**Figure 14**   Carotid arteriogram revealing a chronic subdural hematoma on the left.

10. Kahn, E. A., Crosby, E. C., Schneider, R. C., and Taren, J. A.: Correlative Neurosurgery. Springfield, Ill., Charles C Thomas, 1969.
11. McLaurin, R. L., and Intor, F. T.: Acute subdural hematoma. Review of ninety cases. J. Neurosurg., 18:61, 1961.
12. McLaurin, R. L., King, L. R., Elam, E. B., and Budde, R. B.: Metabolic response to craniocerebral trauma. Surg. Gynec. Obstet., 110:282, 1960.
13. Poppen, J. L.: Chronic subdural hematomas. Geriatrics, 10: 49, 1955.
14. Schwartz, C. W.: Leptomeningeal cysts from a roentgenological viewpoint. Amer. J. Roentgen., 46:160, 1941.
15. Taveras, J. M., and Ransohoff, J.: Leptomeningeal cysts of brain following trauma. J. Neurosurg., 10:233, 1953.
16. Webster, J. E., Dawson, R., and Gurdjian, E. S.: The diagnosis of traumatic intracranial hemorrhage by angiography. J. Neurosurg., 8:368, 1951.
17. Woodhall, B., Devine, J. W., Jr., and Hart, D.: Hemolateral dilation of pupil, hemolateral paresis and bilateral muscular rigidity, in diagnosis of extradural hemorrhage. Surg. Gynec. Obstet., 72:391, 1941.
18. Zingesser, L. H.: Scanning in diseases of the subdural space. Seminars Nucl. Med., 1:41, 1971.

# INTRACRANIAL INFECTIONS

## Robert H. Wilkins, M.D.

The number of patients with infections amenable to neurosurgical treatment is relatively small, but because of the wide variety of infectious agents and the different pathologic lesions they can incite, this area remains a challenge for the neurosurgeon.

### Cranial Osteomyelitis, Epidural Abscess, Subdural Empyema[3, 5, 8]

A cranial bone may be the site of hematogenous spread of a bacterial infection from another area of the body, but more often it becomes involved by adjacent spread from an infected paranasal sinus, by a penetrating wound, or by an operative infection involving a craniotomy flap. Pott's puffy tumor is such a frontal osteomyelitis, with marked overlying soft tissue swelling, that is secondary to frontal sinusitis.

Treatment is centered around the surgical removal of the infected bone, with simultaneous treatment of any coexisting sinusitis. Appropriate systemic antibiotics are administered, and an adequate margin of normal bone is removed with the specimen to minimize the risk of recurrent infection. A cranioplasty may be performed later for cosmetic and protective reasons, but at least a year should be allowed to pass, during which there is no evidence of inflammation in the area, before the plate is inserted. Otherwise, this large foreign body will serve as a focus for a further inflammatory response.

An epidural infection is usually a well confined bacterial abscess associated with one or more of the previously mentioned infections, and it is drained at the same time the coexisting osteomyelitis or sinusitis is treated. A subdural infection, on the other hand, is usually an empyema rather than an abscess, since the developing infection easily dissects open the subdural space to cover the surface of an entire cerebral hemisphere. Subdural empyema may begin by the extension through the dura mater from without, or through the arachnoid from within; or it may result from the operative infection of a subdural hematoma. In any event, a subdural empyema is usually treated by immediate evacuation through multiple trephine openings in order to avert an almost certain fatality. Drains are left in the subdural space through these burr holes, to be removed days later, after all drainage has ceased.

### Meningitis[1, 5, 6]

Bacterial meningitis as such is not a surgical disease, and all but the most resistant or unusual forms will usually respond to systemic antibiotics. But if recurrent bouts of meningitis occur, the neurosurgeon may become involved in the search for and treatment of cerebrospinal fluid rhinorrhea, a midline cranial or spinal dermal sinus tract, or some other portal of entry for organisms into the central nervous system.

Also, in a certain number of patients recovering from meningitis, effusions will develop in the subdural spaces over the cerebral hemispheres, or hydrocephalus due to the obstruction of subarachnoid pathways concerned with the normal absorption of cerebrospinal fluid will occur. Subdural effusions ordinarily occur in infants, and frequently may be cured by repeated aspiration with needle and syringe through the coronal suture. Occasionally large unilateral or bilateral craniotomies are necessary for evacuation of the effusions and removal of coexisting subdural membranes that are formed by the same inflammatory process, and rarely the subdural fluid must be shunted into other areas of the body, such as the heart or peritoneal cavity.

### Encephalitis, Cerebritis, Brain Abscess[3-5, 7]

The neurosurgeon may be fooled into exploring and resecting an area of severe viral or allergic encephalitis, thinking it is a malignant glioma. Herpes simplex, for example, may cause a necrotic and cystic mass in the temporal lobe that closely resembles a brain tumor. However, even if the correct diagnosis is suspected preoperatively, biopsy of the lesion may be of value for verification. Furthermore, resection of such a lesion, or some type of decompressive operation, may also be necessary if steroids and other medical measures are inadequate to control the severe elevations of intracranial pressure that frequently accompany viral or allergic encephalitis.

The term cerebritis is usually reserved to describe the focal area of cerebral inflammation that immediately precedes the development of a bacterial brain abscess. Such areas of cerebritis may arise from:

1. Natural extension of an infection through the meninges. In this way, mastoiditis may lead to an abscess in the ipsilateral temporal lobe or cerebellar hemisphere, or frontal sinusitis may produce a frontal lobe abscess.

2. Hematogenous spread from some other site, especially either from the lungs, pleura, or heart, or from other areas of the body via congenital

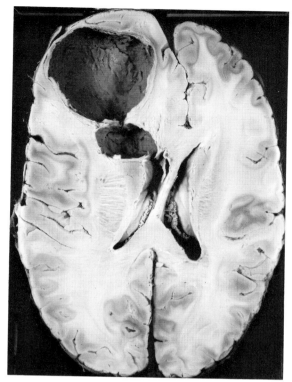

**Figure 15**   Brain abscess, left frontal lobe. A "daughter" abscess, posterior to the main lesion, had ruptured into the left lateral ventricle as the terminal event in this case.

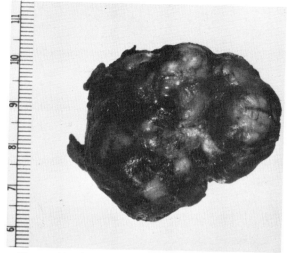

**Figure 16**   Operative specimen of a totally excised brain abscess.

heart defects that permit the pardoxical embolism of infected material. Brain abscesses that originate in this manner are distributed to the various areas of the brain in proportion to the vascular supply, so a large number occur in the territory of the middle cerebral arteries.

3. Artificial inoculation through the meninges, as by a compound depressed skull fracture.

Typically, the patient with a brain abscess uncomplicated by meningitis has no systemic signs of infection, such as fever, tachycardia, or leukocytosis. The abscess presents clinically, and by skull x-rays, electroencephalography, brain scan, cerebral angiography, and pneumoventriculography, as an intracranial mass that must be differentiated from a neoplasm, hematoma, or some other type of space-consuming lesion. Bacteriologically, these abscesses contain one or more of a variety of organisms. Anaerobic or microaerophilic bacteria can be discovered frequently if appropriate techniques are employed, but even so, a large percentage of brain abscesses are found to be sterile.

The neurosurgeon ordinarily prefers to delay operating on a brain abscess until its wall has become dense enough to withstand surgical manipulation without rupturing. For this reason he often waits for about 2 weeks, while the patient receives intravenous antibiotics, before attempting a total excision of the abscess. However, be-

cause of the degree of inflammation and reactive cerebral edema, the surgeon may be forced into operating earlier to prevent cerebral herniation and death. Under these circumstances, excision of the necrotic and poorly defined area of cerebritis may not be technically feasible; aspiration and drainage may be preferred. Aspiration and drainage may also be the treatment of choice of a well encapsulated abscess if it is located in a vital area of the brain that might be irreparably damaged by an attempt at total excision of the abscess. Under these circumstances, Thorotrast or colloidal barium sulfate may be injected into the abscess cavity after its aspiration so that its size may be followed radiographically.

No matter which operative technique is used, there is a high incidence of seizures among survivors of abscesses of the cerebral hemispheres, which justifies the prophylactic administration of anticonvulsants in most of these patients.

### Other Types of Intracranial Infections[2, 5]

Tuberculosis, sarcoidosis, and infections with various fungi sometimes cause a basal meningitis that obstructs the outflow of cerebrospinal fluid from the fourth ventricle. The resultant hydrocephalus may require a shunt. If an intracerebral or intracerebellar tuberculoma or fungal granuloma is formed, it may require excision like any other brain tumor, provided that the patient also receives appropriate drug therapy to combat his systemic illness.

The parasitic infections, especially echinococcosis and cysticercosis, present a problem to neurosurgeons in some countries, but are too seldom seen in the United States to justify further discussion here.

### SELECTED REFERENCE

Ojemann, R. G., ed.: Clinical Neurosurgery. Volume 14. Baltimore, Williams & Wilkins Company, 1967.

*This excellent volume contains 18 papers by a variety of distinguished authors covering all aspects of intracranial and intraspinal infections. It constitutes a relatively recent review of the entire field, complete with numerous references.*

## REFERENCES

1. Dodge, P. R., and Swartz, M. N.: Bacterial meningitis—a review of selected aspects. II. Special neurologic problems, postmeningitic complications and clinicopathological correlations. New Eng. J. Med., 272:954, 1003, 1965.
2. Fetter, B. F., Klintworth, G. K., and Hendry, W. S.: Mycoses of the Central Nervous System. Baltimore, Williams & Wilkins Company, 1967.
3. Gurdjian, E. S.: Cranial and Intracranial Suppuration. Springfield, Ill., Charles C Thomas, 1969.
4. Kiser, J. L., and Kendig, J. H.: Intracranial suppuration. A review of 139 consecutive cases with electron-microscopic observations on three. J. Neurosurg., 20:494, 1963.
5. Ojemann, R. G., ed.: Clinical Neurosurgery. Volume 14. Baltimore, Williams & Wilkins Company, 1967.
6. Swartz, M. N., and Dodge, P. R.: Bacterial meningitis—a review of selected aspects. I. General clinical features, special problems and unusual meningeal reactions mimicking bacterial meningitis. New Eng. J. Med., 272: 725, 779, 842, 898, 1965.
7. Victor, M., and Banker, B. Q.: Brain abscess. Med. Clin. N. Amer., 47:1355, 1963.
8. Wright, R. L.: Postoperative Craniotomy Infections. Springfield, Ill., Charles C Thomas, 1966.

## SPINAL TUMORS

### M. Stephen Mahaley, Jr., M.D.

Spinal tumors can be conveniently divided into three major categories based upon location: extradural, intradural-extramedullary, and intramedullary. The most common extradural tumors are the malignant metastatic carcinomas, most frequently from the lung in males and from the breast in females. Intradural-extramedullary tumors include benign meningiomas and nerve sheath tumors. Intramedullary neoplasms are usually gliomas: ependymomas or astrocytomas. All of these lesions occur with about equal frequency in males and females except meningiomas, which are more common in females. As regards metastatic carcinoma, the upper dorsal region seems to be the level of highest frequency. Not included in this discussion are certain congenital lesions, such as angiomas, dermoids, lipomas, and syrinx, or infectious processes such as tuberculoma, abscess, and gumma.

### Symptoms and Signs

Pain, fairly constant but worse at times on reclining, is a common early symptom because of the frequency of nerve root involvement and traction placed upon meningeal and vascular structures. The site of spine pain may locate the lesion itself, and the radicular component may identify the spinal root(s) involved. As a root is compressed or destroyed by tumor growth, the appropriate neurologic deficit of numbness, weakness, and reflex change may become apparent. When spinal cord compression or destruction occurs, particularly in the cervical or lumbar segments, a lower motor neuron deficit may be observed at the level of the lesion. More significantly, though, a myelopathy will be evident in terms of weakness and numbness distal to the lesion, with hesitancy or incontinence. On examination, a motor and sensory level may be evident with bladder signs of autonomic nervous system dysfunction. An absolute and total neurologic deficit of this type is certainly a late consequence of spinal tumors, and the prognosis for significant recovery of neurologic function when such a deficit has been present for more than a short while is very poor. For this reason, it is imperative that spinal tumors be accurately diagnosed early and that therapy be begun before a complete neurologic deficit develops.

### Diagnosis

Plain spine films may reveal changes indicative of neoplasia. Metastatic tumors frequently cause erosion of the vertebral body or pedicles or both, with collapse or compression fracture of the body in some instances. With intradural tumors, the entire spinal canal over several segments may be widened. The routine chest film may reveal an unsuspected primary neoplasm, or such may be found by physical examination of the breast, lymph

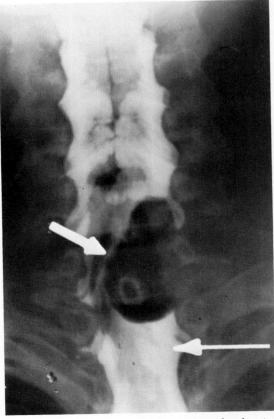

**Figure 17** Myelogram showing an intradural, extramedullary meningioma at the seventh cervical segment. The thin arrow shows a broad dye column on that side of the spinal canal with the halftone shadow of the cord displaced toward the opposite side. The broad (upper) arrow shows the medial border of the tumor mass itself.

nodes, or prostate gland. When an obvious bony change corresponding to the clinical spinal level of disease is not seen, lumbar puncture and myelography become essential. When the Queckenstedt test reveals a block, only 1 to 2 ml. of Pantopaque will be needed to outline the lower level of the lesion. Cerebrospinal fluid removed should be examined for protein content and the presence of inflammatory or neoplastic cells. Characteristic myelographic defects are seen on anterior-posterior views in Figure 17, helping to differentiate the extradural, intradural-extramedullary, and intramedullary lesions. The skin of the back lateral to the midline should be marked at the level of the lesion under fluoroscopic control during myelography for subsequent localization of the skin incision at surgery.

### Treatment

The most common extradural neoplasm is metastatic carcinoma.[1] When this is fairly obvious by virtue of a known primary lesion and appropriate radiographic spine changes produced by the lesions, a decision has to be made as to whether surgery would likely accomplish any useful purpose. If there is no neurologic deficit but adequate evidence of bony infiltration, then one may elect to treat with radiation therapy or chemotherapy. When there is a complete neurologic deficit that has been present for more than a few days and there is evidence of a primary carcinoma elsewhere, then it is often decided that surgical decompression would not likely restore neurologic function or otherwise aid the patient. However, when there is any doubt as to the metastatic origin of the tumor or when the neurologic deficit is only partial or recent, then surgical biopsy and decompression may yield two important results: diagnosis is certain and decompression may permit improvement of the neurologic status at least for a time or until adjunctive therapy can be instituted.

As regards intradural-extramedullary tumors, surgery is essential. A profound neurologic deficit from a benign meningioma compressing the spinal cord may show amazing improvement after tumor removal, which is usually curative as well. The same is true with nerve sheath tumors. Intramedullary tumors require surgery for diagnosis and may be totally resected (ependymomas) or may be only partially resectable (astrocytomas) owing to poor demarcation of neoplasm from surrounding cord tissue. When total resection is impossible or doubt is present regarding any remaining tumor, then postoperative radiation therapy is considered.

Rehabilitative therapy plays an important role in the subsequent management of many of these cases. Great care must often be given to the problem areas such as bladder care and prevention of pressure sores when a neurologic deficit is present. Physical and occupational therapy will assist in the functional recovery of the patient, and occasionally psychiatric assistance is required.

### REFERENCE

1. Veith, R. G., and Odom, G. L.: Extradural spinal metastases and their neurosurgical treatment. J. Neurosurg., 23:501, 1965.

## RUPTURE OF LUMBAR INTERVERTEBRAL DISCS

*Barnes Woodhall, M.D.*

Low back pain and sciatica may well be the price that the human animal has paid for his unique ability among animals to stand on his own feet and walk without falling down. Both Bradford and Spurling[1] and Hanreats[3] in their respective monographs have described the early and modern history of these health problems, and this unique ability of the human animal has been pointed out by LaBarre.[4] Sporadic reports over some decades suggested the true relationship between disc rupture and sciatica but these were either confused or overlooked by the established feeling that these small protrusions from the disc were true tumors called "chondroma." In 1934, Mixter and Barr resolved this issue with a convincing demonstration that a protruding portion of a degenerated intervertebral disc was the common cause for sciatica.[6] Within 6 years, some 49 fresh reports confirming this paper were available. One later report in monograph form is highly readable.[8]

The causation of ruptured disc has been variously attributed to trauma, an inherited connective tissue defect, and aging. As to the factor of aging, Hanreats charts the highest incidence of lumbar disc protrusions at about the third decade and suggests that certainly the common dehydration of aging is not a precipitating factor. These data lead him to suspect a predisposition and he describes a number of families with such a predisposition. Any experienced neurosurgeon might describe similar familial trends. Connective tissue is the product of the metabolism of cells derived from primitive mesenchyme, in large part from fibroblasts. In terms of biochemistry, mixtures of polymeric materials derived from this cell are characteristic of cartilage, tendons, intervertebral discs, arteries, the corium of the skin, and various fluids and secretions. A slow but growing understanding exists concerning the relationship between chemical components and biologic functions in this field. One simple mucopolysaccharide is known, hyaluronic acid. Its molecular weight is grossly reduced in rheumatoid arthritis and restored to normal values with cortisone. In ruptured discs, as compared to normal discs from persons of the same age, the concentration of hyaluronic acid is markedly reduced.[5] The total polysaccharide content is reduced from 30 per cent of the dry weight in normal human samples to 5 per cent of the dry weight in herniated samples. The chondroitin sulfate moiety of the polysaccharide fraction is reduced to a larger extent than is the keratosulfate. The collagen content of the herniated samples rises to 60 per cent of the dry weight from a normal

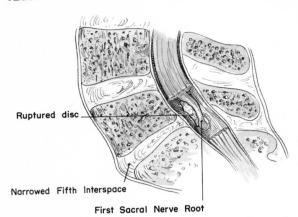

Ruptured disc ——————

Narrowed Fifth Interspace

First Sacral Nerve Root

**Figure 18** Diagram of cross section of lumbosacral spine illustrating a fragment of disc tissue rupturing through the posterior longitudinal ligament and compressing the first sacral nerve—a simple variant of this syndrome.

value of 30 per cent. Ultracentrifuge patterns of chondroitin sulfate from herniated samples show increased polydispersity; the keratosulfate fraction appears similar to the normal. A small but detectable amount of chondroitin B was isolated from herniated samples.[2]

These changes are qualitatively similar to those seen as a result of aging. Are these changes then the result of premature aging secondary to repetitive or acute trauma, weight bearing in the erect human form, or predisposition?

As noted before, the most common cause of low back pain with radicular involvement is a ruptured disc at either the fourth or the fifth lumbar

interspace (Fig. 18). In the classic syndrome intermittent attacks of low back pain are usually associated with pain radiating down the posterior aspect of the thigh and calf. The pain is aggravated by coughing and sneezing. Numbness may involve the foot and lower leg and motor weakness or reflex and sensory changes may occur. Other findings can be classified as mechanical. These consist of scoliosis, paravertebral muscle spasm, limitation of forward bending, limitation of straight-leg raising, positive Lasègue's sign, sciatic tenderness, and positive popliteal compression tests. These may occur with a protrusion at either the fourth or fifth interspace and are never helpful in localizing the involved root. Neurologic findings such as reflex changes or motor weakness may be indicative of the level of the involved nerve root.

Scoliosis, paravertebral muscle spasm, and flattening of the lumbar curve are protective mechanisms that splint the back to prevent further compression of the tense nerve root. Limitation of straight-leg raising, positive Lasègue's sign, and positive popliteal compression tests result from stretching the already tense spinal nerve over the protruded disc.

The neurologic signs result from compression of the spinal nerve and consequent changes within the nerve. A ruptured disc at the fifth lumbar interspace with involvement of the first sacral nerve root may weaken the gastrocnemius and soleus muscles, resulting in weakness of plantar flexion, which is best tested by requesting the patient to walk or stand on tiptoe; the ankle jerk may be decreased or absent and numbness and decreased sensation to pinprick may involve the lateral aspect of the leg and the fourth and fifth toes.

Involvement of the fifth lumbar nerve root at the

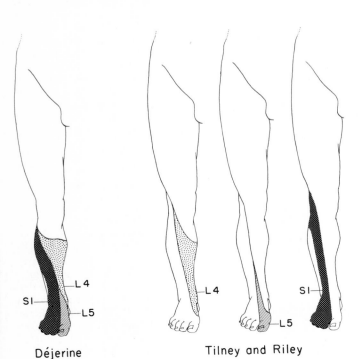

Déjerine

Tilney and Riley

**Figure 19** Commonly accepted variations in the sensory pattern of disc protrusions at the third, fourth, and fifth lumbar interspaces, involving lumbar roots 4 and 5 and sacral 1.

fourth lumbar interspace produces weakness of the anterior tibial, peroneal, and extensor hallucis longus (with weakened dorsiflexion of foot and big toe). Weakness of the extensor hallucis longus may be detected when dorsiflexion of the foot and toes is attempted. The big toe on the involved side is not flexed as much as that of the uninvolved side. The knee jerk may be decreased and numbness and decreased sensation to pinprick may involve the anterolateral aspect of the leg, the dorsum of the foot, and the big toe (Fig. 19).

Although some 90 per cent or more of ruptured discs appear at the fourth and fifth lumbar interspaces, a few may occur at the third or second interspaces. Multiple protrusions may occur and massive protrusions may give the clinical picture of cauda equina paraplegia with bilateral leg pain, marked motor weakness, saddle anesthesia, and urinary retention. In terms of differential diagnosis, metastatic carcinoma of the spine, spinal cord tumors, carcinoma of the cervix and rectum, spondylolisthesis, various gradations of lumbar spondylosis, infections, and Marie-Strümpell arthritis all may simulate the clinical picture of a ruptured disc.

Unless the clinical history and neurologic-mechanical findings are classic for a single-space ruptured disc, myelography with Pantopaque is required. Shapiro has devoted a small monograph to this diagnostic tool. Progress, from the use of spinal air by Dandy, to the serendipity of Sicard and Forestier's finding of Lipiodol, to the development of newer media, forms a tidbit of neurosurgical history.[9] A number of short-term, personalized records of results of intervertebral disc surgery make rather pleasant reading. In one such unpublished study of 1000 cases, there were but 84 instances of operative failures (recurrent sciatica), with 54 recurrences at the same interspace, 9 disc ruptures at another interspace, scar fixation of the nerve root in 5 cases, intractable sciatica, cause not established by requiring spinothalamic cordotomy, in 2 cases, and 14 clinical recurrences treated conservatively. The true story and the life history of this difficult clinical syndrome may well be established by the recent 20 year follow-up study by the Veterans Administration of patients treated in World War II by a number of reasonably competent neurosurgeons.[7]

## SELECTED REFERENCES

Bradford, F. K., and Spurling, R. G.: The Intervertebral Disc with Special Reference to Rupture of the Annulus Fibrosus with Herniation of the Nucleus Pulposus. Springfield, Ill., Charles C Thomas, 1944.
*This is a small monograph of personal experience by surgeons who, quite early after the report by Mixter and Barr, contributed strongly to the understanding of the disc syndrome. The early brief chapters on embryology, anatomy, physiology, and pathology serve as an introduction to the clinical studies. Case reports and 258 references up to 1941 embellish this very readable production.*

Hanreats, P. R. M. J.: The Degenerative Back and Its Differential Diagnosis. New York, Elsevier Publishing Company, 1959.

*This book qualifies as a treatise on the subject. With the exception of some deficiencies in modern biochemistry, it is a thoughtful, very well documented study that points directly to one conclusion: "The syndromes often thought to point to the existence of hernia nucleus pulposus were certainly not, we found, pathognomonic for this affliction." This is a meticulous enterprise and, in part at least, requires some experience on the part of the reader to aid the process of full digestion.*

## REFERENCES

1. Bradford, F. K., and Spurling, R. G.: The Intervertebral Disc with Special Reference to Rupture of the Annulus Fibrosus with Herniation of the Nucleus Pulposus. Springfield, Ill., Charles C Thomas, 1944.
2. Davison, E. A., and Woodhall, B.: Biochemical alterations in herniated intervertebral discs. J. Biol. Chem., 234:2951, 1959.
3. Hanreats, P. R. M. J.: The Degenerative Back and Its Differential Diagnosis. New York, Elsevier Publishing Company, 1959.
4. LaBarre, W.: The Human Animal. Chicago, The University of Chicago Press, 1954.
5. McClure, C., Holland, H. C., and Woodhall, B.: A method for the quantitative determination of hyaluronic acid in the human intervertebral disc. Science, 119:189, 1954.
6. Mixter, W. J., and Barr, J. S.: Rupture of the intervertebral disc with involvement of the spinal canal. New Eng. J. Med., 211:210, 1934.
7. Nashold, B. S., and Krubec, Z., eds.: Lumbar Disc Disease: A 20 Year Clinical Follow-Up Study. St. Louis, C. V. Mosby Company, 1972.
8. Semmes, R. E.: Ruptures of the Lumbar Intervertebral Disc. Springfield, Ill., Charles C Thomas, 1964.
9. Shapiro, R.: Myelography. Chicago, Year Book Medical Publishers, 1962.

# CERVICAL DISC LESIONS

## *Guy L. Odom, M.D.*

For a clear understanding of the problem of cervical disc lesions, they must be divided into several categories: (1) the lateral soft disc protrusions; (2) the foraminal spur (hard disc); (3) the midline soft disc, and (4) the midline hard disc (cervical spondylosis or osteoarthritic bony proliferation). The symptoms, surgery, and results of therapy cannot be grouped together.

## UNILATERAL SOFT DISC PROTRUSIONS

This syndrome was first described by Semmes and Murphey[15] in 1943 and since then has become recognized as the leading cause of neck and radicular arm pain. Although numerous reports have appeared in the literature, very little has been added to their original description.

The most common cervical disc lesion is the lateral soft disc protrusion. In large series,[10, 11, 14] approximately 80 per cent of the lesions are soft lateral discs, with lateral hard discs and midline hard and soft discs making up the balance. The majority of these lesions (90 per cent) are located at either the fifth or sixth cervical interspace,[5, 10] are aggravated by movement (wryneck), and are followed by subscapular, anterior chest (precordial), and radicular arm pain. A characteristic complaint is that the pain is aggravated by hyperextension of the neck.[5, 10-12, 15, 16] The anterior chest pain on the left may be confused with angina pectoris; in fact, two of the first four cases reported by Semmes and Murphey[15] were treated for angina before the correct diagnosis was established.

**Ruptured Intervertebral Disc at the Fifth Cervical Interspace, with Compression of the Sixth Cervical Nerve Root.** The pain, paresthesias, or numbness may extend into the thumb. The biceps reflex may be decreased or absent, and there may be weakness of the biceps muscle. The area of sensory impairment will vary, but may correspond to the distribution of the pain or paresthesias, with involvement of the thumb or the thumb and the second digit.

**Ruptured Intervertebral Disc at the Sixth Cervical Interspace, with Compression of the Seventh Cervical Nerve Root.** The pain and paresthesias may extend into the second and third digits, the triceps reflex may be decreased or absent, and the triceps muscle may reveal decrease in tone and marked weakness.

**Ruptured Intervertebral Disc at the Fourth Cervical Interspace, with Compression of the Fifth Cervical Nerve Root.** The pain or paresthesia seldom extends into the digits, and is usually located over the region of the deltoid. Reflux changes are rare, but the biceps reflex may be decreased. The muscle most commonly involved is the deltoid and at times there may be profound weakness of this muscle.

**Ruptured Intervertebral Disc at the Seventh Cervical Interspace, with Compression of the Eighth Cervical Nerve Root.** The pain or paresthesia may extend into the fourth and fifth digits, the deep reflexes of the extremity are not involved, and muscle weakness is usually restricted to the intrinsic muscles of the hand.

### Roentgenograms

X-rays of the cervical spine should include anterior-posterior, lateral, and oblique views. The films are never diagnostic but may reveal reversal of the cervical curvature, narrowing of the intervertebral space, and foraminal spurs. Odom and associates[11] found that abnormal changes in the x-rays coincided in only 30 per cent of the cases with myelographic defects due to soft disc protrusions.

Pantopaque myelography has proved a reliable diagnostic procedure as to localization of the protrusion or spur.[14] The myelographic defect may vary from a small filling defect of the nerve root to a large cut involving the dural sac (Fig. 20).

### Discography

Cervical discography has been reported as a helpful diagnostic procedure by Cloward,[2] Robin-

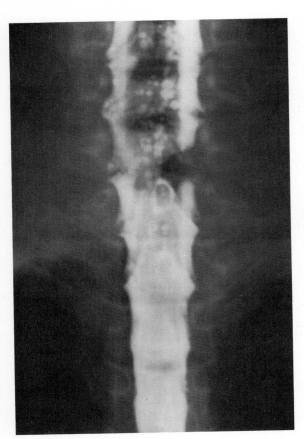

**Figure 20** Pantopaque cervical myelogram with filling defect due to a unilateral ruptured intervertebral disc between sixth and seventh cervical vertebrae on the right.

son et al.,[13] and Dohn.[6] The procedure is performed by injecting 0.2 to 0.3 ml. of a water-soluble contrast medium into the nucleus pulposus of one or more intervertebral discs. If the contrast medium remains within it the disc is normal, but if it extrudes the disc is ruptured or degenerated. We have never considered this procedure to be a helpful diagnostic aid.

### Treatment

A period of conservative therapy should be tried for all patients unless they have marked motor weakness. The patient is placed in halter traction and receives physical therapy and sedation. We have not been impressed by the number of patients in whom conservative therapy has succeeded if the diagnosis has been confirmed by myelography. It is strongly recommended that all patients treated conservatively be checked periodically for motor weakness.

Indications for operation include failure to respond to conservative therapy and development of motor weakness.

### Surgery

POSTERIOR APPROACH. Operation is performed with the patient in the sitting position with the neck flexed. Endotracheal anesthesia is used and the patient is hyperventilated moderately to avoid the negative phase of respiration because of the potential hazard of air emboli when patients are operated upon in the sitting position. A skin incision is made from the third cervical vertebra to the tip of the spinous process of the seventh cervical vertebra. The muscles are separated subperiosteally from the spinous processes, the lamina, and facets. When exposing the sixth interspace, the laminae of the fifth, sixth, and seventh cervical vertebrae should be exposed in order to obtain an adequate lateral exposure. The medial portion of the inferior facet is then removed by rongeurs. The high-speed air drill is used to remove an additional portion of the inferior facet and the medial portion of the superior facet of the corresponding vertebra (Fig. 21A). Gauze packing should be avoided in the wound when the high-speed air drill is used and the ligamentum flavum should be left intact during this part of the procedure. A technique should be developed to leave a thin rim of bone over the nerve root which is then removed with a curet (Fig. 21C). It is always wise to shift from the ordinary burr to the diamond-head burr when the removal is close to the nerve root. After the nerve root is exposed, the ligamentum flavum is removed by sharp dissection from between the corresponding lamina. As the liga-

**Figure 21** *A,* Unilateral exposure of laminae of C6 and C7 on the right with beginning removal of facets. *B,* Removal of ligamentum flavum. *C,* Exposure of nerve root with removal of small portion of laminae of C6 and C7. Additional bone over nerve root removed with curet. *D,* Disc material forced out from beneath nerve root and dura.

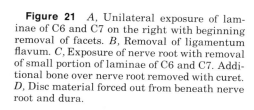
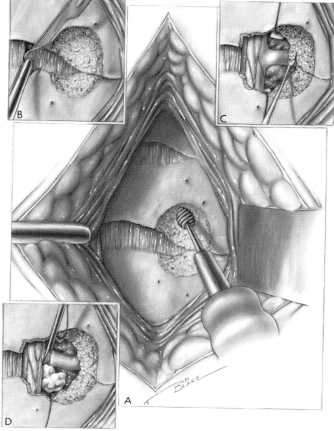

mentum flavum is elevated, the underlying extra-dural veins are carefully separated from the ligamentum flavum and small cottonoid patties are placed in the extradural space above and below the nerve root in order to compress the veins. A small portion of the lateral lower portion of the upper lamina and the upper lateral portion of the lower lamina is removed with rongeurs. The removal should be sufficient to obtain an adequate exposure above and below the dural sleeve of the nerve root. The anterior portion of the spinal canal is then palpated with a blunt dissector and the nerve root is retracted upward or downward to determine whether there is a posterior lateral protrusion of the disc. It must be stressed that the dura should never be retracted during the procedure if damage to the spinal cord is to be avoided. When a protrusion is encountered, an incision is made in the thinned-out anulus over the dome of the protrusion and this will permit soft disc to bulge immediately through the incision. Pressure is then placed on the adjacent part of the anulus with the blunt dissector and additional disc material is milked through the opening (Fig. 21D). Care should be taken to carry the inspection well out into the foramina. All free fragments of disc material are removed but no attempt is made to curet the interspace as is done in the lumbar area. The wound is closed in anatomic layers. The patient is permitted out of bed on the first postoperative day and is usually out of the hospital on the seventh or eighth postoperative day.

FORAMINAL SPUR. A similar approach is used for the foraminal spur syndrome but a more extensive facetectomy is performed, exposing the nerve root farther out into the intervertebral foramen. If the spur is large and the root is very tight, the diamond burr is used to drill a hole just below the nerve root in the superior lateral margin of the vertebra and above the nerve root in the inferior lateral margin of the vertebra above. With a small curet it is then possible to break off the thin spur without traumatizing the nerve root.

ANTERIOR APPROACH. Those interested in the anterior approach for the removal of cervical intervertebral disc are referred to the procedures described by Cloward,[2] Robinson et al.,[13] and Kempe.[9]

## UNILATERAL FORAMINAL SPURS (HARD DISC)

The clinical syndrome produced by the foraminal spur is identical to that produced by soft disc protrusion and usually cannot be differentiated until the lesion is exposed at surgery. Semmes and Murphey[15, 16] believe that the radicular pain due to disc lesions is produced by soft protrusion and that radicular arm pain is not associated with foraminal spurs (hard disc). The postoperative results are not as good as with soft disc protrusions. Haft and Shenkin[7] report excellent or good results in 83 per cent of patients and Odom et al.[5] in 76 per cent.

## CERVICAL MYELOPATHY SECONDARY TO CERVICAL SPONDYLOSIS

Brain et al.[1] must be given credit for clarifying the syndrome of cervical myelopathy associated with cervical spondylosis. They stressed the fact that cervical cord and nerve root involvement due to degenerative disc disease was not uncommon in the older age group and that the neurologic symptoms were due to cord compression by the bony ridge or interference with blood supply to the cord. Holt and Yates[8] studied 120 cervical spines removed at autopsy from elderly patients and found some degree of degeneration of the intervertebral disc in 110 cases, and in 46 of these it was severe. The degeneration is most common in the mid-cervical area.

The symptoms may vary from patient to patient owing to the fact that the ridging or degenerative changes may occur at one or multiple levels in the cervical area. Brain et al.[1] reported single lesions in 18 cases and multiple lesions in 20. The onset may be with weakness or paresthesias in the upper or lower extremities and occasionally radicular upper extremity pain. The deep reflexes are hyperactive, with a decrease in the biceps or triceps reflex if the sixth or seventh cervical nerve root is involved by a foraminal spur.

The syndrome may be confused with amyo-

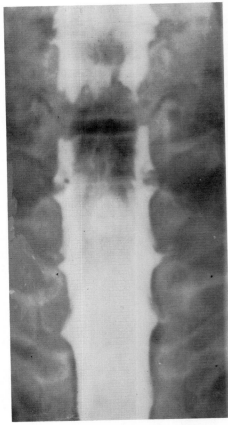

**Figure 22** Pantopaque cervical myelogram with transverse defect secondary to cervical spondylosis.

trophic lateral sclerosis, neoplasm, and syringomyelia.

X-rays of the cervical spine are helpful but more than 50 per cent of the patients in this age group may have degenerative changes in the cervical discs that are of no clinical significance.

Pantopaque myelography is essential to determine whether the diameter of the spinal canal is compromised by a bony ridge associated with a degenerative disc (Fig. 22). The degree of cord involvement is associated with the variation in the diameter of the cervical canal. The diameter of the canal may also be impinged upon posteriorly by the ligamentum flavum with extension of the neck. For this reason, precautions must be taken to avoid hyperextension of the neck during myelography.

### Surgery

The surgery of cervical myelopathy secondary to cervical spondylosis has been the subject of much debate during the past decade concerning posterior laminectomy vs. anterior discectomy and fusion. In cases with a single ridge the procedure of choice seems to be an anterior approach, with removal of bony ridge and interbody fusion, whereas if there are multiple levels, a posterior laminectomy with dural graft is the operation of choice. The laminectomy should extend two vertebral levels above and below the most caudal and rostral ridge. In multiple ridges, it is usually necessary to remove five or six laminae.

## SELECTED REFERENCES

Brain, W. R., Northfield, D., and Wilkinson, M.: The neurological manifestations of cervical spondylosis. Brain, 75:187, 1952.
*These authors must be given credit for clarifying the problem of cervical myelopathy associated with cervical spondylosis. The article contains an excellent review of the literature prior to 1952, and a superb discussion of symptomatology, pathology, and surgical results.*

Cloward, R. B.: The anterior approach for removal of ruptured cervical disks. J. Neurosurg., 15:602, 1958.
*This author is responsible for popularizing the anterior approach to cervical discs. His operative technique for the removal of cervical intervertebral discs by an anterior approach, followed by vertebral body fusion, is given in detail.*

Scoville, W. B.: Types of cervical disk lesions and their surgical approaches. J.A.M.A., 196:479, 1966.
*The author presents a review of 741 consecutive operable cervical disc lesions, of which 607 (82 per cent) were soft discs and 95 (13 per cent) were hard lateral discs, a total of 95 per cent being unilateral disc lesions. He is a strong advocate of the posterior approach for removal of unilateral disc lesions.*

## REFERENCES

1. Brain, W. R., Northfield, D., and Wilkinson, M.: The neurological manifestations of cervical spondylosis. Brain, 75:187, 1952.
2. Cloward, R. B.: The anterior approach for removal of ruptured cervical disks. J. Neursurg., 15:602, 1958.
3. Connolly, E. S., Seymour, R. J., and Adams, J. E.: Clinical evaluation of anterior cervical fusion for degenerative cervical disc disease. J. Neurosurg., 23:431, 1965.
4. Crandall, P. H., and Batzdorf, U.: Cervical spondylotic myelopathy. J. Neurosurg., 25:57, 1966.
5. Davis, C. H., Odom, G. L., and Woodhall, B.: Survey of ruptured intervertebral discs in the cervical region. N. Carolina Med. J., 14:61, 1953.
6. Dohn, D. F.: Anterior interbody fusion for treatment of cervical disk conditions. J.A.M.A., 197:897, 1966.
7. Haft, H., and Shenkin, H. A.: Surgical end results of cervical ridge and disk problems. J.A.M.A., 186:312, 1963.
8. Holt, S., and Yates, P. O.: Cervical spondylosis and nerve root lesions. Incidence at routine necropsy. J. Bone Joint Surg., 48B:407, 1966.
9. Kempe, L. G.: Operative Neurosurgery. Volume 2, Posterior Fossa, Spinal Cord and Peripheral Nerve Disease. New York, Springer-Verlag, 1971.
10. Murphey, F.: Fourth Annual R. Eustace Semmes Lecture, Southern Neurosurgical Society Meeting, January 23, 1971.
11. Odom, G. L., Finney, W. H. M., and Woodhall, B.: Cervical disk lesions. J.A.M.A., 166:24, 1958.
12. Peet, M. M., and Echols, D. H.: Herniation of the nucleus pulposus. Arch. Neurol. Psychiat., 32:924, 1934.
13. Robinson, R. A., Walker, A. E., Ferlic, D. C., and Wiecking, D. K.: The results of anterior interbody fusion of the cervical spine. J. Bone Joint Surg., 44A:1569, 1962.
14. Scoville, W. B.: Types of cervical disk lesions and their surgical approaches. J.A.M.A., 196:479, 1966.
15. Semmes, R. E., and Murphey, F.: The syndrome of unilateral rupture of the sixth cervical intervertebral disk with compression of the seventh cervical nerve root. A report of four cases with symptoms simulating coronary disease. J.A.M.A., 121:1209, 1943.
16. Semmes, R. E., and Murphey, F.: Ruptured intervertebral disks: Cervical, thoracic and lumbar, lateral and central. Surg. Clin. N. Amer., 34:1095, 1954.
17. Stoops, W. L., and King, R. B.: Chronic myelopathy associated with cervical spondylosis. Its response to laminectomy and foramenotomy. J.A.M.A., 192:281, 1965.

# PERIPHERAL NERVE INJURIES

*Barnes Woodhall, M.D.*

The modern historical era of peripheral nerve surgery began with Weir Mitchell's book recounting his experiences in the Civil War, published in 1872.[5] This volume also contains a number of earlier accounts including Paré's record of lance wounds of peripheral nerves. It is fair to say that wars and their wounds account for the majority of laboratory and clinical studies in this special field of surgery.

The basic problem in peripheral nerve repair can be stated quite simply. The surgeon must understand and then adjust the conflict between two forces, one, the continuing and virtually irresistible drive of axonal regeneration, and two, an equally significant barrier at the point of injury, derived from both mesenchymal tissue efforts at local repair and degeneration of all components of the distal nerve segment, distal receptor organs, and distal muscle, skin, and bone tissues.

An appreciation of the finer details of nerve structure is essential when one proposes to suture a divided nerve segment. The term *epineurium* designates the thin but relatively tough sheath of connective tissue that surrounds the aggregated fascicles of a nerve. This is the structure that the surgeon attempts to suture, by one means or another, to restore the continuity of nerve segments. It fuses with the interfascicular connective tissue that binds the nerve fascicles together and carries the larger blood vessels and the vasa nervorum. The interfascicular tissue may contain various

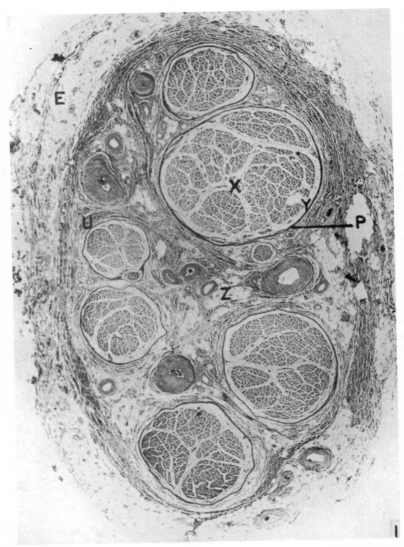

**Figure 23** *1*, There is some vascular pathologic change and intrafascicular edema in this cross section of a common peroneal nerve. E represents the epineurium and P the perineurium. V shows thicker sheaths blending with interfascicular tissue and the perineurium. × 22.5.

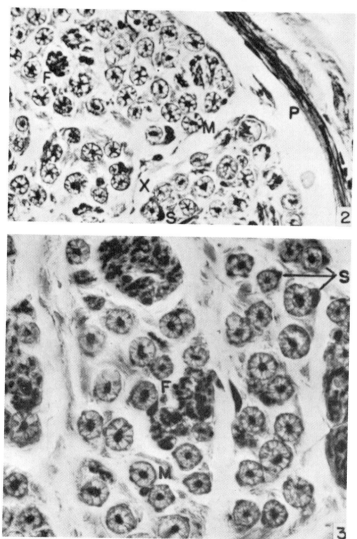

**Figure 23** *Continued* 2 and 3, Cross section at × 600 *(2)* and × 1000 *(3)*, with myelinated fibers (M) and clusters of amyelinated fibers (F). In a few places Schwann cells are seen around the myelinated fibers. (From Lyons, W. R., and Woodhall, B.: Atlas of Peripheral Nerve Injuries. Philadelphia, W. B. Saunders Company, 1949.)

amounts of fat. Longitudinally oriented blood vessels are present beneath and on the epineurium and traverse the interfascicular space. They may represent a large vessel such as the arteria concomitans of the median nerve, and nerves are also fed by irregularly spaced segmental vessels such as that common to the ulnar nerve in the region of the medial epicondyle. The surgeon makes use of their longitudinal orientation to prevent rotation of nerve segments preparatory to suture. Hemorrhage from these vessels poses a technical problem as well.

Each fascicle is surrounded by a thin sheath of laminated connective tissue, the *perineurium.* The internal architecture of the fascicular pattern of a nerve is highly variable, being influenced by the site in any nerve trunk at which it may be examined, by the merging of sensory and motor axons, and by the migration of an emerging nerve branch. The surgical significance of fascicular pattern has been overemphasized since the usual longitudinal extent of an injury plus the removal of damaged nerve ends will make improbable the suture of true mirror images.

Within each fascicle are numbers of myelinated and amyelinated nerve fibers, the latter often occurring in clusters, which vary in size and number depending upon their function and the cross-area of the individual nerve. The *axon,* protected by its myelin sheath and its component parts, is derived from a centrally placed neuron. Its axoplasm is fluid, viscous, and granular; it moves centrifugally with a force that cannot be denied and represents, as a mass, the structure that the surgeon hopes by his efforts to link up with a motor endplate or a sensory end organ. This task, from the point of view of the microanatomist, appears to be virtually an impossible one (Figs. 23 and 24).

The student of peripheral injury must understand as well the metabolic response to injury and regeneration as this occurs at three levels: (1) the anterior horn cell of the spinal cord and the dorsal nerve root ganglion cell, (2) the proximal nerve stump, and (3) the distal nerve segment and associated end organs.[2] A knowledge of the gross anatomy of the peripheral nervous system and of the characteristic clinical signs of injury to major peripheral nerves is another primary prerequisite to peripheral nerve repair. This may be obtained from specialized monographs devoted to the subject.[3, 7, 8] Beyond these points, the student enthralled by pathologic processes may care to peruse a reference volume on normal and pathologic anatomy.[4]

### The Acute Pathology of Peripheral Nerve Injury

When the intact human nerve is transected at the operating room table by a surgical cutting instrument, the nerve ends retract some 4 per cent of their normal length between points of fixation. The thin epineurium is intact about its severed circumference, the proximal fascicles pout for a distance of perhaps 1 mm. beyond the epineurium,

and there is hemorrhage from divided vessels at the point of severance. In the majority of accidental nerve injuries, the application of force is vastly different from that implied in surgical division by a cutting instrument. The application of force through the media of kitchen knives, clasp knives, broken glassware, pottery, and water faucets, beer bottles, window and automobile glass, steel fragments, broken bones, and civilian-type gunshot wounds implies the additional factor of stretch, with resulting damage over a considerable portion of the affected nerve segments.

When such accidental nerve injuries are visualized at emergency operation, much more complicated injuries may be seen, which may be placed in four broad categories: (1) complete nerve division, (2) partial nerve division, (3) a contused or swollen nerve segment in continuity, and (4) a relatively normal-appearing nerve. In complete nerve division, the epineurium is frayed and may be split longitudinally in either proximal or distal nerve segment. Hemorrhage occurs from the divided nerve ends and within the nerve substance as well, at varying distances from the point of severance. In partial nerve division, intact fascicles may herniate through lateral epineural lacerations. Intact fascicles become edematous at the point of maximal force. The divided fascicles retract within the intact cuff of epineurium. The extent of neuronal damage is difficult to assess, both in partial nerve division and in those cases in which the epineurium is quite intact and the nerve trunk is swollen and hemorrhagic. At a time period of 3 weeks to 1 month after injury, the extent of the injury to a peripheral nerve becomes much more apparent, largely as a result of peripheral nerve regenerative and healing processes.

The acute peripheral nerve wound may in addition be associated with fracture, vascular injury, tendon injury, and loss of skin. Neither the surgeon nor the patient may be fully prepared for the disciplined effort of meticulous nerve repair. This is the time for recognition of the extent of the injury, control of hemorrhage, closure of the wound to insure normal healing, appropriate splinting, and support of denervated muscles. In essence, it is the first step in preparation for an elective procedure at a time period 3 to 4 weeks after injury. Three alternatives to this procedure are indicated. The first has to do with preservation of the extremity in cases of major vascular injury. In such instances, vessel repair is mandatory as a primary procedure. The second alternative is found in rare cases of traumatic limb amputation in which replantation of the limb or finger seems feasible. The third alternative to deferred nerve suture is found in accidental section of nerves in the operating room or in simple, clean wounds involving small nerves such as the digital nerve.

### Favorable Prerequisites for Deferred Nerve Repair

1. The patient, his wound, and the surgeon are well prepared for definitive nerve repair. The pa-

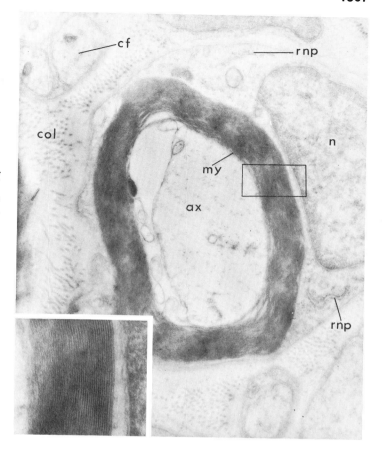

**Figure 24** Electron micrograph of cross section of normal rat sciatic nerve. Note the rnp particles, the axon (ax), the myelin (my), the C fiber (cf), the collagen (col), and the Schwann cell nucleus (n). × 32000. The insert illustrates the concentric and periodic myelin sheath. × 88000. (From Boone, S. C., and Woodhall, B.: J. Surg. Res., 4:413, 1964.)

tient has been evaluated in terms of fitness for local or general anesthesia. The raw, primary wound has healed without infection. The surgeon has now available a reasonably accurate diagnosis supported by electromyography, and he has escaped the errors of misidentification common to primary nerve repair.

2. As Ducker has pointed out, the spinal cord neuron has re-established its metabolic function and is prepared to support, after 2 weeks, the multiple sprouting of axons in the proximal stump. By the same time token, the neurolemmal tubules of the distal segment are free of debris and open for the downgrowth of new fibers (Fig. 25).

3. After 3 weeks, repair and regenerative processes have clearly defined the proximal neuroma and the distal glioma in completely severed nerves (Fig. 26). In so-called neuromas in continuity, intraneural injury can be identified by palpation as nodules and such injuries are in prime condition for proximal and distal electrostimulation. If the primary wound exploration has not disclosed complete nerve division, local anesthesia is preferable for deferred exploration so that sensory stimuli can be evaluated by the patient.

4. Suture line tension must be avoided, and the clean, well healed primary wound at 3 weeks post injury allows free access to the techniques of overcoming nerve defects after resection of pathologic proximal and distal nerve ends. These include free mobilization of nerve segments, transposition, and limb posturing.

In substance then, at 3 weeks after the primary injury, the surgeon and his patient both stand on a very firm foundation. The surgeon can assume the stance of a radical exploration with real hopes of understanding the exact extent of injury to peripheral nerve and other structures. At the same time, lacking evidence of complete nerve division, the surgeon can assume a conservative operative approach, close the wound, and further monitor the degree and usefulness of spontaneous regeneration.

The third time period commonly used in peripheral nerve repair is 3 months after injury, or so-called late repair, when degenerative changes in the distal nerve segment and in all tissues of the denervated extremity will progressively prejudice the quality of peripheral regeneration. Without firm objective evidence of spontaneous regeneration this wait-and-see policy is to be condemned. The long-term results of peripheral repair conducted at various time intervals after injury and other data related to nerve regeneration under the influence of various types of trauma may be found in Sunderland's book[8] and in a Veterans Administration study published some years after the end of World War II.[11]

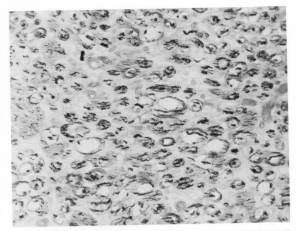

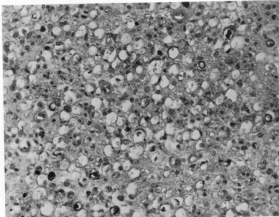

**Figure 25** *Top,* Proximal cross section following resection of proximal neuroma 4 weeks post injury. Note open tubules and regrowth of axons. *Bottom,* Distal cross section from same case. Note open tubules free of debris with minimal connective tissue change. (From Woodhall, B.: Surg. Clin. N. Amer., *31*:1369, 1951.)

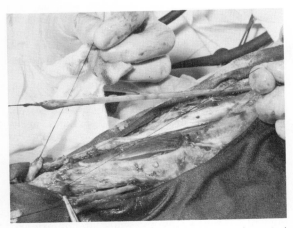

**Figure 26** Deferred median nerve operation at 4 weeks for complete nerve division. Note proximal neuroma at right and distal glioma at left, with wide exposure for mobilization of nerve segments. (From Woodhall, B.: Surg. Clin. N. Amer., *31*:1369, 1951.)

## The Technique of Repair

The additional armamentarium for nerve repair is not formidable. It includes a nerve stimulator delivering short faradic stimuli of variable intensity, fine forceps for handling delicate epineurium, sharp No. 11 scalpels for nerve segment section, both 0.003 inch tantalum swedged sutures and No. 5 swedged ophthalmic silk sutures, and perhaps gelatin sponge for curbing hemorrhage and surrounding the region of the nerve suture. More recently Ducker and his associates under the stimulation of their own experiments and studies during the Vietnam war have advocated the use of Silastic cuffs to cover the suture line.[1]

It is advisable to cleanse the entire extremity in any acceptable technique. Drape it in such a manner that all muscle movements and joint positions may be observed or passively attained. The use of a tourniquet rests with the experience or customs of the operating surgeon.

The skin incision is planned to encompass and then resect the original injury scar, and to include any potential longitudinal extension that may be necessary for mobilization purposes. It is marked in a series of gentle curves and placed transversely across joint creases. The nerve segment may lie quite superficially at the point of injury and dissection is more safely commenced to expose the proximal and distal nerve segments. As the proximal nerve segment is identified and followed toward the point of injury, in a region where motor branches arise, the proximal nerve segment should be stimulated to ascertain the presence of intact nerve branches that may arise just proximal to the lesion and may be embedded in scar tissue. Proximal nerve stimulation may also elicit a peripheral response through the point of injury, strongly suggesting the occurrence of a neuroma in continuity. A normal distal nerve segment is then identified and dissected toward the point of injury.

When the anatomically complete or practically complete nerve division of lacerating wounds is found, the potential nerve defect should be measured that might exist after resection of the pathologic nerve ends and then the surgeon must survey the possibilities of overcoming this defect by the methods at his disposal. In almost every instance, this will require extensive mobilization of distal and proximal nerve segments. This must be done with careful effort to preserve both the blood supply and the integrity of branches. In order, the second choice for making up nerve defect has to do with posturing the extremity, flexing of the hand on the wrist, flexing of the elbow, or flexing of the foreleg on the thigh. The third choice of making up nerve defect has to do with transposition of the nerve segment, and this is virtually always indicated with lesions of the ulnar nerve in the region of the elbow and with median nerve injuries in the region of the heads of the pronator teres. Actual transplantation of the nerve segments medially may be necessary with extensive nerve defects in the radial nerve at the midarm level, and removal of the head of the fibula may be indicated in extensive defects of the peroneal nerve in the upper foreleg. Critical resection lengths have been established for the major peripheral nerves beyond which nerve suture rarely shows regeneration. Fortunately such defects are rarely obtained in civilian-type injuries.

It is well to mark the position in the extremity of the respective nerve segments by single epineural sutures of fine silk placed at corresponding points of the nerve circumference. This prevents undue rotation of the mobilized and resected nerve ends at the time of suture. Various ingenious nerve clamps have been devised for sectioning of nerve segments but a clean deliberate cut with a sharp No. 11 scalpel is equally satisfactory. The proximal section may be made at the base of the proximal neuroma and should be reviewed if any residual neuroma is present. The distal section should always err on the side of generosity. If necessary, at this time the proposed suture line bed may be revised.

A number of epineural sutures should be used just sufficient to provide accurate apposition of the epineurium without undue buckling of the nerve segments. Stay sutures are inadvisable except under conditions of unusual tension.

Immobilization of the suture point in a light plaster cast for 3 to 4 weeks, with control of postured joints, promotes wound healing and may prevent suture line disruption. Such disruption may occur without obvious cause and may be detected by x-ray visualization of the suture line, if tantalum wire or marking sutures have been used. The actual technique of this end point, the suture, is of far less import than the principles of treatment outlined earlier in this report. With the mobilization of the extremity, the continuing protection against the development of deformities, intermittent use of electrical diagnostic measures, and the use of orthopedic transplants to correct muscle function are some parts of the approach to postoperative care. These can be found in major treatises.

Although this account has to do primarily with incised or compound nerve injuries, mention should be made of the involvement of major nerve trunks by traction, by concomitant bone injury, by compression, and by certain complications of vascular injury. All four represent acute conditions with unique pathologic sequelae and should receive the benefit of specific therapy.

Traction or stretch injuries, particularly of the brachial plexus and of the peroneal nerve, occur in the former instance with vehicular accidents and in the latter with forced adduction of the thigh on the lower leg. In all forms of traction palsy, force is directed along the longitudinal extent of the nerve segment with disruption of all constituents of the nerve segment. Intraneural hemorrhage and mesenchymal repair lead to collagenization of a nerve trunk over many centimeters of its length and make resection and repair rarely possible. In the common brachial plexus palsy, myelography of the cervical segment of the spinal cord may demonstrate actual avulsion of nerve roots. If no evidence of regeneration is present after 24 months in brachial plexus palsy, amputation of the upper extremity is often indicated. The peroneal type of traction palsy is best treated with a drop-foot brace and similar rehabilitation measures.

Simple bone fracture with peripheral nerve injury is a common combined injury, and the most common example is fracture of the humerus with radial nerve paralysis. Seddon has estimated that the chances are 5 to 1 in this combined injury that the radial nerve component will represent axonal degeneration without significant disruption of the supporting tissues of the nerve trunk.[6] Regeneration will therefore follow the customary course of axonal growth, roughly 1 mm. a day. In the usual spiral fracture of the humerus, reinnervation of the most proximal muscle, the brachioradialis, should occur therefore within 4 to 5 months after injury. In this particular nerve, with its relatively rough motor function and great capacity for regeneration, it is safe to observe such a combined injury for this period of time. In instances of peripheral nerve injury, the distance from the assumed point of nerve injury to the motor nerve entrance of the next muscle in line of innervation should be estimated. If function cannot be detected clinically or by electrodiagnostic data at the assumed time for reinnervation, exploration is mandatory.

An evaluation of sensory recovery is peculiarly important in the disabling median nerve injury that may accompany anterior displacement of the distal fragment of the humerus in supracondylar fractures of that bone. A similar situation is found at the wrist, where anterior displacement of either of the forearm bones may compromise the rather close confines of the median nerve at this point. Dislocation of the hip and shoulder may stretch or compress major nerve trunks. Spontaneous recovery is the rule. Fracture of the ramus of the pubis may lacerate the sciatic nerve, and if paralysis of this nerve is associated with radiating pain upon pressure over the area of injury, exploration is indicated. Fracture of the clavicle may be followed by brachial plexus palsy if excessive callus forms during healing. Rather common syndromes designated as the carpal tunnel syndrome, tardy ulnar palsy, and the thoracic outlet syndrome are well documented instances of chronic compression syndromes of nerve tissue. The details of their recognition and treatment are available in major treatises. The student should be aware of another common syndrome of accessory nerve division following simple surgical procedures such as lymph node biopsy in the posterior cervical triangle. This is accompanied by disabling and often unrecognized paralysis of the trapezius muscle.[10] In virtually all peripheral nerve injuries, the surgeon is confronted with some form of accompanying pain and the strange and eclectic history of the treatment of pain deserves special and concentrated attention.[9]

## Summary

An effort has been made from a number of biologic points of view to suggest that the repair of peripheral nerve injury secondary to the usual lacerating wounds of civilian life is not a surgical emergency. On the other hand, this documented biologic evidence suggests that primary emergency nerve suture is followed by a high incidence of failure of functional nerve regeneration. A sequence of primary wound debridement and closure, followed by early deferred nerve repair as an elective procedure, has been proposed as the best answer to the majority of these common problems. One of the most respected modern peripheral nerve surgeons, Mr. H. J. Seddon, has stated the premise in clear terms: if he himself were to suffer a peripheral nerve wound, he would suggest that his surgeon defer definitive surgery until he (the patient), the surgeon, and the wound were all in fit shape for such an important matter.

## SELECTED REFERENCES

Ducker, T. B., Kempe, L. G., and Hayes, G. J.: The metabolic background for peripheral nerve surgery. J. Neurosurg., 30:270, 1969.

*This is a superb summary of neuronal metabolism and metabolic responses in the proximal and distal nerve segments that accompany peripheral nerve injury. Such metabolic alterations are related to the time of surgical repair and are derived from personal investigations and from pertinent literature (73 references).*

Haymaker, W., and Woodhall, B.: Peripheral Nerve Injuries. Principles of Diagnosis. 2nd ed. Philadelphia, W. B. Saunders Company, 1953.

*This is a relatively simple and highly usable treatise, derived from experience with war injuries, but from its basic design valuable as an approach to the understanding and treatment of civilian-type injuries. It is a primer on the nature of a peripheral nerve injury, its diagnosis, and its surgical anatomy.*

Lyons, W. R., and Woodhall, B.: Atlas of Peripheral Nerve Injuries. Philadelphia, W. B. Saunders Company, 1949.

*This is another basic neuropathologic reference volume concerned with definitions, normal peripheral nerve anatomy, and the pathologic changes in complete nerve division, neuromas in continuity, nerve sutures, and nerve grafts. Gross and light microscopic photographs are used to illustrate the material.*

Seddon, H. J., ed.: Peripheral Nerve Injuries. London, The Nerve Injuries Committee of the Medical Research Council, Her Majesty's Stationery Office, 1954.

*Another superb, inclusive, and readable record of British wartime experience in this field, an experience readily transferred to civilian-type injuries. The chapter on nerve grafting and the histopathology of nerve grafts represents a good introduction to that subject.*

Sunderland, S.: Nerves and Nerve Injuries. Baltimore, Williams & Wilkins Company, 1968.

*This is a monumental enterprise, the result of activities in the laboratory and the clinic spread over the years 1940 to 1957. It is clearly a reference book but an adequate table of contents and a superb index allow the student ready access to any particular problem. Part VIII under the heading of "individual nerves" is uniquely valuable to the student for the understanding of both open and closed nerve injuries. There are countless references but the volume is fundamentally the work of a man of considerable scholarship.*

White, J. C., and Sweet, W. H.: Pain and the Neurosurgeon. A Forty-Year Experience. Springfield, Ill., Charles C Thomas, 1969.

*A virtual repository of total knowledge and a 40 year personal experience of the senior author in the neurosurgical methods of relieving pain. The first 48 pages are concerned with pain following peripheral nerve injuries but the student at least should continue with those pages concerned with "pain following amputation" and "other varieties of peripheral neuralgia."*

Woodhall, B., and Beede, G. W.: Peripheral Nerve Regeneration. A Follow-Up Study of 3656 World War II Injuries. Washington, D.C., Veterans Administration Monograph, U.S. Government Printing Office, 1956.

*This is one of several monographs published by the Veterans Administration after World War II. As its Introduction states, "This monograph is not a textbook of peripheral nerve surgery. . . . From the data presented in the body of the monograph, certain surgical conclusions have been reached or, when necessary, restated so the informed surgeon can treat a new peripheral nerve injury with a firm concept of the result he will attain under the diverse and many factors that influence such an injury." It is not easy reading but neither is regeneration an easy subject.*

## REFERENCES

1. Ducker, T. B., and Hayes, G. J.: Experimental improvements in the use of silastic cuff for peripheral nerve repair. J. Neurosurg., 28:582, 1968.
2. Ducker, T. B., Kempe, L. G., and Hayes, G. J.: The metabolic background for peripheral nerve surgery. J. Neurosurg., 30:270, 1969.
3. Haymaker, W., and Woodhall, B.: Peripheral Nerve Injuries. Principles of Diagnosis. 2nd ed. Philadelphia, W. B. Saunders Company, 1953.
4. Lyons, W. R., and Woodhall, B.: Atlas of Peripheral Nerve Injuries. Philadelphia, W. B. Saunders Company, 1949.
5. Mitchell, S. W.: Injuries of Nerves and Their Consequences. Philadelphia, J. B. Lippincott Company, 1872.
6. Seddon, H. J.: Nerve lesions complicating certain closed bone injuries. J.A.M.A., 135:691, 1947.
7. Seddon, H. J., ed.: Peripheral Nerve Injuries. London, The Nerve Injuries Committee of the Medical Research Council. Her Majesty's Stationery Office, 1954.
8. Sunderland, S.: Nerves and Nerve Injuries. Baltimore, Williams & Wilkins Company, 1968.
9. White, J. C., and Sweet, W. H.: Pain and the Neurosurgeon. A Forty-Year Experience. Springfield, Ill., Charles C Thomas, 1969.
10. Woodhall, B.: Operative injury to the accessory nerve in the posterior cervical triangle. Arch. Surg., 74:122, 1957.
11. Woodhall, B., and Beede, G. W.: Peripheral Nerve Regeneration. A Follow-Up Study of 3656 World War II Injuries. Washington, D.C., Veterans Administration Monograph, U.S. Government Printing Office, 1956.

# CONGENITAL ABNORMALITIES

*M. Stephen Mahaley, Jr., M.D.*

Congenital aneurysms and arteriovenous malformations have been discussed elsewhere as vascular lesions. Many of the remaining congenital abnormalities represent midline cranial or spinal problems, and it has been postulated that they stem from a common basic embryonic defect, a permeability abnormality in the rhombic roof of the fourth ventricle.

### Hydrocephalus

The production, movement, and reabsorption of cerebrospinal fluid is now recognized as an extremely complex interaction between bulk flow, active transport, and facilitated diffusion. It is subject to a variety of physiologic and pathologic influences.[3]

Two types of congenital hydrocephalus are recognized: communicating and noncommunicating, referring to whether or not the ventricular fluid communicates with the subarachnoid space. The noncommunicating variety may take the form of a stenosis or occlusion of the aqueduct of Sylvius or an impermeable rhombic roof. A child with hydrocephalus evident at birth classically has enlargement of the head, a wide and tense fontanelle, prominent venous channels in the scalp, and downward displacement of the globes within the orbits ("setting-sun" appearance). The head circumference should be carefully measured and the child examined for other congenital abnormalities, since multiple lesions are not uncommon. Transillumination of the head in a totally dark room should be attempted, since this finding in patients with anencephaly or extreme loss of cortex indicates a grave prognosis and usually interdicts surgery. X-rays of the skull are often helpful as regards the relative proportions of the various cranial fossae and the general configuration of the cranium. A transcoronal ventriculogram permits estimation of the thickness of the cortical mantle and may illustrate the actual site of obstruction of cerebrospinal fluid flow (Fig. 27). Arnold-Chiari malformations[2] and Dandy-Walker syndromes[1] probably represent variations on this same theme, the differences relating to specific mechanical displacements of structures in the posterior fossa.[5]

Surgical correction generally takes the form of a shunt procedure, the ventriculoatrial shunt being most commonly used at this time.[6] The decision to perform this procedure has to take into account the severity of the hydrocephalus, the presence or absence of other more serious congenital anomalies, and the general medical condition of the patient. The decision is often as difficult to make as it is to set down hard and fast rules for making it. The shunt, once performed, is subject to complications. Obstruction of the ventricular or atrial end of the shunt or infection of the shunt mechanism can necessitate removal or revision. Elective revisions have been recommended as the child grows and bony lengthening displaces the cardiac catheter,[6] and considerable work has been done regarding the management of the infected shunt.[4,7] The majority of these children are shunt-dependent after surgery, although clinical trials are now attempting to develop shunt independence, as part of the neurosurgical treatment.[8]

### Meningomyelocele and Encephalocele

These lesions represent congenital midline defects with absence of bony covering (spina bifida or cranium bifidum), protrusion of a meningeal sac through this opening (meningocele), and oftentimes a herniation of nervous tissue into the sac (myelocele and encephalocele). If the meningeal sac is extremely thin over the surface, leakage of cerebrospinal fluid may be present at birth or develop shortly thereafter, permitting bacterial contamination and meningitis. Occasionally the meningeal sac is deficient in the midline, thus exposing the underlying nervous tissue, with free

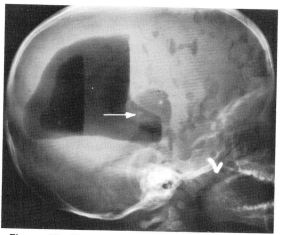

**Figure 27** Ventriculogram, showing hydrocephalus secondary to aqueductal occlusion (arrow). Air (dark areas) is seen to fill part of the enlarged lateral and third ventricles, with the dilated proximal part of the aqueduct attached at the floor of the third ventricle.

flow of cerebrospinal fluid (rachischisis); this condition is most often accompanied by the severest of neurologic deficits and represents the most difficult to manage neurosurgically.

Each child should be examined carefully to ascertain the extent of neurologic involvement at and below the level of the lesion; leg movements, response to pain, and anal sphincter tone are commonly impaired. The meningeal sac (Fig. 28) should be transilluminated to see if nervous tissue can be outlined. Other congenital anomalies should be sought, especially hydrocephalus.

The decision regarding surgical closure of these defects is often a difficult one because of (1) the small size of the patient, (2) the severity of the neurologic deficit often present, and (3) the associated congenital anomalies that may exist. If the patient with a meningocele is known to be hydrocephalic, then the hydrocephalus problem should be treated first and the meningocele later. If the midline defect is severe and leaking spinal fluid, with absence of neurologic function below the level of the lesion, the case may be considered hopeless, although there are those who would disagree and would insist on early surgical correction of almost all such defects.[9] If the midline defect is covered by healthy skin, then there may be no need for early surgery, the advantages to delay being severalfold: a chance to observe the patient longer for any evidence of hydrocephalus, time for the patient to outgrow the newborn period prior to being subjected to a surgical procedure, and the opportunity to carefully evaluate neurologic function as the child gets older. When a meningocele shows areas of extremely thin epidermis or when a small leak of cerebrospinal fluid is seen or suspected, surgical closure is advised at an early date, unless the seriousness of the neurologic deficit weighs against attempted repair. The primary aims of surgical repair are: (1) protection of underlying nervous tissue, (2) prevention of menin-

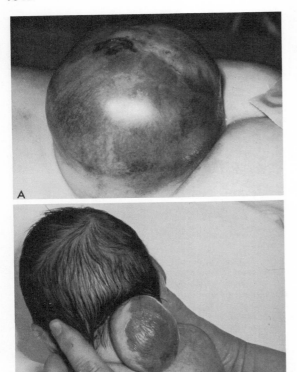

**Figure 28** *A,* Lumbosacral meningocele, with buttocks to the right. *B,* Craniocervical meningocele.

gitis, (3) improvement of the mechanical inconvenience and cosmetic unpleasantness of a midline defect and mass, and (4) in a broad sense, improvement of the quality of existence of the patient.

### Syringomyelia and Hydromyelia

These congenital abnormalities refer to the presence of a pocket of fluid trapped within the cord substance (syringomyelia) or central canal (hydromyelia) more or less isolated from normal pathways of spinal fluid flow. These lesions may also stem from basically a permeability problem at the level of the rhombic roof during embryonic development.[5] However, the typical symptoms of a suspended sensory deficit to pain and temperature, a lower motor neuron dysfunction at the level of the lesion, and distal long tract signs may not appear until later in life, apparently as a result of gradual enlargement of the fluid pocket during life. The lesion is most commonly seen in the lower cervical and upper dorsal spinal areas but may extend the entire length of the spinal cord and occasionally into the brain stem.

Diagnosis may be aided by evidence of widening of the spinal canal on plain spine films and by myelographic evidence of an intrinsic mass lesion of the cord. Treatment involves creation of a communication between the fluid cavity and the subarachnoid space and, in cases of hydromyelia in which a communication exists with the fourth

ventricle, plugging of the cervical canal opening at the obex.

### Craniosynostosis

Premature closure or fusion of one or more of the cranial sutures results in a form of craniosynostosis.[10] The cranium will appear short in the anterior-posterior direction when the coronal suture alone is fused (brachycephaly) or narrow in the lateral dimension with sagittal suture closure (scaphocephaly). These single suture premature closures are largely cosmetic problems. Premature fusion of several or all (oxycephaly) cranial sutures can result in brain damage and visual loss as development occurs within an unnaturally rigid enclosure. The problem of oxycephaly must be distinguished at birth from that of microcephaly, in which the primary defect is one of congenitally poor brain development with secondarily small head. X-rays of the skull are helpful, since microcephaly will usually show overlapping, unfused sutures at birth while oxycephaly will show fused sutures and often a thinning of the calvarium due to increased intracranial pressure. It is usually advisable to correct a craniosynostosis problem surgically as soon after birth as possible. The earlier prematurely fused sutures are opened, the better the chance for a more normal shape to the head and lesser the likelihood of impairment to the underlying developing brain.

### Dermal Sinus and Dermoid

These congenital defects result from persistence of somatic ectoderm in the vicinity of the midline mesodermal elements (muscle and bone) or the neuroectoderm (brain, spinal cord, or cauda equina). The dermal sinus consists of a cutaneous

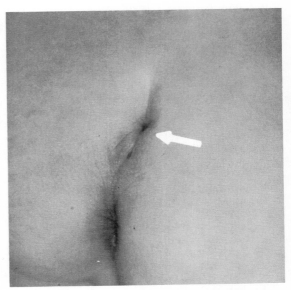

**Figure 29** Dermal sinus. The characteristic cutaneous opening of a dermal sinus (arrow) is seen in the midline above the sacral area and just cephalad to the anal opening.

opening which is usually quite small, located in the sacral (Fig. 29) or suboccipital areas, and connecting to the deeper midline structures by virtue of a sinus tract. The lining of this sinus contains dermal elements (sweat glands, hair follicles, and sebaceous glands) along its length and periodically extrudes debris via the surface orifice. This tract may terminate as a cul-de-sac inside the spinal canal and is then referred to as a dermoid, or a dermoid may exist in the spinal canal without apparent connection with the surface skin. A sinus tract or dermoid extending into the spinal canal may rupture and create meningitis. Indeed, a child with recurrent unexplained bouts of meningitis due to Staphylococcus or *Escherichia coli* should be examined carefully for the possible presence of a dermal sinus. An intraspinal dermoid may present with signs and symptoms of an intraspinal tumor. Careful examination of the midline skin may reveal the sinus opening or an overlying skin angioma or tuft of hair. X-rays of the spine or skull may reveal a bony opening through which a sinus tract passes. It is generally advised that any such midline tracts be explored and excised, with the exploration carried into the spinal canal when necessary to resect an extradural or intradural dermoid.

### Diastematomyelia

Another of the congenital midline spinal defects consists of the presence of a spicule of bone arising perpendicularly from the dorsal surface of a vertebral body, usually in the lower thoracic spine, and often extending superiorly to the overlying laminal arch. This bony spicule effectively divides the spinal canal, cord, and surrounding meninges and acts as a source of traction on these structures as the child grows, resulting in leg weakness, numbness, and incontinence. A plain spine anterior-posterior x-ray may reveal the bony spicule, and a myelogram usually demonstrates division of the subarachnoid space by the bone. Surgical resection of the spicule can usually be accomplished without difficulty, often with improvement in the neurologic symptoms.

### REFERENCES

1. Benda, C. E.: Dandy-Walker syndrome or so-called atresia of foramen megendie. J. Neuropath. Exp. Neurol., 13:14, 1954.
2. Chiari, H.: Uber Veranderungen des Kleinhirns infolge von Hydrocephalie des Grosshirns. Deutsch. Med. Wschr., 17:1171, 1891.
3. Davson, H.: Physiology of the Cerebrospinal Fluid. London, J. & A. Churchill, 1967.
4. Fokes, E. C., Jr.: Occult infections of ventriculo-atrial shunts. J. Neurosurg., 33:517, 1970.
5. Gardner, W. J.: Myelocele: rupture of the neural tube? Clin. Neurosurg., 15:57, 1968.
6. Matson, D. D.: Neurosurgery of Infancy and Childhood. 2nd ed. Springfield, Ill., Charles C Thomas, 1969.
7. Perrin, J. C. S., and McLaurin, R. L.: Infected ventriculo-atrial shunts. A method of treatment. J. Neurosurg., 27:21, 1967.
8. Ransohoff, J.: Personal communication.
9. Sharrard, W. J. W., Zachary, R. B., Lorber, J., and Bruce, A. M.: A controlled trial of immediate and delayed closure of spina bifida cystica. Arch. Dis. Child., 38:18, 1963.
10. Taveras, J. M., and Wood, E. H.: Diagnostic Neuroradiology. Baltimore, Williams & Wilkins Company, 1964.

# NEUROSURGICAL RELIEF OF PAIN

*Blaine S. Nashold, Jr., M.D., and*
*Harry Friedman, M.D.*

Not everyone has a soul of fire, and, in actual human life, even in the case of the great mystics, the struggle against pain exacts a high price.

　　　　　　　　　　　　　　　　　　—Lerche

Pain is not a simple sensory event but a complex neural and psychologic phenomenon that involves the entire nervous system. Humans differ remarkably in their individual reaction to pain and suffering, and when severe pain is unrelieved, a state of suffering may intervene that threatens the very existence of the person. Our understanding of the anatomy and physiology of pain perception in man has evolved slowly simply because pain is a private matter and direct observations in man have their limitations. Someone has said that in order to totally relieve pain the nervous system must be destroyed, and yet we know that section of the dorsal roots and spinal cordotomy are time-honored neurosurgical operations that can relieve pain.

Although the free nerve endings of the C fibers are considered the primary receptors that signal pain, recent physiologic evidence indicates that these free nerve endings also function as receptors for other kinds of sensation. At the peripheral end, fine cutaneous afferent activity appears to be a necessary condition for the sensation of pain. Although the functional localization of pain is important, recent physiologic work emphasizes spatial and temporal mechanisms that are involved in the coding of sensory experience within the central nervous system.

The success of spinal cordotomy in relieving pain is related to the anatomic organization of pain and thermal fibers in the lateral spinothalamic tract. Edinger delineated the spinothalamic tract in 1889 but its function was not known until 1905 when Spiller noted the loss of pain and temperature in a patient with a discrete tuberculoma in the anterior quadrant of the spinal cord.[1, 7] Martin, in 1912, at the urging of Spiller, carried out the first thoracic cordotomy.[8] Although the lateral spinothalamic tract is of considerable importance in the transmission of painful and thermal sensations, recent anatomic evidence indicates additional pathways are available for the transmission of pain. The lateral spinothalamic tract is a phylogenetically recent pain pathway with its input directly into the sensory thalamus. Pain transmission over the spinothalamic route has a rapid transit time to the thalamus where higher levels of integration occur through the thalamocortical connections. A definite topographic scheme of the body's sensory image exists within the cord and the thalamus, the input from the facial region being medial to that from the body, and from the leg regions, lateral. Pain resulting from electrical stimulation of the spinothalamic pathways is usually experienced by the patient as a sharp, well demarcated sensation referred to a localized region of the body.

In contrast to this, the diffuse pain pathways appear to have multiple routes through the spinal cord with distribution to the midbrain, thalamus, and hypothalamus; these spinoreticular pathways are phylogenetically older than the newer lateral spinothalamic tracts and have been designated the paleothalamic system. They may be crossed or uncrossed tracts, which are composed of short chains of neurons that make several synaptic connections at successive rostral levels in the central nervous system. Pain transmitted via these routes appears to be slower in transit to higher levels and the sensation experienced by alert patients during stimulation is ill defined and unpleasant, being diffusely localized to the regions in the central parts of the body, including the head, chest, or abdomen.

Pain can be thought of as either a primary or secondary symptom. In most cases it is a secondary symptom usually originating from some underlying pathologic change, correction of which will relieve the pain. However, when the pathologic state cannot be eradicated, as may be the case in metastatic malignant disease, the pain may be relieved by a specific neurosurgical operation.

Pain as a primary symptom results from physiologic or pathologic involvement of the pain pathways within the central nervous system. A painful dysesthesia occurring after surgical cordotomy,

tractotomy, or thalamotomy is an example of a primary pain syndrome. Other examples include the pain of the thalamic syndrome or painful phantom limb. Central pain syndromes often occur after trauma, vascular occlusion, tumor, degenerative disease in the central nervous system (multiple sclerosis), or infections (herpes zoster). The patient describes this kind of pain as intense, burning, crushing, or tearing and it can be aggravated by the slightest sensory stimulation. An emotional upset will intensify the patient's pain, as can psychiatric disturbances. These patients often become drug addicts and undergo permanent personality changes. Numerous theories have been proposed to explain central pain as the presence of hyperirritable neurons at the site of injury in the diffuse pain tracts, the diversion of noxious impulses from the spinothalamic tract into the paleothalamic system, or the release of the thalamus from cortical inhibition.

Neurosurgical treatment of central pain has not been completely successful although tractotomy and thalamotomy have been used in a limited number of patients.

## NEUROSURGICAL OPERATIONS FOR PAIN

The neurosurgeon must consider certain facts before recommending an operation to relieve pain. The neurosurgical operation must not be done as a last resort or in desperation. Most failures to relieve pain are due to delay in surgical treatment. The neurosurgeon should be consulted early, before the occurrence of drug addiction or suffering. Long-established pain leads to a state of suffering

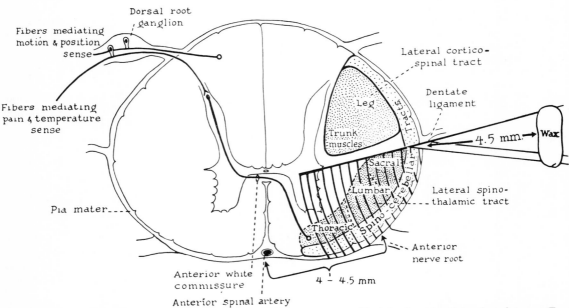

**Figure 30** Cross-sectional drawing of thoracic cord showing extent of incision in anterolateral cordotomy. (From Kahn, E. A., Bassett, R. C., Schneider, R. C., and Crosly, E. C.: Correlative Neurosurgery. 1955. Courtesy of Charles C Thomas, Publisher, Springfield, Ill.)

that is to be avoided. Ideally the benefit from the operation should last for the lifetime of the patient.

Neurosurgical operations for the relief of pain can be divided into four types: (1) anatomic interruption pathways subserving pain or the destruction of sensory integration regions in the central nervous system (rhizotomy, cordotomy, tractotomy, thalamotomy, cingulotomy); (2) sympathectomy for the relief of causalgia and sympathetic dystrophy; (3) pituitary ablation to relieve pain from metastatic tumors under hormonal influence; (4) electroanalgesia to relieve pain, by stimulation of peripheral nerves or the dorsal column of the spinal cord.

The simplest operation for pain relief is a section, avulsion, or alcohol injection of a peripheral nerve. It has the advantage of relieving pain originating from a small localized area. In trigeminal neuralgia, injection or avulsion of one of the peripheral branches of the fifth nerve may give several years of relief. When the pain recurs or involves larger areas of the face, the gasserian ganglion may be sectioned or lightly traumatized by rubbing, adding additional long periods of relief. One disadvantage of sectioning a peripheral nerve is the return of the pain with its regeneration. The sensory loss from a dorsal rhizotomy involves a larger area but at least three to four of the nerve roots must be sectioned to produce an analgesic zone equal to one dermatome. Dorsal rhizotomy may be useful in relieving pain originating from the neck, shoulder, thorax, or abdominal wall but it is usually unsuitable if the pain involves the arm or leg since total loss of sensation in these regions often reduces the usefulness of the limb.

Spinal cordotomy still remains the most useful operation for the relief of widespread pain in the torso and extremities (Fig. 30). It is especially helpful when the pain originates from thoracic or abdominal regions. The surgical section is performed opposite the site of the pain in the anterolateral quadrant of spinal cord at least six cord segments above the origin of the pain, to allow for some degree of postoperative regression of the sensory level. The analgesia resulting from a cordotomy covers the opposite half of the body with the level beginning several segments below the cord section. For the most complete relief of pain, the entire lateral spinothalamic tract must be sectioned, since an incomplete cut, for example, may result in the sparing of sensation in one region or another with the persistence of the pain. An open surgical cordotomy has a mortality of 10 per cent and the cord section can be done at two different spinal levels, usually cervical (C1–C3) and thoracic (T1–T2), and in the case of the cervical operation the analgesic level reaches up to the clavicle, involving the arm to varying degrees but with the densest analgesia over regions of thorax, abdomen, and leg. A thoracic cordotomy produces contralateral analgesia beginning in the lower thorax (Fig. 31). A well executed unilateral lumbar cordotomy should result in good pain relief in 85 per cent of cases, whereas with a high cervical cordotomy relief occurs 50 per cent of the time. After unilateral cordotomy as a rule complications are few, with normal bladder, bowel, and sexual function. Postoperative complications such as an ipsilateral hemiparesis or monoparesis can occur if the surgical incision involves the nearby corticospinal tract. A bilateral cordotomy performed either in the cervical or thoracic cord has higher overall operative risks and the postoperative deficits are greater; most of these operations should be restricted to patients with widespread carcinoma whose life expectancy is limited. Bilateral cordotomy at either level seriously interferes with the bladder, bowel, and sexual function.

Percutaneous cervical cordotomy, introduced by Mullan in 1963, has proved useful in patients who could not withstand the operative rigors of an

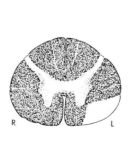

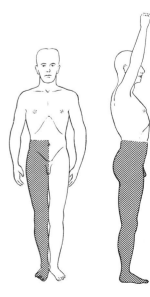

**Figure 31** Extent of analgesia after thoracic cordotomy. Area of cord involved is shown in section on the left.

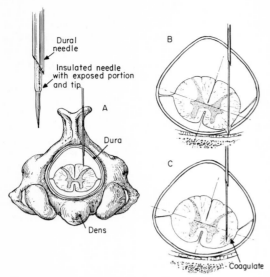

**Figure 32** Percutaneous cordotomy using posterior approach; anterior and lateral introduction of needle also are possible.

open cordotomy.[3] The percutaneous cordotomy is done with local anesthesia, with roentgenographic control of a coagulating needle which is guided into the anterolateral quadrant of the spinal cord between the first and second cervical vertebrae (Fig. 32). The direction and depth of the needle are controlled by roentgenograms and electrical stimulation can be used to test the location of the needle tip within the cord tissue. The lateral spinothalamic tract can be coagulated unilaterally or bilaterally by means of a high-frequency electrical current. Such operations can be done quickly by experienced surgeons with a minimum of surgical trauma. It is, however, a blind operation, so the surgeon must exercise great care not to misplace the lesion and cause additional neurologic deficits. One risk of the percutaneous technique is that the high bilateral cervical cord lesions may interfere with breathing and after surgery patients have died in their sleep of respiratory failure. A percutaneous cordotomy is best suited for a poor-risk patient with a short life expectancy. Long-term chronic pain is best not treated by the percutaneous technique because of the occurrence of late failures and the risk of recurrence of the original pain or even more serious risk of a postoperative painful dysesthesia.

Pain involving overlapping areas of the head, neck, or arm can be difficult to control by a single surgical operation owing to the overlapping of the cranial and cervical nerves in the head and neck. Stereotactic operations at midbrain or thalamic levels have relieved these widespread cranial and cervical pains. A stereotactic medullary tractotomy can be performed to selectively interrupt pain involving the individual divisions of the trigeminal nerve. The first open surgical section of the spinothalamic tracts in the midbrain was performed by Walker in 1942, producing an analgesia

of the opposite half of the body.[9] However, the open medullary or mesencephalic tractotomies were associated with a high mortality (7 per cent) and morbidity, with one serious drawback being the risk of a postoperative dysesthesia. Since 1947, using the human stereotactic instrument, Spiegel and Wycis and others have coagulated the mesencephalic pain tracts by introducing a small probe into the mesencephalon via a frontal burr hole (Fig. 33).[6] The mortality rate has been reduced to 1 per cent, with good relief of pain, and although postoperative dysesthesias still occur, they are less frequent. Postoperatively there is usually loss of upward gaze and occasional diplopia which may complicate recovery.

Stereotactic lesions in the thalamus or the cingulum have been successfully employed to relieve widespread pain causing suffering. A unilateral thalamic lesion (centrum medium or parafascicular nucleus or both) is often sufficient for relief of the pain of extensive carcinoma. The relief is thought to be due to interruption of sensory integration at higher levels in the central nervous system. A thalamic lesion does not alter the threshold for pain and no analgesia occurs despite the relief of the patient's pain. An added risk of the

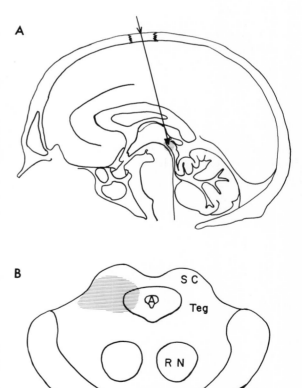

**Figure 33** *A*, Sagittal section of brain shows target tract to midbrain. *B*, Cross section of mesencephalon at superior colliculus. Area of therapeutic lesion shown on the right.

thalamic operation may be an interference with memory or speech mechanism and in some patients the relief of the pain is short-lived.

When suffering is the most prominent clinical feature in a patient with intractable pain it can best be relieved by a medial dorsal thalamic or cingulate gyrus lesion interrupting the cingulum. The beneficial effect of the thalamic lesion is thought to be due to the interruption of the thalamofrontal connections, while a cingulate lesion exerts its effect by interfering with some circuits in the limbic system. Frontal leukotomy can no longer be recommended as an operation for the relief of pain.

### Painful Phantom Limb

The loss of an arm, leg, or breast or the penis will result in a phantom sensation. The neural organization of one's conscious awareness of his own body scheme requires a period of learning when the sensory patterns of the body schema are organized within the sensory cortex. A person with congenital absence of a limb has no phantom sensation. After an amputation, the phantom image seems fixed in the person's awareness. The patient's awareness of the traumatic circumstances surrounding the loss of his limb appears to exert some influence on whether or not he may experience the phantom sensation. Normally the phantom sensation will fade away by retracting into the end of the stump, but the patient is often aware of its posture and may even be able to move the missing fingers or toes. Before an amputation a wise surgeon forewarns his patient about the possible postoperative occurrence of the phantom sensation.

When the phantom sensation is accompanied by pain, surgical treatment may be necessary. The presence of pain intensifies and prolongs the phantom sensation and when the pain is relieved the phantom fades. A painful phantom often follows a traumatic avulsion of the brachial plexus that tears the nerve roots from their attachment to the spinal cord. The arm becomes insensitive and flaccid and the pain is described as burning, tearing, or crushing, and its intensity seems to heighten the patient's awareness of his phantom limb. Injury to the substantia gelantinosa in the spinal cord at the point where the dorsal roots are avulsed may be the site from which the pain originates. A high cervical cordotomy, stereotactic mesencephalic tractotomy, or thalamotomy has relieved the pain, while resection of the arm or leg area of the parietal sensory cortex relieves neither the pain nor the phantom. Amputation of the painful arm after brachial avulsion is of no value in relieving the pain.

### Surgical Sympathectomy for Relief of Causalgia and Sympathetic Dystrophy

Causalgia is a syndrome characterized by severe "burning pain" and autonomic dysfunction that occurs after partial injury to large nerve trunks. The first detailed clinical description appeared in 1864 when Mitchell, Morehouse, and Keen examined Civil War veterans with gunshot wounds of the arm or leg that had injured major nerve trunks.[2] The etiology of this disorder is unknown but the symptoms are more likely to occur after injuries to large peripheral nerves such as the brachial plexus, or the median or sciatic nerve. Usually the nerve lesion is incomplete with only a partial sensory loss in the involved painful limb. The physiologic basis for the pain and its association with autonomic dysfunction is not understood but some have postulated that the burning dysesthesia results from short-circuiting of C fiber impulses or the shunting of efferent sympathetic impulses via the injured somatic nerve which in turn activates the pain fibers. If the disorder persists for too long a time without relief, drug addiction and psychoneurosis may complicate the surgical treatment. The burning pain of causalgia (hyperpathia) usually involves the hand or foot, with the skin of the extremity becoming smooth and glossy in appearance along with loss of the hair. The vasomotor disturbances appear with sweating and coldness involving the limb. The patient becomes irritable, fearful, and protective of his injured limb, and as time passes without relief of his pain, he withdraws from social contacts and avoids bright lights and loud noises, and the slightest emotional problem will aggravate his pain. He may find temporary relief by bathing his painful limb in tepid running water. The symptoms are dramatically relieved by a block of the sympathetic nerves to the involved limb and a cure results after surgical sympathectomy.

The second group of painful disorders associated with pain and autonomic dysfunction is sympathetic dystrophy which occurs after trauma of a less specific degree to extremities or joints. The pain is not usually burning as in causalgia but vasomotor disturbances can occur, with vasospastic phenomena, cyanosis, sudomotor dysfunction, and trophic skin changes in the involved limb. Diagnostic sympathetic nerve block often relieves the symptoms and surgical sympathectomy may be curative. Psychoneurosis is not uncommon in these patients and their disorder is oftentimes complicated by personal problems associated with litigation or compensation claims. Ill advised surgery may tend to magnify the entire symptom complex.

### Relief of Pain by Pituitary Ablation

Bone pain caused by metastases from breast or prostatic tumors will dramatically subside after ablation of the pituitary gland. The relief of pain is probably related to a reduction or loss of the effects of pituitary growth hormone, which has a direct stimulating effect on these tumors. As the pain subsides, the tumor nodules also diminish in size and the lesions in the bone seen on the roentgenogram often resolve with recalcification. Pituitary ablation should be considered only after oophrectomy in women, or following the removal of the gonads in males. Hypophysectomy exerts its best effect in premenopausal women and the most satisfactory results are noted if the pituitary gland is

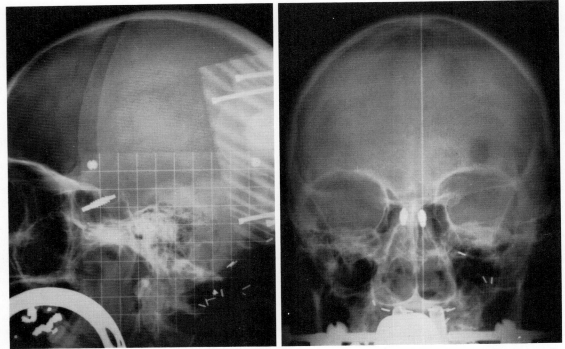

**Figure 34** Skull x-rays of female patient with intractable pain from metastatic breast cancer. Yttrium pellets introduced transsphenoidally for pituitary ablation.

completely ablated to produce a significant drop in the levels of the growth hormone. Complete surgical removal of the pituitary can be accomplished through a subfrontal craniotomy but recently stereotactic ablations have been carried out by introducing lesion probes into the sella turcica (Fig. 34). The overall operative risks are less following the stereotactic operation and the gland can be destroyed by either freezing, heat coagulation, or implanting radioactive yttrium. Postoperatively these patients must be maintained on hormone replacement, often combined with Pitressin if diabetes insipidus appears. Pituitary ablation can be followed by many pain-free months during which time the patient's overall condition improves and life becomes bearable.

### Relief of Pain by Electroanalgesia

In 1967, Wall and Sweet found that during stimulation of a peripheral nerve, pain sensation was reduced over the distribution area of the stimulated nerve.[11] They proposed that the electrical activation of A fibers of the peripheral nerve in some way interfered with the perception of the painful stimulus, probably at the spinal cord level. Wall had already shown, in animals, that when the activity of the larger A fibers in peripheral nerves was increased by electrical stimulus there occurred a concomitant inhibition of the smaller pain fiber activity within the spinal cord.[10] Later, Shealy et al. noted that stimulation of the dorsal column of the cat, which is made up entirely of the large A fibers, reduced the animal's reaction to noxious stimuli.[5] The term "electroanalgesia" was

coined although the neurophysiologic mechanism responsible for the pain relief was not known. Sweet originally employed the electrical stimulation technique to successfully relieve pain originating from an injured peripheral nerve. A pair of platinum electrodes is placed in contact with the nerve trunk above the level of the injury and a miniature RF receiver, which is attached to the stimulating platinum electrodes, is buried beneath the skin. The patient carries out self-activation of the painful nerves by an electrical signal transmitted through the skin of the RF receiver by a small portable RF generator. The patient can vary either the frequency or strength of the stimulating current in order to find a level of stimulation that relieves his pain. Later, in 1970, Shealy and Mortimer reported on the implantation of stimulating electrodes to activate the dorsal columns of the spinal cord in patients with pain from widespread carcinoma.[4] The device was inserted through a laminectomy at either the cervical or thoracic level but always above the segmental level of the body from which the pain originates. Self-activation of the dorsal columns by the patient resulted in his experiencing a paresthesia over the painful region with reduction of the pain. The technique, although still new as a mode of treatment, seems promising and its greatest potential is based on the concept that the nervous system is not physically disrupted but the "ongoing" neural activity related to pain perception is in some way altered by the introduction of an extrinsic electrical impulse, thereby preserving the physical integrity of the central nervous system.

## SELECTED REFERENCES

Cassinari, V., and Pagni, A. C.: Central Pain: A Neurosurgical Survey. Cambridge, Mass., Harvard University Press, 1969.
*A concise monograph of the physiologic and clinical aspects of central pain.*

Knighton, R. S., and Dumke, P. R.: Pain. Boston, Little, Brown and Company, 1966.
*International symposium on new concepts of pain, stressing both clinical and research aspects.*

Spiller, W. G.: The occasional clinical resemblance between caries of the vertebral and lumbothoracic syringomyelia, and the location within the spinal cord of the fibres for the sensations of pain and temperature. Univ. Penn. Med. Bull., 18:147, 1905.
*Classic paper on the functional role of the lateral spinothalamic tracts by a founder of American neurology.*

Sternbach, R. A.: Pain: A Psychophysiological Analysis. New York, Academic Press, 1968.
*An overview of pain and suffering from the psychiatric and psychologic point of view.*

White, J. C., and Sweet, W. H.: Pain and the Neurosurgeon. A Forty-Year Experience. Springfield, Ill., Charles C Thomas, 1969.
*A 40 year experience of the neurosurgical treatment with detailed clinical data combined with anatomic and physiologic correlations.*

## REFERENCES

1. Edinger, L.: Vergleichend-enturick-lungsgeschichtliche und anatomische Studien und Bereiche des Central-nerven-systems: II. Uber die Fortsetzung der hintern Ruckenmarks wurseln Zum Gehirn. Anat. Anz., 4:121, 1889.
2. Mitchell, S. W., Morehouse, G. R., and Keen, W. W.: Gunshot Wounds and Other Injuries of Nerves. Philadelphia, J. B. Lippincott Company, 1864, p. 164.
3. Mullan, S., Harper, P. R., Hekmatpanah, J., Torres, H., and Dobbin, G.: Percutaneous interruption of spinal pain tracts by means of a strontium⁹⁰ needle. J. Neurosurg., 20:931, 1963.
4. Shealy, C. N., Mortimer, J. T., and Hagsfors, N.: Dorsal column electroanalgesia. J. Neurosurg., 32:560, 1970.
5. Shealy, C. N., Mortimer, J. T., and Reswick, J. B.: Electrical inhibition of pain by stimulation of the dorsal columns. Anesth. Analg., 46:489, 1967.
6. Spiegel, E. A., Wycis, H. T., Marks, M., and Lee, A. J.: Stereotactic apparatus for operation on the human brain. Science, 106:349, 1947.
7. Spiller, W. G.: The occasional clinical resemblance between caries of the vertebral and lumbothoracic syringomyelia, and the location within the spinal cord of the fibres for the sensations of pain and temperature. Univ. Penn. Med. Bull., 18:147, 1905.
8. Spiller, W. G., and Martin, E.: The treatment of persistent pain of organic origin in the lower part of the body by division of the anterolateral column of the spinal cord. J.A.M.A., 58:1489, 1912.
9. Walker, A. E.: Relief of pain by mesencephalic tractotomy. Arch. Neurol., 48:865, 1942.
10. Wall, P. D.: Control of impulses at the first central synapse in cutaneous pathways. In: Eccles, J. C., and Schade, J. P., eds.: Physiology of Spinal Neurons. Progress in Brain Research. Volume 12. New York, Elsevier, 1964.
11. Wall, P. D., and Sweet, W. H.: Temporary abolition of pain in man. Science, 155:108, 1967.

# NEUROSURGICAL TREATMENT OF EPILEPSY

*Blaine S. Nashold, Jr., M.D.*

Epilepsy can be defined as a paroxysmal, excessive, neuronal discharge within the brain originating from either cortical or subcortical regions. Although the brain is the site of the dysfunction there occurs a sudden disruption of function of the body or mind and the symptoms produced by the epileptic seizure are a reflection of the part of the brain involved.

The epileptic neuron exhibits an instability of its cellular membrane and the abnormal neuronal discharge is due to excessive depolarization with possible fluctuation in activity associated with repolarizing and hyperpolarizing mechanisms. Although these intrinsic neuronal mechanisms are of prime importance, extrinsic factors affect the irritable neurons, such as excessive afferent bombardment from distant regions of the brain, or systemic metabolic changes may alter the local chemical milieu of the hyperirritable neurons.

Epilepsy is a serious social and medical problem and it is estimated that 1 in 200 persons suffers from seizures, although an accurate figure on the exact numbers of persons who have an attack at some time in their lives is unknown. The incidence of epilepsy is increasing; this increase is largely due to the survival of persons who would have died of brain injuries or other cerebral abnormalities acquired in early life. This has been brought about by the use of antibiotics and the improvements in medical care that have saved many children who might have died of meningitis, brain abscess, encephalitis, severe head injury, or brain tumor. It should be noted that seizures may result from any pathologic process that is capable of affecting the structure and function of the brain; therefore, the causes of seizures are numerous, and include congenital anomalies, disorders occurring during intrauterine life, birth injuries, infections, trauma, vascular anomalies, metabolic and nutritional disturbances, tumors, degenerative diseases, and specific genetic disorders. In man, surgical treatment is usually reserved for those patients who exhibit intractable focal epilepsy originating from either trauma, infection, or vascular anomalies. Traumatic epilepsy can be severe and persistent, regardless of the kind of injury or the length of the interval between injury and the onset of seizures. Trauma is a common source of epilepsy and the insult to the brain may occur either at birth or later in life. It has been estimated that the overall incidence of post-traumatic epilepsy in the American veteran of World War II is 28 per cent, whereas it is 11 per cent in men who sustained a closed head injury associated with varying degrees of concussion. In a group of 1000 civilians who sustained an uncomplicated blunt head injury, the overall incidence of epilepsy was 1 per cent; however, the incidence increased to 50 per cent if the dura and brain were penetrated.

### Clinical Classification of Epilepsy

Various clinical classifications of seizures have been proposed; the most recent, by the International League Against Epilepsy, divides seizures into three types:

1. *Partial seizures* beginning locally, usually without loss of consciousness. The clinical types in this group include the focal motor and jacksonian seizures with somatosensory or autonomic symp-

toms or both, partial seizures with affective or cognitive symptoms, psychosensory illustrations, and hallucinations, and the electroencephalographic abnormality is usually focal.

2. *Generalized or major seizures* beginning bilaterally symmetrically or without local onset. The clinical types include absences and myoclonic, atonic, and akinetic seizures, and the electroencephalographic abnormality is either a 3 per second spike wave or polyspikes and wave discharges.

3. *Unilateral seizures, clonic, tonic,* without impaired consciousness, with focal spikes and waves or focal slow waves recorded in the electroencephalogram.

The modern foundations for the surgical treatment of epilepsy were laid at the end of the nineteenth century by two Englishmen, John Hughlings Jackson and Victor Horsley. It was Jackson who formulated the concept that epileptic seizures originate from hyperirritable neurons in the central nervous system, and he also showed that the pattern of the clinical seizure depends upon its anatomic location in the brain, and stressed the importance of carefully recording in the clinical history the sequence of events during the epileptic seizure. In 1886, at the urging of Jackson, Victor Horsley performed the first subpial cortical resection of the "hinder end of the superior frontal sulcus" in a 22 year old Scotsman who had suffered from focal seizures caused by a depressed skull fracture sustained as a child.[2]

Later, Foerster showed the value of systematic electrical stimulation of the cerebral cortex in patients with post-traumatic focal epileptic seizures and he successfully performed surgical excision of the cortical scar in these patients with significant relief of their post-traumatic epilepsy.[1] It was Penfield and Jasper who introduced the careful clinical analysis of seizure disorders combined with extensive cortical stimulation and simultaneous electroencephalographic recordings carried out prior to the surgical excision of the epileptic focus.[4] Krynauw, in 1950, performed the first cerebral hemispherectomy for intractable seizures due to infantile hemiplegia.[3] At the present time stereotactically implanted cortical and subcortical electrodes are being used to evaluate the electrographic abnormalities of subcortical epilepsy prior to the placement of a stereotactic lesion.

It has been estimated that about 5 per cent of epileptics may be considered as candidates for surgical treatment. Psychomotor seizures originating from a unilateral temporal focus can be relieved by surgical excision of the anterior temporal lobe in about 75 per cent of patients. It is important that every epileptic patient be given an adequate trial (2 to 3 years) of anticonvulsant medication directed by a neurologist before the final decision to operate is made.

### Clinical Evaluation of Seizures for Surgery

A detailed historical account of the patient's seizure pattern is the first important step in the clinical analysis. The reports of the seizure pattern as observed by the patient's family or the medical staff often add important clues that will aid in the cerebral localization of the epileptic focus. The kind of aura experienced by the patient must be determined, along with the physical and psychologic factors that influence the duration of the attacks and the occurrence of postictal phenomena. The nature of the aura gives an important clue as to the possible location of the irritable epileptic focus in the brain. For example, olfactory and epigastric sensations, dreamy states, fear, and automatisms point to involvement of the mesial temporal lobe, while more complex sensory or motor behavior may suggest involvement of the brain stem. Visual and auditory hallucinations or illusions may originate from temporoparietal association cortices, while complex motor behavior may point to involvement of the supplementary motor cortex in the frontal lobe. It is also important to discover which extrinsic factors seem to precipitate or modify a patient's seizure; examples of such factors are the effects of bright lights, noises, or cutaneous stimuli that may activate reflex sensory seizures. The psychologic changes occurring before, during, or after a seizure often give important clues as to the location and severity of the brain involvement. Seizures may be influenced by normal metabolic changes such as hypoglycemia or the hormonal alteration in women associated with their menstrual periods.

Clinical tests should include roentgenography of the skull, electroencephalography, brain scanning, carotid Amytal test, and psychologic testing. The plain roentgenogram of the skull of an epileptic may reveal an old depressed skull fracture, or in the case of a patient with temporal lobe epilepsy or infantile hemiplegia the cranial vault may be deformed or smaller on the side of the damaged hemisphere. The pneumoencephalogram may reveal a porencephalic cyst, enlarged ventricles, or focal dilation of the temporal horn, indicating the area of the brain lesion, and in addition angiography can give valuable information as to the extent of vascular anomalies.

The most important single clinical test for the evaluation of epilepsy is electroencephalography. Multiple scalp electroencephalograms are necessary prior to surgery, plus specialized electroencephalographic recordings such as those using nasopharyngeal electrodes in the patient with temporal lobe seizures. The recording electrodes can be placed directly on the surface of the cortex or implanted stereotactically in the deeper regions of the brain (Fig. 35). The electroencephalographic recordings from these electrodes give valuable information on the degree and extent of epileptic involvement in the deeper brain regions that may not be evident from routine scalp electroencephalogram (Fig. 36). Drugs, sleep, or photic or direct electrical stimulation may be necessary to activate the electroencephalographic focus. Prior to the surgical excision direct electrocortical recordings can be made on the surface of the exposed cerebral cortex to aid in the delineation of the size and

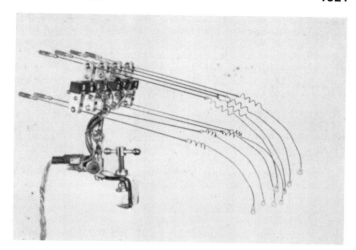

**Figure 35**   Electrodes used by Penfield for direct electrocorticogram on exposed brain. (From Penfield, W., and Jasper, H.: Epilepsy and the Functional Anatomy of the Human Brain. Boston, Little, Brown & Company, 1954.)

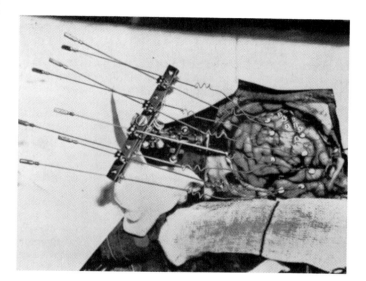

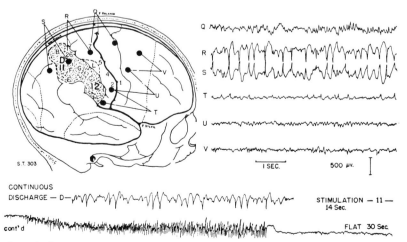

**Figure 36**   Focal cortical seizures. Note after-discharge following stimulation within the area of high-voltage rhythmic spikes. The onset of the patient's attack was reproduced at points 11 and 12. (From Penfield, W., and Jasper, H.: Epilepsy and the Functional Anatomy of the Human Brain. Boston, Little, Brown & Company, 1954.)

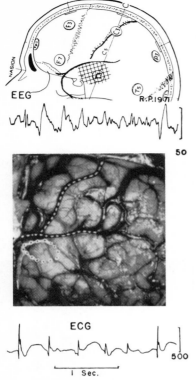

**Figure 37** Spike focus, first temporal convolution. Localization of spike focus on border of tumor. Upper picture shows electroencephalographic abnormality recorded from scalp. The lower picture shows exposed temporal lobe with the spikes recorded from area outlined in black dots. (From Penfield, W., and Jasper, H.: Epilepsy and the Functional Anatomy of the Human Brain. Boston, Little, Brown & Company, 1954.)

shape of the epileptic focus (Fig. 37). Confirmation of the location of the epileptic focus must depend not only on the information from the clinical history but also on the corroborating findings from the radiologic and electroencephalographic evaluation.

The indications for consideration of surgical resection of an epileptic focus are as follows:

1. The attacks should be numerous and resistant to treatment.

2. The attacks should constitute a significant family and social handicap.

3. The epilepsy should have been present for at least 2 years.

4. Careful clinical evaluation should give reasonable evidence of an objective abnormality of the brain as judged by one or all of the following: skull roentgenogram, pneumoencephalogram, angiogram, or electroencephalogram.

5. Repeated electroencephalograms must show the persistence of the focus and its fixed location and this location in the brain should be confirmed by radiographic or angiographic studies and the clinical history.

6. One must deal with a mature brain, which

means waiting a longer time before operating for epilepsy in young children or adolescents; however, temporal lobe epilepsy occurring in adolescents may be an exception to this rule, since relief occurs in about 75 per cent of these patients regardless of their age.

7. The presence of psychiatric disturbance warrants serious consideration for sugery.

### Surgical Treatment of Temporal Lobe or Psychomotor Epilepsy

The surgical treatment of unilateral temporal lobe epilepsy has been highly successful with relief in about 75 per cent of the patients. This means that in most patients anticonvulsants can be stopped 1 year after temporal lobectomy. Brain injury sustained either at birth or postnatally may be a source for temporal lobe epilepsy since it is thought to produce sclerosis of the mesial temporal structures. The cause of this pathologic sclerosis, however, may be unknown in certain patients and the brain tissue removed at surgery may reveal microscopic arteriovenous anomalies or hamartomas. It is well known that the higher rates of cure after surgery for epilepsy occur in those patients in whom a definitive pathologic lesion can be demonstrated in the excised brain tissue.

The epileptic phenomena reported by patients during temporal lobe seizures include auditory illusions, hallucinations, feelings of fear, visual illusions, amnesia, déjà vu phenomenon, and olfactory sensations. During or after the seizure the patient may exhibit aggressive behavior, automatism, memory changes, or simple alterations in awareness.

Two kinds of temporal lobe seizures have been recognized. Uncinate seizures originate from the region of amygdaloid nucleus in the mesial part of the temporal lobe. The person experiences olfactory hallucinations and somatic sensations such as strange feelings in the head, chest, or neck along with a visceral aura with rising or falling epigastric sensation. There may be unilateral or bilateral tonic motor effects during and especially after the seizure, and the patient remains confused, exhibiting automatic and irrelevant behavior in the period of postictal amnesia. Lateral temporal cortex seizures originate from the lateral temporal cortex and are more complex in their behavioral expression, with auditory phenomena, changes in physical or perceptual events, fear, illusion, déjà vu, and postictal behavioral disorders (Fig. 37). Electrical stimulation of the abnormal epileptic cortex in the region of the temporal lobe focus at the time of operation or with depth electrodes may set off the patient's seizure pattern, and greatly aid in its location.

### Infantile Hemiplegia with Intractable Epilepsy

Intractable epilepsy due to infantile hemiplegia can be successfully relieved by surgical excision of the diseased cerebral hemisphere plus the basal ganglia. The hemiplegia may be caused by an acute cerebral insult occurring at or just after birth, and whether or not birth trauma, vascular occlusion, or vital infection may be primarily responsible for the development of this type of epilepsy is not known. In some patients the brain injury probably results from an acute occlusion of the middle cerebral artery. The pathologic consequence of this massive cerebral insult is the development of widespread cerebral scarring followed by intractable epilepsy. The epileptic attacks often involve the hemiplegic side but generalized seizures also can occur and are very resistant to medical therapy. These children, when they are examined, exhibit hemiatrophy of the body opposite the injured hemisphere. The cranial cavity on the side of the cerebral insult is often smaller and skull roentgenogram may show an elevation of the bones of the sphenoid or petrous pyramid, while the pneumoencephalogram reveals a dilated or deformed ventricular system. Angiography often demonstrates a threadlike atrophic middle cerebral artery, which carries a minimum of blood to the injured cerebral hemisphere, and its blood supply often comes via collateral circulation from either the anterior or posterior cerebral arteries. An insult to the left cerebral hemisphere does not usually affect speech development if it occurs before the patient is 5 years of age, and resection of the damaged left hemisphere causes no speech defect. These children often show some degree of mental retardation which may improve after surgery as a result of removal of the adverse influence on brain function of the epilepsy combined with anticonvulsant drugs. In addition to these physical signs, the electroencephalographic observations are of importance in the diagnostic evaluation. The electroencephalographic abnormalities originate from widespread epileptic foci in the damaged hemisphere. They are often greater in the central regions of the brain but isolated epileptic activity may occur in other lobes of the brain as well as in the opposite cerebral hemisphere. The occurrence of bilateral electroencephalographic abnormalities does not contraindicate surgery since the epilepsy in the uninvolved hemisphere often subsides after removal of the damaged brain tissue.

At surgery the diseased cerebral hemisphere and the basal ganglia are removed and pathologic examination of the brain tissue reveals intense scarring in the cortex and white matter, with intense astrocytosis and obliteration of the cerebral blood vessels. Children tolerate the operation well, but occasionally defective absorption of cerebrospinal fluid may follow the hemispherectomy, requiring correction by a ventricular shunt. After surgical excision of the hemisphere, little motor or sensory defect is superimposed on the hemiplegic side and the reduction of seizures is usually immediate, with improvement of the electroencephalographic pattern from the remaining brain. Anticonvulsant medication can often be reduced; this improves the child's alertness and his I.Q. No brain is better than bad (epileptic) brain, and

so every effort should be made to relieve the seizures in these children.

### Stereotactic Treatment of Epilepsy

Spiegel and Wycis were the first to use stereotactic methods to treat epilepsy; they noted improvement of myoclonic seizures in a few persons following coagulation of the basal ganglia.[5]

The childhood epilepsies often originate from the subcortical regions of the brain. The most common disorders are centrencephalic epilepsy (petit mal), myoclonic jerking, and reflex sensory signs. Patients in this group are among the most resistant to treatment. Stereotactic techniques using implanted electrodes in the thalamus, brain stem, and basal ganglia are now being used to investigate these disorders in an effort to devise surgical treatments. Temporal lobe seizures associated with emotional instability or hyperactive aggressive behavior have been relieved by stereotactic lesions in the amygdaloid region. There occurs a normalization of the patient's behavior even though his seizure pattern may not be significantly altered. At times better control of the attacks can be achieved with lesser amounts of anticonvulsants. Reduction in the number of major motor seizures (grand mal) have followed stereotactic lesions in the Forel-H field and thalamic lesions, which are believed to block the conduction pathways of the epileptic spread to deeper regions of the brain stem responsible for the major clonic and tonic seizure with loss of consciousness. These newer stereotactic approaches to the surgical treatment of epilepsy still have limited clinical application but they have increased our understanding of the distribution of epileptic activity in the subcortical regions of the brain.

### SELECTED REFERENCES

Krynauw, R. A.: Infantile hemiplegia treated by removal of one cerebral hemisphere. J. Neurol. Neurosurg. Psychiat., 13:243, 1950.
*The first neurosurgical report of hemispherectomy for relief of intractable seizures.*

Penfield, W., and Jasper, H.: Epilepsy and the Functional Anatomy of the Human Brain. Boston, Little, Brown and Company, 1954.
*A detailed analysis of seizures disorders using extensive electroencephalographic evaluation and direct electrical stimulation of the brain at the time of excision of the epileptic focus. The modern foundation of the neurosurgical treatment of seizures is based on these observations.*

Spiegel, E. A., and Wycis, H. T.: Stereoencephalotomy. Part 2: Clinical and Physiological Application. New York, Grune and Stratton, 1962.
*The first detailed analysis of seizure disorders and their treatment using stereotactic technique.*

Taylor, J., ed.: Selected Writings of John Hughlings Jackson. Volumes 1 and 2. New York, Basic Books, 1958.
*A collection of Jackson's papers on epilepsy and epileptiform convulsions in volume one, and his observations on the evaluation and dissolution of the nervous system in volume two. Jackson's concepts of the functioning of the central nervous system are still the basis for modern neurologic thought.*

### REFERENCES

1. Foerster, O.: Zur operativen Behandlung der Epilepsie. Deutsch. Z. Nervenheilk., 89:137, 1926.

2. Horsley, V.: Brain surgery. Brit. Med. J., 2:670, 1886.
3. Krynauw, R. A.: Infantile hemiplegia treated by removal of one cerebral hemisphere. J. Neurol. Neurosurg. Psychiat., 13:243, 1950.
4. Penfield, W., and Jasper, H.: Epilepsy and the Functional Anatomy of the Human Brain. Boston, Little, Brown and Company, 1954.
5. Spiegel, E. A., and Wycis, H. T.: Stereoencephalotomy. Part 2: Clinical and Physiological Application. New York, Grune and Stratton, 1962.

## STEREOTACTIC NEUROSURGERY

*Blaine S. Nashold, Jr., M.D.*

Clarke and Horsley in 1906, seeking a method of producing localized lesions in the cerebellar nuclei of animals with minimal damage to the cerebellar cortex, devised the first animal stereotactic instrument.[4, 5] Since then the stereotactic technique has been used extensively in neurophysiologic and neuroanatomic laboratories, and much of our knowledge of brain function has been based on data gathered by this technique; one of the greatest advantages of stereotactic neurosurgery has been the use of small exploring probes that can be safely introduced into the thalamus, midbrain, or cerebellum.[10]

In 1947, Spiegel and Wycis applied the stereotactic technique to man and so began the exploration of these deeper regions of the brain in patients suffering from epilepsy, involuntary movement disorders, and psychiatric disturbances.[18] A breakthrough occurred in Parkinson's disease with relief of tremor and rigidity following lesions of the globus pallidus and, later, thalamic lesions.[3]

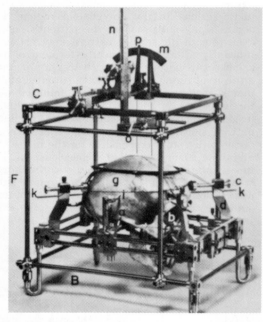

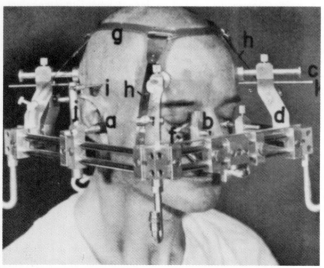

**Figure 38** Human stereotactic instrument devised by Spiegel and Wycis. Upper picture shows complete stereotactic instrument and electrode carrier. Lower picture shows baseplate attached to patient's head, electrode carrier applied later after place of burr hole in skull. (From Spiegel, E. A., et al.: Science, 106:349, 1947.)

Cooper has carried out extensive thalamic surgery for the therapeutic relief of parkinsonian tremor, intention tremor, and other involuntary movements, and low mortality and good clinical results.[19] The overall mortality of stereotactic operations is less than 2 per cent and the morbidity averages 2 per cent. The serious complications include hemiplegia, aphasia, hyperkinesis, ocular dysfunction, convulsive seizures, altered mentation, and hypothalamic dysfunction.

The basic principle in the use of stereotactic surgery is that of localizing a point in space and defining its position with respect to or relative to some suitable frame of reference. The precise location of the point can be defined numerically or graphically. Most stereotactic frames use a right-angled reference system after the cartesian coordinate system of the French mathematician and philosopher Descartes. The cartesian system is convenient to use, and it is relatively easy to construct a physical system on these principles that allows the surgeon to locate the tip of the probe or electrode at a particular point in space, defined by its three coordinates. Furthermore, the position of the tip can easily be changed by any desired amount in any one of the three mutually perpendicular directions.

### Stereotactic Surgical Technique

The neurosurgical techniques necessary for stereotactic operations require the use of a precision stereotactic instrument that can direct probes into various subcortical regions through a small burr hole in the skull (Fig. 38). The intracerebral target is determined from the coordinates of a special stereotactic atlas of the human brain with sections in the coronal, sagittal, and horizontal planes (Fig. 39). At the time of operation localization of the intracerebral target is made from the outline of the ventricular system on an x-ray film. Specific internal landmarks in the brain are used, such as the anterior and posterior commissure, which can be visualized. Then the position of the brain target can be determined from the measurements on the x-ray film and these coordinates can be translated to the stereotactic frame to direct the introduction of the brain probe.

The normal anatomic variations of the human brain, often altered by central nervous system diseases, may cause a certain degree of imprecision in exact target localization; however, these variations can be minimized by using electrical stimulation or electroencephalographic recordings of the brain tissue in or near the target area. The cerebral target can therefore be identified by its anatomic, physiologic, and electrical characteristics, and, for example, activation or suppression of parkinsonian tremor following electrical stimulation or cooling of the thalamus can be a useful technique to localize the position of therapeutic lesion in the thalamus that will relieve the tremor.

Electrographic recordings from the thalamic and midbrain nuclei have not been as helpful in the precise nuclear localization as expected; how-

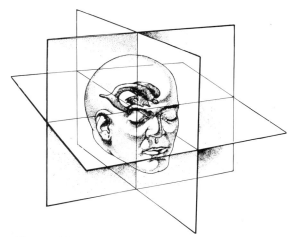

**Figure 39** Intersecting planes used to determine intracranial target area during stereotactic surgery. (From Todd-Wells Manual of Stereotactic Procedures.)

ever, evoked electrical responses produced by the stimulation of a peripheral nerve have been employed for localization in the sensory regions of the central nervous system. The implantation of depth electrodes adds to the understanding of distribution and characteristics of the epileptic activity originating from these deeper cerebral regions but as yet no definitive method of treatment has evolved for relief of epilepsy of subcortical origin.

The ideal technique for producing a therapeutic lesion in the central nervous system of man has as yet not been perfected, however. At present three methods are employed: use of the mechanical leukotome, thermal coagulation, and freezing coagulation. Each of these techniques has certain advantages and disadvantages which must be considered by the stereotactic surgeon, but currently coagulation by heat and by cold are most popular methods and the clinical results from the two seem about equal. The current era of brain exploration and mapping compares with the earliest efforts of Horsley, Foerster, and Penfield, who pioneered the exploration of the cortical mantle in man.

### Complications of Stereotactic Surgery

The immediate operative complications of stereotactic surgery include acute subdural hygroma, subdural hematoma, and intraventricular hemorrhage, which are due to tapping the lateral ventricles or passage of the probe through the brain. Late complications are related to the effects produced by the lesion and may include hemiparesis or speech defects of varying degrees (2 per cent), hyperkinetic movements (2.5 per cent) due to misplaced lesions, convulsive seizures (rare), and change in mentation (transient).[14]

### Disorders Treated with Stereotactic Surgery

Treatment has been carried out in persons with a variety of involuntary movement disorders due to extrapyramidal disease, for relief of painful syndromes, for palliation of epilepsy and mental disturbances, for injection of radioactive material into brain tumors, for thrombosis of intracranial aneurysms, and for the recovery of foreign bodies from the depths of the brain.[12, 20, 21]

To date, patients with parkinsonism represent the largest group treated by stereotactic surgery. The etiology of parkinsonism is unknown and the nature of the pathophysiology is still obscure although recent evidence points to a biochemical disturbance of catecholamine metabolism in the basal ganglia or subthalamic region. In some parkinsonian patients the dopamine content in the basal ganglia may be reduced and replacement with L-dopa administered orally has dramatically relieved the akinesia and rigidity. Tremor, when it is a major disabling symptom, can best be relieved by a therapeutic lesion in the ventrobasal complex of the thalamus with periods of relief from tremor lasting as long as 8 to 10 years in about 70 per cent of the patients.

Athetosis, chorea, dystonia, spasmodic torticollis, and ballismus are also serious disabling involuntary movements that are under active study and treatment by the neurosurgeon using stereotactic techniques.[6] These hyperkinetic disorders are usually nonprogressive. Their pathophysiology remains obscure and current efforts at drug therapy have been disappointing. Chorea, ballismus, and dystonia can be successfully reduced by stereotactic lesions localized to the ventrolateral thalamus and the adjacent subthalamic region. Athetosis and spasmodic torticollis have not been successfully relieved by stereotactic thalamic lesions. Recently therapeutic lesions involving the dentate nucleus of the cerebellum have been reported to reduce athetoid movements but these operations are still in a stage of experimental development.[9, 15]

**Mental Disorders.** Spiegel and Wycis, interested in improving the surgical techniques of frontal leukotomy, developed the first human stereotactic instrument for making lesions in the medial dorsal thalamus of psychotic and psychoneurotic patients.[17] They noted long-lasting relief in the patients with anxiety and depression who have previously failed to respond to psychotherapy, drug, or shock treatments alone or in combination. Localized stereotactic lesions made in the mesial temporal lobe in epileptic patients with severe behavioral disorders have resulted in an amelioration of the behavior disorder but have not always altered the epilepsy. Severely hyperkinetic children have been relieved by bilateral amygdaloid lesions without alteration in their intelligence or general ability to function.[13] Recently patients with violent and aggressive behavior have shown improvement after a stereotactic lesion was made in the posteromedial hypothalamus.[16] Bilateral lesions of the cingulate gyrus of the frontal lobes have successfully relieved certain patients with affective disorders, severe psychosis, and intractable pain.[2, 8] Greater use of these techniques to treat and investigate mental disorders can be expected in the future.

**Brain Tumor.** The stereotactic techniques have had limited use in exploring brain tumors either by tapping deep-lying cystic tumors for the recovery of brain biopsies or for introduction of radioactive materials into cystic lesions. Stereotactic transfrontal or transsphenoidal hypophysectomies to destroy the anterior pituitary gland will satisfactorily relieve pain due to metastatic cancer from the breast or prostate. The symptoms of acromegaly can be arrested by stereotactic ablation of the pituitary gland.[21]

**Other Uses of Stereotaxy.** Although the method is new, certain intracranial aneurysms or arteriovenous anomalies may be treated by stereotactic surgery. A special probe is introduced through a burr hole to the site of the vascular anomaly. Obliteration of the aneurysmal sac may be done with heat or with a recent ingenious technique that employs a magnetic probe placed on the dome of the aneurysm.[1, 11] A suspension of iron particles is then injected into the sac of the aneurysms; the iron particles are held in the aneurysm by the magnet, resulting in coagulation and obliteration of the sac. The method may prove useful in those lesions inaccessible to direct surgical attack or could be used in poor-risk surgical patients to tide them over the critical period of time during the first 2 weeks after rupture of the aneurysm when rebleeding may occur and is often fatal.

Stereotactic neurosurgical techniques are new and still in early stages of development. New applications in the treatment of neurologic disorders can be expected in the future, along with the enriching of our knowledge of the function of the human subcortex, a hope expressed by Clarke and Horsley five decades ago.[4]

## SELECTED REFERENCES

Alksne, J. R., Fingerhut, A. G., and Rand, R. W.: Magnetically controlled metallic thrombosis of intracranial aneurysms. Surgery, 60:212, 1966.
*The use of stereotactic method employing magnetic thrombosis of intracranial aneurysms.*

Clarke, R. H., and Horsley, V.: On a method of investigating the deep ganglia and tracts of the central nervous system. Brit. Med. J., 2:1799, 1906.
*The first report in 1906 of the development and design of the stereotactic instrument for lobotomy.*

Narabayashi, H., Nugao, T., Saito, Y., Yoshida, M., and Nagahata, M.: Stereotaxic amygdalotomy for behavioral disorders. Arch. Neurol., 9:1, 1963.
*The modification of abnormal human behavior by specific stereotactic lesions in the amygdaloid nucleus of the temporal lobe.*

Spiegel, E. A., and Wycis, H. T.: Stereoencephalotomy Part II: Clinical and Physiological Applications. New York, Grune and Stratton, 1962.
*The first detailed clinical use of stereoencephalotomy in the treatment of involuntary movements, pain, mental disorders, and epilepsy.*

Spiegel, E. A., Wycis, H. T., Marks, M., and Lee, A. J.: Stereotactic apparatus for operation on the human brain. Science, 106:349, 1947.
*The first report in 1947 of the development of a human stereotactic instrument.*

## REFERENCES

1. Alksne, J. R., Fingerhut, A. G., and Rand, R. W.: Magnetically controlled metallic thrombosis of intracranial aneurysms. Surgery, 60:212, 1966.
2. Ballantine, H. T., Jr., Cassidy, W. L., Flanagan, N. W., and Marino, R., Jr.: Stereotactic anterior cingulotomy for neuropsychiatric illness and intractable pain. J. Neurosurg., 26:488, 1967.
3. Bertrand, C., and Martinez, N.: Experimental and clinical surgery in dyskinetic disease. Confin. Neurol., 22:375, 1962.
4. Clarke, R. H.: Atlas of Photographs of the Frontal Sections of the Cranium and Brain of the Rhesus Monkey. Baltimore, The Johns Hopkins Hospital Reports, Special Volume, 1920.
5. Clarke, R. H., and Horsley, V.: On a method of investigating the deep ganglia and tracts of the central nervous system. Brit. Med. J., 2:1799, 1906.
6. Cooper, I. S.: Relief of juvenile involuntary movement disorders by chemopallidectomy. J.A.M.A., 164:1297, 1957.
7. Cooper, I. S.: Clinical and physiologic implications of thalamic surgery for dystonia and torticollis. Bull. N. Y. Acad. Med., 41:870, 1965.
8. Foltz, E. L., and White, L. E.: Pain relief by frontal cingulotomy. J. Neurosurg., 19:89, 1962.
9. Heimburger, R. F.: Dentatectomy in the treatment of dyskinetic disorders. Confin. Neurol., 29:101, 1967.
10. Horsley, V., and Clarke, R. H.: The structure and functions of the cerebellum examined by a new method. Brain, 31:45, 1908.
11. Mullan, S., Raimondi, A. J., Dobben, G., Vailati, G., and Hekmatpanah, J.: Electrically induced thrombosis in intracranial aneurysms. J. Neurosurg., 22:539, 1965.
12. Mullan, S., Vailati, G., Karasick, J., and Malis, M.: Thalamic lesions for control of epilepsy. Arch. Neurol., 16:277, 1967.
13. Narabayashi, H., Nugao, T., Saito, Y., Yoshida, M., and Nagahata, M.: Stereotaxic amygdalotomy for behavioral disorders. Arch. Neurol., 9:1, 1963.
14. Nashold, B. S., Jr.: Operative complications due to stereotactic surgery. Confin. Neurol., 30:325, 1968.
15. Nashold, B. S., Jr., and Slaughter, D. G.: Stimulation and lesions of the deeper regions in the cerebellum of man. J. Neurosurg., accepted for publication.
16. Sano, K., Yoshioka, M., Ogashiwa, M., Ishijima, B., and Ohyl, C.: Posteromedial hypothalamotomy in the treatment of aggressive behavior. Confin. Neurol., 27:164, 1965.
17. Spiegel, E. A., and Wycis, H. T.: Stereoencephalotomy. Part II: Clinical and Physiological Applications. New York, Grune and Stratton, 1962.
18. Spiegel, E. A., Wycis, H. T., Marks, M., and Lee, A. J.: Stereotactic apparatus for operation on the human brain. Science, 106:349, 1947.
19. Stellar, S., and Cooper, I. S.: Mortality and morbidity in cryothalamectomy for parkinsonism. J. Neurosurg., 28:459, 1968.
20. Sugita, K., Sato, O., Takaoka, Y., Mutsuga, N., and Tsugane, R.: Successful removal of intracranial air-gun bullet with stereotaxic apparatus. J. Neurosurg., 30:177, 1969.
21. Wycis, H. T., Baird, H. W., III, and Spiegel, E. A.: Long range results following pallidotomy and pallidoamygdalotomy in certain types of convulsive disorders. Confin. Neurol., 27:114, 1966.
22. Zervas, N. T.: Technique of radiofrequency hypophysectomy. Confin. Neurol., 26:143, 1965.

# 42

# DISORDERS OF THE MUSCULOSKELETAL SYSTEM

I

## Fractures and Dislocations

*William A. Larmon, M.D.*

The surgeon must understand the normal anatomy and physiology of the musculoskeletal system if he is to restore maximal function when the system is affected. The pathology of fractures, dislocations, sprains, tissue injuries, and disease must be recognized in order to plan a logical course of treatment. The surgeon must realize that injury to the spine or extremities affects the entire body, not just the part, and his efforts to restore function should be based upon this broad concept of trauma.

### PATHOLOGY OF FRACTURE

When a bone breaks, a chain of reactions follows, which must be understood by the surgeon if he is to treat the injury intelligently. First, bleeding occurs at the fracture site, from the bone as well as from the associated soft tissue injury. The amount of hemorrhage varies; it may be severe and life-endangering, or moderate. Shock may develop rapidly from loss of blood. Bleeding may be internal, into the soft tissues about the fracture, or external, from associated wounds. Hidden bleeding must be recognized and blood volume restored before definitive treatment of the fracture is undertaken. When the bleeding stops a hematoma is formed about the fracture. This hematoma later becomes an important part of the healing process (Fig. 1).

The second event in a fracture is loss of skeletal stability, often followed by obvious deformity. The type and location of the fracture determines the degree of deformity and loss of stability of the part.

### THE HEALING PROCESS OF FRACTURE

When a fracture is reduced and immobilized, the repair process begins immediately. An aseptic inflammatory reaction occurs at the fracture site, often accompanied by a fever and local increase in temperature. The blood vessels near the fracture dilate and produce an active hyperemia. Permeability of the vascular bed increases, allowing edema fluid to accumulate in the tissues. This edema and the hematoma produce varying degrees of swelling and ecchymosis. Within 48 hours, the products of the inflammatory exudate begin to organize. The adjacent muscles and ligaments lose elasticity and become indurated and firm.

Local chemical changes take place rapidly. The pH of the fluids about the bone ends becomes

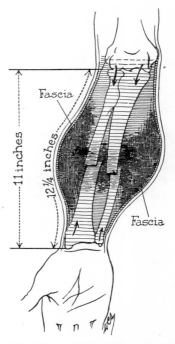

**Figure 1** Typical condition following a fracture. A hematoma has formed. There is deformity and loss of skeletal stability, and the fascial compartment of the extremity is distended.

slightly acid for the first 10 days to 2 weeks. This acid environment forces calcium salts into solution about the bone fragments, so that some absorption of bone takes place. Fibrin strands form in the hematoma; invasion of the blood clot and damaged tissue by white blood cells begins; and the debris of injury is absorbed. New capillaries grow into the hematoma from the surrounding soft tissues and bone ends. Fibrous tissue is laid down, as in all wound healing.

After 10 to 14 days, the local pH becomes alkaline, and the concentration of alkaline phosphatase increases at the fracture site. Bone-forming cells become active. Calcium salts form in the remains of the hematoma, and osteoid tissue is elaborated by bone-forming cells from the periosteum and endosteum, or possibly by metaplasia of other soft tissue cells. In some instances, the fibrous tissue cells that unite the bone fragments may undergo changes resembling those of cartilage. These cells may calcify, may be invaded by new blood vessels and may be absorbed, and new bone may be laid down by the bone-forming cells. All of these processes of new bone formation may take place in the same fracture area. This process is called callus formation and is the method by which bone heals.

After the fracture has been bridged by callus, remodeling of the bone begins. The architecture of the trabecular pattern of the particular bone is re-established by the process. Excess callus is absorbed and new bone is laid down in the predetermined trabecular pattern.

## REHABILITATION OF SOFT PARTS

When the fracture has healed, the soft tissues must be rehabilitated. Inevitably, some scar tissue remains in damaged muscles, ligaments, and associated structures. Scar tissue is inelastic, binding muscle to bone and ligaments to joints; since scar tissue contracts in any wound healing process, deformities may occur. Muscles long immobilized atrophy and, in some instances, shorten, and lose power and tensile strength. Muscles not only act to move the levers of the skeleton, but also by contraction aid in the dynamics of blood circulation. The careful restoration of muscle, ligament, and joint function is essential for movement of the body parts, but is also necessary for proper circulation in the extremities.

## PRINCIPLES OF FRACTURE TREATMENT

Treatment of musculoskeletal injuries follows logically once the underlying pathology of injury and repair is understood.

### Immobilization

Adequate immobilization of a fracture varies with the type and location of the break. Some fractures are stable and require little additional support; others are unstable, tending to shorten,

angulate, and rotate with any motion of the part. Complete immobilization of the fracture area promotes the repair process and minimizes damage and scar formation.

### Reduction of Fractures

Adequate reduction varies with the type and location of the fracture and the age of the patient. The closer the bone ends are approximated, the less will be the gap for repair. Bone ends may be placed side to side or end to end, as long as good contact is made between the fragments. When reduction of a fracture is delayed, organization of the inflammatory exudate reduces the elasticity of the soft tissues. Early reduction of a fracture, while structures are still pliable and muscles are not in spasm, lessens the trauma of reduction. Although immobilization of the fracture and the damaged soft parts is essential, all uninvolved structures should be allowed to function as normally as possible. Use of undamaged muscles and ligaments prevents atrophy of these structures, maintains strength and tone, and aids circulation.

## THE MECHANISM OF FRACTURE

Fracture may be produced by direct or indirect violence. Fractures produced by direct violence result from a direct blow or crushing force. Often, there is considerable soft tissue damage over the fracture site and the bone has a tendency to shatter or crush. Indirect violence fractures are the result of forces transmitted through the bone to an area of weakness where fracture typically takes place. Fractures may also be produced by violent contraction of muscle. An example of this is the fracture of the patella produced by the sudden contraction of the quadriceps muscle.

## TYPES OF FRACTURE

Fractures may be open or closed. A closed fracture does not communicate with the outside air, although adjacent wounds of the skin may be present. An open fracture is accompanied by a wound that communicates through the skin or mucous membrane to the air. The latter is usually a much more serious problem, because the danger to infection of the wound and bone is present.

*Simple* fractures have only one fracture line and produce two fragments, while comminuted fractures have more than one break and produce more than two distinct fragments. Different types of bone break in characteristic ways, and the fractures of childhood differ in some ways from those in the adult.

Cancellous bone may crush, producing a *compression* or *impacted* fracture, usually with comminution. An impacted fracture is one in which the bone ends are driven together by the force producing the fracture, so that they are firmly united. This happens most often at the areas where cancellous bone and cortical bone come together, near the metaphysis or epiphysis.

Cortical bone of the diaphysis may break transversely, or the break may be oblique or spiral when rotatory or shearing force plays a role in the mechanism of fracture.

Fractures of the shaft of diaphysis of the bone in children may be produced by bending force. The bone of a child before puberty is more pliable and is surrounded by a tougher, heavier periosteum than that in the adult. Bending or compression force applied to this type bone may produce a greenstick fracture. In this fracture, the convex side of the bone pulls apart while the concave side compresses, but does not break completely.

Spontaneous fatigue fractures, or *march fractures,* occur from repeated trauma of a force that is insufficient to cause fracture as an isolated injury, but that can break a bone when repeated often enough. It is thought that when bone is "overloaded" for a sufficient period, the crystalline structure alters and produces a weak spot in the bone.

*Pathologic* fractures are those which occur in a diseased part of the bone. Most frequently, this happens in areas of cancer metastasis, but it can take place in Paget's disease, fragilitas ossium, osteoporosis, or osteomalacia.

*Epiphyseal* fractures or separations take place through the epiphyseal plate of the growing bone. These injuries are usually caused by shearing force. The epiphysis is displaced from the metaphysis by disruption of the cartilage of the epiphyseal plate. The damage produced to this structure may arrest or alter the growth of the bone. The prognosis is uncertain, and the parents of the injured child should always be warned that growth disturbances may occur.

## FRACTURE DEFORMITY

Displacement and deformity of fracture fragments occur from the force producing the fracture and the pull of muscles after the fracture. The bone may shorten when fracture fragments slide past each other. This deformity is usually increased by pull of muscles in the long axis of the extremity.

Angulation of the fragments may occur as a result of bending force or unequal muscle pulls. The angulation is termed anterior, posterior, medial, or lateral, depending upon the position of the apex of the triangle produced by the deformity.

*Rotational* deformity occurs when the fracture fragments rotate out of their normal longitudinal axis. This may be caused by rotational strain producing the fracture, by gravity, or by the unequal pull of muscles attached to the fragments of the fracture.

### Correction of Fracture Deformity

To obtain maximal functional restoration of a bone or joint, these deformities must be corrected. The degree of correction necessary for proper function varies with location of the fracture and the age of the patient. Moderate degrees of angula-

tion and shortening may be acceptable, but rotational malalignment must be corrected as fully as possible. The growing bones of the child will, in many instances, correct angular deformity by the normal remodeling process of growing bone. In the adult, this does not take place, so that the degree of angulation acceptable after reduction of the fracture varies with age. Shortening of a bone of minor degree may be acceptable and, in many instances, is even desirable in both the adult and child. In some fractures, good bone contact cannot be maintained without slight shortening. It may be necessary to accept this deformity if union of the bone is to be obtained.

When fractures occur in children, the hyperemia of healing usually causes stimulation of longitudinal growth. If the fracture is reduced with the fragments in end-to-end apposition, this stimulation of growth may produce a bone longer than normal after healing. Rotational deformity is never corrected by growth and is unacceptable in either the child or the adult.

Fractures of joint surfaces are always serious injuries. Malaligned joint surfaces block motion and produce excessive wear of the articular cartilage. Inevitably, some damage is done to the cartilage cells. This eventually leads to traumatic arthritis. Every effort must be made to restore joint surfaces by perfect reduction.

Often, associated ligament injuries are not recognized. Failure to restore damaged ligaments may produce an unstable joint. Although the fracture heals, the instability of the joint may be quite as disabling as a poorly aligned joint.

### Malunion

When a fracture unites in poor position, it is termed a malunion. Depending upon the degree of residual deformity, function of the part is altered. This may be severe and disabling, or slight and only of cosmetic significance. The disability may be apparent immediately following healing of the fracture, or it may be slowly progressive over the span of several years. Rotatory malunion of the forearm bones immediately limits pronation or supination, but may not affect wrist or elbow motion, and there may be no increase in the trouble over the years. Moderate angulation of a healed fracture of the shaft of the femur may produce no immediate disability; however, the alteration of the weight-bearing line through the knee joint may cause stress and strain, which eventually leads to traumatic arthritis in the knee and destroys the joint. The surgeon must be mindful of these factors that influence the short- and long-term functional results of fractures.

## METHODS OF REDUCTION

Reduction of fractures is accomplished by closed or open methods, and fractures are held in reduction by external or internal fixation devices. Reduction is accomplished by manipulation or traction, or both. When a bone is angulated, but the fragments remain in end-to-end contact, the simple manipulation of straightening the bone may be all that is necessary. However, if the bone ends are displaced and overriding, traction is necessary to restore length and possibly overcome angulation. In addition, manipulation may be necessary to approximate the fragments as closely as possible.

A fundamental principle of reduction is to align the fragment that can be controlled with the fragment that cannot be controlled.

When satisfactory reduction cannot be accomplished by closed manipulation and traction, an open surgical procedure may be necessary. In this instance, the fracture is exposed through an appropriate incision and the bone fragments are approximated under direct vision by traction and manipulation with instruments applied directly to the bone.

### Cast Fixation

Reduction of the fragments is maintained by some type of fixation device. This may be a simple splint or plaster cast, suspension traction, or screws, plates, and rods applied directly to the bone. As a general principle, a joint proximal and distal to the fracture must be immobilized in order to maintain reduction by the cast method.

It must be remembered that a cast applied shortly after a fracture occurs may not be large enough in a few hours to accommodate the inevitable swelling of the parts. The peripheral circulation must be watched carefully after the application of a cast. Elevation of the part helps to prevent excessive swelling by aiding return blood flow with the help of gravity.

Should the circulation become inadequate, the parts exposed at the end of the cast may become cold and cyanotic or pale and anesthetic. Pain at first may be severe. This condition demands immediate relief before permanent damage occurs. The cast may be split to allow for expansion, or it may be necessary to remove it and apply another of adequate size.

### Traction Fixation

Another method for the maintenance of reduction is traction. Traction is a force applied distal to the fracture in the long axis of the bone and always demands countertraction, or a force in the opposite direction proximal to the fracture. Enough force must be applied to create sufficient traction to reduce the fracture and maintain reduction. Traction with countertraction accomplishes several things in reduction and the maintenance of reduction. First, it overcomes the shortening by counteracting the contraction of muscles. Second, it neutralizes the displacing or angulating force of muscles. This may be aided by placing the part in a position that lessens the deforming force of the muscles.

There are several methods of applying traction to a limb. The most common is skin traction. If prolonged or heavy traction is needed, skeletal traction may be more useful. When traction is used to maintain reduction, the part must be either suspended in an appropriate supporting splint, or a traction and countertraction device must be incorporated in a cast to maintain the traction force.

If excessive traction force is applied, the bone ends will be pulled apart, causing a gap in the fracture. This condition is termed distraction and is a contributing factor in delayed union and nonunion.

### Internal Fixation

Internal fixation devices consist of screws, plates, rods, pins, wires, and bands designed to hold the fracture in reduction by direct application to the bone. An open operation is necessary in most instances for the application of these devices. The hazard of increased damage to bone and soft parts as well as potential infection of the wound must be carefully considered by the surgeon before the operation is done. These difficulties must be weighed against the inadequacy of reduction by other methods. Open reduction of fractures in children is rarely indicated, and internal fixation is almost never needed. Unnecessary operations on growing bones should be avoided.

### Prosthetic Replacement of Bone

Occasionally, parts of certain fractured bones are replaced by metal prostheses. This may be necessary when the bone is completely destroyed, or when other factors enter into the problem. The intracapsular fracture of the neck of the femur is the one most frequently requiring a prosthesis.

Occasionally, a portion or all of a bone may be excised if adequate restoration of the bone cannot be accomplished. This may be done with a shattered patella, where no amount of reconstruction can produce a smooth articular surface with the femur. The extensor tendon mechanism, however, must be restored.

## DELAYED UNION AND NONUNION

The time necessary for healing of a fracture varies with the age of the patient, the location of the fracture, the degree of tissue damage, the amount of movement of the fragments, the presence or absence of infection, the blood supply to the part, and the gap between fragments. Although average times of healing of fractures can be determined for different age groups, there is always some variation. If the healing time is considerably longer than normally expected, the condition is termed delayed union. This does not mean that the bone will not eventually heal, but it does mean that healing may take many weeks longer than usual. The reason for the delayed union may not be readily apparent. In some instances, inadequate local chemical response to the fracture may play a part.

Nonunion of a fracture exists when the repair process comes to a complete halt. Many of the factors producing delayed union may contribute to the production of nonunion. However, the two most common causes are absence of adequate blood supply and, more important, failure to immobilize the fracture properly. Although some callus may form, the process stops before the gap in the fracture fragments has been bridged. The fragments are united by mature, inactive fibrous tissue scar. A false joint, or pseudoarthrosis, may develop.

When x-ray films are made, an established nonunion shows certain characteristics. The sharp edges of the fragments become blunted and rounded. The bone ends may show varying degrees of sclerosis or increased density. This, coupled with the obvious gap between fragments, usually means a nonunion is present. As in delayed union, bone grafting is usually the method of choice for re-creating the conditions for healing in nonunion.

## BONE GRAFTING

There is considerable clinical and experimental evidence that a bone graft does not grow of itself. In reality, the major portion of the graft may die, as it is deprived of its blood supply; a few surface bone cells may, however, remain alive. The significance of bone grafting to obtain union lies in the fact that the repair process is stimulated. The graft brings the building blocks of calcium and phosphorus to the fracture site. In addition, the graft forms a lattice, or network, through which new bone may grow once the repair process has been restarted. Slowly, the graft is resorbed and new bone is laid down in its place.

Two types of grafts are used: *homogenous* and *autogenous*. In either, the bone may be primarily cortical or cancellous bone. The supply of autogenous graft material is, of course, limited. Cortical graft may be taken from any of the long bones; however, the tibia and fibula are the most frequently used. Cancellous bone is usually obtained from the ilium and ribs.

## OPEN FRACTURE

An open fracture is an emergency. Whether it is a finger or major leg bone, the open wound presents problems that demand immediate care. It must be assumed that an open fracture is contaminated, and the bone and surrounding tissues are exposed to infection. Infection destroys tissue and delays healing; it may lead to crippling or death when uncontrolled.

In addition to the bone injury in open fractures, there may be extensive damage to the nerves, blood vessels, muscles, and tendons. Often, there is serious loss of skin. Excessive blood loss may be encountered. Crushing, tearing, and laceration of the soft parts may produce profound shock. Often, the violent forces of high-speed automobile accidents produce multiple fractures and serious injury to other systems.

Only after thorough evaluation and stabilization of the patient's physiologic status should definitive surgery of the open fracture be attempted. The primary objective of surgical treatment is to convert a contaminated wound into one that is surgically clean. Success depends upon performing debridement before bacteria have invaded the tissues. Ideally, no more than 6 hours should elapse between injury and surgery. Traction must be maintained, either manually or by one of the devices attached to a fracture operating table, while preparation for debridement is carried out.

As the first step, the area around the wound is cleaned. The wound is covered with sterile sponges while the skin is washed with soap and water and shaved. After the patient has been draped, the wound is explored. Devitalized or damaged skin edges are cut away, with as much skin conserved as possible. It may be necessary to enlarge the wound for adequate inspection and debridement. Irrigation with physiologic saline is carried out. The wound must be painstakingly searched for contaminated tissue, debris, and blood clots. More important, however, is removal of devitalized tissue, which is a potential breeding ground for bacteria. Particularly, muscle must be removed when devitalized, as it is the most likely source of gas bacillus infection. All bone fragments attached to viable soft tissue must be preserved; however, small detached fragments may be removed.

Nerves, tendons, and blood vessels exposed in the wound should be inspected and damage to these structures estimated. Rarely, it may be necessary to replace or repair a damaged major blood vessel, if the viability of the extremity is jeopardized. Damaged nerves must be preserved. When debridement is complete, the surgeon must decide whether to repair severed nerves and tendons immediately or defer this procedure.

If internal fixation of the fracture is desirable, the surgeon must know that he has converted the wound into a surgically clean one before this is done. Internal fixation should not be used if there is actual or potential infection.

Lastly, the surgeon must decide whether to close the wound primarily or secondarily. If the surgeon is certain the wound is surgically clean, that bacteria have not invaded the tissue, and that he will have adequate opportunity for postoperative observation, he may elect to close the wound immediately. However, if the surgeon believes that these conditions are not met, wound closure may be delayed until the threat of infection has passed, usually in 3 to 7 days.

## FRACTURES AND DISLOCATIONS OF THE UPPER EXTREMITY

When treating fractures of the upper extremity, one must be mindful of its specialized functions. The bones, joints, and muscles of the shoulder girdle, arm, and forearm are designed to place the end organ—the hand—in multiple positions for use. These movements must be smooth, coordinated, and stable. Slight malalignment of the shaft fragments may not alter this function greatly;

however, limitation of joint motions of these lever arms may reduce the effectiveness of the hand to a marked degree.

## THE HAND

### Fractures of the Phalanges

**Distal Phalanx.** Fractures of the distal phalanx are of two types: those involving the tuft and shaft of the bone, and those involving the joint and tendon attachments. Crushing injury is the usual mechanism of tuft and shaft fractures. The fracture is often comminuted. Subungual hematoma and soft tissue contusion and laceration are common. Prevention of infection of the subungual hematoma or lacerations is imperative. The finger should be prepared with soap and water scrubbing, as in compound fractures. If the fingernail is almost completely avulsed, it may be gently removed. If it is intact, the subungual hematoma should not be disturbed. A pressure dressing of sterile fluff gauze and elastic bandage may provide adequate protection and immobilization. After a week, this may be replaced with a protective metal splint to hold the finger in the position of function for 2 weeks longer. Firm, painless, fibrous union is usually present by this time, and the fingers can be used.

BASEBALL FINGER. If the distended distal phalanx is struck and forced into flexion when the extensor tendon is taut, an avulsion fracture of the attachment of this tendon occurs, or the tendon ruptures. The distal phalanx droops in flexion and cannot be actively extended. The treatment for both injuries is the same. This is one of the few instances in which the finger joint must be immobilized in hyperextension until there is no tendency for the distal phalanx to droop. This may be done with a plaster or metal splint. Immobilization varies from a minimum of 3 weeks to usually a maximum of 6 weeks.

**Middle Phalanx.** Fractures of the middle phalanx involve the condyles of the distal joint, the shaft, or the proximal joint. One or both condyles may be fractured by a blow to the extended finger. The usual fracture line is similar to an inverted V. The condyles split off at an angle to the shaft and are displaced medially and laterally. Angulation of the finger distal to the fracture is the important deformity to correct. Since the pull of the flexor and extensor tendons forces the distal phalanx against the fractured condyles, perpetuating the deformity, it may be necessary to apply continuous traction to the distal phalanx. At the same time, angulation is corrected.

Within 3 weeks, fibrous union will hold the fragments in reduction. The traction is removed and gentle motion is started.

Fractures of the shaft of the middle phalanx may angulate volarward or dorsalward, depending upon the relation of the fracture to the insertion of the sublimis tendon. Fractures distal to the insertion angulate volarward. Fractures proximal to the

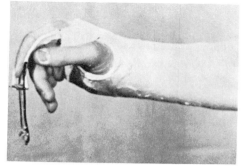

**Figure 2** For all unstable finger and metacarpal fractures, traction is made on the flexed finger.

flexor sublimis tendon insertion angulate dorsalward. If the fracture is stable, correction of the angulation by manipulation is done. Immobilization of the finger is accomplished by a curved metal or plaster volar splint. Comminuted, oblique, or spiral fractures that are unstable may require traction in the position of function to maintain length of the finger (Fig. 2).

**Proximal Phalanx.** Fractures of the proximal phalanx of the finger occur in three locations: at the condyles of the joint, in the shaft, and at the base of the bone. The mechanism is often a direct blow, but fracture may be produced by compression force applied to the phalanx or by medial or lateral angulating force.

Fractures of the condyles are similar to those in the middle phalanx, and are treated the same way. Fractures of the shaft of the bone assume a characteristic volar angulation. Reduction is obtained by traction and manipulation. Immobilization in the position of function is necessary to counteract the deforming pull of the extensor tendons (Fig. 3). Immobilization should continue for 3 weeks.

Fractures of the base of the phalanx are often impacted with medial or lateral angulation. This angulation is a result of the force producing the fracture. The fingers overlap on flexion if this deformity is allowed to persist. The fracture must be disimpacted by traction and manipulation before reduction can be obtained. Immobilization is similar to that used in other fractures of this

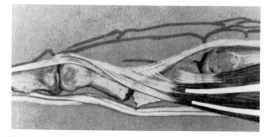

**Figure 3** The insertion of the lumbrical and interosseous muscles into the extensor tendons of the finger causes palmar angulation of fractures of the proximal phalanx.

phalanx. It is important to recognize and correct rotation deformity in all finger fractures. Rotation of the bone in the long axis of the finger results in overlapping of fingers when they are flexed.

### Fractures of the Thumb

**Phalangeal Fractures.**    Fractures of the phalanges of the thumb are similar to those in the fingers, except that the extensor mechanism is different and does not produce the volar angulation to the marked degree found in the fingers. Phalangeal fractures are treated in the same manner as those in the fingers.

**Metacarpophalangeal Dislocations.**    Dislocation of the metacarpophalangeal joints in the hand occurs most frequently in the thumb, and is the result of hyperextension injury to this joint. The volar joint capsule tears, the proximal phalanx dislocates onto the dorsum of the first metacarpal, and the head of the metacarpal protrudes through the rent in the volar capsule (Fig. 4).

Longitudinal traction is made on the thumb. If reduction of the dislocation does not occur easily, the thumb is hyperextended while traction is continued in the long axis of the metacarpal. If the manipulation fails, open reduction is necessary. The thumb is immobilized for 3 weeks in a forearm cast or padded dorsal splint, with the thumb held in 30 to 45 degrees of flexion at the metacarpal phalangeal joint to prevent redislocation. Metacarpophalangeal dislocations of the fingers are produced by similar mechanism and are treated in the same way as those in the thumb.

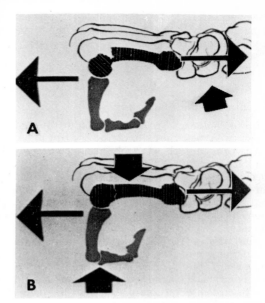

**Figure 5**    *A,* Traction is made on the long axis of the metacarpal with the finger flexed. *B,* While traction is maintained and pressure is applied over the shaft, the metacarpal head is forced dorsalward. Rotation should be checked following reduction. The fingers must not overlap or spread excessively.

### Fractures of the Metacarpals

**Metacarpal Neck.**    Fractures of the metacarpals occur at the neck, shaft, and base of the bone, and are produced by direct or indirect violence. Fractures involving the neck are most commonly produced by striking a blow with the clenched fist. When the fracture occurs, the head is carried into the palm along with the finger. Often the fracture is impacted.

Reduction must be done by forces applied directly to the head of the bone. The finger is flexed to 90 degrees at the metacarpophalangeal joint. Traction is exerted on this finger in the long axis of the metacarpal bone. While traction is applied, pressure is applied over the dorsum of the shaft and the flexed finger is forced dorsalward, carrying with it the distal metacarpal fragment (Fig. 5).

The position is maintained by a molded plaster splint for not longer than 3 weeks. After 3 weeks, the plaster splint is replaced by a removable metal splint which holds the finger in the position of function for 2 more weeks. Active joint motion is started during this period.

**Metacarpal Shaft.**    Fractures of the shaft of the metacarpal bones angulate dorsally because of the bowstring-like pull of the interosseous muscles (Fig. 6). Transverse stable fractures may be reduced by simple manipulation, forcing the distal fragment dorsalward while counterpressure is made at the apex of angulation. A snug-fitting plaster cast is applied, extending from the metacarpal heads to just below the elbow. Unstable spiral oblique and comminuted fractures of the

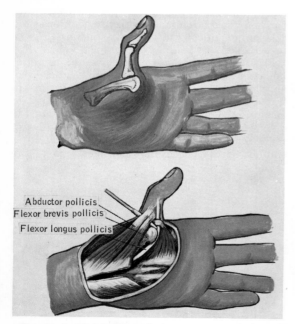

Abductor pollicis
Flexor brevis pollicis
Flexor longus pollicis

**Figure 4**    Dislocation of the metacarpophalangeal joint of the thumb may result in the flexor tendon or joint capsule trapping the metacarpal head and prevent reduction by closed methods.

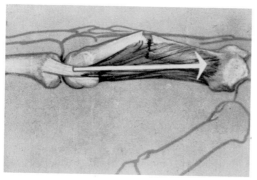

**Figure 6** The bowstring-like action of the interosseous muscles produces volar angulation of fractures of the metacarpal shaft. The head of the bone is forced into the palm and the dorsal angulation interferes with the extensor tendons.

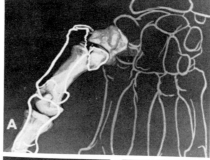

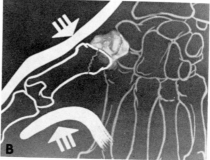

**Figure 7** *A,* Displacement in fracture of the base of the first metacarpal, with involvement of the joint surface, is shown superimposed on the normal anatomy. *B,* The forces applied in reduction of this fracture, together with longitudinal traction, are illustrated; the molding of the cast is shown in white.

metacarpal bones shorten as well as angulate. Reduction and maintenance of reduction must be accompanied by continuous traction to overcome the constant pull of the muscles. The period of traction is usually 3 to 4 weeks, with cast immobilization continuing for another 2 weeks.

**Metacarpal Base.** Fractures of the base of the metacarpal bones are usually the result of direct violence to the hand. Often crushing injuries produce comminution of the fragments. There is little tendency for displacement. In many instances, reduction of the fracture is not necessary; simple splinting or cast immobilization for 4 weeks is often all that is needed.

BASE OF THE FIRST METACARPAL. Fractures at the base of the metacarpal bone of the thumb differ from those at the base of the fingers. The bone is much more mobile because of the saddle-shaped articulation with the greater multangular bone. Two major types of fractures are common, and both are most often produced by indirect compression force.

The bone may break transversely or obliquely near the base, or the fracture may involve the joint surfaces. When the joint surfaces are not fractured, the deformity is usually one of dorsal angulation because of the pull of the thenar flexor muscles. If the fracture is stable, reduction by hyperextension of the thumb followed by cast immobilization is done. When the fracture is unstable, traction may be necessary.

Fracture of the carpometacarpal joint of the thumb can cause serious disability of the hand. Compression force drives the curved articular surface of the metacarpal bone against the greater multangular bone. The fracture occurs through the ulnar palmar aspect of the joint. A small fragment in this area remains attached to the multangular bone. The metacarpal bone dislocates dorsally and radialward on the greater multangular bone. The displacing pull of the short thenar, long flexor, and extensor muscles of the thumb maintains the displacement (Fig. 7).

Reduction of the fracture-dislocation is accomplished by traction and hyperextension of the

metacarpal, with pressure applied over its base in a palmar and ulnarward direction. A cast that maintains this position and pressure point is applied from the distal interphalangeal joint of the thumb to just below the elbow. If the reduction cannot be maintained in nearly an anatomic position, continuous longitudinal traction is applied to the thumb. Occasionally, fractures and dislocations of the hand cannot be reduced or retained in reduction by these closed methods, and open operation with internal fixtures may become necessary.

## THE WRIST

Any bone in the wrist may be fractured by direct trauma; however, the navicular and lunate bones are the most commonly injured, usually by indirect violence. The lunate bone seldom is fractured, but frequently is dislocated. The navicular bone is seldom dislocated but is often fractured. The two bones may be injured simultaneously.

### Fractures of the Navicular Bone

The usual mechanism of injury is a fall on the outstretched hand. One of the two anatomic areas in the bone is most frequently injured: the tubercle or the waist. At the tubercle, carpal ligaments attach and, when they are pulled taut, the tubercle of the bone may be avulsed. At the waist, nutrient vessels enter the bone, producing an area of weak-

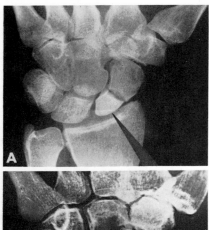

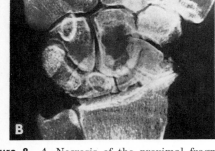

**Figure 8** *A,* Necrosis of the proximal fragment in nonunion of the navicular bone is illustrated. *B,* Traumatic arthritis with destruction of the carpus following nonunion of the navicular is the result of neglect in diagnosis and treatment.

ness. Fractures through this area are usually transverse with little or no displacement. This fracture is much more serious, as nonunion is likely. In addition, the blood supply to the bone may be damaged, depriving one of the fragments of nutrition, with subsequent necrosis (Fig. 8).

All too often, the fracture is not diagnosed. The tendency is to diagnose the injury as a sprain and neglect treatment. This error can lead to nonunion and eventual traumatic arthritis of the wrist. All sprains of the wrist should be treated as fractures of the navicular bone until proved otherwise. The wrist and thumb should be immobilized in a plaster cast from the distal phalanx of the thumb and palmar flexion crease of the fingers to just below the elbow. The fingers are allowed free movement, but the thumb must be completely immobilized in the position of function. The bone heals slowly and may take 6 to 9 months, or a year, to heal. The plaster cast must be changed often enough to maintain maximal immobilization. Nonunion of the bone may require bone grafting. Necrosis of one of the fragments may require bone grafting, or excision of all or part of the bone.

Fractures of the tubercle usually heal rapidly and immobilization for 6 to 8 weeks is usually sufficient.

### Injuries to the Lunate Bone

The lunate bone, like the navicular, is almost completely covered by cartilage, except for the small ligament attachments on the dorsal and volar aspect of the bone. For this reason, the bone is seldom fractured through the body; however, avulsion fractures at the ligament attachment may occur. Displacement of these tiny fragments is usually minimal, and splint immobilization of the wrist for 3 weeks is all that is necessary.

Anterior dislocation of the lunate bone may occur when the wrist is forcefully hyperextended in a fall. The lunate rotates forward, causing rupture of the dorsal ligaments and, in some instance, the volar ones, and dislocating into the carpal tunnel. The flexor tendons of the fingers

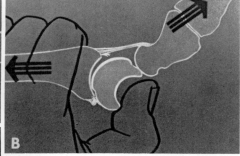

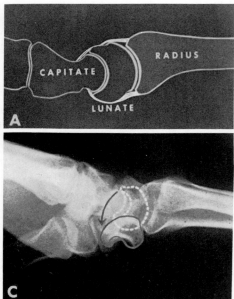

**Figure 9** *A,* Ligamentous attachments to the almost completely cartilage-covered lunate bone are shown. Avulsion fractures of these ligaments may occur. *B,* Reduction of anterior dislocation of the lunate is accomplished by traction, dorsiflexion, and direct pressure. *C,* Lateral roentgenograms are essential for diagnosis.

and the median nerve are compressed, and flexion of the wrist is blocked. Closed reduction of a dislocated lunate is possible if done within the first few days after injury. Strong, steady traction is made while the wrist is dorsiflexed. This is done to open as widely as possible the space formerly occupied by the lunate. The bone is then pressed into position as the wrist is flexed while traction is maintained (Fig. 9). X-ray examination is carried out before the wrist is immobilized in flexion. The ligaments usually heal within 3 weeks when gentle active wrist motion may be started. If closed reduction fails, an open operation must be performed to replace or remove the bone. If the blood supply to the bone has been completely disrupted, the bone should be removed. Immobilization following open reduction is similar to that used following closed manipulation.

### Perilunar Dislocation

Perilunar dislocation is a rare but serious injury to the wrist joint. The mechanism is one of hyperextension of the wrist. The volar carpal ligaments rupture and all of the carpal bones along with the hand dislocate dorsally, with the exception of the lunate, which maintains its normal relationship to the radius. Reduction of this dislocation is accomplished by traction plus hyperextension to engage the head of the capitate bone with the lunate, followed by flexion. The reduction is usually stable and the hand and wrist are placed in a short forearm cast in the position of function for 3 weeks.

### Colles' Fracture

One of the most common of all fractures, Colles' fracture, occurs at the distal radius, usually as the result of a fall on the extended hand. The fracture occurs typically about 1/2 to 3/4 inch above the articular surface. The distal fragment is displaced dorsally, and the articular surface is tilted toward the back of the hand. This displacement limits flexion at the wrist, and produces the typical "silver fork" deformity of this fracture.

A second major displacement occurs as the force producing the fracture continues: this is shortening of the radius with displacement of the distal fragment to the radial side of the wrist. This displacement disrupts the distal radioulnar joint, and, if uncorrected, prevents normal pronation and supination at the joint. Finally, the displacement in Colles' fracture may injure the median nerve as it is pressed against the sharp edge of the proximal fragment. Numbness and paresthesia of the thumb and index and middle fingers are produced, and there may be weakness of opposition of the thumb.

Careful and accurate reduction of a Colles' fracture is important. The first step is to break up the impaction usually found in these fractures. The surgeon applies traction and bends the patient's wrist backward, at the same time pressing downward and forward on the distal fragment. Once the fragments are disengaged, pressure with the thumb on the distal fragment will correct the posterior displacement. While the surgeon maintains traction and pressure with the thumb, the patient's

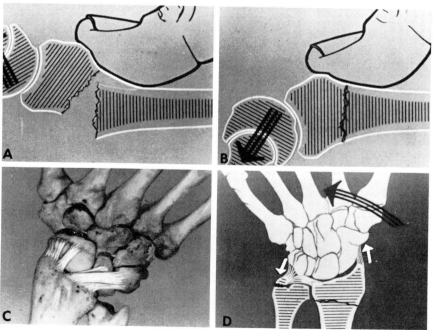

**Figure 10** *A,* Following disimpaction of the fracture, the surgeon creates pressure on the distal fragment with his thumb in order to force it palmarward while longitudinal traction is maintained. *B,* When the distal fragment has been moved forward, the wrist is flexed, tensing the dorsal carpal ligaments. *C,* Traction through these ligaments tilts the articular surface palmarward. *D,* Ulnar deviation of the hand lengthens the radius and replaces the ulnar styloid process or reduces the radioulnar joint disruption by traction through the radial collateral ligaments.

hand is brought into flexion and ulnar deviation (Fig. 10). The wrist is immobilized in flexion and ulnar deviation. To minimize swelling and disabling stiffness in the fingers, the hand should be elevated for the first 3 to 4 days after reduction. The patient should be made to understand that, if full function of his hand is to be regained, he must actively exercise his fingers from the moment the plaster is dry and throughout the healing period. Sufficient healing usually takes about 6 weeks.

### Displacement of the Distal Radial Epiphysis

In the growing child, forces that produce Colles' fracture in the adult often cause displacement of the distal radial epiphysis. The deformity is the same; the displacement takes place through the epiphyseal plate. This is a serious injury because the growth from the epiphyseal plate may be arrested, resulting in a short radius. The parents of the child should be warned about the possibility of arrested growth of the bone. Fortunately, this complication does not often occur. The reduction is performed by traction and pressure over the epiphysis. It is done gently to avoid further damage to the epiphyseal plate. The immobilization is like that used for Colles' fracture, and should continue for 4 to 6 weeks.

In the treatment of all fractures of the wrist and hand, several basic essentials should be kept in mind. Fractures of the hand and fingers should be immobilized in the position of function. Should serious stiffness develop, the patient would at least retain the ability to grasp objects with the hand, and the thumb would still be in a position of apposition to the fingers. Swelling should be kept under control by compression and elevation of the injured part. Early and consistent motion of the fingers not immobilized will help prevent stiffness of the hand. If the arm is immobilized in a sling, there is the additional danger of stiffening of the shoulder. This should be counteracted by exercises for the shoulder.

## THE FOREARM

In treating fractures of the forearm, restoration of the normal relationship of the radius and ulna is essential if maximal function is to be achieved. These two bones articulate at the proximal and distal radioulnar joints. The integrity of both joints is essential for normal rotation. It is obvious that, if one bone in the forearm breaks and angulates or shortens, these joints must be disturbed. Restoration of these joints must be accomplished if proper function is to be achieved.

### Fractures of the Ulna

Fractures of the shaft of the ulna are often the result of direct violence. A blow against the ulna may cause a fracture in any portion of the bone. Since the bone is subcutaneous along the extensor surface of the forearm, the injury may produce an open fracture rather easily. Angulation of the fracture is usually toward the radius, because the elasticity of the interosseous membrane tends to pull the two bones together. The triceps muscle tends to extend the proximal fragment, causing dorsal angulation. Angulation may be difficult to correct, more so if comminution of the fragments is present. Traction and manipulation are attempted and, if successful, the arm and forearm are immobilized in a cast extending from the distal palmar flexion crease to just below the axilla with the elbow flexed to 90 degrees and the forearm in midpronation and supination (Fig. 11).

Recurrence of angulation in the cast occurs frequently. If the angulation cannot be corrected or recurs in the cast, open reduction with internal fixation must be done. This is most easily accomplished with an intramedullary rod placed through the entire length of the bone. The fracture usually heals in 8 to 10 weeks. This method should not be employed in children while the bones are still growing. Slight angulation of the ulna in the growing child will correct the growth of the bone.

### Fractures of the Shaft of the Radius

Any fracture in the shaft of the radius accompanied by shortening of the bone involves the distal radioulnar joint. The distal fragment of the radius, together with the hand, is displaced upward. Since the ulna remains stationary, the ligaments are stretched or torn and the distal articula-

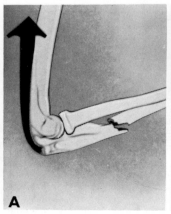
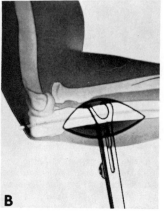

**A**     **B**

**Figure 11** *A,* The pull of the triceps muscle tends to extend the proximal fragment and may produce dorsal angulation of the fracture. The cast must be molded carefully along the ulna to counteract the angulation force of the triceps muscle. *B,* When the ulna cannot be held in reduction by a cast, open reduction must be performed. An intramedullary rod is used for fixation.

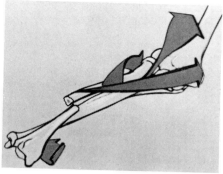

**Figure 12** When the fracture occurs below the insertion of the pronator teres, the pronator teres tends to counteract the supinator, and the proximal fragment remains in midpronation and supination. When the fracture occurs above the insertion of the pronator teres, the proximal fragment is held in supination by the biceps and supinator brevis muscles.

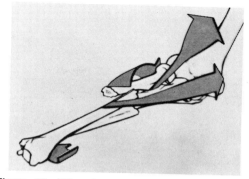

**Figure 13** When both bones of the forearm break above the insertion of the pronator teres, the proximal fragments are held in supination by the supinator brevis and biceps muscles. The pronators hold the distal fragments in pronation. The pull of the flexor and extensor muscles causes shortening.

tion is disrupted. Unless the normal relationship is re-established between the articular surfaces of the radius and ulna, pronation and supination will be limited.

In all fractures of the radial shaft, the interosseous membrane tends to draw the ends of the fragments toward the ulna. When the fracture is low in the shaft, this type of angulation is greatly aggravated by the cross-pull of the pronator quadratus, assisted by the brachioradialis. To counteract this displacement, traction should be exerted mainly on the radial side of the hand, and the hand should be in ulnar deviation when the arm is immobilized.

The rotational displacement in fractures of the shaft of the radius depends upon whether the fracture is above or below the insertion of the pronator teres. When the fracture is above the insertion of that muscle, the proximal fragment is held in supination by the biceps and supinator brevis. The two pronator muscles, however, pull the distal fragment into pronation. When the fracture occurs below the insertion of the pronator teres, that muscle serves to counteract the supinators, so that the proximal fragment is held in a position midway between pronation and supination. In order to align the fragments, the distal fragment must be rotated to midposition (Fig. 12).

The arm is immobilized with the elbow at a right angle. In many fractures of the lower radius, it may be impossible to prevent angulation and overriding by closed methods, particularly if the fracture is oblique or comminuted. If this occurs, open reduction with internal fixation is required to maintain reduction. Plate and screw fixation is particularly suitable for the radius when it is important to prevent rotary movement of one fragment upon the other.

### Fractures of Both Bones of the Forearm

When both bones of the forearm are fractured above the pronator teres insertion, just as when the radius alone is fractured at that level, the upper fragments are held in supination by the biceps and supinator brevis. The lower fragments, controlled by the two pronators, move into the pronated position. The pull of the extensors and flexors for the hand and wrist produces pronounced overriding (Fig. 13).

The method of reduction is similar to the one used for reducing a fractured radius. If the fractures are comminuted, or unstable, internal fixation is required. Frequently, an intramedullary rod is used to fix the ulna, since the bone is relatively straight and has little tendency to rotate. Plates and screws applied to the radius maintain fixation and prevent rotation.

### Monteggia's Fracture-Dislocation

Monteggia's fracture-dislocation is characterized by a fracture of the shaft of the ulna and a dislocation of the head of the radius at the elbow. The fracture-dislocation may occur as a result of a direct blow warded off by the forearm, with the elbow flexed. The force of the blow fractures the ulna and

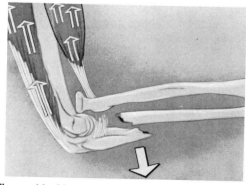

**Figure 14** Monteggia's fracture is characterized by fracture of the ulna with dislocation of the head of the radius. The biceps muscle pulls the radius upward while the triceps extends the ulna. The long forearm muscles produce overriding and shortening.

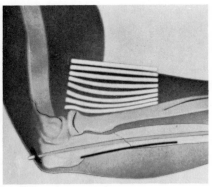

**Figure 15**   Reduction of the head of the radius is maintained by flexion of the elbow. The ulna requires firm splinting to prevent angulation by the triceps muscle. Internal fixation of the ulnar fragments with an intramedullary rod may be necessary to maintain reduction.

carries through to the radius. Although the radius is not fractured, it is torn loose from the orbicular ligament and dislocates upward and forward. More often the fracture results from indirect violence caused by a fall on the extended hand in which violent pronation force is applied to the forearm. The radius reaches the maximal degree of pronation and lies across the shaft of the ulna in the midforearm. The ulna acts as a lever forcing the head of the radius forward or laterally. The orbicular ligament ruptures and the head of the radius dislocates forward. The support of the radius is lost, and the force is transmitted to the ulna which fractures usually in the middle or upper one-third of the bone (Fig. 14).

The displacement of the radius may injure the motor branch of the radial nerve as it passes through the supinator brevis muscle. The median and ulnar nerves and the brachial artery and its branches may be injured. It is important to examine carefully the neurovascular condition of the forearm and hand.

In treating this injury, the surgeon should first attempt a closed reduction. Longitudinal traction is applied with the arm in extension. Once the ulna has been reduced, the head of the radius is pressed back to its normal position, and the arm flexed beyond a right angle. This flexed position holds the radial head firmly in reduction. However, such flexion places a pull on the triceps, which tends to angulate the ulna. This bone, therefore, requires firm splinting. When this injury occurs in children, the reduction is usually stable. In the adult, however, often the ulna can be maintained in position only by internal fixation (Fig. 15).

## THE ELBOW

In treating fractures about the elbow, the surgeon must recognize the mechanics of joint function and must realize the importance of the related soft tissue anatomy.

One of the important characteristics of the elbow

is the angle at which the forearm bones meet the humerus when the elbow is extended. This carrying angle, as it is called, is normally about 16 degrees. With the arm at the side and the elbow fully extended, this angle throws the hand away from the body. If the ulnar nerve is stretched around an abnormal angle, an ulnar nerve palsy may follow. It is important that the carrying angle be carefully checked before a fracture may be considered reduced.

As the elbow joint functions in flexion and extension, the two forearm bones move together as one unit, describing parallel arcs. This is possible because the two condyles of the humerus have a common axis. If a fracture is allowed to heal with the condyles malaligned, the radius and ulna no longer move about a common axis. This effectively blocks the range of motion in the joint. Accurate realignment of the joint surfaces, therefore, is essential if normal function in the elbow is to be restored.

### Supracondylar Fractures of the Humerus

A supracondylar fracture of the humerus, which occurs frequently in children, is caused by a fall on the hand with the elbow flexed. The fracture occurs at the thinnest part of the humerus, from front to back just above the condyles. The force of the fracture displaces the condyles posteriorly. The triceps, biceps, and brachialis contract and hold the fragment in this displaced position and draw it upward. Medial or lateral shearing force may displace the condylar fragment inward or outward. Rotational forces may rotate the condyles medially or laterally to a moderate degree.

As with all fractures, reduction should be undertaken as soon as possible. Traction is made manually. First, the elbow is extended, so that the triceps is relaxed. Traction is applied longitudinally. The fingers of one hand are placed on the anterior surface of the arm, and the thumb on the posterior surface, beneath the lower fragment of the humerus. When the fragments have been drawn past each other, the thumb and fingers are used to press the fragments into alignment. The elbow is then flexed to 105 degrees. This stretches the triceps and locks the fragments into place (Fig. 16).

After the reduction is complete, the surgeon checks it by gently flexing the forearm. If the elbow easily flexes to 105 degrees, anterior-posterior alignment has been achieved. At this point, the pulse is again palpated to make sure that the radial artery is undamaged. The arm is then fully extended and an estimate is made of the carrying angle and the rotational alignment of the lower fragment with the upper. A final evaluation of the reduction can be made by fully supinating the hand and placing the arm in as much flexion as swelling will allow. If the fracture has been reduced correctly, the index finger will point approximately to the tip of the shoulder.

The arm can be immobilized by one of several devices. A posterior molded plaster splint applied

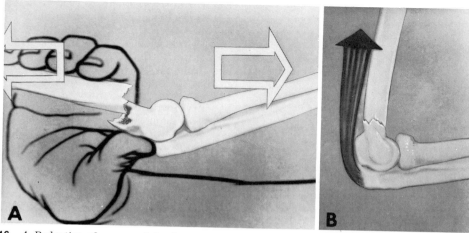

**Figure 16** *A*, Reduction of supracondylar fractures of the humerus is accomplished by traction and manipulation. *B*, With the elbow flexed, the taut triceps muscle holds the reduced condyles in position.

from the axilla to the palm is a simple and effective method for maintaining position.

The surgeon must watch with the greatest care for signs of impaired circulation in the forearm and hand during the first few days after reduction. There is always a threat of a *Volkmann's contracture* following a supracondylar fracture. If the radial pulse disappears or if the signs of circulatory failure appear, the extremity must be extended at the elbow immediately. Often this change of position allows decompression of the blood vessels with return of adequate circulation. It may be necessary to suspend the arm in Dunlop's traction if the swelling is excessive to maintain the reduction as well as the circulation. If the circulation does not return immediately, the deep fascia of the forearm and elbow must be incised to decompress the blood vessels. As soon as the fracture is healed, the patient is allowed to re-establish motion with his own muscles without forceful manipulation.

### Condylar Fractures of the Humerus

Fractures between the condyles may break off either the trochlea or the capitellum, or the condyles may split from the shaft of the humerus, forming a Y- or V-shaped fracture. Displacement of either condyle blocks the arc of motion in flexion and extension; therefore, it is necessary to obtain exact alignment of the condyles. The fractures can be reduced by straight traction on the arm, with lateral pressure over the medial condyle or medial pressure over the lateral condyle. Angulation of the forearm is performed to correct deviation of the forearm. The fingers are used to mold the fragments into accurate position. With the fingers still holding the fragment in position, the arm is then flexed to 90 to 110 degrees. Pressure with the thumb completes the alignment.

In fractures of the capitellum, because of the pull of the extensor muscles, the fragment is rotated outward 90 degrees or more. The articular

surface then lies against the fractured surface of the trochlea and manipulation fails to correct this rotary displacement. It is important to recognize this deformity in the adult, but more so in the child. If this rotational deformity is not corrected and the fracture reduced accurately, nonunion is almost certain. In the child, marked growth disturbance occurs, characterized by angulation at the elbow, which increases the carrying angle and slowly produces ulnar nerve palsy. Open reduction should be performed promptly in either the child or adult if the deformity cannot be corrected. The fragments are fitted together under direct vision and held in reduction by two small pins driven through the capitellum into the humerus. The pins are removed when the fracture heals.

### Fractures of the Medial Condyle and Trochlea of Humerus

Fractures of the trochlea and of the medial condyle of the humerus are produced by a mechanism similar to that in fractures of the lateral condyle, except that the angulating force is lateral. The ulna transmits the force to the trochlea, which splits away from the capitellum and is displaced upward. The carrying angle is decreased or reversed. The upward displacement is maintained by the pull of the brachialis and triceps. The fragment is rotated forward by the flexor muscles of the wrist and hand, as well as by the pronator teres, which originates on the medial epicondyle. There is less tendency for the fracture to rotate medially away from the humerus because of the hingelike connection with the ulna, which stabilizes the fracture in this plane.

### Y and T Fractures of the Condyles

Y and T fractures of the condyles of the humerus are combinations of the two previously mentioned fractures, and usually occur in adults. Comminution of fragments frequently makes reduction difficult. Since the stabilizing influence of one intact condyle is lost when both break from the humerus, some type of continuous traction is necessary to maintain reduction. This may be supplied in suspension traction, or by the weight of a hanging cast. Open reduction with internal fixation is occasionally required if the fragments cannot be molded into position by traction applied through the joint capsule.

### Fractures of the Olecranon Process

Either direct or muscular violence may cause a fracture of the olecranon process. Such fractures occur in a transverse direction and extend into the joint. The triceps, which is attached to the olecranon, pulls the proximal fragment upward. Flexion of the elbow separates the fragments farther. Since it is extremely difficult to overcome the pull of the triceps by any closed method, fracture of the olecranon can best be reduced by surgery.

Internal fixation may be obtained by suturing the fragments together with wire, or by an intramedullary rod placed through the olecranon into the medullary canal of the ulna. Because joint surfaces are involved, accurate restoration of these surfaces is paramount for ideal function. When marked comminution of the olecranon fragment prevents accurate reduction, it may be necessary to excise the fragments and suture the triceps tendon to the ulna. A compression dressing and sling are used for a week while reaction from the trauma and surgery subsides. Then gentle active motion is begun to avoid stiffness and adhesions within the joint.

### Fractures of the Head of the Radius

Fracture of the head of the radius occurs as the result of a fall on the outstretched arm, with the elbow in slight flexion. The force is transmitted upward along the shaft of the radius to the head, driving the head against the capitellum. Some-

times, this type of injury results in very minor damage, producing simple longitudinal fissures in the head. Also, the fracture may occur through the neck, just below the head. Such fractures are usually impacted, and there may be very little displacement. When a fracture in this area results in very little angulation or displacement, it can be treated conservatively with splinting. Motion may be started within a week. However, if the head of the bone is angulated so that the articular surface does not fit the capitellum, or the radioulnar joint is disrupted, reduction must be done. Failure to correct marked angulation will result in faulty flexion and extension, as well as limited pronation and supination. Since the head of the radius is devoid of ligamentous attachment, traction and manipulation by angulation have little effect upon it. Direct pressure with the thumb over the radial head accompanied by pronation and supination may correct angulation; however, open reduction is often necessary (Fig. 17).

In the child, moderate angulation will be corrected by growth and may be accepted. A mechanism similar to that which produces the radial neck fractures may cause the proximal radial epiphysis to slip. The displacement may be lateral, forward, or backward. Closed manipulation reduction should be attempted. If the displacement is great, open reduction may be done gently, forcing the fragments into alignment under direct vision. The radial head must never be removed in a growing child because serious growth disturbance in the forearm will result.

Often, in the adult, the fragile rim of the radial head is broken into several fragments. When the injury is severe, it seriously interferes with the rotation of the forearm. These fragments cannot be manipulated back into position, and they serve as irritants in the joint. Therefore, it is advisable to remove the head of the radius. In the adult, this may be done without serious loss of function. It is essential, however, to start motion in the elbow

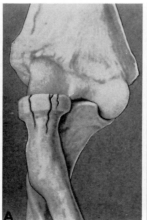 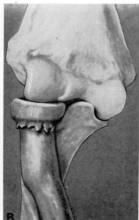 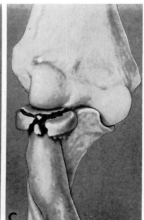

**Figure 17** *A,* Longitudinal fissure fractures may occur in the head of the radius without displacement. *B,* The head of the radius may be impacted on the neck, with varying degrees of displacement. *C,* Fractures with marked displacement of fragments may require removal of the entire radial head.

within a few days after the operation to prevent adhesions.

Several basic principles apply in the treatment of most of these fractures about the elbow. One is to so reduce the fracture that the normal carrying angle at the elbow is maintained. Another is to align the fragments so that in flexion and extension the radius and ulna move in concentric arcs. Just as important as proper alignment is the maintenance of smooth joint surfaces. Circulatory impairment and nerve damage are ever present dangers, and must be evaluated and cared for properly.

Finally, it should be kept in mind that the elbow joint is prone to stiffness after fracture or operative procedures. Motion should be started as early as possible, but such motion should not be strenuous. It is best to let the force of the patient's own muscles provide the required resistance.

## THE HUMERUS

The glenohumeral joint is constructed to allow maximal motion in all planes. For this reason, it is a loose joint. The ball-like head of the humerus rests against the small shallow saucer of the glenoid fossa, and the two structures are approximated by the flexible joint capsule. It is obvious that stability of the joint must come from the synchronous action of the complex shoulder girdle muscles. Fractures and dislocations of the humerus thus are influenced to a great extent by these complex muscle actions. Characteristic deformities occur with fractures of the bones of the shoulder girdle because of these muscles. It follows logically that maximal restoration of function depends upon the integrity of the muscles, tendons, and ligaments of the area, and that early restoration of function of these parts in treatment is essential.

These muscles may be divided into two main groups. On the anterior aspect, there are the adductor-internal rotators. On the posterior aspect of the shoulder are located the abductor-external rotator muscles. The most important single factor in the distribution of muscle pull is the uneven power of the abductors and external rotators compared to the adductor-internal rotator group. The abductors exert their power over the head of the humerus. This limits their leverage in lifting the weight of the arm. The stronger adductors, however, exert a much greater force. They are assisted by gravity and have the advantage of better leverage. This unequal power is even more important in the healing process than in reduction. Ideally, fixation of fractures of the humerus should be in abduction and moderate external rotation. This ensures contraction of the weak abductors and protects the bursae and other structures from adhesion at the shoulder joint. In treatment, this ideal position is not always practical.

A second anatomic factor of great importance is the presence of neurovascular structures in the axilla and upper arm. These nerves and vessels are endangered particularly by fractures of the surgical neck of the humerus and fractures of the shaft just below the insertion of the deltoid.

### Fractures of the Shaft of the Humerus

Fractures of the shaft of the humerus are divided generally into those occurring below the deltoid insertion and those occurring above it. The area may be further divided into fractures above and below the pectoralis major, but above the deltoid insertion. Such fractures may be caused by the indirect force of a fall or the direct force of a blow to the humerus.

There is little displacement in the typical fracture below the deltoid insertion, in which the abductors as well as the adductors are attached to the upper fragment. They serve to balance each other. The distal fragment is controlled principally by gravity and by the long muscles of the arm—the triceps and biceps. Since their pull is upward, parallel with the bone, they have very little displacing effect except to produce shortening. Since the elbow is held at a right angle, the biceps is relaxed. The triceps produces anterior angulation by acting like a bowstring along the back of the humerus. Another hazard occurs when the patient moves his body and tenses the shoulder muscles. This tends to abduct the proximal fragment, causing lateral angulation, particularly if the traction is not enough to overcome the upward pull of the long muscles (Fig. 18).

Another complication in fractures just below the deltoid insertion is injury to the radial nerve. The winding course of the nerve around the bone at the level of the fracture predisposes it to injury. This nerve may be damaged either by sharp fragments of the bone or by the trauma which originally caused the fracture. Sometimes, no involvement of the radial nerve is evident when the fracture is

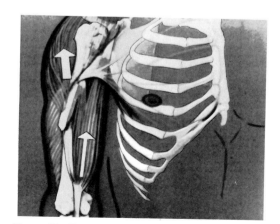

**Figure 18**  Fractures that occur from below the deltoid muscle insertion to above the humeral condyles exhibit similar deformities. The long muscles of the arm cause shortening. The fracture may angulate laterally or medially, as the proximal fragment remains in neutral position. Since the biceps is relaxed with the elbow flexed, the triceps muscle may act as a bowstring posteriorly, producing moderate anterior angulation.

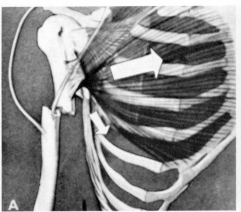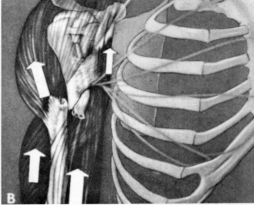

**Figure 19**  *A,* Fractures below the insertion of the pectoralis major but above the deltoid produce medial angulation of the proximal fragment, because the pull of the adductors is stronger than the force of the abductors. *B,* The long muscles of the arm cause shortening, and the deltoid may pull the distal fragment outward.

examined originally, but becomes apparent much later as a gradual weakening of extension of the hand and fingers. This means that the nerve has been damaged subsequently by growing callus or angulation. Callus may be abundant surrounding the nerve, squeezing it and causing a slowly progressive paralysis. When this happens, the nerve must be freed from the callus by neurolysis. If radial nerve palsy is found immediately or develops later, the wrist and fingers must be supported to prevent overstretching of the paralyzed forearm extensor muscles.

The hanging cast is used to supply traction as it is in fractures above the deltoid insertion. Suspension traction may be necessary in fractures that cannot be maintained by splints or casts. Occasionally, reduction cannot be accomplished by closed methods. This is usually due to interposition of muscle between the bone fragments. If the separation of fragments is excessive, open reduction with internal fixation with screws and plates or intramedullary rod is done.

When the fracture occurs above the pectoralis major insertion, the strong adductor muscles hold the distal fragment in adduction and internal rotation. The weak external rotator-abductor muscles exert very little counterpull, and the proximal fragment remains in neutral position. The characteristic displacement is thus medial angulation and displacement of the distal fragment on the proximal, with moderate shortening and overriding.

Fractures between the insertion of the pectoralis major and the deltoid muscles present the opposite deformity. The strong pull of the pectoralis major overcomes the abductor muscles, and the proximal fragment is angulated medialward. The deltoid and long muscles of the arm produce shortening and slight outward displacement of the distal fragment. Usually, a hanging cast will effect and maintain reduction in either fracture; occasionally, however, open reduction and internal fixation are necessary (Fig. 19).

## Fractures of the Surgical Neck of the Humerus

Fractures of the surgical neck of the humerus are usually caused by indirect violence. They frequently occur as the result of a fall on the outstretched arm. Such fractures are frequently comminuted. Because the fracture occurs in an area of cancellous bone, the fracture is often impacted. After the fracture occurs, the upper fragment is held in abduction and slight forward flexion by the supraspinatus. This in effect tips the head of the humerus so that the articular surfaces face backward and medial. The rotators, however, are fairly evenly balanced, so that this fragment is held midway between external and internal rotation. The strong adductors pull the distal fragment inward and somewhat forward. If the distal fragment is displaced medially far enough, the sharp edge of the bone may damage the nerves and blood vessels (Fig. 20). In effecting reduction, the principle is followed of aligning the distal fragment, which can be controlled, with the head of the bone, which cannot. Traction is made toward the foot of the table with only a small amount of abduction, not more than 25 degrees. The free hands of the operator then manipulate the shaft and head fragments into alignment. To maintain reduction, various splints or casts may be applied.

Fortunately, most fractures of the surgical neck of the humerus are impacted in fairly good position. It is better to accept a moderate amount of deformity and start early motion of the shoulder than to attempt anatomic reduction. Since the joint is a loose one, and the head of the humerus contacts the glenoid cavity over a small area, malalignment has very little effect on ultimate function. However, prolonged immobilization with the arm at the side does produce marked disability through adhesions and shortened muscles. The shoulder is immobilized by placing the extremity in a sling and bandaging the arm to the side by a swathe dressing about the chest. This is

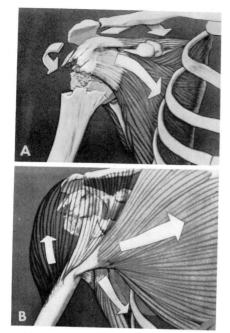

**Figure 20** Because the bone of the surgical neck of the humerus is cancellous, fractures in this region are often comminuted and impacted. *A,* The head of the bone is held in neutral rotation, but is tipped medially and backward by the pull of the external rotator and abductor muscles. *B,* The distal fragment is displaced medially by the adductor muscles, and may threaten the neurovascular structures.

maintained for 3 to 5 days, until the acute pain has subsided. Gentle pendulum exercises are then started. The fracture usually heals in 6 weeks. If a well controlled program of exercise has been instituted early, the patient should have fairly good shoulder motion by this time. However, it may take many months of active exercise to obtain maximal function.

### Epiphyseal Displacement

Epiphyseal separation of the head of the humerus may occur in an infant following the trauma of delivery, or in growing children from indirect violence. Since the ossification center is not present in the humeral epiphysis at birth, x-ray films fail to reveal the nature of the injury. In the growing child, the injury is rare from the age of infancy until about the eighth year. In older children, up to about 13 years of age, epiphyseal separations and fractures are more common. X-ray studies after the ossification center appears in the humeral head readily reveal the injury.

In the infant, the symptoms are pseudoparalysis of the arm coupled with swelling and obvious pain when the part is handled. Occasionally, crepitation can be elicited on manipulation. X-ray films made a week after injury reveal proliferating callus about the upper humerus. Simple immobilization

with a swathe about the chest and arm is usually all that is needed in the infant. The minor displacements are usually corrected by growth. Rarely, the epiphysis is rotated completely around so that the epiphyseal plate faces into the glenoid. This injury is manifested only later by disturbed growth of the humerus when it is too late to restore the bone. Fortunately, the injury is rare. It is, however, almost impossible to diagnose early, and a short humerus always results from the growth disturbance.

In older children, the epiphyseal separation is often coupled with fracture of the metaphysis in the subtrochanteric region. The head of the humerus is often rotated inward with the distal fragment angulating laterally and upward. Reduction is accomplished by downward traction and maintained with a hanging cast. Anatomic reduction is unnecessary because growth will correct the deformity in time. The younger the child, the greater the deformity that may be accepted.

### Fractures of the Neck of the Humerus with Anterior Dislocation

This fracture-dislocation is a result of violence with the humerus abducted posteriorly. The force of the fall and the extreme abduction drive the greater tuberosity against the acromion process. As abduction of the humerus increases, the acromion acts as a fulcrum; the head of the humerus is forced out of its position in the glenoid, stretching and tearing the capsule. This dislocation is increased by the downward and forward pull of the pectoralis major. As the force of the fall exerts its full impact, the head is trapped under the pectoralis major and a fracture occurs through the surgical neck. It is this combination of fracture and dislocation that makes the injury so difficult to treat (Fig. 21).

If closed reduction is attempted by traction and manipulation of the arm, the shaft is usually pulled away from the head completely. This interrupts the blood supply from the shaft to the

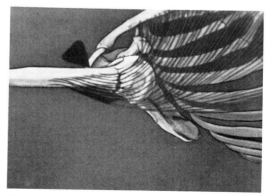

**Figure 21** When the humerus is forcefully abducted, the acromion process acts as a fulcrum, forcing the head of the humerus downward and forward, rupturing the anterior inferior joint capsule. The head is trapped under the pectoral muscle, which causes the neck of the humerus to fracture.

head. Necrosis of the head of the bone may follow, resulting in permanent disability. Because of the dangers resulting from closed manipulation of this type of fracture-dislocation, open reduction is often advisable.

After open reduction, or careful closed reduction of fracture-dislocation of the humerus, the arm is immobilized with the sling and swathe bandage for a few days. Exercise is then started similar to that used for fracture of the neck of the humerus.

### Dislocation of the Glenohumeral Joint without Fracture

Dislocations of the humerus at this joint are among the most common dislocations in the body. Most dislocations take place anteriorly and inferiorly; less commonly, the dislocation occurs posteriorly. The mechanism is similar to that producing the fracture-dislocation of the humerus.

Frequently, the injury occurs in teenagers or in young adults engaged in vigorous athletics. Often, the dislocation in this age group occurs with apparently little force applied to the abducted, extended arm. This may happen when there is a defect in the joint capsule, such as deficient or absent glenohumeral ligaments or an excessively relaxed joint capsule. When the head of the humerus is forced out of the joint, the capsule usually tears away from the rim or labrum of the glenoid. Deformity of the shoulder is usually obvious, and the elbow cannot be approximated to the side of the body. Active abduction of more than a few degrees is impossible. Pain is usually severe. The circulation and integrity of the nerves of the extremity must be determined and an x-ray examination should always be made before reduction is attempted.

Several methods of reduction are available to the surgeon. One of the simplest methods is to place the patient prone with the arm hanging over the edge of a table. With adequate sedation, the traction supplied by the weight of the arm relaxes the spasm of the muscles holding the head in the dislocated position. Reduction may occur spontaneously after 10 to 15 minutes, or additional traction may be necessary, supplemented by gentle internal and external rotatory manipulation.

If this method fails, it may be necessary to apply more traction. The patient is placed supine and, with adequate sedation or a general anesthetic, traction is made on the arm in 30 degrees of abduction. Countertraction is supplied by the surgeon's foot placed against the side of the chest just below but not in the axilla. It is obvious that this form of countertraction should not be used if ribs are fractured on the side of the dislocation.

The joint is immobilized with the arm at the side and the forearm across the chest with the humerus internally rotated to allow the torn joint capsule to approximate the glenoid. Although this position allows the strong adductor-internal rotator muscles to shorten, it is the only position in which the anterior joint capsule is relaxed. The position is maintained for 6 weeks in patients under 35 years of age. Teenagers and young

adults are prone to recurring dislocations of the shoulder; for this reason, the immobilization must be uninterrupted for this period. Motion is regained slowly after this time by gradually increasing shoulder exercise. In persons over 35, recurrent dislocation of the shoulder is much less likely, and immobilization for 3 weeks is usually adequate for healing. Some slight loss of abduction and external rotation may persist in patients in the older age groups.

## FRACTURES AND DISLOCATIONS OF THE CLAVICLE

Fracture of the clavicle is one of the most common fractures from infancy through the first three decades of life, but may occur at any age. Most fractures of the clavicle are caused by the compression force of a fall on the outstretched arm, but occasionally they are the result of a direct blow to the bone. Because of the structure of the bone, it most frequently breaks in the middle one-third and, fortunately, buckles and angulates upward and away from the subclavian vessels and brachial plexus. When the fracture is completely through the bone, overriding and shortening occur. The proximal fragment is held upward by the sternomastoid muscle while gravity and the pectoral muscles pull the distal part downward and forward. Reduction of the fracture is accomplished by bracing the shoulder girdle backward and upward accompanied by manipulation of the bone ends.

The type of fracture varies with the age of the patient. In infants and children up to about the age of 10 years, the fracture is usually of the greenstick type. In adolescents and persons in the next two decades, the fracture is complete and often simple. In the older age persons, the fracture is often comminuted.

Children 10 years of age and younger with greenstick fractures usually do not require reduction of the fracture. The shoulder is immobilized for comfort with a figure-of-eight bandage. Growth will correct the angulation.

Older children and adults require reduction of the fracture if there is overriding or marked angulation of the fragments. This is most easily done after a local anesthetic has been injected into the fracture hematoma. With the patient sitting on a stool, the shoulders are braced backward. The ends of the bone are manipulated into position. A figure-of-eight bandage is applied with adequate padding in the axillae. The bandage must be tightened each day.

Occasionally, the fracture in the adult cannot be held in reduction, particularly if there is comminution. If the deformity is objectionable or symptoms of pressure on the nerves and vessels are present, open reduction with internal fixation with an intramedullary rod may be necessary.

Most fractures of the clavicle in adults heal sufficiently in 4 to 6 weeks to allow removal of the figure-of-eight dressing. Stiffness of the shoulder is usually not a problem, as the arm has been used during the healing time. Rarely, nonunion of the clavicle follows fracture. This condition is treated by intramedullary rod fixation and appropriate bone grafting.

### Dislocation of the Sternoclavicular Joint

The sternoclavicular joint is occasionally dislocated by a fall on the arm or shoulder. Most often the dislocation is anterior. The sternomastoid tends to pull the clavicle upward while the weight of the shoulder and pectoral muscles displaces it medially. Occasionally, dislocation takes place backward behind the sternum. This displacement may force the end of the clavicle against the trachea or great vessels, and cause difficulty in breathing or interfere with circulation. It may require immediate reduction. In either displacement, reduction is accomplished by bracing the shoulders backward; however, the reduction cannot be maintained by closed methods because of the unstable joint surfaces. Open reduction with repair of ruptured joint capsule must be done soon after the injury. Temporary wire fixation may be necessary while healing of the capsule takes place.

Neglected or old dislocations of this joint do not need treatment if the condition is painless. However, the deformity is noticeable, and many patients request that something be done for cosmetic reasons. The proximal 2 inches of the bone may be resected without interfering with shoulder function. This procedure is usually more satisfactory than late reconstruction of the joint.

### Dislocation and Subluxation of the Acromioclavicular Joint

This dislocation, or partial dislocation, results from a fall on the point of the shoulder. The shoulder and arm, fixed to the ground by the weight of the body, pull the arm downward. The momentum of the falling body carries the trunk and thus the clavicle upward. The joint capsule is torn and the main stabilizing ligament, the coracoclavicular ligament, either partially or completely tears. The degree of rupture of this ligament determines whether the dislocation is complete or partial (Fig. 22).

When the patient stands, the distal clavicle is prominent above the acromion, which is pulled downward by the weight of the arm. When the patient lies down, the dislocation may reduce and no deformity may be apparent on inspection of the shoulder. For this reason, x-ray examination must be made with the patient upright, preferably holding a weight of 5 pounds in the hand, which accentuates deformity.

Upward pressure on the bent elbow in the long axis of the humerus effects reduction, while downward pressure is made on the clavicle. Various methods of strapping have been devised to maintain reduction by continuous exertion of these forces. Unfortunately, the force needed to maintain reduction by this method may produce skin necrosis over the elbow or clavicle, and the method is generally unsatisfactory. Recent injuries are best treated by open reduction with repair of the coracoclavicular ligament and joint capsule. Some type of internal fixation is needed while the ligaments are healing.

Old complete dislocations are rarely painful. Partial dislocation or subluxation, however, may lead to painful traumatic arthritis. If the patient does not object to the appearance of the shoulder, and it is painless, the complete dislocation may be accepted, without serious impairment of shoulder function. However, if pain or deformity is to be corrected, either in complete or partial dislocation,

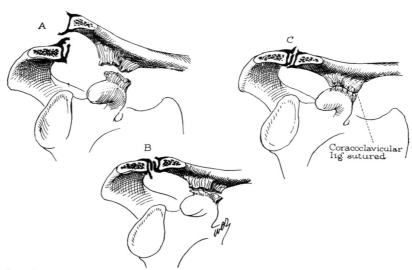

**Figure 22** *A,* Complete rupture of the joint capsule of the acromioclavicular joint and the coracoclavicular ligament must occur before the joint can dislocate completely. *B,* The joint capsule may fold into the joint and prevent reduction. *C,* The coracoclavicular ligament must be repaired to maintain reduction of the dislocation.

the distal 1 to 1½ inches of clavicle may be resected. Elimination of the joint relieves pain, and the resection reduces the deformity without interfering with shoulder function.

## FRACTURES OF THE SCAPULA

The scapula is a triangular, flat, thin bone divided posteriorly into a supraspinous and infraspinous portion by the spine of the scapula. Two other processes, the acromion and the coracoid, also rise from the scapula. The scapula is completely covered by muscles except at the glenoid, where the joint capsule arises. The mobility of the bone provides for absorption of shock during falls on the upper extremity. For this reason, the body of the bone is seldom fractured by indirect violence. The mechanism of fracture of the body of the scapula is usually a direct blow, and the fracture is often comminuted. Since the bone is covered by muscles, the fragments are seldom displaced. However, the force necessary to produce the fracture is considerable and related injuries to the thorax and upper extremity are common.

Fractures of the neck, glenoid, and acromion and coracoid processes may be produced by direct or indirect violence. Occasionally, the acromion process is fractured and displaced downward by a fall on the point of the shoulder. Rarely, the coracoid process may be avulsed by violent contraction of the coracobrachialis muscle, which displaces the avulsed fragment downward. If the acromion process is depressed enough to interfere with scapulohumeral motion, it may be removed. Avulsion of the coracoid process is usually treated conservatively by immobilization for a short period, followed by active exercise. Reattachment by open reduction is seldom necessary.

The treatment for most fractures of the scapula is simple immobilization with a sling and swathe bandage about the chest until the acute pain subsides. After a few days, gentle circumduction exercises, are begun; gradually, shoulder girdle motion is regained. As in all shoulder injuries, early active use is necessary to prevent adhesions and muscle contractures.

## FRACTURES AND DISLOCATIONS OF THE LOWER EXTREMITY

The primary functions of the lower extremities are weight bearing and locomotion. For this reason, the bones, joints, muscles, and ligaments are more massive in construction than in the upper extremity. Since stability is necessary for walking, running, standing, and squatting, the motions of the major joints are more limited. While the motion of the knee joint is similar to that of the elbow, allowing primarily flexion and extension, the motions and construction of the hip and ankle joints differ from those of the shoulder and wrist joints to provide the required stability.

The center of gravity of the body is located in the midline at the second sacral segment; the hip joints lie lateral to this point, and the femur slants toward the midline in its downward course to compensate for this difference. A slight knock-knee effect is produced by this alignment. Since the knee and ankle cannot abduct or adduct to compensate for deformities from fractures that produce medial or lateral angulation, disturbances of this weight-bearing alignment are critical. In the lateral plane of the body, the weight-bearing line of the body passes almost directly through the hip joint. The alignment of the femur and tibia is thus almost in a straight line to the foot. Anterior or posterior angulation may be compensated for by flexion and extension of the hip, knee, and ankle.

Rotational deformity always throws one or more joints out of alignment, and cannot be accepted if proper function is expected. Fractures of the lower extremity that heal with malalignment produce abnormal stress and strain on the joints. In time, traumatic arthritis develops in the hip, knee, or ankle.

Shortening of one extremity produces a pelvic tilt. The spine then articulates with the sacrum at an angle. A compensatory scoliosis must develop in the spine to bring the trunk back to the middle. This produces strain in the joints involved, and may lead to backache and traumatic arthritis.

Because of the forces placed upon the joints on weight bearing, fractures deforming joint surfaces produce wear-and-tear changes in the joints much more rapidly than in the upper extremity. Usually, a painful traumatic arthritis results.

Rehabilitation of the muscles of the lower extremity is imperative if normal function is to be achieved following injury. Muscles atrophy and may shorten with prolonged immobilization. Characteristic deformities develop. At the hip, the strong adductor and flexor muscles tend to shorten, producing a flexion adduction contracture. At the knee, flexion contracture is produced by shortened hamstring muscles while contracture of the calf muscles produces equinus deformity of the foot and ankle. Strength of the atrophied opposing muscles must be rebuilt while the shortened muscles are stretched by means of appropriate exercises. Failure to strengthen the muscles causes limping at the hip and buckling and instability of the knee.

### THE HIP JOINT

Fractures about the hip joint are classified as intracapsular and extracapsular. To treat the special problems that arise in dealing with these fractures, the anatomy peculiar to the hip must be understood.

The blood supply to the head of the femur comes from three sources: through the medullary vessels of the neck, through the ligamentum teres, and through the visceral capsular vessels. Fractures of the neck of the bone disrupt the nutrient vessels

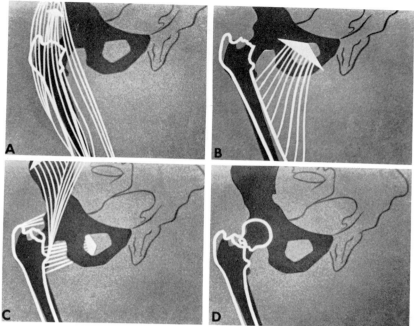

**Figure 23** *A*, Shortening of the bone in fractures of the hip is produced by the long thigh muscles, the rectus femoris, sartorius, and hamstrings. *B*, The adductors produce adduction and shortening. *C*, The abductor muscles and external rotator muscles, aided by the iliopsoas, tend to abduct, externally rotate, and flex the distal fragment in certain hip fractures. *D*, Fractures about the hip result in shortening, adduction, and external rotation as the result of muscle contractions and gravity.

of the medullary canal completely, and may damage or tear the capsular vessels. The nourishment of the head of the bone is then left to the inadequate resources of the artery of the ligamentum teres. Bleeding into the tight confines of the joint capsule may produce a tamponade effect and further impair the circulation to the head. When the blood supply to the head is completely cut off, this fragment undergoes necrosis. Dead bone does not aid in the healing process and must be replaced by the process of creeping substitution. In this process, dead bone is absorbed and new laid down. The process is slow and may be incomplete. Nonunion and destruction of the head of the bone is the plague of the surgeon and the patient.

The neck of the femur progresses outward and downward at an angle of 140 to 145 degrees, placing the shaft of the femur lateral to the joint. This lateral placement of the shaft in relation to the joint may produce shearing force on intracapsular fractures, delaying or preventing healing. The angle of the fracture through the neck in relation to the horizontal plane determines the amount of shearing force. Fractures that are more vertical are subject to more shearing force than those which approach the horizontal.

Since the internal rotators of the hip work at a mechanical disadvantage, they are overcome by the external rotators and gravity. Thus, the leg assumes a typical deformity of shortening and external rotation in fractures of the femur about the hip (Fig. 23).

A general classification divides fractures into two main groups, intracapsular and extracapsular. Because shearing force plays such an important role in healing, these fractures have been classified by Pawles by the angle of the fracture to the horizontal. If the fracture line through the neck is nearly horizontal, impacting force may be exerted by the pull of the thigh muscles. However, as the fracture line becomes more vertical, more shearing force is exerted by these muscles and the prognosis for healing becomes progressively worse.

Fractures outside the hip joint capsule may involve either the greater or lesser trochanter as avulsion-type fractures. More frequently, however, the fracture line runs between the greater and lesser trochanter—the intertrochanteric fracture. Fractures of the shaft of the femur at the lesser trochanter are called subtrochanteric fractures.

### Intracapsular Fractures

Subcapital fractures may be impacted, or complete and displaced. The fracture impacted in good position may show no deformity and, although painful, may allow considerable motion at the hip joint. Indeed, the patient often walks upon the leg for a variable period until the pain forces him to seek medical help. If the head is in valgus position, impacted upon the neck, and there is no anterior or posterior displacement of the neck-head relationship, the fracture may be treated without immobilization or fixation but with no weight bear-

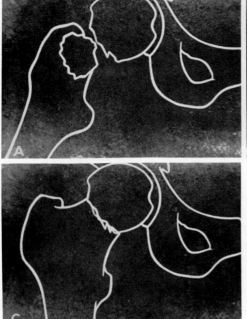
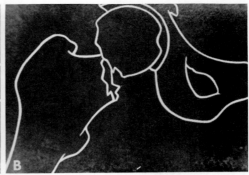

**Figure 24** *A,* Traction is made on the leg to bring the forward-facing and shortened neck down to the level of the head or slightly below it. *B,* The femur is internally rotated 45 degrees to bring the fractured neck under the head. *C,* Traction is then reduced to allow the head and neck to come together.

ing on the leg. Muscle tension tends to promote the impaction. If the head fragment is in varus position, or the head is tipped forward or backward, the impaction is insecure, and, with absorption of bone during healing, the fracture may displace completely. In this instance, reduction and internal fixation should be done.

Complete and displaced fractures of the femoral neck present the typical deformity of shortening and external rotation of the leg. All motion is painful and may be accompanied by spasmodic contractions of the thigh and hip musculature. The degree of shortening varies.

**Reduction of Subcapital and Midcervical Fractures.** Reduction is accomplished by traction and countertraction with the leg in external rotation and neutral or slight abduction. The traction is most easily accomplished on a fracture operating table which insures accurate, stable control of the leg. Countertraction is applied against the perineum by a post placed between the legs and attached to the table. As traction is applied, the forward-facing neck fragment is brought downward to the level of the head or slightly below it. The leg is then internally rotated completely, usually about 45 degrees. This maneuver brings the forward-facing neck back to its normal position in relation to the head. The leg is then brought from slight abduction to almost neutral position to place the neck under the head. Traction is reduced to allow the fragments to come together (Fig. 24).

Accurate x-ray examinations in the anteroposterior and lateral views are essential to control reduction and for the application of internal fixation.

A variety of nails, screws, and pins have been devised for internal fixation of femoral neck fractures. They are all designed to hold the head fragment securely to the neck of the femur. The number and variety attest to the variability of success in accomplishing this.

Since the majority of subcapital and midcervical fractures occur in the elderly, these patients do not tolerate prolonged bed rest or inactivity. Complications involving the lungs, genitourinary system, and circulatory system are common if the patient is not made active as early as possible. Internal fixation, while securing immobilization of the fracture, also allows early non-weight-bearing ambulation and exercise. Exercise of the leg is started immediately to prevent contracture and muscle atrophy. The patient should be instructed in the use of a walker, which provides purposeful exercise, but weight must not be borne upon the leg until union is complete. Healing rates vary, and may be as short as 3 months or as long as a year.

If the fracture line is unfavorable for healing or if the survival of the head is questionable in the elderly patient, the surgeon may elect to replace the head of the bone with a prosthesis.

### Intertrochanteric Fractures

Three major types of intertrochanteric fractures are encountered: undisplaced, displaced, and comminuted. The prognosis for healing is good in all, but the instability produced by the comminuted type often leads to deformity and permanent disability.

Undisplaced fractures require no reduction, but

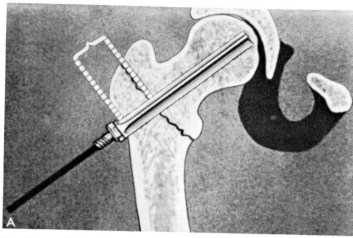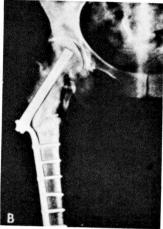

**Figure 25** *A*, The trochanteric fragment does not offer enough holding surface for a nail. *B*, A plate must be attached to the femur with screws to secure adequate internal fixation.

are often treated by internal fixation to insure against displacement while healing. Reduction is performed by a method similar to that used in intracapsular fractures, except that internal rotation only to the neutral position is required and abduction is maintained. If the extremity is internally rotated completely, the fracture line closes in front but opens in back, and the neck may be forced into more posterior angulation. If abduction is not sufficient, coxa vara may persist. Maintenance of reduction may be provided by the continuous suspension traction of Russell or by internal fixation. Undisplaced fractures heal rapidly, usually within 2 months by any method of treatment. Displaced and comminuted fractures may heal in this time, but often require 3 or 4 months. Often it is undesirable to keep elderly patients in bed for the time necessary for healing. For this reason, open reduction with internal fixation is more commonly done (Fig. 25).

Nonunion is rare and is usually due to inadequate fixation or interposition of soft tissue. The condition is treated by bone grafting.

### Dislocation of the Hip Joint

Traumatic dislocation of the hip is produced by extreme indirect violence. Usually, the hip and knee are flexed when the force is applied to the distal end of the femur. The force is transmitted through the head against the posterior capsule and rim of the acetabulum. If the femur is in adduction, the head may be forced laterally out of the socket, with tearing of the ligamentum teres and the capsule. If the femur is in a more neutral position or abduction, the force is exerted against the posterior acetabular rim which may be fractured and driven backward, allowing the head to dislocate. The dislocated head of the femur may displace upward on the ilium, or if the hip is flexed to a greater degree, it may fall into the sciatic notch of the pelvis injuring the sciatic nerve. Posterior dislocation usually produces shortening, internal rotation, and adduction of the femur.

Less frequently, anterior dislocation is produced by a violent twisting injury with the thigh in extreme abduction. This mechanism forces the head over the shallow inferior rim of the acetabulum and through the joint capsule. Rotational force then dislocates the head forward, where it may come to lie in the obturator foramen or be displaced upward onto the pubis. The leg is usually externally rotated and abducted, but shortening may be absent.

The final resting place of the head determines the classification of the dislocation. Thus, the dislocation may be posterior iliac or sciatic, or anterior pubic or obturator. Central dislocation occurs when the floor of the acetabulum fractures and the head of the femur is driven into the pelvis.

Reduction is accomplished by reversing the forces that produced the dislocation. Several manipulative procedures have been described by Allis, Bigelow, and Stimson. The method of Allis is most commonly used and is performed with the patient supine. The hip and knee are flexed and the thigh is adducted. Longitudinal traction is made behind the bent knee. Gentle internal and external rotation movements are performed until the head of the femur slips into the acetabulum. When no fracture is present, the reduction is usually accompanied by a snap and is stable. When the posterior rim of the acetabulum is fractured, the head of the femur may slide easily into the acetabulum, and it may be difficult to tell when the dislocation is reduced. The hip is then extended and abducted and externally rotated moderately. A plaster hip spica cast is applied to prevent redislocation and is maintained for 3 weeks or longer. If the acetabular fragment cannot be replaced and the hip is stable, the dislocation is treated similarly. However, if the dislocation is unstable, it may be necessary to fasten the fragment into position with screws during open reduction.

Anterior dislocations are reduced by traction in a similar position of flexion at the hip and knee.

The femur is slowly abducted to near 90 degrees. This brings the head of the femur downward near the inferior acetabular notch. Internal rotation is performed gently when the thigh is adducted and extended, forcing the head of the bone through the inferior rent in the capsule. Immobilization may be accomplished by strapping the legs together to prevent abduction and external rotation for 3 weeks.

After reduction and immobilization of either anterior or posterior dislocation, the patient should use crutches for at least 2 months from the time of dislocation. Active exercise of the hip, thigh, and leg should be done regularly to rehabilitate the muscles and regain joint motion.

Aseptic necrosis of the head of the femur follows this injury all too frequently. For this reason, the patient should remain on crutches for 2 months after the dislocation. During this time, disuse atrophy of the adjacent bone may reveal the relative increase in density of the head of the femur, indicating aseptic necrosis, on x-ray examination. When necrosis of the head of the femur is established, bone grafting is done to re-establish the blood supply. Additional reconstructive procedures may be necessary if necrosis continues, or if it occurs later with the development of arthritis of the joint.

## THE FEMUR

### Fractures of the Shaft of the Femur

Fractures of the shaft of the femur are classified by location, since the displacing pull of muscles, and thus the deformity produced, varies with the level at which the fracture occurs. These areas are the subtrochanteric, or upper one-third of the femoral shaft, the middle segment, and the supracondylar and condylar area of the bone.

The abductors, flexors, and external rotator muscles are unopposed when the femur breaks in the upper one-third, and the proximal fragment assumes this position of abduction, flexion, and external rotation. The distal fragment is pulled medially and angulated laterally by the action of the adductor magnus inserting along the entire medial femoral shaft. The quadriceps and hamstring muscles produce shortening.

Fractures in the midportion of the bone have a similar deformity but the external rotation and abduction of the proximal fragment is less, since more of the adductor musculature is attached to this fragment.

Supracondylar fractures are influenced primarily by the gastrocnemius muscles, which pull the distal fragment posteriorly. The long thigh muscles attaching below the knee cause shortening.

**Fractures of the Upper and Middle Thirds of the Femur.** Problems relating to fractures of the upper and middle thirds of the femur are similar in many respects. In fractures of the upper third of the femur, the two fragments are subject to characteristic deformities from the pull of strong muscle groups. The proximal fragment is abducted by the gluteal muscles, flexed by the iliopsoas, and rotated by the external rotators; it assumes a flexed, externally rotated, and abducted position. At the same time, the adductor muscles, assisted by the hamstrings and quadriceps muscle group, cause shortening and medial displacement of the distal fragment. The reduction is accomplished by traction on the distal fragment with the knee

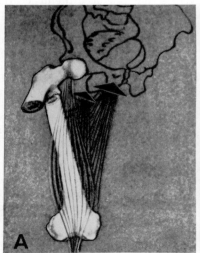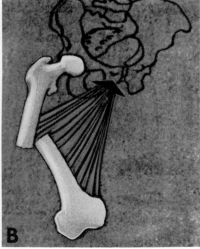

**Figure 26**  *A,* The proximal upper one-third fragment of the femur is abducted, externally rotated, and flexed by the action of the abductor, external rotator, and iliopsoas muscle groups. The distal fragment of the femur is adducted and shortened by the action of the adductor and hamstring muscles, as well as the rectus femoris. The distal femoral fragment must be abducted, flexed, and externally rotated to align it with the proximal fragment. *B,* Fractures of the midshaft of the femur angulate and shorten, as do fractures of the upper one-third; however, abduction of the proximal fragment is less, since part of the adductor muscle system remains attached to this fragment.

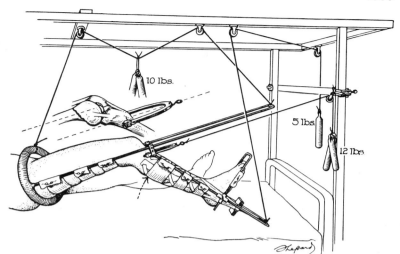

**Figure 27** The Thomas splint with Pearson attachment is used for suspension of femoral fractures. Skeletal traction is made through the upper tibia.

flexed to relax the hamstring muscles. The distal fragment is abducted to align it with the proximal fragment and externally rotated as much as necessary to effect proper alignment (Fig. 26).

If the fracture occurs in the middle of the shaft, there is frequently a similar angulation and shortening. However, the displacement of the proximal fragment is less since more of the adductor muscles are attached to it. The fracture is reduced in the same manner as one occurring higher on the femur.

The problem of reducing these fractures is of small moment compared with the problems of maintaining the reduction. Probably the most useful device for maintaining reduction is the Thomas splint with the Pearson attachment. Traction is frequently skeletal. A pin or wire through the upper end of the tibia, or through the distal end of the femur, allows traction to be made by pulling directly on the bone (Fig. 27). In addition to providing suspension and traction, the apparatus can be adjusted to control abduction, flexion, and rotation.

These fractures usually require at least 10 to 12 weeks for healing. Because of this prolonged time in bed, open reduction with internal fixation is often done. The method that has become popular since World War II is the Küntscher intramedullary rod. Properly applied, the method immobilizes fractures of the midportion of the bone well, and allows early ambulation and mobilization of the joint.

**Supracondylar Fractures of the Femur.** Supracondylar fractures present a different set of problems from those occurring higher on the femur. The distal fragment is usually pulled backward by the force of the gastrocnemius and hamstring muscles. At the same time, the contraction of the quadriceps, which is attached to the tibia, tends to make the fragments override (Fig. 28). The bone ends may threaten the popliteal nerves and vessels with resulting paralysis or massive hemorrhage.

Reduction demands relaxation of the gastrocnemius muscle. To accomplish this, the knee is flexed 90 degrees and the foot is plantar flexed. Traction is then made in the long axis of the femur. The bone ends are manipulated by direct pressure of the surgeon's hands. Maintenance of reduction is best accomplished by suspension skeletal traction. Open reduction with internal fixation is occasionally necessary. These fractures usually heal in 10 to 12 weeks. Knee motion should be started early in the course of treatment to prevent adhesions within the joint.

### Fractures and Epiphyseal Displacement of the Femur in Children

Fractures of the femur in children are classified as upper, middle, and lower one-third injuries. Slipped or displaced femoral epiphyses may involve these structures at the proximal or distal end of the bone. At puberty, slipping and dis-

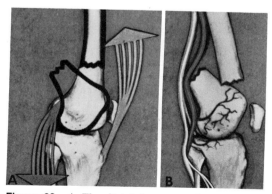

**Figure 28** *A*, The distal fragment of supracondylar fracture of the femur angulates posteriorly because the gastrocnemius muscle arises upon the condyles and pulls the fragment backward. *B*, The displacement of the distal fragment may damage the popliteal nerves and blood vessels.

placement of the epiphysis of the head of the femur is a definite and not uncommon syndrome.

Displacement of the head of the femur through the epiphyseal plate may occur with a single acute, twisting injury, but often the process is slow and insidious. The condition occurs most often in obese male children at or about puberty. Characteristically, the head of the femur rotates backward and downward while the neck rotates forward. In the acute injury, pain and limitation of motion are obvious, and x-ray examination readily reveals the displacement. When gradual slipping occurs, the only symptom may be a painless limp, and meticulous roentgenologic examination may be necessary to detect the beginning displacement. The degree of displacement in either case determines the details of treatment.

The acute, traumatic, slipped, proximal femoral epiphysis should be replaced by traction and internal rotation in moderate abduction. The reduction may be maintained by a spica hip cast, or by internal fixation with pins of small diameter. Often the epiphyseal plate closes after the injury and growth ceases. When this does not occur, the hip must be protected from weight bearing for months or recurrence of the deformity is common.

Gradual slipping of the proximal epiphysis is called adolescent coxa vara. The etiology is not clear. The symptoms may be minimal. The condition is often bilateral. The surgeon must watch the opposite hip carefully for signs of displacement until the epiphysis has closed. The treatment may be conservative or surgical, and the choice depends upon the degree of deformity and the stage of development when the condition is discovered. If the slipping is minimal but acute, internal fixation with multiple small-diameter pins may be done to prevent increasing deformity. When the deformity is found later, the epiphyseal plate may be closing. The small deformity is accepted. It may be necessary to correct more pronounced deformity by osteotomy of the neck or subtrochanteric region, followed by appropriate internal fixation. Weight must not be borne until the epiphysis closes.

**Fractures of the Femoral Neck in Children.** Fractures of the neck of the femur are rare in children. The prognosis is poor, as it is in the adult. Nonunion, coxa vara, and aseptic necrosis are frequent complications. Reduction with internal fixation with small pins is usually necessary, and is one of the few instances when internal fixation is indicated in the child. Healing may require many months, and weight bearing cannot be resumed until union is firm.

**Fractures about the Trochanters and Upper Third of the Femur in Children.** Fractures between the trochanters, or at the level of the lesser trochanter, are usually oblique or transverse. The deforming pull of the muscles produces coxa vara. It must be remembered by the surgeon that deformity produced by fractures above the lesser trochanter is not corrected with growth. Any deformity that results from the fracture is permanent. Every effort should be made to correct the coxa vara deformity.

**Fractures of the Middle Third of the Femur in Children.** Fracture of the middle third of the shaft of the femur occurs in all age groups of children, and this is the common location of femoral fractures in infants. In young children the fracture line tends to be transverse or oblique. In older children approaching puberty, particularly those over the age of 13 years, the fractures tend to resemble those in the adult. The deformity produced is similar to that in the adult.

Reduction and maintenance of reduction is best done by continuous traction. Rotational alignment must be accurate, but slight angulation may be acceptable in younger children, because it is corrected with growth. Shortening, or side-to-side apposition, is desirable in younger children. Stimulation of longitudinal growth always takes place following this fracture, and end-to-end apposition always results in a longer leg, which is just as undesirable as one too short.

In infants and children up to the age of 4 years, Bryant's overhead suspension traction is often used. The child should not weigh more than 40 pounds if this method is employed. Both legs must be suspended by skin traction from an overhead frame. Sufficient traction is applied to lift the buttocks just off the bed. A restraint is used about the trunk to help maintain alignment. Sufficient traction is usually produced to overcome angulation, but it allows some overriding of the fragments. When Bryant's traction is used, the patient must be watched carefully for signs of skin irritation and circulatory embarrassment. Circulatory im-

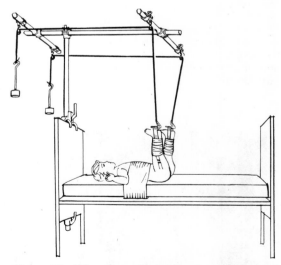

**Figure 29** When Bryant's traction is used for treatment of fractures of the femur in childhood, both legs should be suspended. In addition, skin traction should not encircle the leg, as this may contribute to strangulation of the circulation. Volkmann's ischemic contracture can result when traction is applied improperly. Catastrophic circulatory failure may occur if the patient is not watched every hour. (From Schmeisser, G., Jr.: Clinical Manual of Orthopedic Traction Techniques. Philadelphia, W. B. Saunders Company, 1963.)

pairment seems to occur more readily in the un-fractured leg, and can lead to Volkmann's contracture or catastrophic gangrene. Should signs of circulatory embarrassment develop, the constriction must be removed immediately (Fig. 29).

Children over the age of 4 years and weighing more than 40 pounds are best treated in the Russell suspension traction. Suspension and traction must be maintained until union is firm. In the infant, this time may be as short as 3 weeks, but becomes longer in older children.

Open reduction of shaft fractures of the femur in children is practically never indicated and internal fixation is to be condemned.

**Fractures of the Lower Third of the Femur in Children.** Fractures in the lower one-third of the bone may require traction with the extremity placed in 90 degrees of flexion of the hip and knee to prevent posterior angulation. This may be accomplished by modified Russell traction. Care must be exercised to prevent injury to the peroneal nerve.

**Slipped Lower Femoral Epiphysis in Children.** Slipping of the lower femoral epiphysis is usually produced by forces that hyperextend the knee. The epiphysis is displaced and angulated forward on the metaphysis. Medial or lateral displacement may accompany this major deformity. As in the case of supracondylar fractures in the adult, the displacement may damage the popliteal vessels and nerves. Prompt manipulative reduction is needed. Traction is made on the bent knee while pressure is made backward on the epiphysis and forward on the metaphysis. If the manipulation is unsuccessful and circulatory failure is impending, open reduction with gentle replacement of the epiphysis is warranted. The periosteum must not be stripped from the bone near the epiphyseal plate during the process, as growth arrest may result. The leg is placed in a plaster cast following reduction with the knees in moderate flexion and maintained in this position for 3 or 4 weeks. If the displacement cannot be corrected when the injury is found after several days, open reduction should not be done, because at this stage forceful manipulation will only increase the danger of growth arrest. The knee is immobilized and growth of the bone is allowed to correct the deformity. If the deformity is not corrected with growth, osteotomy may be done later.

Partial growth arrest of the epiphysis may result in knock-knee or bowleg deformity. In young children, it may be necessary to correct this by repeated osteotomy. In older children, when most of the growth of the extremity has been obtained, completion of the closure of the epiphyseal plate with correction of the deformity may be done surgically. A slight amount of shortening is acceptable, but the remaining growth potential in the opposite leg must be carefully estimated before this is done.

## THE KNEE JOINT

The stability of the knee depends upon an intricate set of ligaments, functioning synchronously with the activating muscles. These ligaments allow the hingelike action of flexion and extension, but prevent forward, backward, and side-to-side movement. The surrounding muscles and their tendons provide stability in varying degrees of flexion and extension. The rounded condyles of the femur, resting upon the two saucer-like plateaus of the tibia, provide minimal bony contact, ensuring friction-free movement. The patella, articulating with the femur between the condyles, acts like a pulley, increasing the power of the extensor muscles. Normal function depends upon the synchronous action of all of these parts. Injuries to any one of the components affects the others.

### Fractures of the Femoral Condyles

Fractures of the femoral condyles are produced by indirect compression force transmitted up the leg, or by force causing lateral or medial deviation, or by direct violence. One or both condyles may break. The fracture line usually runs from the superior portion of the condyle downward into the intracondylar notch; when both condyles are fractured, the fracture line may be Y- or T-shaped. When one condyle is fractured, it is usually driven upward and outward by the force producing the fracture. This produces a knock-knee or bowleg deformity, depending upon which condyle is broken. The fragment is then rotated backward by the downward pull of the gastrocnemius muscle. If the force continues, the leg deviates to such a degree that the collateral ligaments are damaged by stretching. The popliteal nerves and vessels may be endangered by sharp fragments of bone displaced into this area. Circulation and the status of the nerves must be determined before reduction is attempted.

Since the ligaments and joint capsule remain attached to the fragment, these structures are used to exert traction on the condyle in reduction. The opposite condyle acts as a fulcrum, as force is applied deviating the leg to correct the deformity. If the lateral femoral condyle is fractured, the medial one serves as the fulcrum. The tibia is angulated toward the midline of the body while pressure is exerted laterally against the medial lower femur. This manipulation pulls the displaced condyle downward. If the fragment remains laterally displaced, widening the condyles, it is forced back into position by compressing the condyles with the surgeon's hands or a C clamp. The knee is then flexed to relax the pull of the gastrocnemius, and by direct manipulation the backward displacement is corrected. Fractures of the medial condyle are reduced by the same method, with the forces applied in the opposite direction.

Since the femoral condyles are not spheres but are elongated from front to back, and the medial one is larger than the lateral, accurate replacement of the fracture is essential if the joint is to function properly. Backward rotation of one condyle disturbs the axis of flexion and extension, and some of the motion will be lost.

Immobilization in a long leg cast, molded to

maintain the leg in the corrected position, may hold a stable fracture in position. The unstable fracture may require suspension traction or operation securing the fragment to the femur with internal fixation.

### Intracondylar Fractures

Most often, both condyles are fractured from the shaft of the femur. Considerable force is necessary to produce the fracture and comminution of the bone is commonplace. The force producing the fracture drives the condyles upward. The bone splits at the intracondylar notch. The fracture lines then run upward or transversely to form a Y or T. As the force continues, the condyles are displaced upward; the shaft of the femur acts like a wedge forcing them apart. The pull of the quadriceps and hamstring muscles maintains the shortening. The gastrocnemius may rotate the fragments posteriorly. The neurovascular structures are threatened.

Reduction is accomplished by traction and manipulation making use of the intact ligaments and joint capsule. Traction is made in the long axis of the femur with the knee flexed to relax the gastrocnemius. As the fragments are pulled downward by the traction exerted through the collateral ligaments, they are molded together by compression. Maintenance of reduction must be obtained by suspension skeletal traction through the upper tibia. When comminution is not severe, open reduction may be done when the fracture cannot be accurately reduced by closed methods.

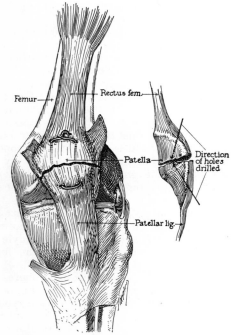

Femur — Rectus fem.
Patella — Direction of holes drilled
Patellar lig.

**Figure 30** Separated fractures of the patella must be reduced by open methods and held by internal fixation. The extensor retinaculum must be repaired.

These fractures heal in 8 to 12 weeks, but weight bearing must not be allowed until the union is complete. Motion, however, must be started as early as possible.

### Fractures of the Patella

A patella can be fractured by indirect or by direct violence. In a fall, the patient may have the good fortune to land on his feet. He is betrayed, however, by a tensed quadriceps muscle acting on a partially flexed knee. The indirect force of the muscle contraction causes the fracture. If the force is continued, the retinaculum tears and the patellar fragments separate. The extensor mechanism is disrupted. The patella may survive this hazard, to be fractured by the force of the direct blow as the knee strikes the ground. There may be a simple fracture with little displacement of the fragments if the anterior capsule is not torn. Often, however, there are varying degrees of comminution in the fractures caused by direct violence.

Treatment is directed toward the re-establishment of the extensor mechanism and the creation of a smooth, anatomically accurate articular surface for the patella. When the fracture is transverse or longitudinal without separation, the extensor mechanism remains intact through the retinaculum. This situation can be treated conservatively. The leg should be kept in full extension. A posterior splint will provide the needed immobilization. Almost all fractures of the knee are accompanied by an effusion of blood and synovial fluid into the joint. Aspiration under local anesthesia contributes to the patient's comfort. If a cast is applied, it should extend from the ankle to the groin. The patient whose leg is thus immobilized may start weight bearing as soon as the cast is dry. The cast is bivalved within a week, and active flexion and extension exercises are begun.

When there is separation of the two major fragments of the patella, the damage can be repaired only through operative treatment. The patella is fitted accurately together and held by a wire suture placed through or around the fragments. The retinaculum is repaired. Following repair, a cylinder cast or posterior molded splint is applied. Weight bearing may be started as soon as the patient is comfortable. Active motion is started as soon as the wound has healed, usually within a week or 10 days. However, the posterior splint is used for at least 3 weeks while the tendon and retinaculum heal (Fig. 30).

The fall that damages a patella may cause such comminution that the fragments cannot be repaired surgically to produce a smooth articular surface. It may be advisable to excise the patella entirely. This procedure impairs the function of the knee less than the presence of a badly damaged patella.

### Fractures of the Tibial Plateau

These fractures may involve one or both condyles of the tibia; however, the most frequent is the fracture of the lateral plateau. In fractures of the

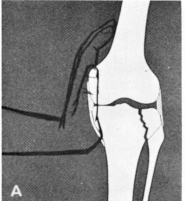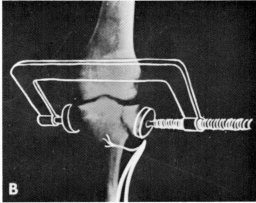

**Figure 31** *A,* When a large single fragment of the tibial plateau is depressed, it may be reduced by using the medial condyle as a fulcrum. Pressure is made on the medial aspect of the knee while the tibia is deviated medially. The joint capsule is pulled tightly, drawing the condyle upward. *B,* The laterally displaced fragment is then forced medially with a C-shaped clamp.

lateral plateau, a blow to the lateral side of the leg forces the knee into valgus or knock-knee position. The medial collateral ligament and cruciates may rupture. If they hold, they produce a fulcrum upon which the lateral femoral condyle acts as a wedge against the lateral tibial plateau, forcing it downward. The articular surface is almost always involved.

Less frequently, a similar fracture occurs in the medial tibial condyle, usually the result of a fall with the knee in the varus or bowed position.

With a fall from a height, the tibia is driven upward against the femoral condyles, the flaring tibial articular surface is compressed. Occasionally, the fracture lines may resemble an inverted T.

All of these fractures produce some damage to the articular surface of the tibia and medial or lateral instability with disturbance of the weight-bearing line. Often, there is some damage to the collateral or cruciate ligaments, and frequently the semilunar cartilages are torn and displaced. Treatment must re-establish as level and smooth an articular surface as possible, free from internal derangement.

When a single large fragment is present, reduction may be accomplished by forcing the knee into the opposite position from the deformity. The displaced fragment is then forced medially by compression with a C clamp. The leg is immobilized in a long leg cast from the uppermost thigh to the toes. The force of reduction is maintained as the plaster sets (Fig. 31).

If the fragment cannot be maintained in reduction, the fracture site should be opened and internal fixation used to hold the fragments securely. Often the central articular surface of the lateral tibial condyle is depressed into the cancellous bone.

With severe depression and disruption of the joint surface, open reduction may be necessary to create stability. Motion must be started early to prevent intra-articular adhesions; however, the joint should be immobilized in extension for 2 or 3 weeks in a cast or splint to allow the reaction to the operation to subside and the fragments to be stabilized with fibrous tissue. Weight bearing cannot be allowed until firm union is present, or compression of the condyle will cause recurrence of the deformity.

### Dislocations of the Knee Joint

Dislocations of the knee joint are produced by extreme direct or indirect violence. The dislocations are classified by the displacement of the tibia on the femur; thus, anterior, posterior, medial, and lateral dislocations describe the location of the tibia in relationship to the femur. The medial, lateral, collateral, and cruciate ligaments, along with the joint capsule, must be torn to allow dislocation. Tearing and displacement of the semilunar cartilage may accompany the injury, producing symptoms of internal derangement of the joint following reduction. The popliteal nerves and vessels may be damaged by any dislocation of the knee, as may the peroneal nerve. Impairment of circulation demands immediate reduction. Occasionally, torn joint capsule or displaced hamstring tendons may fold into the joint or catch in the intracondylar notch and prevent reduction.

Reduction of posterior and medial or lateral dislocations is usually best accomplished with the knee flexed to relax the hamstring muscles. Traction is made on the tibia in the flexed position. The dislocations are usually easily reduced, but are unstable because of the torn ligaments. In recent years, immediate surgical repair of the torn ligaments has been advocated for damage to these structures by sprains, subluxations, and dislocations of the knee. The end results have been more stable, useful knees when immediate ligament repair is done. Cast immobilization for 3 weeks is followed by vigorous active exercise to re-establish motion and restore the power of the muscles.

The quadriceps muscle must be brought to maximal efficiency by means of early active exercise to provide stability of the knee.

## THE TIBIA AND FIBULA

### Fractures of the Shaft of the Tibia and Fibula

The shape and subcutaneous location of the tibia in the leg make this bone particularly vulnerable to injury. Fractures at the junction of the middle and lower one-third of the tibia are common. The bone on the anteromedial surface is covered only with skin and subcutaneous tissue. Direct trauma or angulation easily produces open fractures.

The tibia is well supplied with blood near the knee and ankle. The blood supply to the midsection of the bone, however, is scanty. The precarious blood supply to the distal one-half of the shaft of the tibia makes for slow healing. The incidence of delayed healing and nonunion is high.

As in the forearm, the muscles are confined within tight fascial compartments. Volkmann's ischemic contracture is an ever present danger and occurs much more frequently than is realized. The peroneal nerve, winding about the proximal end of the fibula, lies superficially. It is easily injured by a direct blow. The muscles of the leg lie parallel to the bone on the posterior and lateral aspect. They produce shortening and slight anterior angulation of the fracture fragments of the tibia (Fig. 32).

Fractures of the tibia and fibula may involve one or both bones. The force may be indirect violence such as a twisting injury or a fall from a height, or direct violence such as that encountered when an automobile bumper strikes the leg. Indirect-violence fractures are usually coupled with a twisting force, producing a spiral or oblique fracture of the bone. Direct-violence fractures may be simple, transverse, or comminuted and segmental fractures. If only one bone breaks, the other acts as an internal splint, and shortening is minimal; however, angulation of an objectionable degree may occur.

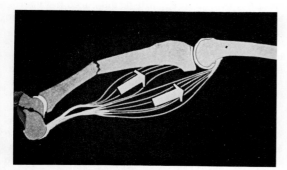

**Figure 32** The triceps surae group of muscles lies posterior to the tibia and produces anterior angulation of the fragments. Flexing the knee and foot helps to relax this muscle and lessens the angulating force.

### Fractures of the Fibula

Isolated fractures of the fibula usually occur from a direct blow or from injuries associated with the ankle joint. Since the bone does not transmit body weight, and since it is firmly bound to the tibia by the interosseous membrane, shaft fractures are usually displaced only slightly. When the stability of the ankle joint is not impaired, treatment of the fracture is simple. Reduction is seldom necessary. An Ace bandage and crutches are all that are needed until the pain subsides, when full weight bearing may be resumed.

Fractures that involve the peroneal nerve at the upper portion of the bone are usually stable. The damage is done at the time of injury and treatment of the bone has little effect upon nerve recovery. The dorsiflexor and peroneal muscles, however, must be protected from overstretching with a dropfoot brace while the nerve recovers. A walking cast may provide some stability and comfort, and allow the patient to move about.

### Fractures of the Upper Third of the Tibia

Fractures just below the condyles are often caused by direct violence. The automobile bumper is ideally suited to produce this fracture. Displacement depends upon the direction of the force administered to the bone. Comminution of fragments is common and open wounds often accompany the injury. The fracture is often stable if marked comminution is not present. Usually, the force that fractures the tibia also breaks the fibula. This force may damage the peroneal nerve. The status of the nerve should be established by testing the power of the dorsiflexors of the foot and toes before reduction is attempted. Reduction is usually accompanied by traction and manipulation followed by immobilization in a long leg cast. The prognosis for healing is usually good.

### Fractures of the Middle and Lower Thirds of the Tibia

When the fibula remains intact, an internal splint is present. This usually prevents shortening, but angulation and displacement may be present. When both bones break, the fractures may be stable if the fracture is transverse or there are jagged edges on the tibial fragments that may be engaged during reduction to provide longitudinal stability. The closer the fracture is to the ends of the bone, the greater will be the effect of the angulation on joint alignment. Thus, a fracture 3 inches above the ankle may angulate to a much greater degree than one in the midshaft with a similar displacement. This principle is true for all long-bone fractures.

If longitudinal stability is present, or can be created by end-to-end reduction, shortening of the bone is not a problem. However, angulation and rotation must be corrected by manipulation. When reduction has been accomplished, a plaster cast is applied from the toe to just below the knee. Rotational alignment is then checked by extending the knee to 45 degrees. A line drawn from the anterior

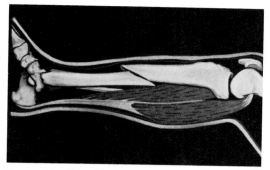

**Figure 33** Unstable fractures shorten and angulate because of the pull of the triceps surae muscles. Continuous traction may be necessary to neutralize the muscle pull.

iliac spine through the patella to the foot should pass between the first and second toes. The cast is then extended above the knee to the upper thigh, with the knee in 20 to 30 degrees of flexion. Rotational alignment can be maintained only in the long leg cast with the knee bent.

### Unstable Fractures of the Tibia and Fibula

Unstable fractures of the tibia and fibula are usually spiral, oblique, comminuted, or segmental. One reduction of these fractures followed by plaster cast immobilization may be tried. If the reduction cannot be maintained, some form of traction or internal fixation may be necessary (Fig. 33). Since healing is slow and nonunion is frequent in middle and lower one-third fractures, many surgeons add bone grafts obtained from the ilium at the time of open reduction. Nonunion is not uncommon and is treated by appropriate bone grafting.

### Tibial Fractures in Children

Fractures of the tibia in children vary with the age of the child. In infants and children up to about 6 years, the most frequent fracture is spiral in nature in the middle or lower one-third of the bone. The injury is produced by a twist to the bone and may occur when the child catches his foot between the bars of the crib. The fibula usually is not broken and provides an internal splint. Displacement is usually minimal and cast immobilization for a few weeks may be the only treatment required. In children from 6 to 13 years of age, the fractures tend to be transverse, caused by direct violence. Both bones may be broken. Reduction and cast immobilization usually produce satisfactory results.

## THE ANKLE

The ankle joint is one of the most frequently injured areas of the body. Since it is the connecting link between the stable leg bones and the mobile foot, it is subjected to a great variety of forces in walking, running, and standing. Abnormal or

excessive forces produce injuries to the bones and ligaments, usually by indirect violence. Fractures about the ankle are classified according to the force that produces them. The talus may be rotated medially or laterally, inverted or everted, pushed backward or forward or medially or laterally, or compressed directly upward. A combination of these forces may take place, producing a variety of fractures, dislocations, and sprains. Since the malleoli are attached to the talus by the joint capsule and collateral ligaments, the fragments follow the displacement of the foot on the leg bones. An understanding of the mechanism of the fracture and the anatomy involved is essential for intelligent management of these injuries. Reduction is based upon reversal of the forces that produced the fracture.

### External Rotation Fractures

External rotation fractures of the lateral malleolus are among the most frequent ankle fractures. In a fall, the talus is rotated on its long axis laterally or the leg bones are rotated medially. The lateral anterior border of the talus impinges against the anterior articular surface of the fibula. The fibula is twisted in its long axis by this force. The deltoid ligament is stretched while the anterior tibiofibular ligament is torn. The fibula then breaks in a spiral manner at the malleolus. The shaft of the fibula maintains its relationship to the tibia while the malleolar fragment follows the foot into external rotation. If the force continues, the deltoid ligament may rupture, allowing the talus to displace laterally on the tibia (Figs. 34 and 35). If rotary force is coupled with lateral displacement of the talus, the ligaments binding the fibula to the tibia along with the deltoid ligament may tear without fracture of the malleoli. This mechanism produces a diastasis between the tibia and fibula, widening the ankle mortise.

Reduction is accomplished by applying the re-

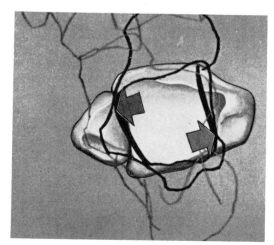

**Figure 34** External rotation of the talus in the ankle mortise forces the lateral border of the talus against the lateral malleolus.

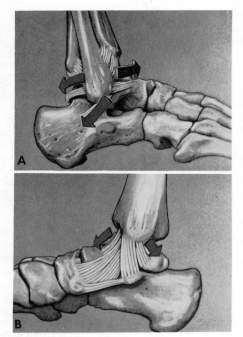

**Figure 35** *A,* As the external rotation force continues, the fibula breaks in a spiral manner and is rotated outward. If the force continues, the deltoid ligament ruptures and the talus may displace laterally. *B,* Reduction is accomplished by medial rotation of the talus. The collateral ligament attaching to the talus pulls the fragment into position.

verse of the force that produced the fracture. The foot is internally rotated on the long axis of the tibia and displaced medially. Since the lateral collateral ligament attaches the distal fragment to the talus, it pulls the fragment into position as the talus is replaced in the ankle mortise. Frequently, the deltoid ligament stretches but does not tear completely. When this occurs, spontaneous reduction may take place when the force producing the fracture abates. X-ray examinations in this instance reveal the fracture of the fibular malleolus

without displacement. The fracture may be quite stable.

Immobilization is accomplished with a cast extending from the toes to the knee if the fracture is stable, but if on examination the fibular fragment rotates easily into the displaced position, the cast should extend above the bent knee to prevent the rotation. Weight may be borne on a walking heel as soon as the pain subsides. The fracture usually heals sufficiently in 6 weeks to allow removal of the cast.

### Eversion or Abduction Fractures

Eversion or abduction fractures are produced by forces that displace the foot in this direction or displace the leg bones in the opposite direction on the foot fixed to the ground. The talus, tipping in the ankle mortise, is forced against the lateral malleolus, which breaks transversely, usually near or above the joint line. If it remains intact, traction on the medial malleolus by the ligament may produce a transverse avulsion fracture of the medial malleolus at or below the joint line. Such a fracture is called a bimalleolar fracture. If the force continues, the talus may dislocate completely from the tibia, carrying the fracture fragments with it. The tendons of leg muscles follow the foot and tend to hold the foot in the displaced position (Fig. 36).

Reduction is accomplished by longitudinal traction to overcome the shortening produced by the muscles of the leg. The foot is then forced medially and inverted. If the medial malleolus has remained intact, or is fractured below the joint line, the talus is forced against this buttress of bone, so that the lateral displacement is reduced. Inversion of the foot pulls the lateral malleolar fragment downward and inward through the intact collateral ligament. The ruptured deltoid ligament usually falls into position. However, if the tibial malleolus has been fractured, it must be forced upward by the hands of the surgeon to secure reduction. The foot is held in neutral dorsiflexion and plantar flexion.

If the fracture of the medial malleolus occurs at

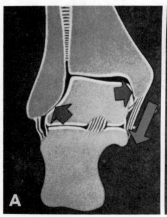
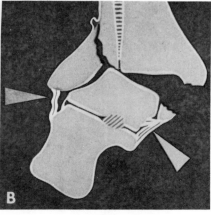

**Figure 36** *A,* Eversion or abduction fractures are produced by the wedging action of the talus against the malleoli. *B,* The talus forced against the lateral malleolus produces the fibular fracture, while traction on the deltoid pulls the medial malleolus from the tibia. If the force continues, the talus may dislocate.

the joint line, the buttress of bone is lost, and the talus may be displaced too far medially. This is an unstable fracture and may require internal fixation of the medial malleolus to re-establish stability. A cast extending above the flexed knee is molded to maintain the force of reduction. Since the medial malleolus heals more slowly than the lateral, immobilization is necessary for 8 to 12 weeks (Fig. 37).

Often a fold of periosteum and ligament is interposed into the medial malleolar fracture. This tissue prevents accurate replacement of the malleolus. Open reduction is then necessary, as nonunion almost always occurs.

### Trimalleolar Fractures

The same mechanism of abduction fracture when coupled with posterior and upward displacement of the talus may cause a fracture of the posterior lateral articular surface of the tibia in addition to the malleolar fractures. The fragment is displaced upward and posteriorly. It is called a trimalleolar fracture. Varying amounts of the tibial articular surface are involved—only the posterior lip of the bone or a third or more of the posterolateral articular surface. The amount of bone and the degree of displacement dictate the treatment. If less than one-fourth of the posterior articular surface is involved in the fracture, there still remains an adequate stable weight-bearing surface on the tibia. However, if more than this amount of bone is displaced, accurate replacement is essential, as instability and irregular joint sur-

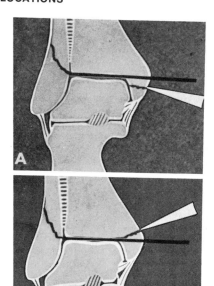

**Figure 37** *A,* If the medial malleolus is fractured below the joint line, the remaining portion acts as a buttress for stable reduction. *B,* If the fracture is above the joint line, the buttress effect is lost and the reduction may be unstable.

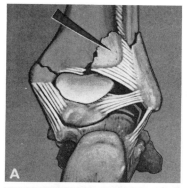

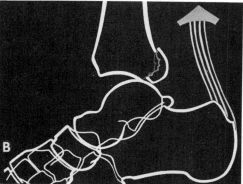

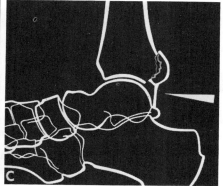

**Figure 38** *A,* A triangular fragment of bone may be fractured posterolaterally from the tibia. *B,* The fragment is displaced backward and upward as the talus is pulled backward by the triceps surae. *C,* The foot is pulled forward and dorsiflexed to make traction on the fragment through the joint capsule.

face will eventually cause traumatic arthritis (Fig. 38).

Following reduction of the malleolar fractures, the foot is pulled forward and placed in dorsiflexion. Since the posterior joint capsule is attached to this fragment, traction is made on the fragment by the joint capsule as the reduction is carried out. This position must be maintained during the immobilization period. When more than one-fourth of the articular surface is fractured and cannot be anatomically replaced, open reduction with internal fixation is necessary.

### Inversion or Adduction Fractures

Inversion or adduction fractures are produced by forces that force the foot into this position or the leg bones laterally on the inverted fixed foot. The talus acts as a wedge against the medial malleolus and produces a fracture, usually at the joint line. The fracture line runs upward and medially. The foot is displaced in this direction, depending upon the degree of the force. The lateral collateral ligament stretches, ruptures, or avulses the lateral malleolus, usually below the joint line. Dislocation may be complete. Contraction of the leg muscles maintains the displacement (Fig. 39).

As in other fractures about the ankle, reduction is accomplished by reversal of this force. Traction is made in the long axis of the leg while the foot is displaced laterally and everted. If the fibula fracture is below the joint line, it will afford a stable lateral wall against which the talus may be fixed. However, if it fractures above this point, the reduction will be unstable and the medial malleolus may require internal fixation to maintain reduction.

### Comminuted Fractures

Direct compression forces, such as a fall from a height, produce comminuted fractures of the articular surface of the tibia. The talus acts as a wedge, forcing the articular surface of the tibia upward and the malleoli apart. Comminution is often ex-

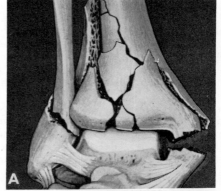
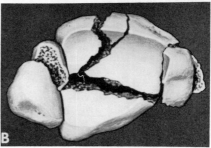

**Figure 40** Compression fractures of the tibial articular surface usually produce marked comminution and damage to the joint. *A*, Lateral view. *B*, Inferior view.

treme. The foot may be displaced in any direction. Since the major forces are directly upward against the tibia, the joint capsule remains, for the most part, intact.

Reduction is accomplished by traction on the foot with appropriate manipulation to align the major fragments. Often central articular fragments are driven upward and impacted in the

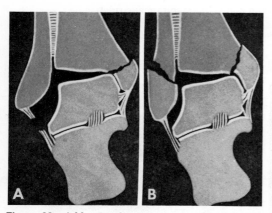

**Figure 39** Adduction fractures are produced by forces that tip the talus against the medial malleolus. *A*, Fracture of the medial malleolus occurs at the joint line and runs upward. *B*, The fibular collateral ligament may rupture, or may cause the fibula to fracture.

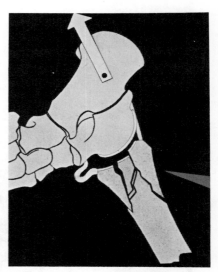

**Figure 41** Traction is made through the joint capsule and must be maintained while union occurs. A central fragment may remain displaced.

cancellous bone of the tibia. No amount of traction or manipulation can bring these isolated fragments into alignment, and a rough joint surface is inevitable in many instances (Fig. 40). Traction through the os calcis by skeletal means is usually necessary. Immobilization is usually necessary for 3 months and weight must not be borne upon the joint until union is complete in 3 to 6 months (Fig. 41).

It is surprising how often a joint that has been destroyed by this fracture may function well for varying periods. Eventually, however, traumatic arthritis produces a painful joint, and arthrodesis is often necessary.

## THE FOOT

### Fractures of the Body of the Talus

Fractures of the talus may involve the body or neck of the bone. Since the majority of the body is cartilage-covered, this adds strength to this part of the talus, and fractures are not common. However, falls from a height may occasionally compress the bone between the os calcis and the tibia, producing vertical or longitudinal fractures. There is usually little displacement with this type fracture; however, with extreme violence, the posterior fragments may be squeezed out of the ankle mortise.

Reduction is accomplished by heavy traction on the foot in neutral position with the knee flexed to relax the triceps surae muscles. The posterior fragment may be manipulated by direct pressure accompanied by slight dorsiflexion of the foot to open up the posterior joint space. If anatomic reduction cannot be achieved, and the fracture involves two large pieces of bone, open reduction with internal screw fixation should be done.

### Fractures of the Neck of the Talus

Fractures of the neck of the talus are usually the result of a fall in which the foot is forced into extreme dorsiflexion. The anterior lip of the tibia acts as a fulcrum on the neck as maximal dorsiflexion is reached. The force shears the neck vertically from the body of the talus and displaces the head of the bone upward. Displacement may be minimal; however, the consequences of this fracture may be serious. The major blood supply to the bone enters through a series of nutrient arteries at the neck. The fracture deprives the body of the talus of its major blood supply and septic necrosis of the bone may follow.

Reduction is accomplished by plantar flexion of the foot with manipulation of the foot to align the fragments. Cast immobilization is usually sufficient to hold the reduction. Although healing of the fracture takes place in 2 or 3 months, the necrosis of the body of the bone may be evident within this time. Relative increased density of the bone on x-ray examination usually heralds this unfortunate event. Weight bearing cannot be allowed until revascularization of the body of the talus has occurred. This may require many months. During this period, active foot and ankle

exercises should be carried out to prevent stiffness of the joints and atrophy of the muscles. If revascularization of the bone is incomplete, some deformity of the bone may occur when weight bearing is resumed. Eventually, a painful arthritis develops in the ankle and subtalar joints, requiring arthrodesis of these joints.

### Subtalar and Talonavicular Dislocation

Dislocation of the foot from the talus is an unusual injury produced by extreme twisting violence. The talus remains in the ankle mortise while the foot usually displaces laterally at the talocalcaneal and talonavicular joints. Minor avulsion fractures about the margins of these joints may complicate the dislocation. The deformity of the foot is obvious and inversion and eversion cannot be performed, although dorsiflexion and plantar flexion may be possible to a limited degree. The prominence of the head of the talus in the dorsum of the foot may impair the circulation to the skin, demanding immediate reduction.

Reduction is accomplished by traction on the heel and forefoot in the long axis of the leg, accompanied by pressure on the os calcis directed medially. The dislocation is usually reduced without difficulty. Occasionally, interposition of soft tissue prevents reduction by manipulation, and an operation must be performed to clear this obstruction. Immobilization in a plaster cast extending from the toes to the knee is necessary for 4 to 6 weeks. After this time, weight bearing may be gradually resumed in a shoe that supports the long arch of the foot. Some loss of motion and pain can be expected from fibrosis about the subtalar joint for many months.

### Fractures of the Os Calcis

Fractures of the os calcis are usually caused by a fall from a height in which the heel strikes the ground and absorbs the major force. Since the os calcis is cancellous, the bone compresses and comminution of the fragments with impaction is usually the result. However, a variety of fractures occur. If, in falling, the patient lands on the forefoot and the tense triceps surae pulls upward on the bone at the attachment of the Achilles tendon, splitting the bone longitudinally, a "duckbill" fracture is produced. If the heel is forcefully inverted or everted, the sustentaculum may be sheared off or the anterior part of the bone may be avulsed by the interosseous ligament. Occasionally, a vertical fracture occurs that shears off the medial or lateral tuberosity of the calcaneus without other involvement of the bone. These forces, coupled with adduction or abduction of the forefoot, may drive the cuboid bone against the articular surface of the os calcis, producing fractures into the calcaneocuboid joint (Fig. 42).

Although healing of the bone occurs within 2 or 3 months, the prognosis for normal function of the foot is poor. Months of disability often follow the injury and some permanent disability is usual. Several factors contribute to this dismal prognosis.

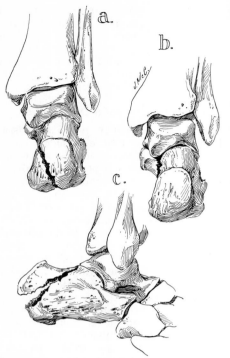

**Figure 42**  *a,* Vertical tuberosity fracture of the os calcis. *b,* Fracture of the sustentaculum. *c,* Duckbill fracture of the os calcis.

The damage to the subtalar joint and peroneal tendons, loss of the long arch, and widening of the os calcis with impingement against the lateral malleolus all contribute to the disability. Secondary to these changes, chronic irritation in the subtalar joint and ligaments produces reflex spasm of the peroneal muscles. This reaction produces a painful spasmodic flat foot. Injuries to the os calcis produce rapid swelling in the foot. Distention by hemorrhage and edema produces bleb formation in the skin, with the hazard of infection. This complication can often be avoided by the prompt application of a compression dressing and elevation of the foot. When the major body of the os calcis is fractured, the tuber joint angle is often lost, and this produces flattening of the arch of the foot. This angle is the one made by the tuberosity in relation to the subtalar joint. Normally, the angle is about 45 degrees (Fig. 43). Loss of the long arch of the foot reduces the shock-absorbing quality of the foot and reduces the effectiveness of the forefoot lever in the push-off phase of walking. Uncorrected, these two factors produce a shuffling, flat-footed limp. Widening of the os calcis causes impingement against the lateral malleolus and pinching or fibrosis of the peroneal tendons and sheaths. Derangement of the subtalar joint leads to painful fibrosis and traumatic arthritis with loss of the ability to invert and evert the foot, and produces pain on walking on uneven surfaces.

Reduction of this fracture is directed to restoring the normal configuration of the bone, reducing the widening, re-establishing the tuber joint angle and long arch of the foot, and correcting the deformity of the subtalar joint as much as possible. Practically, this is almost impossible to accomplish. A long leg cast is applied with knee flexed and the foot in moderate plantar flexion, and is molded snugly about the os calcis. Weight bearing cannot be permitted until healing is complete, usually a minimum of 3 months.

The complication of a painful subtalar joint is the usual cause of the prolonged disability. If the joint is damaged beyond repair and pain is persistent, subtalar arthrodesis is necessary. Because of the prolonged disability following reduction and cast immobilization, some surgeons ignore the deformity of the fractured os calcis and rely on early mobilization to prevent fibrosis. A compression dressing is applied and the leg elevated until the pain and swelling subside. Exercise of the foot and ankle is then started, and the patient is allowed to bear partial weight with crutches as soon as this can be tolerated. The eventual result of

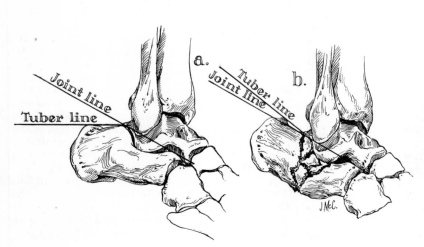

**Figure 43**  *a,* The tuber joint angles of the os calcis measures about 45 degrees. *b,* When the os calcis fractures and the subtalar joint is crushed, the tuber joint angle is reduced, lost, or reversed.

this treatment is uncertain. In some instances, the disability time is shortened; in others, the usual complications arise, necessitating arthrodesis or removal of bone beneath the lateral malleolus.

### Fracture and Dislocation of the Midtarsal Bones

Fractures and dislocations of the navicular, cuboid, and cuneiform bones are usually caused by direct, crushing violence, although a fall from a height may produce dislocations in this area. Since the complex of these bones is bound together by a strong envelope of ligaments, displacement is minimal. Often the fractures are mere avulsions of small fragments of bone at ligament attachments.

Reduction by direct molding of the fragments to eliminate sharp prominences of the dorsum of the foot is all that is necessary in most instances. A compression dressing for a week or two with no weight bearing, followed by heat, massage, and exercise is the usual treatment for these fractures.

Dislocations may take place between any of these bones. The most common dislocation occurs between the talonavicular and calcaneocuboid joints with lateral displacement of the forefoot.

Reduction is usually easily accomplished by traction on the forefoot accompanied by medial or lateral pressure. Maintenance of the reduction may be difficult and may require temporary pin fixation traversing the joints for a few weeks. Weight bearing cannot be allowed until the torn ligaments heal, about 4 to 6 weeks.

Dislocation of the midtarsal and metatarsal bones is an uncommon injury resulting from direct crushing violence. The displacement is usually lateralward and may spare the first metatarsal cuneiform joint. Accurate reduction may be hindered by interposition of the joint capsules and ligaments. The reduction is often unstable. Open reduction with removable pin fixation across the joints is often required.

### Fractures of the Metatarsal Bones

Fractures of the metatarsal bones may take place at the base, shaft, or neck, and articular areas of these bones, and are produced by direct or indirect violence.

A common fracture takes place at the base of the fifth metatarsal bone. This fracture is produced by the indirect violence of turning the forefoot inward while the foot is in equinus position. High-heel shoes are frequently the source of this mechanism, and the fracture is more common in women for this reason. The attachment of the peroneus brevis tendon and the joint capsule hold a triangular fragment of the bone to the cuboid bone, while the shaft of the bone is angulated medially. The fracture takes place through the triangular prominence of the base of the metatarsal. Displacement is minimal and no reduction is necessary; the remaining ligaments hold the fragments together. A compression dressing and walking with crutches is necessary for a few days until the

pain subsides. Weight bearing may be resumed in a well fitted oxford as soon as it is tolerated.

Fractures of the shaft of the metatarsal bones are usually due to direct crushing injury. The interosseous muscles bind and hold the bones firmly together so that displacement is usually not great. Theoretically, the displacing pull of the muscles is similar to that affecting fractures in the hand metacarpals; practically, angulation and shortening is less serious. Simple manipulation by direct pressure followed by a compression dressing or cast usually results in reasonably good reduction. Marked angulation must be corrected to allow proper weight bearing in the metatarsal heads. No weight bearing is followed until the pain and swelling subside, usually for 3 to 6 weeks.

Fractures of the metatarsal necks angulate and displace into the plantar aspect of the foot, producing an objectionable prominence on the weight-bearing surface. The displacement must be corrected by manipulation or a painful callus will develop over the bony prominence. Cast immobilization may be necessary to hold the fragments in reduction. The fractures are stable in 4 to 6 weeks, when weight bearing may be resumed. Undisplaced fractures may be treated by a compression dressing and crutches.

### Fractures of the Toes

Fractures of the toes are produced by crushing or stubbing injury. The proximal phalanx of the small toes is most frequently broken. The most common deformity is lateral displacement of the fifth toe. The injury is painful but not serious. Reduction of any deformity is accomplished with traction and manipulation. Immobilization is most easily accomplished by strapping the toe to the adjacent one, which provides a convenient splint. Weight bearing in a cut-out shoe is permitted immediately. Subungual hematoma often accompanies the fracture, and should be protected from contamination by an appropriate sterile dressing.

## FRACTURES OF THE PELVIS

The pelvis, composed of the two innominate bones and the sacrum, is a rigid bony ring containing the hip joints and housing the pelvic viscera. The two halves of the pelvis are joined by strong ligaments at the symphysis pubis and at the two sacroiliac joints. These ligaments, although preventing motion, lend some elasticity and shock-absorbing properties to the otherwise rigid bony ring. The major portions of the bones serve as muscle attachments which control the trunk and lower extremities. The pelvic viscera, including the bladder, ureters, and urethra, the rectum and sigmoid colon, and the great vessels and nerves, may be injured by fractures in this area.

Fractures are classified as avulsion fractures of muscle attachments, fractures of the ring of the pelvis without displacement, fractures of the ring of the pelvis with displacement, fractures of the acetabulum, and fractures of the sacrum and coccyx.

### Avulsion Fractures

Avulsion fractures of the pelvis are caused by the indirect force of muscle contractures. Avulsion fractures most often occur at the ischium and anterior, superior, or inferior iliac spines. Occasionally, avulsion of a small piece of bone occurs at the crest of the ilium.

These injuries are caused by the sudden contraction of the muscle and most frequently occur in athletic endeavors. Reduction of the fragment is usually not necessary, since the displacement is small and union takes place readily. Rest in bed for a few days, following by the application of heat, often eases the pain. Weight bearing can begin in a week or two. Open reduction is not necessary.

### Pelvic Ring Fractures without Displacement

Fractures of the pelvic ring without displacement can occur through any portion of the bones, but most often involve the pubic or ischial rami. The injury is common in older people, the result of a fall that compresses the pelvic ring. Slight comminution of the fragment may be present. Since the sacroiliac joints are not disrupted and the symphysis pubis is not separated, the fracture is stable and the weight-bearing function of the pelvis is not altered (Fig. 44).

Injury to the urinary tract is uncommon with this type of fracture; however, a urine specimen must be obtained and examined for blood. Bed rest for a week or two until the pain subsides may be followed by walking with full weight bearing as soon as this is tolerated. A binder or belt about the pelvis during this time may give the patient some comfort.

### Pelvic Ring Fractures with Displacement

Fracture of the pelvis with displacement must involve at least two areas of the pelvic ring before deformity occurs. Usually, considerable violence is necessary to produce these fractures. Shock is frequent and may be severe. Hidden blood loss in the retroperitoneal spaces may be considerable, and injury to the pelvic viscera is common. The displacement may alter the shape of the pelvis to a degree that is incompatible with proper weight bearing. In the female, distortion of the pelvis may preclude the normal delivery of children.

In all pelvic fractures with displacement, the bladder and urethra must be investigated for injury. If the patient cannot void, passage of a catheter into the bladder should be attempted. If blood is found in the voided specimen of urine, or that obtained by catheterization, rupture of the bladder must be considered. When these injuries are not recognized, urinary extravasation occurs. Untreated, this complication can result in death. Prompt diversion of the urinary stream must be done. Possible injuries to the rectum and sigmoid colon must be investigated. Sharp spicules of bone may penetrate or tear these structures. A rectal examination should be done. Shock must be treated by blood replacement and other appropriate therapy before reduction of the fracture is attempted.

### Segmental Fractures Involving One-Half of the Pelvis

More serious disruption of the pelvis occurs when the bone fractures through the rami of the pubis and at or near the sacroiliac joints. This section of the pelvis may displace inward, outward, or upward or rotate anteriorly. If the force compresses the pelvis, the anterior fracture or disruption of the sacroiliac joint acts like a hinge. If

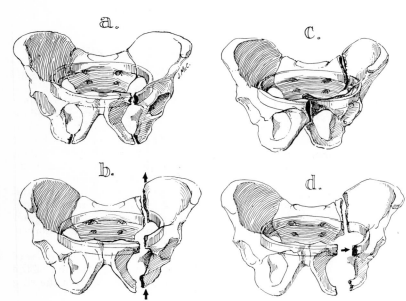

**Figure 44**  *a*, Stable fractures of the pelvic ring involve only one segment of the bone. No displacement is possible if the remainder of the ring remains intact. Weight may be borne as soon as pain subsides. *b*, Unstable fractures of the pelvis involve two segments of the pelvic ring. The flank muscles tend to pull the fragment upward. *c*, When the fracture is due to compression force, the pelvic ring may be constricted. *d*, When the force tears the pelvic bones apart, the pelvic ring opens.

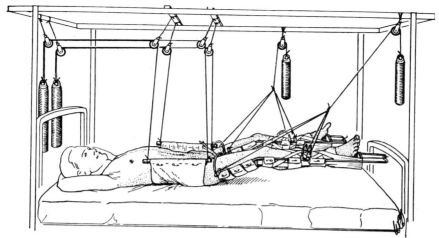

**Figure 45** Pelvic sling with suspension traction may be necessary to maintain reduction of unstable pelvic fractures.

the force is outward on this half of the pelvis, the reverse deformity occurs. The pelvis opens ante-riorly like a clam shell on the hinge of the poste-rior fracture. In either instance, the flank and ab-dominal muscles tend to pull this half of the pelvis upward. If, in the mechanism of injury, the thigh is hyperextended, the rectus femoris and hip joint capsule rotate this half of the pelvis forward, and this displacement may be combined with any of the others.

Fractures that open the pelvis ring are reduced by traction to counteract the upward displacement by the flank and abdominal muscles, then closed by compression force. The reduction may be done by several methods. The least traumatic reduction is achieved by placing heavy, continuous suspen-sion traction on both legs. This may be effectively applied with Russell's traction. Forty or fifty pounds of traction may be necessary on the affected side to pull the displaced half of the pelvis down-ward. This amount of force usually requires skele-tal traction through the lower femur. Compression force may be necessary to close the opened pelvic ring by a sling suspending the pelvis. Compression force is regulated by the degree that the sling is opened or closed over the patient. This method of suspension traction allows the necessary nursing care with minimal discomfort to the patient (Fig. 45). Union is usually complete in 3 months, when weight bearing with crutches may be gradually resumed.

When there is no upward displacement, it may be possible to close or open the pelvic ring by placing the legs in long leg casts with a bar con-necting the casts at the knees. This bar is a ful-crum, and, by forcing the lower ends of the casts together or apart, the upper portions of the casts force the hips together or pull them apart. This force, transmitted through the hip joints, opens or closes the pelvis. Longitudinal traction may be made when it is necessary by placing the casts in suspension traction.

### Fractures of the Acetabulum

Fractures that involve the acetabulum are serious injuries, because the weight-bearing func-tion of the hip is usually deranged. A fall directly upon the trochanter transmits force to the thin floor of the acetabulum through the head of the femur. The head, acting like a ramrod, fractures the floor of the acetabulum and displaces it in-ward. The displacement may be minimal or the entire head of the femur may penetrate into the pelvis. If there is no displacement, and the head of the femur remains in normal contact with the superior weight-bearing portion of the acetabulum, no reduction is necessary. The leg is placed in Buck's extension or suspension traction until the acute reaction to the injury has subsided. Active exercise of the hip is started when the pain abates. Weight bearing is not allowed until union is firm, in about 8 weeks.

When the head of the femur is displaced inward, reduction must be attempted to place the head in proper relationship with the weight-bearing sur-face of the acetabulum. As with all joint fractures, the articular surface must be reconstructed as per-fectly as is possible. Closed reduction is attempted in suspension traction. Strong longitudinal trac-tion may reduce the displacement. However, if this fails, lateral traction is added, either with skeletal traction through the trochanter or by a sling placed about the thigh. This combination of downward and lateral traction must be continued until the fractures unite, or displacement will recur. Occasionally, satisfactory reduction can-not be obtained by traction alone and open reduc-tion may be necessary.

Following central protrusion of the acetabulum, the blood supply to the head of the femur may fail and aseptic necrosis of this bone may produce trouble later. Incongruous joint surfaces may lead to traumatic arthritis requiring reconstructive surgery.

After union is obtained, weight bearing is

started gradually with crutches while active exercise is done to rehabilitate the hip musculature and re-establish motion.

### Fractures of the Sacrum and Coccyx

**Sacrum.** Fractures of the sacrum are usually transverse through the lower segments of the bone, and are produced by direct forces. Longitudinal fractures at the sacroiliac joint may accompany pelvic fractures that are segmental and displace upward. Transverse fractures are most often produced by a fall on the buttocks, and frequently are undisplaced and difficult to identify on x-ray films. When more force is applied, the lower fragment is angulated into the pelvis. If displacement is present, it may be corrected by direct manipulation.

A binder placed about the pelvis may give the patient comfort, and heat applied locally after the first few days may help to relieve pain. The patient cannot sit comfortably for several weeks, and sitting should be avoided when the fracture has been displaced.

Rarely, the sacrum is shattered by direct crushing force, damaging the cauda equina and sacral nerves. If the manipulation of the fragments does not relieve pressure on these vital structures, surgical decompression of the sacral canal may be necessary. Permanent bowel and bladder dysfunction may follow the injury.

**Coccyx.** Fractures of the coccyx are produced by falling upon the bone or by manipulation at childbirth. More often, pain is produced in the region by a sprain of the sacrococcygeal ligaments and the joints of the coccyx. Coccygodynia, or pain in the coccygeal region, may persist for many months following injury. Gentle manipulation by the surgeon's fingers may reduce actual displacement or dislocation rather easily. The normal irregular configuration of these bones is unaffected by manipulation. Sprains, dislocations, and fractures of the coccyx should be protected from the pressure of sitting for many weeks. The patient should be taught to sit forward on the ischial tuberosities to relieve pressure on the coccyx. Occasionally, an inflated ring-like cushion may allow sitting without pressure on the injured structures.

## FRACTURES AND DISLOCATIONS OF THE SPINE

The strength and flexibility of the spine depend upon the integrity of the vertebral bodies, the apophyseal joints, a variety of heavy ligaments, the shock-absorbing resilience of the intervertebral disks, and a finely coordinated muscular system. Contained within the protecting bony spinal canal are the spinal cord and the cauda equina, and emanating from it are the segmental peripheral nerves.

Since the bone of the vertebrae is cancellous, it is prone to compression and impacted fractures. The neural arch forms a protective bony ring through which the spinal cord passes. When injury occurs and the neural arch is displaced by fracture or dislocation, the spinal cord or cauda equina may be compressed and injured. The spinous and transverse processes are subject to avulsion fractures by muscle contractions, and the pull of tense ligaments when the spine is injured.

Alterations of the spinal curves and loss of mobility produce deformity and cause stress and strain in the spine following injury. When a vertebral body is crushed, the mechanism of fracture is usually forced flexion of the spine. A wedge-shaped deformity of the vertebra is produced with the apex of the wedge forward. Because alterations in the curves of the spine in one area shift the center of gravity of the body forward or backward, other areas automatically compensate for this by increasing or decreasing their curves. When this is excessive, strain is produced on the ligaments and joints, and pain may develop in the compensatory area of the spine as well as at the fracture site.

Every patient who complains of pain in the neck or back following injury must be considered to have a fractured spine until proved otherwise. The reason for this rather rigid principle is to prevent injury to the spinal cord by careless handling of the patient.

Most spinal fractures and dislocations are caused by indirect violence that forces the spine into extremes of flexion, extension, rotation, or lateral bending. The most common injuries are produced by flexion. These flexion injuries often are caused by falling from a height, landing on the feet, or by slipping and falling in a sitting position, or by the forced flexion of rapid deceleration of an automobile accident. Less frequently, the spine is injured by falling or diving on the head or shoulders. The most common site is the lower dorsal–upper lumbar area; next in frequency are the mid and lower cervical regions. Usually, the superior aspect of the vertebra is driven downward by the vertebra above, compressing the upper half of the vertebra into the lower half. If the force stops at this point, the fracture is stable and there is no danger to the spinal cord. If one-third or less of the height of the anterior body is lost, no correction is necessary. If more deformity than this exists, it may be necessary to reduce the fracture to prevent painful compensatory strain in other areas of the spine from developing. However, the age of the patient and the location of the fracture determine the course of treatment.

Whenever the body of the vertebra is fractured, bleeding occurs from the bone, forming a hematoma about the spinal column. If the fracture is the common wedge-shaped compression, the bleeding takes place anteriorly away from the spinal canal and the cord is not usually endangered. However, the sympathetic ganglionated trunk, located on the anterolateral surface of the vertebra, is disturbed and a paralytic ileus may result, which may cause more immediate trouble than the fracture.

When this type fracture occurs in the cervical region, the hematoma and associated edema accompanying the strain and tearing of the ligaments of the neural arch may slowly compress the spinal cord. These patients must be observed carefully for signs of central nervous system involvement.

If the force producing the compression is in the long axis of the spine, a bursting type fracture is produced. The body of the vertebra is squashed and expands in diameter, pancake fashion. With this type compression fracture, the spinal canal may be distorted by bone or hematoma and pressure may be exerted upon the spinal cord, demanding decompression.

Treatment of simple wedge-shaped compression fractures, following evaluation of the injury, requires placing the patient supine on a firm bed. Mild sedation may be given.

When the fracture is in the cervical region, traction is applied to the skull by tongs for immobilization and reduction. If the deformity is slight, a cloth head halter may be applied and 6 to 10 pounds of continuous traction made with the neck in moderate hyperextension, although it is not as effective as tong traction. Turning movements of the head may be eliminated by placing padded sandbags on each side of the head. This method of treatment makes use of the intact anterior longitudinal ligament of the spine in reduction. Since this ligament is attached along the anterior surface of the vertebral body, it buckles but does not tear as the compression force produces the wedge-shaped fracture. When the posterior elements of the vertebra are intact, the apophyseal joints act like a hinge when the spine is extended. This maneuver tightens the anterior longitudinal ligament which in turn pulls the compressed anterior body apart. The deformity is thus reduced, and if the vertebra is maintained in this position new bone fills in the gap created anteriorly in the body.

In the cervical area, traction may be continued for 4 to 6 weeks after reduction, when a cervical collar or brace may be applied to maintain the neck in extension for an additional 3 months. When the fracture occurs in the thoracic or lumbar region, the same principle of hyperextension of the spine is used for reduction; however, traction is not necessary. Reduction may be accomplished slowly by placing the fracture site in the spine over the apex of a triangle created in the mattress. When the pain has subsided and paralytic ileus and other injuries have been controlled, the patient may be placed in a body cast or brace to maintain the hyperextended position. He may become ambulatory as soon as he is comfortable. The cast or brace may be used for 4 to 6 months while the fracture site fills in with new bone. Often, some deformity of the vertebra recurs, even with perfect anatomic reduction and adequate immobilization.

Reduction may be accomplished by manipulation in younger people, if it is not accomplished by traction. Following reduction of the fracture, a body cast is applied to maintain the position. Older people do not well tolerate manipulative reduction, prolonged bed treatment, or immobilization in a massive body cast. It is better to place the patient in bed for a few days until the pain subsides, accept the deformity, and begin ambulation in a supporting corset as soon as possible.

### Fracture with Forward Dislocation of the Spine

If the flexion force that produces the wedge compression continues, the ligaments of the apophyseal joints and neural arch may rupture or the posterior elements fracture. This allows forward dislocation of the vertebra. The inferior facet of the cephalad vertebra slips forward over the superior facet of the lower vertebra and may lock in this position. This deformity distorts the spinal canal and the cord or cauda equina may be injured. The fracture-dislocation is unstable and unprotected movement of the patient may increase the deformity and further damage the central nervous system.

The cervical region is most frequently involved in this injury. The lumbar region, similar in mobility to the cervical region but stronger, is less often the site of fracture-dislocation. The thoracic region is more rigid and the configuration of the neural arch, along with the supporting thorax, prevents fracture-dislocation except with extreme violence. The spinal cord, nerve roots, and cauda equina may escape damage, or damage may be minimal, if the displacement of the vertebra is minor. With pronounced displacement, damage to these structures may be severe, permanent, and life-endangering. Continued pressure on the spinal cord or cauda equina whether by displaced fragments or hematoma and edema must be relieved as soon as possible by laminectomy.

In the cervical region, the injury is treated by heavy skull-tong traction with the head and neck in neutral position. Extension and flexion and rotation must be avoided, as the fulcrum of the posterior elements of the spine is lost. Flexion may allow the vertebra to slip forward, increasing the deformity of the spinal canal. Extension forces the lamina of the upper vertebra to move forward against the cord or cauda equina like a guillotine. Rotary or lateral displacement may produce impingement on the central nervous system by distortion of the neural canal.

The amount of traction needed in the cervical region to effect reduction may be 25 pounds or more. Skeletal traction through the skull by appropriate tong devices must be used. Neutral position then maintains the reduction until the ligaments heal, usually in 6 weeks. A cast extending from the pelvis to the occiput and chin is used for 3 months.

### Fractures of the Odontoid

Fractures of the odontoid process are extremely serious injuries. The mechanism of fracture is usually violent acute flexion of the head from a fall on the back of the head or from striking the head in a diving accident. The atlas remains in normal relationship to the occiput. The odontoid process, attached to the atlas by the transverse ligament, is displaced forward on the body of the axis because the fracture usually occurs at the base of the odontoid process. Stability between the two bones is lost, and the head may slide forward, backward, or to the side, producing varying degrees of cord pressure. The displacement may reduce spontaneously. The neurologic lesion may be minimal or severe.

The diagnosis can be made only by adequate x-ray examination. During the examination, the head must be supported, since any shift of the head or neck may compress the spinal cord. If the patient survives the injury, and there is no displacement, he may be placed in head-halter traction with sandbag immobilization for a short period. However, the fracture should be immobilized in a Minerva jacket as soon as possible. The plaster cast extends from the head to the pelvis to secure adequate fixation. The plaster jacket should be used for 4 to 6 months. If displacement is present or a neurologic deficit exists, skull-tong traction should be used until the damage to the spinal cord is stabilized. When the patient's condition will allow it, immobilization by plaster cast is done.

Nonunion of the odontoid process is not uncommon, and may follow an undiagnosed or even an adequately treated fracture. The fracture may be missed on the original examination, as the fracture may be hairline. Later, following absorption of bone at the fracture site, the fracture may be easily detected by x-ray examination. Many years may elapse before minor signs of spinal cord compression are evident to the patient. Nonunion of the odontoid process should be treated by fusion of the occiput to the second cervical vertebra to prevent spinal cord damage by slow displacement or subsequent injury.

### Fracture-Dislocations of the Lumbar Spine

Flexion force that continues after compression of the vertebral body has occurred may result in fracture or dislocation of the posterior elements of the spine in the thoracolumbar region. Since these structures are stronger in the lower spine than in the cervical region, greater violence is needed to produce the displacement, and complicating injuries to the thorax and abdominal contents are common. The lower spinal cord or cauda equina is frequently injured. The area of contact of the apophyseal joints is greater in the lumbar and lower thoracic region than in the upper spine; thus, slipping forward of one facet upon the other is usually accompanied by fractures of these elements. Two major types of injuries occur when vertebrae are displaced in this region of the spine. The inferior facets may break or the fracture may occur through the pedicles. In either case, the spinal canal is distorted and the spine is unstable, endangering the cauda equina and spinal cord.

The degree of displacement varies from minor to major, but any malalignment of the posterior border of the vertebra with the adjacent vertebrae indicates damage to the posterior elements of the spine, and thus instability. This finding on x-ray examination always contraindicates hyperextension during treatment, because further damage may be done to the contents of the neural canal.

When a major neurologic deficit is found, surgical decompression of the cord or cauda equina is usually indicated. When major displacement has occurred, it may be impossible to reduce the deformity. Spinal fusion may be necessary to create stability.

If abnormal neurologic findings are minimal, or if complications prevent laminectomy, the patient should be placed on a Bradford frame, or a posterior plaster shell or bed should be applied. This provides enough stability to allow nursing care while the problems are evaluated and resolved. When the physiologic processes of the patient have stabilized, it can be determined if laminectomy and spinal fusion is needed, or whether a cast will afford sufficient immobilization. It may be wiser to accept some deformity in the absence of neurologic impairment to allow the fracture to heal, and perform arthrodesis of the spine later if pain should arise from the altered mechanics.

### Fractures of the Transverse Processes

Fractures of the transverse processes as isolated injuries are most often found in the lumbar spine. Occasionally, fractures of the thoracic and cervical regions occur, but they are usually associated with other fractures of the vertebrae. The lumbar transverse processes serve as muscle attachments for the psoas and perispinal muscles. When these muscles suddenly contract, the transverse processes may be avulsed. The injury is not serious but is painful. All spine motions produce pain and are restricted. Muscle spasm may distort the normal curves of the back. No reduction is necessary. The muscles reattach, and although nonunion is common it does not produce symptoms.

Treatment is simple. Bed rest with heat and sedation lessen muscle spasm. When the pain subsides, the patient is fitted with a supporting corset and allowed to be ambulatory. Back-strengthening muscle exercises are started early in the healing process. Disability from the injury should not exceed 2 or 3 months.

### Fractures of the Spinous Processes

Fractures of the spinous processes result from direct force or from traction of the interspinous ligament when the spine is flexed. A direct blow to the spine may fracture any of the spinous processes; however, avulsion by the interspinous ligament most frequently affects the cervical vertebrae. Treatment is similar to that for transverse process fractures; rest and support until the pain subsides are followed by exercise.

### Rehabilitation of the Muscles Controlling the Spine

All injuries to the spine affect the muscles that control the spine. Rehabilitation of these muscles must be instituted following the injury if maximal comfortable function is expected. Muscles atrophy and shorten when they are not used. Bed rest or cast-and-brace immobilization promotes the atrophy of disuse. Weak muscles fatigue and ache, and shortened muscles prevent motion. When the spine fracture is stable, exercise should be started as soon as pain subsides. If the fracture is unstable, the exercise program must be delayed until sufficient healing has stabilized the spine.

## REFERENCES

1. American College of Surgeons, Committee on Trauma: Early Care of the Injured Patient. Philadelphia, W. B. Saunders Company, 1972.
2. Bado, J. L.: The Monteggia Lesion. Translated by I.V. Ponsetti. Springfield, Ill., Charles C Thomas, 1962.
3. Blount, W. P.: Fractures in Children. Baltimore, Williams & Wilkins Company, 1955.
4. Cave, E. F.: Fractures and Other Injuries. Chicago, Year Book Publishers, 1958.
5. Charnley, J.: The Closed Treatment of Common Fractures. 3rd ed. Baltimore, Williams & Wilkins Company, 1961.
6. Clark, J. M. P.: Modern Trends in Orthopaedics. Third Series: Fracture Treatment. Washington, D.C., Butterworth, 1963.
7. Clark, J. M. P.: Modern Trends in Orthopaedics. Fourth Series: Science of Fractures. Washington, D.C., Butterworth, 1964.
8. Conwell, H. E., and Reynolds, F. C.: Key and Conwell's Management of Fractures, Dislocations and Sprains. 7th ed. St. Louis, C. V. Mosby Company, 1961.
9. Crenshaw, A. H.: Campbell's Operative Orthopaedics. 5th ed. St. Louis, C. V. Mosby Company, 1971.
10. DePalma, A. F.: The Management of Fractures and Dislocations: An Atlas. 2nd ed. Volumes I and II. Philadelphia, W. B. Saunders Company, 1970.
11. Duchenne, G. B.: Physiology of Motion. Translated by E. B. Kaplan. Philadelphia, J. B. Lippincott Company, 1949.
12. Frankel, V. H., and Burnstein, A. H.: Orthopaedic Biomechanics. Philadelphia, Lea and Febiger, 1970.
13. Frast, H. M.: Bone Remodeling Dynamics. Springfield, Ill., Charles C Thomas, 1963.
14. Hampton, O. P., Jr., and Fitts, W. T., Jr.: Open Reduction of Common Fractures. New York, Grune & Stratton, 1959.
15. MacConall, M. A., and Basmajian, J. V.: Muscles and Movements, A Basis for Human Kinesiology. Baltimore, Williams & Wilkins Company, 1969.
16. Magnuson, P. B., and Stack, J. K.: Fractures. 5th ed. Philadelphia, J. B. Lippincott Company, 1949.
17. Science of Fractures. Series. Washington, D.C., Butterworth, 1964.
18. Watson-Jones, R.: Fractures and Joint Injuries. 4th ed. Volumes I and II. Baltimore, Williams & Wilkins Company, 1957.
19. Wiles, P.: Fractures, Dislocations and Sprains. Boston, Little, Brown and Company, 1960.

# II

# Amputations and Limb Substitution

*William A. Larmon, M.D.*

A multitude of conditions demand amputation of parts of the extremities in order to maintain life or improve function. These problems arise in all age groups. The infant born with defective limbs, the child and adult with malignant tumors or irreparable trauma, and the elderly suffering from vascular failure may all require removal of parts of the extremities. The surgeon must know the conditions that can benefit from amputation, and the details of technique that ensure the most efficient use of the remaining parts.

The surgeon's responsibility to the patient does not end with the removal of deformed or diseased tissue. He must be prepared to restore the person to maximal efficiency through the use of appropriate prosthetic devices. In addition to the knowledge of these factors, he must support the patient through the period of emotional adjustment to the loss of a part and the adaptation to an altered way of life.

Amputation may be required when there is irreparable damage from trauma or its sequelae, failure of circulation from peripheral vascular disease or embolic occlusions, tumors, infection, trophic changes secondary to neurologic disease, and congenital or acquired deformities.

When amputation is not an emergency, the surgeon must discuss the problem in detail with the patient. He must explain the need for the operation, the postoperative care, and the final function that can be obtained through the use of an appropriate prosthesis. The improvement in prosthetic devices in recent years has been remarkable, and, in most instances, substitutes for the missing part can achieve a considerable measure of usefulness.

## TYPES OF AMPUTATION

Two major types of amputation are performed: open and closed. Both are accomplished with tourniquet control, except in peripheral vascular disease, when tourniquet pressure may injure diseased blood vessels.

### Open or Guillotine Amputation

When spreading infection is established or is a potential hazard, open amputation is indicated. The amputation allows adequate drainage of damaged tissue until the danger of spreading infection is passed. Since this operation is performed at the most distal level of viable tissue, and the scar after healing will not tolerate a prosthesis, secondary revision of the stump is practically always necessary.

The amputation is performed by a circular incision about the part, thus the term "guillotine amputation." When the skin and subcutaneous tissue is incised, it is allowed to retract. The deep fascia and muscle are incised in progressive layers as the muscle retracts. The bone is sectioned at the level of final muscle retraction. Nerves and major blood vessels are ligated and sectioned at this same level. Because the retraction of tissue occurs in layers, as the limb is sectioned by progressive circular incision, the end of the stump resembles a cone with the apex at the bone level.

Postoperatively, the wound remains open while skin traction is applied to prevent further retraction of the soft tissues. A sheath of stockinet is glued to the skin, dressings are applied to the open surface, and continuous traction is made on the stockinet sleeve. As the wound granulates and heals, the skin edges are drawn toward the bone end by scar contraction. A circular scar adherent to the bone with inadequate soft tissue cover is formed, necessitating revision of the stump.

Revision of the stump need not wait until healing is complete, but the granulating surface must be clean and healthy before the final amputation is done. If complete healing of the wound is desired before definitive surgery is undertaken, it may be hastened by applying split-thickness skin grafts to the granulating surface. The purpose of reamputation, or stump revision, is to provide adequate soft tissue coverage for the bone at a level practical for the use of a prosthesis. When reamputation at a higher level is not practical, local revision of the scar is done. The scar tissue must be completely excised. Usually, the bone must be resected at a slightly higher level. The soft tissues are then closed to provide adequate bone cover with a minimal scar at the end of the stump.

### Closed or Flap Amputation

When infection is not a hazard, primary closure of the wound may be performed. The best available site for the amputation is chosen. The incision is made to produce two flaps of skin and subcutaneous tissue resembling an open fish mouth. Usually, the flaps are of equal length, but special problems may demand unequal flaps to bring the scar anterior or posterior to the bone end. After reflection of the flaps, the deep fascia is incised at a similar level; the muscle is divided by a circular cut, and in most instances allowed to retract. The periosteum is incised and the bone sectioned transversely at the level of the retracted muscles. Periosteal tags are removed to prevent spur formation, but the periosteum is not stripped from the bone end, as was once advocated.

The major blood vessels are separated and ligated individually to prevent the formation of arteriovenous fistulas. The nerves are pulled downward, sectioned, and allowed to retract above the level of the cut muscle. This is done to prevent

the nerves from adhering to the terminal scar, where they may be subjected to pressure and tension. Severed nerves heal by the formation of a neuroma. If the neuroma forms in the scar tissue of the distal stump, it may be painful. Local or phantom limb pain may prevent the use of a prosthesis. When the neuroma forms above the distal scar in its normal compartment, it is usually painless.

The wound is closed by approximating the deep fascia over the bone and remaining muscle; excessive muscle tissue over the bone end should be avoided. Suturing the deep fascia pulls the muscle downward sufficiently to allow proper attachment to the bone and helps to prevent muscle ends from adhering to the skin. Muscles that become attached to the scar of the flaps distort the stump when the limb is moved. Friction is produced within the socket of the prosthesis, and skin problems may arise from this complication. It may be prevented by suturing the cut muscle to the sides of the bone through holes drilled in the bone; this is a more recent advance in amputation surgery. The subcutaneous tissue is closed with a minimal number of sutures. The skin should be closed under normal tension except in peripheral vascular disease, in which case there should be no tension.

Drains are inserted in the corners of the wound to allow escape of serum from the sectioned structures. Even in the presence of careful hemostasis, a certain amount of serum accumulates, and, if not drained, interferes with wound healing. The drains are removed after 48 or 72 hours. Suction drainage may be used.

A voluminous pressure dressing is used to supply uniform compression over the stump except in peripheral vascular disease. Amputations for vascular problems are dressed loosely to prevent strangulation of tissues with a precarious blood supply.

## POSTOPERATIVE CARE

Dressings are changed infrequently after removal of the drains; however, the outer elastic bandages should be adjusted as often as needed to ensure uniform pressure. Amputation stumps heal slowly, particularly in peripheral vascular disease. The skin sutures should remain in place for at least 2 weeks. Primary healing of the wound is desirable to minimize scar tissue. Wound breakdown or separation must heal by secondary intention, producing a scar that may be fragile and subject to irritation when the prosthesis is used. Splints may be applied during the healing time to prevent flexion contractures, particularly in peripheral vascular disease. Proper bed posture is an aid in preventing contractures, particularly with lower extremity amputations. Patients who have had amputations below the knee tend to keep the knee flexed to lessen the pull on the severed gastrocnemius muscle. This must be counteracted by a splint until the wound heals and the irritation of the muscle subsides. Following removal of the splint, the patient must straighten the knee completely numerous times during the day to prevent a flexion contracture.

Patients who have had amputations above the knee tend to flex and abduct the thigh. Short stumps are more prone to this deformity. These people must lie face down several times a day to stretch the thigh into complete extension at the hip. They must not use a pillow to elevate the distal stump for comfort, and they must not sit in bed with the hip flexed for long periods. They must be taught to adduct the thigh actively and maintain it against the other leg most of the time to prevent abduction contracture.

When the skin has healed, the process of shrinking the stump begins. After amputation, the subcutaneous fat and muscle atrophy, and the stump shrinks in circumference. This process must be completed before the prosthesis is fitted. Proper bandaging must be done to speed this process, prevent the accumulation of edema, and aid in shaping the amputation stump. Elastic bandages are used, and the patient must be instructed in the correct method of wrapping the part. The bandage must be reapplied several times during the day to maintain firm pressure. The process of shrinking usually takes about 3 months.

Exercises to strengthen and prevent contracture of the muscles controlling the stump may be started when the wound has healed. Massaging the stump serves no useful purpose and may irritate sensitive neuromas; it should not be used in the postoperative care. Pounding the stump with the assumption that this process toughens it is to be condemned. Only damage to healing tissue is produced by this antiquated custom.

Ambulation should begin early. The upper extremity amputee may be out of bed in a few days if other injuries permit it. The lower extremity amputee should begin ambulation in a walker after the wound has healed, if his general condition will allow it. Dependency of the amputated upper or lower extremity should be avoided until the wound has healed; for this reason, assisted walking is delayed in lower extremity amputees until this is accomplished.

A recent development in amputation surgery is the immediate fitting of a prosthetic device at the completion of the operation. A socket made of plaster is applied to the fresh stump over appropriate padding. An adjustable skeleton-like prosthesis is attached to the socket through a coupling that allows removal as well as adjustment of alignment of the device. The patient is encouraged to begin partial weight bearing the following day. Several advantages are claimed for this method. Uniform compression of the stump prevents excessive edema. Physiologic use of the remaining part lessens the feeling of loss of the extremity by the patient and muscle atrophy is lessened. There is less likelihood of contractures and the patient becomes ambulatory more quickly. This makes possible earlier fitting and use of the permanent prosthesis.

# AMPUTATIONS OF THE LOWER EXTREMITY

Amputations of the lower extremity alter to varying degrees the ability to stand, walk, and run. The lower extremities are a system of bony levers articulated at the ankle, knee, and hip joints. The levers activated by muscles assume the necessary positions for balance and ambulation almost automatically. These muscles, bones, and joints, acting synchronously, provide shock-free movement of the body from place to place. Loss of any part of this mechanism interferes with balance, propulsion, and stability. Prosthetic devices have been evolved to substitute for the various missing parts. The degree of successful use of these devices depends upon the level of amputation and the skill of the surgeon and prosthetist.

## Amputation of Toes and Forefoot

Amputation of one or more toes has little effect on ambulation except for a slight loss of push-off power. Balance is usually not affected and the gait is usually unaltered. The amputation is performed through a racquet-shaped incision. Any part of the toe may be amputated, or more commonly the toe is disarticulated at the metatarsophalangeal joint (Figs. 1 and 2).

Amputations through the metatarsal bones affect push-off power in walking to a moderate degree; however, balance of the foot is maintained and minimal disability is encountered. Whenever possible, the metatarsal bones should be sectioned transversely, all at approximately the same level. The plantar flap is made longer than the dorsal one if possible to produce a dorsal scar. Although a terminal scar is satisfactory, a plantar scar should be avoided (Fig. 3).

Satisfactory amputations that maintain balance of the foot may be performed to the level of the base of the metatarsal bones. Little power or balance is lost in walking or standing, and a limp is usually not evident. A prosthesis is not necessary, but the shoe must be fitted with a sponge material to help preserve its contour.

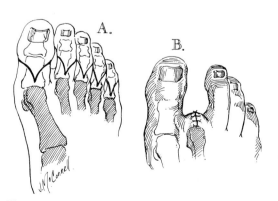

**Figure 1** Amputation of all or part of a toe is performed with racquet-shaped incisions.

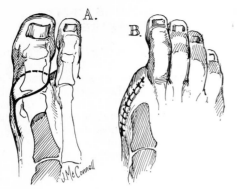

**Figure 2** When the great toe is amputated with the metatarsal head, a modified incision is used to reduce the prominence of the remaining bone.

## Midtarsal Amputation

For many years, amputation through the midtarsal joints was condemned because imbalance in the remaining muscles produced an equinovarus deformity of the hindfoot and an unsatisfactory stump. Since the peroneal tendons are sectioned and the tibialis anticus is usually detached, the triceps surae muscles of the calf produce the equinus deformity of the remaining foot. Ankle motion is thus unopposed plantar flexion. Inversion and eversion at the subtalar joint is usually lost. The tibialis posticus muscle may remain active if the navicular bone is present, pulling the heel into varus. In this position, weight is borne on the end of the irregularly shaped stump. Invariably, the stump is painful and breakdown of the skin is a common complication.

In recent years, an attempt has been made to salvage this amputation by arthrodesis of the ankle joint. The talus is fused to the tibia in 5 to 10 degrees of dorsiflexion. In this position, a full-

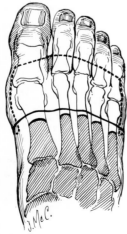

**Figure 3** A longer plantar flap is used when amputations are made through the metatarsal bones. The foot remains balanced, and no prosthesis is necessary.

weight-bearing stump is created. The balancing levers of the foot are lost, however, and there is no active push-off phase on walking. A high shoe with a filler in the forefoot is used to create a substitute forefoot lever.

## Amputation at the Ankle: Syme's Amputation

When the major portion of the foot must be removed, Syme's amputation is preferred. The amputation demands a heel flap free from infection and scarring, possessing adequate sensation and circulation. A transverse anterior incision is made at the ankle joint to the malleoli. A vertical incision is then made directly downward from the anterior tip of the medial malleolus around the bottom of the foot, then upward to the tip of the lateral malleolus. The talus is disarticulated from the tibia, and the talus and os calcis are dissected from the heel flap. The malleoli and articular surface of the tibia are then resected at the level of the joint line.

When the wound edges are brought together, the scar lies anteriorly and the heel flap forms a cushion over the end of the bone. This is a true end-bearing stump with only slight loss of leg length. The patient is able to walk "barefoot" without a prosthesis when necessary. The normal shock-absorbing and propulsive force provided by the foot and ankle is lost with this amputation. The prosthesis must, in some measure, substitute for this loss if near-normal standing and walking are to be achieved. The socket of the prosthesis encases the leg to just below the knee and is molded to the crest of the tibia to prevent rotation of the artificial foot. Since the space for the ankle joint in the prosthesis is limited, a complete hinge joint cannot be used. Shock-absorbing properties are provided by a special foot with a rubber heel and an ankle joint recessed into the foot. This joint allows a slight amount of dorsiflexion and plantar flexion. The forepart of the foot is flexible and dorsiflexes passively at the push-off phase of walking.

During the swing and stance phases of walking, the lower extremity rotates internally and externally on its long axis. When the foot is fixed to the ground, this rotary action of the leg is absorbed in the subtalar joint. With Syme's amputation and those at a higher level, this action of the subtalar joint is lost. The stump tends to rotate within the socket of the prosthesis. A loose-fitting socket allows excessive rotation, producing friction and skin irritation. Thus, the socket must fit the stump accurately to minimize this problem. A properly aligned and accurately fitted prosthesis should permit smooth, pain-free walking and standing.

## Amputations through the Leg

When amputation is demanded above the ankle, the site of election below the knee is chosen. This amputation should produce a stump 5 to 7 inches long below the knee joint. Stumps longer than 7 inches are difficult to fit with a prosthesis and are subject to circulatory failure. Stumps shorter than

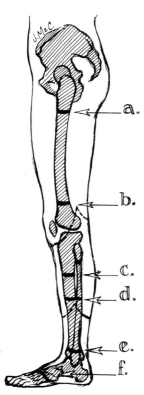

**Figure 4**   Disarticulation of the hip can be fitted successfully with the Canadian hip prosthesis. *a,* Amputation in the upper thigh must produce a stump at least 2.5
to 3 inches below the perineum to allow fitting with a
suction-socket prosthesis. All length to this level should
be saved. *b,* Supracondylar amputation is done just above
the flare of the condyles. *c,* All length to a level 2.5 inches
below the insertion of the hamstrings should be saved.
*d,* The site of election of amputation below the knee
should produce a stump 5 to 7 inches long; however,
stumps as short as 2 inches below the knee can be fitted
with a prosthesis. Knee joint disarticulation and Gritti-
Stokes amputations produce an end-bearing stump.
*e,* The level of the Syme amputation at the ankle joint.
*f,* The level of midtarsal amputation.

5 inches are less powerful in operating the prosthesis because the lever arm of the stump is reduced; however, amputations as short as 2 inches
below the knee can be fitted successfully with a
prosthesis (Fig. 4).

Flaps of skin and subcutaneous tissue are made
of equal length anteriorly and posteriorly. The
length of the flaps can be estimated as two-thirds
to three-fourths the radius of the leg at the site of
amputation. After the flaps are reflected, the bone
and muscle are sectioned at the base of the flaps.
The fascia covering the gastrocnemius muscle is
preserved to the level of the skin flap. The anterior
crest of the tibia is beveled to eliminate this sharp
point of bone. The fibula is resected 1 to 1½ inches
higher than the tibia. Section of both bones at the
same level has been advocated by some surgeons.
When the tibia is less than 3 inches in length, the

distal end of the remaining fibula tends to angulate outward, as there is insufficient interosseous
membrane remaining to hold it in position. This
angulation produces pressure against the side of
the socket that is difficult to relieve. The head of the
fibula may be removed, but the lateral collateral
ligament and the biceps tendon must be reattached
to the tibia. The peroneal nerve should be sectioned above the knee joint.

Removal of the head of the fibula reduces some
of the resistance to rotation of the stump in the
socket and, for this reason, is objectionable. In
recent years, attempts have been made to retain
the head of the fibula in its normal position by
creating a bony bridge between the fibula and
tibia.

When the amputation is completed, the muscle
is sutured to the bone, the fascia of the gastrocnemius muscle is sutured anteriorly over the
tibia, and the skin flaps are closed. The scar is
terminal or slightly posterior.

Several types of prosthetic devices are used for
below-knee amputations, depending upon the
length and condition of the stump. The conventional prosthesis consists of a foot articulating
through a hinged ankle joint to the shank or shin
piece which contains the socket. Attached to the
socket are two metal side bars which connect to
hinges at the knee joint. The hinges are connected
to a leather thigh corset through additional metal
side bars. The stump is retained and stabilized in
the socket by this harness. To aid in active extension of the knee, an elastic band may be attached
to the front of the shin piece and stretched to a belt
about the patient's pelvis. This elastic band reinforces the action of the quadriceps muscle in extending the knee.

Weight is borne by the flaring tibial condyles,
not the end of the stump. Since this is an area not
normally adapted for weight bearing, the socket
must fit accurately to distribute the weight over
the largest area available. The stump must be
firmly supported by the socket, but the blood
vessels posteriorly must not be constricted. Pressure in the popliteal space produces edema in the
end of the stump, which may cause breakdown of
the skin.

Another type socket has been used more recently: the patellar tendon weight-bearing socket.
This prosthesis is a little higher in front and dis-
tributes some of the weight to the patellar tendon.
It is fastened in place by a simple leather strap
placed about the thigh just proximal to the
patella and attached to the prosthesis. The hinge
bars and thigh corset are thus eliminated.

The usual socket is made of willow wood, which
is hard and unyielding. In order to provide some
cushioning for the stump, soft liners have been
made of various materials. Prosthetic sockets of
this type are called soft sockets, and are particularly useful when bony prominences are difficult
to fit. The exceptionally short stump is difficult to
retain in the socket when walking. The hamstring
muscles attaching to the tibia below the knee joint
tend to lever the stump out of the socket when the

knee is flexed. This action produces intolerable friction between the stump and socket. To counteract this tendency, the slip socket has been devised. This mechanism consists of a socket suspended within the shank by a spring or elastic bands from the side bars. The socket thus remains more firmly attached to the stump while the up-and-down excursion is absorbed by the suspension mechanism within the shank. Occasionally, the below-knee stump will not tolerate full weight bearing. When this occurs, the thigh corset may be extended upward and an ischial seat attached to it, to transfer some of the body weight to the ischium.

Even a short knee stump is invaluable in transmitting proprioceptive joint sense so necessary for balance. Whenever possible, the knee joint should be conserved, particularly in the bilateral lower extremity amputee.

Fitting and alignment of all parts of the prosthesis must be done accurately to minimize shock, friction, and excessive pressure. When this is accomplished, the patient should be able to walk comfortably without limping.

### Amputation through the Knee Joint or Lower Femur

Disarticulation through the knee joint has been performed for many years. Certain advantages and disadvantages have made this site for amputation controversial. The advantages are a longer lever controlled by musculature that is relatively undamaged and a fully end-bearing stump. The disadvantages are a bulbous stump, at times difficult to fit with a prosthesis, and the more distally placed knee hinge.

The amputation is performed through flap incisions made longer and wider than usual. The anterior flap must extend to the tibial tubercle. The patellar tendon and joint capsule are reflected with the anterior flap. The hamstring tendons are clamped and sectioned individually. The vessels and nerves are treated as in other amputations. The hamstring tendons are then sutured to the patellar tendon in the intracondylar notch and the deep fascia and skin is closed.

Weight is borne on the end of the stump through the patella. The socket for the prosthesis is usually made of leather or plastic. The socket extends up the thigh as a laced corset. Metal side bars connect the corset to the knee hinges and shank. Because of the bulbous nature of the stump, it may be possible to suspend the prosthesis from the thigh corset without pelvic-band suspension. Alignment of the knee joint is difficult, as the hinges must be located at the sides of the prosthesis. Stability and control of extension is accomplished by placing the hinges slightly posterior to the weight-bearing line. Elastic bands may be used to control flexion and extension.

A modification of the knee-joint disarticulation is the Gritti-Stokes amputation. Originally, the amputation was devised to prevent the spread of infection into the thigh. The incisions are similar to those in the knee-joint disarticulation except that the posterior flap is shorter. The femur is

sectioned transversely at the flare of the condyles. The articular surface of the patella is removed and the patella is placed in contact with the end of the femur. The tendinous and ligamentous structures are closed to hold the patella against the femur. If union of the patella to the femur occurs, a satisfactory end-bearing stump is produced. However, the patella often slips off the end of the femur and fails to unite. The irregularity produced at the end of the stump may be unsuitable for weight bearing. To avoid this complication, the procedure has been modified by removing the patella and suturing the tendon over the bone. Although full end bearing may not be obtained by this method, a partial ischial and end-bearing stump may be produced.

### Thigh Amputations

The site of election for thigh amputation is from the supracondylar region to 10 to 12 inches below the tip of the greater trochanter. Above this level, all length possible should be saved. Long thigh stumps are more powerful than short ones; muscle balance is maintained and control of the prosthesis is positive. When the thigh lever is short, power is lost in the adductor and hamstring muscles. The short thigh stump tends to flex and abduct. Although stumps as short as 3 inches from the perineum can be fitted with a thigh prosthesis, the control of the prosthesis is much more difficult than with a long stump. Conserve as much thigh length as possible above the supracondylar level.

The anterior and posterior flap incisions are made of equal length. The length of the flaps is estimated as two-thirds the radius of the thigh at the level of amputation. Amputation then proceeds as previously described.

This type of amputation demands ischial weight bearing. Two major types of prostheses are used: the suction socket and the conventional pelvic-band suspension socket. The suction socket is quadrilateral in shape to accommodate the muscle groups of the thigh and to provide an ischial seat. The limb is held in place by negative pressure or suction created by a valve mechanism located in the lower end of the socket. The conventional socket is more conical in shape, but in recent years has been modified to a more quadrilateral shape. The socket is secured to the stump by a thigh hinge suspended from a pelvic band or shoulder harness.

Since the center of gravity of the body is medial to the hip joint, the pelvis must be stabilized by the abductor muscles of the hip in walking and standing on one leg. These muscles, arising on the ilium above the hip joint and inserting laterally on the trochanter, act as guide wires to hold the pelvis level. If the foot were not fixed to the ground, this same force used to stabilize the pelvis would abduct the leg. This occurs in the amputation stump in walking and standing; the abduction is counteracted by pressure of the stump against the lateral wall of the socket when the prosthesis is in contact with the ground. If the stump is long, the pressure is distributed over a wide area. If the stump is short, the pressure is concentrated near the end of the bone. Thus, not only is a long thigh lever stronger but pressures against the stump in walking are less. When the thigh is flexed, it tends to rotate inward. If the prosthesis is not properly aligned, excessive friction occurs at the ischial seat because of this internal rotation.

The socket is attached to a knee block, which contains the knee-joint hinge and a braking mechanism to control knee-joint motion. When the amputation is through or above the knee joint, balancing, propulsive, and shock-absorbing action of the knee joint is lost. The limb substitute must provide controlled, stable knee motion. Obviously, active flexion and extension and propulsive power cannot be obtained from the prosthesis. The control of these actions must be obtained from the remaining thigh and hip musculature.

Many mechanical knee joints have been devised. None of them fulfills all of the functions of the human knee. In normal walking, two major events happen in the knee. During the stance phase, as the heel strikes the ground, the knee flexes slightly as part of the shock-absorbing mechanism. It continues to flex slightly until the foot is flat on the ground. As the heel rises and the foot dorsiflexes, the knee straightens through the push-off phase of walking. As the toes leave the ground, the knee is again flexed. The knee of the artificial limb cannot maintain stability and allow flexion during the stance phase of walking; otherwise the knee would buckle and the patient would fall. Thus, the knee hinge must be placed posterior to the weight bearing line of the prosthesis, and the knee must remain extended during the stance phase of walking. The loss of this shock-absorbing power must be compensated for by the ankle joint and foot mechanism.

As the toes leave the ground, the hip and knee flex to allow the toes to clear the ground as the leg swings forward. Normally, the knee flexes to about 65 degrees and is checked by contraction of the quadriceps muscle. At this point, the quadriceps extends the knee gradually during the forward swing of the leg. Just before the heel strikes the ground, the hamstring muscles contract to slow the knee action to prevent it from snapping into extension. This action is lost in above-knee amputations, and the smooth flexion and extension of the prosthetic knee must be accomplished mechanically. As the thigh stump is flexed, the mechanical knee must flex easily and smoothly to allow the foot to clear the ground. As the thigh continues to flex, the prosthesis swings forward. When flexion of the thigh ceases, the pendulum-like action of the prosthesis below the knee continues until full extension of the knee is reached. A braking mechanism must be incorporated in the mechanical joint to slow the extending leg smoothly, duplicating the action of the hamstring muscles. The prosthetic foot and ankle are designed to provide a stable, yet flexible, shock-absorbing base for the artificial leg.

Proper adjustment and alignment of the parts of the artificial foot and ankle is essential for successful action of the entire prosthesis.

## Hip Disarticulation

Hip-disarticulation amputation is usually performed for malignant lesions, or irreparable high-thigh trauma. Fortunately, the operation is not indicated frequently, since lack of a thigh stump makes control of a prosthesis difficult. Two major types of incisions are used; both avoid scars about the ischium.

The first is a racquet-shaped incision. The handle of the racquet centers over the anterior iliac spine and curves medially and downward about 5 cm. below the perineum. The incision is carried across the posterior thigh to about 8 cm. below the greater trochanter, then upward to join the racquet handle. The femoral artery is ligated and the leg elevated to empty it of blood. Following this, the femoral vein is ligated. The adductor, hip rotators, rectus femoris, iliopsoas, and sartorius are all sectioned at their tendinous attachments. The femoral obturator and sciatic nerves are pulled down and sectioned. Some surgeons believe these nerves should be injected with local anesthetic before section to lessen shock. The fascia lata is sectioned below the insertion of the tensor fascia lata muscle. The gluteus maximus is divided from its insertion on the linea aspera. Sectioning all muscles through tendinous areas lessens blood loss.

The hip joint capsule is then sectioned about the acetabular rim. The head of the femur is dislocated and the leg completely detached. The wound is closed by approximating the gluteus maximus tendon to the adductor muscle origins. The deep fascia is sutured and the skin is closed to produce a vertical anterior scar.

The second type of incision results in an anterior transverse scar. This incision begins over the femoral vessels about 1 inch below the inguinal ligament. The incision then curves medially 4 inches below the pubic tubercle and sweeps posteriorly to create a long posterior flap, then forward to the point of origin. The general steps in completing the disarticulation are essentially the same as for the racquet incision.

Before the development of the Canadian hip prosthesis, the tilting-table and saucer-type prostheses were used. These prostheses were conventional above-knee limbs attached by a hinge to a saucer or bucket suspended from the patient by shoulder and pelvic straps, the stump balanced on the saucer or fitted into the bucket of the tilting-table prosthesis. The hip was locked in extension during walking and unlocked for sitting. A very awkward gait was almost always found. The patient moved the prosthesis forward by elevating the pelvis and rotating it forward. After the heel contacted the ground and the knee was extended, he vaulted over the prosthesis. Considerable effort was required to operate the artificial leg and instability was always a problem. Overstressed hinges at the hip joint produced frequent mechanical failures.

The Canadian prosthesis socket is made of plastic and encases the pelvis as well as the stump.

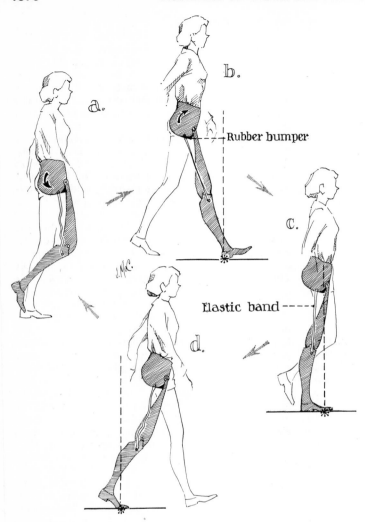

**Figure 5** *a,* With the Canadian hip prosthesis, the hip joint is anterior, on the socket. *b,* As the leg swings forward, an elastic band from the socket to the anterior skin piece stabilizes the knee in extension. As the amputee walks over the prosthesis, the alignment of the joints provides stability. *c,* At the push-off phase, the elastic band is relaxed, allowing the knee to flex. *d,* The back of the thigh piece strikes a rubber bumper on the socket, forcing it forward, and starting the swing phase again.

Three points of fixation are obtained: the ischium and both iliac crests. This provides firm fixation of the socket to the patient and positive control of the socket by the pelvis. Instead of lifting the pelvis and rotating it violently forward to swing the leg, the patient simply tilts the pelvis backward. The bumper on the socket contacts the thigh piece and the leg swings forward, more nearly simulating the normal gait (Fig. 5).

## AMPUTATIONS OF THE UPPER EXTREMITY

Amputation of the upper extremity is usually necessitated by trauma, occasionally by malignant lesions, and rarely by peripheral vascular disease. The upper extremity consists of an end organ, the hand, moved about by a system of jointed levers: the forearm, arm, and shoulder.

As the levers and joints of the upper extremity are lost at higher levels, the problem of activating and placing the terminal device in positions for function are increased. Lever arms must be incorporated in the prosthesis and joints must be provided that the amputee can control. It is apparent that higher amputations compound the problems of terminal device function. The terminal device must be secured to the remaining parts of the arm by a socket. A harness, usually placed about the shoulders, is used to activate the hook or hand by appropriate cables. Depending upon the function needed, the cable may be pulled taut by arm or shoulder-girdle movements. For example, the hook in the below-elbow prosthesis may be opened by arm flexion at the shoulder. When the amputation is above the elbow, the mechanical elbow joint is controlled by a second cable attached to the shoulder harness. When the patient shrugs the shoulder up and down, this cable may flex or extend the elbow or lock or unlock it in the desired position. Another cable is then used to open and close the terminal device by arm or shoulder motion. Many harnesses have been devised and the successful use of an upper extremity prosthesis depends upon a proper harness. The harness must be comfortable and transmit forces to the prosthesis efficiently through the appropriate cables.

Research and development of electrically activated prosthetic devices may eventually eliminate the need for harness control.

### Amputation of Hand

The primary functions of the hand are sensory perception and prehension. Use of the hands to express and transmit feelings of emotion is a secondary function. The organ is a complex miracle of mechanical perfection. Loss of sensation, movement, or parts of the hand always produces disability. Loss of the entire hand is catastrophic, as there is no adequate substitute. Every effort must be made to preserve any functional part of the hand. Amputation of the entire hand is reserved for irreparable lesions.

When the hand is lost, many of its functions cannot be replaced by any prosthetic device. The primary loss that cannot be replaced is sensory perception. Knowing this, the surgeon must attempt to replace prehension as efficiently as possible. This function is provided by a terminal device, usually a split hook or hand. Six basic types of prehension are defined by Schlesinger: cylindrical, spherical, hook, tip, palmar, and lateral grasp. Cylindrical grasp is used in holding the handle of a shovel. Spherical grasp is used to hold a large ball. Hook grasp is used in carrying a suitcase. Tip grasp is used in holding and threading a needle. Palmar grasp is used in holding a pen or pencil. Lateral grasp opposes the thumb against the side of the index finger, as in tearing a page from a magazine.

Coupled with these basic types of prehension is the ability to vary the pressure applied and the rapidity of opening and closing. For example, the force required to hold and swing a golf club is entirely different from that used in holding a paper cup. The carrying of a suitcase requires only stationary hook grasp, while sorting small items requires rapid opening and closing motions.

In attempting to substitute these motions, voluntary opening or voluntary closing terminal devices are used. The patient may elect to use a device that he can close voluntarily, by using the remaining levers of the upper extremity to activate the device, regulating to a degree the pressure applied. He may find it better in particular functions to be able to open the device voluntarily, while closing is performed by a spring mechanism that exerts uniform pressure. Recent development in electrically driven hands and hooks may make possible positive opening and closing of the devices.

The cosmetic hand with less function but a more natural appearance than the split hook may be desirable in certain conditions.

The type of terminal device must be adapted to the age, coordination, and functional demands of each patient. The selection of this important replacement part needs thoughtful study by the patient, physician, and prosthetist.

### Amputation through the Wrist

When the major portion of the hand must be amputated, the surgeon must determine the site for amputation, dependent upon available skin coverage and maximal function that can be obtained from the stump. When adequate palmar skin is present, all or part of the carpal bones may be retained. This amputation demands a long palmar flap and a short dorsal one to ensure a proper, tough cover over the carpal bones. The hand may be disarticulated at the metacarpocarpal joints or through the carpus. Carpal bones allow some flexion and extension of the distal stump, and this may be useful when a prosthesis is not used. Pronation and supination of the forearm are preserved. When the stump has good cover, it may be fitted with a terminal device attached to a forearm plastic socket. The terminal device is activated by a cable attached to a shoulder harness. Electric motors activated by contraction of the muscles of the forearm through contact points on the socket may eventually replace the cable.

### Wrist Disarticulation

Although amputation through the carpal bones has occasionally been possible, it is not often that this is practical. Disarticulation at the radiocarpal joint is the much more common site for total hand amputation. For many years, this site was thought unfavorable because of poor stump coverage, circulatory failure, breakdown of skin, and difficulty in fitting a prosthesis. Since World War II, improved surgical technique and prosthetic development have made this area of amputation desirable. When the stump can be covered by good palmar skin, the amputation has many advantages. When the end of the stump cannot be covered adequately, the amputation is useless.

Full pronation and supination is preserved by this amputation, and the forearm lever is strong. A simple short socket of laminated plastic encases the stump. Because of the flaring end of the radius, the fit is usually secure and about two-thirds of the available pronation and supination is transmitted to the terminal device. When necessary, flexible hinges may be attached to a cuff about the arm above the elbow. The cable activating the terminal device is attached to a shoulder harness.

### Forearm Amputation

If the wrist disarticulation cannot be done, the site of election in the forearm is the junction of the lower and middle thirds of the forearm. This level of amputation creates an adequate lever and preserves about two-thirds of the available pronation and supination. The stump is long enough to fit the socket securely without interference of flexion at the elbow by the socket. From this level upward, amputation may be done to within $1\frac{1}{2}$ inches of the insertion of the biceps tendon. As the stump becomes shorter, leverage and pronation and supination are lost progressively. The socket for the short prosthesis may interfere with flexion by impinging against the biceps tendon. All

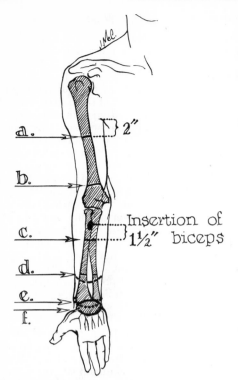

**Figure 6**   Amputation levels through the upper extremity. *a,* It is possible to fit a stump as short as 2.5 inches below the axillary fold with an above-elbow prosthesis. *b,* Supracondylar amputation provides an adequate lever for control of the prosthesis. Above this level, all length possible should be saved. *c,* Amputation through the site of election in the forearm is in the lower one-third of the forearm. *d,* Above this level, all length possible must be saved, although amputation as short as 1.5 inches below the biceps insertion can be fitted with a forearm prosthesis. Disarticulation through the elbow joint helps prevent rotary displacement of the socket. *e,* Disarticulation of the wrist through the radiocarpal joint produces an excellent stump, and preserves maximal pronation and supination. *f,* Above this level, transcarpal disarticulation may occasionally be useful.

length must be preserved above the site of election compatible with good amputation technique (Fig. 6).

Anterior and posterior skin flaps of equal length are made. A terminal scar is formed. A terminal device with an adjustable wrist fixture is fitted to the forearm socket. The socket is attached to a cuff about the arm above the elbow by metal elbow hinges to hold the stump in place. Attempts have been made to supply active pronation and supination by fitting the socket inside a cylindrical forearm piece which attaches to the elbow hinges and cuff. The socket is attached to the terminal device. The strength of the prosthesis may be reduced by the procedure, and the prosthesis may be subject to mechanical failure. If this type of prosthesis is impractical, a coupling is placed at the terminal device, which may allow the patient to predetermine the angle at which the hook operates.

### Short Below-Elbow Amputation

When most of the forearm must be sacrificed, the elbow joint should be saved if possible. However, the most proximal useful stump measures $1\frac{1}{2}$ inches below the insertion of the biceps tendon. The amputation is performed like the amputation in the lower one-third of the forearm. The biceps tendon, however, is freed from its attachments to increase the relative length of the stump. The prosthesis for this stump must be short to allow elbow flexion, yet long enough to hold the stump securely. This may be accomplished with a special prosthesis. A socket is fitted to the stump and, in turn, this small socket is attached to a forearm piece by a gear mechanism incorporated in the elbow hinges. When the stump moves one degree, the forearm piece moves two degrees. Thus, it is possible to flex the forearm piece fully while flexing the stump half this distance. Power is lost by this gear mechanism, however, and it may be necessary to reinforce this by a cable from the shoulder harness.

### Elbow Disarticulation

When the forearm is disarticulated at the elbow or the amputation occurs at a higher level, a mechanical elbow joint is required to place the forearm and terminal device in useful positions. This device must allow free voluntary flexion and extension activated by the shoulder harness. It should also provide positive locking in multiple degrees of flexion for stability.

For many years, the amputation through the elbow joint produced a stump too long to fit the standard elbow-joint mechanism. In recent years, external locking elbow joints have become available, making the amputation practical.

An advantage to elbow-joint disarticulation is that the flaring humeral condyles provide some rotational stability for the above-elbow socket. A disadvantage is the problem of adequate skin coverage and padding of bony prominences. Flaps are made of equal length when skin is available, but may be fashioned in any way that will allow proper cover after disarticulation.

The triceps tendon is sutured to the biceps and brachialis muscles over the joint surface. The lateral extensor muscle stump is trimmed to form a thin pad when it is drawn across the front of the joint and sutured to the medial epicondyle. The skin flaps are then closed.

### Supracondylar Amputation

Although amputation may be done through the condyles of the humerus, the most frequent site is about 2 or $2\frac{1}{2}$ inches above the joint line. Equal skin flaps are made. The triceps tendon is sectioned as low as possible. The wound is closed by suturing the triceps tendon over the end of the bone to the fascia of the biceps muscle. The skin flaps are closed with interrupted sutures.

### Short Arm Stumps

Amputation may be carried out to within $2\frac{1}{2}$ inches of the anterior axillary fold. Above this level, the conventional above-elbow socket will not retain the stump; a shoulder cap must be used, which limits effective arm motion.

As much length as possible should be preserved in amputations above the supracondylar level. The technique is similar to that for amputations lower in the arm. The triceps muscle is tapered from front to back to provide a thin musculofascial cover for the bone.

The prosthesis for arm amputations contains the usual forearm and terminal device but provides a mechanical elbow attached to the socket. Many joints have been designed. Essentially, these joints allow full flexion and extension but no pronation or supination. Flexion is controlled by a cable attached to the shoulder harness. Extension is usually activated by gravity. A positive locking mechanism is provided, by either a shoulder cable or locking lever. The elbow must be locked to permit the cable to act on the terminal device.

Shoulder-joint disarticulation should be avoided whenever possible. The head of the humerus helps to round out the shoulder and reduces the bony prominence of the acromion process. Amputations that must be done above $2\frac{1}{2}$ inches distal to the axillary fold are fitted with a prosthesis suspended from a plastic shoulder caplike socket. Arm motion at the shoulder is lost, and use of the prosthesis is limited. However, elbow flexion and extension is possible by shoulder motion, as is activation of the terminal device. Scapulothoracic motion may also help position the terminal device.

Stump socks of wool are used by most amputees, except those using the suction socket. The sock absorbs perspiration, lessens friction between the stump and prosthesis, and provides a cushion. The sock must fit the stump without wrinkles and must not constrict the circulation.

Careful hygiene of the stump must be followed to prevent skin problems. Stump socks must be washed frequently. The stump should be washed with an antimicrobial soap daily and thoroughly dried. Any skin lesions or abrasion must be treated promptly.

## REFERENCES

1. Advisory Committee on Artificial Limbs: Artificial Limbs. National Academy of Sciences, National Research Council, Washington, D.C. January, May, and September, 1954; January, May, and September, 1955.
2. Aitken, G. T., and Frantz, C. H.: Management of the Child Amputee. The American Academy of Orthopaedic Surgeons. Instructional Course Lectures, 17:246, 1960.
3. Alldredge, R. H., and Thompson, T. C.: The technique of Syme amputation. J. Bone Joint Surg., 28:415, 1946.
4. American Academy of Orthopaedic Surgeons: Orthopaedic Appliances Atlas. Artificial Limbs. Volume II. Ann Arbor, J. W. Edwards, 1960.
5. Burgess, E. M.: Sites of amputation election according to modern practice. Clin. Orthop., 37:17, 1964.
6. Burgess, E. M., and Romano, R. L.: The management of lower extremity amputees using immediate postsurgical prostheses. Clin. Orthop., 57:137, 1968.
7. Clippinger, F. W.: Immediate Post Surgical Fitting of Prostheses in Children. Inter-Clin. Inform. Bull., 5:7, Sept., 1966.
8. Committee on Prosthetic Research and Development: The Geriatric Amputee. Publication 919. National Academy of Sciences, National Research Council, Washington, D.C., 1961.
9. Dederich, R.: Plastic treatment of the muscles and bone in amputation surgery. A method designed to produce physiological conditions in the stump. J. Bone Joint Surg., 45-B:60, 1963.
10. Klopsteg, P. E., and Wilson, P. D.: Human Limbs and Their Substitutes. New York, McGraw-Hill Book Company, 1954.
11. Larmon, W. A.: Amputations and prostheses. Surg. Clin. N. Amer., 29:223, 1949.
12. Nathan, L., and Davidoff, R. B.: A multidisciplinary study of long term adjustment to amputation. Surg. Gynec. Obstet., 120:1274, 1965.
13. Prosthetic Research Board: Artificial Limbs. National Academy of Sciences, National Research Council, Washington, D.C. Vol. 3, No. 1, 1956; Vol. 4, No. 1, 1957; Vol. 5, No. 1 and No. 2, 1958; Vol. 6, No. 1, 1961; Vol. 6, No. 2, 1962; and Vol. 7. No. 1, 1963.
14. Slocum, D. B.: An Atlas of Amputations. St. Louis, C. V. Mosby Company, 1949.
15. Swanson, A. B.: Improving the End Bearing Characteristics of Lower Extremity Amputations Stumps—A Preliminary Report. Inter-Clin. Inform. Bull., 5:1, Feb., 1966.

# III

# Infections and Neoplasms of Bone

*William A. Larmon, M.D.*

Infection of bone consists of two major types: hematogenous and exogenous. Hematogenous osteomyelitis is produced by bacteria carried to the bone by the bloodstream. Exogenous osteomyelitis is produced by direct contamination of the bone through a wound. The courses of the two types of infection are different, as are the prognosis and treatment.

Since the introduction of chemotherapy and antibiotic drugs, the course and prognosis of bone and joint infections have changed. Before these therapeutic tools were available, bone infection was a serious malignant disease; crippling and death were commonplace. Today, the prognosis is brighter; crippling is less frequent and death occurs infrequently. However, to maintain this prognosis, the surgeon must be alert to prevent infection when he can, diagnose it promptly, and treat bone infection intelligently when it occurs.

Hematogenous osteomyelitis is primarily a disease of infancy and childhood; it is rare in the adult, while exogenous osteomyelitis may occur at any age. The anatomy and blood supply of the growing skeleton account for the difference in age distribution of the disease.

## ANATOMY OF BONE

Growing long bones are made up of an epiphysis, epiphyseal plate, metaphysis, and diaphysis. The epiphysis is separated from the metaphysis by the cartilaginous, avascular epiphyseal plate, from which the diaphysis grows in length. The epiphysis and metaphysis are made up of spongy cancellous bone surrounded by a thin layer of cortex. In the infant the metaphyseal cortex is very thin and fragile. As the child grows, this cortical layer thickens and becomes stronger. The diaphysis is primarily thick cortical bone.

The blood supply to the epiphysis and metaphysis is separate and distinct. Three major vascular systems supply the growing bone. The first is composed of nutrient arteries entering the diaphysis. These blood vessels enter the shaft of the bone, divide, and progress upward and downward to supply the metaphysis and diaphysis. In the metaphysis, the arteries become arterioles and finally capillary loops adjacent to the epiphyseal plate. At the capillary loop, the blood flow is slowed to nourish the developing bone produced by the epiphyseal plate. The blood from these capillary loops is collected in venous sinuses which empty into the veins of the medullary canal.

A second set of blood vessels enters the bone through the periosteum by the haversian canal system. These vessels anastomose with the intramedullary vascular system through very fine blood vessels penetrating the cortex of the bone.

A third set of blood vessels nourishes the epiphysis. These blood vessels are carried about the capsular reflections of the joint and are independent of the metaphyseal vessels. They enter the epiphysis, form a network of fine capillaries adjacent to the growing cartilage which surrounds the epiphysis, and emerge through venous sinuses and veins at the margins of the joint. A tough, heavy layer of periosteum surrounds the diaphysis and metaphysis. The periosteum is firmly attached at the epiphyseal plate, but may extend onto certain parts of the epiphysis. The attachment of the periosteum to the diaphysis and metaphysis is less firm than at the epiphyseal plate.

In the adult, when bone growth has ceased, these anatomic entities are blended into a single unit. The blood supply becomes confluent at the epiphysis and metaphysis as the epiphyseal plate turns to bone. The capillary loops are eliminated, the blood supply to the bone diminishes, the cortex of the metaphysis and epiphysis thickens, and the periosteum of the metaphysis thins and blends with that of the epiphysis. These changes account for the different types of bone infection in infancy, childhood, and adult life.

## OSTEOMYELITIS

### Pathology of Acute Hematogenous Osteomyelitis

Hematogenous osteomyelitis is produced when bacteria carried by the bloodstream lodge and grow in bone. The bacteria that circulate in the blood arise from active foci of infection in other parts of the body. These foci may be produced by many types of bacteria and any system of the body may be involved. Furuncles, infected tonsils, and bowel and urinary tract infections may produce bacteremia. Exanthematous lesions, such as scarlet fever, may also liberate bacteria into the bloodstream.

When bacteria enter the bloodstream, they are carried by the current of arterial blood to all parts of the body. As the flow of blood slows in the capillary beds, the bacteria settle into the tissues as sediment in a stream settles to the bottom in the quiet areas of a river. Undisturbed, these bacteria grow, establish a new colony, and proceed to destroy the surrounding tissue.

The anatomy of the growing bone provides ideal conditions for this chain of events. A large volume of slowly flowing blood is present in the capillary loops and venous sinuses of the metaphysis, and in the quiet area of blood flow bacteria can settle and grow. For this reason, osteomyelitis of the metaphysis is most common in infants and children, in whom this particular anatomic condition occurs.

When bacteria begin to grow, they feed upon the surrounding tissues. In this process, tissue is destroyed. The products of this metabolism, coupled with the inflammatory reaction of the body, produce an abscess or cellulitis. Enzymes and chemicals formed in this process influence the pathologic and clinical course of the disease. Some bacteria are easily killed by the body defenses; others are resistant and proceed to multiply under the most adverse conditions. Some bacteria produce toxic substances that affect the whole body; others produce lytic materials that dissolve and destroy tissue locally. As infection becomes established, a general systemic reaction follows. The temperature is elevated, the white blood cells multiply, and the sedimentation rate rises. There may be chills, malaise, and nausea and vomiting. The patient may become rapidly dehydrated.

A local reaction in the bone also takes place. As the products of bacterial growth and tissue destruction accumulate, the body attempts to isolate the process by building a wall of inflammatory cells. As this occurs, pressure is built up within the bone and pain becomes present in the area. Localization of the pain near a bone end is an important sign in the early recognition of the disease.

When pressure builds up in the unyielding bone, the blood supply to the area is strangled. The blood in the capillary loops and venous sinuses clots, and eventually the arterioles are thrombosed. Bone, thus deprived of its blood supply, dies. This dead bone is called a sequestrum. The size of the sequestrum varies, depending upon the degree of vascular damage. It may be a small area in the metaphysis or the entire shaft of the bone may be affected.

If the infection is controlled by the body, an abscess is formed, containing dead bone and bacteria. The repair process starts with the growth of new blood vessels into the area. The debris is absorbed and capillaries invade the dead bone. Osteoclasts remove the devitalized bone and osteoblasts lay down new bone. However, if the body defenses are inadequate, the destructive process continues. Pus formed in the abscess under pressure ruptures through the cortex, elevating the periosteum from the bone. For a time, the tough periosteum contains the inflammatory secretions and bacteria; however, bacteria may invade the bone through the haversian canals of the diaphysis as the periosteum is progressively stripped from the bone. New foci of infection are thus created and the entire shaft of the bone may become infected. Eventually, the periosteum ruptures, and pus is liberated into the soft tissues. In the infant, the cortex of the metaphysis is fragile and the periosteum is less firmly attached to the epiphyseal plate. When rupture of the abscess occurs, the infection may spread into the joint. Rapid destruction of the joint and epiphyseal plate follows. In older children, this is less likely to occur, because the metaphyseal cortex is thicker and the periosteum more firmly attached to the epiphyseal plate. The infected material usually burrows through fascial planes to the skin. The skin eventually breaks down, so that the pus is discharged on the surface of the extremity. A sinus tract is thus formed.

Although the periosteum is stripped from the bone, the periosteum remains viable. New bone is formed by the periosteum surrounding the dead bone of the metaphysis and diaphysis. This new bone surrounding the sequestrum is called involucrum.

Small pieces of sequestrum may be discharged through the sinus tract; however, larger pieces of dead bone are trapped and held by the involucrum. Bacteria continue to grow in this focus of dead bone, slowly destroying the sequestrum. At this stage, osteomyelitis becomes chronic. Infection with discharge of pus through the sinus tract may continue for many years. Pathologic fractures may occur in areas of weakened bone. Periodically, new abscesses in the bone may cause intermittent acute attacks of osteomyelitis during this phase. Bacteremia may arise from the continued infection and produce abscesses in other bones or organs.

**Pathology of Hematogenous Osteomyelitis in the Adult.** In the adult, hematogenous osteomyelitis is not common. When it occurs, the infection is usually less fulminating than in the child. Since the anatomy of the mature bone is different from that of the growing bone, the infection may arise in any part of the bone. The abscess is often walled off early in the course of the infection and contained usually within a small area of cancellous bone. This abscess may, in time, become sterile, but it continues to produce pain by pressure and inflammatory reaction. This type of abscess in bone of the adult is often called Brodie's abscess.

### Pathology of Exogenous Osteomyelitis

Exogenous osteomyelitis most often occurs after open fractures. The infecting organisms are introduced into the soft tissues and bone through the wound. If an abscess forms, the bone fragments may become devitalized, forming sequestra. Since the tract of the original wound offers a path for exit of secretions, a sinus usually forms in the wound. If drainage is insufficient, bone and soft tissue destruction continues and a systemic reaction may occur. Spread of the infection is by direct continuity, and is usually confined to the devitalized bone ends. Intact bone and periosteum of the adult has great resistance to infection, and, even though exposed, may not become infected. However, when the bone breaks, this resistance is lost at the damaged bone ends. The bone infection is thus usually confined to this area. When internal fixation devices have been used, the infection may spread about these foreign materials; however, the infection is usually not as extensive as in hematogenous osteomyelitis.

### Organisms Producing Osteomyelitis

The organism most commonly involved in producing hematogenous osteomyelitis is *Staphylococcus aureus*. Next in frequency is *Staphylococcus albus* or hemolytic streptococci; however, any organism may invade the bone. The clinical course of the infection depends upon the invasiveness and toxigenic characteristics of the invading organisms. Staphylococci and streptococci may produce severe systemic toxic reactions as well as rapid local destruction of bone, while tuberculosis may produce little systemic reaction and slower, more quiet destruction of tissues.

### Diagnosis of Acute Hematogenous Osteomyelitis

Acute hematogenous osteomyelitis presents varying symptoms and physical findings in the infant, child, and adult. All exhibit some evidence of general systemic reactions. Fever and chills with nausea and vomiting may be the first signs of infection in the infant and child. In the adult, the systemic reaction may be mild. The white blood cell count is elevated.

Local manifestations of infection are different in each group early in the course of the disease. In the infant, the infection is often fulminating. Pseudoparalysis of the part develops rapidly. The joints adjacent to the infection are usually held in flexion. The infant is irritable and cries out when the part is moved. Local pressure applied along the course of the bone may produce evidence of discomfort. With these findings, accompanied by the systemic reaction, osteomyelitis must be suspected, and treatment started promptly if serious destruction of the bone is to be avoided.

X-ray films of the part are usually normal in the infant for the first 3 or 4 days. If the disease is untreated until the bone shows destructive change and periosteal reaction on x-ray examination, the damage has already been done.

The thin cortex of the metaphysis and the loose periosteal attachment allows rupture of the abscess into the adjacent joint within the first few days of infection. The joint and epiphyseal plate are rapidly destroyed and growth disturbance of the bone is inevitable. Permanent disability is always expected when this occurs.

The child 1 year of age and older usually can help localize the process in the bone. Swelling and local heat may be absent at the onset of the infection; however, tenderness about the bone involved is usually present. Tapping the superficial bone with the examining finger helps to localize the area of maximal tenderness. In deeper bones, pressure may still elicit local tenderness near the bone ends. As the disease progresses, swelling and local heat develop. An effusion may develop in the adjacent joint. The joint is usually held in flexion. Although some active and passive motion remains in the joint, the patient may resist attempts to move the part. Muscle spasm may further limit motion. X-ray examination is usually normal for the first week or 10 days.

The adult usually presents milder, ill defined symptoms. He may complain of aching pain in the involved area of infection. Swelling may develop slowly. Any part of the bone may be infected. Effusion and limitation of motion of the adjacent joints are often absent.

### Treatment of Acute
### Hematogenous Osteomyelitis

To be effective, treatment must be instituted early. Blood cultures should be made promptly in an attempt to identify the infecting organism. Any focus of infection in the skin, nose and throat, or other areas should be cultured and sensitivity tests made. X-ray films of the suspected part should be made for comparison with those to be made later.

Antibiotic therapy or chemotherapy should be started immediately. Formerly, penicillin was the antibiotic of choice; however, many staphylococci and streptococci have become resistant to this drug. The tetracycline antibiotics may be given promptly in large doses at least 75 to 100 mg. per kilogram of body weight. These broad-spectrum antibiotics may be used until the organism is identified and sensitivity tests indicate a more specific antibiotic. Intravenous fluids and blood may be necessary to maintain hydration and combat anemia. Electrolyte balance must be watched carefully, particularly if the patient is vomiting. The involved part may be put at rest with a posterior plaster molded splint to immobilize the adjacent joint.

If the infection is controlled early, there may be minimal tissue destruction, and the bone may recover promptly. Antibiotic therapy should continue for 3 to 4 weeks after the temperature is normal to ensure sterilization of the bone.

X-ray examination of the bone 10 to 14 days after the onset of symptoms may show a destroyed area of bone in the metaphysis. The periosteum may be stimulated to produce new bone if it has been separated from the bone. This new bone may be seen on the x-ray film.

If the blood supply to the bone has been damaged, a sequestrum may form even though the infection has been controlled. The x-ray examinations over a period of time will then show the changes associated with the repair process. An involucrum forms about the sequestrum. The sequestrum is slowly absorbed and new bone is produced to replace the dead bone.

Occasionally, an abscess in the bone may rupture into the soft tissues while the antibiotic therapy finally controls the infection. This soft tissue abscess may be sterile. Aspiration and culture of the abscess may reveal that the infection is controlled. Aspiration removes the debris of infection and allows the repair process to proceed more rapidly. This should be done in most instances if the soft tissue sterile abscess is a large one.

Surgical drainage of such an area is usually not necessary if the surgeon is sure that the abscess is sterile. Open drainage in this circumstance permits entrance of new bacteria with the danger of secondary infection. When the infection is not completely controlled, or bone destruction is excessive, surgical treatment may be mandatory. Decompression of the bone and soft tissues may be necessary to prevent continued destruction. Dead bone that harbors bacteria must be removed to allow healing of draining sinuses.

If an abscess forms and the infection remains active in spite of adequate antibiotic therapy, surgical decompression of the infection is demanded. Incision and drainage of the bone is performed by removing a window of cortical bone over the infected metaphysis. The wound is packed open with petrolatum gauze and the part is immobilized in an appropriate plaster cast. The defect is allowed to close by growth of granulation tissue from the depths of the wound. When a major part of the bone is sequestrated, removal of this dead bone may disrupt the continuity of the skeleton. It is necessary to wait until an adequate involucrum has formed before this is done. Drainage is established to prevent added destruction; then the surgeon waits until enough new bone has formed to support the part before removing the sequestrum. This may take several months. When adequate new bone is formed, the sequestrum is removed and the cavity in the bone opened completely. This operation is termed saucerization because the bone cavity is made as shallow and broad as possible by the surgeon. This is done to eliminate overhanging edges and pockets in the bone which might harbor growing bacteria. The wound may be packed open until it is evident that the infection has been controlled; then the cavity is closed with split-thickness skin grafts applied to the granulating bone. Occasionally, it may be possible to remove the dead bone and close the soft tissues immediately. This procedure can be done when infection is inactive and the cavity can be filled with soft tissue to eliminate dead space. Muscle and fat may be used to fill the bone cavity. If the cavity in the bone cannot be filled with soft tissue, the wound must be left open and closed later to prevent growth of bacteria in this cavity.

### Treatment of Exogenous Osteomyelitis

Exogenous osteomyelitis can be prevented by adequate care of open fractures and wounds involving the bone. The proper debridement and cleansing of open fractures is essential to prevent infection. When the wound has been invaded by bacteria because of delayed debridement, the area must be packed open to prevent accumulation of the products of infection. Adequate drainage prevents destruction of bone and soft tissue if infection occurs.

When an open fracture is closed and infection develops, the wound must be opened promptly to establish drainage. Antibiotic therapy must be instituted. Rest for the part is essential. Appropriate splinting must be continued. When the infection is controlled, dead bone and foreign material must be removed to allow healing of the wound. The wound is usually packed open after sequestrectomy and closed secondarily when the infection is eliminated.

## SEPTIC ARTHRITIS

Septic arthritis, or pyogenic infection of a joint, occurs when bacteria invade the joint and grow. The bacteria may reach the joint by the bloodstream by extension from the surrounding tissue, or by direct implantation through a wound into the joint. The most common bacteria causing the infection are the various staphylococci and streptococci; however, any organism may produce joint infection. The condition occurs most frequently in infants and children.

The blood supply to the growing joint is independent of the circulation to the shaft of the bone. The epiphysis and metaphysis, separated by the epiphyseal plate, further isolate the joint and shaft of the bone. Blood vessels enter joints through the capsular attachments about the margins of the joint. These vessels divide, some entering the epiphysis while others form a fine capillary network throughout the synovial membrane. In this capillary bed, bacteria may be trapped. If the local defenses of the body are inadequate, infection occurs.

When the bacteria are introduced into the joint by direct penetration, or by extension from osteomyelitis, the bacteria begin to grow on the surface of the synovial membrane. The synovial membrane becomes thickened and an inflammatory reaction stimulates the synovial membrane to form more joint fluid and an effusion develops. The leukocyte content of the joint fluid increases markedly in response to the infection.

As bacteria begin to invade and destroy the tissue of the joint, proteolytic enzymes are liberated which dissolve the cartilage of the articular surface. This dissolution of cartilage is most marked where the articular surfaces are in contact.

Pressure within the joint rapidly increases. Heat, redness, and swelling of the joint become obvious. A generalized systemic reaction accompanies the joint reaction. Pain is severe. Any motion of the part is resisted, and even shaking the bed may cause extreme pain. Muscle spasm holds the joint flexed. If the condition is treated promptly, the damage to the joint may be minimal. However, if it is unrecognized or inadequately treated, the joint will be destroyed. The cartilage of the articular surfaces is rapidly dissolved, so that the underlying bone is exposed and, in turn, infected and destroyed. If the process continues, the distended joint capsule may rupture, with discharge of the abscess into the surrounding tissues. Sinus tracts may form and communicate with the joint.

Since hyaline cartilage cannot regenerate, it is replaced by scar tissue or fibrocartilage. Dependent upon the degree of cartilage destruction, the joint surfaces are damaged in variable degrees. Minimal surface damage may produce no permanent loss of joint function. However, when the deeper layers are involved, some permanent roughness of joint surfaces is inevitable with some loss of joint function. When bone is exposed, scar tissue forms across the joint surfaces. This scar tissue may produce a fibrous ankylosis of the joint, limiting motion and function. The scar may eventually become bone, completely ankylosing the joint. All of these changes occur rapidly in the joint, demanding prompt diagnosis and treatment if the joint is to be preserved.

Administration of broad-spectrum antibiotics must be started at once. The joint is aspirated and the material sent to the laboratory for culture and sensitivity tests. Microscopic examination of the joint fluid shows a tremendous number of leukocytes. Bacteria may be found in the joint fluid and this may help to establish the type of infection. Treatment cannot wait, however, while the organism is identified by culture.

The part should be splinted to prevent all joint motion. If the aspirated fluid is cloudy but still resembles synovial fluid, the infection may subside with splinting, repeated aspiration, and massive doses of broad-spectrum antibiotics. If the aspirated material is thick pus, the joint should be opened surgically and the pus evacuated. The joint is then irrigated with normal saline solution to remove mechanically the debris of infection. The synovial membrane is closed loosely with interrupted plain catgut sutures, and the wound is packed open. Loose closure of the synovium allows drainage but prevents exposure of the cartilage to the outside environment. This surgical drainage removes the proteolytic enzymes so damaging to cartilage. Reduction of intra-articular pressure restores circulation to the synovial membrane and allows the antibiotics to enter the joint more effectively.

When the organism has been isolated, sensitivity tests may indicate that a specific antibiotic drug may be more effective. This drug should then be used. As in osteomyelitis, drug therapy should continue for 3 or 4 weeks after the temperature returns to normal. During the active phase of treatment, the joint should be splinted in the position that will allow maximal function should ankylosis or loss of joint motion occur. When the temperature has returned to normal and the drainage has stopped, gentle active and passive joint motion may be started. If there is any evidence of reactivation of the infection, splinting of the part must be reinstituted and the joint maintained at rest. Use of the part should be restricted for weeks until the tissues return to as nearly normal a state as possible.

## TUBERCULOSIS OF THE BONES AND JOINTS

Tuberculosis of the bones and joints, an extremely destructive disease, has decreased in frequency in the United States in recent years. The pasteurization of milk, better living conditions, and early diagnosis of pulmonary tuberculosis, along with the development of specific drug therapy, have all contributed to this decline in this joint disease. This once common problem has now become rare as a cause of joint infection.

Tuberculosis affects primarily the epiphyses and joints rather than the metaphyses. The infection differs from pyogenic infection. While pyogenic infection stimulates a walling-off process, tuberculosis infection is primarily destructive with little defense reaction in the surrounding tissues. The infection is secondary to a primary focus elsewhere in the body. This primary infection may be in the lung, bowel, lymph glands, or other organs. The tubercle bacilli are carried to the joint or epiphysis by the arterial circulation. The bacilli lodge in the end-arteries of the epiphysis, or in the synovial blood vessels. Tuberculous abscesses are formed in the bone or synovial membrane. The local reaction to the infection is limited. The course of the disease is usually quite destructive of the involved parts. The process is primarily a lytic one, and new bone is rarely formed.

When the infection becomes established in the epiphysis, bone is destroyed until the abscess communicates with the joint. Discharge of this material into the joint produces synovial infection. The infection may start in the synovial membrane and spread to the bone of the epiphysis by direct erosion and pannus formation. Either method of infection eventually destroys the joint if treatment is delayed or is inadequate.

Frequently, tuberculous pus ruptures through the joint capsule and forms soft tissue abscesses. The pus dissects through fascial planes and the abscess may appear some distance from the infected bone or joint. If the tuberculous infection is controlled by the body, these distant abscesses may become isolated from the original focus of infection. The abscess may calcify slowly and become inactive. If the infection is not controlled, the abscess may, in time, rupture through the skin. A sinus forms and pyogenic bacteria may invade the bone or joint through this tract. This mixed infection adds to the destructive process and complicates treatment.

Although any joint in the body may be infected by the tubercle bacillus, those of the spine are most frequently involved. The joints of the lower extremities are next most frequently infected, while those of the upper extremity the least often involved.

A positive diagnosis of tuberculosis depends upon isolation of the organism from the infected area. Acid-fast staining and microscopic examination may be helpful. The guinea pig test is the most reliable method for establishing the diagnosis.

### Treatment

The treatment of bone and joint tuberculosis is both systemic and local. Infection at the primary site must be controlled, as well as that of the joint. Prior to the introduction of the combined drug therapy of streptomycin, para-aminosalicylic acid, and isonicotinic acid, there was no specific treatment for tuberculosis. Rest of the part and the patient was the essential method of treatment, plus arthrodesis of the joint. Although rest is still essential, the combined drug therapy controls the infection much more rapidly and completely.

Casts and splints and occasionally traction are used to immobilize the joint. Abscesses are aspirated if they are in danger of rupturing. When the infection is controlled, as signified by return of the temperature and sedimentation rate to normal, definitive treatment of the joint may be undertaken. Usually, arthrodesis of the joint is performed. In the spine, this may involve several vertebrae. Although function is limited by this procedure, it is the surest way to prevent recurrence of the infection in the joints. Occasionally, synovectomy has been performed, with debridement of the joint, to salvage some function. However, this excision of the focus of infection cannot always be accomplished completely and reactivation of the infection is a potential hazard. Arthrodesis is still the safest method of treatment. Isolated abscesses are aspirated and occasionally they can be completely excised, if they no longer communicate with the original point of infection. Observation of the patient must continue for years to allow prompt treatment of any reactivation of the disease.

## NEOPLASMS OF BONE

The musculoskeletal system may be affected by tumors arising in any of the component tissues or by metastatic lesions from other organs. Tumors involving the skeleton may occur in primary bone cells or in the hematopoietic elements of bone, in cartilage, and in the fibrous and synovial components. Other tumors may arise in muscle, nerve, blood vessels, and the fat of the musculoskeletal system. These tumors may be benign or malignant. The surgeon must understand thoroughly these pathologic processes to treat these patients intelligently.

Through the years, numerous classifications of these tumors have evolved as knowledge about them increased. The classification of bone tumors is necessary for a clear understanding of the pathologic changes that are possible within the system. The classification devised by Louis Lichtenstein is based upon the origin of the tissue involved, and is the most popular one at present (Table 1).

The accurate diagnosis of these tumors is essential because treatment is primarily a surgical problem. The nature of the tumor determines the extent of the surgical procedure, varying from simple excision to radical amputation.

## TUMORS OF CARTILAGE CELL OR CARTILAGE-FORMING CONNECTIVE TISSUE

### Osteocartilaginous Exostosis or Osteochondroma

The most common type of benign tumor arising from precartilaginous tissue is single or multiple osteocartilaginous exostoses, or osteochondroma. Because these tumors arise from aberrant foci of cartilage, as precartilage cells on the surface of the bone, they may be regarded as congenital anomalies.

The tumor arises most often on the metaphyseal surface of the long bones, but may be found on the flat bones, ribs, vertebrae, and small bones of the hands and feet. The tumors are usually found before the age of 20, and affect males and females about equally.

Symptoms are usually minimal. The patient often becomes aware of a painless mass near a joint by accidental palpation. Occasionally, a painful bursa develops over the exostosis when the mass is subjected to pressure by muscle or tendon action or by weight bearing.

The tumor may be sessile or pedunculated and may vary in size from a small protuberance on the bone to a large, cauliflower-like mass. The mass is composed of a cartilage cap covering an extension of cortex from the parent bone surrounding a center of spongiosa continuous from the spongiosa of the involved bone. The entire tumor is covered by a layer of periosteum. Areas of calcification of the cartilage cap may be evident in the roentgenograms of the tumor.

The microscopic appearance of the tumor is characteristic. The cartilage cap is composed of columns of chondrocytes arranged perpendicular to the underlying cortex. In the growing tumor, a zone of enchondral ossification is present on the surface of the cortex similar to that found in the epiphysis of a growing bone. The spongiosa may contain hematopoietic, fatty, or fibrous marrow. Rests of the cartilage cells may be found scattered throughout the tumor. When the involved bone ceases to grow, the tumor becomes quiescent and the cartilage cap may slowly involute.

In about 2 per cent of tumors of the solitary type, malignant transformation may occur, whereas the incidence of this complication may rise to 11 per cent in multiple osteocartilaginous exostoses. Chondrosarcoma is the usual malignant transformation of the benign tumor. Rapid growth or increasing calcification of the cartilage cap may herald the malignant change; thus, roentgenographic records of the benign tumors should be kept. These changes may occur at any time, but are more likely after the age of 30.

Complete excision of the tumor and periosteal covering flush with the surface of the long bones or section of the tumor with its base from the flat bones is the treatment of choice. Because the incidence of malignant transformation is low, routine resection is not indicated unless the tumor is painful or unsightly or interferes with function; however, careful periodic roentgenologic studies should be made of the tumor. Recurrence of the tumor is rare, but should alert the surgeon to the possibility of malignant change or to the possibility of a primary chondrosarcoma.

### Chondroma (Enchondroma or Enchondromatosis)

Chondromas are benign tumors usually found in the interior of the small bones of the hands and feet, although the tumor may arise in the metaphysis of the long bones or the flat bones of the thoracic cage. When they are centrally located, they are called enchondromas. The lesional cell resembles hyaline cartilage. Often areas of calcification or bone formation are found in the interior of the tumor. Usually, the surrounding cortex is thin, and the tumor may expand the bone to form a fusiform swelling (Fig. 1).

The tumor is usually found in persons between the ages of 10 and 50 years, and is often manifested by pathologic fracture through the weakened cortex or by a painless, firm swelling of the bone. There is no predilection for either sex.

The gross appearance of the tumor is usually pearly white and firm with small scattered areas of yellow, gritty, calcified cartilage. At times, the tumor is rather soft and granular.

The microscopic findings reveal usually uniform cartilage cells with a single small nucleus. Areas of degeneration and calcification are found scattered throughout the tumor in varying degrees. Irregular and multinucleated cells may indicate early transformation of a malignant phase; although rare in the small bones, the larger tumors in the long bones occasionally undergo the change.

Treatment is usually curettement of the lesions of the small bones followed by bone graft replacement. The ribs, sternum, and long bones may re-

**TABLE 1**  CLASSIFICATION OF PRIMARY TUMORS OF BONE*

| Benign Tumors of Bone | | Malignant Counterpart (If Any) | Malignant Tumors of Bone (Arising through Malignant Change or Independently) |
|---|---|---|---|
| Of cartilage-cell or cartilage-forming connective tissue derivation | Peripheral: Osteocartilagenous exostosis (multiple exostosis) | Peripheral chondrosarcoma | Chondrosarcoma |
| | Central: Enchondroma (skeletal enchondromatosis) | Central chondrosarcoma | |
| | Benign chondroblastoma | (Not known) | |
| | Chondromyxoid fibroma | Mesenchymal chondrosarcoma | |
| | Poorly differentiated chondroid tumors | Chondroblastic sarcoma | |
| Of osteoblastic derivation | Osteoma | (Not known) | Osteogenic sarcoma { Central / Parosteal } |
| | Osteoid-osteoma | (Not known) | |
| | Benign osteoblastoma | (Osteogenic sarcoma) | |
| Of nonosteoblastic connective tissue derivation | Desmoplastic fibroma | (Not known) | Fibrosarcoma |
| | Nonosteogenic fibroma | (Not known) | |
| | Least aggressive giant-cell tumors → | More aggressive and malignant giant-cell tumors → | Frankly malignant giant-cell tumors |
| Of mesenchymal connective tissue origin | | | Ewing's sarcoma |
| Of hematopoietic origin | | | Multiple myeloma; Chronic myeloid leukemia; Acute leukemias; Malignant lymphoma { Reticulum-cell sarcoma, "Lymphosarcoma," Hodgkin's disease } |
| Of nerve origin | Neurofibroma / Neurilemoma / Ganglioneuroma | (Malignant schwannoma) | |
| Of vascular origin | Hemangioma / Hemangiopericytoma (glomus) | (Hemangioendothelioma) | Hemangioendothelioma |
| Of fat-cell origin | Lipoma | | Liposarcoma |
| Of notochordal derivation | | | Chordoma |
| Of adamantine or possibly basal-cell derivation | | | So-called adamantinoma |

*From Lichtenstein, L.: Bone Tumors. St. Louis, C. V. Mosby Company, 1965.

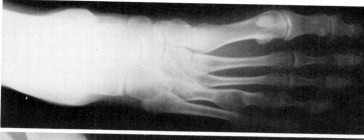
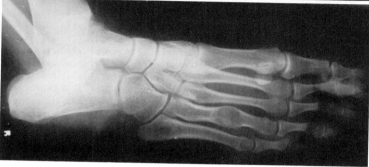

**Figure 1** Enchondroma: An expansile lesion is present in the fourth metatarsal bone. The cortex is thin and expanded but not perforated. (Courtesy of Dr. Harvey White, Chief, Department of Radiology, Children's Memorial Hospital, Chicago, Illinois.)

quire resection of the involved bone followed by reconstructive procedures in the long bones.

### Multiple Enchondromas or Enchondromatosis

These may affect multiple bones, causing varying degrees of deformity. When confined to one side of the body, the condition has been called Ollier's disease, and, when associated with multiple hemangiomas of the skin, Maffuci's syndrome. Removal of multiple lesions is usually impossible, and treatment is directed toward correction of deformity created by growth disturbance. Rarely, these tumors may undergo transformation to malignant chondrosarcoma, demanding radical resection or amputation.

### Benign Chondroblastoma

Chondroblastoma is usually a small benign tumor derived from chondroblasts, and is usually located in the epiphysis of the long bones, but, with growth, may extend into the metaphysis. The size of the tumor varies from a few millimeters up to 6 or 7 cm. in diameter. Often, it is eccentrically placed in the epiphysis, and may lie just beneath the articular cartilage without destroying it. Radiographically and microscopically, the tumor is often confused with benign giant cell tumor of bone.

The most common sites for the tumor are the femur and tibia at the knee joint and the upper end of the humerus, although the tumor may arise in any epiphysis.

The tumor is usually found in patients between the ages of 10 and 20 years, and is more common in males. The ratio is approximately three male patients to one female.

The symptoms are usually pain and swelling about the adjacent joint, frequently of several months' duration.

The roentgenographic appearance is fairly characteristic. An area of rarefaction is found in the epiphysis, eccentrically located, surrounded by a thin area of sclerotic bone. Trabeculae may traverse the tumor, and flecks of calcified tumor are practically always observed. With growth, the tumor may extend into the metaphysis and produce thinning of the cortex.

Grossly, the tumor is firm and grayish pink, with areas of hemorrhage and necrosis and areas of gritty calcification.

The microscopic picture is varied, consisting of areas of chondroblasts, which are clear, distinct cells with oval or round nuclei. The nucleus is often indented. Scattered in areas of the tumor are multinucleated giant cells, which are usually smaller and fewer in number than in the typical giant cell tumor of bone, and occur in areas of hemorrhage. Chondroid material is found in varying amounts, and is a distinctive feature of the tumor. Degeneration of cartilage cells leads to calcification similar to the degenerative change found in cartilage during osseous transformation. These areas may show absorption, hemorrhage, and replacement by connective tissue and collagenous plaques.

The treatment is curettage followed by replacement with bone grafts. When the location allows resection without loss of function, this may be done. Local recurrence is rare, and malignant changes have been reported only in two instances, in which roentgen therapy was used.

### Chondromyxoid Fibroma

Chondromyxoid fibroma is derived from cartilage-forming connective tissue. The tumor is usually found in the metaphyseal region, eccentrically located, and is rare compared to the frequency of other bone tumors. The majority of tumors occur in the second and third decades of life, and there is no predilection for either sex. More than half of these tumors have been reported in the tibia, with the lower femur second, although the small bones of the hands and feet, pelvic girdle, ribs, and scapula may be affected.

Pain and swelling of the metaphyseal area of the bone of several months' duration is the usual complaint of the patient.

Roentgenographically, the appearance of the tumor in the long bones is fairly characteristic. An eccentrically placed, circumscribed, rarefied defect, often involving the cortex, is found in the metaphysis at varying distances from the epiphysis. If the cortex is completely destroyed, a thin shell of periosteal new bone may cover the tumor, which does not invade the surrounding soft tissues. A thin zone of sclerotic bone confines the tumor in the medullary portion of the bone. In the small bone, the rarefied area may appear lobulated and expand the cortex.

Grossly, the tumor is firm and distinctly lobulated, and white or yellow-tan in contrast to the bluish white of chondromas. Microscopic sections of the tumor reveal spindle-shaped cells arranged loosely in a matrix of myxoid intercellular substance. At the periphery of the tumor lobules, the cells may be more densely packed. As the tumor matures, areas of myxomatous matrix may show collagenization or chondroid formation.

The tumor is apparently completely benign, and cure is usually effected by complete curettage with bone grafting or local resection.

### Chondrosarcoma of Bone

Chondrosarcoma may arise centrally in the bone or peripherally from the cartilage cap of osteocartilaginous exostosis. The central lesion may arise from an enchondroma by malignant transformation, or may arise as a primary tumor.

The peripheral chondrosarcomas are usually made up of actively growing, mature hyaline cartilage, whereas the central tumors may show less differentiation.

The long bones are primarily affected—the femur, tibia, and humerus particularly, however, the ribs, scapula, and innominate bones are frequently the site of this tumor. It is rare for malignant transformation to occur in single enchondromas of the bones of the hands and feet. The condition is much more likely to occur when multiple enchondromas are present.

These tumors have a slight predilection for males—about 60 per cent. The majority of tumors appear in those between the ages of 30 and 60. This history often reveals that the patient has been aware of a painless swelling of a long bone or the presence of an osteocartilaginous exostosis for a considerable period of time. The patient may have noticed the mass slowly enlarging or becoming mildly painful. The time interval of pain and swelling may be relatively short in rapidly developing central tumors. In general, however, the tumors are slow-growing, and do not produce

much discomfort. Metastasis occurs late in most chondrosarcomas, but local extension into blood vessels is common. These lesions growing into the larger vessels may grow along the interior of the vessel for great distances from the primary tumor, eventually reaching the heart and lungs by this route. Metastasis to the periphery of the lungs can occur in late stages of the disease or in the highly malignant tumors. Metastatic lesions to the lymph nodes are rare.

Physical examination may indicate the presence of an osteocartilaginous exostosis, or may simply indicate an enlarged long bone. The mass may be mildly tender, but the skin is not red or warm. When the tumor is near a joint, the joint may be swollen with some limitation of motion.

The roentgenologic findings in the central tumors usually show irregular mottling with calcification and fuzzy destruction of the cortex. If the cortex has been perforated by the tumor, the extension of the tumor into the soft parts may produce an abnormal shadow overlying the bone.

Roentgenographs of the peripheral chondrosarcoma show much more blotchy densities than in the benign osteochondromas, and the areas of calcification in the cartilage may extend away from the tumor in irregular, stringy patches.

The histologic appearance of chondrosarcoma may be subtle, but malignancy is indicated when many cells contain plump nuclei, more than an occasional cell contains two such nuclei, and giant cartilage cells with one or more nuclei are found. In the more advanced tumors, frank sarcomatous changes are evident.

Because metastasis generally occurs late in this tumor, wide resection of the lesion or amputation may effect a cure. Central tumors of small size may be resected widely, followed by reconstructive procedures; however, if it appears that complete eradication of the tumor cannot be accomplished by this method, amputation should be performed.

In peripheral chondrosarcoma arising from osteocartilaginous exostosis wide resection should include the soft tissue over the tumor as well as the bone containing the base. Inoperable tumors may be treated with roentgen therapy, but the tumor is radioresistant, and the results have been disappointing.

## TUMORS OF OSTEOBLASTIC DERIVATION

### Osteoid-Osteoma

This tumor of bone is composed of a small, oval or round nidus of osteoid tissue and new bone deposited within a bed of highly vascularized, osteogenic connective tissue. The tumor may occur in medullary or cortical bone, and is most often found in the bones of the lower extremities, but may occur in any bone.

For many years, the origin of this lesion was controversial, but it is now regarded by most authorities as a true neoplasm of bone. There is a slight tendency for the tumor to occur more frequently in males. The age distribution is from 5 to

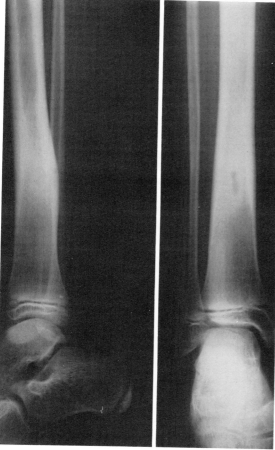

**Figure 2** Osteoid-osteoma: The nidus is seen as a rarefied area surrounded by sclerotic bone on the posterior aspect of the tibia in the lower one-third. (Courtesy of Dr. Harvey White, Chief, Department of Radiology, Children's Memorial Hospital, Chicago, Illinois.)

30 years, with the preponderance of lesions occurring in adolescents or young adults.

The primary symptom is pain, most noticeable at night and relieved to a degree by aspirin. Occasionally, slight heat or redness may be noted. Characteristically, the lesion is quite painful to pressure.

The roentgenographic evidence of the tumor is characteristic, but varies with the location of the tumor in cancellous or cortical bone. When the lesion occurs in cancellous bone, an area of rarefaction with a central area of dense bone may be seen, surrounded by a thin zone of sclerosis. When the lesion is in the cortical area, dense sclerosis extends in the cortex for a considerable distance from the nidus. The nidus often lies on the inner aspect of the cortex, and is observed as a rarefied area with or without a dense central area. In cortical bone, laminagraphs may be necessary to distinguish the nidus in the sclerotic bone. The radiographic appearance may be confused with that of bone abscess or chronic sclerosing osteomyelitis (Fig. 2).

Grossly, when the specimen can be removed intact, the lesion stands out as a reddish circumscribed area in the bone with surrounding sclerosis and adjacent periosteal reaction. Microscopically, the lesion appears to be a circumscribed area of osteoid with areas of calcification and atypical bone formation within a vascular background of osteoblastic connective tissue.

Surgical removal of the lesion is the only effective treatment. The relief of symptoms is immediate and lasting. If the nidus is incompletely removed, pain recurs and a secondary operation becomes necessary.

### Benign Osteoblastoma

This benign tumor, composed of osteoblasts and osteoid tissue in avascular stroma, has been called by various names—osteogenic fibroma and giant osteoid-osteoma. There is some resemblance to osteoid-osteoma; however, the tumor is usually larger, and there is less tendency to form sclerotic bone. The lesion is often expansile, enlarging the bone and thinning the cortex.

The limb bones are most commonly affected in the shaft of metaphyseal regions, and the vertebrae and skull may also be affected. Usually, the neural arch of the vertebra is involved rather than the body.

There is no great difference in the incidence of the tumor in male or female. The majority of these lesions occur in teenagers or children, and the remaining one-third occur in adults.

Symptoms are usually pain in a slowly enlarging bone of months' or several years' duration. When the lesion occurs in the spine, pain and neurologic deficit may be evident as the tumor encroaches on the spinal cord.

The roentgenographic appearance is usually a radiolucent area within an expanded, thin cortex usually without periosteal new bone formation. There may be a thin wall of sclerosis surrounding the tumor in the medullary portions. Calcification or dense areas of bone may be seen in the interior of the lesion (Fig. 3).

Grossly, the tumor appears reddish, and is gritty and quite vascular. The microscopic appearance is quite variable, but consists primarily of osteoid and proliferating osteoblasts with calcification of osteoid in patches. The stroma may often consist of highly vascular fibrocytic tissue. Giant cell macrophages may be found in relation to newly formed, mineralized matrix. The lesions may be confused with giant cell tumors or osteogenic sarcoma. Because the lesion is benign, care in microscopic interpretation must be exercised to prevent inadvertent radical surgery in the mistaken belief that one is dealing with an osteogenic sarcoma.

Thorough curettement or resection of accessible lesions is the preferred treatment. Decompression of the skull and spinal cord must be done as completely as is necessary to relieve the symptoms. When the tumor cannot be removed completely, roentgen therapy is of value.

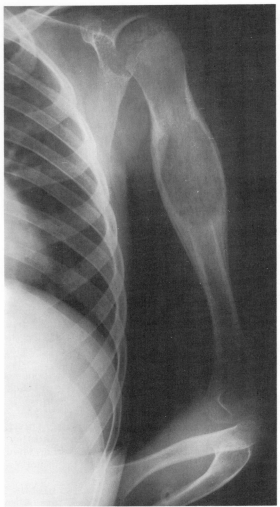

**Figure 3** Benign osteoblastoma: Expansile lesion of the humerus. Thin cortex and periosteal new bone formation with a fine line of sclerosis about the margins of the lesion characterize this particular tumor. (Courtesy of Dr. Harvey White, Chief, Department of Radiology, Children's Memorial Hospital, Chicago, Illinois.)

### Osteogenic Sarcoma

Osteogenic sarcoma apparently arises from primitive bone-forming mesenchyme. Of the malignant tumors of bone, it is second only to myeloma as the most common malignant neoplasm. The tumor is made up of anaplastic connective tissue forming tumor osteoid and bone, but may also form tumor cartilage, which, in turn, ossifies. The tumor may be primarily osteolytic or osteoblastic, depending upon how much tumor bone is formed. These tumors are highly malignant, metastasizing to the lungs by way of the bloodstream early in their development. Five year survival after treatment averages only about 10 per cent.

The tumor seems to affect males more often than females. The most frequent occurrence of the tu-

mor is between 10 and 25 years of age, but it may occur at any age. The older people afflicted with osteogenic sarcoma are most frequently the victims of malignant transformation of Paget's disease, and the incidence of this change may be as high as 10 to 15 per cent.

The most common locations for this tumor are the lower end of the femur, upper tibia, and upper end of the humerus but other bones may be affected as well.

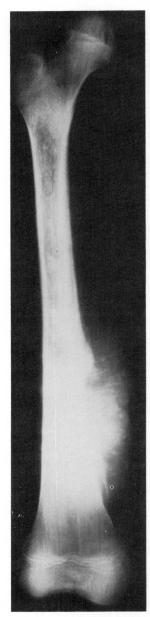

**Figure 4** Osteogenic sarcoma: Dense bone is present throughout much of the shaft of the femur. The tumor has perforated the cortex and the "sunburst" effect of new tumor bone is seen. (Courtesy of Dr. Harvey White, Chief, Department of Radiology, Children's Memorial Hospital, Chicago, Illinois.)

The usual presenting complaint of the patient is pain and enlargement of the affected part. When the tumor is growing rapidly, weight loss, anemia, and elevated alkaline phosphatase blood levels may be found. Usually, the patient is aware of trouble for a few weeks to several months before seeking treatment.

Usually, the tumor arises in the interior of the bone, but rapidly destroys the cortex, elevating the periosteum, which may form nontumorous new bone where it is stripped from the shaft. Tumorous bone then forms about the shaft of the bone. Upon perforating the periosteum, the tumor invades the surrounding muscle, or may invade the adjacent joint.

The roentgenographic appearance is not always characteristic, but perforation of the cortex and formation of tumorous bone beneath the periosteum should indicate the possibility of the serious tumor. The degree of sclerosis or osteolysis depends upon the amount of new bone and bone destruction that is taking place (Fig. 4).

The gross appearance of the tumor varies with the degree of osteoblastic or osteolytic activity. When the tumor is primarily osteoblastic, the interior of the bone may be very sclerotic; however, if the tumor is actively growing outside the cortex, it may be softer and more vascular. The osteolytic tumors are usually softer and cystic with areas of hemorrhage and necrosis. In the medullary cavity, the tumor may extend for a considerable distance, and may be patchy in distribution, occupying areas of normal bone. Thus, it may be difficult to determine the extent of the tumor roentgenographically.

The histologic appearance varies considerably. The criteria for diagnosis of osteogenic tumor are the presence of a sarcomatous stroma and the direct formation of tumor osteoid and bone. Tumor cartilage undergoing ossification may or may not be present.

When the diagnosis has been confirmed by biopsy, treatment is radical amputation. The level of amputation should be well above the tumor, and should be done between tourniquets placed above the tumors. Hindquarter and forequarter amputation may be necessary for tumors extending into the upper femur and humerus. The value of roentgen therapy or chemotherapy is still not determined.

### Ossifying Parosteal Sarcoma

This tumor arises on the surface of the bone in contradistinction to osteogenic sarcoma, which arises centrally. The neoplasm apparently arises from slow-growing bone and cartilage-forming periosteal and parosteal connective tissue. The most frequent site of this tumor is the posterior aspect of the femur near the knee joint. Although the tumor is malignant, it is slow-growing, but may eventually perforate the cortex and invade the medullary canal. Metastasis to the lung occurs late in the course of the tumor.

Block resection of the tumor is recommended, except when the tumor is recurrent; amputation should then be performed.

## TUMORS OF NONOSTEOBLASTIC CONNECTIVE TISSUE

### Nonosteogenic Fibroma of Bone

This lesion, consisting of spindle cell connective tissue, has also been called nonossifying fibroma, metaphyseal fibrous defect, and fibrous cortical defect. It occurs in the shafts of long bones of the extremities, seemingly sparing the other bones of the skeleton. It occurs usually in those between the ages of 10 and 20, but may occasionally be found in younger children. There seems to be no sex predilection.

Symptoms are minimal or may be absent. The lesion is often found accidentally when roentgenograms are made of an extremity following trauma. Occasionally, pathologic fracture may bring the condition to the attention of the surgeon.

The roentgenographic appearance is characteristic in most instances. The lesion usually appears as a sharply delineated, eccentric, lobulated area of rarefaction, usually involving the cortex. The cortex may bulge outward on the surface, but new bone formation is not evident. The lesion may occupy the entire width of the small tubular bones. Calcification in the interior of the lesion is lacking.

Grossly, the tumor is yellow or yellow-brown and of rather rubbery consistency. Microscopically, there are whorls of spindle-shaped connective tissue cells with occasional areas of small, multinucleated giant cells and foam cells.

Surgical excision is elective unless the lesion is painful or likely to cause pathologic fracture. Curettage of the lesion followed by bone grafting is usually all that is necessary to effect a cure.

### Giant Cell Tumor of Bone (Osteoclastoma)

Giant cell tumors of bone arise from the non-bone-forming, supporting connective tissue of the marrow. They may be benign or malignant. It has been stated that 50 per cent of these tumors recur after excision and 15 to 20 per cent are malignant or undergo malignant transformation. Thus, the tumor must be regarded as a potentially dangerous one.

The tumor typically arises in the epiphyseal end of the long bones; the lower femur, upper tibia, and lower radius are the most frequent sites in that order. The lesion may arise in any bone, but it is rare in the innominate bone, ribs, and skull.

These tumors affect females twice as often as males. The greatest incidence of the tumor is in those between 15 and 40 years, but the tumor may occur in older patients. It is rare in young children.

The roentgenographic appearance of giant cell tumors is not always characteristic, but the location of the tumor in the ends of the bone is significant, as these tumors always arise in this location. The lesion produces rarefaction, and is often eccentrically located with thinning and expansion of the cortex without periosteal new bone formation. Eventually, the cortex may be destroyed.

The gross appearance of the tumor varies with

the amount of necrosis, degeneration, and hemorrhage within the lesion. Early, the tumor is dark red or reddish brown. As hemorrhage occurs, patches of bright red or black appear and cystic areas develop. The tumor is destructive of bone, and may perforate through the periosteum, but the cartilage of the articular surface is not destroyed, although it may be distorted by loss of bony support or fracture.

The microscopic appearance of the tumor varies with the amount and degree of hemorrhage and degeneration. In unaffected areas, the tumor is made up of spindle-shaped stromal cells which are moderately vascularized with multinucleated giant cells and collagen fibrils interspersed throughout the tumor cells. In areas of degeneration, osteoid trabeculae and new bone may be found. The more cellular and atypical the stromal cell type, the more likely the tumor is to recur or metastasize.

The treatment of choice is total excision of the tumor; however, the size and location of the tumor and the cytologic picture may warrant thorough curettement and replacement by bone grafts. When the tumor appears frankly malignant or has recurred several times, amputation may be the only method of controlling the lesion. The results of roentgen therapy are debatable.

### Fibrosarcoma of Bone

Fibrosarcoma of bone is a malignant fibroblastic tumor that does not form osteoid or bone. The tumor is usually less malignant than osteogenic sarcoma, as indicated by a 5 year survival rate of 25 per cent. The tumor is less frequently found than osteogenic sarcoma or chondrosarcoma. It is primarily a bone-destructive lesion.

There is no sex predilection, and the age of occurrence is from the second through the sixth decades of life. Thus, the tumor occurs in a much older group of patients than primary osteogenic sarcoma.

The most frequent locations are the interior of the ends of long bones, primarily the femur, tibia and humerus.

There is no characteristic roentgenographic appearance of the lesion, except for bone destruction.

Symptoms are pain or pathologic fracture and a slowly enlarging swelling. The symptoms may be present for a few months to many years.

Grossly, the tumor appears to be made up of fibrous tissue that is destroying bone, and may be confused with nonossifying fibroma or fibrous dysplasia of bone.

The microscopic appearance varies from rather mature fibroblasts to rather anaplastic fibroblasts. There is no true osteoid or bone formation, although occasionally calcification may be found.

When the diagnosis has been established by biopsy, radical amputation is indicated. Although these tumors grow at varying rates and exhibit varying degrees of malignancy, they are all potentially life-endangering, and should be treated as such.

## TUMORS OF MESENCHYMAL CONNECTIVE TISSUE ORIGIN

### Ewing's Sarcoma

Ewing's sarcoma of bone is a highly malignant, multicentric, small round cell sarcoma. The origin of the cell is not clearly defined but it may be of undifferentiated mesenchymal origin. Clinically and cytologically, the lesion is easily confused with reticulum cell sarcoma, neuroblastoma, and metastatic cancer. The lesion is primarily bone-destructive; however, periosteal new bone formation is a common feature of the lesion as it perforates the cortex of the bone. Either multiple primary foci of tumor or early metastatic spread to other bones produces multiple lesions of the skeleton. The solitary lesion may be confused with the inflammatory reaction of osteomyelitis as reflected by bone destruction and periosteal new bone formation.

The tumor may appear to originate in any bone, but is common in the trunk bones and long bones. The lesion arises in the metaphysis or more toward the center of the shaft, but apparently excludes the epiphysis.

The neoplasm is more common in males, and the age distribution is from infancy to about 25 years.

Pain is the usual symptom localized to the area of the tumor. When the pelvic girdle is involved, referred pain in the distribution of the sciatic nerve may occur. Local tenderness to palpation is usual. There may be visible swelling of the part, and occasionally dilated veins are found in the skin over the tumor. Local increase in temperature of the area is common. Weight loss, fever, anemia, and leukocytosis with an elevated sedimentation rate may confuse the clinical picture with osteomyelitis. When these findings predominate, the likelihood of a rapidly fatal course is increased.

The radiographic findings reveal mottled bone destruction with extensive involvement of the shaft of the long bones. Periosteal new bone may occur in layers, producing an onion-peel-like picture, which was considered pathognomonic of the disease, but is now recognized to occur in other conditions and only occasionally in Ewing's sarcoma. Multiple bone involvement is almost inevitable (Fig. 5).

Grossly, the tumor is gray-white, glistening, and, in many instances, soft to almost liquid in consistency. Hemorrhage, degeneration, and cyst formation in the tumor are common findings. At the time of biopsy, the liquid portion of the tumor may resemble pus, further misleading the surgeon to think that he may be dealing with osteomyelitis; however, careful biopsy should rectify this confusion promptly.

The microscopic findings reveal cellular tumor with little intercellular stroma. Fibrous tissue strands may separate the tumor cells into rather large compartments. The nucleus of the lesional cell is oval or round. The cytoplasm is slightly granular and scanty with indistinct cell outlines. Mitotic figures are numerous. Periosteal new bone

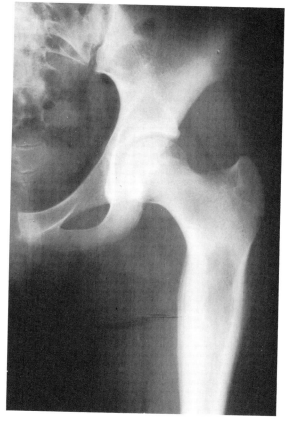

**Figure 5** Ewing's tumor: Irregular destruction of bone in the metaphyseal area and periosteal new bone formation in "onion skin" layers characterize this particular tumor. (Courtesy of Dr. Harvey White, Chief, Department of Radiology, Children's Memorial Hospital, Chicago, Illinois.)

may form where the periosteum has been elevated by the tumor.

The results of treatment either by roentgen therapy or amputation are uniformly poor. Relief of symptoms may be obtained by roentgen therapy for varying periods of from a few months to a year. Eventually, metastasis to lungs and other organs leads to a fatal outcome.

## TUMORS OF HEMATOPOIETIC ORIGIN

### Primary Reticulum Cell Sarcoma of Bone

Primary reticulum cell sarcoma of bone is derived from the reticulum cells of bone marrow. The cell type is similar to that of the reticulum cell sarcoma of lymph nodes; however, the course differs in that solitary lesions of bone accessible to surgical excision have a fairly favorable prognosis when this treatment is accompanied by roentgen therapy.

When it occurs in long bones, the tumor tends to occur in the end or shaft of the bone. The lesion is primarily bone-destructive, and may perforate the periosteum and invade the surrounding tissues. Metastasis to regional lymph nodes is common. There is a predilection for males in the ratio of 3 to 2. The tumor may occur at any age, but is rare in very young children.

There is no characteristic roentgenographic picture. Mottled destruction of bone and areas of sclerosis and cortical destruction with minimal periosteal new bone are the general findings.

Pain with pathologic fracture is the common symptom.

Grossly, the tumor is friable when it invades the soft tissues, and has the appearance of malignant lymphoma.

The predominant lesional cell is the reticulum cell; however, lymphocytes and lymphoblasts may be found in varying amounts in the tumor. There is a tendency for the cells to be in alveolar groupings, separated by the reticulum framework of the tumor. Special strains for reticulum cells may be helpful in differentiating the tumor.

When it has been determined that the lesion is solitary, surgical and roentgen therapy offer a good possibility for a survival rate of 40 to 50 per cent in these patients. Roentgen therapy has been shown to arrest the tumor, but it has not been determined whether amputation in conjunction with this treatment increases the survival rate. The regional lymph nodes should be irradiated.

The other tumors arising from the hematopoietic system include multiple myeloma, chronic and acute leukemia, lymphosarcoma, and Hodgkin's disease. None of these tumors are amenable to surgical treatment as they involve the skeleton in its entirety.

## TUMORS OF NERVE ORIGIN

The types of tumors arising from nerve tissue are neurofibroma, neurolemmoma, and malignant schwannoma. These tumors rarely involve bone, except for neurofibromatosis or von Recklinghausen's disease.

### Neurolemmoma

Neurolemmoma is usually a solitary, encapsulated, benign tumor produced by proliferating Schwann cells. When the nerve is small, the tumor surrounds the nerve, and attempts to remove it may destroy the nerve. In large nerves, the tumor is usually located eccentrically, and it may be possible to remove the tumor without destroying the nerve.

The tumor consists of two types of tissue. One is composed of proliferating masses of Schwann cells arranged in twisted cords, the stroma being reticular, and may resemble tactile corpuscles. The second type is composed of Schwann cells arranged at random in a mucinous reticular stroma.

### Multiple Neurofibromatosis

Multiple neurofibromatosis is characterized by neuromas involving skin, nerve, and bone. When the bone is involved, it is most often by invasion from a subperiosteal nerve. Growth of the tumor may erode the bone and elevate the periosteum, which forms a new bone. When the bone is invaded and extensively involved, cystic areas develop within the bone which may become expansile. Gross deformity of the extremities is not uncommon. Involvement of the spine often produces scoliosis.

Excision of accessible masses may be done; however, correction of deformity in involved bones is the most common surgical procedure.

### Malignant Schwannoma

Malignant schwannoma is a rare tumor, difficult to diagnose because of the variety of tissues that may be formed from the parent cell. Amputation is the treatment of choice if the tumor appears to be highly malignant.

## TUMORS OF VASCULAR ORIGIN

### Hemangioma and Malignant Hemangioendothelioma

Hemangiomas may involve an entire limb, including the bone and soft tissues, or may be an isolated lesion in either. These tumors may be primarily capillary or cavernous hemangiomas. Isolated lesions may be excised when accessible; however, vertebral lesions, when producing symptoms of nerve or spinal cord compression, are probably best treated by irradiation followed by decompression when necessary.

Malignant hemangioendothelioma is a lesion of varying aggressiveness. The tumor is rare. When bone is involved, the tumor tends to destroy bone and expand the cortex. The course of the tumor is unpredictable. At present, resection or amputation is indicated for accessible lesions. The value of radiation therapy is debatable.

## TUMORS OF FAT CELL ORIGIN

### Lipoma and Liposarcoma

Lipoma is one of the common tumors of the soft tissues, but is rare within the bone. The tumor consists of an accumulation of adult fat cells confined by an extremely thin fibrous capsule. The tumor is benign and need be excised only when it becomes unsightly or interferes with function.

Liposarcoma is rare in bone, but not uncommon in the soft tissues. The tumor usually occurs in the fat of the buttock, thigh, lower leg, or the back and shoulder regions. The tumor rarely occurs before the age of 30, and is more common in the fifth decade. It usually grows slowly, producing few symptoms except for local tumefaction. Metastasis tends to occur late in the course of the tumor, although recurrence after resection may be as high as 50 per cent.

The tumor is composed of adult and embryonic fat cells scattered throughout a sarcomatous stroma. Giant cells may be found.

Wide excision of the tumor should be performed. The percentage of 5 year survival may be as high as 85 per cent with adequate resection.

### Chordoma

Chordoma is a rather uncommon tumor arising from neoplastic proliferation of notochordal remnants. It is of low-grade malignancy, but of high recurrence rate, affecting the spine and base of the skull. The tumor is primarily destructive of bone and has a predilection for the ends of the spine, and the sacrococcygeal and spheno-occipital regions. The condition affects males twice as often as females. The tumor is uncommon before the age of 30.

The usual symptom is pain, but encroachment on the central nervous system may produce a variety of symptoms and physical findings.

The roentgenographic appearance is one of midline bone destruction, often accompanied by a soft tissue mass.

Grossly, the tumor is a soft, friable, grayish mass. It appears encapsulated except in the areas of bone destruction.

Microscopically, the tumor may be composed of cavities lined with cuboidal cells resembling epithelium; however, cords, lobules, and sheets of vacuolated cells in a mucinous matrix may predominate.

Wide excision of sacral tumors should be attempted, although recurrence from incomplete removal is common. Inaccessible tumors or recurrent tumors may be treated by high-voltage irradiation.

## TUMORS OF MUSCLE ORIGIN

### Rhabdomyosarcoma

Rhabdomyosarcoma is the most common tumor affecting striated muscle. Three types have been described: orthodox, alveolar, and embryonal. All are malignant tumors; however, survival rate of the orthodox type may approach 50 per cent whereas the alveolar and embryonal types are uniformly fatal.

The orthodox type of rhabdomyosarcoma rarely occurs in patients under 50, whereas the other two types occur in children and young adults. The tumor commonly occurs in the thigh, but may occur in any skeletal muscle. Disparity in cell size and type is characteristic in the orthodox tumor. Elongated, straplike cells, which often contain more than one nucleus, are diagnostic, particularly when cross striations are found. Spider cells, which are large clear cells traversed by threadlike processes, are helpful in the diagnosis when they are found.

The alveolar tumor is composed of embryonic muscle cells divided by fibrous trabeculae.

The embryonal tumor is composed of short spindle cells arranged in interlacing bands mixed with cells resembling lymphocytes.

Metastasis is usually by way of the blood to the lungs.

Wide resection or amputation is the treatment of choice. The tumor is radioresistant.

## TUMORS OF SYNOVIAL ORIGIN

### Malignant Synovioma

Malignant synovioma is a true neoplasm arising from elements of the synovial membrane. Although of rather benign gross appearance and slow-growing in many instances, the tumor is highly malignant. Local recurrence following resection is commonly followed by metastasis to the lungs.

The tumor arises most often in the knee joint or joints of the lower extremity; occasionally the upper extremity is involved.

Grossly, the tumor may appear as fleshy masses in the synovial membrane.

Two main cytologic types are seen microscopically. The sarcomatous type is composed of uniform spindle or fusiform cells with little fibrous supporting structure. Slitlike spaces usually occur lined with tumor cells. In the second type, cells are more cylindrical and are arranged radially about the slits or spaces, forming a pseudoacinar pattern.

Treatment has been unsatisfactory, and long-term survivals are rare. Amputation or radical resection followed by roentgen therapy has not appreciably lowered the mortality rate.

## CONDITIONS SIMULATING BONE TUMORS

Many conditions occur in the skeleton that may simulate bone tumors. Careful roentgenographic studies, appropriate blood studies, and biopsy material usually determine the diagnosis of the true lesion.

The common lesions simulating bone tumors are metastatic carcinoma, fibrous dysplasia of bone, bone cysts, histiocytosis, aneurysmal bone cyst, Paget's disease, and the skeletal changes of hyperparathyroidism. All these conditions must be considered in the differential diagnosis of bone tumors.

## REFERENCES

1. Aegerter, E., and Kirkpatrick, J. A., Jr.: Orthopedic Diseases: Physiology, Pathology, Radiology. 3rd ed. Philadelphia, W. B. Saunders Company, 1968.
2. Allen, A. R., and Stevenson, A. W.: A ten year follow-up of combined drug therapy and early fusion on bone tuberculosis. J. Bone Joint Surg., 49-A:1001, 1967.
3. Anderson, K. J., and Wildermuth, O.: Synovial sarcoma. Clin. Orthop., 19:55, 1961.
4. Bardenheier, J. A., III, Margan, H. C., and Stamp, W. S.: Treatment and sequelae of experimentally produced septic arthritis. Surg. Gynec. Obstet., 122:249, 1966.
5. Barnes, R., and Catto, M.: Chondrosarcoma of bone. J. Bone Joint Surg., 48-B:729, 1966.
6. Bhansali, S. K., and Desai, P. B.: Ewing's sarcoma. Observations on 107 cases. J. Bone Joint Surg., 45-A:541, 1963.
7. Blanche, D. W.: Osteomyelitis in infants. J. Bone Joint Surg., 34-A:71, 1952.
8. Borella, L., Summitt, R. L., and Clark, G. M.: Septic arthritis in childhood. J. Pediat., 62:742, 1963.
9. Bosworth, D. M., and Levine, J.: Tuberculosis of the spine: An analysis of cases treated surgically. J. Bone Joint Surg., 31-A:267, 1949.
10. Buchman, J.: The Rationale of the Therapy of Chronic Osteomyelitis. American Academy of Orthopaedic Surgeons. Instructional Course Lectures, 8:125, 1951.
11. Buchman, J.: Osteomyelitis. American Academy of Orthopaedic Surgeons. Instructional Course Lectures, 16:232, 1959.
12. Cave, E. F.: Tuberculosis of the Spine in Children. American Academy of Orthopaedic Surgeons. Instructional Course Lectures, 5:114, 1948.
13. Chandler, F. A.: Tuberculosis of the Lower Extremity. American Academy of Orthopaedic Surgeons. Instructional Course Lectures, 5:121, 1948.
14. Clowson, D. K., and Dunn, A. W.: Management of common bacterial infections of bones and joints. J. Bone Joint Surg., 49-A:164, 1967.
15. Codman, N. L., Saule, E. H., and Kelly, P. J.: Synovial sarcoma; an analysis of 134 tumors. Cancer, 18:613, 1965.
16. Coley, B. L., Higinbothaus, N. L., and Grasbeck, H. P.: Primary reticulum cell sarcoma of bone. Summary of thirty-seven cases. Radiology, 55:641, 1950.
17. Congdon, C. C.: Benign and malignant chordomas; clinico-anatomical study of twenty-two cases. Amer. J. Path., 28:793, 1952.
18. Curtiss, P. H., Jr., and Klein, L.: Destruction of articular cartilage in septic arthritis. II. In vivo studies. J. Bone Joint Surg., 47-A:1595, 1965.
19. Dahlin, D. C.: Bone Tumors. 2nd ed. Springfield, Ill., Charles C Thomas, 1967.
20. Dahlin, D. C., and Coventry, M. B.: Osteogenic sarcoma. A study of six hundred cases. J. Bone Joint Surg., 49-A:101, 1967.
21. Dahlin, D. C., and Henderson, E. D.: Chondrosarcoma, a surgical and pathological problem. Review of 212 cases. J. Bone Joint Surg., 38-A:1025, 1956.
22. Dahlin, D. C., and Juins, J. C.: Fibrosarcoma of bone. A study of 114 cases. Cancer, 23:35, 1969.
23. Dobson, J.: Tuberculosis of the spine. J. Bone Joint Surg., 33-B:517, 1951.
24. Enzinger, F. M., and Shiraki, M.: Alveolar rhabdomyosarcoma. An analysis of 110 cases. Cancer, 24:18, 1969.
25. Freiberger, R. H., Loitman, B. S., Helpern, M., and Thompson, T. C.: Osteoid osteoma. A report on 80 cases. Amer. J. Roentgen., 82:194, 1959.

26. Geschickter, C. F., and Copeland, M. M.: Tumors of Bone. Philadelphia, J. B. Lippincott Company, 1949.

27. Geschickter, C. F., and Copeland, M. M.: Parosteal osteoma of bone; a new entity. Ann. Surg., *133*:790, 1951.

28. Gilmer, W. S., Jr., Higley, G. B., Jr., and Kilgore, W. E.: Atlas of Bone Tumors. St. Louis, C. V. Mosby Company, 1963.

29. Hodgson, A. R., Skinsnes, O. K., and Leong, C. Y.: The pathogenesis of Potts paraplegia. J. Bone Joint Surg., *49-A*:1147, 1967.

30. Jaffe, H. L.: Osteoid osteoma, a benign osteoblastic tumor composed of osteoid and atypical bone. Arch. Surg., *31*:909, 1935.

31. Jaffe, H. L.: Tumors and Tumorous Conditions of the Bones and Joints. Philadelphia, Lea & Febiger, 1958.

32. Katayama, R., Itami, Y., and Marumo, E.: Treatment of hip and knee-joint tuberculosis. An attempt to retain motion. J. Bone Joint Surg., *44-A*:897, 1962.

33. Lichtenstein, L.: Bone Tumors. St. Louis, C. V. Mosby Company, 1965.

34. Lichtenstein, L., and Sawyer, W. R.: Beign osteoblastoma. A further observation and a report of twenty additional cases. J. Bone Joint Surg., *46-A*:755, 1964.

35. McKenna, R. J., Schwinn, C. P., Soong, K. Y., and Higinbotham, N. L.: Sarcomata of the osteogenic series (osteosarcoma, fibrosarcoma, chondrosarcoma, parosteal osteogenic sarcoma, and sarcomata arising in abnormal bone). An analysis of 552 cases. J. Bone Joint Surg., *48-A*:1, 1966.

36. Orr, H. W.: The treatment of acute osteomyelitis by drainage and rest. J. Bone Joint Surg., *9*:733, 1927.

37. Pack, G. T., and Ariel, I. M.: Tumors of the Soft Somatic Tissues. New York, Paul B. Hoeber, 1958.

38. Phelan, J. T., and Cabrera, A.: Chondrosarcoma of bone. Surg. Gynec. Obstet., *118*:330, 1964.

39. Public Health Service Cooperative Investigation: Evaluation of streptomycin therapy in a controlled series of ninety cases of skeletal tuberculosis. J. Bone Joint Surg., *34-A*:288, 1952.

40. Robertson, R. C.: Acute Infectious Hematogenous Osteomyelitis. American Academy of Orthopaedic Surgeons. Instructional Course Lectures, *5*:136, 1948.

41. Stetson, J. W., DePone, R. J., and Southwick, W. O.: Acute septic arthritis of the hip in children. Clin. Orthop., *56*:105, 1968.

# 43

# REPLANTATION OF THE EXTREMITIES

*G. Rainey Williams, M.D.*

Reattachment of a completely severed extremity, variously described as surgical restoration, reimplantation, or replantation, involves surgical principles and techniques that have been widely accepted for several decades. The principal reason for considering extremity replantation as a separate entity is that the procedure was not successfully performed until 1962. The reservations that prevented performance of an operation for which surgical capability existed for at least 20 years were not instantly overcome, but clinical experience with replantation has increased rapidly and justifies continued review.

## HISTORICAL ASPECTS

Man's long-standing interest in restoration or replacement of severed human parts is amply demonstrated in legend, illustrations,[21] and reports[10] of crude surgical maneuvers. Beginning in 1887, Halsted divided and repaired by suture all structures of the hind limb of dogs except the femoral artery and vein.[12] This was followed by femoral artery and vein ligation at varying intervals, and the formation of edema in the extremity and development of collateral circulation were observed. These experiments were stimulated by Dr. Halsted's interest in postmastectomy edema and were not reported until 1922. In 1903, Hopfner described experiments in which dogs' limbs were amputated and replanted by means of a nonsuture method of vascular anastomosis with maintenance of viability up to 11 days in one animal.[15] Shortly thereafter, Carrel and Guthrie were also able to replant an extremity in a dog with short-term survival.[5] In 1908, Carrel described a dog leg homograft that survived for 22 days.[4] Very few experimental attempts at replantation were recorded between 1908 and the report of Lapchinsky[18] in 1960. Several investigators have subsequently described experimental replantation and have added a substantial amount of information regarding the technique and physiologic effects of extremity replantation.[7-9, 20, 35]

In 1944, a protocol for replantation of amputated human extremities was formulated and published.[11] In 1962 a 12 year old boy presented at the Massachusetts General Hospital shortly after sustaining a traumatic amputation of the right arm below the shoulder. Dr. Ronald Malt, then a resident in surgery, made the decision to attempt replantation, summoned a number of surgical colleagues, and promptly performed the first successful limb replantation. The efforts of a number of laboratory workers and particularly the careful, objective report of successful limb replantation in two patients by Malt and McKhann[22] stimulated world wide interest in replantation. Since 1964, increasing experience with clinical replantation has been reported and this total experience allows identification of problems and increasingly clear definition of the place of extremity replantation in the field of surgery.[21, 33, 34]

## CLINICAL EXPERIENCE WITH REPLANTATION

Public interest in dramatic surgical procedures has resulted in widely distributed and often inaccurate accounts of extremity replantation, leaving the general impression that such procedures are more common and more successful than has been the case. By the end of 1970, approximately 50 major replantation procedures were recorded in the scientific literature. These reports of single cases or very small series vary markedly in descriptive detail and length of follow-up, allowing only general comparison and conclusions. About three-fourths of the reported attempts have been successful in restoring a viable extremity. Early failure after attempted replantation has invariably been due to either circulatory failure (more often venous than arterial) or infection. A few replanted extremities have subsequently been amputated because of faulty reinnervation.

### Age

Replantation has been reported in patients from 20 months[26] to nearly 60 years[16] of age. It is quite clear that the best functional results have been obtained in younger patients. The long period of rehabilitation and the decreasing likelihood of good functional recovery with increasing age suggest that replantation should be attempted only in the most ideal situation in patients over 45 years of age.

## Level of Amputation

Replantation of the upper extremity has been performed at virtually every level between mid-palm and shoulder.[16] Perhaps because of the size of the blood vessels involved, initial success has been somewhat more likely in the higher amputations. However, the ultimate functional recovery is considerably better with more distal wounds. This is in accord with the long-standing observation that nerve regeneration is more complete after distal injuries.

## Etiology of Amputation

Attempts at replantation have followed traumatic amputation due to a wide variety of wounding agents, including automobile accidents, industrial machines, clothes dryers, and assorted sharp instruments (machetes, meat cleavers). Experience indicates clearly that sharp, incised wounds are more favorable for both initial and long-range successful replantation. In general, avulsion wounds have resulted in less complete neural regeneration, and replantation after such wounds should be attempted only under special circumstances. Wounds that would be considered too dirty for primary closure or in which the time interval dictates against primary closure should certainly not be considered acceptable for attempted replantation.

## Time Interval

Successful upper extremity replantation has been reported when circulation was re-established up to 7 hours after injury. In the majority of instances, a period of 3 to 5 hours of ischemia is described. No correlation can be detected between the results of replantation and the period of ischemia up to 7 hours' duration.

## Functional Results

With current techniques, the end result after extremity replantation is never perfect. For practical purposes, the end result is dependent upon the extent of nerve regeneration. Experience with extremity replantation confirms the long-accepted observation that peripheral nerve regeneration is more complete (1) in young persons, (2) in sharply incised wounds, and (3) in more distal wounds. The collected replant material does not permit correlation of either technique or timing of nerve repair with the ultimate degree of regeneration. Most surgeons have followed the suggestion that early, accurate secondary repair of divided nerves is preferable to primary repair in all but the most favorable circumstances. It is also not possible to accurately define functional success in extremity replantation. In general, the procedure is considered successful if the patient and the evaluating physician feel that the extremity function is preferable to that of currently available prostheses (Fig. 1). Using this criterion, the outcome of replantation operations has been termed successful in a high percentage of patients reported.

## Incomplete Traumatic Amputation

It is obvious that the incompletely severed extremity offers virtually the same surgical challenge as complete amputation. Reviews of replantation have customarily not included cases of incomplete amputation because the presence of a viable tissue pedicle introduces so many variables into the assessment of results that even general conclusions become impossible. It is recognized, however, that one of the principal benefits of the recent interest in extremity replantation is a trend to more careful assessment

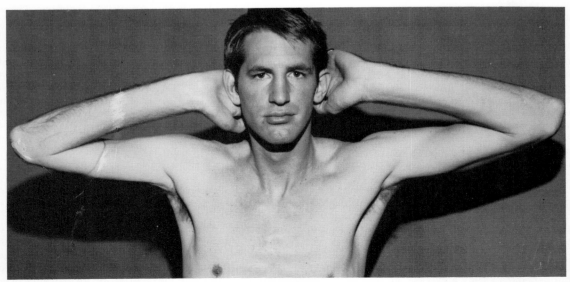

**Figure 1**   Photograph of a patient 14 months after replantation of a severed right arm. (From Williams, G. R.: Monogr. Surg. Sci., 3:53, 1966.)

of the badly injured extremity and the consequent salvage of extremities that might formerly have been amputated.

### Bilateral Replantation

A single instance of bilateral upper extremity replantation is known.[36] The patient was a 12 year old boy who sustained bilateral complete amputation of the upper extremities above the mid-humeral level. Replantation was completed but circulatory failure necessitated amputation of one arm and infection necessitated amputation of the other below the elbow, improving the outlook for prosthetic function. This experience suggests that bilateral replantation is technically feasible and is of interest in that no cardiovascular systemic effects were observed.

### Summary

Experience with upper extremity replantation is encouraging. Better understanding of the basic processes involved and particularly of peripheral nerve regeneration should lead to improved results.

## BASIC CONSIDERATIONS IN REPLANTATION

Extremity replantation involves many basic considerations. Most obvious is the necessity for detailed anatomic knowledge. The traumatic amputation wound is seldom a cleanly incised one and the replantation operation involves more than simply matching up the ends of the divided structures. Even more than with many other operations, surgical restoration of an amputated extremity requires knowledge of wound healing, the factors that influence healing, and the times required for the healing process. Currently, inadequate understanding of the healing process of peripheral nerves is the greatest single cause of imperfect results after replantation. The observation that infection is a major cause of early failure after limb replantation emphasizes the need for knowledge of surgical microbiology and for understanding the methods of minimizing, detecting, and treating bacterial infection. A basic problem shared with other vascular procedures but uniquely complete in replantation is the phenomenon of ischemia and restoration of blood flow. Several important questions regarding ischemia and restoration of flow may be posed. What is the maximal period of ischemia which will allow restoration of function by re-establishing circulation? What factors modify the period of permissible ischemia and, particularly, how can this period be prolonged? What problems are associated with restoration of blood flow and how can these be minimized or prevented?

### Ischemia

When blood flow to an extremity is completely interrupted (as in traumatic amputation), the available oxygen is quickly exhausted and anae-robic metabolism begins. Ultimately, an irreversible state is reached when restoration of blood flow will no longer result in recovery. The length of time between the onset of ischemia and the state of irreversibility varies widely from one tissue to another. Skeletal muscle is the tissue in an extremity that is most sensitive to ischemia, followed by skin, fat, nerves, and bone. In experimental preparation, the ability of skeletal muscle to contract after electrical stimulation diminishes after 2 hours of ischemia and is totally lost after 4 hours.[13] Few gross or microscopic changes can be detected in ischemic muscle until 4 to 6 hours after ischemia is produced although depletion of glycogen and ATP has been described.[27] Most studies of the maximal period of tolerance for ischemia have involved re-establishing flow after varying periods of ischemia in a variety of experimental preparations and studying the morphologic, physiologic, or biochemical changes that occur.[14, 19] When flow is restored in experimental preparations, necrosis of some skeletal muscle cells follows an ischemic period of about 2 hours' duration, and necrosis is very extensive after an ischemic period of 8 hours.[32] There is some species variation in the resistance of muscle to ischemia and presumably this is true of other tissues. In the rat the permissible period of skin ischemia is about 8 hours.[38] It is generally stated that fat, nerve, and bone are more resistant to ischemia but precise experimental definition is lacking. An important observation is that blood usually remains fluid in blood vessels for at least 6 hours after circulation is interrupted.

Basic studies of the effect of ischemia on skeletal muscle and skin, briefly cited in the preceding paragraph, suggest that an extremity replanted with adequate restoration of circulation after 6 to 8 hours should survive with good recovery of skeletal muscle contractility. This has been confirmed by limb replantation experiments in dogs.[35]

For obvious reasons, extension of the tolerable period of limb ischemia is desirable in clinical replantation. The oldest and perhaps most widely used agent to accomplish this is hypothermia. Presumably, hypothermia slows the metabolic processes that lead to an irreversible state. The optimal degree of hypothermia and the exact period of protection that might be offered by hypothermia are not precisely defined. Lapchinsky has reported survival of a replanted, cooled dog leg after 25 hours,[18] and a frozen dog leg has apparently been successfully restored 102 hours after amputation.[6] It seems significant that cooling during the period of ischemia has been shown to minimize some of the events, particularly edema, that follow restoration of circulation.[9]

Clearing the vasculature of the amputated extremity by perfusion should theoretically prevent the intravascular coagulation of blood and might remove some of the metabolic products of anaerobic metabolism. Such clearing has been shown to be useful in prolonging the life of experimental animals after replantation.[9] The efficacy of several perfusates in clearing the microcirculation has been studied, and the most effective was found to be saline with heparin.[23] It is obvious that prolonged perfusion using nonoxygenated solutions has no rationale.

In the field of clinical limb replantation, there is little need for extremity preservation for longer than 12 hours since this time interval permits transportation of the patient for even long distances. Experimental evidence suggests that cooling of the extremity and simple clearing of the circulation will permit replantation after such a time interval. No successful clinical replantation after 8 hours is known. Preservation of amputated extremities for even longer periods using more elaborate perfusion techniques has been accomplished experimentally.[30] It is probable that hyperbaric oxygenation alone or in combination could be used as a preservative measure if longer periods of preservation become desirable. The applicability of the extensive investigations into means of organ preservation is obvious.

### Restoration of Circulation

When blood flow is re-established to an ischemic limb, femoral arterial flow rapidly rises to a level exceeding the preamputation flow in the experimental animal.[37] In addition, there is a marked increase in bleeding from the distal muscle ends and a visible reddening of the skin which has been described as reactive hyperemia. An increase in limb weight occurs rapidly for approximately 2 hours and then increases very slowly for about a week, at which time the edema begins to subside.[9]

Recent studies of the microcirculation of both skin and muscle show that after ischemia of more than a few minutes' duration the restoration of flow in major vessels is not followed by uniform flow in the microcirculation.[38] Rather, the return of flow is patchy, with some areas filling well and others not at all. The distribution of flow improves with time provided the ischemic period is not of too long duration. That distribution of blood flow was not improved with the use of heparin suggests that intravascular thrombosis is not the explanation for the uneven return of flow. The method of investigation did not permit quantitation of flow. The same studies indicate that the formation of edema is not simply due to vascular leakage due to histamine release. Better understanding of these microcirculatory events may lead to methods that will further prolong tissue survival after ischemia. The role of lymphatic interruption in the formation of edema is not clear but there is some evidence that lymph channel reconstruction in the experimental animal reduces the extent of edema.[20]

The principal recognized systemic effect of restoration of blood flow to a replanted extremity is the frequent development of shock. The appearance of shock after replantation is not consistent but it has been described both clinically[24] and experimentally.[18] This shock has been extensively investigated and at least three explanations for its appearance have been suggested. Most evidence suggests that the shock is due to blood and fluid loss into the replanted extremity.[9, 25] Fluid loss into a traumatized extremity was carefully studied by Blalock in classic studies that showed that traumatic shock was not due to a tissue-elaborated toxin.[1] The same conclusion with regard to tourniquet shock[39] and replantation shock[9, 37] was reached after experiments by others. Since shock is not universally encountered after experimental replantation, it seems probable that the original condition of the animal, the blood loss during the amputation, the amount of fluid administration during the procedure, types of anesthesia, and perhaps other factors have served to confuse the experimental results. The concept that a vasodepressor toxic substance is elaborated in ischemic tissue and causes shock on restoration of circulation has had proponents since the work of Cannon.[3] The question is not whether such a substance might be elaborated after prolonged ischemia,[28] but whether the effect is clinically significant under the conditions in which replantation might be attempted. Recent experiments again indicate that it is unlikely that a tissue toxin of significance is elaborated during periods of ischemia of up to 8 hours.[37] Mehl has suggested that shock in the postreplant period is due to fall in pH, and improved survival using an amine buffer in his experiments was impressive.[24] Certainly this work demonstrates the importance of control of pH whether it is the primary cause of shock or secondary to it.

Recent evidence that microemboli to the lung from ischemic areas occur after revascularization[37] is of interest in regard to replantation. The problem has not been specifically studied experimentally but no clinical accounts of respiratory insufficiency following replantation have been identified.

## TECHNICAL CONSIDERATIONS

### The Decision to Attempt Replantation

Replantation should be considered in every instance of upper extremity traumatic amputation. Since the functional result of replantation is imperfect at best and since the procedure entails definite risk to the patient, a number of factors should be carefully considered before a decision is made to proceed with the replant operation. The operation is more strongly indicated in young than old persons, both because of the significance of extremity loss and because the reported results of functional recovery in younger patients have been more favorable. The wound should be one that is acceptable for primary repair. Wounds that are badly contaminated and grossly avulsed should probably be excluded from consideration. The presence of significant associated injury should be carefully ascertained and if present probably constitutes a contraindication to replantation. The time interval between wounding and anticipated restoration of circulation should be less than 8 hours although this is not an absolute figure. If the extremity has been promptly cooled and the circulation can be cleared during the first 8 hours, the time interval may be 12 hours or longer. Finally, the impact of replantation, the expectation of multiple operations, and the necessity for at least 2 years of rehabilitative therapy should be considered in each patient.

Lower extremity replantation is indicated only in exceptional circumstances, such as loss or threatened loss of the other leg. The principal reason for this is that the function of the lower leg is relatively well accomplished by available prostheses. Also of importance is the fact that a shortened, anesthetic lower extremity is a constant and significant handicap during the period between replantation and very unpredictable nerve regeneration. It is obvious that improved methods of managing peripheral nerve injury will alter the indications for attempting to replant lower extremities.

### The Replantation "Team"

All aspects of replantation are integral to other more common surgical procedures, yet experience indicates that preliminary review of the subject by all personnel to be involved will avoid recurring problems and improve the likelihood of success. Laboratory experience with the procedure is strongly recommended.

A single surgeon with one or two capable assistants can perform an extremity replantation. The importance of time and accuracy suggests that the participation of surgeons particularly adept at bone reconstruction may be helpful. Time is gained if sufficient personnel are available to prepare, perfuse, debride, and identify the structural landmarks of the extremity while the amputation wound is being prepared and debrided.

The anesthesiologist should be sensitive to the likelihood of hypovolemia. He should anticipate rapid, sizable blood loss when the extremity circulation is re-established. The problem of replantation shock and acidosis should be recognized and prevented or promptly treated by administration of blood, fluid, bicarbonate, or amine buffers.

The physical facilities and equipment for a replantation operation are widely available. No special instruments are required and the procedure can be performed in any hospital where general, vascular, and orthopedic surgery is done. Specialized facilities are required in the postoperative period, and the availability of physiotherapy and a spectrum of rehabilitative services is highly desirable.

### Steps in Replantation

Control of bleeding from the amputation wound and careful assessment of the general condition of the patient and of the extremity are preliminary to making a decision to attempt replantation. Preoperative x-ray examination of the extremity and the wound is usually indicated. In avulsion injuries, x-ray examination of the cervical spine is indicated to rule out evidence of nerve root avulsion. If such evidence is present, myelography

should be performed prior to attempting what might be a hopeless replantation. The extremity should be cooled by surface cooling in cold water, and when operating room conditions are available, the vasculature of the extremity should be cleared with balanced salt solution to which heparin and an antibiotic have been added. An intravenous infusion set is adequate, and the perfusion is discontinued when venous drainage becomes clear. Occasionally, extraction of thrombus material by means of a balloon catheter may be necessary. Both the extremity and the amputation wound are carefully prepared for replantation. In addition to mechanically cleaning the skin surrounding the wounds, extensive irrigation of the wounds with large volumes of sterile saline is important. Bone stabilization and fixation are initial steps in replantation (Fig. 2). It is essential to shorten the bone by approximately 3 cm. in adults to permit suture of muscles. This shortening may not be necessary when the amputation is distal to sizable skeletal muscles, that is, in the distal forearm or hand. The type of bone fixation depends upon the degree of comminution of the fracture and the anatomic level. A variety of intramedullary devices and plates have been used successfully and evidence does not strongly favor one method over another. When bone fixation is complete, reconstruction of the veins is begun. This is perhaps the most critical technical step in the replantation procedure. As many large veins as possible should be identified and careful anastomoses performed. Gentle dilation of the vein ends and placement of traction stay sutures allow construction of accurate, maximal-size, end-to-end anastomoses.[29] The suture used is very fine synthetic fiber placed with continuous or interrupted technique. Following completion of at least two, and preferably several, venous anastomoses, the arterial anastomosis is performed. In amputations distal to the bifurcation of the brachial artery, both the radial and ulnar arteries should be repaired. Vein grafts from the saphenous system can be used to bridge gaps in either arteries or veins. On release of vascular clamps, hemorrhage from the distal muscle ends should be anticipated. This is apt to be massive, and transfusions will usually be necessary at this time. Establishing hemostasis will involve time, pressure, and patient ligation of multiple bleeding points. At this point, debridement of the amputation wound should be completed, as nonvascularized tissue can be accurately identified for the first time. Thorough debridement is important in preventing infection, and its value cannot be overemphasized.

Management of the divided peripheral nerves is controversial and the reader is referred to the chapter on neurosurgery. In general, it is felt that unless conditions are ideal for primary anastomosis (experienced surgeon, short operation, sharp and clean nerve division), primary repair should not be performed and the nerves should simply be sutured loosely together to permit subsequent identification. Repair of the muscles is then performed by means of interrupted sutures

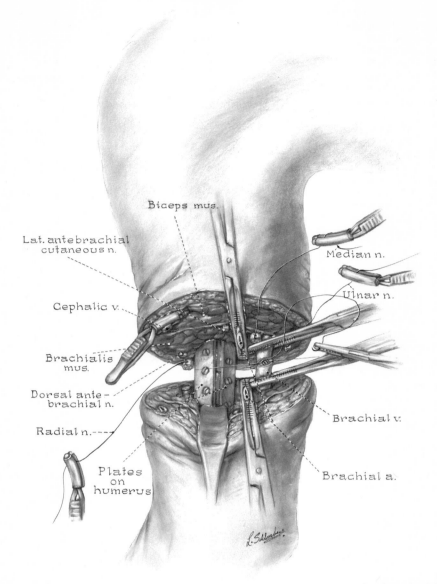

**Figure 2** An illustration of the steps in upper extremity replantation. Bone fixation by plates is visible, the venous anastomosis is being performed, arterial anastomosis will follow, and nerves have been identified for approximation.

in the muscle fascia. Subcutaneous tissue and skin closure are routine. Drainage of the wound is indicated in many instances. If inadequate skin coverage is available, grafting may be necessary, and tendon, bone, nerve, and vessels must be covered by flap tissue. Following the completion of the procedure, the arm should be elevated and protected by padded splinting in a position of function.

### Postoperative Management

Postoperative care of the replanted extremity involves efforts to maintain circulation, protect the extremity against injury, and preserve func-

tional capacity until nerve regeneration occurs. Anticoagulant therapy, fasciotomy, and methods of minimizing edema should be considered in the early postoperative period. The failure of heparin to improve results in experimental replantation and the complications often associated with effective levels of heparin have led to the recommendation that it not be used routinely after replantation. There is experimental evidence that low molecular weight dextran might be useful in maintaining circulation, although its effectiveness after replantation has not been clearly demonstrated. Fasciotomy may be critical in maintaining adequate circulation and should be performed freely but probably not routinely. Edema is controlled principally by elevation, gentle and carefully applied elastic compression, and careful attention to serum protein level. The formation of edema is rapid in the first few hours after replantation and care to avoid constricting dressings in this period is important.

The anesthetic arm is protected by padding, frequent position changes, and skin care. Physiotherapy should be employed very early in the postoperative period to preserve range of motion and joint function in the extremity. Muscle stimulation is added when healing of the wounds is well established. The cooperation, advice, and assistance of a physiotherapy unit is invaluable in the management of these patients and probably essential in obtaining a satisfactory functional result.

The risk of infection is minimized by appropriate selection of patients, careful and complete debridement, good surgical technique, and early, adequate antibiotic therapy. Antibiotic administration is begun prior to the replantation operation and high intravenous doses of broad-spectrum antibiotics are continued for several days. Prophylaxis against tetanus should not be forgotten. Life-threatening infection is an indication for amputation.

Hypovolemia with its attendant cardiovascular and renal problems is the principal threat to the patient in the early postoperative period. Blood replacement prior to and during the replantation procedure should be as complete as possible, and further blood and fluid administration may be required as fluid is sequestered in the extremity in the postoperative period. Careful attention to blood pH, serum electrolytes, and urine output should allow prompt correction of abnormalities before major damage occurs.

The postoperative replantation patient requires far more than the usual psychologic support from the managing team. The attempt to save an extremity will involve a long rehabilitation period, several subsequent operations, and a lengthy period of doubt about the extent of functional recovery. The managing physician and the many ancillary personnel involved in such procedures must realize the importance of establishing good rapport and maintaining support during this long period of treatment.

Most patients will require one or more secondary procedures for nerve repair or grafting and many will require subsequent orthopedic reconstructive procedures. These are not unique to replantation. It is emphasized that most evidence favors early secondary nerve repair. Wound infection is not as destructive to nerve repair as it is to the healing of bone or tendon.

During the long period of convalescence following extremity replantation, frequent review of the course, problems, and outlook by all participating personnel is important. The best interests of the patient are served by appropriate timing of subsequent procedures, recognition of problems, and prompt recognition of failure if it should occur. The difficult decision to amputate a replanted extremity is often made more easily and promptly by a multidiscipline review of the patient's progress.

# REPLANTATION OF AMPUTATED FINGERS

Although an occasional fingertip can be replaced as a composite graft with survival, successful restoration of fingers amputated proximal to the distal interphalangeal joint is rare indeed.[17] The experimental work of Buncke on primates indicated a very modest success rate.[2] A recent report mentions 20 successful finger replantations using vascular anastomoses.[6] The observation that nerve regeneration following digital nerve repair is often nearly perfect and the strong current interest in microsurgical vascular anastomoses lends support to the concept that replantation of fingers should be considered when facilities exist for its performance.

## SELECTED REFERENCES

Malt, R. A.: Clinical aspects of restoring limbs. Advances Surg. 2:19, 1966.
*A well written summary of the state of replantation 4 years after the original successful procedure.*

Malt, R. A., and McKhann, C. F.: Replantation of severed arms. J.A.M.A., *189*:716, 1964.
*This is the original description of the first successful human replantation experience, which more than any other factor stimulated interest in the possibility of extremity salvage by replantation.*

Nabseth, D. C., Mayer, R. F., and Deterling, R. A., Jr.: Experimental basis of limb replantation. Advances Surg. 2:35, 1966.
*This is an extensive review of the pertinent literature concerning the experimental basis for limb replantation, including the authors' investigative experience.*

## REFERENCES

1. Blalock, A.: Experimental shock; cause of low blood pressure produced by muscle injury. Arch. Surg., 20:959, 1930.
2. Buncke, H. J., Jr., and Shulz, W. P.: Experimental digital amputation and reimplantation. Plast. Reconstr. Surg., 36:62, 1965.
3. Cannon, W. B.: Traumatic Shock. New York, D. Appleton and Co., 1923.
4. Carrel, A.: Results of the transplantation of blood vessels, organs, and limbs. J.A.M.A., 51:1662, 1908.
5. Carrel, A., and Guthrie, C. C.: Complete amputation of the thigh, with replantation. Amer. J. Med. Sci., 131:297, 1906.
6. Department of Surgery, Shanghai Sixth People's Hospital, Shanghai (no author listed): Reattachment of traumatic amputation, a summing up of experiences. China Med., 5:392, 1967.
7. Eiken, O., Mayer, R. F., Nabseth, D. C., Apostolou, K., and Deterling, R. A., Jr.: Limb replantation. III. Long-term evaluation. Arch. Surg., 88:66, 1964.
8. Eiken, O., Nabseth, D. C., Mayer, R. F., and Deterling, R. A., Jr.: Limb replantation. I. The technique and immediate results. Arch. Surg., 88:48, 1964.
9. Eiken, O., Nabseth, D. C., Mayer, R. F., and Deterling, R. A., Jr.: Limb replantation. II. The pathophysiological effects. Arch. Surg., 88:54, 1964.
10. Gibson, T.: Early free grafting: the restitution of parts completely separated from the body. Brit. J. Plast. Surg., 18:1, 1965.
11. Hall, R. H.: Whole upper extremity transplant for human

beings: general plans of procedure and operative technic. Ann. Surg., *120*:12, 1944.

12. Halsted, W. S., Reichert, F. L., and Reid, M. R.: Replantation of entire limbs without suture of vessels. Trans. Amer. Surg. Ass., *40*:160, 1922.

13. Harman, J. W.: Histological study of skeletal muscle in acute ischemia. Amer. J. Path., *23*:551, 1947.

14. Harman, J. W., and Gwinn, R. P.: Recovery of skeletal muscle fibers from acute ischemia as determined by histologic and chemical methods. Amer. J. Path., *25*:741, 1949.

15. Hopfner, E.: Uber Gefassnaht, Gefasstransplantation und Reimplantation von amputierten Extremitaten. Arch. Klin. Chir., *70*:417, 1903.

16. Inoue, T., Toyoshima, Y., Fukusumi, H., Uemichi, A., Inui, K., Harada, S., Hirohashi, K., Kotani, T., and Shiraha, Y.: Replantation of severed limbs. J. Cardiovasc. Surg., *8*:31, 1967.

17. Komatsu, S., and Susumu, T.: Successful replantation of a completely cut-off thumb. Plast. Reconstr. Surg., *42*:374, 1968.

18. Lapchinsky, A. G.: Recent results of experimental transplantation of preserved limbs and kidneys and possible use of this technique in clinical practice. Ann. N.Y. Acad. Sci., *87*:539, 1960.

19. LePage, G. A.: Biological energy transformation during shock as shown by tissue analyses. Amer. J. Physiol., *146*:267, 1946.

20. MacDonald, G. L., Jr., Tose, L., and Deterling, R. A., Jr.: A technique for reimplantation of the dog limb involving the use of a mechanical stapling device and a rapid polymerizing adhesive. Surg. Forum, *13*:88, 1962.

21. Malt, R. A.: Clinical aspects of restoring limbs. Advances Surg., *2*:19, 1966.

22. Malt, R. A., and McKhann, C. F.: Replantation of severed arms. J.A.M.A., *189*:716, 1964.

23. Mehl, R. L., Paul, H. A., and Shorey, W. D.: Patency of microcirculation in the traumatically amputated limb — a comparison of common perfusates. J. Trauma, *4*:495, 1964.

24. Mehl, R. L., Paul, H. A., Shorey, W. D., Schneewind, J., and Beattie, E. J., Jr.: Treatment of "toxemia" after extremity replantation. Arch. Surg., *89*:871, 1964.

25. Nabseth, D. C., Mayer, R. F., and Deterling, R. A., Jr.: Experimental basis of limb replantation. Advances Surg., *2*:35, 1966.

26. Rosenkrantz, J. G., Sullivan, R. C., Welch, K., Miles, J. S., Sadler, K. M., and Paton, B. C.: Replantation of an infant's arm. New Eng. J. Med., *276*:609, 1967.

27. Scully, R. E., Shannon, J. M., and Dickerson, G. R.: Factors involved in recovery from experimental skeletal muscle ischemia produced in dogs. I. Histologic and histochemical pattern of ischemic muscle. Amer. J. Path., *39*:721, 1961.

28. Selby, D. M., Haddy, F. J., and Campbell, G. S.: Vasodilator material in ischemic tissues. Surg. Forum, *15*:232, 1964.

29. Shaw, R. S.: Treatment of the extremity suffering near or total severance with special consideration of the vascular problem. Clin. Orthop., *29*:56, 1963.

30. Snyder, C. C., Knowles, R. P., Mayer, P. W., and Hobbs, J. C., II: Extremity replantation. Plast. Reconstr. Surg., *26*:251, 1960.

31. Stallone, R. J., Lim, R. C., and Blaisdell, F. W.: Pathogenesis of the pulmonary changes following ischemia of the lower extremities. Ann. Thorac. Surg., *7*:539, 1969.

32. Strock, P. E., and Majno, G.: Vascular responses to experimental tourniquet ischemia. Surg. Gynec. Obstet., *129*:309, 1969.

33. Williams, G. R.: Replantation of amputated extremities. Monogr. Surg. Sci., *3*:53, 1966.

34. Williams, G. R.: Limb replantation. In: Hardy, J. D., ed.: Human Organ Support and Replacement. Springfield, Ill., Charles C Thomas, 1971.

35. Williams, G. R., Carter, D. R., Frank, G. R., and Price, W. E.: Replantation of amputated extremities. Ann. Surg., *163*:788, 1966.

36. Williams, G. R., Frank, G. R., and Barkett, V. M.: Unpublished data.

37. Williams, G. R., Stamatis, J. J., and Garrett, D. H.: Unpublished data.

38. Willms-Kretschmer, K., and Majno, G.: Ischemia of the skin. Amer. J. Path., *54*:327, 1969.

39. Wilson, H., and Roome, N. W.: Effects of constriction and release of an extremity: experimental study of tourniquet. Arch. Surg., *32*:334, 1936.

# 44

# THE HAND

*Erle E. Peacock, Jr., M.D.*

Until interest in the field was stimulated by the large number of injuries that occurred in World War II, surgery of the hand consisted primarily of incision and drainage of infections and secondary revision of traumatic amputations. A few surgeons were concerned with the possibilities of repairing the hand, but the results, particularly of nerve and tendon restorations, were so discouraging that most surgeons had little interest in the hand once infection was controlled and soft tissue healing accomplished. Control of infection was directed primarily toward saving life or the major portion of a limb. Moreover, lack of detailed anatomic knowledge and antibiotic adjuvants often meant infections were only drained of pus, and highly specialized structures were destroyed by necrotizing inflammation.[11]

## HISTORICAL ASPECTS

Although the introduction of sulfonamides and the pioneer studies of Sterling Bunnell and Sumner Koch in the forties created more interest than previously, it was not until members of the United States Armed Forces suffered an enormous number of major upper extremity injuries during World War II that any large-scale serious emphasis was placed upon reconstructive surgery. Confronted with more than 20,000 major injuries of the upper extremity in otherwise rehabilitatable soldiers, the military organized nine centers in the zone of the interior to concentrate upon reconstruction of injured hands. The problem was finding surgeons with sufficiently comprehensive training in general, plastic, orthopedic, and neurologic surgery to staff the centers. Because trained hand surgeons literally did not exist in the early forties, most patients were seen by four different specialists and often were operated upon by each in turn. The most important lesson learned from this experience was that independent dissection of a hand by each of four surgical specialists, each placing incisions through structures in which he was not particularly interested, often caused serious damage. It was not uncommon for a moderately damaged hand to be operated upon first by a plastic surgeon, with restoration of skin. The skin might be replaced according to cosmetic needs, but without consideration of future incisions or reconstruction of deeper structures. The same obtained for neurosurgical and orthopedic procedures during the first few months of operation of the hand centers.[4]

The most significant step in the history of hand surgery occurred with the emergence in 1945 of a group of relatively young surgeons who had had the unprecedented opportunity in various centers to learn some of the elements of plastic, neurologic and orthopedic surgery as they applied to reconstruction of the upper extremity. As a result, these surgeons were able to perform a number of reconstructive procedures, properly timed and executed, with a predictable final result. Most of the history of

reconstructive hand surgery was written by these men during exciting and challenging disciplines in the surgical sciences. As might be expected, interest centered primarily on replacement or repair of anatomic parts; details of kinetic anatomy were extremely important, and surgical technique for replacing intricate anatomic structures became quite sophisticated. Although static anatomy of the hand was well known prior to World War II, functional and dynamic anatomy had not been studied extensively.

Most of the innovative surgical procedures developed during the forties came as a result of new understanding of the function of complicated structures such as intrinsic muscles and retinacular membranes. Recognition and appreciation of substitution patterns also evolved. By the beginning of the Korean War in 1951, a new group of military surgeons was ready with a series of relatively complicated yet reliable operations for repairing or replacing most of the important structures in the hand.

Future accomplishments, which must occur during the next few decades, are likely to be the result of biologic investigations and therapeutic regimens based upon an ability to control biologic phenomena associated with reaction to injury and healing. Expressed more simply, most of the basic tissues of the hand such as skin, tendon, bone, nerve, and (in some patients under special conditions) joints can be repaired or replaced with high expectation of restoring function. The real frontier of hand surgery is not in the area of replacement or repair of parts. The major obstacle to further progress in restoring function after injury or disease consists of control of pain, fibrosis, and joint stiffness. These serious complications of the healing process loom far more threatening to the successful outcome of reconstructive hand operations as this century draws to a close than did problems of infection or anatomic disruption in the 1940s. More than 25 per cent of industrial and military accidents involve the hand, and until some of the biologic problems created by immobilization and healing are solved, many millions of dollars will be spent annually in the form of compensation payments. It is interesting to note that more than 90 per cent of patients referred to a university hand rehabilitation program are sent because of complications that developed after the patient came under a physician's care.

## CONGENITAL DEFORMITIES

Congenital deformities of the hand and wrist occur in approximately 0.5 per cent of human births. Although environmental stimuli can produce congenital deformities in the extremities of animals, and undoubtedly are responsible for some congenital defects in human beings, the vast majority of congenital deformities in man must be genetically induced. A positive family history is obtainable in more than half the patients studied adequately, while environmental factors have seldom been identified. Any generally noxious agent or factor, such as radiation, vitamin deficiency, or cortisone, administered during a period of maximal growth and differentiation of limb buds will produce a congenital deformity in a high percentage of embryos. The same agent administered during a later period of intrauterine growth, however, will produce a congenital deformity in another organ system, usually the one undergoing the most rapid growth at that time.[21]

### Syndactyly

Syndactyly, persistence of the webbing between digits, is a rather common congenital deformity of the hand, occurring in approximately 0.1 per cent of births. It seems to be more common in males than in females. The web may be complete from metacarpophalangeal joint to fingertip or may be partial, involving only the proximal phalanges. Syndactyly may be accompanied by brachydactylia (short fingers), ectrodactylia (absence of phalanges or metacarpals), or polydactylia (extra digits). Symphalangism (end fusion of the distal phalanges) also is seen with syndactyly and complicates the surgical correction of this condition. The most common form of syndactyly is an incomplete web joining the proximal two-thirds of the ring and long fingers. All of the fingers and the thumb may be joined to produce a complete mitten.

In most patients with syndactyly, the defect should be corrected and the procedure is relatively simple. Only patients who have such a serious anomaly of the deep architecture that separation of digits would not result in improved function should be denied operative correction. Usually, when there is little or no joint function, severe brachydactylia, or symphalangism, it is not worthwhile to separate the digits. The most controversial question in the treatment of syndactyly is the time for releasing the web. Most surgeons agree there is no real advantage in operating upon an infant with syndactyly, and there are several disadvantages in operating upon a tiny hand in which identification of digital nerves and evaluation of joint function and bone development may be inaccurate. In many patients, no serious objection exists to postponing correction of syndactyly until late childhood as far as finger function is concerned. Most surgeons prefer to correct syndactyly in patients between age 2 and 10, however, and a reason for waiting until age 10 is that the major growth period for the hand is completed. Skin grafts are required to correct syndactyly and sometimes growth of transplanted skin is not as rapid as that of surrounding tissue. Failure of a skin graft to grow at the same rate as the rest of the hand results in recurrence of the web and need for a second operation. Most patients are operated upon at approximately 5 years of age, however, and do not require any other procedures.

### Polydactylia

Polydactylia is probably the most frequent congenital anomaly of the hand. Many supernumerary digits are so small or are attached by such a narrow pedicle, however, that surgical consultation often is not required. Most supernumerary digits are abnormal, and unless there is a need for tissue elsewhere in the hand, early amputation is recommended. The mistaken notion that a narrowly attached small digit will undergo further development and become a useful contributor to hand function or appearance has delayed amputation unnecessarily in many patients. Actually, growth and development of the normal parts of the hand invariably exceeds that of the vestigial part; deformity is augmented by growth in some patients. If removal of a supernumerary digit requires extensive bone or soft tissue alteration, such as correction of a bifid thumb, or if selection of the proper digit to remove is difficult, additional delay is justified. If neither of these conditions is involved, and if there is no need for the tissue from the vestigial digit to be used elsewhere, immediate amputation, usually before the infant leaves the nursery, is advisable.

### Congenital Amputation Bands or Annular Grooves

A fairly frequent and interesting anomaly in the upper extremity is an *annular groove*, or congenital amputation band. Similar grooves occur in the lower extremity but are found most often in the hand, wrist, and fingers. Intrauterine autoamputation of a digit apparently can occur; thus the term congenital amputation rings sometimes is used. Usually, there are multiple rings or grooves and the entire hand at the wrist or multiple sites in individual digits may be affected. The conventional explanation for grooves — pressure exerted by amniotic bands or the umbilical cord — is unlikely.

Annular bands or rings usually do not require treatment except for cosmetic reasons. If the groove is not deep or is not located in a prominent place, no treatment is necessary. If digital lymphedema is produced, correction is indicated. Simple excision of the groove and suture of the skin edges will not erase the defect; contraction of the resulting scar invariably re-creates the deformity. Permanent correction requires construction and interdigitation of two lateral flaps as in a typical Z-plasty scar revision. Deep structures such as nerve and tendon are almost never involved, regardless of the depth of the lesion.

### Ectrodactylia

Ectrodactylia (absence of a digit or part of a digit) may involve a complete ray from carpal to fingertip. If a central ray is missing, a deep cleft or "lobster claw" may be produced. Occasionally, parts of the missing ray may be found in such a position that an epiphysis of a misplaced bone lying transversely in the center of the hand may produce growth that expands the hand transversely. Such misplaced bones, usually phalanges, should be removed early so that growth does not produce a worse deformity.

One of the most common ectrodactylia deformities is congenital absence of the thumb. The deformity often is bilateral and may be accompanied by absence of the radius or the pectoralis major muscle or both. A tiny vestigial thumb may be attached to the radial side of the hand by a narrow pedicle without bone or tendon components. Sometimes a vestigial finger, appearing as a supernumerary index finger, also is found. Almost all combinations of absence of the thumb and presence of vestigial index finger or thumb parts have been recorded. Very early, a laxity in the fixation of the index ray to the long axis of the hand can be demonstrated. Normally, the index ray is solidly attached to the lesser multangular bone, and the intermetacarpal ligament is short, permitting only a small amount of movement between index and long metacarpals. The index and long rays literally are the central axis of the hand around which the more movable ring, small, and thumb metacarpals circumduct. Absence of the first ray requires that prehensile function occur primarily between the index and long fingers. In a growing child, considerably laxity in the proximal and distal attachments of the index metacarpal will permit extensive abduction and pronation of the index finger. If pollicization of the index finger is not performed, autopollicization can be improved by merely dividing the transverse metacarpal ligament so that more abduction of the index finger is possible.

If only one thumb is missing, pollicization of the index finger is seldom indicated. One hand with a normal thumb generally is sufficient for most activities if there is no defect in the other hand except loss of the thumb. The normal hand will become dominant if it is not naturally so. If both thumbs are absent or atretic, however, it is usually worthwhile to construct one normally opposable digit; pollicization of the index finger on the dominant hand is the best method for achieving this objective. The procedure cannot be done safely at a very early age, although some highly experienced surgeons have pollicized index fingers on infants with excellent results. The procedure is exacting and tedious, and most surgeons prefer to delay operation until the patient is 3 or 4. It is fairly important to pollicize an index finger before school age, as the relative amount of skin covering the hand changes as subcutaneous fat is lost and adult proportions are reached. The most difficult problem for the surgeon is not transfer of the digit but construction of the highly specialized web between the radial finger and new thumb. The ample skin present in the hands of youngsters during the first 4 years of life is valuable for web construction, and thus operation during early childhood is advised.

## INFECTIONS OF THE HAND

Although loss of life and limb from infections is relatively uncommon since development of antibiotic therapy, severe disability caused by delay in treating infections of the hand remains a serious problem. Accurate diagnosis is essential, and unerring knowledge of fascial compartments may be required if treatment is to be successful in preventing permanent damage.[12] Under the most ideal circumstances, surgical drainage should not be necessary if the infection is diagnosed promptly and treated with antibiotics. Proper care of penetrating wounds and early recognition of cellulitis, before suppuration, can prevent most of the disabling fibrosis accompanying secondary healing and drainage of pus. General principles for early treatment of cellulitis without suppuration include immobilization of joints in a neutral position, bed rest with elevation of the extremity above cardiac level, warm, moist dressings (wet heat is conducted to tissues more efficiently than dry heat), and appropriate selection and administration of antibiotics. The concept that an early cellulitis of the hand is associated with such a serious threat of permanent disability that bed rest and constant elevation are necessary is more prevalent than previously.

Small, localized, superficial infections such as a furuncle or cellulitis can be treated adequately on an ambulatory basis. Deep cellulitis anywhere in the hand is a potentially dangerous threat to hand function, however, and should be treated as aggressively as possible to prevent suppuration and secondary drainage. Some structures such as the highly specialized sheath surrounding flexor tendons with long amplitudes of motion rarely function as a gliding surface again if pus has formed around them. Thus, prevention of suppuration when possible, and the earliest possible drainage of pus when it has already formed, are essential factors in preventing or reducing the amount of fibrosis in a hand invaded by bacteria. Of course, as soon as bacterial invasion has been controlled, motion should be commenced to reduce the disabling effects of fibrosis.

### Paronychia

A superficial infection of soft tissue surrounding a fingernail is called paronychia. Because this infection tends to follow the cuticle around the base of the nail, it is also known as a "run around." A paronychial infection that is only a few hours old often can be aborted by the use of warm applications, rest, and elevation. Once cellulitis at the base of the nail has progressed to suppuration, however, surgical drainage is necessary. Under local nerve block or refrigeration anesthesia, a No. 11 pointed blade is inserted into the subcuticular space and moved along the nail for approximately 2 to 3 mm. The sharp side of the blade is then rotated up, and a quick cut from the inside out opens the attachment of skin to nail sufficiently to provide adequate drainage for most patients. Drainage of this type followed by warm applications, elevation, and rest is sufficient to cure most acute paronychial infections. An acute infection that is not adequately treated may become chronic, with all of the signs and symptoms of a moderately low-grade, chronic soft tissue infection around the base of the nail. Hypertrophy and edema of cuticular tissue occur, and recurring episodes of acute inflammation and drainage are common. Chronic paronychial infections cannot be treated adequately by the type of incision just described. Such an incision may provide drainage and temporary relief for an acute exacerbation of chronic paronychia, but it will not result in permanent cure of a chronic infection. Removal of the nail is necessary to achieve permanent cure of chronic paronychia. If a fungus or other specific wound infection is present, additional measures may be required.

### Felon

A felon is a closed-space infection of the multi-loculated volar compartment at the tip of the digits. The subcutaneous fat in the terminal volar finger pad is attached to the phalanx and overlying skin by fibrous septi, which create a multi-loculated space. If infection is introduced and allowed to proceed to a necrotizing or suppurating stage, the intracompartmental pressure will rise as a result of collection of products of inflammation, necrosis of tissue, and thrombosis of venous and lymphatic channels. The earliest symptom is severe pain which, diagnostically, is throbbing in character, reflecting the arterial pulse wave. Pain is often so severe that sleep is impossible; elevation is the only measure that provides significant relief. Because the distal fingertip normally is red and firm, the usual early signs of inflammation may be obscure. The volar compartment becomes more tense than other fat pads eventually, but the restricting effect of fibrous septi prevents massive edema and enlargement during the early stages of infection. Pressure on the distal tip with a pencil eraser or other blunt object produces intense pain and is a diagnostic test of felon. Conservative treatment is indicated early (within the first 12 to 18 hours), followed by incision and drainage if dramatic response to antibiotics, elevation, and heat is not obtained rapidly. Systemic signs of sepsis such as chills and fever, leukocytosis, and lymphangitis may be present and frequently mean that an unusually virile organism such as the beta hemolytic streptococcus is involved. Drainage is a relatively mutilating procedure because all of the septi must be divided by a lateral through-and-through incision. This usually can be accomplished without extending the incision around the tip of the finger (hockey stick incision); unilateral drainage usually is unsuccessful (Fig. 1).

Drainage of a felon is a major surgical procedure requiring general or regional anesthesia and operating room facilities. Inadequate drainage is frequent, and the secondary complications of further suppuration are awesome. Such complications include thrombosis of digital arteries, leading to osteomyelitis of the distal phalanx and loss of a portion of the digit; invasion of the distal flexor tendon sheath, producing tenosynovitis; and spread of a dangerous infection through thecal channels to other digits or the proximal hand. Prompt institution of antibiotic therapy, elevation, and through-and-through drainage, if dramatic

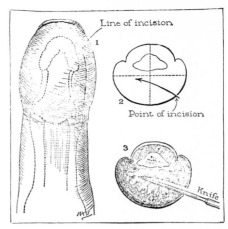

**Figure 1** Drainage of a felon is accomplished by a single hockey stick incision along the side of the phalanx, which is designed to divide the fascial septa. Care must be taken not to carry the incision too far proximally, lest the tendon sheath be opened. (From Koch, S. L.: J.A.M.A., *92*:1171, 1929.)

improvement does not occur, are essential if a catastrophe is to be avoided.[13]

### Bacterial Tenosynovitis

Tenosynovitis is one of the most crippling infections in the upper extremity.[8] Paradoxically, one of the reasons this is so is that the disease is relatively well known and overaggressive treatment following inaccurate diagnosis produces tenosynovitis (and all of the sequelae of surgical treatment) when, in fact, such treatment was not necessary. Fortunately, bacterial tenosynovitis is a rare disease. It is almost always preceded by history of a penetrating wound or cellulitis which should be recognized and treated before the tough digital theca becomes invaded. Unfortunately, however, the surgeon often is preoccupied with the diagnosis of tenosynovitis and opens the tendon sheath through an area of soft tissue cellulitis, thus producing tenosynovitis when it may not have existed before incision. This is a preventable complication. In the middle and proximal phalangeal areas fat and skin are not bound to bone, as in the terminal phalangeal unit; proximal segments undergo relatively enormous swelling when infection is introduced. Thus one should never make the diagnosis of tenosynovitis on the basis of the severity of soft tissue signs. A single test, correctly done, distinguishes between soft tissue cellulitis and intrathecal tenosynovitis, and it must be positive before tenosynovitis is diagnosed.

The test requires passive extension of the distal interphalangeal joint while the proximal finger is gently restrained in a comfortable midflexion position. The proximal digit must not be compressed by the examiner's restraining hand, and pain produced by passive distal interphalangeal joint extension should be different in character and severity from pain produced locally by cellulitis or the examiner's restraint of proximal interphalangeal motion. If severe, lancinating pain is not produced by even a few degrees of passive extension of the distal interphalangeal joint, the diagnosis of tenosynovitis should not be considered, and the tendon sheath should not be opened during drainage of overlying soft tissue. Patients with tenosynovitis usually will have much more systemic reaction than patients with a localized soft tissue cellulitis. An understanding of the anatomic relationships of the tendons and their sheaths is of great importance (Fig. 2).

The treatment of tenosynovitis is aimed primarily at preventing proximal and then distal spread of infection to another digit. Treatment is not aimed at restoring function in the involved digit. Only rarely is significant gliding function possible after a flexor tendon sheath has been opened because of suppurative infection. Tenosynovitis is one of the most dangerous infections in the human body, and extensive drainage is necessary if a more serious or even life-threatening complication is to be avoided. Because opening the sheath is so mutilating to the flexor tendon mechanism, we have treated early tenosynovitis by opening the sheath through a tiny distal incision at the fingertip and making a similar incision proximally in the palm. A tiny catheter is inserted, and if the entire sheath can be irrigated freely, we do not open the sheath but establish through-and-through irrigation with a physiologic solution containing antibiotics. If through-and-through irrigation is not possible, however, the entire sheath must be opened through a midlateral incision. In early cases, some flexor tendon function can be preserved and infection treated adequately by irrigation; it is unthinkable to persist with irrigation treatment if a free flow of fluid is not possible or immediate clinical improvement is not obtained. Failure to irrigate freely or obtain a dramatic clinical response is a strong indication for opening the entire sheath. Of course, proper use of systemic anti-

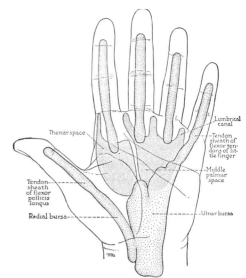

**Figure 2**   The tendon sheaths and fascial spaces of the volar surface of the hand and forearm form definite pathways for the spread of infection. When infectious organisms gain entrance into a tendon sheath, the process soon spreads throughout the whole sheath. When any of the three central digits is involved, the process comes to a momentary halt in the palm. If drainage is not soon provided, the process then ruptures into one of the fascial spaces in the palm: the middle palmar space if the middle or ring finger is implicated, the thenar space if the index finger is the original site. The pathway from the ulnar bursa on the side of the little finger, however, ends in the lower forearm, and an infectious process originating in this bursa ruptures into the retroflexor space here; similarly, a process from the radial bursa extends into the lower forearm. The radial and ulnar bursae usually communicate with each other and, hence, when one is primarily involved, the other is quickly invaded. (From Mason, M. L. In: Sajous: System of Medicine, Surgery and the Specialties. Philadelphia, J. B. Lippincott Company.)

**Figure 3**   The relationship of the tendon sheaths to the fascial spaces in the palm. (From Bell, J. L. In: Davis, L., ed.: Christopher's Textbook of Surgery. 9th ed. Philadelphia, W. B. Saunders Company, 1968.)

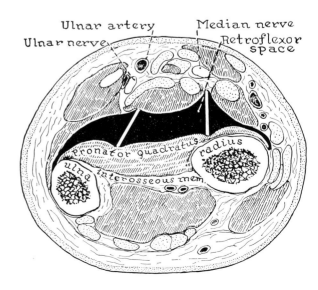

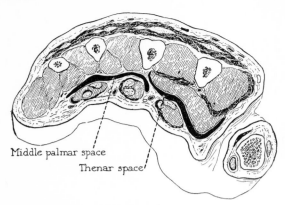

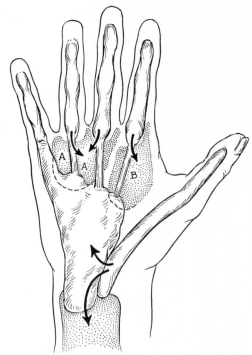

**Figure 4**  The relationship of the radial and ulnar bursae to the retroflexor space in the lower forearm. (From Bell, J. L. In: Davis, L., ed.: Christopher's Textbook of Surgery. 9th ed. Philadelphia, W. B. Saunders Company, 1968.)

biotics is mandatory, and adequate drainage of overlying soft tissue infection must be assured.

### Infection of the Midpalmar Spaces

The two proximal midpalmar spaces, thenar and hypothenar, separated by a tough proximal membrane, are really three spaces in the distal palm where the thenar and hypothenar muscles are separated from the midpalm by fascial compartments (Figs. 3 to 5). The midpalmar space is further subdivided by the creation of tunnels formed by vertical septi of the palmar fascia. These tunnels contain the lumbrical muscles, flexor tendons, and neurovascular bundles. Infection of the various midpalmar spaces is diagnosed from a history of a penetrating injury and signs of inflammation on either the volar or dorsal surface of the hand. Contrary to previous recommendations, drainage is probably best performed by placing an incision directly over the area of most prominent inflammation. Circuitous drainage routes previ-

**Figure 5**  The spread of infection through the various tendon sheaths and fascial spaces of the palm and forearm is shown diagrammatically. (From Bell, J. L. In: Davis, L., ed.: Christopher's Textbook of Surgery. 9th ed. Philadelphia, W. B. Saunders Company, 1968.)

ously recommended to avoid vital structures in the hand or to prevent hypertrophic scars have the disadvantage of sometimes failing to drain an infection adequately. A surgeon who has accurate anatomic knowledge and who plans an incision so that it does not cross lines of changing dimension usually can drain an abscess directly over the point of maximal fluctuation and inflammation. Sometimes through-and-through drainage is

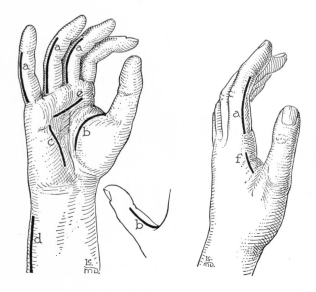

**Figure 6**  Incisions for drainage of the tendon sheath and fascial spaces must be made with the care of anatomic dissection in a bloodless field. The incision in the digit is made on the midlateral side and, since the finger is swollen, it may be difficult to place this incision correctly. The proper location of the incision is indicated by the ends of the transverse creases on the digits, which are never obliterated, regardless of the degree of swelling. (From Mason, M. L. In: Sajous: System of Medicine, Surgery and the Specialties. Philadelphia, J. B. Lippincott Company.)

necessary if a "collar button" abscess is present with a large volar pocket of pus and an extension between the metacarpals and interosseous muscles to the dorsum of the hand. In these patients, the maximal inflammatory reaction may appear to be on the dorsum of the hand where flimsy attachment of skin and loose subcutaneous tissue permit more edema than the tough palmar fascia on the volar surface. Adequate drainage must be followed by proper antibiotic therapy, elevation, and rest. The conventional incisions recommended by Mason are shown in Figure 6.[14] Resumption of active and passive motion as soon as bacterial infection has been controlled is necessary if loss of small joint motion is to be prevented.[7]

### Tuberculosis

Tuberculosis infections in the hand are now uncommon. A pulmonary or other soft tissue infection elsewhere in the body is not necessary for diagnosis of tuberculosis tenosynovitis. Skin, tendon sheath, bones, and joints may be involved. Hematologic dissemination of tuberculosis organisms is responsible for most hand infections. Unfortunately, drug-resistant mutant forms are common, but combination therapy with streptomycin, isoniazid, and PAS usually will control the infection. Approximately 75 per cent of patients can be cured with adequate antibiotic therapy followed by radical excision of involved tissues such as tendon sheath and synovial lining of joints. Of course, normal tendons and nerves must be protected during such dissections.

### Erysipeloid

A chronic, low-grade infection involving the hands of meat handlers, particularly those who handle pork and fish, is known as erysipeloid. The causative organism is usually a fungus known as *Erysipelothrix rhusiopathiae*. Signs and symptoms are only moderately severe, but the disease runs a chronic course of many weeks' duration. Symptoms include itching, burning, and moderate pain; signs are local skin eruption resembling erysipelas and a bluish red discoloration of the skin overlying the swollen area. Specific treatment is not required. Symptomatic treatment is helpful, but avoidance of handling of meat and meat products is the only known permanent cure.

## OTHER DISORDERS

Noninfectious diseases that affect the hand and for which some relief of symptoms can be afforded by surgical treatment include rheumatoid arthritis, Dupuytren's contracture, gout, and scleroderma.

### Rheumatoid Arthritis

Surgical therapy of rheumatoid arthritis has produced one of the most dramatic achievements in hand surgery. Present surgical therapy is based upon biologic observations and measurements incriminating synovial tissues around joints and tendons as the source of the deforming process. The metabolic balance between collagen synthesis and deposition and collagenolysis apparently is upset as a result of the disease process, and collagenolytic activity predominates to the extent that important retinacular structures become attenuated and mutilating deformity occurs. Where tendon and ligaments join bone (Sharpey's fibers), the collagenolytic process seems most active. As a result, lateral stabilizing forces such as joint collateral ligaments and tendon insertions become distracted from bone. Synovial proliferation around long tendons may cause necrosis because of interference with segmental blood supply or abnormal enzyme activity. As far as can be determined now, all of the characteristic deformities of the rheumatoid hand, including swan neck deformity, ulnar deviation, luxation of joints, rupture of tendons, and so forth, are due to extensive collagenolytic activity in proliferating synovium. Major nerve compressions in restricted areas (carpal tunnel syndrome) also may be produced by synovial enlargement.

The most effective treatment to stop progression of the disease and provide relief of pain is synovectomy. Synovectomy can be performed most effectively in the metacarpophalangeal and radiocarpal joints. In interphalangeal joints synovectomy is more difficult and often is incomplete, but in selected patients it can be performed with excellent results. Patients who are subjected to synovectomy usually can be assured of relief of pain and cessation of further progress of deformity in the area operated on. In the judgment of the author, synovectomy should be performed in the metacarpophalangeal joint and wrist joints as soon as the diagnosis of progressive involvement by rheumatoid arthritis is made (Fig. 7). Severe ulnar deviation, dislocated joints, articular destruction, and cosmetic deformities in rheumatoid hands simply are not necessary today. Understandable reluctance of many internists to refer

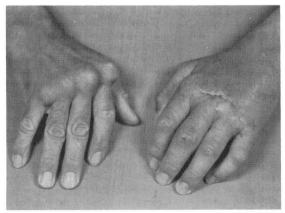

**Figure 7** Rheumatoid arthritis. The patient's right hand (before treatment) shows typical ulnar deviation and luxation of the metacarpophalangeal joints. The left hand (postoperative view) shows correction of ulnar deviation and reduction of metacarpophalangeal dislocations.

patients with rheumatoid disease of the hand will be corrected as knowledge concerning the beneficial effect of removing diseased synovium is more widely disseminated.

Correction of hand deformities does not alter rheumatoid arthritis elsewhere. A patient who may be doomed to wheelchair or crutch existence, however, obtains much benefit from functioning hands. One should not withhold treatment in a small but important area of the body because of inability to understand and control the basic process elsewhere. Although most well-cared-for arthritis patients are being managed satisfactorily without chronic use of steroids, patients who are taking steroids also can be operated upon safely.

In addition to removing diseased tissue and relieving pain in the area operated on, the surgeon occasionally can aid a rheumatoid patient by performing reconstructive procedures. Examples include replacement of destroyed joints with Silastic spacers, arthroplasty, arthrodesis, tendon transfers, and tendon grafts. Age and the total disabling features of the disease detract from extensive reconstructive surgery in many patients, but excellent results can be obtained in selected patients, under carefully controlled conditions.[6]

### Dupuytren's Contracture

The disease that bears the name of Baron Guillaume Dupuytren, one of Europe's most distinguished and productive surgeons of the nineteenth century, is characteristically described as a peculiar hypertrophy of the palmar fascia in the hands of older men. Actually, however, the disease occurs in its most progressive form in younger age groups, particularly in females in the fourth and fifth decades. The cause of the disease is unknown, although it is so often associated with other conditions found in aging populations, such as diabetes, rheumatoid disease, hepatic disease, and grand mal seizures, that cause-and-effect relationship has repeatedly been sought. The disease appears to vary in severity from a small dimple at the base of the ring or small finger to massive hypertrophy and contracture of the entire palmar fascia, creating a severe flexion deformity of metacarpophalangeal and proximal interphalangeal joints. Most often the disease begins as a nodule, band, or dimple on the ulnar side of the hand, and produces a flexion contracture of the ring or small finger or both at the proximal interphalangeal joint. In approximately one-third of patients, prominent nodular hypertrophy and skin dimples develop in the hand or fingers but progression to a significant contracture does not occur. In about 10 per cent of patients, a similar condition can be found in the feet or penis (Peyronie's disease). Knuckle pads (thickening of the dermis and subdermal loose connective tissue on the dorsum of the proximal interphalangeal joints), stenosing tenosynovitis (trigger finger), transient arthritis, and carpal tunnel syndrome also are associated with Dupuytren's contracture

in the hand. Dupuytren's contracture is described as involving primarily the longitudinal and vertical fibers of the palmar fascia. Close examination strongly suggests that the deeper fibers, at least, are normal in appearance, regardless of the plane they traverse. Hypertrophy seems to involve primarily the most superficial fibers or, perhaps, is the result of conversion of subdermal fat to collagenous tissue, which then becomes additive to normal palmar fascia. Histologically, there may be an increased number of fibrocytes and chronic inflammatory cells, particularly in the progressive nodular form of the disease. The most pronounced finding, however, is an increase in collagen. The abnormal collagen exists as grossly discernible fibers; microscopic and ultrastructure studies have not revealed anything unusual about fiber and fibril anatomy. The collagen is firmly cross-linked, as measured by cold saline extractions; no abnormalities in amino acid content or x-ray diffraction patterns have been described. It seems likely, therefore, that the fundamental abnormality is derangement of the metabolic balance between collagen synthesis and deposition and collagenolytic activity. In many respects, this is the antithesis of rheumatoid arthritis, in which collagenolytic activity appears to predominate.

A popular hypothesis for the pathogenesis of Dupuytren's contracture suggests that in genetically predisposed persons repeated trauma produces microwounds in the subcuticular area, resulting in "overhealing" and formation of a sort of keloid in the subcutaneous tissue. It should be emphasized, however, that the only evidence that trauma is related to the process is the rather constant identification of hemosiderin in the early nodules of patients and experimental animals. Moreoever, the lesion can be produced experimentally in monkeys by chronic injury of the subdermal fascia. It is of interest, however, that Dupuytren's contracture is practically unknown in blacks and in those performing heavy manual labor.

Treatment may be either expectant or surgical. In patients who have only nodular or skin-puckering disease without severe deformation of the skin or disabling contractures, no therapy is needed. The most important factor is whether progression of contraction and skin involvement are occurring. Surgical extirpation of involved fascia is best performed before joints have become permanently fixed in a flexed position and before skin is so severely involved that wound healing is jeopardized and a skin graft is required. In at least a third of the cases, contractures are relatively stable after the first signs appear, however, and accurate measurement of rate of progression is desirable before surgery is recommended.

Excision of involved palmar fascia is an interesting exercise in wound healing. The hands of these patients do not tolerate long periods of immobilization and chronic inflammation. Uncomplicated wound healing without infection, hematoma, dehiscence, or skin replacement is highly desirable. Generally, it is advisable to perform multiple small operations to rid a small area completely of abnormal fascia rather than to try to remove all of the palmar fascia in one stage and risk a serious wound complication. The aim should be therapeutic removal of an affected area rather than prophylactic excision of all palmar fascia. Only rarely will the entire palmar fascia become involved. The disease characteristically affects selected areas, and it is only these that should be treated. Occasionally in young females and mesomorphic men with rapidly progressive disease, a type of Dupuytren's contracture is encountered that sometimes is referred to as "malignant" Dupuytren's contracture. The word malignant relates to the rapidly recurring nature of abnormal fascia or hypertrophic scar or both. These patients usually require excision of all overlying skin to control the disease, and sacrifice of a digit may be necessary to provide a local pedicle flap. Such patients also have a high risk of development of a chronically painful hand or Sudeck's atrophy. Most can be treated satisfactorily by removing only the area of fascia that is affecting skin or producing contracture.[10]

### Gout

Patients with gout and large tophi in the fingers sometimes can be helped by excision of the tophi. It is possible to remove tophi without excising them in some patients, but extremely large deposits usually should be removed through a relatively small incision after medical treatment has been instituted. Wound healing may be poor, and recurrence is to be expected unless adequate control of the primary condition is achieved. Hemorrhage in the cavity occupied by uric acid crystals is a common postoperative complication. Suction drainage and occlusive dressings are needed to obtain primary healing in most patients.

### Scleroderma

The end result of scleroderma in the hands usually is autoamputation of fingers. Terminal digital ischemia and vasculitis produce severe pain which often can be relieved by sympathectomy, but this operation does little to increase effectively the circulation, especially after sclerodermal changes become pronounced. The operation can be useful in relieving pain, and successful response to a sympathetic block is a good indication that sympathectomy may be of aid. Early amputations to prevent chronic wound healing and extension of the ulcerative process can delay loss of tissue. Avoidance of trauma to digits, superb wound care when ulcers develop, and early conservative amputations to prevent extension of infection and necrosis are helpful.

### Stenosing Tenosynovitis

A peculiar but surprisingly frequent nonbacterial inflammation involving tendons is called *trigger finger* or *trigger thumb*. The names are descriptive of the restriction and sudden release of a long flexor tendon passing through a digital

theca or other restricted area, such as the passage of the flexor profundus through the flexor sublimis. The condition can be congenital or acquired. Congenital lesions are painless and involve the thumb (flexor pollicis longus) primarily and are bilateral in 5 per cent of patients. Signs relate to a 90 degree flexion position of the interphalangeal joint. Passive extension of the joint may be difficult or even impossible in some infants. Usually, however, passive extension meets firm resistance and then the joint suddenly snaps into normal extension. Active flexion is normal, but after the digit has been flexed to approximately 90 degrees, active extension is not possible and passive extension meets resistance until it is forcibly overcome. Acquired stenosing tenosynovitis may occur in any digit, although the fingers are involved much more often than the thumb. The condition usually is not bilateral, and it is seen frequently in association with other connective tissue disorders such as rheumatoid arthritis or Dupuytren's contracture. In addition to resistance to extension and snapping release, there is palpable crepitation over the proximal end of the digital theca in the palm, and an audible click often can be detected when forced passive extension overcomes resistance to gliding function.

Congenital and acquired stenosing tenosynovitis should be treated by making a small incision over the proximal end of the tendon sheath and, under direct vision, incising the sheath for approximately 1 cm. Good exposure is essential to avoid injury to the flexor tendons or digital nerves. Although insertion of a bistoury and blind incision of the proximal tendon sheath have been recommended, the incidence of damage to tendons and nerves argues strongly against further consideration of such practice. Exposure of the tendon sheath can be accomplished under local anesthesia but should be done under tourniquet hemostasis and in an operating room with proper instruments and assistance. Under such conditions, a surgeon is always impressed with the incorrect terminology for the disease. As soon as the tendon and beginning of the sheath are visible, it is obvious that the condition has been incorrectly named. There is no visible abnormality of the tendon sheath other than mild inflammation, and this only in severe cases when unusual force has been applied during passive extension. The lesion lies within the tendon, and grossly it appears to be a bulbous enlargement that acts as a ball trying to pass through the opening of a tunnel. The lesion is circumscribed and probably is the result of degeneration and repair in the center of the tendon. Because injury to a flexor tendon in the sheath area is a serious complication and incision of the sheath produces instant relief, there is insufficient tissue from affected tendons for adequate study.

One of the reasons for performing incision of the sheath under local anesthesia is that occasionally incision of the proximal sheath will not result in immediate relief. In these patients, further exploration of the flexor mechanism can be expected to reveal that the enlargement of the tendon is more distal than usual and that the tendon is restrained during passage through the sublimis tendon. Enlargement of the passage through the sublimis tendon until it connects with the normal split of the terminal insertion will correct the condition. Distal lesions usually are the result of incomplete division of a profundus tendon following a penetrating injury. Deformation of the gliding surface is caused by failure of the tendon to heal and remodel within the sheath. By having the patient under a local anesthetic only, the surgeon can be satisfied that unobstructed active flexion and extension are possible before the wound is closed. Missing a distal enlargement or opening the sheath inadequately has occurred when patients have been operated upon under general anesthesia. Passive motion is not an adequate test.[5]

A third type of stenosing tenosynovitis seems to be more correctly named, as the tendon sheath is visibly involved. The condition is seen occasionally where long tendons pass beneath a firm retinacular band such as within the common sheath for the extensor pollicis brevis and abductor pollicis longus on the radial side of the wrist. The amplitude of motion of these tendons is relatively small, and there is no restriction to motion or snapping phenomena. The condition is a sterile inflammation of the internal surface of the sheath and is called *de Quervain's disease* when the extensor pollicis brevis and abductor longus tendons specifically are involved. Pain is the major symptom; ulnar deviation of the wrist intensifies the pain and is diagnostic of de Quervain's disease. Opening the sheath results in escape of cloudy fluid and exposure of inflamed synovial tissue.

Treatment of de Quervain's disease is injection with cortisone or incision of the sheath. Treated early, the condition often responds dramatically to injection of cortisone into the distended tendon sheath. Relief may be complete after several days' immobilization following such an injection. Recurrence is frequent, however, and surgical incision of the sheath usually is required for permanent cure. The operation also can be performed under local anesthesia but should be done under tourniquet hemostasis and in an operating room with adequate preparation. Damage to the sensory branch of the radial nerve lying on the sheath is a frequent and unnecessary complication. Although the radial nerve supplies sensation to an insignificant portion of the hand, injury produces neuromas and some of the most stubborn pain problems in the upper extremity. Repair of the nerve always should be done if it is inadvertently injured. For 3 or 4 weeks after incision of the sheath, a troublesome "rolling" sensation of the liberated tendons occurs during flexion and extension of the wrist. This painless, but definitely abnormal, sensation disappears as internal healing and remodeling of scar tissue occur.[22]

### Burns

Burns of the hand are of special significance because of the danger of loss of small joint func-

tion. The prolonged healing required for treatment of thermal burns elsewhere in the body often produces results in the hands that may be even worse than loss or damage of skin secondary to radiant energy. Treatment, therefore, is governed by need to reduce the period of immobilization to an absolute minimum. This means that treatment of hands often takes precedence over treatment of burns elsewhere. It also means that general principles applicable to large body burns do not always apply to treatment of the burned hand.

Thermal burns are classified according to thickness of skin involved. The diagnosis of a first-degree burn (erythema) or a third-degree burn (eschar) usually is not difficult. Second-degree burns generally are classified as partial-thickness burns that produce vesicles. This definition is not particularly helpful to the surgeon considering various methods of treatment. Of more importance in a second-degree burn is the extent of dermal damage. It is desirable that enough viable skin remain so that regeneration of epithelium will produce a satisfactory cover; otherwise, skin replacement is necessary. Unfortunately, there is no unerring test that gives precise data on the prognosis of healing, but a few signs are helpful. A cherry red color (frequently mistaken for erythema and interpreted as evidence of intact circulation), if it does not blanch and reappear on mild pressure, indicates carbon monoxide-fixed hemoglobin in tissue and is a sign of irreparably damaged skin that must be replaced. Burned skin elevated above the surface of normal skin is edematous and contains open channels and cellular elements capable of producing healing without replacement. Burned skin that is below the surface of adjacent skin usually is too badly damaged to become edematous and should be replaced. Heat-tanned collagen is crosslinked too extensively to become overhydrated and will not swell as normal collagen does.

The most important question is whether burned skin can be treated conservatively and allowed to heal by epithelial regeneration, scar synthesis, and wound contraction or whether it should be replaced immediately. This decision should be made at the earliest possible moment.

Skin replacement requires 10 to 21 days of immobilization; many hands, particularly if edematous and in middle-aged or older patients, will not tolerate more than 2 weeks of immobilization without permanent loss of proximal interphalangeal joint function. Thus, the wait-and-see-what-happens test, often utilized successfully in burns elsewhere, may result in permanent loss of hand function even though skin replacement ultimately is successful. The problem, of course, exists primarily in deep second-degree burns in adults. Children most frequently burn the volar surface of their hands by grasping or crawling upon a hot surface. Adults usually burn the dorsal surface when something falls on the hands or by protecting the face against flame. Fortunately, children with volar burns can and should be treated conservatively. If obvious nonviable eschar is produced, it should be excised and replaced with a skin graft at the earliest possible moment. The difficult, deep second-degree burn in which it is not possible to be certain of the depth can be treated with a surface antibacterial agent in children and allowed to heal spontaneously over a prolonged period of time. The reasons for doing so are that in children joint stiffness does not develop during prolonged immobilization and that preservation of small islands of viable skin on the volar surface is worthwhile because of the need for sensation that small islands provide. A uniform full-thickness burn of the skin of the palm and volar surface of the fingers is relatively rare. Any islands of unburned skin that can be salvaged make conservative treatment worthwhile.

Different reasoning is utilized in a deep second-degree burn of the dorsum of the hand in an adult. In this situation, there is no particular advantage in saving islands of unburned tissue, and the cosmetic and functional effects of healing by scar synthesis, contraction, and epithelialization are unsatisfactory. Even though deep dorsal burns eventually may heal by natural processes, the type of cover produced may not be satisfactory and the effects of prolonged immobilization are potentially disastrous. In adults with dorsal burns in which there is any question about the injury being a mixture of third-degree and second-degree, or if the second-degree injury is so deep that fibrous protein synthesis (scar) will be a prominent part of the healing process, immediate excision of burned tissue and replacement with a skin graft is recommended by some. However, it should be emphasized that most surgeons believe conservative treatment is indicated for superficial burns, with early excision reserved for obvious third-degree burns.

The author's reasons for preferring early excision are based upon the biologic effects of prolonged edema and immobilization of collagenous structures. Successful management by early excision is technically demanding, and excision must be performed within a few hours or, at most, a few days after injury. Some previously reported undesirable results following early excision of burned tissue and immediate replacement of skin seem to have been due to a combination of technical errors in obtaining uncomplicated primary healing and misunderstanding of the difference between early excision and primary treatment. Skin grafting in a hand that has been edematous for several weeks produces quite a different result from skin grafting in a hand that has been edematous for less than 24 hours. The exact biologic nature of the difference has not been measured accurately, but it may be associated with the difference between bound water and free water in collagenous tissues. Until the biologic variances that control synthesis and deposition of fibrous tissue throughout an immobilized, edematous hand are better understood, it has seemed advisable to remove damaged tissue as soon as possible, even though some slightly damaged tissue that would have survived may be inadvertently removed. The rationale behind such an approach is that skin so badly damaged that precise diagnosis is impossible probably will not heal satisfactorily and ultimately will require replacement. To be wrong in primary assessment of burn depth and have to resurface a hand after several weeks of immobilization and secondary healing introduces an additional group of biologic reactions which, although not clearly defined now, have predictable results. Avoidance of phenomena such as the possible conversion of fibrin to collagen or spontaneous development of joint arthrodesis can be achieved by shortening the period of immobilization and preventing secondary wound healing. Excision and replacement of all partially damaged skin in the hands of adults is the most predictable and certain way to avoid such sequelae.[17]

*Chemical burns* usually can be treated satisfactorily by extensive washing and neutralization. *Phosphorus* burns require special attention, as small flakes of burning phosphorus become tenaciously adherent to skin and will continue to produce damage for days if every particle is not carefully dissected out of the hand. *Nitric acid* burns tan the surface, giving it an appearance like that of a third-degree thermal burn. These burns usually are not third-degree, however, and will heal primarily without prolonged immobilization. Many acid burns appear to incite abnormal fibrous protein synthesis, and hypertrophic scars may require secondary revision even though primary healing occurred without grafting.

*Radiation* can produce an acute wound but more often produces typical short-wave radiation effect and chronic difficulties. The most common cause for these conditions among physicians—improper use of diagnostic radiation—has almost been eliminated. Treatment of eczema and other benign conditions such as hemangiomas still results in late damage of skin, typified by chronic inflammation, inability to heal, constant pain, recurrent infection, and chronic ulceration. The end result will be carcinoma, and prophylactic removal of all areas of significant radiation effect may be justified on this basis alone. Because most such radiation is soft, unfiltered radiation, the effects usually are superficial; replacement of affected skin with split-thickness grafts produces satisfactory relief of signs and symptoms. Deep effects, however, require a permanent blood-carrying pedicle flap to provide adequate circulation; sacrifice of a digit to contribute a local flap may be needed to restore adequate circulation and permit satisfactory wound healing.[3]

## PENETRATING WOUNDS

The major objective in managing penetrating wounds of the hand is to obtain a healed wound without complications as soon as possible. Regardless of the nature of the injury beneath the skin, there are few exceptions to the general rule that repair of deep structures can be performed as effectively secondarily as primarily. Although an experienced hand surgeon often is able to repair deep structures during primary repair of a compound wound, the inexperienced surgeon should not feel compelled to do so. If doubt exists about whether a nerve, tendon, or bone should be repaired primarily, or if there is any question concerning the adequacy of experience or facilities, only the skin should be closed, and the repair of deep structures should be delayed until primary healing is over and the therapeutic or biologic questions are resolved. The only exception is repair of divided long flexor tendons in the proximal wrist, which must be performed as a primary procedure. The worst complications that result from repairing other long tendons, nerves, and bones, such as dehiscence, malunion or nonunion, are relatively simple to correct. The most common complication of prolonged soft tissue healing—loss of proximal interphalangeal joint motion—may permanently reduce hand function and make secondary reconstruction of an otherwise salvageable structure pointless.

### Fingertip Injuries

The relative frequency of fingertip injuries has made management of these wounds a popular area for postwar application of military reconstructive surgery. When tissue has not been lost, repair of lacerations, molding of fracture fragments, and splinting in a midflexion position are all that is required. The bulbous deformity of the fingertip often resulting when it is struck by a heavy object can be prevented by molding the fingertip in an expertly applied circular dressing rather than splinting it flat against a tongue blade or other splint. Application of a molded circular dressing to a fingertip is fraught with dangerous circulatory complications, however, unless the dressing is applied and cared for expertly.

The objective in treating a partial or complete amputation is to provide a usable surface as rapidly as possible. Production of an amputation scar that makes the fingertip unusable because of inadequate tissue, prominent scar, or prolonged secondary healing may be a more serious disadvantage to the hand than was the subtraction of a fingertip. It is often best to remove enough proximal bone with a rongeur so that the remaining soft tissue can be closed easily without tension, rather than perform a complicated shift of tissue such as a finger flap, local pedicle flap, or distant pedicle flap. Such advice may not be applicable to injuries of prime digits (index finger and thumb), particularly in highly trained persons who use the finger or thumb tip for creative work. The principle is a good one and almost always obtains when treating injuries of the long, ring, and small fingers as well. Sacrifice of a few millimeters of length in an amputation stump to assure full-thickness soft tissue coverage without tension or prominent scar in an opposable surface is indicated in most patients.

When amputation of the tip of a prime digit has occurred and length of the remaining stump is of great importance, a number of sophisticated measures for replacing tissue have been devised. They include bilateral local flaps, island pedicle flap, cross-finger flap, palmar flap, and distant flap. If the bone is not exposed, a simple split-thickness or full-thickness skin graft is an ideal solution. A split-thickness skin graft provides an excellent temporary cover for the wound if the best definitive reconstructive procedure is not obvious or cannot be performed. Use of any local tissue that assures

preservation of highly specialized sensation is superior to shift of distant tissue that creates an anesthetic mound surrounded by circular contracting scar.[18]

### Lacerations and Avulsions

Soft tissue lacerations and avulsions elsewhere in the hand should be treated by primary closure if tissue has not been lost, or by application of a split-thickness skin graft or distant flap when significant tissue is avulsed. It should be remembered that the hand of a child or young adult does not contain excess skin. The integumental envelope may appear redundant on some surfaces when joints are in extreme position; this apparent redundancy, however, is only to permit full joint motion; loss of even a few millimeters of skin in young or middle-aged patients invariably results in restriction of overall hand function. Thus, replacement of skin is always necessary in the reconstruction of an injury characterized by skin loss (Fig. 8).

Although it is often necessary under abnormal conditions, such as the care of large numbers of military casualties under less than optimal conditions, to leave a wound of the hand open for drainage of a potentially infected area, such practice is almost never recommended in normal circumstances. There is seldom any reason why a well trained surgeon should not utilize tourniquet hemostasis and debride any injury as extensively as is necessary to convert a badly contaminated wound into a surgically clean one. Following a massive crushing or penetrating injury, such a procedure may require 2 or more hours. It can and

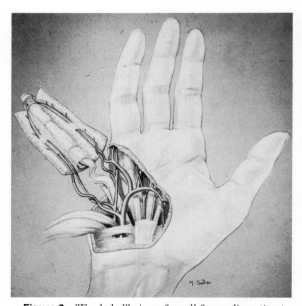

**Figure 8**  "Exploded" view of small finger dissection to show radial orientation of blood supply. An entire finger or any portion of a finger can be nourished by a single neurovascular bundle and transplanted anywhere in the hand or wrist. (From Peacock, E. E., Jr.: Plast. Reconstr. Surg., *25*:298, 1960.)

should be done, however, unless other injuries, other patients, or unacceptable logistic conditions exist. Once a contaminated wound has been converted into a surgically clean one, there is no reason not to close it immediately. The simplest method of closing complicated wounds characterized by loss of skin is by the use of a split-thickness skin graft. If more than split-thickness skin is missing, there is no reason why full-thickness skin or a skin and fat pedicle cannot be utilized during primary treatment. Only inadequate debridement or inadequate preparation of the surgeon for such a procedure militates against restoring skin deficiencies at the time of primary wound closure.

### Nerve Injuries

Nerve injuries in the hand are frequently overlooked because of superficial understanding of the overlap of some nerves and the frequency of abnormal innervation of some muscles, particularly in the thenar group. Sensory defects are relatively easy to diagnose except in inebriated or otherwise uncooperative persons or in small children. In these patients, determination of the presence or absence of sweating can be very helpful when injury to a sensory nerve is suspected. Sweating can be evaluated by drying the skin in a suspected dermatome with ether and then examining it (observation through the +4 lens of an ophthalmoscope is sometimes helpful) for reappearance of small beads of perspiration. If droplets of perspiration appear, division of a sensory nerve to that dermatome is unlikely. If no perspiration can be detected, and surrounding dermatomes perspire normally, division of a sensory nerve is likely. Commonly recommended tests of motor nerve function such as opposition of the thumb as a test of median nerve function or abduction of the fingers as a test of ulnar nerve function are not always reliable. Opposition of the thumb can be performed by at least three well known substitution patterns, and if the long head of the short flexor muscle is innervated by the ulnar nerve, as it is in approximately 40 per cent of persons, opposition may be normal in a patient with complete division of the median nerve. Circumduction of the thumb in a wide 360 degree arc is recommended as a better test for median nerve motor function. It is almost impossible to circumduct the thumb in a symmetric arc if any of the thenar muscles are absent. Froment's sign (ability to maintain a perfect circle with thumb and index finger during strong pulp-to-pulp pinch) is recommended as the best test for evaluating the motor branch of the ulnar nerve. Both tests depend upon function of most of the intrinsic muscles on the radial side of the hand and are more reliable than tests that depend upon utilization of a single motor unit.

Major controversy surrounding repair of lacerated peripheral nerves concerns the optimal time for repair. It might seem that after the experience of the last two decades surgeons would know whether repair of a divided nerve is best done at the time of primary wound repair or delayed until wound healing and secondary scar maturation

have occurred. Not only are there insufficient data to substantiate one recommendation or the other, but it is possible that definitive data will not be available in the near future. The problem is based upon difficulties in making objective measurements in humans and determining subjective reactions in experimental animals. Reaction to injury and axonal regeneration vary considerably between species; the ulnar nerve of the cat and the giant motor axon of a squid, which are most often used to study peripheral nerve conduction, are not completely analogous to peripheral nerves in man. Measurement of sensory return in man is extremely complicated, as apparent return of sensation may be due to several adaptations to injury rather than regeneration of a sensory axon. Apparent return of motor function may be even more difficult to assess because of development of complex substitution patterns. A primate model in which the results of primary and delayed peripheral nerve repairs have been evaluated by electromyographic response recently has provided the best objective evidence upon which therapeutic recommendations can be made.[9]

There are theoretical and practical factors supporting both primary and secondary nerve repair. Theoretically, it should be advantageous to repair a nerve primarily so that motor endplate degeneration and muscular atrophy will not occur over a prolonged period. Theoretically, it is just as advisable to delay repair of a nerve approximately 6 months to permit wallerian degeneration to occur in the distal fragment. The rather marked inflammatory reaction in the distal end of a divided peripheral nerve while phagocytosis of axoplasm and myelin is occurring suggests that regenerating axoplasm from the proximal nerve would have an easier path to travel after cellular reactions are over and only a clean, empty nerve sheath remains. Practically, it is easier technically to orient (circumferentially) and repair accurately a divided nerve immediately after injury. On the other hand, one can determine the exact level of proximal injury (when debriding a nerve preparatory to suture) more accurately after a neuroma has formed.[23]

Most surgeons believe that regardless of the various biologic factors supporting primary or secondary repair enough peripheral nerve restorations have been performed and evaluated in human beings to state that satisfactory results can be obtained by either method. Unfortunately, however, some rather dismal failures also have resulted from both primary and secondary repairs, suggesting that selection of the time to repair a peripheral nerve is only part of the problem in many patients. Technical and temporal advantages of primary repair are so outstanding, however, that most surgeons recommend primary repair of a lacerated nerve in any wound that can be adequately debrided and closed. Two major exceptions must be noted. In high-velocity missile or crushing injuries where the degree of proximal (or distal) injury in the nerve ends cannot be assessed accurately, or when primary tendon repairs also are being performed and the hand would have to be placed in an undesirable position postoperatively if nerves also were coapted, secondary repair is indicated. Otherwise, the practical advantages of a primary repair outweigh the theoretical advantages of a secondary repair. Primate studies support this clinical conclusion.[9]

When the results of either primary or secondary nerve repair are less than predicted, early re-exploration to identify a technically or biologically correctable error is indicated. Such complications include dehiscence, abnormal scar formation, and proximal intraneural neuromas. The results of repair of the median nerve usually are better than results following repair of the ulnar nerve. Anastomosis of pure motor or pure sensory nerves in the hand produces better results than repair of a compound nerve in the wrist or arm. Motor return following a primary repair may be better than sensory return. It is not unusual for sensory return to be incomplete. Protective sensation, at least, should be obtained in all uncomplicated nerve repairs in the distal extremity. Failure to achieve protective sensation means a technical or biologic complication has occurred, but many such complications are correctable by secondary procedures.

Irreparable nerve injury should be treated by redistribution of normally sensitive skin throughout the hand and redistribution of motor units to prevent deformity. Sensation is most important on the ulnar side of the small finger and the radial side of the index finger and thumb. In an irreparable median nerve injury, therefore, sensation from the radial side of the small finger might be transferred to the thumb or index finger, whereas in an irreparable ulnar nerve lesion, sensation from the long or ring finger might be transferred to the ulnar side of the hand. This is accomplished by nerve transfer or island pedicle flaps. Nerve transfer requires a nerve anastomosis; thus, anesthesia is created in one area and only partial sensation can be achieved in another. Island pedicle transfer of normally sensitive skin on a neurovascular pedicle transfers all of the sensory modalities, although a soft tissue defect is created in the donor site and must be resurfaced by a free skin graft.

Deformity is the result of unopposed muscle pull around a joint or series of joints. Dynamic splints substitute elastic or spring force for the paralyzed muscle; stationary splints usually hold a joint in neutral position (Fig. 9). Ultimately, muscle transfers should be performed to redistribute permanently muscle power around joints. Examples include transfer of the flexor carpi ulnaris to paralyzed finger extensors in a radial nerve palsy, transfer of the brachioradialis muscle to provide finger flexion in a high median nerve palsy, transfer of a ring sublimis tendon to the abductor pollicis brevis muscle in a low median palsy, and transfer of a split ring sublimis tendon to paralyzed intrinsic muscles in an ulnar nerve palsy. In each, one of a group of normally functioning muscles is transferred to a group of paralyzed muscles to balance the remaining power in a partially paralyzed extremity.

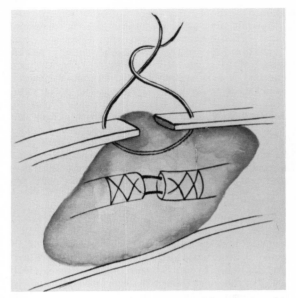

**Figure 9**   Dynamic splint constructed from brass welding rod and plaster. Rubber bands substitute for paralyzed muscles innervated by the radial nerve. Active motion is possible, but the hand returns to a functional position during muscle relaxation. (From Peacock, E. E., Jr.: J. Bone Joint Surg., *34-A*:789, 1952.)

Nerve grafts for large defects generally are unsatisfactory in the proximal extremity and are of only limited usefulness in the distal hand. Pure sensory nerves in the distal palm and fingers can be grafted successfully with autografts from a damaged finger or less important area. It should be remembered that two anastomoses are required when transferring a free graft, and literally only half of the regenerating axons are likely to traverse each anastomosis and reach terminal organs. Work continues on the use of irradiated allografts; data at present are not convincing that great usefulness for irradiated peripheral nerve autografts will be found. Technical details regarding the use of epineural, intraneural, and funicular sutures are covered adequately in technical treatises on this subject.

### Tendon Injuries

Repair of divided tendons has intrigued the reconstructive surgeon more than any other problem in the upper extremity. The problem is primarily one of specialized wound healing in which one set of circumstances is desirable between the ends of an anastomosed tendon and the exact opposite is required surrounding the tendon. Because both sites are only arbitrary areas within the same wound, the problem is a formidable one. Actually, repair of tendons that have relatively small amplitudes of motion (extensor tendons and intrinsic tendons), and of tendons that move in concert with surrounding tendons (flexors in the proximal wrist and midpalm), poses no great problem for an experienced surgeon. Repair of independently acting tendons that change direction in restricted areas (digital sheath and carpal tunnel) and are surrounded by immovable structures such as a phalanx or digital sheath poses a serious problem. Stated more simply, the problem is that a single wound containing repaired tendon, healing soft tissue, and immovable structures (bone, tendon, or sheath) heals by production of a single dense connective tissue scar. Such a scar is desirable to hold the tendon ends together but is highly undesirable if it holds the tendon to fixed objects so that gliding motion is not possible.[19]

**Factors in Tendon Healing.** The reader will not be subjected to a review of the numerous technical procedures that have been designed to solve this problem. Most have as their objective separation of the wound between the tendon ends from the wound surrounding the tendon so that two separate scars will be produced. It is important to state, however, that all such attempts have resulted in failure because of two important biologic factors. One factor is that mature tendons apparently are not endowed with stem cells from the fibroblast series that are capable of synthesizing new collagen. Tendons, of course, are richly endowed with fibrocytes, but fibroblasts are highly specialized cells that are not present in all tissues. In a healing tendon, fibroblasts cannot be transplanted to the wound by circulation or transformation of blood elements. Successful isolation (which can be provided by all sorts of physical and biologic membranes) invariably results in failure of the tendon ends to be amalgamated by newly synthesized collagen. Collagen is needed if strength satisfactory to impart muscle power is to be obtained. Fibroblasts, essential to synthesis of dense connective tissue scar, migrate into the tendon wound from surrounding soft tissue. Generally, mechanical isolation of a tendon anastomosis is not consonant with the general objective of restoring strong union between divided tendon ends.

A second important biologic principle is that the longitudinal blood supply of most long tendons is not sufficient to nourish cells in the center of a tendon without help from segmental vessels in the vincula and mesentery. Segmental blood vessels are specialized, coiled vessels that permit motion of a tendon while nourishing it effectively. The fibrous adhesions that surround a repaired tendon or healing graft contain new blood vessels that ultimately will be long enough to contribute segmental nourishment without restricting motion of the tendon; successful prevention of adhesions by mechanical isolation techniques also prevents development of blood vessels and results in necrosis of part of the tendon. Similarly, early motion that is too vigorous to allow adhesion development also interferes with development of segmental blood supply and may result in replacement of the entire center of a graft with dense, immovable scar tissue.

In all probability, success or failure of tendon repair or tendon grafting is the result of selective remodeling of newly synthesized scar tissue with the result that the gel permeating the entire wound early in the healing process takes on markedly different physical properties at different places in the scar. Between tendon ends and in overlying opposed skin edges, the gel remodels to resemble normal tendon or dermis. Purposefully oriented fibrils and fibers accrue more monomeric particles, and nonpurposefully oriented subunits are removed by collagenolytic enzyme. As a result, tissue between cut tendon and dermal surface becomes remarkably polarized and compact. In these areas, internal crosslinking and external remodeling convert a loose, flimsy gel into dense, compact connective tissue strongly resembling

normal tendon or dermis and clearly organized to withstand longitudinal force without physical deformation.

Newly synthesized connective tissue surrounding a tendon graft or anastomosis must undergo an entirely different type of remodeling if longitudinal motion of the tendon is to occur. Although many surgeons seem to think of this change as a breaking of adhesions to "free the tendon," such reasoning is not consonant with infiltration of cells needed for prolonged wound healing or development of segmental blood supply. Dissection of the healed bed of a functioning tendon graft or anastomosed tendon does not reveal an absence of adhesions. What it does reveal is an entirely different type of scar tissue than is found between tendon ends. Fiber bundles are redundant in length, and the general organization is loose and nonpolarized. Individual fiber bundles are not elastic, but the gross physical weave, like the weave of inelastic nylon fibers to produce elastic nylon hose, permits longitudinal motion of the structure to which they are attached. Microscopic examination reveals lack of polarity of subunits, and the disorganized pattern that characterizes all structures that have viscoelastic properties is present. Dissection of a tendon graft or an anastomosis in which gliding function has failed to develop often reveals exactly the opposite. The newly synthesized collagen surrounding the tendon in many of these patients is remodeled in much the same way as scar tissue between tendon ends. Gross and microscopic examination of various subunits shows internal remodeling resembling dense connective tissue, and the deposition and polarization of collagen appear ideal to resist longitudinal deformation. The result is resistance to longitudinal force, and the tendon remains tightly incarcerated in a healed bed. Such biologic mischief, of course, is not the only cause for failure of a repaired long tendon to provide gliding function, but a majority of properly repaired long flexor tendons that do not regain adequate motion show restriction by fibrous adhesions of this type. Thus, the findings in functioning tendon grafts and anastomoses indicate that the term gliding function is a technical misnomer. Motion in a repaired tendon is not the result of breaking of adhesions and development of a smooth glistening surface that glides over another similar surface. Longitudinal motion is the result of specific changes in the internal assembly of collagen subunits so that lengthening of fibers occurs, probably by longitudinal slipping of various subunits. Secondarily, blood vessels become elongated and coiled to permit extension.

The next obvious question is, What induces newly synthesized and deposited collagen within the same scar to follow different routes at the same time? The answer probably is pivotal to further understanding and control of physical properties of scar tissue. The hypothesis upon which many technical aspects of tendon repair and postoperative rehabilitation are currently based is that newly synthesized collagenous tissue remodels according to the stimulus of inductive influences provided by tissue it has been deposited against. Thus, tissue synthesized against a cut surface of tendon remodels to resemble the internal structure of tendon, and tissue adjacent to loose connective tissue surrounding the longitudinal surface of a tendon or other soft tissue should remodel to resemble that tissue. The implications of these occurrences in an abrasion or cut surface on a tendon graft, healing fracture, damaged sheath, or stationary extension of palmar fascia are obvious. When a tendon anastomosis must lie in a bed containing these structures, the surgeon often finds it advantageous to place a new tendon through the damaged bed so that unscarred, normal, mature tendon and a thin sleeve of loosely organized connective tissue will lie where extensive healing of surrounding structures is occurring.

**Diagnosis of Tendon Injuries.** The diagnosis is often obvious. Absence of motion does not always mean a tendon laceration, and physiologic splinting of an injured digit may not be under cerebral control. With few exceptions, cut tendons do not retract a significant distance, and exploration of a soft tissue wound usually will confirm the suspicion of a divided tendon. Substitution patterns occasionally mislead an inexperienced examiner. For instance, division of the extensor pollicis longus will not be functionally obvious if the metacarpophalangeal joint of the thumb is slightly flexed when the patient is asked to extend the distal interphalangeal joint. The intrinsic thumb muscles are able to extend the tip of the thumb when other thumb joints are flexed. Terminal extension (when all joints are extended) of the distal interphalangeal joint is possible, however, only when the extensor pollicis longus is intact. Extension of all fingers may be possible through the action of an intact extensor communis tendon or of the many lateral decussations that sometimes occur in the extensor mechanism. Independent extension of a digit will be lost after complete division of a proprius tendon. Interruption of the intrinsic tendon connections to the extensor hood may not result in loss of extension when the digit is in a flexed position at the metacarpophalangeal joint. Ulnar luxation of the extensor tendons into the trough between metacarpal heads is responsible for this syndrome.

**Repair of Tendon Injuries.** While most tendon lacerations require either primary or secondary repair, occasionally neither is necessary. Repair of some digital *extensor* tendons may not be indicated in some patients. The extensor tendons have many lateral slips and connections and sometimes more than one tendon may be found supplying a single digit. Repair of an extensor tendon requires 3 weeks of immobilization, which can be dangerous for some patients. Moreover, adherence of an extensor tendon anastomosis to a deep immovable structure can produce a checkrein effect on finger flexion. Thus, if there is no functional deficit, repair of an extensor tendon should not be done simply to restore normal anatomy. Similar reasoning may hold when considering a lacerated wrist flexor such as the palmaris longus. Disability produced by a healing wound and immobilization following repair of some tendons may exceed the benefit of restoring continuity to a motor unit.

As a general rule, *extensor tendons* should be repaired by end-to-end anastomosis at the same time the soft tissue wound is repaired (primary repair). An exception is when a compound fracture also is present and the tendon anastomosis overlies the fracture site. Incarceration of a tendon anastomosis in the callus of a healing fracture produces the checkrein effect already mentioned. Repair of tendons under these circumstances should be delayed or the tendon rerouted by means of a transfer procedure. Three and a half weeks of immobilization is required for healing; the digit should not be placed in a position of extreme extension to remove all tension on the suture line during healing,

as is frequently recommended. Joint damage and adherence to structures in an extreme position make extensor splinting unwise in most patients. Mechanically adequate suturing and rest in a neutral position are recommended. Excess tension on a suture line is best avoided by extending the wrist, not by placing all of the finger joints in extreme extension.

Repair of *flexor tendons* is more complex both biologically and technically than is repair of extensor tendons. The long amplitude of motion—change in direction as the tendon passes alternately through constricted areas and over prominent elevations (volar plates)—requires radically different remodeling of scar than does the small amplitude of motion needed to extend a digit. Technical and judgmental factors, therefore, are critical when managing flexor tendon lacerations. It is impossible to summarize all the factors involved in repair of flexor tendons, but a general statement of principles that have evolved from much experience and that seem to be based upon sound biologic data follows.

Lacerated flexor tendons in the wrist must be repaired primarily or not at all. At the wrist level there are no restraining elements such as vincula, mesotendon, and lumbricals. Proximal muscle retraction and subsequent fibrous fixation make secondary repair impossible in most patients. All other flexor tendon injuries can be restored quite satisfactorily as a secondary procedure, and, in some patients, secondary repair may actually provide a better functional result. The important principle for the beginning student of restorative hand surgery or the surgeon who is unsure of whether primary tendon repair is indicated is that no harm is done by simply closing the skin and delaying tendon repair until later. This does not mean that an experienced hand surgeon working under specified conditions may not be able to repair flexor tendons successfully at any level. It is known that primary repair can produce an excellent result. It is also recognized that a poorly designed or poorly executed primary tendon repair produces incalculable damage. Moreover, it may significantly reduce the possibility of a subsequent successful secondary repair. Except in wrist lacerations, long flexor tendons should be repaired secondarily unless an experienced surgeon, operating under ideal conditions, prefers a primary anastomosis (Fig. 10).

Secondary repairs often take the form of a free graft, and usually there is not enough tendon at a secondary repair to perform a direct anastomosis without undesirable tension. Free tendon grafts are taken from the palmaris longus, plantaris, or toe extensor tendons. In children or in the small finger of adults, the distal end of a divided sublimis tendon may be used to graft the proximal profundus tendon. The main *advantages* of a graft are that the most seriously injured part of the bed (site of the original wound) can be traversed by an intact normal tendon and the anastomoses placed at a more favorable site. The proximal anastomosis usually is placed in the soft, movable fat of the

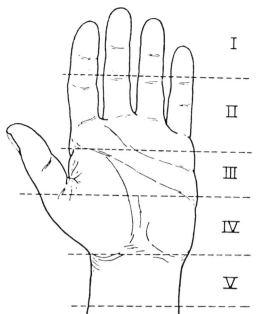

**Figure 10** Five zones in which repair of flexor tendons involves different biologic factors. Treatment of tendon lacerations in Zone I usually is accomplished by advancing the proximal tendon, fusing the distal interphalangeal joint, or performing a full-length tendon graft through the intact sublimis. In Zone II, free tendon grafts are most reliable; primary suture of one tendon can be performed successfully by experienced surgeons. Laceration of tendons in Zone III usually can be treated by primary anastomosis. Treatment of lacerations in Zone IV requires interposition grafts or wide dissection of retinacular structures. Tendon lacerations in Zone V should always be repaired primarily. (From Peacock, E. E., Jr., and Van Winkle, W.: Surgery and Biology of Wound Repair. Philadelphia, W. B. Saunders Company, 1970.)

palm or wrist. The distal anastomosis is an attachment of the graft to the distal phalanx. An oversimplified but helpful principle is that a "good" tendon can be placed in a "bad" (scarred) bed, or a "bad" tendon (site of anastomosis) can be placed in a "good" bed. However, a bad tendon cannot be placed in a bad bed with reasonable expectation of postoperative motion. The proximal palm and wrist are both favorable beds. More central areas involving constriction by sheath, passage of one

tendon through another, or replacement of normal surrounding tissue by scar are bad beds. The undisturbed longitudinal surface of a free graft often is needed to pass successfully through undesirable areas; healing of scarred or anastomosed tendons in such areas usually will result in formation of dense connective tissue adhesions between tendon and an immovable structure.

Special consideration should be given lacerated profundus tendons in the presence of an intact sublimis. Primary repair of a profundus laceration is to be avoided because the anastomosis of the profundus tendon will not pass through the intact sublimis. If the lesion is distal, the proximal tendon often can be advanced to the distal phalanx without putting the finger under too much volar tension. This is a desirable procedure but can be done only if the laceration has occurred within 1 cm. of the insertion of the profundus tendon. If advancement is not possible, a full-length graft is the only procedure that will restore completely normal function. Profundus grafts through an intact sublimis are risky procedures, and valuable sublimis function may be lost if complications occur. Grafting a profundus tendon through an intact sublimis should be done only by an experienced surgeon who can determine, on the basis of previous experience and training, that sublimis function will not be lost. When this is not possible, sublimis function is too valuable to be jeopardized by restoration of a profundus tendon. In many patients, no reconstructive procedure is needed; flexion of the distal interphalangeal joint may not be necessary for normal activity. In some patients in whom no reconstruction of the profundus tendon is performed, a hyperextension deformity may develop in the distal interphalangeal joint. In these patients, fusion of the distal interphalangeal joint in approximately 10 degrees of flexion is indicated. Fusion of the distal interphalangeal joint is an excellent method of treating profundus tendon lacerations when the sublimis is intact. Patients who must place their fingers in restricted passages may be disabled by a 10 degree permanently flexed position; most patients, however, find a 10 degree fusion of the distal interphalangeal joint adequate for all activities.

Immobilization for 3 weeks and gentle resumption of active and passive motion should follow primary or secondary repair or replacement of a

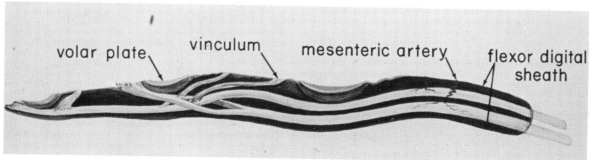

**Figure 11** Diagram of composite tissue graft of the entire flexor mechanism. Flexor tendons, mesotendon, and vincula are enclosed within an intact sheath.

damaged flexor tendon. Little or no active motion will be possible immediately after removal of the splint, but within 6 to 12 weeks full range of motion can be accomplished. The use of drugs, dynamic splints, and mechanical contrivances has not seemed to improve results consistently. Constant supervision of carefully prescribed active and passive exercises by specially trained physical therapists or the patient's surgeon makes an enormous difference. As might be expected, excessive physical therapy or supervision by untrained persons who often have an overzealous approach to reactivation may increase the possibility of an unsuccessful result. Restoration of long flexor tendon motion following repair or replacement has been one of the most difficult and often one of the most disappointing endeavors of reconstructive surgeons. Gradual improvement in results has been achieved by a combination of improvements in operative technique, education and selection of patients, and application of fundamental knowledge of connective tissue biology (Fig. 11).

## NONPENETRATING INJURIES

A wringer injury is one of the most common closed hand injuries, although replacement of roller mechanisms on modern washing machines has reduced the incidence of this potentially dangerous injury. Rolling compression forces occur in accidents other than those involving washing machines, however, and the essential factors that influence treatment of a child's hand that has passed through a washing machine wringer are applicable to other roller or press injuries. Absence of obvious skin avulsions, lacerations, or other damage belies the seriousness of the basic pathologic derangement at the time of initial examination. It is not unusual for patients with injuries of this type to be treated casually at the first examination. When the patient returns several days later with a relatively enormous loss of skin and possibly a deep fibrosis resulting in neurologic palsies, amazement may be expressed that so much damage could occur following this injury. Such events are predictable, however, and relate primarily to the fundamental pathologic lesion, which is destruction of blood vessels traversing the relatively flimsy loose connective tissue between skin and deep fascia on the back of the hand and forearm. Even with no obvious skin damage, circulation to the skin and deep structures may be altered so that tissue loss is unavoidable. Most tissue loss following such an injury is avoidable. Continuous hemorrhage and leaking of plasma during the first 24 hours after injury increases damage to tissue and prevents revascularization and nourishment of devitalized structures. Patients who are known to have suffered roller compression injuries of great force should be confined to bed, and an occlusive dressing should be applied expertly from fingertips to well above the affected area. Treatment of this sort reduces further hemorrhage and maintains the skin in close approxima-

tion to deep tissues as if a free full-thickness graft had been applied. Extremities treated in this manner are often spared large tissue losses. Proper postoperative position and dynamic splinting at the proper time also aid in reducing permanent disability. As soon as any evidence of full-thickness eschar appears, the eschar should be excised and replaced by a free graft. An open wound contributes to prolonged edema and inability of the patient to begin significant motion. If at any time during conservative treatment progressive loss of sensation or distal intrinsic motor function appears, the median and ulnar nerves should be explored. Both nerves are involved in rather restrictive connective tissue compartments; release and transplantation of nerves to an area where extensive fibrosis is not occurring can be influential in preventing sensory and motor disabilities.[16, 20]

*Closed tendon injuries* include rupture of the profundus tendon at the point of insertion into the distal phalanx during forced extension, rupture of the terminal insertion of the digital extensor mechanism at insertion on the dorsum of the terminal phalanx during forced flexion, and attenuation, rupture, or laceration of the dorsal hood of the extensor mechanism as it crosses the proximal interphalangeal joint. Loss of dorsal hood suspension of the lateral bands above the axis of rotation of the proximal interphalangeal joint can be the result of a closed or open injury; sometimes it is secondary to prolonged immobilization in an acutely flexed position. The lesion is called a *boutonniere deformity* and produces flexion of the proximal interphalangeal joint and extension of the distal interphalangeal joint. The deformity is the result of displacement of the intrinsic tendons below the axis of rotation of the proximal interphalangeal joint. In this position, the intrinsic muscles become unopposed proximal interphalangeal joint flexors and overpowering distal interphalangeal joint extensors.

The treatment of avulsion of the insertion of a profundus tendon is immediate operation and advancement of the avulsed tendon to the tip of the finger. All of the vincula, mesotendon, and other attachments may be avulsed with the tendon, which often is found coiled in the palm just distal to the origin of the lumbrical muscle. If the profundus tendon is not retrieved shortly after injury, it will not be possible to pass the profundus through the sublimis tendon and digital sheath. Insertion in the distal phalanx without placing the finger under too much tension also will not be possible. If several weeks have elapsed and reattachment is not possible, replacement of the avulsed flexor tendon with a free full-length tendon graft or fusion of the distal interphalangeal joint is indicated.

When a fragment of bone has been pulled off the distal phalanx by an avulsed extensor tendon (mallet or baseball finger), conservative treatment is sufficient. Splinting the distal interphalangeal joint in hyperextension is all that is required for reattachment of the tendon or avulsed bone fragment, and unless soft tissue of some type intervenes to prevent bone or tendon from re-attaching to the proximal phalanx, hyperextension treatment should produce normal extension after 4 to 5 weeks of immobilization. The most frequent cause of failure of conservative splinting is inadequate technique. It has been recommended in the past that the proximal interphalangeal joint be placed in acute flexion while the distal interphalangeal joint is splinted in extension, in order to place the intrinsic mechanism under minimal strain. It is quite a task to immobilize the proximal interphalangeal joint in flexion and the distal interphalangeal joint in extension and maintain both positions for 4 to 5 weeks. Moreover, damage to the proximal interphalangeal joint frequently occurs when immobilization is prolonged. It is not necessary to immobilize the proximal interphalangeal joint, provided the distal interphalangeal joint is placed in as much hyperextension as possible and maintained for a full 4 weeks. Hyperextension can be obtained by any number of external splints or an internal Kirschner wire. When external splints are utilized, the restraining mechanism often becomes loose and requires replacement at frequent intervals. While the splint is being replaced, the distal interphalangeal joint must be held in rigid extension by an assistant. Even a momentary drop into a flexed position may negate the effect of several weeks of treatment.

Failure to achieve normal extension means that a permanent mallet finger flexion deformity must be accepted or that operative treatment must be utilized. At operation, one frequently finds that the proximal extensor tendon and the distal phalanx are connected by dense connective tissue scar that is insufficient to hold the extensor tendon close enough to the phalanx so that the relatively short range of motion of the intrinsic mechanism will extend the phalanx. The mechanical advantage of the intrinsic mechanism normally is poor owing to the proximity of the insertion to the axis of rotation of the joint. Frequently all that is required to improve the action of the intrinsic mechanism is to divide the attachment of the central slip to the middle phalanx; this will allow the entire mechanism to slip a few millimeters in a proximal direction. This shift restores normal tension on the insertion and allows the extensor mechanism to extend actively the distal phalanx through scar tissue. Such a maneuver may not produce completely normal extension, but by the time operative intervention is resorted to, complete extension may not be possible anyway because of secondary changes in the joint. The full range of passive motion usually can be converted to active motion. Even if all of the range of passive motion cannot be converted to active motion by division of the central slip of the extensor mechanism, recovery of 50 per cent or more of motion usually will suffice for normal activity. The only other alternative is a graft of the extensor mechanism, which requires another 4 weeks' immobilization. It is not worthwhile to attempt to suture the avulsed extensor mechanism directly to the distal

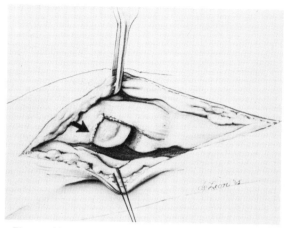

**Figure 12** Typical boutonniere deformity caused by rupture of the extensor mechanism over the proximal interphalangeal joint. Note flexion contracture of proximal interphalangeal joint and hyperextension deformity of distal interphalangeal joint.

phalanx. The tendon is too flat and thin at the point where it passes over the distal interphalangeal joint for an effective repair. A graft almost always is required if scar between tendon and phalanx cannot be utilized.

*Boutonniere* deformities usually require operative treatment (Fig. 12). Occasionally, success has been obtained by splinting, but splinting requires proximal interphalangeal joint immobilization in extension, an extremely hazardous under-

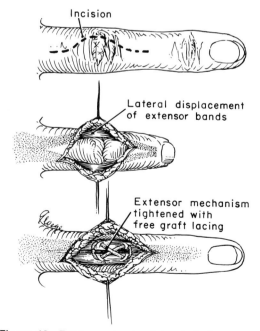

**Figure 13** Diagram showing lateral displacement of extensor bands in a boutonniere deformity. Repair involves lacing the lateral bands in a dorsal position by the use of a free tendon graft. (From Peacock, E. E., Jr. In: Converse, J. M., ed.: Reconstructive Plastic Surgery. Vol. 4. Philadelphia, W. B. Saunders Company, 1964.)

taking in all but very young patients. The danger of permanent stiffness of the proximal interphalangeal joint must always be regarded as less than satisfactory. Exposure of the extensor mechanism in a boutonniere deformity usually reveals either a clean laceration of the extensor hood, which can be reconstructed by merely suturing the lateral bands in a dorsal position, or a severe attenuation of the extensor hood, which makes suture impossible and replacement with a graft necessary. When attenuation has occurred, a palmaris longus or plantaris tendon graft is used to weave the lateral bands into a dorsal position so that they will act primarily as proximal interphalangeal joint extensors (Fig. 13). Extensor hood reconstructive procedures should be performed under metacarpal block regional anesthesia, if possible, so that active and passive extension and flexion of the digit can be checked at the end of the operative procedure. There is not much room for error while adjusting the tension of the extensor mechanism. If it is too tight, flexion of the digit will be lost; if tension is too loose, full extension of all joints will not be possible. Since an accurate method of judging tension in the intrinsic mechanism after a reconstructive procedure is not available, operation under local anesthesia with a full test of function under direct vision is recommended.

## FRACTURES

The most important principle in treating fractures of the hand is recognition that *joint immobility* is the most serious complication of treatment and can be worse than nonunion or malunion. It is therefore possible for the treatment to be worse than the disorder for which it was designed. Fixation must be devised so as not to immobilize important joints. This frequently can be achieved best by internal wire fixation. Kirschner wire fixation has been particularly valuable for phalangeal and metacarpal fractures that otherwise might require immobilization of small joints on either side. When traction is needed because a joint surface is involved or the fracture is badly comminuted, construction and attachment of traction devices should be devised to immobilize only the area of the fracture. Joints on either side should be free at least to move passively. It is important to be certain that Kirschner wires do not pin the lateral bands of the extensor mechanism to a phalanx. Permanent fixation of the extensor mechanism to bone restricts flexion and extension of distal joints. The old banjo-type splint produced many permanently stiff fingers since it applied elastic or spring traction from a fingertip to a distal outrigger and thus immobilized every joint in a ray. Such a splint should not be used except when multiple comminuted fractures throughout the entire digit make any other type of immobilization inadequate. When full-length traction is utilized for the entire ray, the digit should be placed on a curved splint so that trac-

tion is applied while small joints are in a mid-flexion position. As soon as fibrous fixation provides adequate fixation, traction should be discontinued, and splinting, interrupted frequently with cautious passive motion of the proximal interphalangeal joints, should be initiated.[2]

Several frequent and often misdiagnosed fractures in the hand are of special significance. They are fractures of the navicular bone and fracture of the base of the first metacarpal (Bennett's fracture). Navicular fractures are often produced by a fall on the outstretched hand, and they may not show clearly on routine x-rays. Persistent pain in the wrist and sharply localized pain following pressure in the anatomic snuffbox should arouse suspicion of a fractured navicular bone. Special x-ray views to bring out the navicular bone will confirm the diagnosis, often by exposing a hairline fracture. The fracture usually is transverse and may separate one of the fragments from all of its blood supply. Necrosis of the ischemic fragment occurs, and a rather severe arthritis ensues. Early diagnosis is essential to successful treatment. Prolonged immobilization in a snugly fitting cast, changed often to prevent any motion within the cast, is needed. A number of operative procedures have been designed to relieve pain when necrosis occurs. In extremely difficult cases, fusion of the wrist may be needed. Insertion of a bone graft or a plastic substitute for the navicular bone has not been satisfactory for most patients. Excision of the radial styloid does relieve pain sufficiently for normal activity in many patients.

Circumduction of the thumb is an extremely valuable motion for most people. Fracture-dislocation of the base of the first metacarpal (*Bennett's fracture*) is potentially a very disabling injury. Although many patients can be treated satisfactorily by applying traction to the first metacarpal, most patients with this fracture are probably treated best by exposing the fracture, relocating the first metacarpal on the saddle surface of the multangular bone, and replacing the fragment in perfect anatomic position by the use of a Kirschner wire. Early motion is important as soon as soft tissue healing has occurred. Failure to reduce the dislocated metacarpal or to place the dislodged fragment in almost perfect anatomic position will result in a painful and very disabling arthritis with loss of circumduction of the thumb.

## JOINT PROBLEMS

Dislocations should be reduced immediately by closed manipulation when possible. Dislocations of the carpal bones frequently can be diagnosed from a history of severe pain along the median nerve distribution without symptoms in the area of ulnar nerve distribution. Injury to the median nerve is common, and operative replacement of the carpal bones usually is necessary. Dislocation of the thumb metacarpophalangeal and the finger proximal interphalangeal joints may appear simple to reduce but often requires operative relocation because of a large articular surface and a relatively small tear in the joint capsule. After reduction has been achieved, gentle postoperative motion is required if severe disability is to be avoided. Stiffness after a traumatic dislocation usually is permanent. The best way to salvage some function, following dislocation of a proximal interphalangeal joint, is to prevent stiffness from occurring. Even gentle passive motion may be painful and cause an increase in postoperative edema; total immobilization during the healing period almost always results in permanent loss of joint function, however.

The metacarpophalangeal joint of the thumb is not an important joint, and many have less than 60 degrees of motion normally. Finger metacarpophalangeal joints are very valuable joints, and loss of motion is disabling. Fortunately, the metacarpophalangeal joints respond well to surgical manipulation. Dorsal capsulotomy and bilateral collateral ligament excision restore approximately 80 per cent of the normal range of motion to metacarpophalangeal joints. An exception occurs when the capsule becomes adherent to itself or to the articular surface so that the potentially large synovial space required for rotation of the proximal phalanx around the metacarpal head is obliterated. In these patients, capsulotomy and collateral ligament excision will not result in rotatory motion required for permanent metacarpophalangeal joint function. An important prerequisite for successful metacarpophalangeal joint surgery is an intact ulnar motor nerve and normal intrinsic muscle function. After collateral ligaments have been severed, intrinsic muscle action is the only lateral stabilizing force on metacarpophalangeal joints. If intrinsic function has been eliminated by injury to the motor branch of the ulnar nerve, fingers will go into severe ulnar deviation after excision of the collateral ligaments. Experienced hand surgeons occasionally are able to remove only the ulnar collateral ligament in a patient with an ulnar nerve palsy and improve metacarpophalangeal joint function to some extent. No procedure in reconstructive hand surgery is fraught with more danger, however, than collateral ligament excision in the presence of intrinsic muscle paralysis.

Stiff interphalangeal joints respond only moderately well to physical manipulation and very poorly to operative attempts to restore motion (Fig. 14). Occasional reports of success following capsulotomy have encouraged some hand surgeons to operate upon stiff interphalangeal joints. In some patients there apparently is enough volar displacement of the lateral bands of the intrinsic mechanism in the region of the proximal interphalangeal joint so that collateral ligament excision does not produce lateral dislocation. Collateral ligament excision as a method for treating proximal interphalangeal joint stiffness has been disastrous for many surgeons, however; the procedure cannot be recommended as a dependable approach to the serious disability produced by loss of motion in proximal interphalangeal joints.

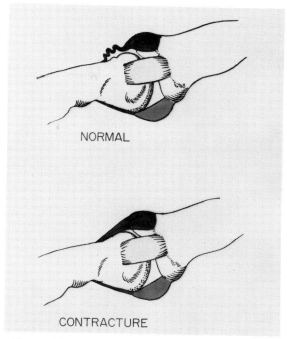

**Figure 14** Diagramatic representation of pathology of interphalangeal joint stiffness. The normally redundant dorsal capsule has remodeled in a shortened position where it prevents flexion. (From Peacock, E. E., Jr.: Ann. Surg., *164*:1, 1966.)

Traction and splinting are more reliable methods of improving interphalangeal joint function.[5]

## PHYSICAL MEDICINE AND REHABILITATION

Incalculable benefit as well as much harm has followed the use of physical medicine adjuvants in restorative hand surgery. Gradual and accurately applied traction is highly effective in inducing and perhaps even controlling secondary remodeling of connective tissue. Nevertheless, application of force sufficient to produce or accentuate an inflammatory reaction resulting in increased fibrous protein synthesis increases disability. The obvious conclusion is that physical agents directed toward increasing hand function, like other therapeutic agents, are both valuable and dangerous. What is needed now is introduction of the science of measurement into this potentially valuable field. Until recently, patient testimony that the hand "felt better" has been the major indication of success of treatment by physical measures. The biologic basis for stretching or heating connective tissue at a particular time after trauma has not been considered, and the actual results of heating, stretching, or in some way manipulating connective tissue have not been measured directly. It is possible to make such measurements now, and an enormous amount of valuable data can be obtained if the proper questions are asked.

Heat is probably used more than any other

agent in physical medicine today. It was only after the question, What is the effect upon the biology of connective tissue of externally applied thermal radiation? was asked that it was learned that thermal radiation does not change fundamental biologic properties of joint tissues and that externally applied heat does not even reach the structures responsible for joint stiffness because of the remarkable effectiveness of skin circulation in dissipating radiant energy. Heat, of course, is a very valuable analgesic, and other forms of administering radiant energy should be studied and possibly utilized to influence the biology of connective tissues. *Ultrasound radiation* can produce significant alterations in the physical properties of collagen. However, energy levels greater than 0.5 watt (present therapeutic limitations) are required. It would not be justifiable to raise energy levels higher than 0.5 watt, however, until we have more data concerning the effect of ultrasound radiation on all of the tissues of the hand. When such data are available, it may be possible to utilize higher energy sources to treat selectively such structures as collateral ligaments or tendon adhesions.

Occupational therapy also has been a valuable asset to reconstructive surgery, although, like physical therapy, it has been plagued with lack of skill in making important measurements. Motivation is one of the most important factors in success or failure of a reconstructive program. Poor occupational therapy can destroy initiative and reduce incentive to subeffective levels. Occupational therapy cleverly designed and adapted to meet specific objectives for individual patients may make spectacular contribution to the overall rehabilitation effort.

## TUMORS

Most epithelial and mesenchymal tumors found elsewhere in the body are found in the hand. Treatment of tumors in the hand is not basically different from treatment of similar tumors elsewhere; the biologic properties of tumors are much the same regardless of their location. In an area such as the upper extremity, where surgeons are primarily interested in reconstruction, however, it is especially important that extirpative surgery be planned primarily on the basis of the biologic characteristics of the tumor and not on the possibilities of later reconstruction. Benign tumors of epithelial origin include epithelial inclusion cysts, mucous cysts, nevi, keratoacanthomas, and warts. Benign tumors of mesenchymal origin include ganglia, xanthomas, fibromas, lipomas, osteomas, chondromas, and neurofibromas. Vascular tumors include lymphangiomas, hemangiomas, and glomus tumors. Malignant tumors include epidermal and basal cell carcinomas, melanomas, synoviomas, chondrosarcomas, fibrosarcomas, muscle tumors, and osteogenic sarcomas.

*Glomus tumors* are unusual tumors that affect the glomus organ or neuromyoarterial body of Masson. These organs, which control arteriovenous fistulas, are the site of tumors that characteristically produce severe pain. Approximately half of the tumors are subungual; pain is usually severe and can be induced by pressure, change in temperature, or vasomotor instability. The tumor, a blue or cyanotic discolored area that is usually not more than 3 or 4 mm. in diameter, may produce erosion of bone or elevation of a fingernail. Complete surgical removal is necessary for cure, but it is often difficult to eradicate a tumor on the first attempt. Definition of the tumor is difficult, and repeated wide excisions of an area may be necessary to remove the lesion completely.

The *ganglion* is probably the most common tumor in the hand and wrist. Some patients relate the onset of a ganglion to trauma, but the usual history is one of spontaneous development of a cystic mass on the volar or dorsal surface of the wrist. Very tiny (1 to 2 cm.) hard nodules that appear and disappear spontaneously on the volar surface of a flexor tendon sheath just over the metacarpophalangeal joints also are likely to be ganglia. Different from other ganglia, however, these lesions always disappear after several months and do not require treatment.

Although pathogenesis of ganglion is not clear, the lesion probably is the result of mucoid degeneration in redundant dense connective tissue of a joint capsule or tendon sheath. No connection with a joint cavity or synovial space around tendons has been demonstrated. The contents are not the same as synovial fluid. The cavity can be either multilocular or unilocular and contains highly viscous, clear fluid. Tiny satellite cysts often can be found around the base of a ganglion in the dorsal or volar capsule of the wrist joint.

Although a ganglion can be made to disappear for several months by aspirating or rupturing it, permanent cure usually requires complete excision. The high rate of recurrence previously reported probably relates more to misunderstanding of the fundamental nature of the lesion than to inadequate surgical technique. Recurrence is rare if the lesion is regarded as an area of mucoid degeneration of dense connective tissue and a large area of dense connective tissue is excised with immobilization of the joint for at least 3 weeks to allow complete regeneration. If only a cyst is excised, however, other tissue that may have been undergoing similar mucoid degeneration will produce another ganglion that may mistakenly be regarded as a recurrence of a previous lesion. After wide excision of an area of carpal retinaculum or wrist joint capsule, it is advisable to immobilize the wrist in a small gauntlet of plaster or leather so that conditions will be optimal for regeneration and remodeling of dense connective tissue. It is very important not to undertake excision of a ganglion under local anesthesia in the office. Wide exposure, tourniquet hemostasis, and careful identification of surrounding structures are necessary for a good surgical result.

*Lymphangiomas* and *hemangiomas* in the hand

are especially vexatious problems. Multiple excisions of hemangiomas at critical places can be rewarding, however. It is impossible in most patients to rid the hand completely of all of the hemangioma, but symptomatic relief in selected areas can be obtained by tedious dissection and reoperation when necessary. Gangrene of the skin can be averted when superficial lesions involve the skin. Radiation should not be utilized in treating hemangiomas; the blood vessels in a typical hemangioma are no more susceptible to radiation than any other blood vessels in the body; irradiation cannot be expected to eradicate the lesion, and radiation effect in overlying skin is a serious complication.

*Lymphangiomas* and *chronic lymphedema* are even more difficult to treat than hemangiomas. Excision of areas of lymphangioma often results in a larger lesion 3 months later. Complete eradication of lymphangioma or lymphedema in an area usually requires excision of all overlying skin and replacement with a pedicle or free graft. In all probability, the fundamental defect in chronic lymphedema is congenital absence of purposefully oriented lymphatic pathways, and because the dermis is involved, skin must be excised as well as deep tissue. In lymphangioma, the propensity for the lesion to recur after partial excision is discouraging, although repeated surgical extirpation of selected symptomatic areas sometimes can be helpful. It is not possible to dissect all of the lymphangioma from most hands, and attempts to do so may result in damage to important structures and a distressing recurrence of the tumor.

One of the most dangerous tumors in the upper extremity is a *subungual melanoma* (melanotic whitlow). These highly malignant tumors usually occur on the thumb as a pigmented, fungating, black mass lying in the sulcus between nail matrix and cuticle. They occur most often in white patients during the fifth decade, and it is rare to find the lesion in blacks. Pigmentation may vary from intense black to nonpigmented lesions. The prognosis generally is poor. Early surgical treatment, consisting of proximal amputation, is mandatory. Although absence of regional lymph node metastases is a favorable sign, the overall 5 year survival rate is less than 20 per cent.

## SELECTED REFERENCES

1. Barsky, A. J.: Congenital Anomalies of the Hand and Their Surgical Treatment. Springfield, Ill., Charles C Thomas, 1958.
   *This book provides a classic description and useful classification of congenital anomalies of the upper extremity. Timing of operative procedures and important points in surgical technique are presented.*

2. Boyes, J. H., ed.: Bunnell's Surgery of the Hand. 4th ed. Philadelphia, J. B. Lippincott Company, 1964.
   *This entire volume is an encyclopedic compendium of experience in reconstructive hand surgery. Chapter 16 on fractures is especially worthwhile.*

3. Brown, J. B., McDowell, F., and Frayer, M. P.: Surgical treatment of radiation burns. Surg. Gynec. Obstet., 88:609, 1949.
   *This classic paper presents the fundamental pathology of radiation injury and the development of surgical procedures for treating it.*

4. Bunnell, S.: Surgery in World War II; Hand Surgery. Washington, D.C., Office of the Surgeon General, Department of the Army, 1955.
   *The history of hand surgery in World War II is thoroughly reviewed. Most of the technical advances made between 1943 and 1947 are included.*

5. Fahey, J. J.: Trigger finger in adults and children. J. Bone Joint Surg., 36:1200, 1954.
   *This is an excellent review of the pathology and treatment of stenosing tenosynovitis in adults and children.*

6. Flatt, A. E.: The Care of the Rheumatoid Hand. St. Louis, C. V. Mosby Company, 1963.
   *Although several new advances in joint reconstruction, including the introduction of Silastic spacers, have occurred since publication of Flatt's book, the basic principles of rheumatoid arthritis surgery in the upper extremity are covered in a scholarly manner.*

7. Flynn, J. E.: Clinical and anatomical investigations of deep fascial space infections of the hand. Amer. J. Surg., 55:467, 1942.

8. Flynn, J. E.: Suppurative tenosynovitis of hand. New Eng. J. Med., 242:241, 1950.
   *These papers record the experience of an outstanding hand surgeon treating a large number of infections at the Boston City Hospital.*

9. Grabb, W. C.: Median and ulnar nerve suture. An experimental study comparing primary and secondary repair in monkeys. J. Bone Joint Surg., 50-A:964, 1968.
   *This is the best controlled study comparing primary and secondary repair of nerves. Although all of the factors have not been controlled, there is strong evidence to support primary repair in humans.*

10. Hueston, J. T.: Dupuytren's Contracture. Baltimore, Williams & Wilkins Company, 1963.
    *This monograph on Dupuytren's contracture is the most encyclopedic work available on the subject.*

11. Kanavel, A. B.: Infections of the Hand. Philadelphia, Lea & Febiger, 1912.
    *This monograph is a classic in the field of hand surgery. Kanavel was the first surgeon to make an intensive study of the spread of infection in the upper extremity. This book should be read by all aspiring hand surgeons.*

12. Kaplan, E. B.: Functional and Surgical Anatomy of the Hand. Philadelphia, J. B. Lippincott Company, 1953.
    *Although the fascia-lined spaces in the hand are not specifically considered from the standpoint of infection, this scholarly presentation of the anatomy of the hand should be a standard reference for surgeons treating infections.*

13. Lowden, T. G.: Infection of digital pulp space. Lancet, 1:196, 1951.
    *The peculiar anatomic configurations of skin, subcutaneous fat, and fascial septi in the digital pulp space are covered in this paper.*

14. Mason, M. L.: Infections of the hand. In: Sajous: System of Medicine, Surgery and the Specialties. Philadelphia, J. B. Lippincott Company.

15. Peacock, E. E., Jr.: Some biochemical and biophysical aspects of joint stiffness: Role of collagen synthesis as opposed to altered molecular bonding. Ann. Surg., 164:1, 1966.
    *The pathology of joint stiffness secondary to immobilization is analyzed. Changes in dense connective tissue are reviewed.*

16. Peacock, E. E., Jr., Madden, J. W., and Trier, W. C.: Transfer of median and ulnar nerves during early treatment of forearm ischemia. Ann. Surg., 169:748, 1969.
    *The effect of fibrosis in the forearm upon median and ulnar nerves is analyzed. The recommendation that median and ulnar nerves be transferred from injured muscle is based upon biologic changes in the forearm during partial ischemia.*

17. Peacock, E. E., Jr., Madden, J. W., and Trier, W. C.: Some studies on the treatment of the burned hand. Ann. Surg., 171:903, 1970.

*The authors analyze various factors involved in treating burned hands conservatively, as opposed to early excision of burned tissue.*

18. Peacock, E. E., Jr., Madden, J. W., and Trier, W. C.: Transplantation of fingertips. Ann. Surg., *173*:812, 1971.
*Modern methods of transplanting fingertips in reconstruction of amputation stumps are reviewed.*

19. Peacock, E. E., Jr., and Van Winkle, W.: Surgery and Biology of Wound Repair. Philadelphia, W. B. Saunders Company, 1970.
*This monograph relates modern wound healing biology to practical problems of tissue repair in humans. Chapter 8 on tendon repair covers in detail the principles outlined in the present text.*

20. Posch, J. L., and Weller, C. N.: Mangle and severe wringer injuries of the hand in children. J. Bone Joint Surg., *36-A*:57, 1954.
*The basic problems in compression injury of the upper ex-*

*tremity are described superbly, and treatment is outlined in detail.*

21. Warkany, J.: Etiology of congenital malformations. Advances Pediat., *2*:1, 1947.
*This paper provides a review of various experimental and clinical factors involved in development of congenital malformations.*

22. Wharton, G. W.: De Quervain's disease. J.A.M.A., *204*:341, 1968.
*The basic pathology and modern therapy of de Quervain's disease are covered.*

23. Wise, A. J., Topuzlu, C., Davis, P., and Kaye, I. S.: A Comparative analysis of macro- and microsurgical neurorrhaphy technics. Amer. J. Surg., *117*:566, 1969.
*A comparative analysis of epineural and funicular repair of peripheral nerve injuries is presented. Adequate controls are lacking, but the experimental design was the best that could be contrived when the work was done.*

# 45

# SURGICAL DISORDERS
# OF THE SKIN

*Kenneth L. Pickrell, M.D.*

In the average adult, the skin has a superficial area of 10,000 to 18,000 sq. cm.; it accounts for about 15 per cent of the total body weight. Its thickness varies from 1.5 to 5 mm., depending upon the location, age, sex, race, and state of nutrition. It is thinnest on the eyelids, penis, and labia minora, and thickest on the palms, soles, shoulders, and back. Infants and the very old have the thinnest skin. Sweat glands are abundant almost everywhere except the glans penis and labia minora. Sebaceous glands are profuse on the face, neck, and back; they are absent on the palms and soles. Sexual differences are involved in the distribution of hair, mainly on the face, neck, chest, and pubis.

The skin as an organ is vulnerable to a wide variety of diseases and conditions. Aging is accompanied by loss of elasticity and wrinkling. Degenerative changes result from excessive exposure to the sun and radioactive elements (see Fig. 4). Reactions to chemicals and drugs are common.

## MICROBIOLOGY OF THE SKIN

Resident bacteria are found chiefly in the stratum corneum (keratin layer) and the openings of the pilosebaceous apparatus. Gram-positive cocci of several types are found essentially everywhere. A number of diphtheroids are widely distributed, especially in moist areas; gram-positive rods are found in moist areas also. *Pityrosporon ovale* is classified as a resident fungus.[11] The number of resident bacteria is said to remain relatively constant unless altered by antibiotics or temperature. Those with oily skin have larger numbers of organisms, and more organisms are present in hot, humid weather. Despite the superficial position of the resident bacteria, it is virtually impossible to sterilize the skin. Body odor is influenced by the bacterial flora. Resident gram-positive bacteria act on the eccrine (sweat) and apocrine (scent) secretions to produce the characteristic odor of the axilla. The use of deodorants that contain aluminum salts reduces the number of gram-positive organisms, thereby reducing or eliminating the odor. The normal pH, 4 to 6, of the skin retards the growth of many skin organisms; streptococci are more affected than staphylococci. The pH of the skin is largely the result of lactic acid from sweat and amino acid residues from keratinization.[20] Intact skin presents a formidable defense against entry by pathogenic organisms, but traumatized skin (burns, penetrating wounds, crush injuries, and so forth) presents a favorable site and environment for their growth.

## SKIN PERMEABILITY

One of the major functions of the skin is to provide a barrier: from inside out and outside in. A very effective barrier is provided against loss of electrolytes, proteins, carbohydrates, lipids, and significant amounts of water from the internal environment. *Percutaneous absorption* is the passage of substances from the outside of the skin through the epidermis and dermis into the circulation. Well absorbed substances are lipid-soluble substances, phenolic and arsenical compounds, hormones, gases, vitamins (A, D, K), insecticides, and so forth. Absorption through the palms and soles is poor because of the thick keratin layer. Skin absorption can be increased by increasing the temperature and moisture.

## REGULATION OF BODY TEMPERATURE

Sweating is a major function of the skin because of its role in regulation of body temperature by evaporative cooling. Each liter of sweat is capable of removing 540 calories of heat from the body.[11] The most important stimuli for sweating are heat, muscular exercise, and a neuroendocrine reaction (fright, cold sweat). Thermoreceptors in the skin are stimulated by an increase in temperature (summertime). Similarly, thermoreceptors in muscle are stimulated by increased temperature of blood from working muscles. The heat center in the hypothalmus induces sweating when the temperature of blood circulating through it is elevated. *Emotional sweating* affects primarily the glands of the face, neck, palms, and axilla. *Reflex sweating* after eating spicy or hot foods affects primarily the face. Sweat glands are innervated by sympathetic nerves of both cholinergic and adrenergic type.[19]

Sweat is hypotonic with a pH range of 3.8 to 6.5 and a specific gravity of 1.001 to 1.006. It contains little or no protein, fat, acetone, or alkaline phosphatase. There are significant amounts of sodium, chloride, calcium, and iodide.[11] In *congenital ectodermal dysplasia* sweat glands are sparse and show lack or absence of function. Affected persons do not sweat adequately and hence they cannot cool their bodies in a hot environment.

Sweating from the skin must not be confused with the *circulation of fluid in the skin*, for in the latter there are three structures with membrane function: (1) dermal capillaries and lymphatics, which are concerned with escape and reabsorption of fluid and metabolites; (2) the basal membrane, which is permeable to water and most electrolytes; and (3) the barrier layer of keratin (stratum corneum), which is essentially impermeable to electrolytes but allows some passage of water and permits free passage of carbon dioxide.

## HISTOLOGY OF THE SKIN

### Epidermis

The epidermis is an avascular cellular structure that varies in thickness from 0.06 mm. on the eyelids to 0.8 mm. on the palms and soles. The border between the epidermis and the dermis is irregular because numerous cone-shaped dermal papillae reach or push upward and indent the inner surface of the epidermis. The ridges of epidermis separating the papillae appear in histologic sections as pegs and therefore are referred to as *rete pegs*, although the term *rete ridges* might be pref-

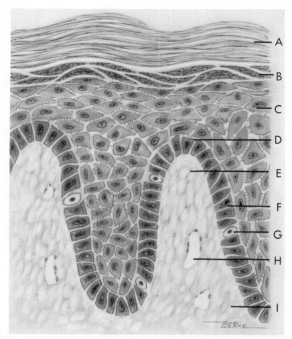

**Figure 2**   Drawing of normal epidermis from dorsum of hand, high magnification. Four layers are recognized: A, stratum corneum or keratin or horny layer; B, stratum granulosum or granular layer; C, stratum malpighii or prickle layer (note the presence of intercellular bridges); D, basal layer, which divides the epidermis from the dermis (an additional layer, stratum lucidum, not shown, is present between the granular and keratin layers, but it is conspicuous only in the epidermis of the palms and soles); E, papillae of dermis; F, mitotic figures, which can be seen in basal and prickle layers; G, melanocytes, clear cells, scattered in the basal layer; H, capillaries; I, collagen and elastic tissue.

erable (Figs. 1 and 2). If one could separate or peel off the epidermis from the dermis, it would look like the inside of an egg carton.

**Layers of Epidermis.**   The epidermis is divided into four layers of cells: (1) the basal layer, (2) prickle layer or stratum malpighii, (3) granular layer or stratum granulosum, and (4) the horny layer of keratin or stratum corneum (Fig. 2). An additional layer, the stratum lucidum, is present between the granular and the horny layers, but it is conspicuous only in the epidermis of the palms and soles. The cells in the various layers represent different stages in the gradual evolution and maturation of the basal cells into cornified cells and do not actually represent different types of cells.

BASAL LAYER.   The basal layer divides the epidermis from the dermis; two types of cells are present: basal cells and melanocytes. The basal cells are columnar in shape with their long axis vertical. These cells are active metabolically and mitotically and are the source of keratinocytes. It is from this layer that basal cell cancer develops. Basal cells frequently contain melanin, especially in dark-skinned persons; the pigment is transferred to them from the melanocytes. Mitotic

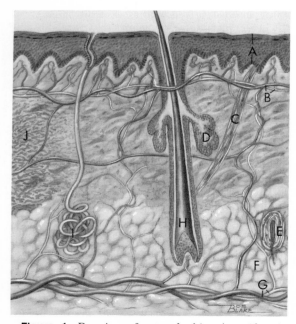

**Figure 1**   Drawing of normal skin: A, epidermis; B, capillaries; C, arrectores pilorum muscle; D, sebaceous gland; E, pacinian corpuscle; F, adipose tissue; G, blood vessels and lymphatics; H, hair; I, eccrine sweat gland; J, collagen, which gives substance to the skin.

figures may be present, denoting regeneration. In the normal epidermis, the cells of the prickle layer show more mitoses than cells of the basal layer. *Melanocytes* are of neural origin and are wedged in between the basal cells.

PRICKLE LAYER. The prickle layer (stratum malpighii) is located immediately above the basal layer. The cells are larger and more spherical and are connected by prickles or intercellular bridges which are formed by opposing protrusions of the cell membrane of neighboring cells. These prickles or intercellular bridges hold them together but do not represent avenues of passage of material from one cell to another. Between the cells, however, is a potential space, which in life appears to contain intercellular fluid and makes possible the exchange of nutrients and waste. As the cells pass upward, they become more egg-shaped with their long axis parallel with the skin surface. This is the layer from which squamous cancer arises.

GRANULAR LAYER. The granular layer (stratum granulosum) comes next and it is three to four cells thick. The cells are flattened with their long axis parallel to the surface. The cytoplasm contains basophilic granules called *keratohyalin* and the nucleus is undergoing degeneration. In areas of imperfect keratinization, *parakeratosis*, the granular layer is absent. The granular layer is normally absent from mucous membrane, in the lips, mouth, and vagina. The mucous membrane in the mouth normally possesses no granular cells and no horny cells. Here the epithelial cells in their migration from the basal layer to the surface first become vacuolated, and then shrink and desquamate.

STRATUM LUCIDUM. The stratum lucidum comes next; however, it is well developed only on the palms and soles.

HORNY, KERATIN LAYER. The horny layer (stratum corneum) is the outermost layer and is composed of anuclear dead cells, keratin, surface lipids, and dirt. This layer is responsible for the "bathtub ring." The cells of the horny layer normally desquamate in an orderly fashion; desqua-

mation and cell production are geared so that one controls the other. The stratum corneum remains at approximately the same thickness unless the balance is disturbed.

Under normal conditions, it takes approximately 26 to 28 days for an epithelial cell to migrate from the basal layer to the surface. Mitoses occur mainly in the basal and prickle layers. The *mitotic index*, the number of dividing cells per 1000 cells, varies from 2 to 8 or higher, depending upon the number of desquamated cells, since the thickness of the epidermis remains quite constant. Mitotic activity is greatest during rest and sleep; it is reduced during activity, in a cool environment, and during stress and starvation. Methotrexate and other anticancer drugs depress division of cells not only in the skin but in other organs also.

**Epidermal Appendages.** Hair and nails are keratinizing appendages; the other appendages are glandular—the eccrine, apocrine, and sebaceous glands.

*Eccrine* (sweat) glands are present everywhere in the skin, being most numerous on the palms and soles and decreasing in concentration from the head and neck to the extremities. The secretory cells are large, cylindrical cells that contain glycogen, which disappears on sweating (Fig. 2).

*Apocrine* (scent) glands are located chiefly in the axilla, groins, labia, scrotum, and pararectal areas. They are tubular glands that are located in the deep derma; the duct usually opens into a hair follicle above the sebaceous gland. Since the ducts do not open directly onto the surface, and since the secretory part of the gland is approximately 10 times larger than the secretory coil of eccrine glands, infections are extremely resistant to local antibiotics and emollients (see hidradenitis, Fig. 22).

*Sebaceous* glands are present everywhere except in the palms and soles. Their greatest concentration is on the head and face. Sebaceous glands are composed of several lobules. They are alveolar, holocrine glands; that is, they have no lumen and their secretion is formed by decomposition of their cells. They usually empty into the

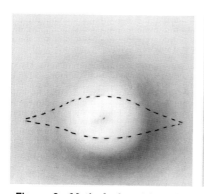 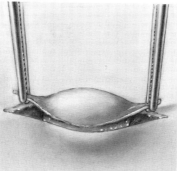 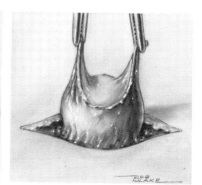

**Figure 3** Method of excision of sebaceous cyst. Sebaceous cysts are intimately fused with the skin, and in the very center the obstructed orifice and duct can be seen. Since the skin is usually very thin because of underlying pressure, one should use rather wide elliptical incisions, the ends of which then serve as handles to remove the cyst without rupture.

upper part of the hair follicle. Cyst formations are common; cancer forming in sebaceous cysts is rare; the author has never seen a case in 35 years. Sebaceous cysts are most common in adolescence and early adult life (Fig. 3). Cysts in the lower forehead, root of the nose, and brow areas must be differentiated from dermoid cysts, which may have an intracranial extension, and encephaloceles (see Fig. 21).

### Dermis (Cutis, Corium)

The dermis constitutes the bulk of the skin; it is thickest on the nape of the neck (where sebaceous cysts and carbuncles are common), back, palms, and soles. It is intimately related to the epidermis which it supports and nourishes and into which the epidermal appendages grow.

The dermis is composed of three types of fibers: collagen, elastic, and reticulum; it also contains blood vessels, lymphatics, nerves, cells, and ground substances (see Fig. 2).

*Collagen* forms about 95 per cent of the connective tissue of the dermis. The bundles and fibers are held together by amorphous ground substance. It is generally accepted that collagen is formed extracellularly by the action of fibroblasts. Collagen bundles are only slightly extensible, but since they are wavy, they permit some stretching of the skin. A few fibroblasts are interspersed between the collagen bundles (see keloids, Fig. 6).

*Elastic fibers* entwine among the collagen bundles. Elastic fibers are wavy and therefore only small portions are seen in histologic sections. Selective tissue stains must be used, such as Verhoeff's stain. There is progressive loss of elastic fibers in actinic (solar) keratoses (see Fig. 4).

*Reticulum fibers* are not visible with routine stains but stain with silver, as Foot's stain. They probably represent immature or young collagen fibers (precollagen), and are the first fibers to form during wound healing. They are replaced gradually or transformed into true collagen.[15] Large numbers of reticulum fibers are present in mesodermal tumors, such as histiocytomas, sarcomas, and lymphomas.

*Dermal blood vessels* consist of capillaries, arterioles, and venules arranged in numerous anastomoses and arcades, abnormalities of which result in hemangiomas (see Fig. 17). There is prompt vascular response in infections (heat, redness), shock, and trauma (vasodilatation in burns and vasoconstriction in lacerations and injuries due to cold and so forth).

A special vascular structure, *the glomus*, occurs most abundantly in pads and nail beds of the fingers and toes. The glomus is concerned with temperature regulation and represents a special short-circuit device connecting an arteriole with a venule. The glomus cells are in intimate association with a rich network of nonmyelinated nerve fibers.[8]

*Lymphatic vessels* begin as fluid spaces between the cells of the epidermis, which then circulate between the collagen bundles as loops in the papillae, leading down through the dermis into the subcutaneous tissues and lymph channels. The response of the lymphatics to trauma and infection (lymphangitis) is prompt and marked. Distant dissemination of cancer is most often due to invasion of the lymphatics, less often by vascular or hematogenous invasion.

*Muscles of the skin* are mainly involuntary or smooth muscles. The arrectores pilorum when they contract produce "gooseflesh." The tunica dartos of the scrotum and the muscle fibers in the nipple and areola contract markedly when exposed to cold. The facial muscles of expression and the platysma muscles of the skin of the neck are striated or voluntary muscles.

# PATHOLOGIC PROCESSES OF THE EPIDERMIS

Localized hyperplastic lesions of the skin are of importance to the surgeon because they may be mistaken for cancer or melanoma. Certain terms are common in skin pathology and need to be defined. *Acanthosis* is a hyperplastic thickening of the prickle cell layer, the rete malpighii, and is a frequent finding in neurodermatitis and psoriasis. *Hyperkeratosis* is thickening of the stratum corneum, the keratin layer, as seen in senile keratoses and warts. It is associated with increased thickening of the granular layer. *Parakeratosis* signifies imperfect keratinization with retention of nuclei in the horny layer, a common finding in psoriasis and in inflammatory dermatoses. *Dyskeratosis* applies to changes in the epidermis suggestive of developing malignancy, including loss of cell polarity and increase in the number of mitoses, changes that are summed up in two descriptive words: atypicality and jumbling, the latter referring to the loss of normal, orderly cell arrangement. *Pseudoepitheliomatous hyperplasia* is a wild, but benign, overgrowth of the prickle cell layer which is seen frequently in infectious granulomas.

## HYPERPLASIA

### Seborrheic Keratosis

This hyperplasia is a benign basal cell papilloma. The lesions are frequently multiple and occur on the forehead, cheek, nape of the neck, and upper back, usually in persons over 50 years of age. The lesions are raised, soft, and greasy, and sometimes wartlike. They may be markedly pigmented and look like a scorched lima bean stuck on the surface. The lesions show little tendency to malignant change. They may be removed by excision, dermabrasion, or curettage in the clinic or office.

### Solar (Actinic, Senile) Keratosis

This lesion, in the beginning, is small and firm, and occurs frequently on the face, posterior neck, and hands in older persons with little skin pigment (redheads and blonds, persons with blue eyes) who have been exposed excessively to the sun (farmers, ranchers, commercial fishermen,

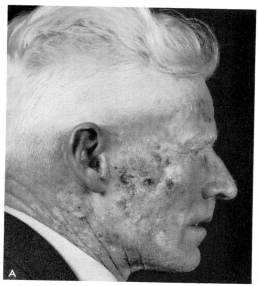 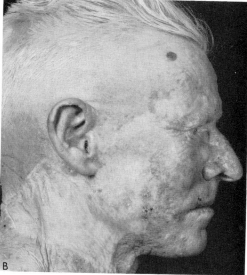

**Figure 4** *A*, A 45 year old commercial fisherman with extensive actinic changes in the skin frequently referred to as *farmer's* or *sailor's disease*. There were many hyperkeratoses and early squamous cell cancers in his thin, dry skin after prolonged exposure to the sun and wind. *B*, The forehead, lateral cheeks, and neck were resurfaced with heavy split grafts. Postoperative photograph taken 3 years later shows beginning changes occurring on the nose and maxillary rim of the graft. (See Fig. 16, xeroderma pigmentosa.)

and "sun worshipers"). The condition is a premalignant one, with a strong tendency to develop into squamous cancer (Fig. 4). Surgical excision and pathologic examination is recommended so that an accurate diagnosis can be made.

### Leukoplakia

This lesion of mucous membranes (lips, mouth, vagina) is analogous to the senile keratosis of the skin. As the name, white patch, implies, it takes the form of white patches of thickened mucous membrane (Fig. 5). It is often associated with chronic irritation, either physical (sharp, jagged teeth) or chemical (snuff, smoking, alcohol). Intraoral lesions are frequently multiple and are decidedly premalignant, of the squamous cell type. The irritating factors should be stopped and if prompt regression does not occur, the lesions should be excised, and skin grafted if necessary to close the mucous membrane defect without tension.

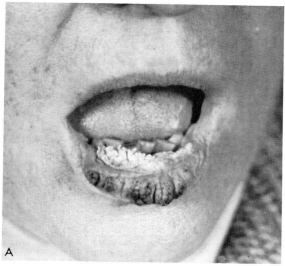 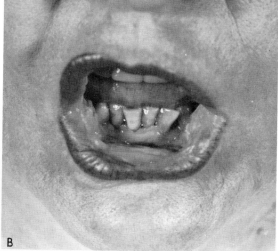

**Figure 5** *A*, A 54 year old woman, an excessive cigarette smoker of many years, with extensive leukoplakia and squamous papillomas of the cutaneous and buccal surfaces of the lip. The lesions were excised widely and grafted. *B*, Postoperative photograph taken 1 year later.

### Verruca Vulgaris (Verruca Juvenilis)

The common wart is the result of invasion of the epithelial cells by a specific virus. Warts occur in childhood through adolescence and early adult life and affect chiefly the fingers and hands. The warts occur in crops because of autoinoculation. Although the condition may be painful and troublesome owing to cracks, fissures, and bleeding, and psychologic trauma may be severe, the condition is self-limited and the lesions will eventually disappear without any residual scarring. Excision is of doubtful value. Dermatologic assistance by electrodesiccation or freezing with liquid nitrogen may be helpful.

### Verruca Plantaris (Plantar Wart)

Verruca plantaris is the most troublesome of all warts. Located on the sole of the foot, over the metatarsal heads or the os calcis, the wart is usu-ally covered by a thickened, cornified epithelium. Compression by the pressure of the weight of the body in standing is very painful. Corrective shoes and orthopedic appliances may be helpful. If the condition persists, excision and either the use of a split-thickness graft or the rotation of a contiguous flap may be necessary. Plantar wart must not be confused with a corn or callus, both of which are due to pressure and friction. In the corn or *clavus*, keratinization is developed as a dense localized plug.

## BENIGN TUMORS OF FIBROUS TISSUE

### Keloid

Keloid, from the Greek root *chēle* (crab's claw), is a dense fibrous tumor of the skin that occurs after injury. That the fibrous tissue represents an

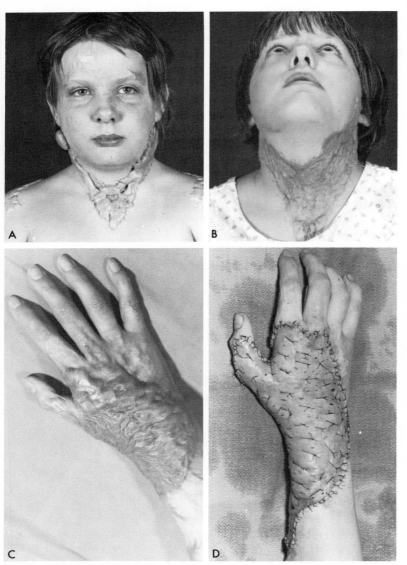

**Figure 6** *A*, An 11 year old girl with extensive keloids of the neck resulting from flame burns 2 years previously. The keloids had extended above and beyond the original areas of injury. Since it was impossible for her to extend her head, the keloids were excised and skin from the buttock was grafted. *B*, Postoperative photograph 1 year later shows some wrinkling of the graft but no recurrence of the keloid. *C*, Extensive keloids of the hand of a 27 year old woman resulting from flaming paraffin-plastic burns 1 year previously. *D*, The entire keloid was excised and skin, 0.015 inch thickness, was grafted from the buttock.

overgrowth is evident from the fact that a keloid extends not only above the surface of the skin but also laterally to involve areas that were not affected by the original injury. This characteristic is the chief finding in the clinical differentiation of keloids from hypertrophic scars. The color of a keloid may vary from red (when it may still be in an active phase) to pink (when its activity is subsiding) to white, when it is mature or quiescent. Telangiectatic vessels usually traverse the surface. Pruritus may be profound and very difficult to control.

**Etiology.** There is a strong individual predisposition and a family tendency in some instances. Black and other dark-skinned persons are particularly vulnerable. Some areas of the body are more susceptible than others: sternum, deltoid region, lateral cheeks, ears, and neck. Thermal burns of the face and neck and grease burns of the hands will frequently result in keloids (Fig. 6).

**Treatment.** Since the lesion may recur following excision, and possibly in greater extent, it must be looked upon as a locally recurrent, yet benign, tumor. If the keloids are young, less than 3 months, and are still in an active phase, benefit may be obtained from radiation.[19] In 3 to 6 months the lesions become organized; the cells mature and are less radiosensitive. Intralesional injection of steroids may reduce itching and result in some softening; however, our results have been far from impressive.

If the keloid is small, as in those which follow piercing of the ear lobe, it may be excised, but should receive two radiation treatments of 200 R, one treatment the day of excision and a similar treatment when the sutures are removed, usually around the sixth day. The results are excellent for small keloids when this regimen is followed.[5]

When the keloids are large and involve important functional areas, such as the face, neck, hands, and forearms, surgical excision and split-thickness grafting then becomes a procedure of necessity (Fig. 6). Wide excision, beyond the keloid into normal skin, and grafting will frequently give a pleasing result. The split-thickness graft should be taken from the thigh or buttock, not the abdomen, and it should be thin, 0.010 to 0.012 (dermatome setting), to lessen the possibility of a keloid developing in the donor area. In a true keloid, former, "prophylactic" irradiation, in small doses, may be given over the donor area in 3 to 4 weeks. The effect of radiation is to produce rapid maturation of the fibroblasts with diminution of the vascularity of the fibrous tissue. It should be reserved only for use as an early postoperative measure. However, a word of caution: in certain persons, despite meticulous attention to lines of elasticity of the skin and to techniques of excision and suture, development of hypertrophied scars or keloids may follow even minimal trauma. Consult Peacock and Van Winkle's excellent volume on *Surgery and Biology of Wound Repair*.[15]

### Fibroma

A pure fibroma is rare. Nearly all tumors known as fibromas are qualified in some way by such terms as dermatofibroma (which is not just a fibroma of the skin), neurofibroma (which is more than a fibroma of nerve), fibroadenoma, and so forth.

Two types are described: The hard fibroma, *fibroma durum*, occurs primarily on the face and extremities as an elevation of the skin. The soft fibroma, *fibroma molle*, is a soft, pedunculated tumor of connective tissue that differs from a papilloma of the skin in that the bulk of the tumor is its subepithelial portion. Neither fibroma molle nor fibroma durum is regarded as a premalignant lesion though the point of origin of

**Figure 7** *A*, Pachydermatocele in a 38 year old man which had grown to its present size in 10 years. He also had many peripheral nodules that had not grown. These tumors are soft but not compressible. They are extremely vascular but no bruit is heard. The tumor was excised in one operation. *B*, Postoperative photograph taken 1 year later.

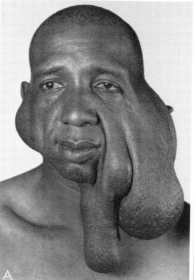
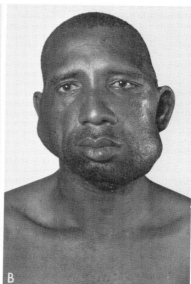

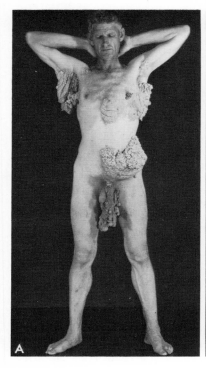
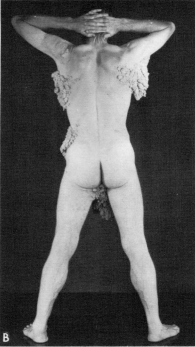

**Figure 8** Diffuse neurofibromatosis of von Recklinghausen's disease. The cutaneous tumors of this 45 year old man ranged from small nodules to large hanging masses which were excised and grafted in stages.

fibrosarcoma of the skin and subcutaneous tissues is a matter of speculation. Either one may occur in conjunction with von Recklinghausen's disease, or neurofibromatosis. The distinction between a soft fibroma and a well differentiated fibrosarcoma may be difficult for the pathologist, unless he knows the clinical history.

*Pachydermatocele* is a type of pendant fibroma of the skin and subcutaneous tissue that occurs in association with von Recklinghausen's disease. The lesions are present from birth but may increase markedly in size. Their tissue weight may cause distortion of regional soft tissues, and underlying bones may be enlarged because of their vascularity. The term "pachydermatocele" comes from the thick, corrugated appearance not unlike that of the skin of an elephant (Figs. 7 and 8). Surgical excision, in stages if the tumor is large, is advised. The tumor may be extremely vascular because of loose areolar tissue and abundant large vascular sinuses. These sinuses have no contractility, as do normal blood vessels, and control of hemorrhage may be difficult.

### Lipoma

Lipomas are among the commonest and the most benign of tumors. They usually occur singly, but may be multiple. The tumor consists of normal fat, arranged in lobules and separated by fibrous septa and enclosed in a very delicate capsule. Although often of small size the tumor may grow tremendously, but still remains benign. It forms a soft, painless mass that moves readily over the fascia. The overlying skin is frequently dimpled owing to fibrous bands passing from it down be-

tween the lobules. The fat of which the tumor is composed is not affected by purposeful reduction or the general wasting of disease. Surgical excision is recommended if the lipoma is large; small ones are only a nuisance. Complete extirpation cannot be guaranteed because of the very thin capsule, since the boundary between the lipoma and the surrounding normal adipose tissue may be indistinct and deceptive.

### Xanthoma

Xanthoma is the name applied to a group of conditions rather than to a single type of tumor. Three types are recognized: *Xanthelasma* is characterized by a small, yellow patch in the medial aspects of both upper and lower eyelids. It usually occurs in persons over middle age and frequently in those with abnormal cholesterol or fat metabolism. Therefore, xanthelasma of the eyelids is not a tumor, but rather a cutaneous manifestation of an abnormal cholesterol-lipid metabolism. The lesions are readily amenable to surgical excision; however, they may recur because of the underlying faulty metabolic process. On pathologic examination, there is a deposit in the tissues of a finely divided lipoid substance, cholesterol ester. *Xanthoma multiplex* is a condition in which groups of yellow nodules are scattered over the trunk and extremities, occurring most often in young people, and usually associated with a disturbance of cholesterol metabolism, hypercholesterolemia or lipemia. It may be associated with diabetes mellitus and biliary obstruction. The nodules are not true tumors. *Heterogeneous xanthomatous masses* are fibromas of the tendon sheaths of the hand and forearm. They may be associated with trauma or infection. All of the lesions have a characteristic bright yellow color which gives the condition its name. Most authorities hold that the color is due to the presence of the cholesterol ester.[2, 10] As stated, xanthomas are probably not true tumors in the strict sense of the term: they may represent more of a granuloma than a neoplasm. Xanthomatous changes, however, may be encountered in giant cell tumors of bone and other connective tissue tumors.

### Gardner's Syndrome

Gardner's syndrome is usually an inherited disorder characterized by fibrous skin tumors, cystic skin lesions, osteomatosis, dental abnormalities, and polyposis of the colon. Fibromas and cystic lesions, usually epidermal inclusion cysts, appear in childhood. They are usually multiple, though variable in number, and most numerous on the face, scalp, and trunk. Benign osteomas tend to develop, especially in the membranous bones of the face and skull. Dental abnormalities consist of supernumerary teeth, missing teeth, odontomas, and dentigerous cysts with abnormalities of the maxilla and mandible. Multiple adenomatous polyps may appear later in the colon and rectum, and may become malignant.

### Rhinophyma

Rhinophyma, from the Greek *rhis* (nose) and *phyma* (growth), is a disease process rather than a neoplasm. The disease is also known as pseudo-elephantiasis nostrum, acne hypertrophica, cystadenofibroma, whiskey-rum nose, and many other names. This slowly growing tumor involves only the lower half of the nose and usually spares the skin of the maxillary regions (Fig. 9). Rhinophyma starts as a hypertrophy of the sebaceous glands and subcutaneous tissue. Large lobulated masses of soft tissue develop in which are located large dilated pores. Telangiectatic vessels may course over the humpy surface, giving the nose a red appearance; hence the name whiskey-rum nose. However, the condition is entirely unrelated to alcohol; in fact, in an analysis of approximately 70 personal patients, there was not a single excessive drinker in the group.[13] Sebum may accumulate between the hypertrophied lobules and produce a foul odor; but the main complaint of the patient is the unsightliness of the nose. The condition itself is benign, but cases of basal and squamous cell epitheliomas developing in the area of involvement have been cited. Rhinophyma occurs primarily in men.

**Treatment.** Some investigators feel that acne rosacea may be a precursor of rhinophyma; if so, early dermatologic treatment may be beneficial. But once the rhinophyma is fully developed, no treatment other than surgery is of value. The simplest technique, which is very effective, is to shave down the hypertrophied tissues to a normal nose level with a No. 10 or 15 scalpel or an ordinary safety razor blade. The precedure may be performed under local infiltration or block anesthesia. Bleeding points are electrocoagulated. Nitrofurazone (Furacin) dressings are changed daily. Re-epithelialization will take place promptly and the transition between the "new nose" and the adjacent skin becomes almost undetectable (Fig. 9).

### Pseudoxanthoma Elasticum

Pseudoxanthoma elasticum is a congenital disorder of the elastic fibers or an "elastotic degeneration of collagen." The skin, eyes, and vascular

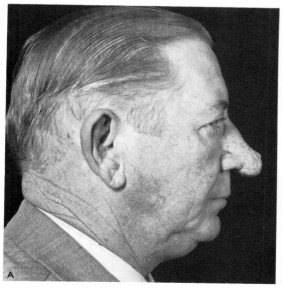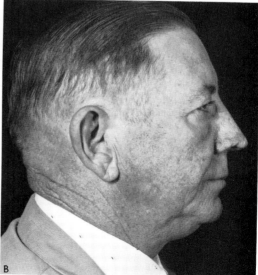

**Figure 9** *A,* A 60 year old engineer whose nose began to enlarge about 10 years prior to admission. The nose was shaved down and sculptured in one operation under local anesthesia. *B,* Postoperative photograph taken 1 year later.

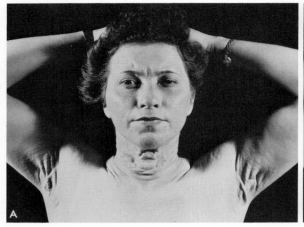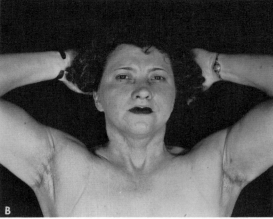

**Figure 10**   *A,* Characteristic appearance of pseudoxanthoma elasticum with pendulous reduplication of the flexural folds of the neck and axilla due to loss of elastic tissue. When the skin was stretched, the exaggerated folds remained unchanged for a considerable time. The color and texture of the skin was similar to a chamois. The deformity was corrected by excision of the redundant tissues after extensive undermining. *B,* Postoperative photograph taken 3 years later.

system are affected. The skin lesions consist of yellow papules and plaques, which are arranged in a crepelike pattern parallel to the folds of skin which may hang in drapelike folds on the neck, axilla, and groin (Fig. 10). In the eyes, angioid streaks of the fundi are found, with progressive impairment of the vision. The cutaneous lesions and the angioid streaks constitute the *Grönblad-Strandberg syndrome.* Cardiovascular manifestations include decrease or absence of peripheral pulse, intermittent claudication, angina, and cardiac decompensation. Rupture of vessels may lead to gastric hemorrhage or bleeding into the subarachnoid space. Pathologic changes in the skin are diagnostic: in the middle and deep dermis there is considerable accumulation of swollen, fragmented, and irregularly clumped fibers staining as do elastic fibers. The collagen fibers are normal. The angioid streaks probably represent degeneration of elastic fibers of Bruch's membrane in the retina.[7] There is no effective therapy. Plastic surgical removal of the excessive folds of skin has been helpful from the psychologic and cosmetic standpoints.

## MALIGNANT TUMORS OF FIBROUS TISSUE

### Fibrosarcoma

Fibrosarcoma may be the prototype of *sarcoma,* which is a malignant tumor of mesenchymal origin. It is the most frequent of the malignant tumors of soft tissues. Fibrosarcomas and sarcomas of the skin and soft tissues are considered as actually one neoplasm, since those arising in the soft tissues below the skin often invade it.[2,21]

The tumor may occur at any age, and may grow in a slow, persistent fashion for some years, without causing the patient concern. The common sites are the trunk and lower extremities. The gross appearance may be dangerously deceptive, for a desmoplastic reaction in the surrounding tissue may cause the formation of a false capsule, from which the tumor may be shelled out. However, this statement should not be interpreted as a degree of benignity of the tumor, for it is highly malignant. *Microscopically* the tumor is composed of spindle-shaped fibroblasts separated by varying amounts of collagen; the cells and fibers tend to run in bundles which either curve gently and interlace or bind almost at right angles.

The tumor spreads principally by invasion; therefore, there is the ever present danger of recurrence due to incomplete removal of the primary lesion. Involvement of the lymph nodes is rare. In the poorly differentiated forms, distant metastasis may occur by hematogenous invasion. Fibrosarcomas of the skin are almost all well differentiated, with superficial rather than deep spread. Nodularity in the operative incision may be the first clue to recurrence, and a more radical extirpation is indicated immediately.

There are many other types of sarcoma which originate in and attack literally every body system and organ: bone, tendon sheaths, nerve, brain, breast, pleura, retroperitoneum, uterus, and so forth.

### Liposarcoma

Liposarcoma is the second most common malignant tumor arising in the subcutaneous tissues. The most common sites are the lower extremity: leg and buttock. Like the benign lipoma, the tumor may reach tremendous size. The lipoma, however, never develops into a liposarcoma. On cut surface, liposarcoma is soft and may be mucoid. Like the fibrosarcoma, it is dangerous because of its tendency to infiltrate and invade locally, rather than to metastasize.

## Myxosarcoma

Myxosarcoma is a cutaneous and subcutaneous malignant disease characterized by multiple semicystic lesions that have a bluish color and occur most frequently on the extremities. The diagnosis presumes the acceptance of primary myxoma as a true tumor, in contrast to the theories that explain myxoma as a development by mucoid change of fibromas and neurofibromas.[2,10] The tumor is characterized as low in degree of malignancy. *Microscopically* it is differentiated from fibrosarcoma by the formation of mucin-containing matrix in which the spindle-shaped cells of sarcoma are found. The lesions are best treated by wide excision; local recurrence may occur; metastases are rare.

## Angiosarcoma

Angiosarcoma (malignant hemangioma, hemangioendothelioma, hemangiopericytoma) is a malignant tumor of angioblastic origin, occurring in any region of the body. The tumors are soft in consistency and blue in color owing to the presence of large vascular sinuses, rupture of which may cause external hemorrhage. Angiosarcomas may grow very rapidly and are highly malignant. Surgical excision may be unsatisfactory because of the large size and mass of vascular tumor. Radiation therapy may be a necessary and valuable adjunctive treatment. If the lesion involves an extremity, amputation may become a procedure of necessity.

## Rhabdomyosarcoma

Since these tumors extend directly to the skin, they are considered here, briefly, with tumors of the skin. They may occur in any body area. They may be confused with liposarcoma and fibrosarcoma. The author has seen two cases in which the tumor involved the lips. The tumor develops within or is attached to striated muscle. Since the tumor is resistant to radiation, wide surgical excision is the treatment of choice. Spread takes place through both the blood and lymph systems.

## Leiomyosarcoma

Leiomyosarcomas occur on any part of the surface by direct extension to the skin from the underlying tissue. Some pathologists feel that these tumors arise in the smooth muscles of blood vessels or from the arrectores pilorum. Occasionally they behave as benign tumors; however, they usually resemble fibrosarcomas in their clinical manifestations and course.

## Kaposi's Sarcoma

Kaposi's sarcoma is a malignant tumor of the skin that usually starts on the hands or feet as multiple nodules that are reddish to purple in the early stages (Fig. 11). There is considerable controversy regarding its pathogenesis: the neurovascular system, the reticuloendothelial system, and the lymphatic system have all been indicated as the primary focus. On microscopic examination, one sees vascularity, pigmentation, elastic fibers, round cell infiltration, and the spindle cells of sarcoma.[7] Kaposi's sarcoma is looked upon as a slowly developing vascular and connective tissue tumor of the skin and subcutaneous tissues which metastasizes via the lymphatics.

## Dermatofibrosarcoma protuberans

Dermatofibrosarcoma protuberans is a fibrous tissue tumor of the skin and subcutaneous tissues which is of low-grade malignancy. The tumor starts as a firm cutaneous or subcutaneous nodule covered with normal epidermis. It may occur on the scalp, torso, and extremities. On microscopic

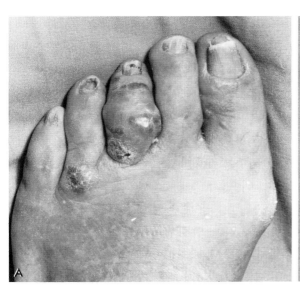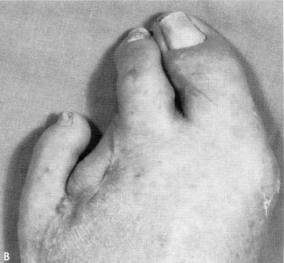

**Figure 11**  *A*, An elderly woman with a 2 year history of expanding mulberry-like lesions of the toes, characteristic of Kaposi's sarcoma. *B*, The third and fourth toes were amputated at the metatarsophalangeal joints to preserve the width of the foot. A plantar flap was used to repair the operative defect.

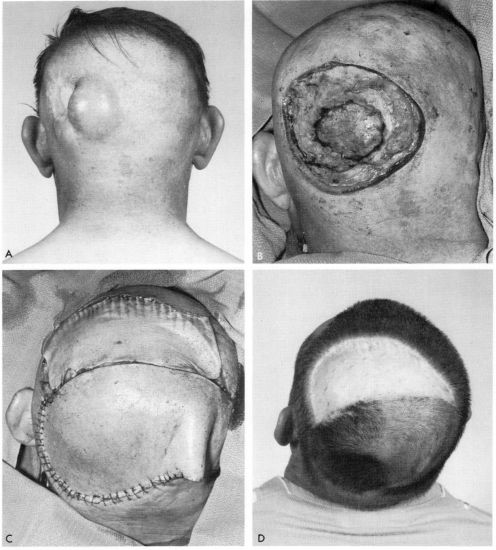

**Figure 12** *A*, A 40 year old man with a recurrent dermatofibrosarcoma protuberans of the occipital area, which had been removed 2 years previously at another hospital. Since the tumor had invaded the skull, a craniectomy was performed. *B*, The large operative defect and dura were covered with a direct transfer scalp flap; a split graft from the buttock was applied to the flap donor area. *C*, Three weeks later the "dog ear" or pedicle was divided and tailored to complete the reconstruction *(D)*.

examination, the picture is that of a fibroma, rich in fibroblasts, which progresses to the characteristic appearance of fibrosarcoma. Wide surgical excision is the treatment of choice; the tumor is radioresistant. Local recurrences may be anticipated unless the primary excision is radical (Fig. 12).

### Lymphangiosarcoma

Lymphangiosarcoma is a rare tumor that may occur in lymphedematous extremities or the scalp. The tumor may develop in the lymphedematous arm after radical mastectomy for cancer. The tumor appears as an ecchymotic area with

induration and overlying vesiculation. Nodularity develops and the local appearance of the tumor is quite similar to that of Kaposi's sarcoma. The tumor is highly malignant; either radical excision of the area or amputation of the extremity is necessary to effect a cure.

### Neurosarcoma

Neurosarcoma (neurofibrosarcoma, neurogenic sarcoma, malignant neurolemmoma) represents malignant degeneration of neurofibroma or of neurolemmoma. The tumor invades the skin from the underlying tissues. The author has recently seen two young patients with large neck masses which were diagnosed as malignant plexiform neurofibromas and it was thought that they represented malignant transformation of von Recklinghausen's disease since there were other stigmata of the disease present. The tumor grows rapidly by local invasion. Radiation therapy may be helpful.

### Von Recklinghausen's Disease

Von Recklinghausen's disease (neurofibromatosis) is characterized by brown macules (café au lait spots) and soft pedunculated and sessile cutaneous neurofibromas (see Figs. 7 and 8). The tumor represents a diffuse proliferation of peripheral nerve elements; according to Anderson, "the tumors of this group may contain nerves with sheaths, nerves without sheaths, sheaths without nerves (containing Schwann cells) and about all this there are masses of fibrous tissue."[2] The lesions may be single and localized (but are not encapsulated), but much more often they are multiple. When numerous, they constitute the classic neurofibromatosis of von Recklinghausen. There may be literally hundreds of neurofibromas growing from cutaneous nerves; there may also be involvement of the spinal and intercostal nerves with dumbbell-like extensions into the chest. The deeper growths are prone to malignant change. In the common cutaneous form, soft nodules in the skin are distributed widely over the body. When proliferation occurs inside the nerve sheaths, rendering the nerve thick, tortuous, and ropelike, the condition is known as *plexiform neuroma*; it occurs frequently in the neck, involving the cervical nodes. Peculiar soft overgrowths of connective tissue may occur, causing the skin to hang in great folds, perhaps with enlargement of an extremity—a condition known as *elephantiasis neuromatosis*.

On microscopic examination, the characteristic tissue has a tangled structure; the tissue does not show palisading or whorls. Superimposed upon this reticular mass is a varying amount of tissue of the Schwann type showing palisades and whorls. With special stains, nerve fibrils can be seen passing through the mass; this never occurs in neurolemmoma.[7]

# CANCER OF THE SKIN

Cancer of the skin occurs primarily on exposed areas; because of its accessibility, especially on the face, it offers an unparalleled opportunity for early diagnosis and treatment. When a lesion attracts attention early and is readily accessible to observation and treatment, its nature and course are more likely to be understood than those of tumors arising in deeply situated organs. From the viewpoint of early recognition, skin cancers are in particularly favorable position. However, in spite of the intensive educational crusade against cancer during the past decade, one is still confronted with a relatively large group of pa-

tients with active lesions who, in many instances, have been "followed and treated" for long periods.

Too much emphasis cannot be placed on the importance of early biopsy and complete eradication of the cancer. Inadequate therapy, whether with surgery or irradiation, only results in residual and recurrent cancer, which may require an extensive or a destruction operation for cure. Furthermore, oft repeated procedures may actually accelerate the growth of the tumor. This has been stressed by cancer surgeons and radiation therapists. I share and repeat the statements of my mentors, principally Dr. Robert Ivy, Dr. Jerome Webster, Dr. Hayes Martin, and the late Drs. John Staige Davis, Ferris Smith, and Vilray Blair: It is not so much the lack of treatment or the selection of the type of treatment that has handicapped the recurrent cancer patient, but the lack of conviction and the use of temporizing methods or puttering treatment that have lowered the quality of our results. Further, every extensive cancer did not become so overnight, but it began as a small, seemingly insignificant lesion, which continued to increase progressively in size. Cutaneous cancer accounts for 50 to 60 per cent of all types of malignant lesions seen by the family physician. This section is presented for the student and young physician and not the specialist. It is hoped some of the following guides will be of help.

**Predisposing Factors.** Skin cancers tend to develop more frequently in blond persons, and those with thin, dry skin. They occur rarely in the yellow races of the Orient and the olive-skinned Italians, Spanish, and South Americans, and almost never in the black race. However, those persons (predominantly men) with "Scotch-type" skin (blond hair and beard, blue eyes, thin skin) who, because of their outdoor occupations or habits (farmers, ranchers, commercial fishermen, sailors, and "sun worshipers"), are exposed for long periods to intense sun and wind frequently do incur skin cancers; however, the precursor is usually an area of hyperkeratosis (see Fig. 7).

**General Statements about Skin Cancer.** Squamous cell cancer may develop in areas of postradiation dermatitis. Ulcerations occurring in old burn scars are favorite sites for the development of squamous cell cancer. While skin cancers may occur at any age, there is a definite predilection for men over 50 years of age. Basal cell cancers of the face are much more common than squamous cell cancers, accounting for more than three-fourths of all cases in some reports.[15]

All cancers arising on the mucous membrane surface of the lip are squamous cell (see Fig. 13). Numerically, most epitheliomas of the skin of the face are basal cell, at least in their beginning, but some of these may change later to squamous cell. However, there is an exception—those lesions which develop in hyperkeratoses on the skin of men who have had a lifetime exposure to sun and wind are squamous cell from the beginning. On the face of an individual, one lesion may develop into a basal cell cancer, while a neighboring lesion may be a squamous cell cancer. Squamous cell cancers metastasize. Basal cell cancers do not metastasize, but they should be regarded as elusive and invasive and are highly malignant locally (see Fig. 14).

**Pathologic Considerations.** The characteristic histologic feature of the malignant cell is its power of unlimited multiplication, in contrast to the orderly migration and maturation of epithelial cells as outlined previously. Structurally, these cells are anaplastic and may tend to revert to embryonal form (undifferentiated). Generally speaking, the more they differ from the normal cell and structure, the nearer they approach the embryonal type, the more malignant is the lesion. When the variation is slight, the degree of malignancy may be low; when the variation is marked, the degree of malignancy may be high. On this basis of differentiation of cells, that is, their ability to resemble and mimic the cells from which they originated, Broder grouped cancers into four grades:[2,6,16] Grade I is least malignant since less than 25 per cent of the cells are undifferentiated (75 per cent or more are normal). Grade IV cancers are the most malignant, because most of the cells are undifferentiated and only 25 per cent or less resemble the parent cell. In between are Grades II and III, Grade II being less malignant and Grade III more malignant. It should be emphasized, however, that this is a microscopic-pathologic classification of cell differentiation and that virulence and evident activity of growth are by no means synonymous, either clinically or by Broder's grading system.

### Squamous Cell Cancer

This tumor, commonly known as epidermoid carcinoma, occurs wherever squamous or transitional epithelium is found. In this chapter we are concerned with squamous cell cancer of the skin, but it may develop in mucous membranes lined by stratified squamous epithelium, such as the tongue, mouth, and esophagus. A favorite site is the junction of skin and mucous membrane, such as on the lip, nostrils, eyelid, penis, and vulva.

Squamous cell cancer develops frequently in areas of previous skin change: from solar keratoses or hyperkeratoses, old burn scars (*Marjolin's ulcer*), an ulcer of long standing, or radiation dermatitis. The difference between an early squamous cell cancer and a keratosis may not be apparent clinically and therefore the lesion should be biopsied or excised or both.

Typical squamous cell cancers, such as occur on the lower lip, may be preceded by an area of leukoplakia or what was thought to be a "fever blister." The transformation from a benign lesion to a squamous cancer may be detected as a slight thickening or a small nodule. Ulceration occurs and is frequently followed by the development of a crusty overgrowth (Fig. 13) in a bulky or papillomatous, cauliflower-like growth which, at the same time, may burrow into the deeper tissues. Pain is not prominent until late in the disease. Squamous cancers are quite malignant from the beginning and may metastasize quite early to the regional lymph nodes. This is particularly true of squamous cancers arising in the mucous membranes of the mouth, tongue, parotid, and pharynx; in fact, a metastatic mass in the neck may be the "prime mover" to get the patient to his physician. If the lesion in question is large and the clinical diagnosis is in doubt, a small portion may be removed, usually without local anesthesia, for histologic study. If it is small, the entire lesion may be removed by excisional biopsy under local anesthesia.

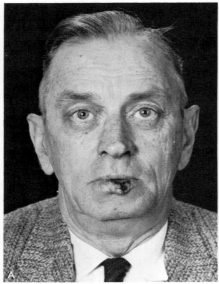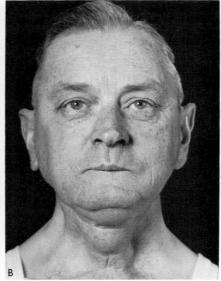

**Figure 13**  *A*, A 55 year old man with a squamous cell cancer of the lip of 1 year's duration. The greater part of the lower lip was removed and reconstructed with cheek advancement flaps. A two-stage bilateral neck dissection was performed to remove metastatic nodes. *B*, Postoperative photograph taken 10 years later.

**Pathology.** Squamous cell cancers invade the dermis early as solid columns of epithelial cells. The cells show varying degrees of atypia including variation in size, shape, and depth of staining, numerous mitoses, and so forth. Abnormal keratinization is manifested by whorls of keratin or horny pearls near the surface. As the cancer invades the dermis, the squamous cells may be arranged in a concentric manner, as "cell nests" or "epithelial pearls," which, although highly characteristic of squamous cell cancer, may be absent in rapidly growing tumors and in the esophagus, where cornification does not normally occur. A well known feature to pathologists is an infiltration of the dermis by chronic inflammatory cells, particularly plasma cells, just deep to the neoplastic epithelium.[7]

**Treatment.** All lesions should be biopsied. It is essential that an accurate pathologic diagnosis be established. It is imperative that the tumor be removed or destroyed completely. Many dermatologists treat small lesions by electrodesiccation. I personally feel that squamous cell cancers are best treated by wide excision. Even rather extensive lesions may be removed with local or block anesthesia supplemented by intravenous diazepam (Valium). Before any treatment is undertaken, an x-ray of the chest and a careful examination of the regional lymph nodes of the neck should be made.

### Basal Cell Cancers

Basal cell cancers should be regarded as elusive, treacherous, and highly, locally malignant, even though they do not metastasize to distant parts (Fig. 14). These lesions are deceptive: they appear and behave like benign lesions in their early stages, but unless removed widely, they will recur and destroy everything in their path of invasion.

Basal cell cancers arise most frequently in the midportion of the face, the so-called seborrheic areas. They develop at an earlier age than squamous cell cancers. The lesions may arise in otherwise normal skin, de novo, and without a prodromal keratosis as frequently occurs in squamous cell cancer. Early lesions rarely show rapid growth; in fact they appear to be quite indolent. There is no pain or discomfort and hence it not infrequently happens that patients defer seeking advice until the disease is well advanced.

The appearance of an early lesion is quite characteristic (Fig. 14): it may resemble an intracutaneous button, in that there is a firm, slightly elevated edge which may surround the lesion partially or completely. The edge may be pearly or gray-blue in color and may have a scalloped appearance. In early lesions, the ulceration in the center is shallow. The lesion is somewhat indurated, and so it looks and feels like a button. However, striking variations in the clinical picture may be encountered. While slow growth and progression is the general rule, any rapid change should be acted upon promptly, for it may be in-

dicative of change from a basal cell lesion to a basosquamous or a pure squamous cell cancer.

I refer to the primary lesion, described in the previous paragraph, as a *button-type basal cell cancer*. However, there are two other types which should be borne in mind. The *field-fire basal cell cancer* is usually a large, flat lesion with an active edge surrounding a central scarred area. It may be serpiginous and the peripheral manner of spread has been compared to that of a fire in a field. The edges are active and spreading, whereas the central area may seem, often falsely, to have burned itself out. This field-fire type of cancer may actually be due to the coalescence and spread of several multicentric lesions.

The third type of basal cell cancer is the highly invasive *rodent ulcer*. This is the most difficult lesion to eradicate and, therefore, one of the most dangerous. The surface lesion may appear quite innocuous; however, there is usually extensive invasion in and beneath the skin—hence the designation *submarine or iceberg type of progression and spread*. What is actually seen on the surface may bear little resemblance to what is found beneath it. Favorite and dangerous sites for the development of basal cell cancers are the nose and along the lower eyelid and inner canthus (Fig. 14). In these special locations basal cell cancers seem to have a definite predilection for burrowing deeply, and unless they are removed early and completely, they may cause widespread destruction or even death.

**Pathology.** The microscopic appearance consists of solid masses of darkly stained cells that extend downward from the basal layer into the dermis and subcutaneous tissues. The columns extend down to a uniform level; their ends have an expanded club-shaped appearance—a geographic arrangement of bays, capes, and promontories. The peripheral nuclei maintain a palisade arrangement.[7]

**Treatment.** It is advisable to perform a biopsy to verify the clinical impression. Small lesions may be treated by excisional biopsy. Irradiation is quite effective in the treatment of early lesions, but much less effective when the lesions are advanced. We believe that wide surgical excision is the treatment of choice. If the surgeon receives pathologic clearance that all margins are free of tumor, on the basis of frozen section studies, primary repair may be undertaken immediately. When in doubt, one should wait for final pathologic clearance before reconstructing the defect. This is doubly important if a free graft or a flap is to be used, and is especially true with basal cell cancers around the orbit.

The physician who treats cancer is, in reality, treating a patient with cancer. Cancers are malignant and a life is at stake. Each far advanced cancer was at one time a small, perhaps seemingly insignificant lesion. Our aim should be to educate the public so that they will seek advice early. Then the remainder is up to us and is our responsibility. The final result depends on how early the patient seeks advice and the adequacy of the treatment administered. Our aim should be to

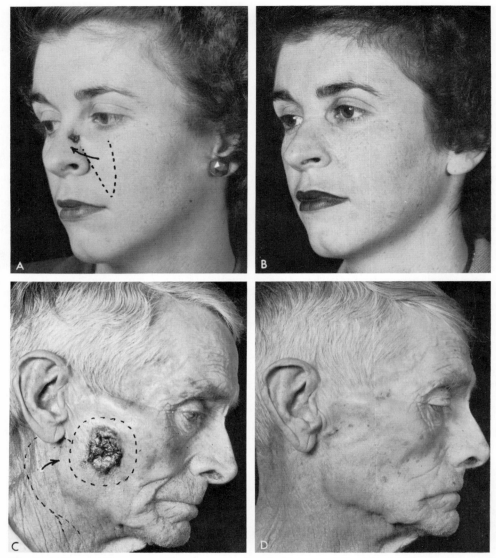

**Figure 14**   *A,* A 25 year old woman with a burrowing basal cell cancer of the side of the nose of 1 year's duration. At operation, the cancer was found to extend into the interior of the nose and to involve the maxillary process. The operative defect was reconstructed with an interpolated flap from the nasolabial crease, as shown. The flap was subsequently trimmed and tailored. *B,* Postoperative photograph taken 5 years later. *C,* An elderly man with a large epithelioma of the cheek. The lesion was excised widely, as indicated, and the operative defect was repaired with a direct transfer flap from the neck. *D,* Postoperative photograph taken 1 year later.

eradicate the lesion completely and, at the same time, to leave a minimum of disturbance of function and disfigurement.

## MISCELLANEOUS SKIN LESIONS

*Intraepithelial cancer or carcinoma-in-situ* is seen frequently on the skin. The layers of the epidermis show evidence of dyskeratosis—cellular "unrest" and malignant transformation, with acanthosis, loss of polarity, and increased mitosis. There is no invasion of the dermis and the neoplastic change is confined to the epidermis.

*Pseudoepitheliomatous hyperplasia* is, in essence, the reverse of carcinoma-in-situ. It is a benign proliferation of the epidermis, the result of chronic irritation. Elongated pegs of epithelium, seemingly frustrated in its attempt to cover the surface, grow downward.

In *Bowen's disease* the picture is one of modified carcinoma-in-situ, the anaplasia being less marked. It is a relatively inactive form of cutaneous malignant disease. The lesion is usually solitary and may be mistaken for a solar keratosis or an early basal cell epithelioma. Excisional biopsy is recommended.

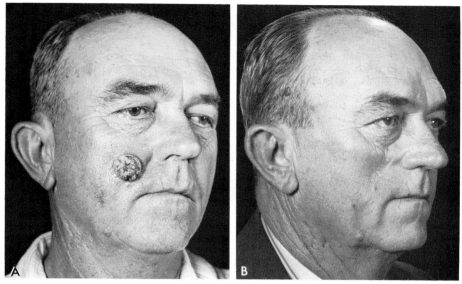

**Figure 15**  *A,* A 52 year old man with a characteristic keratoacanthoma: the lesion grew to its present size in 2 months; it was round, elevated, dome-shaped, cherry red, and friable. Since the lesion is benign, radical excision is not necessary. *B,* Postoperative photograph taken 1 year later.

*Keratoacanthoma* resembles squamous cell cancer both clinically and histologically, although it is a benign lesion (Fig. 15). An important characteristic is the fact that the tumor, which is usually single, may grow with extreme rapidity, to 2 cm. or more in a month. It is a round, elevated, dome-shaped lesion that is cherry red and friable. There is no discomfort. Some investigators feel that the causative agent may be a virus. The major differentiation is between it and squamous cell cancer. Its rapid growth and its mushroom-like appearance should not be relied upon implicitly; therefore, biopsy is necessary. Surgical removal is recommended, although radical excision is not necessary.

*Adenoacanthoma* or *pseudoglandular squamous cell carcinoma* has a predilection for the skin of the face and ears. The surface has a verrucous appearance; the lumina are filled with desquamated cells—this may be seen both clinically and on histologic study. The lesions are confined to the surface and have little tendency to metastasize. Surgical excision is recommended.

*Cylindroma* or *adenoid cystic carcinoma* is a circumscribed but poorly encapsulated infiltrating tumor, taking origin in the subcutaneous tissues, most commonly from the ducts of the parotid (Stenson's) and submaxillary (Wharton's) glands. The growth is slow but relentless and invasion and metastasis may occur. Histologic examination is characteristic: there are anastomosing cords of small dark cells which are arranged around tubules in a "Swiss cheese" pattern.

*Xeroderma pigmentosum* is a rare disease of children who show extremely abnormal sensitivity to sunlight. The condition begins in early life with hyperpigmentation of the exposed parts which then deepens; atrophy and tightening of the skin is followed by ectropion of the eyelids and lips. Both squamous and basal cell cancers develop and metastasis may occur. We have resurfaced the entire face of a boy, shown in Figure 16, with split- and full-thickness grafts.[22] However, the condition recurred in the grafted areas within 5 years, even though protective measures were taken: sun screen ointments, wide-brim hats, long sleeves, gloves, and so forth. The prognosis is poor; few patients survive their adolescence. Radiation therapy is contraindicated since the skin is already damaged severely. The basic vulnerability is inherited in a recessive pattern. The two sexes are equally susceptible. Clinically this condition in childhood resembles severe radiodermatitis in the adult.

*Calcifying epithelioma of Malherbe* is usually a solitary, well circumscribed, indurated tumor firmly attached to the skin but freely movable over the deep tissues. It occurs most frequently on the face and upper extremities, and in the author's experience, children show a definite predilection. Microscopically the lesion consists of fragments of what have been termed "mummified basal epithelium" with varying amounts of calcium. Anderson[3] feels that it is probably not a true neoplasm, but a mummified epidermal cyst.

### Hemangiomas (Vascular Nevi)

*Nevus* is a general term to designate pigmented neoplasm of vascular and epidermal origin. In infants and children, nevi make up the largest group of benign tumors.

The *hemangioma* or *vascular nevus* has its origin in the angioblastic layer of embryonic mesoderm. It is a tumor of independently growing vascular channels. Small hemangiomas have little connection with the surrounding vascular

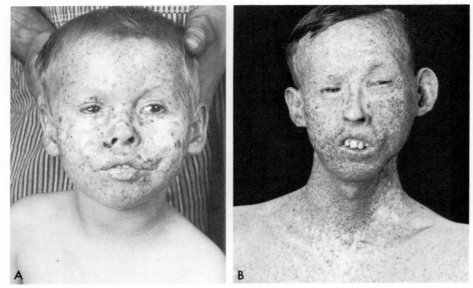

**Figure 16** *A*, A 4 year old boy with advanced changes in the skin of the face and neck characteristic of xeroderma pigmentosa. Many cancers, both basal and squamous cell, were present. In stages, the entire skin of the face—forehead, eyelids, nose, lips, and cheeks—was removed and resurfaced with split- and full-thickness grafts; however, the same condition recurred in the grafts in spite of protective measures: limited exposure, wide-brim hat, sun screen lotions, and so forth. *B*, Postoperative photograph taken 10 years later, patient 17 years of age. (From Woolf, R., et al.: Plast. Reconstr. Surg., *24*:214, 1959.)

tree; large and extensive tumors have "feeder" vessels which may be tremendous. Hemangiomas are classified pathologically into two groups: capillary and cavernous (Fig. 17).

*Capillary hemangiomas* are very common in infancy and childhood and are of two varieties. The *strawberry hemangioma* (hemangioma simplex) is composed of masses of capillaries lined with embryonic endothelium. The *congenital port-wine stain* is lined with adult-type endothelium. The strawberry hemangioma looks somewhat like a strawberry that has been cut in half and placed on the skin, cut side down. They are usually bright red, raised above the surface, and quite circum-

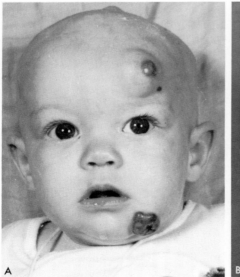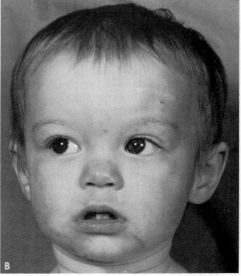

**Figure 17** *A*, A 4 month old child with rapidly growing hemangiomas of the chin and forehead. She also had large vascular nevi on the elbow and back. All were excised. The hemangioma on the chin was of the capillary variety; that on the forehead was of cavernous origin; those on the elbow and back were juvenile hemangioendotheliomas. While the classification of hemangiomas is a pathologic one, it may be difficult to ascribe an exact diagnosis from the clinical appearance. *B*, Postoperative photograph taken 6 months later.

scribed. Their growth may be very rapid—from the size of a pea to several centimeters in 4 to 6 weeks. Port-wine stains are present at birth, may vary in coloration from pink to purple, and are usually flat and not raised, except slightly, above the surrounding skin surface. Pressure will cause blanching; however, the color will return immediately when the pressure is released. They do not grow or increase in size in themselves, although their dimension increases with the normal growth and development of the part. They frequently follow roughly the distribution of the trigeminal nerve of the face, along the frontal, maxillary, and mandibular branches; however, they have nothing to do with the nerve. Generally port-wine stains do not cross the midline of the face. Hemangiomas are not painful until ulceration occurs.

*Cavernous hemangiomas* are soft, bluish, compressible tumor masses which on pathologic examination are composed of large, thin-walled venous sinuses. They may reach tremendous size gradually over a period of months. Because of their thin epithelial covering, ulceration or bleeding may occur. Frank hemorrhage may be difficult to control because of the lack of supporting stroma to permit the normal vascular retraction and clotting mechanism to work effectively. Cavernous hemangiomas rarely undergo complete regression.

**Treatment.** Many small hemangiomas in infants will regress and disappear; pediatricians will verify and confirm this statement. The regression is due to fibrosis, possibly initiated by trauma. These are frequently referred to as sclerosing hemangiomas. In them, the capillaries become partially or completely obliterated. The surgeon usually does not see these. However, a large number of hemangiomas will grow with extreme rapidity and can be quite alarming because of their location in rather critical areas: eyelids, nose, lips, cheeks, neck, hands, and vulva. For a physician to give assurance to already anxious parents that the hemangioma will regress or disappear may invite medicolegal trouble, for their course is extremely variable. We believe that early excision is the treatment of choice. This avoids the possibility of uncontrollable growth and the resulting deformity, and also the fear and apprehension of the parents. A fine surgical scar is far to be preferred to a rapidly growing, ulcerated hemangioma whose future course remains in doubt (Fig. 17).

Although radiation has been used in the treatment of hemangiomas, there are distinct disadvantages and contraindications which must be kept in mind. Radiation should not be given over the penis, testicles, vulva, or ovaries, or over epiphyseal growth centers, especially of the fingers, toes, jaws, and tooth buds because of the danger of interference with these growth centers. The ocular lens is very susceptible to radiation; therapy over hair-bearing areas will produce permanent alopecia, and unless the normal skin is shielded and protected, radiation dermatitis may result as a late complication.

The port-wine stain may be cosmetically one of the most deforming of all vascular nevi when it involves the face. There is no uniformly successful method of treatment. Excision and resurfacing with skin grafts may be desirable when the stain is deep red or purple; however, grafts from another part of the body to the face will not have the same color and texture and the seam or edge, where the grafts join the normal skin, may be quite visible even when cosmetics are used. Tattooing with insoluble dyes has been quite successful in some instances when the discoloration is not marked. The recent improvements and better methods have been reported by Thompson.[22] Dermabrasion and electrodesiccation has been disappointing in our experience. Port-wine stains are totally radioresistant since the endothelial lining is of adult variety. The use of Cover-Mark is recommended in women; men do not like to use cosmetic agents.

While hemangiomas are considered benign lesions, on rare occasions malignant change may occur. *Three malignant entities have been described:* metastasizing hemangioma, hemangiopericytoma, and hemangioendothelioma. *Hemangioendotheliomas* in children increase in size with great rapidity, and because of this fulminating rate of growth, closely resemble a true malignant tumor. *Hemangiopericytomas and metastasizing hemangiomas* are uncommon in children, and when they do occur, the tumor is more orderly in arrangement and metastasizes later than its adult counterpart.

### Pigmented Nevi (Moles)

The common mole and its variants constitute the second broad category of cutaneous tumors of congenital origin. They are among the most common tumors of childhood and adult life. The exact origin of the pigmented nevus is still argued: Masson's neurogenic theory and Allen's epidermal theory are the two most widely accepted concepts. Masson feels that the nevus cell is derived basically from the tactile end organs of nervous tissue within the dermal and basal layers of the epidermis. Allen's epidermal theory suggests that the nevus arises from the basal layers of the skin by a process of "abtrophung" or dropping off of cells containing the enzyme melanogenase from the basal layer. The argument is of academic-pathologic interest only and it does not influence the treatment.[2,17,18]

*The classification of pigmented nevi is a pathologic one;* it should be emphasized that the clinical appearance of nevi is deceiving and unreliable. In general, they fall into five major groups: (1) intradermal nevus, (2) junctional nevus, (3) compound nevus, (4) blue nevus, and (5) juvenile melanoma. All are present during childhood, but many, particularly the junctional nevi, do not become apparent until puberty.

*Intradermal nevus*, the common mole, may assume a wide variety of sizes, shapes, and colors. It occurs anywhere except on the palms, soles, and genitalia. On histologic section it is composed of masses or cords of nevus cells which contain varying amounts of pigment. As the term implies, the intradermal nevus is located beneath the basal cell layer in the dermis. It does not possess malignant potential.

The *junctional nevus* may occur anywhere, particularly on the hands, feet, and genitalia. They may not become apparent until puberty, when they may appear quite suddenly and in multiples. The junctional nevus varies in size, shape, and degree of pigmentation. Clinically it is not always possible to distinguish a junctional nevus from an intradermal nevus or common mole, except by its location. Histologically, it is composed of irregular masses of cells within the epidermis, in or above the basal cell layer, which have lost some degree of cohesion. This loss of cohesion is manifest by the formation of "clear cells" either within the epidermis or in the prolongations of the epidermis.[7] Although the lesion is benign, the presence of junctional activity may be the forerunner of malignant change. Some girls and women regard a mole of the face as a beauty spot. Any change in size or coloration demands immediate removal.

The *compound nevus* is generally manifest in infancy as a large pigmented lesion which may occupy the face (Fig. 18), extremity, or trunk. In the latter location, it is frequently referred to as a bathing trunk nevus, for the greater part of the trunk may be involved. Microscopically, it is an intradermal lesion with superimposed areas of junctional change. While it is considered a benign lesion, the author has had two children as patients in whom there was rapid and devastating malignant change resulting in death.

The *blue nevus* is an uncommon tumor similar to the mongolian spot of childhood. It occurs about the face, the dorsum of the hands, the feet, and the buttocks. Pathologically, the cells are spindle-shaped. Unlike the mongolian spot, the blue nevus does not fade or disappear. While the blue nevus is a benign lesion, malignant change may occur.

*Juvenile melanoma* occurs only in the prepubertal child; it varies markedly in size, shape, and color. On microscopic examination it is identical with malignant malanoma; however, the clinical course does not correspond with the histologic picture, for it is considered by Pack[14] and other authorities to be a benign lesion.

**Treatment.** Surgical excision is the treatment of choice of pigmented nevi. Pathologic evidence of the benign nature of the lesion and the adequacy of removal is proof positive of clinical safety. Malignancy cannot occur in a mole that has been completely excised. The crux of the problem, however, lies in the decision as to which nevi should be removed. The author feels that any pigmented lesion occurring in an area of chronic stress and irritation such as the shave area of the face and neck and the belt or bra line and those occurring on the palms, soles, and genitalia all should be removed, for the best treatment of melanoma is the prophylactic removal of its precursor. In addition, any pigmented lesion that has changed in size or character, with increased pigmentation, satellite lesions, or other changes, should be removed immediately under block or local anesthesia, with the anesthetic injected at some distance from the lesion. Procrastination may be fatal.

### Lymphangioma

Lymphangiomas are true tumors of lymph vessels, analogous in some ways to hemangiomas, which are tumors of blood vessels. They are much less common than hemangiomas. They are usually

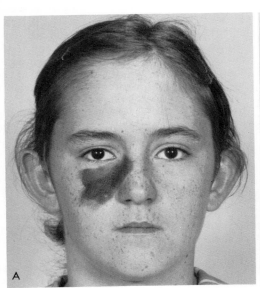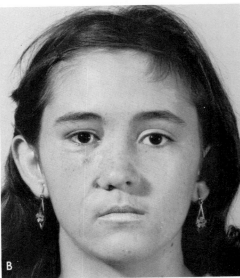

**Figure 18** *A*, A 13 year old girl with a benign compound nevus of the right side of the nose and maxillary region. In three stages, the nevus was excised and the cheek was advanced superiorly. *B*, Postoperative photograph taken 3 years later.

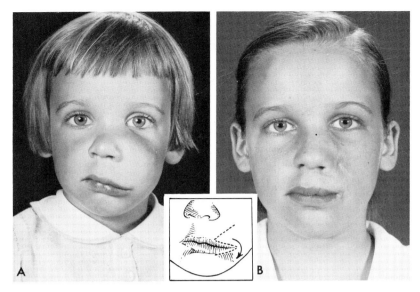

**Figure 19** A, A 4 year old girl with a diffuse, noncystic lymphangioma of the maxillary region, cheeks, and lips, producing severe asymmetry and macrostomia. The tumor was first removed through incisions in the nasofacial and nasolabial creases. The lips were then repositioned with interpolated flaps, using the Z-plasty principle, as shown in the inset. B, Postoperative photograph taken at 10 years.

present at birth and constitute a proliferation of lymph vessels to form a wormlike mass. Lymphangiomas are common on the face and neck (Figs. 19 and 20) and also in the tongue where they are the cause of macroglossia.

Lymphangiomas are of three clinical types: simple or capillary, cavernous, and cystic. Capillary lymphangiomas occur superficially and present a shiny, wartlike surface which may be reddish purple in color. Pressure on the excrescences may yield a serous fluid. The skin of the face and mucous membranes of the lip and tongue are favorite sites.

Cavernous lymphangiomas, like cavernous hemangiomas, are more deeply situated and consist of a loose framework of connective tissue in which are numerous single or multiple communicating lymphatic cysts. These tumors are found most frequently in the neck and axilla.

Cystic hygromas may represent a late stage of the cavernous type. Some authorities feel that cystic hygromas are at the outset cavernous lymphangiomas that have become dilated with lymph because of either a change in drainage or an alteration in the function of their endothelial lining. These are cystic tumors which may reach tremendous size, involving the lower face, with extension into the neck on one or both sides, and downward beneath the clavicle into the pectoral region and axilla. Since they occur frequently in the newborn in the face and neck (Fig. 20) an immediate tracheostomy may be necessary to prevent suffocation.

**Etiology.** It is generally agreed that lymphangiomas develop from embryonic sequestrations of lymph buds which continue to grow and increase progressively in size and, as shown, may reach tremendous proportions.

**Treatment.** If the lymphangioma involves the face and neck, a tracheostomy may be a life-saving procedure. Since cystic hygromas are fre-

quently multiloculated with cysts which may vary tremendously in size, aspiration with a Luer syringe and a lumbar puncture needle of large bore may result in "tapping" or decompressing some of the larger cysts, as a temporary measure. Surgical excision is recommended. When the tumor mass is well localized, operation is a procedure of choice, as to time. When the mass is large, diffuse, and infiltrating, operation becomes a procedure of necessity. If remnants are left behind, the condition will recur. Cystic hygromas are not radiosensitive.

### Cysts

*Sebaceous cysts* (epidermal inclusion cyst, wen) are cutaneous swellings that develop as the result of blocking of the anatomically constricted necks of the sebaceous glands by sebum. They are lined by flattened epidermal cells. The scalp, face, neck, and retroauricular areas are favorite locations. Surgical excision is the treatment of choice (see Fig. 3). To prevent recurrence, the entire cyst must be removed without rupture. Redness over the cyst area is evidence of infection and is a contraindication to excision. Infected areas should be treated by incision and drainage, with definitive excision at a later time. Multiple cysts in the retroauricular area require the removal of a large ellipse of cyst-bearing skin.

Milia (whiteheads) are minute, multiple, white cutaneous cysts that occur commonly on the forehead, nose, and cheeks. They develop from mechanical blocking of the outlet of sebaceous glands. They may occur in skin grafts, especially if the remnants of the original skin are present, and also after dermabrasion procedures for acne and post-acne scarring. They respond nicely to incision with a No. 11 scalpel or needle.

*Dermoid cysts* are congenital lesions located near embryonic lines of fusion. Those of the face are

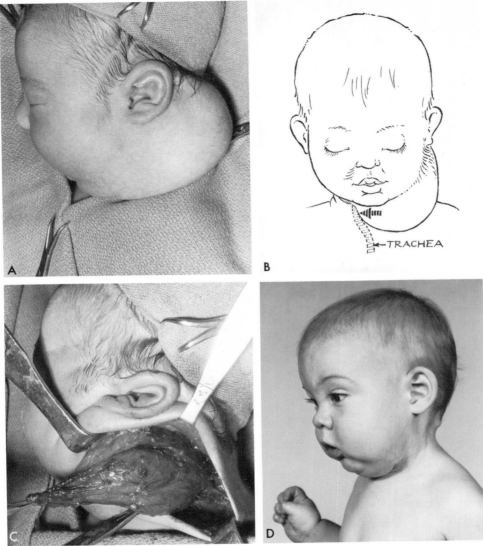

**Figure 20** *A*, A 3 day old infant with a large cystic lymphangioma (hygroma) of the neck producing tracheal deviation, compression, and obstruction, as shown in *B*. *C*, The tremendous lymphangiomatous mass extended beneath the sternum and to the right side of the neck. *D*, Postoperative photograph taken at 9 months shows no residual tumor.

regarded as cysts originating from faulty fusion of the embryonic facial processes. They occur commonly on the forehead, base of the nose, and brow areas (Fig. 21) on the scalp, especially the occiput, over the abdomen and back, in the median raphe of the scrotum and perineum, and in the ovaries. The cysts are usually soft and elastic; they do not exhibit adherence to the skin as sebaceous cysts do. The tumors contain various epidermal structures including hair and sebaceous material. They are lined by stratified squamous epithelium and are benign. Surgical excision is recommended on an inpatient basis under general anesthesia, even for the small cysts of the brow area. On occasions, the presenting cutaneous cyst is but the outer manifestation of an hourglass dermoid cyst with intracranial extension.

*Mucous retention cysts* occur primarily on the buccal surface of the lower lip as a soft, fluctuant mass. The overlying mucous membrane is normal unless the cyst has been bitten or traumatized. Surgical excision under local or block anesthesia is recommended. A sticky mucoid fluid occupies the cyst.

*Synovial cyst* is a degenerative cyst of the finger occurring most frequently over the distal interphalangeal joint and adjacent nail bed. The cysts appear suddenly as dome-shaped painless swellings and contain a clear to yellow viscid fluid. They arise from the joint capsule or tendon sheath. Fluid re-collects after drainage; therefore, excision under block anesthesia is recommended. A small skin graft is usually necessary since the tissues cannot be reapproximated.

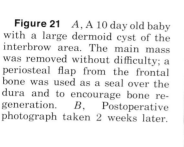
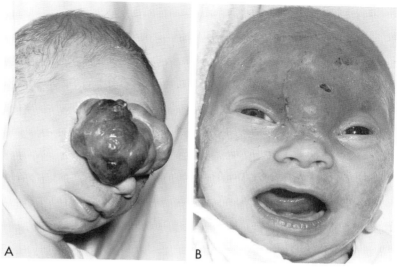

**Figure 21**  *A*, A 10 day old baby with a large dermoid cyst of the interbrow area. The main mass was removed without difficulty; a periosteal flap from the frontal bone was used as a seal over the dura and to encourage bone regeneration.  *B*, Postoperative photograph taken 2 weeks later.

*Ganglia* are small, round, tense, subcutaneous swellings occurring most commonly over the wrist but also over the tendon sheaths of the hands and feet. They progress slowly and are mildly painful. They may result from trauma, either accidental or occupational. They contain a glycerin-jelly-like fluid. Microscopically the wall of the ganglion is composed of collagenous tissue and may or may not be lined with synovial cells. Surgical excision with block anesthesia and tourniquet, using a transverse incision, is recommended. At operation ganglia are found to be adherent to the synovium or to a tendon sheath and frequently extend down in between the wrist bones. The complete excision of a ganglion requires an operative assistant to retract the margins of the wound, tendons, and deep structures; the dissection can be a difficult one. The entire cyst must be removed as protection against recurrence.

*Hidradenitis* (apocrinitis) is a chronic, cicatrizing, suppurative process involving the apocrine (scent) glands. A better term is apocrinitis, since hidradenitis refers more generally to an inflammation of the sweat glands. The disease is most common in the second and third decades and is three times more common in women than in men. The axilla (Fig. 22) is affected much more frequently than the groin and perineum. Many conditions have been incriminated as contributing to the development of the disease: hyperhydrosis

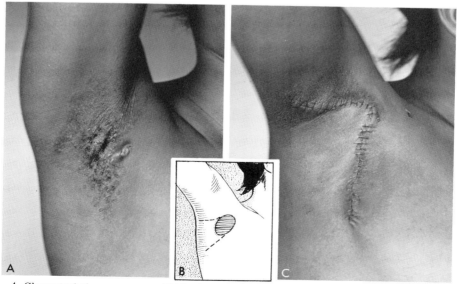

**Figure 22**  *A*, Characteristic appearance of hidradenitis suppurativa of the axilla with multiple draining sinuses. The use of local antibiotics and emollients is of limited value because of the deep-seated infection. *B*, Operative defect following excision of all of the axillary sweat glands and outline of posterolaterally based advancement flap. *C*, Result 7 days after primary closure.

(excessive sweating), poor hygiene, the use of chemical depilatories and deodorants, trauma from shaving, and so forth. Locally, duct obstruction by keratin plugging, followed by rupture of the apocrine glands into the dermis and subcutaneous tissue, coupled with superimposed infection, is the mechanism of development of this progressive, chronic process. Because of the anatomic arrangement of the duct orifice, which opens into a hair follicle above the sebaceous gland, infections are extremely resistant to emollients and local antibiotics. Pain is severe; disability in bilateral cases may be marked.[3]

In cases that are refractive to medical management, wide excision becomes a procedure of necessity. If the operative defect cannot be closed primarily (use catgut subcutaneously because of infection), one may use an advancement flap or free graft. The axilla thereafter will be dry since the eccrine (sweat) glands have been removed also (Fig. 22).

## SELECTED REFERENCES

Burian, F.: Plastic Surgery Atlas. New York, Macmillan Company, 1968.
*A splendid three-volume atlas written by the late Professor Burian, Chairman of the Institute of Plastic Surgery, Prague.*

Conley, F.: Cancer of the Head and Neck. Washington, D.C., Butterworth, 1967.
*A collection of papers presented at the International Workshop on Cancer, New York City, May 10–14, 1965.*

Converse, J. M., ed.: Reconstructive Plastic Surgery. Philadelphia, W. B. Saunders Company, 1964.
*An exhaustive five-volume work covering the entire field of reconstructive plastic surgery.*

Gaisford, J. C.: Symposium on Cancer of the Head and Neck. St. Louis, C. V. Mosby Company, 1969.
*A splendid collection of papers on head and neck cancer by more than 50 authors.*

Grabb, W. C., and Smith, J. W.: Plastic Surgery, A Concise Guide to Clinical Practice. Boston, Little, Brown and Co., 1968.
*A concise but exhaustive guide for both the student and surgeon in practice.*

MacComb, W. S., and Fletcher, G. H.: Cancer of the Head and Neck. Baltimore, Williams & Wilkins Company, 1967.
*An excellent volume written by an outstanding head and neck cancer surgeon and an outstanding radiologist.*

Martin, H.: Surgery of Head and Neck Tumors. New York, Paul B. Hoeber, Inc., 1957.
*A profusely illustrated atlas on head and neck cancer by a world authority from Memorial Hospital, New York.*

May, H.: Plastic and Reconstructive Surgery. 3rd ed. Philadelphia, F. A. Davis Company, 1971.
*A magnificent volume on general reconstructive plastic surgery.*

McGregor, I.: Fundamental Techniques of Plastic Surgery. 4th ed. Baltimore, Williams & Wilkins Company, 1968.
*A primer on plastic surgery principles and techniques recommended especially for students and house officers.*

Pack, G. T., and Ariel, I. M.: Treatment of Cancer and Allied Diseases. Volume III. 2nd ed. New York, Hoeber Medical Division, Harper and Row, 1962.
*A fine book on all types of neoplastic disease; concise and to the point.*

Paletta, F. X.: Pediatric Plastic Surgery. St. Louis, C. V. Mosby Company, 1967.
*An excellent little book. Pediatric patients are not just small people, for their treatment demands knowledge that is applicable directly to them.*

Stark, R. B.: Plastic Surgery. New York, Harper and Row, 1962.
*An excellent volume dealing with the general principles of excisional and reparative surgery.*

Thompson, D. E., Frost, H. M., Hendrick, J. W., and Horn, R. C.: Soft tissue sarcomas involving the extremities. Southern Med. J., 64:33, 1971.
*An excellent review of the literature and the authors' experiences providing an up-to-date categorization of sarcomas and histologic criteria.*

Ward, G. E., and Hendrick, J. W.: Diagnosis and Treatment of Tumors of the Head and Neck. Baltimore, Williams & Wilkins Company, 1950.
*Among the first of the books to be devoted exclusively to cancer of the head and neck; a classic.*

## REFERENCES

1. Allen, A. C.: A reorientation on the histogenesis and clinical significance of cutaneous nevi and melanomas. Cancer, 2:28, 1949.
2. Anderson, W., Boyd, S.: Pathology for the Surgeon. 8th ed. Philadelphia, W. B. Saunders Company, 1967.
3. Armstrong, D., and Pickrell, K. L.: Axillary hidradenitis suppurativa. Plast. Reconstr. Surg., 36:200, 1965.
4. Callaway, J. L. (Chairman and Professor of Dermatology, Duke University Medical Center): Personal communication.
5. Cavanaugh, P. (Director, Radiation Therapy, Duke University Medical Center): Personal communication.
6. Conway, H.: Tumors of the Skin. Springfield, Ill., Charles C Thomas, 1956.
7. Fetter, B. (Professor of Pathology, Duke University Medical Center): Personal communication.
8. Freier, D. T., and Lindenauer, S. M.: Subcutaneous glomus tumor. Amer. J. Surg., 120:359, 1970.
9. King, G. D., and Salzman, F. A.: Keloid scars. Surg. Clin. N. Amer., 50:595, 1970.
10. Lever, W. F.: Histopathology of the Skin. Philadelphia, J. B. Lippincott Company, 1961.
11. Lewis, G. M., and Wheeler, C. E.: Practical Dermatology. 3rd ed. Philadelphia, W. B. Saunders Company, 1967.
12. Masson, P.: Pigmented nevi; Nerve Tumors. Les Naevi Pigmentoires, Tumeurs Nerveuses. Ann. Anat. Path., 3: 417, 1926.
13. Matton, G., and Pickrell, K. L.: The surgical treatment of rhinophyma; an analysis of 57 cases. Plast. Reconstr. Surg., 30:403, 1962.
14. Pack, G. T.: Prepubertal melanoma of the skin. Surg. Gynec. Obstet., 86:374, 1948.
15. Peacock, E. E., Jr., and Van Winkle, W., Jr.: Surgery and Biology of Wound Repair. Philadelphia, W. B. Saunders Company, 1970.
16. Pickrell, K. L., and Georgiade, N. G.: Surgical treatment of early carcinoma of the face. Postgrad. Med., 27:406, 1960.
17. Pickrell, K. L., and Georgiade, N. G.: Plastic surgery conditions in infancy and childhood. Postgrad. Med., 27:704, 1960.
18. Pickrell, K. L., and Masters, F. W.: Tumors of the head and neck in infancy, childhood and adolescence. Plast. Reconstr. Surg., 12:10, 1953.
19. Pickrell, K. L., Kelley, J. W., and Marzoni, F. A.: The surgical treatment of pseudoxanthoma elasticum. Plast. Reconstr. Surg., 3:700, 1948.
20. Pillsbury, D. M., Shelley, W. B., and Kligman, A. M.: Dermatology. Philadelphia, W. B. Saunders Company, 1957.
21. Thompson, D. E. Frost, H. M., Hendrick, J. W., and Horn, R. C.: Soft tissue sarcomas involving the extremities. Southern Med. J., 64:33, 1971.
22. Thompson, H. D., Douglas, L., and Monroe, I.: Surgical tattooing: An experimental study (Part II). Plast. Reconstr. Surg., 39:291; 1967; also 37:536, 1966.
23. Woolf, R., Kepes, J., Georgiade, N., and Pickrell, K.: Xeroderma pigmentosa. Plast. Reconstr. Surg., 24:214, 1959.

# 46

# GYNECOLOGY: UTERUS, OVARIES, AND VAGINA

*Charles B. Hammond, M.D.*

## INTRODUCTION AND HISTORY OF GYNECOLOGY

Gynecology is that branch of medicine which deals with diseases of the female genital tract. In practice, however, it includes some aspects of internal medicine, obstetrics, and endocrinology as well as multiple other areas of interest that are common to any surgical specialty.

The art and practice of gynecology dates to the ancient Egyptians, the time of the Old Testament, and the early Greeks when most thoughts and practices of gynecology were vested in superstition and based on empiricism derived from observation. Rules concerning menstruation and sexual conduct are recorded in Lev. 15:19-32. Soranus, Hippocrates, and Galen taught about diseases of the uterus and observed mental attitudes and traits in women that they related to the uterus and its humors. The visible events of female physiology were so steeped in folklore and myth that it was not until the emergence of scientific medicine in the Middle Ages that gynecology actually profited from objective observation of the human body. Gynecology advanced as medical science as a whole prospered, but at perhaps a slower pace because of the persistence of the fantasies surrounding human reproduction, many of which remain in the twentieth century.

Modern gynecologic surgery dates from 1809 when Ephraim McDowell of Kentucky performed the first ovariotomy for a large ovarian cyst. The operation was a success and laid the foundation for abdominal and pelvic surgery. Many others provided significant discoveries: In 1817, Langenbeck reported the first vaginal hysterectomy. In 1842, Long and, in 1846, Morton introduced ether anesthesia. In 1849, Mattauer and, in 1852, Sims described successful closure of vesicovaginal fistula, a common complication of obstructed labor in that time. In 1860, Hodge described the vaginal pessary for support of the prolapsed uterus. In 1861, Pasteur noted living organisms lead to fermentation and tissue destruction. In 1867, Lister conceived and published his principles of antisepsis. In 1878, Freund performed the first successful abdominal hysterectomy for cancer of the uterus. In 1884, Tait reported excellent success with abdominal operation for ruptured ectopic pregnancy. In 1895, Röntgen discovered x-rays. In 1898, The Curies discovered radium; Kelly described the operative cure of bladder and urethral prolapse and published a two-volume text of operative gynecology.

The twentieth century began with Wertheim describing a radical operation for cancer of the cervix and Landsteiner discovering the major human blood groups. Other contributions include: In 1903, Cleaves treated the first patient with cancer of the cervix with radium. In 1908, Hitschmann and Alder demonstrated the cyclic physiologic changes of endometrium. In 1921, Sampson described pelvic endometriosis and published his theory of "retrograde menstruation." In 1923, Allen and Doisy isolated estrogen. In 1928, Aschheim and Zondek discovered human chorionic gonadotropin. In 1929, Allen and Corner isolated progesterone. In 1935, Stein and Leventhal described the polycystic ovary syndrome. In 1936, Hamblen first induced human ovulation with gonadotropins of nonhuman primates; Colebrook and Kenny first used antibiotics (sulfanilamides) to treat human puerperal infections. In 1941, Papanicolaou and Traut published the classic monograph on vaginal cytology for cancer screening. In 1949, Barr discovered the sex chromatin body; Li, Simpson, and Evans isolated human follicle-stimulating hormone. In 1951, Brunschwig reported exenterative pelvic surgery for advanced or recurrent cervical cancer. In 1956, Li, Hertz, and Spencer first cured metastatic choriocarcinoma with chemotherapy; Tijo and Levan identified the normal human karyotype as 46 chromosomes. In 1958, Gemzell reported successful ovulatory induction with human gonadotropins; Pincus introduced oral contraceptives.[18, 19]

The accomplishments of these men, plus many others, have enabled gynecology to become a broadly based discipline. While this chapter is not intended to be a complete treatise on the diagnosis and management of gynecologic disorders, it is hoped it will provide a summation of the current and accepted knowledge of the specialty. Ideally, it will stimulate the reader to more in-depth study regarding specific problems.

## EMBRYOLOGY AND ANATOMY

A knowledge of embryology is necessary for proper understanding of gynecology, particularly as it relates to problems as congenital malformations, hermaphroditism, endocrine interrelationships, and generative

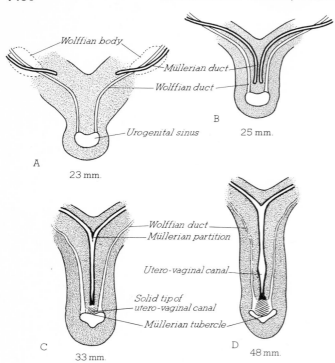

**Figure 1** Relationships of müllerian and wolffian ducts during early genital development. (After Koff, A. K.: Contributions to Embryology. Washington, D.C., Carnegie Institute of Washington, *24*:61, 1933.)

neoplasms. The external genitals develop from the genital tubercle, a group of cells found at the caudal end of the body (Fig. 1). The urogenital sinus develops from part of the ventral entodermal cloaca. The lower portion of the vagina originates from the genital tubercle and provides an invading epithelium which covers the external genitalia, the vagina, and the vaginal part of the cervix. Externally, the clitoris forms first, then the labia minora, and finally labia majora. The hymen forms from the unfolding of the urogenital sinus. As the urogenital sinus unfolds it joins the müllerian tubercle developing cephalad as the upper vagina. At this stage the urethra acquires a separate orifice.

The urogenital ridge is formed on each side of the posterior body cavity. From these primordial cells develop the ovaries, the wolffian ducts and bodies, and the müllerian ducts. The müllerian ducts develop into the tubes, uterus, cervix, and upper vagina. To form these latter three structures the müllerian ducts must fuse in the midline, and aplasia of one duct or failure of fusion may result in several congenital malformations. The ovaries develop from coelomic epithelium covering the surfaces of the wolffian bodies. This epithelium forms early into a sex gland anlage and at this stage histologic sexual differentiation is not evident. When ovarian development occurs primordial follicles appear and remain inactive until gonadotropic stimulation begins at puberty. The wolffian ducts are the forerunner of the male reproductive system and undergo regressive changes in the female which cause them to become vestigial. Remnants of the wolffian ducts persist in the normal female as ductal structures which may become manifest clinically as Gartner's duct cysts, usually seen in the vagina, parovarian cysts, and as hydatid of Morgagni.[5]

### The External Genitalia (Fig. 2)

The female external genitals, or vulva, include the mons veneris which is a fat pad over the pubic symphysis

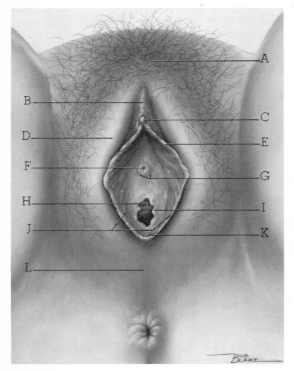

**Figure 2** The external genitalia. A, Mons pubis. B, Prepuce. C, Clitoris. D, Labia majora. E, Labia minora. F, Urethral meatus. G, Skene's ducts. H, Vagina. I, Hymen. J, Bartholin glands. K, Posterior fourchette. L, Perineal body.

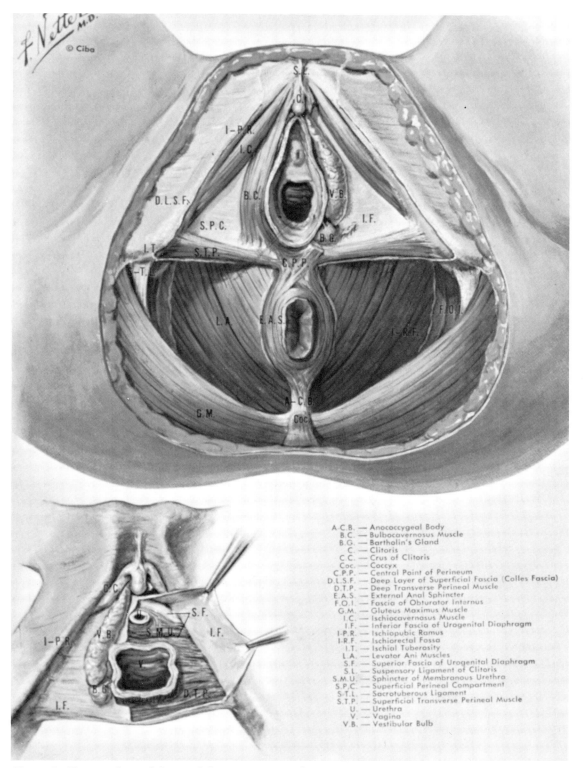

A.C.B. — Anococcygeal Body
B.C. — Bulbocavernosus Muscle
B.G. — Bartholin's Gland
C. — Clitoris
C.C. — Crus of Clitoris
Coc. — Coccyx
C.P.P. — Central Point of Perineum
D.L.S.F. — Deep Layer of Superficial Fascia (Colles Fascia)
D.T.P. — Deep Transverse Perineal Muscle
E.A.S. — External Anal Sphincter
F.O.I. — Fascia of Obturator Internus
G.M. — Gluteus Maximus Muscle
I.C. — Ischiocavernosus Muscle
I.F. — Inferior Fascia of Urogenital Diaphragm
I-P.R. — Ischiopubic Ramus
I-R.F. — Ischiorectal Fossa
I.T. — Ischial Tuberosity
L.A. — Levator Ani Muscles
S.F. — Superior Fascia of Urogenital Diaphragm
S.L. — Suspensory Ligament of Clitoris
S.M.U. — Sphincter of Membranous Urethra
S.P.C. — Superficial Perineal Compartment
S.T.L. — Sacrotuberous Ligament
S.T.P. — Superficial Transverse Perineal Muscle
U. — Urethra
V. — Vagina
V.B. — Vestibular Bulb

**Figure 3**   The muscles and fascia of the perineum. (© Copyright 1954, 1965, CIBA Pharmaceutical Company, Division of CIBA Corporation. From The CIBA Collection of Medical Illustrations by Frank H. Netter, M.D.)

into which the labia majora blend. It is covered with skin which contains sweat glands and hair follicles. The labia majora are the most lateral structures of the external genitalia and do not acquire full growth until puberty. After menopause, atrophy may occur. These structures are covered with skin which contains sweat glands, hair follicles, and sebaceous and sudoriferous glands beneath the squamous epithelium. The underlying tissue is adipose and the round ligaments insert into the upper ends of the labia majora. The labia minora are medial to the majora and are covered with skin containing sweat glands but no hair follicles. The labia minora extend from the clitoris anteriorly and continue to the perineum. Anteriorly they pass over the top of the clitoris to form the prepuce and join below the clitoris to form the frenulum. Growth and configuration of the labia minora are influenced by estrogen. The clitoris is composed of two roots which traverse the pubic rami to unite beneath the symphysis in the clitoridal body and terminate in the upper portion as the glans, which is exposed. The covering of the glans is modified cutaneous

tissue. The clitoris contains two corpora cavernosa and is erectile.

The urethral meatus is situated below the clitoris and above the vaginal orifice. Lateral to this meatus open Skene's ducts which lead from paraurethral glands. Bartholin glands are located at four and eight o'clock at the vulvovaginal orifice, and are compound racemose glands that connect to the surface by a single tubule lined by transitional epithelium. The gland acini are lined by a single layer of cuboidal epithelium. In its normal state the gland usually cannot be seen or palpated. The hymen divides the external and internal genitalia and may be a fibrous structure. The aperture varies greatly in size and shape and may be imperforate.

### The Muscles and Fascia of the Perineum (Fig. 3)

The superficial fascia of the perineum consists of outer and deep layers, both continuous with the layers of the anterior abdominal wall; the outer layer is called

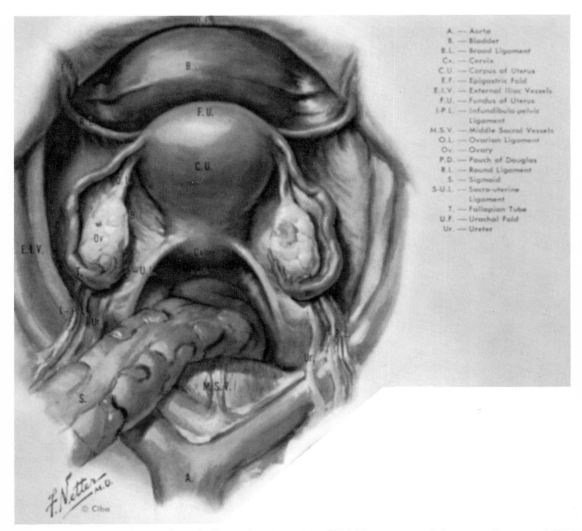

A. — Aorta
B. — Bladder
B.L. — Broad Ligament
Cx. — Cervix
C.U. — Corpus of Uterus
E.F. — Epigastric Fold
E.I.V. — External Iliac Vessels
F.U. — Fundus of Uterus
I-P.L. — Infundibulo-pelvic Ligament
M.S.V. — Middle Sacral Vessels
O.L. — Ovarian Ligament
Ov. — Ovary
P.D. — Pouch of Douglas
R.L. — Round Ligament
S. — Sigmoid
S-U.L. — Sacro-uterine Ligament
T. — Fallopian Tube
U.F. — Urachal Fold
Ur. — Ureter

**Figure 4** The internal genitalia. (© Copyright 1954, 1965, CIBA Pharmaceutical Company, Division of CIBA Corporation. From The CIBA Collection of Medical Illustrations by Frank H. Netter, M.D.)

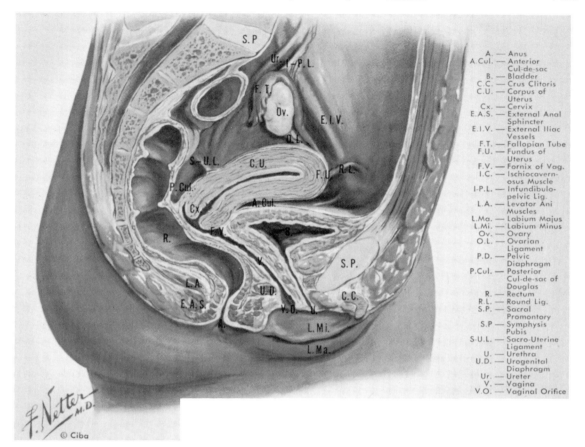

**Figure 4**  *Continued.*

Cruveilhier's fascia and is continuous with Camper's fascia of the anterior abdominal wall; the deep layer of the superficial perineal fascia is called Colles' fascia and is continuous with Scarpa's fascia of the abdomen. The outer layer of superficial fascia forms the greater part of the labium majus and is continuous with the superficial fascia of the thigh. The deep layer of superficial fascia, Colles' fascia, is a strong membrane adding support to the urogenital structures. This fascia is firmly attached laterally to the medial surface of the thigh being continuous with the fascia which covers the saphenous vein opening. It becomes attached to the deep fascia along the posterior border of the superficial transverse perineal muscle and blends on either side into the median raphe of the perineum.

The deep perineal fascia consists of obturator fascia, infra-anal fascia, and fascia of the bulbocavernosus, ischiocavernosus, and transverse perineal muscles. The obturator fascia forms the lateral wall of the ischiorectal fossa, and meets the infra-anal fascia deep in the fossa. The infra-anal fascia is the fascia of the levator ani and coccygeus muscles. The deep transverse perineal muscle is covered on both sides by fascia and the three structures constitute the urogenital diaphragm. The urethra and vagina perforate this diaphragm which stretches as a wall across the space between the ischiopubic rami. The deep layer rests between the deep transverse perineal muscle and the pubococcygeal portions of the levator ani sling.

The perineal muscles divide into deep and superficial portions, sphincter urethrae, and bulbocavernosus and ischiocavernosus muscles. The superficial transverse perineal muscles arise from the ischial tuberosity on either side and insert into the central perineal tendon. They blend with the anal sphincter muscle and with fibers from the bulbocavernosus muscles. The bulbocavernosus muscles surround the vaginal orifice and have a sphincteric contractile effect arising anteriorly from the clitoris and inserting posteriorly into the perineal body. The ischiocavernosus muscles arise from the medial borders of the ischial rami and clitoris, and course posteriorly and laterally to insert into the ischial tuberosity. The sphincter muscle of the urethra is attached to the periurethral structures and fans laterally on either side to attach to the pubic rami. The deep transverse perineal muscle lies below the superficial muscle and attaches in the midline of the perineal body.

### The Internal Genitalia (Fig. 4)

**The Vagina.** The vagina is a muscular tube lined with stratified squamous epithelium that is histologically similar to the mucosa of the cervix and vulva. It does not contain glands or hair follicles but individual cells produce mucus. The superficial layer is not keratinized. During menstrual life the vagina has transverse folds called rugae. After menopause the vaginal walls become thin and atrophic, reflecting the lack of estrogen as seen in the childhood years. The adult vagina measures 12 to 13 cm. in depth, and in nulliparous women there is coaptation of the anterior and posterior walls. The vaginal axis is toward the sacral promontory and the cervix is suspended at the upper end, surrounded by the anterior, posterior, and lateral fornices. The upper two-thirds of the vagina is supported by the paravaginal fascia and the paracervical tissues, the lower one-third by the perineal body.

**The Cervix.** The inferior portion of the uterus, the cervix, is a fibromuscular organ covered with stratified squamous epithelium. The portio vaginalis of the cervix arises in the vaginal fornices and ends at the external cervical os at the entrance of the endocervical canal. This squamocolumnar junction is the most common site of origin of squamous cell carcinoma. The endocervical canal is lined by columnar epithelium, and racemose glands, lined with similar epithelium, are in the fibromuscular stroma. Such glands, if obstructed, may form nabothian cysts on the cervical surface. The nulliparous cervical os is round but parturition changes this to a horizontally flattened orifice. The cervix is the most common site of genital malignancy in women.

**The Uterus.** The uterus is a hollow, fibromuscular-walled organ between the bladder and rectum and consists of cervix and fundus. The organ is pear-shaped, and in nonpregnant women measures approximately 8 cm. in length and weighs 30 to 100 gm. The fallopian tubes and the cervical canal communicate with the uterine cavity which is lined by the endometrium. The endometrium proliferates in response to estrogen and becomes secretory with progesterone, and bleeds as it sloughs when hormonal support is withdrawn or inadequate. The uterine fundus is covered by peritoneum except in its lower anterior portion, where the bladder is contiguous with the lower uterine segment and the peritoneum is reflected, and laterally where the folds of the broad ligament are attached. The uterus is supported by condensations of endopelvic fascia and fibromuscular tissue laterally at the base of the broad ligaments, the cardinal ligaments, and the uterosacral ligaments. The round ligaments arise from the cornual areas, pass through the external inguinal ring, and insert in the upper labia majora. The broad ligaments support laterally and the uterovesical fold anteriorly. None of these last three provide major uterine support.

**The Oviducts.** The fallopian tubes arise from the superior portion of the lateral borders of the uterus, superior to the attachment of the round ligaments, and are patent. The distal ends, the fimbriae, open into the abdominal cavity and the proximal ends into the uterine cavity. The tubes are lined by a single layer of low columnar epithelium, some ciliated, arranged in a branching or "frond" pattern. This structure is divided into interstitial, isthmic, ampullar, and fimbriated portions. The wall is thin with two muscular layers and an outer layer of peritoneum within the upper borders of the broad ligament.

**The Ovaries.** The normal ovary is a white, almond-shaped structure measuring 2 by 3 by 3 cm., and is located on the posterior surface of the broad ligament and inferior to the fallopian tube. The nerves, lymphatics, and blood vessels enter the ovary at the point of attachment to the broad ligament, the hilus. Lateral support of the ovary is the infundibulopelvic ligament which extends to the pelvic sidewall and medial support is to the uterus by the utero-ovarian ligament. The ovary has a cortex and medulla. Germinal epithelium, a single layer of cuboidal cells, covers condensed fibrous tissue called the tunica albuginea. Follicles originate within the ovarian cortex and are composed of the basic embryonic complement; no new follicles are formed after birth. The medullary portion of the ovary is occupied by blood vessels, lymphatics, nerves, and connective tissue and contains remnants of wolffian body precursors. The ovary is an endocrine and a generative organ. Parafollicular granulosa cells produce estrogen and, after ovulation and corpus luteum formation, progestins. Androgens are produced by stromal cells, particularly in the hilus.

**The Urinary System.** The kidneys and ureters arise from the metanephros and a diverticulum from the wolffian duct in both sexes. The ureters vary from 28 to 34 cm. in length, the right about 1 to 2 cm. shorter than the left. The ureter is not of uniform caliber. The abdominal part of the ureter lies behind the peritoneum on the medial part of the psoas muscle and is crossed obliquely by the ovarian vessels. It enters the pelvis by crossing either the termination of the common, or the commencement of the external, iliac vessels. The pelvic ureter runs at first downward on the lateral wall of the pelvis, then medially and forward toward the lateral aspect of the cervix about 1.5 cm. from the exterior of the cervix. In this course it is accompanied by the uterine artery. The uterine artery then crosses over the ureter and ascends between the leaves of the broad ligament to enter the uterus laterally. Blood supply of the ureter arises from branches of the renal, ovarian, hypogastric, and inferior vesical arteries.

In the female, the uterus, cervix and upper vagina are behind the bladder and it is separated from the uterus by the vesicouterine fold. Below this peritoneal fold the bladder is connected to the cervix and upper vagina by areolar tissue. The bladder is stabilized by ligamentous attachments at its inferior portion or base, near the exit of the urethra, and at the vertex. The remainder is free to move. The basal attachment is to the internal investing layer of deep fascia on the pubic bone by strong fibrous bands. The arterial supply of the bladder is the superior, middle, and inferior vesical arteries, derived from the anterior hypogastric artery, the obturator and inferior gluteal arteries, and the uterine and vaginal arteries.

The female urethra is a narrow membranous canal about 4 cm. long extending from the internal to the external urethral orifice. It is placed behind the symphysis, embedded in the anterior vaginal wall, and its direction is obliquely downward and forward. The resting diameter is about 6 mm. The urethra perforates the fasciae of the urogenital diaphragm where it acquires longitudinal folds. Many small paraurethral glands open into the urethra.

### The Rectosigmoid Colon

The sigmoid colon forms a loop that averages 40 cm. in length and normally lies in the pelvis. It begins vertically from the left side of the pelvis as the continuation of the descending colon, passes transversely across the front of the sacrum to the right side of the pelvis, curves on itself and turns toward the left to reach the midline at the level of S3 where it bends inferiorly and terminates in the rectum. The colon is completely surrounded by the peritoneum and forms a mesentery which diminishes in length from the center. The sigmoid loop is fixed at its junctions with the two other parts of the colon and the central portion has considerable mobility. The rectum is continuous with the sigmoid colon. From its origin at the third sacral vertebra, the rectum passes downward, lying in the sacrococcygeal curve, and extends in front of, and below, the tip of the coccyx. It then turns posteriorly into the anal canal. The rectum is approximately 12 cm. long and is dilated near its distal end to form the rectal ampulla. The peritoneum is applied to the upper two-thirds of the rectum, covering it at first anteriorly and laterally, but more inferiorly covering its anterior surface only. The distal 5 cm. is devoid of

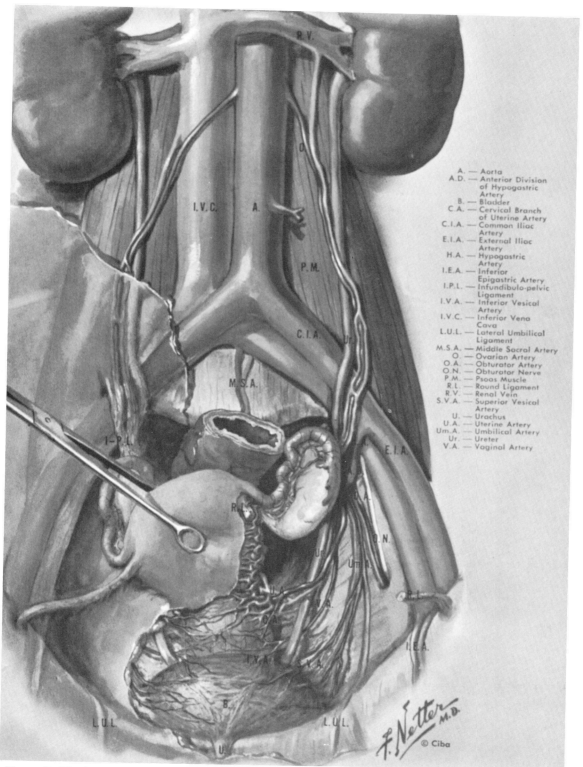

**Figure 5** Blood supply of the pelvis. (© Copyright 1954, 1965, CIBA Pharmaceutical Company, Division of CIBA Corporation. From The CIBA Collection of Medical Illustrations by Frank H. Netter, M.D.)

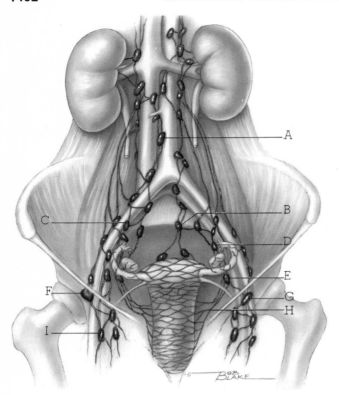

**Figure 6** Lymphatics of the pelvis. A, Aortic. B, Sacral. C, Common iliac. D, Hypogastric. E, Obturator. F, Deep inguinal. G, Cloquet's node. H, Parametrial. I, Superficial inguinal.

peritoneal covering. The arterial supply of the rectum is derived from the superior hemorrhoidal branch of the inferior mesenteric artery. The anal canal is supplied by the middle hemorrhoidal branch of the hypogastric artery, the superior hemorrhoidal branch of the inferior mesenteric artery, and the inferior hemorrhoidal branch of the internal pudendal artery.

### The Blood Vessels of the Pelvis (Fig. 5)

The ovarian arteries arise from the front of the aorta just below the renal arteries. The left ovarian vein empties into the left renal vein; the right ovarian vein empties into the vena cava just inferior to the renal vein. The ovarian vessels follow a downward course and pass between the layers of the infundibulopelvic ligament and the broad ligament to reach the ovary. Small branches divide to supply the ureter and fallopian tube. The main branches unite with the uterine vessels on the side of the uterus and small branches supply the round ligaments.

The iliac vessels originate as the common iliac arteries from the aorta at the L4 vertebral level and slightly to the left of midline. Each is about 5 cm. long, and just below the S1 level divides into the internal iliac (hypogastric) artery and the external iliac artery. The common iliac veins closely follow the arteries and join inferiorly and to the right of the aorta to form the vena cava. The external iliac vessels lie on the lateral walls of the pelvis above the psoas muscles, behind the peritoneum, to pass beneath the inguinal ligaments through the femoral canal to become the femoral artery and vein. The inferior epigastric vessels arise from the external iliacs immediately superior to the ligament. The hypogastric (internal iliac) vessels pass inferiorly and posteriorly along the border of the great sciatic notch. The hypogastric vessels are 3 to 4 cm. in length before they

divide into anterior and posterior branches. The anterior branch provides the main blood supply to the bladder and forms the middle hemorrhoidal, obturator, internal pudendal, inferior gluteal, uterine, and vaginal arteries. The uterine artery arises from the anterior branch of the hypogastric artery and passes medially on the levator ani muscle toward the junction of the cervix and the uterus. At the level of the internal os the vessels turn superiorly and follow a tortuous route between the leaves of the broad ligament to join the ovarian arteries. An inferior branch of the uterine artery turns inferiorly on either side to form the cervical arteries. The vaginal artery arises from the hypogastric artery below the level of the uterine artery and sends branches to the vagina, bladder, and rectum. The internal pudendal artery is the most caudal extension of the hypogastric artery and supplies the external genital organs. This vessel emerges from the pelvis between the piriformis and coccygeus muscles, crosses the ischial spine, and passes through the lesser sciatic foramen to enter the perineum. The artery traverses the lateral wall of the ischiorectal fossa and supplies the erectile tissue of the vulva.

### The Lymphatics of the Pelvis (Fig. 6)

The lymphatics of the pelvis parallel the vascular channels. The external iliac nodes are interposed in the drainage pattern of the deep inguinal nodes, the fundus of the bladder and the uterus, cervix, and upper vagina. The external iliac and hypogastric drainage occurs via the common iliac nodes. The hypogastric nodes surround the hypogastric vessels and receive drainage from the cervix, uterine fundus, upper vagina, bladder, urethra, and lower ureter. The obturator nodes reside in the obturator fossa, lateral to and surrounding the obturator nerve, and receive channels from the cervix, uterus, and part of the buttocks. The sacral nodes receive branches from the cervix and uterus and reside in the sacral concavity. The rectal lymphatics course posteriorly to the sacral nodes also. The vulva drainage takes place via subcutaneous ascending lymphatics to the superficial and deep inguinal nodes and femoral nodes which also receive the lymphatics from the lower portions of the vagina and urethra. The lower extremity lymphatics lead to the femoral and inguinal nodes. Cross drainage in this region may occur via Cloquet's node (femoral canal) to deep nodes of the pelvis.

### The Nerve Supply of the Pelvis

The sacral plexus arises from the fourth and fifth lumbar and the first four sacral cord segments. The pudendal nerve originates from the second, third, and fourth sacral segments. The plexus rests in the hollow of the pelvis over the piriformis muscle. The branches of the plexus contain fibers of sympathetic and parasympathetic nerve trunks. The parasympathetic fibers are efferent preganglionic to pelvic viscera, and afferent from the pelvic organs. The sympathetic fibers arise from the hypogastric sympathetic plexus. The levator ani, coccygeus, and sphincter ani muscles receive branches from the pudendal plexus. The pudendal nerve leaves the pelvis through the greater sciatic foramen, crosses the ischial spine, and re-enters the pelvis via the lesser sciatic foramen. It accompanies the pudendal vessels and sends branches to the sphincter ani muscle and sensory fibers to the labia majora, while another branch supplies the perineal muscles. The dorsal nerve of the clitoris also arises from the pudendal nerve.

# PHYSIOLOGY AND ENDOCRINOLOGY

The interactions of physiologic and endocrinologic mechanisms cannot be separated in any adequate summary of the function of the female genital system. Numerous workers have identified the interrelationships between the central nervous system, hypothalamus, pituitary, ovary, and other endocrine systems. Dependence of the pelvic structures, breasts, skin, other organs, and many metabolic processes on estrogen and progesterone has been demonstrated.[5, 6, 8, 13, 14, 16]

### Hypothalamus, Pituitary, and Gonadotropins

The hypothalamus (Fig. 7) serves as the primary control center for reproductive endocrine systems. This system is essentially dormant until late childhood when activation begins and certain hypothalamic cells become capable of releasing short-chain peptides to the anterior pituitary via the hypophyseal portal system. In experimental animals, and probably also in man, these humoral agents, or releasing factors, cause the anterior pituitary to produce and release follicle-stimulating hormone (FSH) and luteinizing hormone (LH). Physiologic, pathologic, and even psychologic problems can alter these interrelationships.

The pituitary gonadotropins, FSH and LH, are necessary for normal ovarian function and, via the hypothalamus, are in turn regulated through feedback mechanisms from ovarian estrogen and progesterone (Fig. 8). FSH arises from the basophilic cells of the anterior pituitary, is transmitted through the blood, and stimulates maturation of the ovarian follicle and parafollicular cells to produce estrogen. FSH, which can occasionally be found in small amounts in the urine of young

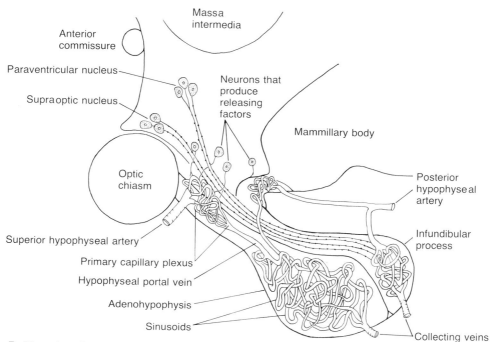

**Figure 7**  Neural and vascular connections from the hypothalamus to the pituitary. (Redrawn from Radford, H. M.: Proc. Aust. Soc. Anim. Prod., 6:19, 1966.)

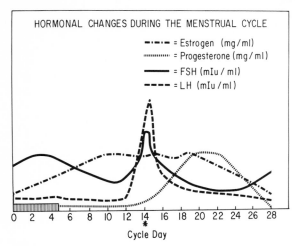

**Figure 8** Hormonal changes during the menstrual cycle. Menses, days 0-5; ovulation, day 14.

girls, increases in amount just prior to puberty, and is found in large amounts in the urine of mature women. After the ovarian failure of menopause, there is a sharp rise in urinary and plasma FSH as the hypothalamus attempts to correct resultant hypoestrogenism. In ovulating women FSH is elevated during the follicular phase of the cycle, then rises sharply at midcycle during ovulation. FSH levels are relatively low during the luteal phase of the cycle. Luteinizing hormone (LH) complements FSH secretion and the two provide a synergistic effect on ovarian function. LH levels are relatively low during the follicular and luteal phases of the menstrual cycle but rise sharply for a 72 hour span surrounding ovulation. Luteinizing hormone, acting on the FSH-stimulated follicle, can cause ovulation. LH also stimulates the interstitial cells of the ovary and may be an integral part of corpus luteum maintenance.

Excessive amounts of sex steroid hormones, estrogen, progesterone, or androgens, will inhibit hypothalamic-pituitary secretion.

### Ovarian Function (Fig. 9)

During infancy and childhood the ovary is dormant, owing to low gonadotropin production, but is capable of being stimulated if these hormones are present. The beginning of puberty and the age of menarche vary considerably between individuals but the usual age for the first menstrual period is from 12 to 15 years. The age of menarche may vary normally from the tenth to eighteenth year. The early menstrual periods are usually irregular and anovulatory. Later, regular ovulatory cycles usually ensue. At puberty there is a spurt in somatic growth, probably due to growth hormone production by the pituitary and the growth effect of increased ovarian estrogen on bone. Later in adolescence higher levels of estrogen result in epiphyseal closure.

Before puberty the primordial follicles develop in the deeper portions of the ovary, and after puberty the maturing follicle migrates to the surface of the ovary. After achieving full maturation, the graafian follicle ruptures and the ovum is extruded into the peritoneal cavity, usually around the fourteenth day of the cycle. With rupture of the follicle, the corpus luteum is formed. It persists for 14 days in a normal cycle. Should pregnancy occur, the corpus luteum will persist for approximately 12 weeks before beginning regression. After ovulation the corpus luteum shows hypertrophy and vascularization of the theca lutein cells. The granulosa cells about the follicle become enlarged and polyhedral and are transformed into lutein cells. Progesterone, produced in small amounts just prior to ovulation, is now produced in large amounts. About 4 days before menses the corpus luteum regresses and loses the ability to produce progesterone unless human chorionic

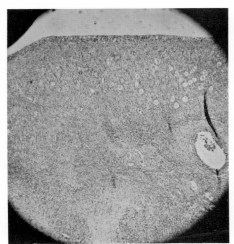
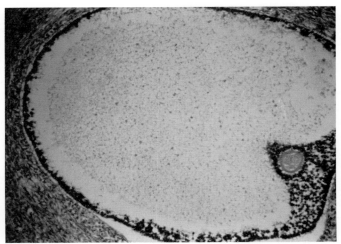

**Figure 9** Human ovary with multiple primordial follicles (left) and a higher-power view of a maturing follicle (right).

gonadotropin from pregnancy sustains corpus luteum function.

Menopause occurs with waning of ovarian function, usually between 45 and 53 years of age. With intrinsic failure of the ovary, there is atresia of the follicles and failure of estrogen production, which is at first sharp but later becomes more gradual, with a minimal amount of estrogen production extending for several additional years. With decline of estrogen the breasts atrophy, the pelvic structures become smaller, and the vaginal mucosa becomes thin and smooth.

### Estrogen

Many studies have demonstrated that oophorectomy performed on the immature female is followed by persistent infantile characteristics of genital tissues. If the gonads are removed from a mature female animal, the uterus and breasts atrophy. The human ovary produces primarily estrone, 17β-estradiol, the most potent naturally occurring estrogen, and estriol. These estrogens are produced primarily in the theca interna cells. Preadolescent girls and women beyond the menopause secrete little estrogen. The adult, cycling woman produces 10 to 55 μg. of the various estrogens each day, with a low level during menses which increases steadily until ovulation. After ovulation there is a slight decline, then significant levels persist until 2 to 3 days prior to menses. The placenta and adrenal gland also produce estrogens.

The estrogens are lipids with the same phenanthrene nucleus as the other steroids, from which they are distinguished by a phenolic ring A (Fig. 10). In addition to natural estrogens, chemicals with estrogenic activity have been synthesized. These include diethylstilbestrol, hexestrol, dienestrol, and, most recently, a group of 17α-ethinyl steroids. The various estrogens are rapidly metabolized by the liver and are conjugated with glucuronic and sulfuric acid. These conjugated compounds are excreted 60 per cent in urine and 40 per cent in bile and feces and by other routes.

The principal physiologic function of estrogen is stimulation of endometrial growth, myometrium, other tissues of müllerian origin, the vulva, and the breast. Estrogen is responsible for uterine and tubal contractility and is the feminizing hormone that at puberty brings about the secondary sex characteristics: mammary growth, primarily of ductal tissue, and the adult female fat pad distribution. A variety of metabolic processes are also influenced by estrogen, notably plasma protein production, bone matrix stabilization, and lipid metabolism.

### Progesterone

Progesterone is the other steroid hormone produced by the ovary (Fig. 10). The corpus luteum begins to secrete this hormone just before ovulation and throughout the luteal phase of the cycle. The placenta and adrenal glands also produce progesterone. It is synthesized in the body from cholesterol via pregnenolone and is converted by the ovary to estrogens and small amounts of testosterone. The production rate of progesterone from the ovary and adrenal glands of a normal adult female is approximately 3 mg. per 24 hours during the follicular phase of the cycle and 22 mg. per 24 hours during the luteal phase. Progesterone is readily synthesized for both oral and parenteral use. Natural progesterone is deactivated by gastric secretions. Synthetic progestins are abundantly available and are useful for treating menstrual disorders and endometriosis and for inhibition of ovulation.

Progesterone is essential for the maintenance of pregnancy; initially it is produced by the corpus luteum and later by the placenta. It has not been of major use as a drug for quieting uterine activity or labor. There is some evidence that progesterone reduces tubal activity. Progesterone is responsible for the acinar and lobular development in the breast and for characteristic changes seen in cervical mucus and in cervical and vaginal cytology. Progesterone is thermogenic and basal body temperatures are 0.2 to 0.8° F. higher in the latter half of the ovulatory cycle.

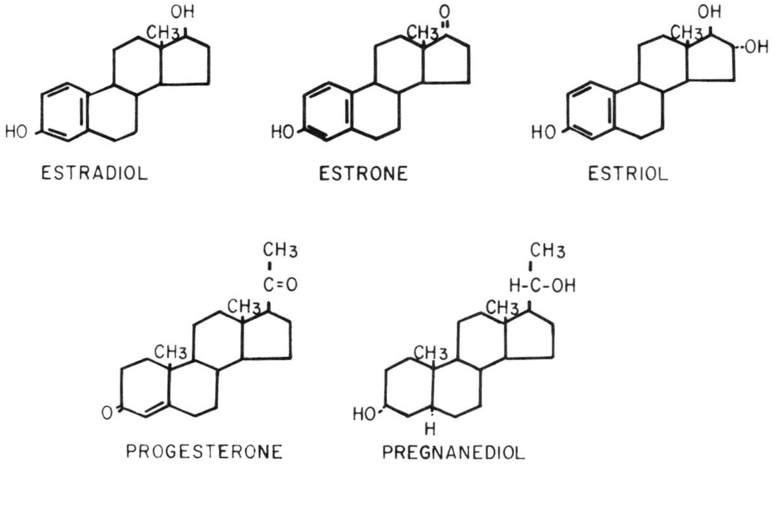

**Figure 10** Structural formulas of three prominent natural estrogens, and progesterone and its main urinary metabolite, pregnanediol.

ESTRADIOL   ESTRONE   ESTRIOL

PROGESTERONE   PREGNANEDIOL

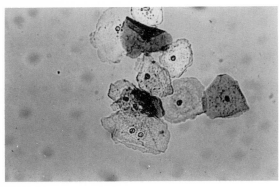 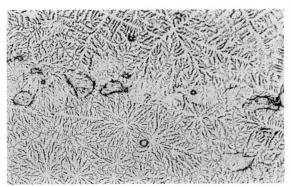

**Figure 11**  Estrogen effect on exfoliated vaginal cells (left) and cervical mucus (right) with the characteristic "fern" pattern.

### Genital Structures

The female genitalia are responsive to estrogen. In the child these structures are immature and thin and begin to mature only with pubescence and the onset of ovarian function. The vulva is thin and not prominent. The vaginal epithelium, which is quite thick at birth because of maternal gestational hormones, rapidly regresses to a thin membrane and pH is neutral. With puberty the vagina thickens, glycogen storage increases, and pH becomes more acid. The cycling woman's vagina normally contains diphtheroids and Döderlein's bacilli, which aid normal vaginal secretion and acidity. After menopause, the vagina again becomes thin and loses the normal rugal pattern, and pH slowly rises. Exfoliated vaginal cells may be stained and microscopically examined for histologic changes that occur with the varying hormonal patterns (Fig. 11).

The cervix of the child is disproportionately larger than the fundus, but after puberty this ratio is reversed. As in the vagina, the cervical epithelium undergoes cyclic changes during the menstrual cycle but these are less than those seen in the endometrium. The racemose glands of the endocervix are dormant in children but initiate secretion of mucus after puberty. Under the dominance of estrogen the cervical mucus increases, is thin and watery, and forms a "fern" pattern when dried (Fig. 11). When progesterone is present cervical mucus is opaque, thick, and tenacious and does not "fern." After menopause cervical mucous production declines as estrogen production declines.

The myometrium of the adult woman normally undergoes spontaneous rhythmic contractions. The uteri of castrates lose this rhythmicity. Hypertrophy of myometrium occurs when higher levels of estrogen are present, and uterine atrophy occurs after menopause. The endometrium reflects generally the levels of estrogen and progesterone. Estrogen causes proliferation of the endometrium and its vascular channels. Progesterone transforms proliferative into secretory endometrium with glandular and stromal features that promote

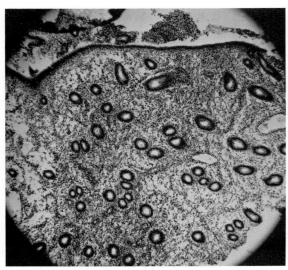 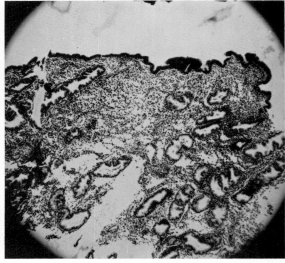

**Figure 12**  Endometrial biopsies demonstrating the proliferative pattern of estrogen dominance (left), and the secretory effects of progesterone after ovulation (right).

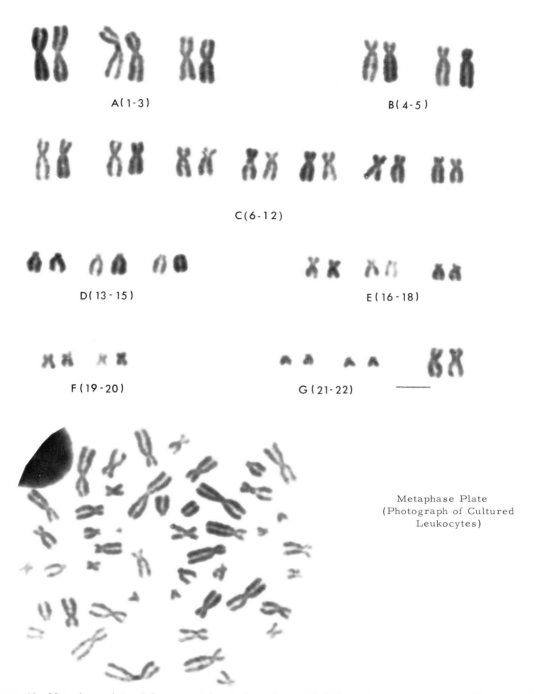

**Figure 13** Metaphase plate of the normal female karyotype with XX sex chromosome pattern. (Courtesy of Dr. A. C. Christakos.)

possible implantation. Endometrial biopsy is a simple office procedure that may allow precise interpretation of ovarian hormonal production (Fig. 12).

The fallopian tube epithelium also reflects ovarian hormonal changes through cyclic modification, maturation, and regression changes. The tubal musculature possesses an intrinsic peristaltic action believed to aid tubal transport. The action of cilia of certain tubal cells may also be involved in transport. Estrogen appears to influence these activities.

## CYTOGENETICS

During the past 15 years observations on the chromosomal etiology of gonadal defects have led to a much better understanding of these problems.[10, 17] In 1938 Turner described seven young girls in whom short stature, sexual infantilism, webbing of the neck, and cubitus valgus were prominent clinical features. These patients were found to have high levels of pituitary gonadotropins, suggesting inadequate ovarian responsiveness, and at laparotomy were found to have either no ovarian tissue or rudimentary streaks of tissue where ovaries should have been. The terms "ovarian agenesis" and "gonadal dysgenesis" were introduced to signify a chromosomally caused gonadal defect.

In 1949 Barr and Bertram demonstrated a characteristic chromatin mass present as a satellite structure on the nuclear membrane of a significant percentage of cells from normal females, but not present on cells of males. This "Barr body" has since been shown to be the condensed chromatin of the second X chromosome of the normal female complement of XX and its detection can aid in the evaluation of "chromosomal sex." Examination of blood smears from females shows that a percentage of polymorphonuclear leukocytes have "drumstick" projections not seen often in males. In 1956 Tijo and Levan accurately identified the normal human chromosomal karyotype as 46, 22 pairs of autosomes and two sex chromosomes. The normal female sex chromosomal complement is XX; that of the male is XY (Fig. 13).

With these discoveries more fundamental studies of chromosomal aberrations as causes of gonadal defects became possible. Recent studies have shown that sex chromosomal aberrations such as Turner's syndrome, Klinefelter's syndrome, and XXX and XXXY patterns are caused by nondisjunction. Other gonadal defects may occur as a result of mosaicism, chromosomal translocation, isochromosome formation, and deletion during the course of meiosis or mitosis. Problems of pseudohermaphroditism in certain patients suggest mutation of sex chromosomes to yield paradoxical function (testicular feminizing syndrome).

It seems clear that chromosomal surveys should be done in a larger group of patients, particularly those with primary amenorrhea in whom abnormal chromosomal constitutions can be expected in up to 40 per cent.

## THE GYNECOLOGIC HISTORY AND EXAMINATION

An adequate history remains a prerequisite for intelligent diagnosis and treatment. All elements of a general medical history are essential to adequate evaluation of pelvic complaints. The gynecologic history should include:

*Present illness:* A chronological story of the patient's problem, relating symptoms, signs, dates, effects of other organ function, and prior investigation or therapy.

*Menstrual pattern:* Age at onset of menses; frequency, duration, and amount of flow; menstrual irregularities; date of the first day of the two most recent episodes of menstrual bleeding; history of pain with menses and its location, character, and duration; any vaginal bleeding between periods or after contact as douching or coitus; and any other major physiologic or pathologic changes associated with menses.

*Vaginal discharge:* Amount, type, color, relation to menses, itching, and previous vaginal infections and therapy.

*Obstetric history:* Each pregnancy should be listed chronologically with comments about duration, complications, delivery, and the puerperium.

*Marital history:* The dates of marriages, contraceptive techniques and duration of use, frequency of coitus, and dyspareunia.

*Other factors:* Sensations of pressure, incontinence, urinary symptoms, bowel complaints, pelvic or abdominal surgery including findings and complications, and a thorough general and endocrine systems review.

The normal woman dislikes a pelvic examination and presents herself for examination with reservation. Gentleness, privacy, and dignity are necessary, and a female chaperone should always be present for assistance, patient reassurance, and protection from possible legal embarrassment. Each step in the pelvic examination should be explained briefly to the patient to gain her confidence and cooperation. The pelvic examination is done with the woman in the lithotomy position with the legs placed in stirrups. Before being placed on the table, the patient should empty her bladder. The chaperone aids in positioning of the patient and drapes her.

The first part of the pelvic examination consists of inspection of the external genitalia for evidence of infection, neoplasia, hypertrophy, atrophy, or trauma. Specific note is made about skin texture, hair patterns, clitoridal size, Skene's ducts, and Bartholin glands. The groins should be examined. The speculum examination is next and a variety of instruments of different sizes and shapes are available. There is no substitute for adequate equipment and lighting. The instrument should be approximately body temperature and lubricated slightly. The vaginal wall and cervix should be inspected for size, shape, and evidence of atrophy, infection, trauma, bleeding, or neoplasia. Specimens can be obtained for cancer cytologic study, hormonal interpretation, and bacteriologic examination. The vagina should be inspected again during withdrawal of the speculum, particularly the anterior and posterior surfaces which may have been covered initially by the blades of the speculum. The patient then performs the Valsalva maneuver while the support of the bladder, rectum, and uterus is visualized and note is made of any stress incontinence.

The examiner then proceeds to the bimanual part of the examination, introducing the first two fingers of one hand into the vagina and palpating above the symphysis

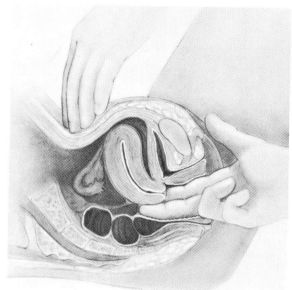

**Figure 14**  Bimanual pelvic examination. The examiner inserts two fingers into the vagina and places the other hand on the lower abdomen. The structures of the pelvis are then outlined between the two hands. (From Nelson, J. H., Jr.: Atlas of Radical Pelvic Surgery. New York, Appleton-Century-Crofts, 1969.)

with the other hand (Fig. 14). The physician attempts to determine the consistency, size, shape, and mobility of the uterus. After the uterus is palpated, the adnexal regions are felt. Next, it is important to palpate the parametrial and paracervical areas. Finally, a combined rectovaginal examination should be done. In children and virgins, a rectal examination may be all that is possible because of the intact hymen. A child's small speculum or Kelly cystoscope may aid visualization and appropriate smears should be obtained.

## LABORATORY AND CLINICAL TESTS

### Cytologic Studies

Approximately 20 per cent of cases of cancer in women arise in the genital tract. The most useful techniques for the early detection of genital malignant diseases are the pelvic examination and Papanicolaou studies. It should be routine to utilize these techniques for all new patients and at yearly intervals at least thereafter. Not only can early malignancy be detected but also premalignant changes may frequently be discovered. Malignant and preinvasive lesions arising from the genital organs exfoliate tumor cells which may traverse the intermediate structures and collect in the vaginal pool and on the surface of the cervix. Malignant cells from the vagina and cervix will be present in 90 per cent of patients with these lesions. If the tumor is of the vulva, it may be missed unless the external genitals are carefully examined and direct scrapings obtained from suspicious areas. For endometrial or uterine smears best results are achieved by passing a fine probe, sound, or small brush into the uterine cavity and obtaining direct smears. Malignant tumors of the tubes or ovaries rarely

exfoliate cells that can be collected on routine pelvic examination.

Exfoliated cells are collected by aspiration or gentle scraping and evenly spread onto glass slides, then immediately fixed in an equal solution of ether and 95 per cent alcohol. Deeper scraping may yield basal cells of different cytologic patterns which may confuse the unwary cytologist. Delay in fixation may allow drying and cytologic alteration. After fixation and Papanicolaou staining, slides should be studied microscopically by an experienced cytologist for cytologic changes compatible with malignancy.

Papanicolau cervical cytology offers a high degree of accuracy, but can be no better than the material collected. If gross infection or blood and mucus are present, care must be exercised to provide sufficient material for study. Such cytologic studies should be used in the detection of

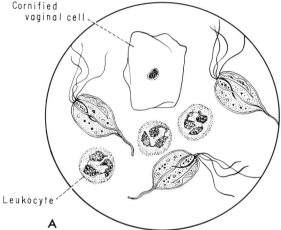

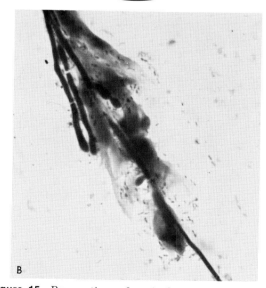

**Figure 15**  Preparations of vaginal secretions showing: *A,* trichomonads, about one-half the size of a cornified vaginal cell but larger than leukocytes, and *B,* the fiber-like mycelia of *Candida albicans.* (From Gynecology: Principles and Practice by Robert W. Kistner. Copyright © 1964, Year Book Medical Publishers. Used by permission.)

premalignant disease or hidden or occult malignant disease, and for follow-up of patients after treatment of malignant disease. *Cytologic studies should never be used as an indication for surgical or irradiative therapy*; rather, they should lead the examiner to diagnostic surgical studies to provide adequate tissue for histopathologic diagnosis.

Fresh vaginal smears also may be of aid in evaluating the hormonal status of the patient. Such vaginal smears are made by obtaining a drop of material from the vaginal pool. For hormonal studies the material is evenly spread on a slide, then stained (Papanicolaou, eosin Y, or Shorr's) and microscopically examined for biologic changes that occur with estrogen or progesterone (see Fig. 11). Such hormonal values are reported as the maturation or cornification index. Vaginal material obtained for study of the etiology of vaginal infection is mixed with saline, placed on a slide, and microscopically examined for the presence of *Trichomonas vaginalis* or *Candida albicans* (Fig. 15). Cultures are required for positive identification of vulvovaginal fungi.

### Cervical Studies

While Papanicolaou cytology is the major tool in the screening for premalignant cervical or vaginal neoplasia, other techniques also may be of use. Gross visualization of the cervix is mandatory and any suspicious areas should be biopsied, usually without anesthesia. The cervix may be painted with an iodine solution, such as Schiller's stain, with which normal cells rich in glycogen stain darkly, whereas neoplastic cells do not take the stain. This technique, as well as colposcopy or colpomicroscopy (microscopic visualization of the cervix in situ), can serve to direct biopsies for histologic diagnosis. If abnormal Papanicolaou smears have been reported, use must be made of either multiple biopsies or cold-knife conization of the cervix, which removes the exocervix, including the squamocolumnar junction, and the endocervical canal (Fig. 16). The important fact is not to miss the diagnosis of invasive carcinoma. Presumption of a benign or premalignant diagnosis on the basis of cytology alone may result in a patient with occult invasive carcinoma receiving inadequate therapy. Cervical mucus also provides information for evaluation of the hormonal status of the patient. Under the influence of estrogen the endocervical epithelium produces clear, watery mucus which can be stretched into long strands. If such estrogen-stimulated mucus is dried on a slide, it will form a crystalline "fern" pattern (see Fig. 11). Cervical mucus is scanty if estrogen is deficient, is maximal just prior to ovulation, and regresses to form a thick turgid plug when progesterone is present. After ovulation the fern pattern is lost.

Cervical smears and cultures are quite important for the diagnosis of gonorrhea, but all too often negative results are obtained because of faulty technique. To properly obtain cervical cultures a vaginal speculum is inserted and the cervix is wiped clean with cotton swabs. Through compressive force of the blades of the speculum on the anterior and posterior cervix, the mucus of the

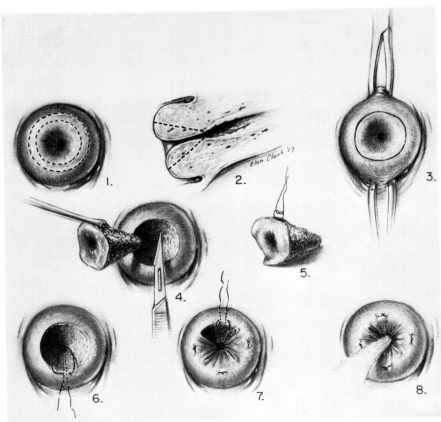

**Figure 16** Technique of cold-knife conization of the cervix. (From Parker, R. T.: Obstet. Gynec. Survey, *24*:691, 1969.)

endocervical glands is "milked" into the endocervical canal. A sterile culture swab is introduced into the endocervical canal, with care not to contaminate the swab with other vaginal secretions. One such swab is spread on a slide, dried, stained with Gram's stain, and examined under high microscopic power for the classic gramnegative intracellular diplococci. Another swab is immediately plated onto Thayer-Martin medium, and then incubated in carbon dioxide for culture identification. One should never inform a patient that she unequivocally has gonorrhea on the basis of a smear, although therapy can be initiated. Diagnosis of this disease without culture identification may be fraught with legal hazard.

### Endometrial Studies

The endometrial biopsy is used to study hormonal effects, fertility, and ovulatory factors and, on occasion, to aid in the diagnosis of malignancy. The procedure is done without anesthesia and discomfort is minimal. By the insertion of a fine curet several samples of endometrium can be obtained for histopathologic examination. Endocrine changes are reflected quite adequately through such endometrial biopsy techniques and, by timing the biopsy to the latter half of the menstrual cycle, the presence of progesterone and ovulation can be detected. For conditions of abnormal bleeding or abnormal genital cytologic findings the endometrial biopsy may provide the tissue for appropriate diagnosis of endometrial or uterine malignant disease, dysfunctional bleeding, polyps, or other abnormalities. If the diagnosis is negative, however, an indicated dilation and curettage should seldom be replaced by endometrial biopsy since the tissue sampled by curettage is considerably greater and diagnosis more accurate.

### Pregnancy Tests

Pregnancy may be detected by a variety of tests that detect the presence of human chorionic gonadotropin (HCG). Most biologic tests have been replaced by immunologic tests which give a positive result with a urinary level of 0.5 to 1.0 IU per milliter, concentrations that are usually achieved 2 weeks after the first missed menstrual period. False-positive pregnancy tests can occur. As HCG and pituitary luteinizing hormone (LH) cross-react, these tests are intentionally set at higher levels to reduce false-positive results from the hypergonadotropinuria of normally timed or premature menopause. To adequately measure normal pituitary gonadotropins, 0.005 IU per milliter or less, sensitive biologic assays on urinary concentrates or the new, highly sensitive radioimmunoassay must be employed.

### Other Studies

Several other diagnostic tests should be mentioned. Hysterosalpingography is a technique by which a cannula attached to the cervix allows the uterine cavity and fallopian tubes to be filled with a radiopaque dye.[6] By appropriate x-ray techniques the endometrial cavity and tubes can be outlined quite adequately. Laparoscopy and culdoscopy are techniques by which the pelvic viscera can be directly visualized by a transperitoneal route and with a minimum of morbidity.

## CONGENITAL ANOMALIES
### Imperforate Hymen

An imperforate hymen may lead to retention of mucus or blood, causing hematocolpos, hematometrium, hematosalpinx, and even hemoperitoneum. Such defects are rarely recognized until after puberty and the onset of menses, and may present as primary amenorrhea, pelvic pain, or a palpable abdominal-pelvic mass. Diagnosis is based on careful examination of the external genitals which reveals a bulging hymen, without communication with the vagina, and a fluctuant pelvic mass that lies anterior to the rectum. With adequate surgical drainage the distended structures will promptly return to normal.

A transverse vaginal septum is rare but may present in similar fashion to that of imperforate hymen. A vertical vaginal septum occurs with failure of müllerian fusion. In both cases the septum can be partial or complete. Therapy, if necessary at all, is surgical excision.

### Defects of Müllerian Fusion (Fig. 17)

Other defects in müllerian fusion can present a spectrum of congenital anomalies. As one tube and half of the uterine fundus, cervix, and upper vagina arise from each müllerian duct, improper fusion can result in duplication of part or all of the system. One abnormality is uterus didelphys with two vaginas, cervices, and uteri, each with a separate tube and ovary. Such patients can present with pelvic pain due to obstruction of outflow of blood from one uterine horn, as an intra-abdominal crisis if pregnancy occurs in a rudimentary uterine horn that cannot expand properly, or as an undiagnosed pelvic mass. Therapy, if indicated, is surgical excision or reconstruction.

### Dysgenesis

There are a variety of defects of the female genital tract due to hypoplasia or aplasia of its various components. Such defects may occur either primarily or as secondary underdevelopment due to lack of estrogen. Congenital absence of both ovaries is rare, but absence of one tube or ovary at birth is not unusual. There are cases of complete absence of the vagina, usually associated with absence of the uterus, and congenital absence of the uterus despite a normal vagina. In these patients the testicular feminizing syndrome should be suspected, in which the gonad is testicular, yet secondary sexual characteristics are feminine. Most of these patients present with primary amenorrhea, and are infertile. Jacobs has shown that 40 per cent of patients with primary amenorrhea have demonstrable chromosomal abnormalities or sex inversions of some type. Buccal smears and karyotypic studies are therefore important. In patients with vaginal agenesis a normally functional vagina can be surgically created by dissection or progressive dilation of the potential space between bladder and rectum. Skin grafting may be required. Such reconstruction should be delayed until just prior to marriage as repetitive dilation is mandatory to retain patency. If the primary defect is due to ovarian abnormalities, replacement of estrogen provides a growth stimulus to the genital structures. In patients with testicular feminization the intra-abdominal gonad should be removed in late adolescence because of the high rates of malignancy during the third and fourth decades of life.

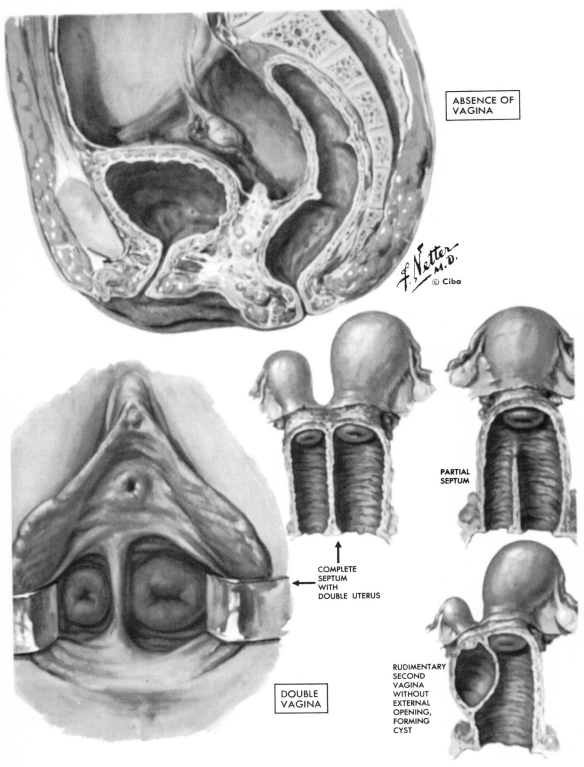

**Figure 17**   Abnormalities of genital formation. (© Copyright 1954, 1965, CIBA Pharmaceutical Company, Division of CIBA Corporation. From The CIBA Collection of Medical Illustrations by Frank H. Netter, M.D.)

### Hermaphroditism

True hermaphroditism, a medical rarity, exists when male and female gonadal tissue is present in the same person. Most hermaphrodites are pseudohermaphrodites, or persons who possess the genitalia of one sex and gonads of the opposite sex. Chromosomal studies are of use in evaluating such patients and the reader is referred to excellent review articles of Miller and Simpson.[10, 17] A male pseudohermaphrodite has testes with the genitalia of a female. An example is the testicular feminization syndrome. A female pseudohermaphrodite has ovaries but the external genitals resemble those of a male. Such persons usually have a combination of anatomic maldevelopment and congenital adrenal hyperplasia. In these patients excess androgen from the hyperfunctioning fetal adrenal cortex results in persistence of the urogenital sinus and marked hypertrophy of the clitoris. The vagina, cervix, uterus, tubes, and ovaries are present but hypoplastic and nonfunctional. Patients with these abnormalities usually present with problems in sexual identification or with primary genital failure at puberty with amenorrhea or male hypogonadism. Therapy is fraught with problems as the patient's personality, age, and psyche must be carefully weighed in relation to anatomy. In some cases it may be best to assist and encourage the patient to continue to live as previously identified, even if gonadal biopsy shows her to be of the opposite sex. In other patients it may be appropriate to reverse the previous sexual identification by surgery and hormone administration.

During the evaluation of patients with congenital anomalies of the female genital system, one should always evaluate the urinary system. Associated urinary anomalies are quite common, occurring in as many as 50 per cent of such patients.

### Wolffian Duct Persistence

Other congenital anomalies of the female genital system consist of those derived from remnants of the mesonephric duct or the wolffian duct and body, which normally regress during female genital development. The most common of these is the parovarian cyst which arises from the upper wolffian duct and may grow as large as 20 cm. There are no symptoms specific to a parovarian cyst to differentiate if from an ovarian cyst. The treatment is surgical excision with preservation of the tube and ovary. A similar cyst, the hydatid of Morgagni, may also develop near the distal end of the fallopian tube. Significant enlargement of these cysts is rare, and only under unusual circumstances is their removal mandatory. Similarly, the wolffian system may give rise to Gartner's duct cysts. As the lower portion of the wolffian duct courses along the lateral vaginal wall, remnants persist and may later form this tubular cystic tumor mass. Only if dyspareunia develops because of excessive size is surgical excision indicated. Finally, remnants of the mesonephric system may remain in the cervix, broad ligament, and ovarian hilus and develop into bizarre varieties of malignant neoplasms. These include clear cell tumors, adenocarcinomas, and mixed tumors.

## THE VULVA

The gynecologist faces an exceptional variety of problems in the area of the external genitals. Trauma, allergy, inflammatory conditions, infection, degenerative changes, and neoplasia give rise to disorders ranging from minor annoyances to major hazards to life.

The vulva is rich in pigment, which increases in pregnancy. Vitiligo of the vulvar skin is no different from the same lesion in other locations, nor does it require treatment. Vitiligo should not be confused with leukoplakia, in which the skin is whitish, but thickened and leathery. Various skin eruptions involving the body as a whole may affect the vulva and appear as do other lesions elsewhere on the body. Varicose veins of the vulva often are found in association with varicosities of the lower extremities, and pregnancy may cause further hypertrophy. Therapy consists of lower extremity and vulvar support and ligation or injection in the nonpregnant state. A severe direct blow to the vulva may be complicated by subcutaneous hematoma formation. Such a hematoma may dissect widely beneath the fascia of the vulva and it is usually necessary to carry out surgical evacuation. It is frequently difficult to isolate bleeding points and packing is often required. Vulvar lacerations should be cleansed and sutured as lacerations elsewhere on the body.

### Glandular Lesions

The vulvar glands are subject to a variety of disorders. Skenitis usually occurs as a consequence of gonococcal infection. In the acute phase an exudate may be expressed from ductal orifices and the patient often has dysuria and other symptoms of urethral irritation. In chronic infections secondary organisms are usually present and on occasion these glands may become abscessed and require surgical drainage. Antibiotic therapy is indicated for both acute and chronic infections. Infections and cysts of Bartholin glands are common. A Bartholin abscess should be treated with heat until fluctuant, and then sharply incised on the mucocutaneous junction between the vagina and vulva. After drainage the margins of the incision are marsupialized with fine interrupted chromic catgut. Bartholin abscesses may occur from gonococcal infection but more commonly other organisms are involved. Antibiotic therapy is indicated in cases of significant cellulitis or systemic symptoms, but drainage remains the treatment of choice. Bartholin cysts may be marsupialized or excised, but the latter procedure is usually associated with significant blood loss. Small asymptomatic Bartholin cysts usually require no treatment unless biopsy is necessary to exclude malignancy. The vulva is also a common site of sebaceous cysts. These may be removed if they become greatly enlarged or secondarily infected. Rarely, one may find vulvar apocrine tumors, hidradenomas, as raised, red, sessile masses less than 5 cm. in diameter. These are treated by wide local excision.

### Vulvitis

Vulvar irritation occurs from a variety of causes, allergic, infectious, degenerative, or neoplastic. Pruritus unaccompanied by vaginal infection or vulvar skin change suggests allergy as the underlying cause. Usually the sensitivity is due to undergarments made of synthetic fibers or washed in harsh detergents. Other contact irritants can include soaps, vaginal lubricants or sprays, rubber condoms, and spermicidal foams or jellies. Other causes of vulvar irritation include pediculosis pubis or mechanical irritation from obesity, clothing, or menstrual pads. Intestinal parasites may remain on the vulva and cause irritation. Systemic diseases as Hodgkin's disease, diabetes mellitus, leukemia, congestive heart failure, and anemia may cause vulvar irritation. Inadequate nutrition, poor hygiene, and vitamin deficiencies also have been associated with vulvar irritation. The basic principles of management of a patient with vulvitis are to search thoroughly for a diagnosis, treat any specific infectious disease, investigate possible allergies, and then keep the area clean and dry and avoid trauma from scratching, harsh soaps, drugs, ointments, or rubbing with a towel.

The most common cause of vulvar irritation is an infectious vulvovaginitis caused by either *Candida albicans* or *Trichomonas vaginalis* or both. The vulva appears swollen and red and may be excoriated and secondarily infected. Mycotic vulvovaginitis is a common problem among diabetics, oral contraceptive users, and persons receiving systemic antibiotics. Diagnosis is based on fresh-preparation identification of yeast or Trichomonas (see Fig. 15). Therapy is discussed in the section dealing with vaginitis. For both types of infection immediate relief is obtained by additional use of topical creams containing hydrocortisone, or nystatin (Mycostatin), as well as the general instructions for nonspecific vulvitis.

Follicular vulvitis may occur and penicillin treatment and local therapy are recommended. Another cause of infectious vulvitis is herpes progenitalis infection with painful vesicular eruptions. Treatment is supportive. Finally, condylomata acuminata, or venereal warts, occur as a presumed infectious vulvitis of viral origin but also are associated with any irritating vaginal discharge. These benign epithelial neoplasms may be few or many, even to covering the entire perineum and extending onto the vagina or cervix (Fig. 18). Therapy is topical use of podophyllin or 5-fluorouracil. Cautery is used for the more extensive forms of the disease but requires an anesthetic.

A variety of venereal diseases may present as vulvar lesions. The primary chancre of syphilis may involve the external genitals although these lesions are usually found on the vagina or cervix.

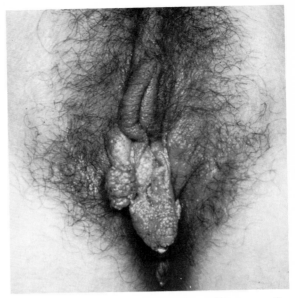

**Figure 18** Condylomata acuminata. These growths may appear anywhere on the vulva. They may be either broad and confluent or papillary. (Courtesy of Mr. C. P. Jones.)

The lesion is a painless, 1 to 2 cm. ulcer with raised, sharp edges and appears 3 to 4 weeks after exposure. The moist, grayish patches that appear in some patients during the secondary stages of syphilis are condylomata lata. Diagnosis of both lesions is made by dark-field examination. Therapy consists of penicillin treatment or a suitable alternate if penicillin sensitivity exists. Granuloma inguinale is a rare infectious disease of the vulva caused by the Donovan bacillus. A scraping of the serpiginous superficial lesion may reveal the intracellular Donovan body. Streptomycin, chloramphenicol (Chloromycetin), and tetracyclines are the most useful agents for this disease. Lymphogranuloma venereum is a disease of viral origin, associated frequently with inguinal adenitis, multiple draining sinuses, and rectal stricture. The diagnosis is made by the Frei skin test. Therapy success depends considerably on the extent of damage present. Chloromycetin and tetracycline are useful, as are the sulfonamides. Surgical repair may be mandatory. Chancroid is caused by the gram-negative Ducrey's bacillus. This disease usually appears as a small papule 2 to 4 days after exposure, and shortly afterward becomes an indurated and punched-out lesion with soft edges and a purulent surface. Inguinal adenitis, often suppurative, is a frequent occurrence. Chancroid is treated with sulfonamides although Chloromycetin, tetracycline, and other broad-spectrum antibiotics may be useful.

### Degenerative Diseases of the Vulva

There are three degenerative diseases of the vulva, all occurring most frequently after menopause. All result in itching, pain, dyspareunia, and frequent secondary infection. These diseases are more commonly seen after vulvar irradiation or premature menopause. The incidence of vulvar carcinoma is increased with these lesions and biopsy should be employed when necessary to rule out neoplasia. Papanicolaou cytology of scrapings is of aid.

Kraurosis vulvae is a disease in which the vulva appears shrunken and dried. Leukoplakia, another degenerative vulvar disease, presents initially as a hypertrophic lesion and later as an atrophic problem. The skin is whitened and leathery. Lichen sclerosus et atrophicus may be difficult to differentiate from either kraurosis or leukoplakia. This is a slowly changing, chronic, localized lesion but, unlike the other two problems, tends to involve the skin of the thighs. In all three lesions an intense pruritus frequently occurs and excoriation with secondary infection is often noted. Approximately 50 per cent of vulvar carcinomas are found in areas of these degenerative lesions and both cytologic smears and biopsy should be frequently used. Treatment of these three lesions is symptomatic with relief of pruritus a primary goal. Topical and systemic estrogens may offer some aid. Local excision is frequently necessary and with more extensive lesions simple vulvectomy may be required

### Carcinoma-in-situ of the Vulva

Bowen originally described a preinvasive cancer of the skin of the vulva and others have noted a high incidence of this disease associated with previous venereal disease. Carcinoma-in-situ of the vulva may appear in a woman who has leukoplakia, kraurosis vulvae, or lichen sclerosus et atrophicus, with or without pruritus. The diagnosis should be made only after adequate histologic study shows the criteria of intraepithelial changes characteristic of epidermoid carcinoma, but without invasion. Treatment should be simple vulvectomy in most instances. In patients with carcinoma-in-situ of the vulva, up to 35 per cent may have a second genital malignant lesion. In approximately 15 per cent of patients with either intraepithelial or invasive carcinoma of the vulva carcinoma of the vagina or cervix later develops. Thus, patients with carcinoma-in-situ of the vulva should be carefully followed.

### Carcinoma of the Vulva (Fig. 19)

Vulvar cancers compose about 3.5 per cent of all genital cancers and the peak incidence occurs in the seventh decade of life. Way reports that among patients with vulvar cancer 20 per cent were between 20 and 50 years old, 26 per cent were in the sixth decade, and 40 per cent were in the 61 to 70 year age range.[20] In approximately half of the patients the cancer develops in areas of pre-existing leukoplakia, kraurosis vulvae, or lichen sclerosus et atrophicus, and others report a high incidence of syphilis and other vulvar venereal diseases among these patients. Most patients with vulvar carcinoma complain of a mass on the vulva or perineum, ulceration or vulvar irritation, or

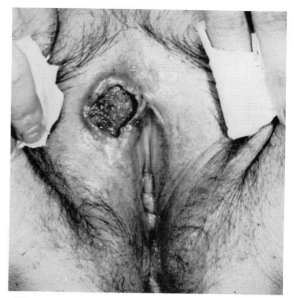

**Figure 19** Carcinoma of the vulva. (Courtesy of Mr. C. P. Jones.)

pruritus. Bleeding and pain may be additional findings. Any firm tumor or ulceration must be biopsied and the biopsy should include the primary lesion and some adjacent normal tissue. There is an average patient delay of 20 months from discovery of some vulvar abnormality.

Carcinoma of the vulva is usually squamous (95 per cent) but adenocarcinoma, melanocarcinoma, basal cell carcinoma, and Paget's disease are reported. Squamous cancer may arise anywhere on the vulva but lesions of the labia majora or labia minora are most frequent. Most squamous cancers of the vulva are rather well differentiated. Adenocarcinoma of the vulva usually arises from Bartholin glands, but may develop from paraurethral glands or embryonic cell nests. Melanocarcinoma is an infrequently found vulvar cancer, as is Paget's disease, a slowly spreading ulcerative eczematoid lesion of the vulvar skin, which is thought to be an adenocarcinoma of the apocrine sweat glands of that region. Basal cell carcinoma of the vulva is most frequently seen on the labium majus but may appear on other structures. Microscopically, basal cell carcinoma shows extensive proliferation of the cells of the basal layer of the epidermis which invade the dermis beneath and usually present as a crater-like ulcer. Unlike other varieties of vulvar cancer, basal cell carcinoma usually does not metastasize but grows deeply into underlying or adjacent tissues. Some basal cell cancers have squamous cell carcinoma elements.

Vulvar cancer tends to spread by local extension and lymphatic metastasis. The frequency and sites of metastasis are dependent upon the size, location, and differentiation of the vulvar lesion. Of those in whom the primary lesion is less than 1.5 cm. in diameter, approximately 12 per cent have positive lymph nodes. However, if the vulvar lesion measures 1.5 to 3.0 cm. in diameter, the incidence of lymph node metastasis is 45 per cent. Way found lymph node metastasis in 62 per cent of cases of anaplastic cancer, but if the primary tumor was well differentiated the incidence of lymphatic metastasis was only 35 per cent. The primary lymphatic drainage of the vulva is via superficial inguinal lymph nodes of that side. From there, the lymphatics drain via Cloquet's node to the external iliac nodes and up the aortic chain. Contralateral vulvar drainage may occur, however, even from well lateralized lesions. The upper vulvar areas, principally around the clitoris, may drain directly to Cloquet's node, which then may be involved with tumor while the superficial inguinal nodes are negative. Vulvar lesions in the perineal, Bartholin, or posterior fourchette areas may involve the rectovaginal septum, rectum, or vagina and may metastasize via the deep pelvic nodes. Way has demonstrated the difficulty of detecting inguinal node metastases by palpation, as many enlarged nodes will not contain metastases while nodes normal to palpation may have tumor cells when microscopically examined.[20] In general, however, if the primary vulvar lesion is small and the superficial inguinal lymphatics and Cloquet's node are negative, it is unlikely that the deeper nodes will be involved. Metastasis may also occur to the skin of the thigh, pubis, groin, and bladder, urethra, upper vagina, or the rectovaginal septum. Blood-borne metastases are unusual.

The treatment of vulvar cancer is surgical. Radiotherapy has been of little use for primary or recurrent disease, and is contraindicated because of the risk of intense vulvar necrosis. Basal cell carcinoma and Paget's disease of the vulva should be treated with wide and deep local excision of the tumor and, if it is large, hemivulvectomy should be done. Removal of regional lymph nodes is not indicated. The prognosis is generally excellent, but these patients should be followed closely for local recurrence. *Such operations as local excision, hemivulvectomy, and simple vulvectomy have proved to be inadequate therapy for the other forms of vulvar cancer.* Most authors have outlined appropriate therapy as including at least a block dissection of the vulva, in continuity, removing the skin, subcutaneous tissues, and lymphatic tissues of the groins, vulva, and perineum as one specimen. Controversy exists as to whether all patients should also have a retroperitoneal node dissection to include removal of the femoral, iliac, and obturator nodes. These procedures are usually done as a one-stage operation, but may be divided, with the deep node dissection performed later. Utilizing the radical vulvectomy and node dissections, one can expect a 5 year cure rate of over 80 per cent in patients without positive nodes, and a 5 year survival of 47 per cent of patients with positive inguinal nodes. Overall, the 5 year cure rate after surgical therapy of cancer of the vulva is approximately 60 per cent. If the vulvar lesion involves the vagina, rectum, or urethra, then pelvic exenteration may be the operation of choice. Recurrence of surgically treated vulvar cancer may occur at the skin margins of the primary operation or in the skin of the groin. Distant metastases may also develop. Therapy of recurrent vulvar cancer with local excision or chemotherapy may provide palliation.

## THE VAGINA

The stratified squamous epithelium of the vagina is histologically similar to epithelium of the cervix and the skin of the vulva, and responds by proliferation to estrogen. The vagina of the child and that of the postmenopausal woman are similar in that the epithelial layer is quite thin, is easily traumatized, and is subject to a variety of infections. The normal adult vagina contains diphtheroids, Döderlein's bacilli, and anaerobic streptococci. This flora converts glycogen of vaginal cells to lactic acid which maintains the vagina with an acid pH and enhances normal secretions.

### Vaginitis

Vaginal inflammation can occur from protozoan, fungal, bacterial, or viral infection and also from deficiencies of estrogen. *Trichomonas vaginalis* is a common protozoan organism causing pruritus, tenderness, and dyspareunia. Trichomonas vaginitis is characterized by a foamy, greenish yellow vaginal exudate; the vaginal walls are erythematous and tender. The diagnosis of this infection is made by high-power microscopic examination of fresh preparations of the vaginal discharge and identification of the flagellated, motile organisms which are the size of leukocytes (see Fig. 15). There is uncertainty about the epidemiology of trichomonas vaginitis, but it is seen most commonly among sexually active women. The male sexual partner may harbor these organisms without symptoms and promptly reinfect the women who has been treated successfully. This infection is also frequently seen in chronically ill and debilitated women and in women with other pelvic infections. Current therapy consists of oral metronidazole (Flagyl) for both sexual partners.

*Candida albicans* is probably the most frequent and bothersome cause of vaginitis. The wide use of antibiotics and oral contraceptives predisposes to this fungal infection, as does diabetes mellitus. Symptoms are vaginal discharge, vulvar and vaginal irritation, and itching. Inspection reveals a "curdy" white vaginal exudate, intense vaginal erythema, and a white watery discharge. Diagnosis is made from fresh preparations of vaginal discharge which microscopically reveal the mycelia as threadlike fibers or budding forms (see Fig. 15). Cultures on Sabouraud's medium may be necessary to identify the etiology of low-grade vaginitis. Therapy consists of the intravaginal application of Mycostatin suppositories each night for 2 weeks, including during the menses if it occurs. There is a tendency for vaginal moniliasis to recur and in these patients one should consider evaluation for diabetes mellitus. If such a patient is taking oral contraceptives, their use may have to be temporarily terminated until the infection is controlled.

Vaginal irritation can occur in the patient with insufficient estrogen to maintain normal vaginal thickness. Infection of this thin, atrophic, easily traumatized vagina is nonspecific and caused by a variety of usually nonpathogenic bacteria. Treatment is replacement of systemic or topical estrogen. *Haemophilus vaginalis* can also cause severe vaginitis. Treatment with sulfonamides or tetracyclines is usually successful after smear or culture diagnosis is made. Herpes simplex virus may result in an intense, painful vaginitis that is associated with a granular surface and vesicular eruptions. The diagnosis is made clinically and by serial serum antibody determinations. Therapy is supportive but, fortunately, the disease usually terminates within 2 to 3 weeks. Gonorrhea is an occasional cause of vaginitis in the child. The diagnosis is made by smear and culture and therapy with penicillin is recommended. Children with vaginitis should be examined for intestinal parasites and intravaginal foreign bodies. Rarely do these last three causes of childhood vaginitis produce similar problems in the adult.

### Dysplasia and Intraepithelial Carcinoma of the Vagina

Dysplasia of the vaginal epithelium may be the source of abnormal genital smears even if the cervix is normal or absent. Treatment consists of replacement with systemic or topical estrogen and regular follow-up. Intraepithelial carcinoma may also develop, most commonly in patients treated previously for other lower genital tract cancers. These lesions may occur at the apex of the vagina in patients after hysterectomy or may be multifocal in areas remote from the vaginal apex. As in dysplasia, intraepithelial carcinoma of the vagina causes no specific symptoms. Diagnosis is suspected from genital cytology and confirmed by biopsy. Therapy can be by irradiation or surgery, either partial or total colpectomy. These lesions justify the close follow-up suggested for patients, even adequately treated, who have had other lower genital tract cancers. Results of therapy are excellent.

### Carcinoma of the Vagina

Primary carcinoma of the vagina is a rare lesion and most are epidermoid in variety. Postcontact bleeding is the usual presenting complaint. Many patients with invasive vaginal carcinoma have previously had other preinvasive or invasive epidermoid lesions of the lower genital system. Primary vaginal cancer may occur in any location, but prognosis is considerably more grave if the lesion is situated anteriorly. The current classification of primary vaginal cancer (International Federation of Gynecology and Obstetrics) includes: Stage I, limited to the vaginal mucosa; Stage II, subvaginal tissue involved, but not to the pelvic wall; Stage III, tumor extended to the pelvic wall or to the symphysis, but not fixed to the symphysis; Stage IV, tumor fixed to symphysis, outside the pelvis, or proved by biopsy to involve the bladder or rectum. Treatment may be by irradiation or surgery. Rutledge's most recent review of radiation therapy of primary vaginal carcinoma describes the type of treatment varying according to the location of the vaginal lesion. In general, it consists of 3000 to 5000 rads of external irradiation followed by 5000 to 3000 rads of intravaginal radium by sources specifically designed to deliver the radiation to the primary lesion. He reports survivors as follows: Stage I, 16 of 22 patients; Stage II, 19 of 25 patients; Stage III, 3 of 14 patients; Stage IV, 3 of 16 patients. Complications of therapy are relatively low, but include radiation cystitis and proctitis. Individualization of therapy was recommended.[15] Exenterative surgery may be used as primary therapy or therapy for recurrence. Results of primary surgical therapy are not as good as those achieved with irradiation, and the operative and postoperative morbidity and mortality are significant.

The vagina may also be the site of other histologic types of cancer, including melanocarcinoma, sarcoma, and mesonephric adenocarcinoma. Melanomas of this organ have an extremely poor prognosis, regardless of therapy utilized. Only 3 of 30 patients reported in the literature have survived 5 years or longer. Surgery should be radical, usually exenterative, and should include removal of the regional lymph nodes. Sarcoma of the vagina, the so-called "sarcoma botryoides," is most frequently seen in children and the prognosis is grave. Irradiation is ineffective and radical surgery is only of limited success. These tumors are thought to be of mixed mesodermal origin. Primary vaginal adenocarcinoma is occasionally seen, showing a variable histologic pattern and thought to be secondary to remnants of the mesonephric duct in one of the lateral vaginal fornices or from paraurethral glands. Treatment is usually surgical although irradiation is frequently of assistance. Such adenocarcinomas may be metastatic.

## DEFECTS OF PELVIC SUPPORT

The major support of the uterus and vagina is provided by the cardinal ligaments, condensations of endopelvic fascia at the bases of the broad ligaments. The round, broad, and uterosacral ligaments are more important in maintaining uterine position than in providing support. Support from the vaginal side of the bladder and rectum is provided by the pubocervical fascia which is not true fascia but condensed connective tissue in the vesicovaginal and rectovaginal septum. The distal vagina is also supported by the perineal body. Overdistention of these supporting structures, usually by childbirth, may give rise to a variety of defects in pelvic support. Frequently, these defects cause few symptoms until atrophy after menopause results in further weakness. Such de-

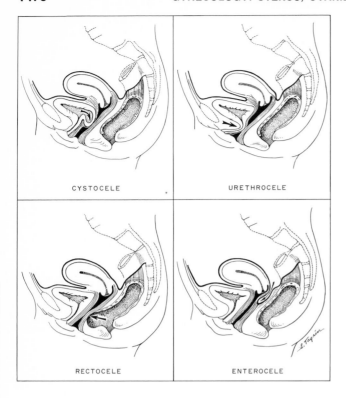

CYSTOCELE

URETHROCELE

RECTOCELE

ENTEROCELE

**Figure 20** Diagrammatic representation of the four most common types of pelvic floor relaxation: cystocele, urethrocele, rectocele, and enterocele. Arrows depict sites of maximal protrusion. (From Gynecology: Principles and Practice by Robert W. Kistner. Copyright © 1964. Year Book Medical Publishers. Used by permission.)

fects include cystocele, urethrocele, rectocele, enterocele, and uterine descensus (Fig. 20).

### Cystocele and Urethrocele; Stress Urinary Incontinence

A cystocele is a herniation of the anterior vaginal wall with secondary relaxation, descent, and protrusion of the bladder floor into the vaginal introitus. Cystocele is usually accompanied by urethrocele, and not infrequently by some degree of uterine descensus or rectocele. The classic symptoms of cystocele are vaginal protrusion and recurrent cystitis which occurs because of incomplete bladder emptying. A large cystocele may be relatively asymptomatic. Surgical repair is indicated not for the size of the cystocele, but rather for its symptoms. A common problem associated with cystocele is urethrocele and together they may produce flattening of the vesical neck, predisposing to stress urinary incontinence. Stress incontinence can be identified by observation of bladder support during Valsalva maneuver. If pressure and elevation lateral to the urethrovesical junction inhibits the incontinence (Marshall test), good results can be expected from surgical repair. Such supporting surgery should be postponed until childbearing has been completed, for delivery after repair will usually be accompanied by return of the defect. The primary surgical repair is usually anterior colporrhaphy, frequently performed with vaginal hysterectomy. This operation includes separating the overlying vaginal mucosa from the bladder and urethra, fol-

lowed by plication of the pubocervical fascia beneath these organs before reclosure of the vaginal mucosa. Elevation and narrowing of the urethrovesical neck are the keys to success of the procedure. Anterior colporrhaphy will provide successful repair in approximately 85 per cent of patients with stress urinary incontinence. Such procedures as the retropubic Marshall-Marchetti-Krantz cystourethropexy or suburethral sling techniques may offer good results for the remaining patients.

### Rectocele

Rectocele is protrusion of the rectal wall toward the vaginal canal. In this condition, the paravaginal tissue which is normally interposed between the vagina and rectum becomes attenuated and lacerated during delivery. Symptoms of rectocele are vaginal protrusion and sacculation of the rectal wall when fecal material is propelled into the anal canal. Defecation may require digital pressure to the posterior vaginal wall to force the feces from the sacculation back into the ampulla. Such problems may be reduced by posterior colpoperineorrhaphy by which the rectovaginal fascia is rebuilt and the pubococcygeus and lower levator ani muscles are joined. Most patients with rectocele also have some associated cystocele or uterine descensus. Thus, vaginal hysterectomy and anterior colporrhaphy must be combined with the posterior repair for best results. In addition, combined repairs may be mutually supporting, as the posterior repair may provide extra support for cystourethrocele. Nonoperative treatment is usually unsuccessful.

### Enterocele

Pelvic enterocele is a herniation of the peritoneum of the cul-de-sac with invagination of the sac into the rectovaginal septum. A sliding hernia may develop in this space, usually created by labor, delivery, or vaginal hysterectomy. An enterocele of considerable size may exist without symptoms, but most will provoke pelvic pressure, pain, and posterior vaginal protrusion. Enterocele may be difficult to separate from rectocele, but combined rectovaginal examination, or examination with the patient in the standing position, will usually clarify the problem. Enterocele may be surgically repaired by vaginal or abdominal approaches, but the gynecologist usually utilizes the former to allow repair of other associated defects. From either approach, surgical repair of enterocele consists of plication of the uterosacral ligaments and obliteration of the cul-de-sac. If there is accompanying rectocele it should be repaired.

### Prolapse of the Uterus

Uterine prolapse, or procidentia and descensus uteri, occurs when the uterus and its adjoining structures herniate through the vaginal canal. Prolapse is described as first, second, and third degree in severity, the latter being protrusion of the entire uterus from the vagina, with the entire vagina inverted as a consequence. While congenital weakness of the supporting tissues may rarely cause uterine prolapse, the most frequent cause is childbirth. The symptoms of uterine prolapse are protrusion of the cervix or uterus through the introitus. Prolapse frequently is associated with cystocele or rectocele and these defects may cause presenting symptoms. Other symptoms include backache, significant pelvic pressure, and ulceration or bleeding of the prolapsed structures. Uterine prolapse cannot be cured by nonoperative means, but can be supported by a pessary in most patients if surgery is not feasible. Uterine prolapse is best approached vaginally for surgical repair since abdominal procedures are usually inadequate. Successful procedures include vaginal hysterectomy and repair of the pelvic diaphragm, procedures that preserve the uterus while resupporting these structures, and total colpocleisis if coital function is never again anticipated.

## BENIGN DISEASES OF THE CERVIX

The portio vaginalis of the normal cervix is covered with squamous epithelium that is similar to that of the vagina. In the nulliparous woman the external cervical os is a centrally located, small, round opening connecting with the endocervical canal. After childbearing, the external os is longitudinally flattened. Mucus-secreting columnar epithelium lines the endocervical canal and its junction with the squamous epithelium of the cervical portio is the squamocolumnar zone.

### Cervicitis

Cervical infection, in one form or another, is one of the most frequently encountered gynecologic lesions. Acute cervicitis is rarely seen except in gonorrhea, in patients with acute vaginitis from *Trichomonas vaginalis* or *Candida albicans*, in patients with puerperal endometritis, or in patients with retained intravaginal foreign bodies. The cervix is erythematous and edematous, and leukocytic infiltration is prominent. Pain and tenderness are rarely prominent symptoms, but a purulent discharge is frequently seen. Diagnosis is made by appropriate smears and cultures (see Laboratory Tests) and therapy with topical or systemic antibiotics usually is curative.

In chronic cervicitis the cervical mucus is mucopurulent and profuse. The histologic changes seen in chronic cervicitis are variable and are present to some extent in nearly all women. Cellular changes such as metaplasia, epidermization, and hyperplasia of the basal cells are frequently seen. Often seen are erosions or eversions of the cervix. An erosion is a true ulcer of the cervix while the eversion is formed by columnar epithelium of the endocervical canal proliferating downward, forming a lowered squamocolumnar line. Orifices of the cervical mucus-secreting glands may become obstructed to form nabothian cysts. A mucopurulent discharge may be the only symptom of chronic cervicitis, although postcontact bleeding, infertility, and, rarely, pain may occur. Diagnosis is based on cytology and biopsy, but one must remember that while cervical cytologic studies are very effective in the discovery of early cervical cancer with an intact surface epithelium, they are much less reliable when an erosion is present. Colposcopy, colpomicroscopy, and iodine staining may be of aid in localizing areas for biopsy. Any suspicious or eroded area should be biopsied before treatment. Therapy of chronic cervicitis is usually by electrodesiccation, by ultrarefrigeration (cryosurgery), or with silver nitrate. Cautery should include the involved exocervix and endocervical canal, and rarely requires an anesthetic. These methods destroy the infection of the columnar area and allow the squamous epithelium to grow over the area. Repeated cautery, surgical conization, and, on occasion, even hysterectomy (if childbearing is ended) may be necessary for severe chronic cervicitis.

### Cervical Polyps

Polyps may arise from the endocervix and are rarely malignant. The usual symptom is postcontact bleeding. They appear as single or multiple, cherry red growths protruding from the external cervical os. Such polyps may be removed by biopsy or dilation and curettage, with cauterization of the pedicle. One must not overlook uterine or other cervical causes of abnormal bleeding which may be the symptom of other, more severe, pelvic disease. Another polypoid hyperplastic lesion, atypical endocervical hyperplasia, may develop in oral contraceptive users. The gross appearance is that of a polyp and histologically it may resemble adenocarcinoma. This is not a malignant lesion, however, and will regress with discontinuation of use of the contraceptive pills.

# CANCER OF THE CERVIX

Invasive carcinoma of the cervix is the most common pelvic malignant disease and accounts for 15 per cent of cancers of women. At birth there is a probability that 2.3 per cent of our female population will eventually have cervical cancer; and it is currently estimated that 10,000 women die in this country each year from these neoplasms. It is encouraging that, during the past 15 years, primarily through early detection, the death rate from cervical cancer has declined from 21.8 to 11.5 per 100,000 population. Invasive carcinoma of the cervix should be a preventable disease as regular examinations and frequent use of today's diagnostic techniques should enable detection of nearly all patients with preinvasive cervical carcinoma, a totally curable disease.

The average age of occurrence of carcinoma of the cervix is 48 years, with the majority of patients between 35 and 55 years of age. However, many authors have reported cervical cancer in women as young as the teens and as old as the eighth decade. Much has been written about the etiology of cervical carcinoma. Epidemiologic studies show peak instances of this disease among women of low socioeconomic status, among those who begin coitus and childbearing at an early age, and among women with multiple sexual partners. Heredity seems to play a small role. The theory of a viral relationship has been advanced, suggesting that a virus transmitted through intercourse is responsible for cervical cancer.[2, 3]

## Cervical Dysplasia

Dysplastic changes may be seen in epithelium exfoliated or biopsied from the cervix. While this is not a diagnosis of malignancy, patients with cervical dysplasia should be followed with cytologic studies every 4 to 6 months for it has been found that carcinoma-in-situ of the cervix will develop in a significant percentage of these patients over the subsequent several years. Dysplasia may resemble carcinoma-in-situ of the cervix, but the abnormal cells do not extend through the full thickness of epithelium. Cervical biopsy should be frequently employed as well as the colpomicroscopic and iodine staining techniques. Recent studies suggest electrocautery, cryosurgery, or biopsy may cure the lesions, and many patients with limited dysplasia do quite well without treatment.

## Preinvasive or Carcinoma-in-situ of the Cervix

Bowen in 1912 described a preinvasive malignant lesion of the skin and in the same year Schottlander, Rubin, and Schiller described preinvasive carcinoma of the cervix. During the next 30 years this interesting lesion was noted only but ultimately it was described as a precursor to invasive carcinoma of the cervix. It remained for Papanicolaou and Traut, in 1941, to develop the cytologic evaluation of exfoliated cells that suggests the need for biopsy and adequate tissue study. Histopathologically, carcinoma-in-situ consists of cellular changes in the squamous epithelium of the cervix that are compatible with cancer, but evidence of invasion in the underlying stroma is absent. Glandular epithelial replacement by neoplastic cells may be mistaken for invasion and it is important that this differentiation be made. Other benign conditions that may confuse diagnosis are atypical basilar hyperplasia and the metaplasia and hyperplasia of glandular elements frequently seen in pregnancy. The peak incidence of carcinoma-in-situ is approximately 35 to 40 years of age. *There are no gross lesions or symptoms of carcinoma-in-situ of the cervix.* The use of Papanicolaou cytology screening and adequate biopsy techniques are discussed in the Laboratory Tests section of this chapter. The diagnosis of carcinoma-in-situ is made by histologic review of biopsy specimens (Fig. 21).

The treatment of carcinoma-in-situ of the cervix is abdominal or vaginal hysterectomy with excision of 2 to 3 cm. of upper vagina. The tubes and ovaries are usually left in place in younger women. Radical hysterectomy and pelvic lymph node dissection is not indicated for this lesion. Results of therapy are uniformly good and 5 year survival approaches 100 per cent.[11] Radiation therapy may be indicated for carcinoma-in-situ but it usually results in ablation of ovarian function and may cause the same side effects as radiation therapy for invasive carcinoma.[9] As carcinoma-in-situ is a disease of younger women the question of allowing continued reproduction prior to hysterectomy has been raised. If the patient has normal smears after conization and desires to have more children, we have allowed her to do so and delivery vaginally. Hysterectomy is recommended after childbearing is ended, even if cytologic findings are benign. If the smears remain positive after conization, hysterectomy is suggested at that time. If abnormal smears are detected during pregnancy, cervical conization is used for diagnosis, or quadrant biopsy in later pregnancy and when there is no obvious lesion present. If carcinoma-in-situ is detected the pregnancy is allowed to continue with vaginal delivery. If invasive carcinoma is present, adequate therapy is begun immediately.[11]

## Microinvasive Cancer of the Cervix

There has been considerable debate as to both the diagnosis and treatment of microinvasive carcinoma of the cervix, a condition in which carcinoma-in-situ exists and there is less than 5 mm. of invasion present. Data showing lack of nodal metastasis have led to treatment of patients as if the lesions were only carcinoma-in-situ. Results of this treatment in microinvasive cancer of the cervix are equally as good as those of full radical surgery or irradiation and morbidity has been much less.

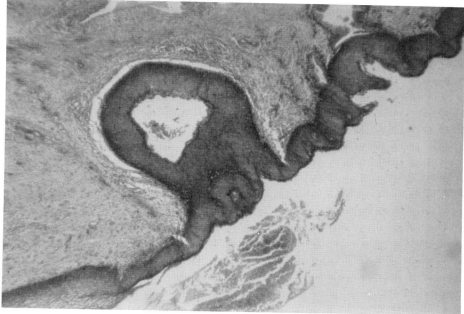

**Figure 21** Carcinoma-in-situ of the cervix. Note sharp demarcation between normal and malignant epithelium (lower border) and the glandular epithelial involvement. (Courtesy of Dr. D. E. D. Jones.)

## Carcinoma of the Cervix

Approximately 95 per cent of cervical cancers are squamous, the remaining 5 per cent usually being adenocarcinoma. Most often the adenocarcinoma arises from the mucus-secreting epithelium of the cervix, but rarely adenocarcinoma may arise in mesonephric duct remnants. Squamous cell, or epidermoid, carcinoma of the cervix usually arises at the squamocolumnar junction. Varying degrees of microscopic differentiation are found. A halo of carcinoma-in-situ is frequently found around the invasive cancer or on the vagina.

There are no symptoms of early carcinoma of the cervix; the first symptoms of bleeding, usually postcontact, or a bloody discharge, do not begin until ulceration is present. More advanced cervical cancers cause symptoms referable to invasion of adjacent organs (bladder, rectum, ureter) or to distant metastasis. Pain is a sign of advanced cervical cancer.

Although cytologic findings and clinical appearance may strongly suggest carcinoma of the cervix, the diagnosis can be made only by histopathologic study. In the presence of an obvious exophytic lesion, as is found in more than 80 per cent of patients with even early cervical cancer, tissue may be easily obtained by punch biopsy. If the lesion is endophytic, or if the punch biopsy shows carcinoma-in-situ, or less, conization may be mandatory to fully evaluate abnormal cytologic studies. Broken and ulcerated epithelium and proliferating tissue that bleeds easily upon touch are most valuable clinical signs, particularly when such lesions involve the squamocolumnar junction. Colposcopy and staining techniques may aid direction of biopsies.

If treatment of cervical cancer is adequate, the single most important factor in prognosis is the extent of disease when therapy is begun. For this reason each patient should have a careful pelvic examination, cystoscopy, proctoscopy, intravenous pyelography, and x-rays of the chest and bones so that the extent of the disease may be established. Staging of cervical cancer is arrived at by entirely clinical evaluation and is made before treatment is initiated (Fig. 22). Such staging should not be changed at any later time. We currently utilize the classification for clinical staging of cervical carcinoma provided in 1966 by the Cancer Committee of the International Federation of Gynecology and Obstetrics:

Stage 0
    Carcinoma-in-situ (preinvasive or intraepithelial).
Stage I
    Carcinoma confined entirely to the cervix (IA, early stromal invasion; IB, all other Stage I lesions).
Stage II
    Carcinoma extends beyond the cervix but has not reached either the pelvic sidewall or the lower third of the vagina. (IIA, no parametrial involvement; IIB, parametrial involvement is present).
Stage III
    Carcinoma has reached the pelvic sidewall or the lower third of the vagina.
Stage IV
    Carcinoma involves the bladder, rectum, distant nodes, or distant areas.

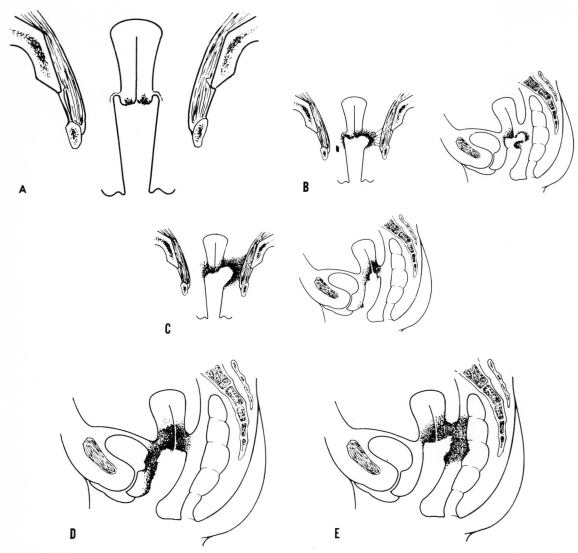

**Figure 22**    Stages of carcinoma of the cervix. *A,* Stage I, the cancer is confined to the cervix. *B,* Stage II, the cancer is confined to the parametrium on one or both sides, and is not fixed to either pelvic wall. Or the cancer involves the upper one-third of the vagina. *C,* Stage III, the cancer has spread to one or both pelvic walls, or has invaded the lower one-third of the vagina. *D,* and *E,* Stage IV, the cancer involves the bladder or the rectum, or it has spread beyond the pelvis. (From Taylor, E. S.: Essentials of Gynecology. 4th ed. Philadelphia, Lea & Febiger, 1969.)

While clinical staging is done before therapy, it is useful to understand the significance of such staging on disease spread. The most common method of tumor spread, and most frequent cause of patient death, is direct extension of cervical cancer to involve the vagina, uterus, parametrium, pelvic sidewall, ureter, bladder, and rectum. More than 50 per cent of patients who die with cervical cancer die of ureteral obstruction and uremia. Fistula formation from ureter, bladder, and rectum is not infrequently seen and bleeding may be a serious complication. Carcinoma of the cervix also has a propensity for lymphatic metastasis. Lymphatic drainage of the cervix is via the hypo-gastric and obturator lymph chains to the iliac and then aortic nodal systems. Vertebral lymphatic metastases may also occur. Morton and others have shown positive lymph node metastases in the following percentages of clinically staged cases of cervical carcinoma: Stage I, 16.5; Stage II, 31.9; Stage III, 46.7; and Stage IV, 80.8.[2] In addition to the clinical staging, the size of the primary cervical lesion has also been shown to influence the frequency with which lymph node metastases are found: less than 1 cm., rare metastases; 1 to 3 cm., 17 per cent with metastases; greater than 3 cm., 52 per cent with lymph node metastases. These latter two factors of lymphatic node metastasis are variable and of little use in the therapy of a given patient. Other studies have shown that lymphatic spread beyond the pelvic nodal chains is present in more than 40 per cent of patients who die of cervical cancer. Autopsy data demonstrate distant metastases in many patients dying of carcinoma of the cervix and nearly every organ may be involved. Most common sites of distant metastases include: liver, 16 per cent; lung, 14 per cent; vertebrae, 9 per cent; and other bony metastases, 9 per cent.

**Treatment of Cervical Cancer.** Carcinoma of the cervix can be effectively treated by surgery or irradiation, *but treatment does not include simple hysterectomy or nonindividualized radiotherapy.* No other major lesion requires more critical selection of techniques and methods of therapy. The present operation for cancer of the cervix (Stages I and IIA) is an extended hysterectomy (Wertheim) which removes the parametrial tissues, the upper third of the vagina, and perhaps the adnexa, and a pelvic node dissection which removes the iliac, hypogastric, ureteral, obturator, and lower aortic lymph nodes. The radical operation for cancer of the cervix has two primary disadvantages: first, there is a 7 to 8 per cent incidence of ureteral or bladder fistula; and second, few surgeons are qualified to undertake the operation and perform it satisfactorily. Certain patients with Stage IV carcinoma, those with only rectal or bladder involvement, may be candidates for primary surgical therapy by pelvic exenteration. The results of primary surgical treatment for cervical cancer are perhaps best demonstrated by Brunschwig's data from 703 patients managed by the choice of operations just noted.[1] That study showed 5 year survivals of: Stage I, 78.8 per cent; Stage II, 53.0 per cent; Stage III, 31.3 per cent; Stage IV, 19.7 per cent. The numbers of patients with Stages III and IV disease were small. The operative mortality was 2.3 per cent and a high rate of postoperative urinary fistulas was reported. Most gynecologists now reserve the primary surgical treatment of of carcinoma of the cervix for those patients with smaller Stage I or early Stage II lesions.

Most clinics favor primary radiation treatment of cancer of the cervix. The purpose of therapy is to deliver to the lesion and to areas of possible pelvic spread sufficient radiation to destroy the cancer and still not cause irreparable damage to surrounding tissues. Most therapists employ a combination of external supervoltage therapy, such as from cobalt-60 units, and intravaginal, contracervical, and intracervical irradiation with radium. In our clinic external cobalt-60 radiotherapy is initially delivered to a dosage of 4000 to 6000 rads to the entire pelvis, over a 4 to 6 week course. This is followed by one or two radium applications to deliver 6000 to 4000 rads to the primary cervical lesion. In Stages I and II disease we tend to deliver the higher dose by radium; in Stages III and IV disease the higher dose is usually administered by external cobalt-60. Total dosage administered by the two routes approximates 10,000 rads. As in surgery, the prognosis with primary radia-

tion therapy for carcinoma of the cervix varies with the clinical stage present at the time therapy is begun. The usually accepted figures for 5 year survival with this type of treatment are: Stage I, 86.4 per cent; Stage II, 60.0 per cent; Stage III, 26.3 per cent; Stage IV, 8.8 per cent.[2, 9]

As with surgery, there are complications of radiation therapy for cervical cancer. These problems include radiation sickness, leukopenia, pelvic infection, proctitis, cystitis, small bowel injuries, vaginal stenosis, menopausal symptoms, radiation necrosis of vagina and cervix, skin reaction, and fistulas. Many of these problems may develop only at long intervals after therapy and management is based on conservatism, exclusion of extant carcinoma, and surgical repair when indicated. Estrogen replacement may alleviate many of the symptoms and does not appear to influence the likelihood of recurrence of carcinoma.

Regardless of the type of therapy utilized, patients with carcinoma of the cervix must be followed frequently and regularly. We speak hopefully of 5 year "cures," but there are significant numbers of patients in whom recurrent disease will develop 10 or 20 years later or who later have other malignant lesions of the genital tract. Follow-up should include frequent cytologic study and appropriate biopsy. Secondary treatment for therapeutic failures, with surgery or further irradiation, have provided limited success. Chemotherapy has been of palliative aid only.

## BENIGN UTERINE DISEASE

Various benign uterine diseases occur, including leiomyoma uteri, adenomyosis, endometrial hyperplasia, and polyps. Abnormal bleeding, uterine enlargement, and pain are the usual symptoms associated with these diseases but the primary difficulty is to achieve an accurate diagnosis.

### Leiomyoma Uteri

Uterine leiomyomas, also called myomas, fibromyomas, or fibroids, are the most common cause of benign uterine enlargement and are seen in 20 per cent of women. The incidence is higher in the Negro race. Leiomyomas originate from the smooth muscle cells of the myometrium and vary in size from microscopic to large enough to fill the entire abdomen. Such tumors may be single but are more often multiple. On cut section these solid tumors have a white, glistening appearance with a characteristic whorl pattern. There is no true capsule but compressed peripheral fibers form a pseudocapsule. Microscopically, smooth muscle cells are arranged in interlacing muscle bundles, interspaced with varying amounts of connective tissue and hyaline material. Such tumors may be submucous, intramural, subserous, pedunculated, parasitic, cervical, or interligamentous (Fig. 23).

The symptoms of leiomyoma vary according to location; some may produce severe complaints, others none at all. The three most common symptoms are abnormal bleeding, pain, and uterine en-

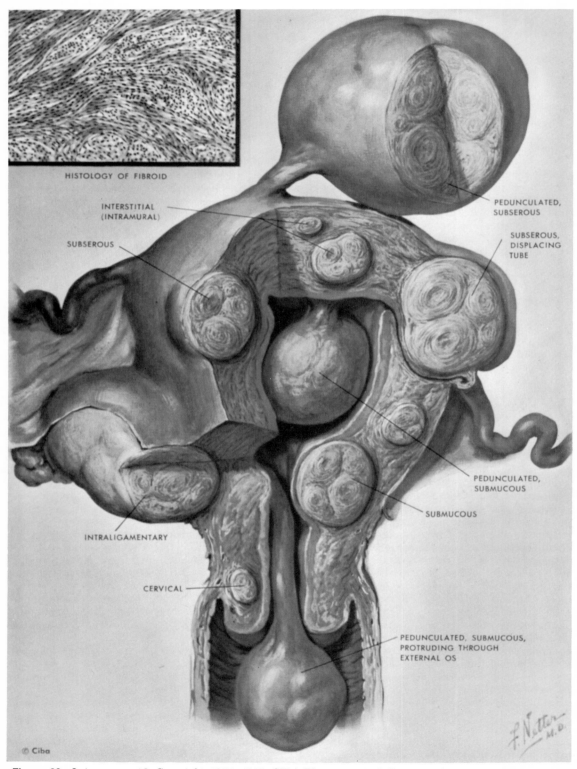

HISTOLOGY OF FIBROID

INTERSTITIAL
(INTRAMURAL)

SUBSEROUS

INTRALIGAMENTARY

CERVICAL

PEDUNCULATED,
SUBSEROUS

SUBSEROUS,
DISPLACING
TUBE

PEDUNCULATED,
SUBMUCOUS

SUBMUCOUS

PEDUNCULATED, SUBMUCOUS,
PROTRUDING THROUGH
EXTERNAL OS

**Figure 23** Leiomyoma. (© Copyright 1954, 1965, CIBA Pharmaceutical Company, Division of CIBA Corporation. From The CIBA Collection of Medical Illustrations by Frank H. Netter, M.D.)

largement. Abnormal bleeding, usually cyclic but profuse and prolonged, is most frequently due to submucous tumors which distort the overlying endometrium and interfere with normal hemostatic mechanisms. Occasionally a submucous or cervical myoma may be extruded and also cause abnormal bleeding. Abnormal bleeding is the most common indication for hysterectomy for leiomyoma, but caution must be taken to exclude other causes as a malignant lesion may coexist with myoma. Often a curettage may be mandatory to make this differentiation. Rapid enlargement is another symptom of concern in patients with leiomyoma, as 1 to 2 per cent of such tumors may undergo sarcomatous change or degeneration of other nonmalignant varieties. Estrogen, including the synthetic estrogens of oral contraceptives, may cause enlargement of myomas. Myomas tend to regress after menopause and any enlargement of these tumors demands prompt removal of the uterus. Slow enlargement of leiomyomas during the menstrual years frequently occurs with a minimum of symptoms. Surgical removal is not mandatory for slow growth or moderate size unless other symptoms occur. Pelvic pressure, frequency of urination, and sciatic or hip pain from pressure on pelvic nerves can be symptoms of uterine leiomyoma. Tenderness in a myoma is usually caused by degeneration or by impairment of the blood supply. Cystic changes and calcification can follow degeneration. Significant pain or tenderness usually warrants hysterectomy. Infertility is not infrequently seen in patients with myomas, nor is abortion, but in the former it is not known whether the infertility or the myoma is primary. The increased rate of abortion is attributed to poor uterine distensibility and compression. While uterine myomas are usually recognized without difficulty in the operating room, their preoperative diagnosis may be quite difficult, especially if the myoma involves primarily one of the adnexa.

The treatment of leiomyoma demands individualization for each patient. Some tumors require no treatment if small and asymptomatic and semiannual examination only is warranted. If a young patient, who desires further childbearing, has symptomatic leiomyomas, then multiple myomectomy is a useful surgical procedure. In larger or more symptomatic myomas in a woman who has completed her reproduction, hysterectomy is the treatment of choice.

### Adenomyosis

Invasion of the myometrium by endometrium, adenomyosis, is a frequent cause of uterine enlargement and pain. Grossly the uterus is enlarged, fibrotic, and thickened and on cut section the areas of endometrial growth and loculated menstruation may be quite apparent.

The classic symptoms and signs of adenomyosis are acquired dysmenorrhea occurring in the 35 to 40 year age group, menstrual irregularities with cyclic, prolonged, and profuse flow, and an enlarged, tender uterus. Treatment is hysterectomy although hormonal suppression (pseudopregnancy regimen with estrogen and progesterone) may provide relief without removal of the uterus.

### Endometrial Hyperplasia and Polyps

Hyperplasia of the endometrium, causing abnormal uterine bleeding, is a common problem of women. Women near menopause, or less frequently in early adolescence, are most frequently affected. The basic problem is anovulation and failure of corpus luteum formation without production of progesterone. Continued stimulation of the endometrium by estrogen brings about proliferation, overgrowth, and cystic hyperplasia of the endometrium. Areas of the thickened endometrium may form polyps. Cycles become irregular with intervals of amenorrhea associated with other intervals of intermenstrual spotting or bleeding. Pelvic examination is usually nonrevealing and curettage produces copious amounts of endometrial scrapings. Microscopic examination shows hyperplasia of the epithelium and stroma. The cells lining the glands are nonsecretory and the stroma often contains cells with frequent mitotic figures. Cystic changes of the glands may be present.

Curettage is useful in diagnosis and for treatment as it removes the hypertrophied endometrium and leaves a fresh surface for endometrial regeneration. Because of the frequency of recurrence of hyperplasia the administration of cyclic progesterone will aid in prevention of recurrence and promote cyclic menses. If endometrial hyperplasia recurs, it may proceed to atypical or adenomatous hyperplasia, and then to carcinoma-in-situ, which may lead to endometrial cancer. Recurrent abnormal bleeding requires repeated curettage for diagnosis and proper therapy.

Adenomatous hyperplasia is diagnosed when there is marked proliferation with the glands being closely packed and the stroma quite dense and hyperplastic. This adenomatous pattern closely resembles adenocarcinoma and is felt to be a precancerous lesion. Diagnosis of this lesion is by curettage. While cyclic progesterone will be of aid for most patients, hysterectomy is probably the treatment of choice for the older patient who has completed her reproduction.

## MALIGNANT DISEASES OF THE UTERUS

### Adenocarcinoma of the Endometrium

Adenocarcinoma of the endometrium, the second most prevalent gynecologic cancer, is seen most commonly among postmenopausal women. The peak incidence occurs in the 50 to 70 year age groups, but one must suspect the condition as early as the third decade if there is bleeding irregularity. Postmenopausal bleeding is the cardinal symptom of endometrial cancer and must be considered as due to malignancy until proved otherwise. Prolonged, profuse, or irregular bleed-

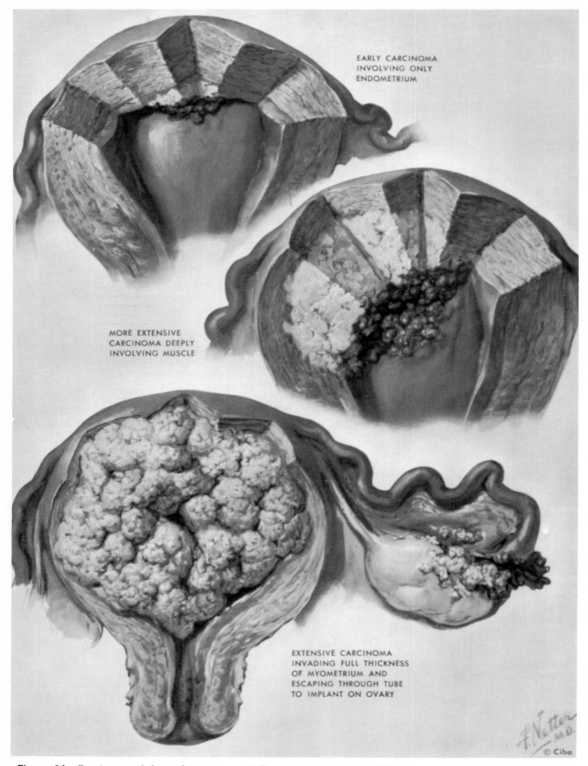

EARLY CARCINOMA
INVOLVING ONLY
ENDOMETRIUM

MORE EXTENSIVE
CARCINOMA DEEPLY
INVOLVING MUSCLE

EXTENSIVE CARCINOMA
INVADING FULL THICKNESS
OF MYOMETRIUM AND
ESCAPING THROUGH TUBE
TO IMPLANT ON OVARY

**Figure 24**  Carcinoma of the endometrium. (© Copyright 1954, 1965, CIBA Pharmaceutical Company, Division of CIBA Corporation. From The CIBA Collection of Medical Illustrations by Frank H. Netter, M.D.)

ing may occur in the premenopausal woman. Papanicolaou cytologic study may yield negative results as the exfoliated cells may not reach the vaginal pool. Cervical stenosis with secondary hematometrium or pyometrium is frequently present and can be identified by passage of an endocervical probe. Fractional curettage is the diagnostic method of choice and only in this fashion can the diagnosis be established as well as the degree of cervical involvement, an important factor influencing therapy. Histologically, adenocarcinoma of the endometrium has wide variations in differentiation and in stromal invasion by the glandular epithelial cells, and, finally, there is a highly undifferentiated type in which neither glandular nor stromal elements can be identified.

Although the etiology of endometrial cancer is unknown, there does appear to be a relationship of these tumors to prolonged estrogenic stimulation, particularly when unassociated with cyclic progesterone. Patients with estrogen-producing ovarian tumors have an increased incidence of endometrial cancer. There is also an increased incidence of endometrial cancer in women who have had endometrial hyperplasia. Other frequently associated findings in patients with endometrial adenocarcinoma are obesity, tallness, diabetes, hypertension, and low parity.

Endometrial cancer is usually a polypoid lesion growing into the endometrial cavity, and only late in the disease does myometrial or cervical involvement occur (Fig. 24). Uterine size is usually normal to slightly increased in women with early cancer of the endometrium. Uterine enlargement and irregularity occur in advanced disease or disease associated with hematometrium or leiomyoma. In addition to direct extension to adjacent structures, adenocarcinoma of the endometrium may spread through the extensive lymphatic anastomosis at the upper uterus between the tube and ovary. Thus, the tubes and ovaries are frequent sites of early metastases. Besides this direct lymphatic extension of endometrial cancer, these tumors may spread by regional and distant lymph node metastasis to the pelvic and aortic nodal chains. The incidence of such lymph node metastasis is rare when only the urine fundus is involved (2 per cent) but frequent if the primary lesion is near the cervical junction (50 per cent). Hematogenous dissemination may also occur and the most frequent sites are the peritoneal surfaces, lungs, liver, and skin. Local recurrence in the apex of the vagina, vaginal walls, and perineum occurs in 10 per cent of patients who have been treated for endometrial cancer.

The usual clinical staging of endometrical cancer includes: Stage 0, preinvasive or carcinoma-in-situ of the endometrium; Stage I, the growth is confined to the uterine body; Stage II, the carcinoma involves the corpus and the cervix; Stage III, the tumor extends outside the uterus but not outside the true pelvis; Stage IV, the carcinoma has extended outside the true pelvis or has involved the mucosa of the rectum or bladder.[2] The location of the primary neoplasm in the uterus, the degree of anaplasia of the cells, and the gross size of the uterus influence the prognosis of the patient and the effectiveness of treatment.

The treatment of adenocarcinoma of the endometrium is primarily surgical. Many clinics supplement the surgical treatment with preoperative intrauterine radium application or preliminary deep x-ray or cobalt-60 therapy to the pelvis. There is considerable disagreement as to whether preoperative radiotherapy enhances survival rates, but it does seem clear that such treatment will reduce vaginal recurrence after appropriate surgical therapy. Nolan has shown that in Stage I disease in which the uterus is small, preoperative radiotherapy does not improve survival, but in other Stage I lesions the survival may be increased by a factor of 10 per cent.[2] If the cervix is involved by endometrial carcinoma, or Stage II disease, preoperative treatment with irradiation followed by radical Wertheim hysterectomy with pelvic lymphadenectomy may be indicated. The survival rate for patients with cancer spread beyond the uterus is poor, regardless of whether surgery, irradiation, or a combination of the two methods is used. Approximately 30 per cent of patients with recurrent or metastatic adenocarcinoma of the endometrium will benefit from large doses of parenteral progesterone (Delalutin or Depo-Provera), usually those with tumors that are well differentiated histologically. Other forms of chemotherapy have been of little aid. External pelvic radiotherapy or transvaginal irradiation and intravaginal radium may provide palliation for locally recurrent adenocarcinoma of the endometrium.

The prognosis for adenocarcinoma of the endometrium is generally good but results of larger series are frequently difficult to compare owing to differences in tumor size, differentiation, stage, and type of treatment. Of those patients selected for surgery because of an operable lesion, with and without preoperative irradiation, approximately 60 per cent will survive 5 years.[2, 9]

### Sarcoma of the Uterus

Sarcomas may arise from the endometrium, myometrium, cervix, a leiomyoma, or uterine blood vessels. These diseases are most frequently seen in the fifth decade and a rare sarcoma of the cervix, sarcoma botryoides, is seen in infants. The incidence of corpus sarcoma is much higher than that of sarcoma of the cervix. As all elements of the uterus are mesodermal in origin, and mesodermal rests may be present, mixed tumors may occur. A wide spectrum of histopathologic types can be found. Rapid uterine enlargement is a prominent sign of uterine sarcoma and abnormal bleeding may or may not be present. Pain, anemia, and weight loss are late symptoms. Pulmonary metastases frequently occur early. Surgical excision of the uterus, tubes, and ovaries is the recommended treatment for sarcoma of the uterus. The prognosis after treatment varies with the type and extent of the original tumor. The sarcomas arising in myomas generally appear to be of low malignancy and thus have a relatively good prognosis, with 45 to 50 per cent of patients with operable lesions surviving. There are very few survivors among patients with the other types of uterine sarcoma despite appropriate surgery for patients with operable lesions. Radiotherapy may offer benefit. We are currently exploring a combination approach, with extirpative surgery and combination chemotherapy with simultaneous methotrexate, actinomycin D and chlorambucil, followed by external pelvic irradiation with cobalt-60. The initial results are encouraging but warrant further investigation.

## PELVIC INFECTION

### Acute Pelvic Infection

Acute pelvic infection may occur after pelvic surgery or result from other causes, but by far the most frequent etiology is gonorrhea. The initial symptoms of gonorrhea usually occur within 3 to 6 days after inoculation and consist of urethritis, skenitis, bartholinitis, cervicitis, and vaginal discharge. Tubal involvement is usually a later symptom and does not occur until after a menstrual period. At this time the gonococcus spreads rapidly from the endocervix, across the endometrium, and involves the endosalpinx. It is in the fallopian tube that the major infection and damage occurs. The tube becomes acutely inflamed and edematous, and its lumen fills with a purulent exudate. The tubular, peritubular, ovarian, and pelvic peritoneal surfaces are rapidly involved. Pelvic abscess may develop.

The signs and symptoms of acute pelvic infection are those of pelvic peritonitis with bilateral lower abdominal pain and tenderness, temperature of 38 to 39° C., and signs of peritoneal irritation with direct and rebound tenderness and muscle spasm. On pelvic examination one may be able to express pus from the paraurethral glands or cervix, exquisite tenderness is present with cervical manipulation and in the adnexal areas, and there is a thickened, doughy feeling in the tubular areas. Bilaterality of pain is an important point in differentiating acute pelvic infection from appendicitis and the fever of the former disease is usually higher. The diagnosis of acute pelvic infection is made by cervical smear and culture (see Laboratory Tests).

Therapy is based on the degree of peritonitis and fever. If significant peritonitis is present or the temperature is greater than 38.5° C., hospitalization is indicated and intravenous antibiotic therapy recommended. Treatment in this situation consists of administration of penicillin, streptomycin, or ampicillin. This intensive treatment, plus analgesia, elevation of the head to encourage pelvic localization of pus, and parenteral fluid replacement, is continued until the acute symptoms have subsided, and then oral therapy is begun and continued on an outpatient basis for a week. Total therapy should include more than 5 million units of penicillin so as to adequately treat unrecognized syphilis which the patient may have contracted at the same time as the gonorrhea. If the presenting symptoms are not severe, one can treat the patient entirely as an outpatient. The patient should be examined twice weekly to follow her progress and exclude pelvic abscess. Surgery is not indicated for acute pelvic infection unless pelvic abscess drainage is required. If the abdomen is opened for an erroneous preoperative diagnosis but acute pelvic infection is found, no further surgery is indicated and the abdomen is closed and antibiotic therapy initiated. If significant pelvic contamination with pus is present, cul-de-sac drains are inserted.

### Pelvic Abscess

This condition may follow acute pelvic infection, pelvic surgery, septicemia, puerperal endometritis, appendicitis, or peritonitis of any cause. The abscess may be localized in the cul-de-sac, or between the leaves of the broad ligament, or it may be tubo-ovarian in location. If gonorrhea is the primary etiology, the purulent exudate will usually not contain the organism since it is short-lived in such conditions. Secondary organisms such as colon bacilli, anaerobic organisms as bacteroides, streptococci, and staphylococci may be present in large quantities. The signs and symptoms of pelvic abscess are elevation of temperature and pulse, pelvic or lower abdominal pain, and leukocytosis. If the abscess is anteriorly placed, as in an interligamentous pelvic abscess, one may discover a tender, fluctuant mass on abdominal examination. Pelvic examination is usually quite helpful. A cul-de-sac abscess bulges into the posterior vaginal fornix and displaces the cervix anteriorly. Interligamentous abscesses may bulge into the lateral fornix and displace the cervix to one side. Treatment of pelvic abscess consists of surgical drainage. Posterior colpotomy is performed to drain a pelvic abscess localized in the cul-de-sac, any loculations are digitally opened, and large drains are left indwelling. Antibiotics should be used after surgery. Other pelvic abscesses may be drained vaginally, but may require anterior extraperitoneal drainage or abdominal exploration for removal of involved structures and drainage. If a pelvic abscess ruptures intra-abdominally, there is significant morbidity and mortality from disseminated infection. In that event the uterus, tubes, and ovaries should be removed and adequate drainage and antibiotic coverage instituted.

### Chronic Pelvic Infection

Included among chronic pelvic infections are chronic salpingo-oophoritis, pyosalpinx, hydrosalpinx, and tubercular salpingitis. Chronic salpingo-oophoritis is one of the major complications of gonorrhea. The patient may have few complaints. Since the endosalpinx was intensely involved in the acute infection the tube may be agglutinated. Pyosalpinx is one of the chronic destructive lesions of gonorrhea in which the tube is dilated, closed, and filled with pus. Hydrosalpinx results from pyosalpinx in which the purulent material is replaced by a serous fluid. Chronic oophoritis may develop after ovarian surface involvement and often the tube and ovary are involved in a single inflammatory process. The classic pattern of chronic pelvic infection is one of quiescent intervals interspaced with flares of more acute inflammation. After the initial infection, usually gonococcal, anaerobic organisms invade and involve these tissues. Tuberculous salpingitis is now a fairly rare problem in this country and the process usually involves the endometrium and adjacent structures as well. The dense adhesions of pelvic viscera to bowel and omentum are outstanding features of this disease and these structures may be covered with a caseous exudate.

Chronic pelvic infection may be treated medically or surgically. The important elements of medical therapy are rest, heat, and antibiotic therapy. Sedation and analgesia will usually be required. Penicillin, ampicillin, streptomycin, and tetracycline are the oral antibiotics utilized. Those patients who have recurrent pain or abnormal uterine bleeding from reduced ovarian function from chronic pelvic infection are often difficult to relieve of symptoms. This disease is a common gynecologic complaint and surgical therapy is often required. The only cure for chronic, recurrent pelvic infection is surgical removal of the uterus, tubes, and ovaries. Surgery should always be delayed, if possible, until maximal medical control has been obtained. Estrogen replacement is indicated for the younger woman if both ovaries are removed.

## BENIGN DISEASES OF THE OVARY

Benign ovarian tumors may be solid or cystic and may represent a "functional" process or neoplasia. While these growths are usually small, they may persist or become massively enlarged. The judgment as to the necessity of surgical removal should be based on size, duration of symptoms, the interval of persistence of the smaller lesions, and the age of the patient. Most classifications of such benign tumors include ovarian cysts, non-neoplastic and neoplastic, and solid ovarian tumors.

Many authors report that more than 90 per cent of ovarian growths discovered in women less than 30 years old are benign. In the 30 to 50 year age group, 80 per cent are benign. After 50 years of age approximately half of such ovarian growths are malignant. Others, excluding the frequently seen follicle and corpus luteum cysts, report the likelihood of the various benign ovarian growths as: endometrial cysts, 33 per cent; simple cysts, 26 per cent; serous and mucinous cystadenomas, 19 per cent; dermoids, 15.2 per cent; others, 2 per cent.[2] The most frequent sign of benign ovarian growths is slow abdominal enlargement. Other symptoms are pain and tenderness from torsion of the pedicle and interference with the blood supply.

Less than 10 per cent of such growths are associated with aberrations in the menstrual cycle. Amenorrhea or irregular bleeding may accompany follicle or corpus luteum cysts, polycystic ovaries, or endometrial cysts. Unless quite large, most benign ovarian tumors rarely cause pressure on adjacent pelvic structures. Most commonly, such ovarian growths are asymptomatic and discovered on routine pelvic examination.

The benign, non-neoplastic ovarian cysts are usually of "functional" origin. The follicle cyst represents failure of a developing follicle to rupture or regress and rarely exceeds 8 cm. in diameter. Corpus luteum cysts occur from hemorrhage into the corpus luteum and these blood-filled cysts have the yellow granular color of the normal corpus luteum while the follicle cyst is filled with clear fluid. Both usually regress over a 4 to 8 week period. The theca lutein cyst and the luteoma of pregnancy are also functional cysts resulting from the high levels of circulating chorionic gonadotropin of normal pregnancy and trophoblastic disease. They regress after pregnancy is terminated. Germinal inclusion cysts occur in the cortex of the ovary and represent inward growth of the germinal epithelium which has undergone cystic change. These cysts are thought to be the origin of the neoplastic serous cystadenoma. Polycystic ovaries are enlarged with multiple small follicular cysts and leuteinization of the stroma, and have a thickened capsule. The etiology is unknown but may relate to tonic elevation of luteinizing hormone.

The benign neoplastic ovarian cysts are most frequently the endometrial cyst or "chocolate" cyst of pelvic endometriosis (Fig. 25) or the simple cyst. These may achieve large size, especially the latter. Serous and mucinous cystadenomas arise from neoplastic changes in germinal epithelium and often reach considerable size. These cystic tumors are multilocular, have smooth capsules, and usually replace the entire ovary. Histologic examination reveals an adenomatous pattern or tall columnar cells producing mucin, respectively. The benign teratoma, or dermoid cyst, is a common

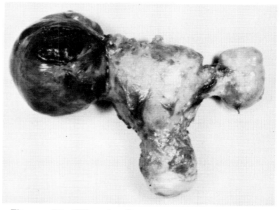

**Figure 25** "Chocolate" cyst, endometrioma of the ovary with attached hysterectomy specimen.

ovarian tumor, benign in more than 99 per cent of patients. The gross appearance is that of a smooth-coated, gray tumor which usually replaces the ovary. Microscopically, ectodermal and mesodermal structures are found with hair, teeth, bone, and cartilage present. Approximately 25 per cent of dermoids are bilateral and, thus, if one ovary is involved, the other should be opened and inspected.

The solid benign ovarian tumors include the Brenner tumor, which is thought to arise from Walthard inclusion rests in the cortex of the ovary. This tumor grossly resembles the ovarian fibroma, another benign solid tumor. Ovarian fibromas are occasionally the cause of Meigs' syndrome with concomitant sympathetic hydrothorax and ascites. Other solid ovarian tumors include the rare androgen-producing Leydig cell tumor, or hilus cell tumor, and the neuroma, angioma, papilloma, and fibroadenoma. The most important decision facing the surgeon who finds a solid ovarian tumor is to differentiate benign from malignant.

The treatment of benign ovarian growths is primarily surgical removal with conservation of all normal ovarian tissue possible. The functional cysts, follicle and corpus luteum, should regress in a relatively short interval and do not require surgery unless rupture and hemorrhage have occurred. These will not infrequently be found during surgery for other reasons and do not require treatment. The majority of the other benign cystic and solid ovarian tumors will usually replace or destroy any remaining ovarian tissue in the involved gonad, and oophorectomy, preserving the tube, is often indicated. Endometrial or "chocolate" cysts are an exception, and after all involved ovarian tissue is resected one attempts to leave even a small amount of normal ovarian tissue for future fertility. In any event, bilateral oophorectomy is rarely indicated in the young woman unless one is *sure* malignancy is present. If there is any doubt, the abdomen should be closed even if reoperation is needed at a later date. In general, we have felt that if an undiagnosed ovarian mass is larger than 6 cm., or if it persists without diminution in size for longer than 3 months, exploration should be done. Acute torsion or significant hemorrhage may require immediate surgery.

## OVARIAN CANCER

The incidence of cancer of the ovary varies considerably in different reports because of the wide range of criteria accepted for making this diagnosis. Among the adenomatous tumors there is a broad group of borderline cases. Most series report that ovarian cancer accounts for 4 to 6 per cent of all cases of malignant disease in the female. Most investigators report incidences of histologic types as serous cystadenocarcinoma, 60 per cent; pseudomucinous carcinoma, 15 per cent; solid undifferentiated adenocarcinoma, 10 per cent;

granulosa cell carcinoma, 6 per cent; dysgerminoma, 2 per cent; and other rare types (arrhenoblastoma, teratoma, mesonephroma), 7 per cent. The ratio of benign ovarian tumors to malignant ovarian tumors is 4 to 1, until the peak incidence of ovarian cancer at 40 to 60 years of age, when the ratio is 1 to 1.[2]

The International Federation of Gynecology and Obstetrics has adopted the following clinical classification, based on clinical studies and surgical exploration, for staging primary carcinoma of the ovary:[9]

Stage I
  Growth limited to the ovaries.
Stage II
  Growth involves one or both ovaries with extension of the cancer to other areas within the pelvis.
Stage III
  Growth involves one or both ovaries with widespread intraperitoneal metastasis to the abdomen.
Stage IV
  Growth involves one or both ovaries with distant metastasis outside the peritoneal cavity.

Several factors need to be stressed in regard to ovarian cancer. First, the delay in diagnosis is reprehensible: 50 per cent of ovarian cancers are neglected by the patient and 25 per cent by the physician who does not examine the patient in more than 60 per cent of cases. Second, 30 to 50 per cent of ovarian cancers are inoperable at the time of diagnosis and in only 20 per cent can the tumor be entirely removed surgically. Third, only 11 per cent of patients have suspicious or positive Papanicolaou cystologic findings. Fourth, as expected, the survival is greater the earlier the stage of the disease at the time of diagnosis. As the overall survival of ovarian cancer has improved only slightly in the past 20 years, we must strive for earlier diagnosis.[2, 12]

Ovarian cancer occurs more frequently in Caucasians and the mean age at diagnosis is 51 years. Fifty-eight per cent of patients are postmenopausal. Childbearing may have some effect in reducing the likelihood of ovarian cancer. It is suggested that a family history of cancer, exposure to pelvic irradiation, and previously existing benign ovarian tumors may increase the likelihood of development of cancer of the ovary.[2, 12]

### Signs and Symptoms

The signs and symptoms of ovarian cancer may be only those of an enlarging tumor in the pelvis. Parker reported 56 per cent of his patients complained of pain and 46 per cent of abdominal swelling. He also reported 31 per cent had experienced at least a 10 pound weight change, usually loss, and 22 per cent had either abnormal or postmenopausal bleeding.[12] There may be ascites with unilateral or bilateral hydrothorax. Anemia is fre-

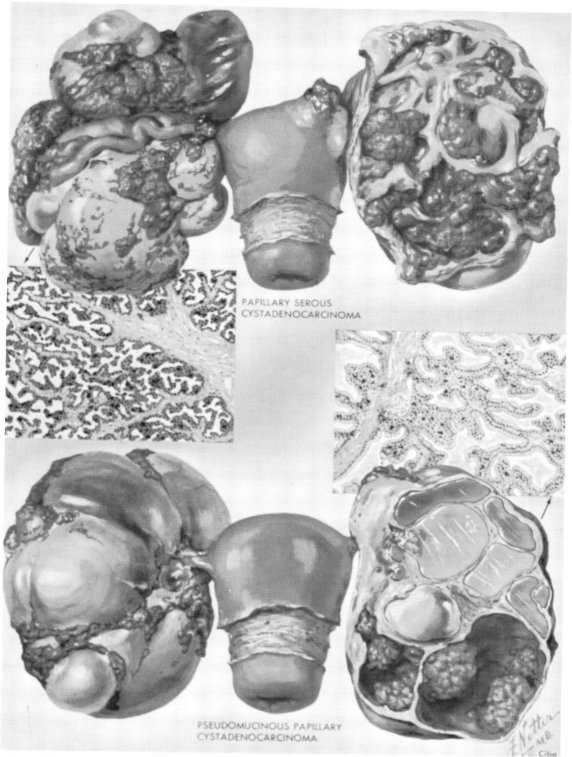

PAPILLARY SEROUS
CYSTADENOCARCINOMA

PSEUDOMUCINOUS PAPILLARY
CYSTADENOCARCINOMA

**Figure 26**  Ovarian carcinoma: primary, cystic, and solid; secondary carcinoma. (© Copyright 1954, 1965, CIBA Pharmaceutical Company, Division of CIBA Corporation. From The CIBA Collection of Medical Illustrations by Frank H. Netter, M.D.)

quently seen in advanced disease. Pelvic examination may reveal firm nodular implants of metastatic tumor in the cul-de-sac and pelvic viscera. As noted, there are often no early symptoms of ovarian cancer. Every women should have an annual pelvic examination before age 40 and more frequently thereafter. The diagnosis is made histopathologically and the differential between benign and malignant ovarian tumors cannot be made until operation. The gross examination of the tumor at surgery is usually helpful, as papillary growths on the surface of a cystic or semicystic tumor, or papillations on the inside of the tumor, are suggestive of malignancy (Fig. 26). Solid ovarian tumors that are lobulated or have hemorrhagic areas in the capsule are usually malignant. Peritoneal cell washings should be obtained with any suggestive ovarian tumor.

### Treatment

The reader is referred to the many excellent reviews on the various types of therapy for ovarian cancer.[2, 7, 9, 12] Results of all therapy, however, remain poor and various proponents report limited success with a variety of therapeutic regimens. There is general agreement that total abdominal hysterectomy, bilateral salpingo-oophorectomy, and possibly omentectomy should be carried out, even if some tumor is left behind. As the 5 year survival for Stage I ovarian cancer is only 60 per cent, and only 20 per cent of patients explored have disease as limited as Stage I, most investigators feel supplemental therapy is mandatory for all patients with ovarian cancer. Radiotherapy and chemotherapy have both been used with moderate palliative success. Total pelvic and abdominal irradiation, intraperitoneal radioisotopes, alkylating agents, and combination chemotherapy are of significant palliative aid in nearly half of patients so treated.[7, 9, 12]

## MALIGNANT TROPHOBLASTIC DISEASE

Malignant gestational trophoblastic diseases are relatively rare cancers of women but are of major importance. Even if metastases are present, essentially all patients with these tumors can be cured. It is tragic for a woman to have an erroneous diagnosis of "anaplastic metastatic cancer" made and the diagnosis of trophoblastic malignancy overlooked. As these tumors frequently present with the symptoms of metastases, it is useful for any physician who treats women of reproductive ages to be aware of the patterns of these diseases.

Malignant trophoblastic disease may follow any type of pregnancy, including abortion or term live birth, although more than half the tumors occur after hydatidiform mole. Tissue diagnoses include invasive mole (chorioadenoma destruens), choriocarcinoma, and anaplastic trophoblastic tissue. Irregular uterine bleeding is a common presenting sign, but patients present with amenorrhea, uterine rupture, or the sequelae of distant metastasis to lung, vagina, brain, bowel, kidney, and elsewhere. The anaplastic pattern of the placental trophoblasts, with or without preservation of the pattern of the villus, may be seen histologically. Fortunately, all of these tumors produce a hormone identical to human chorionic gonadotropin (HCG) which can be measured in higher levels by pregnancy tests (positive in 75 per cent of these patients) or by sensitive biologic or radioimmunologic techniques. The finding of a suspicious metastatic lesion, with or without pelvic symptoms, should lead to HCG testing. If the HCG level is elevated and normal pregnancy can be excluded, one should strongly suspect malignant trophoblastic disease.

Considerable assistance for physicians treating patients with suspected malignant trophoblastic disease can be obtained from any of the several trophoblastic disease centers in this country. Treatment consists of intensive chemotherapy with methotrexate or actinomycin D, given alone or in combination with surgery or irradiation. With appropriate and intensive therapy essentially all patients with these diseases can be cured, even when metastases are present.[4]

## AMENORRHEA

Amenorrhea is defined as the absence of menses at the time a women should be menstruating and may be classified as primary or secondary. Most investigators feel a patient should be without menses for at least 6 months before the diagnosis of amenorrhea is made. Amenorrhea occurs physiologically in pregnancy and lactation. Menstruation is based on the interaction of the central nervous system, hypothalamus, pituitary, ovary, uterus, and other glands and their hormones (see Physiology and Endocrinology).

Primary amenorrhea, in which the patient has never had menses, may occasionally be due to abnormalities of central nervous system or pituitary gland, but much more commonly occurs from gonadal, adrenal, or uterine defects. Most girls will begin menses by 18 years of age and failure of menstruation by this age warrants careful examination, chromosomal testing, hormonal assays, and, on occasion, visualization of the gonad. Gonadotropin assays will frequently provide the appropriate direction for further study as these levels are increased in cases of ovarian failure or abnormal function and are usually reduced with central nervous system or pituitary gland diseases. Congenital absence of the uterus always, and endometrial disease frequently, result in amenorrhea while gonadotropins are normal.

Secondary amenorrhea, or cessation of menses, may be due to a variety of problems. Space-occupying lesions of the central nervous system, hypothalamus, or pituitary result in absence or low levels of gonadotropins and amenorrhea. Pituitary tumors or infarction can also yield similar results. Skull films, visual field examinations, appropriate contrast studies, and hormonal studies

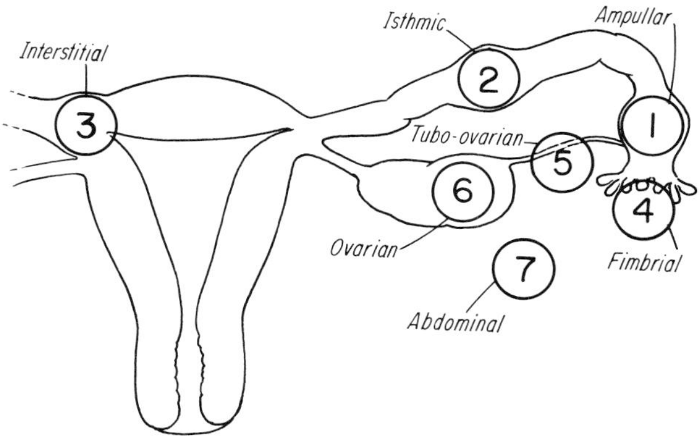

**Figure 27** Ectopic pregnancy. Diagram shows the various implantation sites numbered in order of decreasing frequency of occurrence.

may aid in making these diagnoses. However, one must always remember the symptom of amenorrhea may precede the diagnosis of such lesions by a span of years and prolonged follow-up is mandatory. Psychiatric illnesses may interfere with gonadotropin release and result in amenorrhea. Ovarian problems as polycystic ovaries and premature ovarian failure may cause secondary amenorrhea and in these patients gonadotropins will be normal and elevated, respectively. Acquired failure of endometrial responsiveness may also cause secondary amenorrhea, as can significant dysfunction of the thyroid or adrenal glands. Treatment is based on the appropriate diagnosis.

## ECTOPIC PREGNANCY

An ectopic pregnancy is one in which the ovum implants and develops outside the normal location, the uterine cavity. Ninety-five per cent of ectopic pregnancies are tubal, with the greatest percentage of these occurring in the dilated ampulla, that portion of the distal tube immediately proximal to the fimbriated end. Less common sites of ectopic pregnancy are abdominal, ovarian, and interligamentary (Fig. 27). Abdominal ectopic pregnancy usually occurs after tubal abortion with secondary reimplantation elsewhere in the abdominal cavity. The incidence of all types of ectopic pregnancy is approximately 1:150 births.

Despite the fact that the ovum is implanted outside the uterine cavity, the uterine endometrium is converted into a decidua similar to that of normal pregnancy. The size and consistency of the uterus also changes in ectopic pregnancy. The cervix and body of the uterus soften and the corpus may enlarge to a size compatible with a 6 to 8 week intrauterine pregnancy. All of these changes are due to the production of placental hormones from the ectopic embryo. As ectopic placental function declines, as usually occurs in tubal pregnancy, the hormonal support declines and irregular uterine bleeding begins. The decidua is usually discharged in fragments, but may on occasion be expelled intact as a decidual cast.

The duration and eventual outcome of tubal ectopic pregnancy are determined primarily by the area of tube involved. If the ovum implants in the relatively large ampullary region of the tube, the pregnancy will usually continue longer than one in the narrow isthmus. Local bleeding from trophoblastic invasion continues and increases, and blood dissects the ovular sac from the tubal wall. With complete separation, the ovular sac is usually extruded from the end of the tube and, unless a major vessel is involved, bleeding terminates. More often, however, the process is prolonged and repeated bleeding episodes yield a pelvic hematoma. In other areas of the tube, the tubal wall is less distensible and the lumen is narrower and tubal rupture is inevitable as the trophoblasts invade and blood collects. Ectopic pregnancies in the narrow isthmic segment usually rupture in 6 to 8 weeks, while those in the interstitial portion, where the tube traverses the uterine wall, continue for 14 to 16 weeks before rupture. Rupture is usually into the peritoneal cavity and is accompanied by sudden and significant bleeding. Tubal pregnancies may regress spontaneously with either the ovum dying at an early age or being extruded from the tubal ostium without significant bleeding.

The classic symptoms of ectopic pregnancy are a history of infertility or pelvic disease, light vaginal bleeding beginning within 2 to 4 weeks after the first missed period, and sharp and fleeting lower abdominal pain. Eventually the patient experiences sudden severe abdominal pain and shock as the tube ruptures. On examination one usually notes the signs of early pregnancy such as cyanosis and softening of the cervix and uterine enlargement. The most important pelvic finding prior to tubal rupture is a unilateral tender mass. In patients with pelvic hematoma the cul-de-sac may be "doughy" and distended. Signs of peritoneal irradiation may be present. Fever is a rare finding but progressive anemia is frequently observed. Pregnancy tests are positive in about one-half of patients with unruptured tubal pregnancy, the discrepancy being due to low levels of chorionic gonadotropin produced by the functional restricted placenta.

The diagnosis of an unruptured tubal pregnancy

is not difficult to make when classic symptoms are present but, unfortunately, the symptoms are frequently atypical and the pelvic findings misleading. A high index of suspicion is one's most valuable adjunct. Culdocentesis, or large-gauge needle perforation of the cul-de-sac, may reveal considerable old dark blood and strongly suggest pelvic hematoma. Laparoscopy or culdoscopy may allow visualization of the ectopic embryo. Posterior colpotomy, or vaginal incision into the cul-de-sac, not only allows accurate diagnosis, but the skillful operator can remove the embryo in approximately 50 per cent of tubal pregnancies through this incision. Although it is usually possible to diagnose tubal pregnancy with reasonable accuracy, problems such as uterine abortion, salpingitis, appendicitis, or ruptured corpus luteum or follicular cysts may produce signs and symptoms causing confusion in diagnosis. In uterine abortion the period of amenorrhea is usually longer, the amount of vaginal bleeding is greater, and pain is less severe, more midline, and cramping in nature. No adnexal mass or tenderness is present. Salpingitis and appendicitis usually present with signs of infection and there has been no amenorrhea or irregular bleeding. Ruptured cysts, particularly those of the corpus luteum, usually are not associated with prolonged amenorrhea. Follicular cysts tend to rupture at midcycle. In both varieties an occasional patient may require surgical exploration for control of hemorrhage.

The treatment of ectopic pregnancy consists of surgical removal of the involved tube and replacement of blood loss. Prompt blood replacement and surgical intervention are mandatory, but the patient's condition should be stabilized prior to surgery if at all possible. General anesthesia should be used. Abdominal pregnancy is treated by removal of the fetus and ligation of the umbilical cord near its insertion into the placenta. Owing to the intense vascularity of the placenta, it is usually best to leave it in situ. Prognosis with prompt management is good and mortality from ectopic pregnancy has been reduced to 1 to 2 per cent. Recurrence of ectopic pregnancy in the remaining tube occurs in about 10 per cent of patients.

## SELECTED REFERENCES

*The following books were utilized heavily in the preparation of this chapter, and a number of the illustrations were drawn from them. For detailed and factual information about gynecology, the reader is recommended to them all:*

Brewer, J. I.: Textbook of Gynecology. 4th ed. Baltimore, Williams & Wilkins Company, 1967.

Kistner, R. W.: Gynecology, Principles and Practice. Chicago, Year Book Medical Publishers, 1964.

Nelson, J. H.: Atlas of Radical Pelvic Surgery. New York, Appleton-Century-Crofts, 1969.

Novak, E., Jones, G. S., and Jones, H.: Textbook of Gynecology. 8th ed. Baltimore, Williams & Wilkins Company, 1970.

Parsons, L., and Ulfelder, H.: An Atlas of Pelvic Operations. Philadelphia, W. B. Saunders Company, 1968.

Taylor, E. S.: Essentials of Gynecology. 4th ed. Philadelphia, Lea & Febiger, 1969.

Willson, J. R., Beecham, C. T., and Carrington, E. R.: Obstetrics and Gynecology. 2nd ed. St. Louis, C. V. Mosby Company, 1963.

## REFERENCES

1. Brunschwig, A., and Daniel, W. W.: The surgical treatment of cancer of the cervix uteri. Amer. J. Obstet. Gynec., 75:875, 1958.
   *Dr. Brunschwig and the group at Memorial Hospital in New York became leading proponents for the radical surgical treatment of gynecologic malignant disease. This group popularized exenterative surgery and proved it a useful operation. Techniques, results, and complications are reviewed.*

2. Corscaden, J. A.: Gynecologic Cancer. 3rd ed. Baltimore, Williams & Wilkins Company, 1962.
   *This text, now in its third edition, is one of the standards about gynecologic malignancy. Cancers of the vulva, vagina, cervix, uterus, tube, and ovary are discussed in detail. Etiology, epidemiology, natural history, diagnosis, and therapy are well reviewed. The bibliography is excellent.*

3. Fluhmann, C. F.: The Cervix Uteri and Its Diseases. Philadelphia, W. B. Saunders Company, 1961.
   *Diseases of the cervix are reviewed in detail in this book, including cervical cancer. The illustrations and material are excellent. Any student of gynecologic disease should utilize this valuable text.*

4. Hammond, C. B., and Parker, R. T.: The diagnosis and treatment of trophoblastic malignancy. Obstet. Gynec., 35:132, 1970.
   *The authors review the history of trophoblastic malignancy, including the work of Hertz's group at the National Institutes of Health who popularized chemotherapeutic treatment. The article reviews the experience at Duke University in more than 100 patients with these cancers, approximately half with metastases. More than 93 per cent of patients were cured. Methods of chemotherapy and the roles of surgery, combination chemotherapy, and arterial chemotherapy are discussed.*

5. Huffman, J. W.: The Gynecology of Childhood and Adolescence. Philadelphia, W. B. Saunders Company, 1968.
   *This textbook has been long needed by gynecologists and other physicians who care for pelvic problems of the young girl. The chapters dealing with embryology, endocrinology, oncology, and functional disorders are exceptionally strong.*

6. Israel, S. L.: Diagnosis and Treatment of Menstrual Disorders and Sterility. 5th ed. New York, Hoeber Medical Division, Harper & Row, 1967.
   *As the title suggests, this book primarily deals with sterility and its multiple causes. Menstrual dysfunction is also quite adequately reviewed. The reader is referred to it for further details regarding these problems.*

7. Julian, C. G., and Woodruff, J. D.: The role of chemotherapy in the treatment of primary ovarian malignancy. Obstet. Gynec. Survey, 24:1307, 1969.
   *In 1969, this excellent journal began a monthly, detailed review article and this paper is from that series. The detail, clarity, and bibliography are excellent. It summarizes the current knowledge and therapy for chemotherapy of ovarian cancer, a tumor particularly responsive to this form of treatment.*

8. Kupperman, H. S.: Human Endocrinology. Philadelphia, F. A. Davis Company, 1963.
   *This three-volume set on human endocrinology contains considerable detail about reproductive endocrinology. Concise and detailed information is presented about the physiology and biochemistry of this system.*

9. M. D. Anderson Hospital and Tumor Institute: Cancer of the Uterus and Ovary. 11th Annual Clinical Conference. Chicago, Year Book Medical Publishers, 1969.
   *This institution is well known for its contributions to gynecologic oncology. The details about treatment and follow-up of results for cancers of the cervix, uterus, and ovary are quite good, particularly the sections on radiotherapy and chemotherapy.*

10. Miller, O. J.: The sex chromosome anomalies. Amer. J. Obstet. Gynec., part 2, *90*:1078, 1964.
    *This article is one of the first detailed summaries of chromosomal aberrations that can result in gonadal and extragonadal defects. The article is commended for its clarity and completeness.*

11. Parker, R. T.: The clinical problems of early cervical neoplasia. Obstet. Gynec. Surgery, part 2, *24*:691, 1969.
    *This article presents the problems, findings, therapy and results in more than 1000 patients with early cervical neoplasia. The entire issue of the journal is devoted to various problems with these diseases and the reader will profit from its detailed study.*

12. Parker, R. T., Parker, C. H., and Wilbanks, G. D.: Cancer of the ovary. Amer. J. Obstet. Gynec., *108*:878, 1970.
    *Ovarian cancer remains a diagnostic and therapeutic problem of major proportion. This article reviews the past 20 years experience with these diseases at Duke University. The influence of histopathologic diagnosis, clinical staging, positive cell washings, and ascites are discussed. The effects of surgery, radiotherapy, and chemotherapy are reviewed.*

13. Richardson, G. S.: Ovarian Physiology. Boston, Little, Brown and Company, 1967.
    *This monograph discusses in considerable detail what is currently known about ovarian physiology and is suggested for better basic understanding of this subject and its influence on gynecologic disease.*

14. Rogers, J.: Endocrine and Metabolic Aspects of Gynecology. Philadelphia, W. B. Saunders Company, 1963.
    *This relatively small book is highly recommended for one who desires a rapid but reasonably detailed review of the endocrinologic and metabolic problems that the gynecologist encounters. Clarity is excellent and the bibliography is adequate.*

15. Rutledge, F. N.: Cancer of the vagina. Amer. J. Obstet. Gynec., *97*:635, 1967.
    *Primary vaginal carcinoma remains a poorly responsive malignant lesion, regardless of the therapy chosen. This article reviews the experience at the M. D. Anderson Hospital with radiotherapy for this tumor and the results are the best reported.*

16. Sherman, R.: Human Ovulation Induction. Springfield, Ill., Charles C Thomas, 1969.
    *Anovulation and amenorrhea are perplexing problems for both diagnosis and therapy, particularly if fertility is desired. With the advent of newer drugs capable of allowing ovulation induction, this timely text reviews the problems, studies, findings, and treatment schedules that offer the best chance of success.*

17. Simpson, J. L., and Christakos, A. C.: Hereditary factors in obstetrics and gynecology. Obstet. Gynec. Survey, *24*:580, 1969.
    *This excellent review article summarizes the more current chromosomal aberrations that can result in gonadal and extragonadal defects. The bibliography is most adequate.*

18. Speert, H.: Obstetric and Gynecologic Milestones. New York, Macmillan Company, 1958.
    *This book, subtitled "Essays in Eponymy," explores the discoveries and men who have contributed to this specialty. It is recommended to all practitioners of this area of medicine and to any student of medical history.*

19. Taylor, E. S.: Essentials of Gynecology. 4th ed. Philadelphia, Lea & Febiger, 1969.
    *This general textbook of gynecology was particularly useful to the author. The organization, graphic material, and detail of presentation are excellent.*

20. Way, S.: Carcinoma of the vulva. Amer. J. Obstet. Gynec., *79*:692, 1960.
    *The names of Taussig, Bassett, Twombly, Collins, and others all come to mind during any discussion of vulvar cancer. Dr. Way must certainly be included among those who have made major contributions to our knowledge of these diseases and their surgical treatment. This article summarizes his experience.*

# 47

# THE URINARY SYSTEM

*John T. Grayhack, M.D.*

The production, transport, storage, and discharge of liquid waste by the human body is accomplished by an integrated system which includes functions varying from delicately controlled, highly complex cellular mechanisms to those of a rather gross muscular conduit. The kidneys, ureters, bladder, and urethra are located extraperitoneally in the abdomen and pelvis (Fig. 1). The embryologic development of the upper urinary tract is complex.[1] The adult renal parenchyma, the metanephros, arises from the mesoderm of the nephrotome after sequential lysis of the pronephros and the mesonephros. Fusion of the ureter, which arises from the wolffian duct, with the mesoderm of the nephrogenic cord is necessary for the normal development of collecting tubules and functioning nephrons. As the kidney matures, it migrates upward from the region of the fourth to the first lumbar vertebra and rotates so that the original dorsal border becomes the convex lateral border. The superior pole of the left kidney may lie as high as T10 or as low as L2. X-ray measurements indicate a length of $12.6 \pm 0.8$ cm. by a width of $5.9 \pm 0.4$ cm. in females and a length of $13.2 \pm 0.8$ cm. by a width of $6.3 \pm 0.5$ cm. in males. The right kidney is slightly lower than the left and slightly smaller. The arterial blood supply is derived from the aorta; the venous blood flow enters the vena cava.

The kidney is divided into the peripherally situated cortex, which contains the glomeruli and portions of the tubules, and the centrally located medulla, composed primarily of portions of the tubules and the collecting ducts (Fig. 1A). The initial step in urine formation is the physical process of filtration accomplished in the glomerulus of the nephron. The glomerular filtrate is modified in the tubules by reabsorption of solute and water as well as secretory activity. The urine is delivered from the papilla through the collecting ducts into the minor calyx. The urine that enters the calyx is normally excreted essentially unmodified. The calyces, pelvis, ureter, and bladder are lined by transitional epithelium. Transport of urine is accomplished with development of pressures exceeding 35 cm. $H_2O$ by a coordinated contraction of the smooth muscle surrounding the epithelium. The volume of urine retained in the pelvis is small. Once urine enters the ureter peristaltic activity results in its prompt delivery to the bladder. Unlike the pelvis and the ureter, the bladder, which derives its arterial blood supply from branches of the hypogastric artery, is a reservoir

with the capacity for storage of urine for hours. Periodic integrated contraction of this smooth muscle reservoir results in normal micturition with minimal postvoiding residual urine. The mechanism of normal voiding and its neurogenic control are discussed briefly in the section on neurogenic bladder.

Historically, operative procedures for removal of bladder calculi were undoubtedly carried out by the ancients. In the middle ages, itinerant lithotomists who retained the secrets of their art for their family carried out this procedure. However, the development of urology as a recognized, respected surgical specialty depended primarily on the introduction of specialized roentgenographic and endoscopic diagnostic techniques. Specialized therapeutic procedures were conceived and improved once diagnoses could be established with regularity. Similarly, proper treatment today demands accurate diagnosis. This in turn requires a painstaking history, a complete physical examination, a careful examination of the urine with employment of special tests as indicated, and utilization of appropriate x-ray, isotope, and endoscopic studies. All are essential to establish a diagnosis.

A patient may have a life-threatening disease of the genitourinary tract with few if any symptoms. However, the following symptoms are suggestive of urinary tract disease.[7, 45]

*Nocturia,* awakening at night to void, is unnecessary for the normal person. Nocturia may be caused by lower urinary tract disease, such as bladder neck obstruction, neurogenic dysfunction, infection, and calculus; metabolic disorder, such as diabetes mellitus or diabetes insipidus; congestive heart failure; renal failure; and habitual excessive fluid or drug intake.

*Frequency:* The normal person voids three to five times a day. Increased frequency may be due to organic or psychogenic causes. Diurnal frequency in the absence of nocturia suggests a functional disorder.

*Polyuria* means larger than normal total urine volume and is characteristic of metabolic disorders, renal disease, and excessive fluid intake.

*Oliguria* is utilized to describe diminished urine volume; usually 400 ml. is considered the minimal obligatory urine output.

*Anuria* is complete suppression of urine formation.

*Urgency* is a precipitous desire to void, making control difficult or impossible.

*Dysuria* means pain or discomfort on urination.

When it is severe, it is called strangury. Bladder spasm or tenesmus often follows voiding in the presence of an irritated or infected bladder.

*Hesitancy* denotes undue delay and difficulty in initiating voiding.

*Intermittency* is the term used to describe the interrupted urinary stream thought to be due to detrusor fatigue in the presence of bladder neck obstruction. Usually there is an associated decrease in size and force of the urinary stream.

*Incontinence* is involuntary loss of urine. It is further characterized as true when caused by abnormalities such as sphincter injury or fistula; as paradoxical or overflow when resulting from urinary leakage from an overdistended bladder; as stress when associated with coughing or straining, or as urgency when it is preceded by a desire to void as may occur with neurogenic dysfunction or inflammatory lesions.

*Pyuria* is used to denote the presence of pus in the urine. It is due to inflammation and may be associated with an undesirable odor.

*Crystalluria* due to precipitated urinary solutes is similar in gross appearance to pyuria.

*Hematuria* may be gross or microscopic, painless or painful. Hemoglobinuria, beeturia, red bladder dyes, and the brick-dust color of uric acid crystals may be confused grossly with hematuria. Hematuria may be further characterized by its relationship to the act of micturition. Initial hematuria is noted only at the beginning of urination and usually is secondary to pathologic change distal to the neck or the bladder. Terminal hematuria is noted at the end of urination and is secondary to pathologic change in the region of the trigone, bladder neck, and posterior urethra such as a calculus, bladder neoplasm, or prostatitis. When blood is passed throughout urination, the descriptive term total is utilized. The common causes for hematuria vary with age and sex (Table 1). Although there are more than 100 causes for hematuria, consideration of tumor of the bladder, tumor of the kidney, stone, tuberculosis, acute hemorrhagic cystitis, trauma, and blood dyscrasia as causes of gross hematuria in the adult is a useful diagnostic framework. Benign prostatic hypertrophy is probably the commonest cause of bleeding in males over the age of 55. Blood dyscrasias have assumed greater importance with the increased use of anticoagulants.

*Lithuria* is used to describe the passage of urinary calculi.

*Pneumaturia,* passing gas in the urine, may be due to an enterovesical fistula, gas-forming organisms, or urologic instrumentation.

*Pain* from a renal lesion may vary from a dull, aching flank discomfort to a severe, sharp flank pain radiating into the lower abdomen or the gluteal region. The pain may be episodic or persistent. Often, it is associated with anorexia, nausea, and vomiting. No relationship is evident to the intake of food or to movement. Occasionally, as in the presence of ureteral reflux, the pain may be precipitated by voiding, or as in the occasional rare instance in which renal ptosis is obstructing, by the assumption of an erect position. In general, renal pain is as likely to awaken a patient as to occur during waking hours. Usually, with severe discomfort the patient tends to move about restlessly and to indicate the site of discomfort by grasping the flank between his thumb and forefingers. Renal disease may be responsible for bizarre abdominal complaints.

Pain from ureteral colic often causes flank discomfort associated with severe abdominal discomfort, nausea, and vomiting. As the site of the calculus or clot responsible for the discomfort progresses inferiorly, the pain tends to radiate into the lower abdomen, the genitalia, and occasionally the thigh. If a calculus lodges at the ureterovesical junction it may also cause associated frequency, urgency, and dysuria.

Pain from bladder disease is often dull and aching and confined to the suprapubic area. It may, as in the case of an acute infection, be severe and associated primarily with voiding or a desire to void. Discomfort of the glans penis, particularly at the end of voiding, often results from a lesion in the region of the neck of the bladder.

All patients with urologic complaints deserve a complete physical examination, including a neurologic evaluation. Inspection of the abdomen in the presence of a distended bladder may disclose a lower midline mass tending to flatten rather than accentuate the lower abdominal crease. Neither the distended bladder nor the hydronephrotic kidney is easy to delineate on palpation. Palpation of the kidney should usually be initiated with the patient supine and with one examining hand on the flank and the other hand anteriorly on the

**TABLE 1** COMMON CAUSES OF HEMATURIA IN VARIOUS AGE GROUPS
LISTED IN ORDER OF FREQUENCY

| Male and Female | | | Male | | | Female | | |
|---|---|---|---|---|---|---|---|---|
| *1–5* | *5–10* | *11–30* | *31–40* | *41–50* | *51–60* | *31–40* | *41–50* | *51–60* |
| Inf. | Gl. Neph. | Inf. | Inf. | Bl. Neo. | Bl. Neo. | Inf. | Inf. | Bl. Neo. |
| Gl. Neph. | Inf. | Cal. | Bl. Neo. | Cal. | B.P.H. | Cal. | Cal. | Inf. |
| | | Bl. Neo. | Cal. | Inf. | Cal. | Bl. Neo. | Bl. Neo. | Cal. |
| | | | | | Inf. | | | |

Inf.—Inflammatory lesion; Gl. Neph.—glomerulonephritis; Cal.—calculus; Bl. Neo.—bladder neoplasm; B.P.H.—benign prostatic hypertrophy.

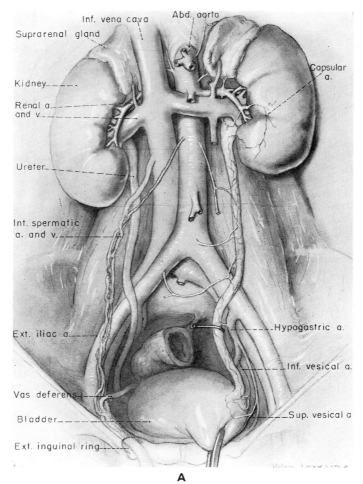

Figure 1   *A,* Gross anatomic relationships of the organs composing the urinary tract.
*Illustration continued on opposite page.*

abdomen. Utilization of both the lateral margin and tips of the fingers of the anterior examining hand is an aid in the examination. Observation of the changes in position of a palpable mass with respiration and change to a lateral or erect position of the patient is of value in identifying the mass, as is recognition of a landmark such as the renal hilum. In a child, a hydronephrotic kidney can occasionally be seen by transillumination. Sudden pressure in the costovertebral angle may elicit pain in the diseased kidney; this does not require delivery of a blow to the flank. On many occasions the site of maximal abdominal tenderness is best localized by examination with a single finger or by having the patient cough or strain and identify the site of discomfort. Pressure over a full bladder often precipitates a desire to void. Percussion will often assist in recognition and delineation of an enlarged kidney or a distended bladder.

Accurate diagnosis is usually dependent on judicious utilization of the many laboratory studies now available. This in turn requires an understanding of the tests and their limitations.

*Urinalysis*[30] should be preceded by cleansing of the genitalia, particularly in the female. In the male a two- or three-glass urine specimen assists in localizing the abnormality found in the urinary sediment. The first glass should contain the initial 30 to 60 ml. and the third glass, if employed, the final 30 ml. of voided urine. In the female, midstream urine should be utilized; if properly collected, the sample is likely to reflect the findings in the urinary tract, particularly if negative. Under some circumstances, catheterization is required in the female to obtain a representative specimen. Assessment of findings on urinalysis and urine culture is discussed in the section on infection.

Evaluation of total and often individual renal function is of importance in patients with suspected or proved disease of the urinary tract.[21, 33] Clinically, evaluation of total renal function is achieved by measurement of the degree of retention in the blood of endogenous wastes such as *urea* or *creatinine* and excretion of these substances or of exogenous chemicals such as *inulin, para-aminohippurate,* or *phenolsulfonphthalein.* The blood urea nitrogen is a less accurate indicator of

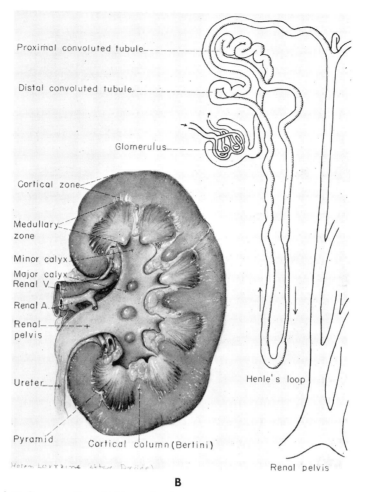

Proximal convoluted tubule

Distal convoluted tubule

Glomerulus

Cortical zone

Medullary zone

Minor calyx

Major calyx
Renal V.

Renal A.

Renal pelvis

Ureter

Henle's loop

Pyramid          Cortical column (Bertini)

Renal pelvis

Helen Lorraine after Dodson

**B**

**Figure 1**  *Continued. B,* Cross section of kidney showing gross anatomic relationships. Inset, Diagrammatic representation of the nephron shown joining a collecting duct. (From Dodson, A.I. In: Campbell, M. F., ed.: Urology. Philadelphia, W. B. Saunders Company, 1954.)

renal function than the serum creatinine level. Although both substances are excreted primarily by glomerular filtration, the amount of the former available for excretion is variable. For example, excessive protein breakdown following hemorrhage may result in a marked increase in total urea production. Creatinine is produced in essentially constant amounts. The blood urea level often seems more indicative of the clinical status of the patient, although urea itself is a nontoxic substance. In clinical practice, the creatinine clearance and phenolsulfonphthalein excretion tests are popular. The latter apparently reflects primarily renal blood flow. It correlates well with the creatinine clearance and has the advantage that it can be performed rapidly by the physician with little specialized equipment. The creatinine clearance test is a satisfactory measure of glomerular filtration rate and may be performed in most hospital laboratories. Inulin clearance, an extremely accurate measure of glomerular filtration, is utilized as an investigative tool. Para-aminohippurate is secreted by the proximal tubule and is a measure of renal plasma flow. All excretory tests are dependent on total urine collection for accuracy and may yield inaccurate results in patients with significant residual urine unless this is corrected. Knowledge of the concentrating ability of the kidney is of value in assessing renal functional status and in studying patients with possible diabetes insipidus. Individual renal function may be assessed crudely by cystoscopic observation of concentration of a chromogen such as indigo carmine excreted by each ureter or more accurately by the insertion of ureteral catheters bilaterally and collection of individual urine for clearance studies—split function studies.[53]

In addition, the *radioisotope renogram* may be utilized to indicate the functional status of the individual kidney in a qualitative fashion (Fig. 2). This test is carried out by placing a scintillation counter over each renal area and measuring the

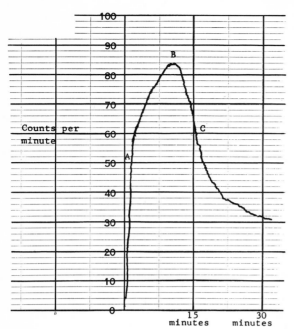

**Figure 2** Normal renogram. The initial vascular spike (A) is the result of blood-borne radioactivity supplemented by tubular function. The accumulation or tubular phase (B) represents the excess of tubular secretion over excretion. The excretory phase (C) is dependent on the ability of the pelvis and ureter to transport the radioactive substance from the renal area.

accumulation of radioactivity following the intravenous injection of an organic iodide labeled with isotopic iodine, either $^{131}$I or $^{125}$I. Efforts to permit quantitation of this test are continuing.

Development of special instruments, useful in both diagnosis and treatment, has greatly benefited the patient with genitourinary disorders. *Catheters* of varying construction have been utilized since ancient times. They are employed to bypass and relieve obstruction, to measure residual urine, to introduce and remove solutions or other substances, or to collect specimens. These hollow tubes come in varying sizes and are made of a variety of materials (Fig. 3). Properly utilized for a reasonable indication, they can provide important information and may be lifesaving; employed indiscriminately in an unskilled fashion, they can cause serious complications.

*Cystometry* (Fig. 4), a method of assessing the pressure response of the bladder to distention, may be performed by infusing fluid through a urethral or suprapubic catheter and recording the pressure response. Bladder capacity and voiding pressure may be noted. This method is of value in evaluating neurogenic dysfunction.

A *bougie* (Fig. 5) is an acorn-tipped instrument usually utilized for calibration of the urethra.

*Sounds* are metal instruments of various shapes primarily employed to dilate the urethra. A *filiform* is a thin threaded guide used to bypass a difficult stricture or tortuous area of the urethra and act as a guide for larger, less flexible sounds or catheters.

Direct visualization of the bladder and urethra has been achieved by development of an excellent group of endoscopic instruments (Fig. 6). In general, the *cystoscope* combines a hollow tube or sheath with a light source and a lens system. Employment of water as an irrigating fluid distends the portion of the lower urinary tract being studied and permits visualization. Proper combinations of instruments permit complete inspection of the lower urinary tract. In addition the instruments may be utilized to pass other diagnostic

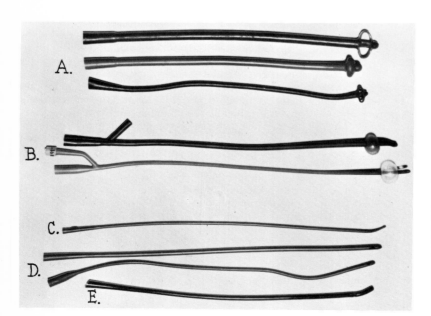

**Figure 3** Types of catheters. *A* and *B* represent self-retaining catheters made of rubber. *A* shows a Malecot and two de Pezzer catheters. *B* shows a coudé and conical-tip Foley catheter. *C* is a red rubber coudé catheter. *D* shows a polyvinyl and red rubber Nélaton catheter. *E* is a woven silk coudé catheter. Many other materials and shapes are utilized in the manufacture of catheters for special purposes.

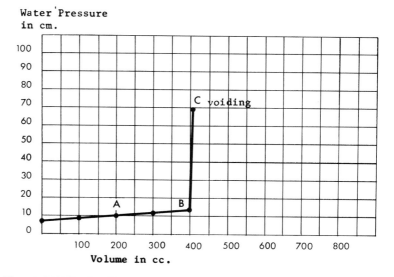

**Figure 4** Normal cystometrogram. Pressure response is recorded to gradual or intermittent filling of the bladder. First desire to void (A) is usually at 150 to 250 ml. Sensation of discomfort (B) precedes voiding. Voiding pressure is usually 40 cm. $H_2O$ or more. Residual urine determination and testing of sensation of bladder to heat and cold are carried out as part of the test. The initial pressures may be set at 0 or utilized as a zero point as in this drawing.

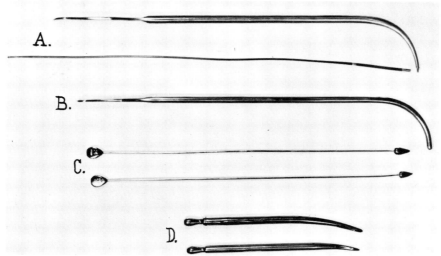

**Figure 5** Urethral instruments. *A*, Filiform and LeForte (following) urethral sounds. *B*, Van Buren urethral sound. *C*, Otis bougie à boule. *D*, Walther female dilator-catheter. Many other specialized instruments exist for diagnostic and therapeutic manipulation of the urethra.

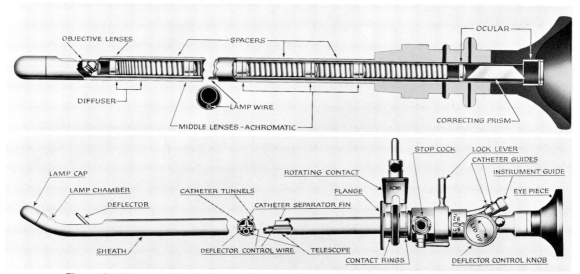

**Figure 6** Diagram of typical cystoscope. (Courtesy of American Cystoscope Makers, Inc.)

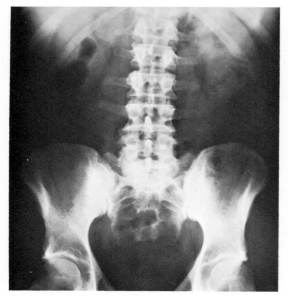

**Figure 7**   KUB. The renal and psoas shadows are visible as well as the bony structures. An estimate of renal size as well as evaluation of renal shape and position is possible. Small radiodensities in the left side of the pelvis represent phleboliths.

aids such as ureteral catheters and may be employed for a number of therapeutic purposes such as ureteral stone extraction and fulguration of bleeding areas or bladder neoplasms.

The *resectoscope* is an endoscopic instrument that permits excision of prostatic and bladder tissue through the urethra. The tissue is excised with a movable wire loop by employing a high-frequency current; bleeding is controlled by fulguration.

Roentgenographic study of the urinary tract has been a great asset in increasing accurate diagnosis of genitourinary disorders.[14] A scout film of the abdomen taken with a soft tissue technique (KUB—kidneys, ureter, bladder) may demonstrate normal structure—e.g., the size, shape, and position of the kidney, the psoas shadow, and the bony structures of the pelvis and lumbar spine (Fig. 7). In addition, significant abnormalities such as soft tissue masses or radiopacities representing possible calculi may be seen. Visualization of the various portions of the urinary tract by employing contrast media has added to the value of x-ray as a diagnostic tool. These studies should always be preceded by a plain film to permit accurate interpretation.

The *intravenous pyelogram* (Fig. 8) is a technique for achieving visualization of the urinary tract that employs the intravenous injection of an organic iodide and is dependent on renal function. The contrast medium is excreted primarily by glomerular filtration and concentrated because of reabsorption of water. The collecting system of the kidney is visualized as an opacity because of the absorbed x-rays. Visualization can usually be improved by increasing water reabsorption as occurs

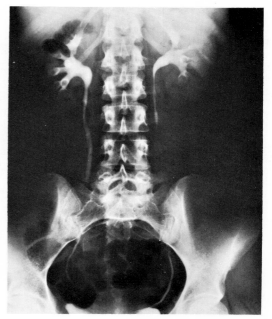

**Figure 8**   Intravenous pyelogram. Excellent visualization of the renal collecting system is achieved bilaterally. The distal collecting tubules are faintly visualized near the tip of the papilla, causing a fanlike effect within some of the minor calyces. The calyces do not lie in one plane, so that they may be seen in an "end-on" view at times. The patchy visualization of the ureter is the result of normal peristaltic activity.

in a dehydrated patient. Administration of large amounts of contrast medium increases the amount filtered and may achieve visualization even in patients with some degree of impaired renal function.

The *nephrotomogram* (Fig. 9) is an x-ray study

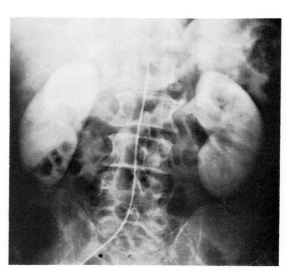

**Figure 9**   Nephrogram. Opacification of the renal parenchyma resulting from functional accumulation of contrast medium by kidney. Tomogram technique is unnecessary in this postaortogram study because of absence of interfering shadows.

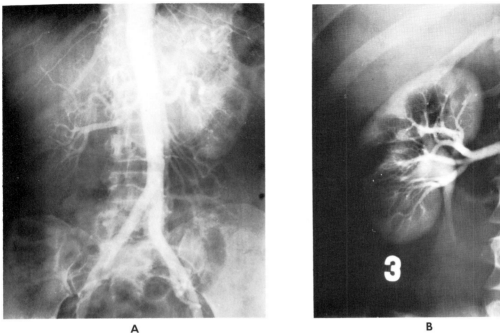

A                                                   B

**Figure 10** *A*, Brachial angiogram performed by retrograde pressure injection of contrast medium through a needle inserted in the brachial artery. Both main renal arteries and major branches are visualized. Visualization of other abdominal vessels decreases clarity of renal vessels to some degree. *B*, Selective renal arteriogram by retrograde technique.

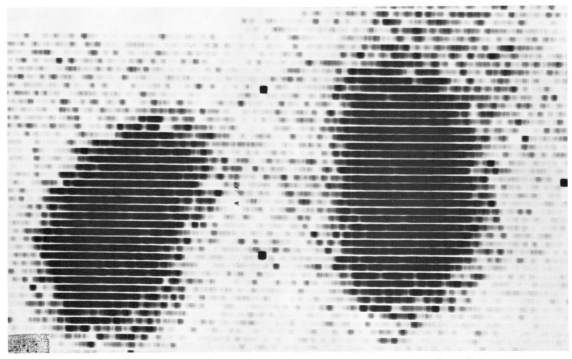

**Figure 11** Mercury-203 renal scan. Functioning renal tissue concentrates the radioisotope.

that combines the prolonged injection of large amounts of an organic iodide contrast medium with tomography. The contrast medium is concentrated homogeneously by functioning renal tissue. Nonfunctioning vascular tissue such as a neoplasm shows irregular pooling of the medium; avascular tissue such as a cyst lacks opacification. Use of a body-sectioning x-ray technique such as tomography aids visualization by reducing interfering shadows overlying an organ.

*Aortography* (Fig. 10) is an x-ray technique utilized to visualize the renal arteries. It is dependent on delivery of a sizable concentrated bolus of contrast medium to the renal arterial system and is independent of function. The contrast medium is commonly introduced through a needle placed in the lumbar aorta from the back, through a catheter threaded into the lumbar aorta from the femoral artery, or through a needle inserted in the brachial artery. The retrograde catheter technique is favored by most and has the advantage of allowing selective catheterization of individual renal arteries (Fig. 10*B*).

X-ray studies utilizing intravascular injection of contrast media introduce the risk of various allergic reactions, including anaphylactic shock. Damage to the arterial system or the kidney may also occur after intra-arterial injection. The possibility of these infrequent complications must be recognized.

A *radioactive renal scintiscan* (Fig. 11) may be carried out by injecting a radioisotope-labeled

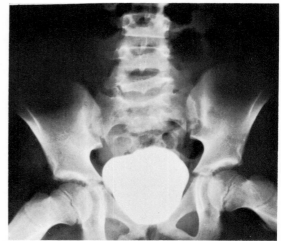

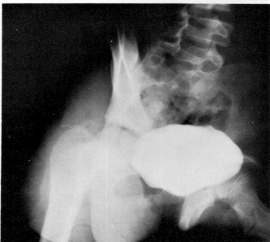

**Figure 13** Retrograde cystogram. Anteroposterior and oblique views of bladder filled with opaque medium instilled in a retrograde manner. Note that the bladder wall is smooth, filling defects are absent, and the contour is nearly symmetric.

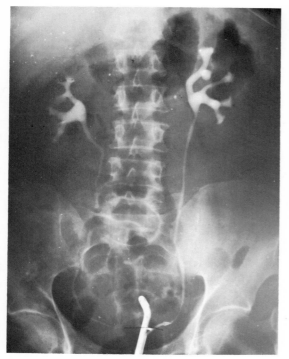

**Figure 12** Retrograde pyeloureterogram obtained by instillation of an organic iodide through an acorn-tip ureteral catheter.

compound such as chlormerodrin $^{203}$Hg or $^{197}$Hg which is concentrated throughout the functioning renal tissue. Areas composed of nonfunctioning tissue, such as cyst or tumor, fail to concentrate the isotope. The routine renal scan provides information similar to that obtained with a nephrotomogram. Modifications of the method to allow assessment of individual renal function are currently being evaluated.

Combinations of instrumentation and instillation of contrast media have the advantage of permitting complete visualization of the portion of the urinary tract being studied without relying on function. They are disadvantageous in that instrumentation must be possible and that it introduces risk, although minimal, of infection, bleeding, or perforation.

The *retrograde pyelogram* (Fig. 12) is accomplished by the instillation of contrast media

**TABLE 2**  COMPOSITION OF URINARY CALCULI*

Urinary pH usually acid; urine usually sterile:

| | |
|---|---|
| Calcium oxalate, $CaC_2O_4$ | 33% |
| Calcium oxalate + apatite | 34% |
| Uric acid, $C_5H_4N_4O_3$ | 6% |
| Cystine, $(-SCH_2CH(NH_2)-COOH)_2$ | 3% |

Urinary pH usually alkaline; urine usually infected:

| | |
|---|---|
| Apatite | 3% |
| Carbonate, $Ca_{10}(PO_4\ CO_3OH)_6(OH_2)$ | |
| Hydroxyl, $Ca_{10}(PO_4)_6(OH)_2$ | |
| Magnesium ammonium phosphate, $MgNH_4PO_4$ | 19% |
| Pure (0.3%) + Mixed (18.5%) | |
| Calcium hydrogen phosphate, $CaHPO_4$ | 2% |

*Data from Prien, E. I., and Prien, E. I., Jr.: Amer. J. Med., *45*:654, 1968; hydrated state of crystals is ignored in formula presented.

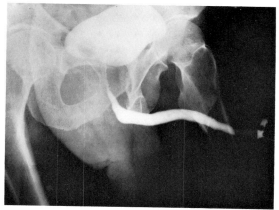

**Figure 14**  Retrograde urethrogram. Oblique view of the urethra of a male with a bladder neck contracture as it is being filled with a viscous radiopaque medium.

through a small catheter inserted in the ureter or wedged into the ureteral orifice.

The *retrograde cystogram* (Fig. 13) is made by gravity instillation of contrast media through a catheter into the bladder. This study has considerable value in demonstrating ureteral reflux and in delineating abnormalities such as bladder diverticula and urinary extravasation. X-rays taken as the patient voids the contrast medium may disclose ureteral reflex, or bladder neck or urethral disease.

A *retrograde urethrogram* (Fig. 14) accomplished by instilling a thick contrast medium in the urethra may also be of assistance in demonstrating urethral lesions such as strictures and diverticula.

## CALCULOUS DISEASE OF THE URINARY TRACT[7, 9, 49, 50]

Calculous disease of the urinary tract has been the object of diagnostic and therapeutic effort since ancient times. A urinary calculus is usually composed of a crystalline component and an organic matrix. Table 2 lists the common crystalline compositions of calculi received from patients and the frequency with which they are found. The organic matrix is a mixture of mucoprotein and mucopolysaccharide. The factors initiating calculus formation are controversial. However, a typical calculus can be made to form artificially without an organic matrix. On the other hand, so-called matrix calculi with crystalloids present in minute traces form clinically. Currently, the crystalloid component is thought to be critical under ordinary circumstances.

Areas of high incidence of stone formation are recognized throughout the world. The etiologic factors in this phenomenon are unknown. In general, stone formation is facilitated by factors that increase solute concentration in the urine, alter urinary pH, and provide a nidus for precipitation. Recognized abnormalities contributing to stone formation are stasis; infection with alteration in

pH and nidus formation; immobilization impairing transport of urine and altering calcium metabolism; dehydration; metabolic disorders, e.g., hyperparathyroidism, hyperuricemia, cystinuria, and oxalosis; hypercalciuria secondary to neoplasm or sarcoidosis, or occurring without apparent cause; vitamin D intoxication; prolonged ingestion of excessive quantities of milk and absorbable alkali, the so-called milk-alkali syndrome; abnormal renal function altering urine composition, e.g., renal tubular acidosis or Fanconi syndrome; and a foreign body, e.g., catheter.

The patient with urinary tract calculi may present with any one or a combination of symptom complexes: pain, severity, and site being dependent on the site and effect of the calculus; systemic or local symptoms of infection including fever, chills, frequency, dysuria, urgency, and pain; hematuria; anuria, if complete obstruction of the only functioning or both kidneys develops; or uremia characterized by nausea, vomiting, diarrhea, mental confusion, somnolence, muscular irritability, and weight loss.

Physical findings in the presence of an uncomplicated urinary calculus are minimal. There may be slight abdominal or costovertebral angle tenderness and muscle spasm with guarding over the site of a ureteral calculus. If infection or obstruction is present, characteristic physical findings may be evident.

Urinalysis usually discloses the presence of erythrocytes but not always. Leukocytes may be present with or without associated bacteria. The pH of the urine may assist in reasonable speculation regarding the composition of the calculus once its presence is established. Calcium oxalate, uric acid, and cystine calculi usually are found in acid urine. Crystals such as the hexagonal crystal of cystine may be present. Determination of calcium or cystine excretion and culture of the urine may aid in evaluation of cause or complications of calculous disease.

The diagnosis depends primarily on indirect

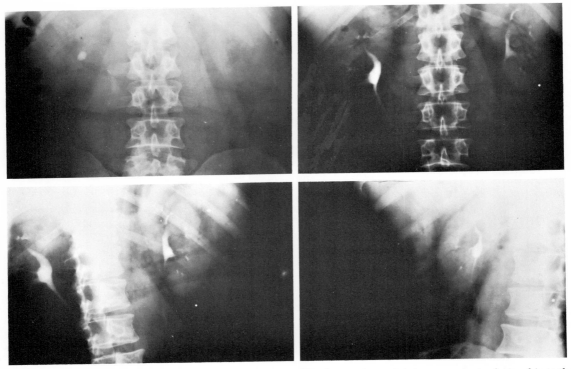

**Figure 15**   Renal calculus. Radiopacity in renal area on KUB; the opacity maintains a constant relationship to the renal collecting system in all views of the intravenous pyelogram, supporting the diagnosis of renal calculus.

methods of evaluating the urinary tract, namely, roentgenography. The plain film of the abdomen usually discloses a radiopacity due to the calculus (Fig. 15), provided that the size and composition of the stone permit sufficient absorption of the x-rays to cause this, and that surrounding or overlying structures permit its recognition. The radiopaque stones are primarily those containing a heavy metal, such as calcium or magnesium; cystine calculi are radiopaque presumably because of their sulfur content. Uric acid calculi are radiolucent and therefore not seen on a plain film. Not all radiopacities seen on x-ray of the abdomen are urinary calculi. It is necessary to establish a constant relationship of the opacity to the urinary tract to justify the presumptive diagnosis of uri-

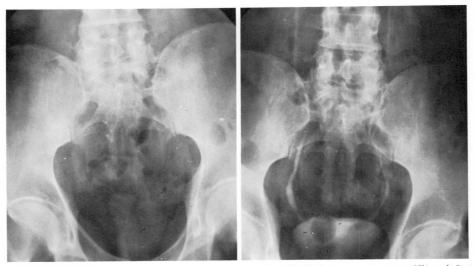

**Figure 16**   Radiolucent bladder calculus not evident on scout film (KUB) but appearing as a filling defect in the cystogram of the intravenous pyelogram.

nary calculus. To achieve this, visualization of the urinary tract by intravenous or retrograde pyelography is necessary. Radiolucent calculi cause a filling defect on pyelography (Fig. 16). Calculi may be diagnosed by other indirect methods such as the clank resulting when a urethral sound strikes a bladder stone or the scratch resulting on a waxed ureteral catheter when it bypasses a ureteral calculus, but these methods are primarily of historical interest. On the other hand, direct visualization of bladder calculi by cystoscopy is commonly employed and is extremely useful. Extension of endoscopic techniques for visualization of calculi in other areas is being investigated.

The therapy of urinary calculi may consist mainly of observation to prevent serious complications from occurring. Medical therapy utilizing such rational measures as forcing fluid and alteration of urinary pH in uric acid and cystine calculi may be initiated. Drugs such as allopurinol in patients with uric acid calculi and penicillamine in patients with cystine calculi may be given to reduce production or excretion of components of the calculus. Chemotherapeutic and antibiotic agents are useful in the prevention and treatment of urinary infection. Surgical procedures may be urgently necessary to correct the complication resulting from the presence of urinary calculus. Surgical removal of calculi may be accomplished by various techniques, both endoscopic and open. Obstruction, infection, and recurrent or persistent pain are the usual indications for surgical intervention.

Between 10 and 20 percent of patients with urinary calculi develop so-called "malignant stone disease," a life-threatening process.

## URINARY TRACT INFECTION[1, 17, 25, 27, 34, 45, 47]

*Bacteriuria* may be defined as significant presence of pathogenic bacteria in the urine. Bacteriuria is usually thought to be indicative of a urinary tract infection. However, if an infection in the urinary tract is defined as a tissue reaction resulting from the presence of a foreign organism, bacteriuria and urinary tract infection need not always be synonymous.

In any consideration of urinary tract infection, the resistance of the normal urinary tract to infection must be emphasized. Consequently, persistence or recurrence of urinary tract infection must be assumed to be associated with a local or systemic abnormality. Systemic abnormalities such as malnutrition, diseases causing severe liver dysfunction, or diabetes mellitus may contribute significantly to the development and persistence of infection. The local factors usually considered are urinary stasis and the presence of a calculus, essentially a foreign body (Fig. 17). Urinary stasis may result from obstruction, neuromuscular dysfunction, or a congenital or acquired abnormality such as ureteral reflux. The presence of any foreign body such as an indwelling catheter

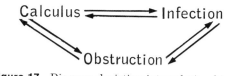

**Figure 17**  Diagram depicting interrelationship of obstruction, stone formation, and urinary tract infection.

or a calculus acts as a nidus for continued infection and makes eradication of infection extremely difficult if not impossible. Trauma is a third local factor which is employed experimentally to permit development of infection and which has probable clinical significance in the urinary tract infections developing after instrumentation and in the common occurrence of so-called "honeymoon cystitis."

Bacteria do not enter the urinary tract by normal filtration. The routes by which they do enter the urinary tract are *hematogenous,* as in the coccal infections of the kidney; *ascending,* as in the presumed entrance of bacteria into the bladder via the female urethra or into the kidney from the bladder; *direct extension,* as in the bladder infection at times associated with a diverticulitis of the colon; and *lymphatic.* The organisms infecting the urinary tract are commonly gram-negative bacilli. However, infections of the urinary and adjacent genital organs may be caused by parasites such as Echinococcus, primarily in the kidney, and *Schistosoma, haematobium* and *mansoni,* primarily in the bladder; by Protozoa, such as Trichomonas, primarily in the prostate and the female urethra, and by *Entamoeba histolytica;* by yeast, usually occurring in debilitated patients treated repeatedly with antibiotics; by the tubercle bacillus, and by other specific organisms such as the Gonococcus which causes an anterior urethritis in the male. The common bacterial organisms causing urinary tract infection are *Escherichia coli, Pseudomonas aeruginosa, Aerobacter aerogenes, Proteus vulgaris,* Staphylococcus, Streptococcus, *Alcaligenes faecalis,* and Paracolon organisms. Among these, Proteus is recognized for its ability to split urea with liberation of ammonia. The resulting alkalinization may be important, not only in stone formation, but also in permitting persistence of infection. Subcellular forms of bacteria such as protoplasts may play a role in the persistence of urinary tract infections.

The patient presenting with an acute urinary tract infection has symptoms related to the site and severity of the infection. Acute pyelonephritis is usually associated with flank pain, chills, fever, and often nausea and vomiting. Acute cystitis is associated with frequency, dysuria, urgency, suprapubic pain, and hematuria. The patient with a chronic urinary tract infection may experience the symptoms associated with acute urinary tract infection chronically or periodically or may be virtually asymptomatic until renal failure develops.

The physical findings in urinary tract infection vary with the site and severity of the infection.

Marked flank tenderness and muscle spasm are characteristic of acute pyelonephritis. The patient with chronic pyelonephritis may have only equivocal flank tenderness or no abnormal physical findings. Occasionally, a physical finding makes a diagnosis highly probable, as in the beading of the vas deferens or the scrotal fistula seen with tuberculosis of the vas deferens and epididymis.

Examination of the urine is the most important tool employed in establishing a diagnosis of urinary tract infection. Gross inspection of the urine may yield valuable clues. As an example, the first portion of the voided urine of the patient with prostatitis usually contains shreds.

The number of white blood cells that must be present on microscopic examination of the urine to cause suspicion of a urinary tract infection is not clearly established. If the uncentrifuged urine is employed, 10 white cells per 20 high-power field must be regarded with suspicion. If a 10 ml. random midstream urine sample is centrifuged at 2500 rpm for 5 minutes, one or two white blood cells per high-power field requires further evaluation. One or more red blood cells per high-power field must be regarded as abnormal. White cell casts in the urinary sediment are a significant abnormality and are indicative of renal infection, past or present, until this presumption has been disproved. Visualization of bacteria on a wet smear or on Gram stain of the urine is an excellent indicator of bacteriuria. Occasionally, as in the gonococcal infections, the stained smear remains the practical method of establishing a diagnosis.

A persistently alkaline urinary pH or the finding of abnormal amounts of protein may be the result of urinary tract infection, although other causes warrant equal consideration.

The urine culture is the definitive laboratory test for establishing the presence of bacteria in the urine and the diagnosis of urinary tract infection. Identification of the bacteria is of value in directing therapy and sensitivity testing is of even greater assistance. Normal urine is sterile. The sterility is maintained in the bladder but because the urethra frequently contains a few bacteria, the urine collected after passage through the urethra often contains bacteria. Passage of a catheter through the urethra also occasionally yields a contaminated urine and is not entirely free of risk. The problem, then, is to obtain a urine sample that satisfactorily reflects the status of the bladder urine and to obtain this with a minimum of risk. Urine may be obtained by voiding, catheterization, or suprapubic aspiration. A voided urine sample should be obtained after satisfactory cleansing of the genitalia by utilizing a two- or three-glass collection technique for urine to be examined microscopically and by employing a midstream specimen for culture. The voided urine reflects the bacteriologic status of the urinary tract more accurately in the male than in the female. In either sex it has a great significance if it is sterile and free of abnormality on examination of the sediment. In an attempt to assess the significance of finding bacteria in the urine, quantitative

techniques have been employed to count numbers of bacteria present. Because urine is an excellent culture medium and because the bladder is a reservoir usually emptying at 3 to 4 hour intervals, one can predict that bacteria present in the bladder will multiply and be present in great numbers in the urine. Observations have confirmed this postulation. Further, on studying urine samples obtained by both catheter and voided techniques there seem to be two groups, one with little or no bacterial growth, and a second with more than 100,000 colonies per milliliter. The finding of a colony count exceeding 100,000 organisms per milliliter is employed clinically to increase the probability to over 90 per cent that bacteria found in the urine are representative of the state of the bladder urine. However, with a voided urine, particularly in the female, this may represent contamination or mishandling of the specimen. Furthermore, a urinary tract infection may be present with a colony count of less than 1000 colonies per milliliter. Routine use of the catheter increases the reliability of the urine sample, particularly in the female. However, catheterization of a patient with a sterile urinary tract may introduce a urinary tract infection. Therefore, as much reliable information as possible should be obtained from the voided specimen. Catheterization is a valuable tool and should be employed when indicated. Separate microscopic and culture studies of urine obtained by voiding or catheterization from various portions of the urinary tract may assist in identification of the sites of infection.

Biopsy may yield isolated evidence of infection of a genitourinary organ in rare instances. The x-ray studies of the upper urinary tract may be characteristic of a urinary tract infection such as tuberculosis and occasionally chronic pyelonephritis. The presence of characteristic anatomic changes makes a diagnosis highly probable even in the absence of bacteriologic confirmation on examination of the urine.

Although infection of any portion of the urinary tract constitutes a risk to other organs and both ascending and descending infection occur, isolated infection of an organ such as the bladder or prostate does occur and is relatively common. Although the possible effect on renal function is of primary concern, not all or even the majority of urinary tract infections are pyelonephritis. In addition to local effects of a urinary tract infection, the systemic effects of a chronic infection, such as weight loss, weakness, and easy fatigability, may be evident. Furthermore, the bacteria in the urinary tract are a potential cause of bacteremia, septicemia, and occasionally bacteremic shock.

Once the diagnosis of infection is established, the fact that a single urinary tract infection in the male, or a recurrent infection in the female, is likely to be related to an underlying systemic or local cause must be emphasized. Stasis, stone, diabetes, and other abnormalities must be sought by repeated examination.

Treatment should be directed at elimination or control of the underlying causes for the infection, elimination of the bacterial agent by employment of antibiotic or chemotherapeutic agents indicated by culture, and re-examination at intervals following treatment to be certain that the infection has been eliminated.

# OBSTRUCTION OF THE URINARY TRACT[8, 17–19, 38, 42]

Obstruction to the free egress of urine in response to normal contracture of the musculature of any portion of the urinary tract results in a series of events that may eventually result in destruction of the portions of the urinary tract above the obstructive site. The sequence of events following an obstruction may usually be divided into the following stages:

**Trauma.** The site of the obstruction and the areas above it may show hemorrhagic areas. The urine above the site may increase both in volume and hemoglobin content.

**Muscular Hypertrophy.** Muscular hypertrophy is presumably related to development of increased pressure required to overcome obstruction. The portion of the urinary tract just above the obstruction shows these changes first. In the urinary bladder, the hypertrophied muscle associated with a distal obstruction is evident on gross inspection as prominent ridges called trabeculae.

**Dilatation and Destruction.** Dilatation resulting in anatomic changes such as hydroureter, hydronephrosis, and caliectasis, which are recognized as a consequence of obstruction, may be marked. With progression there is usually replacement of functioning muscle or nephrons by fibrous tissue.

## Etiology

The causes of an obstructive lesion in the urinary tract may be *congenital* or *acquired, intrinsic* or *extrinsic* (Fig. 18). The obstruction may be partial or complete. The effects of an obstructive lesion depend on the site, degree, and duration of the obstruction. Any obstructive lesion below the site of the ureteral orifices is likely to affect the functional status of both kidneys and to subject them both to any complications that may occur.

With regard to the development of hydronephrosis, the kidney is unique in that even after total obstruction urine formation continues (Fig. 19). After the development of an obstructive lesion,

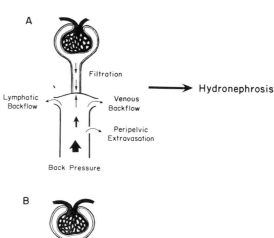

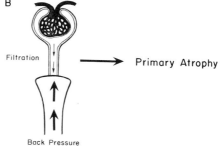

**Figure 18** Causes of urinary tract obstruction. (From Hinman, F., Jr. In: Campbell, M. F., and Harrison, J. H., eds.: Urology. 3rd ed. Philadelphia, W. B. Saunders Company, 1970.)

**Figure 19** *A* represents the mechanism by which hydronephrosis is thought to develop; if reabsorption failed, as shown in *B*, it is postulated that a small contracted kidney would result from primary atrophy.

the intraluminal pressure above the site of obstruction rises rapidly. One would suspect that as this pressure reached filtration pressure glomerular filtration would cease and tubular secretion would be minimal. However, active reabsorption of urine occurs by pyelovenous, pyelolymphatic, tubulovenous, and tubulolymphatic routes and by peripelvic extravasation. This permits continued urine formation by filtration. Although there is an immediate increase in renal blood flow with an acute obstruction, this rapidly diminishes to levels well below normal. The resulting anoxia adds to the tissue destruction resulting from the back-pressure. This sequence of events, continued secretion of urine with gradual destruction of tissue, probably accounts for the dilatation of the kidney usually found as the result of ureteral obstruction. Otherwise, primary atrophy would be expected. Experimentally, respiration of cortical tissue falls markedly within 48 hours after obstruction but the respiration of medullary tissue is unaltered. Anaerobic glycolytic ability of the cortical tissue increases markedly in the same period after occlusion.

### Clinical Symptoms

The patient with urinary tract obstruction may present with one of the following symptom complexes: obvious symptoms related to obstruction, as in the patient with bladder neck obstruction presenting with hesitancy, intermittency, decrease in size and force of the urinary stream, frequency, and nocturia; symptoms related to the primary pathologic disturbance causing the obstruction, as in the patient presenting with hematuria from stone or bladder tumor; symptoms related to the presence of an abdominal mass, such as the epigastric distress that may accompany a hydronephrosis, and symptoms resulting from the complication of the obstruction, as in the patient presenting with nausea, vomiting, diarrhea, muscular irritability, mental confusion, and somnolence as the result of renal failure, or in the patient presenting with chills, fever, and flank pain as the result of infection of an obstructed kidney.

The significant physical findings in a patient with obstruction may be those associated with the lesion causing the obstruction, such as the enlarged prostate causing bladder neck obstruction. They may be due to the enlarged distended organ, such as the palpable midline abdominal mass associated with dullness on percussion characteristic of a distended bladder. They may be the result of the development of a complication of an obstruction, such as the flank tenderness and muscle spasm associated with infection of the obstructed kidney.

Unfortunately, there are no findings characteristic of obstruction on urinalysis or blood chemistry studies. The findings on urinalysis may be due to the primary pathologic disorder, such as red blood cells seen with a calculus, or to a complication such as bacteria or pyuria seen with a urinary tract infection. Similarly, findings of elevated serum creatinine, blood urea nitrogen, serum phosphorous, and serum potassium associated with decreased serum calcium, characteristic of renal failure, raise the question of the presence of an obstructive lesion but do not assist in establishing this diagnosis.

The diagnosis of an obstruction in the urinary tract is dependent on one of the following: demonstration of abnormal retention of urine by recovery by catheter, by visualization of dilatation and delayed drainage by intravenous pyelography, or by showing abnormal retention of contrast medium instilled in a retrograde fashion; demonstration of the obstructing lesion by cystoscopic visualization of the obstructing prostatic tissue or x-ray visualization of the calculus, or demonstration by cystoscopy or cystogram of secondary disorder usually due to obstruction such as trabeculation and diverticulum of the bladder.

Treatment is directed toward relieving the obstruction (Fig. 20). This is often easily accomplished by as simple a maneuver as passage of a catheter. The effects of even long-standing obstruction including renal failure are potentially reversible with this relief. Whereas provision for unobstructed drainage of the urinary tract is essential, correction of the cause of obstruction is frequently elective.

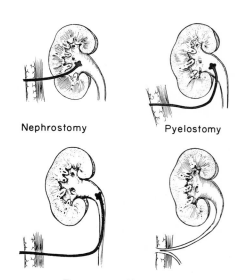

Nephrostomy        Pyelostomy

Temporary  Ureterostomy

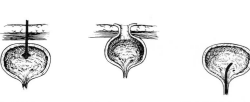

Cystostomy        Vesicostomy        Urethral Catheter

**Figure 20**   Representative methods of achieving temporary diversion of urine at various sites in the urinary tract.

# DISEASES OF THE KIDNEY AND URETER

## ANOMALIES OF THE KIDNEY[2, 3, 10, 52]

Anomalous development of the upper urinary tract can be life-threatening in the patient with renal hypoplasia or polycystic renal disease, or may predispose to acquired disease, as in partial ureteral duplication. Urogenital malformations account for 35 to 40 per cent of all congenital abnormalities and are frequently one of multiple abnormalities. In some patients, an association of particular defects exists, such as aneurysm of cerebral vessels with polycystic kidney and nerve deafness with congenital renal parenchymal failure. Anomalies of the genital organs and kidney frequently coexist. The complex embryologic development of the kidney with serial maturation of the pronephros, mesonephros, and metanephros, the independent development of the collecting system prior to joining the renal parenchyma, and the ascent and rotation from a pelvic to a flank position provide multiple opportunities for maldevelopment of the upper urinary tract. The renal anomalies are usually classified as anomalies of number, including bilateral agenesis, unilateral agenesis, and supernumerary kidney; anomalies of position, including simple ectopia such as pelvic kidney, crossed ectopia with or without fusion, and nephroptosis or movable kidney; anomalies of form, including horseshoe, disk, L-shaped, lump, hourglass, lobulated, and round kidney; anomalies of rotation; anomalies of volume and structure, such as hypoplasia, congenital hypertrophy, solitary cyst, multicystic disease, parapelvic cyst, sponge kidney, and polycystic disease; and anomalies of the renal pelvis, including duplication or so-called double kidney, and congenital hydronephrosis.

All these lesions have clinical importance. Knowledge that a patient without an abdominal scar may have been born with only one kidney can be critical even if the incidence of this abnormality is one in 1200. Recognition that a palpable mass may be a functioning renal mass can prevent serious errors in diagnosis and treatment. The relative frequency of urogenital abnormalities requires consideration of this possibility in patients with abdominal complaints or physical findings of an obscure nature. These lesions may become manifest at any age. Employment of modern diagnostic techniques should permit uniformly accurate assessment of the anatomic status of the upper urinary tract.

## CYSTIC DISEASE[1, 2, 11, 17, 24, 46]

*Solitary cysts* of the kidney are probably the most common renal mass recognized clinically. They are thought to result from a malunion or obstruction of the tubules when the etiology is congenital, and from tubular obstruction associated with localized vascular insufficiency when the lesion is acquired. Solitary renal cysts are bluish, thin-walled, smooth masses characteristically containing a clear serous fluid with small quantities of albumin, chlorides, globulin, urea, cholesterol, epithelial cells, and leukocytes. They are rarely seen before adulthood and are most common in the fourth, fifth, and sixth decades. Renal cysts are often asymptomatic. They may be associated with slight flank discomfort, mild gastrointestinal complaints, or infrequently with hematuria. Even less commonly, the cyst may be associated with excessive production of erythropoietin and consequent polycythemia. Infection of the cyst is a possibility. Demonstration of a thin-walled avascular mass on nephrotomography and arteriography makes a diagnosis of solitary cyst highly probable, but not certain. Aspiration of the cyst and instillation of contrast medium increases the probability of accurate nonoperative diagnosis. Definite diagnosis is dependent on observation of the characteristic gross and histologic appearance in the absence of neoplasm. The treatment of solitary renal cyst is partial excision of the cyst wall with oversewing of the remaining edge. If nonoperative differentiation of solitary cyst and renal neoplasm were certain, many would not require operative therapy.

*Peripelvic cyst* is essentially a simple serous cyst located in the hilum of the kidney. It characteristically exerts lateral pressure on the collecting system and shows no evidence of renal parenchymal distortion on aortography or nephrotomography.

*Medullary sponge kidney* is a term applied to describe a dilatation of the distal collecting tubules of the kidney. This anatomic deformity probably results from either a developmental defect or an acquired abnormality. The characteristic dilated tubules seen at the renal papilla on intravenous pyelography suggest the diagnosis. Tuberculous lesions of the kidney may mimic the changes seen in medullary sponge kidney. Rarely the lesion may be localized to one segment of the kidney and partial resection may be employed because of complications such as persistent infection or calculous disease.

*Medullary cystic disease* of the kidney is an infrequent lesion often associated with renal failure and salt losing. At present this disease has no surgical significance.

*Multicystic renal disease* usually presents as an abdominal mass in infancy. Older patients may complain of dull abdominal pain. The lesion consists of multiple thin-walled cysts resembling a bunch of grapes. There is no associated renal parenchyma. The ureter is characteristically rudimentary and not connected with the cystic mass. Unfortunately, an abnormality of the opposite kidney may be associated with this lesion.

*Congenital polycystic disease* is an inherited renal abnormality. The adult variety is probably transmitted as a mendelian dominant, the infant variety as a recessive. The disease must be considered bilateral. Pathologically, Oasthanondh and Potter have described four types of polycystic disease: Type I, due to hyperplasia of interstitial portions of the collecting tubules; Type II, due to inhibition of ampullary activity resulting in marked reduction of the number of generations of tubules derived from the ureteral bud; Type III, consisting of multiple developmental renal defects; and Type IV, due to urethral obstruction. In polycystic disease the kidneys are usually several times larger than normal and studded with cysts of varying sizes. Cysts of the liver and pancreas and aneurysms of the circle of Willis are recognized as associated lesions infrequently.

Clinically, the disease becomes manifest either in infancy or in early adulthood. Some patients with polycystic disease have a normal life expectancy. The symptoms calling attention to polycystic disease are pain, hematuria, abdominal mass, and the symptoms of renal failure or hypertension. The physical examination characteristically discloses palpable, irregular enlarged renal masses bilaterally. Hypertension is common. Urinalysis characteristically shows proteinuria; pyuria and hematuria may be present. Evidence of renal failure may become apparent on testing as the disease progresses. The diagnosis is made from the history, the physical findings, and the demonstration on intravenous or retrograde pyelography of bilateral renal enlargement with flattening of the minor calyces, elongation of the infundibula, and other evidences of multiple space-occupying lesions (Fig. 21). Progressive renal failure is the rule in recognized disease in the adult.

Hematuria, infection, obstruction, and calculous disease occasionally require surgical intervention in these patients. All attempts to preserve renal function permanently have been unsuccessful to date. The disease presents a continuing challenge because many of the patients have satisfactory renal function when first seen. At present, they constitute a group for whom renal transplantation is often ultimately advised.

## CONGENITAL OBSTRUCTION OF THE UPPER URINARY TRACT[2, 18, 19]

Although obstruction at the ureterovesical junction and other sites may have a congenital basis, congenital obstruction of the upper urinary tract occurs most frequently at the ureteropelvic junction. Obstruction at the ureteropelvic junction may be due to an aberrant renal vessel, adhesions, intrinsic stenosis, and perhaps a functional abnormality of this segment, either alone or in combination. The lesions may be bilateral. The patient with a congenital ureteropelvic junction obstruction usually presents with intermittent flank pain, often associated with nausea and vomiting, hematuria, or evidence of a urinary tract infection. In children, an abdominal mass is commonly palpable. The lesion may not become symptomatic until early adulthood or late in life. The diagnosis

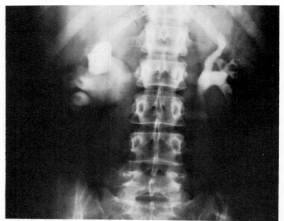

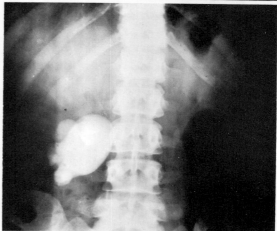

**Figure 22** Intravenous pyelogram demonstrating typical deformity of hydronephrosis resulting from ureteropelvic junction obstruction. Note abrupt absence of contrast medium below this site.

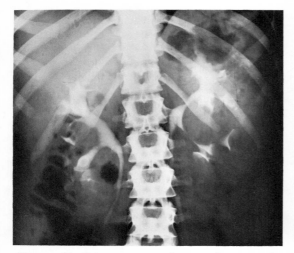

**Figure 21** Intravenous pyelogram demonstrating typical configuration of polycystic renal disease. Note enlarged renal shadow, flat minor calyces, and deformity and elongation of infundibulum.

is usually established by x-ray studies demonstrating the dilatation of the pelvis or calyces characteristic of a hydronephrotic kidney and the site of obstruction at the ureteropelvic junction (Fig. 22). Functional impairment may be sufficiently great to prevent visualization by intravenous pyelography.

Decisions to operate on the patient with a congenital obstruction are guided by the presence of functional impairment, complications such as infection or stone, and symptomatic complaints related to the obstruction. Whether removal of the hydronephrotic kidney or repair of the obstruction is the preferable course depends on assessment of the probable degree of function retained in the diseased kidney, as well as the status of the opposite kidney. Of course, the age and general condition of the patient are important. A number of ingenious techniques have been devised to permit repair of a stenotic ureteropelvic junction with a high degree of success.

## ANOMALIES OF THE URETER[2, 3, 10, 52]

Anomalies of the ureter and kidney are often associated. However, the ureteral anomalies are usually considered separately to facilitate presentation. The following is a commonly employed classification: anomalies of number—agenesis, duplication, triplication; anomalies of form, caliber, and structure—aplasia, congenital stricture, congenital valves, megaloureter, congenital diverticula; and anomalies of origin and termination—ectopia, ureterocele, blind ending, ureteropelvic defect, postcaval ureter.

From a clinical standpoint, the anomalies of origin and termination are of primary importance. *Ureteral ectopia* in the female may be the cause of a disturbing clinical symptom complex which requires knowledge of its existence to permit its recognition and treatment. The patient presents with a history of constant dribbling incontinence with intermittent normal voiding. Usually, the offending ectopic ureter is in the upper segment of a duplicated collecting system. The extravesical source of the urinary leak can be demonstrated by instilling a colored fluid into the bladder and observing the persistent loss of clear urine. The site of the extravesical orifice can often be demonstrated. Removal of the portion of the kidney supplying the aberrant ureter is the common method of treatment.

*Ureterocele* is a cystic dilatation of the lower end of the ureter. The ureteral orifice is narrowed. The intravesical dilatation of the ureter is covered externally by bladder mucosa and lined internally by ureteral mucosa. The lesion is of importance because it may be a cause of significant obstruction to the ipsilateral ureter and also because it may give rise to mechanical obstruction to the bladder neck with its attendant complications, particularly renal failure. The lesion can often be recognized by a characteristic cobra-head deformity of the lower ureter on intravenous pyelog-

raphy. Cystoscopic examination yields the definite diagnosis.

## NEOPLASMS[12, 23, 40]

Renal neoplasms may be benign or malignant, primary or secondary. A satisfactory classification is presented in Table 3. Clinically, carcinoma of the kidney, the so-called hypernephroma, is the common (80 to 85 per cent) primary adult malignant disease. Nephroblastoma, Wilms' tumor, is the common primary renal tumor of infancy and childhood. Metastatic involvement of the kidney by lesions such as lymphosarcoma, leukemia, and carcinoma of the breast occurs with greater frequency than the clinical recognition would indicate.

### Renal Cell Carcinoma

Carcinoma of the kidney occurs predominantly in persons in the 50 to 70 year age group and very infrequently in those under 30 years of age. Males are affected about twice as frequently as females. Each kidney is involved with about equal frequency. Histologically two cell types are recognized, clear and granular. In addition, a variable degree of differentiation of the tumor cells can be recognized which permits histologic grading of the tumor. The ultimate prognosis is better with the more differentiated (Grade I) tumor than with the undifferentiated (Grade IV). Metastasis from renal cell carcinoma is both hematogenous to the lungs, liver, and bone in addition to the renal vein, and lymphatic to the regional lymph nodes. Although a renal cell carcinoma can be induced in the male hamster with estrogen and in the rat with dimethylnitrosamine, no etiologic relationship has been established for the human renal cell carcinoma.

The common symptoms associated with primary renal tumor are the triad of hematuria, mass, and flank pain. Any of these may be present alone. When all three are present the lesion is usually far advanced. In addition, fever is often associated with renal carcinoma and either erythrocythemia or anemia may be. The primary renal lesion is often silent and found only when systemic symptoms such as weakness, fatigue, anorexia, and weight loss signal the presence of a neoplasm.

**TABLE 3**  ABBREVIATED CLASSIFICATION
OF RENAL TUMORS

Tumors of mature renal parenchyma—adenoma, adenocarcinoma

Tumors of immature renal parenchyma—nephroblastoma (Wilms' tumor)

Tumors of renal pelvis—transitional cell, squamous cell

Other primary renal tumors—hemangioma, hamartoma, fibroma, leiomyoma, sarcoma

Secondary renal tumors—carcinoma of breast, sarcoma

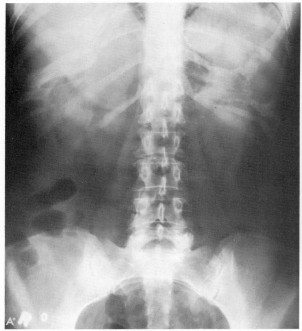

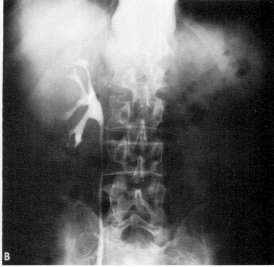

**Figure 23**   *A*, KUB demonstrating a mass at the lower pole of the right kidney. *B*, Retrograde pyelogram demonstrating deformity of collecting system by a mass occupying the midportion of the right kidney.

Physical examination may reveal a flank mass which is firm and nodular. The lesion may be so sizable that it is fixed and definite identification of its association with the kidney is impossible.

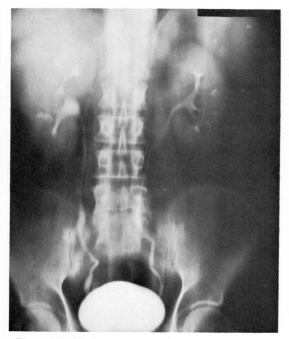

**Figure 24**   Nephrotomogram demonstrating an opacified mass at the upper pole of the right kidney. Opacification following injection of contrast medium indicates vascularity of a mass and is typical of a neoplasm.

Clinical recognition of a renal mass is primarily dependent upon x-ray studies. The plain film of the abdomen may show evidence of distortion of the renal outline (Fig. 23*A*). Retroperitoneal carbon dioxide injection or tomograms may serve to demonstrate this more clearly. The intravenous pyelogram may reveal nonfunction, usually due to obstruction of the renal vein, or may show distortion of the collecting system compatible with the presence of a space-occupying lesion in the renal parenchyma (Fig. 23*B*). The nephrotomogram is of considerable assistance in further identifying the renal mass and in indicating the vascularity of the lesion (Fig. 24). The aortogram identifies the abnormal arterial and venous pattern frequently seen with a renal carcinoma (Fig. 25).

Those x-ray studies which simply indicate the presence of a mass do not establish the presence of a renal carcinoma. Any lesion that occupies space in the kidney, such as a carbuncle, a tuberculous granuloma, or a simple cyst, may cause similar distortion. Of these, the simple serous cyst is seen with five to eight times the frequency of a renal neoplasm. The renal cyst is avascular so that demonstration of blood supply to the mass on nephrotomography or aortography makes the diagnosis of renal neoplasm highly probable. Unfortunately, the demonstration of an avascular lesion does not eliminate the possibility of the presence of a tumor that has undergone necrosis, a well recognized phenomenon.

The presence of symptoms such as hematuria or pain increases the probability that a renal mass is a neoplasm. Attempts to utilize urinary enzymes to assist in establishing the diagnosis have been inconclusive. Histologic study of the lesion is

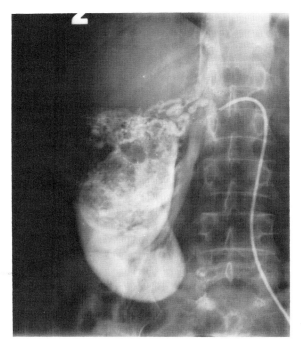

**Figure 25** Aortogram demonstrating extreme vascularity with pooling of contrast medium in the right kidney typical of renal cell carcinoma. Rapid visualization of veins is characteristic of arteriovenous fistula.

required to establish its nature. Although needle biopsy and examination of aspirated material have been utilized for this purpose, the presumed danger of spread by these techniques has made them unpopular. At present, open exploration and biopsy, if necessary, are utilized in most instances to establish the diagnosis.

The established method of treatment for carcinoma of the kidney is excision of the kidney with its surrounding fat, Gerota's fascia, and adherent peritoneum. The regional nodes and ipsilateral adrenal gland are removed systematically by some. The desirability of occlusion of the renal vessels prior to manipulation of the renal neoplasm has been repeatedly emphasized on theoretical grounds. Prior to nephrectomy, the presence of a contralateral kidney with life-sustaining functional ability is essential. Knowledge of the absence of demonstrable metastases at common sites is important. X-ray therapy prior to or following nephrectomy may be therapeutically useful. The chemotherapeutic agents and hormones such as progesterone must be regarded as having no established role in the treatment of this disease.

Except for isolated experiences with highly select groups, the 5 year survival rates for patients with renal carcinoma subjected to nephrectomy have approached 50 per cent in recent communications. The 10 year rate approximates 30 per cent in these studies. Renal neoplasm is one of the tumors known to undergo spontaneous remission of metastatic lesions. This regression has

occurred after nephrectomy in a few patients. The lesion is also known occasionally to follow an indolent course with metastases developing as late as 20 years after removal of the primary growth.

### Carcinoma of the Renal Pelvis and Ureter

Carcinoma of the renal pelvis is most common in the fifth, sixth, and seventh decades. Males are affected four times as often as females. Each kidney is affected with equal frequency. Bilateral tumors occur in less than 5 per cent of the patients. The common pelvic neoplasm is a transitional cell one, although adenocarcinoma and squamous cell tumors occur. The prognosis with the latter lesion is uniformly bad. Transitional cell carcinoma tends to be associated with development of multiple lesions in the ureter and bladder either because of multicentric origin or because of metastatic spread or implantation. Other sites of metastases are lung, liver, bone, and lymph nodes. As with bladder tumors, the greater the degree of infiltration of the tumor, the poorer the prognosis. All tumors, even the typical papilloma, are to be regarded as potentially malignant.

Hematuria is the common symptom in a patient with a tumor of the renal pelvis. Pain may accompany the passage of a clot or tissue fragment in the ureter. Physical examination commonly reveals no abnormality. The diagnosis is suspected by the demonstration of filling defects on intra-

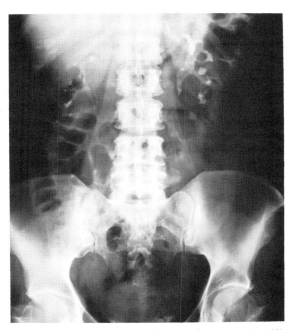

**Figure 26** Intravenous pyelogram demonstrating filling defect of left renal pelvis compatible with transitional cell tumor. Similar deformity may be caused by blood clot and nonopaque calculus. Retrograde pyelogram confirmed the filling defect. Exploration revealed a transitional cell carcinoma of the renal pelvis.

venous or retrograde pyelography (Fig. 26). In a pyelogram of good quality these defects may represent tumor, a nonopaque calculus, blood clot, or air. Urinary cytology and repeat x-ray studies carried out after passage of 2 to 3 weeks often help to differentiate these.

The treatment of choice in the presence of a normal contralateral kidney is nephroureterectomy with removal of a cuff of adjacent bladder. If a portion of the ureter remains, neoplasm develops in about 50 per cent of the patients. The 5 year survival rate after nephroureterectomy is approximately 50 per cent. Occasionally, local resection, or destruction of a transitional cell neoplasm of the pelvis or ureter, has apparently resulted in long-term survival without recurrence.

### Nephroblastoma of the Kidney (Wilms' Tumor)

Nephroblastoma of the kidney is a mixed tumor containing epithelial, muscular, and connective tissue elements. In a recent survey, 89 per cent were recognized before or at 6 years of age, 64 per cent being identified before 4 years of age. An occasional nephroblastoma is seen in an adult. There is no predilection for sex or side. Metastasis occurs by direct invasion of organs such as the liver, spleen, and intestine or by blood-borne spread to the lung, bone, and occasionally brain. Bilateral tumors do occur, perhaps as often as 5 per cent of the time.

An abdominal mass discovered in an infant by a parent or an examiner is the frequent presenting complaint in the presence of a Wilms' tumor. About 20 per cent of the abdominal masses noted in infancy arise from the genitourinary tract; about one-third of these represent malignant neoplasm. Pain and vomiting are occasionally associated with a Wilms' tumor. Gross hematuria is an infrequent complaint, being present in about 15 per cent of the patients. Fever of an irregular character and degree may be present.

On physical examination, the characteristic mass noted on palpation is usually spherical, of variable consistency from soft to rubbery, and confined to the flank. The desirability of avoiding repeated palpation of the flank in the presence of Wilms' tumor has been emphasized by many surgeons. Hypertension has been noted in association with Wilms' tumor in from 60 to 95 per cent of the patients.

The diagnosis is established by the studies employed to establish the presence of a renal cell carcinoma, although aortography is employed with less regularity in the child. Nonfunction on intravenous pyelography is unusual in Wilms' tumor, as is calcification of the mass seen on x-ray. The collecting system is usually distorted by the mass. Hydronephrosis is usually differentiated from Wilms' tumor by the x-ray studies. Neuroblastoma, another common retroperitoneal tumor of infancy and childhood, is more difficult to identify; these tumors show a much higher incidence of calcification. Tuberculosis, retroperitoneal lymph gland tumors, and pancreatic, splenic, and hepatic enlargement may cause confusion.

The basic treatment of Wilms' tumor is nephrectomy. The tumor is very radiosensitive; x-ray therapy is employed preoperatively infrequently and postoperatively commonly. In addition, the nephroblastoma is responsive to the administration of chemotherapeutic agents, the most widely used at present being actinomycin D. Various combinations of surgery, x-ray therapy, and chemotherapy are currently being evaluated.

The prognosis with current therapeutic techniques is difficult to estimate. The reported control in Wilms' tumor varies considerably. Recently combinations of therapeutic modalities have resulted in prolonged survival of a number of patients with metastatic disease and an overall control rate approximating 80 per cent.[15] There is no question that a Wilms' tumor treated before the patient is 1 year of age has a better prognosis than one treated after this age. The high control rate reported for patients less than 1 year of age may be due in part to inclusion of tumors now recognized as benign. Survival for a period equal to the time required for the initial tumor to become clinically manifest (age plus gestation period) has been utilized as an indicator of control of the neoplasm by Collins. A 2 year survival period seems to be of equal value.

## RENAL INFECTIONS[1, 17, 27, 31, 34, 45, 47]

Renal infections are commonly divided on the basis of the infecting organism into *nonspecific*, which includes the common pathogenic organisms, and *specific*, which includes tuberculosis, actinomycosis and echinococcosis. Routes of entry of infection include hematogenous, lymphogenous, ascending, and direct extension.

*Pyelonephritis* is the term applied to the common diffuse parenchymal infection of the kidney. As the name implies, both the pelvis and parenchyma are involved. The exact incidence of pyelonephritis is difficult to determine. Clinically, it is definitely recognized in less than 1 per cent of hospital admissions. Histologic evidence of chronic pyelonephritis has been reported to be present in 2.8 to 9 per cent of autopsies. The incidence of an active lesion is high at death but the significance of this observation is questionable. In younger groups, the lesion is found predominantly in women; in the older age groups, men are more often affected. The common infecting organisms are *Escherichia coli, Pseudomonas aeruginosa, Aerobacter aerogenes, Proteus vulgaris,* Staphylococcus, Streptococcus, *Alcaligenes faecalis,* and Paracolon organisms.

The kidney with acute pyelonephritis is a swollen, tense organ with multiple subcapsular whitish areas. The mucous membrane of the pelvis and calyces may be edematous and erythematous. Microscopically, there are accumulations of leukocytes with some lymphocytes and plasma cells scattered between and within tubules but usually sparing the glomerulus. The patient with acute pyelonephritis may first note the onset of frequency, dysuria, and urgency followed by the onset of chills, high fever, and flank pain, often associated with nausea and vomiting. At other times the chills, fever, and flank pain occur initially, often followed by frequency, urgency, and dysuria. Characteristically, the patient has a tachycardia and appears ill. Flank tenderness is often marked. When bacilluria on wet smear, stain, or culture is accompanied by symptoms of chills, high fever, flank pain, and the findings of flank tenderness, the urinary tract infection present is presumed to have affected the kidney. A moderate leukocytosis is usually present.

Treatment is administration of a chemotherapeutic or antibiotic agent selected initially on the basis of findings on smear and continued or changed on the basis of culture and sensitivity studies when they become available. General supportive measures such as the maintenance of fluid balance initially by the administration of intravenous fluids, and then by encouraging copious oral intake, and use of analgesics or antipyretic agents are essential. Urinary output and body weight should be observed. As in all patients with a bacteremia due to a urinary tract infection, bacteremic shock may develop in a few of these patients. The response to therapy of a patient with an uncomplicated pyelonephritis is usually prompt. Following the subsidence of the acute episode or during it, if it does not respond promptly, a search for local and systemic causes of the infection should be initiated. In addition to looking for evidence of obstruction and calculous disease, the possibility of ureteral reflux should be considered, especially in patients with repeated episodes of acute pyelonephritis. If urinary stasis is present, relief, at least by catheter drainage, may be required to allow control of the infection. Subsequently, correction of the primary cause of the stasis, such as removal of an obstructing stone or relief of an intrinsic ureteral stenosis or bladder neck obstruction, may be accomplished. Evidence that the pathogenic bacteria have been eradicated should be sought by culture rather than by relying upon absence of symptoms as evidence of cure of the infection.

*Chronic pyelonephritis* may be associated with a predisposing cause or may occur without a contributory abnormality which can be recognized with current techniques. Grossly, the kidney with chronic pyelonephritis is a pale, firm, shrunken organ with scarred, irregular surface depressions and adherent capsule. Etiology of an end-stage or contracted kidney is difficult to identify with certainty. The pelvis and calyces may be normal or thickened and fibrotic.

Microscopically, lymphocytes, plasma cells, monocytes, and neutrophils may be present. Fibrosis of the medulla and cortex with involvement of the glomeruli may be seen. The tubules may be normal or dilated with their lumen containing colloid-like casts. Varying degrees of sclerosis may

occur in the arteries. Fever, chills, flank pain, frequency, dysuria, and urgency, symptoms of recurring or persistent urinary tract infection, may be present. Or, the patient may be essentially asymptomatic until nausea, vomiting, diarrhea, gastrointestinal bleeding, muscular irritability, drowsiness, weakness, and fatigue, symptoms of renal failure, develop. Urinalysis may show white cell casts, white blood cells, red blood cells, and protein alone or in combination.

Diagnosis is complicated by the occasional absence or intermittent presence of bacteria from the urine in patients with long-standing disease. Recognition of the infecting organisms by smear or culture is essential to establish the diagnosis of urinary tract infection. Similarly, isolation of the organism from ureteral urine supports the involvement of the upper urinary tract in the infectious process. X-ray changes of reduced renal size, irregular renal contour, calyceal blunting or clubbing, and infundibular narrowing are often sufficiently suggestive to make the diagnosis highly probable. Renal biopsy may assist in establishing the diagnosis of chronic pyelonephritis. In this type of chronic infection, search for and correction of a contributory cause such as bladder neck obstruction secondary to benign prostatic hypertrophy or neurogenic bladder dysfunction assumes great importance.

Treatment is directed to control or elimination of the bacterial infection by prolonged administration of antibiotic or chemotherapeutic agents indicated by culture. Repeated urine cultures are utilized to guide therapy. Careful, repeated evaluation of renal function is essential to permit evaluation of the effects of therapy. The importance of repeated search for underlying local or systemic cause for the infection cannot be overemphasized. Occasionally, chronic pyelonephritis may be unilateral; if the infection cannot be eliminated, nephrectomy may be necessary. Similarly, unilateral chronic pyelonephritis may occasionally be a cause of renovascular hypertension which may be alleviated by nephrectomy.

A form of renal damage in which the tip of the papilla is partially or completely destroyed occurs in association with diabetes and obstruction. The necrotic papilla often sloughs. This condition, known as *papillary necrosis*, has recently been recognized in association with other abnormalities, such as sickle cell trait and massive prolonged intake of analgesics, particularly phenacetin.[29] The sloughing papilla can obstruct and necessitate measures to relieve the obstruction.

Urinary tract infection and pyelonephritis are recognized complications of *pregnancy*. The incidence of recognized pyelonephritis in pregnancy approximates 2 per cent. The hydroureteronephrosis which is commonly present, particularly on the right side, is an important contributory factor. These upper tract changes are thought to be due to mechanical pressure on the ureter and to some degree of ureteral hypotonia. There is an accompanying increase in vascularity and some edema of both upper and lower urinary tracts. Recent observations indicate that ureteral reflux may play a role in the etiology of pyelonephritis of pregnancy. The diagnosis is established as in the nonpregnant female. Treatment is similar to that usually employed but may include use of the knee-chest position or in unusual circumstances insertion of a ureteral catheter to reduce urinary stasis. Postpartum evaluation is essential in these patients. Evidence of persistence of infection or any deviation from expected course demands a search for etiologic factors not related to pregnancy.

*Staphylococcic infections* of the kidney are generally hematogenous and are usually related to a focus elsewhere in the body. The infection is primarily in the cortex of the kidney. It may subside or progress to multiple abscesses, carbuncle formation, or if rupture into the perinephric space occurs, a perinephric abscess.

Symptoms vary considerably with the stage of the infection and the patient's status. Generally chills, high fever, lumbar or abdominal pain, and generalized malaise and weakness are present. Tenderness in the renal area and occasionally an enlarged kidney may be evident on physical examination. Leukocytosis is usually marked. The urine may show a few red and white cells on microscopic examination. Isolation of the organism is characteristically difficult. Both urine culture and smear should be utilized.

X-ray studies may show evidence of renal enlargement, obliteration of the psoas shadow, and curvature of the spine away from the infected kidney. The intravenous or retrograde pyelogram may show deformity characteristic of a space-occupying lesion or may show little deviation from normal. With perinephric involvement, either directly or indirectly, fixation of the kidney develops which prevents normal movement on respiration or the assumption of an erect position. This finding can be demonstrated by lack of blurring of the renal image on x-ray during respiratory movement.

Treatment is primarily by antibiotic therapy if the lesion is confined to the kidney. Often sensitivity studies are not available and selection of the antibiotic is empiric. If a perinephric abscess is present, or if the response to therapy is poor, suggesting a persistent renal abscess, surgical drainage is necessary. Nephrectomy is rarely required.

*Perinephric abscess* may develop from causes other than staphylococcic infection of the kidney. The infection of the perinephric space may be metastatic or may result from a suppurative process in adjacent organs. It may be secondary to renal infection other than a cortical abscess, such as calculous pyonephrosis. Physical, laboratory, and x-ray findings are similar to those of renal abscess, except that distortion of the renal collecting system is often absent. In general, the patients have symptoms for a prolonged period before a diagnosis is established. Perinephric abscess should be considered in any patient with prolonged

sepsis of unknown etiology. Needle aspiration of the perinephric space may assist in establishing the diagnosis. Treatment is by incision and retroperitoneal drainage. If renal disease is present and severe, primary or secondary nephrectomy may be necessary.

*Tuberculosis of the urinary tract* is a hematogenous disease which, in the United States, usually is secondary to pulmonary tuberculosis. The primary tuberculous lesion may heal, whereas the renal tuberculosis progresses. The initial renal lesions are in the renal cortex and in the glomeruli. The medulla is involved secondarily. Initial bilateral involvement is thought to be the rule. Bilateral or unilateral healing of the disease follows the initial hematogenous dissemination in some patients. Once the medulla is involved, the disease tends to progress and cavitation in the region of the renal papilla occurs. Renal tuberculosis is found in males more often than females. Its highest incidence is in the third decade.

The symptoms associated with renal tuberculosis are those of secondary tuberculous cystitis. Hematuria, dysuria, frequency, urgency, and nocturia draw attention to the presence of this urinary tract infection. Flank pain, usually mild but occasionally of a severe degree, may also be present. Physical examination may disclose evidence of genital tuberculosis, such as a scrotal fistula, beading of the vas deferens, or irregular nodular involvement of the prostate and seminal vesicles. The findings on urinalysis may vary from gross hematuria and pyuria to minimal microscopic hematuria and pyuria or in some instances to a normal urine. Bacteriologic studies of the urine, including smear, culture, and guinea pig inoculation, permit accurate diagnosis. Usually three pooled morning urine samples, or concentrates of 24 hour urine samples, are utilized for study. Repeated bacteriologic studies are often necessary to establish the diagnosis.

Active, diffuse tuberculosis may be present without x-ray evidence. The classic changes noted on intravenous pyelogram are calcification, evidence of a renal mass, ulceration of the papilla, causing a moth-eaten appearance, and stricture formation in the infundibulum. A nonfunctioning mass of putty-like calcium deposits is characteristic of the autonephrectomy seen as a result of a far advanced tuberculous infection. Tuberculosis of the ureter secondary to renal tuberculosis may result in stricture formation or in a dilated fibrotic ureter that becomes almost "lead pipe" in character and that has a gaping "golf hole" type of orifice. Tuberculosis of the bladder is characterized by ulceration and tubercle formation.

Currently, the majority of patients with urinary tuberculosis are treated with antituberculous drug therapy. Usually, this includes streptomycin, isoniazid, and para-aminosalicylic acid. Variations in this drug regimen may be necessitated by the patient's tolerance or by the development of a drug-resistant organism. Nephrectomy for persistent active unilateral tuberculous infection, or because of secondary infection of a poorly functioning kidney, is occasionally necessary. Similarly, surgical correction of a ureteral stricture following therapy is occasionally necessary, as is a procedure to enlarge the small contracted bladder which may sometimes persist after treatment. In general, tuberculosis of the ureter and bladder are secondary to renal tuberculosis and even prior to institution of chemotherapy they would subside once the renal tuberculosis had been eliminated. Genital and urinary tuberculosis are commonly associated.

## RENAL AND URETERAL CALCULI[7, 9, 49, 50]

Calculi may occur in the kidney at any age but are more common in the third and fourth decades. They may be single or multiple, impacted or free. The calculi may be confined to the tubules at the tip of the papilla as in nephrocalcinosis (Fig. 27), may be a cast of the collecting system as in a staghorn calculus (Fig. 28), or may be in any of a variety of shapes. In about 15 per cent of patients the calculi are bilateral. They may result in renal destruction by causing obstruction, infection, or both.

Renal calculi may cause pain, hematuria, or symptoms of vague abdominal distress. They may be entirely asymptomatic even when large and causing serious renal damage. Characteristically, renal calculi cause severe, sharp flank pains which are often acute in onset and present intermittently.

The pain may radiate into the lower abdomen or buttocks and is often associated with nausea, vomiting, and gross or microscopic hematuria. The patient usually moves about restlessly seeking relief. At other times, gross hematuria or routinely discovered microscopic hematuria may be the only indication of the presence of the calculus. Not infrequently, the symptoms or urinary findings of a urinary tract infection will lead to evaluation leading to the diagnosis.

Physical findings in patients with renal calculi may be entirely normal or may yield nonspecific evidence of renal disease, such as tenderness, muscle spasm, or a palpable mass. Tenderness and muscle spasm are usually minimal even when present. On microscopic examination of the urine sediment, hematuria is present in about 75 per cent of patients even in the absence of colic. Pyuria and bacilluria may be present. Occasionally, characteristic crystalluria is noted. Observations of the urinary pH may assist in directing attention to the composition of the calculus. The diagnosis is usually dependent on x-ray demonstration of the calculus. In the presence of a calcium-containing stone, a radiopacity maintaining a constant relationship to the kidney and its collecting system will usually be demonstrated on plain film of the abdomen and intravenous or retrograde pyelogram. If the calculus is composed of uric acid, or another nonopaque substance, its presence will be evident only as a filling defect on visualization of the urinary tract with contrast media.

Treatment of renal calculi is dependent on their

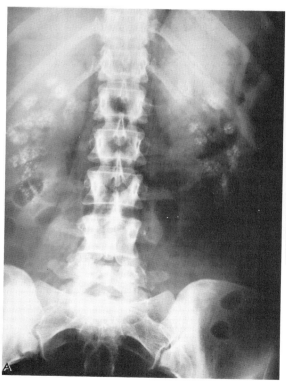

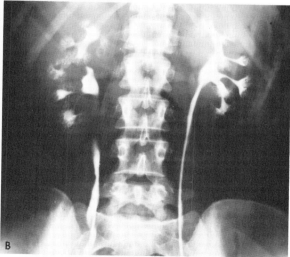

**Figure 27** Nephrocalcinosis. *A,* Typical stippled calcification of kidney, demonstrated on pyelography. (*B*) to be associated with collecting ducts in the tip of the papillae.

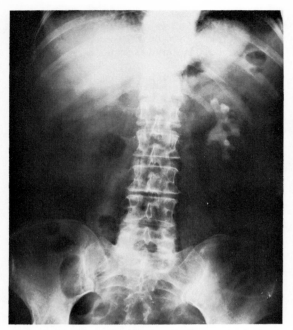

**Figure 28** Staghorn calculus. Radiopaque calculus is seen to be a cast of the collecting system of the left kidney.

size, composition, and the presence or absence of symptoms or complications such as infection or obstruction. A cause for the calculus is always sought and an attempt made to correct it. Observation utilizing analgesics for relief of acute episodes of pain, forcing fluids, and employing such measures as alkalinization and administration of allopurinol in known uric acid calculi, or alkalinization and d-penicillamine in known cystine calculi, may be indicated. If life or renal function is threatened, or if symptoms are severe with little hope of spontaneous passage of the calculus, removal by incising the renal pelvis or the renal parenchyma or both may be indicated. If the kidney is destroyed, if infection is confined to one stone-bearing kidney, or if the condition of the patient dictates, unilateral nephrectomy may be the desirable course. The recovered stone should always be analyzed to serve as a guide for future therapy.

Ureteral calculi are presumed to arise in the kidney and pass into the ureter. Their composition is essentially the same as that of renal calculi. They occur primarily in middle age and with equal frequency on each side. Men are affected about twice as frequently as women. Pain, either typical colic or indefinite or indistinct abdominal discomfort, is present in the overwhelming majority of patients. Hematuria, symptoms of infection, or anuria may also cause the patient to seek aid. The local physical findings are usually limited to minimal localized tenderness. Flank tenderness and guarding may be noted when obstruction is present.

Urinalysis shows red blood cells in most pa-tients with ureteral calculi. A ureteral calculus may be present in the absence of abnormality on urinalysis but this finding should increase suspicion that a presumed diagnosis of ureteral calculus is in error. The diagnosis is established by x-ray studies. Demonstration of a constant relationship of a presumed stone to the urinary tract is essential. Most ureteral calculi pass spontaneously. They tend to impact at the ureteropelvic junction, the area over the iliac vessels, or in the lower third of the ureter, particularly in the ureterovesical area. Relief of pain of ureteral colic often requires large amounts of narcotics. Nausea and vomiting may necessitate fluid replacement. If symptoms are prolonged, they may be relieved by bypassing the calculus with a catheter. Similarly, catheter drainage of an obstructed kidney may be necessary to permit control of infection. Persistent obstruction, infection, and severe recurrent pain are the general indications for operative removal of ureteral calculi. Instrumental removal of stones is frequently accomplished with a variety of baskets and catheters; most limit the use of baskets to stones in the lower third of the ureter.

The operative approach employed for ureterolithotomy is dependent on the site of the impaction of the calculus. Every effort should be made to recover all stones and analyze them. A search for an etiologic factor, such as hyperparathyroidism, should be made routinely. Measures such as elimination of infection and obstruction and encouraging fluid intake should be undertaken to prevent recurrence.

## VASCULAR DISEASE OF THE KIDNEY[17, 35, 48]

Diseases of the renal artery have been recognized with increasing frequency since aortography became a relatively safe, readily available diagnostic tool. These arterial lesions have clinical importance if they are a cause of bleeding, contribute to renal functional impairment, or cause alteration in renal blood supply sufficiently severe to stimulate excessive production of renin and consequent hypertension.

### Aneurysm of the Renal Artery

Arteriosclerotic saccular aneurysm of the renal artery is commonly asymptomatic. Occasionally, rupture of the aneurysm causes massive hemorrhage or the aneurysm may be associated with hypertension. Typically, these lesions are recognized as faintly calcified ringlike shadows near the hilum of the kidney. If the lesion is small, asymptomatic, and seemingly completely surrounded by calcification, treatment is not necessary. If bleeding or hypertension secondary to the aneurysm occurs, or if the aneurysm has a significant uncalcified portion, resection of the aneurysm or nephrectomy may be desirable. Bleeding is rarely associated with a calcified aneurysm. In addition to the saccular aneurysm the renal artery may be the site of a dissecting aneurysm, poststenotic aneurysm, multiple microaneurysms, or a fusiform aneurysm. When present, they are often associated with fibrotic stenosis of the renal artery in hypertensive patients.

### Arteriovenous Fistula

Arteriovenous fistula, either extrarenal or intrarenal, is also being recognized with increasing frequency. Trauma, accidental or surgical, including needle biopsy, and neoplasm are the common causes of the acquired fistula. Some are thought to be congenital in origin. Pain, hematuria, and symptoms related to hypertension and congestive failure may be presenting complaints. A localized bruit is the outstanding physical finding. The diagnosis is made by rapid visualization of the renal veins on aortography. The treatment has shifted in recent years toward a reconstructive approach rather than nephrectomy.

### Occlusive Disease

Occlusive disease of the renal artery has assumed clinical importance with the recognition that it is a cause of hypertension. It has become increasingly apparent that renovascular hypertension may run almost any course. However, a renal cause should be particularly suspected in patients with hypertension of abrupt onset, in patients under 35 years of age, in patients with malignant hypertension of abrupt onset, in patients with symptoms of atherosclerosis preceding the onset of hypertension, and in patients with an epigastric bruit.

Atherosclerosis is the commonest cause of occlusive lesions of the renal artery. These lesions are usually well localized and characteristically occur near the orifice of the renal artery, although other sites are affected. The second group of occlusive arterial lesions is characterized by constriction of the arterial lumen by fibrous replacement of a portion of the arterial wall. These lesions were formerly designated fibromuscular hyperplasia but actual hyperplasia of the smooth muscle of the media is uncommon. Medial fibroplasia is the more appropriate term for the common fibrous replacement of the muscle of the media. This lesion occurs eight to nine times more frequently in women than in men. About one-half of the patients have bilateral lesions, which are characteristically located in the middle and distal thirds of the renal artery. The remainder of the fibrous lesions are designated intimal or subadventitial fibroplasia because of the location of the collagen. Each constitutes about 10 per cent of this group. Subadventitial fibroplasia also occurs mostly in young women and usually involves the right renal artery predominantly.

An abdominal bruit is the only physical finding suggesting the presence of renal artery stenosis. Establishing the diagnosis of a significant renal artery lesion is dependent on laboratory studies. The intravenous pyelogram may show a discrepancy in renal size of 1 cm. or more, a delay in the appearance or absence of contrast medium, or a late hyperconcentration of contrast medium on the side of the arterial lesion. The radioactive renogram is almost always abnormal on the affected side but the nature of the abnormality may be variable. The aortogram will show evidence of an anatomic lesion of the artery which may or may not have functional significance. Differential renal function studies assist in determining this and also provide information of considerable value in formulating plans for treatment. The characteristic physiologic changes associated with significant narrowing of the renal artery are a reduction in glomerular filtration rate, an excessive tubular reabsorption of water, and an even greater reabsorption of sodium. As a consequence, the urine from a kidney with a significant renal artery lesion is reduced in volume, shows a slight decrease in sodium concentration, and marked increase in the concentration of creatinine, inulin, and para-aminohippurate which are filtered or secreted high in the tubule and not reabsorbed. The demonstration of these characteristic changes in the urine from the kidney with a renal artery lesion makes an abnormality of this organ a highly probable cause of hypertension. Currently, determination of renin levels in the renal venous effluent of each kidney and in the systemic blood seems to be the most reliable method for identifying a kidney responsible for hypertension. Segmental artery disease and renal infarct may also cause hypertension.

Treatment of renovascular hypertension is dependent on the general condition of the patient, the nature of the renal artery disease, and the bilateral status of the renal parenchyma. When surgical correction is indicated, reconstruction of the renal artery, bypass of an arterial lesion, partial nephrectomy, and nephrectomy all are utilized depending on these findings. Relief or marked improvement in the hypertension may be expected in about three-fourths of the patients treated when properly selected.

Renal failure as a consequence of major renal artery disease has been recognized infrequently. This possibility warrants consideration in patients with renal failure of unknown etiology despite its infrequent occurrence because the possibility of reversal of the renal malfunction exists.

### Renal Vein Thrombosis

Renal vein occlusion has been recognized infrequently in the past, and then almost always in infants. The infants usually present with evidence of systemic illness, hematuria, and an abdominal mass. Blood studies often show a diminished platelet count. Adults present with lumbar or abdominal pain, occasionally an enlarged kidney, and occasionally symptoms and findings compatible with the nephrotic syndrome. Cardiac failure is a frequent associated finding. As methods of visualizing the renal veins become more accurate and available, diseases of the renal vein are being recognized more frequently. In children nonoperative treatment is apparently associated with a significant incidence of renal functional recovery. In adults, medical and surgical treatment have been employed too infrequently to assess their relative merits.

### RENAL AND URETERAL TRAUMA[20, 41, 43, 44]

Renal trauma may be secondary to a penetrating injury or to a blunt force. Penetrating injuries of the abdomen usually require exploration and, therefore, constitute less of a problem in diagnosis than does blunt abdominal trauma. Although renal trauma usually follows severe injury and is often associated with injury of other organs, seemingly minor falls or blows may occasionally produce severe renal injury. Aside from the direct effect of force on the kidney, injury may apparently result from the forceful whiplike movement of the kidney on its pedicle. Although spontaneous renal rupture occurs infrequently, the kidney diseased by reason of obstruction or tumor is more easily injured by trauma than is a normal kidney.

The types of renal injury are depicted in Figure 29. Depending on the type and extent of injury, the immediate complications of renal injury are those related to blood loss and urinary extravasation. Rarely, in bilateral injury or injury of a single kidney, acute renal failure may be a primary result of the renal trauma.

Hematuria is the primary finding in trauma to the urinary tract. It is often gross but may be microscopic or absent. Abdominal pain is usually present, located in the flank or upper abdomen, and variable in severity. Physical examination may

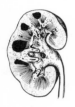

Contusion (Minor)

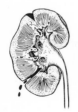

Laceration With & Without
Urinary Extravasation (Major)

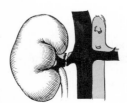

Pedicle Injury (Critical)

**Figure 29** Diagram representing the various types of renal injury. Laceration with urinary extravasation usually requires drainage. Pedicle injury demands prompt control of hemorrhage.

disclose evidence of shock as well as local tenderness, swelling, and ecchymosis. Usually, muscle spasm is marked in the flank and upper quadrant of the abdomen. A mass is usually not palpable early in injuries other than renal pedicle injuries. An expanding mass with recurrent evidence of severe blood loss is evidence of a type 3 or pedicle injury.

The diagnosis is usually made by the finding of hematuria associated with the physical findings suggesting renal trauma and evidence of renal malfunction or distortion on pyelography. In addition to providing evidence of renal abnormality, the intravenous pyelogram provides invaluable evidence of the presence of a contralateral functioning kidney. Other x-ray studies such as aortography, nephrotomography, or mercury scan may be indicated to delineate the extent and nature of the trauma. The possibility that the hematuria noted may be related to lower urinary tract injury must be kept in mind and investigated, usually with a cystogram, in any questionable instance.

If a diagnosis of renal pedicle injury is suspected by the clinical course of the patient, prompt exploration and control of the hemorrhage are indicated. Even in these circumstances demonstration of a contralateral functioning kidney by intravenous pyelography is usually possible by temporary restoration of the blood pressure and a single film taken after injection of contrast medium on the way to the operating room. Other renal injuries associated with blunt trauma usually do not require immediate intervention. Bed rest, analgesics for relief of pain, and observation coupled with investigation of renal status as indicated by the patient's course constitute the usual treatment. Aside from hemorrhage, the presence of urinary extravasation or development of infection may necessitate surgical intervention. If an operative procedure is performed, it may vary from simple drainage to partial or total nephrectomy. Usually, a delay of 2 to 3 days after trauma before exposure of the kidney simplifies the surgical procedure. The majority of patients with renal injury can be treated without operative intervention. Upper urinary tract extravasation is better tolerated than lower urinary tract extravasation and is not subjected to drainage by all urologists. Secondary hemorrhage from renal parenchymal injury may occur and dictates caution in allowing the patient out of bed. In many instances in patients with multiple injuries, the ideal treatment of the renal injury must be compromised.

### Ureteral Injury

Ureteral injury is an uncommon complication of penetrating or blunt trauma. In penetrating trauma, symptoms from other injuries usually mask any symptoms due to ureteral involvement. In blunt trauma, evidence of urinary tract involvement is so slight that diagnosis of ureteral injury is delayed. Tenderness and muscle spasm due to urinary extravasation and development of signs of infection usually cause x-ray evaluation of the

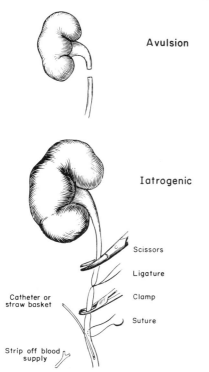

**Figure 30** Diagrammatic representation of various types of ureteral injury.

difficult to differentiate from acquired diverticulum and is recognized infrequently. The presence of muscle fibers in the diverticular wall, thought to be characteristic of congenital lesions, is probably not a valid differential feature. The symptoms of a congenital and an acquired diverticulum are similar.

*Exstrophy* of the bladder is an embryologic catastrophe in which there is an absence of the lower abdominal and anterior vesical walls. The posterior bladder wall is exposed. There is an accompanying epispadiac deformity of the urethra and separation of the pubes. This abnormality occurs in about 1 in 50,000 births, with males predominating 3 to 1. Muecke has produced the defect experimentally in the chicken by utilizing a plastic graft to interfere with normal cloacal membrane regression. In addition to the social inconvenience occasioned by total incontinence, upper urinary tract infection is common and often leads to death. Attempts to reconstruct the bladder are frequently unsuccessful and diversion of the urine by placing the ureters in the large bowel, or in an isolated loop of ileum with an external orifice, is necessary (Fig. 31). Retained exstrophic epithelium has been the frequent site of adenocarcinomatous change in the past.

*Urachal abnormalities* vary from persistent fistula due to the failure of closure of the allantoic duct to cyst formation, persistent umbilical sinus,

urinary tract. Intravenous or retrograde pyelography discloses the urinary extravasation and often identifies the site of injury. Drainage of extravasated urine and relief of obstruction are essential. Reconstruction of the disrupted ureter may be attempted by a number of techniques. In the past the resultant damage associated with injury and delay in recognition has made nephrectomy a frequent necessity. The ureter is subject to iatrogenic injury with much greater frequency than it is to injury from external trauma. These injuries result from both open surgical and endoscopic surgical technique. Some of the more common types are seen in Figure 30. These may result in silent destruction of the kidney from unilateral hydronephrosis or in acute renal failure if a single ureter or both are ligated. Urinary extravasation with eventual infection and fistula between the ureter and the skin, vagina, or uterus is more common. In treating iatrogenic ureteral injuries, both relief of obstruction and drainage of extravasated urine must be achieved promptly. Reconstruction of the defect may then be attempted as indicated by the general and local condition of the patient.

## THE BLADDER

### ANOMALIES[2, 3, 10, 52]

*Agenesis* and *duplication* of the bladder occur but are very rare. *Congenital diverticulum* is

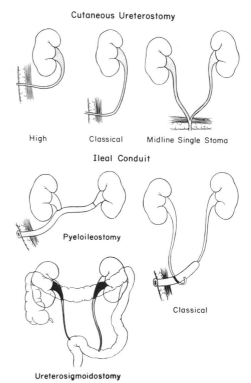

**Figure 31** Methods of permanent supravesical diversion.

or a diverticulum of the dome of the bladder due to failure of fusion of a portion of the duct.

*Ureteral reflux* may be congenital in origin. The responsible defect is a maldevelopment of the trigone of the bladder with the trigone being large and the ureter being laterally placed with a short intramural tunnel. At times, these defects are accompanied by a thin-walled bladder with a large capacity, so-called *megacystis syndrome*.

## Tumors of the Urinary Bladder[22, 32, 51]

Malignant tumors of the urinary bladder account for about 3 per cent of the deaths from cancer in the United States. Males are affected approximately 2.5 to 4 times as often as females. Epithelial tumors are rare in children but may occur at any age in adults. The peak incidence is in the sixth and seventh decades in both males and females. The overwhelming majority of bladder neoplasms are epithelial in origin. Grossly, they are commonly exophytic, protruding into the vesical lumen. They may vary from a papillary configuration with a narrow stalk and multiple frondlike projections to a sessile serpiginous growth. Ulceration and encrustation with calcium salts may occur. Approximately 40 per cent of the tumors involve the trigone and an additional 45 per cent the posterior and lateral bladder walls. Multiple tumors are common, being present in approximately 25 per cent of the patients on diagnosis, and becoming evident in as many as 50 per cent of the patients with a so-called benign papilloma in a 5 year period.

Classification of the epithelial tumors of the bladder has been and is confusing. Histologically, these tumors are primarily transitional or squamous in cell type. Undifferentiated carcinoma, adenocarcinoma, and mucus-forming adenocarcinoma are also recognized. Some utilize a designation of benign papilloma for well differentiated epithelial tumors; others prefer to utilize the term Grade I carcinoma because patients with these tumors show a tendency to reappearance of neoplasm as well as to development of a more advanced neoplasm. Grading of the tumor on the basis of cellular differentiation has clinical significance; the most differentiated tumors are designated Grade I and the undifferentiated or poorly differentiated, Grade IV. Degree of cellular differentiation varies throughout a tumor approximately 50 per cent of the time. The transitional, squamous, or undifferentiated cell type of the tumor is commonly maintained throughout.

The demonstration by Jewett and Strong that depth of infiltration of a bladder tumor is related to the presence of recognizable metastasis at autopsy was an important observation (Fig. 32). They observed no evidence of metastasis in patients with invasion confined to the submucosa, and metastatic spread in 14 per cent of patients with invasion confined to the muscularis, and in 74 per cent of the patients with invasion of the perivesical tissue. Subsequent clinical experience

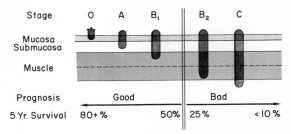

**Figure 32**   Staging of bladder tumors (after Jewett). Solid vertical bars indicate depth of infiltration. If lymph node or prostatic involvement is demonstrated, "D" classification is utilized by some.

has tended to confirm the potential survival without evidence of neoplasm in patients with superficially infiltrating lesions and the poor prognosis of patients with deeply infiltrating lesions.

Nonepithelial tumors of the bladder are mesenchymal in origin and may be benign such as fibroma or leiomyoma, or malignant such as sarcoma. Metastases to the bladder are unusual.

Bladder cancer is known to be associated with exposure to two chemicals, beta-naphthylamine and xenylamine. In addition, a higher incidence of bladder tumors is recognized in smokers than in nonsmokers. Bladder infestation with *Schistosoma haematobium* is also recognized as predisposing to the development of a bladder neoplasm.

Gross hematuria is the presenting complaint in about 70 per cent of the patients with bladder neoplasm. The hematuria is usually total but may be initial or terminal. Microscopic hematuria is present in an even greater proportion of patients. Symptoms of vesical irritability, such as urgency, frequency, and dysuria, constitute the other common group of complaints in patients with bladder tumors.

Physical examination is usually normal in the patient with a bladder tumor unless the lesion has spread beyond the bladder. The diagnosis of a bladder neoplasm warrants serious consideration in any patient with gross or microscopic hematuria, or recurrent episodes of vesical irritability. Presence of a filling defect on the cystogram of the intravenous pyelogram or on a retrograde cystogram should increase the suspicion of a bladder tumor. Definitive diagnosis is dependent on cystoscopic visualization of a mucosal abnormality and biopsy with confirmation of the presence of a neoplasm on histologic examination. Studies of urinary cytology may yield evidence of neoplastic change not identified by cystoscopy. Efforts to utilize drug-induced fluorescence with ultraviolet light to aid in cystoscopic identification of bladder tumors not readily identified by routine light cystoscopy have been of limited value. In any patient with a bladder neoplasm, the kidneys and ureters should be visualized to eliminate the possibility that a transitional cell neoplasm of the upper urinary tract is seeding the bladder.

Once the diagnosis of bladder neoplasm is established, clinical staging of the neoplasm is important to permit rational therapy and prognosis. Staging is based on the pathologic observations correlating tumor spread with degree of tumor invasion as confirmed and modified by clinical experience. The gross appearance of the bladder tumor assists in staging, with the more advanced lesions tending to have a broader, flatter base with evidence of fixation of the bladder wall. Similar fixation of the bladder wall may be evident on retrograde cystography. The single most important observation in staging is the depth of infiltration of the bladder tumor. To allow assessment of the infiltration, an adequate biopsy of the tumor and of the muscle at its base, as well as deep biopsy of any other suspicious area in the bladder and prostate, is essential. If biopsy indicates infiltration limited to the superficial portion of the muscle, prognosis is good. Infiltration deep in the muscle is associated with a poor prognosis. Bimanual examination under anesthesia is also of value in clinical staging. Induration of any type indicates a poor prognosis but this is particularly true if the induration extends beyond the bladder. If histologic evidence of invasion of the prostate or involvement of the iliac lymph nodes is obtained, the prognosis for cure becomes so poor that vigorous therapeutic attempts are usually avoided in favor of palliative procedures. In general, evidence of lymphatic invasion on biopsy is a poor prognostic sign as is evidence of ureteral obstruction. Squamous carcinomas often are of a higher stage than indicated by biopsy.

Therapy of bladder tumors may be curative or palliative. The results achieved with any type of therapeutic approach seem more related to the stage of the tumor at the initiation of therapy than to the therapy itself. Untreated, the majority of the patients with carcinoma of the bladder die directly or indirectly from their disease. Renal failure from obstruction and infection is a prominent cause of death. Carcinomatosis is also common, with frequent involvement of the regional nodes, liver, lungs, and vertebrae in that order. Uncontrolled hemorrhage from the bladder tumor also contributes to mortality.

Attempts to eradicate the neoplasm employ surgery or radiation therapy. Operative procedures utilized in the treatment of bladder tumors are directed to the local destruction or excision of the neoplasm or to removal of the entire bladder. The procedures utilized in local destruction of the neoplasm include:

1. Transurethral fulguration or transurethral excision and fulguration carried out with an endoscopic instrument per urethram; this is limited by size and location of the lesion.

2. Suprapubic excision and fulguration through a cystotomy incision; the excision is followed by local destruction.

3. Segmental resection of bladder with or without ureteral reimplantation. Location and extent of the tumor have limited the utilization of partial excision of the bladder, as has the tendency for tumors to be multiple. Current techniques for ureteral reimplantation have permitted more enthusiastic employment of this technique when adequate resection requires sacrifice of the intravesical ureter.

4. Various techniques for local application of radon packs, radon seeds, and radioactive suture materials.

5. Instillation of chemotherapeutic agents has been utilized with some success in noninvasive tumors.

6. Cystectomy is employed in the treatment of higher-stage neoplasms, multiple recurrent tumors, or failures by locally destructive techniques. It is rarely employed in the presence of metastases to iliac nodes or the prostate unless some local complication, such as bleeding, dictates the palliative removal of the bladder. Cystectomy necessitates diversion of the urine. Utilization of an ileal conduit to divert the ureteral urine to the skin (see Fig. 31) affords the best long-term results currently. However, the surgical procedure involves moderate risk. For this reason diversion of the ureter to the skin is employed at times. Placement of the ureters into the intact large bowel is also employed. It has the advantage of providing urinary continence. The disadvantages of this technique are its frequent failure to preserve renal function and the development of hyperchloremic acidosis in some patients from the reabsorption of urine by the bowel.

Palliation of the patient with bladder neoplasm may be a very difficult problem. The local complications of hemorrhage, frequency, pain, and ureteral obstruction may necessitate utilization of the procedures employed in an attempt to eradicate the neoplasm. Locally destructive procedures or urinary diversion often provides required relief.

## INFLAMMATORY LESIONS OF THE BLADDER[31, 45]

Bacterial cystitis is characterized by urinary frequency, nocturia, urgency, and dysuria. In women acute hemorrhagic cystitis is probably the commonest cause of hematuria. As in any urinary tract infection, cystitis may be secondary to upper or lower urinary tract disease or to a systemic illness and requires thorough evaluation if recurrent or persistent in the female. Males should be evaluated after a single episode. Classically, the diagnosis is based on the symptoms, the finding of a two-glass pyuria, and the identification of bacteria by smear or culture.

The symptoms of *tuberculous cystitis* are those of bacterial cystitis. Hematuria is often present. The small contracted bladder is rarely seen at present. Tuberculous cystitis is usually secondary to tuberculosis of the upper urinary tract.

*Interstitial cystitis*[6] is an inflammatory disease of the bladder, the etiology of which is unknown. It occurs predominantly in women. Frequency, nocturia, urgency, dysuria, and lower abdominal pain are prominent symptoms. The physical examination reveals no abnormality. The urinalysis and urine culture are normal. The diagnosis is established by the demonstration, on cystoscopy carried out under anesthesia, of an extremely small bladder capacity and evidence of ulceration and cracking of the bladder wall with hydraulic distention. Hydraulic distention of the bladder is also therapeutic, temporarily increasing bladder capacity. Other therapy has included instillation of various mild caustic solutions into the bladder. Occasionally, intractable discomfort and frequency necessitate use of a patch of bowel to increase bladder capacity and on occasion diversion of the urine has been necessary.

## URETERAL REFLUX[2, 52]

Despite development of high voiding pressures by the detrusor muscle, urine does not normally reflux from the bladder into the ureters on voiding. The oblique submucosal course of the intravesical ureter combined with normal ureteral peristalsis is thought to prevent backflow of urine from the bladder into the ureter. Ureteral reflux has come to be recognized as an important abnormality of the urinary tract contributing to persistent or recurrent infection. The role of reflux in the production of renal damage in the absence of infection is equivocal. The recognized causes of ureteral reflux are congenital deformity, bladder outflow obstruction, neurogenic dysfunction, surgical alteration of the intravesical ureter, and infection. It is important to recognize that infection may be the result as well as cause of ureteral reflux. Patients with reflux commonly present with symptoms of persistent or recurrent urinary tract infection. Occasional intermittent flank pain with voiding may be present. Although reflux may be identified by cystoscopic techniques employing a chromogen or by isotope studies, the voiding cystourethrogram and the retrograde cystogram have permitted recognition of this phenomenon with ease (Fig. 33). Ureteral reflux has been recognized with greater frequency in children than in adults, and in females than in males. In some patients, reflux may subside with elimination of a contributory cause, such as infection or obstruction. In others, institution of simple techniques, such as double and triple voiding, coupled with treatment of infection, eliminates infection and prevents renal damage. When the intravesical ureter is abnormal, restoration of the normal anatomic relationship of the bladder and the tunneled intravesical ureter may be achieved by any of a number of techniques, usually employing reimplantation of the ureter. With elimination of reflux, the control of infection is usually possible.

## BLADDER CALCULI[49]

In the United States, bladder calculi are a disease of the adult male. In other parts of the world,

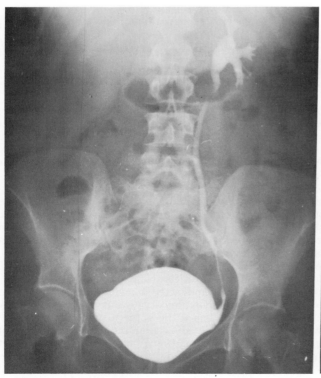
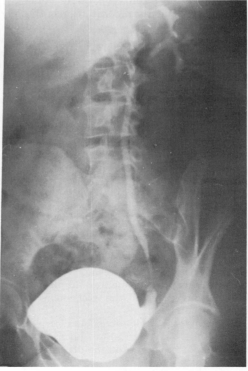

**Figure 33** Ureteral reflux on left demonstrated on cystogram study in adult female with recurrent left pyelonephritis.

children are primarily affected. Calcium oxalate stones are the commonest type found in the bladder. They may assume a mulberry or jackstone configuration. Many patients present with symptoms of urinary tract infection. Dull or sharp pain, aggravated by movement and relieved by rest, and hematuria are the common complaints in the absence of infection. The pain may be referred to the tip of the penis. Occasionally, the patient experiences periodic retention from the ball valve action of the calculus or passes calculi per urethram. The physical examination rarely aids in establishing a diagnosis. The urinalysis characteristically shows red blood cells and may disclose white blood cells. Only about half of the bladder calculi are visible on x-ray, either because of their size, composition, or overlying structures. Characteristically, stones lying free in the bladder lie in the midline. Whenever bladder calculi are present in the adult, the possibility of urinary stasis either on an obstructed or a neurogenic basis becomes paramount. Other causes of calculus formation also warrant consideration. Treatment consists in removal of the stone either by endoscopic or open surgical techniques. Often, smaller calculi may be removed by irrigation through an endoscopic sheath. Fracture of the calculus may be carried out by either a blind or a visual technique to facilitate its transurethral removal. If an open surgical technique is utilized, the suprapubic route is usually employed. After removal of the calculi, prevention of recurrence is dependent on correction of the underlying cause for their development.

## Bladder Diverticulum[31, 45]

A bladder diverticulum is an outpouching of the bladder wall. It may be congenital or acquired. Differentiation on the basis of etiology is often difficult; it seems probable that congenital abnormality may play a role in the diverticula developing as the result of obstructive lesions. The majority of bladder diverticula are associated with and probably secondary to obstruction at or distal to the bladder neck. Neurogenic bladder dysfunction may also lead to their formation.

Diverticula of the bladder may be single or multiple, small or large. They form most commonly in the region of the ureteral orifices on the posterior or lateral bladder wall. The diverticular wall usually consists of bladder mucosa with few, if any, investing muscular fibers. The patient with a bladder diverticulum usually presents with symptoms of bladder neck obstruction such as hesitancy, intermittency, weak urinary stream, and nocturia. None of these symptoms suggests that the bladder neck obstruction has been complicated by the development of a diverticulum. The presence of a urinary tract infection or bladder calculus may result from the stasis of urine occasioned by a nonemptying diverticulum and cause symptoms leading to its discovery. Occasionally, an asymmetric lower abdominal cystic mass will be evident on inspection or palpation of the abdo-men of a thin patient but the physical examination rarely aids in establishing the diagnosis.

Cystoscopic visualization of the orifice or base of the diverticulum and visualization of a smooth asymmetric outpouching of the bladder wall on retrograde cystogram are useful in establishing the diagnosis. Indirect visualization of the diverticulum by the cystogram is particularly important, because it allows an assessment of the size, the presence or absence of pathologic change on the wall, and the ability of the diverticulum to empty.

Since bladder diverticula are usually secondary to obstruction at or below the bladder neck, relief of this obstruction is essential to their treatment. If the size or configuration of the diverticulum does not permit it to empty despite relief of obstruction, or if complications of stasis such as stone or persistent infection are present, measures to ensure emptying are required. Under these circumstances the diverticulum is usually excised and the bladder wall reconstructed to eliminate the defect permitting its development. Occasionally, the presence or suspicion of a neoplasm in a diverticulum is an indication for its removal.

## Bladder Trauma[36, 37, 39]

Perforation of the urinary bladder is a surgical emergency requiring prompt recognition and treatment. Spontaneous perforation is extremely rare and almost always associated with disease of the bladder, such as infection or neoplasm. Bladder rupture may result from blunt and penetrating wounds of the abdomen. A full bladder predisposes to rupture. Injuries of the bladder and urethra are associated with fractures of the pelvis with sufficient frequency to warrant consideration in patients with this type of trauma. Instrumentation and endoscopic operative procedures have assumed major importance as a cause of bladder perforation. Because a peritoneal injury may accompany the bladder injury, the extravasation may be intraperitoneal, extraperitoneal, or both. The inferior extension of the extravasated urine is usually limited by the urogenital diaphragm.

Severe abdominal pain and hematuria or inability to void are common symptoms. Tenderness, rebound tenderness, and muscular rigidity are commonly seen with perforation of the bladder. Shock is not uncommon. However, the symptoms and signs of bladder rupture may be insignificant and insidious if the possibility is not considered. Although procedures such as measuring return of instilled irrigating fluid and cystoscopy may assist in recognition of perforation of the bladder, they are often misleading. The retrograde cystogram is the most useful and reliable diagnostic tool (Fig. 34). It should always be preceded by a plain film of the abdomen because the extravasated contrast medium can be difficult to recognize in an intraperitoneal perforation.

Once the diagnosis of ruptured bladder is made or strongly suspected, treatment should be

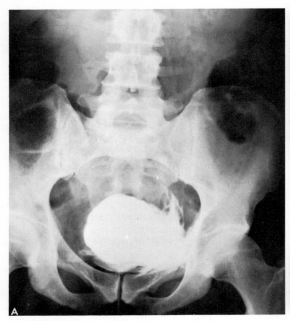 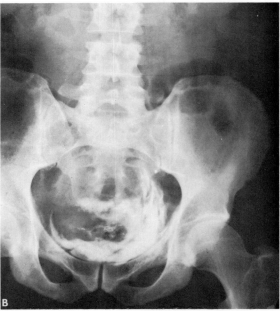

**Figure 34**   Retrograde cystogram demonstrating extravasation. *A,* Filling phase; *B,* postevacuation.

prompt because mortality increases markedly with delay. The essential therapeutic maneuver is institution of adequate suprapubic drainage. Repair of the bladder defect, although desirable, is unnecessary if adequate drainage is achieved. Repair of the peritoneal rent in patients with intraperitoneal extravasation should be carried out if possible.

## NEUROGENIC BLADDER[4, 5, 24, 28]

The adult urinary bladder is an integrated smooth muscle viscus that will normally act as an asymptomatic reservoir for 300 to 500 ml. of urine and will respond to the desire to expel this stored urine promptly with uninterrupted forceful flow. Normal function is dependent on an intact musculature and a complex control mechanism that involves both automatic and somatic nerves.

The syncytium of smooth muscle that forms the main spherical body of the bladder, the fundus, encompasses the bladder neck as it passes into the posterior urethra. The bladder neck–urethral component of this muscular complex is assisted by a generous complement of elastic tissue in the urethra in its definite but poorly understood role in maintaining urinary incontinence. The striated muscle of the urogenital diaphragm and levator ani surrounding the midurethra in the female and the distal prostatic and membranous urethra in the male also play a significant role in urinary control.

The smooth muscles of the bladder and urethra receive sympathetic and parasympathetic nerve fibers (Fig. 35). The sympathetic fibers originate from T9 to L5 and course through the hypogastric

nerves to the pelvic plexus. The parasympathetic fibers originate from S2 to S4 and course through the pelvic nerves to the pelvic plexus. The striated muscle of the urogenital diaphragm is innervated by the medulated fibers of the pudendal nerve, also originating from S2 to S4. All peripheral nerves contain both motor and sensory fibers. The afferent fibers carry pain, temperature, and proprioceptive sensation; the latter are related to fullness and desire to void. The important motor neurons to the smooth muscle of the bladder are parasympathetic in origin. In fact, the sympathetic innervation plays no unique role in either the sensory or motor phases of micturition in man. The reflex center for micturition is in the sacral spinal cord segments 2, 3, and 4 (Fig. 35). Except in the untrained infant, this center is usually subject to control of the cerebral cortex.

Normally, smooth muscle is in a state of tension which is independent of central nervous system innervation. Stretching will cause a shortening of the muscle with resultant increases in tension. Even if the extrinsic nerve supply is completely divided, the bladder can store and evacuate a limited amount of urine. However, controlled accumulation of urine, as well as its timely complete evacuation, usually requires nervous control.

Initiation of *normal micturition* may be associated with a desire to void stimulated by proprioceptive impulses from bladder filling or may be volitional. With the former, release of cerebral inhibition is associated with a short latency period before detrusor contraction is initiated. The detrusor contraction shortens the urethra and increases the caliber of the urethral lumen. Relaxation of the external (striated muscle) sphincter is mediated through the pudendal nerve. The pelvic

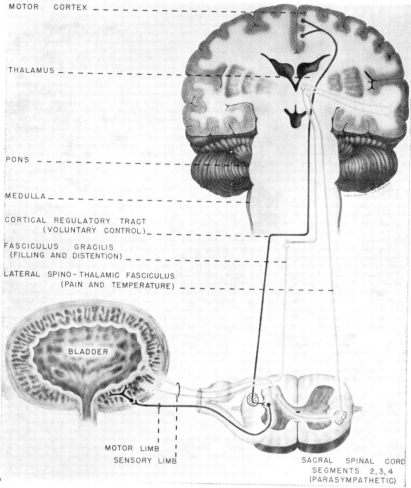

**Figure 35** Diagram of major nerve pathways of importance in controlling bladder function. (From Lapides, J. In: Campbell, M. F., and Harrison, J. H., eds.: Urology. 3rd ed. Philadelphia, W. B. Saunders Company, 1970.)

floor relaxes and sustained detrusor tone results in an uninterrupted flow of urine. Terminally, contraction of the external sphincter, bulb, and perineal musculature occurs. Attempts to void on command are associated with a longer detrusor latency period and a temporal association of pelvic floor relaxation with shortening and opening of the urethra.

Although all micturitional disturbances are manifested ultimately by detrusor dysfunction, in some, such as those related to overstretching of the bladder, direct detrusor injury may be the cause. The majority are associated with anatomic, functional, or pharmacologic interference with the primary or secondary reflex arc. The frequent combination of factors makes exact, clinically useful classification of micturitional disorders associated with neurogenic or detrusor abnormality difficult.

In assessing the individual patient with a micturitional disturbance a careful history is essential. Particular attention should be given to the following: (1) evidence of systemic disease such as diabetes or syphilis; (2) a history of utilization of drugs with recognized parasympatholytic effect such as atropine, methantheline (Banthine), or selected tranquilizers; (3) a history suggestive or diagnostic of neurologic disease. The physical and general neurologic examination may provide evidence helpful in recognizing the possibility of and characterizing a neurogenic bladder dysfunction. Absence of rectal sphincter tone suggests a defect in the primary reflex arc. Failure of the rectal sphincter to contract with painful stimulus of the glans penis or clitoris (bulbocavernosus reflex) tends to support this supposition.

Assessment of the functional status of the upper urinary tract, by determination of endogenous serum creatinine or blood urea levels, and of the individual anatomic and crude functional status of the kidneys by use of intravenous urography is important to patient survival and care but adds little to the determination of the nature of the bladder dysfunction. A voiding cystourethrogram may disclose a bladder diverticulum or ureteral reflux and aids in assessment of the status of the bladder neck and the urethra. Visualization of the latter assists in localizing the site of anatomic or functional obstruction. Cystoscopy and panendoscopy are useful in evaluating the bladder and urethra. Trabeculation associated with neurogenic dysfunction is variable in degree. In a bladder with deficient sensation (e.g., tabes dorsalis), trabeculation is minimal and patchy. In traumatic cord lesions, pronounced trabeculation and cellule formation may be present, depending on the degree of detrusor coordination and the duration of the abnormality. The presence of bladder lesions such as diverticula or calculi can have a marked influence on bladder function. Endoscopic procedures permit recognition of obstructing prostatic tissue and

evaluation of the functional status of the external sphincter.

The most important objective observations with regard to bladder function and neurologic disease are provided by knowledge of the bladder capacity and of efficiency of voiding or achieving bladder emptying, and by observation of variation in sensation, bladder pressure, and contraction in response to filling (cystometrogram). An effort should be made to determine the amount of urine usually voided and the residual urine. Bors suggests 250 ml. rather than 300 ml. as a minimal normal capacity. He advocates considering residual urine in relation to bladder capacity (normal up to 20 per cent of capacity in upper motor neuron lesion and 10 per cent of capacity in lower motor neuron

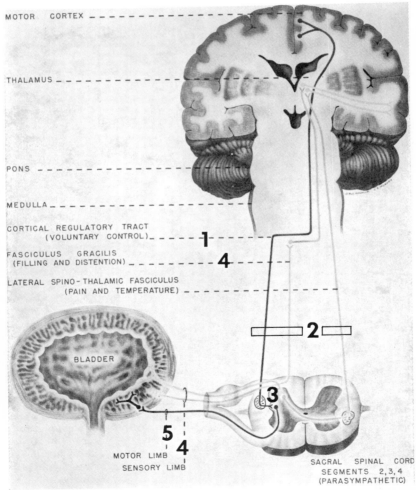

**Figure 36** *1*, Site of typical lesion resulting in an uninhibited neurogenic bladder; lesion anywhere along the corticoregulatory tract, including an intracranial site, can be responsible. *2*, Complete transection of spinal cord above reflex center, a typical cause of a reflex (automatic) bladder. *3*, Lesions involving both limbs of the reflex arc produce an autonomous neurogenic bladder. *4*, Interruption of the sensory limb of the lower reflex arc or the long afferent tracts to the brain results in sensory paralytic bladder. *5*, Lesions of the lower motor neurons or motor fibers result in a motor paralytic bladder. (Modified from Lapides, J. In: Campbell, M. F., and Harrison, J. H., eds.: Urology. 3rd ed. Philadelphia, W. B. Saunders Company, 1970.)

lesion) rather than as an absolute amount. After the residual urine is measured, the exteroceptive sensation of the bladder is tested by instillation of cold and hot water. If a neurologic lesion involves the upper motor neurons but not the conus or cauda equina, part or all of the sterile ice water is expelled promptly. Cystometry (see Fig. 4) consists of intermittent (50 ml. per minute) or continuous infusion of water at body temperature through a catheter with observation of first desire to void (150 to 250 ml.), feeling of fullness (350 to 450 ml.), and pressure response of the bladder. The intravesical pressure increases minimally until bladder capacity is reached; no spontaneous detrusor contractions are evident. On instruction to void the normal patient generates a pressure exceeding 50 cm. $H_2O$ and often voids around the catheter. Administration of 2.5 mg. of bethanechol (Urecholine) subcutaneously increases the pressure response to filling up to 15 cm. $H_2O$ in adults with a normal bladder and to a much greater degree in patients with a sensory- or motor-paralytic bladder. In addition to these tests sphincter resistance can be measured by determining the pressure required to overcome the sphincteric contraction. Electromyographic studies of the urinary and rectal sphincter have been utilized as investigative tools and have been informative.

Depending on degree and duration, overdistention of the bladder causes functional and probable anatomic changes in the bladder musculature and should be avoided at all times. Recognition of the undesirable effect of overdistention on bladder function is particularly important immediately after spinal cord injury. During this period (designated *spinal shock*) the bladder acts as a denervated organ and is unable to empty. Prevention of overdistention is essential and can be accomplished by intermittent urethral catheterization, indwelling urethral catheter, or suprapubic cystostomy. The method utilized will depend on the skill and availability of personnel and on the patient's condition. Every effort should be made to avoid urinary tract infection. Periodic catheter changes and sterile irrigation of the bladder to prevent stone formation are important aspects of care. Detrusor function is monitored periodically until return of voiding seems likely, at which point the catheter is removed.

A number of factors influence the type of neurogenic dysfunction resulting from a nerve lesion. The location of the nerve lesion is important. Lesions of the reflex arc (lower motor neuron) leave the detrusor more or less on its own (Fig. 36). Lesions above the sacral reflex center (upper motor neuron) affect the modification of the voiding reflex mediated through the sacral reflex center. Incomplete, selective (sensory or motor), and combinations of upper and lower motor lesions occur clinically, making exact correlation of bladder function difficult and often unpredictable. However, a loose classification of neurogenic bladder dysfunction that usually correlates with the major aspects of the neurologic lesion is useful (Table 4).

The *uninhibited neurogenic bladder* results from decreased cerebral inhibition of bladder reflexes due to a defect in the corticoregulatory tract (Fig. 36, *1*). In the normal infant, urination occurs whenever vesical or other regional stimuli reach a sufficient height to act through a lower motor neuron reflex arc. As the child grows older, bladder training allows the cerebral cortex to exercise an inhibitory effect over this simple reflex arc so that reflex emptying can be delayed. Inhibition is obtained first during the waking hours and subsequently becomes so patterned that it is present even during sleep so that enuresis ceases.

In some children, however, the cerebral inhibitory control does not become developed, perhaps as a result of deficient pathways or from psychologic defect, and the child continues to have uninhibited contractions (Fig. 37). There is then urinary frequency during the daytime and enuresis at night. The characteristics of this type of bladder are normal or increased tone and decreased capacity without residual urine.

Two types are recognized: congenital and acquired. In patients with the congenital type, administration of atropine in dosage sufficient to atropinize a child, if effective, is diagnostic of the uninhibited neurogenic bladder and, in addition, is therapeutic. Patients with the acquired type, that is, those with cerebral or high cord damage, are less susceptible to this form of treatment although tranquilizers with parasympatholytic effects such as imipramine produce beneficial effects at times.

The *reflex (automatic) neurogenic bladder* typically results from complete transection of the cord at a level above the conus (Fig. 36, *2*). It may also result from a disturbance of the suprasegmental arc that simulates transection of the cord. The result is a reflex arc running from the bladder to the sacral cord, synapsing and running back to the bladder. The bladder, then, is an organ controlled

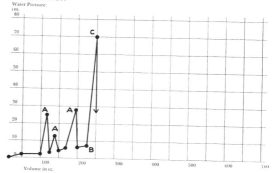

CYSTOMETROGRAM

UNINHIBITED NEUROGENIC BLADDER

A. DESIRE TO VOID.

B. STRONG DESIRE TO VOID.

C. VOIDED AROUND CATHETER.

MANY SMALL CONTRACTIONS, NOT CONTROLLED BY PATIENT, ENDING IN STRONGER CONTRACTION AND VOIDING.

**Figure 37**

**TABLE 4** CHARACTERISTICS OF NEUROGENIC BLADDERS

| I. Uninhibited | II. Reflex (Automatic) | III. Autonomous | IV. Sensory (Atonic) | V. Motor |
|---|---|---|---|---|
| | *Site of Lesion* (see Fig. 36) | | | |
| Cerebral or high cord (underdeveloped central control) | A and B: Upper neuron | A and B: Lower neuron | Dorsal columns | Anterior horn cells |
| | *Characteristics* | | | |
| Voiding reflexes to filling are not suppressed | A, Spastic (imbalanced): Bladder takes part in general hypertonicity<br>B, "Normal" (balanced): Bladder independent of control but reflex arc functions well | A, Flaccid (imbalanced): No external nervous control, but atonic<br>B, "Normal" (balanced): No external nervous control, but bladder tone adequate for urethral resistance | Loss of sensation allowed excess filling, ending in flaccidity and atony | Sensation normal, but motor paralysis |
| | *Disease Process* | | | |
| A, Congenital: Delayed development of inhibitory pathway<br>B, Acquired: Hemiplegia, brain tumors, multiple sclerosis | A and B: Transection of cord | A and B: Transection of conus or cauda equina | Tabes, pernicious anemia, multiple sclerosis, diabetes, syringomyelia | Poliomyelitis |
| | *Symptoms* | | | |
| Enuresis, urgency, and frequency; occasional incontinence | A: Reflex, involuntary voiding without sensation<br>B: Same; occasional trigger zones cause voiding | A: Overflow incontinence<br>B: Continence by periodic forceful evacuation | Painless overflow incontinence | Painful overflow incontinence |
| | *Tone* | | | |
| Normal or increased | A: Increased<br>B: Normal or increased | A: Decreased<br>B: Decreased | Decreased (late) | Increased (early) |
| | *Capacity* | | | |
| Decreased | A: Decreased<br>B: Normal or increased | A: Increased<br>B: Increased | Increased | Increased (late) |
| | *Residual Urine* | | | |
| 0 | A: 20–50 cc.<br>B: 0–50 cc. | A: ± 300 cc.<br>B: ± 30 cc. | 500 cc. + | 300 cc. + |
| | *Treatment* | | | |
| Atropinization (parasympathetic block) | A: 1, Remove irritants (infection, calculi); 2, sacral neurotomy; 3, alcohol subarachnoid block<br>B: None | A and B: 1, Presacral neurectomy; 2, pudendal block; 3, TUR; 4, Credé (5, Urecholine) | 1, Preserve bladder tone; 2, evacuate with straining (3, presacral neurotomy if sphincter tight; 4, pudendal block; 5, Urecholine) | Catheter drainage expectantly |
| | *Results* | | | |
| Good in children | A: Fair if treatment prolonged.<br>B: Good | A: Poor<br>B: Fair | Poor | Good |

by a simple reflex. The lesions that cause this syndrome are usually injuries to the thoracic or lumbar cord that result in paraplegia. Characteristically the bulbocavernosus reflex is present and hyperactive.

The diagnosis of reflex neurogenic bladder rests upon locating the site and degree of injury and determining the type of bladder function that results. The bladder empties by reflex activity arising either from intrinsic stimuli from the bladder wall or from extrinsic stimuli that provoke mass movement. The patients have no real sensation of vesical filling, but the increasing size of the bladder as the urine accumulates produces sensations within the abdomen that they may interpret as fullness of the bladder. Urination occurs without warning as soon as the reflex arc is closed by summation of afferent stimuli.

Two major types of reflex bladders are recognized. The more usual is the spastic type; the other is the so-called normal reflex neurogenic bladder. The former is seen in patients with spasticity of the extremities. It is characterized by small capacity with more or less residual urine. The spasticity and small capacity necessitate frequent urination that is precipitant and inconvenient (Fig. 38). The goal of therapy is a so-called normal reflex neurogenic bladder. If this is obtained, bladder capacity may be as high as 300 cc. Visceral sensation of bladder filling may be enough to give the patient opportunity to reach a convenient place for voiding. Residual urine is low.

The therapeutic aim is first to remove all irritative foci, since the bladder is a purely reflex organ with sensory stimuli arising within the bladder wall itself, both from the mucosa and from the muscle as a stretch reflex. Bladder infection and calculi increase the sensory component of the reflex arc and cause increased stimuli for contraction.

A period of observation and restudy of several months is necessary to re-evaluate the effect of

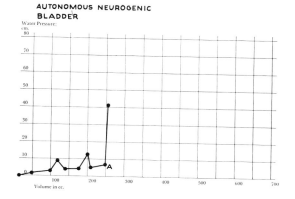

CYSTOMETROGRAM

A. STRAIN TO VOID.

NO SENSATION OF FILLING.
VOIDS BY STRAINING AND LITTLE REFLEX ACTIVITY.

Figure 39

eliminating these sources of sensory stimuli. If spasticity persists, blocking of the sensory nerve impulses is necessary and may be accomplished either by alcohol block or by sectioning the sacral roots. Intradural alcohol injection of the lower spinal cord blocks all long reflexes and produces an autonomous neurogenic bladder. The result is greater capacity and relative freedom from the inconvenient reflex voiding of the reflex bladder. A more direct approach is to block the sensory roots of the third, fourth, and fifth sacral nerves to cut off the sensory components arising from the irritable bladder and so interrupt the reflex arc. The bladder is then free to relax and to attain a normal capacity. In addition, the irritative stimuli arising from the posterior urethra are cut off, releasing the reflex spasm of the sphincter. Thus, sphincteric tone is more nearly normal. These procedures may assist patients with reflex bladders to regain almost normal control.

The *autonomous neurogenic bladder* results from section of the cauda equina and conus, usually by trauma, but occasionally by inflammatory lesions and often from such congenital anomalies as meningocele with spina bifida. In contrast to a lesion across the spinal cord above the conus, a lesion through the cauda equina leaves the bladder autonomous (Fig. 36, 3; Fig. 39), possessing little or no outside reflex arc. It acts merely by the intrinsic reflex arc through the detrusor ganglia.

The bulbocavernosus reflex is usually absent and saddle anesthesia is present. Bladder sensation is diminished and coordinated reflex stimulus to the detrusor is absent. The bladder fills against the intrinsic detrusor tone and urination is irregular and incomplete. Depending on the degree of resistance at the vesical neck, the patient will be able to void more or less of the bladder contents

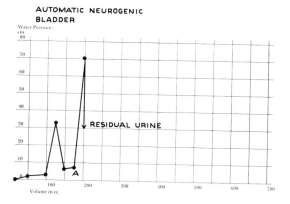

CYSTOMETROGRAM

A. UNABLE TO RESIST VOIDING.

REFLEX CONTRACTIONS, UNCONTROLLED, DURING FILLING, ENDING IN FORCEFUL, INCOMPLETE EMPTYING.

Figure 38

by increasing abdominal pressure or by the use of manual pressure over the bladder. The capacity of the bladder may be as great as 350 ml., but the amount of residual urine is, of course, also quite high.

Treatment of these patients is directed at balancing urethral resistance against intravesical pressure. For emptying to occur, the ineffective detrusor contractions, supplemented by the pressure of the abdomen and the hand, must overcome urethral resistance. If urethral resistance is too high, retention of urine will result. On the other hand, if urethral resistance is too low, incontinence occurs.

Several measures have been proposed to decrease urethral resistance, since the strength of detrusor contraction can seldom be affected directly by therapy, even by such agents as the parasympathomimetic drugs.

Pudendal nerve block and section, either unilateral or bilateral, will cause partial paralysis of the external sphincter. Transurethral resection of the prostatic urethra, especially when definite obstructive elements are seen with the panendoscope, will quantitatively reduce urethral resistance. Often more than one resection must be done to secure a good result, since initial overenthusiasm can result in total incontinence.

The *sensory neurogenic bladder* occurs after interruption of the sensory side of the lower reflex arc or the long afferent tracts to the brain (Fig. 36, 4). Tabes dorsalis, occasionally pernicious anemia and multiple sclerosis, and syringomyelia are followed by this dysfunction. The patient does not know when his bladder is full because the afferent stimuli are cut off, so that after a time gross overdistention occurs, which results in atony. This atonic bladder devoid of motor power is the end result of the sensory defect. The bladder has a large capacity and urination occurs by overflow during straining. Incontinence often brings these patients to the physician. They are able to empty their bladders only by forceful abdominal pressure and manual compression. A cystometrogram would show a low filling pressure with a very large capacity and no contractions of any sort. Cystoscopically, fine trabeculations are seen. The neck of the bladder is open and relaxed, as are the other portions of the detrusor. The external sphincter is not involved by the atony, and so its resistance is the cause of the retention of urine and overflow incontinence.

The object of treatment is primarily preventive. If the patients are seen early, before bladder tone is destroyed, they can be instructed to void at predetermined intervals, perhaps every 2 or 3 hours. Their bladders then will not become overdistended. After overdistention and atony have occurred, the object of therapy can only be to reduce the amount of residual urine and hope for return of bladder tone. The patient should be instructed to strain at each voiding and supplement the straining by manual pressure on the bladder. Bethanechol chloride (Urecholine) may be of some assistance in increasing detrusor activity. In very severe cases, a period of drainage by an indwelling catheter will occasionally reduce capacity to a more normal level and restore some tone. The fundamental disease process should be treated. Transurethral resection of the bladder neck is of little value to these patients since the bladder neck is already widely open. Section of the pudendal nerve, either unilaterally or bilaterally, in certain cases will promote reduced urethral resistance because of partial paralysis of the normally active external sphincter and so will decrease the amount of residual urine.

The *motor neurogenic bladder* is the result of loss of the motor side of the reflex arc (Fig. 36, 5). It is seen with poliomyelitis, trauma, and tumor. Sensation is normal and so distention is painful, but overdistention occurs because the bladder is unable to contract as a result of loss of efferent stimuli to the detrusor. The cystometrogram is normal initially except for absence of detrusor contraction. Treatment consists of prompt institution of catheter drainage to avoid overdistention and atony while recovery of the nerve lesion occurs. If a partial motor lesion persists, use of bethanechol (Urecholine) may assist in restoration of function. If a complete motor lesion persists, the outlook for functional recovery is grave.

In summary, the initial treatment of the bladder with a neurogenic dysfunction should be directed to minimizing bladder damage by preventing overdistention by catheter drainage, avoiding or minimizing infection, and reducing the risk of stone formation by encouraging ambulation and high fluid intake. Subsequent to this the nature of the bladder dysfunction should be clarified by careful assessment of the neurologic state of the patient and his bladder. Return of the bladder to a stable functional state may require many months after injury. The ultimate goal of therapy is a functional state of the bladder that will insure preservation of renal function and will permit the patient to lead as normal an existence as possible while accomplishing this. A combination of preventive and active therapeutic measures is often necessary to achieve this desired goal. Active therapy may include such diverse measures as administration of drugs to control infection and modify neuromuscular response, mechanical modification of the bladder neck and external sphincter utilizing transurethral techniques, and various blocking and surgical procedures to modify the nerve supply to the bladder. Both the temporal and quantitative aspects of these measures are important to the results obtained. At times preservation of renal function or other serious complications from an unmanageable bladder require abandoning the organ and diverting the urine.

# SELECTED REFERENCES

Campbell, M. F., and Harrison, J. H., eds.: Urology. 3rd ed. Philadelphia, W. B. Saunders Company, 1970.
*This three-volume standard reference text in urology contains 70 chapters written by recognized authorities. The detailed written text is well illustrated. An excellent list of selected references is appended to each chapter to assist the interested student.*

Emmett, J. L., and Witten, D. M.: Clinical Urography. 3rd ed. Philadelphia, W. B. Saunders Company, 1971.
*This three-volume reference work describes the diagnostic techniques commonly employed in urology and illustrates the radiographic findings in various pathologic states.*

Glenn, J. F., and Boyce, W. H., eds.: Urologic Surgery. New York, Hoeber Medical Division, Harper & Row, 1969.
*This multiauthor text presents modern concepts of indications for and complications of various surgical therapeutic endeavors as well as detailing the surgical technique. Preoperative and postoperative care is discussed.*

Grayhack, J. T., ed.: Year Book of Urology. Chicago, Year Book Medical Publishers.
*This reference book is published yearly. It contains abstracts of significant works contributed to each of the major areas of urology during the year. References to major recent contributions in a field are available by consulting several Year Books in sequence.*

# REFERENCES

1. Allen, A. C.: The Kidney: Medical and Surgical Disease. 2nd ed. New York, Grune and Stratton, 1962.
2. Amar, A. D., Culp, O. S., et al.: Malformations: Encyclopedia of Urology. Berlin, Springer-Verlag, 1968.
3. Arey, L. B.: Developmental Anatomy. 7th ed. Philadelphia, W. B. Saunders Company, 1965.
4. Bors, E.: Neurogenic bladder. Urol. Survey, 7:177, 1957.
5. Bors, E., and Comarr, A. E.: Neurologic Urology. Baltimore, University Park Press, 1971.
6. Bowers, J. E., and Lattimer, J. K.: Interstitial cystitis. Surg. Gynec. Obstet., *105*:313, 1957.
7. Boyce, W. H.: Surgery of renal calculi. In: Glenn, J. F., and Boyce, W. H., eds.: Urologic Surgery. New York, Hoeber Medical Division, Harper & Row, 1969, p. 77.
8. Bricker, N. S.: Obstructive uropathy. In: Strauss, M. B., and Welt, L. G., eds.: Diseases of the Kidney. Boston, Little, Brown and Company, 1963, p. 728.
9. Butt, A. J.: Treatment of Urinary Lithiasis. Springfield, Ill., Charles C Thomas, 1960.
10. Campbell, M. F.: Urology in infancy and childhood. In: Campbell, M. F., and Harrison, J. H., eds.: Urology. 3rd ed. Philadelphia, W. B. Saunders Company, 1970, p. 1379.
11. Dalgaard, O. Z.: Bilateral polycystic disease of the kidneys. Acta Med. Scand., Supp. 328, 1957.
12. Deming, C. L., and Harvard, B. M.: Tumors of the kidney. In: Campbell, M. F., and Harrison, J. H., eds.: Urology. 3rd ed. Philadelphia, W. B. Saunders Company, 1970, p. 885.
13. Dodson, A. I.: Anatomy and surgical approach to the urogenital tract in the male. In: Campbell, M. F.: Urology. Philadelphia, W. B. Saunders Company, 1954, p. 1.
14. Emmett, J. L., and Witten, D. M.: Clinical Urography. 3rd ed. Philadelphia, W. B. Saunders Company, 1971.
15. Farber, S.: Chemotherapy in the treatment of leukemia and Wilms' tumor. J.A.M.A., *198*:826, 1966.
16. Grayhack, J. T., and Graham, J. B.: Surgery of the kidney. In: Glenn, J. F., and Boyce, W. H., eds.: Urologic Surgery. New York, Hoeber Medical Division, Harper & Row, 1969, p. 37.
17. Heptinstall, R. H.: Pathology of the Kidney. Boston, Little, Brown and Company, 1966.
18. Hinman, F.: Principles and Practice of Urology. Philadelphia, W. B. Saunders Company, 1935.
19. Hinman, F., Jr.: The Pathophysiology of urinary obstruction. In: Campbell, M. F., and Harrison, J. H., eds.: Urology. 3rd ed. Philadelphia, W. B. Saunders Company, 1970, p. 313.
20. Hodges, C. V., Gilbert, D. R., and Scott, W. W.: Renal trauma. J. Urol., *66*:627, 1951.
21. Holland, J. M., Grayhack, J. T., and Del Greco, F.: The kidney. In: Preston, F. W., and Beal, J. M., eds.: Basic Surgical Physiology. Chicago, Year Book Medical Publishers, 1969, p. 455.
22. Jewett, H. J.: Tumors of the urinary bladder. In: Campbell, M. F., and Harrison, J. H., eds.: Urology. 3rd ed. Philadelphia, W. B. Saunders Company, 1970, p. 1003.
23. King, J. S., Jr., ed.: Renal Neoplasia. Boston, Little, Brown and Company, 1967.
24. Kropp, K. A., Grayhack, J. T., Wendel, R. M., and Dahl, D. S.: Morbidity and mortality of renal exploration for cysts. Surg. Gynec. Obstet., *125*:803, 1967.
25. Kunin, C. M.: Epidemiology and natural history of urinary tract infection in school children. Bull. N. Y. Acad. Med., *40*:767, 1964.
26. Kuru, M.: Nervous control of micturition. Physiol. Rev., *45*:425, 1965.
27. Lattimer, J. K., Uson, A. C., and Melicow, M. M.: Tuberculous infections and inflammation of the urinary tract. In: Campbell, M. F., and Harrison, J. H., eds.: Urology. 3rd ed. Philadelphia, W. B. Saunders Company, 1970, p. 443.
28. Lapides, J.: Neuromuscular vesical and ureteral dysfunction. In: Campbell, M. F., and Harrison, J. H., eds.: Urology. 3rd ed. Philadelphia, W. B. Saunders Company, 1970, p. 1343.
29. Lindvall, N.: Renal papillary necrosis. Acta Radiol., Supp. 192, 1960.
30. Lippman, R. W.: Urine and the Urinary Sediment: A Practical Manual and Atlas. Springfield, Ill., Charles C Thomas, 1969.
31. Lousley, O. S., and Kerwin, T. J.: Clinical Urology. Baltimore, Williams & Wilkins Company, 1944.
32. Marshall, V. F., et al.: Bladder Tumors: A Symposium. Philadelphia, J. B. Lippincott Company, 1956.
33. Merrill, J. P.: The Treatment of Renal Failure. 2nd ed. New York, Grune and Stratton, 1965.
34. O'Grady, F., and Brumfield, W., eds.: Urinary Tract Infections. New York, Oxford University Press, 1968.
35. Poutasse, E. F.: Surgical treatment of renal hypertension. Amer. J. Surg., *107*:97, 1964.
36. Prather, G. C.: Injuries of the bladder. In: Campbell, M. F., and Harrison, J. H., eds.: Urology. 3rd ed. Philadelphia, W. B. Saunders Company, 1970, p. 852.
37. Prather, G. C., and Kaiser, T. F.: The bladder and fracture of the bony pelvis. The significance of a "tear drop bladder" as shown by cystogram. J. Urol., *63*:1019, 1950.
38. Rao, N. R., and Heptinstall, R. H.: Experimental hydronephrosis: A microangiographic study. Invest. Urol., *6*:183, 1969.
39. Reynolds, C. J.: The diagnosis and a new treatment of traumatic rupture of the posterior urethra. Southern Med. J., *35*:825, 1942.
40. Riches, E.: Tumors of the Kidney and Ureter. Edinburgh, E. & S. Livingston, 1964.
41. Rusche, C., and Morrow, J. W.: Injuries to the ureter. In: Campbell, M. F., and Harrison, J. H., eds.: Urology. 3rd ed. Philadelphia, W. B. Saunders Company, 1970, p. 811.
42. Schirmer, H. K. A., et al.: Renal metabolism with proximal or distal ureteral occlusion. Surg. Gynec. Obstet., *123*:539, 1966.
43. Scholl, A. J., and Nation, E. F.: Injuries of the kidney. In: Campbell, M. F., and Harrison, J. H., eds.: Urology. 3rd ed. Philadelphia, W. B. Saunders Company, 1970, p. 785.
44. Scott, R., Jr., Carlton, C. E., Jr., and Goldman, M.: Pene-

trating injuries of the kidney: An analysis of 181 patients. J. Urol., *101*:247, 1969.

45. Smith, D. R.: General Urology. Los Altos, Calif., Lange Medical Publications, 1966.

46. Spence, H. M., et al.: Cystic disorders of the kidney—classification, diagnosis, treatment. J.A.M.A., *163*:1466, 1957.

47. Stamey, T. M.: Localization and treatment of urinary infections: Role of bactericidal urine levels as opposed to serum levels. Medicine, *44*:1, 1965.

48. Stewart, B. P., Dustin, H. P., Kiser, W. S., Meaney, T. F., Straffon, R. A., and McCormack, L. J.: Correlation of angiography and natural history in evaluation of patients with renovascular hypertension. J. Urol., *104*:231, 1970.

49. Straffon, R. A., and Higgins, C. C.: Urolithiasis. In: Campbell, M. F., and Harrison, J. H., eds.: Urology. 3rd ed. Philadelphia, W. B. Saunders Company, 1970, p. 681.

50. Symposium on Stones. Amer. J. Med., *45*:649, 1968.

51. Wallace, D. M., ed.: Tumors of the Bladder; Vol. 2. Monographs of Neoplastic Disease at Various Sites. Edinburgh, E. & S. Livingston, 1959.

52. Williams, D. I.: Urology in Childhood. Berlin, Springer-Verlag, 1958.

53. Winter, C. C.: Radioisotope diagnostic tests in urology. In: Campbell, M. F., and Harrison, J. H., eds.: Urology. 3rd ed. Philadelphia, W. B. Saunders Company, 1970, p. 2940.

# 48

# THE PROSTATE, SEMINAL VESICLES, PENIS, AND TESTES

*James F. Glenn, M.D.*

## HISTORICAL ASPECTS

The development of genitourinary surgery constitutes an important and provocative chapter in surgical history. Painful and disabling conditions of the genitourinary system were recognized by the ancients; early Egyptian hieroglyphics depict phimosis and bladder calculi. Anatomic interest in the lower urinary tract and the male genital system was defined in early Greece; Herophilos of Chalcedon, the Father of Anatomy, described the genital organs in 300 B.C. and is credited with naming the prostate, a term indicating that the gland guards or stands before the bladder. Lower urinary tract obstruction was recognized as a principal cause of bladder stone, and both suprapubic and perineal vesicolithotomy were practiced without benefit of anesthesia in the earliest civilizations, attended by extreme morbidity and mortality due to infection, hemorrhage, and injury of the gastrointestinal system. The lithotomists or "cutters for stones" were recognized in the Hippocratic Oath which declares, "I will not cut persons laboring under the stone, but will leave this to men who are practitioners of this work."

Early catheters were devised of straws, quills, and hollow instruments of horn, bone, and various metals. Ultimately, catheters of rubber and synthetic substances permitted comfortable instrumentation and alleviation of urinary obstruction. Diagnostic evaluation of the lower genitourinary tract evolved with cystoscopic techniques; in 1879, Nitze developed the cystoscope employing Edison's incandescent bulb. Discovery of the roentgen ray in 1895 added another modality of diagnosis, and radiographic contrast materials such as colloidal silver, introduced by von Lichtenberg in 1906, allowed further urographic evaluation of the urinary tract. Excretory urography was discovered serendipitously by Rowntree and associates in 1923,[15] and Swick, working in von Lichtenberg's laboratories in 1929 and 1930, employed a pyridine ring iodine compound, "uroselectan," for successful excretory definition of the urinary tract.

Little clinical attention was given to disorders of the prostate before 1900. Indeed, a classic text of 1858, Morland's *Diseases of the Urinary Organs*, deals extensively with kidney disorders, stones, inflammatory conditions of the bladder, urethral abnormalities, and other urologic difficulties, but states only that "an enlarged prostate may be mistaken for stricture." The first total prostatic enucleation was probably accomplished in St. Peter's Hospital by Sir Peter Freyer of London in the latter part of the nineteenth century. Shortly before the turn of the century, Hugh H. Young accomplished successful "operative removal of the enlarged prostate that was causing the obstruction to urination. At operation a finger was inserted through the opening into the bladder and found a large rounded mass projecting about three inches into the bladder cavity. With the assistance of a gloved finger in the rectum, it was not difficult to shell out this great mass from within the prostatic capsule, thereby removing the obstruction—my first prostatectomy."[25] Perineal prostatectomy was probably first accomplished in this country by Goodfellow. A transurethral cold "punch" operation was the forerunner of modern transurethral prostatic resection, the latter introduced by Davis and others in the early 1930s. The retropubic approach to open surgical prostatic enucleation is the most recent addition to the armamentarium of the urologic surgeon.

Modern perception of disorders of the male genitourinary system includes an advanced understanding of the physiology of the genital system, the endocrinology of sexual disorders, and the biochemistry of diseases of the prostate, seminal vesicles, and external genitalia. Recognition of the enzymatic and hormonal capabilities of the male genital system has permitted more accurate diagnosis and definitive therapy in a host of threatening conditions including carcinoma of the prostate, testicular tumors, benign prostatic hypertrophy, and male genital infections.

## ANATOMY

The organs of the male genital tract include the prostate gland and seminal vesicles, the penis and its incorporated urethra, and the scrotum and scrotal contents. The male genitourinary system functions for purposes of copulation and reproduction, hormone production, and urinary excretion.

The prostate gland, seminal vesicles, and Cowper's glands produce secretions that serve to lubricate the system and provide a vehicle for storage and passage of spermatozoa. In addition, the prostate gland is essen-

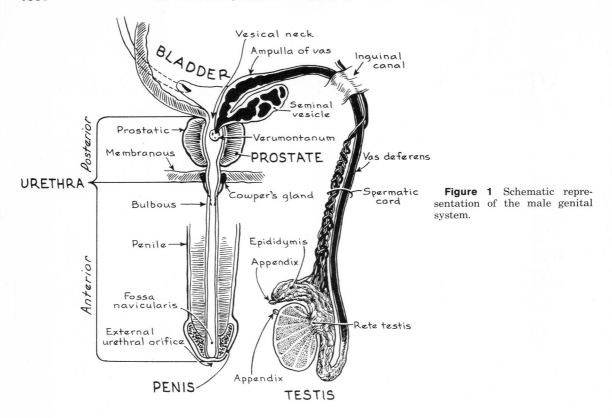

**Figure 1** Schematic representation of the male genital system.

tial to normal erectile capacity of the penis. The penis, composed of two vascular erectile bodies, the corpora cavernosa, also incorporates the corpus spongiosum, which contains the male urethra. The paired testes produce both male hormones, predominantly testosterone, and spermatozoa, the former in the interstitial cells and the latter in the seminiferous tubular portions. The epididymides, lying in intimate contact with the testes, serve as the collecting system for sperm which are transported along the efferent tract composed of the vasa deferentia and ejaculatory ducts, emptying into the posterior urethra at the verumontanum of the prostate.

### Prostate Gland

The prostate is a fibromuscular glandular organ that surrounds the vesical neck and proximal portion of the male urethra. The prostate of the normal young adult male is approximately 20 gm. in weight and consists of two portions, an anterior group of glands intimately associated with the urethra and a posterior portion of more fibromuscular character. Embryologically, the gland derives from five epithelial evaginations of the posterior urethra which constitute alveolar glands emptying into the urethra.

The inferior vesical and internal pudendal arteries provide the blood supply to the prostate, entering the gland posterolaterally at the vesical neck. Venous drainage of the prostate gland is complex and diffuse with plexuses over the anterior and lateral aspects of the gland which drain into the internal iliac veins. The nerve supply of the prostate derives from the pelvic plexus of the autonomic system. Intercommunicating lymphatics of the prostate, bladder, seminal vesicles, vasa defer-

entia, and rectum provide drainage into the internal and external lymphatic systems.

Of considerable surgical importance is the difference in embryologic origin of the anterior and posterior portions of the gland. The anterior portion, consisting of periurethral glandular structures, gives rise to the hyperplasia and hypertrophy of benign enlargement and bladder outlet obstruction in older men. The posterior segment, a musculoglandular structure, is the most frequent site of origin of prostatic carcinoma. Anatomic, physiologic, endocrinologic, and enzymatic variations between the anterior and posterior segments of the gland are incriminated as factors contributing to the difference in propensity for disease.

The prostate lies immediately beneath the bladder, and in the presence of prostatic enlargement, the adenomatous hyperplastic gland is separated from the bladder only by mucosa and fibromuscular strands of the vesical neck. The gland is supported anteriorly by the puboprostatic ligament, inferiorly by the urogenital diaphragm or external urinary sphincter, and posteriorly by the rectal wall which is separated from the prostate by an obliterated pelvic reflection of peritoneum, the dual-layered Denonvilliers' fascia. In the presence of adenomatous hyperplasia and hypertrophy of the prostate, the fibromuscular outer portion of the gland is compressed and distended peripherally, constituting the surgical capsule of the prostate. A distinct cleavage plane is recognized between the adenoma and the surgical capsule in benign enlargement.

Traditionally, urinary control is attributed to the involuntary function of the internal sphincter or vesical neck and the voluntary control of the external sphincter

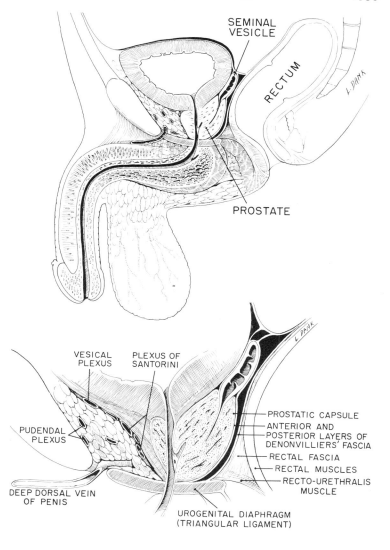

**Figure 2** The anatomic relationships of the prostate gland. (From Brendler, H. R. In: Glenn, J. F., and Boyce, W. H.: Urologic Surgery. New York, Hoeber Medical Division, Harper & Row, 1969.)

or urogenital diaphragm. It is probable that advanced benign prostatic hypertrophy may irreparably compromise the sphincteric action of the vesical neck, and prostatic surgery may further compromise function of the internal sphincter mechanism. Diffuse, infiltrating carcinoma of the prostate may interfere with action of the vesical neck or the external sphincter.

### Seminal Vesicles

The seminal vesicles are paired monotubular convoluted structures, lying beneath the base of the bladder and under the trigone. Posteriorly, they are invested by Denonvilliers' fascia which separates them from the anterior wall of the rectum. The two seminal vesicles fuse medially with the ampullae of the vasa, forming the ejaculatory ducts which open at the verumontanum. The seminal vesicles secrete a mucoid vehicle for spermatozoa and elaborate fructose; a high free fructose level in seminal vesicle fluid is apparently necessary to maintain viability of spermatozoa. The muscular wall of the seminal vesicle is contractile, and ejaculation is accompanied by muscular contraction which expels the ejaculate through the ejaculatory ducts into the posterior urethra.

### Cowper's Glands

Cowper's glands are small paired glands lying between the layers of the urogenital diaphragm at the junction of the bulbous and membranous portions of the urethra. The ducts of Cowper's glands empty into the bulbous urethra, proving an alkaline secretion which serves as a lubricant during sexual activity. Inflammatory and neoplastic diseases of Cowper's glands are extremely rare, and while they are important to normal sexual activity, they have little clinical significance.

### Penis

The penis serves the dual function of copulation and excretion of urine by the male. It consists of two parallel erectile compartments known as the corpora cavernosa, which are situated dorsolaterally, as well as the corpus spongiosum penis which invests the urethra and terminates distally in the glans penis, also an erectile body. Each corpus cavernosum and the corpus spongiosum are enveloped in fascial sheaths, and all three corpora are surrounded by the dense fibrous Buck's fascia.

The principal blood supply of the penis is through the

dorsal arteries which course over the superior surface of the corpora cavernosa, lying deep to Buck's fascia. The principal blood supply is derived from the internal pudendal arteries, while venous drainage is through the dorsal veins of the penis communicating with the prostatic plexuses. Penile erection is induced by engorgement of the erectile tissue of the corpora, principally the corpora cavernosa. The exact mechanisms of erection are not fully understood, but competence of the pelvic blood supply and autonomic nervous system are essential. The corpora cavernosa take origin from the ischiopubic rami as the crura, these fusing in the perineum. Further fixation of the penis is provided by the suspensory ligament which connects the root of the penis to the pubis.

Lymphatic drainage of the penis is abundant, and that from the shaft of the penis, the corpora cavernosa, and the skin passes to the superficial and deep inguinal nodes, communicating thence to the iliac nodes. Lymphatic drainage of the glans penis parallels that of the urethra to the subinguinal, external iliac, and deep pelvic nodes, while lymphatics from the urethral mucosa drain to the hypogastric nodes. Skin of the penis differs from other skin in its paucity of sebaceous glands, its elasticity, and the extensive blood supply. These factors contribute to ready healing and permit extensive surgical reconstruction. The redundant foreskin, subject to extensive inflammatory involvement, may become constricted distally to produce phimosis, or proximal to the glans to produce paraphimosis.

### Male Urethra

The male urethra consists of two major portions, the posterior urethra and the anterior urethra, each with two subdivisions. Beginning most proximally at the neck of the bladder, the posterior urethra consists of the prostatic portion and the membranous urethra. The prostatic urethra is analogous to the entire urethra of the female and is liberally invested with periurethral glands which are subject not only to enlargement, but also to acute and chronic infectious processes. The verumontanum opens in the floor of the prostatic urethra proximal to the apex of the prostate gland. The membranous urethra lacks periurethral glands, though Cowper's glands are located in the urogenital diaphragm lateral to the membranous urethra, the site of external or voluntary sphincteric action. The prostatic and membranous portions of the urethra are relatively fixed by the puboprostatic ligaments and the inherent stability of the urogenital diaphragm, while the urethra distal to the urogenital diaphragm is relatively mobile. In instances of pelvic injury including fracture, rupture or transection of the urethra is quite common at the junction of the membranous posterior urethra and the bulbous anterior urethra.

The anterior urethra includes the bulbous or perineal portion of the urethra, beginning at the urogenital diaphragm and extending to the penoscrotal junction, and the distal penile or pendulous urethra. The bulbous urethra exhibits a larger caliber than the remainder of the male urethra, and is richly invested with periurethral glands, often the site of gonococcal infection with subsequent fibrosis, cicatrix, and stricture. The penile or pendulous portion of the anterior urethra begins at the penoscrotal junction and extends distally to the external urethral meatus, just proximal to which a bulbous enlargement, the fossa navicularis, constitutes a nozzle-like effect which produces a unified urinary stream. The pendulous urethra is also invested with periurethral glands which may be the site of infection, and the narrow caliber of the pendulous urethra renders it more sensitive to irritation by a catheter.

### Scrotum

The scrotal sac, consisting of two lateral compartments fused in the midline, encloses the testes, the epididymides, and the terminal portions of the spermatic cords. The dartos muscle is intimately attached to the corrugated skin of the scrotum, rich in sebaceous glands, providing for muscular contraction of the scrotal sac in response to temperature changes or sexual excitation. The principal function of the scrotum is to provide for maintenance of temperature control of the testes, since spermatogenesis is optimal at a temperature several degrees lower than that within the abdominal cavity. The alternate contraction and relaxation of the scrotum, in conjunction with similar contraction and relaxation of the cremasteric muscles of the spermatic cord, allow for maintenance of testicular temperature within a narrow and precise range. The blood supply of the scrotum arises from the femoral, internal pudendal, and inferior epigastric arteries, with venous drainage paralleling the arterial supply and emerging laterally. Lymphatic drainage of the scrotum is into the superficial and deep inguinal nodes, communicating with the femoral system. The loose character of scrotal skin permits accumulation of large quantities of lymph, extravasated urine, or blood, and in the presence of such accumulations, venous and lymphatic drainage are compromised, predisposing to gangrene or other serious infectious processes.

### Testes

The testes are the essential organs of male reproduction, two in number, ovoid in form, averaging 4 to 5 cm. in length and 2.5 to 3.5 cm. in width in the normal adult male. Posteriorly, the testes are intimately attached to the epididymides and the terminal portions of the spermatic cord. The factors that control the descent of the testes from the abdominal cavity into the scrotum are probably hormonal. A poorly defined fibrous structure, the gubernaculum testis, is possibly associated with descent which occurs during the latter phases of gestation. The peritoneum anterolateral to the testis evaginates into the scrotum and, following descent of the testicle, this processus vaginalis is obliterated, leaving around the testicle two layers of peritoneum which become the tunica albuginea, investing the testicle itself, and the tunica vaginalis, providing a cushioning sac around the testis.

Since the testis arises from the wolffian body on the genital ridge in close proximity to the kidney, it is not surprising that the blood supply of the testis arises from the aorta just beneath the renal arteries. Further blood supply follows the course of the vas deferens and may be sufficient to maintain testicular viability in instances in which the spermatic artery is divided. Venous drainage of the testis is through the multiple veins of the pampiniform plexus to the spermatic vein which emerges from the upper end of the cord. On the right, the spermatic vein empties into the vena cava below the right renal vein, while on the left the spermatic vein empties into the main renal vein. Increased hydrostatic pressure, particularly on the left, may result in dilatation of the pampiniform venous plexus, producing varicocele. Lymphatic drainage of the testis is through the spermatic cord to the common iliac and para-aortic nodes, the latter communicating across the midline and with the mediastinal and supraclavicular chains. Testicular nerves derive from the aortic and renal plexuses which in turn communicate with the solar plexus. Traumatic injury of the testicle may produce acute abdominal pain because of these interdigitating pathways, and intra-abdominal disease may cause referred pain in the testis.

Histologically, there are two principal portions of the

testis: the seminiferous tubules which are responsible for spermatogenesis, and the interstitial or Leydig cells which elaborate androgenic hormones, predominantly testosterone. Because of the required relative hypothermia necessary to spermatogenesis, seminiferous tubule function may be impaired in the cryptorchid or maldescended testis, while hormonal function may be unimpaired, even in the intra-abdominal undescended testicle.

### Epididymides

The epididymides are cordlike structures lying along the posterior aspect of each testis, the head of each epididymis resting upon the superior extremity of the testis and the tail attached to the inferior extremity of the testis. The medial surface of each epididymis attaches to the terminal portion of the spermatic cord through which blood, nerve, and lymphatic supply is received. A dozen or more tubular efferent ducts take origin from the rete testis, providing the system for collection of sperm. Sperm are then transmitted into the vasa deferentia which are continuations of the ducts of the epididymides, passing up the spermatic cord and retroperitoneally to the ampullae of the seminal vesicles with which they conjoin to form the ejaculatory duct on each side. The principal blood supply of the epididymis is from the spermatic artery which also supplies the testis, but the deferential artery, arising from the superior or inferior vesical artery, follows the course of the vas deferens and also provides some of the vascular supply of the epididymis. Venous drainage corresponds to the arterial supply, and the lymphatic drainage of the epididymis parallels that of the testis. The prime function of the epididymides is to provide a conduit for spermatozoa, but the epididymides also contribute to maturation of spermatozoa, sperm recovered from the body or tail of the epididymis exhibiting a greater degree of maturation and fertilizing capacity than those recovered from the head of the epididymis. Senescent deterioration of interstitial cells with concomitant decrease in androgen production will result in involution of epididymal epithelium.

### Spermatic Cord

The spermatic cord, suspending each testicle with its attached epididymis, comprises the vas deferens, the spermatic artery, the pampiniform plexus of veins, the lymphatic drainage system of the scrotal contents, and the autonomic nerve supply to the testicle and its appendages. The cord is surrounded by fibers of the cremasteric muscle which assist by contraction and relaxation in maintenance of optimal testicular temperature as well as providing for testicular retraction with sexual excitation or in the primitive fright reaction.

The vasa deferentia are tubular structures of 2 to 3 mm. in diameter, providing a narrow lumen for transport of spermatozoa which are propelled by contraction of longitudinal smooth muscle fibers. Vasectomy, an operation for purposes of sterilization or prevention of retrograde infection of epididymides and testes, is accomplished by division of the vas, with or without excision of a small segment of each ductus deferens, and ligation of each divided end of the tubular structure. Successful restoration of continuity of the vasa — vasovasostomy — may be accomplished by meticulous surgical reanastomosis, a procedure that may be successful even after many years of interruption of continuity.

The pampiniform plexus is subject to venous dilatation and stasis, varicosities of this system being termed varicocele. Because of the complexity of the venous drainage in this plexus, direct surgical intervention for venous ligation is tedious; a more direct approach is to the single spermatic vein at the level of the internal inguinal ring where the pampiniform plexus becomes confluent into a single channel. Division of the venous drainage at this point is successful in preventing further stasis and will obviate the varicocele.

The processus vaginalis, the evaginated portion of the peritoneum, may not be obliterated after descent of the testis and may persist in part, producing hydrocele of the spermatic cord, or in toto, permitting partial or complete indirect inguinal hernia. In instances of incomplete or maldescended of the testis, the processus vaginalis remains patent, and orchidopexy must be accompanied by simultaneous repair of the potential or overt hernia.

## PROSTATE GLAND

While all of the intricacies of the prostate gland have not yet been defined, clinical observation and basic investigation have elaborated prostatic function and provided insight into management of the various disorders that can affect this unique male organ. Normal prostatic function is apparently dependent upon androgens, principally testosterone, which is metabolized to dihydrotestosterone and androstenediol, substances of similar androgenicity. The prostate is capable of elaborating specific enzymes, principally lactic dehydrogenase and acid phosphatase. The interrelated physiologic and endocrinologic functions of the prostate are responsible for normal sexual function and provide certain clues to the etiology of benign prostatic enlargement as well as carcinoma of the prostate.

### CONGENITAL ANOMALIES

Complete absence of the prostate gland in an otherwise normal male has not been observed. However, failure of normal development and maturation of the prostate may be associated with the intersex states and male gonadal failure. Congenital contracture of the vesical neck at the point of juncture of prostate and bladder may cause severe urinary obstruction. Congenital valves of the prostatic urethra — mucosal folds which may be diaphragmatic or alar — occur relatively frequently and cause profound obstructive uropathy in some cases; early diagnosis and prompt treatment by endoscopic or open surgical removal of valves can prevent ultimate and inevitable renal failure. Congenital müllerian cysts predispose to obstruction and infection, presenting as midline masses beneath the gland and base of the bladder, treated by open surgical removal.

### TRAUMA

Fracture of the bony pelvis may often result in laceration and transection of the membranous urethra just distal to the prostate, and urinary extravasation as well as bleeding may displace the prostate and bladder superiorly. Occasional penetrating wounds of the prostate due to gunshot wounds or perineal straddle injuries have been reported. The most common cause of prostatic injury is inexpert urethral instrumentation, generally in the course of urethral dilation in treatment of stricture, though injury at the time of rectal surgery is occasionally encountered. The usual concomitant of prostatic injury is damage to the external urinary sphincter, which lies in proximity to the distal portion of the gland, with fibrosis, stricture, and possible secondary sphincter damage.

## PROSTATIC INFECTIONS

Problems of prostatic infection constitute a significant fraction of urologic practice. Infectious agents that may involve the prostate gland include the spectrum of gram-negative organisms that most frequently involve the urinary tract, gram-positive cocci, gonococci, various mycotic organisms, mycobacteria, trichomonads, and Candida species. The usual route of infection is ascending through the urethra, the potential for such exogenous infection being enhanced by stricture, diverticulum, or other abnormality of the urethra, though hematogenous and lymphatic routes of access have been incriminated, and descending infection through the urinary tract may occur, as with tuberculosis, which almost always involves first the kidney and later the organs of the lower genitourinary tract.

### Acute Prostatitis

Suppurative acute prostatitis is generally a disease of younger men, but may be seen from pubescence throughout the life span. The organisms most commonly involved are the gram-negative group, principally *Escherichia coli.* Acute gonococcal prostatitis is relatively uncommon, but the involvement of the periurethral glands by gonorrhea predisposes to inflammation and stricture which invite secondary gram-negative infection in the prostate. Stamey and others have demonstrated both bacteriostasis and a bactericidal effect of prostatic fluid, indicating that there are natural defense mechanisms inherent in the prostate gland.[21] Simple prostatic congestion may predispose to acute prostatitis. The usual symptoms of acute prostatitis include urgency and frequency of urination with severe dysuria and stranguria. There may be perineal aching and rectal discomfort, the patient sometimes complaining of a feeling of constipation. Chills and fever and even bacteremia may ensue. Edema may predispose to acute urinary retention. Examination discloses an exquisitely tender prostate which is diffusely indurated and enlarged. Urinalysis will usually reveal pyuria and often the offending organisms can be cultured. Prostatic massage should be accomplished most gently if at all, seeking to avoid bacteremia. Prostatic

secretions will be filled with purulent debris, and the stained smear may reveal bacteria.

Instrumentation should be avoided in the acute phase of prostatitis unless there is associated urinary retention which demands catheterization. Vigorous antibiotic therapy with a broad-spectrum agent such as ampicillin or one of the cephalothin group should be initiated, pending culture and sensitivity studies. Bed rest, intermittent hot sitz baths, antipyretics, and restriction of sexual activity are necessary supportive measures. Antibiotic therapy should be continued for not less than 2 weeks, followed by a course of supplemental sulfonamides or chemotherapeutic agents in association with follow-up examination and prostatic massage.

### Prostatic Abscess

Prior to the era of antibiotic therapy, prostatic abscesses were frequent sequelae of acute prostatitis, but are encountered less frequently today. Surgical drainage of prostatic abscess is required and may be accomplished by transurethral incision and resection, perineal incision and drainage, aspiration, or massage. Transrectal drainage of prostatic abscess is effective and is attended by surprisingly few complications, spontaneous healing of both the prostate and the rectal wall occurring in the majority of cases.

### Chronic Prostatitis

Chronic inflammation of the prostate gland may ensue as sequel of acute prostatitis or may occur as a complication of prostatic enlargement and obstruction. Presenting symptoms usually consist of dull aching perineal discomfort with minimal but recurring symptoms of lower urinary tract irritation, frequency and urgency with symptoms of fullness and irritability. Occasionally, urethral discharge occurs. Many patients may have chronic prostatitis without symptoms. Chronic prostatitis predisposes to associated urethritis, cystitis, vasitis, epididymitis, and even orchitis.

On examination, the prostate gland may be essentially normal in size and consistency, enlarged and boggy, or irregularly indurated and tender to palpation. Urinalysis may reveal red cells, white cells, and bacteria, or may be entirely within normal limits. Prostatic secretions, elicited by gentle massage accomplished by a sweeping motion of the examining finger over the lobes of the prostate from lateral to medial, followed by antegrade stripping of the prostatic urethra in the midline, contain pus cells with or without demonstrable bacteria. Normal prostatic secretions will contain 5 to 10 per cent pus in the cellular elements of prostatic secretion, but greater numbers of pus cells and particularly leukocytes trapped in mucoid clumps confirm the diagnosis of chronic prostatitis.

The treatment of chronic prostatitis is often less than satisfactory. Antimicrobial agents may or may not be effective, and unless the symptoms are extremely severe and a positive culture can be elicited, antibiotics are usually avoided.

Sulfonamides, nitrofurans, or other chemotherapeutic agents may be employed for chronic therapy along with urinary analgesics such as phenazopyridine (Azo-pyridon). Regular and periodic prostatic massage is probably the most beneficial modality of treatment, and must be accomplished over periods of several weeks or months. Hot sitz baths may offer symptomatic relief, and regular sexual intercourse will encourage normal drainage of inspissated secretions. Surgical intervention is not often indicated, by prolonged and severe chronic prostatitis may lead to fibrosis, scarring, contracture of the vesical neck, and prostatic calculi, these conditions sometimes requiring intervention by transurethral prostatic resection.

### Prostatic Calculi

Calculi may occur in the glandular acini and ducts of the prostate gland, most often as the result of chronic inflammatory reaction with cellular necrosis, inspissation of debris, and deposition of calcific deposits. While prostatic calculi may be scattered through the gland, they most often occur near the periphery of the prostate, lying in a cleavage plane between the adenomatous periurethral glands and the fibromuscular capsule; the stony hard induration produced may be mistaken for prostatic carcinoma. Bacteria may be trapped in the interstices of prostatic calculi, contributing to perpetuation of prostatitis. Treatment is dictated by the clinical course: if the patient is asymptomatic and the urine is negative, no treatment is required, but associated obstructive or irritative symptoms, persistent urinary infection, or severe pain may necessitate prostatectomy, accomplished transurethrally or by open surgery.

### Tuberculous Prostatitis

Tuberculosis of the prostate gland does not occur as an isolated entity. Genitourinary tuberculosis is always secondary to a primary infection, either pulmonary or gastrointestinal. Tubercle bacilli are transmitted hematogenously, usually to the kidney and thence to the ureter, bladder, prostate, and other genitourinary organs. However, it has been suggested that primary hematogenous spread to the prostate may occur. Symptoms may be totally absent or may be those of chronic obstruction and infection. Digital examination of the prostate may disclose stony hard induration, reminiscent of carcinoma or prostatic calculi. The diagnosis is established by demonstration of tubercle bacilli in the urine or prostatic biopsy with characteristic histologic findings of caseation necrosis and the other stigmata of tuberculosis. Medical management is indicated, employing various combinations of streptomycin, para-aminosalicylic acid, isoniazid or other effective antituberculous drugs. Occasionally, total prostatectomy is indicated, but this procedure is almost universally accompanied by impotence and since the disease affects young males predominantly, surgical removal of the prostate is not the desirable modality of treatment.

### Granulomatous Prostatitis

Chronic prostatitis may predispose to a severe multifocal, abacterial inflammatory process which is thought to be due to extravasation of prostatic excretions into the interstitium of the prostate gland, initiating the histiocytic granulomatous reaction. Examination of the prostate reveals irregular induration that mimics prostatic carcinoma. Symptoms of urinary urgency, frequency, and perineal pain usually bring the patient to the attention of the urologist. The palpatory findings of diffuse irregular prostatic induration generally demand prostatic biopsy—transperineal or transrectal needle biopsy or possible open perineal biopsy—in order to establish the diagnosis and rule out the possibility of carcinoma. Prostatic massage and treatment of associated bacterial infection constitute the primary methods of treatment, but transurethral resection of the prostate may be required for alleviation of symptoms.

### Miscellaneous Prostatic Infections

Other inflammatory processes in the prostate gland are encountered less frequently. Blastomycosis and actinomycosis have been reported as causes of chronic prostatitis, and treatment of these conditions may require surgical extirpation of the prostate gland. Moniliasis involving the urethra and prostate is usually alleviated by simple urinary acidification with concomitant treatment of the involved sexual partner. *Trichomonas vaginalis* may infest the prostate gland and produce symptoms and findings similar to those of chronic nonspecific prostatitis, the diagnosis being established by identification of trichomonads in the urine or prostatic secretions. Fortunately, a 10 day course of oral metronidazole of both sexual partners will usually eradicate Trichomonas infestation.

## BENIGN PROSTATIC HYPERPLASIA

Benign prostatic overgrowth is the most common cause of bladder outlet obstruction in men over 50 years of age.[12] While exact mechanisms of prostatic hyperplasia are incompletely appreciated, it is recognized that adolescent development of the glandular acini and the fibromuscular matrix of the prostate is stimulated by gonadotropins and the androgens of the interstitial cells of the testes. After the age of 40, androgen production diminishes and glandular hypertrophy and hyperplasia of the prostate occur, progressing with advancing age. Typically, the glandular elements surrounding the prostatic urethra centrally—analogous to the periurethral glands of the female urethra—undergo spheroidal proliferation. The true acinar glands of the prostate and the fibromuscular capsule of the gland are displaced peripherally and compressed as the adenomatous hyperplasia progresses. A lobular pattern of growth is observed, the hyperplastic process involving the two lateral lobes of the gland

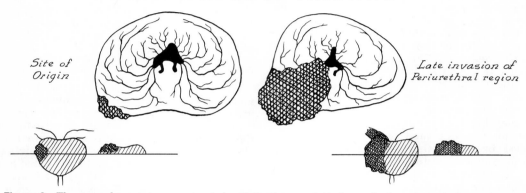

**Figure 3**  The normal prostate as contrasted with benign prostatic hyperplasia and prostatic carcinoma.

or the median lobe, situated centrally and proximally beneath the bladder neck and trigone.

As the enlargement progresses, the prostatic urethra may become elongated and the caliber of the prostatic portion of the urethra may actually increase. However, the adenomatous process causes compression of the prostatic urethra, restricting the free flow of urine, sometimes associated with actual mechanical intrusion of a median lobe at the vesical outlet, predisposing to difficulty in initiating the urinary stream, maintaining it, and completing the act of bladder emptying. Mechanical pressure phenomena then may include upward displacement of the base of the bladder, fishhooking of the lower ureters due to trigonal displacement, hypertrophy of the bladder wall with trabeculation, cellule formation, and even diverticula of the bladder. Complete bladder outlet obstruction may result in decompensation of the detrusor muscle and total urinary retention.

The symptoms of benign prostatic hyperplasia are those of mechanical obstruction and the consequences of urinary stasis. In the early stages of prostatic enlargement, the patient complains of diminished size and force of the urinary stream, and as obstruction progresses, there is increasing frequency of urination, probably due to pressure of the enlarging gland beneath the trigone of the bladder. Nocturia is a similar index of the mechanical pressure of the enlarging prostate. It should be noted that nocturia normally occurs in older patients, both men and women, partially as a result of the inability of the kidney to concentrate urine with resultant excretion of larger nocturnal volumes. However, nocturia more than once or twice nightly in the elderly male suggests mechanical pressure of prostatic enlargement as well as the possibility that the bladder is emptying incompletely with each voiding. Later, the patient with prostatic obstruction may note hesitancy and intermittency of the urinary stream, occasioned by intermittent fluttering occlusion of the prostatic urethra by the hypertrophic lateral lobes. Terminal dribbling suggests both residual urine and pooling of urine within the prostatic urethra.[4]

Urinary bleeding may first bring the patient to the attention of the physician. Hematuria may result from prostatic enlargement with engorgement of the small mucosal vessels covering the adenomatous gland, ruptured as a consequence of straining to urinate. With progressive residual urine, infection may occur with purulent cystitis; about half of the men suffering urinary retention as a consequence of prostatic obstruction will exhibit infection. Similarly, vesical stasis of urine can predispose to the formation of bladder calculi with severe symptoms of dysuria and stranguria.

Occasionally, patients may have few symptoms of bladder outlet obstruction, the syndrome of so-called "silent prostatism." Residual urines of 1000 ml. or more may produce a palpable lower abdominal mass before the patient experiences any particular symptoms and it is not uncommon to observe bilateral hydroureteronephrosis and evidence of impending renal failure with azotemia and electrolyte imbalance.

The diagnosis of prostatic hypertrophy with bladder outlet obstruction is suggested by the history and is confirmed by careful physical and ancillary examinations. Rectal examination will reveal varying degrees of prostatic enlargement, most often symmetric, with the prostate rubbery in consistency. As enlargement progresses, the gland protrudes posteriorly, compressing the anterior rectal wall and sometimes producing symptoms of constipation. The size of the gland may bear little relationship to the degree of symptomatic difficulty incurred by the patient, a small gland often completely obstructing the bladder outlet

while a large prostate three or four times normal size may produce few if any obstructive symptoms. Palpation of the distended bladder suggests incomplete emptying with significant residual urine. Cystourethroscopy will confirm the presence of prostatic enlargement and permit assessment of the degree of occlusion of the bladder neck or prostatic urethra, and the degree of bladder trabeculation and cellule or diverticulum formation.

General physical evaluation of the patient with benign prostatic enlargement is mandatory, with emphasis upon evaluation of renal function. Azotemia may occur insidiously with bladder outlet obstruction, and the usual measurements of blood urea nitrogen, serum creatinine, and creatinine clearance provide indices of renal functional capacity. The time-honored phenolsulfonphthalein (PSP) test provides a basis for evaluation of renal function as well as the degree of urinary retention; a flat curve of PSP excretion during the 2 hour interval of observation suggests severe renal

## PERINEAL PROSTATECTOMY

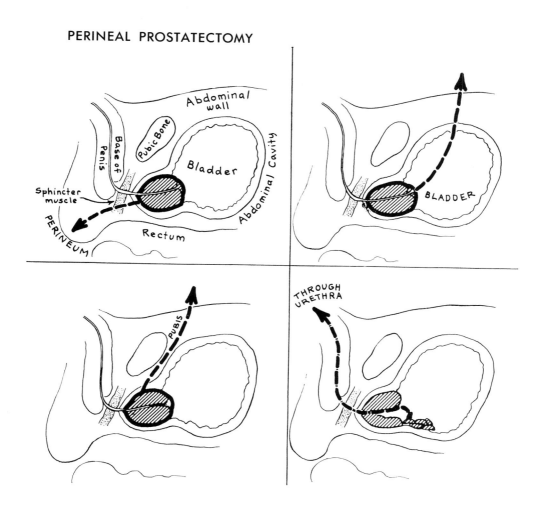

**Figure 4**  The four basic surgical enucleative procedures for benign prostatic hypertrophy: perineal prostatectomy, suprapubic prostatectomy, retropubic prostatectomy, and transurethral resection of the prostate.

functional impairment, while a rising curve suggests the dilutional effect of significant residual urine.

Conservative and medical measures of managing benign prostatic enlargement with bladder outlet obstruction are generally unsuccessful. Prostatic massage is of little value unless there is substantial congestion with retention of prostatic secretions. Urethral dilation is useless unless there is associated urethral stricture and should be avoided because of the danger of introducing infection. Anticholinergic drugs which induce hypotonicity of smooth muscle may effectively control symptoms of urinary frequency, but impose the risk of precipitating urinary retention. Occasionally, estrogens in small dosage may induce minimal improvement in the urinary stream, presumably through the mechanism of some prostatic shrinkage, but in general hormonal measures have been ineffective in benign prostatic hypertrophy.

The decision for surgical intervention in benign prostatic enlargement is reached after evaluating a variety of factors.[18] Indications for surgery include residual urine of more than 100 ml., particularly when there is associated azotemia of any degree; persistent or recurrent urinary infection, refractory to usual therapeutic methods; gross hematuria on more than one occasion; acute urinary retention; or chronic urinary retention with overflow dribbling. To these classic indications for surgery, most urologic surgeons would add the factors of patient comfort and desire for surgery; nocturia more than two or three times nightly will interfere with rest, diurnal urinary frequency may pose a significant disability, the patient may be significantly concerned about the prospects of urinary retention, or it may be suspected that the enlarged prostate may be compromising sexual function, as it sometimes does.

There are four standard surgical procedures for removal of the obstructing enlarged portion of the prostate galnd. None of these procedures constitutes total prostatectomy; all of them are designed for removal of the adenomatous hyperplastic portion of the gland, lying centrally and periurethrally. Hence, these procedures should most properly be termed prostatic adenectomy rather than prostatectomy since the true prostate, compressed laterally into a fibromuscular and acinar surgical capsule, is retained after removal of the central adenomatous elements.

### Suprapubic Prostatectomy

Historically, the suprapubic or transvesical method of enucleating the prostatic adenoma was the first to be generally employed. While utilized with less frequency today, this procedure still constitutes a fundamental method of surgical treatment in benign prostatic hyperplasia. A suprapubic incision, either vertical or transverse, gives access to the anterior surface of the bladder which is then opened to give exposure of the vesical neck and the underlying prostate, a low transverse

bladder incision being employed for better visualization. The mucosa surrounding the bladder neck is incised and a cleavage plane is then established between the adenomatous elements and the peripheral surgical capsule. At the apex, the prostatic adenoma is amputated from the urethra, and the enucleated adenomatous elements embrace the mucosa of the prostatic urethra. The fibromuscular surgical capsule that remains will contract to relatively normal configuration, and the inner aspect of the capsule will be epithelialized by growth of mucosa down from the trigone and bladder neck and up from the membranous urethra below, this process requiring several weeks or months. Hemostasis may be enhanced by direct fulguration and by mattress sutures, particularly at the posterolateral aspects of the vesical neck, the site of entry of the principal arterial supply. A urethral catheter is introduced and some surgeons prefer to inflate the balloon within the prostatic fossa, effecting tamponade against further bleeding. A second suprapubic mushroom catheter is usually employed as well. Surgical mortality rates of 1 to 5 per cent are generally recognized[3] and the morbidity of suprapubic prostatectomy tends to be somewhat higher than that incurred with the other operative approaches to benign prostatic hyperplasia. However, suprapubic or transvesical prostatectomy remains a useful procedure, particularly when there is a very large median lobe or intrusion of the prostate well within the bladder cavity, since this approach affords maximal exposure within the bladder.

### Perineal Prostatectomy

Perineal enucleation of the hyperplastic prostate was popularized at the turn of the century by

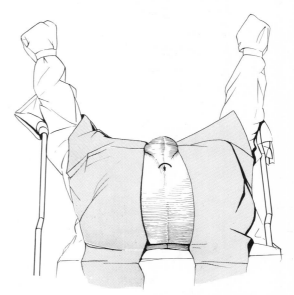

**Figure 5** Position of patient and standard incision for perineal prostatectomy. (From Brendler, H. R. In: Glenn, J. F., and Boyce, W. H.: Urologic Surgery. New York, Hoeber Medical Division, Harper & Row, 1969.)

Young. Perineal prostatectomy is particularly suitable to the large, low-lying prostate. The patient is placed in the extreme lithotomy position, giving access to the perineum where a transverse incision in the shape of an inverted U is made anterior to the rectum. The rectum is separated from the posterior aspect of the prostate. The prostatic capsule is incised, and sharp and blunt dissection is employed to free the adenoma from the interior of the prostatic surgical capsule. The adenoma is amputated from the urethra distally and at the bladder neck. Hemostasis is effected with absorbable suture material at the vesical neck. A Foley catheter is inserted into the bladder through the urethra and the capsulotomy opening is closed to re-establish continuity. A rubber wick or drain is employed in the perineal incision. Catheter drainage is generally maintained for 7 to 10 days. The perineal procedure carries a lower mortality and morbidity than suprapubic prostatectomy,[2] but hospitalization is usually somewhat longer. The procedure offers the advantage of good control of bleeding, and it is thought that the extreme lithotomy position promotes venous return and minimizes operative vascular complications.

### Transurethral Prostatic Resection

The emergence of endoscopic transurethral surgery was dependent upon the development of adequate lens systems, the incandescent bulb, and later fiberoptics, the refinement of electrical current for purposes of cutting and coagulation, and the ingenious combination of these advances into instruments satisfactory for surgical purposes. Transurethral prostatectomy has become the most commonly employed form of surgical treatment of benign prostatic hyperplasia with obstruction. Endoscopic resection of the enlarged prostate is most suitable in the smaller prostatic adenomas, those under 40 or 50 gm. in total resectable weight. It is best to resect the smaller fibrotic glands rather than attempting difficult open surgical enucleative procedures.

The patient is placed in lithotomy position and the urethra is calibrated with progressive urethral sounds. The resectoscope sheath is introduced into the bladder and the working element is positioned. Under direct vision, the wire loop is employed to cut away fragments of the obstructing adenoma. These fragments are subsequently evacuated from the urinary bladder. Constant irrigation is required employing a nonelectrolytic isotonic irrigant of satisfactory optical properties such as commercially available solutions of glycine, urea, or mannitol-sorbitol mixtures. Saline cannot be employed since it is an electrolyte solution which will dissipate the electrical current, and glucose cannot be utilized because of its stickiness. An isotonic solution must be employed since fluid extravasated into the circulation may cause hemolysis with subsequent acute tubular necrosis. The electrical current passed through the wire loop may be modified as a high-frequency, high-amplitude cutting current or as a low-frequency, low-amplitude coagulating current for control of bleeding. An adequate resection is concluded when the fibers of the surgical capsule of the prostate have

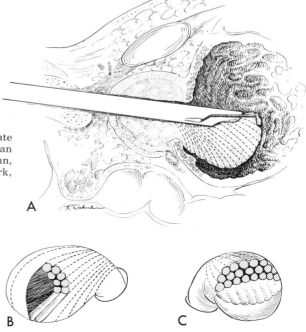

**Figure 6** Transurethral resection of the prostate gland, here depicting resection of an enlarged median lobe of the prostate. (From Thompson, I. M. In: Glenn, J. F., and Boyce, W. H.: Urologic Surgery, New York, Hoeber Medical Division, Harper & Row, 1969.)

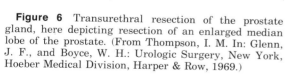

been visualized in all quadrants and there is no residual obstructing adenomatous tissue. Hemostasis is insured and a balloon catheter is left indwelling for 3 or 4 days. Operative mortality is minimal, usually only 0.1 to 0.5 per cent; hospitalization is generally a matter of a week or less; and morbidity and complications are minimal in patients properly selected for transurethral prostatic surgery.

### Retropubic Prostatectomy

The retropubic route to prostatic enucleation was popularized by Millin[13] and is ideally suited to the rather high-lying larger gland with little if any intravesical component. The patient is operated on in the supine position and a transverse suprapubic incision is preferred. The anterior surface of the prostate is exposed and the surgical capsule is incised transversely. Under direct vision, enucleation of the adenomatous portion of the gland is initiated by sharp dissection and completed bluntly. The adenoma is amputated from the urethra distally and from the bladder neck proximally. With a retractor in the prostatic capsulotomy, the vesical neck is visualized and hemostasis is achieved by fixation sutures of absorbable material. The prostatic fossa is fulgurated when necessary. A catheter is passed through the urethra and into the bladder and the capsulotomy is closed with absorbable suture. The procedure is modified by some surgeons who prefer to employ a vertical capsulotomy, extending the incision superiorly on the anterior surface of the bladder to gain added exposure of the bladder neck and the interior of the bladder itself. There are no contraindications to such an incision which transects the region of the vesical neck, and exposure may be improved by this approach, particularly when there is a median lobe extending intravesically. In general, only a single urethral catheter is employed, and this is usually removed 5 to 7 days postoperatively. Problems of postoperative urinary incontinence are minimal with retropubic prostatectomy, morbidity is approximately equivalent to that of transurethral resection though hospitalization may be somewhat longer, and the operative mortality is only slightly greater than that of transurethral surgery, considerably less than that reported with suprapubic prostatic enucleation.

Long-term complications following prostatic surgery for benign adenomatous hyperplasia are relatively minimal. Since the surgical capsule is retained, sexual potency is usually unaltered, sometimes even improved, by these enucleative procedures. Urinary incontinence may occur as a permanent result of any form of prostatectomy for benign enlargement, but tends to be more prevalent after perineal prostatectomy and transurethral resection. Even here, the incidence of true and total urinary incontinence is minimal, probably no more than 1 per cent. The retained surgical capsule may afford an opportunity for regrowth of further adenomatous tissue, possibly requiring a second operative procedure. Retained

adenomatous elements similarly may regrow and reobstruct. It has been estimated that 10 per cent of patients undergoing transurethral resection may have recurrent prostatic obstruction at a later date, necessitating another operative intervention, while recurrent adenomatous obstruction is seen with less frequency after the open procedures.

## MEDIAN BAR OBSTRUCTION

Median bar is the term applied to the fibrous obstruction that can occur on the inferior vesical lip posteriorly, most often of congenital origin. If the fibrotic process extends entirely around the vesical neck, the condition is termed contracture of the vesical neck, which may be the result of chronic prostatitis. Not infrequently, patients may exhibit contracture of the vesical neck after previous prostatic enucleation of one sort or another, and such obstruction can demand secondary operative intervention. It should be reiterated that even the small prostate may obstruct and that diagnosis of median bar formation or contracture of the vesical neck can be established only by cystoscopic examination. Treatment of median bar or contracture of the vesical neck may be accomplished endoscopically or by open surgical revision. Endoscopic methods include transurethral resection with the electroresectoscope or with the cold-knife Thompson instrument, while some authorities—Keitzer and Turner-Warwick—recommend transurethral incision of the vesical neck with the cold knife. Severe compromise of the vesical outlet by median bar or contracture may be managed by suprapubic revision of the bladder neck, often employing the Bradford Young Y-V-plasty. Repeated instrumentation and dilation of the contracted vesical neck is ineffective and may predispose to fibrosis which aggravates the obstruction.

## CARCINOMA OF THE PROSTATE

Adenocarcinoma of the prostate gland is the most common malignant disease of men over 65 years of age. As a cause of death, carcinoma of the prostate is surpassed only by cancer of the stomach and colon in men. Autopsy studies by Rich have established the fact that prostatic cancer, occult or overt, is present in about 15 per cent of men over the age of 50 years.[19] It is estimated that the prevalence rate of prostatic carcinoma may be up to 20 cases per 100,000 population at the present time, and as the geriatric population increases, so must we expect an increase in prevalence of prostatic carcinoma. Squamous cell carcinoma of the prostate remains a relatively rare occurrence, and sarcoma of the prostate, still rarer, is generally seen only in the first two decades of life.

The etiology of prostatic carcinoma remains unknown. Alterations in the estrogen-androgen balance of a person have been incriminated, but

# BENIGN HYPERPLASIA OF THE PROSTATE

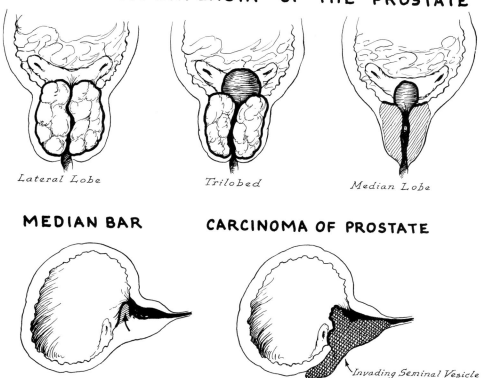

*Lateral Lobe*                *Trilobed*                *Median Lobe*

## MEDIAN BAR          CARCINOMA OF PROSTATE

*Invading Seminal Vesicle*

**Figure 7**  Vesical outlet obstruction may be occasioned by benign prostatic hyperplasia, median bar formation, or prostatic carcinoma.

clinical definition of hormonal imbalance as an etiologic factor remains to be accomplished. No definite carcinogens potentially responsible for prostatic carcinoma have been identified. Sexual activity is apparently not a factor, prostatic carcinoma having been observed in both celibate groups and those men with histories of extensive sexual activity. Infection, nonspecific or venereal, has not been incriminated as a causative factor. Metabolic alterations in the prostate may play a role; in benign prostatic hypertrophy, marked increases in the concentration of both zinc and magnesium have been observed, while in prostatic carcinoma there is a considerable increase in zinc concentration alone.

Prostatic carcinoma most often has its origin in the posterior capsular region of the gland, that segment of the gland which originates as the posterior element of the five embryologic components of the gland. Scott and others have observed definite differences between the dorsal and ventral portion of the prostate in experimental animals, particularly the rat, and it may be that similar biologic and metabolic differences occur in various segments of the human prostate. Recent studies of McNeal suggest that there is no particular predilection for carcinoma in the posterior lobe. Investigators are agreed that adenocarcinoma of the prostate does originate in glands that are

metabolically and biologically active rather than those which are atrophic, and the acinar elements in the fibromuscular surgical capsule of the peripheral prostate are frequently of an atrophic nature. There are variations in biologic behavior of prostatic cancers among those persons in whom the malignant lesion is peripheral as opposed to those who have a more centrally located paraurethral tumor, suggesting that different groups of glandular elements within the prostate may give rise to tumors of varying malignant potential.

Prostatic tissue may elaborate a variety of enzymes including acid phosphatase and lactic dehydrogenase. Nearly 40 years ago, it was recognized that phosphatases with principal activity in the acid range were produced in significant quantities in the prostate gland, and it was subsequently realized that tissue of prostatic origin, such as metastatic adenocarcinoma of the prostate, had similar capacity to elaborate acid phosphatase.[10] Measurement of serum acid phosphatase has become a standard modality in the identification of prostatic carcinoma, an elevation in the serum level signifying either advanced local disease or appreciable metastatic activity. Since acid phosphatase is richly concentrated in normal prostatic tissue as well, even prostatic examination or massage may elevate the serum level for up to 36 hours after rectal palpation.[9]  Acid phosphatase is prevalent in other tissues as well, notably the erythrocyte, and tartrate fractionation of acid phosphatase is capable of differentiating that fraction of the enzyme which is of prostatic origin, though current studies would indicate that total serum acid phosphatase determination is at least as sensitive an index of prostatic carcinoma, either locally or metastatic. Normal levels of serum acid phosphatase do not rule out prostatic carcinoma, since those patients with small local lesions will not exhibit phosphatase elevations, prostatic tumors of a low order of metabolic activity may not produce such elevations, and even patients with advanced osteoblastic metastatic disease may on occasion display normal serum acid phosphatase values.

Lactic dehydrogenase (LDH) activity in human serum probably reflects glycolytic activity in all body organs and tissues. Prout and his co-workers have demonstrated alterations in the pattern of the five isozymes of LDH in patients with advanced and progressive prostatic carcinoma. It is suggested that the observed elevations of LDH isozymes IV and V in patients with advanced prostatic carcinoma reflect increased glycolytic activity within the tumor itself or in its metastatic foci. Most interesting has been the observation of reversion to normal of these elevated isozymes when adequate hormonal control measures have been initiated.[17] Serial estimation of LDH and its isozymes may thus provide an accurate laboratory method for assessment of therapeutic efficacy in the management of prostatic carcinoma.

The prostate gland is also known to be a source of fibrinolytic factors. Normal seminal fluid has significant fibrinolytic activity, possibly enhancing motility of sperm, attributed to the release of fibrinolytic activators from prostatic epithelium. Plasminogen, the precursor of plasmin, is a fibrinolytic protease found in many tissues including the prostate. In prostatic carcinoma, increased fibrinolytic activity predisposes to spontaneous bleeding and hemorrhage, particularly after prostatic surgery. Prostatic carcinoma may predispose to increased production of plasminogen, though the source of fibrinolytic activity in the blood of patients with prostatic carcinoma has not yet been identified.

It has been estimated that prostatic cancer must be present for 2 to 5 years before it becomes clinically evident by rectal palpation. Growth rate of prostatic carcinoma seems to follow a logarithmic curve, and as the tumor increases in size, there is a concomitant increase in the ability to violate the natural tissue planes and penetrate into the periprostatic areas, predisposing to metastatic disease. On this basis, it has been suggested that only those tumors of more than 1 cc. in volume and having significant biologic potential will metastasize.

Unfortunately, early symptoms of prostatic carcinoma are generally lacking. Since the majority of prostatic tumors occur in the periphery of the gland, encroachment on the urethra is a late manifestation of the disease. Irritative obstructive symptoms therefore do not signal the presence of the cancer, and it is only in advanced prostatic carcinoma that lower tract symptoms occur. Occasionally, patients may present with bone pain, usually lumbosacral, as a manifestation of metastatic disease long before local urologic symptoms occur. At the present time, there are no satisfactory screening methods for prostatic carcinoma other than routine and regular rectal examination. In the examination of 5856 men in the Cancer Detection Clinic of the University of Minnesota, 75 unsuspected carcinomas of the prostate were detected.[8]

In essence, the diagnosis of prostatic carcinoma must be based upon suspicion. Every man over the age of 50 should have mandatory rectal examination, and the finding of areas of induration and irregularity should suggest the diagnosis. Characteristically, prostatic carcinoma is stony hard in consistency and must be differentiated from focal tuberculosis, granulomatous prostatitis, and prostatic calculi. The isolated prostatic nodule should be regarded with the highest suspicion and other appropriate diagnostic maneuvers should be undertaken, including serum acid phosphatase determination, bone survey, possible

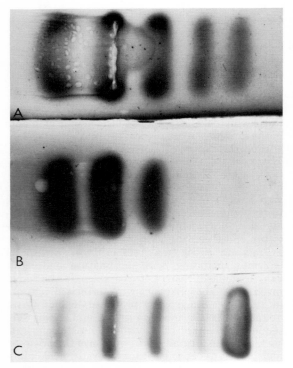

**Figure 8**  Alterations in the electrophoretic pattern of the enzyme lactic dehydrogenase (LDH) occur with prostatic carcinoma. *A,* From left to right, elevations of the isozymes IV and V are noted in a patient with active prostatic carcinoma. *B,* After hormonal therapy isozymes IV and V disappear. *C,* With exacerbation of prostatic carcinoma elevations of isozymes IV and V, particularly the latter, are observed. (Courtesy of Dr. George R. Prout, Jr.)

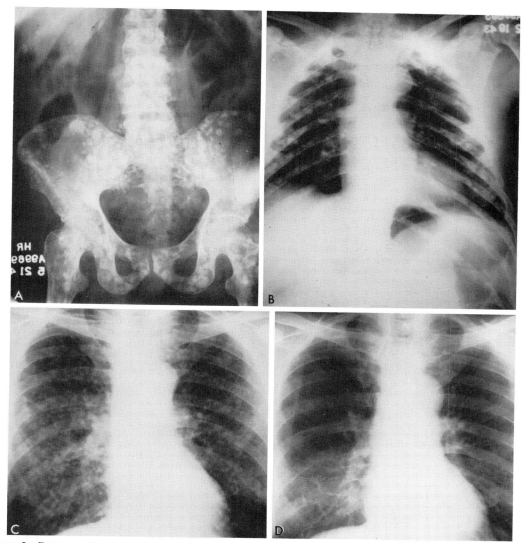

**Figure 9**  Patterns of metastatic prostatic carcinoma include *(A)* multiple osteoblastic bony lesions, particularly in the pelvis and lumbar spine; *(B)* nodular pulmonary lesions and osteoblastic metastases in the ribs; and *(C)* miliary pulmonary metastases which regress *(D)* after adequate hormonal management.

marrow aspiration for tumor cells, and an appropriate form of biopsy. In advanced cases of local disease, there is usually little doubt as to the diagnosis. The prostate becomes nodular and irregular with extension of the indurated process beyond the confines of the gland, culminating in fixation of the prostate to the surrounding structures. At this stage of the disease, the patient is usually experiencing significant symptoms.

Definition of the stage of prostatic disease is aided by ancillary clinical and laboratory determinations. Bone survey may disclose metastatic lesions, classically osteoblastic in character, though poorly differentiated prostatic tumors occasionally produce osteolytic bone lesions. Bones most often involved are those of the pelvis and lower spine, though ribs, skull, and the long bones may also be involved. Even in the absence of radiographically demonstrable metastatic

lesions, prostatic tumor cells may be evident in the bone marrow, and sternal or iliac aspiration may not only confirm the diagnosis but indicate an advanced stage of prostatic carcinoma. Serum acid phosphatase determination constitutes a necessary step in diagnostic evaluation, since an elevated acid phosphatase frequently indicates metastatic activity, precluding cure by radical prostatic surgery. Intravenous urography and cystourethrography are useful radiographic techniques in evaluating degrees of lower tract obstruction due to advanced prostatic carcinoma. Cystourethroscopy is negative at early stages, but is useful in assessing the degree of bladder outlet obstruction occasioned by advanced prostate cancer.

The metastatic patterns of prostatic carcinoma are unique and interesting. Most common manifestations of metastatic disease are bony lesions in the sacrum and lumbar spine, but it is thought

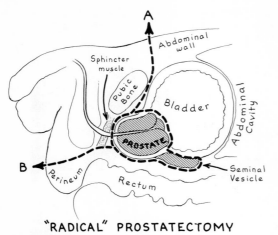

## "RADICAL" PROSTATECTOMY

**Figure 10**   Schematic representation of radical prostatectomy, removing the prostate, seminal vesicles, and contiguous tissues by the retropubic method (A) or by radical perineal prostatectomy (B).

that earlier metastases occur in the iliac nodes, prompting some surgeons to advocate abdominal exploration as a method of assessing extent and stage of disease. Paradoxical metastases to the brain and skull with no intervening metastatic lesions in the lung or other bones may occur via Batson's plexus, the spinal venous system that communicates directly with the periprostatic veins. Pulmonary lesions may be isolated nodular metastatic defects or diffuse multiple seedlike lesions reminiscent of miliary tuberculosis. In advanced stages of the disease, metastatic adenocarcinoma of the prostate may be observed in virtually every organ including such unlikely sites as the testes, the skin of the scrotum, and the adrenal glands.

The treatment of prostatic carcinoma is, fortunately, a relatively bright page in the annals of cancer therapy. Observations by Huggins and his associates more than 30 years ago led to recognition of the androgen dependency of prostatic tumors and the corollary therapeutic response of these tumors to estrogen administration. These observations and subsequent investigations demonstrated the efficacy of hormonal management and provided the basis for the first genuinely effective chemotherapeutic approach to malignant disease. In addition, cure of prostatic carcinoma through surgery in the early stages of the disease has been practical for more than half a century. Most recently, advanced radiotherapeutic technique has provided yet another approach to control and possible cure of prostatic cancer.

### Surgical Treatment

The potential for surgical cure of early carcinoma of the prostate was demonstrated shortly after the turn of the century. The efficacy of radical perineal prostatectomy has subsequently been elaborated by Jewett, Dees, and others. Clearly, radical prostatectomy, involving removal of the entire prostate and the seminal vesicles, can

constitute cure only when the malignant process is confined to these tissues with no contiguous or distant spread. It is estimated that as many as 10 per cent of patients presenting with prostatic carcinoma are in an early stage that is amenable to radical surgery. In general, the indications for radical prostatectomy include the isolated or localized prostatic malignant process, anticipated life expectancy of 10 years or more, good general condition of the patient with no significant ancillary disease, and the absence of demonstrable metastatic lesions as evaluated by radiologic survey, marrow aspiration, and normal serum acid phosphatase. Radical prostatectomy may be accomplished by the classic perineal methods of Young or Belt, and in recent years the retropubic approach to radical prostatectomy has been found successful by many. Complications of radical prostatectomy include impotence, a 2 to 5 per cent incontinence rate, and a surgical mortality of approximately 5 per cent. However, the efficacy of radical prostatectomy is apparent in various reports, Dees recording a 60 per cent 10 year survival following radical perineal prostatectomy as compared with a 22 per cent 10 year survival with palliative therapy and a 30 per cent 10 year survival with hormonal manipulation measures.[5]

### Hormonal Management

While hormonal manipulation cannot afford cure of prostatic carcinoma, excellent and prolonged control can be achieved. The survey by Nesbit and Baum in 1950 documents the enhancement of survival of patients with prostatic carcinoma undergoing endocrine therapy.[14] The oral administration of exogenous estrogens, bilateral orchiectomy, or a combination of orchiectomy and estrogens may be employed, the latter approach offering the most significant palliation and effective method of control. Alyea, reporting experience with castration and simultaneous initiation of estrogens, given as diethylstilbestrol, 0.5 to 1.0 mg. daily by mouth, observed a 30 per cent 10 year survival, irrespective of stage and grade of disease at the time of diagnosis.[1] It has been observed that total orchiectomy, indeed even scrotal evisceration, may be necessary to achieve the desired results, since residual tunics of the testis may be responsible for further androgen production. Since the adrenal gland is also responsible for production of a significant fraction of total-body androgens, bilateral adrenalectomy has been employed as an additional endocrinologic palliative measure in control of advanced prostatic carcinoma. Surgical or radiotherapeutic ablation of the pituitary may be similarly effective in palliation of advanced disease. The administration of exogenous cortisone or its derivatives may result in "medical adrenalectomy" with suppression of endogenous adrenal function, such therapy having the added advantages of inducing an anabolic state, producing a sense of well-being and a moderate euphoria, and diminishing the discomfort of advanced metastatic disease without the trauma of major surgery. Other measures of hormonal manipulation include the utilization of progestational agents and cyproterone acetate as additional modalities of treatment in advanced prostatic carcinoma. Recently, utilization of estrogens in dosage of 5 mg. per day and more has been subjected to some criticism on the basis of evaluation by a Veterans Administration cooperative research group; patients receiving larger doses of estrogens exhibited a substantial increase in mortality rates, predominantly from vascular complications of thrombosis involving cerebral and cardiac vessels, and it has been recommended that hormonal therapy be withheld until the disease becomes symptomatic.[23] This view, however, is not universally shared, and retrospective analyses fail to support the view that estrogen therapy increases the mortality rate for patients with prostatic carcinoma. At the present time, it is generally held that bilateral orchiectomy with simultaneous institution of estrogen therapy in modest dosage is the procedure of choice in advanced prostatic carcinoma that is beyond the realm of surgical cure. To such hormonal manipulation may be added the other modalities noted, and there is also the potential for secondary radical prostatectomy following adequate local response and regression of prostatic cancer. Finally, the implementation of hormonal measures does not preclude the utilization of radiation therapy as an adjunctive modality of treatment.

### Radiation Therapy

Prior to the advent of cobalt equipment and high-voltage apparatus, standard radiation therapy was effective only in the diminution of bone pain due to metastatic disease. A significant addition to the therapeutic armamentarium was the introduction of radioactive gold solution for interstitial radiation of the prostate and surrounding tissues; Flocks, reporting on 4000 cases of prostatic carcinoma, indicated a 40 per cent improvement in the 5 year survival rate among patients treated by such interstitial instillation of radioactive gold through perineal exposure of the gland.[7] Additional efforts to treat metastatic disease include the utilization of radioactive isotopes of phosphorus and strontium which are selectively absorbed by metastatic bone lesions of high metabolic activity. Most recently, carefully planned radiotherapy of prostatic carcinoma, employing external sources, has been advocated. Such radiation therapy may, of course, be employed for locally inoperable disease, as an adjuvant to hormonal therapy, and possibly as a primary therapeutic method in localized malignancy though such utilization has yet to be demonstrated to be as effective as the radical surgical approach. Complications of radiation therapy include inflammatory reaction with cystitis, urethritis, and proctitis, as well as potential stricture or slough.

## SEMINAL VESICLES

The seminal vesicles, lying posterior to the bladder and uniting distally into the ejaculatory ducts which empty into the prostatic urethra, are paired tubular structures, functioning to produce mucous secretions that serve as the vehicle for sperm. The seminal vesicles are relatively inert, functioning as a reservoir for semen until ejaculation occurs, at which time muscular contraction causes the expulsion of ejaculate. Abnormalities of the seminal vesicles are relatively uncommon. Rarely, one of the seminal vesicles may be congenitally absent or exhibit cystic anomalies, usually associated with ipsilateral absence of kidney and ureter. Because of the secluded and protected location of the seminal vesicles, they are infrequently involved in trauma.

The most common clinical problems related to the seminal vesicles are those of inflammation and involvement by malignancy, due to the intimate connection of the seminal vesicles with the prostate and the base of the bladder. Chronic lower urinary tract infection may cause seminal vesiculitis, usually seen in association with chronic prostatitis, and obstruction of the ejaculatory ducts at the ampullae may predispose to abscess of the seminal vesicle. Diagnosis of such inflammatory disease is made by digital rectal examination; the dilatation and induration of the seminal vesicles can be readily appreciated, while the normal seminal vesicle is difficult to palpate. Massage and stripping of the seminal vesicles will produce purulent debris, confirming the diagnosis.

Primary carcinoma of the seminal vesicles is extremely rare. However, the communication of the seminal vesicles with the prostate, lying within the same fascial planes and subserved by the same lymphatic system, predisposes to early spread of prostatic cancer to the seminal vesicles. For this reason, radical prostatectomy demands the removal of the contiguous seminal vesicles. The surgical approach to the seminal vesicles may be perineal, retropubic, or transperitoneal, the method selected depending upon diagnosis; benign cysts of the seminal vesicles are best approached abdominally, while removal of the seminal vesicles with the prostate in cases of prostatic carcinoma is most readily accomplished by perineal exposure.

## COWPER'S GLANDS

Cowper's glands are paired secretory organs lying in contiguity with the bulbomembranous urethra, draining through ducts in the floor of the bulbous urethra. They function to produce the clear mucoid secretion that serves as a lubricant to sexual function and implements ejaculation. Normally, Cowper's glands are not palpable, but occasionally infection may supervene, usually secondary to urethritis, predisposing to enlargement which is palpable on rectal examination distal to the prostate in a paraurethral position. Diagnosis of infected Cowper's glands is established by expression of pus per urethram, and treatment is usually conservative, though transurethral or perineal incision and drainage may be required. Carcinoma of Cowper's glands is extremely rare, but produces perineal pain, difficult urination, and a stony hard mass that presents rectally and perineally. Rectal fistulae may occur. Radical surgery is indicated.

# PENIS

The penis serves the dual function of incorporating the male urethra and serving as the male organ of copulation. There are three erectile tissue compartments of the penis, the two corpora cavernosa situated dorsolaterally and the corpus spongiosum which invests the urethra and terminates distally in the glans penis. The loose integument of the penis permits elasticity for erection. The mechanism of erection relates to both psychic and nervous stimuli which produce engorgement of the corpora cavernosa and, to some extent, the corpus spongiosum. Neurophysiologic studies indicate that there is a center localized to the medial frontal lobe that is a positive locus for penile erection. Certain anterior thalamic nuclei and the mamillary bodies may be involved.

## CONGENITAL ANOMALIES

It is fortunate that congenital anomalies of the penis are rare, since abnormalities of the genitalia may be the cause of severe anxiety and psychologic distress, not only to the patient but to the parents of the newborn male as well. Rare anomalies of the penis include duplication (double penis) and congenital absence of the penis in an otherwise normal male, the latter condition probably treated best by sex conversion surgery since there are no adequate surgical methods for construction of a satisfactory erectile phallus. Microphallus may be managed successfully.

### Phimosis

The normal foreskin of the penis provides a covering for the glans, the redundant portion of the foreskin being termed the prepuce. In many newborn males, the prepuce cannot be retracted satisfactorily, infection and inflammatory reaction result, and edema, fibrosis, and scarring cause constriction of the foreskin or phimosis. In severe cases of phimosis, trapped preputial secretions predispose to balanitis (inflammation of the glans) and balanoposthitis (inflammation of both the glans and the foreskin). Obstruction to urination may occur and urinary infection can result. Further, such chronic inflammation is thought to predispose to penile malignant disease. Accordingly, prophylactic infant circumcision has been widely practiced for many years, though the universal necessity for such routine circumcision has been questioned. When phimosis leads to such complications, dorsal slit of the foreskin may be required as an emergency measure, and circumcision should be accomplished at an appropriate time. Very often, phimosis is accompanied by meatal stenosis, and a urethral meatotomy may be effected at the time of circumcision. If the constricted foreskin becomes retracted and trapped proximal to the glans, severe swelling and even necrosis of the glans may ensue, a condition known as paraphimosis. Emergency surgical intervention is essential if the paraphimotic prepuce cannot be reduced manually; dorsal slit of the constricted foreskin is the procedure of choice.

### Congenital Curvature

The most common congenital curvature of the penis is chordee, a fibrous constricting band along

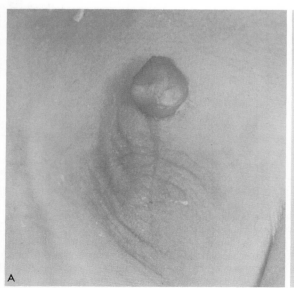
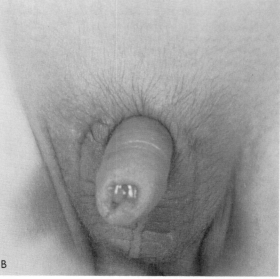

**Figure 11**   Congenital microphallus (A) is a distressing condition, but will respond to local application of testosterone preparations, response generated within 3 months as seen in (B).

the ventral aspect of the penis which is usually associated with hypospadias, the congenital defect of the distal urethra. Epispadias, congenital absence of the upper portion of the urethra, causes dorsal deflection and curvature of the penis. In addition, abnormalities of the investing Buck's fascia may cause asymmetry of the penis with deviation.

## TRAUMA

Trauma to the penis is relatively uncommon, but can cause total sexual disability. In pelvic fracture, rupture of the urethra will produce extravasation of blood and urine into the penile tissues; treatment is directed toward correction of the urethral rupture. In the erect state, the penis is subject to dislocation or even fracture, the latter condition being one of rupture of one or both of the corpora cavernosa with severe bleeding and hematoma. Immediate surgical intervention is required to repair the laceration of the investing fascia. Rupture of the veins of the penis may produce severe hemorrhage, usually best managed by catheter drainage and compression dressings. Lacerations of the penile skin and the glans are not uncommon as a consequence of masturbation, manipulation, or sexual activity, the frenulum of the penis occasionally tearing with sexual intercourse. Avulsion of the skin of the penis and of the scrotal skin may result when clothing is caught in various types of machinery, the loose integument of the genitalia being avulsed rather readily. Split-thickness skin grafts to the penile shaft take well and the cosmetic and functional results of such repair are satisfactory.

## PENILE INFECTIONS

The penis is subject to infectious involvement by the various venereal diseases as well as other pathogenic bacteria and viruses. The abundant blood supply of the penile skin predisposes to excellent healing of such lesions. However, furunculosis of the penis may lead to severe cellulitis and even infection of the erectile corpora of the penis, cavernositis, most frequently due to urethritis of gonorrheal or nongonorrheal origin. Incision and drainage with appropriate antibiotic therapy constitute the treatment of choice.

### Balanoposthitis

Inflammation of the glans penis and the prepuce constitutes balanoposthitis, most frequently the result of retained secretions and bacterial infection beneath the redundant prepuce, particularly when phimosis is present. Local irritative symptoms vary according to the severity of the infection, and it is thought that such chronic infections may predispose to squamous cell carcinoma of the penis. Dorsal slit of the foreskin, local measures, and antibiotics are employed initially, with circumcision the definitive method of treatment.

### Condylomata Acuminata

Condyloma acuminatum is a cauliflower-like growth known as venereal wart, occurring singly or multiply on the prepuce, glans penis, and within the urethra itself. The lesions are of viral origin, usually associated with poor local hygiene, and may be transmitted from one sexual partner to another. In cases of redundant foreskin, circumcision may be beneficial in preventing recurrence. The standard method of treatment is application of 25 per cent podophyllum in benzoin on several successive occasions. Occasionally the venereal warts may achieve such size that surgical excision is necessary. Other methods of management include desiccation with dry ice, electrofulguration, and application of solutions of thio-TEPA. In advanced cases, the differential diagnosis lies between condylomata acuminata and carcinoma of the penis.

### Herpes Progenitalis

Small reddened areas of the glans, prepuce, and dorsal surface of the penile shaft may become vesiculated, rupturing to leave superficial ulcerations, foci of secondary infection. This common viral infection is best managed by local cleansing and applications of bland ointments, sometimes incorporating anti-inflammatory agents.

### Venereal Diseases

The principal venereal diseases to involve the penis itself are syphilis and chancroid. The primary lesion of syphilis is an ulcer or chancre, crater-like in appearance, usually occurring around the corona of the glans penis. Dark-field smear of the lesion will reveal *Treponema pallidum*. Similar chancres may be caused by sporotrichosis and tularemia, but these lesions do not usually involve the penis. The penile lesion of chancroid is a soft ulcerated area, again usually on the distal portion of the penis, later associated with inguinal buboes. Gonorrhea does not produce external penile lesions, the primary involvement being of the urethra and the paraurethral glands. Granuloma inguinale and lymphogranuloma venereum involve the inguinal lymphatics.

## PENILE MALIGNANT DISEASE

Squamous cell carcinoma of the penis is the usual malignant lesion, though basal cell carcinoma and others have been described. Benign lesions such as nevi, hemangiomas, and papillomas are readily managed by local excision. Squamous cell carcinoma of the penis constitutes a more difficult challenge. It is usually seen in males of the lower socioeconomic strata, most commonly in uncircumcised men, and is a disease of filth, often the sequel of chronic balanoposthitis. Infant circumcision confers almost total immunity, though very rare cases of penile carcinoma have been reported in circumcised persons. The lesion is slow-growing and very often is obscured by the redundant foreskin. Patients tend to present with

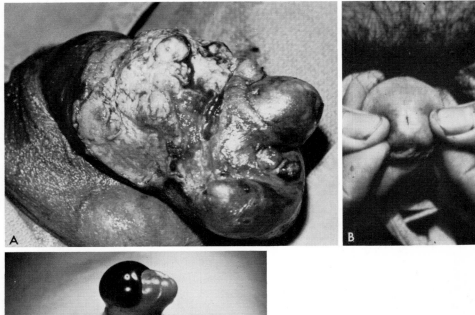

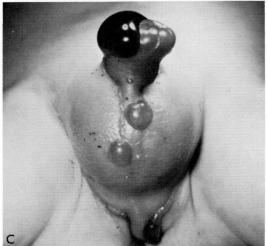

**Figure 12** Penile lesions include *(A)* fungating squamous cell carcinoma; *(B)* balanitis xerotica obliterans with blanching, fibrosis, and stricture of the urethral meatus; and *(C)* phimosis with extravasation of urine.

lesions in advanced stage. Persky and his associates have proposed clinical staging as follows: Stage I, limited to the glans penis or prepuce; Stage II, invasion of the corpora but without metastases; Stage III, invasive with positive regional nodes; and Stage IV, with distant metastases. Cure and survival are virtually 100 per cent in the Stage I patients, about 50 per cent in Stage II and Stage III, and nil in Stage IV.[6]

Diagnosis is established by biopsy. Treatment consists of partial or total penectomy; a proximal margin free of tumor of at least 1.5 cm. is desirable. Inguinal node dissection, with exicision of both superficial and deep inguinal groups, is advocated when palpable nodes persist after amputation. Lymphadenopathy may result from the secondary infection seen in most advanced penile carcinomas. Radiation therapy in squamous cell carcinoma of the penis is relatively ineffective, but may be employed in treatment of known inguinal metastatic disease; the primary lesion should always be treated surgically. Chemotherapeutic efforts have been without avail.

## SPECIAL CONDITIONS

Certain peculiar disorders of the penis or of penile function deserve special consideration, particularly since etiologic factors remain obscure in these disorders.

### Peyronie's Disease

Localized plastic induration of the fibrous investments of the penile shaft was first described by the French surgeon Peyronie more than 100 years ago. Despite adequate description and an abundance of clinical observation, the etiology of the condition is unknown.[20] A firm fibrotic thickening of the fascia of the corpora cavernosa is observed, usually involving the dorsolateral aspects of the penile shaft or the intracavernous septum between the corpora cavernosa, histologically similar to keloid or Dupuytren's contracture. The fibrous plaques themselves may be painless, but there is often compromise of erectile capability of the penis with deviation of the penis on erection and pain as a consequence of this derangement.

Patients usually note the lesion by self-examination, and they may have experienced significant deviation which interferes with intromission and coitus. Progression is slow, and spontaneous remissions are observed. Treatment is unsatisfactory; surgical excision is often unsuccessful, since recurrence of the plaquelike induration is common after excision of plaques. High doses of alpha-tocopherol (vitamin E) and the oral use of potassium para-aminobenzoate (Potaba) as a fibrinolytic agent have been recommended, but successful resolution has been the exception rather than the rule. Systemic steroid therapy has not been beneficial, but local injection of high-potency corticosteroids such as dexamethasone has been reported to soften and resolve the plaques; the therapy itself—requiring weekly injections over a period of several months—is exquisitely tedious and painful. Perhaps the most effective modality of treatment at the present time is localized radiation therapy, employing 300 R in a single dose which is repeated at 3 month intervals to a total of 900 to 1200 R.

When the diagnosis of Peyronie's disease has been established, it is perhaps most important to reassure the patient that the process is not malignant. In most instances, the disease process is self-limiting with slow if any progression. Radiation therapy may alleviate any discomfort and though there may be some penile deviation with erection, sexual disability is not the rule.

### Priapism

Prolonged pathologic and painful erection of the penis is termed priapism in recognition of the Greek god of sexual excess, Priapus. Pelvic venous thrombosis predisposes to priapism, and such thrombosis is observed with metastatic malignant diseases of various sorts, leukemia, pelvic trauma, sickle cell disease or trait, trauma to the corpora, or spinal cord injury. In a majority of patients, no definite etiologic factor can be identified, and both local neural and vascular abnormalities have been incriminated as possible causes. Prompt recognition and therapy are essential, since prolonged unrelieved priapism will almost inevitably lead to subsequent permanent impotence. Immediate sedation and analgesia will sometimes alleviate priapism. Continuous spinal anesthesia has been advocated and is occasionally effective in the early hours of the condition. Classic treatment consists of insertion of large-bore needles for aspiration and detumescence, but unless pelvic venous congestion is simultaneously relieved, turbidity will recur. Thrombosis of the corpora occurs only late in the course of priapism, and accordingly venous bypass operations may be effective. The superficial saphenous vein may be employed for a corporosaphenous shunt, unilaterally or bilaterally, and a cavernospongiosum shunt may also be an effective surgical maneuver since the corpus spongiosum is rarely obstructed in priapism. A proteolytic enzyme from pit viper venom has been reported to cause rapid reduction in plasma fibrinogen, effective in one patient with priapism.

### Impotence

While it is recognized that the aging process will diminish not only the libido but the capacity for erection as well, many men will remain potent throughout a lifetime of 90 years or more. Potency in the elderly male may be related to psychologic factors as much as to general health. Arteriosclerotic cardiovascular disease may compromise circulation to the corpora. Diabetes and other systemic disorders producing generalized neuropathies may diminish ability for erection. Impotence may be one of the earliest signs of the Leriche syndrome, thrombotic obstruction of the iliac arteries, and the condition may be relieved by appropriate vascular surgery. Spinal cord injury may impair the capacity for erection, as may prostatic surgery, particularly perineal prostatectomy which apparently compromises the pudendal nerves in some men undergoing such surgical treatment of benign prostatic enlargement. It should be noted that the vast majority of potent males undergoing prostatectomy remain potent postoperatively, irrespective of the surgical method employed. Radical perineal prostatectomy for malignant disease universally results in impotence. Finally, certain drugs such as the phenothiazines may impair erections and produce impotence, presumably by the adrenergic blocking effect of medication. Despite knowledge of this spectrum of potential causes of impotence, a majority of males who are otherwise healthy and who complain of an isolated problem of impotence must usually be categorized as having idiopathic or psychologic difficulties; psychiatric consultation is mandatory when the various physical causes of impotence have been eliminated.

### Ejaculatory Disorders

One of the most distressing sexual disabilities of the young and middle-aged male may be premature ejaculation. Intromission may be scarcely achieved before ejaculation occurs, terminating the sexual act to the frustration of the patient and the partner. Certain organic and psychic factors can be incriminated; chronic prostatitis can increase irritability and predisposition to ejaculation, and long abstinence with attendant sexual excitation can initiate premature ejaculation. In most instances, however, the problem relates to inadequate sexual technique in the marital unit, and careful consultation and counsel may aid in overcoming premature ejaculation.

Another disorder of sexual function is retrograde ejaculation occasionally seen as a consequence of neuromuscular disturbance of the vesical neck secondary to diabetes, spinal cord injury, and other causes of neuropathy, but most often due to surgical alteration of the vesical neck. Prostatectomy by open or endoscopic means, transurethral resection of the bladder neck, vesical outlet reconstructive procedures, and even retroperitoneal surgery with autonomic nerve damage may diminish the capacity for closure of the bladder neck, an essential ingredient of normal ejaculation, with consequent retrograde flow of ejaculate into the bladder. Once such surgical abnormality is incurred, little can be done to overcome retrograde ejaculation. In some instances, gradual narrowing of the bladder neck over a period of a year or two after prostatectomy will promote more normal ejaculation. Fortunately, retrograde ejaculation in no way diminishes sexual gratification, but it may, of course, be the cause of infertility since sperm are deposited in the bladder rather than expelled through the urethra.

## MALE URETHRA

The posterior portion of the male urethra, embryologically analogous to the female urethra, consists of the prostatic and membranous portions passing through the central portion of the prostate gland and the urogenital diaphragm or external voluntary urethral sphincter. Distal to this area, also known as the triangular ligament, lies the anterior urethra, consisting of the bulbous portion and the penile or pendulous portion. The prostatic urethra is most often involved secondarily by diseases that primarily affect the prostate gland, such as carcinoma and prostatitis. The membranous urethra within the triangular ligament which attaches to the pubic arch is a frequent site of rupture since the prostatic and membranous urethra are relatively fixed in position with the remainder of the urethra somewhat mobile, predisposing to a shearing tear of the urethra at that point. The bulbous and penile portions of the urethra are invested with paraurethral glands which are often the site of infection, and the anterior urethra is rarely sterile in contrast to the posterior urethra, bacteria gaining entry to the distal portions of the urethra through the external meatus.

## CONGENITAL ABNORMALITIES

Urethral meatal stenosis can usually be recognized by inspection and is suspected when the urinary stream is of poor caliber. Such stenosis may predispose to infection and may be a cause of enuresis. Treatment of meatal stenosis is by meatotomy. Other congenital strictures of the urethra may also be seen, often in the bulbous urethra. Open surgical repair may be favored in longer strictures, while lesser areas of involvement may be satisfactorily handled by internal urethrotomy and prolonged catheter drainage to provide stenting of the urethra in an open position during the phase of healing.

### Urethral Valves

Congenital valves of the urethra usually cause severe obstructive uropathy with decompensation of the urinary bladder, hydroureteronephrosis, supervening infection, and consequent renal failure unless prompt and adequate treatment is instituted. Valves are mucosal or fibrous folds obstructing urethral urinary flow, usually occurring in the distal portion of the prostatic urethra at the level of the verumontanum, taking an alar

configuration and sweeping from the verumontanum to the lateral wall of the prostatic urethra or occurring as a diaphragm-like constriction of the urethra. Transurethral electroresection or destruction by fulguration is most often employed, but a retropubic transprostatic open exposure may effect surgical cure of valves. The sequelae of obstruction by urethral valves may be so severe that permanent urinary diversion is required, generally accomplished in the form of an ileal conduit, an isolated segment of ileum to which the ureters are attached at the proximal end, the distal end being brought out in the right lower quadrant as a urinary ileostomy.

### Hypospadias

Varying degrees of failure of complete development of the distal urethra may be observed, termed hypospadias. The urethra may terminate just proximal to the glans (glanular hypospadias), at some point along the penile shaft (penile hypospadias), at the anterior margin of the scrotum (penoscrotal hypospadias), or in the perineum with bifid scrotum (perineal hypospadias). Associated with this defect is severe ventral curvature of the penis or chordee which results from a fibrous band occurring in the projected course of the urethra. The embryologic defect is a failure of closure of the urethral groove. In extreme cases, particularly if there is associated bilateral testicular maldescent, the configuration of the genitalia may be so ambiguous that an intersex state results. Early and accurate diagnosis is imperative. Virtually all degrees of hypospadias demand surgical repair, for cosmetic as well as functional reasons. A classic approach is to accomplish release of chordee and penile straightening as one procedure, followed at a later date by a one- or two-stage urethroplasty. A

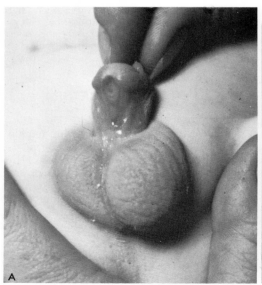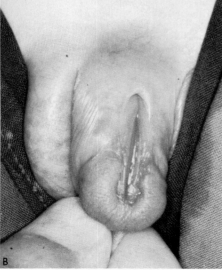

**Figure 13**   Urethral abnormalities include *(A)* hypospadias and *(B)* epispadias.

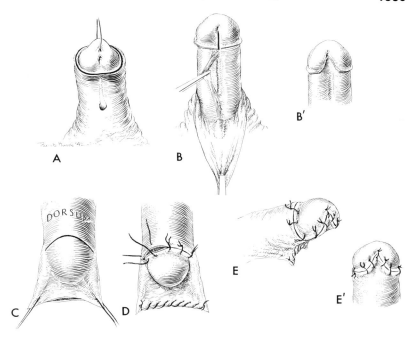

**Figure 14** Nesbit technique of release of chordee, excising the fibrous band with transposition of dorsal foreskin to ventral surface of penile shaft. (From Creevy, C. D. In: Glenn, J. F., and Boyce, W. H.: Urologic Surgery. New York, Hoeber Medical Division, Harper & Row, 1969.)

tremendous variety of operative procedures have been advocated, and all may be successful. Most recently, both Hodgson and Horton have advocated one-stage operations for release of chordee and simultaneous urethroplasty, and both of these procedures may be successful in the majority of cases. The principal difficulty encountered in surgical repair of hypospadias with associated chordee relates to achieving adequate penile straightening, imperative before urethral reconstruction is effected. The commonly employed types of urethroplasty involve construction of a skin tube from the original orifice to the coronal margin or tip of the glans. Since hypospadias and chordee are universally associated with splaying of the glans and hooded redundant dorsal foreskin, the glans can be reconstituted in conjunction with the urethroplasty, and the redundant dorsal foreskin can be mobilized and brought ventrally for covering of any defect created. The operative complications of urethroplasties of all sorts include fistula and stricture, both of which may be managed by relatively minor secondary surgical procedures.

### Epispadias

Failure of development of the anterior wall of the urethra and concomitant failure of dorsal fusion of the penile corpora result in epispadias. Complete vesical exstrophy, a rare condition, is always accompanied by epispadias; epispadias alone with some degree of urinary continence is more commonly seen, perhaps as often as once in 30,000 live male births. The urethral opening may lie anywhere from the vesical neck to the glans, but if it is distal to the prostatic urethra, urinary continence and control may be satisfactory. The severe cosmetic deformity and the associated dif-

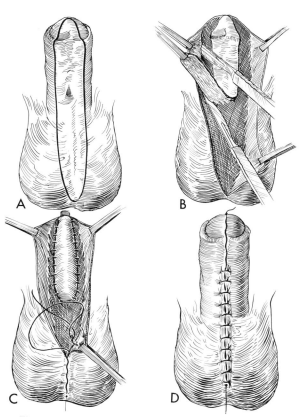

**Figure 15** One technique for urethral reconstruction in hypospadias, this method the Crabtree urethroplasty, a similar procedure having been employed by Horton and Devine. (From Creevy, C. D. In: Glenn, J. F., and Boyce, W. H.: Urologic Surgery. New York, Hoeber Medical Division, Harper & Row, 1969.)

ficulty in controlling the urinary stream demand surgical correction, usually accomplished in infancy. Plastic reconstruction of the penis, closure and ventral inversion of the urethra, and reconstruction of the bladder neck by the Young-Dees method is usually satisfactory. Unless there is complete failure of urinary control, urinary diversion is not necessary. While early repair is desirable, the child is usually better able to cooperate in achieving urinary control after the age of 3 years.

## TRAUMA

Traumatic injury of the urethra most commonly occurs in association with pelvic fracture. Shearing injuries induced by external force cause rupture at the urogenital diaphragm in the region of the membranous urethra. Urinary extravasation is noted, often with extensive pelvic hemorrhage. The prostate and bladder may be displaced superiorly, well away from the distal urethra. Catheterization is impossible in such circumstances, and open surgical repair or suprapubic urinary diversion should be accomplished promptly, though primary perineal reconstruction may be most advantageous in some circumstances. The diagnosis of urethral rupture must be suspected in every instance of pelvic injury and unless the patient is able to void clear urine in a normal fashion, catheterization may be undertaken in an aseptic fashion to determine the patency and competence of the urethra. If the attempt at catheterization is unsuccessful, urethrograms may establish a diagnosis. Untreated urethral rupture, whether partial or complete, can result in urethral stricture and possible urinary incontinence. Penetrating injuries of the urethra are also observed, most commonly due to gunshot wound or stab wound. Immediate urethral reconstruction and urinary diversion by suprapubic cystotomy are advocated. Similarly, straddle injuries to the perineum may cause urethral rupture which usually demands prompt surgical intervention or prolonged catheter stenting of the urethra. Iatrogenic perforation or rupture of the urethra may occur in the course of instrumentation, cystoscopy or urethral dilation. Pre-existing urethral strictures due to trauma or gonococcal urethritis predispose to difficult instrumentation and potential perforation of the urethra, often followed by the establishment of urethral diverticulum or false urinary passage. Periurethral abscess and attendant complications may ensue unless urethral injury of this sort is recognized. In instances of iatrogenic injury, suprapubic cystotomy for catheter drainage should be initiated along with the usual conservative supportive measures.

## INFECTIONS

The urethra is subject to both gonococcal and nonspecific infections. Congenital abnormalities of the urethra such as stricture of stenosis, acquired strictures of the urethra of any cause, urethral

diverticulum, or any other structural abnormality will predispose to development of urethritis and will complicate management. Associated anatomic abnormalities should be treated surgically to effect maximal control of urethral infections.

Acute gonococcal urethritis results when gonococci are introduced into the urethra, finding an appropriate milieu in the relatively hypoxic recesses of the periurethral glands which invest the bulbous and penile portions of the urethra. Characteristic symptoms of gonococcal urethritis include burning on urination, frequency of urination, and a urethral discharge which is usually creamy white in character, exhibiting the typical gram-negative diplococci on the stained smear. Anaerobic culture of the urethral discharge will confirm the diagnosis. Treatment of acute gonococcal urethritis is with penicillin, ampicillin, or relatively large doses of the tetracyclines. Secondary associated gram-negative infections may demand employment of adjunctive antibiotic therapy. Untreated acute gonococcal urethritis may lead to urethral stricture through the mechanism of fibrosis and cicatrix formation, and such gonococcal strictures then dispose to the establishment of posterior urethritis and prostatitis which are refractory to usual methods of management. Gonococcal stricture may be treated by urethral dilation periodically until the stricture is relieved, or by internal urethrotomy with the Otis urethrotome or a similar instrument, with stenting of the urethra for a period of several weeks with an inlying catheter to prevent reoccurrence of the stenotic area.

The term nonspecific urethritis refers to those infections in which no evidence of gonorrhea can be found. Nonspecific urethritis may be due to bacterial infection or to viral infection. The typical complaint of the patient with nonspecific urethritis is of a clear viscid urethral discharge, particularly in the early morning, associated with some degree of urinary frequency and burning discomfort on urination. Prostatitis may or may not accompany the urethritis. Treatment is usually with one of the tetracyclines.

## URETHRAL MALIGNANT DISEASE

Carcinoma of the male urethra is rare, only several hundred cases having been documented in the English literature. Those malignant lesions occurring in the distal penile portion of the urethra are most often squamous cell carcinoma, while the more proximal tumors are transitional cell lesions. Symptoms of urethral malignant disease are hematuria, dysuria, stranguria, frequency, and ultimate urinary retention. The diagnosis is established by endoscopic visualization of the lesion and appropriate biopsy, either cystoscopically or by urethrotomy and excision under direct vision. Spread of malignancy is via lymphatics of the corpus spongiosum into the deep pelvic nodes and by venous channels. Since the diagnosis is usually established late in the course of the disease, the prognosis is poor despite radical surgical intervention. Depending upon the location of the lesion, partial urethrectomy with or without penectomy may be effective. Radiation therapy and chemotherapeutic measures are unproven as effective therapeutic modalities. It is interesting that a high percentage of patients with carcinoma of the urethra give a history of previous venereal disease or urethral stricture.

## SCROTUM

The loose skin of the scrotal sac is peculiarly adapted to house the testes, epididymides, and spermatic cords. Spermatogenesis is dependent upon critical temperature regulation and requires temperature several degrees lower than that within the abdominal cavity. Contraction of the dartos in response to cold provides added insulation for the testis, while relaxation in warm weather permits cooling to a temperature 5° to 8° lower than that within the abdomen, an optimal condition for spermatogenesis. The spermatic cords are supplied by the cremaster muscle which contracts and relaxes in coordination with the dartos muscle.

Most common anomalies of the scrotum are associated with other developmental abnormalities such as absence of a testis or cryptorchism in which case one compartment of the scrotum may fail to develop, a condition termed hemiabsence of the scrotum. In conjunction with complete perineal hypospadias, the scrotum may be bifid as a consequence of failure of fusion of the two compartments in the midline. Rarely, partial or complete penoscrotal transposition may be observed, all or a part of the scrotum fusing anteriorly and superior to the penis; surgical correction of penoscrotal transposition is neither complicated nor difficult and should be accomplished at an early age.

While the scrotal contents are delicate and subject to damage by even minimal trauma, the scrotum itself is not often severely injured. Blunt blows and penetrating injuries may, however, involve the scrotum, and hematomas may develop readily since scrotal skin is rather loose and provides little hemostatic pressure effect. Partial or complete avulsion of the scrotal skin may result from injury by various types of agricultural and industrial machinery with power belt apparatus, clothing usually becoming enmeshed in the power drive with resultant tearing and avulsion of the loose skin of the genitalia. If any scrotal skin remains, the testes may be recovered. Frequently, all scrotal skin is avulsed and it is necessary to bury the testes and cords in the loose subcutaneous tissues of the inner aspect of each thigh. Penetrating and perforating injuries of the scrotum should be treated vigorously, since infection may lead to gangrene and slough.

Infections of the scrotum are usually secondary to infection of the testicles or its appendages or to urinary infection with fistula formation as seen with severe urethral stricture. Extravasation of urine may lead to extensive scrotal cellulitis and multiple fistulas through the scrotum and surrounding areas, the so-called "watering-pot perineum." The scrotum so involved is best treated by multiple incisions for drainage, with the use of many rubber wicks. Urinary diversion is mandatory, and a suprapubic cystotomy is preferable to an inlying urethral catheter. Scrotal gangrene may result from such infection, but may also be caused by mechanical, chemical, or thermal injury, and is treated by appropriate antibiotic therapy, surgical drainage, and hyperbaric oxygenation.

Localized scrotal swelling may be caused by edema associated with cardiac failure, renal disease, blood dyscrasias, ascites, or abdominal neoplasms that interfere with venous and lymphatic

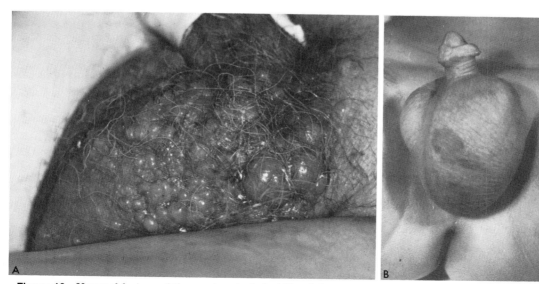

**Figure 16**   Unusual lesions of the scrotum include *(A)* nodular metastatic cutaneous implants of prostatic carcinoma, and *(B)* hemangioendothelioma of the scrotum.

return from the scrotum. Similarly, large inguinal hernias may sometimes embarrass venous and lymphatic return, predisposing to edema formation. Simple edema must be differentiated from elephantiasis, classically caused by the filariae, *Wuchereria bancrofti*, and usually associated with elephantiasis of the lower extremities. Idiopathic elephantiasis, Milroy's disease, may also involve the scrotum. Finally, inguinal node dissections or inguinal radiation therapy, employed in treatment of metastatic malignant lesions of the penis or other organs, may cause severe chronic scrotal edema. Any of these conditions of edema or elephantiasis may demand generous reduction scrotoplasty in order to effect mechanical improvement of the physical disability involved.

Tumors of the scrotum are uncommon, though benign neoplasms such as fibromas, adenomas, lipomas, and hemangiomas are occasionally seen. More commonly observed are multiple sebaceous cysts of the scrotum, sometimes demanding repeated surgical excision or incision and drainage when infection supervenes. Hemangioendothelioma of the scrotum may assume tremendous proportions and demand surgical removal. Carcinoma of the scrotal skin has been associated with prolonged exposure to chemical carcinogens and has been termed "chimney-sweeps' cancer" because of the association with that occupation; coal tar derivatives are liposoluble in the sebaceous glands of the scrotal skin. Treatment of scrotal malignant lesions requires wide local excision, sometimes associated with orchiectomy, and inguinal lymphadenectomy; radiation and chemotherapeutic agents are relatively ineffective.

# TESTES

The testes, suspended in the scrotal compartments by the spermatic cords, serve a dual function, producing spermatozoa and secreting male hormones, predominantly testosterone. Impairment of spermatogenesis may occur without affecting androgen production, while the secretion of male hormones may be compromised without significant interference with spermatogenesis.[24] Most often, the two functions of the testes may be compromised simultaneously, as with severe epididymo-orchitis or the atrophy seen after hernia repair with compromise of the vascular supply of the testis. Testicular blood supply is derived from the internal spermatic arteries which arise from the aorta below the renal arteries, and course down to the internal inguinal ring and then along the spermatic cord. Venous return is accomplished through the pampiniform plexus which merges into a single spermatic vein on either side.

## CONGENITAL ANOMALIES

The most common congenital anomalies of the testes relate to anomalous location, though congenital absence of one or both testes may be ob-

served. The testes develop within the abdominal cavity, differentiating from the primitive gonadal ridge in the early weeks of fetal life. Normally, the testis begins its migration and descent through the inguinal canal at the end of the first trimester of gestation, but various mechanical and hormonal events may impede or alter normal descent. The gubernaculum, previously thought to provide a fibroelastic cord for guidance of the testis into the scrotal compartment, probably adds little mechanical assistance in this process. It seems most likely that the inherent functions of the testis itself are primarily responsible for the necessary ductal differentiation and descent of the normal testis.

### Anorchism

The classic experiments of Jost indicate that the primitive gonad must differentiate as a testis in order to produce androgens which are the stimulus to normal male (wolffian) ductal development. In the complete absence of testes, female (müllerian) ductal development will differentiate in feminine configuration. However, one testis may fail to develop, frequently in association with ipsilateral agenesis of kidney and ureter; monorchism is seen most often on the right and is termed the "right-sided syndrome." Rare persons are seen who exhibit no evidence of viable testicular tissue, though the external genitalia are fully differentiated in masculine configuration. In these cases, internal male ductal structures, the vasa deferentia, can be identified, usually extending to the internal inguinal ring and terminating blindly in fibrous tissue. Such persons are apparently normal males, though with a completely empty scrotum; puberty is delayed and incomplete with persistent elevation of gonadotropin levels and inadequate plasma testosterone levels. It is postulated that such persons with complete anorchism did indeed have normal testes at an early stage of gestation, but that sometime after the sixteenth week of fetal life the testes atrophied, possibly because of mechanical torsion or other interference with testicular blood supply in the course of the descent. Surgical exploration is required to establish the diagnosis, and a gratifying therapeutic response to continuing exogenous testosterone therapy will be observed: sexual maturation, cessation of growth, increased libido, and masculine redistribution of body fat and muscle mass are concomitants to treatment.

### Cryptorchism

The term cryptorchism, derived from the Greek *cryptos* or hidden, should be reserved for those testes which are truly obscure, usually within the abdominal cavity and not palpable on examination. Testes lying in the course of normal descent in the inguinal canal or in ectopic locations can usually be palpated and are not truly hidden. Cryptorchid or intra-abdominal testes are observed unilaterally or bilaterally in 1 to 10 per cent of male infants. Again, the cause of cryptorchism is obscure, but a selective hormonal deficiency of the testis is suspected as a factor in such failure of descent. Occasionally, a truly cryptorchid testis will descend spontaneously at puberty or in response to parenteral chorionic gonadotropin therapy, but this is not the rule and surgical exploration with orchidopexy generally is required. The cryptorchid abdominal testis will fail in its spermatogenic function, though it may secrete adequate amounts of androgens. Spermatogenic failure is progressive, and transposition of an intra-abdominal testis to the scrotum should be accomplished before the age of 5 years to insure production of normal quantity and quality of spermatozoa. In cases of unilateral cryptorchism, the matter of surgical exploration is less critical, but in bilateral cryptorchism early surgical intervention is necessary. Exploration may be accomplished through an extraperitoneal inguinal incision, but more adequate exposure is obtained through an abdominal approach, particularly if bilateral cryptorchism exists. Cryptorchid testes are usually found retroperitoneally deep within the pelvis and in proximity to the internal inguinal ring, but may be located almost anywhere within the lower abdomen, even up in the renal fossa. It is necessary to isolate the testis with its vas and vessels, mobilizing these structures completely.[16] When the spermatic artery is short, it may be possible to bring the testis through the abdominal wall at Hesselbach's triangle, rather than through the inguinal canal which necessitates a more devious course. Finally, since the testis may derive some blood supply from the small vessels coursing along the vas deferens, it may be feasible to divide the spermatic vessels and depend upon this collateral blood supply, permitting scrotal placement of the testis. When it is impossible to bring the testis to a palpable location within the scrotum or low in the inguinal canal, it is generally thought best to remove the testis since there is a very high incidence of carcinoma in abdominal testes, the incidence perhaps being as much as 20 times greater than that of carcinoma in a normally descended testis. When cryptorchism is diagnosed after the age of 10 or 12 years, orchiectomy may be the preferred treatment since such testes will rarely exhibit normal function despite adequate scrotal placement.

### Incomplete Descent

Incomplete descent or maldescent of the testis is the term reserved for those cases in which the testis is arrested at some point in its normal course of descent and is palpable on careful examination. The usual sites of arrest are at the internal inguinal ring, within the inguinal canal, or at the external ring. Most often, there is an associated congenital indirect inguinal hernia, since the processus vaginalis has not been obliterated at its proximal extent; there is potential for inguinal hernia, and the accumulation of normal peritoneal fluid dependently within the processus vaginalis produces communicating hydrocele. Since function of a testis in the inguinal region is less compromised than that of the abdominal cryptorchid testis, treatment may depend on other associated factors. The presence of overt hernia prompts

earlier surgical correction, and bilateral maldescent constitutes cause for earlier surgical intervention. Some authorities recommend the use of chorionic gonadotropin in dosage of up to 2000 units twice weekly for 6 weeks as a stimulus to testicular descent, but in the truly arrested testis, such treatment is generally ineffective. Further, prolonged chorionic gonadotropin therapy may lead to premature pubescence and growth arrest. A brief course of chorionic gonadotropin therapy may, however, be employed in preparation before orchidopexy and herniorrhaphy, since such stimulation may improve the vascular supply and augment the potential of surgical success. Exploration is accomplished through a high inguinal incision, exposing the entire cord to the internal inguinal ring. The testis and cord are completely freed from the surrounding structures; the patent processus vaginalis is identified, opened, stripped from the cord, and excised, so that the neck of the peritoneal sac is closed; and the spermatic vessels are carefully dissected extraperitoneally in order to afford maximal cord length. The testis is then positioned in the scrotum and fixed with an external traction suture of heavy silk (Bevan technique) or attached to the fascia of the inner thigh, later to be released at a second operation (Torek procedure).

### Hypermobile Testis

In many young males thought to be cryptorchid, the testis or testes are merely highly mobile, retracting into the inguinal canal in an inaccessible position owing to hyperactivity of the cremaster muscle. The simplest means of evaluation is to have the patient sit in a tub of hot water for up to 15 minutes; hypermobile testes will descend into the scrotum and will be normally palpable under such conditions. At puberty, hypermobile testes tend to situate normally within the scrotum, there is rarely any associated hernia, and surgery can be avoided.

### Ectopic Testis

Occasionally, one or both testes may undergo vicarious excursion in the course of descent, coming to lodge in ectopic positions. The exact cause of such wandering ectopia is obscure, but must relate to mechanical factors. Favorite sites of testicular ectopia are symphyseal, prepubic, femoral, crural, penile, or perineal positions. Surgical correction should be accomplished for cosmetic reasons as well as to insure normal testicular function and patient comfort.

## TRAUMA

Surprisingly, the testes are relatively protected against trauma despite their external position. The primitive cremasteric reflex constitutes a part of the "fight or flight" mechanism, and the testes are retracted to a protected inguinal position under extreme stress. Even in instances of avulsion of skin of the genitalia, the testes, appendages, and cords are usually undisturbed, remaining inviolate within their fascial coverings. Blunt external trauma may result in testicular hemorrhage and infarction, usually requiring surgical intervention. Penetrating wounds should be treated by surgical exploration and may be quite bizarre in character; rotary lawn mowers have been known to sweep up coat hangers, wires, and nails which impale the testes in shish-kebab fashion. Torsion of the spermatic cord may occur as a result of external trauma, compromising blood supply and threatening viability of the testis, but such torsion is usually of spontaneous variety. Surgical intervention in instances of testicular trauma should be accomplished promptly since the risk of surgery is minimal and early surgical repair can prevent subsequent infarction, atrophy, and loss of testicular function.

### INFECTIONS

Pyogenic infections of the testis are almost always secondary to spread of infection through the male ductal system, the vas deferens and epididymis. Chronic urinary tract infection, particularly suppurative prostatitis and seminal vesiculitis, predisposes to the spread of bacteria via the vas into the epididymis and the testis. It is rare to observe pyogenic orchitis without associated epididymitis, while epididymitis may occur with virtually no involvement of the associated testis. In rare instances, systemic bacteremia may result in embolic metastatic foci of infection within the testis.

Orchitis may result from viral infection in association with mumps, usually not until after the patient has reached pubescence. Mumps orchitis produces severe local inflammatory reactions with excess accumulation of fluid within the compartment of the tunica vaginalis, the acute hydrocele of mumps. Supportive treatment is generally indicated, and aspiration of the hydrocele is usually avoided since there is a risk of introducing bacteria and initiating a secondary infection which can result in testicular atrophy. Mechanical support to the scrotum with an adhesive bridge, bed rest, analgesics, and antipyretics constitute the first line of treatment. Smallpox, varicella, measles, influenza, and other similar infections may occasionally induce a secondary orchitis.

Tuberculous orchitis is almost always secondary to tuberculous epididymitis, the primary focus within the urinary tract generally being within the kidneys, sometimes in the prostate. Genitourinary tuberculosis of all sorts is responsive to intensive antituberculous medical management, and surgery is reserved for advanced cases of localized tuberculosis; epididymectomy, vasectomy, or epididymo-orchiectomy may be required in some cases. Syphilitic gummas may occur within the testis, and surgical removal is almost always required, since chronic draining fistulas are the rule. Fungus infections such as blastomycosis and actinomycosis of the testis are rarely observed but

usually necessitate orchiectomy and continuing medical management.

The patient with an acute testicular infection is quick to appear for examination and treatment, since the condition is exquisitely painful. On physical examination, a swollen and tender testis may be observed, usually in conjunction with epididymal induration. There is increased local heat and an acute inflammatory hydrocele may be associated. Orchitis must be differentiated from testicular tumor with hemorrhage and from torsion of the spermatic cord, both conditions demanding immediate surgical intervention.

### INFERTILITY

The inability of a couple to produce offspring is termed infertility or sterility. It is estimated that up to 10 per cent of marriages in this country are initially barren, approximately half of this number responding to various therapeutic measures. Infertility may be attributed to the male in as many as 50 per cent of these barren marriages. Adequate evaluation of the marital unit for sterility demands assessment of the male partner and thorough evaluation of the possible factors involved. Infertility and sterility should not be confused with impotence, the latter term applied to the inability to achieve or sustain satisfactory erection for sexual intercourse.

The principal cause of male infertility is a spermatogenic defect, estimated to account for 95 per cent of cases of male infertility or sterility. Most males with such spermatogenic defects will produce sperm in some quantity, though there are usually diminished numbers of sperm and those produced are of inadequate quality, exhibiting malformations and diminished motility. Oligospermia, by definition, indicates a sperm count of less than 20 million per milliliter, and under such conditions fertility can rarely be expected. The principal causes of defective spermatogenesis include congenital inadequacy of the seminiferous tubules; testicular damage as a consequence of pyogenic infection, mumps orchitis, trauma, or infarction; Klinefelter's syndrome; hormonal defects as in hypopituitarism; and cryptorchism. Other causes of oligospermia may relate to transport of spermatozoa. Chronic prostatitis and seminal vesiculitis may result in fibrosis that impedes transport and delivery of sperm. Infection spreading into the vasa deferentia may induce fibrosis and stricture, even to the point of total occlusion of one or both vasa. Tuberculosis affecting the genitourinary system may induce similar inflammatory changes with obstruction to the conductive mechanism. Chronic suppurative prostatitis, particularly with coliform organisms, may result in impedance of sperm motility, an apparent absolute effect as demonstrated by Teague and associates. Abnormal fructose metabolism in the seminal vesicle may predispose to inadequate storage capacity and diminished numbers of spermatozoa available for fertilization.

Azoospermia, complete absence of spermatozoa in the ejaculate, may be the result of total occlusion of the sperm transport system, vasa, seminal vesicles, or ejaculatory ducts. Congenital absence of the vas and seminal vesicles may occur as an isolated anatomic defect, and congenital absence of the vasa is the rule in males with cystic fibrosis. Gonococcal epididymitis and vasitis may cause complete stenosis and azoospermia. Trauma to the vasa in the course of inguinal hernia repair or orchidopexy may result in complete obstruction. Finally, previous bilateral vasectomy, accomplished for elective sterilization or medical purposes, will quite naturally result in azoospermia.

In some instances, infertility may be due to mechanical factors with no defects in spermatogenesis or delivery of spermatozoa. Surgery of the vesical neck, particularly transurethral resection, open wedge resection, or plastic reconstruction and treatment of congenital contracture may result in an inability of the vesical neck to close with ejaculation, causing the ejaculate to be passed in retrograde fashion into the bladder rather than out through the urethra. Cystoscopic evaluation is helpful in identifying such causes of infertility.

Physical evaluation of the infertile male should include a careful and painstaking examination of the genitalia, particularly to assure that the testes are of normal size and consistency, that the epididymides and vasa are present and normal, and that there is no evidence of chronic inflammatory disease of the external genitalia. Prostatitis should be ruled out by digital examination, prostatic massage, and smear of prostatic fluid. Appropriate cultures will constitute the basis for antibiotic therapy, sometimes effective in alleviating chronic infection as a cause of infertility. Cystourethroscopic examination and radiographic studies including vasograms, accomplished by catheterization of the ejaculatory ducts or direct injection of the vasa, will help to rule out obstructive phenomena in the transport system.

Specimens of ejaculate should be examined for numbers and quality of spermatozoa. The ejaculate may be collected by masturbation technique or at the time of intercourse with a condom. The specimen should be examined within 2 to 3 hours after collection. The normal volume ranges up to 5 ml. with an average of 3.5 ml. Fifty to 100 million spermatozoa per milliliter constitutes a normal count, and approximately 60 per cent of these spermatozoa will exhibit good motility and normal adult forms. When azoospermia exists or when there is an inadequacy of the ejaculate, testicular biopsy may be indicated, accomplished by the techniques described by Heller and Nelson. Identification of normal architecture of the seminiferous tubules and normal spermatogenesis strongly suggest the probability that obstructive or inflammatory phenomena are being overlooked, while inadequacy of the spermatogenic elements suggests congenital or hormonal deficits.

In general, treatment of male infertility is neither encouraging nor rewarding. In cases of mechanical obstruction such as previous vasectomy, vasovasostomy may be highly effective. Inflammatory lesions of the vasa and epididymides may be corrected by epididymovasostomy. Little can be done to stimulate spermatogenesis, though administration of thyroid preparations has been advocated and may on rare occasions improve the numbers and quality of sperm. Occasionally, chronic administration of testosterone may result in the rebound phenomenon, an increase in numbers of spermatozoa following discontinuation of testosterone. Gonadotropins are of little therapeutic value. Orchidopexy cannot be expected to improve spermatogenesis if the patient is beyond the age of 10 or 12 years. Most recently, varicocelectomy has been advocated in treatment of oligospermia. It is suggested that varicocele causes defective spermatogenesis on the basis of increased intrascrotal temperature and possible backflow of inhibiting adrenal hormones which reflux from the adrenal and renal veins down the left spermatic vein. High inguinal ligation of the left spermatic vein occasionally may result in an increased sperm count and often results in improved sperm motility, according to MacLeod, and impregnation rates as high as 44 per cent have been reported for patients undergoing such surgical treatment of varicocele when infertility is a problem.

## TESTICULAR TUMORS

Neoplasms of the testis itself are almost universally malignant; only those rare fibromas of the tunica vaginalis constitute the benign tumors of the testis. In contrast, extratesticular tumors within the scrotum are almost always benign, such as the adenomatoid tumors of the epididymis and cord. Because of this sharp distinction in the potential of neoplasms within the scrotum, diligent physical examination is necessary in distinguishing the site of origin of a scrotal mass. Malignant neoplasms of the testes may be of germinal or nongerminal origin, the latter tumors arising from the interstitial cells and known as interstitial cell tumors, Leydig cell tumors, or androblastomas. These are relatively rare tumors, producing excessive quantities of androgenizing hormones which may cause virilism and precocious puberty in young males, impotence and gynecomastia in adults, and feminizing changes in the male that are analogous to those alterations observed with ovarian arrhenoblastomas in the female. Interstitial cell tumors of the testis must be differentiated from adrenal rest tumors, cells of adrenal origin being of very similar histologic character. It has been suggested that many cases of testicular tumors identified as interstitial cell neoplasms may indeed have represented unrecognized rests of hyperplastic adrenal tissue. The malignant germinal tumors of the testis arise from the totipotential cells of the seminiferous tubules and constitute a serious threat to the male population, accounting for 2 per cent of all malignant tumors, the dominant cause of death from genitourinary malignant disease in the younger adult male population. Testicular tumors are seen at all ages, but predominate in persons between the ages of 20 and 35 years. Germinal testicular tumors are categorized according to degree of cellular differentiation, which parallels malignant potential.

### Seminoma

The most common of testicular malignant lesions, accounting for 35 to 50 per cent of germinal tumors, seminomas are uniform in gross and histologic appearance, characterized by slow growth and late invasion. Metastases spread via the testicular lymphatics and dominate in the iliac, aortic, and renal hilar nodes. Because of the relatively slow growth of these tumors, they may be appreciated and removed surgically prior to the development of metastases. Metastatic seminoma is responsive to radiation therapy with 5 year survival rates in the range of 90 per cent.

### Embryonal Carcinoma

Of somewhat more malignant potential, embryonal carcinoma may also be seen in the younger age group, and is usually thought to be the most common testicular tumor of childhood. The histologic pattern of embryonal carcinoma is of a less differentiated form than that of seminoma and invasion and metastases occur earlier in the course of the disease. Because of relatively rapid growth of the tumor, hemorrhage and necrosis are common. Metastases to the abdominal lymphatics and the lungs may occur as an early event.

### Teratocarcinoma

Pure teratoma of the testis is relatively uncommon. Most such tumors are teratocarcinomas, embracing elements of seminoma, embryonal carcinoma, or choriocarcinoma. Tumors of the teratoma category may contain all types of tissue, and careful histologic evaluation of testicular teratocarcinoma must be accomplished since the clinical behavior of the tumor will depend upon the most malignant element present. Prognosis of teratocarcinoma admixed with seminoma is much better than that of a teratocarcinoma with elements of embryonal or choriocarcinoma.

### Choriocarcinoma

Fortunately, choriocarcinomas account for only a small number of the germinal cell tumors. The tumor is rapidly invasive, trophoblasts invading the venous system early in the course of the disease. Metastasis may be both blood-borne and via lymphatics, and has usually occurred at the time of diagnosis. Unlike choriocarcinoma in the female, which responds well to methotrexate, choriocarcinoma in the male is relatively unresponsive to chemotherapeutic measures. The prognosis is extremely poor, and the 5 year survival despite all combinations of surgical, radiation, and chemotherapeutic efforts is only about 1 per cent.

The earliest symptom of testicular tumor is a mass in the testicle, unfortunately unrecognized by most patients until there is associated pain, usually of a dull aching character. Hemorrhage within the testicle may follow minimal trauma, suggesting that traumatic injury is related to the tumor, which is probably not the case. Some of the more malignant tumors may produce hormones, measured as gonadotropins, which will induce gynecomastia. In other instances, the more malignant tumors, relatively small in the primary location, may induce an abdominal mass as an early manifestation of disease.

The successful treatment of testicular tumors demands scrupulous physical examination, a high index of suspicion, and the willingness to accomplish prompt scrotal exploration when the diagnosis is suggested. The typical testicular neoplasm is stony hard in character with a suggestion of weightiness on palpation. When the suspicion of testicular tumor is raised, extensive laboratory evaluation should be deferred and surgical exploration should be accomplished as a primary event. The approach is through a high inguinal incision, exposing the spermatic cord at its emergence from the internal inguinal ring where it is isolated. Rubber-shod clamps are applied and the testicle with its surrounding attachments can be mobilized for inspection and biopsy, and if diagnosis of testicular neoplasm is confirmed, high inguinal orchiectomy is accomplished, removing the entire cord with the involved testicle.

After orchiectomy, further diagnostic studies may be undertaken Planograms of the chest may reveal pulmonary metastatic disease. Lymphangiograms, inferior vena cavagrams, and intra-

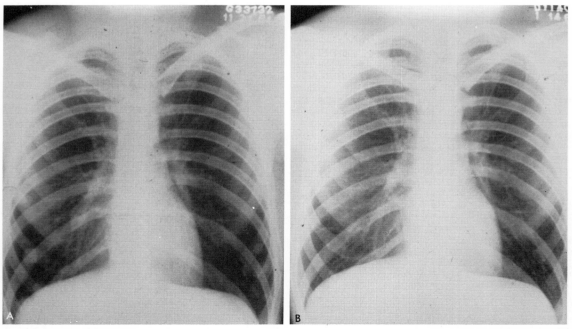

**Figure 17**  Metastatic testicular carcinoma, in this instance embryonal cell tumor, may manifest as pulmonary metastases *(A)* and may respond or resolve *(B)* as a consequence of intensive systemic chemotherapy. (Courtesy of Dr. John E. Dees.)

venous urograms may give evidence of metastatic tumor. Gonadotropin levels may be assayed by 24 hour urine collection, elevations of gonadotropins being observed most commonly with choriocarcinoma, less frequently with embryonal or teratocarcinoma, and rarely if ever with pure seminoma. Bone survey may rule out skeletal metastases, a relatively uncommon event in most testicular tumors, the metastatic pattern being lymphatic and visceral.

Further treatment of testicular tumors following orchiectomy is dictated by the results of such evaluation and by the philosophy of the urologic surgeon. In most instances, it is felt that abdominal node dissection is of little value when pulmonary metastases have been demonstrated. Further, choriocarcinoma dictates against radical retroperitoneal lymphatic dissection since its metastatic pattern is vascular in character. In other instances of testicular neoplasm, radical retroperitoneal node dissection, usually through a transabdominal approach and less commonly through bilateral thoracoabdominal exposures, is advocated as an effective modality in the control of the malignant process. Since metastatic seminoma is highly radiosensitive, many authorities question node dissection in treatment of seminoma. However, it must be pointed out that any seminoma may contain a microscopic focus of a more malignant germinal element and that metastases may reflect embryonal carcinoma, teratocarcinoma, or even choriocarcinoma which will not respond so favorably to radiation therapy. Finally, empiric radiation therapy of the abdominal and mediastinal lymphatic regions should not be condoned unless there is known metastatic disease, proven only by surgical exploration.

Because of these considerations, it is the usual practice to accomplish transabdominal radical peritoneal lymph node dissections in all instances of testicular tumor except choriocarcinoma and except when generalized metastatic disease is recognized. The efficacy of surgical node dissection has been elaborated by Staubitz and others, irrespective of ancillary radiation therapy or chemotherapy.[22] When node dissection is accomplished and there is no histologic evidence of metastatic disease, no further treatment is given. Survivals in this group of patients, irrespective of the histologic classification of the primary tumor, are extremely good. On the other hand, when positive nodes are identified or removed at surgery, radiation therapy is advisable, treating the abdomen, mediastinum, and supraclavicular areas.

When lymphatic metastases of testicular tumors respond poorly to chemotherapeutic measures, some patients with visceral metastatic disease, particularly pulmonary metastases, may respond in dramatic fashion to chemotherapeutic efforts. The most effective antitumor drugs in treating metastatic embryonal carcinoma and teratocarcinoma include actinomycin D, methotrexate, and chlorambucil which may result in regression and 5 year cure of metastatic testicular malignant lesions. Isolated pulmonary metastases may be treated by local radiation or by surgical resection. The ultimate prognosis in testicular malignant disease, a dire condition in the young male, thus depends upon the stage of the disease at diagnosis, the histologic character of the tumor, and the vigor with which therapeutic measures are pursued. Follow-up should extend over a minimum of 5 years with regular and periodic examination, urinary chorionic gonadotropin determinations, and other modalities of evaluation, in the hope of identifying recurrence of disease and initiating appropriate therapeutic measures.

## EPIDIDYMIDES

The epididymides are coiled ductal structures posterolateral to the testes with which they communicate through the rete testis, collecting spermatozoa for maturation and transport up the vasa deferentia. The upper end of the epididymis, globus major or head, accumulates sperm which are relatively immotile, sperm becoming more motile as they pass through the body and tail, globus minor, of the epididymis which communicates with the vas. The most common abnormalities of the epididymis are inflammatory in character. Rarely, congenital absence of the epididymis and vas may be observed, though such absence is usually associated with unilateral anorchism. Occasionally, there may be a defect in fusion of the epididymis and the testis. Traumatic injuries of the epididymis are not of great clinical importance but accompany testicular injuries. Infectious epididymitis is common, particularly after puberty, but is relatively rare in the prepubescent male.

Acute nonspecific epididymitis is nongonococcal and nontuberculous, secondary to suppurative infection which usually has its origin in the prostate and seminal vesicles, spreading in retrograde fashion to the epididymis. Hematogenous and lymphatic spread of infection from a distant focus may occur but is probably quite rare. The inflammation is diffuse through the epididymis and may or may not involve the testicle concomitantly. The patient complains of severe pain and acute swelling with chills and fever and other systemic symptoms which may include headache, nausea, and vomiting. Symptoms of urinary infection such as frequency, urgency, burning, dysuria, pyuria, and hematuria may be present. The epididymis and surrounding structures including the spermatic cord may be thickened by edema, swollen, and exquisitely tender to palpation. It is important to differentiate testicular swelling from epididymitis, since a mass in the testicle almost always indicates testicular tumor, and to differentiate acute epididymitis from torsion of the spermatic cord, in which the testicle generally lies high in the scrotum or even in the inguinal canal; torsion demands immediate surgical exploration, while epididymitis is treated by conservative measures. Other conditions that may confuse the diagnosis include inguinal hernia and acute hydrocele. Treatment of epididymitis consists of bed

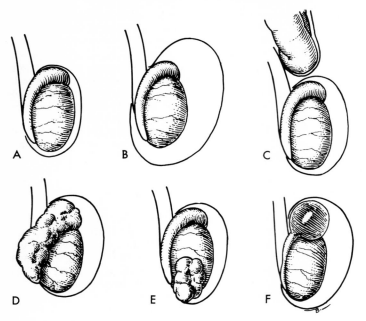

**Figure 18** Common scrotal masses can be differentiated with knowledge of normal anatomy *(A)*, as compared with *(B)* hydrocele of the tunica vaginalis, *(C)* inguinal hernia penetrating the scrotal compartment, *(D)* epididymitis causing induration and enlargement of the epididymis but not the testis, *(E)* testicular tumor causing an irregular mass intrinsic to the testis, and *(F)* spermatocele or epididymal cyst arising extrinsic to the testis.

rest, elevation and support of the scrotum, application of cold packs, antipyretics, and appropriate antimicrobial agents, sometimes administered intravenously. Occasionally, suppurative epididymitis may localize into an abscess and drain spontaneously, but surgical intervention should be avoided in most instances. Acute epididymitis usually proceeds to some degree of chronic epididymitis, continuing over a period of several weeks. In past years, acute epididymitis was a common concomitant of all forms of prostatic surgery. However, utilization of routine preoperative vas ligation is extremely effective in preventing such epididymal infection, and the utilization of broad-spectrum antibiotics further diminishes the propensity for such disabling infection.

Chronic epididymitis is usually the sequel of acute epididymitis but may arise insidiously with few localizing symptoms except mass and slight tenderness. The demonstration of associated prostatic infection is an adjunct to differential diagnosis, but tumor must always be suspected when there is a relatively painless chronic enlargement of the epididymis. The most common neoplasms of the epididymis are benign and include adenomatoid tumors, leiomyomas, and cysts. Spermatocele is a diverticulum of the epididymis, containing cloudy fluid with spermatozoa, unilocular or multilocular, often confused with hydrocele since both spermatocele and hydrocele can be transilluminated. The differential diagnosis of spermatocele and hydrocele is aided by localization of the mass: hydrocele generally surrounds the testis, while spermatocele is more eccentric in location.

Other epididymal abnormalities are less common. Gonococcal epididymitis, once seen with relative frequency, is less common now though gonorrhea continues to exist in epidemic proportion. It is probable that earlier treatment of gonorrheal urethritis diminishes the tendency to development of subsequent gonococcal prostatitis, seminal vesiculitis, vasitis, and epididymitis. Similarly, tuberculous epididymitis is rare today. Tuberculous epididymitis results in indurated asymmetric enlargement of the epididymis with nodular thickening and relatively little tenderness. Caseation necrosis may ensue, sometimes involving the scrotal wall and skin with ulceration and fistula formation. In such cases, epididymoorchiectomy with excision of the involved portion of the scrotal wall is usually necessary. Other granulomatous reactions in the epididymis may be observed in association with syphilis or as a consequence of escape of spermatozoa with development of sperm granuloma, sometimes painful and requiring excision of the mass.

## SPERMATIC CORDS AND TUNICS

The spermatic cord, composed of vas deferens, spermatic artery, venous plexus, lymphatics, autonomic nerves, and investments of cremaster muscle, terminates in the testis, which is covered by the fibrous tunics, the tunica albuginea testis, which is the capsule of the testicle, and the tunica vaginalis, which constitutes a sac partially surrounding the testis and epididymis. The entire spermatic cord is subject to inflammatory diseases, usually the result of trauma or pyogenic bacteria, termed funiculitis. The principal abnormality of the cord is torsion. Neoplasms of the spermatic cord are extremely rare, but sarcoma, usually rhabdomyosarcoma, and both invasive and metastatic malignant lesions from other structures may involve the cord. Benign tumors of the cord include adenomatoid tumor, lipoma, fibroma, and cysts, particularly hydrocele of the cord, a remnant of the processus vaginalis.

## TORSION

Torsion of the spermatic cord, an axial rotation, is probably the result of an abnormally high attachment of the tunica vaginalis around the terminal cord, allowing the testicle to twist freely within the compartment, the so-called "bell clapper" deformity. When rotation of the testicle on the end of the cord exceeds 90 degrees, there may be compromise of blood supply which causes exquisite pain and results in gangrene and subsequent atrophy of the testicle unless torsion is treated immediately. Incomplete torsion may result in partial strangulation, effects of which may be overcome if surgical intervention is accomplished within about 12 hours, while severe torsion with total compromise of blood supply will result in loss of the testes unless surgery is effected within about 4 hours.

Torsion is usually seen in young males and most often occurs spontaneously, even during sleep. Physical and sexual activity may predispose to torsion and aggravate it by contraction of the cremaster muscle. There is rapid onset of severe pain and swelling accompanied by nausea, vomiting, abdominal pain, and even fever. On examination, the testicles seem to ride rather high in the scrotal compartment. The differential diagnosis is between torsion and epididymitis, and it should be remembered that epididymitis is almost always accompanied by evidence of prostatitis and pyuria. With torsion, the entire testicle and appendages are involved in the swelling process, while with epididymitis the prominent induration is within the epididymis and not the testes.

Torsion must always be suspected with acute onset of scrotal pain, and prompt surgical intervention is necessary.[11] In 17 of 19 patients with torsion operated upon the day of onset of symptoms, viable testes were salvaged, while any delay in surgery will diminish the prospects for salvage. When torsion is treated on one side, the contralateral scrotum should be explored; the tunica vaginalis should be opened and inverted around the testis as with hydrocele repair, and steps should be taken to surgically correct any additional defects such as deficit attachment of the epididymis to the testes.

The appendix epididymis and the appendix testis (hydatid of Morgagni) are vestigial remnants of ducts attached to the head of the epididymis and to the superior pole of the testes, respectively. These small cystic structures may become twisted, producing acute and severe pain with generalized scrotal edema. Little permanent damage or disability is incurred by torsion of these appendages, but because of diagnostic confusion, it is generally advisable to explore the scrotum when any doubt exists.

## INFECTION

Infection of the spermatic cord is relatively uncommon as an isolated process, usually being an associated complication of epididymitis and prostatitis. However, isolated inflammation of the vas may occur, and the entire spermatic cord may become inflamed. Because of the rich blood supply and ample lymphatic drainage, funiculitis will generally resolve with no permanent abnormality. Vasitis may proceed to chronic inflammatory and fibrotic reaction with beading of the vas, a particularly common complication of genitourinary tuberculosis.

## VAS DEFERENS

The vasa deferentia are the conduits for spermatozoa from epididymis to seminal vesicles and prostate. Thus, normal vasa are necessary to human reproduction. Since a single testis is capable of producing sufficient numbers of sperm for purposes of fertility, a single normal intact vas is all that is necessary to insure the reproductive capacity of the male. The most common anomaly of the vas is congenital absence, seen almost universally in males with cystic fibrosis. There are other isolated incidences of unilateral ductal failure with absence of the vas deferens.

While the vas is responsible for transit of spermatozoa, it may also serve as a conduit for retrograde passage of bacteria and infection of the scrotal contents, such retrograde infection being the principal cause of epididymo-orchitis. The prevalence of epididymo-orchitis in association with prostatic obstruction and prostatic surgery has prompted the employment of prophylactic vasectomy for more than 40 years. Most urologists accomplish such vasectomy in the course of prostatic surgery, though preliminary vasectomy may also be advocated as an initial step prior to surgical management of prostatic obstruction.

Vasectomy is not a new procedure, though it is gaining increased public acceptance as an elective sterilization measure at the present time. It has been estimated that up to nearly 40,000 elective vasectomies were accomplished by American urologists for purposes of voluntary sterilization in 1967, and it may be projected that even greater

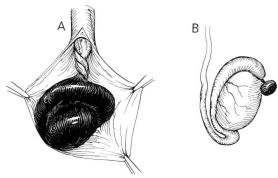

**Figure 19** Torsion of the testis *(A)* is a result of twisting of the spermatic cord, usually within the tunica vaginalis; the appendix testis may also become twisted *(B)*.

numbers of such procedures are being accomplished today. As an outpatient procedure under local anesthesia, a 1 cm. incision is made over each vas or a single midline incision may be employed. The vasa are isolated, ligated, and sometimes electrocoagulated, and a small section is removed between the points of ligation. It is desirable to isolate the divided ends of the vasa in different fascial planes to prevent spontaneous recanalization. It must be remembered that spermatozoa distal to the point of ligation and stored within the seminal vesicles and prostate remain viable for several weeks. Spermatozoa disappear from the ejaculate at the rate of 50 to 70 per cent of remaining sperm with each ejaculation, and most sexually active males will have emptied all viable sperm from the reservoirs after 10 or more ejaculations. Microscopic examination of a freshly collected specimen of ejaculate should be accomplished 6 to 8 weeks after the procedure. The patient should not be pronounced surgically sterile until a negative specimen of ejaculate has been observed.

Such elective vasectomy is gaining legal as well as public acceptance. It is incumbent upon the urologic surgeon to insure that the letter of the law is met in accomplishing such sterilization operation. Conference with both the patient and spouse should be mandatory, with written request for the procedure signed by both. A waiting period should be required before the procedure is done and it must be made clear that a follow-up examination of ejaculate is essential. It should also be explained to the couple that vasectomy must be considered a permanent sterilization measure, though there is increasing success in microsurgical reconstruction of the vasa provided an extensive segment of the vas has not been removed.

## VARICOCELE

Varicocele is the term applied to dilatation and tortuosity of the veins of the pampiniform plexus, most commonly observed on the left. It has been stated that varicocele may be an indicator of left renal tumor since the left spermatic vein system drains into the renal vein and obstruction at that point could produce dilatation of the veins of the left cord; however, varicocele is uncommonly found to be associated with renal tumor. Most varicoceles are idiopathic, though there may be a defect in the valve system of the spermatic vein, particularly on the left where the vein takes a longer course. Varicocele rarely causes symptoms but there may be a heavy, dragging, aching sensation in the scrotal compartment. Discomfort or infertility may prompt surgical repair, accomplished by varicocelectomy which is a tedious dissection and ligation of the multiple venous channels of the cord, or by high ligation of the spermatic vein through an incision at the level of the internal inguinal ring, giving ready access to the single vein. Following such ligation, venous collateral circulation is assumed by the deep pelvic venous system.

## HYDROCELE

The tunica vaginalis, derived from the peritoneum as the processus vaginalis at the time of testicular descent, is a secretory membrane. Fluid is generated by the serous surface of the tunica vaginalis, fluid formation being enhanced by inflammation or trauma. Fluid within the tunica vaginalis is resorbed at a constant rate through the extensive venous and lymphatic systems of the spermatic cord. Hydrocele, the excessive accumulation of this serous fluid, results when there is increased production or decreased resorption, the latter condition usually being idiopathic.

Congenital hydrocele may result from failure of obliteration of the processus vaginalis, and fluid formed within the peritoneal cavity may gravitate into the tunica vaginalis. Such congenital hydroceles may fluctuate in size depending upon position of the child, and there may sometimes be an associated palpable inguinal hernia; whether a hernia exists or not, the potential for herniation is present. Occasionally, spontaneous closure of the processus vaginalis will occur during infancy and surgical intervention may not be necessary. Even in instances of complete obliteration of the processus vaginalis along the spermatic cord, there may be excessive accumulation of fluid in the tunica vaginalis in the newborn, sometimes requiring aspiration or early surgical intervention for fear of mechanical compression and compromise of testicular viability. Congenital hydrocele, particularly with associated hernia, demands surgical repair, accomplished through a high inguinal incision, giving access to the internal inguinal ring at which point the hernia sac or processus vaginalis is ligated.

In older persons, hydrocele is frequently the re-

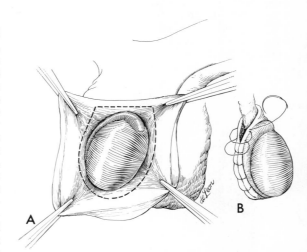

**Figure 20**  Repair of hydrocele involves incision of the tunica vaginalis with excision of its redundant wall *(A)* and inversion of the remaining wall *(B)* around the epididymis and terminal portion of the spermatic cord. (From Bunce, P. L. In: Glenn, J. F., and Boyce, W. H.: Urologic Surgery. New York, Hoeber Medical Division, Harper & Row, 1969.)

sult of epididymo-orchitis or trauma. If there is active pyogenic infection, the hydrocele may become infected, demanding surgical incision and drainage. Compromise of venous and lymphatic return along the cord may occur with a large inguinal hernia or as a result of herniorrhaphy with fibrosis of the inguinal canal obstructing venous and lymphatic drainage. Large intra-abdominal and pelvic masses may similarly compromise return and predispose to hydrocele. While small hydroceles may require no treatment, the swelling may assume such proportions as to cause severe discomfort and interfere with physical and sexual activity. Hydrocelectomy is accomplished by scrotal exploration with excision of redundant tunica vaginalis and retroversion of the remaining sac around the epididymis and terminal portion of the cord. A permanent cure may be expected by this procedure. Aspiration and injection of sclerosing materials is condemned because of the risk of infection.

## INGUINAL LYMPHATICS

The superficial and inguinal lymphatic intervals constitute the principal drainage system for the external genitalia. There is interdigitation of lymphatic drainage between the superficial inguinal nodes and the deep inguinal groups, which communicate with the hypogastric and iliac nodes. Lymphatics of the penis, penile skin, and scrotum drain to the superficial inguinal group, while drainage from the urethra is to the inguinal and hypogastric nodes and that from the glans penis is to the external iliac group. Inflammatory lymphadenitis occurs with many infections of the external genitalia and is usually treated conservatively with antimicrobial agents, bed rest, and other supportive measures. Suppuration may necessitate incision and drainage. Inguinal buboes may result from chancroid, the soft chancre that usually occurs primarily on the corona of the glans penis.

### Lymphogranuloma Venereum

Probably of viral origin though possibly due to L-forms, lymphogranuloma is also known as lymphopathia venereum and lymphogranuloma inguinale. Transmission of infection is by sexual intercourse, either genital or anal. Severe adenitis is sometimes associated with elephantiasis of the genitalia. Diagnosis is established by intradermal Frei test and complement fixation, though these are not positive early in the course of the disease. There may be spontaneous remission, but therapy is usually effective with sulfadiazine, tetracyclines, and chloramphenicol. Surgical excision of the involved node groups may be required, particularly if secondary infection supervenes.

### Granuloma Inguinale

Granuloma inguinale is a superficial ulcerative skin lesion associated with inguinal adenitis, due to the encapsulated gram-negative Donovan body

which is transmitted by sexual contact and is related to the Friedländer and Klebsiella groups of organisms. Granuloma inguinale is seen more commonly in the south and among the Negro population. Multiple painless granulomatous lesions cause extensive scarring which may necessitate surgical excision. Streptomycin and tetracyclines are effective in controlling the infectious process.

## INTERSEX AND TRANSSEXUALISM

The intersex state is that condition in which there is ambiguity of the external genitalia or inadequate and incomplete differentiation of gonadal and ductal structures. Transsexualism, on the other hand, refers to surgical or social conversion of an individual to the opposite sex on a voluntary basis. Intersex is thus a congenital abnormality, while transsexualism may represent a psychosocial disorder.

### INTERSEX STATES

The most common mode of presentation of the intersex patient is by request for sexual differentiation in the neonatal nursery. Ambiguity of the external genitalia necessitates prompt and definitive assignment of sex, reassurance of parents, and early mobilization of medical and surgical measures required to constitute the appropriate sex of the child. On occasion, the intersex patient may be seen as a rather late event, often because of microphallus, undescended testes, labial fusion, or clitoral hypertrophy noted as late as pubescence. The interested reader is referred to a number of definitive texts and monographs dealing with the various types of intersex.

#### True Hermaphroditism

The true hermaphrodite is the person with gonadal tissue of both sexes, manifesting as ovary and testis, ovary and ovotestis, testis and ovotestis, or two ovotestes. In such instances, relatively rare, ductal development may also be ambiguous, with male wolffian ductal structures ipsilateral to the testicular tissue and feminine müllerian ductal structures ipsilateral to the gonad with ovarian differentiation. Chromosomes are generally normal in number and buccal smear reveals XX or XY patterns. The dominant gender role, as dictated by external genital development, should be pursued and supported by medical and surgical measures. When the external genitalia exhibit severe ambiguity, it is generally best to seek a feminine role for the patient, removing male gonadal tissue and ductal structures, effecting reduction phalloplasty if necessary, and constructing a vagina when the patient reaches marriageable age if there is no vaginal canal present. As for other forms of the intersex state, satisfactory cosmetic and functional results may be achieved with the external genitalia, restoring the patient to a fully satisfactory male or female role as the conditions warrant. Endocrine abnormalities usually do not coexist, but complete removal of gonadal tissue as in instances of bilateral ovotestes may demand lifelong supportive endocrine therapy in the form of appropriate estrogens or androgens.

#### Adrenogenitalism

The adrenogenital syndrome may occur in males or females, more commonly the latter. Congenital adrenal hyperplasia with excessive production of androgenizing steroid precursors, such as the 17-ketosteroids and pregnanetriol, results from one of several basic enzymatic defects within the gland, compromising the capability of the adrenal to synthesize cortisone and cortisol. Deficiencies of corticosteroids prompt excessive production of adrenocorticotropic hormone by the pituitary, stimulating the already hyperplastic adrenal glands to still further production of androgenizing precursors. The usual enzymatic defect is a deficiency of 11 $\beta$-hydroxylase or 21-hydroxylase. Associated hypertension may be observed, and one-third or more of children so affected may exhibit a salt-losing tendency with severe vomiting and dehydration, often mistaken for the syndrome of pyloric stenosis. In the male, precocious puberty is observed as a result of the androgenizing influence: early appearance of pubic hair, growth of genitalia to adult proportions, increased muscle mass, and early epiphyseal closure leading to the terms "infant Hercules" and macrogenitosomia praecox. In the female, similar androgenizing changes occur with hypertrophy of the clitoris to the point that it simulates a penis, growth of pubic hair, fusion of the labia in the midline obscuring the urethra and the vaginal introitus behind the single perineal opening or urogenital sinus, and other stigmata including acne, hirsutism, voice changes, and the musculoskeletal changes also seen in the male. Adrenogenitalism is the most common cause of intersex, girls so affected presenting at birth with ambiguous genitalia. The diagnosis is established by demonstration of a normal female chromatin pattern (XX) and an elevation of urinary 17-ketosteroids and 17-hydroxysteroids. Accurate assessment of urinary steroids may be accomplished in the first week of life and appropriate definition of sex is essential during the neonatal period if subsequent emotional trauma is to be avoided. Urologic investigation of the female with adrenogenitalism should include cystourethroscopy through the urogenital sinus; introduction of the examining instrument into the vaginal introitus will permit identification of cervix, virtually certain evidence that there is a normal uterus. Once the diagnosis is established, appropriate exogenous cortisone therapy should be initiated, suppressing further pituitary activity and diminishing endogenous adrenal output of androgens. When adequate control is effected, surgical correction of the external genitalia can be accomplished; subtotal phallectomy and labioplasty will result in satisfactory cosmetic appearance of the external female genitalia. Pubic hair, seen in the older patients with adrenogenitalism, may be removed periodically with one of the liquid depilatories. Abdominal exploration is unnecessary when appropriate diagnostic measures have been accomplished, and adrenal surgery is undesirable since adequate suppression can be achieved by medical management.

### The Male Intersex

Differentiation of the external genitalia to a completely masculine configuration is apparently dependent upon the fetal testes, elaborating testosterone or some other substance, sometimes referred to as müllerian-inhibiting factor. If the fetal testes fail before genital differentiation has been completed during the first trimester of gestation, ambiguous external genitalia will result. Occasionally, mechanical developmental defects may account for genital ambiguity in the male, and often such genital abnormalities are associated with massive congenital deformities of the gastrointestinal system as well. The most common ambiguity of the male external genitalia is the association of cryptorchism or incomplete testicular descent with perineal hypospadias and severe penile chordee. A male chromatin pattern (XY) can be demonstrated and there are no associated endocrinopathies.

Cystourethroscopic evaluation is helpful since identification of a verumontanum is evidence of normal internal male ductal structures. Release of chordee and bilateral orchidopexy can be accomplished at an early age, and urethroplasty should be effected before the child reaches school age.

### Maternal Virilization

In the past, it was common practice to treat abortion and habitual abortion with androgenizing drugs such as testosterone. While this mode of therapy is less frequently employed today, occasional instances of virilization of females are still observed. The administration of androgenizing agents to the mother has little or no effect on the male fetus, though there may be some precocious genital growth. In the female, the clitoris may be stimulated to considerable enlargement, assuming penile proportions. Some degree of labial fusion may also be observed, though usually the urogenital sinus is not fully formed and the urethra and vaginal introitus can be visualized. Since the influences are terminated at the end of gestation, there is no progression of the deformity. External genital reconstructive procedures are effected as with adrenogenitalism, but no continuing therapy is necessary.

### Gonadal Dysgenesis

The dysgenetic testis results in varying degrees of ambiguity of the external genitalia. In males with dysplastic testes, diagnosis may not be suspected until a normal age of pubescence at which time failure of development of secondary sex characteristics points to testicular inadequacy, as with Klinefelter's syndrome. The diagnosis of gonadal dysgenesis should be approached with caution, since delayed pubescence may be a simple genetic characteristic, not indicative of any serious underlying disease process. In the male child approaching puberty with small penis and testes gonadal dysgenesis should be suspected, but the diagnosis is dependent upon testicular biopsy and should be confirmed by complete endocrine evaluation. Gonadotropins will become elevated at puberty, inducing increase in testosterone production. Measurement of urinary gonadotropins and plasma testosterone is effective in defining hypogonadal states; persistent elevation of gonadotropins with inadequate levels of testosterone supports the diagnosis of hypogonadism. Management is by medical measures.

### Anorchism

The complete absence of viable testicular tissue is a rare event. Unilateral failure of testicular development, monorchism, is not uncommonly observed, and is usually unattended by any genital or developmental abnormalities. Certain males are observed, however, to lack identifiable testicular tissue though ductal and external differentiation in normal male fashion has occurred, as indicated in the discussion of testicular anomalies. Administration of exogenous androgens in the form of depo-testosterone will result in inhibition of gonadotropins, redistribution of body fat in masculine configuration, increased muscle mass, closure of epiphyses and cessation of growth, pubescence of the external genitalia, growth of pubic and axillary hair, and some increase in beard growth. Libido is markedly improved by such treatment. Silastic testicular prostheses may be introduced into the empty scrotal compartments.

## TRANSSEXUALISM

Transsexual patients are persons who are usually normal anatomic males or females without endocrinologic abnormality. For various psychosocial reasons, frequently related to events in childhood, these persons cast themselves in roles of the opposite sex and request surgical transformation. While such surgical sex conversion has been accomplished abroad and with relative discretion in the past, current public attitudes of permissiveness have allowed a more scientific approach to the problems, both psychiatric and surgical. A number of centers in this country are now actively engaged in transsexual investigation and treatment. It is much more common for males to seek conversion to female body characteristics, and such surgical conversion involves penectomy, castration, reduction scrotoplasty, and vaginoplasty as well as estrogen administration and subsequent augmentation mammoplasty by implantation of silicone prostheses. In a careful and detailed evaluation of 121 male transsexual patients followed after surgery, the result was deemed highly satisfactory in 68 per cent, and a satisfactory emotional and social readjustment in such patients is felt to be 10 times more likely than an unsatisfactory outcome. Sex conversion surgery for female transsexuals is, at present, less satisfactory. Reduction mammoplasty and complete hysterectomy are feasible, and the vaginal canal can be obliterated. Unfortunately, an erectile penis cannot be constructed, though tube skin flaps can be developed to effect a cosmetic phallus. Construction of a distal urethra through this phallus constitutes yet another surgical challenge. Since the functional status of the genitalia in such instances will be less than satisfactory, it may be anticipated that psychosocial adjustment of female transsexual patients will be less satisfactory than with their male counterparts.

## SELECTED REFERENCES

Creevy, C. D.: The correction of hypospadias: A review. Urol. Survey, 8:1, 1958.
*The problem of hypospadias, the incompletely developed urethra, has challenged surgeons for centuries. The term hypospadias itself derives from the Greek roots meaning "under" and "to tear." This superb review, replete with lavish drawings, defines and elaborates the theory and practice of hypospadias repair. While a few of the more recent modifications of technique are not included, this survey constitutes basic information for the interested surgeon.*

Federman, D. D.: Abnormal Sexual Development: The Genetic and Endocrine Approach to Differential Diagnosis. Philadelphia, W. B. Saunders Company, 1967.
*The complexities of sexual differentiation and the intersex states are thoroughly presented in this compendium of current information. The normal processes of sexual differentiation are emphasized, the chromosomal and endocrinologic abnormalities associated with intersex are elaborated, and a rational approach to diagnosis and treatment of the intersex patient is presented.*

Rubin, P., ed.: Cancer of the urogenital tract: Testicular tumors. J.A.M.A., 213:89, 1970.
*This symposium, one of a series of multidisciplinary forums on malignant disease of the genitourinary system, constitutes a review and progress report relative to testicular tumors. Pathologic classification of testicular tumors, diagnostic methodology, and various aspects of treatment are emphasized with attention directed toward results of various forms of therapy. Eight authorities in the involved disciplines participate in this colloquium.*

Rubin, P., ed.: Cancer of the urogenital tract: Prostate cancer. J.A.M.A., 210:322, 1072, 1969.
*This symposium on carcinoma of the prostate is presented in two parts, one dealing with confined and localized cancer of the prostate gland and the second with advanced and metastatic prostate cancer. Ten authorities deal with incidence and detection of prostate cancer, radical surgery, hormonal manip-*

*ulation, conservative therapy by transurethral resection, ancillary hormonal measures, and the role of radiation therapy including both interstitial irradiation and definitive external radiotherapy.*

Weyrauch, H. M.: Surgery of the Prostate. Philadelphia, W. B. Saunders Company, 1959.
*This volume, more than a monograph, is a lucid and complete exposition of diseases of the prostate and prostatic surgery. The available methods of surgical management of prostatic obstruction are stressed with emphasis upon selection of the appropriate operation for the given patient. Philosophic and technical details are of particular interest to urologic surgeons.*

## REFERENCES

1. Alyea, E. P.: Early or late orchiectomy for carcinoma of the prostate? J. Urol., 53:143, 1945.
2. Bennett, A. H., and Harrison, J. H.: A comparison of operative approach for prostatectomy, 1948 and 1968. Surg. Gynec. Obstet., 128:969, 1969.
3. Campos Freire, J. G.: Transvesical prostatectomy with primary closure of the bladder. Urol. Int., 7:300, 1958.
4. Castro, J. E., Griffiths, H. J. L., and Shackman, R.: Significance of signs and symptoms in benign prostatic hypertrophy. Brit. Med. J., 2:598, 1969.
5. Dees, J. E.: Radical perineal prostatectomy for carcinoma. J. Urol., 104:160, 1970.
6. Fegen, P., and Persky, L.: Squamous cell carcinoma of the penis: Its treatment with special reference to radical node dissection. Arch. Surg., 99:117, 1969.
7. Flocks, R. H.: Clinical cancer of the prostate: A study of four thousand cases. J.A.M.A., 193:89, 1965.
8. Gilbertsen, V. A.: Cancer of the prostate gland: Results of early diagnosis and therapy undertaken for cure of the disease. J.A.M.A., 215:81, 1971.
9. Glenn, J. F., and Spanel, D. J.: Serum acid phosphatase and the effect of prostatic massage. J. Urol., 82:240, 1959.
10. Gutman, A. B.: The development of the acid phosphatase test for prostatic carcinoma. Bull. N. Y. Acad. Med., 44:63, 1968.
11. Leape, L. L.: Torsion of the testis: Invitation to error. J.A.M.A., 200:93, 1967.
12. Lytton, B., Emory, J. M., and Harvard, B. M.: The incidence of benign prostatic obstruction. J. Urol., 99:639, 1968.
13. Millin, T.: Retropubic prostatectomy. J. Urol., 59:367, 1948.
14. Nesbit, R. M., and Baum, W. C.: Endocrine control of prostatic carcinoma. J.A.M.A., 143:1317, 1950.
15. Osborne, E. D., Sutherland, C. G., Scholl, A. J., and Rowntree, L. G.: Roentgenography of urinary tract during excretion of sodium iodide. J.A.M.A., 80:368, 1923.
16. Prentiss, R. J., Weickgenant, C. J., Moses, J. J., and Frazier, D. B.: Undescended testis: Surgical anatomy of spermatic vessels, spermatic surgical triangles and lateral spermatic ligament. J. Urol., 83:686, 1960.
17. Prout, G. R., Jr., Macalalag, E. V., Jr., and Denis, L. J.: Alterations in serum lactic dehydrogenase and its isozymes in patients with prostatic carcinoma after hormonal therapy. Surg. Forum, 15:486, 1964.
18. Ray, E. H., Sr.: Bladder neck obstruction due to prostatic hyperplasia: Diagnosis, treatment, and postoperative care. Amer. Surg., 31:325, 1965.
19. Rich, A. R.: On frequency of occurrence of occult carcinoma of the prostate. J. Urol., 33:215, 1935.
20. Smith, B. H.: Peyronie's disease. Amer. J. Clin. Path., 45:670, 1966.
21. Stamey, T. A., Fair, W. R., Timothy, M. M., and Chung, H. K.: Antibacterial nature of prostatic fluid. Nature, 218:444, 1968.
22. Staubitz, W. J., Magoss, I. V., Grace, J. T., and Schenk, W. G., III: Surgical management of testis tumors. J. Urol., 101:350, 1969.
23. Veterans Administration Cooperative Urological Research Group: Treatment and survival of patients with cancer of the prostate. Surg. Gynec. Obstet., 124:1011, 1967.
24. Wershub, L. P.: The Human Testis: A Clinical Treatise. Springfield, Ill., Charles C Thomas, 1962.
25. Young, H. H.: Hugh Young: A Surgeon's Autobiography. New York, Harcourt, Brace and Company, 1940.

# 49

# DISORDERS OF
# THE LYMPHATIC SYSTEM

*Harry S. Goldsmith, M.D., and Gordon F. Schwartz, M.D.*

Although knowledge of arteries and veins has been documented far back into history, the lymphatic system was not described until the seventeenth century, even though Hippocrates and Aristotle had previously reported "white blood" and the existence of structures containing a clear fluid. In 1622, Gasper Asellius, Professor of Anatomy at Milan, noted ramifying cordlike structures in the canine mesentery that discharged a milky fluid when cut. Twenty-five years later, in 1647, Pecquet noted the thoracic duct, and Rudbeck, in 1653, accurately described the lymphatic system in detail. The existence of lymphatic valves, which he reported, was all but forgotten until Ryschius rediscovered them in 1721. By the end of the eighteenth century, the scientific world not only had accepted the presence of the lymphatic system, but also agreed that lymphatics absorbed various substances in their course from the periphery of the body to the thoracic duct and eventual confluence with the venous system.

## COMPARATIVE ANATOMY

A true lymphatic system is found only in vertebrate animals. Lower animals with less well differentiated cardiovascular systems rely upon the venous system to perform the functions of the absent lymphatic system. Among the vertebrates, only birds and mammals possess a lymphatic system consisting of narrow, ramifying vessels endowed with valves.

The lymphatic system of all mammals parallels that of man and is characterized by a single major connection between the lymphatic and venous systems, at the jugular region. Lymph flow, which is normally centripetal and unidirectional, usually traverses at least one lymph node before draining into the thoracic duct. Afferent lymphatic channels drain from the periphery of the body to lymph nodes, and efferent vessels emerge from the nodes to form confluent main collecting channels. Groups of nodes are situated in relatively constant positions to collect lymph from a particular organ or region and, therefore, are aptly designated as regional lymph nodes. The higher the phylogenetic scale, the greater is the number of lymph nodes encountered, although the age and size of the animal also influence this number. A characteristic of mammalian lymphatics is a valve system which is present even in small lymphatic tributaries and which insures the unidirectional flow necessary for the maintenance and regulation of normal lymph flow.

## EMBRYOLOGY

Paired jugular lymph sacs are recognizable in the 6 week human embryo. These sacs enlarge and coalesce with adjacent endothelial pockets to form chains of small sacs, which are the forerunners of the major collecting lymphatics. By 9 weeks of gestation, the basic pattern of the main lymphatic channels becomes noticeable, as lymph sacs give rise to small endothelial channels, which develop into lymphatic vessels. Coincidentally, connective tissue invades and permeates the lymphatic sacs. It is by these maneuvers that the main lymphatic channels and their tributaries become delineated.

Pouchlike protuberances from the lymphatic trunks differentiate into lymph nodes, with contiguous connective tissue becoming compressed around the periphery of each node to form its capsule. Afferent lymphatic vessels develop at the periphery of the lymph node through which lymph flow enters, later exiting via the efferent lymphatic vessel on the contralateral side.

## GENERAL ANATOMY

The lymphatic system is divided into three major components: (1) a network of *capillaries*, which serves to collect lymph from the various tissues and organs; (2) *collecting vessels*, which carry the lymph from the capillaries to the great veins at the root of the neck via the thoracic duct; and (3) *lymph nodes*. Other lymphoid organs, which resemble lymph nodes and are part of the reticuloendothelial or lymphoreticular system, are the tonsils, adenoids, spleen, and thymus. Lymphatic vessels that drain the small intestine are called lacteals. They are identical to other lymphatic vessels except that during the process of digestion they contain a thick, white fluid called chyle.

### Lymphatic Capillaries

These small structures are necessary for maintaining fluid equilibrium within the interstitial space of the body. Lymphatic capillaries have been demonstrated in all areas of the body except for the central nervous system, cornea, inner ear, cartilage, and splenic pulp. Plexuses of these capillaries are especially extensive in the dermis and in the mucous membranes of the respiratory and digestive systems. There appears to be a direct relationship between the number of lymphatic and vascular capillaries in a particular area; i.e., the better the blood supply, the better the lymphatic drainage.

### Collecting Lymphatics

Small lymphatic capillaries eventually enlarge into collecting lymphatics. These collecting lymphatics parallel blood vessels and drain through regional lymph nodes in their course toward the thoracic duct and, ultimately, the systemic circulation. As the lymphatics become confluent and extend centrally toward the thoracic duct, they normally traverse at least one, but often as many as eight to ten lymph nodes or node groups. Exceptions to this rule exist in the thyroid gland, esophagus, heart, and adrenal glands, where draining lymphatics may empty directly into the thoracic duct without passing through a lymph node.

Walls of collecting vessels possess intimal, medial, and adventitial layers, with the media containing elastic fibers and smooth muscle in proportion to the size of the lymphatic. Lymphatic

vessels have their own vasa vasorum, with larger lymphatics having their own artery and vein, which in turn are surrounded by small lymphatics. The large lymphatic channels contain neural elements from the vagus nerve, lesser splanchnic nerves, and para-aortic sympathetic nerves.

### Lymph Nodes

Lymph nodes, varying in size from a few millimeters to more than a centimeter, are interposed throughout the course of the collecting lymphatic channels. These lymph nodes are encapsulated and oval or bean-shaped, with an indentation along the concave surface (Fig. 1).

Lymph is brought to individual lymph nodes by afferent lymphatics which pierce the capsule's convex surface. Lymph flows into the subcapsular, cortical, and medullary sinuses within the lymph node, prior to exiting via the efferent lymphatic channel. Most commonly, there are several afferent lymphatics that carry lymph to a node, but usually only one efferent vessel.

Trabeculae, which are extensions of the capsule penetrating the nodal substance, divide the interior of the lymph node into interconnecting cavities which contain reticular tissue. The major cellular component of the lymph node is the lymphocyte, but all elements of the blood may be found in various proportions. These cells aggregate at the nodal periphery into large nodules, or follicles, making up the cortex of the node. Within

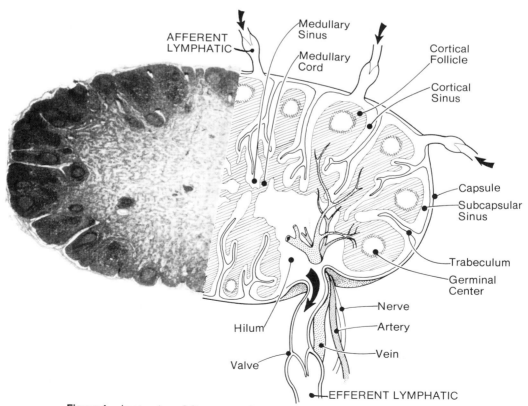

**Figure 1**  Anatomic and diagrammatic representation of a normal lymph node.

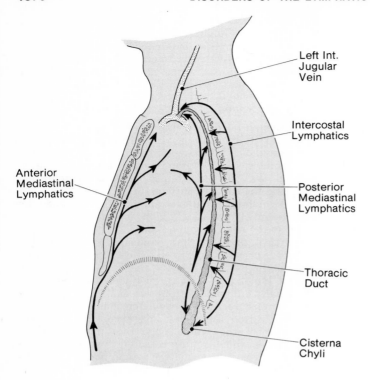

**Figure 2** Supradiaphragmatic patterns of lymphatic drainage.

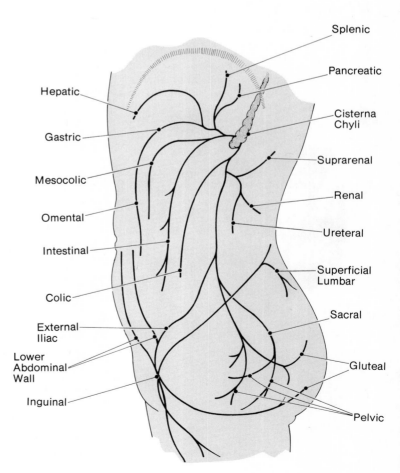

**Figure 3** Subdiaphragmatic patterns of lymphatic drainage.

the central portion of the node or medulla, lymphocytes are arranged in anastomosing cords continuous with the cortex. These medullary cords are rich in small lymphocytes, plasma cells, and macrophages. In the normal lymph node, these cells exist in equilibrium with one another, the proportion of each changing with age, diet, and hormonal milieu. At present there is no information as to how this equilibrium is controlled.

Lymph flows within the intranodal sinuses between cortical follicles and medullary cords. Within the cortical follicles, there are two distinct areas, the germinal center, which contains cells that are less densely packed and are histologically characterized by having a pale-staining and voluminous cytoplasm with abundant nuclear mitoses, and a darker-staining outer zone composed of smaller cells. The germinal center has been implicated as the site of antibody production and phagocytosis and the source of new lymphocytes.

### Lymph Flow

Almost all the lymph collected throughout the body is returned to the systemic circulation by way of the thoracic duct. The thoracic duct originates as the cisterna chyli at the level of the second lumbar vertebra. The cisterna chyli receives lymph from the lower extremities, pelvic viscera and parieties, renal and suprarenal nodes, and the deep lymphatics of the abdominal wall. In addition, it also receives lymph from the stomach, intestines, pancreas, spleen, and the caudal and ventral surfaces of the liver (Figs. 2 and 3).

Immediately below the diaphragm, the cisterna chyli becomes the thoracic duct, which extends superiorly through the aortic hiatus of the diaphragm. Emptying into the caudal end of the thoracic duct are descending lymphatic trunks from intercostal and posterior mediastinal nodes. The thoracic duct ascends behind the aortic arch and left subclavian artery, rising in an arch behind the clavicle. It then crosses the subclavian and vertebral vessels, and the thyrocervical trunk, before finally emptying into the venous system at the angle of the junction of the left subclavian and internal jugular veins. The right jugular and subclavian lymphatic trunks drain into the right lymphatic duct, which in turn enters the right subclavian vein near its junction with the right internal jugular vein.

## PHYSIOLOGY

The lymphatic system has two functions: (1) the uptake, transportation, and return of fluid and macromolecules from the interstitial space to the systemic circulation; and (2) protection of the host by providing a filtering system that resists infection and impedes the spread of neoplastic disease.

Ten per cent of the arterial capillary filtrate is not reabsorbed by the venous capillaries but enters the lymphatic system, to be returned to the circulation via the thoracic duct. In addition to this fluid transfer, the lymphatic system is almost totally responsible for the reabsorption of protein from the interstitial space, since only a small portion of filtered protein diffuses back into venous capillaries.

The absorption of protein-laden filtrate begins in small lymphatics, which are characterized by having openings of several micra between individual cells within the endothelial wall of the lymphatic vessel. These open intercellular junctions are superimposed upon one another, providing a valvelike action to the endothelial cells of the lymphatic wall, thus favoring the entry of fluid and large molecules into the vessel but preventing the egress of protein filtrate from these lymphatics. The spaces between individual cells become progressively smaller as the lymphatic channels enlarge, which further restricts the flow of large molecules back into the interstitial space.

Lymph is a reflection of the composition of tissue fluid in a particular area of the body. Peripheral lymph protein concentration is usually 2 gm. per 100 ml., intestinal lymph 3 to 4 gm. per 100 ml., and liver lymph protein sometimes exceeds 5 gm. per 100 ml. Thoracic duct lymph, a mixture of lymph from all areas of the body, has a protein concentration of approximately 3 to 5 gm. per 100 ml. Because the lymphatic system is also a major vehicle for fat absorption from the gastrointestinal tract, thoracic duct lymph, especially following meals, may contain a small percentage of fat in the form of protein-coated fat droplets called chylomicrons.

The total flow of lymph passing through the thoracic duct under basal conditions is estimated at 120 ml. per hour, so that the total amount of lymph returned daily to the bloodstream approximates the total plasma volume. Lymph return, therefore, plays an important role in the maintenance of the normal blood volume.

Normal interstitial fluid pressure is subatmospheric, approximately −7 mm. Hg. This negative interstitial pressure represents the mean pressure, with the actual pressure within the interstitial compartment varying considerably during movement of the tissues. Elevation of interstitial fluid pressure toward a more positive pressure forces fluid into the lymphatics and increases the rate of lymph flow. However, when the interstitial fluid pressure reaches atmospheric pressure, this increased pressure in the interstitial compartment compresses the adjacent lymphatics and retards lymph flow.

In addition to its function as the prime regulatory mechanism for the absorption of interstitial fluid protein and intestinal fat, lymphatic tissue is the body's major defense system. This system, which includes lymph nodes, tonsils, adenoids, spleen, and thymus, has the major responsibility for filtering bacteria, red blood cells, tumor emboli, and inanimate particles. Malignant cells or infecting organisms are removed because of the mechanical inability of tumor cells to traverse the intact lymph nodes, or by phagocytosis within the lymph nodes by reticuloendothelial cells. Viruses are apparently filtered quite inefficiently, and it has been suggested that the lymph node may serve as a center for viral replication and subsequent dissemination.

The role of the lymphatic system as a mechanism of defense against infection and neoplasia includes the production of specific immunity. Lymphoid tissue is the source of both the lymphocyte, which is necessary for cell-mediated immunity, and the plasma cell and its precursors, which are thought to be involved in the elaboration of immunoglobulins and humoral antibodies.

Malignant cells are carried to regional lymph nodes after gaining access to afferent lymphatic channels. Abundant anastomoses among lymphatics may account for the appearance of metastases in distant nodes even before proximal node involvement. If malignant cells are not destroyed after entering a lymph node, the cells continue to multiply and ultimately obstruct the efferent lymphatic channel. Continuing tumor growth within the lymph node may lead to tumor cell embolization via collateral lymphatic pathways. Occasionally, malignant cell emboli drain directly into the thoracic duct or through lymphaticovenous communications into the vena cava.

The relationship between the lymphatic system and the spread of neoplastic disease was proposed by Virchow, who first noted left supraclavicular adenopathy in patients with gastrointestinal malignant disease. It was this observation that implicated the thoracic duct as the means by which cellular emboli arising from a primary tumor were deposited in distant lymph nodes.

## REGIONAL LYMPH NODE ANATOMY

### Head and Neck

Lymph nodes are found symmetrically on both sides of the head and neck, lying in circular and vertical chains (Fig. 4). The lymph nodes that are positioned in a circular fashion are the following: (1) *Occipital nodes*—These nodes drain the back of the scalp and are situated under the deep fascia, midway between the external occipital protuberance and the mastoid process. (2) *Posterior auricular nodes*—These nodes lie on the mastoid process under the deep fascia and drain the temporal area, the back of the pinna, and the external auditory meatus. (3) *Anterior auricular nodes*—These nodes lie in front of the tragus and drain the scalp and pinna. (4) *Parotid nodes*—These nodes are buried under the deep fascia and lie within the substance of the parotid. The location of these nodes explains the rationale for including a superficial parotid dissection for malignant lesions of

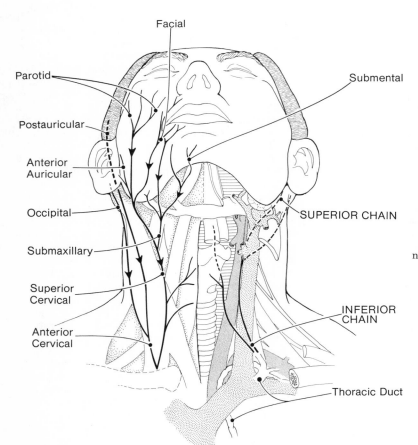

**Figure 4**  Lymphatics and lymph nodes of the head and neck.

the face that have shown evidence of spread to the cervical lymph nodes. An example of this would be a melanoma of the cheek with palpable neck nodes. The parotid nodes drain the nasopharynx, external auditory canal, inner ear, and eyelids. (5) *Facial lymph nodes* — These nodes are divided into superficial and deep groups, in relation to the anterior facial and internal maxillary vessels, and drain the face, pharynx, and mucous membrane of the cheek. (6) *Submaxillary nodes* — These nodes lie within the fascia of the submaxillary gland and drain the side of the nose, cheek, angle of the mouth, upper lip, portion of the lower lip, gum, and side of the tongue. In order to be certain that these lymph nodes are removed, it is necessary to resect the submaxillary gland. (7) *Submental nodes* — These nodes lie lateral to the midline in the submental triangle. They receive drainage from the lower lip, especially on the ipsilateral side, the apex of the tongue, and the floor of the mouth. (8) *Superficial cervical lymph nodes* — These nodes lie along the external jugular vein on the sternomastoid muscle and drain the parotid area and lower portion of the external ear. (9) *Anterior cervical lymph nodes* — These nodes lie close to the midline of the neck and have a superficial and a deep group. They drain the larynx, thyroid gland, and trachea. The "Delphian" node is a member of this node group, which, when enlarged, is highly suspicious for carcinoma of the thyroid.

The vertical chains of lymph nodes in the head and neck area follow the carotid sheath from the base of the skull to the mediastinum. These nodes are extremely important clinically in the treatment of head and neck tumors, because they ultimately receive a majority of the lymphatic drainage from the head and neck. These vertical nodes are divided into superior and inferior groups by the bifurcation of the common carotid artery, at the level of the upper border of the thyroid cartilage. Several nodes of the inferior group lie between the trachea and esophagus near the recurrent laryngeal nerve and drain the thyroid gland. Efferent vessels from these nodes enter the thoracic duct on the left side, and, on the right side, enter the confluence of the subclavian vein and internal jugular vein.

The basic mechanism for the spread of cancer of the head and neck is by tumor embolization via lymphatic vessels into regional lymph nodes. If a tumor embolus cannot be destroyed within a lymph node, it may grow and overwhelm the filtering capacity of the involved lymph node. Tumors of the head and neck are known for their propensity to remain localized to the primary area and within regional lymph nodes. Eventual dissemination of the tumor occurs as a relatively late stage of the disease. These concepts, based on the recognition and importance of lymphatic drainage pathways in the head and neck, have led to the present surgical maneuvers which attempt to remove both the primary lesion and regional lymph nodes in an "en bloc" in-continuity fashion.

## Breast

Knowledge of the lymphatic pathways from the breast is extremely important in understanding the natural history and rationale of proposed treatment for patients with mammary carcinoma (Fig. 5). The breast lymphatics begin around the lobules, with collecting channels following mammary ducts centripetally to the areolar area and to the subareolar lymphatic plexus. There is also a network of cutaneous lymphatics, both superficial and deep, within the skin of the breast, with unidirectional lymph flow to the axilla.

Coursing from the subareolar plexus toward the axilla are large medial and lateral collecting trunks which pass around the outer edge of the pectoralis major muscle and penetrate the axillary fascia, prior to terminating in several groups of axillary lymph nodes. In addition to these two large trunks, there are collecting lymphatics between the pectoral fascia and the breast, which perforate the pectoralis major muscle and follow the course of the thoracoacromial vessels. These lymphatics eventually drain into the nodes at the apex of the axilla. Additional lymphatic drainage pathways are present on the posterior aspect of the pectoralis major muscle, composing the transpectoral lymphatic route, and occasionally in the superior portion of the breast, forming the retropectoral lymphatic route. Between the pectoralis major and minor muscles, along the transpectoral route, lie the interpectoral or "Rotter's" nodes. From the apical, or subclavicular, nodes of the axilla, efferent lymphatic trunks emerge, run cephalad behind the clavicle, and empty into the venous system at the confluence of the internal jugular and subclavian veins.

Lymph nodes within the axilla vary in number, but meticulous pathologic clearing techniques may yield as many as 30 to 60 or more lymph nodes. The lymphatics of the breast drain into five lymph node groups within the axilla: (1) The *external mammary group*, which lies along the medial wall of the axilla and is contiguous with or within the fascia overlying the interdigitations of the serratus anterior muscle, from the sixth rib cephalad to the axillary vein. Occasionally, this group may include several paramammary nodes along the lateral edge of the pectoralis major muscle. (2) The *scapular group*, which lies along the subscapular and thoracodorsal vessels, from the lateral thoracic wall to the axillary vein. (3) The *central group*, which lies in the center of the axilla. These nodes are the largest within the axilla and are the ones most often clinically palpable. (4) The *axillary vein group*, which is found along the inferior surface of the lateral aspect of the axillary vein. (5) The *subclavicular group*, which is at the apex of the axilla and is often referred to as the apical group of nodes. These nodes are found at the point where the subclavian vein disappears behind the subclavius muscle. They are clinically important because of their proximity to the edge of the surgical field in most techniques of radical mastectomy, and because the efferent

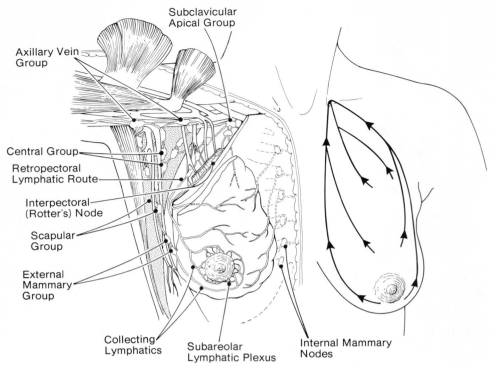

**Figure 5**  Lymphatic drainage of the breast.

lymphatics from the other groups of axillary lymph nodes empty into this subclavicular group.

In addition to axillary lymphatic drainage pathways, the breast is drained by the internal mammary system of lymphatics and lymph nodes, which receives efferent lymphatics primarily from the central and medial portions of the breast. These lymphatics pass through the pectoralis major muscle prior to emptying into the internal mammary nodes, which are situated at the edge of the sternum on the endothoracic fascia within the intercostal spaces. The internal mammary lymph nodes are small, and their efferent lymphatics drain into the thoracic duct on the left, into the lymphatic duct on the right, and, infrequently, directly into the jugular-subclavian confluence by lymphaticovenous anastomoses.

### Thorax

The lymphatic vessels and nodes of the thorax may be divided into two major groups, those of the thoracic wall, or parietes, and those of the intrathoracic viscera (Fig. 6). The parietal nodes include *intercostal, diaphragmatic,* and *internal mammary* nodes. The intercostal nodes drain the posterolateral chest wall and, depending upon their location, empty into the thoracic duct or right lymphatic duct or both superiorly, or into the cisterna chyli inferiorly. Lymph nodes that lie along the diaphragm receive afferent channels from the diaphragm and from the superior surface of the liver. The internal mammary nodes have already been discussed in the preceding paragraph.

The thoracic visceral nodes consist of three groups—the anterior mediastinal, the posterior mediastinal, and the tracheobronchial nodes. The *anterior mediastinal* nodes receive afferent lymphatics from the thymus, pericardium, and internal mammary nodes. Their efferent lymphatics unite with the tracheobronchial lymphatics to form the right and left bronchomediastinal lymphatic trunks. The *posterior mediastinal* nodes receive afferent lymphatics from the esophagus, posterior pericardium, and superior surface of the liver. Their efferent lymphatics drain into the thoracic duct, with a few channels joining the tracheobronchial nodes. The *tracheobronchial* nodes are divided into four subgroups: (1) tracheal nodes, which lie on both sides of the trachea; (2) bronchial nodes, which lie in the angle between the trachea and bronchi, and between the two major bronchi; (3) pulmonary nodes, which lie within the lung parenchyma in relation to the larger bronchioles; and (4) bronchopulmonary nodes, which lie at the hilum of each lung. Afferent lymphatics empty into all four of these groups from the lungs, bronchi, thoracic trachea, and pericardium. Their efferent trunks join with the internal mammary and anterior mediastinal lymphatics to form right and left bronchomediastinal trunks, which usually end at the jugular-subclavian confluence on the ipsilateral side, separate from the orifices of thoracic or right lymphatic ducts. Occasionally, however, they do drain directly into the thoracic duct or right lymphatic duct. Lymphatic vessels within the pulmonary parenchyma originate in superficial or deep lym-

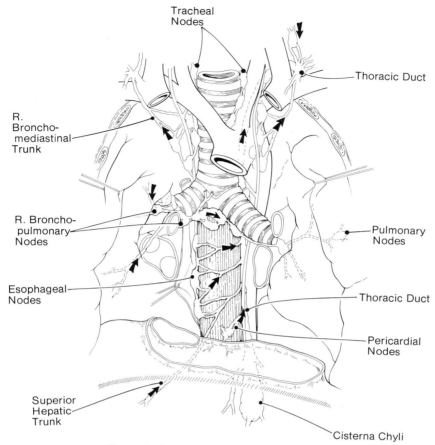

**Figure 6**   Lymphatic anatomy of the thorax.

phatic plexuses beneath the visceral pleura and accompany the pulmonary blood vessels before finally emptying into the tracheobronchial nodes. Connections between the superficial and deep plexuses within the lung seldom occur except at the hilum.

Esophageal lymphatic vessels form a circumferential plexus around the esophagus. These lymphatics freely anastomose with one another prior to forming confluent collecting vessels draining into the posterior mediastinal lymph nodes. The cardiac lymphatics are divided into superficial and deep plexuses, the former being subjacent to the visceral pericardium, and the latter, beneath the endocardium. The superficial plexus receives lymph from the deep plexus prior to forming right and left collecting trunks, which then pass cephalad behind the pulmonary artery to end in the tracheobronchial lymph nodes.

### Stomach and Duodenum

Gastric lymphatics are continuous with esophageal lymphatics at the proximal stomach and the duodenal lymphatics at the pylorus. There are four principal lymphatic pathways and nodal groups draining the stomach (Figs. 7 and 8). The first group is the *superior gastric* lymphatics and

nodes, which receive afferent lymph from both sides of the proximal stomach before draining into the celiac para-aortic lymph nodes. The second is the *pancreaticolienal* system, which drains the lateral portion of the body and fundus of the stomach. Afferent lymphatics from these areas of the stomach accompany the short gastric and left gastroepiploic vessels before entering the pancreaticolienal lymph nodes. Efferent channels from these nodes drain into the para-aortic lymph nodes. The third set of gastric lymphatics and nodes is the *inferior gastric* group, which receives lymph from the medial half of the greater curvature of the stomach. Nodes of this group lie between the two layers of the greater omentum along the distal margin of the greater curvature. Efferent lymphatics from these lymph nodes pass to the subpyloric lymph nodes and eventually empty into the para-aortic celiac nodes. The *subpyloric* system drains the pyloric area. Efferent lymphatics from these nodes drain into the hepatic and superior gastric nodes, prior to emptying into the para-aortic nodes.

Afferent lymphatics from the duodenum drain into the pancreaticoduodenal lymph nodes, which lie inferiorly and posteriorly between the head of the pancreas and the duodenum. Efferent lym-

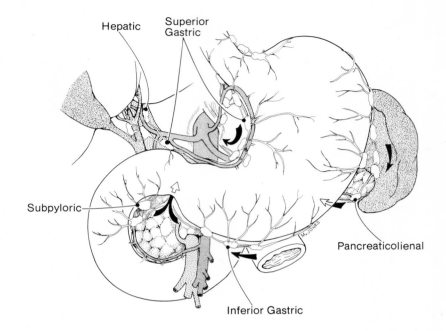

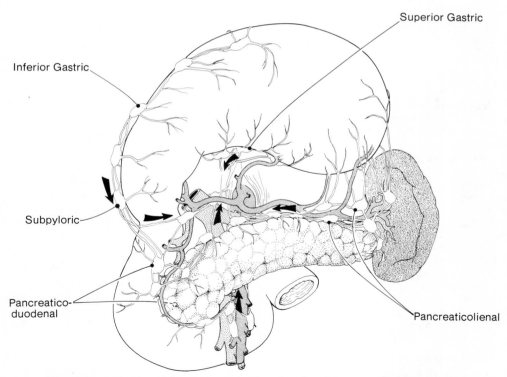

**Figures 7 and 8** Lymphatic drainage and lymph nodes of the stomach and duodenum.

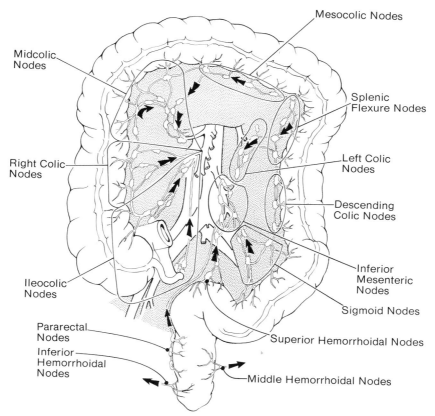

**Figure 9**  Lymphatic drainage and lymph nodes of the colon.

phatics from these nodes run cephalad to the hepatic nodes, and caudad to the para-aortic nodes at the origin of the superior mesenteric artery.

### Intestinal Lymphatics

The afferent lymphatics draining the small intestine are called lacteals and, following digestion, contain white fluid called chyle. These lacteals run between the layers of the mesentery to numerous mesenteric lymph nodes, which are arranged in groups along the course of the superior mesenteric artery. The efferent vessels from these lymph node groups drain to the para-aortic nodes.

Lymphatics of the cecal and appendiceal region are extensive, perhaps because of the abundant lymphatic tissue present with the appendiceal wall. Drainage from this area ascends by way of the ileocolic lymph nodes, which are arranged along the distal ileum, the appendix, and the cecum, and which extend proximally to the trunk of the ileocolic branch of the superior mesenteric artery. These nodes drain into the paraortic nodes (Fig. 9).

Lymphatics of the ascending and transverse colon drain to the right colic and mesocolic lymph nodes before entering the superior mesenteric nodes and ultimately the para-aortic nodes. Lymphatics of the splenic flexure, descending colon,

and sigmoid colon enter a small group of lymph nodes that lie along the left colic and sigmoidal arteries and also enter another group of nodes within the sigmoid mesocolon related to the superior hemorrhoidal artery. These lymphatics eventually end in the para-aortic lymph nodes near the origin of the inferior mesenteric artery.

The rectum, anal canal, and anus drain via different pathways in spite of their close anatomic proximity. The lymphatics of the rectum traverse the pararectal nodes, which are almost contiguous with the rectum, before entering the para-aortic nodes. Lymphatics of the anal canal accompany the middle and inferior hemorrhoidal arteries and terminate in the hypogastric lymph nodes. The lymphatics of the anus accompany those of the skin of the perineum and drain primarily into the superficial inguinal lymph nodes.

### Liver

Lymphatics contiguous with the falciform ligament drain both right and left lobes of the liver via two lymphatic trunks, one that accompanies the inferior vena cava through the diaphragm, and another that runs caudad and anteriorly, ending in the upper hepatic nodes which parallel the common bile duct at the porta hepatis. Lymphatics from the inferior surface of the liver drain into the porta hepatis and then to the celiac para-aortic nodes.

Deep lymphatics of the liver end in the hepatic lymph nodes, but occasionally drain cephalad in association with the hepatic veins, ending in a small group of lymph nodes at the vena cava. Lymphatics from the gallbladder and common bile duct drain to the hepatic nodes and the pancreaticoduodenal nodes. The cystic node, or "Calot's node," which lies adjacent to the common bile duct, is a member of the hepatic group of lymph nodes and is often encountered during operations for biliary inflammation and neoplasm. It should be identified when repair of the common bile duct is attempted since its relationship to the duct is almost constant.

### Pancreas

Pancreatic lymphatics follow the same course as the blood vessels supplying the pancreas. These lymphatics drain into the pancreaticolienal lymph nodes, where they join other lymphatics from the spleen or empty directly into the celiac lymph nodes.

### Pelvic and Retroperitoneal Lymphatics

There are both superficial and deep lymphatics in the pelvis. The former follow superficial blood vessels as they converge to the superficial inguinal lymph nodes, while the deep lymphatics parallel retroperitoneal blood vessels. The external iliac nodes drain the infraumbilical abdominal wall, the medial thigh, the external genitalia, the cervix or prostate gland, and the fundus of the bladder. The internal iliac nodes receive lymphatics from the pelvic viscera, the deeper structures of the perineum, and the buttock. The efferent lymphatics of both internal and external iliac lymph nodes are received by the common iliac nodes, which eventually drain into the para-aortic nodes.

Lumbar lymph nodes are numerous and are arranged laterally on the right and left side of the lumbar region, and centrally as the celiac, superior mesenteric, and inferior mesenteric nodes. These lumbar nodes receive efferent lymphatics from the iliac, gonadal, renal, and suprarenal lymph nodes. The efferents from the lumbar nodes either enter the cisterna chyli or connect with the lower end of the thoracic duct after piercing the diaphragm. Efferent lymphatics from the para-aortic nodes pass directly into the cisterna chyli.

### The Extremities

Lymphatics of the upper extremity, both superficial and deep, follow the course of the major arm veins and pass directly to the axilla. The ulnar or basilic lymphatic vessels occasionally traverse the epitrochlear lymph nodes, and the radial, or cephalic, lymphatics occasionally drain to deltopectoral nodes. Axillary lymph nodes and lymphatics are described in the section on lymphatic drainage of the breast.

The superficial lymphatics of the leg follow the course of the greater saphenous vein medially and lesser saphenous vein laterally. Deep lymphatics of the lower extremity are not numerous, but when present, accompany the deep vascular structures. Popliteal nodes drain these deep lymphatics as well as lymphatics from the lateral aspect of the leg.

Inguinal lymph nodes are divided into superficial inguinal and subinguinal lymph nodes at the level of the confluence of the saphenous vein and the femoral vein. The superficial inguinal nodes drain the skin of the external genitalia, perineum, buttock, and the lower abdominal wall. Medial superficial lymphatics of the leg usually continue without interruption to the subinguinal group of lymph nodes, which are divided into superficial and deep systems. The deep subinguinal nodes receive the deep lymphatic trunks from the femoral vessels and from the penis or clitoris. Efferent lymphatic vessels from the inguinal lymph nodes drain above the inguinal ligament cephalad into the external iliac lymph nodes.

# LYMPHANGITIS

Lymphangitis results from the introduction of bacteria into the subcutaneous tissues following an abrasion or superficial laceration of the skin. Because these cutaneous openings are the usual portals of entry, it is the superficial rather than the deep lymphatic system of the skin that is involved. The hands and feet are the most common sites for bacterial penetration and subsequent septic foci. Any organism can be the source of lymphangitis, but the most common are the beta-hemolytic streptococcus and *Staphylococcus aureus,* in that order.

Once bacteria invade and permeate the subcutaneous tissues, organisms can penetrate and progress rapidly along the lymphatic vessels. The affected lymphatics become surrounded by exudate and hyperemic areas, with the vessels gradually becoming clogged by desquamated endothelial cells, white blood cells, and coagulated lymph. The infection continues to spread along lymphatic channels until it reaches a regional lymph node. If the regional lymph node cannot contain the infection, bacteria may advance centrally to the next lymph node or may empty directly into the circulation, with resulting bacteremia or septicemia or both.

The clinical appearance of acute lymphangitis is characterized by the formation of fine, red lines, which usually spread up the arm or leg to the axillary or inguinal lymph nodes, without stopping at the epitrochlear or popliteal nodes. The erythema is the result of the inflammatory action of the invading pathogen as it progresses up the lymphatic channel. Movement of the involved extremity not only can cause discomfort but also aids in milking bacteria along the lymphatic channel. Regional lymph nodes usually become enlarged and tender within 12 to 24 hours after the first sign of infection. When there is extensive lymphatic involvement, the patient may become flushed, dehydrated, and quite ill.

Treatment of lymphangitis requires immobilization, elevation of the affected extremity, moist dressings, and appropriate antibiotics. Broadspectrum antibiotics should be administered until culture and sensitivity reports are available. Surgical drainage of an area of lymphangitis is seldom required, since it is not a suppurative process. An incision into an area of inflammation can only aggravate the condition and disseminate infection. There are occasions, however, when the primary focus of infection, for example, a paronychia, should be incised, in order to afford local drainage and diminution in the number of organisms being disseminated throughout the lymphatic system.

Recovery from acute lymphangitis is usually complete, without residual lymphatic obstruction or abnormality of the lymphatic vessel. However, chronic or recurrent infection of lymphatic vessels leads to chronic lymphangitis, which may then lead to permanent damage of lymphatic structures and subsequent lymphedema.

## LYMPHANGIOGRAPHY

Kinmonth, in 1955, selected the word "lymphangiography" to describe the intralymphatic injection of contrast material to visualize lymphatic vessels and the intervening lymph nodes. Earlier attempts at visualizing lymphatic vessels and nodes by injecting radiopaque material directly into a palpable lymph node had been less successful.

### Technique

Following the intradermal injection of a supravital dye, such as Direct Sky Blue, a fine polyethylene catheter is secured within a stained lymphatic vessel via a surgical "cutdown." The lymphatics ordinarily used are on the dorsum of the foot for abdominal and thoracic lymphatic visualization, on the back of the hand or in the antecubital space for outlining axillary and subclavian pathways, and over the mastoid process for cervical lymphangiograms. The contrast material used for intralymphatic injection is Ethiodol, an iodine solution in an ester of poppy seed oil. This material is injected into the lymphatic at the rate of 0.1 ml. per minute, the speed of injection regulated by a constant-rate infusion pump. The maximal amount of Ethiodol used is usually 10 ml. per leg or 5 ml. per arm. Serial radiographs in several projections are taken, up to 24 hours following injection, to outline lymphatic flow, lymphatic channels, and lymph nodes.

### Radiographic Appearance

Normal lymphatic vessels parallel the venous system, the major channels following the course of the greater and lesser saphenous veins in the lower extremity and the basilic vein in the upper extremity. As the dye flows toward progressively larger collecting vessels, lymph nodes are visualized as contrast material passes through them.

Lymphangiograms of the lower extremity usually show 10 to 12 lymphatic channels entering the inguinal lymph nodes. The efferent channels from the inguinal nodes are fewer in number but are of considerably larger caliber than the afferent vessels. Valves are conspicuous. Above the inguinal area, radiographs disclose iliac pathways and external, internal, and common iliac lymph nodes. Paravertebral channels carry the contrast material to the lumbar region where paravertebral or para-aortic nodes may be seen on delayed (24 hour) x-rays (Fig. 10).

The cisterna chyli and the thoracic duct are difficult to visualize radiographically. If demonstration of these structures is clinically indicated, it is necessary to massage the lower extremities and repeatedly flex and extend the hips following the injection of Ethiodol. Simultaneously, the

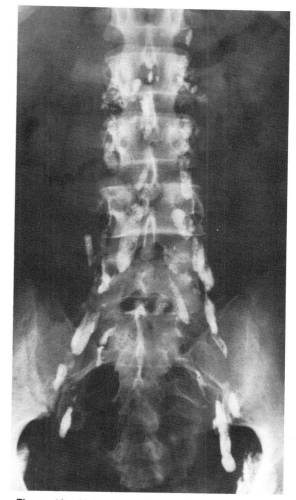

**Figure 10** Abdominal radiograph obtained 24 hours after the intralymphatic injection of oily dye, showing normal lymph node arrangement and architecture. External, internal, and common iliac nodes and lumbar para-aortic nodes are well visualized.

groin and lower abdomen are massaged in order to propel contrast material in a cephalad direction. Using this technique, approximately one-fifth of subjects may demonstrate flow of dye as high as the cervical lymph nodes.

A normal lymph node on a lymphangiogram exhibits a homogeneous internal architecture with a fine reticular or granular appearance. There may be a normal filling defect in the central portion at the hilum, but the contrast material is evenly distributed throughout the remainder of the node. Serial films disclose the contrast material entering the node from the peripheral afferent lymphatics, filling its central portion, and finally leaving the node via the efferent lymphatic. Customarily, nodes are more numerous when they are of smaller size, and conversely, they may be quite large where few in number.

### Application

Initially, lymphangiography was employed primarily to differentiate among the several types of lymphedema. The uses of this technique have expanded greatly in the past decade, and include the following: (1) the study of unilateral and bilateral peripheral edema; (2) the diagnosis, prognosis, and staging of lymphomas and other lymphoproliferative diseases; (3) the evaluation of patients with chylous effusions; (4) the diagnosis of intra-abdominal, pelvic, and thoracic masses; and (5) as a guide to the surgeon in performing complete regional lymphadenectomy.

The greatest clinical experience has been gained in lymphangiography of the lower extremities, in which retroperitoneal lymphatics and nodes are visualized throughout their course. Pathologic conditions studied by this technique have included lymphatic infections and infestations, granulomatous diseases, metastatic cancer, and malignant lesions of the reticuloendothelial system, such as Hodgkin's disease and lymphosarcoma.

### Complications

Occasional complications accompany lymphangiography. These are attributable either to the local effects of the surgical incision required to isolate and cannulate a peripheral lymphatic, or to a systemic reaction to the contrast material. Transient pyrexia is seen in approximately half the patients, with nausea, vomiting, headache, chills, or arthralgias reported in one-fifth of patients. Wound infection has been noted in less than 10 per cent of patients undergoing lymphangiography. Complications of increasing magnitude are iodine sensitivity and anaphylaxis. Lymphangiography will cause an elevation of the serum protein-bound iodine (P.B.I.) for as long as 18 months.

The complication unique to lymphangiography is pulmonary embolization of the contrast material. The oily dye enters the pulmonary circulation via the thoracic duct, subclavian vein, and right heart, as well as by lymphaticovenous shunts below the thoracic duct. Clinical symptoms are evident in approximately 10 per cent of patients undergoing lymphangiography, and radiographic evidence of oil emboli in the lung may occur in almost half these patients (Fig. 11).

When pulmonary embolization of contrast ma-

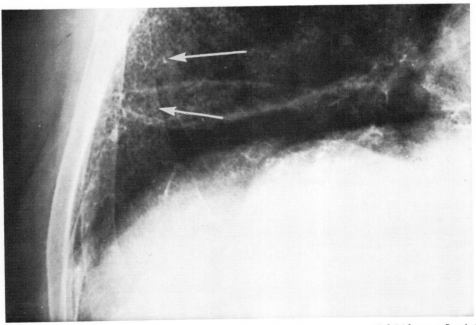

**Figure 11** PA chest radiograph showing pulmonary embolization of contrast material 24 hours after intralymphatic injection into the dorsum of the foot. The fine, reticular pattern of contrast within the pulmonary parenchyma is characteristic.

terial occurs, an alveolar-capillary block is produced in the pulmonary parenchyma. Patients in whom serial studies of pulmonary function have been done after lymphangiography show a decrease in carbon monoxide diffusion capacity of 25 per cent within 2 to 4 hours. This returns to normal over the next 2 to 3 days. Arterial $pO_2$ drops significantly during the first 4 hours following injection of the oily material, followed by a rapid return to normal. Measurement of vital capacity and maximal breathing capacity indicates no significant impairment of these ventilatory functions.

## CHYLOUS EFFUSIONS

Chylothorax, chylous ascites, and chyluria are infrequently encountered clinical problems, each characterized by an effusion derived from disruption of a major lymphatic vessel. These effusions are usually rich in lipids and are milky white in color. Generally, the recognition of chylothorax or chylous ascites is made only at the time of thoracentesis or paracentesis by discovering the characteristic milky fluid instead of the serous fluid encountered with the majority of effusions. Chyluria is easily documented, since few patients could ignore the passage of milky white urine.

### Chylothorax

Chylothorax may follow injury to the thoracic duct, either by penetrating or closed thoracic trauma. The latter includes vertebral fracture, thoracic contusion, or indirect trauma to the thoracic duct from sudden hyperextension of the vertebral column. If there is lymphatic congestion within the mediastinum, as for instance in patients with tuberculosis, lymphoma, metastatic tumor, or filariasis, a relatively minor injury can be the precipitating factor in the disruption of the thoracic duct. When chylothorax develops secondary to malignant disease, the primary tumor is usually located in either the posterior mediastinum or the retroperitoneal region. Penetrating trauma includes direct injury to the thoracic duct by knife or gunshot, or iatrogenic injury occurring during an intrathoracic diagnostic procedure or at the time of thoracotomy.

The symptoms and signs of chylothorax are identical to those of any pleural effusion. The chylous nature of the pleural effusion is detected at the time of thoracentesis. This fluid is sterile, is usually abundant in volume, and has a high lipid content.

When a chylous pleural effusion is encountered, in the absence of an obvious cause, an extensive work-up should be undertaken, since treatment is determined by the underlying pathologic condition. This work-up may include lymph node biopsy, mediastinoscopy, and other studies to determine the presence of a lesion within the chest. Lymphangiography is the technique by which the actual site of the leak in the thoracic duct may be visualized.

Repeated thoracenteses or closed catheter drainage of the pleural cavity may be required. Frequently, these techniques control further leakage from the thoracic duct. However, thoracotomy may be necessary to ligate the thoracic duct if these maneuvers fail to control the effusion. Thoracic duct ligation may be required, even in the presence of extensive neoplastic invasion, if chylothorax is a severe problem.

### Chylous Ascites

Chylous fluid is infrequently present within the peritoneal cavity at the time of birth, if an embryologic abnormality exists in the development of the lymphatic system. Usually, however, chylous ascites follows intra-abdominal lymphatic block in the area of the cisterna chyli, or less frequently, a lymphatic block within the thorax. Although chylous ascites may follow lymphatic blockage due to parasites or large inflammatory lymph nodes, the most common cause is metastatic cancer. Neoplastic invasion is reflected by dilatation of distal lymphatic vessels, lymphatic valvular insufficiency, and reversal of lymph flow. The dilated walls of distended lymphatics eventually weaken and are susceptible to rupture by minor trauma. Lymphorrhea may occur, from either the lymphatics at the site of obstruction or intestinal subserosal lymphatics. Lymphangiography in the presence of chylous ascites may demonstrate compression or distention of the lumbar collecting trunks.

Radiation therapy may prove helpful if the chylous effusion is secondary to lymph node obstruction from a radiosensitive neoplasm, such as Hodgkin's disease. Unfortunately, the treatment of chylous ascites due to invasion of lymphatic channels by metastatic tumor is rarely successful. Most often, repeated paracenteses are indicated to enhance patient comfort.

In addition to the usual causes of chylous effusions, an exudative enteropathy has been described that is manifested by malabsorption, low serum calcium, increased gastrointestinal protein loss, and chylous ascites. This entity has been linked to dilatation and ectasia of the intestinal mucosal lymphatics rather than lymphatic obstruction or an abnormality of subserosal lymphatics.

### Chyluria

The passage of intestinal lymph in the urine, implying a communication between the urinary collecting system and the lymphatic system, is rarely encountered in the Western hemisphere. The etiology of chyluria in the overwhelming majority of cases is parasitic infestation by *Wuchereria bancrofti*, but other parasites, including Echinococcus, Ascaris, Cysticercus, and Plasmodium (malaria), have been implicated. Chyluria of nonparasitic etiology is extremely rare, but when it does occur, it usually follows trauma, or implies obstruction to the thoracic duct or cisterna chyli or both by enlarged lymph nodes, metastatic tumor, pyogenic abscess, or tuberculosis.

The pathophysiology of chyluria was described by Ackerman in 1863 and confirmed by lymphangiographic studies within the past decade. Initially, partial obstruction occurs within the lymphatic vessels between the bowel and either the cisterna chyli or the thoracic duct. This obstruction leads to increased intralymphatic pressure, causing lymphangiectasis, which in turn leads to valvular incompetence and retrograde flow of chyle. Because of the fragile nature of lymphatic vessels, their close association with the renal collecting system, and lack of adequate perirenal collateral lymphatic vessels, lymphaticorenal shunts occur, resulting in chyluria.

The passage of cloudy or milky fluid in the urine may be intermittent rather than continual, since remissions of long duration can occur. The degree of chyluria is directly related to patient activity, with increased exercise causing increased lymph flow and increased chyluria. A high-fat diet also tends to increase the passage of lymph in the urine. Associated pyelonephritis occurs in a high percentage of cases of chyluria.

Lymphangiography confirms obstruction to the flow of lymph and may demonstrate not only dilated lymphatic channels with backflow toward the renal lymphatics, but even the exact site of the fistula.

The best therapy for chyluria is treatment of the pathologic process responsible for it, which, in most cases, implies the administration of antifilarial drugs. Bed rest and low-fat diet have been advocated during the course of therapy to minimize lymphatic flow.

Surgery has been advised for refractory cases of chyluria. Although controversy still exists, the surgical treatment of choice appears to be the meticulous removal of the lymphatics surrounding the renal pedicle combined with renal decapsulation. This operation has resulted in the cure of approximately 75 per cent of patients with chyluria.

## TUMORS OF THE LYMPHATICS

### Lymphangioma

Lymphangioma is a benign tumor of lymphatic origin encountered most frequently in young children. This tumor, commonly called cystic hygroma, is composed of soft, cystic masses which develop from lymph sacs originating from embryonic outpouchings of the venous system. Most of these lesions are found in the neck, few are located in the axilla, and the remainder are scattered throughout the body (Fig. 12). The posterior triangle of the neck is the most common single location. There is no racial or sexual predilection.

The majority of cystic hygromas appear within the first year of life, and almost 90 per cent are evident before the second year. The tumor may be large in size and, occasionally, a rapid increase in the dimensions of the mass is noted after an upper respiratory infection, probably as a result

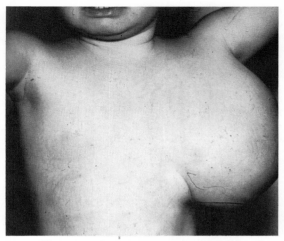

**Figure 12**   Lymphangioma of the axilla.

of lymphatic rupture subsequent to coughing. Another cause of sudden enlargement is hemorrhage within the lesion.

Lymphangiomas are classified into three pathologic groups: (1) *simplex,* which consists of small lymph capillaries; (2) *cavernous*, which is composed of larger lymph capillaries; and (3) *cystic,* which is the classic cystic hygroma. All three types usually coexist within the same tumor and are usually grouped together and called cystic hygroma.

Lymphangiomas contain multiple, multilocular, cystic masses, ranging in size from 0.1 to 5.0 cm. in diameter. Cysts within the larger cyst may or may not communicate. Walls are thin and delicate, and the cysts are filled with clear fluid. The endothelial lining of the cyst glistens, resembling peritoneum.

The characteristic appearance of cystic hygroma is that of a soft, cystic mass which appears fluctuant and lobulated and which is readily transilluminated. Aspiration of the cyst yields thin, watery, serous fluid, i.e., lymph. A large cystic hygroma may cause dysphagia or dyspnea, and the rare tumor that is present in the floor of the mouth may embarrass respiration (Fig. 13). Chylothorax and chylopericardium have been infrequently reported complications. Occasional cystic hygromas extend into the mediastinum, where they may be demonstrated by chest radiography.

The only effective treatment for cystic hygroma is surgical removal. Although spontaneous regression is unlikely in large lesions, most small hygromas eventually disappear, as evidenced by the scarcity of patients in their late teens or thereafter who exhibit these lesions. Spontaneous regression occurs by irritation of the endothelial lining of the cyst wall, resulting in scarring and eventual obliteration.

There does not appear to be any justification for early operation for this condition except in the presence of airway obstruction, repeated inflammation, or rapid enlargement. It is unnecessary and unwise to operate on an asymptomatic hygroma, exposing crucial structures in a very small neck to great surgical risk. Operation should be deferred until the patient is older, so that if surgery is still necessary, it may be performed with less chance of injury to important structures.

A cystic hygroma has no clear-cut boundaries but is simply a collection of lymphatic channels which, at their periphery, blend into the normal surrounding structures. An attempt to remove all the lymphatics, especially when they interdigitate with major nerves and vessels, may be hazardous. At operation, as much macroscopic tumor as possible should be excised, and the divided lymphatic trunks that remain should be ligated.

### Lymphangiosarcoma

In 1948, Stewart and Treves first reported the development of lymphangiosarcoma arising in the presence of postmastectomy lymphedema of the arm. This tumor is rare, occurring in less than 0.5 per cent of patients who undergo mastectomy, and in an even smaller number of patients who have lymphedema of the lower extremity. The origin of these tumors is most likely related to lymphedema, which has been present in all reported cases. The duration of the edema is variable and has ranged from 1 to 24 years, with a mean duration of 9 years. Although most reported cases of lymphangiosarcoma have been noted in lymphedematous arms following mastectomy and radiotherapy for mammary carcinoma, this tumor has also been associated with lymphedema secondary to nonmalignant inflammatory diseases, surgical procedures, or radiation therapy alone. Despite the history of radiotherapy in a majority of patients in whom lymphangiosarcoma has developed, radiation has been considered a major

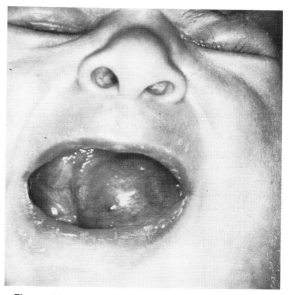

**Figure 13**  Lymphangioma of the floor of the mouth, necessitating urgent operation because of respiratory embarrassment.

cause for the development of lymphedema, rather than an apparent carcinogen per se.

Lymphangiosarcoma first appears as a blue to reddish purple discoloration or nodule in the skin. Later, small satellite nodules may form and coalesce around the original lesion (Fig. 14). The main tumor mass, as well as the satellite nodules, may ulcerate. Lymphangiosarcoma spreads by direct bloodstream invasion, resulting in visceral metastases early in the course of the disease.

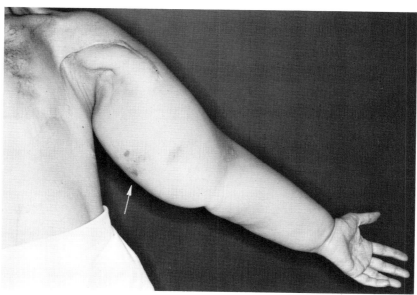

**Figure 14**  Fifty-one year old woman with 12 year history of lymphedema following radical mastectomy and radiotherapy for mammary carcinoma. Arrow denotes purple, coalescent cutaneous lesions characteristic of lymphangiosarcoma. Biopsy confirmed the diagnosis. The patient succumbed to widespread metastases less than 2 years later despite interscapulothoracic amputation, radiotherapy, and chemotherapy.

Histologically, this malignant tumor shows marked lymphangiomatosis in the subcutaneous and dermal layers. Lymphatic channels are lined by endothelial cells that have foci of large, hyperchromatic, proliferating cells with bizarre, papillary, intraluminal projections. The multiple foci of abnormal cells suggest a possible multicentric origin of the tumor.

The lethal nature of lymphangiosarcoma, regardless of the treatment employed, has resulted in a pessimistic outlook. Methods of treatment have included radiation therapy, wide excision with subsequent radiotherapy, interscapulothoracic amputation with or without accompanying radiation therapy, high humeral amputation, and shoulder disarticulation, all of these with or without chemotherapy using a variety of tumoricidal agents, alone or in combination.

With these methods, only an occasional patient has survived 5 years. Half the patients are dead within 2 years of the time the appearance of the first cutaneous lesion is noted, and the mean survival time following initial definitive therapy is less than 18 months.

Because of the poor results, regardless of therapy, it is difficult to be enthusiastic about recommending any specific type of treatment. The apparent multicentricity of the disease suggests that early amputation, followed by systemic chemotherapy, might provide the best chance for survival.

## LYMPHOPROLIFERATIVE DISORDERS

Malignant lymphomas or primary lymphatic neoplasms include Hodgkin's disease, lymphosarcoma, reticulum cell sarcoma, Burkitt's lymphoma, follicular lymphoma, and mycosis fungoides.

Hodgkin's disease, lymphosarcoma, and reticulum cell sarcoma account for the overwhelming majority of primary malignant lymphatic diseases and have been the subject of considerable controversy regarding classification, staging, and treatment. These neoplasms vary in clinical severity and histologic appearance, but their histologic characteristics do not necessarily correlate with their clinical course. Generally, lymphosarcoma and reticulum cell sarcoma have simple histologic patterns, with primarily a single type of proliferating cell that gradually replaces the architecture of the lymph node. Hodgkin's disease exhibits varying numbers of lymphocytes, granular cells, plasma cells, monocytes, fibroblasts, and characteristic Reed-Sternberg cells.

### Hodgkin's Disease

Hodgkin's disease is a malignant process of lymph nodes that is considered unicentric in origin and is characterized by the presence of Reed-Sternberg cells with a variable proliferation of lymphocytes and histiocytes. The Reed-Sternberg cell is a large cell with abundant cytoplasm, multiple or multilobed nuclei, and prominent nucleoli.

Hodgkin's disease is clinically characterized by painless enlargement of a lymph node or group of lymph nodes, usually unilateral and frequently located in the cervical region. The disease spreads by involvement of adjacent lymph nodes so that symptoms are noted only when there is rapid enlargement of lymph nodes or when an involved lymph node impinges upon other structures. The interval between initial lymph node enlargement and progression of the disease to adjacent areas is variable, usually being much longer than that observed in lymphosarcoma or reticulum cell sarcoma.

Systemic symptoms occur early in Hodgkin's disease, fever being most prevalent. The allegedly pathognomonic Pel-Epstein fever, of alternating periods (days to weeks) of high and normal temperatures, is uncommon. If fever is an early symptom, the prognosis of the disease is allegedly poor. Lassitude, weight loss, night sweats, pruritus, and anemia with lymphopenia are additional systemic symptoms. Jaundice can occur as a result of either parenchymal liver involvement or pressure on the porta hepatis by an enlarged node, resulting in bile duct obstruction. Splenomegaly occurs in half the cases. An interesting symptom that occasionally occurs in Hodgkin's disease is pain in an involved lymph node following the ingestion of alcohol. This pain appears shortly after the alcohol is drunk and persists approximately 1 hour, the time necessary for partial oxidation of the alcohol.

Hodgkin's disease is more prevalent among Caucasians than other races, and twice as many males are affected as females. The age distribution of the disease is bimodal—a peak between 15 and 34 years of age, and a second peak over the age of 50. Extranodal Hodgkin's disease is seen infrequently, except for cutaneous manifestations which may occur in as many as one-fourth of patients. These manifestations include hyperpigmentation, subcutaneous nodules, and erythematous eruptions.

In 1944, Jackson and Parker classified Hodgkin's disease into three histologic categories, Hodgkin's paragranuloma, granuloma, and sarcoma, in increasing order of aggressiveness. This classification has limited usefulness, since an overwhelming proportion of cases fall into the granuloma category. Lukes and Butler later reclassified Hodgkin's disease into four histologic types: (1) *Lymphocyte predominance,* made up of occasional Reed-Sternberg cells and abundant lymphocytes and histiocytes. This type may have a diffuse or nodular pattern, and corresponds to the old paragranuloma group. (2) *Nodular sclerosis,* identified by bands of doubly refractile collagen that separate the lymph node into islands of lymphoid tissue. Reed-Sternberg cells are easily visualized. (3) *Mixed cellularity,* which represents the classic Jackson-Parker granuloma. This type consists of a variety of cells including plasma cells, eosinophils, fibroblasts, and abundant Reed-Sternberg cells. (4) *Lymphocyte depletion,* characterized by few normal lymphoid cells and considerable fibrosis. Reed-Sternberg cells vary in number. In the old Jackson-Parker classification, this description corresponds to the sarcoma group.

The diagnosis of Hodgkin's disease is made by histologic study of a biopsied lymph node. It is desirable to remove an entire lymph node not recently involved by inflammation, so that the pathologist has an opportunity to study nodal architecture in addition to cellular morphology.

Therapy and prognosis for patients with Hodgkin's disease are determined by accurate clinical staging. In 1966, an international committee proposed a classification for the clinical staging of Hodgkin's disease, which subsequently has been universally accepted. Based on the anatomic distribution of sites of involvement, this classification divides Hodgkin's disease into four distinct stages: *Stage I* limits the disease to one anatomic region or two contiguous anatomic regions on the same side of the diaphragm. *Stage II* is present when two anatomic regions are involved, or if disease exists in two noncontiguous regions on the same side of the diaphragm. *Stage III* describes the disease when it is localized to lymph nodes on both sides of the diaphragm, but does not extend beyond the involvement of lymph nodes, spleen, and/or Waldeyer's ring. *Stage IV* implies the presence of secondary disease, i.e., extralymphatic involvement, such as of bone marrow, liver, skin, gastrointestinal tract, lung parenchyma, or pleura.

Hodgkin's disease is further subdivided into "A" or "B" (for example, Stage IIB), describing either the absence or presence, respectively, of systemic symptoms. Fever, night sweats, and pruritus are the systemic manifestations, the presence of any of which justifies a "B" subclassification. However, weight loss, malaise, anemia, fatigue, leukocytosis, leukopenia, cutaneous anergy, alcohol pain, and elevated sedimentation rate are also systemic manifestations of Hodgkin's disease, but are not of sufficient significance to relegate the patient to a "B" subgroup.

To insure the accurate clinical staging of Hodgkin's disease, the following studies are desirable: (1) careful clinical history and physical examination with special attention to the presence or absence of systemic symptoms; (2) complete blood count, including differential count, hematocrit or hemoglobin, platelet count, and erythrocyte sedimentation rate; (3) chest radiographs in PA and lateral projections, plus tomograms if hilar adenopathy exists; (4) bone survey radiographs; (5) intravenous pyelogram; (6) liver function studies, including Bromsulphalein retention, alkaline phosphatase, and radioisotopic liver scan; (7) bone marrow examination, including needle biopsy of the marrow rather than simple aspiration; (8) documentation of cutaneous anergy; and (9) lymphangiography.

Until recently, hematologists and radiologists had believed that, once the tissue diagnosis of Hodgkin's disease was made, lymphangiography would confirm the clinical stage of the disease process. There is no question that lymphangiographic patterns do exist in patients with Hodgkin's disease (Fig. 15), but, despite these characteristic lymphangiographic findings, occasionally the radiographic abnormalities are indistinguishable from those encountered in pyogenic or fungal infections, other metastatic malignant diseases, or reactive hyperplasia (Figs. 16–18). Normally, however, the lymphangiographic findings in Hodgkin's disease occur in the following sequence. Initially, lymph nodes appear normal, but may be slightly enlarged, round, oval, or elongated, with well demarcated peripheral sinuses. Droplets of contrast material are evenly distributed within the nodes. As Hodgkin's disease progresses, the nodes become destroyed by the malignant process, so that the resulting lymphangiogram becomes more characteristic. Lymph nodes no longer retain all the contrast material, and radiolucent filling defects become evident. Isolated neoplastic areas may produce lacuna-like filling defects which resemble moth-eaten areas of various sizes and shapes. Continued destruction of the lymph node architecture results in a coarse, foamy, cystic mottling of the lymph node pattern, caused by

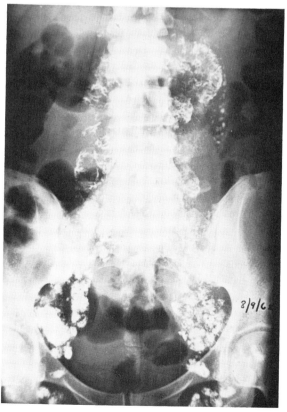

**Figure 15** The lymphangiographic appearance of Hodgkin's disease involving the inguinal, iliac, and para-aortic lymph nodes. All the nodes are enlarged, with filling defects or a foamy, lacy pattern of dye distribution, or both.

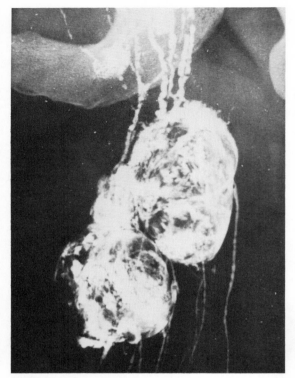

**Figure 16** Enlarged inguinal lymph nodes demonstrated on 24 hour film following intralymphatic injection of oily dye, showing central and peripheral filling defects due to metastatic melanoma.

the contrast material being displaced to the periphery. Stasis of the entire lymph circulation may also occur. Hodgkin's disease eventually may obliterate the entire lymph node so that the contrast material is seen only in a few delicate lymphatic vessels, which skirt the involved lymph node, which is no longer itself visualized.

Because staging of Hodgkin's disease has become so important in determining both therapy and prognosis, surgeons are now called upon more frequently to define the exact clinical stage of disease. Previously, the surgeon's role was merely the removal of a lymph node for histologic examination. Occasionally, laparotomy was performed in patients with hepatomegaly or abnormal liver function tests, an equivocal lymphangiogram, or splenomegaly. Other infrequent indications for laparotomy were recurrence of Hodgkin's disease after treatment, or suspicion of subsequent tumor extension following initial assessment of the disease. In those patients who underwent laparotomy, it was found that the clinical extent of disease, evaluated by lymphangiograms alone, was underestimated in almost half the patients, and in one-fourth of the patients, it was necessary to restage the disease as a result of the operation.

With this retrospective evidence as a basis, several centers elected to initiate prospective studies, in which all patients with Hodgkin's disease would undergo laparotomy for clinical

staging prior to initial therapy. Several significant observations have resulted. Abdominal involvement by Hodgkin's disease occurred in one-fifth of the patients with normal lymphangiograms in whom no abdominal involvement was suspected. Another 20 per cent of patients with equivocal lymphangiograms, but no evidence of hepatomegaly or splenomegaly, also proved to have intra-abdominal Hodgkin's disease. Splenic involvement was difficult to ascertain before operation. Almost half of the patients with palpable or radiographically enlarged spleens failed to show splenic involvement at operation. One-third of the patients with clinically normal spleens were found, at laparotomy, to have splenic involvement with Hodgkin's disease. Liver involvement rarely occurred without concomitant splenic disease. Preoperative lymphangiographic prediction of abdominal node involvement was inconclusive, since 15 per cent of patients with negative or equivocal lymphangiograms were subsequently found to have abdominal nodal disease, and 20

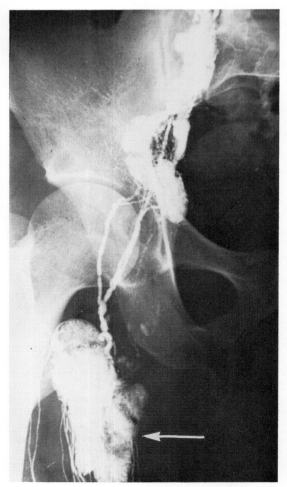

**Figure 17** Enlargement of lymph nodes due to inflammation. Filling defects (arrow) caused by abscess formation within the node can be mistaken for neoplastic invasion.

per cent of patients with positive lymphangiograms did not have intra-abdominal Hodgkin's disease.

As a result of this experience with laparotomy as part of the initial work-up, surgery is at present advised for all patients with Hodgkin's disease, except those unequivocally in the Stage IV group. The maneuvers suggested at the time of surgery are as follows: (1) splenectomy, (2) liver biopsy, (3) removal of representative splenic, mesenteric, and para-aortic lymph nodes, and (4) affixing of radiopaque clips to the sites of the removed lymph nodes, to the splenic vascular pedicle, and at the boundaries of abdominal disease when present. In women of childbearing age, the ovaries are sutured in the midline posteriorly to bring them out of the field of intended radiation therapy. Splenectomy is performed not only to allow its histologic examination, but also to remove a large target from the field of radiation therapy, thus decreasing possible secondary complications of left lower lobe radiation pneumonitis or radiation nephritis.

Radiation therapy is the treatment of choice for Hodgkin's disease, and it is important that large fields be treated in continuity to avoid missing involved lymph nodes. The "mantle" field technique, as reported by Kaplan, is most commonly employed. This technique uses parallel opposing anterior and posterior fields, which are shaped to encompass all the nodes on both sides of the neck, from the mastoid tip to the supraclavicular fossa, the intraclavicular regions, both axillae, and the hilar and mediastinal nodes down to the diaphragm. Not only should the field of radiation therapy be extensive, but the dosage should be delivered with high-voltage equipment. Today's practice of using megavoltage therapy spares tissues which previously had been injured by comparable doses of low-voltage radiotherapy. Radiation burns of the skin and significant pulmonary restriction, due to radiation pneumonitis, have been minimized. In addition, severe leukopenia and thrombocytopenia have occurred less frequently since these present-day methods of radiation therapy have been employed.

Prior to the advent of clinical staging for Hodgkin's disease, prognosis was predicted by histologic classification. Clinical staging, however, has proved more accurate than histologic classification in determining the natural history of the disease, with patients in the lowest clinical stage having the best prognosis.

Present techniques of high-voltage radiation therapy have not been used long enough to assess accurately long-term survival rates. Current results suggest that a majority of patients with Stages I and II disease, even in the "B" subgroup, are clinically free of disease for periods in excess of 5 years, with as many as 50 to 60 per cent of patients surviving 10 years. Patients in Stage III have a 20 to 40 per cent 10 year survival rate. Patients with Stage IV disease have only a 10 to 20 per cent chance of surviving 5 years.

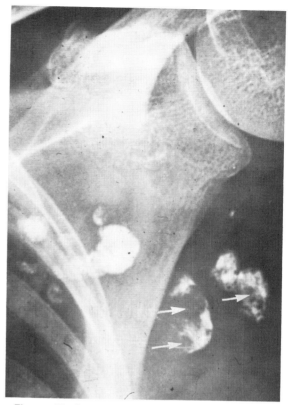

**Figure 18** Lymphangiographic appearance of axillary lymph nodes enlarged and partially replaced by metastatic mammary carcinoma. Arrows indicate foci of tumor within nodes.

Patients with Stages III and IV Hodgkin's disease are frequently treated not only by radiation therapy but also with chemotherapy, using agents alone or in combination with one another. The drugs that are most often used are vincristine, nitrogen mustard, cyclophosphamide, and corticosteroids. These drugs, in addition to a variety of others, are constantly being evaluated in order to improve the efficacy of chemotherapy.

### Lymphosarcoma and Reticulum Cell Sarcoma

Lymphosarcoma and reticulum cell sarcoma occur most frequently among Caucasians and involve males twice as often as females. Lymphosarcoma is two to four times more frequent than reticulum cell sarcoma. Although these tumors originate primarily within lymph nodes, 20 to 40 per cent of patients with lymphosarcoma and 30 to 60 per cent of patients with reticulum cell sarcoma have extranodal disease. Despite the usual spread of these diseases by contiguous involvement of adjacent nodes, distant metastases are frequent, and this fact has led to speculation that these neoplasms may be multifocal in origin.

Histologic sections of lymphosarcoma and reticulum cell sarcoma show a thickened capsule around matted nodes. The normal follicular pattern is lost, and there is diffuse replacement by sarcomatous cells. In lymphosarcoma, lymphocytes are present in varying degrees of maturity, whereas in reticulum cell sarcoma the cells are mainly reticulum cells. In both diseases, cells invade nodal sinuses and may extend through the node capsule into the surrounding tissues. Mitoses are frequent.

Clinically, patients with lymphosarcoma or reticulum cell sarcoma show early lymph node enlargement, which may be either unicentric or multicentric. The patient who complains of abdominal or back pain, stridor, or dyspnea may well be manifesting mediastinal or retroperitoneal nodal involvement, both of which are early symptoms in the course of these diseases. One-fifth of patients with lymphosarcoma or reticulum cell sarcoma present with a systemic complaint as the first symptom of the disease.

After the initial localized symptoms occur, the disease progresses, and widespread visceral involvement is common. Effusions, both pleural and intra-abdominal, occur frequently. Hepatic parenchymal invasion or hilar node enlargement may result in jaundice. When splenomegaly occurs, it usually is late in the course of the disease. Bone lesions are demonstrated in one-tenth of patients, being observed most frequently in vertebrae, femora, ribs, pelvis, and skull.

The diagnosis of lymphosarcoma or reticulum cell sarcoma is made by lymph node biopsy. Inguinal nodes should be avoided as biopsy material whenever possible since these nodes frequently have acute and chronic inflammatory changes which add to the difficulty of accurate histologic evaluation.

Lymphosarcoma and reticulum cell sarcoma are clinically staged by means of the same criteria as are used for Hodgkin's disease. However, alternate criteria are used to allow for the frequent primary extranodal origin of both lymphosarcoma and reticulum cell sarcoma. Primary extralymphatic disease without regional lymph node enlargement is considered Stage I—for example, lymphosarcoma of the stomach, without nodal involvement. If regional node enlargement accompanies the primary extranodal disease, it is considered Stage II. When local invasion has occurred beyond the primary extralymphatic site, the disease is relegated to Stage IV even if generalized lymph node enlargement is not present.

The early stages of lymphosarcoma and reticulum cell sarcoma are usually treated with high-voltage radiation therapy. Even in the presence of advanced disease, palliative radiation therapy is indicated for such conditions as bone pain or tumor compression of a nerve.

A variety of chemotherapeutic agents are used in the treatment of advanced lymphosarcoma and reticulum cell sarcoma, the most popular being nitrogen mustard, cyclophosphamide, chlorambucil, vincristine, and corticosteroids. When effusions occur, a variety of intracavitary agents may be employed, including quinacrine (Atabrine), nitrogen mustard, phosphorus-32, or ThioTEPA.

Prognosis is related to clinical stage of disease, Stages I and II demonstrating as high as 40 to 45 per cent long-term survival following therapy. Stages III and IV imply a more pessimistic outlook.

### Burkitt's Lymphoma

In 1958, Burkitt described an unusual variety of lymphosarcoma among native children in tropical Africa. He observed that this tumor accounted for almost half of all childhood malignant diseases in this part of the world. It was also noted that this tumor has a high incidence of maxillary and mandibular involvement, common association with abdominal or retroperitoneal masses, which implies ovarian or renal invasion, and infrequent involvement of the spleen or lymph nodes.

Epidemiologic data indicated that this tumor, which has since become known as Burkitt's lymphoma, occurred in areas of Africa where the temperature rarely fell below 60° F., and the rainfall was always in excess of 20 inches per year. These data suggest that Burkitt's lymphoma is infectious in origin and is transmitted by an insect vector. Another hypothesis for the etiology is that this tumor is a response to a viral infection, since two viruses have been isolated from patients with Burkitt's lymphoma, a reovirus type 3, encountered in up to 25 per cent of the patients studied, and a herpes group Epstein-Barr virus, which has been grown in tissue cultures of the lymphomatous cells.

Burkitt's lymphoma is highly sensitive to chemotherapeutic agents and, on occasion, large mandibular or maxillary lesions have rapidly disappeared following administration of systemic drugs. This disease is apparently less virulent than other malignant diseases of lymph nodes, demonstrating frequent long-term remissions.

### Follicular Lymphoma

This infrequently encountered disease was initially called giant follicle lymphoblastoma because of multiple follicle-like nodules within lymphoid tissue. It was thought to have a relatively benign course but occasionally, after an indeterminate length of time, become transformed into lymphosarcoma, reticulum cell sarcoma, or Hodgkin's disease. Since all the lymphomatous diseases may histologically exhibit a follicular or a diffuse pattern at some time in their course, it is questioned whether follicular lymphoma is truly a separate entity or simply a different manifestation of the natural history of lymphoproliferative growth.

The clinical picture of follicular lymphoma occurs twice as often in men as in women, usually after the age of 40, and is characterized by extremely large lymph nodes, occasionally exceeding 5 cm. in diameter. Although systemic symptoms in this condition are rare, enlargement of liver, spleen, and retroperitoneal nodes is the rule. Diagnosis is made by lymph node biopsy, which usually shows prominent lymphoid follicles which are widely distributed throughout the node and not confined only to the cortex. The treatment of choice in follicular lymphoma is radiation therapy. If splenomegaly or hypersplenism is a problem, splenectomy or corticosteroids or both are recommended.

### Mycosis Fungoides

This uncommon disease is a variant of lymphoma, in which the first manifestation is a cutaneous eruption. There are three characteristic periods defined in the natural history of this disease: (1) the premycotic period, during which the patient may complain of a nonspecific skin eruption; (2) the stage of infiltration and plaque formation, during which an intradermal infiltrate is noted; and (3) the tumor stage, wherein cellular aggregates within the skin form tumors which invade the subcutaneous tissues. Histologically, these tumors look like lymphosarcoma or reticulum cell sarcoma.

Histologic diagnosis may be made if a cutaneous lesion is biopsied in either the infiltrative or the tumor stage of the disease. However, in the premycotic period, histologically and clinically the lesions resemble psoriasis, eczema, or other benign skin eruptions.

Lymph node enlargement may occur in the infiltrative and tumor stages, but biopsy of an enlarged lymph node may not be diagnostic, because all degrees of lymphoreticular proliferation may be encountered. Lymph node morphology may remain normal despite the presence of disseminated mycosis fungoides.

Although the premycotic stage may last as long as 20 years, prognosis in mycosis fungoides is very poor. Treatment includes local therapy to the cutaneous lesions with nitrogen mustard, topical corticosteroids, or radiation therapy, alone or in combination, with or without associated systemic chemotherapy.

## LYMPHEDEMA

Lymphedema of the extremities has been known since antiquity and long recognized as a consequence of lymphatic obstruction. The classification of lymphedema differentiates the primary, or idiopathic, type from secondary lymphedema, which results from the absence, obstruction, or interruption of lymphatic channels (Table 1).

### Primary Lymphedema

Primary, or idiopathic, lymphedema is divided into three subgroups based upon the age at which it becomes apparent. Lymphedema congenita indicates lymphedema present at birth or shortly thereafter (Fig. 19). Of all patients affected by primary lymphedema, less than 10 per cent are in the congenital category. Within this group of patients with congenital lymphedema exists a unique subgroup, originally described by Milroy in 1892 as having "chronic hereditary edema." He identified 22 patients with this condition in a 97 member family representing six generations. These

**TABLE 1** CLASSIFICATION OF LYMPHEDEMA*

A. Primary
 1. Congenita
 2. Praecox
 3. Tarda
B. Secondary
 1. Infection and infestations
  a. Parasitic
  b. Pyogenic
  c. Fungal
 2. Mechanical, chemical, and physical trauma
  a. Abrasions or lacerations
  b. Burns
  c. Chemical irritation
  d. Radiation therapy
 3. Granulomas
  a. Lymphogranuloma venereum
  b. Syphilis
  c. Tuberculosis
  d. Sarcoid
 4. Postphlebitic
 5. Surgery
  a. Removal of lymph nodes
  b. Removal of lymph vessels
 6. Neoplastic invasion of lymph nodes
 7. Dependency edema

*Modified from Nomenclature and Criteria for Diagnosis of Diseases of the Heart and Blood Vessels. New York Heart Association, 1953.

patients had a family history of congenital edema of the limbs. Kinmonth and his associates reported 107 patients with primary lymphedema, 12 of whom had congenital lymphedema, but only two in whom it was also hereditary. Therefore, the classic requirement that "Milroy's disease" be both hereditary and congenital makes its actual occurrence today extremely rare.

If primary lymphedema occurs between early childhood and the third decade of life, it is called lymphedema praecox. The largest number of patients with primary lymphedema fall into this category, with females predominating over males in the ratio of three to one.

Those patients with lymphedema occurring after the age of 30 have lymphedema tarda.

It is unlikely that the three classifications of primary lymphedema listed here characterize three separate pathophysiologic states. It is more likely that the natural history of progressive lymphatic insufficiency is divisible into three different periods. If at birth there is an insufficient number of normal lymphatic channels, early lymphedema, i.e., lymphedema congenita, results. If a patient is born with lymphatics that are marginal in quality or quantity, repeated trauma throughout childhood may damage a significant number of these lymphatics, so that lymphatic drainage eventually becomes compromised. If this lymphatic inadequacy becomes evident about the time of puberty, the condition is considered lymphedema praecox. If the damage to lymphatic channels does not become manifest until later in life, the patient is placed in the lymphedema tarda group.

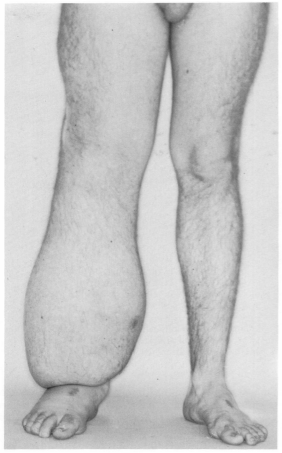

**Figure 19**   Congenital lymphedema. Twenty-four year old white male with progressive swelling of the right lower extremity noted since birth. (From Goldsmith, H. S., and De los Santos, R.: Surg. Gynec. Obstet., *125*: 607, 1967.)

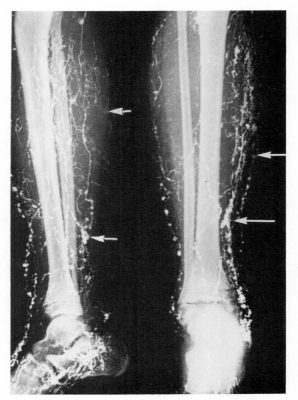

**Figure 20**   Lymphedema. Fourteen year old girl with progressive lymphedema of the right leg. Lymphangiogram demonstrates dermal backflow (upper arrows) and hypoplastic lymphatics with lymphangiectasia (lower arrows) in both lateral (*left*) and AP (*right*) projections.

Prior to the advent of lymphangiography, it was assumed that primary lymphedema was most likely due to the absence of lymphatic channels. However, lymphangiography has demonstrated that lymphatic aplasia is relatively infrequent, but that hypoplasia and other lymphatic defects are responsible for the majority of cases of primary lymphedema. Kinmonth and his associates demonstrated hypoplastic lymphatics in 55 per cent of patients with primary lymphedema, but aplasia in only 14 per cent. Twenty-four per cent of patients exhibited hyperplastic, or dilated, lymphatics. An additional radiologic finding in occasional patients with primary lymphedema is reflux of contrast material from collecting lymphatic vessels to the superficial dermal plexus of lymphatics, so-called "dermal backflow" (Fig. 20).

Another small group of patients with primary lymphedema have broad, tortuous lymphatics with incompetent or absent valves, a condition designated as "lymphangiectasia." There is no familial tendency in this group, and neither

sex predominates. These patients frequently have capillary angiomas over their limbs and trunks.

One-third of patients with gonadal dysgenesis (Turner's syndrome) have primary lymphedema of the lower extremities at birth, caused by hypoplastic distal lymphatic vessels. This group represents a very small portion of the total number of patients with primary lymphedema.

### Secondary Lymphedema

Secondary lymphedema results from the obstruction or interruption of previously normal lymphatic channels. This interference with lymph flow results in the back-up of lymph within distal lymphatic channels, which eventually becomes reflected in increased tissue fluid in the interstitial space. The distention of the interstitial space by this increased tissue fluid puts traction on connective tissue fibers attached to lymphatic capillaries. The lymphatic valves thus become incompetent and can no longer prevent the pull of gravity from exerting its downward and peripheral effect upon the lymph column. A cycle of lymph stasis, interstitial fluid overload, and lymphatic valve incompetence becomes established.

The most common cause of secondary lymphedema is parasitic infestation by the mosquito-borne nematode, *Wuchereria bancrofti*. The mosquitoes that carry this parasite deposit the filarial larvae subcutaneously. The larvae migrate via blood and lymphatic vessels to various sites throughout the body, where they mature into adults and produce microfilaria. The adult worms live primarily in lymphatic vessels and nodes, where repeated episodes of inflammation and infection can cause lymphatic obstruction, which in turn can result in massive lymphedema or elephantiasis.

The presumptive diagnosis of acute filariasis depends upon characteristic clinical findings in conjunction with a history of exposure to mosquitoes in an endemic area. Clinically, the patients manifest chills, fever, and malaise, which may last several weeks. Specific target areas most susceptible to inflammation are the epididymis, spermatic cord, testis, retroperitoneal lymphatics, and renal pelvis. Acute symptoms result from an allergic response to the products of living and dead worms. However, microfilariae are often demonstrable in the blood without clinical symptoms.

In temperate climates, secondary lymphedema is usually due to the surgical interruption or removal of lymphatics, radiation therapy, or malignant disease. The most common surgical procedure associated with secondary lymphedema is radical mastectomy, which, in up to one-quarter of patients, is followed by edema of the ipsilateral upper extremity. The temporal relationship between this operation and the onset of lymphedema is quite variable, with edema of the arm developing at any time from the early postoperative period to many years thereafter.

Radical groin dissection is another operative procedure frequently followed by edema of the ipsilateral extremity. Since any interference with *per primam* wound healing increases the likelihood of subsequent lymphedema, meticulous attention to wound care is particularly important in this operation.

Halsted first called attention to the relationship between infection and the subsequent development of lymphedema. Infection superimposed upon surgically interrupted lymphatics leads to further compromise of remaining lymphatic channels. Radiation therapy, by injuring the lymphatic endothelium, can also result in secondary lymphedema.

Malignant disease may present with secondary lymphedema as its first manifestation. Carcinoma of the cervix, with widespread pelvic involvement causing lymphedema of a lower extremity, is an example.

### Treatment

Conservative measures enable the majority of patients with lymphedema to lead a relatively normal life. Recommendations for treatment include elevation of the involved extremity, prevention of infection, weight reduction, fluid and salt restriction, and local therapy using compression bandages or pulsatile air pressure devices. If fluid retention is difficult to control, diuretics may be necessary, especially in the premenstrual period.

Acute lymphangitis is particularly threatening to patients with or predisposed to the development of lymphedema. Even a minor abrasion or infection can lead to severe systemic manifestations, such as chills, high fever, and septicemia. Recurrent episodes of lymphangitis are invariably associated with progressive lymphedema, which becomes increasingly more difficult to treat effectively. Any patient with lymphedema who has had more than one bout of lymphangitis is a candidate for long-term antibiotic prophylaxis. Such therapy will render 80 per cent of patients free from further attacks of lymphangitis.

Fortunately, only a small proportion of patients with lymphedema require surgical treatment. The classic indications for surgery are the following: (1) increasing size of limb despite aggressive medical treatment, (2) significant functional impairment, (3) serious skin changes, (4) recurrent bouts of infection despite adequate attempts at prophylactic antibiotic therapy, and (5) severe emotional disturbances because of the appearance of the involved limb.

The large number of different operations devised to correct lymphedema are modifications of three basic procedures: (1) an attempt to stimulate the formation of new lymphatic channels, (2) the removal of large segments of lymphedematous tissue, and (3) the transfer of normal lymphatics into a lymphedematous extremity. The first of these procedures, namely the subcutaneous implantation of threads or tubes of foreign materials to stimulate lymphatic growth, has not been effective and has generally been discarded.

The second category of procedures is based on the excision of large volumes of diseased tissue, not only to improve patient appearance but in an effort to encourage anastomoses between remaining superficial lymphatics and those deep to the excised fascia. This type of operation was popularized by Kondoleon and Charles and subsequently modified by others. Unfortunately, none of these procedures has been consistently successful in alleviating the cosmetic and functional disabilities of patients with lymphedema.

New surgical techniques designed to transfer normal lymphatic channels from a healthy area into a lymphedematous limb are gaining in popularity. Thompson has suggested an operation that buries an intact dermal flap to aid in lymph drainage. This is accomplished by excising skin and subcutaneous tissue in a longitudinal plane along the edematous extremity, leaving a 1 inch wide dermal flap. This long flap is tucked into the deep tissues and sutured in place. Theoretically, the intact lymphatics within the buried flap will act as a conduit for lymphatic drainage.

Another operation advocated as a means for re-establishing centripetal lymphatic flow is the transposition of the intact omentum, with its own rich lymphatic and blood supply, into the lymphedematous extremity. It is technically possi-

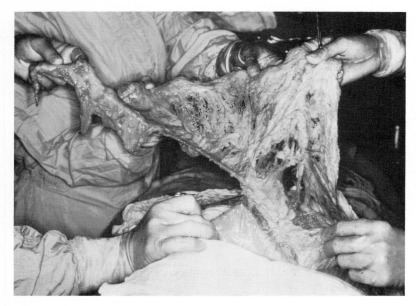

**Figure 21**  Omentum being removed from the greater curvature of the stomach. The omentum can be lengthened to reach the most distal part of any extremity, yet retain its viability. (From Goldsmith, H. S., De los Santos, R., and Beattie, E. J., Jr.: Ann. Surg., *166*:573, 1967.)

ble to tailor the omentum sufficiently to allow its transfer from the peritoneal cavity into any involved limb (Fig. 21). Connections between omental lymphatics and deep lymphatics of an affected limb have been demonstrated lymphangiographically, and the procedure can be clinically successful (Fig. 22).

Each advocate of a particular procedure for treating lymphedema tends to be enthusiastic about the results of his favorite operation. This enthusiasm for a single procedure makes it difficult for an investigator to alternate various operations among the few patients with lymphedema he is called upon to treat. It is, therefore, difficult, at the present time, to draw valid conclusions from available published data as to the operation of choice for the individual patient with lymphedema.

## ACKNOWLEDGMENT

The authors wish to thank Dr. K. F. Lee, Professor of Radiology, Jefferson Medical College, for the lymphangiograms used in this chapter.

## SELECTED REFERENCES

Glatstein, E., Guernsey, J. M., Rosenberg, S. A., and Kaplan, H. S.: The value of laparotomy and splenectomy in the staging of Hodgkin's disease. Cancer, *24*:709, 1969.
  *This important current reference presents a study in a series of patients that forms the basis for the expanding use of exploratory laparotomy and splenectomy in "staging" patients with Hodgkin's disease. This approach is well supported by early data, but, as the authors emphasize, further investigation is needed to define and confirm its eventual clinical usefulness.*

Kaplan, H. S.: Clinical evaluation and radiotherapeutic management of Hodgkin's disease and the malignant lymphomas. New Eng. J. Med., *278*:892, 1968.
  *This is a classic presentation on the radiotherapeutic management of Hodgkin's disease and other lymphomas.*

Kinmoth, J. B., Taylor, G. W., Tracy, G. D., and Marsh, J. D.: Primary lymphedema. Brit. J. Surg., *45*:1, 1957.
  *This is an excellent discussion of primary lymphedema.*

Pomerantz, M.: Lymphangiography. Surg. Clin. N. Amer., *49*:1451, 1969.
  *This is a review of the various techniques and clinical indications for the use of lymphangiography together with the results.*

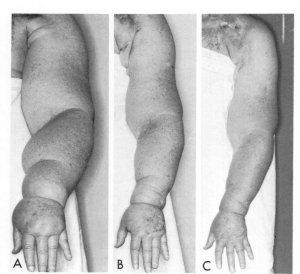

**Figure 22**  Composite picture of a patient before and after omental transposition for lymphedema. *A,* Preoperative; *B,* 12 months after operation; *C,* 18 months after operation. (From Goldsmith, H. S.: Surg. Clin. N. Amer., *49*:407, 1969.)

# REFERENCES

1. Aisenberg, A. C.: Hodgkin's disease—prognosis, treatment, and etiologic and immunologic considerations. New Eng. J. Med., 270:508, 1964.
2. Collette, J. M., Jantet, G., and Schoffeniels, E., eds.: New trends in basic lymphology. Experientia, Suppl. 14, 1966.
3. DeVita, V. T., Serpick, A. A., and Carbone, P. P.: Combination chemotherapy in the treatment of advanced Hodgkin's disease. Ann. Intern. Med., 73:881, 1970.
4. Glatstein, E., Guernsey, J. M., Rosenberg, S. A., and Kaplan, H. S.: The value of laparotomy and splenectomy in the staging of Hodgkin's disease. Cancer, 24:709, 1969.
5. Goldman, J. M.: Laparotomy for staging of Hodgkin's disease. Lancet, 1:125, 1971.
6. Goldsmith, H. S.: Lymphangiosarcoma in the lymphedematous extremity. Ca, 17:213, 1967.
7. Goldsmith, H. S.: The treatment of post-surgical lymphedema. Surg. Clin. N. Amer., 49:407, 1969.
8. Goldsmith, H. S., De los Santos, R., and Beattie, E. J.: Relief of chronic lymphedema by omental transposition. Ann. Surg., 166:573, 1967.
9. Guyton, A. C.: Textbook of Medical Physiology. 4th ed. Philadelphia, W. B. Saunders Company, 1971, Chapter 21, The lymphatic system, interstitial fluid dynamics, and edema.
10. Hugo, H. E.: Recent advances in the treatment of lymphedema. Surg. Clin. N. Amer., 51:111, 1971.
11. Kadin, M. E., Glatstein, E., and Dorfman, R. F.: Clinicopathologic studies of 117 untreated patients subjected to laparotomy for the staging of Hodgkin's disease. Cancer, 27:1277, 1971.
12. Kaplan, H. S.: Clinical evaluation and radiotherapeutic management of Hodgkin's disease and the malignant lymphomas. New Eng. J. Med., 278:892, 1968.
13. Kinmonth, J. B., Taylor, G. W., and Harper, R. K.: Lymphangiography—a technique for its use in the lower limb. Brit. Med. J., 1:940, 1955.
14. Kinmonth, J. B., Taylor, G. W., Tracy, G. D., and Marsh, J. D.: Primary lymphedema. Brit. J. Surg., 45:1, 1957.
15. Lewis, S. R., and Smith, J. R.: Lymphedema. In: Converse, J. M., ed.: Reconstructive Plastic Surgery. Philadelphia, W. B. Saunders Company, 1964.
16. Mayerson, H. S.: The physiologic importance of lymph. In: American Physiological Society: Handbook of Physiology. Section 2, Circulation. P. Dow, ed. Baltimore, Williams & Wilkins Company, Volume 2, 1963.
17. Mayerson, H. S., ed.: Lymph and the Lymphatic System. Springfield, Ill., Charles C Thomas, 1968.
18. Mayerson, H. S.: Three centuries of lymphatic history—an outline. Lymphology, 2:143, 1969.
19. O'Brien, P. H., Sherman, J. O., Brand, W. N., and Scarff, J. E.: Lymphangiography. Surg. Gynec. Obstet., 126:131, 1968.
20. Pomerantz, M.: Lymphangiography. Surg. Clin. N. Amer., 49:1451, 1969.
21. Rosenberg, S. A.: Report of the committee on the staging of Hodgkin's disease. Cancer Research, 26: Part I, 1310, 1966.
22. Rusznyak, I., Foldi, M., and Szabo, G.: Lymphatics and Lymph Circulation. New York, Pergamon Press, 1960.
23. Ruttiman, A.: Progress in Lymphology. Stuttgart, Georg Thieme Verlag, 1967.
24. Viamonte, M., Koehler, P. R., Witte, M., and Witte, C.: Progress in Lymphology, II. Stuttgart, Georg Thieme Verlag, 1970.
25. Yoffey, J. M., and Courtice, F. C.: Lymphatics, Lymph, and the Lymphomyeloid Complex. New York, Academic Press, 1970.

# 50

# DISORDERS OF VEINS

*John Ludbrook, Ch.M., F.R.C.S., F.R.A.C.S.*

## FUNCTIONAL AND SURGICAL ANATOMY

The description that follows concentrates on the anatomic features of veins (particularly of the lower limbs) that are relevant either to their function or to the disorders that affect their function. The emphasis is thus somewhat different from that found in most anatomic texts.

### Wall Structure

All veins that are visible to the naked eye, from venules to the venae cavae, have certain features in common. They possess *smooth muscle* in their walls, unless they are rigidly enclosed by bone or by the cranium. The more dependent a vein is in the standing posture (and thus the higher the hydrostatic blood pressure within it), the thicker is its wall in relation to the diameter of its lumen. The smooth muscle layer is thicker in the actively contractile subcutaneous veins than in the almost inert deep veins (Fig. 1). In the great veins of the trunk, the smooth muscle is arranged as a long spiral, while in the contractile subcutaneous veins of the limbs it is nearly circular in disposition. The density of *innervation* of veins by sympathetic constrictor fibers is approximately proportional to the smooth muscle content of the vein wall. Sensory endings (pain receptors, and perhaps mechanoreceptors) are present in subcutaneous veins. The *vasa vasorum* of veins, unlike those of arteries, do not communicate with the lumen.

### Valves

Most veins possess valves: two frail cusps attached to a point of thickening of the vein wall (the valve ring). There is a dilatation of the vein wall immediately downstream from the valve ring (the valve sinus). There are some general rules about the frequency distribution of valves, about the direction in which they face (Fig. 2). They tend to be located immediately distal to a point of entry of a major tributary, and the orifices of the major tributaries themselves usually bear valves. In the limbs, valves usually direct blood flow from distal to proximal, and from superficial to deep. Notable exceptions are the perforating veins of the hands, feet, and forearm, in which flow is from deep to superficial. Valves occur with greater frequency distally in a limb than proximally. Valveless veins of note are the innominate veins, common iliac veins, venae cavae, renal veins, hepatic veins, and portal, mesenteric, and splenic veins.

### Gross Anatomy of the Limb Veins

Each limb has three anatomically and functionally distinguishable sets of veins:

1. *Subcutaneous* (superficial). These have relatively thick, muscular walls. The major trunks run in tunnels, created by a condensation of the superficial fascia and lined by areolar tissue. Each limb has two major superficial systems of veins that intercommunicate free with each other as well as with the deep veins. Each superficial system ends by penetrating the deep fascia to enter a major deep vein.

2. *Deep* (intermuscular, intramuscular). These have thin, scantily muscled walls. The intermuscular veins accompany named arteries, taking the form of a plexus below the level of the elbow or knee, and forming a single major vein toward the root of the limb.

3. *Perforating* (communicating) veins. These, too, are thin-walled. They pass through the deep fascia to link the superficial and deep sets of veins.

In the *lower limb*, the *great saphenous vein* (Fig. 3) begins at a point midway between the medial malleolus and the tendon of the tibialis anterior muscle, and ends by passing through an opening in the deep fascia (fossa ovalis) to enter the femoral vein at a fairly constant site 3 cm. lateral to, and 3 cm. below, the pubic tubercle. The trunk of the great saphenous vein is sometimes reduplicated (particularly in the lower thigh), and there may be a double entry into the femoral vein. In the last 5 cm. of its course the great saphenous vein receives a variable number of subcutaneous tributaries: *pudendal, epigastric, circumflex iliac,* and *medial* and *lateral femoral.*

In the leg, the great saphenous vein is closely accompanied by the *saphenous nerve*. Just below the knee it usually receives a major tributary (sometimes called the *posterior arch vein*): this collects blood from a complex of

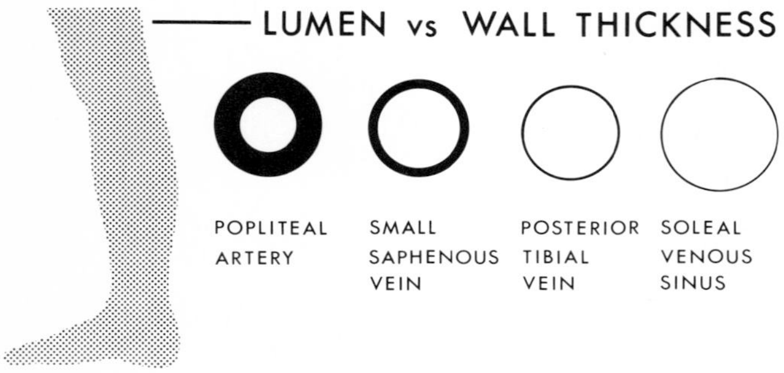

LUMEN vs WALL THICKNESS

POPLITEAL ARTERY · SMALL SAPHENOUS VEIN · POSTERIOR TIBIAL VEIN · SOLEAL VENOUS SINUS

**Figure 1** Relation of wall thickness to lumen diameter for an artery, subcutaneous vein, intermuscular vein, and intramuscular vein in the leg. (After Ludbrook, J.: Aspects of Venous Function in the Lower Limbs. 1966. Courtesy of Charles C Thomas, Publisher, Springfield, Ill.)

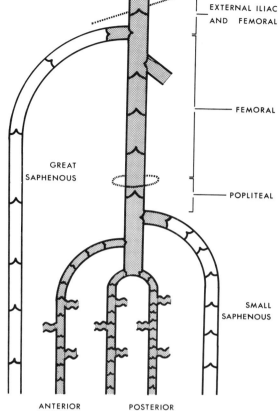

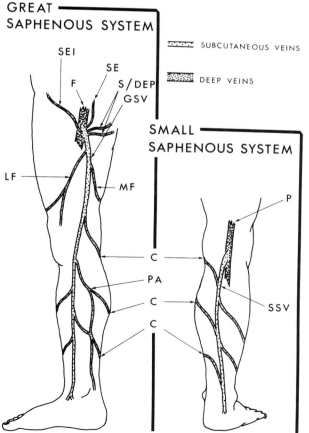

**Figure 2** Frequency distribution of valves in the veins of the lower limb, based on averaged data from published reports. (After Ludbrook, J.: Aspects of Venous Function in the Lower Limbs. 1966. Courtesy of Charles C Thomas, Publisher, Springfield, Ill.)

**Figure 3** Diagrammatic representation of the courses and tributaries of the saphenous veins. *GSV* = great saphenous vein; *SSV* = small saphenous vein; *F* = femoral vein; *P* = popliteal vein; *SEI, SE, S/DEP, LF, MF* = superficial circumflex iliac, superficial epigastric, superficial and deep external pudendal, lateral femoral, medial femoral tributaries; *PA* = posterior arch vein; *C* = short saphenous–great saphenous communicating veins.

veins overlying the posteromedial aspect of the calf, and has multiple communications with the deep system. Both below and above the knee the great saphenous vein receives tributaries that run upward and medially from the *small saphenous vein.* Throughout its course the great saphenous vein is closely accompanied by *lymphatic trunks.*

Below the knee, numerous *perforating veins* (Fig. 4) join tributaries of the great saphenous vein to the deep veins of the leg. The most important from the surgical point of view is the medial set, which joins the posterior arch complex of veins to the venae comitantes of the posterior tibial artery, and the anteromedial set running close to the periosteum of the tibia. An anterolateral set enters the anterior tibial vein. In the thigh, a perforating vein often joins the great saphenous vein (or a tributary) to the femoral vein (or its subsartorial tributary).

The *small saphenous vein* (see Fig. 3) begins at a point midway between the Achilles tendon and the posterior border of the lateral malleolus. It passes almost vertically to the middle of the popliteal fossa, accompanied by the *sural nerve* and by lymphatics. It penetrates the deep fascia at about the middle of the leg. It usually enters the deep system (the popliteal vein) in the middle of the popliteal fossa, but the precise level is variable. A posterolateral set of *perforating veins* (see Fig. 4) joins its tributaries to the peroneal vein, while less constant perforating veins enter calf muscle veins.

At the root of the lower limb there are alternative routes for venous drainage from the skin, by way of the *internal pudendal vein* (scrotum, vulva), and through the *gluteal veins* (thigh below the gluteal crease): ultimately these drain into the internal iliac vein.

The *popliteal vein* is formed from the plexiform *venae comitantes* of the three main branches of the popliteal artery, and then is joined by the veins draining the gastrocnemius and soleus muscles to constitute a single (or sometimes double) vessel behind the artery. The gastrocnemial and soleal veins are so large and tortuous that the latter have been termed *soleal venous sinuses.* At the groin the *femoral vein* lies a little behind, as well as medial to, the corresponding artery. It receives its large deep femoral tributary(ies) just below the point of entry of the great saphenous vein.

Another point of surgical import is the formation of the *inferior vena cava* by the junction of the two *common iliac veins.* The terminations of the latter are closely applied to the back of the right common iliac artery, which indents the left common iliac vein.

## PERFORATING VEINS IN THE LOWER LIMB

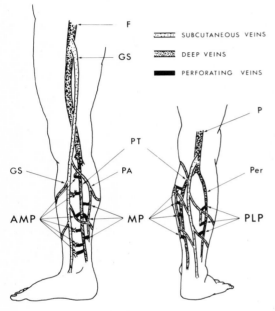

SUBCUTANEOUS VEINS
DEEP VEINS
PERFORATING VEINS

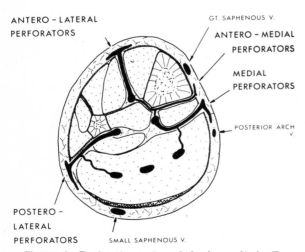

ANTERO - LATERAL PERFORATORS

GT. SAPHENOUS V.

ANTERO - MEDIAL PERFORATORS

MEDIAL PERFORATORS

POSTERIOR ARCH V.

POSTERO - LATERAL PERFORATORS

SMALL SAPHENOUS V.

**Figure 4** Perforating veins of the lower limb. *Top,* Medial and posterior views of the leg. *F* = femoral vein; *GS* = great saphenous vein; *PA* = posterior arch vein; *PT* = posterior tibial vein; *P* = popliteal vein; *Per* = peroneal vein. *AMP* = anteromedial perforators; *MP* = medial perforators; *PLP* = posterolateral perforators. *Bottom,* Schematic cross section at junction of middle and lower thirds of the leg.

## VENOUS FUNCTION

There are four general ways in which veins function: (1) as conduits, (2) in thermal regulation, (3) as capacity vessels, (4) and as musculovenous pumps. In individual regions or tissues of the body variations in structure of the veins, and in the nature of the tissue that surrounds them, allow one or more of these functions to be dominant.

### Conduit Function

The total cross-sectional area of the veins draining a region is some two or three times greater than that of the corresponding arteries. The resistance to blood flow in the venous system is thus comparatively low, and postcapillary vessels contribute normally only about 10 to 15 per cent of the total resistance to cardiac output (Fig. 5). However, maximal dilatation of precapillary and capillary resistance vessels (as in violent muscle exercise) may relocate the site of maximal vascular resistance from precapillary arterioles to postcapillary venules, the latter acting as governors that prevent an uncontrolled increase in cardiac output.

The venous system is in two senses a low-pressure one. Because the precapillary resistance vessels lie upstream, the *hydraulic pressure* of blood as it enters the venous system is normally low (less than 15 mm. Hg); and because of the relatively large cross-sectional area of veins, the *hydraulic pressure gradient* between venous capillaries and the right atrium is small (less than 10 mm. Hg).

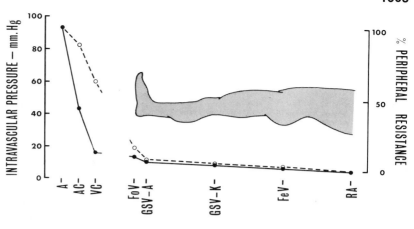

**Figure 5** Hydraulic pressure gradients in the lower limb, at rest (solid line) and with maximal arteriolar dilatation (broken line). Constructed from published data. *A* = artery; *AC* = arterial capillary; *VC* = venous capillary; *FoV* = subcutaneous foot vein; *GSV-A* = great saphenous vein at ankle; *GSV-K* = great saphenous vein at knee; *FeV* = femoral vein; *RA* = right atrium. (After Ludbrook, J.: Aspects of Venous Function in the Lower Limbs. 1966. Courtesy of Charles C Thomas, Publisher, Springfield, Ill.)

There is a second major determinant of venous pressure in man, which is a consequence of his two-legged gait. On the hydraulic pressure is superimposed a *hydrostatic pressure* (Fig. 6), equivalent to the gravitational effect of an unbroken column of blood extending to the right atrium. At rest, any part of the venous system that is below the level of the right atrium is exposed to a positive hydrostatic pressure equivalent to the vertical distance from the atrium. Yet the converse does not apply: at points above this phlebostatic axis the hydrostatic pressure is not negative, because the pliable vein walls collapse together and prevent a siphon effect.

At a tertiary level, other *transient pressure changes* may be superimposed on the steady-state hydraulic and hydrostatic pressures. Centrally, there are pressure waves corresponding to cardiac action ("a," "c," and "v" waves), and to respiratory variations in intrathoracic pressure. In the limbs, there are pressure transients from the action of the musculovenous pumps (see later).

### Thermoregulatory Function

The specialized anatomic features of cutaneous and subcutaneous veins are closely concerned with the regulation of body temperature (Fig. 7). The dermal venules, subdermal venous plexuses, and subcutaneous veins constitute an effective and important means for heat exchange with the environment (the others being the pulmonary microvasculature and sweat glands). The size of, and rate of blood flow in, the dermal venules of the hands, feet, head, and neck is inversely proportional to the magnitude of the *tonic sympathetic vasoconstrictor discharge* to skin resistance vessels. The cross-sectional area of the muscular subcutaneous veins is also under *direct sympathetic control*, and there is as well a *direct temperature effect* on their smooth muscle. The juxtaposition of *deep arteries and veins* in the limbs constitutes a passive countercurrent heat conservation-loss mechanism, while the *disposition of venous valves in the hands and feet* ensures that all blood entering these extremities leaves by way of subcutaneous veins, and can thus exchange heat with the environment.

### Capacity Function

It is thought that about 80 per cent of the blood volume is contained by low-pressure blood vessels: systemic veins, the right heart and pulmonary vasculature, and the left atrium. Some two-thirds of the blood volume is contained by the systemic venous system (from venules to the great veins), and most of this by deep veins.

A feature of these thin-walled, collapsible, low-pressure, venous capacity vessels is that large changes in the volume of their contents induce only small pressure changes (at least over a wide, physiologic range). This is in contrast to the elastic behavior of the high-pressure arterial vessels. A consequence is that the considerable blood volume changes that may be occasioned by hemorrhage and transfusion, and the redistributions of blood occasioned by exercise, take place almost entirely within the low-pressure "compartment" of the circulation.

This pressure-volume characteristic of capacity vessels tends to assure a relatively constant filling pressure for the heart. Moreover the whole-body geometry of these vessels is such as to ensure this constancy in face of a variety of body postures, and without the need for other than fine-control active regulatory mechanisms (to which reflex control of tone in superficial veins makes a modest contribution).

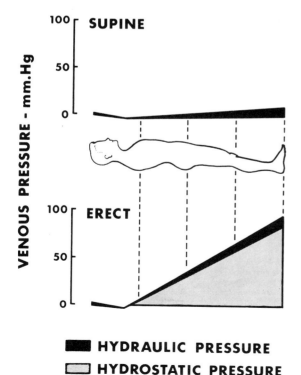

**Figure 6** Schematic representation of hydraulic and hydrostatic venous pressure gradients in the supine and erect postures.

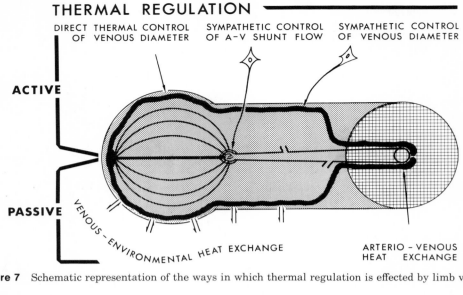

**Figure 7** Schematic representation of the ways in which thermal regulation is effected by limb veins.

### Musculovenous Pumps

The valved deep veins of the limbs, and their investing muscles, constitute reciprocating pumps. The most specialized of these are in the legs, where the musculature is enclosed by a dense covering fascia (permitting the generation of high intramuscular pressures during contraction), and where the calf muscles contain large venous sinuses (which act as pump chambers). This specialization seems to be a peculiarly human characteristic, presumably associated with man's adoption of the upright posture and his ability to run.

*Muscle contraction* raises the pressure in the muscles of the leg by up to 250 mm. Hg. The intramuscular veins

are completely emptied, and the intermuscular veins greatly compressed (Fig. 8). The valves of the perforating and deep veins direct a flush of blood up the thoroughfare deep veins, causing a modest and transient rise of pressure in the latter. During the phase of *muscular relaxation* there is a sharp pressure fall in the deep veins, then a rising slope while they refill with blood from the muscle circulation, the distal deep veins, and the subcutaneous veins (by way of perforating veins). When *rhythmic muscle contraction-relaxation* (as in walking) is continued, there is a fall of mean pressure in the superficial veins (Fig. 9) to a new steady level (from 90 to about 20 mm. Hg at the ankle), and also a fall in mean deep venous pressure (from 90 to about 40 mm. Hg at the ankle).

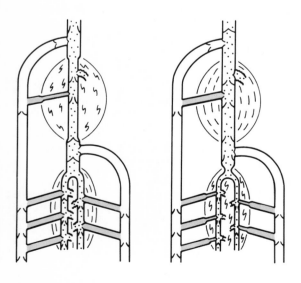

**Figure 8** Schematic representation of the behavior of the lower limb veins and their valves during reciprocal thigh and calf muscle contraction-relaxation, as in walking.

☐ SUPERFICIAL

▨ COMMUNICATING  (ϟ) MUSCLE CONTRACTION

⬚ DEEP  (⎮⎮) MUSCLE RELAXATION

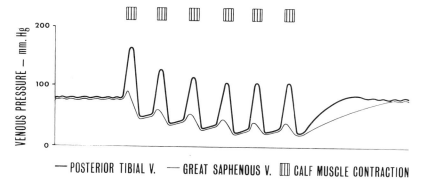

**Figure 9** Diagrammatic representation of the behavior of deep and subcutaneous venous pressures in the lower third of the normal leg during intermittent calf muscle contraction, as in walking.

There are at least three recognizable effects of the musculovenous pumps of the leg. They constitute a genuine form of peripheral heart, or rather, *peripheral supercharger:* calf muscle blood flow can be boosted by nearly 50 per cent over that possible from cardiac action alone. The rhythmic action of the limb muscle pumps also results in a steady-state *blood volume reduction* in the lower limbs, allowing the redistribution of some 200 ml. of blood during ambulation (mainly to the pulmonary vascular bed). A third function is to minimize the accumulation of *tissue fluid* in the lower limbs, which would otherwise be considerable in the upright posture if there were a continuously maintained high subcutaneous venous pressure. Clinical manifestations of disorders of the lower limb muscle pumps occur if free outflow is obstructed (that is, there is *deep vein obstruction*), or if there is *incompetence of the valves* of the subcutaneous or perforating veins.

## INVESTIGATION OF THE VENOUS SYSTEM

While enlightened physical examination remains the mainstay of diagnosis for most disorders of veins, certain special investigations — especially phlebography — are sometimes invaluable. Nevertheless, tests on the venous system are more susceptible to observer and interpretive errors than most.

### Physical Examination

Physical diagnosis of venous disorders is as much a matter of pattern recognition as of systematic clinical logic. However, special mention should be made of tests for *venous valvular incompetence* (Fig. 10), both because of their historic interest and because they sometimes allow of very accurate conclusions. Retrograde flow in the saphenous veins or their varicose tributaries may be seen as the patient stands up. This is made more evident if a proximal venous tourniquet has been applied with the patient supine and the veins empty, and then released when he is erect (Trendelenburg test). Segmentally placed tourniquets may identify incompetent perforating veins, by retrograde filling of the superficial veins in an isolated limb segment when the patient exercises (*Ochsner-Mahorner test*). *Retrograde pressure waves,* or even the *thrill* of retrograde flow, can be felt by the fingers in response to coughing (varicose veins, varicocele). An alternative technique is to tap the vein proximally, and sense the pressure wave by means of a distally placed finger.

### Phlebography

The main uses of this technique are in detecting venous obstruction (especially by thrombus), and venous valvular incompetence (especially of perforating veins). In the case of the lower limb the usual technique is to make the radiocontrast injection into a dorsal vein of the foot, with the patient semierect, so that both superficial and deep veins fill from below up (*ascending phlebography*). A tourniquet above the ankle may be used to encourage filling of the deep veins. Activation of the calf pump by static exercise may also help fill deep and perforating veins (*exercise phlebography*). When no suitable veins are available, injection of radiocontrast material into the medullary cavity of the great trochanter will regularly demonstrate the iliac veins, and into the ankle malleoli or os calcis, the deep veins of the leg (*intraosseous phlebography*).

To demonstrate the upper femoral vein, iliac veins, and inferior vena cava, *direct injection* into one or both femoral veins is usually necessary. The performance of a Valsalva maneuver, or rapid foot-down tilting, helps to arrest the contrast medium, and if the femoral venous valves are incompetent the contrast medium may be forced distally to outline the whole length of the femoral vein (*descending phlebography*). Inaccessible deep veins can be demonstrated by sophisticated *orthograde* techniques (splenic portography, transhepatic hepatic phlebography), or by *retrograde catheterization* (renal, adrenal, hepatic veins).

### Radionuclide Techniques

Gamma detection after the injection of iodine-131-labeled fibrinogen, plasminogen, antifibrinogen, and antithrombin has been used to identify the location at which a thrombus is being formed. However, the most widely used radiopharmaceutical (and apparently the most reliable) has been [125]I-labeled fibrinogen, with a half-life of 60 days. Incorporation of the labeled fibrinogen into a developing thrombus is identified by means of a hand-held gamma detector and rate meter. Indices of a thrombus are the development of asymmetry

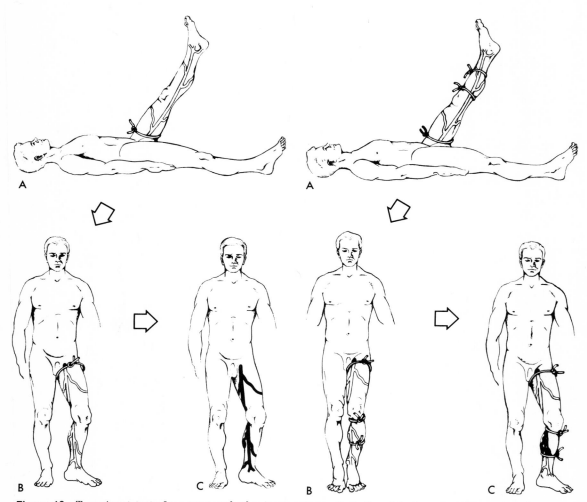

**Figure 10**  Tourniquet tests for venous valvular incompetence. Left, Trendelenburg test for great saphenous incompetence. Right, Ochsner-Mahorner test for perforating vein incompetence.

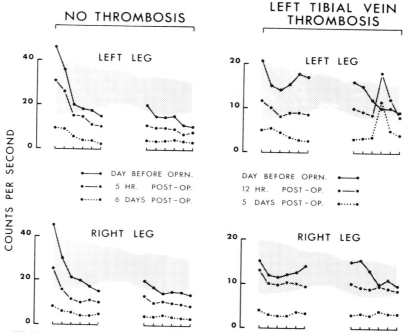

**Figure 11**  The $^{125}$I-fibrinogen test for deep leg vein thrombosis, showing the temporal and spatial pattern of gamma emission in two patients in the perioperative period. *Left,* Normal pattern. *Right,* pattern of development of a left tibial vein thrombosis. (After Flanc, C., Kakkar, V. V., and Clarke, M. B.: Brit. J. Surg., 55:742, 1968.)

in the gamma emission pattern of the two limbs, or of a rising gamma emission at one point compared with the precordial count (Fig. 11). The results of the test correlate excellently with phlebography, but it is only applicable to the lower limb below midthigh level. This test has proved invaluable in epidemiologic surveys and clinical trials of preventive measures and treatment.

### Venous Pressure and Flow

*Venous pressure measurements* have had only a limited clinical application. Obstruction to a vein usually causes only a small pressure rise distally, unless an increase in blood flow is provoked (as by exercise in the case of a limb). Though venous pressure measurement is probably the most accurate way of detecting perforating vein incompetence in the lower limb (see Figs. 9 and 18), it is rarely used as a routine diagnostic technique.

Qualitative measurement of femoral vein flow by the external application of a *Doppler effect ultrasonic flowmeter* has been used as a screening test for iliofemoral venous thrombosis, and to detect the reverse flow that occurs on exercise at the site of incompetent perforating veins. *Thermography* has also been used for this purpose, incompetent perforating veins appearing as "hot spots."

# PATHOGENESIS AND CLINICAL PATTERNS OF VENOUS DISEASE OF THE LIMBS

The possible ways in which veins and their contained blood react to disease or injury are very

limited. Chief among them are thrombosis, obstruction, dilatation, and hemorrhage. Causative of these reactions are a number of more or less well understood pathogenic mechanisms. Resulting from these pathologic reactions of veins are a variety of clinical manifestations, determined mainly by the location of the affected veins.

## VENOUS THROMBOSIS

The sequence of events was quite clearly described by Eberth and Schimmelbusch in 1888; their classic description has scarcely been bettered since. The initial phase is the same as that in any other blood vessel: adherence of platelets to the endothelium, and the buildup of a platelet aggregate. Superimposed on the aggregate there is deposited a mesh of fibrin, the two constituting a *white thrombus.* In a vein (in contrast to an artery) the white thrombus tends to occlude the lumen, and to arrest the flow of blood in a segment between tributaries. The stagnant blood in the vein clots as if in a test tube, forming a mesh of red cells, platelets, and fibrin. This *red thrombus* exhibits other features of a test-tube clot, in that it tends to retract, and may undergo lysis.

The further behavior (Fig. 12) of a venous thrombus is the result of two competing processes. On the one hand it tends to be rapidly dissolved over a matter of days from the action of *fibrinolysins* that are normally present in the thrombus, in the vein wall, and in the plasma. It is during this phase that large portions of a thrombus may break

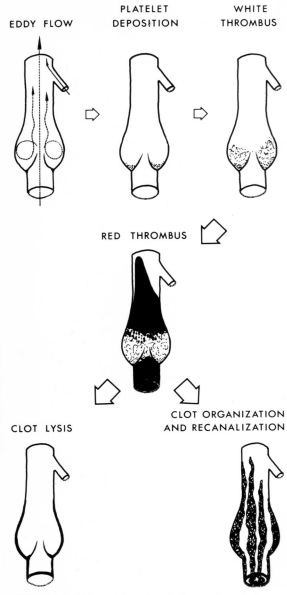

EDDY FLOW  PLATELET DEPOSITION  WHITE THROMBUS

RED THROMBUS

CLOT LYSIS  CLOT ORGANIZATION AND RECANALIZATION

**Figure 12**   The pattern of evolution and resolution of a venous thrombus.

ized thrombus tends to become *recanalized* over a period of weeks, usually by multiple small channels. The *venous valves* are important in this whole process: first, because the initial platelet aggregate tends to occur in a valve sinus (presumably because of eddy currents), and second, because if the process of organization and recanalization has an opportunity to occur, it incorporates and then destroys the valve cusps and their function.

The etiology of venous thrombosis is complex. It is classically represented as resulting from the action of Virchow's triad: (1) reduced blood flow, (2) blood hypercoagulability, and (3) endothelial damage. Over the past century opinion has swung to favor one or other of these three factors as pre-eminent. Yet in clinical practice it is only rarely that any one of the triad can be clearly implicated.

### Subcutaneous (Superficial) Venous Thrombosis

In clinical practice a specific cause for superficial venous thrombosis can often be identified. In the case of the upper limb it is most often the result of an intravenous infusion, occasionally of bacterial cellulitis. A common association in the lower limb is with varicosity of the affected vein. Sometimes there has been a precipitating local blunt injury, and much less often infection. When recurrent thrombosis at different sites occurs (thrombophlebitis migrans), a systemic cause may be identifiable at the time or later.

Thrombosis of a subcutaneous vein is always accompanied by a vigorous inflammatory reaction. For this reason an alternative descriptive term— *superficial thrombophlebitis*—is often used. The patient almost always experiences pain, the skin over the affected vein is reddened, edematous, and hot, and there is often fever. In lean patients the thrombosed segment of vein can usually be clearly felt, but when the subcutaneous fat is thick (particularly in the lower limbs) the venous origin of the inflammatory process may be disguised. The true diagnosis may (but should not) be confused with such conditions as bacterial cellulitis, acute gout, or any one of a number of other less common inflammatory processes.

Thrombi in subcutaneous veins rarely if ever escape as emboli, even in the case of the large veins of the lower limb (because of the firm inflammatory adherence of the thrombus to the vein wall). Nevertheless, pulmonary embolism does occur in association with superficial lower limb venous thrombosis. This contradiction is explained by concomitant deep vein thrombosis, either from extension of the thrombus through perforating veins, or merely from enforced inactivity. Thus there is a good case for seeking phlebographic evidence of deep vein involvement in patients with extensive subcutaneous venous thrombosis of the lower limbs. In the absence of deep vein involvement, the treatment of superficial venous thrombosis is usually symptomatic: pain relief, local heat, compression bandaging, and continued ambulatory activity.

off and be swept as *emboli* to lodge in the pulmonary arterial tree. At the same time, a much slower process of *inflammation* in and around the wall of the vein, followed by *fibroblastic organization* of the thrombus, is going on. Provided an individual thrombus does not embolize, its fate may vary from complete dissolution, leaving the structure of the vein almost unimpaired (when the thrombus and the area of its attachment are small, and fibrinolysis is active), to its conversion into fibrous tissue (when the thrombus and its area of attachment are large, and fibrinolysis is weak). The terms *phlebothrombosis* and *thrombophlebitis* are sometimes used to describe these two patterns of pathologic (and clinical) behavior. An organ-

### Deep Vein Thrombosis in the Lower Limb

The clinically important form of venous thrombosis is that which occurs in deep veins, and particularly in those of the lower limb. The mode of action of the initiating mechanisms is still largely speculative, though a number of clear associations are recognizable. There is usually a background of inactivity, whether from confinement to bed, to an airplane seat, or to a chair in front of the television. Similar contributory causes are surgical operation and heart failure. Autopsy studies have identified thrombi in the deep veins of about 80 per cent of those who have died after more than 1 week's recumbency from disease or injury. Studies with $^{125}$I-labeled fibrinogen have shown that leg vein thrombosis develops in the intraoperative and postoperative period in about 35 per cent of middle-aged patients undergoing major operation. A similar incidence has been found among those who suffer acute myocardial infarction. Autopsy and phlebographic studies have shown that the two favored sites are the deep veins of the lower leg (soleal venous sinuses, the popliteal vein and its tributaries), and the so-called iliofemoral venous segment (common and external iliac veins, femoral vein at the groin). Thrombosis at either site may occur in isolation, or thrombosis may occur at both sites, usually independently but sometimes by propagation (Fig. 13).

These may (or may not) be simple blood flow phenomena. Following operation, there is a reduction in the transit time from ankle to groin of sodium-24 injected into the great saphenous vein, maximal at about the tenth postoperative day. Plethysmographic measurements have confirmed a reduction in calf blood flow. However, recent evidence from $^{125}$I-fibrinogen studies suggests that in patients who incur deep vein thrombosis in association with surgical operations the thrombotic process often commences on the operating table. There is thus a gross discrepancy between the reported time of maximal postoperative venous flow reduction and the time at which most venous thrombi commence to form.

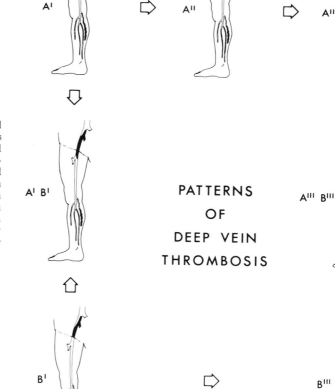

**Figure 13** Spatial and temporal patterns of deep lower limb venous thrombosis. Commencing in a soleal venous sinus ($A^I$), a thrombus can extend to the tibial veins ($A^{II}$), and popliteal vein ($A^{III}$). Commencing in the iliac veins ($B^I$), a thrombus can extend to the femoral vein ($B^{III}$). An iliofemoral thrombus can coexist with a leg vein thrombus, independently ($A^IB^I$) or by extension from above or below ($A^{III}B^{III}$).

PATTERNS OF DEEP VEIN THROMBOSIS

There are certain other proven associations with deep vein thrombosis. The incidence is high in thrombocytosis, especially in polycythemia vera or after splenectomy. There have been reports of increase in the platelet count and adhesiveness, elevation of levels of fibrinogen, prothrombin, and other plasma clotting factors, and diminished plasma fibrinolytic activity, following operation. However, that platelet adhesiveness increases has been seriously challenged, no clear correlation between the magnitude of these changes in the individual patient and the occurrence of venous thrombosis has emerged, and the reported changes again tend to be maximal at about the tenth postoperative day.

*Estrogen administration,* whether therapeutic (carcinoma of prostate) or in the form of the contraceptive pill, is associated with a statistically greater risk of venous thromboembolism. Remote *malignant neoplasms* (especially bronchial, pancreatic, and renal) may be associated with bizarre and widespread episodes of superficial and deep venous thrombosis. This *thrombophlebitis migrans* may also occur in Buerger's disease, and in a variety of systemic disorders from ulcerative colitis to disseminated lupus erythematosus. It is clear that no single causative agency of deep vein thrombosis has yet been identified, though on balance it seems that there is a multifactorial, systemic disturbance of the coagulation mechanism, expressed most evidently in the slow-flow veins of the lower limbs.

The traditional symptoms of *leg (calf) vein thrombosis* are mild pain or tightness in the calf, particularly when the patient is sitting, standing, or walking. The corresponding signs are slight ankle edema, calf muscle tenderness which can be pinpointed by deep finger palpation, and pain when the foot is passively dorsiflexed (Homan's sign). It has belatedly become evident that these signs are grossly unreliable. Extensive calf vein thrombosis may (and commonly does) induce no symptoms or signs whatsoever, and conversely the traditional symptoms and signs may be due to other causes.

If it be important to establish the diagnosis beyond doubt (as is the case if prolonged and potentially hazardous therapy is contemplated, or if pulmonary embolism is suspected), phlebographic confirmation or denial of the diagnosis is essential.

In its florid form, *acute iliofemoral venous thrombosis* is easily recognizable. Sometimes there is premonitory mild soreness in the iliac fossa or groin, and a low-grade fever (even to the point of mimicking appendicitis or diverticulitis). When the main vein becomes completely occluded the entire lower limb becomes swollen. If the patient is bedridden, this swelling may be of gradual onset and insignificant. If he is ambulant, it is common for the limb to become acutely swollen, and tightly uncomfortable, over a matter of minutes or hours. To examination, the limb is uniformly swollen up to the groin, and deeper in color than normal. Subcutaneous veins may be visibly fuller, particularly in the groin where they are acting as collaterals. To palpation, all tissue layers are edematous: not only is there pitting subcutaneous edema, but the muscle compartments are palpably turgid. Thus the limb exhibits the signs of acute venous outflow obstruction, and this has occurred either because external and internal iliac veins are both occluded, or because the main femoral vein and its deep femoral tributary are both blocked. Rarely, thrombosis of the deep system of veins may be so extensive, and so limiting to blood flow, as to threaten or cause *gangrene* of the toes, feet, or even leg (while the arterial tree remains demonstrably patent).

At an earlier stage a large, long, clinically silent thrombus may have been present in the iliac veins, adherent at only one spot and allowing flow past it. This may never be detected; it may extend and become adherent to produce the classic syndrome just described, or it may break loose as a potentially lethal embolus. The more extensive use of phlebography has revealed that such *silent thrombi* are remarkably common. When acute venous outflow obstruction occurs, there is usually no doubt as to the diagnosis. There are nevertheless strong indications for phlebography (or possibly Doppler flowmetry), in order to exclude a contralateral, silent, potentially lethal iliofemoral thrombus.

The three common sequels to lower limb deep vein thrombosis are pulmonary embolization (see Chapter 39), continuing obstruction to venous flow, and damage and malfunction of venous valves. *Malfunction of valves* occurs from damage caused by recanalization of a thrombus. It is clinically recognizable only when thrombosis has affected the deep and perforating veins of the leg. The manifestations are varicose veins or leg ulceration or both. *Continuing venous obstruction* is recognizable only when the thrombus occludes a major vein (iliac, femoral, popliteal) and undergoes organization rather than lysis. Edematous swelling of the limb is the chief clinical manifestation.

The aims of *prophylactic and therapeutic measures* for deep vein thrombosis are to prevent the condition itself or to prevent its sequelae, whether the latter be remote (pulmonary embolism) or confined to the affected limb (chronic venous outflow obstruction; venous valve damage and leg ulceration). Great and increasing emphasis has been placed on prophylaxis for at least three decades. The simple reason is that the incidence of the disorder in at-risk (e.g., hospital) populations is so high that the alternative approach of detect and cure is impractical. The three approaches used have been attempts to nullify one or other of the three elements of Virchow's triad. Almost all clinical trials that have used a clinical end point are of little more than historic interest, because of the low diagnostic accuracy inherent in clinical symptoms and signs. Only the demonstration of deep vein thrombosis by phlebography, or by gamma detection of [125]I-labeled fibrinogen, is acceptable.

It has been hard to accept mechanical *endothelial damage* as a cause for human deep vein thrombosis, and there is no evidence that prophylactic measures such as elevation of the calves from the operating table are effective.

Attempts have been made to increase the velocity of deep vein *flow*. Lower limb elevation and compression bandages probably do this, and early postoperative ambulation and leg exercises may do so. Neither approach has been shown to be effective. A more recent approach is based on evidence that venous thrombosis is commonly initiated on the operating table. Repetitive electrical stimulation of the calf muscles has been claimed to lower the incidence of leg vein thrombosis. Indeed, this claim must in the meantime stand, for while some reports have failed to corroborate it, a trial in which [125]I-fibrinogen uptake was used as the index of thrombosis has supported it.

The third approach has been to diminish *blood coagulability*. Well controlled clinical trials have demonstrated that heparin or prothrombin depressants (coumarins, indandiones) lower the incidence of pulmonary embolism (but only by inference of deep vein thrombosis) in high-risk groups of patients with myocardial infarction, with fractured neck of femur, or undergoing gynecologic procedures. The anticoagulants were used in full therapeutic dosage and with careful control: the latter may not be so readily attainable in everyday practice. Dextran infusions (mean molecular weight 70,000) in the peroperative period have been shown to be superior to warfarin in preventing deep vein thrombosis in gynecologic patients, and effective in preventing deep vein thrombosis in patients with fractured neck of femur (though other studies have not shown dextran to be effec-

tive). Low-dose heparin therapy has been tried prophylactically, as have inhibitors of platelet adhesiveness (dipyridamole, hydroxychloroquine). These can not yet be accepted as being of proven value, if only because of the design of the trials.

In summary, the need is great for discovery of a safe and effective means of preventing deep vein thrombosis in all predisposed patients. The most that can be said is that a reduction in incidence can be achieved in certain exceptionally high-risk groups by means of anticoagulant drugs, but at the risk of side effects such as bleeding. Attempts are being made to identify the patient at high risk (or in whom venous thrombosis is occurring) by blood measurements of fibrin degradation products, by a rapid fall in blood [125]I-fibrinogen level, or by the more elaborate procedure of measuring [125]I-fibrinogen uptake in the legs. If the high-risk patient can be identified, clinicians will feel more secure in offering him prophylaxis with potentially dangerous drugs.

From the 1940s to the 1960s the established method of *treatment* for deep vein thrombosis was by administering *anticoagulant drugs:* heparin by intravenous (and sometimes subcutaneous) injection, or prothrombin depressants by mouth. The new anticoagulant agent arvin, a fibrinogen depressant obtained from the Malayan pit viper, has not yet been used extensively. The rational basis of the therapy has been to attempt to stop progression of the thrombotic process. No scientifically controlled trials have been carried out which provide direct proof of benefit from anticoagulants in deep vein thrombosis, but most clinicians have believed this therapy to be beneficial. Because epi-

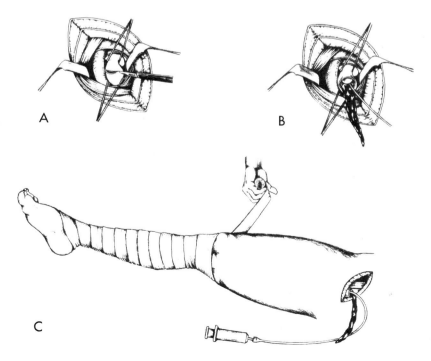

**Figure 14** The steps in iliofemoral venous thrombectomy. *A*, Exposure, taping, and incision of the femoral vein. *B*, Extraction of proximal thrombus with a Fogarty balloon catheter. *C*, Removal of distal thrombus with a combination of Fogarty catheter and pressure bandaging.

sodes of recrudescence of thrombosis are common, there has been a tendency to maintain therapy for increasing periods of time (3 to 12 months).

A more recent development has been the use of *fibrinolytic agents,* in an attempt to actually dissolve the clot (and thus avoid valve damage, or continuing obstruction from organized thrombus). The most commonly used agent has been purified *streptokinase,* given systemically or locally. Clinical trials have suggested that it is superior to heparin in resolving venous thrombi, though with a greater risk of bleeding episodes. Similar evidence has accumulated for the use of *urokinase,* although it is not yet available for general distribution.

There were isolated reports of *surgical removal* of venous thrombi by Laewen (1937) and Leriche and Geisendorf (1939), before Mahorner and his colleagues introduced iliofemoral venous thrombectomy in its modern form in 1957. Recent thrombi in the iliac and femoral veins can be removed via the femoral vein at the groin, under local or general anesthesia, by means of a balloon-tipped (Fogarty) catheter (Fig. 14). Technically, and in terms of end result, the operation of venous thrombectomy is most suitably performed within 7 to 10 days of the recognition of the condition. Unfortunately, the rather dramatic removal of large quantities of thrombus has not been matched by quality of the end result. Follow-up phlebographic studies have demonstrated rethrombosis or gross valvular damage in a very high proportion of patients, and comparisons of operation and drug therapy have not greatly favored operation. Nevertheless, the operation has a definite place in patients with threatened or actual venous gangrene, and possibly in the young, previously well patient in whom an iliofemoral thrombosis develops suddenly and inexplicably.

### Other Forms of Venous Thrombosis

In the upper limb, *axillary-subclavian* vein thrombosis is worthy of note. The etiology of this condition is distinct from that of deep lower limb venous thrombosis. The typical victim is a well muscled young man who has recently taken up an unaccustomed, vigorous occupation, or has engaged in some form of violent upper limb exercise: hence the term "effort thrombosis." It seems highly probable that the initiating factor is injury to the vein wall as it crosses the first rib. Treatment is by anticoagulant or fibrinolytic drugs, or by thrombectomy. However, the end result tends to be continuing venous obstruction, with limb swelling during exercise.

*Inferior vena caval thrombosis* may rarely occur as a neonatal phenomenon, with swelling (and sometimes venous gangrene) in both lower limbs. In adults, the condition may also occur spontaneously, usually as an extension of bilateral iliac vein thrombosis. The commonest cause of caval thrombosis in adult life is probably *surgical caval interruption* for thromboembolism. *Renal vein thrombosis* may occur as an isolated incident, manifest as a form of nephrotic syndrome. *Hepatic vein thrombosis* may occur apparently spontaneously, in association with polycythemia vera (Budd-Chiari syndrome), or with a caval diaphragm and caval thrombosis. The main manifestations are disturbances of liver function, together with gross hepatomegaly and ascites. *Thrombosis of the portal vein* can occur in neonatal life, supposedly by extension of septic thrombophlebitis in the umbilical vein. Extensive collateral development occurs, both locally (cavernous transformation of the portal vein) and at a distance (gastroesophageal varices). Thrombosis of the portal and even splenic and superior mesenteric veins may occur in adult life in association with liver cirrhosis, and rarely as spontaneous events. Acute thrombosis of *mesenteric or omental veins* may cause an apparent or real abdominal emergency, with pain resulting from local inflammation, segmental paralysis of the gut, or even venous gangrene.

*Superior vena caval* or innominate vein thrombosis most often results from compression, usually by a bronchial cancer or its lymph node metastases, less often by other superior mediastinal tumors (thyroid, thymus, lymphoma). It is recognizable by swelling of the neck and face and readily visible engorgement of the subcutaneous veins of the head and neck.

Occasionally, particularly in association with septic abortion, puerperal sepsis, or tubal infection, *septic thrombi* occur in the pelvic veins. Together with signs of major venous obstruction there is high fever from septicemia, and sometimes septic pulmonary emboli occur via the iliac or ovarian veins. Septic thrombi can occur at other sites: the *cavernous sinus* from propagated facial infection, and as an iatrogenic disease from infection at the variety of sites at which *intravenous catheters* are placed.

## VENOUS OBSTRUCTION

Whether occlusion of the lumen of a vein results in any clinical manifestation depends on the anatomic location of the affected vein and on the length of vein involved. These two factors are important in determining whether there are sufficient alternative venous pathways (collateral veins) to allow continuing venous outflow at low pressure.

Obstruction (or operative excision) of subcutaneous veins rarely results in recognizable dysfunction, because of the great number of superficial and perforating veins that can act as collaterals. Conversely, there are certain critical segments of the deep venous system in which occlusion does result in abnormalities of pressure or flow. Examples of the latter are the cavernous sinus, the subclavian vein, the superior vena cava, the suprarenal inferior vena cava, hepatic veins, the portal vein, the right renal vein, and the iliofemoral venous segment. The consequence of venous occlusion at these critical sites is edematous swelling of

# NORMAL

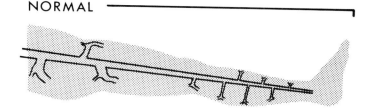

# LEG VEIN THROMBOSIS

- SHORT SEGMENT
- MANY COLLATERALS
- MINIMAL EDEMA

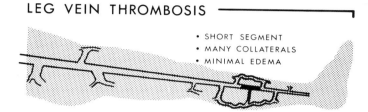

# ILIO-FEMORAL VEIN THROMBOSIS

- LONG SEGMENT
- LIMITED COLLATERALS
- GROSS EDEMA

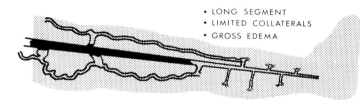

**Figure 15** The obstructive effects of leg vein thrombosis versus iliofemoral vein thrombosis.

the tissues in the venous watershed, dilatation of collateral veins (which may be visible if subcutaneous), and organ-specific dysfunctions such as convulsions (cavernous sinus), proteinuria (renal vein), ascites (hepatic or portal veins), and skin ulceration (lower limb veins).

The most common cause for clinically significant venous obstruction is thrombosis, whether acute (and completely occluding the lumen) or recanalized (as multiple, small, high-resistance channels).

*Iliofemoral venous thrombosis* that has been so extensive as to produce generalized lower limb swelling almost always results in chronic venous outflow obstruction no matter how aggressive the treatment. The manifestations of this are edematous swelling of all tissue layers of the lower limb (Fig. 15), a greater depth of color of the skin and sometimes a bluish hue, and visible and palpable subcutaneous collateral veins running from the groin onto the abdominal wall (and thence to the axilla or opposite groin). Walking or running increases the swelling and turgor, and sometimes results in a bursting, deep pain (venous claudication). Chronic venous obstruction and the edema of lymphatic obstruction are sometimes confused. A successful search for collateral veins provides a very strong index of suspicion that the limb swelling is venous in origin, though phlebography may be necessary to establish the nature and extent of the venous occlusion.

The obstruction that may result from extensive thrombotic occlusion of veins in the *lower leg* (Fig. 15) is manifest less as chronic edema (which is often mild) than as varicose subcutaneous veins and associated skin changes such as eczema, fat necrosis, or ulceration.

Uncommonly, *nonthrombotic venous obstruction* may occur. This is a misnomer, as external compression of a vein is likely to lead to secondary thrombosis. Recognition of this form of venous obstruction demands an awareness of some of the causes. In general, these are either benign lesions growing in a restricted compartment or malignant neoplasms. Among the benign lesions are aneurysms of the aorta, or iliac, femoral, or popliteal arteries; popliteal cysts, or benign neoplasms within the popliteal fossa; and rarely giant abdomino-pelvic tumors such as uterine fibroids, ovarian cysts, and the pregnant uterus. Among the malignant neoplasms is cancer of the sigmoid colon, ovary, or uterine cervix. Miscellaneous causes include retroperitoneal fibrosis and surgical misadventure.

Some success has been attained by *surgical treatment* of patients with chronic iliac or femoral vein obstruction. The most versatile technique has been to use the great saphenous vein to create a bypass. An advantage of this method is that only one anastomosis is necessary, and so, it is hoped, the risk of thrombosis is reduced. It also places the

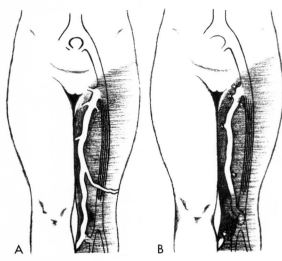

**Figure 16** Popliteal-femoral saphenous bypass operation for femoral vein obstruction.

valves in the direction of flow, though whether they remain competent is less certain. The technique was first used as a crossed bypass in patients with iliac vein obstruction, but has also been employed as a popliteal-femoral bypass (Fig. 16). It has been reasonably successful in cases of non-thrombotic venous occlusion (neoplastic invasion, accidental or surgical damage), but much less so in post-thrombotic obstruction. Post-thrombotic stenosis, particularly of the left common iliac vein where it passes behind the right common iliac artery, has been treated by local *venoplasty* but the results have usually been disappointing. A similar technique has been used to relieve *postmastectomy swelling* of the arm when this is due to axillary vein stenosis.

The cause of superior *vena caval obstruction* (with or without thrombosis) is most often a malignant neoplasm, and radiotherapy may relieve symptoms. However, a number of ingenious resective and bypass procedures have been employed to overcome the venous engorgement of the head and neck.

Nonoperative forms of treatment—elastic stockings, massage, and diuretics—are purely palliative and no more than modestly successful.

## VARICOSE VEINS

Dilated veins commonly assume a varicose form. In most circumstances when the diameter of a vein is abnormally increased, so is its length between fixed points; that is, it becomes tortuous as well as thin-walled. The direct consequences of the dilation are either *cosmetic* (subcutaneous varicose veins) or a greatly increased risk of *hemorrhage* (gastroesophageal varices). The cutaneous *ulceration* associated with lower limb varicose veins is a consequence of the cause of the varicose veins:

malfunction of the musculovenous pumps of the leg.

*Obstruction* is one cause for venous dilatation—in this circumstance, of collateral veins: hence, portal vein obstruction (gastroesophageal varices), and iliofemoral or inferior vena caval obstruction (groin-abdominal wall collaterals). Rarely, dilatation may result from a prolonged and great increase in systemic or regional venous pressure, due to a nearby *arteriovenous fistula* or to *tricuspid valve incompetence:* in these circumstances the dilated veins usually pulsate. However, by far the commonest causes for varicose veins of the lower limb are more or less well defined disorders of the *musculovenous pumps*.

### Primary Varicose Veins

This is a rather unsatisfactory term that is used to describe a clearly identifiable disease pattern affecting the subcutaneous veins of the lower limb. The condition is familial, though in rather a vague way: the mode of inheritance has been variously described as autosomal dominant, autosomal recessive, and sex-linked recessive. It is expressed more commonly in women than in men, and it is commoner among populations with high living standards. The underlying defect is clearly inborn, for the condition can often be recognized shortly after adolescence. It is not clear whether the primary defect is of the venous valves themselves, of the vein wall, or (more probably) of both. At all events, incompetence of subcutaneous venous valves is an invariable accompaniment. A plausible explanation, though it has not been completely proved, is that one inborn defect is absence or hypoplasia of the external iliac venous valve. The evidence for this is that primary varicose veins are invariably associated with incompetence of this valve, and that in a high proportion of young people with a family history of varicose veins (but who have not yet themselves been affected) this valve is incompetent. It is supposed that transient pressure rises from exertion and coughing expand the saphenofemoral junction, rendering incompetent the terminal saphenous valves. This process spreads downward in a fashion that is sequential, but that affects the tributaries of the great saphenous vein in a random manner. Thus any, or all, of its tributaries may be picked out to become varicose (Fig. 17). The small saphenous vein and its tributaries are less often affected, and then either because of incompetent subcutaneous communications between it and a varicose great saphenous vein, or because the femoral and popliteal (deep) venous valves have become incompetent (Fig. 17). Tributaries of the internal iliac vein (vulva, back of thigh) may also become varicose by a similar process (Fig. 17).

An alternative explanation that has been advanced is that the disorder is one of abnormally increased blood flow through the superficial veins, leading to dilatation in an analogous fashion to that which occurs in the case of collateral veins or an arteriovenous fistula. Two mechanisms for such an increase in blood flow have been suggested.

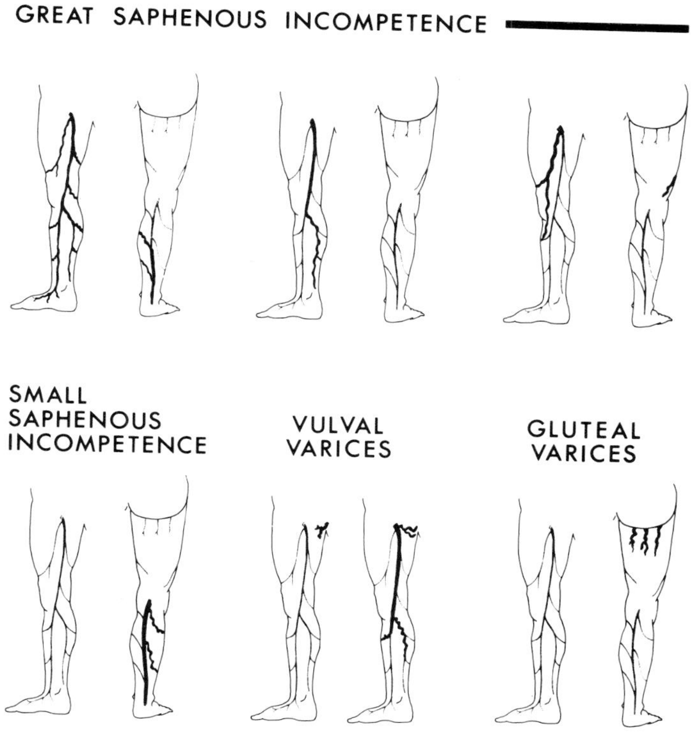

## GREAT SAPHENOUS INCOMPETENCE

**Figure 17**   Patterns of primary varicose veins. *Top,* Great saphenous incompetence resulting in gross varicose veins (*left*) of great and small saphenous systems; (*center*) of the posterior arch vein; (*right*) of the lateral femoral cutaneous vein. *Bottom,* Primary small saphenous incompetence; vulval varices, from (*left*) internal pudendal incompetence or (*right*) great saphenous incompetence; gluteal varices from internal iliac incompetence.

**SMALL SAPHENOUS INCOMPETENCE**     **VULVAL VARICES**     **GLUTEAL VARICES**

One is that there are multiple microscopic arteriovenous shunts present in the skin. The other is that valvular incompetence in perforating veins occurs as the primary defect, causing a rerouting of deep venous blood through subcutaneous veins. On present evidence, neither of these latter explanations is as satisfactory as that of sequential valvular incompetence.

Another association with primary varicose veins has been suggested: an *aberration of endocrine function,* or an abnormal response to normal endocrine secretion. There is some evidence to support this view. The sex difference in incidence is evident before childbearing. Increase in size of varicose veins is often apparent in the first trimester of pregnancy, before vena caval obstruction by the pregnant uterus is demonstrable. A cyclic premenstrual exacerbation of varicose veins is quite common. Indeed, it is difficult to escape the conclusion that overlying the genetic basis is an endocrine effect, whether estrogenic or other, that accounts for the sex difference in incidence.

The *clinical manifestations* are chiefly cosmetic, and the demand for treatment is closely related to the sophistication of the female society, and to current fashions in clothing. The physical manifestations are not so clear-cut. Among them are aching of the legs after standing, night cramps, and swelling of the ankles. However, some care must be taken in the interpretation of these symptoms. Those in the age group that most commonly seeks medical attention for this condition (35 to 45 years) tend to notice aching legs even in the absence of varicose veins. Night cramps afflict a cross section of the otherwise normal population. In older age groups there is a variety of causes for leg pain, ranging from arterial obstruction to degenerative hip or knee joint disease. While increased tissue fluid accumulation does occur in this condition, frank pitting edema usually has some other cause. Any or all of these symptoms may be blamed by the patient (and by his unwary doctor) on visible varicose veins.

There are definite complications of primary varicose veins. They are more susceptible to thrombosis, and to laceration or blunt rupture, than normal veins. When the varicose condition is of long standing, and especially when venous dilatation is gross, skin eczema or ulceration may occur. There is a clear association between these changes and failure of the calf muscle pump to lower subcutaneous venous pressure, just as there is clear evidence that correction of the pump defect is the major prerequisite to reversal of the skin changes. In the case of primary varicose veins, subcutaneous venous pressure fails to fall on exercise because the saphenous vein and its varicose tributaries have become wide-bore pipelines connecting the central venous pool to the skin of the leg (Fig. 18).

Gross varicose veins may have a capacity of several hundred milliliters. As a result, such patients tend to have greater postural swings of right atrial pressure, heart rate, cardiac output, and arterial pressure than normal, sometimes to the point of postural syncope.

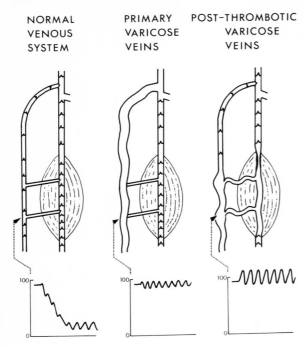

NORMAL          PRIMARY        POST-THROMBOTIC
VENOUS          VARICOSE       VARICOSE
SYSTEM          VEINS          VEINS

**Figure 18**  The causes of high subcutaneous venous pressure in association with leg ulcers. *Top,* The valvular defects. *Bottom,* The resulting ambulatory venous pressure patterns.

The differentiation of primary varicose veins from the post-thrombotic variety is not always easy. Features characteristic of the former are an early age of onset (15 to 25); the ability to trace the varicose veins back to the saphenofemoral junction (and rarely the saphenopopliteal junction) by inspection, palpation, or percussion; and the ability to completely prevent reflux filling of the varicose veins by the Trendelenburg tourniquet test.

### Post-thrombotic Varicose Veins

This is a useful descriptive term for the syndrome of perforating vein valve incompetence. It is presumed that prior deep vein thrombosis has resulted in a degree of deep vein obstruction, combined with damage to the valves of the deep and perforating veins. In only about half of such patients has the preceding thrombotic episode been overt, but it is now apparent that clinically unrecognized deep vein thrombosis is a rather common event in the population. In the case of perforating vein incompetence, the distending force that is exerted on the wall of the subcutaneous vein is provided by muscle contraction, which squirts jets of blood at high pressure into the superficial system (see Fig. 18): the incompetent perforating veins have become the line of least resistance for the output of the musculovenous pump. Rarely, complete *absence of deep and communicating vein valves* occurs as a congenital familial defect.

When there has been a history of florid venous thrombosis in the past, diagnosis is simple. Otherwise, the features to be described must be sought. These patients tend to be a little older than those

with primary varicose veins. Post-thrombotic varicose veins are rarely as large as the primary type, and are often partly concealed by overlying eczema, subcutaneous fat necrosis, or ulceration. In theory, it should be possible to detect incompetence of the valves in affected perforating veins by means of the Ochsner-Mahorner test. In practice, because of the small size or obscurity of the varices, the result of this test is often equivocal. To complicate matters, there is often dilatation of the great saphenous vein or its tributaries, whether as a chance association, because these have acted as collateral veins round a deep venous block, or even merely from carrying the blood that is pumped in a retrograde direction from deep to superficial veins.

It has been suggested that a "flare" of intracutaneous varices over the medial malleolus is diagnostic of post-thrombotic varices, but this is not necessarily true. It has also been suggested that the dilated perforating veins can be localized by feeling the holes in the deep fascia through which they pass; but the apparent holes are more often a rim of subcutaneous fat necrosis surrounding a subcutaneous varix.

Various special tests to identify incompetent perforating veins have been described, including thermography, Doppler flowmetry, phlebography. Interpretation of even the latter is susceptible to observer error, and diagnosis is most accurately made on a basic of pattern recognition by an experienced clinician.

### Miscellaneous Forms of Varicose Veins

When varicose veins are associated with an increase in girth (but not length) of the entire limb, care should be taken that these are not *collateral veins*, resulting from chronic deep venous obstruction (usually post-thrombotic, and usually in the iliofemoral segment).

Gross varicose veins that appear before the age of 16 to 20 years may represent one of the rarer forms of congenital anomaly. Multiple *congenital arteriovenous fistulas* often do not become evident till the growth of puberty, when a manifestation may be varicose veins of unusual distribution, which may show arterial pulsation, and over which the skin temperature is raised. A rare cause of juvenile varicose veins is congenital, often *hereditary, absence of deep vein valves.*

In adult life there are other vascular blemishes that are usually, though by no means always, associated with primary varicose veins. Fans of *dilated intracutaneous veins* may appear in irregular patches on the lower limb. These are ugly, and are not significantly improved by the usual methods of treating varicose veins. Small (less than 1 cm.), raised, discrete, red, painful vascular anomalies are sometimes associated with varicose veins, and have been termed *angiectids.* They occur only in women, and have as their characteristic that they enlarge and become extremely painful during the premenstrual period and especially during pregnancy. They are presumed to be endocrine-determined microscopic arteriovenous fistulas. Dilated veins in the region of an *acquired arteriovenous fistula* are easily recognizable from a history of injury, increased skin temperature over the pulsating veins, and an audible local machinery murmur. The pulsating veins of gross *tricuspid valve incompetence* are widespread over the body.

### Venous ("Varicose") Leg Ulcers

Apart from their association with varicose veins, these ulcers have several other distinctive features. The patient is more often obese than of normal weight for height. The ulcer is almost invariably located in the lower third of the leg—the "gaiter" area—and most often above the medial malleolus. It will invariably heal, or show signs of rapid healing, if the patient is put to bed with the affected leg elevated above heart level. The ulcer may be moderately painful when the patient is standing, but rapid and complete pain relief is to be expected from leg elevation. The appearance of the ulcer is not especially characteristic. Its size can vary from a square centimeter to the entire circumference of the lower half of the leg. While the shape is usually regular, it too is highly variable. The skin surrounding the ulcer is commonly eczematous, and almost invariably shows brown pigmentation (due both to a melanocytic reaction and to iron-containing macrophages). This skin and the edge of the ulcer are generally edematous. The wall of the ulcer can be sloping, or at the other extreme, undermined. The floor always shows pink-red granulations when the overlying slough is removed. Recurrent ulceration is associated with progressive loss of subcutaneous tissue, and a visible loss of circumference of the affected por-

tion of the leg (indeed, a firm plaque of subcutaneous fat necrosis often precedes frank ulceration). When fat necrosis is associated with proximal swelling from chronic venous obstruction, the term "inverted bottle leg" is appropriate. The natural history of a venous ulcer is a cycle of healing and recurrence, unless cure of the underlying defect in the musculovenous pump is effected. With whichever form of varicose veins the ulcer is associated, there is the same underlying physiologic disturbance: failure of subcutaneous venous pressure to fall during ambulatory activity (see Fig. 18). Healing of the ulcer can be maintained only if this fall can be restored to near normal.

*Primary varicose veins* can be causative of ulceration, but only when the primary varicose veins are gross and have been evident for many years, and even then the ulceration runs rather a benign course. At least half of all venous ulcers are associated with post-thrombotic *incompetent perforating veins* (Fig. 19). Conversely, clinically recognized florid deep leg vein thrombosis is associated with a very high risk that ulceration will develop in later years. It is remarkable that in this case the varicose veins themselves are often not prominent, and indeed may sometimes be invisible beneath the base or edematous edges of the ulcer. They can nevertheless be detected when the patient is standing, by the spongy compressible quality of the tissues that lie deep to the subcutaneous scarring.

Provided the classic characteristics of venous ulcers are borne in mind, there should not be confusion with the many other forms of leg ulcer that can occur. Nevertheless a great many patients have had actual or supposed varicose veins eradicated for nonvenous forms of ulceration, with at best no improvement, and at worst disastrous consequences. Simple *mechanical injury to the skin* of the lower third of the leg, particularly when there has been full-thickness skin loss, may be slow to heal. *Factitious ulcers* usually show surrounding scratch marks caused by the fingernails. Generalized *atopic dermatitis* is often most floridly expressed in the lower third of the legs. *Ischemic ulcers* from obliterative arterial disease are usually located on the toes or foot. However, concurrence of varicose veins and arterial disease is not uncommon, and in this circumstance an apparent venous ulcer may not heal unless arterial reconstruction is performed. A rare and bizarre ulcer is associated with the names of *Martorell* and *Hines and Farber.* It is an extremely painful, shallow, serpiginous, creeping ulcer, usually on the lateral side of the leg. The original descriptions associated these ulcers with arterial hypertension, but this is not a constant feature. The importance of these ulcers lies in the pain they produce, and in their tendency to recur whatever form of treatment is employed. Other unusual ulcers may be associated with *disseminated lupus erythematosus, macroglobulinemia,* and other systemic disorders that affect blood or blood vessels. *Malignant neoplastic lesions* of the skin (particularly melanoma, squamous cell cancer, and

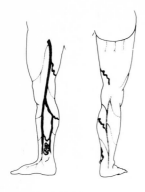

**GROSS GREAT SAPHENOUS INCOMPETENCE**

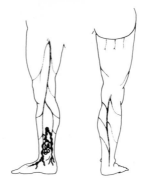

**INCOMPETENT ANTERO - MEDIAL PERFORATORS**

**Figure 19**  The venous pattern in venous ulceration.

Kaposi sarcoma) may occur in the presence of varcose veins and may be mistaken for varicose ulcers. Very occasionally a *squamous cell cancer* may develop at the site of—and apparently as a result of—a very long-standing varicose ulcer.

## Treatment of Varicose Veins and Venous Ulcers

There is a single rational basis for the treatment of varicose veins. It is to interrupt the valveless

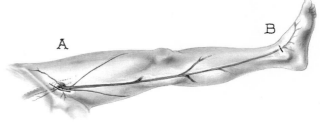

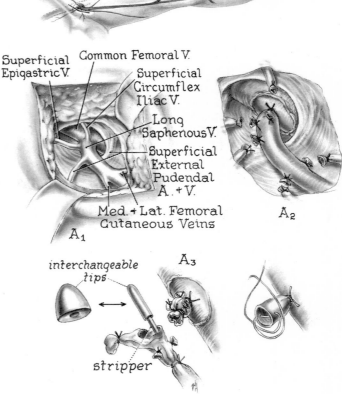

**Figure 20**  The procedure of flush saphenofemoral ligation. *A*, Groin incision. $A_1$, Exposure of the saphenofemoral junction and the terminal saphenous tributaries. $A_2$, Ligation and division of the tributaries. $A_3$, Transfixation-ligation of the great saphenous vein, and the appearance of the Myers stripper passed up from *B*. (From Venous Disease of the Lower Extremities, by A. D. McLachlin. Copyright © 1967, Year Book Medical Publishers. Used by permission.)

pathways between the subcutaneous and deep systems of veins, in order to correct the abnormality of the musculovenous pumps and in the hope that venous blood flow will be rerouted through channels with normal valves. The only controversy is as to how this should be done.

Trendelenburg has the reputation for having first devised a logical operation for *primary varicose veins* in 1891, when he undertook ligation of the great saphenous vein at midthigh level. Perthes pointed out 4 years later that in many of these patients the varicose veins had recurred, and suggested that the site of ligation should be flush with the femoral vein, above the point of entry of the subterminal great saphenous tributaries. It is not clear who first systematically practiced this operation, though the credit is usually given to Homans (1916). Thus one essential component of any procedure for primary great saphenous varicose veins is division of the great saphenous vein flush with the saphenofemoral junction, and division of the tributaries that enter its last 5 to 7 cm. in order to minimize the chance of reconnection of the superficial and deep systems (Fig. 20). An entirely analogous procedure is performed at the saphenopopliteal junction if there is primary varicosity of the small saphenous vein and its tributaries (see Fig. 22).

This procedure by itself will rarely lead to a good cosmetic result, however. The pressure fall in the subcutaneous veins on exercise is restored, but while the patient is standing still the normal hydrostatic pressure still obtains in the persistently varicose subcutaneous veins. Thus a further component of treatment must be to obliterate the varicose veins themselves. This is variously done by multiple ligations through small incisions (to induce thrombosis), by excision of the varicose veins through long incisions, or by injection of sclerosants at a later date. The method of choice depends to some extent on the sex and age of the patient, and the perfection of cosmesis desired.

The third component of a satisfactory operation is to remove the great (or small) saphenous vein itself. This further reduces the risk of reconnection with the deep system at the groin or popliteal fossa. The technique used is to pull, or strip, out the saphenous vein from the ankle to the saphenofemoral or saphenopopliteal junction (Figs. 20–22). This concept was first described by Keller (1905) and Mayo (1906), and perfected by Myers (1947) by the use of an intraluminal braided or cabled wire leader that is passed up the lumen of the vein, and to which is attached a hemiolivary head.

Some care is necessary in the design of the appropriate operation for varicose veins of *small saphenous distribution.* Most stem from saphenofemoral incompetence, as a result of valve incompetence in the subcutaneous veins that link great and small saphenous systems (see Fig. 3). Thus the three-component operation must be applied to both systems. It is much more rarely that "primary" small saphenous incompetence occurs as an isolated event.

The surgical treatment of *post-thrombotic varicose veins* is similar in principle, but different in detail. Every incompetent perforating vein must be identified and divided: the main problem is that of identification, which requires considerable experience. At physical examination the location of incompetent perforating veins can be strongly suspected from the presence of visible and palpable "blowouts" of the subcutaneous veins. Phlebography may help to enumerate and locate perforating veins, especially if radiopaque skin markers are taped over the clinically suspected sites of incompetent perforators. Thermography and Doppler flowmetry have also been used.

When the skin is normal, or relatively normal, it is usual to seek the perforating veins superficial to the deep fascia, and to ligate and divide them in this plane. When there has been ulceration of the skin, and subcutaneous fat necrosis has given a wooden consistency to the tissues, it is preferable to seek them in the subfascial plane. On the medial side of the leg a vertical incision is made 2 to 3 cm. behind the subcutaneous border of the tibia, through which the medial, anteromedial, and even the posterolateral perforating veins can be located and divided (Fig. 23). Linton introduced this technique in 1938 as an incision from tibial tubercle to medial malleolus, and the author believes that this is preferable to the more limited exposure later suggested by Cockett. The less-often incompetent anterolateral perforating veins can be explored through an incision over the anterior tibial compartment.

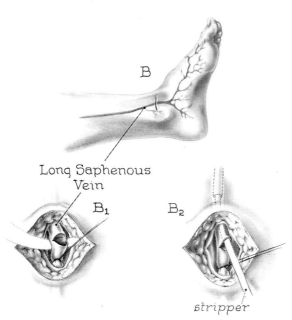

**Figure 21**   Introduction of the Myers stripper into the great (long) saphenous vein at the ankle. (From Venous Disease of the Lower Extremities, by A. D. McLachlin. Copyright © 1967, Year Book Medical Publishers. Used by permission.)

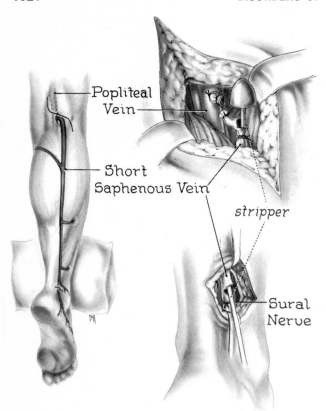

Popliteal Vein

Short Saphenous Vein

*stripper*

Sural Nerve

**Figure 22**  The procedure of flush saphenopopliteal ligation and division, and of small (short) saphenous vein stripping. (From Venous Disease of the Lower Extremities, by A. D. McLachlin. Copyright © 1967, Year Book Medical Publishers. Used by permission.)

**Figure 23**  The Linton technique of subfascial exposure, ligation, and division of the anteromedial perforating veins of the leg. (From Venous Disease of the Lower Extremities by A. D. McLachlin. Copyright © 1967, Year Book Medical Publishers. Used by permission.)

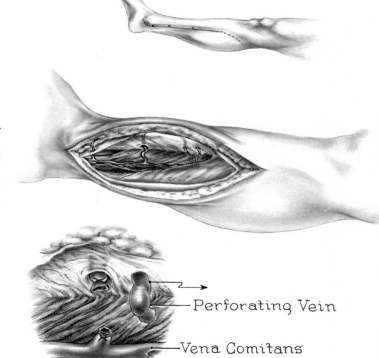

Perforating Vein

Vena Comitans

*Sclerosant injection therapy* is sometimes used as an alternative, or adjunct, to surgery. Ever since the technique was described in the Hippocratic writings, the popularity of this form of therapy has waxed and waned. Fegan has drawn attention to a very important prerequisite to successful sclerotherapy: if the blood is emptied out of the injected venous segment by elastic bandage compression which is continued without interruption for 6 weeks, the inflamed endothelial surfaces adhere by direct contact rather than by way of organized thrombus, and the chance of recanalization of the vein is greatly reduced. Using "continuous compression sclerotherapy" as the sole form of treatment, and 3 per cent sodium tetradecyl sulfate in benzyl alcohol as the sclerosing agent, he has claimed excellent and long-lasting results in both primary and post-thrombotic varicose veins.

*Venous leg ulcers* can be invariably healed by bed rest with lower limb elevation, accelerated if necessary by free split-skin grafts. Indeed, they can often be healed without hospitalization if firm bandage compression of the leg is maintained at all times when the patient is upright. The maintenance of healing depends on the extent to which the underlying venous abnormality can be corrected. This is always possible in the case of primary varicose veins, less often so in post-thrombotic varices. In the latter case, if the ulcer is a first one, if it has been present for no more than a few months, if the patient is not obese, and if only one or two perforating veins are incompetent, excellent results are obtainable by surgery. The less these conditions are met, the less the chance that anything approaching cure is possible, without the requirement that the patient wear an elastic support for the remainder of his life.

## VENOUS HEMORRHAGE

If *varicose veins* are perforated by injury, severe hemorrhage may result. The injurious agent may be chemical (gastroesophageal varices), infective (chronic venous ulceration), or mechanical (accidental, felonious, or surgical wounds). Hemorrhage is profuse either because the arterial inflow to the region finds this the line of least resistance for outflow (collateral veins), or because there is a wide pipeline to a central venous reservoir (low limb varicose veins).

The control of hemorrhage from veins is often more difficult than that from arteries. The wide lumen of a vein, and its often scanty musculature, means that spasmodic constriction at the site of injury is weak, and that an occluding thrombus is easily dislodged. Security from continuing or recurrent hemorrhage is achieved only by suture closure of a side defect, or by double ligation. The major practical problem is that of controlling hemorrhage until one of these definitive procedures can be performed. Some special maneuvers can be used in special circumstances. In the limbs, elevation or external counterpressure will eliminate or counteract hydrostatic pressure.

## SELECTED REFERENCES

### Venous Anatomy and Function

Hollinshead, W. H.: Anatomy for Surgeons. New York, Hoeber Medical Division, Harper & Row, 1969.
*Contains a fine and current account of the gross anatomy of the venous system, especially the lower limb veins (Volume 3).*

Alexander, R. S.: The peripheral venous return. In: American Physiological Society: Handbook of Physiology, Section 2, Circulation. Ed. W. F. Hamilton and P. Dow. Baltimore, Williams & Wilkins Company, Volume 2, p. 1075.
*An excellent account of, and reference source for, the wall structure, valves, and nerve and blood supply of veins.*

Ludbrook, J.: Aspects of Venous Function in the Lower Limbs. Springfield, Ill., Charles C Thomas, 1966.
*A surgically oriented account of structure and function of veins generally, but with particular reference to those of the lower limbs.*

Mark, A. L., and Eckstein, J. W.: Venomotor tone and central venous pressure. Med. Clin. N. Amer., 52:1077, 1968.

Webb-Peploe, M. M., and Shepherd, J. T.: Veins and their control. New Eng. J. Med., 278:317, 1968.
*Taken together, these two review articles give excellent accounts of the physiologic and clinical significance of the venous system as a whole.*

### Investigation of the Venous System

Ludbrook, J., ed.: The venous system. In: Karner, P. I., ed.: Standardization of Cardioangiological Flow Methods. 1972.
*Current methods of investigating the venous system by radiology, radionuclides, pressure, volume, and flow measurements, and venous tone measurement.*

### Venous Thrombosis

Haller, J. A.: Deep Thrombophlebitis: Pathophysiology and Treatment. Philadelphia, W. B. Saunders Company, 1967.

Kakkar, V. V.: The problems of thrombosis in the deep veins of the leg. Ann. Roy. Coll. Surg. Eng., 45:257, 1969.

Browse, N., Flute, P. T., and Mavor, G. E.: Clinical progress: deep vein thrombosis. Brit. Med. J., 4:676, 1969.
*Three good reviews of current methods of diagnosis, prophylaxis, and treatment of lower limb deep vein thrombosis.*

### Varicose Veins

Dodd, H., and Cockett, F. B.: The Pathology and Surgery of the Veins of the Lower Limb. Edinburgh, E. & S. Livingstone, 1956.
*A classic account of varicose vein surgery, which is only just beginning to date (new edition in preparation).*

Myers, T. T.: Results and technique of stripping operation for varicose veins. J.A.M.A., 163:87, 1957.
*A clear description of the Mayo Clinic approach to the operative treatment of primary varicose veins.*

McLachlin, A. D.: Venous Disease of the Lower Extremities. Chicago, Year Book Publishers Inc., 1967.
*An excellent, well illustrated, and well referenced account of the pathophysiology and operative treatment of varicose veins (and other venous disorders).*

Fegan, G.: Varicose Veins: Compression Sclerotherapy. London, Heinemann Medical Books, 1967.
*Details of the principles and technique of the modern injection treatment, as applied to 1171 patients.*

### Classic Descriptions of Venous Disease

Franklin, K. J.: A Monograph on Veins. Springfield, Ill., Charles C Thomas, 1937.
*The pre-eminent source book for information on venous structure and function published prior to 1937.*

Berberich, J., and Hirsch, S.: Die röntgenographische Darstellung der Arterienen und Venen am lebenden Menschen. Klin. Wschr., 2:2226, 1923.
*The first account of phlebography.*

Dos Santos, J. C.: La phlébologie directe. Conception, technique, premiers résultats. J. Int. Chir., 3:625, 1938.
*The introduction of phlebography as a diagnostic tool.*

Nanson, E. M., Palko, P. D., Dick, A. A., and Fedoruk, S. O.: Early detection of deep vein thrombosis of the legs using I[131]-tagged human fibrinogen: a clinical study. Ann. Surg., *162*:438, 1965.
*The first systemic study of human deep vein thrombosis using a radionuclide-labeled clotting factor.*

Eberth, C. J., and Schimmelbusch, C.: Die Thrombose nach Versuchen und Leichenbefunden. Stuttgart, 1888.
*The first clear account of the mechanism of intravascular thrombosis.*

Virchow, R. L. K.: Thrombose und Embolie. Frankfurt, 1856.
*The classic enunciation of the three etiologic factors in the production of venous thrombosis.*

Laewen, A.: Thrombectomy in venous thrombosis and arteriospasm. Int. Abstr. Surg., *65*:348, 1937.

Leriche, R., and Geisendorf, W.: Résultats d'une thrombectomie précoce avec résection veineuse dans une phlébite grave des deux membres inférieurs. Presse Méd., *47*:1301, 1939.
*The earliest two accounts of thrombectomy for iliofemoral venous thrombosis.*

Mahorner, H., Castleberry, J. W., and Coleman, W. O.: Attempts to restore function in major veins which are the site of massive thrombosis. Ann. Surg., *146*:510, 1957.
*The first "modern" account of venous thrombectomy.*

Fogarty, T. J., Cranley, J. J., Krause, R. J., Strasser, E. S., and Hafner, C. D.: Surgical management of phlegmasia cerulea dolens. Arch. Surg., *86*:256, 1963.
*The introduction of the balloon-tipped catheter for venous thrombectomy.*

Palma, E. C., and Esperón, R.: Vein transplants and grafts in the surgical treatment of the postphlebitic syndrome. J. Cardiovasc. Surg., *6*:94, 1960.
*An early account of the crossed saphenous vein bypass for iliac venous obstruction.*

Trendelenburg, F.: Ueber die Unterbindung der Vena saphena magna bei Unterschenkelvarican. Bruns. Beit. Klin. Chir., *7*:195, 1891.

Perthes, G.: Ueber die Operation der Underschenkelvaricen nach Trendelenburg. Dtsch. Med. Wschr., *21*:253, 1895.
*Trendelenburg's account of midthigh great saphenous ligation, and Perthe's follow-up of the patients containing the suggestion of flush saphenofemoral ligation.*

Keller, W. L.: A new method of extirpating the internal saphenous and similar veins in varicose conditions; a preliminary report. N.Y. Med. J., *82*:385, 1905.

Mayo, C. H.: Treatment of varicose veins. Surg. Gynec. Obstet., *2*:385, 1906.
*The first accounts of stripping for varicose veins.*

Homans, J.: The operative treatment of varicose veins and ulcers, based upon a classification of these lesions. Surg. Gynec. Obstet., *22*:143, 1916.
*The paper that put flush saphenofemoral ligation on the map.*

Edwards, E. A.: The treatment of varicose veins: anatomical factors of ligation of the great saphenous vein. Surg. Gynec. Obstet., *59*:916, 1934.
*An excellent historic review of varicose vein treatment from Hippocrates to Homans.*

Linton, R. R.: The communicating veins of the lower leg and the operative technique for their ligation. Ann. Surg., *107*:582, 1938.
*The first clear account of the surgical anatomy and significance of perforating veins, and of subfascial ligation.*

Cockett, F. B.: The pathology and treatment of venous ulcers of the leg. Brit. J. Surg., *43*:260, 1955.
*The extension and publicization of Linton's work, and alternative surgical approaches to perforating veins.*

Martorell, F.: Las ulceras supramaleolares por arteriolitis de los grandes hipertensos. Actas Inst. Policlínico, *1*:6, 1945.

Hines, E. A., Jr., and Farber, E. M.: Ulcer of the leg due to arteriolosclerosis and ischemia occurring in the presence of hypertensive disease (hypertensive-ischemic ulcer). Proc. Mayo Clin., *21*:337, 1946.
*First descriptions of hypertensive-ischemic ulcers.*

# 51

# PULMONARY EMBOLISM

*David C. Sabiston, Jr., M.D., and Walter G. Wolfe, M.D.*

Pulmonary embolism is a serious complication of a variety of medical and surgical disorders. Despite an improved understanding of this condition, its incidence continues to rise and more than 50,000 patients die annually of its effects in the United States. Although pulmonary embolism is especially apt to follow surgical procedures, most series indicate that the majority of cases are *nonsurgical*, the condition developing as a complication of a serious *medical* disorder, such as congestive heart failure, pulmonary disease, carcinomatosis, and many others. In the recent past, considerable attention has been given the fact that a high percentage of persons over the age of 40 are found to have pulmonary embolism at autopsy. Although in many the pulmonary embolus is *incidental* to death, in numerous others it either *contributes* to or is actually the principal *cause* of death.

## HISTORICAL ASPECTS

It has long been recognized that thrombi may be found in the pulmonary arteries at autopsy. However, early pathologists regarded these thrombi as being *primary*, that is, arising in situ in the pulmonary arteries. In 1819 Laennec[38] described "pulmonary apoplexy," which now appears to have been pulmonary embolism. He described a typical hemorrhagic infarct and reported that "it looked like liver." In 1829 Cruveilhier[15] made the gross observation that "all arterial branches which lead to those lesions were filled with clots that branched according to the vascular tree."

Rudolf Virchow,[77] the father of modern pathology, was the first to demonstrate convincingly the *embolic* origin of the pulmonary thrombi. He noted that patients with pulmonary embolism had concomitant thrombosis in the systemic veins, usually in the legs or pelvis. When challenged as to whether or not such thrombi could indeed pass through the heart and into the lungs, Virchow placed pieces of muscle or rubber or thrombi recovered from patients into the veins of dogs and demonstrated their subsequent appearance in the lungs. He also emphasized age differences in the emboli and suggested that they might break off at different times and embolize in different stages of development. In addition, Virchow noted that the emboli that arrived from a distant source could be differentiated from in situ thrombi occurring *distal* to the emboli. It was his belief that the latter occurred as a result of stasis (Fig. 1). Regarding this array of contributions, William H. Welch, the American pathologist, was to state, "Between the years of 1846 and 1856 Virchow constructed the whole doctrine of embolism upon the basis of anatomical, experimental and clinical investigations which for completeness, accuracy and just discernment of the truth must always remain a model of scientific research in medicine."[82]

## PATHOGENESIS OF VENOUS THROMBOSIS

The experimental and clinical studies that Virchow conducted on pulmonary embolism more than a century ago led to the conclusion that there were three primary factors in the pathogenesis of pulmonary embolism. These have since become known as Virchow's *triad*: (1) *stasis* or reduction of blood flow in the veins, (2) *injury* to the intimal surface predisposing to thrombosis, and (3) a state of *hypercoagulability*. These factors, either singly or in combination, are still thought to be of primary importance in the formation of thrombi in the systemic veins. When such thrombi become

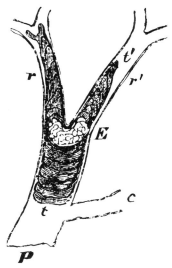

**Figure 1** Illustrations taken from Virchow's original drawing depicting a pulmonary artery (*P*) occluded with an embolus (*E*). In addition, in situ thrombosis (*t*) is present which extends to the first proximal branch (*C*). A thrombus also is formed distal to the clot (*r'* and *t'*). Thus, there are two types of thrombi present: (1) the thrombus that comes from a distant source and is a true *embolus*; and (2) the thrombus that forms in situ as a result of the stasis produced by the embolus. (From Virchow, R.: Die Cellularpathologie. Berlin, A. Hirschwald, 1858.)

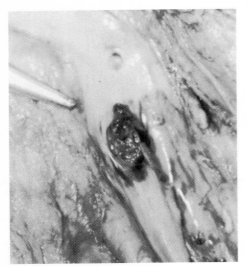

**Figure 2** A primary thrombus forming in the valve pocket at the mouth of the deep femoral vein. (From Hume, M., Sevitt, S., and Thomas, D. P.: Venous Thrombosis and Pulmonary Embolism. Cambridge, Mass., Harvard University Press, 1970.)

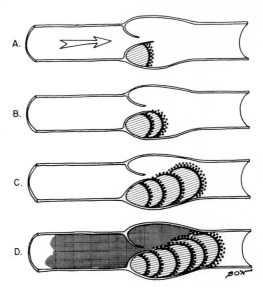

**Figure 3** Diagrammatic illustration showing propagation of a deep thrombus arising in a valvar pocket with deposition of successive layers (*A, B,* and *C*) and retrograde extension of the thrombus after venous blockage by propagation (*D*). (From Hume, M., Sevitt, S., and Thomas, D. P.: Venous Thrombosis and Pulmonary Embolism. Cambridge, Mass., Harvard University Press, 1970.)

detached from the venous wall, they are swept into the circulation and pass through the heart into the lungs.

One of the more important of the factors producing thrombus formation in the systemic veins is *stasis.* It has been demonstrated that radiopaque contrast medium injected into the deep veins of the leg may take a prolonged time to clear when the patient remains in the horizontal position.[43] Moreover, Allison[3] has demonstrated that this medium in postoperative patients may remain in the calf veins up to 25 minutes after injection. Similarly, patients ill for any reason are less apt to move the extremities, and thus a situation is created that favors intravenous thrombosis.

Sites especially vulnerable to stasis and thrombosis are the sinuses of the venous valves. Here, local stasis permits the accumulation of sufficient amounts of clotting factors to initiate the primary thrombus (Fig. 2). Platelets also become adherent to the pockets created by the valves and a thrombus develops. The thrombus grows by successive deposition of aggregated platelets, leukocytes, and fibrin. From this source, propagation of the thrombus may occur upstream or the process may spread retrograde as proximal obstruction develops (Fig. 3).

*Injury* is another factor favoring thrombosis. Thus, soft tissue injury either by blunt trauma or as a result of operative procedures is known to be associated with an increased incidence of venous thrombosis. *Hypercoagulability* has been defined as "the existence of an excessive amount or activity of one or more procoagulant substances, or a decrease in anticoagulant factors."[1] Thus, during pregnancy, a time when thrombosis is prevalent, the concentrations of fibrinogen, prothrombin,

factor VII, Stuart factor, Christmas factor, and antihemophilic factor all are elevated,[2] and the risk of venous thrombosis is correspondingly increased.

## PATHOLOGIC ASPECTS

In 1851 Wharton Jones first described the detachment of a thrombus from an injured vessel in the web of a frog's foot and noted that the vessels became "blocked up by a mass composed of apparently colourless corpuscles and fibrin . . . a portion . . . becoming detached and carried away."[33] During the past decade, there has been an increased awareness of the fact that pulmonary embolism (especially microscopic occlusion of the smaller vessels) is quite common. The importance of pulmonary embolism at postmortem examination is emphasized clearly by a study demonstrating evidence of old or fresh pulmonary emboli in *64 per cent* of all persons over the age of 40.[22] Moreover, the *clinical diagnosis* of pulmonary embolism is frequently difficult to establish and its presence is often recognized for the first time at autopsy.

Although *reflex* responses are of importance in the physiologic changes following pulmonary embolism, primary emphasis should be placed upon the *mechanical* factors of arterial occlusion. This feature is well demonstrated in a classic pathologic study of 100 consecutive patients with *fatal* pulmonary embolism in which 85 had occlusion involving *one* pulmonary artery and, in addition, emboli in the *opposite* lung.[24, 25] Of the evidence supports the importance of *mechanical* occlusion in the cardiodynamic sequelae of massive pulmonary embolism (Fig. 4). These data are in agreement with similar observations upon reduction of pulmonary blood by other causes including arterial ligature, intravascular balloons, pulmonary resection, and various forms of emboli.[9,10,69] Following injection of experimental pulmonary emboli, reduced function of the embolized lung occurs immediately, but pulmonary function returns to near normal within several weeks.[42,61] Similarly, marked histologic changes occur in these thrombi, with intravascular resolution and ultimate disappearance. Such resolution can be confirmed by serial pulmonary radioactive scans, arteriography, pulmonary function studies, and gross and microscopic evaluation. The gradual dissolution can be serially demonstrated (Figs. 5 and 6).

Clinical observations also confirm the resolution of large pulmonary emboli with or without the use of anticoagulants or fibrinolysins (Fig. 7). These observations have demonstrated convincingly that the *natural history* of pulmonary embolism in most instances is one of spontaneous resolution.[21,61,63] This relatively new concept has become of increasing significance in a more complete understanding of the principles of diagnosis and management.

Pulmonary embolism occurs in *children* as well as in adults and in one study was found to be present in approximately 1 per cent of all children examined at autopsy, usually as a secondary manifestation of serious illness such as a respiratory infection, phlebitis, systemic infection, congenital heart disease, or rheumatic heart disease.[32] Although pulmonary embolism in children is rarely diagnosed before death, its clinical manifestations are similar to those in adults.

The emboli generally found at postmortem examination are 1.0 to 1.5 cm. in diameter, apparently having arisen in sizable veins. Their length ranges up to 50 cm. or more,[29] and they often break up after arrival in the lungs into multiple small portions with occlusion of multiple branches of the pulmonary arteries. Generally, the right pulmonary artery and its branches are more commonly involved than the left, and the *lower* lobes are preferentially involved.

The *source* of pulmonary emboli is primarily the systemic venous circulation, and the prevailing evidence indicates that the majority of emboli arise from the *iliac* and *femoral* veins (Table 1).[23,44,52,57,59,65] While the smaller leg veins such as those of the calf may be involved, it is not as likely that such will cause serious clinical manifestations of pulmonary embolism. In other words, only thrombi produced in veins the size of the iliac or femoral vein are large enough to produce serious symptoms in most patients.

Rarely, a venous thrombus may pass through an intracardiac opening (patent foramen ovale, atrial septal defect, or ventricular septal defect) and embolize a systemic organ.[67] This is termed *paradoxical embolism* and is more apt to occur

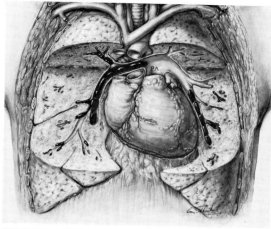

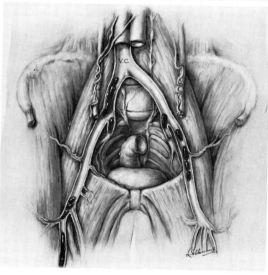

**Figure 4**   Illustration of the findings in a patient with massive pulmonary embolism at the time of postmortem examination. Multiple thrombi are present in the iliofemoral system. The right pulmonary artery and its branches are totally occluded by emboli. The left lower lobar pulmonary artery is also occluded. Under these circumstances, the entire output of the right ventricle must pass through the left upper lobe, which greatly increases pulmonary resistance and right ventricular work. The sudden development of this degree of pulmonary arterial occlusion produces a clinical state of severe shock since the left ventricle receives a much diminished amount of blood to supply the systemic arterial circulation. In otherwise normal patients, 50 per cent or more of the pulmonary arterial circulation must be occluded before serious cardiovascular manifestations are produced. (From Sabiston, D. C., Jr., and Wolfe, W. G.: Ann. Surg., *168*:1, 1968.)

100 patients, only 15 had emboli restricted solely to one lung, and 12 of these were more than 54 years of age and thus members of an age group with an appreciable incidence of underlying cardiac and respiratory disease. Moreover, in patients with massive pulmonary embolism in whom embolectomy is performed, it is usual to find emboli in more than one pulmonary artery.[4,60] This

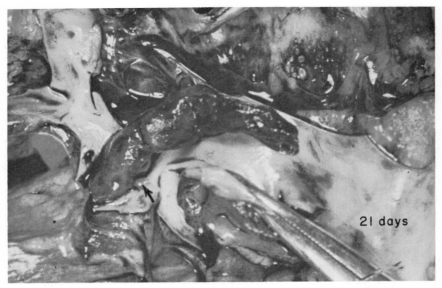

**Figure 5**   A large pulmonary embolus (originally produced experimentally in the inferior vena cava) is shown in the pulmonary artery 21 days after embolization. (From Sabiston, D. C., Jr., and Wolfe, W. G.: Ann. Surg., *168*:1, 1968.)

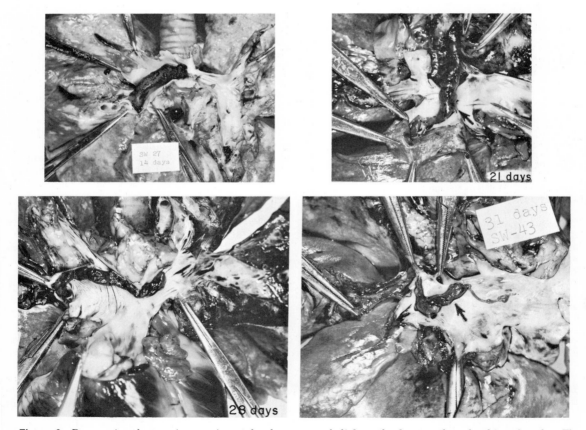

**Figure 6**   Progressive changes in experimental pulmonary emboli from the fourteenth to the thirty-first day. The attachments are demonstrated at the tip of the arrow at 21 days. The diameter of the embolus is definitely less by the twenty-eighth day. The embolus at 31 days demonstrates the variability in resolution in different parts of the thrombus. One end of the thrombus has been reduced to a small fragment while the remaining part is larger. (From Sabiston, D. C., Jr., and Wolfe, W. G.: Ann. Surg., *168*:1, 1968.)

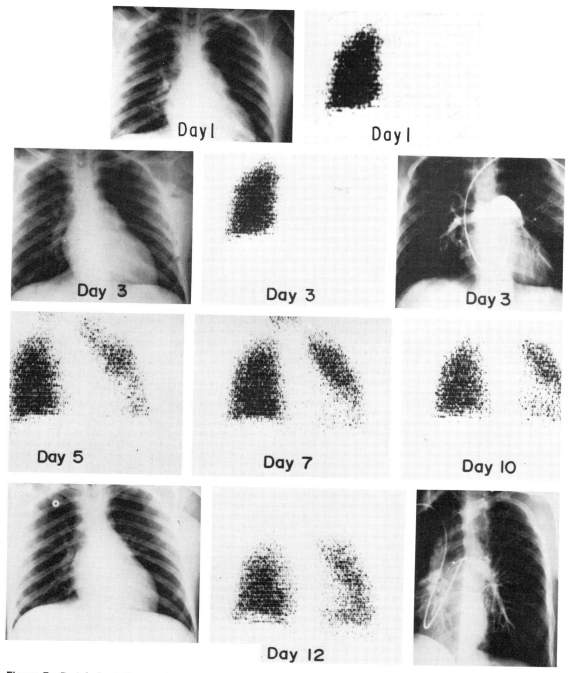

**Figure 7** Serial chest films and scans following a massive pulmonary embolus to the left pulmonary artery in a 25 year old female after a pelvic operation. On the fifth postoperative day, discomfort was noted in the left chest with dyspnea. A plain chest film taken on this day (day 1) showed diminished vascular markings (Westermark's sign). A radioactive pulmonary scan showed no evidence of pulmonary flow to the entire left lobe. Beginning on the third day after the embolus, the scan and arteriogram both show evidence of flow to the left lung. In subsequent scans and pulmonary arteriograms, resolution of the thrombus occurred with progressively increasing amounts of flow by the twelfth day.

**TABLE 1**   SITE OF ORIGIN OF VENOUS THROMBI*

| References | Cases with Thrombosis at Necropsy | Per Cent of Cases with Thrombi in | | | | |
|---|---|---|---|---|---|---|
| | | Iliac Veins | Femoral Veins | Popliteal Veins | Soleal Veins | Any Deep Calf Vein |
| Rossle[59] | 94 | — | 49 | — | — | 92 |
| Neuman[52] | 100 | — | 22 | — | — | 87 |
| McLachlin and Paterson[44] | 34 | 9 | 82 | — | — | 41 |
| Gibbs[23] | 149 | — | 42 | — | — | 65 |
| Sevitt and Gallagher[65] | 81 | | 70 | 33 | 67 | 74 |
| Roberts[57] | 58 | 14 | 43 | 41 | 86 | 95 |

*From Hume, M., Sevitt, S., and Thomas, D. P.: Venous Thrombosis & Pulmonary Embolism. Cambridge, Mass., Harvard University Press, 1970.

when right ventricular and right atrial hypertension is present.

In addition to the iliofemoral and pelvic veins, other possible sources of venous thrombi include the inferior vena cava, the subclavian and internal jugular veins, and the cavernous sinuses of the skull. Some have emphasized that as many as one-fifth of pulmonary emboli arise from sources other than veins drained by the inferior vena cava.[27]

It is important to stress the fact that pulmonary *embolism* and *infarction* are not synonymous. Whereas pulmonary embolism is of common occurrence, pulmonary infarction is much less frequent. Pathologically, an infarct is generally a circumscribed area of local hemorrhage and demonstrates *necrosis* of the lung parenchyma. The majority of the patients with embolism do not show these features. Generally, infarcts are located peripherally in the lungs, most often in the lower lobes, and are less than 5 cm. in diameter. In one series, the proportion of infarcts to emboli was 1 to 10.[70]

## PREDISPOSING FACTORS

Present evidence indicates that females are more likely to have pulmonary embolism than are males. A British study reports that in females pulmonary embolism is responsible for 110 deaths per million, as contrasted to 77 deaths per million in males.[56] There is little doubt that *age* plays an important factor and pulmonary embolism is clearly a disorder affecting the middle-aged and elderly. This relationship between age and incidence of thromboembolism is shown in Figure 8. There is evidence that *blood type* affects the incidence of pulmonary embolism. In a cooperative study involving the United States, Sweden, and Great Britain, the ABO distribution of subjects with thrombosis or embolism was compared with control data. The results showed a higher frequency of Group A subjects as compared with controls (the A:O ratio—normal is 0.8 to 1.0—ranging in different subgroups from 1.4 to 4.6). In this study the highest

ratios were in women using oral contraceptives.[31] The significance of these findings is not fully apparent, although it may be related to the fact that patients with Group O blood have lower levels of factor VIII than those with Groups A and B, and as a corollary, it is known that patients with Group O blood are more apt to bleed as a complication of peptic ulcer than those of Groups A, B, and AB.[39] Bed rest and lack of exercise in general are well established antecedent causes of pulmonary embolism causing a twofold or greater incidence.[5] The presence of heart disease, especially congestive heart failure or atrial fibrillation, is particularly conducive to the development of pulmonary embolism. The presence of *cancer*, particularly cancer of the pancreas and prostate and carcinomatosis, is associated with a high incidence of pulmonary embolism.[13] The role of surgical procedures, especially extensive ones, is significant. In one study, thrombi were detected in 15 per cent of patients after relatively *minor* surgical procedures, whereas they were present in 44 per cent of those undergoing *major* operations.[20]

It has long been recognized that there is a higher risk of pulmonary embolism during pregnancy and the

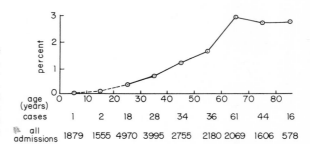

**Figure 8**   Graph showing the relationship of age to occurrence of thromboembolism. The ordinate represents the percentage of all hospital admissions in which a diagnosis was made clinically or at necropsy. The abscissa indicates age by decade. (From Hume, M., Sevitt, S., and Thomas, D. P.: Venous Thrombosis and Pulmonary Embolism. Cambridge, Mass., Harvard University Press, 1970.)

puerperium. Pressure from the gravid uterus may act to retard venous flow from the limbs and pelvis. Infection in the postpartum patient may also give rise to septic thrombophlebitis and embolism. *Oral contraceptives* have been shown to be positively associated with the presence of pulmonary embolism in studies in both the United States and Great Britain. In a British study[45,76] the results showed that the risk of venous thrombosis or pulmonary embolism was increased threefold in women receiving oral contraceptives and about sixfold in women who were pregnant or in the puerperium.

## PHYSIOLOGIC RESPONSES TO PULMONARY EMBOLISM

The pulmonary arteries receive the total output of the right ventricle, and a characteristic and impressive feature of the pulmonary circulation is its *low* vascular resistance. This fact enables flow in the pulmonary vascular bed to be increased severalfold with minimal elevation of pulmonary arterial pressure. Despite numerous experimental and clinical studies, opinion remains divided concerning the relative importance of *reflex* versus *mechanical* effects in pulmonary embolism. The occasional finding of a small pulmonary embolus in a patient after sudden death has been cited as evidence that intraluminal occlusion of a relatively small pulmonary artery can produce death, presumably as a result of reflex mechanisms. Currently, such an explanation would rarely be accepted except under very unusual circumstances.

Experimental pulmonary embolism has been produced by many methods. The physiologic changes appear to be related to the *size* of the emboli and can be divided into those that produce *microembolism* (obstruction of terminal small arteries and arterioles) and those that produce *macroembolism* (occlusion of the larger pulmonary vessels). Considerable reduction in the diameter of the main pulmonary artery or the primary branches is required to reduce pulmonary blood flow significantly or to produce pulmonary hypertension proximal to the obstruction. It has been shown that large experimental thrombi produced in the inferior vena cava and transferred to *either* the right or left pulmonary artery 10 to 14 days later produce a minimum of cardiovascular and respiratory responses.[42] Specifically, occlusion of one pulmonary artery produces only minimal and generally insignificant changes in the central venous pressure, right ventricular pressure, pulmonary artery pressure, aortic pressure, cardiac output, total oxygen consumption, and the electrocardiogram *despite* occlusion of half the pulmonary arterial circulation. From these studies it is concluded that this type of embolism produces minimal circulatory effects that can be attributed specifically to reflex action.

Normal man usually tolerates pneumonectomy quite well. Tidal volume and oxygen consumption at rest following resection of a lung have been shown to be little changed.[10] Similarly, occlusion of one pulmonary artery by ligature or an intraluminal balloon is accompanied by few cardiodynamic changes. Patients have tolerated balloon occlusion well for periods up to 2 hours,[9] and even during exercise with similar occlusion, pulmonary arterial pressure is increased only 12 to 50 per cent while cardiac output may increase as much as threefold. Arterial occlusion of this type closely simulates the obstruction produced by large pulmonary emboli. Emphasis should be placed on the fact that such studies have been conducted in otherwise normal subjects. The presence of underlying cardiac or respiratory insufficiency is quite likely to alter this response appreciably. For example, in patients with heart disease, exercise during temporary unilateral occlusion of the right or left pulmonary artery by a balloon catheter produces a marked elevation in pulmonary arterial pressure.[69] Cardiac output does not increase significantly with exercise, and an increase in arteriovenous oxygen difference occurs. Available data suggest that resection of less than one lung is followed by only minor changes in the pulmonary arterial pressure, whereas removal of greater amounts of pulmonary tissue produces an elevation of pulmonary arterial pressure.[81]

Experimental data suggest that embolization of the lung with small particles (100 $\mu$ or less) creates *reflex* effects including tachypnea, pulmonary hypertension, and systemic hypotension that may lead to death. However, it is currently thought that microembolism of the lung is infrequently encountered as a clinical problem. Embolization with larger particles requires considerably more blockage of the pulmonary arterial system to produce significant effects. Thus, in general, the conclusion has been drawn that arterial emboli produce pulmonary hypertension by *mechanical* obstruction, while vasoconstriction is produced by arteriolar embolism and is mediated by *reflex* changes.[19] Such studies suggest that the clinical manifestations of pulmonary embolism are usually produced primarily by occlusion of the larger pulmonary arteries, a concept supported by both clinical and pathologic studies.

*Cyanosis* is a recognized finding in clinical pulmonary embolism and hypoxemia is almost always present. The *cause* of reduced oxygen tension in the arterial blood has elicited considerable discussion. A number of possible etiologic factors have been advanced and include: (1) alveolar hypoventilation, (2) ventilation-perfusion abnormality, (3) decreased diffusing capacity of the lungs, (4) pulmonary edema, (5) venoarterial shunting, and (6) rapid transit of blood through the capillary bed without adequate time for oxygenation. It is apparent that a combination of these factors may be responsible, as is implied in experimental studies.[37]

Clinical evidence of *reflex bronchoconstriction* in pulmonary embolism is a subject of considerable interest.[7] Repeat pulmonary function studies after injection of intravenous heparin showed a prompt improvement in the maximal expiratory flow rate or a reduction in lung resistance.[26] Such observations are cited as further evidence of a *humoral* factor. Humoral factors mediated by platelets may be of importance in the genesis of cardiopulmonary disturbances in patients with pulmonary embolism. It is known that platelets are a concentrated source of biologically active amines. In experimental studies evidence has been obtained that 5-hydroxytryptamine (serotonin) is liberated from platelets in the process of blood coagulation and that it produces bronchoconstriction.[12]

In summary, a combination of experimental and clinical evidence suggests that a variety of factors contribute to the changes that occur following embolism. The majority of evidence favors a primary *mechanical* basis for the physiologic changes with the belief that the blockage of the emboli themselves produces the most serious changes. It is quite clear that the *pre-embolic* status significantly affects the clinical manifestations, and the presence of pre-existing cardiac or respiratory insufficiency is of great importance. If the latter is present, lesser degrees of pulmonary embolism cause greater clinical responses. Evidence clearly exists for the presence of *reflex changes,* although these are in general of secondary importance. The vasoactive amines, probably arising from the emboli themselves, appear to exert a significant role.

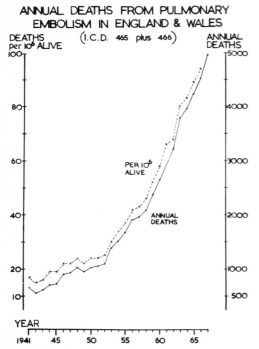

**Figure 9** Graph illustrating increase in annual deaths from pulmonary embolism in England and Wales. (From Hume, M., Sevitt, S., and Thomas, D. P.: Venous Thrombosis and Pulmonary Embolism. Cambridge, Mass., Harvard University Press, 1970.)

## INCIDENCE

Current statistics indicate that the incidence of pulmonary embolism is increasing, and the risk of death from pulmonary embolism following surgical procedures from a collected series is 0.11 per cent.[16] An English study over a 10 year period (1952 to 1961) showed a progressive rise in incidence,[51] and a similar rise has been observed in Germany.[46] The data for the increase in England are shown in Figure 9. Although most statistics indicate a definite increase in the incidence of thromboembolism, the causes for this increase remain unclear. Factors that are cited as being responsible include: (1) the increase in older members of the population, (2) larger numbers and greater magnitude of operative procedures, and (3) increased recognition.

## DIAGNOSIS OF PULMONARY EMBOLISM

### Clinical Manifestations

Pulmonary embolism is notorious for the similarity of its clinical manifestations to those of other cardiorespiratory disorders. This makes difficult the establishment of an accurate *clinical* diagnosis. The characteristic symptoms of dyspnea, chest pain, hemoptysis, and hypotension may be present in the classic example, but experience has shown that these are not sufficiently specific to permit a definite diagnosis. The following points bear emphasis: (1) many patients have underlying cardiac disease; (2) dyspnea and tachypnea are the most frequent clinical findings; (3) accentuation of the pulmonary second sound is common, whereas the more classic signs of hemoptysis, pleural friction rub, gallop rhythm, cyanosis, and chest splinting are present in only a quarter or less of patients; and (4) clinical evidence of venous thrombosis is the exception and occurs in only one-third of patients.[62]

### Laboratory Findings

The *plain chest* film may show diminished pulmonary vascular markings at the site of the embolus (Westermark's sign).[83] This is an inconstant and frequently equivocal sign, although it may be of aid.[73] It is apparent that the symptoms and physical signs of pulmonary embolism are frequently insufficient to establish an accurate diagnosis.

Specific serum *enzyme* changes may be helpful although are seldom conclusive. The triad of an elevated serum lactic dehydrogenase (LDH) activity, increased serum bilirubin, and a normal serum glutamic oxalacetic transaminase (SGOT) activity is often present.[79] Serum LDH is frequently elevated and the bilirubin is increased in approximately two-thirds of patients. While determination of serum enzyme activity is helpful in diagnosis in patients with massive embolism and acute cardiovascular changes, the time factor is often critical and a more rapid means of diagnosis is necessary.

The *electrocardiographic* changes have been studied extensively. While the electrocardiogram can be helpful, there is an increasing appreciation of the fact that it cannot be depended upon for an objective diagnosis. It is probable that not more than 10 to 20 per cent of patients who subsequently are proved to have pulmonary embolism show *any* electrocardiographic changes, and of these, a still smaller number show identifiable diagnostic abnormalities.[40] Electrocardiographic alterations include disturbances of rhythm (atrial fibrillation, ectopic beats, heart block), enlargement of P waves, S–T segment depression, and T wave inversion (particularly in leads III, $AV_F$, $V_1$, $V_4$, and

$V_5$). The most common abnormality is S–T segment depression, a result of myocardial ischemia from a reduced cardiac output and arterial pressure as well as increased right ventricular pressure.

**Imbalance of Pulmonary Ventilation and Perfusion.** The ventilatory dead space is increased in pulmonary embolism.[58] Occlusion of a major pulmonary arterial branch causes a decrease in gas exchange in the corresponding segment of the lung while alveolar ventilation continues. In a ventilated but underperfused segment of lung, the composition of the alveolar air tends to approach that of inspired air, with a low partial pressure of carbon

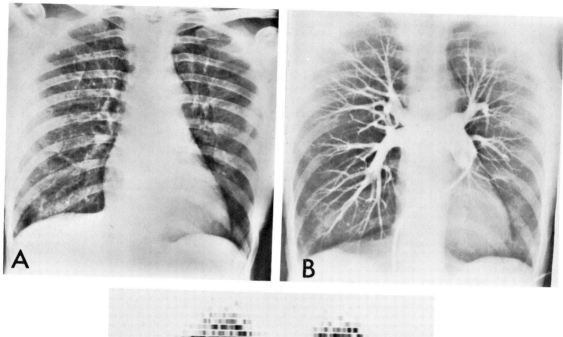

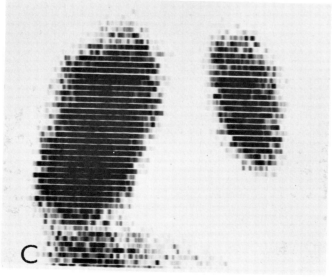

**Figure 10** Films from a patient with pulmonary embolism involving the left lower lobar pulmonary artery. *A,* Slight diminution of the vascular markings to the left lower lobe is noted in comparison with those in the right lower lobe on the plain chest film (Westermark's sign). *B,* Pulmonary arteriogram illustrating occlusion of the right lower lobar pulmonary artery. *C,* Pulmonary scan showing absence of perfusion of the left lower lobe. (From Sabiston, D. C., Jr., and Wagner, H. N., Jr.: Ann. Surg., *160*:585, 1964.)

dioxide. This air is mixed with that from the normal areas of the lung during expiration but reduces the mean alveolar carbon dioxide tension to a degree that can be detected in the expired air. Arterial carbon dioxide tension remains at a nearly normal level because of the presence of normal lung tissue. The difference between the arterial and alveolar carbon dioxide tensions therefore may be of aid in the diagnosis of pulmonary embolism.

**Pulmonary Arteriography.** Pulmonary arteriography is an excellent technique for demonstration of embolism. Knowledge of the normal pulmonary angiographic appearance provides a background for the evaluation of morphologic and physiologic disturbances of flow in the pulmonary vessels.[68] The arteries in the lower areas of the lung are normally larger than those in the upper portions since they serve a larger volume of lung tissue. Major branches are readily identifiable by comparison with normal anatomic charts of the pulmonary arteries. Such vessels usually follow the branching pattern of the bronchi. Occasionally, total obstruction of the main pulmonary artery is found, usually in association with marked symptoms. In most instances, the obstruction involves lobar or segmental branches (Fig. 10). The filling defect may be sharply delineated, usually manifest as a convex shadow with a blunt end or an irregular taper. The defect should remain *constant* on several successive films in the series, and the flow may be sluggish as shown by a small pool of contrast medium that may persist in the artery above the obstruction well into the venous phase of the angiogram. When pulmonary arteriography is performed later in the course of embolism, contrast medium may pass around the obstruction, causing delayed opacification of the artery distally. The pattern in some areas may show avascular segments that represent the result of unresolved thromboembolism.

**Pulmonary Scanning.** Wagner and associates[80] introduced radioisotope pulmonary scanning in 1964, and the technique has since been widely employed. The principle of the method is measurement of intravenously injected particles labeled with iodine-131, chromium-51, or technetium-99m. Macromolecules of human serum albumin (10 to 100 $\mu$ in diameter) become lodged in the pulmonary capillary bed following intravenous injection. It is thus possible to delineate the distribution of pulmonary arterial blood flow and reveal areas of decreased perfusion. It must be emphasized that lesions present on the plain chest film (such as pneumonitis, atelectasis, emphysematous bullae, or neoplasm) will uniformly demonstrate *scanning defects; therefore, these areas must be excluded from consideration.* Under these circumstances it is essential that misinterpretation be avoided by review of a simultaneous plain chest film. This technique has been found to be particularly useful in the patient with massive pulmonary embolism, especially if the plain chest film is essentially normal.

Inhalation scanning with the use of xenon-133

has been of additional aid in the interpretation of the perfusion pulmonary scan. This allows the differentiation of underperfused and underventilated areas in the lungs. It is also recognized that pulmonary embolism produces bronchoconstriction, therefore reducing the amount of air delivered to the embolized portion of the lung. Moreover, areas of the lung without pulmonary embolism may also show bronchoconstriction with reduced ventilation.

## MANAGEMENT

Before specific therapy for pulmonary embolism is initiated, it is essential that an *objective* diagnosis be established. The two most important and reliable means of diagnosis are pulmonary *scanning* and *arteriography*. Since scanning is a simple, safe, and reliable technique, it is generally preferred. It causes the patient little inconvenience and has no appreciable risk.

### ANTICOAGULANTS

Anticoagulants form the primary basis of therapy in the majority of patients. The scanning and arteriographic features of an appropriate patient for treatment with anticoagulants are shown in Figure 6. Heparin is usually employed initially, and its effect when administered intravenously is immediate. Heparin interferes with blood coagulation in at least two ways: (1) by preventing the activation of factor IX (Christmas factor) by factor XI (thromboplastin antecedent) in the early coagulation sequence; and (2) by acting as a potent antithrombin in the presence of heparin co-factor. Therefore it inhibits both the *intrinsic* and *extrinsic* coagulation mechanisms. In its antithrombin effects, heparin inhibits the conversion of fibrinogen to fibrin by thrombin and in high doses prevents the action of thrombin on platelets. Heparin is largely excreted in the urine and awareness of the renal state is important. Also, the enzyme heparinase is present in the liver, a site of some degradation.

The therapeutic level of heparin is accomplished by maintaining the clotting time twice to three times normal (20 to 35 minutes, assuming a normal clotting time of 8 to 12 minutes). The amount required varies. In general, 15,000 units should be given intravenously as the initial dose with 5000 to 10,000 units each 4 to 6 hours thereafter to maintain the desired clotting time. At the beginning of therapy, a continuous intravenous heparin drip is the most reliable method of obtaining and controlling the extended clotting time. Later the heparin may be given subcutaneously. Heparin therapy prevents both extension of the thrombus in the venous system and the formation of distal in situ thrombi in the pulmonary arteries. Some employ quite high doses of heparin (100,000 units daily) with good results.[6, 35] The Lee-White clotting time is usually used, but other methods including partial thromboplastin time on plasma have been advocated.[71]

The duration of heparin therapy is dependent upon the individual patient and the clinical course. In general, 8 to 10 days of heparin with extension of clotting time to two to three times normal is recommended since this approximates the time necessary for the venous thrombi to become firmly adherent to the vessel wall. During this period, a moderate amount of thrombolysis also occurs. Customarily, oral coumarin anticoagulation is begun several days prior to the cessation of heparin therapy in order to allow the required time for adequate prolongation of the prothrombin.

The oral anticoagulant coumarin drugs have indirect and delayed action on the blood clotting mechanism. These agents act upon the liver and inhibit the production of four of the factors involved in the transformation of prothrombin to thrombin — factors XII, IX, and X and prothrombin itself. The sum of these effects has been termed "hypoprothrombinemia." The coumarin drugs are rapidly absorbed from the gastrointestinal tract and are concentrated primarily in the liver. Although short-acting, intermediate, and long-acting agents are available, one of the more commonly used is warfarin sodium. It has only a slight cumulative effect. The average loading dose on the first day is 15 to 30 mg. and on the second day 10 to 20 mg. The maximal effect is usually reached in 1½ to 2 days, and the average daily maintenance dose is usually between 5 and 10 mg. (ranges from 2 to 20 mg.). The duration of coumarin therapy is controversial, but most believe it should be continued for a minimum of 6 weeks and some advocate up to 6 months or longer. In any event, it is apparent that the local responses and subsequent course of the patient are the primary indicators. The recovery time required after maximal effect is 2 to 4 days. Administration of vitamin K counteracts the effect of the coumarin and should be employed if bleeding complications occur.

## THROMBOLYTIC AGENTS

Considerable effort has been directed toward finding suitable thrombolytic agents for use in the treatment of venous thrombosis and pulmonary embolism. In the body *plasminogen* is the inactive precursor of *plasmin*, the active fibrinolytic enzyme. Under normal circumstances, plasminogen is present in the blood and tissues. Exercise, stress, and shock cause plasminogen to be activated by plasmin through a labile activator present in many tissues and especially in venous endothelium. Plasmin activity in the blood stream is prevented by inhibitors, both by an antiactivator and by antiplasmins. Two thrombolysins, streptokinase and urokinase, have been studied extensively. Both act by transforming plasminogen to plasmin. Streptokinase is a soluble product of the metabolism of *Streptococcus pyogenes* (Lancefield Group A) and is available in a highly purified form. Since patients who have had previous streptococcal infections may be allergic to streptokinase, it can produce toxic reactions (pyrexia, dyspnea, tachycardia, and anaphylaxis). Urokinase is a strong thrombolytic agent found in human urine. In an effort to document its effects, the National Heart and Lung Institute is conducting a national cooperative study of urokinase. The initial results have demonstrated that urokinase combined with heparin therapy, as compared to heparin therapy alone, significantly accelerates the resolution of pulmonary thromboemboli at 24 hours as shown by pulmonary arteriograms, lung scans, and right-sided heart pressure measurements. *However*, no significant differences in recurrence rate of pulmonary embolism or in the 2 week mortality were noted. Bleeding was a prominent complication and occurred in 45 per cent of the patients receiving urokinase as contrasted to 27 per cent of those given heparin alone. It was concluded that since the urokinase regimen did not usually achieve complete or nearly complete thrombolysis, and especially because of its hemorrhagic potential, further studies with urokinase are necessary before specific therapeutic recommendations can be made.[75]

## PREVENTION

Much attention has been directed toward prophylaxis against thrombosis with the hope that this complication might be eliminated. However, no proven method or combination of methods currently exists for total prevention of thromboembolism. Several factors are considered of importance, including (1) physical activity, (2) elevation of the lower extremities, (3) stocking compression of the legs, and (4) prophylactic anticoagulation in selected patients.

A number of observers have recommended early ambulation and physical activity following operations or during bed rest for other illness. In a study undertaken to evaluate the role of exercise, postmortem vein dissections showed that thrombi were found in only 18 per cent of patients who had been given exercises before death, as compared with 53 per cent in controls (nonexercised and nonambulatory).[30] Other studies have been less confirmatory, including one in which the [125]I fibrinogen method for detection of leg vein thrombi was employed. The patients in this study group underwent an intensive regimen including vigorous leg exercises both before and after surgery, elevation of the foot of the bed, and the continuous use of elastic stockings. Despite such intensive efforts, the overall results fell short of those desired, with thrombosis being detected in 25 per cent of the patients on the regimen as compared with 35 per cent in controls. It is interesting that in *older* patients undergoing major surgery the incidence of thrombosis was 24 per cent compared with 61 per cent in the controls. Therefore, in the elderly this regimen appeared to have a significant prophylactic effect.[20] Prophylactic anticoagulation is also of proven benefit in certain patients following trauma and orthopedic problems including fracture of the hip.[29, 65]

## SURGICAL MANAGEMENT

When anticoagulant therapy fails, several surgical procedures may be useful. It was originally thought important to interrupt the superficial femoral veins in the groin by ligature to prevent thrombi from passing into the inferior vena cava, but this procedure is rarely, if ever, indicated. An analysis of a great deal of data has shown that femoral vein ligation is less effective in preventing subsequent emboli than the use of anticoagulants alone. Moreover, if surgical interruption is clearly indicated, interruption of the inferior vena cava is preferred.

### Venous Thrombectomy

The direct removal of venous thrombi by thrombectomy has had a number of advocates.[17,28,41] It has been employed both to reduce and to prevent chronic venous insufficiency, which often follows thrombosis, as well as to reduce the likelihood of pulmonary embolism. Favorable results following venous thrombectomy have been reported, but other surgeons have warned of a high incidence of post-thrombectomy thrombosis.[34] Massive pulmonary embolism has occurred during the course of iliofemoral thrombectomy. Most advocates of venous thrombectomy recommend immediate anticoagulation with heparin and its continuous use postoperatively to prevent recurrent thrombosis, but most observers view thrombectomy as seldom indicated.

### Interruption of the Inferior Vena Cava

With proper clinical indications, interruption of the inferior vena cava has been advocated by a number of authors for patients with pulmonary embolism. Some prefer total ligation[53] while others prefer the plication technique,[72] the "filter" or "screen" method,[18] or the use of plastic clips.[47,50] Interruption of the inferior vena cava does not *completely* prevent subsequent embolism. Evidence of recurrent pulmonary embolism after ligation in as many as 20 per cent of patients has been reported.[27] Failure to ligate the ovarian vein in females is also a cause of subsequent embolism. The portion of the inferior vena cava between the ligature and the renal veins, the veins of the upper extremity and neck, the right atrium, and the right ventricle have each been shown to be the source of recurrent pulmonary emboli. Clinical evidence of this type further emphasizes the importance of considering all systemic veins as well as the right heart as potential sources of pulmonary emboli.

In summary, controversy exists at present concerning the indications for inferior vena caval interruption. One group of authors recommends the use of inferior vena caval interruption quite frequently, usually after the first attack of pulmonary embolism, irrespective of its severity. In their series, the long-term complications appeared minimal.[54] An opposing view is presented in a report of another series of cases in which the complications of inferior vena caval interruption were quite significant and the results from point of view of mortality and control of pulmonary embolism were less than desired.[55] From an analysis of recent literature, there appears to be little doubt that there has been a trend away from the use of inferior vena caval interruption. The use of the

"umbrella filter," which may be passed under local anesthesia from the jugular vein and opened in the inferior vena cava just below the renal vessels, has also been advocated but not widely adopted.[48]

### Pulmonary Embolectomy

The first pulmonary embolectomy was performed in 1908 by Friedrich Trendelenburg,[74] Professor of Surgery at the University of Leipzig. He first approached this difficult problem in the laboratory by removing a large embolus from the pulmonary artery of a calf. In the original report, Trendelenburg described three patients upon whom embolectomy was performed, the longest living 37 hours and dying of hemorrhage from an internal mammary artery. In 1924, Kirschner,[36] a pupil of Trendelenburg, was the first to perform pulmonary embolectomy successfully with a long-term survivor. Despite the logical concept of Trendelenburg and the brilliant feat of Kirschner in performing it, it is generally recognized that far more patients have succumbed from embolectomy *without* extracorporeal circulation than have survived it.

In a series of 43 Trendelenburg operations performed between 1957 and 1963, there were only seven survivors, indicating again the high mortality associated with this procedure in the *absence* of cardiopulmonary bypass.[78]

In 1961, Sharp[66] was the first to use extracorporeal circulation in pulmonary embolectomy. This technique is the one generally preferred since it permits the operation to be conducted deliberately with concomitant oxygenation of body tissues.

**Indications.** An increasing appreciation of the natural history of pulmonary embolism and its characteristic tendency for spontaneous lysis, a process that is clearly augmented by the administration of anticoagulants and thrombolytic agents, has brought about a reduction in the number of patients considered to be appropriate candidates for embolectomy. At present, the primary indication for pulmonary embolectomy is *persistent and refractory hypotension* in a patient with massive embolism documented by either a lung scan or pulmonary arteriography. The findings from a patient in whom pulmonary embolectomy was necessary are shown in Figure 11. The immediate treatment of such patients is supportive, and many will respond to oxygen, heparinization, vasopressors, and inotropic agents. Clearly, every effort should be made to manage the patient by these means. The use of a vigorous regimen of this type has demonstrated that a number of patients previously thought to require embolectomy will respond favorably. Depending upon the severity of the clinical condition, one to several hours may be taken in an effort to restore satisfactory cardiopulmonary status. If administration of the agents described is effective in maintaining a blood pressure of 60 to 80 mm. Hg as demonstrated by a continuous intra-arterial recording, embolectomy may be deferred, particularly if renal and cerebral function is maintained.

**Technique.** A median sternotomy provides excellent exposure of the main pulmonary artery. The pericardium is opened and cardiopulmonary bypass is established. The main pulmonary artery is exposed and incised, and it is usually free of emboli although partially obstructing ones may be present. The emboli are removed from the right and left pulmonary arteries and their major branches. A Fogarty catheter may then be passed, with inflation of the balloon and withdrawal, to recover emboli from the smaller pulmonary arterial branches. Finally, copious irrigation with saline of the pulmonary arterial tree on both sides can be accomplished. During this portion of the procedure, general compression of

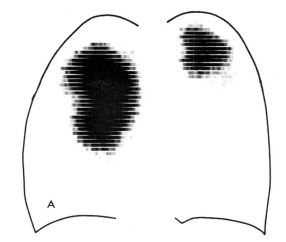

**Figure 11**  Illustrations from a patient with massive pulmonary embolism on the twelfth postoperative day following an orthopedic operation and accompanied by intractable shock. *A*, The pulmonary scan shows massive occlusion of the right lower and middle lobar pulmonary arteries as well as nearly all of the pulmonary arterial circulation to the left lung. *B*, Emboli removed from both pulmonary arteries at the time of embolectomy. (From Sabiston, D. C., Jr. In: Gibbon, J. H., Jr., Sabiston, D. C., Jr., and Spencer, F. C., eds.: Surgery of the Chest. 2nd ed. Philadelphia, W. B. Saunders Company, 1969.)

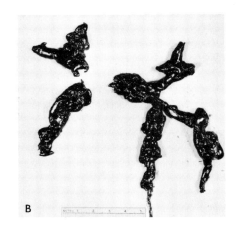

both lungs with the hand forces peripheral emboli back toward the central arteries for aspiration. Following closure of the pulmonary artery, cardiopulmonary bypass is gradually discontinued, and the heart and lungs are allowed to resume their normal function. Most observers agree that after closure of the median sternotomy the inferior vena cava should be interrupted with one of the appropriate methods (ligation, plication, or clip) in order to prevent further emboli. In some patients with severe cardiovascular collapse, partial cardiopulmonary bypass from the femoral vein to the femoral artery for immediate resuscitation may be necessary before the operative procedure is begun. If extracorporeal circulation is not available, an approach to either the right or left pulmonary artery can be made. In most patients with massive pulmonary embolism, one or the other pulmonary artery is primarily affected. Thus, the side with the major amount of embolus can be approached *without* the necessity for extracorporeal circulation. An anterior thoracotomy in the third interspace is quite appropriate for good exposure of the pulmonary artery. It can then be dissected to its origin, clamped, and opened for removal of the emboli while circulation and pulmonary function in the opposite lung are allowed to continue.[8,11,65]

**Results.**  In a collected series of 137 patients undergoing pulmonary embolectomy, the procedure was performed with cardiopulmonary bypass in 115 patients and without it in 22. Thrombi were found in *both* pulmonary arteries in 110 patients, whereas unilateral

thrombi were found in only 20 patients. Fifty of the 115 patients operated on with bypass survived (43 per cent) although the ultimate mortality (late deaths) reduced final survival to 32 per cent. Of the 22 patients operated on without use of extracorporeal circulation, 7 had emboli in one pulmonary artery and unilateral embolectomy was performed. Each of these 7 patients survived, but only 2 of the 15 remaining patients (with bilateral emboli) survived. It is of further interest that in 7 patients the diagnosis was in error, and at the time of operation no emboli were found; all 7 patients died after operation. *These latter findings emphasize quite strongly the necessity of establishing an objective diagnosis of pulmonary embolism prior to operation, either by lung scan or by pulmonary arteriography.*[14]

## CHRONIC PULMONARY EMBOLISM AND COR PULMONALE

Although embolic occlusion of the pulmonary arteries is most often an acute phenomenon, recent attention has been directed toward chronic pulmonary embolism associated with cor pulmonale. This is now a well established disorder, and despite its grave prognosis little attention has been given to its treatment.

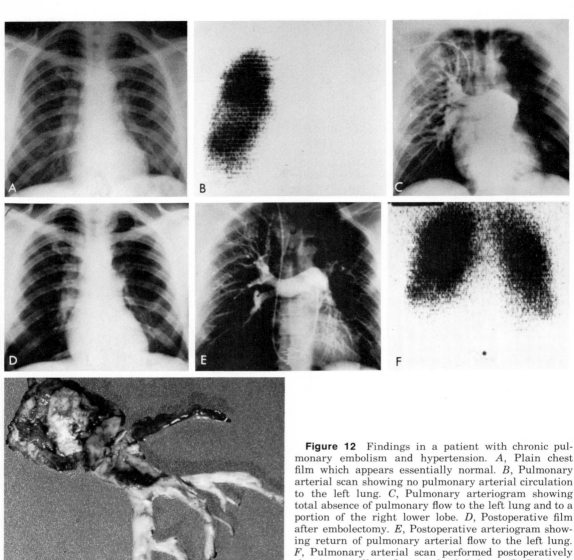

**Figure 12** Findings in a patient with chronic pulmonary embolism and hypertension. *A*, Plain chest film which appears essentially normal. *B*, Pulmonary arterial scan showing no pulmonary arterial circulation to the left lung. *C*, Pulmonary arteriogram showing total absence of pulmonary flow to the left lung and to a portion of the right lower lobe. *D*, Postoperative film after embolectomy. *E*, Postoperative arteriogram showing return of pulmonary arterial flow to the left lung. *F*, Pulmonary arterial scan performed postoperatively showing excellent flow to the left lung. *G*, Specimen removed from the left pulmonary artery and its branches which microscopically was shown to be a well organized thrombus. (From Moor, G. F., and Sabiston, D. C., Jr.: Circulation, *41*:701, 1970.)

In the recent past the diagnosis has been made with increasing frequency, and is in part a result of the more widespread use of pulmonary scanning and arteriography. The clinical manifestations of chronic pulmonary embolism are primarily dyspnea with evidence of pulmonary hypertension.

Firm indications should be present for surgical intervention. The patient clearly should have considerable dyspnea and preferably no serious additional cardiac or respiratory problems. Studies should demonstrate occlusion of the right or left main pulmonary artery and not solely occlusion of the smaller distal branches. The findings from a patient with chronic pulmonary embolism and hypertension successfully treated by embolectomy are shown in Figure 12. At present the results obtained appear to establish a firm role for operative treatment in selected cases of chronic pulmonary embolism and hypertension.[49] This is particularly important in view of the poor prognosis of patients treated nonoperatively.

## SELECTED REFERENCES

Cross, F. S., and Mowlem, A.: A survey of the current status of pulmonary embolectomy for massive pulmonary embolism. Circulation, Supp. 1, *35*:86, 1967.
*This paper presents the data obtained from a collective survey of patients undergoing pulmonary embolectomy from a large number of centers. Emphasis is placed on the necessity for an objective diagnosis (either by scan or by arteriography). A comparison is made between the use of extracorporeal circulation and the Trendelenburg technique of pulmonary embolectomy. This represents an unusually large series for analysis.*

Gorham, L. W.: A study of pulmonary embolism. Parts I and II. Arch. Intern. Med., *108*:8, 189, 1961.
*These companion papers emphasize the gross pathology of pulmonary embolism. Special emphasis is given the fact that in most patients with fatal embolism a substantial amount of the pulmonary arterial bed is occluded, generally more than half. This is one of the best pathologic studies in the literature.*

Hume, M., Sevitt, S., and Thomas, D. P.: Venous Thrombosis & Pulmonary Embolism. Cambridge, Mass., Harvard University Press, 1970.
*This monograph represents an updated source of the most recent information on the pathology, predisposing factors, mechanisms of thrombosis and clinical features of thromboembolism. The authors are a surgeon, a pathologist, and an internist each of whom has a particular interest in blood coagulation and thrombosis. The bibliography is extensive, and the pathophysiology of thromboembolism is described in detail. This monograph can be highly recommended.*

Marshall, R., Sabiston, D. C., Jr., Allison, P. R., Bosman, A. R., and Dunnill, M. S.: Immediate and late effects of pulmonary embolism by large thrombi in dogs. Thorax, *18*:1, 1963.
*In this experimental study, a variety of physiologic measurements were determined following pulmonary embolism. The study emphasizes the paucity of changes that occur when only one pulmonary artery is occluded and illustrates the wide margin of pulmonary reserve.*

Moor, G. F., and Sabiston, D. C., Jr.: Embolectomy for chronic pulmonary embolism and hypertension. Case report and review of the problem. Circulation, *41*:701, 1970.
*The use of pulmonary embolectomy for chronic pulmonary embolism and hypertension is reviewed. The diagnostic features, indications for operation, operative technique, and results are presented.*

Ochsner, A. A., Ochsner, J. L., and Sanders, H. S.: Prevention of pulmonary embolism by caval ligation. Ann. Surg., *171*:923, 1970.
*The authors of this paper describe an increasing utilization of inferior vena caval ligation in the treatment of pulmonary embolism. A strong position is taken concerning the necessity of ligation, and it represents what is probably the most outspoken view supporting inferior vena caval interruption.*

Piccone, V. A., Jr., Vidal, E., Yarnoz, M., Glass, P., and LeVeen, H. H.: The late results of caval ligation. Surgery, *68*:980, 1970.
*The data in this paper emphasize the numerous and frequent complications following inferior vena caval interruption. Moreover, recurrent embolism after interruption is appreciable. These studies indicate the increasing reluctance to employ inferior vena caval interruption unless firm indications are present.*

Sabiston, D. C., Jr., and Wolfe, W. G.: Experimental and clinical observations on the natural history of pulmonary embolism. Ann. Surg., *168*:1, 1968.
*In this paper the natural history of pulmonary emboli in the experimental animal and man is discussed. The gross and microscopic features and their changes with the passage of time are illustrated. The gradual resolution of the emboli and final disappearance in most instances are confirmed by serial scans and pulmonary arteriograms.*

Sasahara, A. A.: Pulmonary angiography in the diagnosis of thromboembolic disease. New Eng. J. Med., *270*:1075, 1964.
*The use of pulmonary angiography is critically appraised in this paper. The indications and diagnostic features of pulmonary angiography are well reviewed. For a detailed consideration of pulmonary arteriography, this paper is an important one.*

Sasahara, A. A., and Stein, M.: Pulmonary Embolic Disease. New York, Grune & Stratton, 1965.
*This monograph is an excellent source of detailed information on all aspects of pulmonary embolism. It is composed of contributions of numerous authorities in the field and is highly recommended.*

Sevitt, S., and Gallagher, N. G.: Prevention of venous thrombosis and pulmonary embolism in injured patients: Trial of anticoagulant prophylaxis with phenindione in middle-aged and elderly patients with fractured necks of femur. Lancet, *2*:981, 1959.
*The studies described in this paper are classic for objective documentation of the value of prophylactic anticoagulation in high-risk patients. The authors are highly respected, and the data presented have led to a general use of prophylactic anticoagulants for special indications in a number of centers.*

Wagner, H. N., Jr., Sabiston, D. C., Jr., Ilio, M., McAfee, J. G., Meyer, J. K., and Langan, J. K.: Regional pulmonary blood flow in man by radioisotope scanning. J.A.M.A., *187*:601, 1964.
*In this paper the original experimental and clinical studies introducing the technique of radioactive pulmonary scanning are described.*

## REFERENCES

1. Alexander, B.: Blood coagulation and thrombotic disease. Circulation, 25:872, 1962.
2. Alexander, B., Meyers, L., Kenny, J., Goldstein, R., Gurewich, V., and Grinspoon, L.: Blood coagulation in pregnancy. Proconvertin and prothrombin, and the hypercoagulable state. New Eng. J. Med., 254:358, 1956.
3. Allison, P. R.: Pulmonary embolism and thrombophlebitis. Brit. J. Surg., 54:466, 1967.
4. Baker, R. R.: Pulmonary embolism. Surgery, 54:687, 1963.
5. Barker, N. W., Nygaard, K. K., Walters, W., and Priestley, J. T.: A statistical study of post-operative venous thrombosis and pulmonary embolism: Predisposing factors. Proc. Mayo Clin., 16:1, 1941.
6. Bauer, G.: Clinical experiences of a surgeon in the use of heparin. Amer. J. Cardiol., 14:29, 1964.
7. Boyer, N. H., and Curry, J. J.: Bronchospasm associated with pulmonary embolism. Arch. Intern. Med., 73:403, 1944.
8. Bradley, M. N., Bennett, A. L., III, and Lyons, C.: Successful unilateral pulmonary embolectomy without cardiopulmonary bypass. New Eng. J. Med., 271:713, 1964.
9. Brofman, B. L., Charms, B. L., Kohn, P. M., Elder, J., Newman, R., and Rizika, M.: Unilateral pulmonary artery

occlusion in man. Control studies. J. Thorac. Surg., 34:206, 1957.

10. Burnett, W. E., Long, J. H., Norris, C., Rosemond, G. P., and Webster, M. R.: The effect of pneumonectomy on pulmonary function. J. Thorac. Surg., 18:569, 1949.

11. Camishion, R. C., Pierucci, L., Jr., Fishman, N. H., Fraimow, W., and Greening, R.: Pulmonary embolectomy without cardiopulmonary bypass. Amer. J. Surg., 111:723, 1966.

12. Comroe, J. H., Jr., Van Lingen, B., Stroud, R. C., and Roncoroni, A.: Reflex and direct cardiopulmonary effects of 5-OH-tryptamine (serotonin). Amer. J. Physiol., 173:379, 1953.

13. Coon, W. W., and Coller, F. A.: Some epidemiologic considerations of thromboembolism. Surg. Gynec. Obstet., 109:487, 1959.

14. Cross, F. S., and Mowlem, A.: A survey of the current status of pulmonary embolectomy for massive pulmonary embolism. Circulation, Supp. 1, 35:86, 1967.

15. Cruveilhier, J.: Anatomie Pathologique de Corps Humain. Paris, J. B. Bailliere, 1829–42.

16. DeBakey, M. E.: A critical evaluation of the problem of thromboembolism. Int. Abstr. Surg., 98:1, 1954.

17. DeWeese, J. A., Jones, T. I., Lyon, J., and Dale, W. A.: Evaluation of thrombectomy in the management of iliofemoral venous thrombosis. Surgery, 47:140, 1960.

18. DeWeese, M. S., and Hunter, D. C., Jr.: A vena cava filter for the prevention of pulmonary embolism: A five-year clinical experience. Arch. Surg., 86:852, 1963.

19. Dexter, L.: Cardiovascular responses to experimental pulmonary embolism. In: Sasahara, A. A., and Stein, M. eds.: Pulmonary Embolic Disease. New York, Grune & Stratton, 1965.

20. Flanc, C., Kakkar, V. V., and Clarke, M. B.: Post-operative deep vein thrombosis: Effect of intensive prophylaxis. Lancet, 1:477, 1969.

21. Fred, H. L., Axelrad, M. A., Lewis, J. M., and Alexander, J. K.: Rapid resolution of pulmonary thromboemboli in man. J.A.M.A., 196:1137, 1966.

22. Freiman, D. G.: Pathologic observations on experimental and human thromboembolism. In: Sasahara, A. A., and Stein, M., eds.: Pulmonary Embolic Disease. New York, Grune & Stratton, 1965.

23. Gibbs, N. M.: Venous thrombosis of the lower limbs with particular reference to bed rest. Brit. J. Surg., 45:209, 1957.

24. Gorham, L. W.: A study of pulmonary embolism. Part I. Arch. Intern. Med., 108:8, 1961.

25. Gorham, L. W.: A study of pulmonary embolism. Part II. Arch. Intern. Med., 108:189, 1961.

26. Gurewich, V., Sasahara, A. A., and Stein, M.: Pulmonary embolism, bronchoconstriction and response to heparin. In: Sasahara, A. A., and Stein, M., eds.: Pulmonary Embolic Disease. New York, Grune & Stratton, 1965.

27. Gurewich, V., Thomas, D. P., and Rabinov, K. R.: Pulmonary embolism after ligation of the inferior vena cava. New Eng. J. Med., 274:1350, 1966.

28. Haller, J. A.: Thrombectomy for deep thrombophlebitis of the leg. New Eng. J. Med., 267:65, 1962.

29. Hume, M., Sevitt, S., and Thomas, D. P.: Venous thrombosis & Pulmonary Embolism. Cambridge, Mass., Harvard University Press, 1970.

30. Hunter, W. C., Krygier, J. J., Kennedy, J. C., and Sneeden, V. D.: Etiology and prevention of thrombosis of the deep leg veins. Surgery, 17:178, 1945.

31. Jick, H., Slone, D., Westerholm, B., Inman, W. H. W., Vessey, M. P., Shapiro, S., Lewis, G. P., and Worcester, J.: Venous thromboembolic disease and ABO blood type. Lancet, 1:539, 1969.

32. Jones, R. H., and Sabiston, D. C., Jr.: Pulmonary embolism in childhood. Monogr. Surg. Sci., 3:35, 1966.

33. Jones, T. Wharton: Guy's Hospital Reports, 2nd Series, 7:42, 1851.

34. Karp, R. B., and Wylie, E. J.: Recurrent thrombosis after iliofemoral venous thrombectomy. Surg. Forum, 17:147, 1966.

35. Kernohan, R. J., and Todd, C.: Heparin therapy in thromboembolic disease. Lancet, 1:621, 1966.

36. Kirschner, M.: Ein durch die Trendelenburgsche Operation geheilter Fall von Embolie der Arterien pulmonalis. Arch. Klin. Chir., 133:312, 1924.

37. Kovacs, G. S., Hill, J. D., Abert, T., Blesovsky, A., and

38. Gerbode, F.: Pathogenesis of arterial hypoxemia in pulmonary embolism. Arch. Surg., 93:813, 1966.

39. Langman, M. J. S., and Doll, R.: ABO blood group and secretor status in relation to clinical characteristics of peptic ulcer. Gut, 6:270, 1965.

40. Littmann, D.: Observations on the electrocardiographic changes in pulmonary embolism. In: Sasahara, A. A., and Stein, M., eds.: Pulmonary Embolic Disease. New York, Grune & Stratton, 1965.

41. Mahorner, H., Castleberry, J. W., and Coleman, W. O.: Attempts to restore function in major veins which are the site of massive thrombosis. Ann. Surg., 146:510, 1957.

42. Marshall, R., Sabiston, D. C., Alliston, P. R., Bosman, A. R., and Dunnill, M. S.: Immediate and late effects of pulmonary embolism by large thrombi in dogs. Thorax, 18:1, 1963.

43. McLachlin, A. D., McLachlin, J. A., Jory, T. A., and Rawling, E. G.: Venous stasis in the lower extremities. Ann. Surg., 152:678, 1960.

44. McLachlin, J., and Paterson, J. C.: Some basic observations on venous thrombosis and pulmonary embolism. Surg. Gynec. Obstet., 93:1, 1951.

45. Medical Research Council Subcommittee: Risk of thromboembolic disease in women taking oral contraceptives. Brit. Med. J., 2:355, 1967.

46. Meister, H.: Ueber Thrombose und Lungenembolie. Statistische Untersuchungen an 15,130 Sektionen. Frankfurt. z. Path., 70:640, 1960.

47. Miles, R. M., Chappell, F., and Renner, O.: Partially occluding vena caval clip for prevention of pulmonary emboli. Amer. Surg., 30:40, 1964.

48. Mobin-Uddin, K., Bolooki, H., and Jude, J. R.: A new simplified method of caval interruption for the prevention of pulmonary embolus. Circulation, Supp. 3, 40:149, 1969.

49. Moor, G. F., and Sabiston, D. C., Jr.: Embolectomy for chronic pulmonary embolism and hypertension. Case report and review of the problem. Circulation, 41:701, 1970.

50. Moretz, W. H., Rhode, C. M., and Shepherd, M. H.: Prevention of pulmonary emboli by partial occlusion of inferior vena cava. Amer. Surg., 25:617, 1959.

51. Morrell, M. T., Truelove, S. C., and Barr, A.: Pulmonary embolism. Brit. Med. J., 2:830, 1963.

52. Neumann, R.: Ursprungszentren und Entwicklungsformen der Beinthrombose. Virchow's Arch. Path. Anat., 301:708, 1938.

53. Ochsner, A.: Indications for and results of inferior vena caval ligation for thromboembolic disease. Postgrad. Med., 27:193, 1960.

54. Ochsner, A., Ochsner, J. L., and Sanders, H. S.: Prevention of pulmonary embolism by caval ligation. Ann. Surg., 171:923, 1970.

55. Piccone, V. A., Jr., Vidal, E., Yarnoz, M., Glass, P., and LeVeen, H. H.: The late results of caval ligation. Surgery, 68:980, 1970.

56. Registrar-General's Statistical Review of England and Wales. London, Her Majesty's Stationery Office, 1966.

57. Roberts, G. H.: Venous thrombosis in hospital patients: A postmortem study. Scot. Med. J., 8:11, 1963.

58. Robin, E. D., Julian, D. G., Travis, D. M., and Crump, C. H.: A physiologic approach to diagnosis of acute pulmonary embolism. New Eng. J. Med., 260:586, 1959.

59. Rossle, R.: Uber die Bedeutung und die Entstehung der Wadenvenenthrombosen. Virchow's Arch. Path. Anat., 30:180, 1937.

60. Sabiston, D. C., Jr., and Wagner, H. N., Jr.: The pathophysiology of pulmonary embolism: Relationships to accurate diagnosis and choice of therapy. J. Thorac. Cardiovasc. Surg., 50:339, 1965.

61. Sabiston, D. C., Jr. and Wolfe, W. G.: Experimental and clinical observations on the natural history of pulmonary embolism. Ann. Surg., 168:1, 1968.

62. Sasahara, A. A.: Clinical studies in pulmonary thromboembolism. In: Sasahara, A. A., and Stein, M., eds.: Pulmonary Embolic Disease. New York, Grune & Stratton, 1965.

63. Sautter, R. D., Fletcher, F. W., Emanuel, D. A., Lawton, B. R., and Olsen, T. G.: Complete resolution of massive pulmonary thromboembolism. J.A.M.A., 189:948, 1964.

64. Sautter, R. D., Lawton, B. R., Magnin, G. E., and Burns, J. L.: Pulmonary embolectomy. A simplified technique. Wisconsin Med. J. 61:309, 1962.

65. Sevitt, S., and Gallagher, N. G.: Venous thrombosis and pulmonary embolism in injured patients: A trial of anticoagulant prophylaxis with phenindione in middle-aged and elderly patients with fractured neck of femur. Lancet, 2:981, 1961.

66. Sharp, E. H.: Pulmonary embolectomy: Successful removal of a massive pulmonary embolus with the support of cardiopulmonary bypass. A Case Report. Ann. Surg., 156:1, 1962.

67. Silver, D., and Gleysteen, J. J.: Paradoxical arterial embolism. Amer. Surg., 36:47, 1970.

68. Simon, M., and Sasahara, A. A.: Observations on the angiographic changes in pulmonary thromboembolism. In: Sasahara, A. A., and Stein, M., eds.: Pulmonary Embolic Disease. New York, Grune & Stratton, 1965.

69. Sloan, H., Morris, J. D., Figley, M., and Lee, R.,: Temporary unilateral occlusion of the pulmonary artery in the preoperative evaluation of thoracic patients. J. Thorac. Surg., 30:591, 1955.

70. Smith, G. T., Dexter, L., and Dammin, G. J.: Postmortem quantitative studies in pulmonary embolism. In: Sasahara, A. A., and Stein, M., eds.: Pulmonary Embolic Disease. New York, Grune & Stratton, 1965.

71. Spector, I., and Corn, M.: Control of heparin therapy with activated partial thromboplastin times. J.A.M.A., 201:157, 1967.

72. Spencer, F. C., Jude, J., Rienhoff, W. F., III, and Stonesifer, G.: Plication of the inferior vena cava for pulmonary embolism: Long-term results in 39 cases. Ann. Surg., 161:788, 1965.

73. Torrance, D. J.: The Chest Film in Massive Pulmonary Embolism. Springfield, Ill., Charles C Thomas, 1963.

74. Trendelenburg, F.: Ueber die operative Behandlung der Embolie der Lungenarterie. Arch. Klin. Chir., 86:686, 1908.

75. Urokinase Pulmonary Embolism Trial Study Group: Urokinase pulmonary embolism trial. Phase 1 results. A cooperative study. J.A.M.A., 214:2163, 1970.

76. Vessey, M. P., and Doll, R.: Investigation of relation between the use of oral contraceptives and thromboembolic disease. Brit. Med. J., 2:199, 1968.

77. Virchow, R.: Die Cellularpathologie in ihrer Begrundung auf physiologische und pathologische Gewebelehre. Berlin, A. Hirschwald, 1858.

78. Vossschulte, K.: The surgical treatment of pulmonary embolism. J. Cardiovasc. Surg., Supp. 197, 1965.

79. Wacker, W. E. C., and Snodgrass, P. J.: Serum LDH activity in pulmonary embolism diagnosis. J.A.M.A., 174:2142, 1960.

80. Wagner, H. N., Jr., Sabiston, D. C., Jr., Ilio, M., McAfee, J. G., Meyer, J. K., and Langan, J. K.: Regional pulmonary blood flow in man by radioisotope scanning. J.A.M.A., 187:601, 1964.

81. Weideranders, R. E., White, S. M., and Saichek, H. B.: The effect of pulmonary resection on pulmonary artery pressures. Ann. Surg., 160:889, 1964.

82. Welch, W. H.: W. H. Welch's Papers and Addresses. ed. W. C. Burket. Baltimore, Johns Hopkins Press, 1920.

83. Westermark, N.: On the roentgen diagnosis of lung embolism. Acta Radiol., 19:357, 1938.

# 52

# DISORDERS OF
# THE ARTERIAL SYSTEM

## I

## Historical Aspects

*David C. Sabiston, Jr., M.D.*

Much of the history of surgery is a record of its technical advances, and the development of surgical control of the *arterial* system represents one of the most important achievements. It is of particular significance that within the past two decades vascular surgery has reached a state previously thought impossible. The advent of direct surgery of the arteries and the use of autografts, homografts, and arterial prostheses, together with the introduction of extracorporeal circulation, have formed the basis for brilliant accomplishments. Moreover, there is reason to believe that these advances will continue and that much more progress lies ahead.

The beginning of hemostasis in wounds is recorded in ancient Chinese literature, where bandaging and use of styptics were advocated. During the era of Hippocrates, ligation of vessels was rarely practiced, and amputations were done only through the gangrenous extremity at a site where the vessels were thrombosed. Hemorrhage was controlled by the use of elevation, compression, and tamponade and occasionally by hot metal cautery. Celsus advanced beyond the hippocratic doctrine to the point of amputation at the line of demarcation, but here again most of the vessels were thrombosed. At that time he advocated limited use of the ligature. In about A.D. 100, Archigenes was more daring and advanced the scope of amputation materially by proposing that it be performed for "gangrene, necrosis, cancer and certain callus tumors." He advocated preliminary ligation of vessels leading to the site of amputation. Antyllus made a further advance by recommending surgical treatment of aneurysms by proximal ligation of the arteries, and Galen advocated the use of Celtic linen ligatures. Despite these advances, the ligature was *rarely* used for amputations and then only as a last resort, preference being given to the actual cautery to secure hemostasis.

In 1552, Paré used a ligature instead of hot irons to control the hemorrhage in amputating the leg of an officer wounded at the siege of Danvilliers. It was this procedure that prompted Paré to state, "I dressed him and God healed him. He returned home gaily with a wooden leg saying that he had got off cheaply without being miserably burned to stop the bleeding." This operation heralded the beginning of the common use of the ligature for the control of arterial bleeding, and Paré deserves much credit for reintroducing a forgotten principle. An excellent account of the historical facts concerning control of bleeding and the development of ligatures is found in *The History of Hemostasis* by Harvey.[8]

To William Hunter[9] is due recognition for his dissections of aneurysms and early recommendations for arterial ligature. He also was the first to recognize that an arteriovenous aneurysm represented a direct communication between an artery and vein and was not a simple aneurysm. In the next century, Matas[11] first advocated endoaneurysmorrhaphy in the treatment of arterial aneurysms. Another major advance was made by Carrel and Guthrie,[2-4] with their contribution of direct suture anastomosis of arteries. It was for this and pioneering work in the transplantation of organs that Carrel was awarded the Nobel Prize in 1912. In 1910 Lexer[10] reported the substitution of an artery by a saphenous vein autograft, a procedure now commonplace in vascular surgery.

In 1927, Moniz, a Portuguese neurologist, used intra-arterial injection of thorium dioxide to outline the cerebral vessels.[12] About the same time, dos Santos and associates injected a contrast medium directly into the aorta.[13] An aortic abdominal aneurysm was successfully removed and replaced by an arterial homograft for the first time by Dubost in 1951.[6] Following this, thoracic aneurysms were successfully attacked by DeBakey[5] and Bahnson,[1] and these procedures were greatly augmented by the introduction by Gibbon of successful extracorporeal circulation in 1953.[7] The introduction of prosthetic arterial substitutes began in 1952, when Voorhees and Blakemore[14] first used Vinyon-N; additional study with other materials led to the present-day use of Dacron and Teflon.

For references, see page 1642.

# II

# Anatomy

*David C. Sabiston, Jr., M.D.*

The function of the arterial system is delivery of blood from the heart to the tissues. For purposes of convenience, the arteries may be divided into (1) large, (2) medium-sized, and (3) small arteries. Arteries less than 100 $\mu$ in diameter are termed *arterioles*. The histologic characteristics of the arterial wall are largely dependent upon the *size* of the vessel. The *large* arteries must withstand the greatest stress and pressure and therefore contain considerable *elastic tissue* in their walls. The *medium-sized* arteries have less elastic tissue and more *smooth muscle*, and the wall of the small arteries is composed primarily of smooth muscle. At the level of the arteriole, elastic tissue is quite scant or absent. *Collagen* is present in all parts of the arterial system, with the collagen ratio becoming dominant as the arteries become smaller.

The principles of *collateral circulation* are of primary importance in all aspects of medicine, and particularly in surgery. All organs have *some* degree of collateral circulation, although the amount that occurs naturally varies greatly in the different tissues and organs and in the same organs in different subjects. For example, the subclavian artery usually can be ligated safely in the first portion, as in the performance of a subclavian-pulmonary anastomosis for congenital cyanotic heart disease (Blalock operation), since the collateral circulation around the shoulder is excellent. It is rare for ischemic symptoms to follow ligation of the subclavian at this site, and, indeed, frequently with the passage of time a pulse reappears in the radial artery as additional collateral circulation develops. Moreover, three of the four major arteries to the stomach (the left and right gastric and left and right gastric epiploic) can be ligated without significant ischemia in most subjects. With a number of other arteries the extensiveness of collaterals varies considerably from person to person, ligation producing no ill effects in some patients and ischemia in others. Finally, some arteries, such as the coronary, renal, and retinal arteries, have a very inadequate natural collateral circulation. Acute occlusion of these vessels is usually followed by serious changes of ischemia and infarction, and such arteries are referred to as "end-arteries."

The *natural* collateral circulation of a tissue or organ is important in the sequence of events following acute occlusion. In addition, the *time* involved in occlusion of an artery is of great significance. For example, with *slow* and progressive occlusion of an artery, there is ample time for collateral vessels to become *larger*. Generally, as a smaller vessel is subjected to a need for increased flow (primarily due to a pressure gradient), the vessel is apt to become *tortuous*. The latter characteristic is easily and consistently delineated arteriographically, as in chronic occlusion of the abdominal aorta (Leriche syndrome). Under these circumstances, adequate arterial collaterals develop which link the branches above the occlusion with the iliac and femoral systems below. It is surprising to recognize that total occlusion of the entire abdominal aorta may produce minimal symptoms in some patients, whereas in others it results in the characteristic symptoms of intermittent claudication and impotence. Nevertheless, in the Leriche syndrome, it is rare to note gangrene until late in the disease, whereas *acute* occlusion of the abdominal aorta usually produces disastrous effects, with acute appearance of severe ischemia and gangrene of the legs if untreated.

# III

# Physiologic Aspects

*David C. Sabiston, Jr., M.D.*

There are a number of physiologic variables that control flow through the arterial system. It is apparent that the pumping action of the heart and its force are essential for blood flow. Flow is also critically regulated by *resistance* in the peripheral arterial bed. The factors that contribute to resistance to flow through a tube are expressed in Poiseuille's law:

$$P_1 - P_2 = \frac{8L\,Fv}{\pi R^4}$$

L = length
R = radius
F = volume flow
v = viscosity
$P_1 - P_2$ = pressure gradient

In consideration of the entire vascular bed, the total resistance to flow is the sum of the resistances of both the arterial and venous systems. The primary effect on resistance is contributed by those arteries which are 200 $\mu$ or less in diameter. Thus, the force of cardiac contraction, luminal size, and the peripheral resistance are all important in the control of arterial pressure. The sympathetic nervous system may produce *vasoconstriction*, thus increasing peripheral resistance. Hypoxia produces *vasodilation* and may be followed by increased blood flow without an increase in perfusion pressure. Thus, the major factors controlling blood flow reside in the small arteries.

## SELECTED REFERENCES

Green, H. D., Rapela, C. E., and Conrad, M. C.: Resistance (conductance) and capacitance phenomena in terminal vascular beds. In: American Physiological Society: Handbook of Physiology. Section 2, Circulation. Dow, P., and Hamilton, W. F., eds. Baltimore, Williams & Wilkins Company, 1963.
*This is an excellent resource for a complete discussion of the regulation of peripheral blood flow. The anatomic, physiologic, neurogenic, and metabolic aspects of the peripheral circulation are considered in appropriate detail.*

Strandness, D. E., Jr.: Functional characteristics of normal and collateral circulation. In: Strandness, D. E., Jr., ed.: Collateral Circulation in Clinical Surgery. Philadelphia, W. B. Saunders Company, 1969.
*This chapter provides an excellent description of the natural*

*collateral circulation in the various systems and organs of the body. Those features which control the development of collaterals following vascular obstruction and the pathways involved are beautifully presented.*

## REFERENCES

1. Bahnson, H. T.: Definitive treatment of saccular aneurysms of the aorta with excision of sac and aortic sutures. Surg. Gynec. Obstet., *96*:382, 1953.
2. Carrel, A.: La technique opératoire des anastomoses vasculaires et la transplantation des viscères. Lyon Med., *98*:859, 1902.
3. Carrel, A.: Suture of blood-vessels and transplantation of organs. Nobel Lecture, 1912. In: Nobel Lectures in Physiology-Medicine. Volume 1. New York, American Elsevier Publishing Company, 1967, p. 442.
4. Carrel, A., and Guthrie, C. C.: Uniterminal and biterminal venous transplantations. Surg. Gynec. Obstet., *2*:266, 1906.
5. DeBakey, M. E., and Cooley, D. A.: Successful resection of aneurysm of thoracic aorta and replacement by graft. J.A.M.A., *152*:673, 1953.
6. Dubost, C., Allary, M., and Oeconomos, N.: Resection of an aneurysm of the abdominal aorta: Reestablishment of the continuity by a preserved human arterial graft, with results after five months. Arch. Surg., *64*:405, 1952.
7. Gibbon, J. H., Jr.: Application of a mechanical heart and lung apparatus to cardiac surgery. Minn. Med., *37*:171, 1954.
8. Harvey, S. C.: The History of Hemostasis. New York, Paul B. Hoeber, 1929.
9. Hunter, W.: The history of an aneurysm of the aorta, with some remarks on aneurysms in general. Med. Observ. Inquir., *1*:323, 1757.
10. Lexer, E.: Die ideale Operation des arteriellen und des arteriell-venosen Aneurysma. Arch. Klin. Chir., *83*:459, 1907.
11. Matas, R.: An operation for the radical cure of aneurism based upon arteriorrhaphy. Ann. Surg., *37*:161, 1903.
12. Moniz, E.: Injections intracarotidiennes et substances injectables opaques aux rayons. X. Presse Med., *2*:969, 1927.
13. dos Santos, R., Lamas, A., and Caldas, J.: L'artériographie des membres, de l'aorte et de ses branches abdominales. Bull. Soc. Nat. chir., *55*:587, 1929.
14. Voorhees, A. B., Jr., Jaretzki, A., II, and Blakemore, A. H.: The use of tubes constructed from vinyon "N" cloth in bridging arterial defects. Ann. Surg., *135*:332, 1952.

# IV

# Arterial Substitutes

*William W. Krippaehne, M.D.*

The perfect arterial substitute has not yet been developed. Normal arteries have often been classified as the ideal, and autogenous arteries as the best vascular substitute. For long-term survival, however, these vessels leave much to be desired. Their ultimate fate is progression to arterial disease, which at present is the leading cause of death in the United States. Since the most frequent need for arterial substitutes is in patients with degenerate vascular disease, other substitutes warrant further consideration.

An optimal arterial substitute should: (1) have persistent strength, (2) be easily, reliably, and permanently attachable to the host vessel, (3) be resistant to infection, (4) be obtainable in sterile form or easily sterilizable, (5) be available as needed and in appropriate sizes, and (6) have considerable flexibility. Moreover, such substitutes *should not*: (1) leak blood on restoration of flow, (2) participate in degeneration encountered by other vessels, (3) incite abnormal surrounding reaction such as neoplasia, (4) induce thrombus formation either in the graft or at the interface with the blood vessel to which it is attached, and (5) occlude when bent at a flexion crease.

The modern era of arterial vascular substitutes received impetus from experimental studies of Alexis Carrel reported in 1908.[3] He demonstrated that fresh arterial homografts could be safely transplanted for months. Elastic and medial fibers remained viable and intima thickened. Recognizing the difficulty of obtaining arteries, he explored anew the use of veins as arterial substitutes. A careful observer, Carrel quickly recognized that the reported high thrombotic complication rate was partially due to the difference in caliber of vessels. Results improved when he experimented with veins comparable in size to the arteries to be replaced. He further observed that by 14 days the veins had thickened in response to the physical forces of arterial pulsatile flow. Adventitial connective tissues increased, as did the interstitium of the muscular coat. He noted that this process was not uniform. In addition, Carrel pioneered studies of preservation and banking of homografts.[3,4] Microscopic changes in the arterial wall seemed to depend upon the nature of the preservative and duration of refrigeration. In later studies,[4] nonviable grafts killed by heat, formalin, and glycerin rapidly degenerated but did elicit host reaction—building of a surrounding new wall of connective tissue.

Research and clinical trial of many possible replacements soon followed the demonstration that early successful substitution was feasible. Experimental design has resulted in the evaluation of many categories of substitutes: autografts, homografts, heterografts, solid tubes, textile grafts, and composite or compound grafts. At present, evidence suggests that large arteries are best replaced with textiles of desirable specifications and small vessels with autogenous veins of suitable size and wall thickness.

## ARTERIAL AUTOGRAFTS

Arterial autografts are generally accepted as the ideal arterial substitute; however, they are not readily available. Technically, they are easy to handle. Their clinical function is comparable to that of the normal artery. Upon implantation, the wall usually retains viability of all its components. Anastomotic strength at 10 days is approximately 20 per cent, gradually rising to 70 per cent of normal artery tensile strength within 6 weeks.[14] If the arterial graft is thicker than 500 to 600 $\mu$ and revascularization of the vasa vasorum does not occur, the outer layer undergoes avascular necrosis, as has been demonstrated by Berger.[1] Geiringer,[15] Berger,[1] and others found that the inner 350 to 500 $\mu$ receives its nutrition by luminal diffusion. This process as diagrammatically depicted by Berger is shown in Figures 1 and 2. Clot surrounding any graft or suture line may delay revascularization. There is minimal or no luminal thrombus deposition if the endothelium is not damaged and if the procedure is technically correct. Varying amounts of late thrombus formation occur in rough proportion to the degree of degeneration or inflammation in or around the graft wall. A small amount appears initially at suture lines, but is characteristically resorbed within 10 to 20 days. If thrombosis persists, organization by capillaries and fibroblasts contributes to permanent intimal thickening and luminal narrowing. This process is similar to the fibrotic stage of human atherosclerosis.

## VENOUS AUTOGRAFTS

Venous autografts have many advantages as autologous materials. They retain cellular viability and do not show rejection phenomena. They are more readily available than arteries,

**Figure 1** Diagrammatic conception of nutrition to the thoracic aortic wall. Luminal diffusion serves the inner portion of the wall. Vasa vasorum serve the outer portion. A narrower zone, the overlap zone, is served by both mechanisms. At *1*, an intercostal artery emerges. This in turn gives off branches that travel in the outer medial layer of the wall, as well as along the adventitia. At *2*, branches from the adventitial system traverse into the outer media. At *3*, connection may occur to adventitial vessels other than those derived from intercostals. At *4* is shown an adventitial vessel derived from the "nonintercostal" system. (From Berger, K., et al.: Pacif. Med. Surg., 75:367, 1967.)

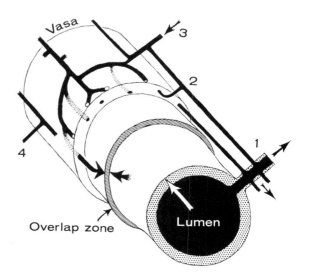

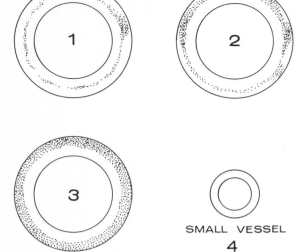

**Figure 2** Diagrammatic summary of luminal diffusion and vasa vasorum zones of influence as observed in canine experiments. Necrosis is indicated by stippled areas. *1*, Results from minor trauma exemplified by aortic-aortic anastomoses, namely, freeing of the vessel ends necessary for sewing them together. This is taken to be an example of overlap zone damage. *2*, Irregular necrosis of outer wall resulting from removal of thoracic aortic segment with intercostals ligated only. *3*. Necrosis of outer wall following removal of aortic segment, plus excision of intercostal ostia. In all three instances the viable luminal diffusion zone remains of about the same order of thickness. *4*, Full wall viability of small transected and reanastomosed vessel, whose wall thickness falls within diffusion zone distance. (From Berger, K., et al.: Pacif. Med. Surg., *75:367*, 1967.)

although not always in the proper size, length, or wall thickness. Wall strength is insufficient for large vessel replacement, as in the aorta or iliac system, but adequate for smaller vessel replacement, as in the extremities or in aortocoronary grafting. The thin walls of veins make them particularly suited for vessel replacement. Luminal diffusion maintains wall nutrition even if the venous microcirculation is interfered with. Vein walls increase in thickness and strength when exposed to the environmental stress of the arterial position (a common biologic phenomenon of body collagen on stretching).

Technically, veins are not as readily sutured as arteries because of thin walls. As anastomoses become smaller, exacting microsurgical techniques are imperative. Vessels of proper diameter are required and endothelial damage must be scrupulously avoided.

In the femoropopliteal system, "long-term" patency rates are reported as high as 85 per cent.[26] A more accurate comparison, recommended by Kouchoukos et al.,[20] is based upon accumulative patency rates. They are higher in cases of aneurysms or trauma than in the presence of obliterative disease with its diminished run-off potential.

The best rates are achieved when all of the popliteal trifurcation is open and least when only one vessel is patent. Grafts smaller than 5 mm. in diameter demonstrate lower rates of patency than do larger vessels. Early studies suggest that autogenous veins are the best material now available for aortocoronary grafting, although some occlude with either fibrosis or thrombosis.

## ARTERIAL HOMOGRAFTS

Arterial homografts were first implanted by Hoepfner in 1903 and studied by Carrel in 1906 to 1908. In early results these grafts appeared functional and similar to autografts. Further investigation with longer evaluation revealed that both fresh and preserved grafts lose viability and undergo degenerative changes.

Grafting of the aorta and the iliac arteries, which are composed predominantly of collagen and elastin with smooth muscle cells, is associated with fewer complications and longer graft survival than grafting of the femoral vessels, which have a larger proportion of smooth muscle. Histologically, grafts in both sites lose endothelium early. Exposed collagen attracts fibrin and cellular elements, including platelets. This mass organizes and endothelializes early at the suture line where host fibroblasts are available to invade. This process proceeds slowly along the wall. The central wall undergoes degeneration and becomes acellular. Over a 1 to 3 year period, the elastin fragments. Walls become thinner owing to loss of the muscular layer. A high degree of patchy ulceration and aneurysmal dilatation occurs in most grafts by 3 years. The degenerative process is more marked in the femoral location because of its larger muscular components. The high antigenicity of smooth muscle also results in greater homograft rejection signs in these vessels. Varying amounts of host collagen are deposited around these vessels and gradually invade the graft's superficial layers.

Gross results show that aortic homografts rupture, thrombose, are subject to development of aneurysms, and occasionally leak at the suture line. Degenerative problems progress with time. Deterling[8] reported that 77 per cent of such grafts were clinically satisfactory at 5 years and 38 per cent at 10 years after operation. Femoral grafts present a similar but worse history, with fewer than a third satisfactory at 3 years. Because of these factors, the arterial homografts have been abandoned in favor of more satisfactory materials.

## ARTERIAL HETEROGRAFTS

Owing to long-term failure of the available smaller-caliber textile grafts and the frequent unavailability of satisfactory veins for femoropopliteal reconstruction, a modified bovine arterial heterograft is receiving increasing interest.[19, 27] This graft is fresh bovine carotid artery, treated with a proteolytic enzyme (ficin) to remove elastic and muscular tissue. The remaining collagen is tanned with a dialdehyde starch solution. The former procedure removes antigenicity and the latter crosslinks collagen, resulting in a strong, stable graft with a negative zeta potential of the inner wall, making it more resistant to thrombus formation[19, 30] Follow-up to 2 years in Keshishian's series revealed a satisfactory patency rate of 77 per cent. Longer-term follow-up will be necessary to determine late results.

## TEXTILE GRAFTS

Since the report of Voorhees[39] in 1952 of the use of Vinyon-N cloth for the repairs of arterial defects, a large number of textiles of different materials, different yarns, and varied fabrications have been studied and implanted by investigators. The most systematic studies are reported by Wesolowski.[44, 45] He defined the optimal specifications for prosthetic vascular grafts. Some important identifiable criteria for evaluation are: biologic healing, handling characteristics, early and late strength, preclotting properties, and absence of any tendencies toward toxicity, allergenic potential, or cancer induction.

### Biologic Properties

An extremely important determinant of the ultimate fate of luminal lining and biologic function of cloth grafts is biologic porosity to capillary and fibroblastic ingrowth. The luminal tissue equivalent of intima results from capillary and fibroblastic ingrowth through the fabric interstices, organizing and replacing the initial luminal thrombus. If porosity to ingrowth is absent, as in tightly woven Teflon prostheses, the graft remains lined by thrombus except at the suture line. With optimal biologic porosity, early ingrowth and early endothelial coverage take place. Several manifestations are evident when porosity is marginal: the pseudointima may calcify or ulcerate or further thrombus formation may occur on its surface. If the secondary thrombus organizes, additional fibrous tissue may appear and result in septum formation.

Porosity has been described by Wesolowski[43] as the amount in cubic centimeters of filtered tap water that will pass through 1 cm. square area of graft wall per minute at a pressure head equivalent to 120 mm. Hg. This method of measurement of porosity correlated with biologic experience. If the porosity is equivalent to 5000 cc. or greater, good pseudointima forms and degenerative calcification of the pseudointima is avoided in the growing pig experimental model. At this porosity, enough change is present in the pseudointima that fibrin deposition may still occur until the porosity reaches 10,000 cc. per minute.

The newly formed tissue lining the fabric grafts (pseudointima) has been studied in great detail by Florey et al.[11] in baboons. It is reported to be composed of connective tissue, fibroblasts, large numbers of smooth muscle cells, some elastic tissue, and small vessels of capillary and arteriolar size. Some of these small vessels have luminal ostia. If biologic healing of the pseudointima is good, the inner coat becomes lined with endothelium. This is thought to result from endothelial proliferation from capillaries permeating the porous grafts.[25]

The body surrounds the textile graft with connective tissue, forming an outer layer often termed neoadventitia. The rapidly developing neoadventitia should remain stable with the pseudointima, which forms in sequential fashion and at a slower rate. Disturbing this process can produce late tearing and degeneration of the fragile vascular-collagen bundles and result in intramural hemorrhage, ulceration of the pseudointima, calcification, narrowing, and new luminal thrombus formation — a phenomenon resembling the fibrotic stage of atherosclerosis of arteries, with loss of the vasa vasorum of any etiology. Late intrawall hemorrhage or inflammation is theorized to change luminal surface charge from negative to positive, inducing negatively charged blood elements to plate on the surface, thrombose, or organize and become additional pseudointima. The result is narrowing of the lumen. This may not be critical in vessels of large size and high flow rate, such as the aorta and iliac arteries, but it can lead to thrombotic failure when applied to the femoropopliteal system or other small arteries or those with poor run-off. If the developing pseudointima is over 400 to 500 $\mu$ in thickness and vascularity is not supplied through graft interstices, luminal diffusion of nutrients is insufficient and late degeneration of neointima may occur.

The amount of inner surface thrombus (fibrin, platelets, varying amounts of entrapped red cells, and leukocytes) formed in a prosthesis appears to be a function of many interacting variables. In successful patent grafts, it is rarely greater than 1 mm. in thickness. In surgical failure cases, the entire lumen is filled with thrombus or, if flow is insufficient, true red clot. Thrombus not lysed becomes predominantly fibrous tissue. As an end result of thrombus formation or its organized form — pseudointima — narrowing occurs. Luminal obliteration is the commonest cause of failure of "normal vessels" as well as of prosthetic devices. Some important factors relating to thrombus formation appear to be:

**Wall Charge and Electrokinetic Phenomenon.** The major advances in understanding of wall characteristics demonstrate that positive wall charge leads to thrombosis. Negative wall charges are antithrombotic.[34] Normal arterial walls are negatively charged. An electrical double layer occurs at all solid-solution interfaces. One measure of the electronegativity "streaming potential"[34] can be obtained between two identical reference electrodes when there is a pressure difference across them due to solution flow. Higher streaming potentials correlate with decreased thrombogenic potentials and greater negative surface charge density on the vessel wall. Implanted prosthetic

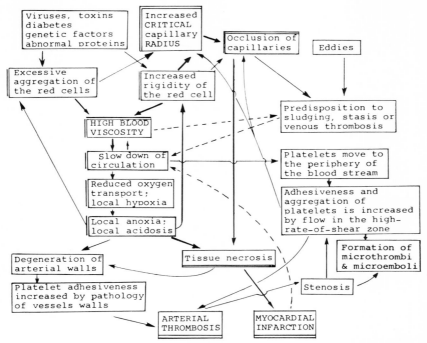

**Figure 3** A diagram representing the hypothesis of the role of rheologic factors in pathogenesis of myocardial infarction and arterial thrombosis. The sequence of events is indicated by arrows (thick full lines, full lines, and broken lines, according to the degree of importance). The upper case type and a double frame indicate more important steps. (From Dintenfass, L.: Amer. Heart J., 77:139, 1969.)

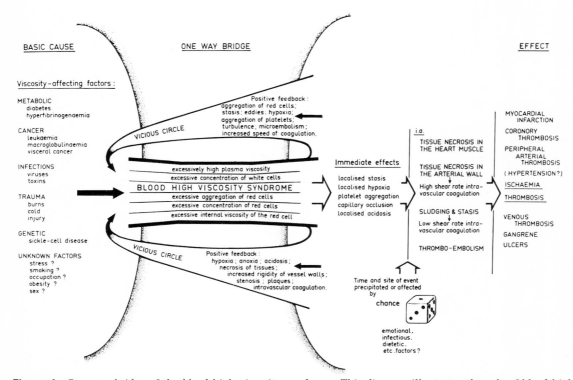

**Figure 4** One-way bridge of the blood high viscosity syndrome. This diagram illustrates the role of blood high viscosity in the development of ischemia, infarction, and thrombosis. The basic causes (left) can affect blood viscosity by increasing plasma viscosity, aggregation of red cells, internal viscosity of the red cell, hemoconcentration, and concentration of white cells. Immediate effects and vicious circles are indicated. (From Dintenfass, L.: Amer. Heart J., 77:139, 1969.)

devices fail unless the wall charge is negative with respect to blood. Changes from negativity toward positive of normal vessels or prosthetic pseudo-intima appear with wall degeneration or surrounding inflammatory processes. This again leads to thrombus formation which, if extensive, leads to acute or chronic occlusion. Studies to further explain and modify this mechanism are in progress by many investigators. Heparin and low molecular weight dextran are known to temporarily and acutely increase wall negativity.[34]

**Rheologic Factors.** Rheologic factors were suggested as a cause of thrombosis over a century ago by Virchow.[38] The diagrams (Figs. 3 and 4) of Dintenfass[10] represent schemata of theoretical sequences in the pathogenesis of thrombosis. Little detailed attention has been paid to this problem and its management in vascular surgery and follow-up care by many surgeons and cardiologists.

**Platelet-Surface Interactions.** Platelets are the prime source of thrombosis of damaged small vessels and needle holes in suture lines with exposed collagen. They are a major component of surface thrombus.[24] With narrowing of vessels having a local high rate of shear, platelets agglutinate and aggregate at the wall to produce thrombus formation. This aggregation also arises at areas of turbulence of the bloodstream. The modification of platelet activity to decrease thrombus formation is being studied in many laboratories. Its clinical usefulness has not been fully explored.[23] Some agents known to decrease platelet activity are aspirin, phenylbutazone, phosphatidylserine, and antiserotonins.

**Fibrin Deposition and Fibrinolysis.** Fibrin deposition occurs in essentially all cases in which prosthetic materials are implanted as vascular substitutes. Deposits have been identified on apparently normal endothelium of experimental animals. Major deposition is found in vessels or grafts as a response to blood vessel and tissue injury or inflammatory processes. Normally these events are followed by fibrinolysis in the majority of cases, although the process may take weeks to months. On the arterial side with end circulation, however, if the process is totally occluding before resolution is possible, anoxia may lead to loss of the extremity. Invasion by fibroblasts precludes further resolution. Fibrinolysis can be markedly enhanced by plasminogen activators such as streptokinase or urokinase given intravenously. No clinical use of these or other agents has been made to modify fibrin deposition on graft surfaces or at suture lines, although they are used to treat thrombotic or embolic disease in nongrafted cases. A review of fibrinolysis is well presented by Sherry.[31] Experimental early use of these agents in porous prostheses has resulted in hemorrhage through the graft.[6]

In clinical practice, the more porous materials such as the Wesolowski "Weaveknit" have maintained higher patency rates under severe conditions. A strict test of this principle is seen by comparing the long-term patency rates of axillofemoral bypass grafts of different materials as reported by

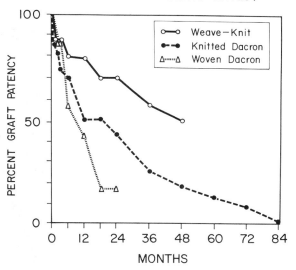

## COMPARISON OF GRAFT TYPES
### (CUMULATIVE PATENCY RATES)

**Figure 5**  Long-term patency rates of axillofemoral bypass grafts in relation to degree of porosity. (From Moore, W. S., and Hall, A. D.: Amer. J. Surg., *122*:148, 1971.

Moore[22] in Figure 5. The least porous grafts demonstrated the poorest results in this model.

The use of porous grafts is contraindicated in patients with platelet defects — major fibrinolytic disorders, severe clotting defects such as may develop in cirrhosis, and noncoagulable states following disseminated intravascular coagulation, such as may result from shock from a ruptured aneurysm. As the plugging of small holes in grafts and at suture lines is primarily a function of platelets, their deficit in numbers or quality makes the use of porous grafts hazardous. Under these conditions, one must accept poorer biologic healing for the priority of lack of hemorrhage during the early postoperative period. In other words, a tight-woven graft should be used.

Biologic healing of grafts is also affected by the graft bed. Extensive clot surrounding grafts or suture lines delays or prevents capillary and fibroblastic ingrowth. This may result in suture line failure, defective pseudointima formation, bleeding through porous grafts, pseudoaneurysm formation, and thrombosis of the graft. Contamination with bacteria may result in graft failure through clotting, dissolution of suture lines with hemorrhage, or continuing sepsis necessitating graft removal.

### Handling Characteristics

To facilitate implantation a graft should be able to conform to differential size between the host vessel and prosthesis — should be "scrunchable," to use Wesolowski's term.[40] Some degree of "crimping" allows for flexion across creases, without buckling or disruption of vascular supply through the graft. The graft should not occlude when twisted moderately.

### Early and Late Strength

Owing to the vagaries of wound healing related to many factors, collagen in and around the graft is not uniform in amounts and strength. Current prostheses are dependent for their strength upon a fabric and suture that maintain strength upon implantation. Materials available with this characteristic are Dacron, Marlex, and Teflon. Nylon, Orlon, Ivalon, Vinyon, and polypropylene lose a majority of their tensile strength after months to years.[17]

### Preclotting Properties

When porous textile grafts are not reliably preclotted, bleeding occurs through the interstices as pressure and flow are restored. If normal blood is used, preclotting is a function of the yarn and interstices between the fibers. Materials impervious to blood do not require preclotting.

### Overview Results

The textile graft has performed well in high-flow systems of large diameter. In replacement for aortic aneurysm, long-term patency rates exceed 90 per cent. Many studies suggest that in cases of aortic occlusive disease endarterectomy may provide superior cumulative patency rates.

## AUTOGENIZED VASCULAR PROSTHESES

An innovative and theoretically attractive concept, pioneered by Hufnagel[18] and studied experimentally and clinically applied by Sparks,[33] is that of "autogenization" of vascular prosthesis. A loose-woven or knitted Dacron material is placed over a mandril and implanted subcutaneously or adjacent to the vessel to be bypassed. The interstices fill with collagen. Within a few weeks, a compound prosthesis develops with high biologic porosity, low implantation porosity, and smooth lining of autologous collagen with good tensile strength. While exposed collagen on the luminal surface has been shown to attract platelets and cause them to adhere as well as to activate clotting through the intrinsic and extrinsic clotting pathways, initial results have not implicated this as a major problem. With slow-flow states, such as poor distal run-off, clotting should theoretically appear in most cases. Perhaps modification of platelet activity by aspirin, phenylbutazone, or dextrans could avoid this problem. The time interval required for endothelial formation, important in small vessels, is not defined. Autogenized vascular prostheses are useful only in elective surgery when sufficient time will permit their growth. Further experience is necessary in order to determine the long-term usefulness of this approach[33] (Figs. 6 and 7).

## COMPOUND GRAFTS

The theoretical advantages of low implantation porosity and delayed high biologic porosity in textile grafts led to the design and investigation of numerous grafts of a mixture of adsorbable-replaceable and nonadsorbable components. The most systematic studies were reported by Wesolowski et al.[42] Two general types of compound materials were tested—one a biologic adsorbable substance applied over stable nonadsorbable mesh, and the other an adsorbable fiber (collagen) interwoven with nonadsorbable fibers. A third category using a very loose Dacron knit with a tanned adsorbable collagen inner liner has also been studied.[21] The most satisfactory grafts experimentally were the mixed fiber grafts. Here biologic healing generally followed the same sequence as with textile grafts of the same biologic porosity. When the adsorbable component was replaced at a slower rate than fibrin, luminal healing was delayed. There are definable advantages to this concept: one can attain optimal biologic porosity of high degree, still maintaining initial bloodtightness, and fibrinolytic or uncoagulable states do not lead to hemorrhage through the grafts. The theoretical advantages of this concept will ensure further attempts toward the development of compound grafts.

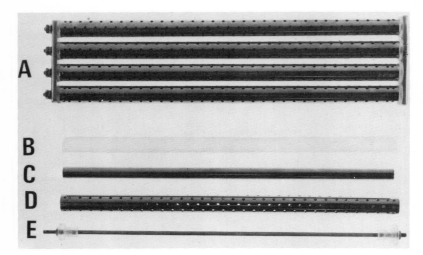

**Figure 6** Tissue die cluster (TDC). A TDC is an assembly of two, three, or four dies. It produces grafts 6.5 inches in length which, when sutured together, form a graft up to 25 inches in length. *A*, TDC; *B*, Dacron knitted tube; *C*, mandril; *D*, ingrowth tube; *E*, tie rod. (From Sparks, C. H.: Ann. Surg., *171*:787, 1970.)

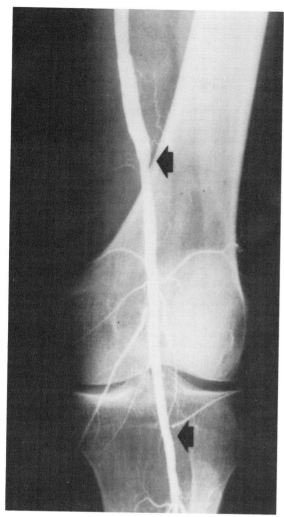

**Figure 7** Arteriogram 18 months after grafting. An endarterectomy was done on the dilated portion. The graft is between the arrows. The branches that seem to come from the graft in actuality originate from the by-passed femoropopliteal artery, which is covered by the grafts.

build up an electrical double layer with the metal being negatively charged. This process produces corrosion of metals and loss of substance.

Another method of producing a negatively charged surface on tubes is reported by Gott.[16] Colloidal graphite is bonded to a material, and treated with benzalkonium chloride and subsequently heparin. This remains firmly bonded and results in a lasting nonthrombogenic surface.

Glass tubes that activate clot formation do not remain patent. Metals and glass, being rigid, are not suitable for any location with movement. Plastic solid tubes with antithrombogenic surfaces are at present not easily, reliably, or permanently attachable to arteries. Use of solid tubes in clinical practice will depend upon further study and experimentation.

The development of prosthetic vascular substitutes has only recently begun. Under most circumstances, the best materials for large artery grafting are probably *porous* cloth prostheses because of the scarce supply of autogenous arteries. Small vessels are best replaced with autologous veins. For obliterative disease of the aortoiliac area, endarterectomized segments of autologous artery of good quality are most often preferable. With further research, new and better arterial substitutes will probably emerge to improve the results of surgical reconstruction.

## SELECTED REFERENCES

Sawyer, P. N., ed.: Biophysical Mechanisms in Vascular Homeostasis and Intravascular Thrombosis. New York, Appleton-Century-Crofts, 1965.
*This report is a valuable contribution by specialists in vascular surgery, hematology, biophysics, and engineering to the understanding of interfacial phenomena in blood cells and vessel walls. Further investigation based upon these studies should provide practical guidelines for the surgical treatment of intramural thrombus formation.*

Wesolowski, S. A., and Dennis, C., eds.: Fundamentals of Vascular Grafting. New York, Blakiston Division, McGraw-Hill Book Company, 1963.
*This monograph contains a summary of most of the important historical, experimental, and clinical fundamentals of vascular reconstructive surgery, including biology of arteries and arterial prostheses, clinical indication, and end results.*

## SOLID-WALL PROSTHESES

At this writing, solid-wall prostheses are not widely accepted in clinical use. Solid-wall plastic materials of similar composition (Teflon, Dacron) to porous materials produce extensive luminal thrombus formation, usually originating at the junction of the tube with the artery. Metal tubes have been investigated. Sawyer's studies[29] indicate that magnesium and aluminum conduits have remained patent for 330 days, stainless steel tubes for 30 to 40 days, and copper tubes for 1 to 7 days. Platinum tubes occlude at 1 to 2 days. Magnesium and aluminum high in the electromotive series have less tendency to electrochemically precipitate blood elements on metal electrodes. Metals high in the series lose positive ions to the solution and

## REFERENCES

1. Berger, K., Savage, L. R., Wood, S. J., and Sameh, A. A.: Endarterectomy and other surgical injuries to cardiovascular walls. Pacif. Med. Surg., 75:367, 1967.
2. Boddy, P. J., Brattain, W. H., and Sawyer, P. N.: In Sawyer, P. N., ed.: Biophysical Mechanisms in Vascular Homeostasis and Intravascular Thrombosis. New York, Appleton-Century-Crofts, 1965.
3. Carrel, A.: Results of the transplantation of blood vessels, organs, and limbs. J.A.M.A., 51:1662, 1908.
4. Carrel, A.: Latent life of arteries. J. Exp. Med., 12:460, 1910.
5. Chopra, P. S., Srinivasan, S., Lucas, T., and Sawyer, P. N.: Relation between thrombosis on metal electrodes and the position of metal in the electromotive series. Nature, 215:1494, 1967.
6. Deaton, H. L., and Anlyan, W. G.: Fibrinolytic therapy in the presence of vascular prostheses. Surg. Forum, 13:227, 1962.
7. de Takats, G., and Vaithianathan, T.: Bodily defenses against thrombosis. Amer. J. Surg., 120:73, 1970.

8. Deterling, R. A., and Clauss, R. H.: Long-term fate of aortic arterial homografts. J. Cardiovasc. Surg., *11*:35, 1970.
9. Dintenfass, L.: Some rheological factors in the pathogenesis of thrombosis. Lancet, *2*:370, 1965.
10. Dintenfass, L.: Blood rheology in pathogenesis of the coronary heart diseases. Amer. Heart J., *77*:139, 1969.
11. Florey, H. W., Greer, S. J., Kiser, J., Poole, J. C. F., Telander, R., and Werthessen, N. T.: The development of the pseudointima lining fabric grafts of the aorta. Brit. J. Exp. Path., *43*:655, 1962.
12. Florey, H. W., Poole, J. C. F., and Meek, G. A.: Endothelial cells and "cement" lines. J. Path. Bact., *77*:625, 1959.
13. Fry, W. J., DeWeese, M. S., Kraft, R. O., and Ernest, C. B.: Importance of porosity in arterial prostheses. Arch. Surg., *88*:836, 1964.
14. Gaylis, H., Corvese, W. P., Linton, R. R., and Shaw, R. S.: The rate of healing of arterial autografts. Surgery, *45*:41, 1959.
15. Geiringer, E.: Intimal vascularisation and atherosclerosis. J. Path. Bact., *63*:201, 1951.
16. Gott, L., Whiffen, J. D., Dutton, R. C., Leininger, R. I., and Young, W. P.: In: Sawyer, P. N., ed.: Biophysical Mechanisms in Vascular Homeostasis and Intravascular Thrombosis. New York, Appleton-Century-Crofts, 1965.
17. Harrison, J. H.: Synthetic materials as vascular prostheses. Amer. J. Surg., *95*:16, 1958.
18. Hufnagel, C. F., Gillespie, J. F., Brea, C., and Franco, W.: Introduction to the concept of "autogenization" of vascular prostheses. In: Wesolowski, S. A., and Dennis, C., eds.: Fundamentals of Vascular Grafting. New York, Blakiston Division, McGraw-Hill Book Company, 1963.
19. Keshishian, J. M., Smyth, N. P. D., Adkins, P. C., Camp, F. C., and Yahr, W. S.: Clinical experience with the modified bovine arterial heterograft. Ann. Surg., *172*:690, 1970.
20. Kouchoukos, N. T., Levy, J. F., Balfour, J. F., and Butcher, H. R.: Operative therapy for aortoiliac arterial occlusive disease. Arch. Surg., *96*:628, 1968.
21. Krajicek, M., Zastava, V., and Chvapil, M.: Collagen-fabric vascular prostheses. J. Surg. Res., *4*:290, 1964.
22. Moore, W. S., and Hall, A. D.: Late results of axillary-femoral bypass grafting. Amer. J. Surg., *122*:148, 1971.
23. Mustard, J. F., Glynn, M. F., Nishizawa, E. E., and Packham, M. A.: Platelet-surface interactions: relationship to thrombosis and hemostasis. Fed. Proc., *26*:106, 1967.
24. Poole, J. C. F., and French, J. E.: Thrombosis. J. Atheroscler. Res., *1*:251, 1961.
25. Poole, J. C. F., Sabiston, D. C., Jr., Florey, H. W., and Allison, P. R.: Growth of endothelium in arterial prosthetic grafts and following endarterectomy. Surg. Forum, *13*:225, 1962.
26. Ray, F. S., Lape, C. P., Lutes, C. A., and Dillihunt, R. C.: Femoropopliteal saphenous vein bypass grafts. Amer. J. Surg., *119*:385, 1970.
27. Rosenberg, N., Henderson, J., Lord, G. H., and Bothwall, J. W.: An arterial prosthesis of heterologous vascular origin. J.A.M.A., *187*:741, 1964.
28. Sauvage, L. R., Wood, S. J., Eyer, K. M., and Bill, A. H.: Experimental coronary artery surgery: preliminary observations of bypass venous grafts, longitudinal arteriotomies, and end-to-end anastomoses. J. Thorac. Cardiovasc. Surg., *46*:826, 1963.
29. Sawyer, P. N., Brattain, W. H., and Boddy, P. J.: In: Sawyer, P. N., ed.: Biophysical Mechanics in Vascular Homeostasis and Intravascular Thrombosis. New York, Appleton-Century-Crofts, 1965.
30. Sawyer, P. N., and Srinivasan, S.: Studies on the biophysics of intravascular thrombosis. Amer. J. Surg., *114*:42, 1967.
31. Sherry, S.: Fibrinolytic agents. DM, May, 1969, pp. 3–32.
32. Shore, E., Foran, R., Golding, A., and Treiman, R.: Femoral-popliteal occlusive disease. Arch. Surg., *102*:548, 1971.
33. Sparks, C. H.: Die-grown reinforced arterial grafts. Ann. Surg., *171*:787, 1970.
34. Srinivasan, S., Aaron, R., Chopra, P. S., Lucas, T., and Sawyer, P. N.: Effect of thrombotic and antithrombotic drugs on the surface charge characteristics of canine blood vessels: In vivo and in vitro studies. Surgery, *64*:827, 1968.
35. Stokes, J. M., Sugg, W. L., and Burcher, H. R., Jr.: Standard method of assessing relative effectiveness of therapies for arterial occlusive diseases. Ann. Surg., *157*:343, 1963.
36. Szilagyi, D. E., McDonald, R. T., Smith, R. F., and Whitcomb, J. G.: Biologic fate of human arterial homografts. Arch. Surg., *75*:506, 1957.
37. Szilagyi, D. E., Smith, R. F., Elliott, J. P., and Allen, H. M.: Long-term behavior of a dacron arterial substitute. Ann. Surg., *162*:453, 1965.
38. Virchow, R.: Gesammelte Abhandlung zur wissenschaftlichen Medizin. Frankfurt, 1856.
39. Voorhees, A. B., Jr., Jaretzki, A., III, and Blakemore, A. H.: The use of tubes constructed from Vinyon "N" cloth in bridging arterial defects. Ann. Surg., *135*:332, 1952.
40. Wesolowski, S. A.: In: DeBakey, M. E., and Spurling, R. G., eds.: Evaluation of Tissue and Prosthetic Vascular Grafts. Springfield, Ill., Charles C Thomas, 1962.
41. Wesolowski, S. A., and Dennis, C.: Fundamentals of Vascular Grafting. New York, Blakiston Division, McGraw-Hill Book Company, 1963.
42. Wesolowski, S. A., Fries, C. C., Domingo, R. T., Liebig, W. J., and Sawyer, P. N.: The compound prosthetic vascular graft: a pathologic survey. Surgery, *53*:19, 1963.
43. Wesolowski, S. A., Fries, C. C., Liebig, W. J., Sawyer, P. N., and Deterling, R. A.: The synthetic vascular graft. Arch. Surg., *84*:74, 1962.
44. Wesolowski, S. A., Fries, C. C., McMahon, J. D., and Martinez, A.: Evaluation of a new vascular prosthesis with optimal specifications. Surgery, *59*:40, 1966.
45. Wesolowski, S. A., Sauvage, L. R., Golaski, W. M., and Komoto, Y.: Rationale for the development of the gossamer small arterial prosthesis. Arch. Surg., *97*:864, 1968.

# V

# Aneurysms

*David C. Sabiston, Jr., M.D., and Others*

*An aneurysm is the dilatation of an artery full of spiritous blood.*

—Fernel, 1581

An aneurysm is a localized or diffuse dilatation of an artery. Most aneurysms are designated as *true* aneurysms and contain all three layers of the arterial wall (intima, media, and adventitia). A *false* aneurysm ("pulsating hematoma") is the term applied when only the adventitia is present, as is often the situation following traumatic rupture of an artery with subsequent aneurysmal for-

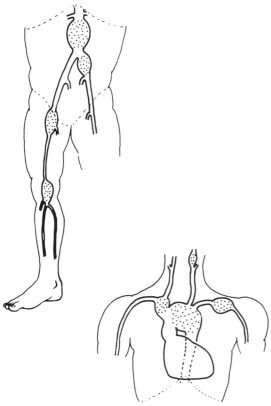

**Figure 1** Common anatomic sites of arterial aneurysms. (From Ludbrook, J., and Elmslie, R. G.: An Introduction to Surgery: 100 Topics. New York, Academic Press, 1971.)

mation. It is further helpful to classify aneurysms into *saccular* and *fusiform* types. The former usually arise from a distinct portion of the wall and possess a mouth, whereas the latter involve the total circumference of the artery and represent a diffuse dilatation. Aneurysms tend to occur at certain anatomic sites, and the most common locations are shown in Figure 1.

Aneurysms may be either *congenital* or *acquired,* the latter being much more frequent than the former. Acquired aneurysms may be caused by arteriosclerosis, trauma, infection (mycotic), syphilis, or medial cystic necrosis. Although aneurysms were once untreatable, nearly all can be managed now by surgical means. Moreover, the results are usually highly satisfactory.

# 1. ANEURYSMS OF THE SINUS OF VALSALVA

Aneurysm of the sinus of Valsalva was first described in 1834,[3] and the first successful repair of such an aneurysm with a fistula was reported in 1953.[1] Since then, a number of these lesions have been described and surgical treatment has been quite satisfactory.

## ANATOMY

The anatomic characteristics of these lesions permit classification into three groups: (1) aneurysms, (2) aneurysms with fistula, and (3) fistula alone. The etiologic factors include bacterial endocarditis, syphilis, rheumatic heart disease, and Marfan's syndrome, or the lesions may be congenital. The condition is more common in the male, with an average age of 40 in one large series.[2] *Multiple* sinus aneurysms represent the most common pattern, usually involving all three coronary sinuses. Fistulas frequently develop from these aneurysms and usually communicate with the heart. The right coronary sinus is most frequently involved, and should a fistula develop, it most often enters the right ventricle and occasionally the right atrium. Most aneurysms arising in the noncoronary cusp rupture into the right atrium (Fig. 2).[2] Aneurysms of the left sinus are uncommon.

## DIAGNOSTIC FEATURES

Patients with this lesion may initially be asymptomatic, but dyspnea and fatigue usually become the predominant symptoms. The stigmata of Marfan's syndrome may be present, and occasionally a history of bacterial endocarditis can be obtained. Cardiac enlargement and an appropriate diastolic murmur occur in the presence of a fistulous rupture into a cardiac chamber. The electrocardiogram usually shows left ventricular enlargement, and S-T segment depression and T wave inversion are frequently observed. The plain chest film may show enlargement of the proximal aorta at its origin, although definitive diagnosis is made by retrograde aortography with injection into the aortic root. With malfunction of the aortic cusp, aortic insufficiency is a common associated finding.

## SURGICAL MANAGEMENT

Patients with this disorder are best managed by surgical correction. The aneurysm should be ex-

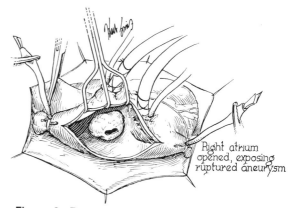

Right atrium opened, exposing ruptured aneurysm

**Figure 2** Demonstration of sinus of Valsalva aneurysm with a fistula to the right atrium. A right atriotomy has been made. Following excision of the fistula, the opening into the atrium is closed directly with sutures. (From DeBakey, M. E., Diethrich, E. B., Liddicoat, J. E., Kinard, S. A., and Garrett, H. E.: J. Thorac. Cardiovasc. Surg., 54:312, 1967.)

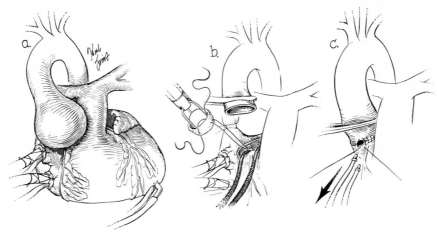

**Figure 3**  *a*, Illustration of patient with aneurysm involving all three sinuses of Valsalva. *b*, Aortic valve replacement for insufficiency of aortic valve. *c*, Closure of proximal aorta following excision of aneurysm and insertion of prosthetic aortic valve. (From DeBakey, M. E., Diethrich, E. B., Liddicoat, J. E., Kinard, S. A., and Garrett, H.E.: J. Thorac. Cardiovasc. Surg., *54*:312, 1967.)

cised, with primary closure of the fistula if present. A prosthetic patch is sometimes required. In some instances, concomitant replacement of the aortic valve is required to correct severe aortic insufficiency (Fig. 3).[2] Complete replacement of a segment of the ascending aorta may be necessary for severe aneurysmal dilatation involving all cusps. The operation is performed with the use of cardiopulmonary bypass. In one series of 33 patients managed surgically, the mortality was only 6 per cent.[2]

### SELECTED REFERENCE

DeBakey, M. E., Diethrich, E. B., Liddicoat, J. E., Kinard, S. A., and Garrett, H. E.: Abnormalities of the sinuses of Valsalva. Experience with 35 patients. J. Thorac. Cardiovasc. Surg., *54*:312, 1967.
*This paper describes the largest single series of patients with aneurysms of the sinus of Valsalva and their management. It is a definitive reference source.*

### REFERENCES

1. Brown, J. W., Heath, D., and Whitaker, W.: Cardioaortic fistula: A case diagnosed in life and treated surgically. Circulation, *12*:819, 1955.
2. DeBakey, M. E., Diethrich, E. B., Liddicoat, J. E., Kinard, S. A., and Garrett, H. E.: Abnormalities of the sinuses of Valsalva. Experience with 35 patients. J. Thorac. Cardiovasc. Surg., *54*:312, 1967.
3. Oram, S., and East, T.: Rupture of aneurysm of aortic sinus (Valsalva) into the right side of the heart. Brit. Heart J., *17*:541, 1955.

## 2. DISSECTING ANEURYSMS OF THE AORTA

*Myron W. Wheat, Jr., M.D.*

### HISTORICAL ASPECTS

Dissecting aneurysms were first characterized in 1761 by Morgagni, who described the magenta-colored appearance of the involved aorta that is produced by the column of blood in the dissecting hematoma just beneath the adventitia. The first comprehensive review of dissecting aneurysms was an analysis of 300 cases by Shennan in 1934.[14] Shennan considered medial degeneration of the aorta to be the basic pathologic defect underlying aortic dissection. In 1935, the first efforts at surgical therapy were reported by Gurin, Bulmer, and Derby,[6] who attempted a localized "fenestration" operation on the right external iliac artery. The operation successfully restored the blood supply to the extremity but the patient died 6 days later in acute renal failure. In 1955, DeBakey, Cooley, and Creech[3] reported the first successful treatment of dissecting aneurysms and first applied the "fenestration" operation to the descending thoracic aorta for dissecting aneurysms (Fig. 4).

### INCIDENCE

Dissecting aneurysms are the most common acute catastrophe involving the aorta. They occur with a frequency of about one per 500 autopsies or about five dissecting aneurysms per million population per year, compared to ruptured abdominal aneurysms, which occur at the rate of about 3.5 per million, and ruptured thoracic aneurysms, which occur at a rate of only one per million population per year.[16]

Dissecting aneurysms occur with the greatest frequency in persons between 50 and 70 and are relatively rare in persons under the age of 40 except in those with a familial predisposition.[7] As many as 50 per cent of dissecting aneurysms seen in patients under the age of 40 may occur in pregnant women.[10] Patients with Marfan's syndrome[11] or congenital heart disease such as coarctation of the aorta or bicuspid aortic valve have an increased incidence of occurrence of dissecting aneurysms.[17]

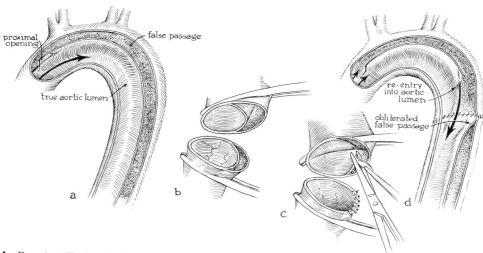

**Figure 4** Drawing illustrating DeBakey, Cooley, and Creech's application of the "fenestration operation." *a*, The site of origin and extent of the dissecting process in the thoracic aorta in Case 5. *b*, The aorta has been divided. *c*, The false lumen has been obliterated distally, and proximally a segment of the inner layer is being excised to create a re-entry passage. *d*, The anastomosis is completed. (From DeBakey, M. E., et al.: Ann. Surg., *142*:586, 1955.)

There appears to be an increased incidence of dissecting aneurysms in the black race and this may be related to their increased frequency of hypertension. In our own series, 60 per cent of the patients were black.[20] Eighty-seven per cent of our patients with acute dissecting aneurysm have had hypertension on admission or a history of hypertension in the past. The disease also appears to be more common in males, with males accounting for as many as 65 per cent of the cases in some series.[20] Therefore, the patient with an acute dissecting aneurysm might be typified as a black male aged 60 with known hypertension.

## PATHOGENESIS

Medial degeneration of the aorta, most commonly of the cystic medial necrosis variety, is the underlying pathologic finding in most patients with dissecting aneurysms.[8] Only about two-thirds of the changes are of the classic Erdheim's cystic necrosis with cystic accumulations of mucoid material, fragmented elastic lamina, and collagen fibers. In fewer than 5 per cent of cases the changes may be related to syphilis or atherosclerosis. Atherosclerotic aneurysms are rare in the ascending aorta, where about two-thirds of the dissecting aneurysms originate. In the distal abdominal aorta, where atherosclerotic changes are more pronounced, and fusiform aneurysms related to atherosclerosis are common, dissecting aneurysms are rare.

### The Intimal Tear

Rupture of the vasa vasorum in the outer one-third of an underlying diseased media has been the major theory of origin of dissecting aneurysms of the aorta in the past.[8] The rupture of the vasa vasorum was believed to produce a hematoma in

the aortic wall which was then propagated until it ruptured into the aortic lumen, admitting systolic blood and pressure to the dissecting hematoma. Although there are a few reported instances in which intramural aortic hematomas have occurred without demonstrable intimal tears, such an explanation seems unlikely in most cases of dissecting aneurysms for the following reasons:

1. The intraluminal pressure in the aorta is greater than that in the vasa vasorum 100 per cent

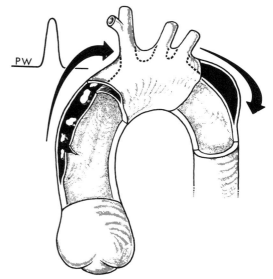

**Figure 5** Diagrammatic representation of pathogenesis of dissecting aneurysms: (1) aortic wall with medial degeneration sets the stage; (2) combined forces acting on aortic wall result in intimal tear, giving aortic bloodstream direct access to weakened media; (3) resulting dissecting hematoma is propagated by pulse wave (PW) of blood produced by each myocardial contraction.

of the time and even if a localized intramural hemorrhage should occur, a significant hematoma of the aortic media would not develop.

2. Since vasa vasorum are present only in the outer third of the aortic wall, all dissections should originate in the outer one-third of the media, but they do not. Such a hypothesis does not fit with the actual findings that in most dissections there is an intimal tear and that the inner layers of the media are more frequently involved than the outer one-third where the vasa vasorum are present.

3. The vasa vasorum hypothesis also does not fit with hydrodynamic data, which demonstrate that the point of greatest stress on the aortic wall is the point nearest the mainstream of the blood, i.e., the intima and inner one-third of the media.[13]

4. If most or all of the dissecting aneurysms immediately involve the outer one-third of the aortic wall and adventitia, many more than 3 per cent of the patients should succumb abruptly from aortic rupture after initiation of the intimal tear, whereas actually only 20 per cent die within the first 24 hours.[8]

A more likely explanation of the pathogenesis of dissecting aneurysms is as follows[21] (Fig. 5):

1. Medial degeneration of the wall of the thoracic aorta sets the stage by decreasing the cohesiveness of the layers of the aortic wall.

2. Repeated motion of the aorta related to the beating of the heart results in flexion stresses, most marked in the ascending and first portion of the descending thoracic aorta, 60 to 100 times per minute (37 million times per year). With each heartbeat, the heart, because of the rigid sternum anteriorly and the vertebral column posteriorly, moves predominantly from side to side, producing this flexing motion in the ascending aorta and in the descending aorta just distal to the left subclavian artery. The extent and frequency of this flexing action can be documented simply by tracing the outline of the thoracic aorta during systole and diastole in the left anterior oblique projection of aortograms and superimposing the two tracings (Fig. 6). Supportive evidence for the tendency of the aortic wall to be disrupted just distal to the left subclavian artery is also available from studies of patients suffering deceleration accidents with traumatic rupture of the aorta. Most of the disruptions occur in the area of the isthmus just distal to the left subclavian artery where mobile aorta becomes fixed descending thoracic aorta.[12]

3. Hydrodynamic forces in the bloodstream related to the pulse wave propagated by each cardiac systole act upon the wall of the aorta, most markedly in the proximal aorta.

4. A combination of the preceding three factors eventually results in an intimal tear, which leads to a hematoma dissecting into the media of the aortic wall for varying depths.

### Propagation of the Dissecting Hematoma

After the intima tears and the dissecting hematoma forms, a second set of forces comes into play, those forces that propagate or extend the dissecting hematoma once it has developed. These forces include: (1) blood viscosity; (2) pressure; (3) velocity (shearing forces); (4) turbulence; and (5) steepness of the pulse wave ($dp/dt_{max}$). On the basis of experimental evidence, it seems that the steepness of the pulse wave is the most important of the forces propagating the dissecting hematoma. Therefore, the forces that cause the dissection to progress and the forces that cause the aorta to rupture must come from the heart.[21]

The major force responsible for continuation of the dissection, the steepness of the pulse wave, involves the pulsatile nature of the blood flow in large arteries. This is known because: (1) the aorta is remarkably resistant to static pressure; (2) static pressure provides no pressure gradients as driving forces to induce shear stresses or other stresses on aortic tissue; (3) experimental models, e.g., aortas made of Tygon tubing with rubber cement intimas, dissect only when flow is pulsatile, and not when flow is nonpulsatile,[13] and experiments with dog aortas show the same relationship to pulsatile flow; and (4) in turkeys, protection from aortic rupture can be accomplished with propranolol, a beta-adrenergic blocking agent, at a dose that does not affect mean aortic pressure but does alter the quality of pulsatile blood flow.[15] Propranolol exerts its main effect directly upon the heart and decreases the steepness of the pulse wave ($dp/dt_{max}$).

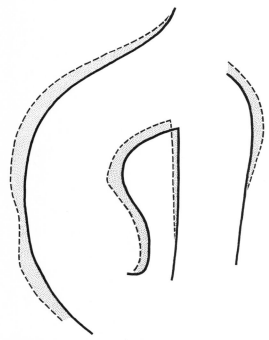

**Figure 6**　Superimposed tracings of aortograms, left anterior oblique projection. Solid lines with heart in systole; dotted lines, diastole. Tracings demonstrate side-to-side and "flexing" motion of ascending and first portion of descending thoracic aorta with each myocardial contraction.

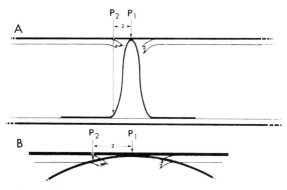

**Figure 7** Steepness of pulse wave as a factor in propagating dissecting hematoma: $P_1$ and $P_2$ represent pressures on aortic wall at these two points; Z, constant and finite, equals length of torn intima and media. Driving force ($\triangle P$) equals $P_1 - P_2$. If pressure curve is flattened, as shown in B, driving force ($\triangle P$) will be less over distance Z than in A, where pressure curve is steep.

### Pressure Differentials at Sites Along the Aortic Wall

An attractive analysis of the forces that cause the progress of the dissection to continue in both a forward and a retrograde direction involves continuous pressure differentials (provided by the pulsatile nature of the blood flow) throughout the aorta. In addition to pressure differences, Womersly, in a mathematical approach to hydrodynamics, considered vessel radius (r), blood density (po), blood viscosity (n), and instantaneous blood velocities in the longitudinal (u) and in a radial (w) direction.[21] He considered the forward driving force the pressure differential along the longitudinal axis (Z) (dp/dz). From Figure 7A, if we assume that Z is finite and represents the effective distance along which, if a force were applied, dissection would occur (e.g., Z = length of the torn intima and media), then the shape of the pressure

pulse would determine the value $\triangle P$ ($P_1 - P_2$). In Figure 7A, the pressure profile at any time is steep, and $\triangle P$, if Z is finite and constant, is greater than in Figure 7B, where the shape of the pressure profile is flatter. In other words, if one could flatten the pressure curve, the driving force $\triangle P$ would be less over the effective length Z. Conversely, if the pressure curve is steep (Fig. 7A), then the force driving the dissecting hematoma is increased.

### Summary of Pathogenesis (see Fig. 5)

1. Medial degeneration in the wall of the thoracic aorta sets the stage by decreasing the cohesiveness of the layers of the aortic wall.

2. Repeated motion of the aorta related to the beating of the heart results in "flexion stresses" most marked in the ascending and first portion of the descending thoracic aorta.

3. Hydrodynamic forces in the bloodstream related to the pulse wave propagated by each cardiac systole act upon the wall of the aorta, most markedly in the proximal aorta.

4. A combination of the preceding three factors eventually results in an intimal tear, which leads to a hematoma dissecting into the media of the aortic wall for varying depths.

The hydrodynamic forces in the bloodstream, which are predominantly related to the steepness of the pulse wave, extend the dissecting hematoma until rupture occurs either: (1) back into the lumen of the aorta, resulting in a spontaneous cure, a rare but documented occurrence; or more likely, (2) into the pericardium or pleural cavity, leading to death in most instances within 30 days.

### CLINICAL MANIFESTATIONS[8]

The patient frequently is a middle-aged black male with known hypertension who suddenly experiences excruciating pain. The pain may be described as knife-like, sharp, and often tearing or ripping in nature and is difficult or impossible to

**Figure 8** Low-power photomicrograph of cross section of carotid artery almost completely occluded by dissecting hematoma (*DH*). *CL* = compressed lumen.

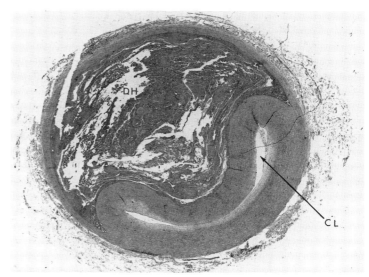

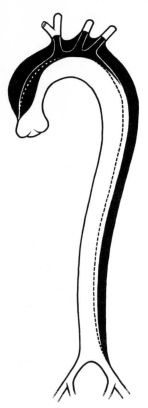

**Figure 9** Diagrammatic illustration of the usual path of the dissecting hematoma (shaded area) originating from an intimal tear in the ascending aorta and re-entering in the region of the left common iliac artery.

relieve with opiates. The pain most commonly is in the anterior chest or in the back between the shoulder blades. This pain does not radiate into the neck or arms as does angina pectoris. There are frequently systolic murmurs over the heart and there may be the murmur of aortic valve insufficiency. Murmurs over major branches of the aorta such as the carotid and subclavian arteries are secondary to partial occlusion of the vessel orifices by the dissecting hematoma (Fig. 8). There may be a significant difference in blood pressure between the two upper extremities, further indicating the partial compression of one subclavian artery, usually the left, by the dissecting hematoma. Even though the patient may appear to be in shock, his blood pressure will usually be in the hypertensive range or he may even show marked hypertension. Occasional patients presenting in frank shock with a low blood pressure may demonstrate a rapid hypertensive response to the transfusion of only one or two units of blood. Once the diagnosis is suspected, the patient should be placed in an intensive care unit and carefully monitored. Consultation with cardiologists should be obtained since the most common problem in diagnosis is differentiation of acute dissecting aneurysm from acute myocardial infarction.

## ROENTGENOGRAPHIC FINDINGS

Chest roentgenograms should be taken as soon after admission to the hospital as possible and will usually show widening of the mediastinum. The mediastinum will bulge to the right in dissection of the ascending aorta and show widening on the left in involvement of the descending thoracic aorta. Earlier chest roentgenograms are very helpful for comparison. The typical path of dissection of the aorta is shown in Figure 9. When the dissection begins in the ascending aorta, it is usually to the right and anterior, beginning just distal to the level of the coronary artery ostia. As the hematoma advances into the arch, it is posterior and superior, and posterior and to the left in the descending thoracic aorta. If the hematoma continues into the abdominal aorta, it is most commonly posterior and to the left with a higher incidence of dissection into the left renal artery and the left iliofemoral system than on the right side.

Mediastinal widening is a highly suggestive but nondiagnostic sign of aortic dissection since neoplastic or inflammatory processes involving the mediastinum can produce similar widening. Calcium in the wall (intima of the aorta) with obvious widening beyond the calcium of at least 4 to 5 mm.

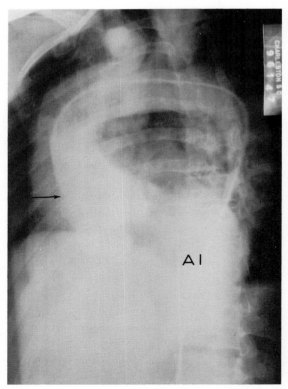

**Figure 10** Aortogram, left anterior oblique projection. Compression of the lumen of the ascending aorta by dissecting hematoma can be seen at the arrow. *A1* indicates 4+ aortic valve insufficiency. (Courtesy of Dr. William H. Lee, Jr., Division of Thoracic and Cardiovascular Surgery, University of South Carolina.)

has been considered diagnostic in the past. The chest roentgenogram also may show a left pleural effusion, which is most frequently serous. The roentgenographic manifestations of dissecting aneurysm on plain films can be summarized as:[5] (1) a change in configuration of the aorta on successive films; (2) aortic wall thickening shown by displacement of intimal calcification; (3) a localized hump in the aortic arch; (4) disparity in the size of the ascending and descending aorta; and (5) mediastinal, lung, and pleural changes.

Since plain chest roentgenograms are not diagnostic, aortography should be performed to either confirm the diagnosis or rule out a dissecting aneurysm. There is essentially no danger of elevating a plaque and initiating a dissection with proper technique for aortography. The aortogram manifestations of dissecting aneurysms are (Fig. 10): (1) splitting of the contrast column; (2) distortion of the contrast column; (3) alternate flow patterns; and (4) aortic valvar insufficiency.

The definitive diagnosis of dissecting aneurysms demands that the aortogram show some compression of the true aortic lumen by the dissecting hematoma.

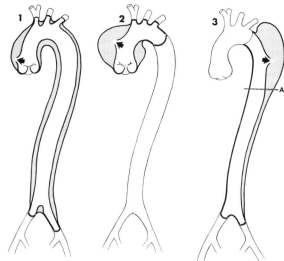

**Figure 11** Classification of dissecting aneurysms of the aorta. Type I: Dissection involves ascending aorta and aortic arch and extends distally for varying distances. Type II: Dissection limited to ascending aorta. Type III: Dissection originates at or distal to left subclavian artery, extends distally for varying distances, and does not involve aorta proximal to left subclavian artery. (Modified from DeBakey, M. E., et al.: Ann. Surg., *142*:586, 1955.)

## SURGICAL TREATMENT

As previously mentioned, the first successful treatment of dissecting aneurysms of the aorta was reported by DeBakey and associates in 1955[3] and used the "fenestration" operation (see Fig. 4). The fenestration operation was an attempt to achieve, by surgical means, re-entry of the dissecting hematoma similar to the spontaneous re-entry known to occur in long-term survivors of aortic dissection. Almost 10 years later DeBakey's group reported the most successful results with surgical treatment of dissecting aneurysms in a group of 179 patients, with an overall survival rate of 79 per cent.[4] A concise classification was presented which has become the one most generally accepted (Fig. 11). This series was heavily weighted by cases of Type III aneurysm (68 per cent) in which the problems are generally less difficult and the operations are predominantly elective in patients with chronic aneurysms. Although no definition of acute was given, the mortality rate was 40 per cent for the acute variety of Type I and 19 per cent for Type III. Fifty per cent of the patients were still alive at the end of 5 years, as contrasted to Hirst's series of patients not treated surgically, of whom only 0.7 per cent were alive at 5 years.[8] DeBakey's results, truly a remarkable accomplishment, established the fact that surgery, particularly for the Type III chronic dissecting aneurysm, can be carried out with a reasonable mortality rate in experienced hands.

In summary, the 15 years following DeBakey's initial successful use of surgery for treatment of dissecting aneurysms have been marked by advances in surgical technique and the application of cardiopulmonary bypass. These advances have resulted in patient survival rates of 70 to 80 per cent for the resection and replacement of chronic dissecting aneurysms, particularly those occurring distal to the left subclavian artery.[1] Although technical advances and experience have improved the results in patients with acute dissections, the mortality rate for the surgical treatment of acute dissection continues to be about 40 per cent or greater in most series.

## PHARMACOLOGIC TREATMENT

As a result of the high mortality rate with the surgical approach to the acute dissecting aneurysm,[9, 18] an alternate approach to the treatment of dissecting aneurysms involving intensive drug therapy was initiated in 1963.[22] Drug therapy is based on the following factors in the natural history of acute dissecting aneurysms of the aorta:[8] (1) In untreated dissecting aneurysms, only 3 per cent of the patients die immediately. The mortality for untreated patients then rises rapidly to 21 per cent in 24 hours, 60 per cent in 2 weeks, and 90 per cent in 3 months. (2) The main cause of death is not the initial intimal tear but is related to extension of the dissecting hematoma with ultimate rupture and death due to hemorrhage or cardiac tamponade or both. (3) It has been documented that acute dissecting aneurysms can occur and resolve through rechannelization or healing and present as incidental autopsy findings many years later.[2] The basic phenomenon in the progression from the intimal tear to death in the acute dissecting aneurysm is extension of the dissecting hematoma. As previously pointed out, there is considerable evidence to support the thesis that the progress of the dissecting hematoma to rupture is due to pulsatile forces initiated by the heart. Therefore, drug therapy rests upon the basis of decreasing the pulsatile nature of the blood pressure to a point at which the dissecting aneurysm, instead of progressing, becomes static and heals or at least remains in a stable condition so that it can be approached operatively on an elective basis.

In our most recent report of the results of drug therapy involving 50 patients with acute dissecting aneurysms admitted to two different hospitals over a 5 year period, there were seven deaths in the acute phase with a survival rate of 86 per cent.[20] Among those patients discharged from the hospital who either died or were followed for at least a year, 84 per cent were alive at 1 year, 70 per cent at 2 years, and 62 per cent at 3 years. The past 8 years have seen intensive drug therapy become an established useful method of treatment for patients with dissecting aneurysms of the aorta, particularly of the acute variety.

## CURRENT STATUS OF SURGERY AND INTENSIVE DRUG THERAPY IN THE MANAGEMENT OF PATIENTS WITH DISSECTING ANEURYSMS OF THE AORTA[21]

### Acute Dissecting Aneurysms, Symptoms Less Than 14 Days

Patients suspected of having acute dissecting aneurysms of the aorta should be placed in an intensive care unit where they can be monitored carefully on a minute-to-minute basis. Other cardiovascular catastrophes such as acute myocardial infarction or cerebral vascular hemorrhage must be ruled out by appropriate studies and consultations. Then:

1. Monitor electrocardiogram and blood pressure, and insert a Foley catheter to follow urinary output.

2. Reduce systolic blood pressure to 100 to 120 mm. Hg (if appropriate). Use trimethaphan (Arfonad), 1 to 2 mg. per milliliter, as an intravenous drip acutely, and if necessary for 24 to 48 hours, with a flow rate to maintain the desired blood pressure (Table 1). Keep the head of the bed elevated 30 to 45 degrees to gain the orthostatic effect of the drugs.

3. Administer reserpine, 1 to 2 mg. intramuscularly every 4 to 6 hours, or propranolol, 1

**TABLE 1**   DRUGS USED IN MANAGEMENT OF DISSECTING ANEURYSM OF THE AORTA

| Drug | Mechanism of Action | Total Effect |
|---|---|---|
| Reserpine | Depletes all catecholamines from all tissue stores. Neurotransmitter (norepinephrine) release diminished after nerve stimulation | *Decreases myocardial contractility.* Sedation, depression, bradycardia (reduces cardiac output), reduces peripheral resistance, stimulates gastric secretion |
| Trimethaphan (Arfonad) | Ganglionic blockade. Direct relaxing effect on vascular smooth muscle. Histamine release | *Reduces cardiac output.* Lowers peripheral resistance, produces ileus, bladder distention, pupil dilatation |
| Guanethidine (Ismelin) | Selectively depletes catecholamines from postganglionic nerve terminals particularly in heart, gut, and blood vessels but not central nervous system | *Decreases myocardial contractility.* Postural hypotension, diarrhea, bradycardia (*reduces cardiac output*), decreases peripheral resistance, no C.N.S. effect |
| Propranolol (Inderal) | Specifically blocks beta-adrenergic stimulation at end organ receptor (blood vessels, heart) | Bradycardia, *decreases myocardial contractility (reduces cardiac output).* Increases peripheral resistance. Mild sedation. Little hypotensive effect |
| Alpha-Methyldopa (Aldomet) | Metabolized to alpha-methylnorepinephrine, a weak neurotransmitter and pressor agent which replaces the more potent norepinephrine at nerve terminal. Other unknown mechanisms | Decreases blood pressure. Sedation, little depression, reduces peripheral resistance, slight bradycardia |
| Thiazides (Diuril, Hydrodiuril) | Decreased tubular reabsorption of $Cl^-$ and $Na^+$; some $K^+$ is lost. Results in salt and/or extracellular fluid volume depletion with possibly, also, a direct cardiovascular effect | Decrease in blood pressure |

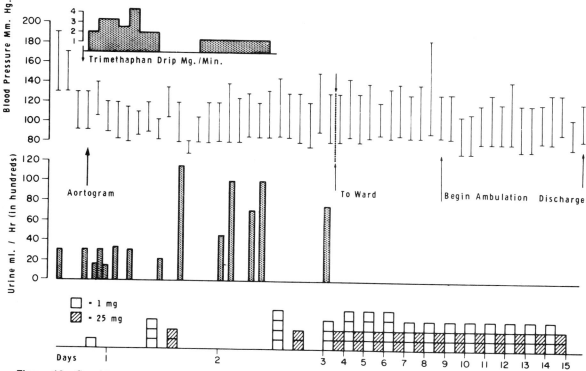

**Figure 12** Graphic representation of clinical course of patient with acute dissecting aneurysm of aorta managed with intensive drug therapy. Trimethaphan drip was begun soon after admission (arrow), with prompt blood pressure response. Open squares = 1 mg. reserpine; shaded squares = 25 mg. guanethidine.

mg. intramuscularly every 4 to 6 hours. (These drugs may also be used in combination.)

4. Give guanethidine, 25 to 50 mg. orally twice a day.

5. Continue to monitor electrocardiogram, blood pressure, pulses, urine output, and stools for blood.

6. Take daily chest roentgenograms to check for mediastinal widening and the presence of pleural fluid.

The management of a typical patient is outlined in chart form in Figure 12. Usually the blood pressure response to trimethaphan is rapid and it can be profound if not carefully regulated. *As a rule when the blood pressure is lowered, the chest and/or back pain are dramatically relieved. The relief of pain is an important clinical guide as to the effectiveness of the drug therapy in arresting the "dissecting hematoma."*

Occasional patients with acute dissection are not hypertensive. The management of these patients is similar but trimethaphan is not used. Instead, these patients are given either reserpine or propranolol to modify the cardiac impulse. Aortograms should be obtained within 4 hours after admission or as soon as reasonably possible in order to confirm or rule out the diagnosis of acute dissecting aneurysm of the aorta. We believe it is important to visualize the aorta from the aortic valve to the abdominal aortic bifurcation in each patient in the initial study. This study then enables the physician to know: (1) the site of the

intimal tear; (2) the extent of the dissecting hematoma; (3) the degree of the involvement of branches of the aorta, particularly the renal arteries; and (4) the presence or absence of acute saccular aneurysms. All of these points are of paramount importance in the management of the patient.

When his condition has stabilized and the trimethaphan has been discontinued, the patient can be transferred to routine floor care and permitted progressive ambulation while regulation of drug dosages is carried out.

Follow-up of the patients with acute dissecting aneurysms treated by drug therapy is one of the most important aspects of this type of treatment. These patients must be followed forever and monitored carefully so that the development of complications of the dissecting aneurysm, which can be anticipated in 25 per cent of chronic cases, will not be missed.

### Subacute and Chronic Aneurysms

Subacute aneurysms, with symptoms for more than 14 days but less than 3 months, and chronic dissecting aneurysms, in which the onset of symptoms occurred 3 months before, are somewhat less urgent problems. Usually the pain has subsided and the patient is in a stable situation. The diagnosis in each instance should be confirmed by aortography and the patient given appropriate doses of drugs such as reserpine and propranolol to adequately control the cardiac impulse and the blood pressure. Surgical intervention is indicated only if there is progressive aortic valve insufficiency, compromise of a significant branch of the aorta, progressive enlargement of the aneurysm, or development of a localized saccular aneurysm.

### Surgical Therapy

Surgery for dissecting aneurysms falls into two general categories, surgery in the acute dissecting aneurysm and surgery in the subacute or chronic dissecting aneurysm.

In the acute situation surgical intervention is indicated when there is: (1) failure to bring the pain or blood pressure under control within 4 hours after admission; (2) impending rupture or significant leaking of the aneurysm; (3) overwhelming aortic valve insufficiency; (4) significant compromise or occlusion of major branches of the aorta such as the carotid or renal arteries or celiac axis; and (5) the presence of an acute saccular area in the aneurysm.

In the subacute or chronic stage, the indications for surgical intervention are: (1) progressive aortic valve insufficiency; (2) development of a saccular aneurysm; and (3) significant compromise of a major branch of the aorta, i.e., claudication of a lower extremity.

In either the acute or chronic stage, if a single branch of the aorta such as a subclavian, iliac, or femoral artery is compromised, a local procedure such as segmental replacement or fenestration is preferred, if feasible, to operation on the main dissection, which requires total-body heparinization and cardiopulmonary bypass.

Patients with dissections of the Type I variety and severe aortic valve insufficiency should be operated upon on an elective basis if possible. Preferably, operation at least 6 weeks after the onset of dissection is desirable in order to take advantage of the scarring and healing around the dissection. At 6 weeks or longer, the aortic wall tissues have toughened to the point that they hold sutures in a realistic fashion and tears and hemorrhaging from the suture lines are not the severe threats they represent in the acute situation.

For dissection involving the aortic root, definitive treatment usually requires replacement of the aortic root and aortic valve and reimplantation of the coronary arteries.[19] This seemingly radical approach is necessary because of the progressive nature of the basic pathologic process present in the wall of the aorta, cystic medial necrosis. If the dissection is distal to the coronary artery ostia and there is no involvement of the aortic valve, replacement of the ascending aorta alone is the procedure of choice. Segmental resection of the dissection and Dacron or Teflon prosthetic replacement is the procedure of choice for dissecting aneurysms in the descending thoracic aorta. There is probably no indication for the use of the fenestration operation in the thoracic aorta today.

## SELECTED REFERENCES

DeBakey, M. E., Henly, W. S., Cooley, D. A., Morris, G. C., Jr., Crawford, E. S., and Beall, A. C., Jr.: Surgical management of dissecting aneurysms of the aorta. J. Thorac. Cardiovas. Surg., 49:130, 1965.
*This report presents the largest series of dissecting aneurysms treated with surgery and also the best results with surgical therapy in this disease.*

Hirst, A. E., Johns, V. J., and Kime, S. W.: Dissecting aneurysms of the aorta. A review of 505 cases. Medicine, 37:217, 1958.
*This is the most exhaustive review of the largest series of dissecting aneurysms in the literature. It should be the starting point as well as basic source for information regarding any aspect — except therapy for dissecting aneurysms.*

Hume, D. M., and Porter, R.: Acute dissecting aortic aneurysms. Surgery, 53:122, 1963.
*This is an excellent clinical review of dissecting aneurysms, stressing the evaluation and status of treatment and in particular the results and status of surgical treatment for acute dissecting aneurysms as of 1963.*

Wheat, M. W., Jr., and Palmer, R. F.: Dissecting aneurysms of the aorta. Curr. Probl. Surg., July, 1971.
*This monograph presents a current general review of the historical background, incidence, pathogenesis, and evaluation and current status of intensive drug therapy and surgical therapy in dissecting aneurysms of the aorta.*

## REFERENCES

1. Austen, W. G., Buckley, M. J., McFarland, J., DeSanctis, R. W., and Sanders, C. A.: Therapy of dissecting aneurysms. Arch. Surg., 95:835, 1967.
2. Conston, A. S.: Healed dissecting aneurysm. Arch. Path., 48:309, 1949.
3. DeBakey, M. E., Cooley, D. A., and Creech, O., Jr.: Surgical considerations of dissecting aneurysm of the aorta. Ann. Surg., 142:586, 1955.
4. DeBakey, M. E., Henly, W. S., Cooley, D. A., Morris, G. C., Jr., Crawford, E. S., and Beall, A. C., Jr.: Surgical management of dissecting aneurysms of the aorta. J. Thorac. Cardiovasc. Surg., 49:130, 1965.
5. Eyler, W. R., and Clark, M. D.: Dissecting aneurysms of the aorta: Roentgen manifestations including a comparison with other types of aneurysms. Radiology, 85:1047, 1965.
6. Gurin, D., Bulmer, J. W., and Derby, R.: Dissecting aneurysm of the aorta; diagnosis and operative relief of acute arterial obstruction due to this cause. New York J. Med., 35:1200, 1935.
7. Hanley, W. B., and Bennett Jones, N.: Familial dissecting aortic aneurysm, a report of three cases within two generations. Brit. Heart J., 29:852, 1967.
8. Hirst, A. E., Johns, V. J., and Kime, S. W.: Dissecting aneurysms of the aorta. A review of 505 cases. Medicine, 37:217, 1958.
9. Hume, D. M., and Porter, R.: Acute dissecting aortic aneurysms. Surgery, 53:122, 1963.
10. Mandel, W., Evans, E. W., and Walsford, R. L.: Dissecting aortic aneurysm during pregnancy. New Eng. J. Med., 251:1059, 1954.
11. McKusick, V. A.: Cardiovascular aspects of Marfan's syndrome; a heritable disorder of connective tissue. Circulation, 11:321, 1955.
12. Pate, J. W., Butterick, O. D., and Richardson, R. L.: Traumatic rupture of the thoracic aorta. J.A.M.A., 203:1022, 1968.
13. Prokop, E. K., Wheat, M. W., Jr., and Palmer, R. F.: Hydrodynamic forces in dissecting aneurysms. Circ. Res., 27:121, 1970.
14. Shennan, T.: Dissecting Aneurysms. Medical Research Council, Special Report Series 193. London, H. M. Stationery Office, 1934.
15. Simpson, C. F., Kling, J. M., and Palmer, R. F.: The use of propranolol for the protection of turkeys from the development of β-aminopropionitrile-induced aortic ruptures. Angiology, 19:414, 1968.
16. Sorensen, H. R., and Olsen, H.: Ruptured and dissecting

aneurysms of the aorta. Acta Chir. Scand., *128*:644, 1964.
17. Strauss, R. G., and McAdams, A. J.: Dissecting aneurysm in childhood. J. Pediat., *76*:578, 1970.
18. Warren, W. D., Beckwith, J., and Muller, W. H.: Problems in the surgical management of acute dissecting aneurysm of the aorta. Ann. Surg., *144*:530, 1956.
19. Wheat, M. W., Jr., Boruchow, I. B., and Ramsey, H. W.: Surgical treatment of aneurysms of the aortic root. Ann. Thorac. Surg., *12*:593, 1971.
20. Wheat, M. W., Jr., Harris, P. D., Malm, J. R., Kaiser, G., Bowman, F. O., Jr., and Palmer, R. F.: Acute dissecting aneurysms of the aorta. J. Thorac. Cardiovasc. Surg., *58*:344, 1969.
21. Wheat, M. W., Jr., and Palmer, R. F.: Dissecting aneurysms of the aorta. Curr. Probl. Surg., July, 1971.
22. Wheat, M. W., Jr., Palmer, R. F., Bartley, T. D., and Seelman, R. C.: Treatment of dissecting aneurysms of the aorta without surgery. J. Thorac. and Cardiovasc. Surg., *50*:364, 1965.

## 3. TRAUMATIC ANEURYSMS OF THE AORTA

*Allan M. Lansing, M.D., Ph.D.*

Traumatic aneurysms of the aorta may occur as a result of penetrating or nonpenetrating trauma. Although penetrating injuries of the aorta are dramatic, steadily rising numbers of automobile accidents have increased the significance of nonpenetrating aortic trauma. The incidence of traumatic rupture of the aorta at autopsy used to be placed at 1 per cent, but more recent estimates suggest that between 10 and 15 per cent of all automobile fatalities are associated with rupture of the aorta.[10, 28]

### PATHOLOGY

When blunt trauma is involved, the site of aortic injury is usually the isthmus of the thoracic aorta, the region of the ligamentum arteriosum just beyond the left subclavian artery.[5, 15, 22, 28] The second most common site is just above the aortic valve, and occasionally the origin of the innominate, left carotid, or subclavian artery is involved. The much rarer injury of the abdominal aorta is briefly discussed at the end of this chapter. The pathogenesis of thoracic aortic injury was first detailed in 1893 by Rindfleisch, who surmised that the aortic arch was fixed by the attachment of the great vessels, whereas the heart and the descending thoracic aorta were more mobile.[24] Thus, sudden deceleration of the body at the time of impact with differential rates of deceleration of the fixed portions of the thoracic aorta and the great vessels causes a tear involving either the intima, the intima and media, or the entire wall.[5] This tear is usually transverse, but may be ragged, stellate, or spiral. The average age of the patient is 27 years, and therefore atherosclerosis is seldom a factor in the aortic injury. Since the adventitia provides about 60 per cent of the tensile strength of the thoracic aorta, survival of the patient until he is admitted to hospital usually depends upon continuity of this tissue.

Other types of injuries are much less common. Crushing injury of the thoracic aorta is extremely rare. Traumatic dissection of the thoracic aorta may also occur.[20] Multiple sites of injury of the aorta have been reported, and other associated injuries, particularly cardiac, are very common and constitute an important factor in determining the survival rate. In fact, in one large series, cardiac injuries were found in 70 per cent of the patients with traumatic injuries of the thoracic aorta.[22]

### PROGNOSIS

The outcome of these injuries has been well documented in an excellent review of 275 patients by Parmley et al.[22] Surprisingly, there is no correlation between the survival rate and the extent of the disruption of the aorta, that is, partial versus complete transection. Fourteen per cent of all patients survived the initial injury and arrived at the hospital: isolated rupture of the aorta was associated with a 20 per cent initial survival rate, whereas the combination of aortic and heart injury resulted in only a 4 per cent initial survival rate. Thus, 80 to 90 per cent of the patients die immediately of exsanguination, whereas in 10 to 20 per cent the leak is temporarily controlled by the adventitia of the aorta or the pleura.

In the patients who survive the immediate injury, delayed rupture of the aorta with massive hemorrhage is the commonest event. In Parmley's series, 66 per cent of those who survive the initial injury die within 2 weeks of aortic rupture, 82 per cent within 3 weeks, and 90 per cent within 10 weeks. In the seven patients of 275 in this series who were still alive at the end of 10 weeks, five died of rupture within a few months and two survived operative repair. According to other reports, in a few patients the picture of pseudo-coarctation appears when a flap of intima develops distal to the injury and produces partial stenosis of the aorta, with resulting hypertension in the arms and diminished blood flow to the lower part of the body.[15, 16, 19] Finally, a few patients live long enough for a traumatic aneurysm to develop, an outcome that is extremely rare; Bennett and Cherry found only 105 cases reported up to 1967.[3] It is estimated that only 2 per cent of the immediate survivors of traumatic aortic rupture live long enough for an aneurysm to develop. Even then, these lesions are rarely stable, only about 20 per cent remaining asymptomatic over 5 years, and nearly all producing symptoms or evidence of expansion at some time.[3] Since there is no way to predict when signs of compression of the neighboring structures, bacterial infection, rupture, or embolism will occur, repair is recommended even when the patient is asymptomatic.

### DIAGNOSIS

The lethal nature of traumatic rupture of the thoracic aorta makes prompt diagnosis extremely

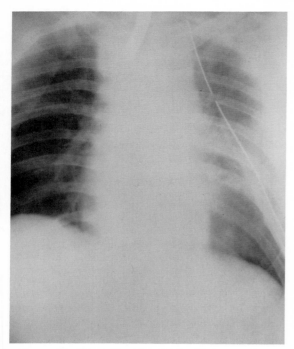

**Figure 13**  Chest film of patient with traumatic rupture of the aorta. Note the widened mediastinum and loss of sharpness of the aortic arch.

gram in all patients with sternal injuries, injuries of the first rib, and fractures of the clavicle that are displaced posteriorly.[6] Aortography is preferable to exploratory thoracotomy since not only will a negative exploration in a patient who is otherwise seriously ill add significantly to his risk, but tears of the intima or media may be missed unless visualized by routine opening of the thoracic aorta.[15, 27]

In those rare patients in whom the diagnosis is missed and who survive to incur a thoracic aneurysm, the lesion is usually discovered later by an incidental chest x-ray, by the development of symptoms of compression of other neighboring structures, or by the occurrence of pain and shock when the lesion ruptures spontaneously (Fig. 15). In a few patients, the mediastinal mass appears within 24 hours of injury and is accompanied by hemothorax, increasing chest pain, and symptoms of dysphagia, tracheal or bronchial obstruction, hoarseness, or hemoptysis.

It is evident that the most important factor in successful treatment is immediate and accurate diagnosis. In the 10 to 20 per cent of the patients who reach the hospital alive, the injury must be recognized and treated as an emergency, and urgent operative intervention must be undertaken. On the other hand, the rare chronic aneurysms may remain stable for many years, but they should be viewed with grave suspicion and should be resected unless other factors contraindicate operation.

important. Since at best only 20 per cent of the victims reach a hospital alive and over 80 per cent of these die of aortic rupture within 3 weeks, the clinician must be constantly aware of the possibility of this injury. The first clue is the *history of a sudden deceleration injury,* which should immediately arouse suspicion. The most important radiologic findings are *widening of the upper mediastinum* and *loss of the sharpness of the contour of the aortic knob* (Fig. 13).[8] The occurrence of both of these radiologic signs demands immediate investigation, since rupture is said to be present in 90 per cent of patients with this combination. It must be admitted that a widened mediastinum does not always indicate rupture, nor will every patient with rupture present with a widened mediastinum. Further, allowance must be made for the fact that an AP supine chest film will frequently give the appearance of a widened upper mediastinum, and hence a PA chest x-ray should be performed if at all possible. The presence of a left pleural effusion may also support the diagnosis, but rib fractures, pneumothorax, contusion of the lung, and other injuries do not help. Despite these limitations, if a deceleration injury has occurred, and if the mediastinum is widened with loss of contour of the aorta, the next step is an aortogram as soon as the patient's general condition and other injuries permit (Fig. 14). A high index of suspicion will lead to more frequent aortography and a lower incidence of positive findings, but the very high mortality when the condition is missed makes this a justifiable emergency diagnostic procedure. In fact, some authorities recommend an arterio-

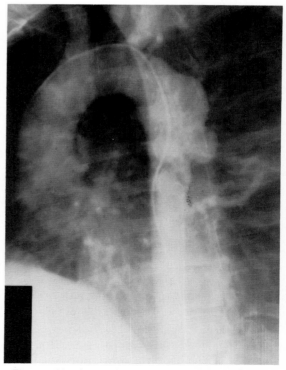

**Figure 14**  Aortogram in patient with traumatic rupture of the aorta.

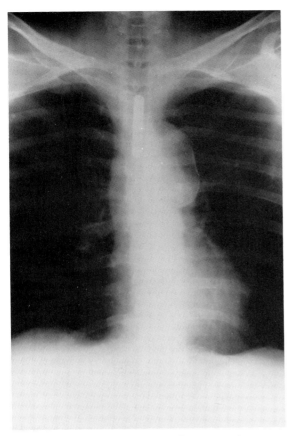

**Figure 15** Chronic aneurysm following aortic trauma. Note the calcification of the wall.

## TREATMENT

Once the diagnosis is established, preparations for operation are made immediately. Resuscitation and supportive measures are instituted during this period, and other critical injuries may have to be treated first or simultaneously. If either the patient's general condition or the hospital facility is unsuitable for immediate repair, pharmacologic treatment to lower the blood pressure and reduce the pulsatile force of ventricular systole may be instituted to delay rupture of the aorta.[2] This is the same regimen that is applied in the non-operative treatment of dissecting aneurysm, and includes the use of trimethaphan, reserpine, and guanethidine.

Since the operative treatment of these injuries will require cross-clamping of the thoracic aorta, the blood supply of the kidneys and spinal cord must be maintained during this period and back-pressure on the brain and heart minimized. Only rarely has thoracic aortic injury been treated in its acute stage without any form of protection. The first protective measure to be employed was hypothermia, but this has been supplanted by some form of left heart bypass, as first proposed by Gerbode.[9] In this technique, a cannula is inserted into the left atrium to drain blood from the heart;

the blood is then pumped back into the femoral artery (Fig. 16). This provides perfusion of the lower part of the body during aortic cross-clamping, but has the disadvantages of requiring the use of heparin, which can result in postoperative bleeding, of occasionally causing sudden rises of left atrial pressure and pulmonary edema, and of requiring a pump and the personnel to run it. An alternative procedure, femoral vein to femoral artery bypass with a pump-oxygenator, avoids the risk of pulmonary congestion and disturbance of left atrial function, but still requires the use of heparin, a heart-lung machine, and technicians. These two methods are the most commonly employed today, but in complicated cases of aneurysms involving the aortic arch total cardiopulmonary bypass and deep hypothermia followed by a period of complete circulatory arrest have been recommended so that dissection is minimized and the aortic defect can be repaired from inside the lumen of the vessel.[7]

Another technique that is available for use in all hospitals, and does not require a pump or the use of heparin, has been popularized by Kirsh et al.[17] They recommend the use of a simple temporary external shunt consisting of a cannula inserted through a purse-string suture into the aorta proximal to the lesion and Tygon tubing to conduct the blood to a distal cannula inserted into the lower thoracic aorta beyond the lesion. The problems of bleeding from the operative area, extensive equipment, specialized personnel, and the need to use the less desirable woven grafts are thus eliminated.

After the method of bypass has been selected, the operative technique is fairly well standardized. The aortic arch is dissected within the pericardium to gain proximal control without entering the hematoma or touching the aneurysm. The aorta is encircled between the left carotid and left subclavian vessels and again distal to the lesion in its descending portion. Bypass is then established, the aorta cross-clamped, and the aneurysm or area of rupture approached directly.

In acute cases, the tissues are usually very friable and, although direct suture repair can occasionally be accomplished, most often the lesion must be treated by resection of the damaged area and insertion of a synthetic graft.[4, 13, 27] If the type of bypass employed requires the use of heparin, a woven graft must be used to prevent massive blood loss through the prosthesis after the clamps are removed from the aorta; otherwise, a knitted graft that will be better incorporated by the body tissues is preferable.

In the case of the chronic aneurysm, the patient's general condition is assessed to determine his life expectancy and complicating factors that might contraindicate surgical treatment. In general, however, these lesions nearly always enlarge or produce symptoms, although it may take many years for them to do so. At the time of operation, bypass using a pump or an external shunt is established, the aorta is occluded in the arch and descending portion, and the aneurysm is opened (see Fig. 16). Often direct suture repair can be

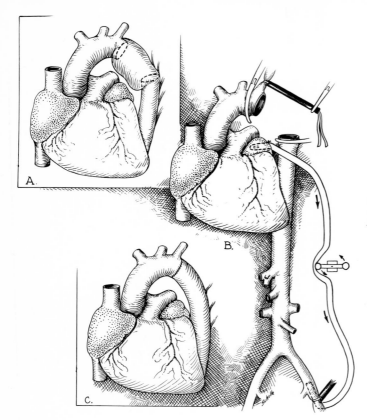

**Figure 16**   Technique of resection of aneurysm following aortic rupture. (From Alley, R. D., et al.: Ann. Thorac. Surg., 2:514, 1966.)

achieved by trimming the neck of the aneurysm and approximating the aorta by sutures after the distal portion has been mobilized.[1, 14] If wide separation of the ends of the aorta prevents this, a synthetic graft is employed to restore continuity. Dissection of the tissues outside the aneurysm is kept at a minimum to decrease the chance of injury to vital structures and to lessen the degree of bleeding from the structures after the repair has been accomplished.

## ABDOMINAL AORTIC INJURY

Rare cases of blunt injury of the abdominal aorta have been reported, usually associated with a longitudinal tear of the aortic wall caused by a compression injury.[22, 28] Only about 5 per cent of the traumatic injuries of the aorta involve its abdominal portion, and aneurysms are very rarely seen. Two cases of abdominal aneurysms resulting from blunt trauma, and one caused by a penetrating injury, have been reported.[11, 23, 25] In only one case has peripheral embolism occurred from a traumatic aneurysm of the abdominal aorta.[25] Traumatic dissection of the abdominal aorta has been reported in two cases with a resulting tear in the intima, formation of a flap, occlusion, and thrombosis of the terminal aorta.[12, 20]

Nonpenetrating injuries of the abdominal aorta are extremely rare and their management is straightforward. If acute thrombosis of the aorta occurs, it must be operated upon immediately. Traumatic aneurysms of the abdominal aorta are treated by standard surgical approaches once they have been recognized. Penetrating injuries of the aorta require immediate operation even if the injury appears to have sealed off. Delay will almost universally result in a secondary fatal hemorrhage or rupture of a false aneurysm.[21]

## SELECTED REFERENCES

Bennett, D. E., and Cherry, J. K.: The natural history of traumatic aneurysms of the aorta. Surgery, 61:516, 1967.
*This is an important review of the natural history of traumatic aneurysms of the aorta. The incidence and site of the lesion, the time of death, and the prognosis in the chronic aneurysm are discussed, with excellent references.*

Freed, T. A., Neal, M. P., Jr., and Vinik, M.: Roentgenographic findings in extracardiac injury secondary to blunt chest automobile trauma. Amer. J. Roentgen., 104:424, 1968.
*The radiologic diagnosis of traumatic injury of the aorta is well described. Emphasis is placed on the findings in routine chest x-rays and the role of arteriography in the diagnosis.*

Gerbode, F., Braimbudge, M., Osborn, J., Hood, M., and French, S.: Traumatic thoracic aneurysms: Treatment by resection and grafting with the use of an extracorporeal bypass. Surgery, 42:6, 1957.
*The technique of left atrial to femoral artery bypass for treatment of traumatic aneurysm of the thoracic aorta was first described in this paper. References to cases of traumatic aneurysm treated by excision are provided.*

Parmley, L. F., Mattingly, T. W., Manion, W. C., and Johnke, E. J., Jr.: Nonpenetrating traumatic injury of the aorta. Circulation, *17*:1086, 1958.
*This is the most complete and authoritative reference for the pathology, clinical aspects, and management of nonpenetrating injuries of the aorta. It is highly recommended.*

Spencer, F. C., Guerin, P. F., Blake, H. A., and Bahnson, H. T.: A report of fifteen patients with traumatic rupture of the thoracic aorta. J. Thorac. Cardiovasc. Surg., *41*:1, 1961.
*This is an excellent report of an early series of 15 cases, seven acute and eight chronic. A fine review of the literature combined with a discussion of the problems makes this worthwhile reading.*

## REFERENCES

1. Alley, R. D., Van Mierop, L. H. S., Li, E. Y., Jagdish, K. R., Kausel, H. W. and Stranahan, A.: Traumatic aortic aneurysm. Four cases of graftless excision and anastomosis. Ann. Thorac. Surg., 2:514, 1966.
2. Aronstam, E. M., Gomez, A. C., O'Connell, T. J., Jr., and Geiger, J. P.: Recent surgical and pharmacologic experiences with acute dissection and traumatic aneurysms. J. Thorac. Cardiovasc. Surg., 59:231, 1970.
3. Bennett, D. E., and Cherry, J. K.: The natural history of traumatic aneurysms of the aorta. Surgery, 61:516, 1967.
4. Bromley, L. L., Hobbs, J. T., and Robinson, R. E.: Early repair of traumatic rupture of the thoracic aorta. Brit. Med. J., 2:17, 1965.
5. Cammack, K., Rapport, R. L., Paul, J., and Baird, W. C.: Deceleration injuries of the thoracic aorta. Arch. Surg., 79:244, 1959.
6. DeMeules, J. E., Cramer, G., and Perry, J. F., Jr.: Rupture of aorta and great vessels due to blunt thoracic trauma. J. Thorac. Cardiovasc. Surg., 61:440, 1971.
7. Dumanian, A. V., Horksem, T. D., Santschi, D. R., Greenwald, J. H., and Frahm, C. J.: Profound hypothermia and circulatory arrest in the surgical treatment of traumatic aneurysm of the thoracic aorta. J. Thorac. Cardiovasc. Surg., 59:541, 1970.
8. Freed, T. A., Neal, M. P., Jr., and Vinik, M.: Roentgenographic findings in extracardiac injury secondary to blunt chest automobile trauma. Amer. J. Roentgen. 104:424, 1968.
9. Gerbode, F., Braimbudge, M., Osborn, J., Hood, M., and French, S.: Traumatic thoracic aneurysms: Treatment by resection and grafting with the use of an extracorporeal bypass. Surgery, 42:6, 1957.
10. Greendyke, R. M.: Traumatic rupture of aorta. J.A.M.A., 195:119, 1966.
11. Griffen, W. O., Jr., Belin, R. P., and Walder, A. I.: Traumatic aneurysm of the abdominal aorta. Surgery, 60:813, 1966.
12. Hewitt, R. L., and Grablowsky, O. M.: Acute traumatic dissecting aneurysm of the abdominal aorta. Ann. Surg., 171:160, 1970.
13. Jahnke, E. J., Jr., Fisher, G. W., and Jones, R. G.: Acute traumatic rupture of the thoracic aorta. A report of six consecutive cases of successful early repair. J. Thorac. Cardiovasc. Surg., 48:63, 1964.
14. Kahn, A. M., Joseph, W. L., and Hughes, R. K.: Traumatic aneurysms of the thoracic aorta. Excision and repair without graft. Ann. Thorac. Surg., 4:175, 1967.
15. Kaufman, J., and Storey, C. F.: Acute traumatic aneurysms of the thoracic aorta: Resection and graft replacement during cardiac massage. Amer. Surg., 34:780, 1968.
16. Kinley, C. E., and Chandler, B. M.: Traumatic aneurysm of thoracic aorta: A case presenting as a coarctation. Canad. Med. Ass. J., 96:279, 1967.
17. Kirsh, M. M., Kahn, D. R., Crane, J. D., Anastasia, L. F., Lui, A. H., Moores, W. Y., Vathayanon, S., Bookstein, J. J., and Sloan, H.: Repair of acute traumatic rupture of the aorta without extracorporeal circulation. Ann. Thorac.Surg., 10:227, 1970.
18. Lim, R. C., Jr., Sanderson, R. G., Hall, A. D., and Thomas, A. N.: Multiple traumatic thoracic aneurysms after nonpenetrating chest injury. Ann. Thorac. Surg., 6:4, 1968.
19. Malm, J. R., and Deterling, R. A., Jr.: Traumatic aneurysm of thoracic aorta. J. Thorac. Cardiovasc. Surg., 40:2, 1960.
20. Ngu, V. A., and Konstam, P. G.: Traumatic dissecting aneurysm of the abdominal aorta. Brit. J. Surg., 52:981, 1965.
21. Parmley, L. F., Mattingly, T., and Manion, W. C.: Penetrating wounds of the heart and aorta. Circulation, 17:953, 1958.
22. Parmley, L. F., Mattingly, T. W., Manion, W. C., and Johnke, E. J.: Nonpenetrating traumatic injury of the aorta. Circulation, 17:1086, 1958.
23. Ricen, E., and Dickens, P. F., Jr.: Traumatic aneurysm of the abdominal aorta of 27 years duration. U.S. Naval Med. Bull., 40:692, 1942.
24. Rindfleisch, E.: Zur Entsteung und Heilung des Aneurysma dissecans aortae. Arch. Path. Anat., 13:374, 1893.
25. Smith, R., III, Perdue, G. D., Jr., Walter, L. G., Jr., and Israle, P. Z.: Posttraumatic aneurysms of the abdominal aorta with recurrent emboli to the superior mesenteric artery: A case report. Surgery, 64:736, 1968.
26. Spencer, F. C., Guerin, P. F., Blake, H. A., and Bahnson, H. T.: A report of fifteen patients with traumatic rupture of the thoracic aorta. J. Thorac. Cardiovasc. Surg., 41:1, 1961.
27. Stoney, R. J., Roe, B. B., and Redington, J.: Rupture of the thoracic aorta due to closed-chest trauma. Arch. Surg., 89:840, 1964.
28. Strassmann, G.: Traumatic rupture of the aorta. Amer. Heart J., 33:508, 1947.

## 4. ANEURYSMS OF THE THORACIC AORTA

*David C. Sabiston, Jr., M.D.*

The ascending, transverse, and descending thoracic aorta may be the site of aneurysms due to a variety of causes. Most are congenital, arteriosclerotic, syphilitic, dissecting, traumatic, or due to cystic medial necrosis (Marfan's syndrome). Syphilitic aortitis destroys the medial layer of the arterial wall and is particularly apt to attack the thoracic aorta. Fortunately, the use of antisyphilitic drugs has reduced this form of the disease greatly. Dissecting and traumatic thoracic aortic aneurysms have been discussed in the preceding sections.

*Cystic medial necrosis* was orginally described by Erdheim.[4] It usually occurs in young males and involves the ascending aorta from the valve to the innominate artery. Necrosis is present in the medial layer, with mucoid-filled cystic spaces. The weakening of the wall thus produced allows aneurysmal dilation to occur, and the aneurysm may subsequently dissect or rupture. If the dissection is directed proximally toward the heart, aortic insufficiency may result. In many patients with cystic medial necrosis, evidence of *Marfan's syndrome* may be present, including skeletal defects, dislocations of the lens, arachnodactyly, a high palate, and pectus excavatum.

Thoracic aortic aneurysms often produce symptoms resulting from pressure on surrounding structures. Substernal discomfort and pain may occur, and obstruction of the trachea and bronchi may lead to a wheeze, cough, or dyspnea. The diagnosis is usually best made by aortography, which demonstrates the site and extent of the lesion.

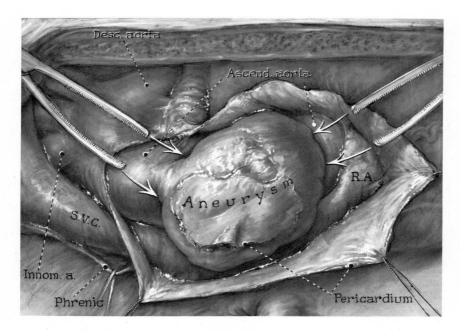

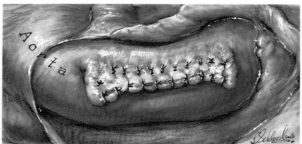

**Figure 17**  Excision of saccular aneurysm of the ascending aorta without extracorporeal circulation. The adjacent aorta is mobilized and the base of the aneurysm clamped with resection of the aneurysm and direct suture of the base. (From Bahnson, H. T.: Surg. Gynec. Obstet., *96*:383, 1953. By permission of Surgery, Gynecology & Obstetrics.)

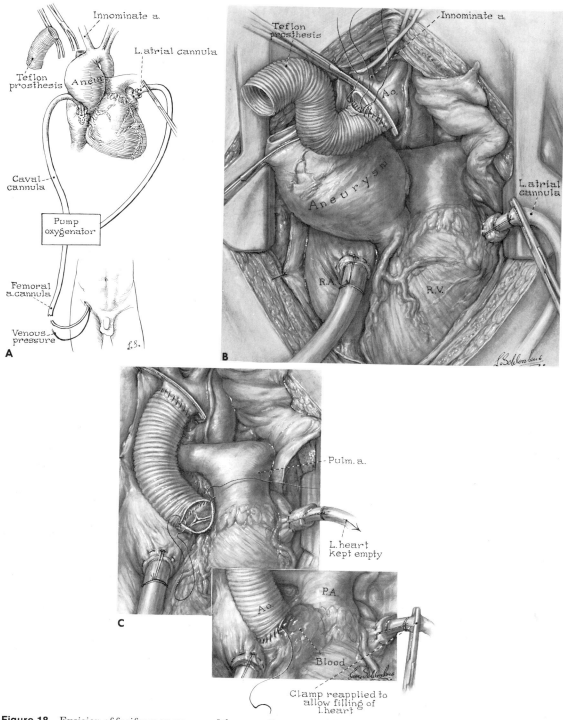

**Figure 18** Excision of fusiform aneurysm of the ascending aorta. *A,* Plan of bypass. *B,* While the distal anastomosis is made, venous blood is not completely removed from the right atrium, and the left atrial suction is used only to prevent excessive pressure in the aneurysm. The coronary circulation is thus maintained intact. *C,* After the aneurysm is excised, all blood is aspirated from both sides of the heart while the proximal anastomosis is completed. When the proximal aorta is opened, the coronary arteries should be perfused. (From Bahnson, H. T., and Spencer, F. C.: Ann. Surg., *151*:879, 1960.)

### SURGICAL THERAPY

Most aneurysms of the thoracic aorta have a sufficiently poor prognosis to justify surgical removal. For saccular aneurysms, this at times may be accomplished without the use of extracorporeal circulation (Fig. 17),[1] although in most patients cardiopulmonary bypass is necessary. Primary anastomosis of the two ends is occasionally feasible, but replacement of a segment of the aorta with a prosthetic graft is usually required (Fig. 18).[2]

### SELECTED REFERENCE

Bahnson, H. T., and Spencer, F. C.: Excision of aneurysm of the ascending aorta with prosthetic replacement during cardiopulmonary bypass. Ann. Surg., *151*:879, 1960.
*A review of the diagnosis and management of aneurysms of the thoracic aorta.*

### REFERENCES

1. Bahnson, H. T.: Definitive treatment of saccular aneurysms of the aorta with excision of sac and aortic suture. Surg. Gynec. Obstet., *96*:383, 1953.
2. Bahnson, H. T., and Spencer, F. C.: Excision of aneurysm of the ascending aorta with prosthetic replacement during cardiopulmonary bypass. Ann. Surg., *151*:879, 1960.
3. DeBakey, M. E., Cooley, D. A., Crawford, E. S., and Morris, G. C., Jr.: Aneurysms of the thoracic aorta: Analysis of 179 patients treated by resection. J. Thorac. Surg., *36*: 393, 1958.
4. Erdheim, J.: Medionecrosis aortae idiopathica. Virchow's Arch. Path. Anat., *273*:454, 1929.

## 5. ANEURYSMS OF THE CAROTID ARTERY

Sir Astley Cooper first introduced proximal ligation of the artery as definitive treatment for carotid artery aneurysm in 1805.[1] Although his first patient died, a second, treated in 1808, lived for 13 years without neurologic deficit. These lesions are the result of atherosclerosis, trauma, and mycotic infection.

The *natural history* of carotid artery aneurysms is generally an unfavorable one. The development of thrombosis in the aneurysms with subsequent embolization to the cerebral and retinal arteries can produce catastrophic complications. In addition, rupture and hemorrhage occur. The development of thrombosis with propagation of the thrombus into the circle of Willis is a major and ever present hazard, especially with lesions involving the *internal* carotid artery.[3] Aneurysms may occur in the common, internal, or external carotid arteries, those in the external carotid artery being the least common.

The usual clinical manifestation is a pulsating mass in the neck with a bruit. The lesion may appear to be inflammatory, and errors have occurred in considering it a cervical abscess. Occasionally, a kink in the carotid or a "U-shaped" artery can simulate an aneurysm. Such disorders of the carotid are usually asymptomatic and require no treatment, although rarely they produce symptoms. Arteriography clearly delineates the size and origin of the lesion, factors that are important in the consideration of surgical therapy.

The *treatment* is excision of the aneurysm, with restoration of continuity either by end-to-end anastomosis or with a graft. Such a procedure removes the hazard of distal embolization and rupture. When located in the internal carotid artery, these lesions are often "false" aneurysms secondary to trauma. The first successful resection of a carotid aneurysm with restoration of the arterial circulation by end-to-end anastomosis was performed by Shea in 1953.[2]

### SELECTED REFERENCE

Raphael, H. A., Bernatz, P. E., Spittel, J. A., Jr., and Ellis, F. H., Jr.: Cervical carotid aneurysms: Treatment by excision and restoration of arterial continuity. Amer. J. Surg., *105*:771, 1963.
*This is a concise review of the diagnosis, pathology, and management of carotid aneurysms. A review of the literature on cervical carotid aneurysms treated by excision and restoration of arterial continuity is included.*

### REFERENCES

1. Cooper, A.: A case of aneurysm of the carotid artery. Med. Chir. Trans., *1*:1, 1809.
2. Shea, P. C., Jr., and Harrison, J. H.: Anastomosis of common and internal carotid arteries following resection of defective portion. Report of a case. Surgery, *34*:895, 1953.
3. Webb, R. C., Jr., and Barker, W. F.: Aneurysms of the extracranial internal carotid artery. Arch. Surg., *99*:501, 1969.

## 6. SUBCLAVIAN ARTERY ANEURYSMS

Aneurysms of the subclavian artery are most often associated with lesions producing the thoracic outlet syndrome. In this situation, the proximal subclavian artery is partially obstructed, and poststenotic dilatation and aneurysmal formation result. Thrombosis may occur, with subsequent embolization to the arterial circulation of the upper extremity. This condition is discussed further in the section on the thoracic outlet syndrome in Chapter 53.

## 7. VISCERAL ARTERIAL ANEURYSMS

Aneurysms of the visceral arteries are more common than is generally appreciated. Although in many instances these aneurysms are asymptomatic, in others they may cause catastrophic results. The fact that these lesions are not rare is

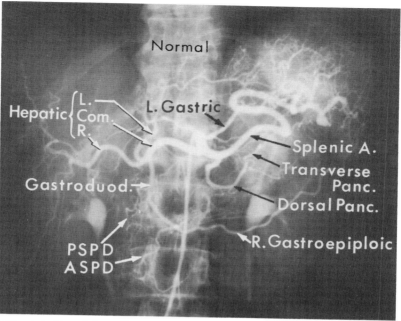

**Figure 19** Selective injection of the celiac axis demonstrating normal anatomy. PSPD: posterior-superior pancreaticoduodenal artery; ASPD: anterior-superior pancreaticoduodenal artery. (Courtesy of Dr. Irwin Johnsrude.)

emphasized by a recent study in which 45 patients with splanchnic arterial aneurysms were seen in one center over a 12 year period.[5] The most important visceral arterial aneurysms are those of the splenic, celiac, hepatic, superior mesenteric, and renal arteries. Aneurysms have also been reported of the gastroduodenal, pancreaticoduodenal, and gastroepiploic arteries. Selective arteriography of the visceral circulation has greatly aided the diagnosis of aneurysms of these arteries (Figs. 19 and 20).

## SPLENIC ARTERY ANEURYSMS

The most common of the visceral arterial aneurysms are those involving the *splenic artery*, representing nearly two-thirds of all such lesions. The first description of a splenic artery aneurysm was by Beaussier in 1770.[1] More than 600 aneurysms of the splenic artery have been reported.[5] These lesions are most commonly found in females, and rupture of the aneurysm during *pregnancy* is a well known complication. The most common *etiology* of these aneurysms is medial degeneration of the arterial wall. They are usually *saccular*, and the wall may contain calcium. Forty-five per cent of females with these aneurysms have had six or more pregnancies.[5] Splenic artery aneurysm may occur in association with fibromuscular hyperplasia involving the renal artery, and atherosclerosis is also a cause of these aneurysms. Congenital aneurysms are rare and are usually multiple. Mycotic lesions, usually the sequel of septic emboli in the spleen after subacute bacterial endocarditis, also occur but are rare.

The *clinical manifestations* of splenic artery aneurysms vary considerably, and many patients are asymptomatic. The most common complaint is that of vague pain in the left upper quadrant with radiation to the left subscapular region. In expanding aneurysms, the symptoms may be

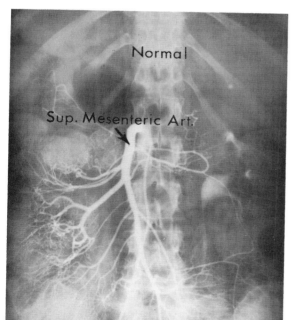

**Figure 20** Selective injection of superior mesenteric artery demonstrating normal anatomy. (Courtesy of Dr. Irwin Johnsrude.)

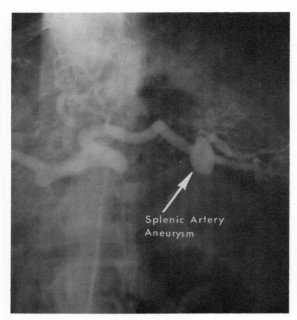

**Figure 21**   Splenic artery aneurysm demonstrated by selective arteriographic injection into the celiac axis. (Courtesy of Dr. Irwin Johnsrude.)

## HEPATIC ARTERY ANEURYSMS

Aneurysm of the hepatic artery was first described by Wilson in 1819,[7] and more than 200 are reported in the literature.[5] The etiology includes arteriosclerosis, infection (mycotic), trauma, and medial degeneration. Periarteritis nodosa is rarely responsible. The most prominent clinical manifestation is right upper quadrant or epigastric pain, frequently similar to that occurring in gallbladder disease. Hematemesis or melena may follow erosion into the gastrointestinal tract, as may fever and jaundice. Free rupture into the peritoneal cavity is the most serious complication of these aneurysms, and only five survivors after this complication have been reported.[5]

When the lesion is diagnosed, surgical extirpation is indicated. In a collected series of 175 patients with this disorder, only 41 were successfully treated, 37 of them in the last decade. Most aneurysms are discovered incidentally at operation, and 80 per cent are extrahepatic and can be identified during abdominal operation, whereas 20 per cent lie within the liver and are not easily palpable.[6] The procedure of choice is *excision* of the aneurysm. If the aneurysm is located proximal to the gastroduodenal artery, the lesion may be simply excised with distal ligation since the collateral circulation through the gastroduodenal artery to the liver is excellent. If the aneurysm involves the hepatic artery *distal* to the gastroduodenal branch, preservation of arterial continuity may be necessary to prevent liver necrosis and requires aneurysmorrhaphy, direct anastomosis, or the use of a venous graft.

more prominent and become acute with rupture. The diagnosis is most often made by the discovery of a calcified lesion on abdominal roentgenograms, with objective demonstration by arteriography (Fig. 21). Physical findings are uncommon, although rarely a tender, pulsatile mass can be felt in the left upper quadrant. Generally, these lesions are small and are not palpable.

The *risk* of rupture of splenic aneurysms is difficult to determine; some reports suggest an extremely high incidence.[4] Among 40 ruptured splenic artery aneurysms recently reported, 10 resulted in death (25 per cent).[5] Operation should be recommended for most splenic artery aneurysms, especially in pregnant patients because of the unduly high risk of rupture. The mortality of rupture during pregnancy is quite high (68 per cent in one group of 65 patients).[5] The procedure of choice is excision of the splenic artery aneurysm, usually with splenectomy.

## CELIAC ARTERY ANEURYSMS

Aneurysms of the celiac artery are relatively uncommon; some 50 examples can be found in the literature. Arteriosclerotic, congenital, mycotic, and traumatic types have been described. When present, the clinical manifestations are primarily those of vague abdominal discomfort. Most of the previously reported cases have been those recognized at the time of rupture. Aggressive *surgical therapy* is recommended, with excision and restoration of continuity either directly or with a graft.

## ANEURYSMS OF THE SUPERIOR MESENTERIC ARTERY

By 1970, 89 cases of aneurysms of the superior mesenteric artery had been reported. The majority (57 per cent) were mycotic in origin, with atherosclerosis, trauma, or medial degeneration being the cause in others. In particular, this lesion should be suspected in patients with subacute bacterial endocarditis in whom abdominal pain develops in association with an expanding, tender mass. These lesions rupture in a high percentage of patients. The first successful treatment was in 1949.[3] Since then, a total of 12 patients have been successfully managed by excision of the aneurysm.[5]

## ANEURYSMS OF THE GASTRODUODENAL AND PANCREATICODUODENAL ARTERIES

Aneurysms of the gastroduodenal and pancreaticoduodenal arteries are rare, with only eight examples reported in the literature. Aneurysms of the gastric and gastroepiploic arteries are more common, with 53 patients having been reported. The majority of these lesions present with rupture, either into the peritoneal cavity or into the upper gastrointestinal tract, presenting with massive bleeding. Ligation of the aneurysm or partial gastric resection has been accomplished in approximately 30 per cent of these patients.

## ANEURYSMS OF THE RENAL ARTERIES

Although once considered rare, aneurysms of the renal arteries are being recognized with increasing frequency. Since the first description in 1770, 345 cases had been reported by 1968.[2] These lesions constitute approximately 1 per cent of all aneurysms and occur most frequently in patients with hypertension. The lesions are located in the main renal artery or the bifurcation of the primary branches in approximately 60 per cent of cases. Approximately 15 per cent of the aneurysms are *intrarenal,* and in about a quarter there is calcification in the wall of the aneurysm. Most of the lesions are due to atherosclerosis or medial necrosis, and occurrence distal to renal artery stricture is not uncommon. *Saccular* aneurysms are the most frequent. The primary risk with these lesions is rupture. The *clinical manifestations* include the symptoms of hypertension and especially headache. Less common are symptoms of upper abdominal and flank pain. A bruit may be heard over the flank, and hematuria may be present. A palpable mass is rare (less than 10 per cent of cases). The definitive diagnosis is made by arteriography. If the renal artery is stenotic, unilateral renal ischemia can be demonstrated on the rapid-sequence pyelogram. The hypertensive mechanism is most apt to be the result of the renin-angiotensin-aldosterone mechanism, whether associated with arterial stenosis or the result of arterial emboli from the aneurysm.

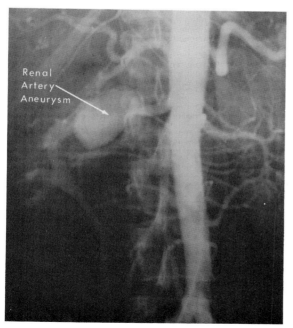

**Figure 22** Aneurysm of the right renal artery. (Courtesy of Dr. Irwin Johnsrude.)

The management of renal artery aneurysms includes careful preoperative demonstration of the size, type, and location of the aneurysm. Rupture is an absolute indication for emergency operation. Those aneurysms without calcification, which represent the majority, are more prone to rupture, are associated with a high mortality, and should be managed surgically. For those aneurysms which are calcified, opinion is divided concerning their treatment, as they are less apt to rupture. At present, the majority favor operation for these lesions, and in most instances it is possible to restore continuity to the renal artery and save the kidney, although nephrectomy may be required.[2] In one series of 22 patients, nine were treated by nephrectomy and nine by aneurysmectomy with arterial repair. Operation is recommended for all except those who are poor surgical risks or who have bilateral intrarenal lesions.

## SELECTED REFERENCES

Cerny, J. C., Chang, C., and Fry, W. J.: Renal artery aneurysms. Arch. Surg., *96*:653, 1968.
  *An excellent description of the diagnosis and management of renal arterial aneurysms in a series of 25 patients.*
Stanley, J. C., Thompson, N. W., and Fry, W. J.: Splanchnic artery aneurysms. Arch. Surg., *101*:689, 1970.
  *A very good review of splanchnic aneurysms. The natural history, diagnosis, management, and results are described.*

## REFERENCES

1. Beaussier, M.: Sur un aneurisme de l'artère splénique dont les parios se sont ossifiées. J. Med. Toulouse, *32*:157, 1770.
2. Cerny, J. C., Chang, C., and Fry, W. J.: Renal artery aneurysms. Arch. Surg., *96*:653, 1968.
3. DeBakey, M. E., and Cooley, D. A.: Successful resection of mycotic aneurysms of superior mesenteric artery: Case report and review of the literature. Amer. Surg., *19*:202, 1953.
4. Owens, J. C., and Coffey, R. J.: Aneurysm of the splenic artery, including a report of six additional cases. Int. Abstr. Surg., *97*:313, 1953.
5. Stanley, J. C., Thompson, N. W., and Fry, W. J.: Splanchnic artery aneurysms. Arch. Surg., *101*:689, 1970.
6. Weaver, D. H., Fleming, R. J., and Barnes, W. A.: Aneurysm of the hepatic artery: The value of arteriography in surgical management. Surgery, *64*:891, 1968.
7. Wilson, J.: Lectures on the Blood, and on the Anatomy, Physiology, and Surgical Pathology of the Vascular System of the Human Body. Read before the Royal College of Surgeons, London, 1819.

## 8. AORTIC ABDOMINAL ANEURYSMS

One of the most common and most dangerous of arterial aneurysms is that encountered in the abdominal aorta. Although recognized for many years, it was not until 1951 that the first aortic abdominal aneurysm was successfully resected by Dubost in France with use of an aortic homograft.[4] Since then, thousands of aortic abdominal aneurysms have been resected, with an appreciable extension of life.

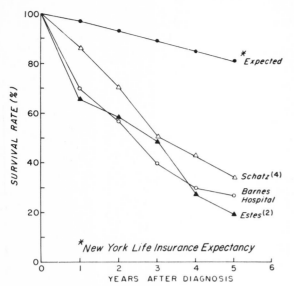

SURVIVAL RATE (%)

YEARS AFTER DIAGNOSIS

*Expected

△ Schatz (4)

○ Barnes Hospital

▲ Estes (2)

*New York Life Insurance Expectancy

**Figure 23** The natural history and survival rates among patients with *untreated* abdominal aortic aneurysms. (From Klippel, A. P., and Butcher, H. R., Jr.: Amer. J. Surg., *111*:629, 1966.)

## PATHOLOGIC ASPECTS

The vast majority—more than 95 per cent—of abdominal aortic aneurysms are due to atherosclerosis. Rarely, trauma, syphilis, mycotic infection, or the Marfan syndrome may be responsible. The majority of the atherosclerotic aneurysms occur in the sixth and seventh decades.

## NATURAL HISTORY

The *fate* of patients with atherosclerotic aneurysms of the abdominal aorta is a subject of prime significance. Careful studies of the *natural history* of untreated abdominal aortic aneurysms have been accumulated in an effort to delineate the role of surgical treatment. In 1950, prior to the advent of surgical therapy, Estes[5] published a classic study of the natural history of abdominal aneurysms in 102 patients. In this group, 64 patients died, and in 63 per cent death was due to rupture.

Only 67 per cent of these patients survived 1 year, 49 per cent survived 3 years, and 19 per cent survived to the fifth year. Similar findings were reported by Schatz[12] and Klippel (Fig. 23).[8] In another study, by Gliedman,[6] emphasis was placed upon patients with *symptomatic* aortic abdominal aneurysms. Thirty per cent of these patients were dead within 1 month after onset of symptoms, and 74 per cent had succumbed by 6 months. The death rate by the end of the first year was 80 per cent. Thus, the survival rate in this group was found to be much lower than that in a group of patients in whom aneurysms were found *incidentally* and were *asymptomatic*. Among the 49 per cent who died, only 4 per cent died from a disease that was entirely unrelated to the aneurysm or its underlying cause. Causes of death included coronary, cerebral, and renal complications of atherosclerosis (Figure 24). Hypertension was present in 47 per cent of the patients.

## CLINICAL MANIFESTATIONS

The majority of abdominal aortic aneurysms are discovered at the time of routine examination and are *asymptomatic*. In the remainder, abdominal symptoms range from vague discomfort in the epigastrium to excruciating pain. Severe pain in the flanks or back suggests leakage or actual rupture of the aneurysm and is usually accompanied by signs of blood loss.

*Physical examination* usually shows the presence of a pulsating mass. The smallest aneurysms are approximately 4 cm. in diameter, but the size may range upward to 20 cm. or more. The aneurysm may be tender to palpation, although this is usually not a prominent symptom. Fortunately, more than 95 per cent of abdominal aortic aneurysms arise *below* the level of the renal arteries, with the inferior mesenteric artery being the only important vessel emerging from the aneurysm. Generally, the latter is either completely occluded or severely stenotic, and this gives rise to prominent collateral circulation to the distal branches of the inferior mesenteric artery. Care should be taken to examine carefully the femoral, popliteal, dorsal pedal, and posterior tibial pulses bilaterally, particularly in reference to possible changes that may occur postoperatively.

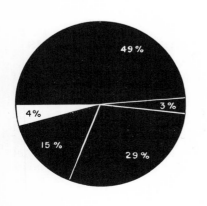

49% = Death from rupture of the abdominal aneurysm.

3% = Death from vascular rupture at another site.

29% = Death due to a disease related to cause of aneurysm.

15% = Death secondarily due to related disease (i.e., a major contributing cause of death.)

4% = DEATH DIRECTLY AND SECONDARILY DUE TO UNRELATED DISEASE.

**Figure 24** Cause of death in 68 patients with an untreated abdominal aneurysm. (From Gliedman, M. L., Ayers, W. B., and Vestal, B. L.: Ann. Surg., *146*:207, 1957.)

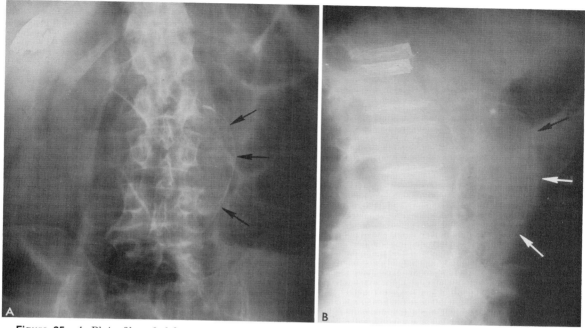

**Figure 25** *A*, Plain film of abdomen of a patient with an abdominal aortic aneurysm. Note the calcium in the wall of the aneurysm outlining its border ("eggshell"). *B*, Lateral film showing calcified wall of the aneurysm.

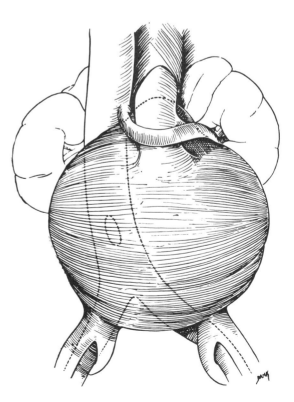

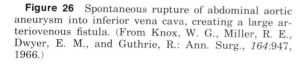

**Figure 26** Spontaneous rupture of abdominal aortic aneurysm into inferior vena cava, creating a large arteriovenous fistula. (From Knox, W. G., Miller, R. E., Dwyer, E. M., and Guthrie, R.: Ann. Surg., *164*:947, 1966.)

### DIAGNOSTIC STUDIES

Plain films of the abdomen frequently show calcification in the wall of the aneurysm, often best observed in the lateral view (Fig. 25). This "eggshell" appearance is essentially diagnostic. Although formerly aortography was used frequently, it is not considered necessary in the vast majority of patients since a firm diagnosis can be made on physical examination and often confirmed on plain films. However, if the aneurysm is thought to involve the renal arteries, aortography is helpful. It is also of aid in the patient with a pulsating abdominal mass in whom neoplasm or cyst must be seriously considered in the differential diagnosis. Arteriography is *essential* for evaluation of the distal circulation in patients who have evidence of obstruction in the iliac, femoral, or popliteal arteries since surgery may also be required for these lesions.

### COMPLICATIONS

The complications that may be associated with untreated aortic abdominal aneurysms are largely dependent upon the size of the aneurysm. Bernstein and associates have emphasized in a collective survey that patients with aneurysms less than 7 cm. in diameter have a lower mortality risk from rupture (4 to 18 per cent), whereas those with aneurysms greater than 7 cm. in diameter have a mortality rate of 72 to 83 per cent.[1] For these reasons, they believe that in *asymptomatic* aneurysms less than 7 cm. in diameter observation without operation may at times be permissible. However, should symptoms appear, resection is indicated. Other complications include *embolism* to the distal iliofemoropopliteal arterial system from thrombus in the aneurysm, rupture into the gastrointestinal tract with hemorrhage, and rupture into the inferior vena cava with creation of an arteriovenous fistula (Figure 26).[9]

### TREATMENT

Most abdominal aortic aneurysms should be managed by excision and restoration of arterial continuity with a prosthetic graft. Rarely, as already mentioned, small aneurysms or those in poor-risk patients may be observed if they are asymptomatic. However, the vast majority of aneurysms should be excised.

#### Operative Technique

Operation for excision of abdominal aortic aneurysm is best accomplished through a midline incision extending from the xiphoid process to the symphysis pubis, which provides excellent exposure. The abdominal aorta is mobilized proximally so that an arterial clamp can be placed across it for total occlusion (Fig. 27).[2] Similarly, the iliac arteries are clamped below. The inferior mesenteric artery is ligated at its origin from the aneurysm and divided. The anterior portion of the aneurysmal wall, including any thrombus present, is then removed. The posterolateral wall of the aneurysm is usually best left in place to prevent unnecessary dissection. The lumbar

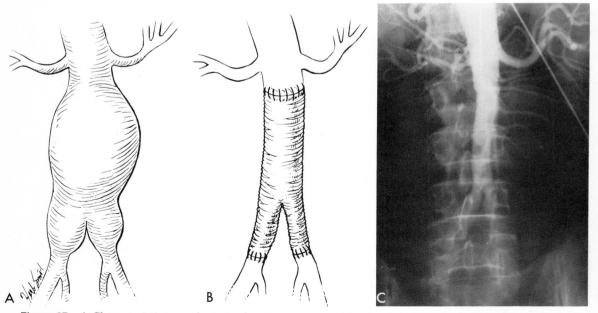

**Figure 27**   *A*, Characteristic type of arteriosclerotic aneurysm arising just below renal arteries and involving both common iliac arteries. *B*, Treatment by resection and replacement with bifurcation Dacron graft. *C*, Aortogram made 5 years after operation, showing restoration of normal circulation. In the majority of patients, it is possible to perform an end-to-end anastomosis to the distal aorta rather than to the iliacs. (From DeBakey, M. E., Crawford, E. S., Cooley, D. A., Morris, G. C., Jr., Royster, T. S., and Abbott, W. P.: Ann. Surg., *160*:622, 1964.)

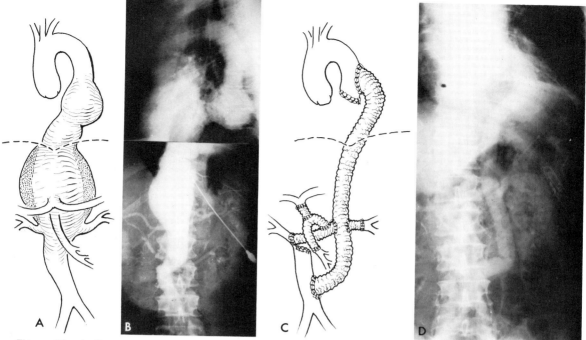

**Figure 28** *A*, Drawing; and *B*, aortogram before operation, demonstrating arteriosclerotic thoracoabdominal aortic aneurysm in a 54-year old male. *C*, Drawing illustrating method of resection and graft placement. *D*, Aortogram after operation, showing satisfactory function of graft replacements. Patient remains well, 5 years after operation. (From DeBakey, M. E., Crawford, E. S., Garrett, H. E., Beall, A. C., Jr., and Howell, J. F.: Ann. Surg., *162*: 650, 1965.)

vessels entering the aneurysm are apt to bleed in a retrograde direction and are controlled with transfixion ligatures. A preclotted prosthetic graft, preferably of knitted Dacron, is then sutured to the aorta above and below. Although silk was formerly used for the anastomosis, plastic sutures are preferable as they do not fragment and their use is less apt to be followed by development of a false aneurysm. Although the proximal portions of both common iliac arteries formerly were resected, this is much less commonly done today. Therefore, a straight graft is usually employed, and the bifurcation type is reserved for use when the iliac arteries are involved in an aneurysm. The results of this operation have been highly satisfactory. Prophylactic antibiotics are often used, although there is little objective evidence that antibiotics are needed.

Rarely, aortic aneurysms are extensive and involve the lower thoracic aorta; these *thoracoabdominal aneurysms* pose difficult problems in surgical treatment. The celiac axis, superior mesenteric artery, and renal arteries may arise from the aneurysm. Therefore, surgical correction requires extensive dissection and mobilization, with tedious restoration of blood flow to each of these critical vessels. By total resection of the aneurysm and stepwise insertion of appropriate grafts, these lesions can be successfully treated (Fig. 28).[3]

In the patient presenting with a *ruptured* aortic abdominal aneurysm, an *emergency* operation should be undertaken immediately. The blood loss should be replaced rapidly, and as soon as the abdomen is entered, it is essential first to control the hemorrhage by proximal compression of the

aorta. Large amounts of blood may be necessary in the resuscitation of these patients, and appropriate attention must be given to the temperature of the infused blood as well as to the administration of calcium. In those recovering from the immediate operative procedure, the effects of renal ischemia constitute the major cause of late deaths. Myocardial infarction may also occur, being precipitated by hypotension. The mortality varies between 30 and 50 per cent in operations for ruptured abdominal aortic aneurysms.[10]

## RESULTS

The *mortality* for elective operations can be as low as 5 per cent, although in a collective review of statistics from nine leading centers the mortality ranged from 5 to 18 per cent.[1] The mortality is primarily due to associated lesions of atherosclerosis that complicate the postoperative recovery, including myocardial infarction, cerebrovascular lesions, and hypertensive cardiovascular-renal disease. Rarely, the prosthetic graft becomes infected. Such an infection is a grave complication, and generally it cannot be eradicated until the plastic graft is removed. This requires the use of additional grafts through uninfected tissues, such as bilateral axillofemoral grafts (Fig. 29).[7] Such has been satisfactorily accomplished with removal of the aortic graft, ligature of the proximal and distal aorta, and institution of drainage. Owing to the extensiveness of the atherosclerotic process,

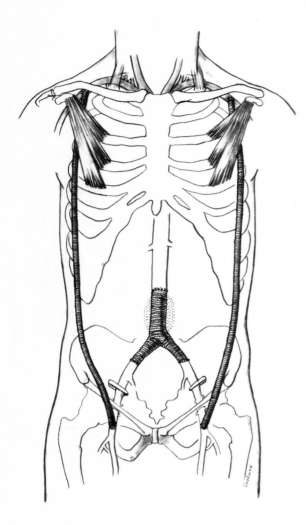

**Figure 29** Diagrammatic illustration of patient with an infected aortic abdominal prosthetic graft treated with bilateral axillofemoral prosthetic grafts passed in subcutaneous tunnels on either side. The infected aortic graft was subsequently removed, with ligation of both iliac arteries and the terminal aorta. (From Hardy, J. D., and Conn, J. H. In: Hardy, J. D., ed.: Critical Surgical Illness. Philadelphia, W. B. Saunders Company, 1971.)

**Figure 30** Life expectancy of patients with abdominal aortic aneurysm in the study of DeBakey et al., compared with that of the normal population adjusted for sex and age and with that of patients in a nonresected series by Estes and Wright and others. (From DeBakey, M. E., Crawford, E. S., Cooley, D. A., Morris, G. C., Jr., Royster, T. S., and Abbott, W. P.: Ann. Surg., *160*:622, 1964.)

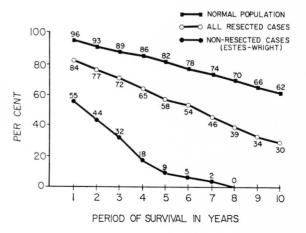

ischemia of the lower extremities may occur after operation and require bypass therapy or embolectomy to remove thrombi in the distal circulation, which may arise from the aneurysm at the time of resection. Another recognized complication is the development of a fistula between the proximal anastomosis and the intestinal tract. These fistulas usually enter the duodenum since it is immediately adjacent. Less commonly, the distal anastomosis is involved, with entry into the small intestine. Such lesions may be successfully managed by subsequent operation and correction.[11]

The long-term results of resection of abdominal aortic aneurysms have been evaluated by DeBakey and associates, who report that 84 per cent of all patients operated on are alive at the end of 1 year, 72 per cent at 3 years, and 58 per cent at 5 years (Fig. 30).[2]

*Iliac* arterial aneurysms frequently occur either unilaterally or bilaterally in association with aortic abdominal aneurysms. Occasionally, an iliac aneurysm occurs as an isolated lesion. Both types should be managed by resection with prosthetic graft replacement.

## SELECTED REFERENCES

DeBakey, M. E., Crawford, E. S., Cooley, D. A., Morris, G. C., Jr., Royster, T. S., and Abbott, W. P.: Aneurysm of abdominal aorta: Analysis of results of graft replacement therapy one to eleven years after operation. Ann. Surg., *160*:622, 1964.
  *Long-term follow-up of the fate of patients with removal of abdominal aortic aneurysms is presented in this paper. The favorable prognosis following surgery is emphasized.*

Estes, J. E., Jr.: Abdominal aortic aneurysm: A study of one hundred and two cases. Circulation, 2:258, 1950.
  *This is an often quoted study of the follow-up of a large group of patients with aortic abdominal aneurysms prior to the advent of surgical treatment.*

## REFERENCES

1. Bernstein, E. F., Fisher, J. C., and Varco, R. L.: Is excision the optimum treatment for all abdominal aortic aneurysms? Surgery, 61:83, 1967.
2. DeBakey, M. E., Crawford, E. S., Cooley, D. A., Morris, G. C., Jr., Royster, T. S., and Abbott, W. P.: Aneurysm of abdominal aorta: Analysis of results of graft replacement therapy one to eleven years after operation. Ann. Surg., *160*:622, 1964.
3. DeBakey, M. E., Crawford, E. S., Garrett, H. E., Beall, A. C., Jr., and Howell, J. F.: Surgical considerations in the treatment of the thoraco-abdominal aorta. Ann. Surg., *162*:650, 1965.
4. Dubost, C., Allary, M., and Oeconomos, N.: Resection of an aneurysm of the abdominal aorta: Reestablishment of the continuity by a preserved human arterial graft, with results after five months. Arch. Surg., *64*:405, 1952.
5. Estes, J. E., Jr.: Abdominal aortic aneurysm: A study of one hundred and two cases. Circulation, *2*:258, 1950.
6. Gliedman, M. L., Ayers, W. B., and Vestal, B. L.: Aneurysms of the abdominal aorta and its branches. A study of untreated patients. Ann. Surg., *146*:207, 1957.
7. Hardy, J. D., and Conn, J. H.: Infected arterial grafts. In: Hardy, J. D., ed.: Critical Surgical Illness. Philadelphia, W. B. Saunders Company, 1971.
8. Klippel, A. P., and Butcher, H. R., Jr.: The unoperated abdominal aortic aneurysm. Amer. J. Surg., *111*:629, 1966.
9. Knox, W. G., Miller, R. E., Dwyer, E. M., and Guthrie, R.: Abdominal aortic aneurysm-vena caval fistula: Report of cardiac function and blood volume following surgical correction. Ann. Surg., *164*:947, 1966.
10. Lawrence, M. S., Crosby, V. G., and Ehrenhaft, J. L.: Ruptured abdominal aortic aneurysm. Ann. Thorac. Surg., 2:159, 1966.
11. Levy, M. J., Todd, D. B., Lillehei, C. W., and Varco, R. L.: Aorticointestinal fistulas following surgery of the aorta. Surg. Gynec. Obstet., *120*:992, 1965.
12. Schatz, I. J., Fairbairn, J. F., II, and Juergens, J. L.: Abdominal aortic aneurysms: A reappraisal. Circulation, 26:200, 1962.

## 9. FEMORAL ARTERY ANEURYSMS

Femoral aneurysms are relatively common and are bilateral in a third of patients. The lesions are primarily due to atherosclerosis and present the hazard of distal embolization from thrombi in the aneurysms. The diagnosis can usually be made by palpation of the femoral artery. A plain roentgenogram is helpful since the aneurysmal wall is frequently calcified. In approximately a quarter of patients, a coexisting aortic abdominal aneurysm is present. In a study of 115 femoral aneurysms in 89 patients at the Mayo Clinic, 86 of the patients were males and 3 were females; the average age of the patient at the time of discovery was 64 years. The anatomic location in this series was common femoral (27 per cent), superficial femoral (26 per cent), iliofemoral (14 per cent), femoropopliteal (13 per cent), and profunda femoris (1 per cent); in the remaining 19 per cent either operation was not performed or anatomic location could not be established by arteriography. A high incidence of aneurysms in other parts of the arterial system was found, as shown in Table 2.[4] Hypertension was present in 54 per cent of patients in this series, ischemic heart disease was present in 18 per cent, and spontaneous rupture occurred in 5 per cent.

### MANAGEMENT

Most femoral arterial aneurysms should be removed, with restoration of continuity of the femoral arterial system. Occasionally, coexistence

**TABLE 2** ASSOCIATED ANEURYSMS IN SERIES OF FEMORAL ANEURYSMS (89 PATIENTS)*

| Location of Associated Aneurysms | No. of Patients | % |
|---|---|---|
| Popliteal artery | 27 | 38 |
| Iliac artery | 20 | 28 |
| Abdominal aorta | 20 | 28 |
| Thoracic aorta | 3 | 4 |
| Posterior tibial artery | 1 | 1 |
| Ulnar artery | 1 | 1 |
| Total | 72 | 100 |

*From Pappas, G., Janes, J. M., Bernatz, P. E., and Schirger, A.: J.A.M.A., *190*:489, 1964.

TABLE 3  SITES OF 139 EXTRAPOPLITEAL ANEURYSMS AMONG 152 PATIENTS WITH POPLITEAL ANEURYSMS*

| Location of Aneurysm | Patients† No. | % |
|---|---|---|
| Abdominal aorta | 53 | 35 |
| Common femoral artery | 40 | 26 |
| Common iliac artery | 28 | 18 |
| Internal iliac artery | 7 | 5 |
| Superficial femoral artery | 4 | 3 |
| Thoracic aorta | 4 | 3 |
| External iliac artery | 2 | 1 |
| Renal artery | 1 | 1 |
| Total affected | 69 | 45 |

*From Wychulis, A. R., Spittell, J. A., Jr. and Wallace, R. B.: Surgery, 68:942, 1970.

†Some patients had more than one extrapopliteal aneurysm.

TABLE 4  COMPLICATIONS OF 111 POPLITEAL ANEURYSMS AT THE TIME OF INITIAL EXAMINATION*

| Complication | Aneurysms† |
|---|---|
| Thrombosis | 65 |
| Venous occlusion | 30 |
| Ulceration, gangrene, or both | 28 |
| Peripheral embolus | 23 |
| Compression of the popliteal nerve | 15 |
| Popliteal thrombophlebitis | 11 |
| Rupture | 6 |
| Infection | 2 |

*From Wychulis, A. R., Spittell, J. A., Jr., and Wallace, R. B.: Surgery, 68:942, 1970.

†Some aneurysms presented more than one complication.

of multiple aneurysms or other serious complications of atherosclerosis constitute a contraindication to operation. The results are good.

## 10. POPLITEAL ARTERY ANEURYSMS

The most common site of peripheral aneurysms is the popliteal artery. Moreover, popliteal aneurysms are unique in that they are associated with an unusually high incidence of distal thromboembolism. In one series of 100 popliteal aneurysms, 23 per cent of 80 patients managed nonsurgically eventually had to undergo amputation,[2] and in another series limb loss was reported as 77 per cent.[3] Nearly all popliteal aneurysms are the result of arteriosclerosis. Rarely, syphilitic, mycotic, and false aneurysms following trauma occur. The size of the aneurysm varies from 3 to 15 cm. in diameter, the majority being 5 to 7 cm. Additional aneurysms in other sites are common and in one series were present in 45 per cent of patients (Table 3).[5] An even larger number of patients (59 per cent) had bilateral aneurysms.

The *diagnosis* is usually obvious on clinical examination from the presence of a pulsatile mass in the popliteal space. The mass may be firm if it is largely filled with thrombus. Calcification of the wall is present in about a quarter of these aneurysms. While some aneurysms are uncomplicated when first recognized, thrombosis is the most serious of the sequelae and occurs in approximately half of patients (Table 4).[5] Other complications include venous occlusion, ulceration gangrene, peripheral emboli, compression of the popliteal nerve, and popliteal thrombophlebitis. Rupture occurs in approximately 5 per cent.

## TREATMENT

Since in a significant number of patients with these aneurysms symptoms develop with the passage of time, operation should usually be recommended. In one series of 94 patients with asymptomatic aneurysms who were followed without surgery, complications developed in 29 per cent.[5] The procedure of choice is excision of the aneurysm with restoration of arterial continuity. Occasionally, it is possible to perform an end-to-end anastomosis of the proximal and distal artery after resection, but a saphenous vein autograft is generally required. If a suitable vein is not available, a plastic graft can be employed. The results of operation are quite good.[1]

## REFERENCES

1. Crichlow, R. W., and Roberts, B.: Treatment of popliteal aneurysms by restoration of continuity: Review of 48 cases. Ann. Surg., 163:417, 1966.
2. Gifford, R. W., Jr., Hines, E. A., Jr., and Janes, J. M.: An analysis and follow-up study of one hundred popliteal aneurysms. Surgery, 33:284, 1953.
3. Linton, R. R.: The arteriosclerotic popliteal aneurysm: A report of fourteen patients treated by a preliminary lumbar sympathetic ganglionectomy and aneurysmectomy. Surgery, 26:41, 1949.
4. Pappas, G., Janes, J. M., Bernatz, P. E., and Schirger, A.: Femoral aneurysms: Review of surgical management. J.A.M.A., 190:489, 1964.
5. Wychulis, A. R., Spittell, J. A., Jr., and Wallace, R. B.: Popliteal aneurysms. Surgery, 68:942, 1970.

# VI

# Thrombo-Obliterative Disease of the Aorta and Its Branches

*David C. Sabiston, Jr., M.D.*

Occlusive disease of the major branches of the aorta is most frequently the result of atherosclerosis. Certain arterial anatomic sites are especially susceptible to development of stenoses or total occlusion, and these are generally at the origins of vessels, where *turbulence* may be present (Fig. 1).[4] When branches of the aortic arch (innominate, carotid, subclavian) become stenotic or occluded, the symptoms produced represent ischemic disturbances due to diminution in blood flow to the cerebral circulation and to the upper extremities. In younger patients, especially women, an obliterative endarteritis, Takayasu's disease ("pulseless disease"), may produce similar symptoms.

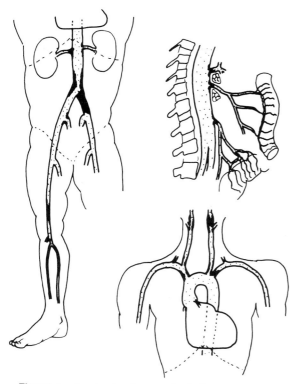

**Figure 1** Anatomic sites particularly apt to become stenotic or occluded by atherosclerosis. (From Ludbrook, J., and Elmslie, R. G.: An Introduction to Surgery: 100 Topics. New York, Academic Press, 1971.)

## CLINICAL MANIFESTATIONS

The subclavian artery is most commonly involved and is followed in incidence by the carotids and innominate artery. The location and extent of a large number of lesions reported in one series are shown in Table 1.[1] The *symptoms* vary depending upon the nature and extent of the obstruction. Moreover, the natural development of *collateral* circulation that follows arterial occlusion and its effectiveness are of prime importance. The symptoms are primarily (1) neurologic, relating to diminished blood flow to the brain, and (2) those producing *ischemia* of the upper extremities causing claudication. The distribution of symptoms is shown in Table 2.[1] The diagnosis is confirmed by *arteriography* with use of multiple roentgenographic exposures to present the films in a series, thus demonstrating the lesion and the collateral blood supply around it.

## SURGICAL MANAGEMENT

The surgical management of patients with occlusive disease is primarily accomplished by bypass grafts (Fig. 2).[1] The preoperative and postoperative obstructions as demonstrated by arteriography are shown, as well as the pressure gradient present before and after correction. The results of surgical bypass treatment are encouraging, as shown in Table 3.[1] In this series, obstruction was incomplete in 168 and complete in 244 of the arteries involved. Regardless of the extent of obstruction, the occlusive process was *segmental* in almost every instance. The surgical treatment most often is a bypass graft, but endarterectomy is at times applicable.

## 1. TAKAYASU'S ARTERITIS

Takayasu's disease, described by a Japanese ophthalmologist in 1908,[6] is a nonspecific arteritis affecting the thoracic and abdominal aorta and its major branches. Relatively rare in the United States, it is quite common in the Orient and usually attacks young females (85 per cent of cases). The arteritis involves all layers of the aortic wall with proliferation of connective tissue

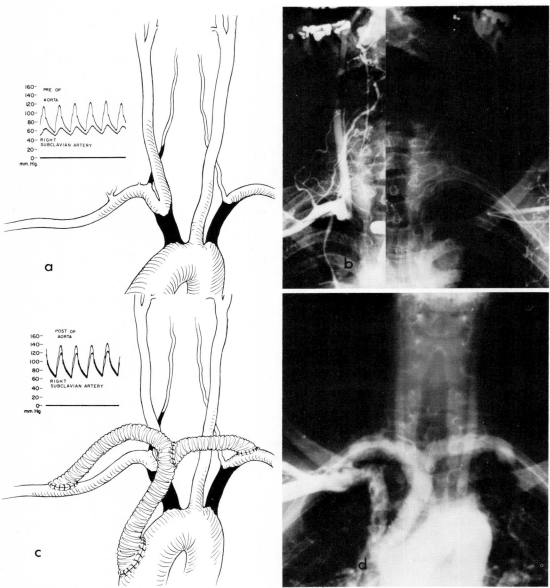

**Figure 2**  Patient with obstruction of innominate and left subclavian arteries, causing cerebral arterial insufficiency, and obstruction of the abdominal aorta and iliac arteries, causing both intermittent claudication and ischemic lesions of the feet. The patient treated first at one operation by ascending aortobilateral subclavian bypass graft, and at a second operation by bilateral aortoexternal iliac artery bypass graft, relieving all symptoms. Diagram (a) and arteriogram (b) with pressure recording made before bypass show location and extent of innominate and subclavian lesions. Diagram (c) and aortogram (d) made 3 years after operation and pressure recordings made at operation after bypass show grafts in place and functioning. Diagram (e) and aortogram (f) made before operation show location and extent of aortoiliac obstruction. Diagram (g) and aortogram (h) made 3 years after operation show graft in place and functioning. The patient is alive and well 5 years after operation. (From Crawford, E. S., DeBakey, M. E., Morris, G. C., Jr., and Howell, J. F.: Surgery, 65:17, 1969.)

*Illustration continued on opposite page.*

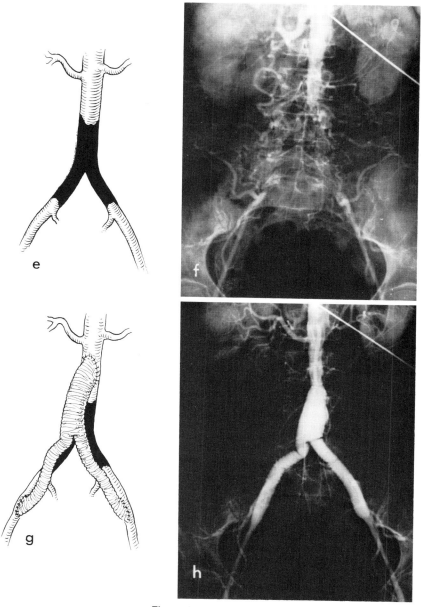

Figure 2 *(continued)*

**TABLE 1**  LOCATION AND EXTENT OF 412 LESIONS IN 299 PATIENTS[*]

| Location | Extent of Obstruction | | Totals |
|---|---|---|---|
| | *Incomplete* | *Complete* | |
| Innominate artery | 40 | 26 | 66 |
| Right common carotid artery | 5 | 19 | 24 |
| Right subclavian artery | 30 | 29 | 59 |
| Left common carotid artery | 24 | 37 | 61 |
| Left subclavian artery | 69 | 133 | 202 |
| Total | 168 | 244 | 412 |

[*]From Crawford, E. S., DeBakey, M. E., Morris, G. C., Jr., and Howell, J. F.: Surgery, *65*:17, 1969.

**TABLE 2**  SYMPTOMS OF OCCLUSION (299 PATIENTS)[*]

| Type of Symptom | No. of Patients | Percent |
|---|---|---|
| Neurological only | 97 | 32 |
| Neurological and upper extremity ischemia | 124 | 42 |
| Upper extremity ischemia | 63 | 21 |
| Systolic ear noise | 3 | 1 |
| No symptoms | 12 | 4 |
| Total | 299 | 100 |

[*]From Crawford, E. S., DeBakey, M. E., Morris, G. C., Jr., and Howell, J. F.: Surgery, *65*:17, 1969.

**TABLE 3**  FUNCTIONAL RESULTS IN 299 PATIENTS WITH OCCLUSION OF GREAT VESSELS OF THE AORTIC ARCH[*]

| Time of Follow-up | Asymptomatic, Improved | | Unimproved | | Worse | | Dead | |
|---|---|---|---|---|---|---|---|---|
| | *No.* | *Percent* | *No.* | *Percent* | *No.* | *Percent* | *No.* | *Percent* |
| Immediate | 268 | 89.6 | 10 | 3.3 | 5 | 1.7 | 16 | 5.4 |
| Late | 274 | 91.6 | 3 | 1.0 | 6 | 2.0 | 43 | 14.4 |

[*]From Crawford, E. S., DeBakey, M. E., Morris, G. C., Jr., and Howell, J. F.: Surgery, *65*:17, 1969.

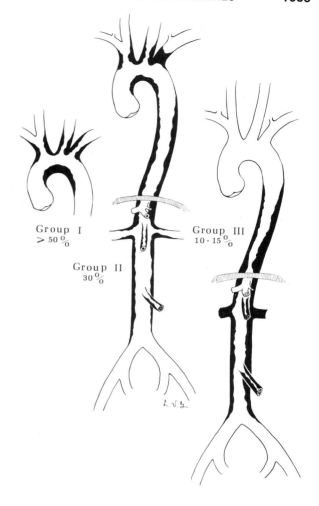

**Figure 3**  Clinical subdivisions of Takayasu's arteritis. The panarteritis may be localized to the aortic arch and great vessels (Group I), the distal thoracoabdominal aorta (Group III), or the entire aorta (Group II). (From Edmunds, L. H., Jr. In: Strandness, D. E., Jr., ed.: Collateral Circulation in Clinical Surgery. Philadelphia, W. B. Saunders Company, 1969.)

and degeneration of the elastic fibers. Granulomatous lesions may be present with associated fusiform or saccular aneurysmal formation. Three types of this disorder are now recognized (Fig. 3).[2]

The *clinical manifestations* of Takayasu's arteritis are at first generalized and include fever, malaise, arthritis, and arthralgia. Pericardial pain, tachycardia, and vomiting may also occur. It has been suggested that the disorder may be an autoimmune disease,[5] and steroids may be beneficial. The later manifestations are those of ischemia of both the cerebral and upper extremity circuits. Surgical treatment of Takayasu's arteritis has often proved disappointing since the endarterectomy site and grafts are apt to reocclude. Operation is occasionally recommended for patients with disabling symptoms.[3]

## REFERENCES

1. Crawford, E. S., DeBakey, M. E., Morris, G. C., Jr., and Howell, J. F.: Surgical treatment of occlusion of the innominate, common carotid, and subclavian arteries: A 10 year experience. Surgery, 65:17, 1969.
2. Edmunds, L. H., Jr.: Trauma and occlusive disease. In: Strandness, D. E., Jr., ed.: Collateral Circulation in Clinical Surgery. Philadelphia, W. B. Saunders Company, 1969.
3. Ekeström, S., and Hansson, L. O.: Surgical treatment of "pulseless disease." Acta Chir. Scand., 128:127, 1964.
4. Ludbrook, J., and Elmslie, R. G.: An Introduction to Surgery: 100 Topics. New York, Academic Press, 1971.
5. Nakao, K., Ikeda, M., Kimata, S., Niitani, H., Miyahara, M., Ishimi, Z., Hashiba, K., Takeda, Y., Ozawa, T., Matsushita, S., and Kuramochi, M.: Takayasu's arteritis. Clinical report of eighty-four cases and immunological studies of seven cases. Circulation, 35:1141, 1967.
6. Takayasu, M.: Case of queer changes in central blood vessels of retina. Acta. Soc. Ophthal. Jap., 12:2554, 1908.

# 2. CAROTID OCCLUSIVE DISEASE

*Vallee L. Willman, M.D.,*
*and Hendrick B. Barner, M.D.*

Considering the prevalence and the awesome presentation of stroke, there is little wonder that it has been described as a clinical entity since biblical times. Stroke has afflicted nine presidents of our nation, and is considered to have influenced decisions of two, Woodrow Wilson and F. D.

Roosevelt, during times of national emergency. The social and emotional impact of stroke on its victims and their families has been vividly described by several victims.[23,33] In addition to causing 200,000 deaths annually in our country, stroke leaves even more people physically and emotionally crippled.[32] It is curious, then, that the importance of extracranial vascular disease as a cause of stroke has become generally recognized only in the past 20 years. Prior to 1950, the major treatises on stroke listed as etiology hemorrhage, thrombosis, and embolus, thrombosis being considered as an intracranial vascular phenomenon and embolus considered as having its origin within the heart. As recently as 1930, discussions on stroke listed hemorrhage as accounting for most instances, with intracranial thrombosis being the next most frequent cause. The failure to recognize extracranial vascular disease as a major cause of stroke is perhaps attributable to an overconcern that existed only a few years ago about the complications of cerebral arteriography, as well as the failure to examine vessels in the neck regularly in postmortem examination.

The possibility of extracranial vascular disease as a basis of stroke was suggested by Savory's

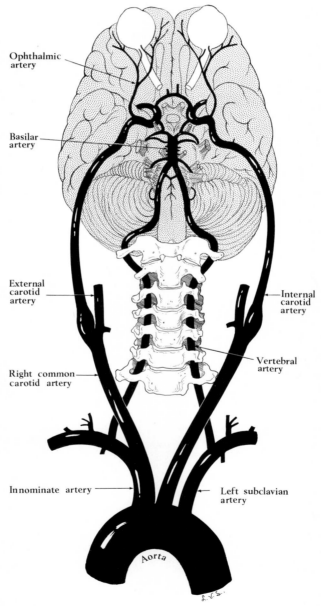

Ophthalmic artery

Basilar artery

External carotid artery

Internal carotid artery

Vertebral artery

Right common carotid artery

Innominate artery

Left subclavian artery

Aorta

**Figure 4**    Diagram of major extracranial components of cerebral and ocular arterial supply. (From Wylie, E. J., and Ehrenfeld, W. K.: Extracranial Occlusive Cerebrovascular Disease. Philadelphia, W. B. Saunders Company, 1970.)

report more than a hundred years ago of a woman with right hemiparesis and extracranial vascular occlusions.[30] Gowers in 1875 described a patient with left eye blindness and right hemiparesis, probably due to carotid occlusion.[21] Hunt in 1914 reported on 20 patients with hemiplegia, four of whom had diminished neck pulses.[24] Among 82 patients with evidence of cerebrovascular disease studied at autopsy, Hutchinson found that in 40 at least half of the lumen of either a carotid or vertebral artery or both was obliterated.[25] It was Fisher in two important reports (1951 and 1954) who drew attention to the relationship of disease of the carotid arteries in the neck and the several clinical patterns of cerebrovascular insufficiency.[18,19] He described both partial and total occlusions of the carotid arteries on the basis of atherosclerosis, noting that the distal vessels were often free of disease. He suggested that operation might become a form of treatment. "It is even conceivable that some day vascular surgery will find a way to bypass the occluded portion of the artery during the period of ominous fleeting symptoms."[18] During the same year (1954), Eastcott, Pickering, and Rob reported on the resection of a stenotic area of the left carotid with relief of the recurrent signs of cerebral ischemia that had plagued the patient.[10] Reports of operative treatment of occlusion and stenosis have since appeared regularly as thousands of patients have been treated. The diagnosis and management of lesions of the extracranial vasculature is now a major interest of vascular surgeons.[39]

The pathophysiology of stroke as a result of carotid artery disease has defied precise description. This is in part due to the complex and variable anatomic circulatory arrangements of the brain, the incompletely understood regulatory mechanisms of brain blood flow, the complex interrelationship of brain circulation with cardiorespiratory function, and the inability to easily assess regional brain blood flow.

The extracranial arterial blood supply of the brain is by four vessels: two internal carotids and two vertebrals. The two vertebrals join high in the neck to form the basilar. Within the cranium the two internal carotids and the basilar communicate rather freely with each other (Fig. 4). The major collateral circulation was described by Willis[37] in 1684 and is generally referred to as the "circle of Willis" (Fig. 5). Because of this arrangement, occlusion of one of the extracranial vessels is generally well compensated for by increased flow through the others. The adequacy of this collateral system, however, is limited at times by developmental or acquired variations.

It is readily understandable that occlusive lesions in the extracranial vessels might reduce total flow to the brain below that level necessary to sustain normal brain function and thus result in stroke. It can be reasoned that lesions in the extracranial vessels progress through a stage in which brain blood flow is marginal, causing some slight aberrations in cerebral function, to the stage of occlusion, which results in clearly

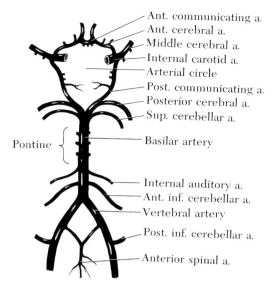

**Figure 5**  Diagram showing the most common configuration of the terminal branches of the vertebral and internal carotid arteries and their interconnections to form the circle of Willis. (From Wylie, E. J., and Ehrenfeld, W. K.: Extracranial Occlusive Cerebrovascular Disease. Philadelphia, W. B. Saunders Company, 1970.)

insufficient blood flow, with brain death and clinical stroke. Several studies have drawn a corollary between the clinical course of patients with stroke and the extent of occlusive lesions in the carotids and vertebrals.[9,17,36] Repetitive angiographic studies have identified the natural tendency for lesions to progress.[3] In addition to continued aggregation of atheromatous material, the severity of obstruction can be enhanced by hemorrhage into the plaque itself or by thrombus formation on an ulcerated area.[38]

What is not easily explainable on the basis of decreased brain blood flow is the occurrence of brain dysfunction with only partially occlusive lesions in one carotid artery. It is well known that in most instances occlusion of one internal carotid artery is well tolerated. Why, then, should signs of cerebral ischemia occur in the presence of a partially occlusive lesion in one carotid?

Several possible explanations have been offered. One is that atherosclerosis is a generalized disease, and in most instances a process found in the internal carotid reflects the presence of multiple lesions throughout the cerebral vascular tree. Although cerebral vascular lesions are frequently multiple, they have not been found diffusely throughout the smaller vasculature of the brain. Indeed, vessels distal to a major stenosis are frequently free of disease. The occurrence of lesions in more than one of the four major extracranial vessels would logically explain variations in compensatory flow when there is flow limitation in one vessel, but it does not quite satisfy as an explanation of cerebral ischemia when lumen narrowing is no more than 50 per cent. Although a 50 per cent constriction of a carotid artery will

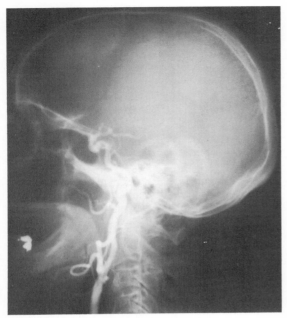

**Figure 6** Left carotid arteriogram of a patient who has had transient ischemic attacks. There is an ulcerative lesion detectable near the origin of the internal carotid artery.

often induce a pressure gradient across the area, experimental observations indicate that a reduction in area of approximately 90 per cent is necessary in order to reduce blood flow.[6,13]

*Transient ischemic attacks* have been attributed to periods of hypotension and low cardiac output,[7,8] yet the episodes have not been reproducible by artificially lowering blood pressure.[14,26] Alteration in brain blood flow due to position has been proposed as a cause of transient ischemic attacks, but again the attacks have not been reproducible.

Embolization from ulcerated atherosclerotic lesions seems to offer the best explanation for transient ischemic attacks. Ulcerative lesions have been described both pathologically and radiographically[29] (Fig. 6). Atheromatous emboli have been observed in retinal vessels[12] (Fig. 7). Fisher has observed an embolus passing through the retinal vessels of a patient who experienced repeated transient ischemic attacks, and he recognized the association of stenosis of the carotid artery on that side.[20] Platelet aggregations have been identified histologically in a patient with carotid occlusion.[27]

A characteristic of transient ischemic attacks that casts some suspicion on the embolic etiology is the tendency for the recurring clinical events to be similar, indicating that the same central nervous system area is repeatedly involved. It is of some importance that another form of repetitive central nervous system insult, that occurring with prosthetic heart valves, also has the tendency to recur in the same anatomic area and is also thought to have embolization as its basis. The flow distribution patterns of blood coursing through the carotids and over atheromatous lesions might well be so constant as to permit a high degree of selectivity for the distribution of emboli to a particular anatomic location.

The usual site of internal carotid artery disease

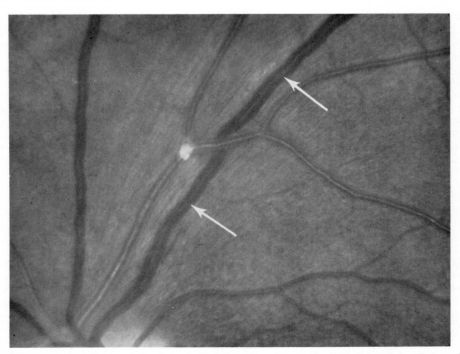

**Figure 7** Atheromatous retinal embolus lodged at a bifurcation. (From Hoyt, W. F. In: Wylie, E. J., and Ehrenfeld, W. K.: Extracranial Occlusive Cerebrovascular Disease. Philadelphia, W. B. Saunders Company, 1970.)

is at and just distal to its origin at the bifurcation of the common carotid. The lesions are typical of atherosclerotic lesions elsewhere in the vascular tree. At times the disease extends centrally to the base of the skull; however, it is most commonly localized to the first 3 cm. of the vessel. The carotid sinus and carotid body are located in this region of the vessel. The effect of the disease process on the function of these receptor sites has not been determined, although there is evidence that carotid baroreceptor function is strikingly modified in patients with symptoms of cerebrovascular disease.[1]

The determination of lesions of the carotid artery is made ultimately by arteriography. Thermography, ophthalmodynamometry, and pulse changes are all aids that can help make the decision for arteriography but will not provide the information necessary to decide on operation. Arteriography is indicated when there are signs and symptoms of cerebrovascular insufficiency in a patient susceptible to improvement by revascularization, or in the presence of a carotid bruit in the asymptomatic patient.

Egas Moniz is credited with introducing arteriography as a means of studying the cerebral circulation.[28] He accomplished this by direct needle puncture of the common carotid artery in the neck. This is a procedure requiring a considerable degree of care and patience and is not without complications. The inconvenience and risk are perhaps reasons why extensive use of cerebral arteriography as a diagnostic measure was slow in developing. Currently, most cerebral arteriography is performed by the introduction of a catheter into the aorta by a percutaneous technique through either the brachial or femoral artery. This allows for visualization of all four of the principal vessels in the neck, a highly desirable goal in evaluating both the need for and the approach to relief of obstructive lesions (Fig. 8).

The technical details of the operative procedure for carotid endarterectomy have undergone many alterations in the past decade and are as yet not standardized. Since stroke and myocardial infarction occurring during the operative period are the greatest risks, careful cardiac evaluation is important, and great attention is directed to maintaining adequate cerebral perfusion at all times. Preoperative medications should be administered cautiously to avoid any depression of ventilation or of cardiac output. Operation under local anesthesia was advised at one time in order to avoid the consequences of general anesthesia as well as to allow for intraoperative evaluation of the patient's motor and mental function. It has now been generally accepted that with local anesthesia there is a greater discrepancy between brain oxygen requirements and supply than with a well conducted general anesthesia,[2, 34] and most operations are now conducted under general anesthesia with endotracheal intubation.[38] Expeditious intubation and maintenance of a high arterial $pO_2$ are probably the most important aspects of the anesthetic management. The proper $pCO_2$

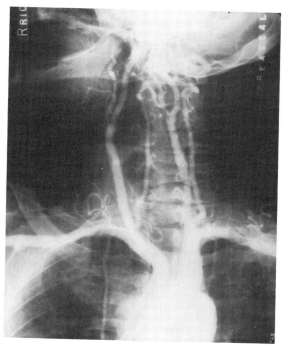

**Figure 8** Contrast material injected into the aortic arch allows visualization of all four extracranial vessels supplying the brain.

maintenance remains debatable.[11, 38] Maintenance of blood pressure at or slightly above the usual preoperative level is considered important in order to maintain optimal cerebral and myocardial circulation. The maintenance of blood pressure involves the avoidance of agents that depress cardiac output or inhibit vasomotion, the meticulous replacement of blood and fluid loss, the vigorous treatment of bradycardia and other cardiac arrhythmias, and the judicious use of vasopressor agents.[38]

The patient is positioned with the head somewhat extended and turned to the side opposite the lesion. In addition to the neck, a site for obtaining a segment of vein is prepared and draped in case reconstruction of the artery requires substitution. One cannot rely on a suitable vein always being available in the neck.

The skin incision is extended through the platysma medial to the sternocleidomastoid muscle. The fascia over the internal jugular vein is opened, and the common facial vein, which courses over the carotid artery, is divided. Care is taken to identify and preserve the descending branch of the hypoglossal nerve and the superior laryngeal nerve (Fig. 9). The common carotid, internal carotid, and external carotid arteries are dissected at levels not involved in the disease process and are then occluded only after the patient has been given heparin intravenously to prevent clotting in any stagnant areas. An incision is made in the anterolateral aspect of the common carotid to a point beyond the plaque. A plane between diseased intima and the media-

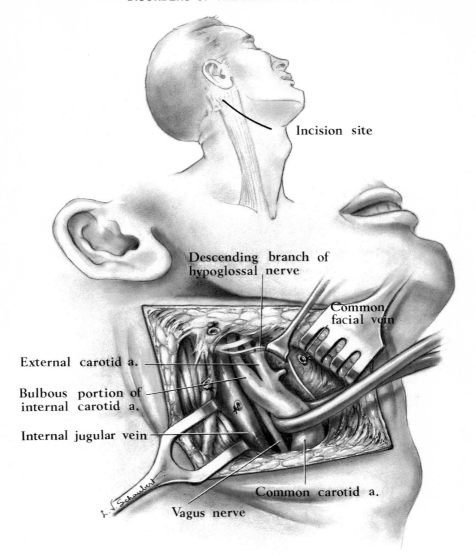

Incision site

Descending branch of
hypoglossal nerve

Common
facial vein

External carotid a.

Bulbous portion of
internal carotid a.

Internal jugular vein

Common carotid a.

Vagus nerve

**Figure 9**   Incision site and exposure of the carotid bifurcation area. (From Wylie, E. J., and Ehrenfeld, W. K.: Extracranial Occlusive Cerebrovascular Disease. Philadelphia, W. B. Saunders Company, 1970.)

adventitia is developed, and the obstructing lesion is removed. The artery is then carefully reconstructed; the vessel is supplemented with a vein patch if there is insufficient tissue for construction of a vessel of a size greater than that distal to the operative site (Fig. 10). Arteriograms are obtained to assess the anatomic result. Many surgeons advise the use of a shunt during the period of occlusion in order to assure blood flow to the brain. Others use shunts selectively, judging the need on the basis of distal artery pressure following occlusion, ipsilateral jugular vein oxygen tension, or the severity of the associated lesions outlined by preoperative arteriography.

Continued surveillance of oxygenation and blood pressure is important postoperatively. The endotracheal tube is removed only when there is evidence of adequate ventilation without support.

Arrhythmias and falling blood pressure are aggressively treated. Both baroreceptor and chemoreceptor function are in danger of alteration by the current operative procedures, which dissect long segments of the arteries. The loss of baroreceptor function does not seem to be of great importance as the loss is compensated for by the several other regulatory mechanisms. Chemoreceptor function, on the other hand, although not altered by unilateral dissection, is measurably altered by bilateral carotid endarterectomy.[34] The loss of carotid chemoreceptor response in the patient with central nervous system damage, altered cardiac dynamics, and pulmonary disease could be intolerable, and the patient's survival might be dependent upon ventilatory support.

The value of operative treatment of carotid

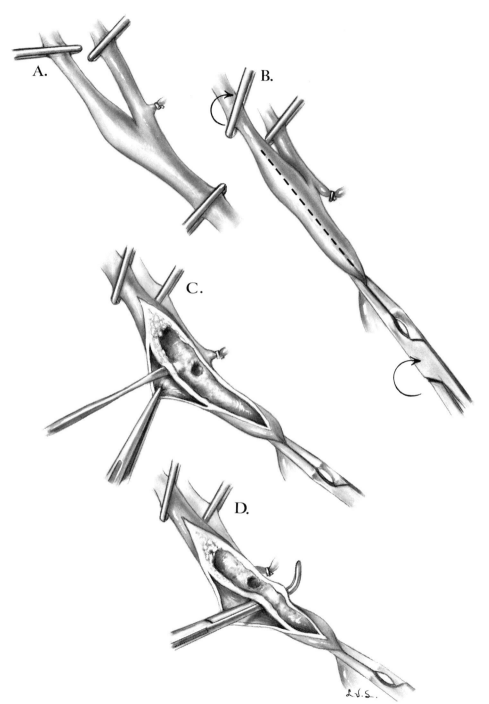

**Figure 10**  Technique of carotid endarterectomy. (From Wylie, E. J., and Ehrenfeld, W. K.: Extracranial Occlusive Cerebrovascular Disease. Philadelphia, W. B. Saunders Company, 1970.)

*Illustration continued on following page.*

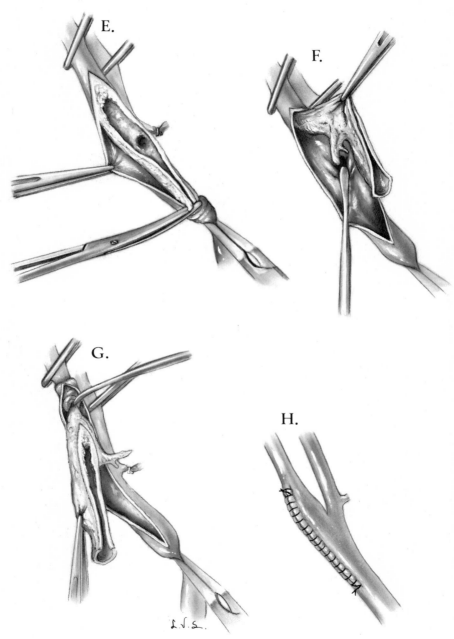

**Figure 10**  (*continued*)

occlusions in relieving symptoms and prolonging life has not been well enough established to gain the procedure unqualified support. A remarkable attempt to evaluate carefully the role of operative treatment has been made by a large group of investigators, working in 24 different institutions, who categorized patients according to a common protocol and randomized these patients for operative treatment and nonoperative management. This effort has resulted in five reports that aid considerably in the clinical approach to the condition.[4,5,15,16,22]

Over a 5 year period (1961 to 1966) 4748 patients entered this collaborative study. Entry was on the basis of symptoms of cerebrovascular ischemia as well as, in some instances, carotid bruits in completely asymptomatic patients. The ischemic patterns were: (1) transient ischemic attacks consisting of sudden onset of distinct neurologic deficit, such as paresis, dysphasia, paresthesia, or vertigo, the symptoms being transitory and clearing within a few hours; (2) steadily progressive deficit from onset that becomes a serious neurologic deficit with progression; (3) single catastrophic episode, with a severe, definitive neurologic deficit that has stabilized.

Eighty per cent of the patients had complete arteriographic study, with visualization of both the intracranial and extracranial circulation. Eighty per cent of those studied had lesions in the extracranial vasculature. This incidence is comparable to that found in recent postmortem studies. The lesions in the majority of instances were accessible to operative treatment. In nearly 70 per cent of the patients with lesions operatively accessible, the lesions were multiple. The existence of multiple lesions obviously complicates a clear relationship between lesions and the clinical pattern.

Severe complications from arteriography occurred in slightly more than 1 per cent of the patients, and clearly were related to more severe neurologic deficit. It was concluded that in patients with severe and progressive brain stem dysfunction angiographic studies should not be done until the clinical course has stabilized.

The large number of anatomic sites of obstruction and the various clinical presentations combine to make for a large number of categories coming under consideration, so that subgroups of this large group of patients are rather small, and firm conclusions are difficult to make. Data from this study suggest, however, that operation undertaken during the acute phase of a stroke, while it is progressing, is quite hazardous, and survival is less likely than if a nonoperative course is followed. During this early period, restoration of normal arterial blood flow to an area of softened brain can result in cerebral hemorrhage.[39] In the circumstance of a stabilized single catastrophic episode, with a single carotid artery involved, operative correction offered an improved chance of survival and lessened risk of recurrent stroke. If both carotids were involved, one occluded and one stenotic, the advantage of operation was prob-

lematic. Operation is clearly of advantage in the clinical condition of ischemic attacks when one carotid artery has a partially occlusive lesion. Both survival and relief of symptoms were improved by operative correction.

Complete occlusion of an internal carotid usually results in thrombosis to the origin of the caroticotympanic arteries at the base of the skull. In this circumstance, endarterectomy and thrombectomy have been infrequently successful in restoring circulation.[31] Such a lesion in conjunction with a stenotic lesion in the other carotid poses a severe threat and so far has not yielded well to treatment. The technically demanding but logical approach of bypassing such an obstruction with a vein bypass graft from the carotid in the neck to the intracranial carotid is certain to be tried with increasing frequency.

As with many therapies, carotid endarterectomy for treatment of cerebral ischemia seems to require proper timing in the course of the disease. Unfortunately, when it is applied late in the disease, when death of a portion of the brain has already occurred, it introduces risks equaling or outweighing the advantages. Applied early in the course of the disease, when it is prophylactic against stroke, it seems to be clearly advantageous. This is the challenge to the surgeon — to apply the procedure with such skill as to essentially avoid risk in the seemingly well patient. Current techniques certainly allow for approaching that goal. The challenge then becomes one of case finding — searching out seemingly well persons who, untreated, are unknowingly under risk of stroke. This is the most promising approach to stroke prevention in the foreseeable future.

## SELECTED REFERENCES

Fields, W. S., North, R. R., Hass, W. K., Galbraith, J. G., Wylie, E. J., Ratinor, G., Burns, M. H., McDonald, M. C., and Meyer, J. S.: Joint study of extracranial arterial occlusion as a cause of stroke. I. Organization of study and survey of patient population. J.A.M.A., *203*:153, 1968.

Hass, W. K., Fields, W. S., North, R. R., Kricheff, I. I., Chase, N. E., and Bauer, R. B.: Joint study of extracranial arterial occlusion. II. Arteriography, techniques, sites, complications. J.A.M.A., *203*:159, 1968.

Bauer, R. B., Meyere, J. S., Fields, W. S., Remington, R., McDonald, M. C., and Callen, R.: Joint study of extracranial arterial occlusion. III. Progress report of controlled study of long-term survival in patients with and without operation. J.A.M.A., *208*:509, 1969.

Blaisdell, W. F., Clauss, R. H., Galbraith, J. G., Imparato, A. M., and Wylie, E. J.: Joint study of extracranial arterial occlusion. IV. A review of surgical conditions. J.A.M.A., *209*:1889, 1969.

Fields, W. S., Maslenikov, V., Meyer, J. S., Hass, W. K., Remington, R. D., and McDonald, M.: Joint study of extracranial arterial occlusion. V. Progress report of prognosis following surgery or nonsurgical treatment for transient cerebral ischemic attacks and cervical carotid artery lesion. J.A.M.A., *211*:1993, 1970.
*These reports are from a study entered into cooperatively by 25 institutions in an attempt to gain a sufficient number of case studies to permit meaningful analysis of the value of treatment in a rather ill defined entity. These are important articles not only for the extensive data and close analyses they contain, but also because this study is an excellent*

*example of a new and important approach to the analysis of clinical information by cooperative effort.*

Wylie, E. J., and Ehrenfeld, W. K.: Extracranial Occlusive Cerebrovascular Disease. Diagnosis and Management. Philadelphia, W. B. Saunders Company, 1970.
*This is a complete, yet concise monograph that expertly considers all the aspects of extracranial vascular occlusion. It is particularly valuable for its elucidation of pathogenesis and discussion of diagnostic methods and selection of patients for operative treatment.*

## REFERENCES

1. Appenzellei, O., and Discaucts, L.: Circulatory reflexes in patients with cerebrovascular disease. New Eng. J. Med., *271*:820, 1964.
2. Bain, J. A., Catton, D. V., Cox, J. M. R., and Spoerel, W. E.: The effect of general anaesthesia on the tolerance of cerebral ischemia in rabbits. Canad. Anaesth. Soc. J., *14*:64, 1967.
3. Bauer, R. B., Boulos, R. S., and Meyer, J. S.: Natural history and surgical treatment of occlusive cerebrovascular disease evaluated by serial arteriography. Amer. J. Roentgen., *104*:1, 1968.
4. Bauer, R. B., Meyer, J. S., Fields, W. S., Remington, R., McDonald, M. C., and Callen, R.: Joint study of extracranial arterial occlusion. III. Progress report of controlled study of long-term survival in patients with and without operation. J.A.M.A., *208*:509, 1969.
5. Blaisdell, W. F., Clauss, R. H., Galbraith, J. G., Imparato, A. M., and Wylie, E. J.: Joint study of extracranial arterial occlusion. IV. A review of surgical consideration. J.A.M.A., *209*:1889, 1969.
6. Brice, J. G., Dowsett, D. F., and Lowe, R. D.: Hemodynamic effects of carotid artery stenosis. Brit. Med. J., *2*:1363, 1964.
7. Corday, E., Rothenberg, S., and Werner, S. M.: Cerebral vascular insufficiency. An explanation of the transient stroke. Arch. Intern. Med., *98*:683, 1956.
8. Denny-Brown, D.: Recurrent cerebrovascular episodes. Arch. Neurol., *2*:194, 1960.
9. Drake, W. E., Jr., and Drake, M. A. L.: Clinical and angiographic correlates of cerebrovascular insufficiency. Amer. J. Med., *45*:253, 1968.
10. Eastcott, H. H. G., Pickering, G. W., and Rob, C. G.: Reconstruction of internal carotid artery in patients with intermittent attacks of hemiplegia. Lancet, *2*:994, 1954.
11. Ehrenfeld, W. K., Hamilton, F. N., Larson, C. P., Jr., Larson, R. F., and Severinhaus, J. W.: Effect of $CO_2$ and systemic hypertension on downstream cerebral arterial pressure during carotid endarterectomy. Surgery, *67*:87, 1970.
12. Ehrenfeld, W. K., Hoyt, W. F., and Wylie, E. J.: Embolization and transient blindness from carotid atheromata. Arch. Surg., *93*:787, 1966.
13. Eklof, B., and Schwartz, S. I.: Effects of critical stenosis of the carotid artery and compromised cephalic blood flow. Arch. Surg., *99*:695, 1969.
14. Fayekces, J. F., and Alman, R. W.: The role of hypotension in transitory focal cerebral ischemia. Amer. J. Med. Sci., *248*:567, 1964.
15. Fields, W. S., Maslenikov, V., Meyer, J. S., Hass, W. K., Remington, R. D., and McDonald, M.: Joint study of extracranial arterial occlusion V. Progress report of prognosis following surgery or nonsurgical treatment for transient cerebral ischemic attacks and cervical carotid artery lesion. J.A.M.A., *211*:1993, 1970.
16. Fields, W. S., North, R. R., Hass, W. K., Galbraith, J. G., Wylie, E. J., Ratinor, G., Burns, M. H., McDonald, M. C., and Meyer, J. S.: Joint study of extracranial arterial occlusion as a cause of stroke. I. Organization of study and survey of patient population. J.A.M.A., *203*:153, 1968.
17. Fields, W. S., Sharkey, P. C., Crawford, E. S., and Morris, G. C.: Correlation of neurologic syndromes with lesions found angiographically. Neurology, *10*:431, 1960.
18. Fisher, C. M.: Occlusion of the internal carotid artery. Arch. Neurol. Psychiat., *65*:346, 1951.
19. Fisher, C. M.: Occlusion of the carotid artery: Further experiences. Arch. Neurol. Psychiat., *72*:187, 1954.
20. Fisher, C. M.: Observations of the fundus oculi in transient monocular blindness. Neurology, *9*:333, 1959.
21. Gowers, W. R.: On a case of simultaneous embolism of central retinal and middle cerebral arteries. Lancet, *2*:794, 1875.
22. Hass, W. K., Fields, W. S., North, R. R., Kricheff, I. I., Chase, N. E., and Bauer, R. B.: Joint study of extracranial arterial occlusion. II. Arteriography, techniques, sites, complications. J.A.M.A., *203*:159, 1968.
23. Hodgins, E.: Episode: Report on an Accident Inside my Skull. New York, Atheneum, 1964.
24. Hunt, J. R.: The role of the carotid arteries in the causation of vascular lesions of the brain with remarks on certain special features of the symptomatology. Amer. J. Med. Sci., *147*:704, 1914.
25. Hutchinson, E. C., and Yates, P. O.: Carito-vertebral stenosis. Lancet, *1*:2, 1957.
26. Kendall, R. E., and Marshall, J.: Role of hypotension on the genesis of transient focal cerebral ischemic attacks. Brit. Med. J., *2*:344, 1963.
27. McBrien, D. F., Braddey, R. D., and Ashton, N.: The nature of retinal emboli in stenosis of the internal carotid artery. Lancet, *1*:697, 1963.
28. Moniz, E.: L'encéphalographie artérielle, son importance dans la localisation des tumeurs cérébrales. Rev. Neurol., *2*:72, 1927.
29. Moore, W. S., and Hall, A. D.: Ulcerated atheroma of the carotid artery: A cause of transient cerebral ischemia. Amer. J. Surg., *114*:800, 1967.
30. Savory, W. S.: Case of a young woman in whom the main arteries of both upper extremities and of the neck were throughout completely obliterated. Med. Chir. Te. Land, *39*:205, 1856.
31. Thompson, J. E., Austin, D. J., and Patman, R. O.: Endarterectomy of the totally occluded carotid artery for stroke: Results in one hundred operations. Arch. Surg., *95*:791, 1967.
32. U.S. President's Commission on Heart Disease, Cancer and Stroke. Washington, D.C., U.S. Government Printing Office, Dec., 1964.
33. Van Rosen, R. E.: Comeback: The Story of My Stroke. New York, Bobbs-Merrill Company, 1962.
34. Wade, J. G., Larson, C. P., Jr., Hickey, R. F., Ehrenfeld, W. K., and Severinhaus, J. W.: Effect of carotid endarterectomy on carotid chemoreceptor and baroreceptor function in man. New Eng. J. Med., *282*:823, 1970.
35. Wells, B. A., Keats, A. S., and Cooley, D. A.: Induced tolerance to cerebral ischemia produced by general anesthesia during temporary carotid occlusion. Surgery, *54*:216, 1963.
36. Whisnant, J. P., Martin, M. J., and Sayre, G. P.: Atherosclerotic stenoses of cervical arteries: Clinical significance. Arch. Neurol., *5*:429, 1961.
37. Willis, T.: Practice of Physick. London, S. Pordage, 1684, Part 6, p. 59.
38. Wylie, E. J., and Ehrenfeld, W. K.: Extracranial Occlusive Cerebrovascular Disease. Diagnosis and Management. Philadelphia, W. B. Saunders Company, 1970.
39. Wylie, E. J., Hein, M. F., and Adams, J. E.: Intracranial hemorrhage following surgical revascularization for treatment of acute stroke. J. Neurosurg., *21*:212, 1964.

## 3. SUBCLAVIAN "STEAL" SYNDROME

*David C. Sabiston, Jr., M.D.*

In 1961, Reivich and associates described a clinical disorder in which cerebral ischemia was produced by the "subclavian steal syndrome." The pathophysiology of this disorder is produced by *stenosis* or *occlusion* of the subclavian artery proximal to the origin of the vertebral artery. Thus, blood may flow from the cerebral circulation and circle of Willis in a *retrograde* direction, down the vertebral artery into the subclavian artery to the arm. This is particularly apt to occur during

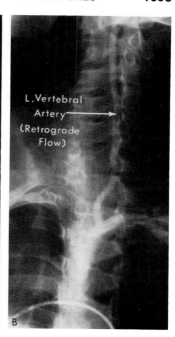

**Figure 11** *A*, Arteriogram with injection into aortic arch showing occlusion of left subclavian artery. *B*, Later phase showing retrograde filling of the left vertebral artery from the circle of Willis.

exercise of the involved arm. The symptoms include claudication in the arm and hand on the involved side, frequently with concomitant signs of cerebral ischemia. A decrease in the pulse and blood pressure is usually present in the involved arm. A bruit is also frequently heard over the lesion in the subclavian artery. Arteriography establishes the diagnosis, and serial films demonstrate the retrograde filling of the vertebral artery from the circle of Willis with flow into the subclavian (Fig. 11).

## SURGICAL MANAGEMENT

Originally, endarterectomy was performed to remove the occluding lesion from the subclavian artery. More recently, a simplified approach with use of a saphenous vein autograft (or plastic graft) from the carotid to the subclavian has been employed (Fig. 12). This procedure is performed

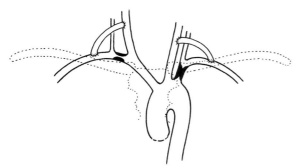

**Figure 12** Total occlusion of the left subclavian artery treated by saphenous vein bypass graft from left carotid artery. A severe stenosis is shown in the right subclavian artery, also treated by a vein graft.

through a simple incision, and the results have been excellent.

## SELECTED REFERENCES

Killen, D. A., Foster, J. H., Gobbel, W. G., Jr., Stephenson, S. E., Jr., Collins, H. A., Billings, F. T., and Scott, H. W., Jr.: The subclavian steal syndrome. J. Thorac. Cardiovasc. Surg., *51:* 539, 1966.
*This paper comprises an excellent presentation of the clinical manifestations, diagnosis, arteriographic findings, management, and results in a group of patients with different anatomic types of arterial obstruction.*

Reivich, M., Holling, E., Roberts, B., and Toole, J. F.: Reversal of blood flow through the vertebral artery and its effects on cerebral circulation. New Eng. J. Med., *265:*878, 1961.
*This is the first description of the subclavian "steal" syndrome and is a classic.*

## 4. THROMBOTIC OBLITERATION OF THE ABDOMINAL AORTA AND ILIAC ARTERIES (LERICHE SYNDROME)

Thrombotic obliteration of the aortic bifurcation was described by Leriche in 1940.[10] In an excellent discussion of this entire subject, Leriche emphasized that the disorder is a chronic process and is associated with a specific symptom complex. Typically, the condition affects males in the 35 to 60 age group.

### CLINICAL MANIFESTATIONS

The symptoms characteristic of thrombotic occlusion of the terminal aorta include (1) extreme

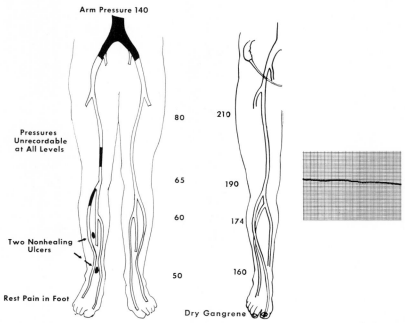

**Figure 13**   *A,* The extensive aortoiliac occlusion, combined with the superficial femoral artery and anterior tibial artery occlusion, reduced limb blood pressures below recordable levels. *B,* The normal ankle pressure of 160 mm. Hg and absent digit pulses placed the arterial occlusion between the ankle and digits. (From Strandness, D. E., Jr.: Collateral Circulation in Clinical Surgery. Philadelphia, W. B. Saunders Company, 1969.)

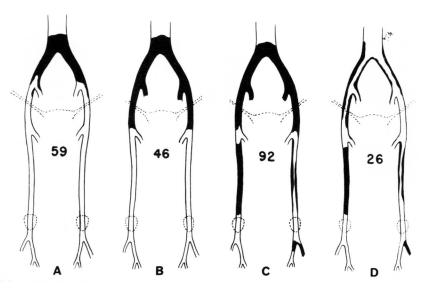

**Figure 14**   Schematic classification of extent of involvement in a series of patients with aortoiliofemoral arterial occlusive disease. (From Perdue, G. D., Long, W. D., and Smith, R. B., III: Trans. Southern Surg. Ass., *82*:330, 1970.)

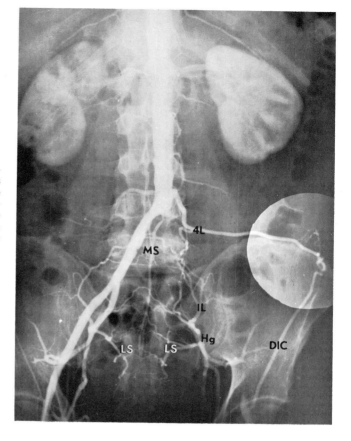

**Figure 15** A 43 year old male with left intermittent claudication. The fourth lumbar (4L) is the origin of a pathway to the femoral via the deep iliac circumflex (DIC) and to the hypogastric (Hg) via the iliolumbar (IL). The middle sacral (MS) and lateral sacral (LS) contribute to a transpelvic anastomosis to the hypogastric (Hg). (From Friedenberg, M. J., and Perez, C. A.: Amer. J. Roentgen., *94*:145, 1965.)

liability to fatigue of both lower limbs, which Leriche described as a *weariness* rather than the typical intermittent claudication; (2) *symmetric atrophy* of both lower limbs without trophic changes of the skin or nails; (3) *pallor* of the legs and feet; and (4) *inability to maintain a stable erection* due to inadequate arterial flow to the penis secondary to hypogastric arterial obstruction. The physical findings include absence of pulses in the abdominal aorta and in all arteries distal to it. The physiologic changes in arterial pressure are shown in Figure 13.[18] Distal sites of segmental occlusion produce a further fall in arterial pressure, with development of ischemic ulcers.

Leriche emphasized that the disease was often well tolerated for 5 and even 10 years, but usually ended in gangrene of one or both extremities. The characteristic pathologic finding is an atherosclerotic lesion in the wall of the abdominal aorta with superimposed thrombosis. The lumen characteristically narrows gradually, and so *acute* symptoms are not apt to occur.[11]

The diagnosis is confirmed by *arteriography,* in which occlusion of the terminal abdominal aorta, and often of both common iliacs, is demonstrated (Figure 14).[14] The occlusion may involve any portion of the abdominal aorta from the renal arteries distally. The collateral circulation that develops is shown in an arteriogram in Figure 15,[7] and the anatomic collateral pathways are shown schematically in Figure 16*A*.[7]

## SURGICAL MANAGEMENT

Although thromboendarterectomy with direct reconstitution of flow is appropriate in some patients, the majority with occlusion of the abdominal aorta are managed by bilateral bypass grafts from the aorta to the common femoral arteries (Fig. 16*B*). It may be necessary to perform a short thromboendarterectomy just distal to the renal arteries to permit a site for the proximal anastomosis. However, it is important not to disturb the aorta any more than necessary and to reduce dissection in this region to the minimum. These precautions prevent the troublesome ejaculatory complications that may otherwise result. It has been shown that thromboendarterectomy and resection of the aorta as definitive procedures for aortic thrombosis produce disturbances in ejaculation in 68 per cent of patients, whereas when bypass is chosen as the primary treatment, only 26 per cent have this difficulty.[13]

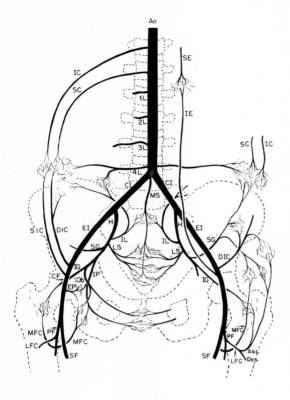

(From Friedenberg, M. J., and Perez, C. A.: Amer. J. Roentgen., *94*:145, 1965.)

**Figure 16A**  Composite line drawing showing schematically the major parietal pathways of collateral circulation in aortoiliofemoral occlusive disease.

| | |
|---|---|
| Ao | Aorta |
| Asc | Ascending branch |
| CF | Common femoral |
| CI | Common iliac |
| Des | Descending branch |
| DIC | Deep iliac circumflex |
| EI | External iliac |
| EP | External pudendal |
| H | Hypogastric |
| IC | Intercostal |
| IE | Inferior epigastric |
| IG | Inferior gluteal |
| IL | Iliolumbar |
| IP | Internal pudendal |
| L | Lumbar |
| LFC | Lateral femoral circumflex |
| LS | Lateral sacral |
| MFC | Medial femoral circumflex |
| MS | Middle sacral |
| Ob | Obturator |
| PF | Profunda femoris |
| SC | Subcostal |
| SE | Superior epigastric |
| SF | Superficial femoral |
| SG | Superior gluteal |
| SIC | Superficial iliac circumflex |

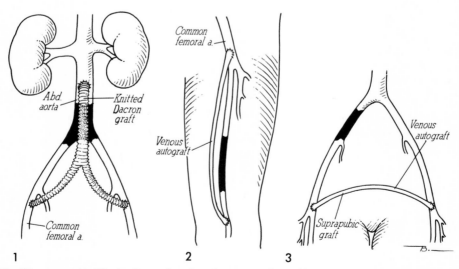

**Figure 16B**  Diagrammatic illustrations of various bypass grafts. *1,* For occlusion of the abdominal aorta, a bypass graft placed proximal to the occlusion can be inserted distally into each of the common femoral arteries in the groin. *2,* For occlusion of the superficial femoral artery, a venous autograft may be placed from the common femoral artery above to the femoral or popliteal artery distal to the obstruction. *3,* For unilateral iliac arterial occlusion, a suprapubic graft can be placed from one common femoral artery to the other in a subcutaneous suprapubic tunnel, Generally, under these circumstances a venous autograft is preferable to a plastic prosthesis, although the latter can be employed.

## 5. ILIAC ARTERIAL OCCLUSION

The iliac arteries may be individually stenosed or occluded. The symptoms are usually those of claudication of the hip and thigh associated with diminished or absence of pulses in that extremity. Arteriography is diagnostic. When symptoms are unilateral, involvement of the opposite leg can often be seen on the arteriogram. Indeed, symptoms may appear in the opposite leg following operation when the patient is able to exercise sufficiently. Bypass grafts from the aorta above to the common femoral artery below are usually indicated.

## 6. FEMOROPOPLITEAL ARTERIAL OCCLUSION

While any segment of the femoral artery may become stenotic or occluded by atherosclerosis, the most common site is the distal superficial femoral artery in the *adductor canal.* Occlusion usually produces claudication of the calf muscles and, less commonly, in the muscles of the thigh, unless the iliac artery is also involved. Progressive occlusion is accompanied by the development of collateral circulation in the involved area, and these collaterals are typically *tortuous* (Figure 17A and B).

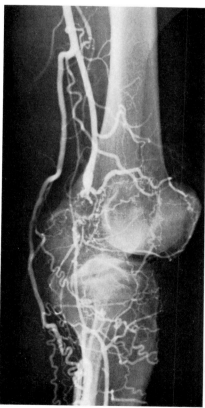

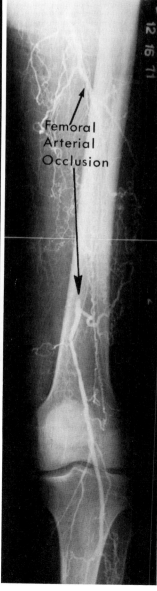

**Figure 17** *A,* Femoropopliteal occlusion. *B,* Femoral arteriogram showing the supreme genicular artery as the major bypassing collateral for a mid-popliteal artery obstruction. *B,* From Radke, H. M.: Strandness, D. E., Jr., ed.: Collateral Circulation in Clinical Surgery. Philadelphia, W. B. Saunders Company, 1969.)
*Illustration continued on opposite page.*

### CLINICAL MANIFESTATIONS

Femoral arterial occlusion presents in its *early* phases with symptoms of claudication. At this time there are few, if any, ischemic changes noted in the limbs. Pallor and absence of hair may be present distal to the arterial lesion, and pulses are absent. With the passage of time, trophic changes, including ulceration and ultimate gangrene, may occur. However, gangrenous changes are present in only a small number of patients with symptoms of claudication, particularly within the first several years of the onset of symptoms.

*Arteriography* is diagnostic and essential to establish the site and magnitude of the obstruction, as well as to demonstrate the patency of the arterial system distally. The latter determines the operability of the lesion (Figure 17*B*).[16]

### TREATMENT

Management of patients with femoral arterial occlusion is dependent upon the magnitude of symptoms. Those patients with minimal symptoms, or those in whom the claudication does not alter the pattern of daily life, are generally not candidates for surgical arterial procedures. However, the presence of severe claudication or of any symptoms that cause the patient to change his life style is generally an indication for revascularization. Originally, endarterectomy was performed, as advocated by Fontaine.[6] Currently, venous autografts (saphenous) are most commonly chosen. Earlier experiences with plastic arterial substitutes led to a relatively high incidence of subsequent occlusion[4] in comparison to the more favorable results with venous autografts. Long-term results with venous bypass grafts have been quite gratifying, with prolonged patency (Fig. 17*C*). Six months after operation in one series, 87 per cent of venous grafts into the femoral arterial system were patent. The cumulative patency rate was 80 per cent at 2 years, 73 per cent at 5 years, and 65 per cent at 7 to 10 years.[2]

Patients who are poor risks for venous bypass grafts may be candidates for axillofemoral grafts.

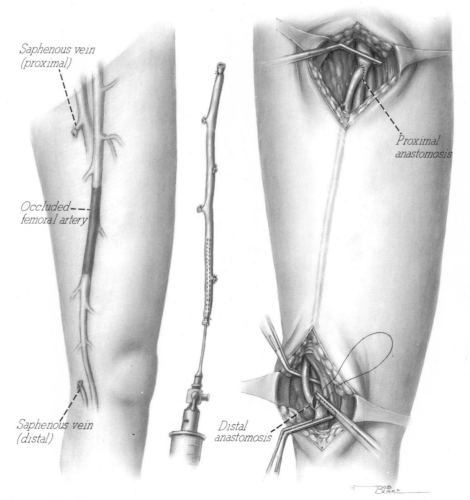

**Figure 17** *Continued.* C, Illustration of occlusion of superficial femoral artery with bypass by a venous autograft in a tunnel along the femoral canal. The vein graft is distended slightly by injection of saline as shown in the center.

In this procedure, performed under local anesthesia, the axillary artery is exposed and a subcutaneous tunnel is created to a point in the femoral system for the distal anastomosis. However, the long-term patency rate is considerably lower with these grafts.

A variety of vasodilators have been recommended in the nonsurgical management of patients with arteriosclerosis obliterans, but there is little objective evidence of their benefit. In a recent study with measurement of femoral blood flow by plethysmography and disappearance rates of radioisotopes, Coffman and Mannick concluded that these agents had little, if any, effect.[1]

Plastic grafts have been used, with relatively good results.[12] This technique is also useful in the treatment of infected grafts. At times, "crossover" vein grafts from the opposite femoral artery through a suprapubic tunnel have also been used. Occasionally, a very aggressive surgical approach for ischemic disease of the leg has been undertaken, with anastomoses to the vessels of the trifurcation of the popliteal artery—namely, the anterior tibial, posterior tibial, and peroneal arteries.[8] Such procedures should be carefully considered prior to their use. As a part of the complete management of patients with peripheral arterial insufficiency, complete cessation of smoking, avoidance of obesity, and regular exercise such as walking are all of importance.

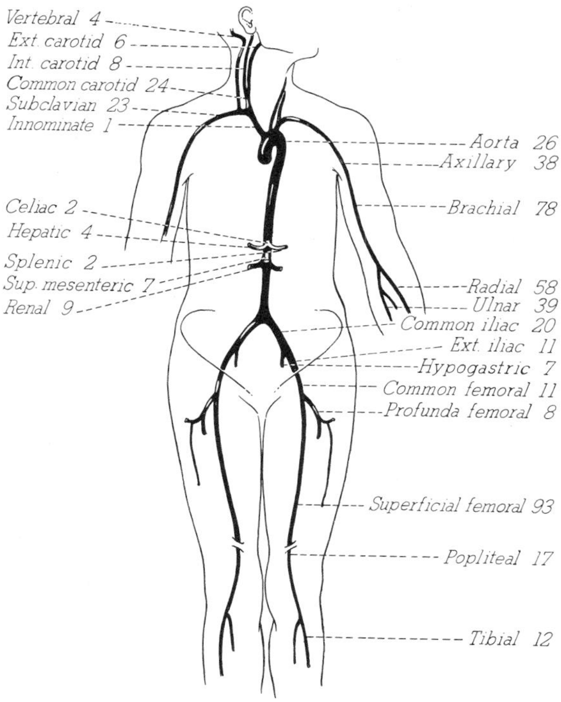

**Figure 18** Distribution of injuries. (From Perry, M. O., Thal, E. R., and Shires, G. T.: Ann. Surg., *173*: 403, 1971.)

## 7. ARTERIAL INJURIES

Arterial injuries are common lesions in both civilian and military life. Until the recent past, direct restoration of arterial continuity was uncommon, and many amputations were performed that would be considered needless today. Although Carrel provided the basis for direct arterial repair early in the century, it was infrequently employed until the 1950s. In World War II, only 81 cases of arterial suture were reported,[3] whereas in the Korean War, a much smaller conflict, many more cases were accumulated and direct repair became widely practiced.[9] One of the chief reasons for the increased emphasis on primary repair was the introduction of the venous *autograft.* Thus, direct suture of bypass grafts replaced ligation of arteries in the treatment of arterial injuries and thereby prevented amputation of extremities.

### PATHOLOGIC ASPECTS

The majority of military arterial injuries are the result of missile wounds; in civilian practice, both gunshot lacerations and stab wounds are quite common. With gunshot wounds, especially those caused by bullets of high velocity, it is important to recognize that, despite a normal appearance of tissue surrounding the injury, the energy released in the immediate vicinity of the missile so severely injures tissue that it may later become necrotic. Thus, debridement of such areas must be more extensive than that required for an incised wound. In civilian life, the most common sites of injury are the extremities. The sites of injury in 508 consecutive patients seen in a large municipal hospital are shown in Figure 18.[15] Of additional importance are the associated lesions that may occur in these injured patients. The incidence of associated injuries in one series is shown in Table 4.[5]

### CLINICAL MANIFESTATIONS

Arterial injuries, especially those which are severe, are frequently accompanied by associated lesions of considerable magnitude. Such patients

**TABLE 4**    INCIDENCE OF ASSOCIATED INJURIES*

| | | | |
|---|---|---|---|
| Veins | 47% | Lung | 4% |
| Nerves | 28% | Stomach | 3% |
| Tendons | 19% | Kidney | 3% |
| Bones | 11% | Diaphragm | 3% |
| Small intestine | 7% | Spleen | 2% |
| Colon | 6% | Duodenum | 1% |
| Liver | 5% | Pancreas | 1% |

*From Ferguson, I. A., Byrd, W. M., and McAfee, D. K.: Trans. Southern Surg. Ass., 72:372, 1960.

**TABLE 5**   CLINICAL SIGNS SUGGESTING ARTERIAL INJURY

1. Diminished or absent distal pulse
2. History of or persistent arterial bleeding
3. Large or expanding hematoma
4. Major hemorrhage with hypotension or shock
5. Bruit at or distal to suspected site of injury
6. Injury of anatomically related nerves
7. Anatomic proximity of wound to major artery

are often in *shock,* owing to either internal or external loss of blood. In addition to injuries of the abdominal organs, fractures and nerve injuries are common and should be carefully sought and identified. *Hematomas* are common at the site of injury, and direct communications of the artery with an accompanying vein may occur. In arterial injuries of the limbs, ischemia characteristically develops distal to the injury. The symptoms and signs associated with such injuries include pallor, coolness, paresthesias, and ultimate anesthesia. Arterial pulses are generally absent distal to the lesion. Of all the signs and symptoms, *loss of sensation* is the most significant, since it is usually associated with severe ischemia, which will progress to gangrene unless the arterial circulation is improved. A listing of the critical signs that suggest arterial injury is shown in Table 5.

## MANAGEMENT

Control of the hemorrhage is the immediate aim of management. Usually this can be accomplished effectively by pressure alone and rarely requires the use of a tourniquet. Tourniquets have probably produced more injuries than they have prevented, and if employed should be carefully padded and released at intervals in order to prevent nerve and soft tissue injury. Following control of the hemorrhage, an evaluation should be made concerning the amount of blood lost either into the tissues or externally, and this should be replaced with blood or appropriate plasma expanders. Because of possible contamination, antibiotics should be administered from the outset, and prophylactic therapy for tetanus (toxoid and human antiserum) should be given when indicated.

As soon as the patient's general condition permits, it is essential that arterial continuity be restored. Experience has shown that approximately 6 to 8 hours is the maximal amount of time an extremity can withstand severe ischemia with ultimate recovery. Arteriography is often helpful in establishing the site and extent of the injury. It is particularly useful in patients with fractures and other associated injuries in whom the site of obstruction may not be well localized by the clinical manifestations.

## SURGICAL MANAGEMENT

The primary aim of surgical management is direct restoration of arterial continuity. This is most often accomplished by direct arterial suture with approximation of the two ends of the injured artery. Most frequently, an end-to-end anastomosis is indicated. Experience has shown that after excision of 2 to 3 cm. of artery, with sufficient proximal and distal mobilization, the vessel can usually be re-established safely. With missile injuries, it is important to debride the defect in order to excise tissue injured by the missile. In those instances in which considerable amounts of the artery have been avulsed, a venous autograft should be employed. The anastomoses are performed with fine plastic sutures (6-0 or 7-0). An everting anastomosis is preferable, either with triangulation of the vessel or with stay sutures at both ends.

Venous injuries are common in association with arterial lesions. *Lateral* venous injuries can be closed directly. Autogenous venous grafts have been recommended for avulsed areas of vein, although in most instances it is preferable to ligate the vein unless it is a large one. The advocates of venous grafts for these injuries believe that although the grafts may ultimately become occluded, they provide time for collateral circulation to develop.[17]

## ANTERIOR COMPARTMENT SYNDROME

An additional entity that may be associated with trauma is the "anterior compartment syndrome." This syndrome is produced by conditions that result in an increase in both fluid and pressure in the closed anterior tibial compartment. It may follow trauma or arterial occlusion by thrombi or emboli, and is known to occur occasionally after femoral cannulation for extracorporeal circulation. The clinical manifestations include pain, an increase in the circumference of the leg, and ultimate paralysis of the anterior tibial and extensor hallucis longus muscles. If it is unrelieved, the contents of the anterior tibial compartment become ischemic and gangrenous. The treatment consists of a fasciotomy over the anterior tibial muscles, permitting decompression. Depending upon the amount of swelling, the skin incision may be closed loosely or, preferably, reapproximated at delayed closure after the edema has subsided.

With the increasing utilization of diagnostic arterial procedures such as cardiac catheterization and arteriography, the incidence of these iatrogenic injuries has increased, and they may require direct arterial surgery or thrombectomy.

The results following direct restoration of arterial continuity have been quite good both in military experience and in civilian practice.[19] The amputation rate has been sharply reduced, being less than 5 per cent in most reported series.

## SELECTED REFERENCES

Darling, R. C., Linton, R. R., and Razzuk, M. A.: Saphenous vein bypass grafts for femoropopliteal occlusive disease: A reappraisal. Surgery, *61*:31, 1967.

*This is an excellent report of 295 consecutive saphenous vein grafts in 240 patients studied at the Massachusetts General Hospital and followed for periods up to 10 years. The follow-up data are well presented, with appropriate evaluations.*

DeWeese, J. A., and Rob, C. G.: Autogenous venous bypass grafts five years later. Ann. Surg., 174:346, 1971.
*This is an important study concerning the patency of venous autografts of different lengths implanted in the legs. The data indicate that short grafts have the best patency rates. An additional point emphasized concerns the cumulative mortality in these patients with the passage of time, with 48 per cent dead at the end of 5 years. Of the deaths, 71 per cent were the result of some form of atherosclerosis.*

Leriche, R., and Morel, A.: The syndrome of thrombotic obliteration of the aortic bifurcation. Ann. Surg., 127:193, 1948.
*This is the initial report of the Leriche syndrome in English. The first cases are described in detail by the authors. Leriche emphasizes the characteristic symptoms and pathophysiology of the condition as well as the fact that it may attack relatively young males.*

## REFERENCES

1. Coffman, J. D., and Mannick, J. A.: Failure of vasodilator drugs in arteriosclerosis obliterans. Ann. Intern. Med., 76:35, 1972.
2. Darling, R. C., Linton, R. R., and Razzuk, M. A.: Saphenous vein bypass grafts for femoropopliteal occlusive disease: A reappraisal. Surgery, 61:31, 1967.
3. DeBakey, M. E., and Simeone, F. A.: Battle injuries of the arteries in World War II. An analysis of 2,471 cases. Ann. Surg., 123:534, 1946.
4. Edwards, W. S., Holdefer, W. F., and Mohtashemi, M.: The importance of proper caliber of lumen in femoral-popliteal artery reconstruction. Surg. Gynec. Obstet., 122:37, 1966.
5. Ferguson, I. A., Byrd, W. M., and McAfee, D. K.: Experiences in the management of arterial injuries. Trans. Southern Surg. Ass., 72:372, 1960.
6. Fontaine, R., Buck, P., Riveux, R., Kim, M., and Hubinot, J.: Treatment of arterial occlusion: Comparative value of thrombectomy, thromboendarterectomy, arterial venous shunt and vascular grafts (fresh venous autografts). Lyon Chir., 46:73, 1951.
7. Friedenberg, M. J., and Perez, C. A.: Collateral circulation in aorto-ilio-femoral occlusive disease: As demonstrated by a unilateral percutaneous common femoral artery needle injection. Amer. J. Roentgen., 94:145, 1965.
8. Garrett, H. E., Kotch, P. I., Green, M. T., Jr., Diethrich, E. B., and DeBakey, M. E.: Distal tibial artery bypass with autogenous vein grafts: An analysis of 56 cases. Surgery, 63:90, 1968.
9. Hughes, C. W.: Arterial repair during the Korean War. Ann. Surg., 147:555, 1958.
10. Leriche, R.: De la résection du carrefour aortico-iliaque avec double sympathectomie lombaire pour thrombose artéritique de l'aorte. Le syndrome de l'oblitération termino-aortique par artérite. Presse Med., 48:601, 1940.
11. Leriche, R., and Morel, A.: The syndrome of thrombotic obliteration of the aortic bifurcation. Ann. Surg., 127:193, 1948.
12. Mannick, J. A., Williams, L. E., and Nabseth, D. C.: The late results of axillofemoral grafts. Surgery, 68:1038, 1970.
13. May, A. G., DeWeese, J. A., and Rob, C. G.: Changes in sexual function following operation on the abdominal aorta. Surgery, 65:41, 1969.
14. Perdue, G. D., Long, W. D., and Smith, R. B., III: Perspective concerning aorto-femoral arterial reconstruction. Trans. Southern Surg. Ass., 82:330, 1970.
15. Perry, M. O., Thal, E. R., and Shires, G. T.: Management of arterial injuries. Ann. Surg., 173:403, 1971.
16. Radke, H. M.: Arterial circulation of the lower extremity. In: Strandness, D. E., Jr., ed.: Collateral Circulation in Clinical Surgery. Philadelphia, W. B. Saunders Company, 1969.
17. Rich, N. M., Hughes, C. W., and Baugh, J. H.: Management of venous injuries. Ann. Surg., 171:724, 1970.
18. Strandness, D. E., Jr.: Chronic arterial occlusion. In: Strandness, D. E., Jr., ed.: Collateral Circulation in Clinical Surgery. Philadelphia, W. B. Saunders Company, 1969.
19. White, J. J., Talbert, J. L., and Haller, J. A.: Peripheral arterial injuries in infants and children. Ann. Surg., 167:757, 1968.

# 8. ACUTE ARTERIAL OCCLUSION

## *Thomas J. Fogarty, M.D.*

Reference to occlusion of the arterial circulation was first made by Harvey in 1628.[7] Labey[8] in 1911 has been credited with the first successful surgical removal of an arterial embolus. Review of the surgical literature indicates that the operative approach to acute arterial occlusion was limited by the inability of the surgeon to remove simply and effectively the embolus and distally propagated thrombus. The introduction of the balloon catheter technique[5] in 1963 simplified the technical aspects of surgery for acute arterial occlusion. Advances in the field of open heart surgery have eliminated some of the sources of arterial emboli, and further reduced mortality by making possible correction of the cardiac disorder.

## PATHOLOGY

Regardless of the source or histologic structure of an embolus, it is the location and secondary events following the impaction that determine the viability of an extremity. Following occlusion, a softer coagulum of blood forms in areas of decreased flow. Linton[10] has emphasized that this propagation of thrombus distal to the embolus is of major importance in the outcome of the disease process. Failure to recognize and to remove atraumatically the distally propagated thrombus may result in less than complete restoration of circulation and possibly in amputation. Surgeons have uniformly relied upon the presence or absence of backbleeding from the peripheral arterial bed as a guide to distal patency. Repeated clinical observations have confirmed that backbleeding is an unreliable guide to distal patency. Discontinuous thrombotic material is present in approximately one-third of the cases (Fig. 19). Under these circumstances, backbleeding may be quite forceful, despite the presence of additional distal thrombotic material. The presence of adequate collateral vessels will result in significant bleeding from the distal segment despite the fact that the more peripheral arterial bed may be totally occluded. Failure to recognize this circumstance will result in less than complete restoration of the circulation.

Arterial emboli most commonly occur in the elderly, seriously ill patient with multiple systemic diseases. Prolonged periods of surgical manipulation and general anesthesia have been considered valid deterrents to operative intervention in such patients. This has been particu-

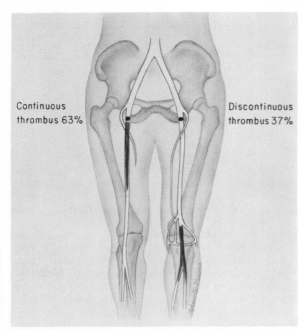

Continuous thrombus 63%

Discontinuous thrombus 37%

**Figure 19**   Anatomic location of distal thrombus as it relates to location of embolus.

larly true when the clinical findings indicated that conservative measures might preserve life at the cost of limb loss or impairment of function. The balloon catheter technique is an operative procedure designed to avoid general anesthesia, reduce surgical trauma, and effectively remove all thrombotic material in a simple manner, regardless of its anatomic location.

## PREOPERATIVE EVALUATION AND CARE

Patients presenting with an acute embolic occlusion should be assumed to have significant underlying heart disease. Table 6 shows the sources of arterial emboli in a series of 300 patients. The large number of patients presenting with arteriosclerotic heart disease reinforces the concept that the heart represents the site of underlying basic pathologic change.

Evaluation of cardiac function should proceed simultaneously with the examination of the peripheral vasculature. Digitalis, antiarrhythmic

**TABLE 6**   SOURCE OF ARTERIAL EMBOLUS IN 300 CONSECUTIVE PATIENTS

| | |
|---|---:|
| 1. Atrial fibrillation | 231 |
|    A.S.H.D.* | 183 |
|    R.H.D.† | 48 |
| 2. Acute myocardial infarction | 50 |
| 3. Arteriosclerotic plaque | 7 |
| 4. Unknown | 12 |

*A.S.H.D. = arteriosclerotic heart disease.
†R.H.D. = rheumatic heart disease.

agents, morphine, diuretics, and heparin are drugs basic to patient care. Utilization of these agents when indicated should not delay surgical intervention.

Appropriate therapy is initiated while emergency preparation for operation is being made. The presence of congestive heart failure, cardiogenic shock, and significant arrhythmias requires intensive care unit monitoring. A Silastic Medicath unit* is placed in the superior vena cava or right atrium through an appropriate vein. In addition to allowing for the rapid administration of drugs and fluids, this permits monitoring of central venous pressures. Central placement of catheters represents a convenient means for the intravenous administration of heparin. Cannulation of the internal jugular vein as advocated by Daily[2] is simple, and has been free of significant complications in our hands.

In the presence of an embolus to a lower extremity, the possibility of simultaneous emboli to mesenteric or renal arteries should always be entertained. Hematuria or abdominal complaints indicative of a possible occlusion require preoperative visualization of these vessels. Involvement of more than one extremity occurs in approximately 10 per cent of the patients and this fact should not be overlooked. Once the diagnosis of an acute arterial occlusion has been made, heparin should be given immediately and preparation for operation initiated.

## INSTRUMENTATION

A balloon catheter has been developed with specific adaptations in its construction for safe, effective extraction of arterial emboli. It consists of a hollow, pliable body in graduated sizes for use in major vessels of any caliber (Fig. 20). At its proximal portion the syringe fitting provides the means for fluid exchange into a soft, distensible balloon placed at the distal tip of the instrument. The catheter is inserted into the acutely occluded vessel as far as possible. The balloon is inflated and withdrawn in the inflated position. By a mechanism of fluid displacement, the balloon maintains uniform, even contact with the vessel wall as it proceeds through areas of narrowing. This mechanism allows for removal of thrombotic material distal to stenotic areas. One surgeon manipulates both the syringe and the catheter during withdrawal. In this way it is easy to judge the amount of traction required for extraction of the occluding material as well as the quantity of fluid necessary to effect alternate inflation and deflation as the instrument proceeds through areas of arteriosclerotic narrowing or vessels of increasing or decreasing diameter.

The concept of a balloon catheter has remained basically the same since its initial introduction. There have been minor changes in the instrument itself directed at increasing its effectiveness and

*Chesebrough-Pond's, Inc., Hospital Products Division, 485 Lexington Avenue, New York, New York 10017.

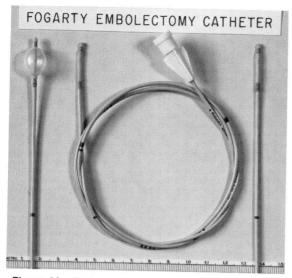

FOGARTY EMBOLECTOMY CATHETER

**Figure 20**   Catheter for extraction of arterial emboli.

reducing the incidence of complications. A variety of balloon configurations and catheter materials have been evaluated. Although the utilization of double-lumen catheters and spiked balloon catheters appears attractive, significant disadvantages have been associated with their use. The utility and effectiveness of the instrument are related to its simplicity. Attempts to incorporate nonessential refinements have thus far not proved advantageous or practical.

Complications secondary to the use of the balloon catheters have been those common to all catheter techniques, and have included cases of plaque dissection, catheter tip separation, and vessel perforation. Vessel rupture can occur if the balloon portion of the instrument is overdistended in small vessels. Experience and a realization of the limitations of the instrument are the most significant factors in reducing the incidence of complications.

## OPERATIVE PROCEDURE

The experience with acute peripheral arterial embolization has clearly indicated that successful management of these patients is related to well defined factors. From a technical standpoint, it must be recognized that there are varying degrees of difficulty encountered in the attempt to reestablish the peripheral circulation. Patients presenting with advanced ischemia with extensive distal propagation of the thrombus and patients presenting with significant chronic occlusive disease present the most difficult technical problems. A careful history and physical examination allow one to identify these situations.

### Operative Preparation

The procedure is initiated with local anesthesia. An anesthetist should be in attendance to monitor

vital signs and administer a general anesthetic if it becomes necessary. The extremity should be surgically prepared from the toes to the nipple line. A bilateral inguinal approach is utilized for aortic emboli and both extremities are prepared. An iliac embolus requires bilateral preparation. The possibility of dislodging a high iliac embolus with occlusion of the opposite extremity exists. This has not occurred in the author's experience, but the possibility is always anticipated by preparation of the opposite extremity so that the pulses may be externally palpated at the time of surgery.

An x-ray cassette should be placed under the extremities. Adequate quantities of blood should be available.

### Technique

The approach to embolic occlusion regardless of the anatomic location has been through a femoral incision (Fig. 21). The common femoral artery, superficial femoral artery, and deep femoral artery are isolated and encircled with Silastic occluding pads* (Fig. 21 inset). The arterial incision is made in relation to the orifice of the superficial femoral artery and deep femoral artery. A distal exploration is carried out initially and catheters should be routinely placed in the superficial and deep femoral arteries. An open deep femoral circulation is capable of providing the margin necessary to maintain viability in many patients with advanced ischemia or in patients who had prior chronic occlusion of the superficial femoral system. Recovery of embolic material from the deep femoral artery, even in the presence of a patent common femoral artery, has been frequent in our experience. The 2F and 3F catheters are most commonly employed for exploration of the deep femoral system, while 3F and 4F catheters have been found suitable for exploration of the femoral-popliteal systems.

If there is uncertainty about adequate distal clot removal, operative arteriograms should be obtained. The presence of additional distal thrombotic material is an indication for a second incision in the medial aspect of the leg exposing the distal popliteal artery and the popliteal trifurcation (Fig. 22). Occluding Silastic pads should be placed about the distal popliteal, the anterior tibial and the posterior tibial arteries (Fig. 22). The 2F or 3F catheter should be introduced selectively into each one of these vessels through a transverse arteriotomy. If these vessels were previously patent and uninvolved in an arteriosclerotic process, a 2F catheter should pass beyond the ankle joint. The course of the catheter can be felt by placing the hand on the distribution of the anterior and posterior tibial arteries (Fig. 22). If the progress of the catheter is impeded at the ankle joint, extension of the foot frequently permits further passage. Inability to pass the 2F catheter beyond the ankle along with the presence of angiographic evidence of obstruction beyond this point requires

---

*Medidyne Industries, 525 Commercial Avenue, Sun Prairie, Wisconsin 53590.

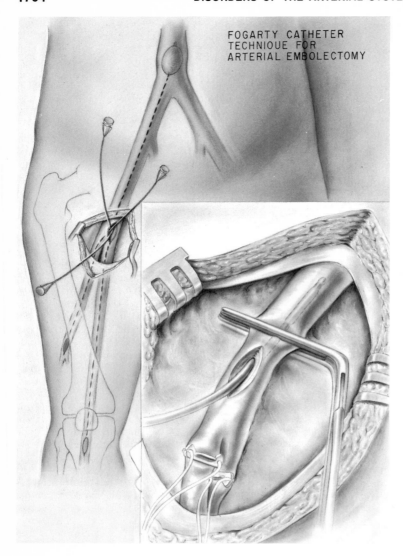

FOGARTY CATHETER
TECHNIQUE FOR
ARTERIAL EMBOLECTOMY

**Figure 21**    Inguinal incisions utilized for extraction of arterial embolus.

direct exposure of the anterior and posterior tibial arteries at the ankle. By direct manipulation of the vessel combined with gentle simultaneous probing of the catheter from the proximal end, it is possible to pass the catheter beyond the point of obstruction without the necessity of an arteriotomy. If an arteriotomy at the ankle level in either of these vessels is required, a vessel opening is made just large enough to allow for introduction of the 2F catheter. The catheter is then threaded distally, inflated, and withdrawn in the inflated condition. This maneuver frequently brings thrombotic material above the small arteriotomy. Additional attempts to extract thrombotic material should be made by the introduction of the 2F catheter into the anterior or posterior tibial vessel at the level of the popliteal arteriotomy. This maneuver avoids the necessity of enlarging the arteriotomy at the ankle level, and decreases the possibility of reocclusion. Following removal of the thrombotic

material, copious irrigation of the distal arterial system should be carried out with a heparinized solution.

In the presence of advanced ischemia, the simultaneous presence of major venous occlusion demands consideration. In a personal series of 300 patients, 8 per cent were found to have concomitant major venous occlusion.[6] The majority of the patients in this group had advanced ischemia with extensive distal propagation of clot on the arterial side. In this situation the vein is explored before the arterial circulation is re-established, and large venous thrombi are removed by means of venous thrombectomy catheters.[4] Prior to suture closure of the vein, the arterial circulation is re-established. After removal of the arterial occlusions, the distal arterial system is irrigated with 200 to 300 cc. of a heparinized solution. The distal venous clamp is removed to allow smaller thrombi to be flushed out during this irrigation. The artery is

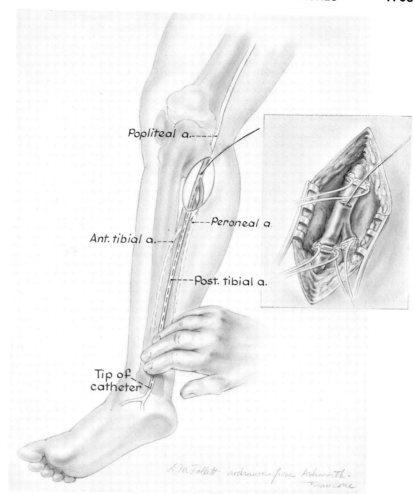

**Figure 22**  Exposure of popliteal trifurcation.

closed first. The vein is flushed once again after re-establishment of the arterial circulation. The venotomy is closed last.

There has been reference in the literature to delaying surgical intervention in patients who present with advanced ischemia.[1] We have not employed this delayed approach, and feel that advanced ischemia secondary to acute embolic occlusion represents a surgical emergency. In these patients heparin is employed at the time of surgery and in the immediate postoperative period.

In those situations in which it is recognized that heparin should be employed in the immediate postoperative period, it has been our policy to anticipate the possible complications of hemorrhage and hematoma at incisional sites and to employ vacuum-type drainage.

Swelling of a revascularized, ischemic extremity can assume considerable proportions and requires treatment. Massive swelling that may embarrass arterial inflow is observed most frequently in those patients who present with advanced ischemia prior to surgical intervention. Capillary damage resulting in fluid exudation into ischemic tissues

is a factor in this swelling. Obstruction of the venous outflow tract aggravates the problem. Failure to control immediately this edema may result in reocclusion of the arterial inflow. Fasciotomy has been required in 10 per cent of the patients who present with acute embolic occlusion. Initial decompression is carried out through small skin incisions as described by Rosato.[12] If immediate improvement is not obtained by this limited fasciotomy, the skin incisions should be extended and the deeper fascial compartments widely opened. Radical decompression requiring fibular resection is rarely necessary in patients who have an acute embolic occlusion. Patman and Thompson[11] have given an excellent review of the technique and indications for fasciotomy.

Immediately following restoration of arterial continuity in extremities with advanced ischemia, significant alterations in electrolytes and acid balance may occur.[3] The venous efflux of ischemic extremities following restoration of arterial continuity was studied in 10 patients (Table 7). These data clearly indicated that, following successful restoration of the circulation, there was a sudden return of very acidotic blood with a high potassium

**TABLE 7** MEAN VALUES OF BIOCHEMICAL DETERMINATIONS ON VENOUS EFFLUX OF ISCHEMIC EXTREMITY BEFORE AND AFTER RESTORATION OF FLOW

| Ten Patients | pH | pO$_2$ | pCO$_2$ | K | CPK |
|---|---|---|---|---|---|
| System venous blood before embolectomy | 7.38 | 38.2 | 36.4 | 4.3 | 77 |
| Venous blood from ischemic leg before embolectomy | 7.31 | 19.3 | 45.8 | 4.7 | 200 |
| Venous blood from ischemic leg 5 minutes after restoration of flow | 6.80 | 34.8 | 77.3 | 7.2 | 653.4 |

content to the heart. This metabolic effect in conjunction with pooling of blood in the revascularized extremity can result in significant hypotension. In 8 of the 10 patients studied, adverse effects were associated with clamp release, in the form of significant electrocardiographic changes or hypotension or both. The necessity of using buffering agents and antiarrhythmic agents should be anticipated at the time of clamp release. Electrolytes should be closely followed in the postoperative period. A high creatine phosphokinase level noted in the venous efflux indicates significant muscle damage.

### EMBOLIC OCCLUSION IN THE PRESENCE OF SIGNIFICANT CHRONIC OCCLUSIVE DISEASE

A careful history and examination of the uninvolved extremity affords a reliable assessment of the peripheral circulation prior to the acute episode. The patient's general condition, his prior level of activity, and the extent of the pathologic change encountered at the time of operation all play an important role in determining the extent of the surgical procedure. In general, it is advisable only to attempt initially to return the circulation to its acute preocclusive state. Definitive reconstructive procedures are delayed until a more critical evaluation of the patient is possible. Major reconstructive procedures may be indicated, however, if the general condition of the patient is good when he is initially seen. Definitive procedures may be carried out, particularly if one is concerned about the viability of the extremity and the patient was active prior to the acute occlusion. Elderly patients in poor general condition are poor candidates for major reconstructive procedures.

**TABLE 8** RECONSTRUCTIVE PROCEDURES PERFORMED AT THE TIME OF ARTERIAL EMBOLECTOMY

| | |
|---|---|
| 1. Common and deep femoral endarterectomy | 14 |
| 2. Femoral-femoral crossover graft | 7 |
| 3. Iliac endarterectomy | 3 |
| 4. Aortofemoral endarterectomy | 3 |
| 5. Aortofemoral graft | 2 |

Local angioplasty of the deep femoral system in these situations is simple and quick and can be done under local anesthesia. Frequently it will provide the margin necessary to maintain viability. Table 8 lists the number of reconstructive procedures carried out in conjunction with arterial embolectomy in a series of 300 patients.[6] Localized endarterectomy and femoral-femoral jump grafts are simple and can be done under local anesthesia. In 15 cases the procedure was performed at the time of initial exploration, and in 14 it was performed as a second procedure carried out during the initial hospital stay. In a total of 21 cases sympathectomy was performed; in 12 it was done in conjunction with a reconstructive procedure.

### UPPER EXTREMITY EMBOLI

The management of emboli to the upper extremity is identical to that described for the lower extremity. Proximal subclavian artery emboli can be simply removed under local anesthesia by retrograde extraction. It should be borne in mind, however, that if the embolus appears to reside close to the origin of the cranial vessels, fragmentation of the embolus may occur during withdrawal, resulting in central nervous system ischemia. Thus far, this has not occurred in our experience but the possibility should be anticipated. If there is serious doubt as to the exact location of the embolus as it relates to the orifices of the carotid and vertebral vessels, preoperative x-ray visualization should be performed.

### RENAL, MESENTERIC, AND CAROTID ARTERY EMBOLI

The principles of management of emboli to these areas are similar to those described for management of peripheral arterial emboli. It should be borne in mind, however, that the external support provided by adjacent tissue is significantly less with vessels supplying the viscera and brain than with the vessels of peripheral vasculature. Considerable care should be taken in introducing the catheter into these vessels. The 2F and 3F catheters are of appropriate size for distal exploration of these vessels, and the catheters are provided with a very flexible tip which significantly diminishes the possibility of perforation of the vessel. Only gentle inflation and traction should be used in removing emboli located in these areas.

Unless emboli to the internal carotid system are seen within the first few hours of onset, surgical intervention should not be considered. Hemorrhagic infarction represents a frequent and often fatal complication when attempts are made to remove emboli to the cerebral circulation, and when they are undertaken after a considerable lapse of time.

## POSTOPERATIVE CARE AND MANAGEMENT

The indications for heparin in the postoperative period should be individualized for each patient. The possible presence of simultaneous venous thromboses and embolization following acute myocardial infarction represent indications for heparinization in the postoperative period.

The specific aspects of postoperative care will relate obviously to the underlying pathologic condition responsible for the embolus, the presence or absence of significant cardiac impairment, and the presence or absence of associated diseases. One's concern with the status of the peripheral vasculature should not impair the management or care of these other critical disorders. Peripheral embolization following myocardial infarction should immediately direct one's attention to the underlying cardiac lesion. Left heart catheterization and coronary artery visualization may be indicated in order to define whether or not a correctible cardiac lesion is present. The presence of significant valvular heart disease obviously deserves diagnostic investigation and surgical correction.

## MORBIDITY AND MORTALITY

The aim of surgical intervention for arterial emboli is to restore the peripheral circulation to its preocclusive state. Evaluation of results is based upon restoration of pulses, relief of symptoms, and return of normal color and temperature. It is sometimes difficult to evaluate results in those patients in whom the condition of the extremity prior to the acute occlusion was unknown. Conditions such as mental confusion, concurrent illness, or death obviously preclude evaluation by exercise tolerance. Evaluation of therapy is best determined by mortality and the amputation rates. The possibility of maintaining a viable, functional extremity following acute arterial occlusion should exceed 90 per cent. The possibility of a successful procedure will obviously relate to the presence or absence of advanced ischemia. The condition of the extremity and not the duration of occlusion represents the primary determinant of operability. Reference to Table 9 indicates that even after prolonged periods of occlusion, successful surgical intervention is possible. Even in the presence of established gangrene, a lower

### TABLE 10  MORBIDITY AND MORTALITY
### 300 PATIENTS, 330 EMBOLECTOMIES

| | |
|---|---|
| Limb salvage | 95% |
| Patient survival | 84% |
| | |
| Cause of death: | |
| Myocardial infarction | 20 |
| Congestive heart failure | 16 |
| Pulmonary embolus | 5 |
| Massive CVA | 4 |
| Renal failure | 2 |

level of amputation can often be achieved following successful embolectomy.

Failure of the initial exploration after an apparent success represents an indication for re-exploration. The most common cause for failure relates to technical factors which on occasion can be corrected if recognized. The possibility, however, of re-embolization to the same extremity should not be overlooked. Its documented occurrence should reinforce a second-look attitude.[6]

A constant physical finding that should be cause for considerable concern after an apparently successful embolectomy is the presence of a water-hammer-type pulse. An apparently stronger than normal pulse has in our experience been associated with a high incidence of reocclusion. Under these circumstances, obstruction is present at the small artery and arteriolar level. Re-exploration should include copious distal irrigation in conjunction with venous exploration.

The mortality associated with acute arterial occlusion has in our experience been unrelated to surgical intervention. Table 10 lists the causes of death in a series of 300 consecutive patients with acute arterial occlusion. All deaths were related to cardiovascular dysfunction. Seventy-seven per cent of the patients died as a direct result of a cardiac cause. It would appear from this study and from the reviews by Levy[9] and Thompson[13] that the mortality associated with arterial embolism relates to the underlying cardiac disorder. These findings reinforce the contention that the recognition and correction of the cause for embolism should represent a very important aspect of the care of these patients. It is only through aggressive treatment of the underlying cardiac lesion that the mortality figures can be improved. With the increasing success of coronary artery surgery, patients in whom emboli develop

### TABLE 9  TIME INTERVAL IN RELATION TO ADVANCED ISCHEMIA

| Age of Embolus | Number of Emboli | Advanced Ischemia* | Amputations |
|---|---|---|---|
| 1-24 hours | 193 | 24 | 3 |
| 24-48 hours | 57 | 21 | 3 |
| 2-90 days | 80 | 39 | 10 |

*Advanced ischemia = early rigor or gangrene.

### TABLE 11  ASSOCIATED CARDIAC PROCEDURES

| | |
|---|---|
| Replacement of S-E ball valve: | |
| Aortic | 2 |
| Mitral | 3 |
| Replacement of mitral valve: | |
| Ruptured papillary | 4 |
| Rheumatic | 12 |
| Resection of ventricular aneurysm | 5 |
| Repair of infarct VSD | 1 |

after myocardial infarction deserve consideration for coronary visualization. The timing of such studies should relate to the general condition of the patient. Revascularization or aneurysmectomy, if indicated, should be done as soon as possible. Table 11 lists the number and kind of associated cardiac procedures carried out in a group of 300 patients who had peripheral arterial emboli. One-half of these procedures represented emergency situations and were carried out at the time of arterial embolectomy. The remaining one-half were semiurgent and all were carried out within 1 month from the time of acute occlusion.

## CONCLUSION

Recognition and appropriate surgical management of the more difficult technical problems associated with acute arterial occlusion result in a decreased morbidity. The mortality associated with embolic episodes is due primarily to severe underlying heart disease. Further reduction in the mortality is made possible by an aggressive surgical and medical approach to the underlying cardiac disorder.

## SELECTED REFERENCES

Fogarty, T. J., Daily, P. O., Shumway, N. E., and Krippaehne, W.: Experience with balloon catheter technic for arterial embolectomy. Amer. J. Surg., *122*:231, 1971.
*The authors report on a series of 330 embolic occlusions occurring in 300 patients. The paper emphasizes the necessity of identifying high-risk areas in terms of morbidity and mortality. An aggressive overall approach to the medical and surgical problems is presented.*

Patman, R. D., and Thompson, J. E.: Fasciotomy in peripheral vascular surgery. Arch. Surg., *101*:663, 1970.
*The authors review their personal experience with 164 patients who required fasciotomy. The indications for fasciotomy and the technique employed are presented. Fasciotomy, performed correctly and with proper indications, is a valuable procedure that can result in an increased limb salvage and a decrease in morbidity. The paper is well written and a variety of clinical situations that may require fasciotomy are detailed.*

## REFERENCES

1. Blaisdell, F. W.: Discussion of: Levy, J. F., and Butcher, H. R.: Arterial emboli: an analysis of 125 patients. Surgery, *68*:973, 1970.
2. Daily, P. O., Griepp, R. B., and Shumway, N. E.: Percutaneous internal jugular vein cannulation. Arch. Surg., *101*: 534, 1970.
3. Fisher, R. D., Fogarty, T. J., and Morrow, A. G.: Clinical and biochemical observations of the effect of transient femoral artery occlusion in man. Surgery, *68*:323, 1970.
4. Fogarty, T. J.: Surgical management of acute vascular occlusion. In: Cooper, P., and Nyhus, L. M., eds.: Surgery Annual. New York, Appleton-Century-Crofts, 1970, pp. 207–221.
5. Fogarty, T. J., Cranley, J. J., Krause, R. J., et al.: A method for extraction of arterial emboli and thrombi. Surg. Gynec. Obstet., *116*:241, 1963.
6. Fogarty, T. J., Daily, P. O., Shumway, N. E., and Krippaehne, W.: Experience with balloon catheter technic for arterial embolectomy. Amer. J. Surg., *122*:231, 1971.
7. Harvey, W.: Exercitatio anatomica de motu cordis et sanguinis in animalibus (An English translation by Chauncey D. Leake). Springfield, Ill., Charles C Thomas, 1931, Chapter 30, p. 37.
8. Labey: Cited by Mosney, M., and Dumont, N. J.: Embolie fémorale au cours d'un rétrécissement mitral pur. Artériotomie. Guérison Bull. Acad. med., *66*:358, 1911.
9. Levy, J. F., Butcher, H. R.: Arterial emboli: an analysis of 125 patients. Surgery, *68*:968, 1970.
10. Linton, R. R.: Peripheral arterial embolism. A discussion of the postembolic vascular changes and their relation to the restoration of circulation in peripheral embolism. New Eng. J. Med., *224*:189, 1941.
11. Patman, R. D., and Thompson, J. E.: Fasciotomy in peripheral vascular surgery. Arch. Surg., *101*:663, 1970.
12. Rosato, F. E., Barker, C. F., Robert, B., and Danielson, G. K.: Subcutaneous fasciotomy. Description of a new technique and instrument. Surgery, *59*:3, 1966.
13. Thompson, J. E., Sigler, L., Raut, P. S., et al.: Arterial embolectomy: a 20-year experience with 163 cases. Surgery, *67*:212, 1970.

## 9. ARTERIOVENOUS FISTULA

*David C. Sabiston, Jr., M.D.*

There are few disorders in clinical medicine that can produce as many pathophysiologic changes as an arteriovenous fistula. This is especially true of large communications between an artery and vein that allow enormous amounts of arterial blood to pass through the fistula into the low-resistance venous bed. Many physiologic changes result from such a fistula in an attempt to compensate for the large and continuous shunt of blood from the arterial circuit.

In 1758, William Hunter recognized for the first time that an arteriovenous aneurysm was characterized by a direct communication between the artery and vein.[6] Until then, these lesions had been interpreted as simple aneurysms. Hunter designated the lesion an "aneurysm by anastomosis," with emphasis upon communication of the two vascular systems. Early surgical attempts to correct these lesions consisted primarily of *ligation* of the involved artery proximal to the fistula. Such a procedure was quite apt to be followed by gangrene of the extremity, since the blood reaching the distal extremity by arterial collaterals drained in a retrograde direction through the fistula into the venous system, thus depriving the limb of any significant arterial flow.[4] By 1886, it was emphatically recommended that the hunterian principle of ligation of the artery *proximal* to the fistula be condemned and that, instead, quadruple ligation of the artery and vein be the procedure of choice.[2] In 1875, Nicoladoni described a patient with an arteriovenous fistula in whom compression of the fistula (with cessation of flow through it) caused a decrease in the pulse rate from 96 to 64 per minute.[10] This phenomenon was described by Branham in 1890 as a "mysterious" slowing of the pulse with obliteration of an acquired femoral arteriovenous fistula.[3] Rudolph Matas called this the "Branham bradycardiac reaction," and it has since borne that name.[5]

Arteriovenous fistulas may be either *congenital* or *acquired*. Congenital fistulas in nearly every organ of the body have been described, but they are most prevalent in the extremities, where more than half of all fistulas have been reported.[15] Other common locations include the brain, lungs, neck, and kidney. Most congenital arteriovenous fistulas are accompanied by large varicose veins in and around the site of the fistula. In fact, the presence of varicose veins at unusual sites, and especially early in life, should lead one to suspect a congenital arteriovenous fistula. A pulsating mass, a continuous murmur, and signs of stasis including edema and phlebitis of the extremities are all common. Cyanosis or erythema of the skin and cutaneous hemangiomas are commonly observed. Generally, surgical excision of these lesions is indicated, and this may be difficult because of the extensive and penetrating nature of these congenital lesions. They produce manifestations similar to those of acquired fistulas.

Congenital *pulmonary* arteriovenous fistulas represent an interesting phenomenon. These lesions may be either single or multiple and are often observed for the first time on routine chest films. In addition, cyanosis, polycythemia, and clubbing of the fingers are apt to be present. These are the result of unsaturated blood flowing directly from the pulmonary artery into the pulmonary venous system without passage through the pulmonary capillary bed.[9]

*Acquired* arteriovenous fistulas are most frequently the result of trauma, following either incised or missile wounds. In addition, iatrogenic fistulas, especially those associated with operations on the renal pedicle and fistulas between the aorta or iliac veins and arteries secondary to intervertebral disc operations, are quite common. Rarely, erosion of an atherosclerotic aneurysm into an accompanying vein may occur, as, for example, erosion of an abdominal aortic aneurysm into the inferior vena cava.

## PATHOPHYSIOLOGY

The pathophysiologic changes that follow establishment of a direct communication between the arterial and venous systems are best demonstrated in the presence of a *large* fistula. Much blood flows through such a fistula since it offers the path of least resistance. Thus, a sequence of changes occurs that is directly related to the shunt of blood from the arterial to the venous circuit. The *cardiac output* increases, the heart rate increases, and the diastolic pressure falls in the presence of *low* peripheral resistance (Table 12). Both blood and plasma volumes increase in an effort to compensate for the increased blood in the venous circuit. The heart becomes larger, primarily because of increase in size of the ventricular cavities. In the presence of large fistulas, a chronic burden is placed upon the heart that may ultimately lead to congestive heart failure. If the fistula is both *acute* and *large*, the heart may not be able to compensate adequately, with resultant pulmonary edema and death. Large experimental fistulas in animals demonstrate this feature quite strikingly.[12]

**TABLE 12**  MANIFESTATIONS OF ARTERIOVENOUS FISTULA

| Systemic | | | |
|---|---|---|---|
| Pulse rate | ↑ | Diastolic arterial pressure | ↓ |
| Cardiac output | ↑ | Peripheral resistance | ↓ |
| Blood volume | ↑ | | |
| Cardiac size | ↑ | | |

| Local |
|---|
| Thrill |
| Continuous murmur |
| Increased arterial collaterals |
| Aneurysmal formation |
| Diminished pulse rate with occlusion |

Physiologic changes occurring in the systemic circulation with an arteriovenous fistula are most marked in the presence of a large fistula and may be minimal to absent with a small fistula. Late manifestations of a large fistula include congestive heart failure, pulmonary edema, and death in untreated patients.

The oxygen saturation of the mixed venous blood is increased since the shunt bypasses the capillary bed, and the central venous pressure is usually increased. The *site* of the fistula in the systemic circulation is of importance since the diameter of the vessel involved is critical. The location of the communication can be determined precisely by arteriography (Fig. 23). Much more blood will flow through a fistula of a given size in a vessel with a large diameter than in one with a smaller diameter. Thus, aortic fistulas of small size can produce more severe symptoms than larger fistulas in the femoral artery or arteries of comparable size. Occasionally, the presence of an arteriovenous fistula is responsible for the development of bacterial endocarditis, and in fact the first patient ever cured of bacterial endocarditis prior to the introduction of antibiotics was managed by surgical closure of an iliac arteriovenous fistula, after which the subacute bacterial endocarditis disappeared.[11]

## LOCAL EFFECTS OF FISTULA

In addition to the systemic manifestations that arteriovenous fistulas create, there are several *local* changes of interest. An *aneurysmal dilatation* is usually present in the artery and vein at the site of the fistula. Since the arterial pressure distal to the fistula is greatly reduced (Fig. 24), an extensive collateral circulation develops from the branches of the artery arising above the fistula to those communicating below. This collateral circulation may become massive and usually results in an increase in both skin and muscle temperature. There are significant changes that occur in the *pressures* in the artery distal to the fistula and in the accompanying vein (Fig. 25).[14] When the fistula is in an extremity, the limb may have *increased length*, a fact confirmed by both experimental[8] and clinical observations.[7] There

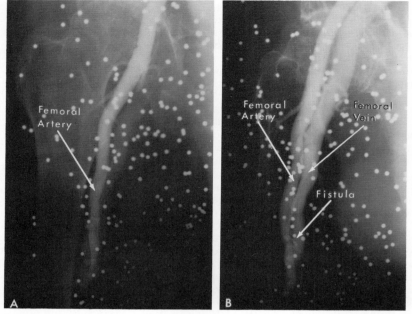

**Figure 23** *A,* Femoral arteriogram in a patient with a gunshot wound of the thigh and a femoral arteriovenous fistula. *B,* The site of the fistula is seen with rapid filling of the proximal femoral vein without filling distally.

is no clear explanation for the stimulating effect of arteriovenous fistulas on bone growth, but it may be related to the fact that bone temperature is increased 1 or 2° C. and to the increased blood supply.

## MANAGEMENT

Since most arteriovenous fistulas are either actually or potentially symptomatic, surgical closure is generally recommended. Rarely, a small fistula may close spontaneously; this is recorded in 5 of 245 patients surveyed in World War II.[13] The site of the fistula can be determined by arteriography, and the surgical management of choice is usually direct repair of both the artery and the vein. If it is not possible to repair the vein satisfactorily, ligation of the vein may be necessary. Rarely, quadripolar ligation of the fistula is necessary. Thus, direct restoration of arterial

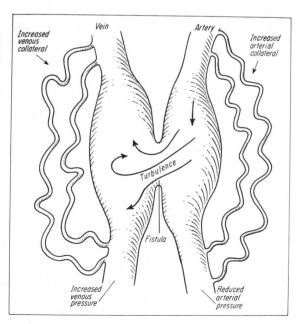

**Figure 24** Diagrammatic illustration of the local changes that occur in the presence of an arteriovenous fistula. The changes shown are proportional to the *size* of the fistula. In a small fistula, these changes may be quite minimal.

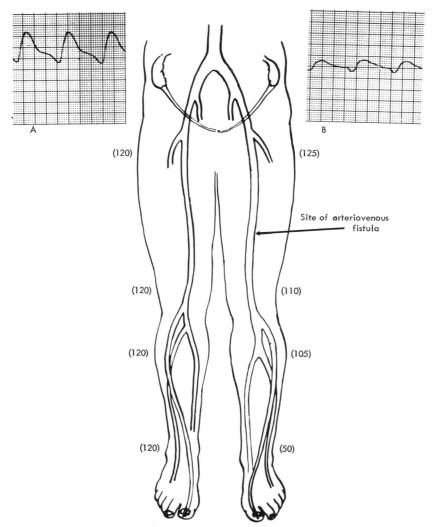

**Figure 25** Plethysmographic record of a 35 year old man with a traumatic superficial femoral arteriovenous fistula. Digit pulse contours are abnormal on the left, and there is a significant depression of the ankle pressure (50 mm. Hg) distal to the fistula (Courtesy of Dr. D. E. Strandness, Jr., Department of Surgery, University of Washington. From Strandness, D. E., Jr., ed.: Collateral Circulation in Clinical Surgery. Philadelphia, W. B. Saunders Company, 1969.)

continuity with closure of the fistula is the procedure of choice in the vast majority of instances. In a recent report, traumatic arteriovenous fistulas in 50 consecutive patients were corrected without a single amputation.[1]

### SELECTED REFERENCES

Holman, E.: Abnormal Arteriovenous Communications. Peripheral and Intracardiac. Acquired and Congenital. Springfield, Ill., Charles C Thomas, 1968.
*This monograph is the definitive one on the subject of arteriovenous fistula. The historical, experimental, and clinical aspects of this interesting disorder are presented in a complete and highly commendable manner.*

Sumner, D. S.: Arteriovenous fistula. In: Strandness, D. E., Jr., ed.: Collateral Circulation in Clinical Surgery. Philadelphia, W. B. Saunders Company, 1969.
*This section in an excellent monograph is an updated source of detailed information on all forms of arteriovenous fistulas.*

### REFERENCES

1. Beall, A. C., Jr., Diethrich, E. B., Morris, G. C., Jr., and De-Bakey, M. E.: Surgical management of vascular trauma. Surg. Clin. N. Amer., 46:1001, 1966.
2. Bramann, F.: Das arteriell-venous Aneurysma. Arch. Klin. Chir., 33:1, 1886.
3. Branham, H. H.: Aneurismal varix of the femoral artery and vein following a gunshot wound. Int. J. Surg., 3: 250, 1890.
4. Breschet, G.: Mémoire sur les aneurysmes. Mem. Acad. Roy. Med. (Paris), 3:101, 1833.
5. Holman, E.: Abnormal Arteriovenous Communications. Peripheral and Intracardiac. Acquired and Congenital. Springfield, Ill., Charles C Thomas, 1968.
6. Hunter, W.: The history of an aneurysm of the aorta, with some remarks on aneurysms in general. Med. Observ. Inquir., 1:323, 1757.
7. Janes, J. M., and Jennings, W. K., Jr.: Effect of induced arteriovenous fistula on leg length: 10-year observations. Proc. Mayo Clin., 36:1, 1961.
8. Janes, J. M., and Musgrove, J. E.: Effect of arteriovenous

fistula on growth of bone: An experimental study. Surg. Clin. N. Amer., *30*:1191, 1950.

9. Moyer, J. H., Glantz, G., and Brest, A. N.: Pulmonary arteriovenous fistulas. Physiologic and clinical considerations. Amer. J. Med., *32*:417, 1962.

10. Nicoladoni, C.: Phlebarteriectasie der rechten oberen Extremitat. Arch. Klin. Chir., *18*:252, 1875.

11. Rienhoff, W. F., Jr., and Hamman, L. D.: Subacute Streptococcus viridans septicemia cured by the excision of an arteriovenous aneurysm of the external iliac artery and vein. Ann. Surg., *102*:905, 1935.

12. Sabiston, D. C., Jr., Theilen, E. O., and Gregg, D. E.: Physiologic studies in experimental high output cardiac failure produced by aortic-caval fistula. Surg. Forum, *6*:233, 1956.

13. Shumacker, H. B.: Arterial aneurysms and arteriovenous fistulas. Spontaneous cures. In: Elkin, D. C., and DeBakey, M. E., eds.: Surgery in World War II: Vascular Surgery. Washington, D. C., Office of the Surgeon General, Department of Army, 1955.

14. Sumner, D. S.: Arteriovenous fistula. Physiology and pathological anatomy. In: Strandness, D. E., Jr., ed.: Collateral Circulation in Clinical Surgery. Philadelphia, W. B. Saunders Company, 1969.

15. Tice, D. A., Clauss, R. H., Keirle, A. M., and Reed, G. E.: Congenital arteriovenous fistulae of the extremities: Observations concerning treatment. Arch. Surg., *86*: 460, 1963.

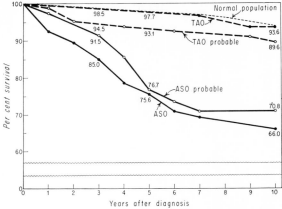

**Figure 26** Widely differing 10 year survival rates in Buerger's disease (TAO) and arteriosclerosis (ASO). Confirmed cases of Buerger's disease show no significant difference from the normal population. (From McPherson, J. R., Juergens, J. L., and Gifford, R. W.: Ann. Intern. Med., *59*:288, 1963.)

## 10. BUERGER'S DISEASE

In 1909, Buerger described a syndrome of vascular occlusion in which the arteries, veins, and nerves of the extremities were involved in an extensive fibrosis with obliterative vasculitis.[1] The *pathologic* aspects include widespread thrombosis in small peripheral arteries and veins, with periadventitial scarring. The changes in the vessels are usually associated with a perineuritis of the accompanying nerve. The *acute* lesion is regarded as an inflammatory one, with microabscesses and organizing thrombi on the vessel wall. Polymorphonuclear leukocytes and giant cells are frequently seen. Microabscesses may result. Frequently, the arteries immediately proximal and distal to the Buerger lesions appear normal.

### CLINICAL MANIFESTATIONS

In the characteristic form, the disease attacks young males, generally between the ages of 20 and 40. The symptoms include intermittent claudication, coldness of the extremities, phlebitis, rest pain, ulceration, and gangrene. The vasospastic symptoms that occur are often of the *Raynaud* type, with blanching and numbness of the digits accompanied by cyanosis and rubor. Pain may be elicited by exposure to cold. Phlebitis is usually superficial, nodular, and migratory. The use of tobacco clearly accentuates the symptoms.

### DIFFERENTIAL DIAGNOSIS

The primary condition from which Buerger's disease must be differentiated is arteriosclerosis obliterans. In general, Buerger's disease is *unlike* arteriosclerosis in that it attacks those in the 20 to 45 years age group, the upper limbs are frequently involved, and phlebitis is common. Gangrene often appears early and may be limited to the digits, with nearby pulses being present. Each of these features is uncommon with arteriosclerosis. The life course in the two diseases is also quite different, as shown in Figure 26.[3]

### ARTERIOGRAPHY

In most patients with Buerger's disease, the main artery (femoral or brachial) is usually essentially normal. The point of occlusion is usually precise, and there is little proximal irregularity. There is no patency of the main artery beyond the point of occlusion, unlike the usual finding in arteriosclerosis.

The prognosis is variable but is much more favorable if the patient stops smoking. There is no doubt that smoking is a crucial factor, and if it is continued, the disease will inevitably progress with rapidity. Abstinence from all forms of tobacco nearly always yields improvement, although it may take several weeks for this to become apparent. Prognosis for *life* is considerably better than that in arteriosclerosis and is more similar to that of the normal population.

### MANAGEMENT

Conservative treatment is generally recommended, with tobacco withdrawal as a prime goal. Heparin, low molecular weight dextran, and steroids have all been recommended but are of questionable value in therapy.

*Surgical* management begins with *sympathectomy,* which is indicated in many instances since it provides freedom from vasoconstrictor activity in the *distal* limb, the portion most often involved. A further benefit of sympathectomy is that it produces anhidrosis, which reduces the incidence of bacterial and fungal infections of the skin. *Amputations* are frequently necessary to control both gangrene and severe pain.

In the recent past, Wessler and associates have questioned the validity of a clinical and pathologic diagnosis of Buerger's disease.[4] It is their view that the manifestations are essentially those of arteriosclerosis and that Buerger's disease is not a distinct entity. This position has been vigorously challenged by McKusick and associates[2] and by others.

## SELECTED REFERENCES

McKusick, V. A., Harris, W. S., Ottesen, O. E., Goodman, R. M., Shelley, W. M., and Bloodwell, R. D.: Buerger's disease. A distinct clinical and pathologic entity. J.A.M.A., *181*:5, 1962.
   *These authors refute the viewpoint of Wessler and associates and instead support the position that Buerger's disease is a definite clinical and pathologic disorder. The features of this disorder are commendably reviewed.*
Wessler, S., Ming, S., Gurewich, V., and Freiman, D. G.: A critical evaluation of thromboangiitis obliterans. The case against Buerger's disease. New Eng. J. Med., *262*:1149, 1960.
   *In this paper, the authors attack the concept that Buerger's disease is a distinct clinical entity. It is their view that the disorder is a severe form of arteriosclerosis obliterans occurring in a younger population.*

## REFERENCES

1. Buerger, L.: The association of migrating thrombophlebitis with thromboangeitis obliterans. Int. Clin., *3*:84, 1909.
2. McKusick, V. A., Harris, W. S., Ottesen, O. E., Goodman, R. M., Shelley, W. M., and Bloodwell, R. D.: Buerger's disease. A distinct clinical and pathologic entity. J.A.M.A., *181*:5, 1962.
3. McPherson, J. R., Juergens, J. L., and Gifford, R. W., Jr.: Thromboangiitis obliterans and arteriosclerosis obliterans. Clinical and prognostic differences. Ann. Intern. Med., *59*:288, 1963.
4. Wessler, S.: Buerger's disease revisited. Surg. Clin. N. Amer., *49*:703, 1969.

## 11. RAYNAUD'S DISEASE

*Donald Silver, M.D.*

In 1862, Raynaud[1] described a process caused by disturbances of the circulation that is characterized by color changes in the skin of the digits and extremities in response to exposure to cold or emotional disturbances and can progress to symmetric gangrene of the digits. Raynaud's disease occurs most commonly in young women and most frequently involves the digits of the upper extremity. It usually begins in a digit or two of each hand but gradually spreads to involve all digits of the hands and, eventually, the feet. Occasionally the toes are involved first.

Classically, an attack begins after exposure to cold or an emotional outbreak and consists of an excessive vasoconstriction response. During the first part of the attack there is intense vasoconstriction, and the induced ischemia causes blanching and pain of the involved digit(s). The vasoconstriction phase is followed by a period of sluggish flow, during which time the digit(s) becomes cyanotic. Finally, vasodilation occurs, and rubor, warmth, and paresthesias of the digit(s) develop. The symptoms are usually mild and intermittent at first, but tend to increase in severity and frequency. Early in her illness, the patient may have difficulty only on the coldest of days or only when her hands are in ice water. Later in her illness, the patient frequently notes that air conditioning, minor degrees of coolness, or minor emotional disturbances may precipitate an attack.

The etiology of Raynaud's disease remains obscure. The symptom complex results from an abnormal vasoconstriction response to the stimuli of cold and emotion. Microscopic studies of the vessels usually do not demonstrate any changes that can be related to the disease process. If the disease continues, there is loss of digital hair, the skin over the digits becomes thin and atrophic, thickening of the nails occurs, and eventually ischemic gangrene of the digit tips occurs.

When an underlying cause of the symptom complex cannot be detected, the patient is said to have Raynaud's disease. Many patients with the classic vasomotor responses have underlying disorders, e.g., scleroderma, lupus erythematosus, dermatomyositis, arteriosclerosis obliterans, thromboembolism, cryoglobulinemia, rheumatoid arthritis, or the thoracic outlet syndrome; in these patients, the condition is called Raynaud's phenomenon. Early in the course of the illness, it is very difficult to distinguish these patients from those with Raynaud's disease. Frequently, careful re-evaluation for several years is necessary before the underlying cause becomes apparent. Raynaud's phenomenon has been associated with certain occupations and is seen in persons who use vibratory tools or use their fingers constantly, i.e., pneumatic hammer operators, lathe operators, typists, and pianists.

Treatment of Raynaud's disease is complicated by the difficulty of distinguishing those patients with the disease from those with the phenomenon. If the underlying disorder or occupation can be treated or changed, patients with Raynaud's phenomenon will usually have diminution of their symptoms and not require additional treatment. When the underlying disorder is progressive and cannot be treated, multiple system failure and death frequently ensue. The Raynaud phenomena in these patients usually do not respond for any length of time to any form of therapy. Treatment for patients with Raynaud's disease consists of cervicothoracic sympathectomy, avoiding cold, protection from trauma, and reducing anxieties. Sympathectomy gives limited, if any, relief to patients with Raynaud's phenomenon. The sympathectomy should be performed early in the course of Raynaud's disease for best results. The author prefers to perform the sympathectomy through a transaxillary incision (Fig. 27); the lower third of the stellate ganglion and the second, third, fourth, and fifth thoracic sympathetic

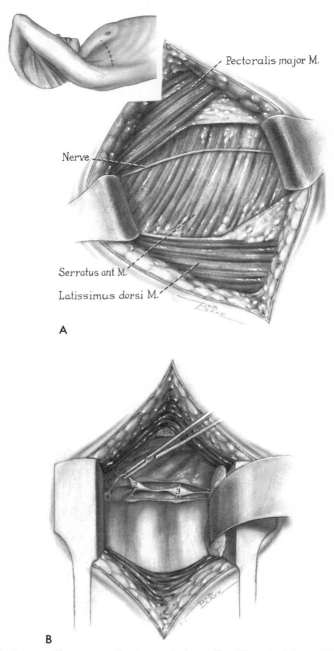

Pectoralis major M.

Nerve

Serratus ant M.

Latissimus dorsi M.

A

B

**Figure 27** Incision for transaxillary sympathectomy. *A,* A small axillary incision exposes the serratus muscle, which is separated in the direction of its fibers. *B,* The chest is entered through the bed of the resected third rib. Retraction of the lung inferiorly and incision of the pleura permits the sympathetic ganglia to be readily visualized and removed. In the figure, the lower portion of the stellate ganglion is coming into view. (From Silver, D. In: Gibbon, J. H., Jr., et al.: Surgery of the Chest. 2nd ed. Philadelphia, W. B. Saunders Company, 1969.)

ganglia are resected. An adequate sympathectomy may also be accomplished through a standard anterior or posterolateral thoracotomy incision.

## REFERENCE

1. Raynaud, A. G. M.: De l'asphyxie locale et de la gangrène symétrique des extrémités. Paris, Rignoux, 1862 (cited in Allen, E. V., Barker, N. W., and Hines, E. A., Jr.: Peripheral Vascular Diseases. 3rd ed. Philadelphia, W. B. Saunders Company, 1962, p. 125.

## 12. CIRCULATORY PROBLEMS OF THE UPPER EXTREMITY

*Donald Silver, M.D.*

### ARTERIAL INSUFFICIENCY

The upper extremities tolerate reductions of arterial flow much better than the lower extremities because of a smaller muscle mass and the intermittent character of the work required of them. The collateral circulation of the upper extremity is almost always sufficient to prevent distal ischemic necrosis. However, in patients with acute arterial insufficiency and insufficient collaterals, and in those whose occupation requires that they constantly use their upper extremities, ischemic symptoms and gangrene of distal parts may develop.

The arterial blood flow to the upper extremity may be reduced by atherosclerosis, trauma, thromboembolism, or tumors. Atherosclerosis of the upper extremity, as elsewhere, is most pronounced at the origin of vessels and at the bifurcation of vessels. Symptomatic occlusions most commonly involve the innominate or subclavian artery. The small arteries of the hand and of the fingers are next most frequently involved, and the brachial, radial, and ulnar arteries least often.

In trauma to an extremity, compression of the vessels may result from bony angulation or bone fragments, from hematomas and edema, and from direct vascular injury. The arteries may be partially or totally compressed or disrupted. If the intima is torn by sudden stretching of an artery, blood flow may then lift it and produce a "flap-valve" obstruction. Penetrating wounds of the arteries may also penetrate the adjacent veins and produce arteriovenous fistulas.

Emboli are an increasingly common cause of arterial insufficiency of the upper extremity. Six to ten per cent of all arterial emboli lodge in the upper extremities. Most emboli arise in the heart, and the incidence of thromboembolic occlusion of the upper extremity parallels the increasing number of geriatric patients, with their cardiac problems. Emboli usually lodge at sites of arterial bifurcation or reduction of arterial diameters. Transbrachial and transaxillary cardiac catheterization also causes thrombotic occlusions of the respective arteries in approximately 0.5 per cent of the cases.[3]

A careful history and physical examination supplemented by appropriate x-rays and angiograms should document the site and extent of the arterial occlusion and give some indication of the etiology of the insufficiency. Asymptomatic or minimally symptomatic occlusions usually require no therapy.

### VENOUS INSUFFICIENCY

The manifestations of venous insufficiency include edema, distention of superficial veins, tightness, aching, and pain. Edema of the upper extremity from venous insufficiency is most often caused by occlusion of the axillary, subclavian, or innominate vein, or the superior vena cava. More distal venous occlusions rarely produce significant edema or chronic symptoms.

Tumors, mediastinal fibrosis, and trauma are the principal causes of thrombosis in the large central veins, although indwelling catheters for prolonged infusions are producing increasing numbers of thromboses of these veins. Thromboses of the distal upper extremity veins most often are associated with intravenous infusions.

The thrombosis of the axillary or subclavian vein that occurs after effort or strain[1] has been called "effort thrombosis." This thrombosis usually occurs in the dominant arm of a young or middle-aged healthy person. It usually occurs immediately after the effort, but its onset may be delayed several hours. A history of mild effort or strain with the arm abducted can be obtained in most cases. Many of the cases of effort thrombosis were probably caused by compression of the axillary vein by either the pectoralis minor tendon or the costocoracoid ligament, or both, when the arms were abducted and, therefore, could be considered a manifestation of the thoracic outlet syndrome. An occasional patient will have edema after effort but will not have thrombosis of the axillary vein, although the axillary and subclavian veins do show areas of compression at the time of phlebography. These patients are thought to have temporary compression of the veins by the edema associated with the effort.

The presence and extent of the venous thrombosis should be documented by phlebography. Most patients with clinically significant thromboses of the veins of the upper extremity should be treated with elevation of the extremity and with heparin (provided there are no contraindications) in sufficient amounts to overcome the circulating thrombin and prolong the clotting time to three times the control value. Heparin is best given as a constant intravenous infusion, maintained a minimum of 8 to 10 days. It is continued longer if symptoms persist. The fibrinolytic agents urokinase and "purified" streptokinase, under current investigation, appear to be useful in lysing these thromboses.

### CAUSALGIA

In 1872, Mitchell coined the term "causalgia"[2] to describe the burning, agonizing pain and vasomotor disturbances that occur in an occasional patient after a peripheral nerve injury. The pain of causalgia varies in intensity and is exacerbated by touching or moving a part, changes in temperature, pressure changes, or local irritants. The pain may become so agonizing that complete cessation of motion of the involved extremity ensues.

Sympathetic blockade is an excellent diagnostic and therapeutic procedure because it usually gives complete relief from pain and allows use of the previously guarded limb. The vasomotor changes also are usually completely relieved by the blockade. In a few patients, lasting relief is provided by a single sympathetic blockade. Others require repeated treatment to obtain complete relief. However, if sympathetic block gives only limited relief, operative sympathetic denervation should be performed with the expectation that complete relief of symptoms will be obtained. Active physical therapy is an important part of the post-sympathectomy management.

## POST-TRAUMATIC REFLEX DYSTROPHY

In some patients, causalgia-like pain develops after a trivial injury in which there is no demonstrable nerve damage. In addition to the pain, there may be edema, vasomotor disturbances, soft tissue dystrophy, and atrophy of the bone in the region of or distal to the traumatic injury. The process may follow minimal trauma, such as a sprain, or an infection, and occasionally occurs after thrombophlebitis, burns, spinal anesthesia, or herniation of nucleus pulposus. The process is called post-traumatic reflex sympathetic dystrophy, or Sudeck's atrophy because of the the description of bone atrophy by Sudeck in 1900.[5]

Treatment consists of treating the local injury with supportive measures—local heat, analgesics, and so forth. Sympathetic blockade may be necessary to control the pain before physical therapy is initiated and may have to be repeated several times. Early sympathetic blockades and physical therapy are the mainstays of therapy. The majority of patients make a complete recovery with these supportive measures. However, if the supportive measures do not completely relieve the symptoms, sympathetic denervation of the involved extremity is indicated. Physical therapy is a very important adjunct during the early postoperative period.

## ACROCYANOSIS

Acrocyanosis is characterized by an almost continuous painless coldness and cyanosis of the distal portions of the extremities. It is caused by constant spasm of the small arteries in response to an overactive vasomotor system. The condition should be easily differentiated from Raynaud's disease by careful history and physical examination. Treatment consists only of protection from cold in mild cases, or sympathectomy, which usually gives complete relief from symptoms, in severe cases.

## ERYTHROMELALGIA

Erythromelalgia is characterized by a burning sensation in the extremities that is associated with local warmth and a reddish or cyanotic color of the skin of the affected part. It occurs most often in middle-aged men and women during times of exposure to increased heat. It may be primary or secondary, occurring in patients with hypertension, polycythemia, or gout. Treatment of secondary erythromelalgia should be directed toward eliminating the underlying disorder. Treatment of primary erythromelalgia is symptomatic, i.e., cooling and reducing body temperature. Sympathectomy of the involved extremity offers favorable to excellent results.[4, 6]

## SELECTED REFERENCE

Allen, E. V., Barker, N. W., and Hines, E. A., Jr.: Peripheral Vascular Diseases. 3rd ed. Philadelphia, W. B. Saunders Company, 1962.
*All students of vascular and related disorders should be familiar with this excellent text. It is an encyclopedia of information concerning vascular diseases. A historical review, discussion of the pathophysiology, and methods for diagnosis and management are presented for each disorder.*

## REFERENCES

1. Matas, R.: Primary thrombosis of the axillary vein caused by strain. Amer. J. Surg., 24:642, 1934.
2. Mitchell, S. W.: Injuries of Nerves and Their Consequences. Philadelphia, J. B. Lippincott Company, 1872.
3. Ross, R. S.: Arterial complications. *Circulation*, Suppl. III, p. 39, 1968.
4. Shumaker, H. B., Jr.: Sympathetic denervation of the extremities. Curr. Probl. Surg., July, 1965.
5. Sudeck, P.: Ueber die acute Entzundliche. Knochenatrophie. Arch. Klin. Chir., 62:147, 1900 (cited in Allen, E. V., Barker, N. W., and Hines, E. A., Jr.: Peripheral Vascular Diseases. 3rd ed. Philadelphia, W. B. Saunders Company, 1962, p. 459).
6. Telford, E. D.: Discussion on peripheral vascular lesions. Proc. Roy. Soc. Med., 37:621, 1944.

## 13. VISCERAL ISCHEMIC SYNDROME: OBSTRUCTION OF THE SUPERIOR MESENTERIC, CELIAC, AND INFERIOR MESENTERIC ARTERIES

*David C. Sabiston, Jr., M.D.*

In 1869, Chiene described complete obliteration of the celiac and mesenteric arteries, with the organs supplied by these vessels receiving blood through collateral circulation.[2] In patients who demonstrate *symptoms* as a result of stenosis or occlusion of these vessels, the term *abdominal angina* is applied.[1] This condition was first successfully treated in 1958.[6]

## PATHOPHYSIOLOGY

Atherosclerosis, with either partial or complete occlusion, is the most common cause of symptomatic visceral arterial obstruction. The lesion is most often at or near the origin of the vessels from the aorta. The obstruction is usually segmental, frequently only several millimeters in length, with a normal or dilated lumen distally. *Fibromuscular hyperplasia* of the celiac axis is another cause of mesenteric angina.[4] In addition, external compression of the celiac artery by the arcuate ligament of the diaphragm may produce compression of the artery with resultant ischemic symptoms.[3, 7] Rarely, mesenteric angina may be produced by abdominal coarctation, a neoplasm, or severe sclerosing pancreatitis, causing reduced blood flow through the celiac or superior mesenteric arteries.

It has long been recognized that slowly progressive occlusion of the mesenteric vessels leads to the development of a prominent collateral circulation. If the obstruction develops rapidly, with inadequate time for sufficient collaterals to develop, intestinal infarction may ensue. Finally, chronic intestinal ischemia may develop when blood supply is sufficient to maintain viability of the small intestine but inadequate when demands are increased, such as after meals. The latter state is called *intestinal angina*.

## CLINICAL MANIFESTATIONS

The symptoms of this condition characteristically occur in the *postprandial* state and consist of abdominal pain, usually associated with a feeling of abdominal distention. Discomfort usually begins 15 to 30 minutes after a meal and may last for 1 to 3 hours. Its severity and duration are related to the amount of food ingested. Nausea, vomiting, and diarrhea may all occur. Reluctance to eat because of the *fear* of pain as well as the pain itself and the malabsorption that may occur in an ischemic intestinal tract often lead to weight loss. The symptoms usually progress and may ultimately become quite severe. Malabsorption in some patients can be documented by a high fat and protein content in the stool. Since the celiac arterial obstruction in median arcuate ligament syndrome may be intermittent, symptoms with this condition are often less characteristic than those associated with atherosclerotic occlusion of the superior mesenteric or celiac arteries, and it is unusual for patients with this syndrome to have diarrhea.[8] Physical examination may demonstrate evidence of weight loss, and a *bruit* is often heard over the epigastrium.

The differential diagnosis includes gallbladder disease, peptic ulcer, pancreatitis, and malignant disease of the alimentary tract. The definitive diagnosis is made by selective aortography, with injection of the celiac and superior mesenteric arteries. In most patients with symptoms, either the celiac or the superior mesenteric artery is occluded and the other is severely stenotic or also occluded. Occasionally, occlusion of one vessel

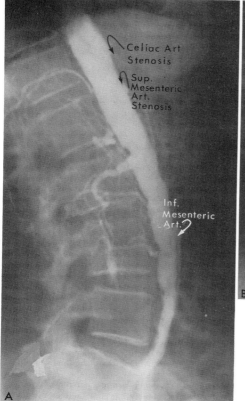

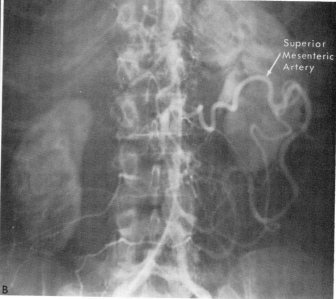

**Figure 28** *A*, Arteriogram in a patient with mesenteric angina. Both the celiac and superior mesenteric arteries are almost totally occluded. Flow can be seen in the inferior mesenteric artery. *B*, Later film in the arteriographic series showing filling of the superior mesenteric artery by retrograde flow from the inferior mesenteric artery. (Courtesy of Dr. Irwin Johnsrude.)

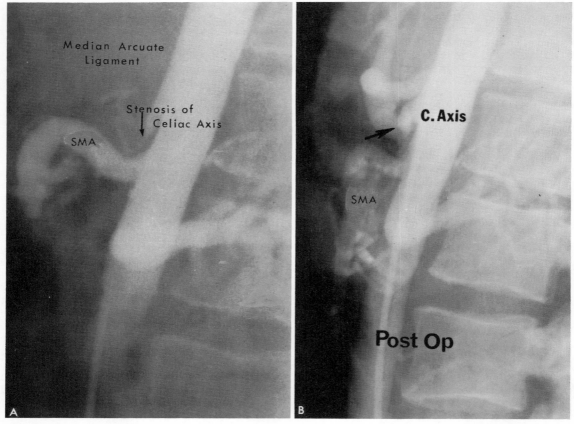

**Figure 29**   *A,* Aortogram in patient with median arcuate ligament syndrome. A severe stenosis at the origin of the celiac axis is apparent. The superior mesenteric artery is quite large. *B,* Postoperative aortogram showing patency of the celiac axis. The patient was relieved of the intestinal angina. (Courtesy of Dr. Irwin Johnsrude.)

alone may produce the symptoms.[8] Arteriography also demonstrates the median arcuate syndrome, with quite proximal occlusion of the celiac artery (Fig. 28).

## MANAGEMENT

In patients with severe symptoms, a direct arterial approach for relief of the stenosis is indicated. Either an abdominal or thoracoabdominal approach may be employed. The use of an autogenous vein to bypass the stenosis is usually the preferred procedure. Other operations that can be employed include thromboendarterectomy, insertion of a synthetic graft, and excision of the stenotic area with reimplantation of the vessel into the aorta. Rarely, the splenic artery may be used for anastomosis distal to the obstruction. It is usually necessary to bypass only one artery, most often the superior mesenteric.[5] In patients with the median arcuate ligament syndrome, the obstruction of the celiac artery can be relieved by division of the occluding ligamentous fibers, and an abdominal or thoracoabdominal approach is used.[8] The results of operation are generally quite good,

with relief of pain and improvement in intestinal absorption (Fig. 29).

## OCCLUSION OF THE INFERIOR MESENTERIC ARTERY

Although atherosclerotic occlusion of the inferior mesenteric artery commonly occurs, it rarely produces symptoms. The collateral circulation in this arterial circuit is so extensive that ischemic symptoms rarely develop. Occasionally, acute obstruction, as by an embolus, may cause infarction of the descending and sigmoid colon and produce acute abdominal pain and tenderness. The treatment is emergency operation with resection of the infarcted colon.

## SELECTED REFERENCES

Rob, C.: Surgical diseases of the celiac and mesenteric arteries. Arch. Surg., *93*:21, 1966.
*This is a very well written account of the various disorders that may produce occlusion of the celiac and mesenteric arteries. Both acute and chronic forms of obstruction are discussed. The appropriate surgical therapy is reviewed and an excellent bibliography is included.*

Stoney, R. J., and Wylie, E. J.: Recognition and surgical management of visceral ischemic syndromes. Ann. Surg., *164*:714, 1966.

*This paper is an excellent reference source for details of the median arcuate ligament syndrome. The diagnosis and surgical management are well presented.*

## REFERENCES

1. Baccelli, cited by Goodman, E. H.: Angina abdominis. Amer. J. Med. Sci., *155*:524, 1918.
2. Chiene, J.: Complete obliteration of celiac and mesenteric arteries: Viscera receiving their blood supply through extraperitoneal system of vessels. J. Anat. Physiol. (London), *3*(second series):65, 1868–1869.
3. Dunbar, J. D., Molnar, W., Beman, F. F., and Marable, S. A.: Compression of the celiac trunk and abdominal aorta. Preliminary report of 15 cases. Amer. J. Roentgen., *95*: 731, 1965.
4. Palubinskas, A. J., and Ripley, H. R.: Fibromuscular hyperplasia in extrarenal arteries. Radiology, *82*:451, 1964.
5. Rob, C.: Surgical diseases of the celiac and mesenteric arteries. Arch. Surg., *93*:21, 1966.
6. Shaw, R. S., and Maynard, E. P., III: Acute and chronic thrombosis of the mesenteric arteries associated with malabsorption: A report of two cases successfully treated by thromboendarterectomy. New Eng. J. Med., *258*:874, 1958.
7. Stanley, J. C., and Fry, W. J.: Median arcuate ligament syndrome. Arch. Surg., *103*:252, 1971.
8. Stoney, R. J., and Wylie, E. J.: Recognition and surgical management of visceral ischemic syndromes. Ann. Surg., *164*:714, 1966.

# 14. THE SURGICAL MANAGEMENT OF RENOVASCULAR HYPERTENSION

*J. Caulie Gunnells, Jr., M.D., and David C. Sabiston, Jr., M.D.*

The fact that obstructive lesions of the renal arteries can produce hypertension is firmly established. Moreover, surgical revascularization of an ischemic kidney is now an accepted procedure in appropriate circumstances and has produced relief of hypertension in a number of patients.

The *normal* blood pressure in the human is known to vary with age. In infants and young children, levels of 70 to 85 systolic with a diastolic pressure of 50 are within the normal range. In adolescents, a blood pressure of 100/75 is accepted as normal, whereas in the adult the upper range of normal is regarded as 140/90. Systemic arterial pressure is controlled by a number of variables, including the cardiac output, blood volume, elasticity of the arterial wall, peripheral resistance, and blood viscosity. It is thought that the most important feature determining significant and sustained renal hypertension is an elevated *peripheral resistance* as typified by the response to the *renin-angiotensin* system.

There are a number of specific causes of arterial hypertension. The forms of hypertension that are *surgically correctable* are those associated with coarctation of the aorta, pheochromocytoma, Cushing's syndrome, primary aldosteronism, and unilateral renal parenchymal disease. In addition, *renovascular* hypertension forms an increasingly important area for surgical therapy.

## PHYSIOLOGIC ASPECTS

Occlusive lesions of the renal arteries are well recognized as a cause of *sustained diastolic hypertension.* The incidence of renal artery lesions and coexistent hypertension has not been established, but estimates suggest their presence in 5 to 15 per cent of the adult population in the United States. In 1898, Tigerstedt and Bergman[14] demonstrated that an extract of kidney which they named renin was capable of producing hypertension in animals. The now famous experiments by Goldblatt in which hypertension was produced by unilateral narrowing of a renal artery clearly documented the role of the ischemic kidney in the development of hypertension, especially when reduction in blood pressure followed removal of the involved kidney.[3] In the Goldblatt experiment, unilateral renal artery clamping resulted in *transient* hypertension, whereas sustained or persistent elevation in arterial pressure was produced either by constriction of both renal arteries or by clamp constriction of one main renal artery with removal of the contralateral kidney. In man, it has been shown that sustained arterial hypertension may result from *unilateral* renal artery obstruction. Following the Goldblatt experiments, Page and Corcoran,[10] Braun-Menendez,[1] and Helmer[6] all contributed to the description of the renin-angiotensin system. A diminished flow of blood to the renal artery, and especially a reduction or damping of the arterial pulse pressure, is thought to represent one of the possible stimuli that elicit the renal pressor mechanism. The accepted relationships of the renin-angiotensin system are shown in Table 13.[11] The reaction of renin with its alpha globulin substrate yielding angiotensin I is ordinarily considered to be the rate-limiting response. This substance is essentially inert, but a plasmolytic converting enzyme splits off two amino acids and forms angiotensin II, an octapeptide. Angiotensin II is a powerful *vasoconstrictor.* It also evokes aldosterone secretion, and thus produces sodium retention. Angiotensin II is rapidly destroyed in the capillary circulation by tissue angiotensinases. *Renin* is the significant precursor, since the alpha globulin substrate is usually in excess and converting enzyme is available throughout the body. Renin is apparently secreted by the kidney in response to a number of stimuli. Renin has a high molecular

**TABLE 13**   THE RENIN-ANGIOTENSIN SYSTEM*

| | + Activators | |
|---|---|---|
| α-Globulin substrate | Renin − Inhibitors ⟶ | Angiotensin I (decapeptide) |
| Angiotensin I | Converting enzyme ⟶ | Angiotensin II (octapeptide) |
| Angiotensin II | Tissue peptidases ⟶ | Inactive peptides |

*From Romero, J. C., and Hoobler, S. W.: Amer. Heart J., *80*:701, 1970.

weight and a half-life in the bloodstream following bilateral nephrectomy of 45 minutes. Its concentration can be measured under suitable conditions of incubation by the amount of angiotensin it produces.

Much speculation has arisen concerning the physiologic role of renin. Originally, its purpose was thought to be the regulation of perfusion pressure to the kidney beyond an obstructed renal artery, although more recently a broader hypothesis supports the concept that renin is the primary stimulus for maintenance of body *sodium balance.*[11] This concept thoroughly explains the two classic conditions in which plasma renin activity (PRA) is increased: (1) decreased renal perfusion pressure, and (2) decreased delivery of sodium and water to the macula densa cells of the distal renal tubule. Examples of the former include renal artery stenosis, systemic hypotension, the upright posture, malignant hypertension, and afferent renal arteriolar vasoconstriction in hemorrhagic shock. Decreased sodium delivery to the distal tubules probably occurs without an obvious change in renal hemodynamics during dietary salt restriction and in certain disease states accompanied by sodium retention.

The *macula densa* theory—that sodium delivery to the distal tubule is a controlling factor in renin release—is now widely accepted, although discrepancies remain. In this hypothesis, it is assumed that the macula densa cell signals the juxtaglomerular (JG) cells to release renin. It is known that patients with renovascular hypertension frequently are found to have a hyperplastic juxtaglomerular apparatus on microscopic examination.[2,15] Angiotensin II is an extremely powerful vasoconstricting substance, with an effect approximately 10 times greater than that of norepinephrine as a pressor agent. Others have supported the *baroreceptor* hypothesis—that renin release occurs with very slight reductions in mean arterial pressure, of the order of 10 mm. Hg.[13] Moreover, the ability to correct or ameliorate this form of hypertension with the induction or injection of antirenin antibodies has added further support to a *humoral* etiology of renovascular hypertension. In addition to the macula densa and baroreceptor hypotheses, the renal nerves[16] and the adrenal medulla and autonomic nervous system[17] have been reported to have important roles in the overall feedback control of renin release by the kidney.

## PATHOLOGIC OBSERVATIONS

The most common cause of renovascular hypertension is *atherosclerosis,* which is the etiologic basis in some two-thirds of the patients with this disorder. The lesions are most apt to occur near the *origin* of the renal vessels from the aorta and

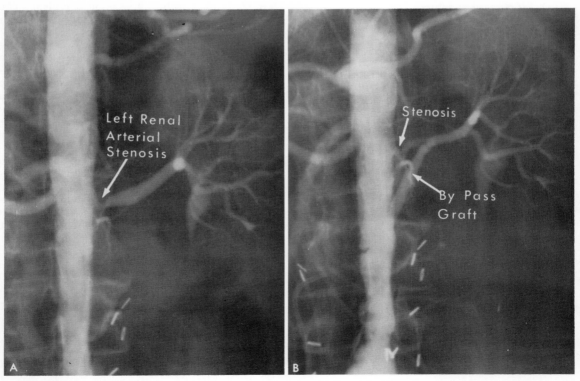

**Figure 30**   *A,* Arteriogram demonstrating severe stenosis of left renal artery in a patient with marked hypertension. *B,* Postoperative arteriogram after insertion of a venous autograft to bypass the stenotic lesion. The hypertension was relieved.

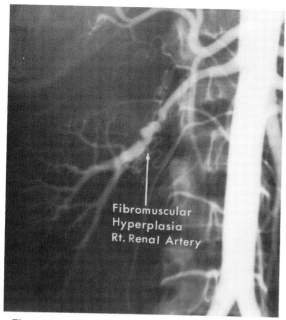

**Figure 31** Arteriogram demonstrating fibromuscular hyperplasia of the right renal artery producing hypertension. Note the characteristic "scalloping."

are *segmental*, usually less than a centimeter in length (Fig. 30). Males are more commonly affected, and bilateral lesions are present in approximately a third of patients.

*Fibromuscular hyperplasia* is another cause of renovascular hypertension and occurs primarily in young women. It is responsible for the disorder in approximately a fourth of patients. The microscopic lesion consists of a thickening of the media with separation and distortion of the muscle fibers by a degenerative process involving myxomatous fibrous tissue. The lesions are apt to be multiple, and the term "microaneurysms" has been used to describe their appearance, which produces a corrugated effect termed the "string of beads" phenomenon observed on arteriograms (Fig. 31).

In one series, an arteriographic diagnosis of fibromuscular hyperplasia of the renal arteries was made in 136 hypertensive patients.[18] In 25 of these, the lesions were minimal, and hypertension was easily controlled with medication. In 31, the lesions were bilateral, either in secondary branches of the artery or in accessory arteries, and were considered inoperable. Major lesions associated with hypertension and considered operable were found in 80 patients. The distribution of lesions determined the selection of operation, and primary nephrectomy was performed in 14 patients with unilateral disease in whom branch or accessory arteries were not amenable to arterial reconstruction. Revascularization procedures were performed in 62 patients with unilateral and 9 patients with bilateral disease of the main arteries. This disorder occurs almost exclusively in the distal three-fourths of the main

renal artery or its primary branches and may not be suitable for surgical correction.[7]

## CLINICAL MANIFESTATIONS

Experience has demonstrated that there are several important *clinical* diagnostic features of renovascular hypertension. These include the onset of sudden hypertension, often prior to the age of 35 or after the age of 55, with the absence of a family history and onset or worsening of the hypertension following an episode of flank pain, and the existence of malignant hypertension after the age of 55. In other words, these features would by atypical for *essential hypertension*, although it must be emphasized that a number of patients with proven renovascular hypertension exhibit none of these features.

Physical examination may reveal the most important diagnostic feature, an abdominal *bruit* located in the epigastrium or upper quadrants. This finding is present in 50 to 80 per cent of patients with *renovascular* hypertension, whereas it occurs in less than 5 per cent of those with essential hypertension. Patients with fibromuscular hyperplasia are more apt to have bruits than those with atherosclerotic lesions. Moreover, in fibromuscular disease the bruits are soft, to-and-fro, or continuous, whereas higher-pitched systolic bruits are more characteristic of atherosclerotic lesions. Patients presenting with these findings are acceptable for thorough renovascular evaluation. The appropriate studies include angiography, split renal function studies, and renal vein renin studies. At the outset it is important to recognize that a general medical evaluation is necessary and that attention should be given to the age of the patient and duration and severity of hypertension, as well as to the presence of coexisting vascular and unrelated diseases. Emphasis must be placed on careful assessment of overall renal function in the selection of candidates for surgery.

## LABORATORY EXAMINATIONS

The initial studies of importance include a urinalysis with culture, serum creatinine determination, chest roentgenography, electrocardiography, serum potassium determination, and assessment of peripheral vein renin activity.

## ANATOMIC STUDIES

### Intravenous Urography

Intravenous urography is a simple and possibly the best screening test for the presence of renovascular hypertension. It establishes the presence or absence of primary parenchymal renal disease. The criteria for a positive minute sequence study include the following changes in the affected or ipsilateral kidney: (1) an initial delay in the appearance time and concentration (nephrogram)

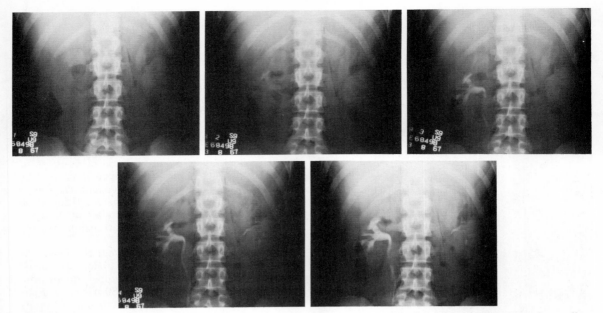

**Figure 32** A positive rapid- or minute-sequence intravenous urogram. The left kidney is significantly smaller and demonstrates a delay in the appearance and concentration of the contrast medium. Paradoxical hyperconcentration is not seen in this study; delayed films not shown, only the serial one minute films for 5 minutes. (From Gunnells, J. C., Jr. In: Earley, L., Sanders, C., Fudenberg, H., Dietschy, J., and Sanford, J., eds.: The Science and Practice of Clinical Medicine. New York, Grune & Stratton, 1972.)

of the contrast medium, followed by a paradoxical hyperconcentration of the dye in the pyelocaliceal system; and (2) a reduction in kidney length greater than 1.5 cm. A representative minute sequence urogram is shown in Figure 32.[4] These criteria support the presence of main-stem renal arterial lesions, and within these guidelines, the minute sequence intravenous urogram correlates at a level of 80 per cent with the angiographic studies in detecting renal artery stenosis. The study produces a false-negative result in approximately 10 per cent of patients and a false-positive result in another 10 per cent of those studied. The urogram has diagnostic limitations with segmental or branch arterial lesions, bilateral renal artery disease, and bilateral parenchymal renal disease of unequal severity, and in certain congenital anomalies of the kidney.

### Radioisotope Renography

The radioisotope renogram has been advocated to delineate renovascular hypertension and is characterized by three phases: (1) "vascular phase"—a rapid ascending slope attributed to renal and extrarenal vascular radioactivity; (2) "functional phase"—a more slowly ascending second segment attributed to tubular activity and intraluminal accumulation of radioactive material; and (3) "excretory phase"—a descending slope considered to represent elimination of radioactive urine from the region of the kidney. This test has several disadvantages, including a number of false-positive and false-negative results, lack of a standardized technique, and

necessity for specialized equipment. In addition, there are technical variables including probe placement, patient position, and state of hydration, and there is no characteristic curve that serves to differentiate renal arterial stenosis from unilateral parenchymal disease.

### Renal Arteriography

The definitive study for the anatomic localization of a renal artery lesion is renal arteriography. This study is indicated in those patients in whom preliminary results suggest renovascular hypertension. The percutaneous retrograde transfemoral technique[12] is quite suitable. In addition to demonstrating the main renal arteries and potential lesions, the study provides important additional information, including the extent of poststenotic dilatation and of collateral circulation, and makes possible evaluation of the renal arterial anatomy. After establishing the fact that a lesion is present, it is then necessary to pursue further studies to determine whether or not the observed lesion is responsible for the hypertension.

## RENAL FUNCTION STUDIES

In addition to obtaining anatomic evidence, assessment of the function of the kidneys is of prime importance. Differential renal studies are important in estimating the degree of unilateral ischemia. Criteria for the physiologic or functional alteration produced by a unilateral renal arterial lesion are based firmly upon animal

**TABLE 14** CRITERIA FOR POSITIVE SPLIT-RENAL FUNCTION STUDIES*

| | Howard | Stamey |
|---|---|---|
| $U_v$ (ml/min) | 50% reduction on involved side | >3:1 decreased flow from involved kidney |
| $U_{Na^+}$ (mEq/L) | 15% reduction from involved side | — |
| $U_{creatinine}$ (mg%) | Increased by 50–100% on involved side | — |
| $U_{PAH}$ (mg/100 ml) | — | 100% or greater concentration from involved kidney |

*Utilizing original proposed criteria; for subsequent additional modifications see text and references. From Gunnells, J. C., Jr. In: Earley, L., Sanders, C., Fudenberg, H., Dietschy, J., and Sanford, J., eds.: The Science and Practice of Clinical Medicine. New York, Grune & Stratton, 1972.

studies with experimentally induced renal lesions. The changes produced consist of a unilateral decrease in glomerular filtration rate, with an increased fractional reabsorption of sodium and water and increased urinary osmolality, and increased urinary concentration of endogenous or exogenous nonreabsorbable solutes. The currently acceptable differential renal function tests (Howard, Stamey, Rapaport, and Birchall) all utilize one or more of these parameters of altered renal function as the basis. The two most widely used techniques are those described by Howard and Stamey. The diagnostic features of these split function studies are shown in Table 14.[4] These studies require bilateral ureteral catheterization and simultaneous evaluation of timed urine samples from each kidney, which are analyzed for volume, sodium, urea, creatinine, and osmolality. The reliability of differential function studies varies considerably; however, a combined experience has reported an operative cure rate of 73 per cent for those patients with positive split function studies. At the same time, an incidence of 49 per cent surgical success is recorded in patients with *negative* studies, and therefore the overall interpretation of this test is of somewhat limited value. In an effort to improve the diagnostic accuracy of these studies, efforts have been made to (1) assess the renal blood flow of the contralateral or normal kidney and exclude from surgery those patients who fail to exhibit a contralateral renal plasma flow of at least 200 to

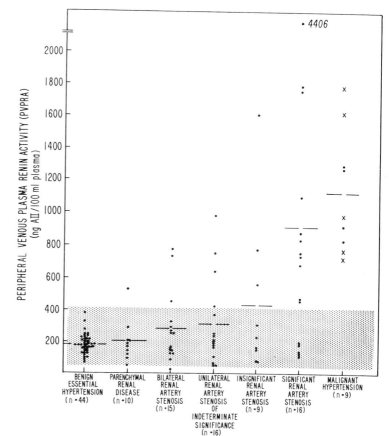

**Figure 33** Peripheral venous plasma renin activity in 111 patients with a wide variety of hypertensive diseases. The four patients with malignant hypertension and parenchymal renal disease are shown in the last column on the right and identified by the closed circles (●); the remaining patients in this column (x) have occlusive renal artery lesion(s) and are also included in columns 3-6. (From Gunnells, J. C., Jr., McGuffin, W. L., Jr., Johnsrude, I., and Robinson, R. R.: Ann. Intern. Med., *71*:555, 1969.)

250 ml. per minute in combination with a positive differential function study; and (2) combine an assessment of the degree of arteriolar nephrosclerosis (renal biopsy studies) with renal plasma flow studies. Despite these additions, the split function tests continue to be fraught with a high incidence of technical failures, postprocedural complications, unreliability in the presence of segmental and bilateral arterial lesions, and unexplained false-positive and false-negative results.

The plasma renin activity (PRA) is of considerable help in segregating those patients in whom a humoral mechanism involving the renin-angiotensin-aldosterone system is causally related to renovascular hypertension. The value of measurement of peripheral venous plasma renin and renal vein renin activity has added greatly to the criteria for selection of patients for operative procedures. Thus far, the most experience and greatest emphasis have been placed upon estimates of *renin* activity rather than that of angiotensin. Problems in methodology have contributed to some of the controversy related to the diagnostic usefulness of these measurements. Current methods for measuring plasma renin activity do not measure renin concentration directly, but only the capacity to generate angiotensin II after an appropriate period of incubation. Most methods utilize the bioassay technique. However, recent experience with a radioimmunoassay for the measurement of angiotensin I and angiotensin II has been described, and this is now being applied clinically. It is worth emphasizing that clinicians must be familiar with the methodology involved, and that careful assessment must be made of the conditions under which renin measurements are obtained. These conditions include the status of body posture, sodium balance, and the presence or absence of pharmacologic agents, all of which may affect renin activity measurements.

The presence of an increased peripheral venous plasma renin activity in conjunction with a normal dietary sodium intake and the absence of diuretic drugs and malignant hypertension provides strong supportive evidence for functional renal arterial stenosis. In contrast, recent evidence[9] suggests that patients with essential hypertension in asso-

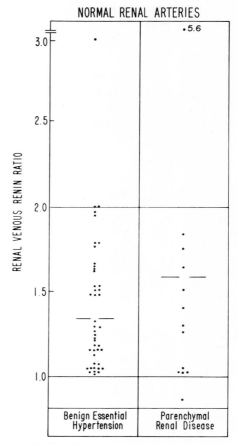

**Figure 34** Renal venous renin ratios in 58 patients with normal renal arteries. (From Gunnells, J. C., Jr., McGuffin, W. L., Jr., Johnsrude, I., and Robinson, R. R.: Ann. Intern. Med., *71*:555, 1969.)

ciation with a low plasma renin activity have a distinctly different, quite benign and indolent clinical course unassociated with the usual vascular complications seen in other types of hypertensive diseases. These and other observations further support the diagnostic and prognostic usefulness of plasma renin activity measurements. An experience with measurements of peripheral

**TABLE 15** MEASUREMENTS OF RENIN ACTIVITY CORRELATED WITH RESULTS OF SURGICAL THERAPY IN 23 PATIENTS*

| Peripheral and Renal Venous Renin Activity | Surgical Success | Number of Patients |
|---|---|---|
| Patients with elevated peripheral venous PRA† and greater than a twofold difference in renal venous PRA | 100% | 11 of 11 |
| Patients with normal peripheral venous PRA and greater than a twofold difference in renal venous PRA | 50% | 4 of 8 |
| Patients with normal peripheral venous PRA and less than a twofold difference in renal venous PRA | 25% | 1 of 4 |

*From Gunnells, J. C., Jr. In: Earley, L., Sanders, C., Fudenberg, H., Dietschy, J., and Sanford, J., eds.: The Science and Practice of Clinical Medicine. New York, Grune & Stratton, 1972.

†PRA = Plasma renin activity

venous plasma renin activity in a wide variety of clinical hypertensive diseases is shown in Figure 33.[5] Since peripheral venous renin activity measurements can be quite variable, the use of *bilateral renal vein renin* measurements alone or in combination has assumed considerable importance. Patients with hypertension and normal renal arteries only *rarely* exhibit a renal vein renin ratio greater than 2 to 1 (Fig. 34),[5] whereas in patients with functionally significant renal artery stenosis, renal vein renin concentrations are at least 1.2 to 2 times higher in the venous blood of the involved or affected kidney than in that of the normal one. The combined use of peripheral vein plasma renin activity and renal vein renin activity measurements in determining or predicting surgical success is summarized in Table 15.[4]

## TREATMENT

Selection of patients for medical or surgical treatment is dependent upon the primary establishment of a strong likelihood that the hypertension is present as a *direct result* of a renal arterial lesion. In addition, one should consider the age and general health of the patient, the natural history of the disease, the feasibility of vascular repair versus nephrectomy, the comparative role of control of the hypertension with drugs, and the surgical mortality.[8] For example, elderly patients with evidence of atherosclerotic lesions elsewhere might have an operative mortality in an excessive

range. Contrariwise, a young patient with a fibro-muscular lesion would be an essentially ideal candidate. The majority of patients are between these two extremes, and most patients thought to have an arterial lesion responsible for the hypertension are candidates for surgery.

The choice of surgical technique is dependent upon the nature of the occluding lesion and the individual preference of the surgeon. Segmental renal artery *resection with reanastomosis* may be feasible when the proximal and distal ends of the vessel are suitable. An anastomosis of the *splenic artery* to the distal renal artery has also been employed with good results. In properly selected patients, the stenosis can be incised and enlarged by a *vein patch angioplasty*. A saphenous vein *autograft* from the aorta to the renal artery distally with a side-to-side anastomosis at both ends is probably the most commonly used and most successful procedure. Occasionally, the renal artery can be *reimplanted* into the aorta following excision of the stenosis. Arterial *autografts* have also been employed successfully, and *endarterectomy* is the procedure of choice of several surgeons with excellent results. The closure may require a patch venous graft or the use of a prosthetic graft. *Prosthetic arterial grafts* from the aorta to the distal renal artery may also be used. *Nephrectomy* may be necessary when obstructing lesions or aneurysms are present in branch or small accessory arteries. It may also be required in patients who have failed to respond to another reconstructive procedure. The various techniques are illustrated in Figure 35.

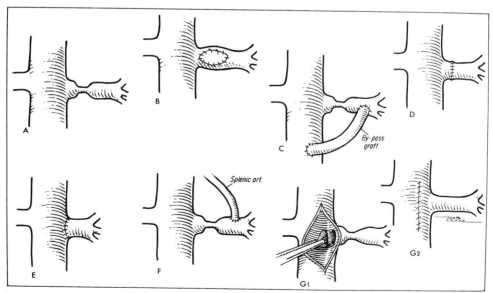

**Figure 35** Diagrammatic illustration of operations designed to relieve renal arterial obstruction in renovascular hypertension. *A,* The stenosis is usually located near the origin of the renal artery. *B,* An endarterectomy performed with the use of a patch graft to prevent narrowing at the time of closure. *C,* In most patients a bypass graft from the aorta to the distal renal artery is the most satisfactory operation. The graft can be either an autogenous vein or artery or a prosthetic graft. *D,* The stenotic area is excised, with end-to-end anastomosis of the renal artery. *E,* The stenosis is excised, with reimplantation of the renal artery into the aorta. *F,* The splenic is divided and its distal end anastomosed to the side of the renal artery beyond the stenosis. *G₁,* The aorta is temporarily opened, with endarterectomy performed from within the aortic lumen. *G₂,* After endarterectomy, the aortic incision is closed.

## RESULTS

Approximately 40 to 50 per cent of patients can be "cured" by surgical revascularization procedures and an additional 25 to 35 per cent "improved"; and the remaining 25 to 35 per cent exhibit essentially no change in their hypertension. The reported overall surgical mortality ranges between 5 and 10 per cent.

## SELECTED REFERENCES

Hunt, J. C., Strong, C. G., Sheps, S. G., and Bernatz, P. E.: Diagnosis and management of renovascular hypertension. Amer. J. Cardiol., 23:434, 1969.

*This review considers a series of 100 patients with renovascular hypertension from the Mayo Clinic. The clinical features, laboratory data, operative procedures, and results are reviewed in detail.*

Wylie, E. J., Perloff, D. L., and Stoney, R. J.: Autogenous tissue revascularization technics in surgery for renovascular hypertension. Ann. Surg., 170:416, 1969.

*This summary describes the results of nephrectomy and revascularization operations for the treatment of renovascular hypertension in 190 patients. The obstructive lesions of the renal artery were caused by fibromuscular hyperplasia in 80 patients and by atherosclerosis in 110. The surgical techniques and results are discussed in detail.*

## REFERENCES

1. Braun-Menendez, F., Fasciolo, J. C., Leloir, L. F., Munoz, J. M., and Taquini, A. C.: Renal Hypertension. Translated by L. Dexter. Springfield, Ill., Charles C Thomas, 1946.
2. Crocker, D. W., Newton, R. A., Mahoney, E. M., and Harrison, J. H.: Hypertension due to primary renal ischemia: A correlation of juxtaglomerular cell counts with clinicopathological findings in twenty-five cases. New Eng. J. Med., 267:794, 1962.
3. Goldblatt, H., Lynch, J., Hanzal, R. F., and Summerville, W. W.: Studies on experimental hypertension. I. The production of persistent elevation of systolic blood pressure by means of renal ischemia. J. Exp. Med., 59:347, 1934.
4. Gunnells, J. C., Jr.: Renal vascular hypertension. In: Earley, L., Sanders, C., Fudenberg, H., Dietschy, J., and Sanford, J., eds.: The Science and Practice of Clinical Medicine. New York, Grune & Stratton, 1972.
5. Gunnells, J. C., Jr., McGuffin, W. L., Jr., Johnsrude, I., and Robinson, R. R.: Peripheral and renal venous plasma renin activity in hypertension. Ann. Intern. Med., 71:555, 1969.
6. Helmer, O. M.: Presence of renin in plasma of patients with arterial hypertension. Circulation, 25:169, 1962.
7. Hunt, J. C., Harrison, E. G., Jr., Kincaid, O. W., Bernatz, P. E., and Davis, G. D.: Idiopathic fibrous and fibromuscular stenoses of the renal arteries associated with hypertension. Proc. Mayo Clin., 37:181, 1962.
8. Kauffman, J. J., Maxwell, M. H., Craven, J. D., and Okun, R.: Hypertension—primary and secondary. Ann. Intern. Med., 75:761, 1971.
9. Laragh, J. H.: Biochemical profiling and the natural history of hypertensive diseases. Circulation, 44:971, 1971.
10. Page, I. H., and Corcoran, A. C.: Hypertension: Review of humoral pathogenesis and clinical treatment. Advances Intern. Med., 1:183, 1942.
11. Romero, J. C., and Hoobler, S. W.: The renin-angiotensin system in clinical medicine. Amer. Heart J., 80:701, 1970.
12. Seldinger, S. I.: Catheter replacement of needle in percutaneous arteriography: New technique. Acta Radiol., 39:368, 1953.
13. Skinner, S. L., McCubbin, J. W., and Page, I. H.: Control of the renin secretion. Circ. Res., 15:64, 1964.
14. Tigerstedt, R., and Bergman, P. G.: Niere und Kreislauf. Skand. Arch. Physiol., 8:223, 1898.
15. Tobian, L.: Relationship of juxtaglomerular apparatus to renin and angiotensin. Circulation, 25:189, 1962.
16. Vander, A. J.: Effect of catecholamines and the renal nerves on renin secretion in anesthetized dogs. Amer. J. Physiol., 209:659, 1965.
17. Winer, N., Chokski, D. S., Youn, M. S., and Freedman, A. D.: Adrenergic receptor mediation of renin secretion. J. Clin. Endocr., 29:1168, 1969.
18. Wylie, E. J., Perloff, D., and Wellington, J. S.: Fibromuscular hyperplasia of the renal arteries. Ann. Surg., 156:592, 1962.

# 53

# DISORDERS OF THE LUNGS, PLEURA, AND CHEST WALL

## I

## The Development of Thoracic Surgery

*Hiram T. Langston, M.D.*

The thorax was the last of the body cavities to become a domain of surgeons because entry into it often resulted fatally. The last organ within this area to be approached surgically was the heart, where the narrow margin between mechanical intervention and death proscribed operation until fairly recently. Primary interest concerns the steps by which the thoracic cavity was broached and the means by which security in doing so was acquired. This is not the story of one man or one incident or even of any concise piece of research, but rather of the contributions from sundry fields of endeavor adopted by surgeons to insure that invasion of the chest for appropriate reasons could be done with ever increasing impunity.

It is clear that the first obstruction to successful intrathoracic surgery was posed by an open and uncontrolled pneumothorax. The ability to render a patient unconscious through narcosis did not alter this problem. It was obvious that the lungs had to maintain function. This problem was attacked in two basic ways. In the earlier attempts, the lung was kept inflated by application of positive pressure at the entry of the airway. In the mid 1890s, Quénu in Paris constructed, for enclosure of the head, a chamber in which increased pressure could be maintained or an anesthetic agent placed. Various tubes copied after those used in the intubation techniques required in laryngeal diphtheria were also adapted to serve a similar purpose. Tight-fitting face masks were at times likewise employed. These earlier attempts were, however, more or less isolated instances, and it seems that no clearly definable program evolved prior to early 1900.

In 1903, Sauerbruch, working with Mikulicz, developed a differential pressure chamber, reversing the approach and proposing to keep the lungs inflated by applying negative pressure to the chest. In this technique, the head remained outside the chamber at atmospheric pressure, and the thorax was enclosed within the chamber wherein subatmospheric pressure was created. This concept spread and such chambers were created to house not only the patient but the entire operating team as well. They were available both in the capitals of Europe and in America (Fig. 1).

In 1909, Meltzer and Auer exploited the concept of endotracheal intubation in a manner comparable to that in use today. They began with a simple tube used to insufflate the lungs and described their method as "continuous respiration without respiratory movements." Although use of endotracheal catheters and even possibly cuffed ones may date back to the experiments of Vesalius, the clinical application of the method for thoracic surgery is credited to Meltzer and Auer.

It is interesting that prior to World War II local anesthesia was frequently a favored technique of thoracic surgeons. The poor control of bronchial secretions and the ever present danger of aspiration during drainage procedures for empyema (particularly if a bronchopleural fistula existed), or of a lung abscess, dictated this technique because it insured that the patient could cough and have control over his own secretions.

Fear of the danger of deep narcosis with its obtunding effect on cough led many to combine nitrous oxide analgesia with local infiltration, particularly in operating upon tuberculosis, even while undertaking such extensive procedures as thoracoplasty. The evolution of various anesthetic agents has been of particular advantage to thoracic surgery.

The diagnostic potential of Röntgen's discovery of the x-ray in 1895 is obvious. The exciting possibilities of this discovery were so quickly recognized that attempts were being made before the end of 1896 to find practical contrast media. Although numerous investigators had studied the tracheobronchial tree of animals and patients,

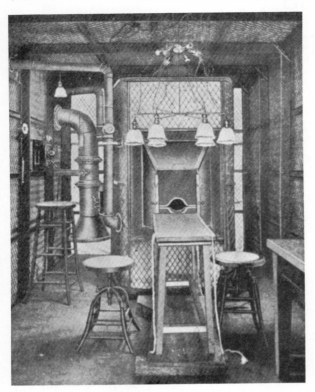

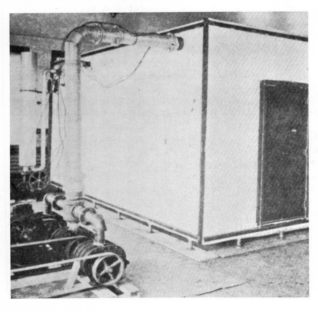

**Figure 1**    The Sauerbruch chamber as it was ultimately developed by Dr. H. Willy Meyer of New York City. The interior of the chamber accommodated the surgeons, the surgical table, and the patient's body below the neck. The patient's head and the anesthetist were enclosed in the smaller chamber shown at the end of the table, which provided positive pressure. This universal chamber then provided both negative and positive factors for control of surgical pneumothorax. (From Miscall, L., ed.: 50th Anniversary Booklet, American Association for Thoracic Surgery. New York, 1967.)

bronchography became an established technique only with the introduction of Lipiodol by Forestier and Sicard in 1922.

Discovery of means of inspecting remote body recesses long challenged physicians but was delayed by the problems of illumination. Visualization of the larynx under reflected light was first accomplished about 1858. It was von Mikulicz who developed esophagoscopy utilizing rigid tubes and reflected light in the early 1880s. He apparently extended this inspection into the stomach. Once direct laryngoscopic examination became feasible, inspection of the airway then followed. Killian is credited with being the "father of bronchoscopy" and demonstrated the clinical value of this method by removing a foreign body from the bronchus in 1897.

Just at the turn of the century, Einhorn devised

an esophagoscope with an auxiliary tube in the wall of the main tube that served as a light carrier to the distal end. In 1904, Chevalier Jackson combined the lighting principle of the Einhorn esophagoscope with the tube of Killian. The amazing skill acquired by the Jacksons, father and son, in the removal of foreign bodies and in the interpretation of changes induced by disease placed endoscopy apart as a highly developed field of specialization.

There is little doubt that the ability to replace blood losses by transfusion has been essential in the development of thoracic surgery and has permitted the specialty to become established. As the hazards and complications of blood transfusion, particularly the transmission of hepatitis, became more evident, greater care in blood utilization developed. Interestingly it was in the environment of thoracic surgery that the feasibility of utilizing the patient as his own donor (autologous transfusion) was demonstrated.

To one who never treated lung abscess, bronchiectasis, or empyema before the advent of penicillin, it is difficult to describe the toxicity, the chronicity, and the fetor of patients in nontuberculous thoracic surgical wards before 1945. The tedium of postural drainage, and of serial bronchoscopies to aspirate secretions and shrink the appropriate draining bronchial orifices by topical applications, and the interminable sessions of tube and dressing changes are difficult to visualize. By eliminating the former risk of flooding the bronchial tree during operation and dispelling the dread of spreading the disease by this means, the antibiotics have truly earned their reputation as "miracle drugs." The various antibiotics, properly selected, can change the course of suppurative pneumonitis from necrosis to resolution and can reduce, if not eliminate, the sputum of the patient with bronchiectasis. The greatly enhanced curability of pneumonia has rendered empyema, bronchiectasis, and lung abscess uncommon entities in daily practice.

In tuberculosis, equally profound changes have been effected by eliminating from surgical consideration most minimal and moderately advanced lesions but preserving from death the victim of advanced disease who then becomes a candidate for surgery. The antituberculous agents have changed the surgical approach in the disease from collapse procedures to resection. By shortening drastically the period of hospitalization, these drugs have eliminated the need for many of the sanatorium beds and have permitted care of this disease in general hospitals or even on an outpatient basis. Since tuberculosis incidence and mortality figures had dropped markedly before the availability of these drugs, control of the "white plague" must be ascribed to factors other than chemotherapy (Fig. 2). This, of course, is in no way to deny the tremendous impact that the antituberculous agents have on the course of the disease.

It seems strange that throughout the succession of wars no concerted opinion with respect to the

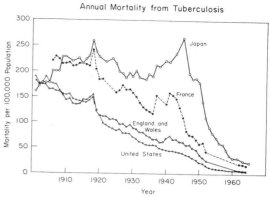

Annual Mortality from Tuberculosis

**Figure 2** This graph illustrates the value of general measures in the control of tuberculosis. It is seen that the mortality rates had been steadily falling in England and Wales as well as the United States long before antituberculosis drugs became available during the mid 1940s to early 1950s. These drugs did, however, accelerate the fall in mortality rates, and this was particularly dramatic in the case of France and Japan, as depicted in this graph. The effect of a breakdown in general control measures during World War I and World War II is highlighted by the experience in the latter two countries. (From Myers, J. A.: Dis. Chest, *51*:500, 1967.)

management of thoracic wounds evolved. It is clear that the ancients understood the significance of a "sucking" chest wound. Advocates of prompt closure recognized the immediate physiologic benefits, but the proponents of leaving such wounds open had in mind the provision of egress for the blood and ultimately the more or less inevitable pus. Many from the latter school did use packing or other means to establish controlled forms of drainage. The apparent lack of physiologic information kept the debate alive well into World War I. It is remarkable indeed that a method of preventing unwanted entry of air into the chest while providing for egress of blood or pneumothorax air took so long to evolve as an accepted practice. The mechanical methods for providing this closed drainage were devised in the latter part of the nineteenth century. The exact credit for this contribution in terms of priority appears to be due Hewitt in 1876 in England, von Bülau in 1891 in Germany, and Subbotin in 1888 in Russia. It is likely that von Bülau applied water-seal drainage as early as 1875 and thus is generally conceded to be the originator of the method.

The treatment of purulent pleural effusions, *empyema*, has followed an evolution similar to the development of the understanding of thoracic physiology. The critical time in this area came in 1918, when the United States was mobilizing its manpower for World War I. The pandemic of "influenza" and its complications attacked the aggregates of soldiers in various army camps. This infection in recruits was often followed by streptococcic pneumonia with a high incidence of empyema. It was the current practice to provide open surgical drainage as soon as the infected effusion was recognized. In the army camps the mortality reached 30 per cent with occasional peaks in some areas of over 70 per cent.

It was undoubtedly the rather satisfactory results achieved in civilian practice with open drainage of empyema that led to a similar practice in the military hospitals. The important difference, however, seemed to be that civilian experience was obtained principally with pneumococcic infections instead of streptococcic infections. The difference in behavior between these two infections helps explain the difference in results obtained by early surgical drainage. The pneumococcus produced a heavy fibrinous exudate and the surgeon had a better chance of entering a localized pleural abscess and much less risk of incurring a total pneumothorax at drainage. Furthermore, the pneumonic process had generally subsided before the onset of the pleural extension. Thus, pneumococcic empyemas were, in the main, postpneumonic. In contrast, the army experience involved empyema that was metapneumonic in time. Thus, when evacuation of this relatively thin pleural fluid was done by surgical drainage, an open and sucking pneumothorax often resulted, in a patient already very ill from pneumonia.

The physiologic studies performed by Graham and Bell as members of the U.S. Army Empyema Commission yielded great clarification of the pathologic physiology of pneumothorax and established the management of pleural empyema. These principles were: (1) drainage, but with the careful avoidance of an open pneumothorax during the period of active pneumonia; (2) early sterilization and obliteration of the cavity; and (3) maintenance of the nutrition of the patient. Open drainage was feasible when sufficient fibrinous deposit had occurred so that an encapsulated space might reasonably be expected. This point in time was suggested by the proportion of sediment to the total amount of a pleural fluid sample aspirated and allowed to settle overnight. Thus, when a sample of pleural fluid in a container taped to the bed showed 75 to 80 per cent sediment and 20 to 25 per cent supernatant liquid, the time for drainage had probably arrived.

The principal problem in chronic pleural disease was the pleural space that persisted without being filled by the expanding lung. In very simplified terms, if the lung would not rise to meet the chest wall, the chest wall would have to be taken to meet the lung. In a rather oversimplified manner, the various steps in accomplishing this can be illustrated by the following examples of thoracoplasties. The simplest is the *Estlander* type. This consists of subperiosteal removal of appropriate lengths of ribs so that the parietal portion of the empyema cavity can collapse centrally and help obliterate the residual cavity. Over large or total empyema cavities, the procedure begins at the first or second rib and extends as far as necessary, being staged as required by the magnitude of the resection.

A further step in insuring the obliteration of the empyema cavity is typified by the *Schede* thoraco-plasty. Here the full thickness of the parietal portion of the empyema space is resected — ribs, intercostal muscles, and parietal empyema wall — so as to saucerize the empyema space and allow the extracostal muscles to fall onto the visceral bed and ultimately obliterate it. This process is mutilating and slow in achieving its ultimate goal which is, of course, final healing and cessation of drainage. The final step is to remove the visceral "peel" of the empyema in order to allow the entrapped lung to balloon out and obliterate the space. This can be combined with resection of the entire empyema sac or merely resection of the visceral coat (Fowler or Delorme) or by crosshatching the visceral peel, permitting the lung to expand through this released area to fill the chest.

During World War II, a renewal of interest in the problems of the pleura took place. During the North African campaign, it became evident to Army surgeons that blood in the pleura does in fact clot. This was contrary to the suggestion that respiratory motion tended to defibrinate blood so that intrapleural blood remained liquid, in contradistinction to extrapleural blood which uniformly clotted. When this pleural clot became infected, the standard approach to management by drainage merely evacuated the center of the clot. The periphery of this clot remained as an organizing pleural peel.

On the conclusion that this was in fact the case, a direct attack on the problem resorted to thoracotomy and evacuation of the clot while also lifting the peel of organized fibrin from the lung surface, thereby allowing the lung to expand. The first such formal decortication was carried out by Burford in 1943. This became the established management for such an organizing hemothorax. Thoracotomy was advocated at 3 to 6 weeks after injury. At that time the "peel" was sufficiently established to permit handling with technical ease, yet had not gone on to sufficient fibrosis to make it a difficult undertaking. When infection was evident (hemothoracic empyema), an earlier thoracotomy was proper. Before this, surgeons had usually carried out a lesser procedure referred to as "turning out the clot." This limited intrapleural maneuver did in fact evacuate the clot but did not necessarily provide for prompt expansion of the lung. Suppuration was not unexpected under these circumstances because the organizing visceral peel tended to perpetuate the pleural space. Complete mobilization of the entrapped lung was carried out even in the face of infection. Although basically this was the same operation as that described by Fowler and Delorme, it was bolder and more efficacious. It was indeed a distinct conceptual contribution. How strange it is that lessons once learned can pass into oblivion to be revived at a later date.

Prior to assured control of open pneumothorax, surgery for neoplasms or suppuration in the mediastinum was undertaken through an extrapleural approach, with displacement of one or both pleurae for access and maneuverability. This was a tedious technique since disruption of the pleura changed the outlook for the procedure very decidedly. Control of surgical pneumothorax, however, permitted a free choice between an extrapleural and a transpleural approach as dictated by the exigences of the surgical problem.

As experience accumulated with resection of lung tissue, tension pneumothorax (incident to insecure bronchial closure) and infection were common causes of death. It emerged that greater likelihood of success existed when the pleural space was obliterated by adhesions so that air leaks and the products of infection could be limited. The efficacy of this circumstance, particularly in suppuration, led to the application of various maneuvers intended to reduce the postoperative pleural space. These included performance of thoracoplasties, the paralyzing of the hemidiaphragm, and production of pleural symphysis before or after the resection.

The induction of a pneumothorax followed by talc poudrage to the healthy lobe surface under visual control through a thoracoscope and prompt (it was hoped) re-expansion of the lung represented the ultimate in a first-stage lobectomy. The chest would be entered at a later date for separation of the diseased lobe and approach to the lung root. The hilar structures were generally managed by massive ligation. The encircling ligature, rubber tubing for example, was often left in place in the anticipation that the lung would slough in 10 days to 2 weeks. The pleural space would be packed. Refinements in means of narrowing the hilum as well as securing it by sutures permitted amputation of the lobe or lung rather than sloughing. Notable was the introduction of hilar tourniquets. These were essentially cord snares used to encircle the hilum so that appropriate suturing of the hilar stump could be safely carried out after the lobe had been amputated. They were applicable to lobectomy as well as pneumonectomy. In suppurative diseases, actual cautery to destroy the infected lung was also employed. This procedure was performed in stages and provided improved drainage of the area of pulmonary disease as well as extirpation of the offending portions of lung. Improved handling of the hilar structures by individual treatment of bronchus, arteries, and veins while under protection of an encircling tourniquet, and the provision of drainage for the pleura, led to improved results. From initial mortality levels of 50 and 60 per cent, Brunn could report a mortality rate of 13 per cent in a small series and Alexander a 16 per cent mortality rate in a somewhat larger group a short time after these procedures became available.

It is difficult to single out those responsible for the earliest successes with lobectomy. Amputation of some portion of lung with survival is recorded even in ancient times, and Tuffier is usually credited with the first successful resection of a tuberculous lesion by partial lobectomy in 1892. The frequency of pulmonary resection increased thereafter. For removal of an entire lung, priorities are somewhat clearer. In 1931, Nissen, working in Germany with Sauerbruch, extirpated a destroyed

left lung in a staged procedure using an encircling hilar ligature of rubber, allowing the lung to slough. In 1932, Haight, working with Alexander in Ann Arbor, likewise extirpated a left lung destroyed by bronchiectasis from a young woman. The resection was staged, the hilum was encircled with rubber tubes, and the lobes were allowed to slough. This represented the first successful pneumonectomy in the Western Hemisphere.

In 1933, Graham in St. Louis removed a left lung for epidermoid carcinoma using a rubber tourniquet for control, amputating the lung, securing the hilum with suture ligatures, and then removing the tourniquet. Although there were postoperative complications, the patient, a physician, survived for 30 years. The first successful resection of a right lung is credited to Overholt in 1934.

The individual ligation technique for lobectomy had apparently been used as early as 1912 by Davies in England but his patient succumbed. This approach was repeatedly used by Churchill for lobectomies after 1938. It was Churchill and Belsey who developed *segmentectomy* for the lingular division of the left upper lobe in cases of bronchiectasis. Shortly after Graham performed his operation, Reinhoff reported pneumonectomy by individual treatment of the hilar structures. Surgical advances spurred the quest for more detailed anatomic information, and even though this did incite anatomists to respond, the practical details of bronchial and hilar anatomy were supplied originally by the surgeons themselves. The greatest utilization of segmental resection in terms of volume came in the management of pulmonary tuberculosis.

Advances in the ability to examine the esophagus by x-ray and endoscopically elicited increasing interest in this organ. The field is still developing. Prior to better control of the physiologic problems with open thoracotomy, attack on diseases in this area was primarily extrapleural and endoscopic.

The first successful resection (with long survival) of esophageal carcinoma was performed by Torek in 1913. When reporting the successful resection of a carcinoma of the esophagus with intrathoracic esophagogastrostomy 25 years later, Adams and Phemister could find only some 30 limited successes in the interim.

Prior to the advent of antimicrobial drugs, the control of pulmonary suppuration was difficult. The medical management of bronchiectasis or lung abscess was not highly rewarding and surgical therapy was fraught with hazards. Neither approach offered great dependability of results. In the care of lung abscess, the various medical and supportive measures were applied, in the hope that the process would stabilize. If adequate drainage was not provided via the bronchial communication, external drainage was the approach of choice. After appropriate localization of the abscess and selection of the site where it contacted the chest wall and where pleural fusion was most likely, one or more ribs were resected, usually under local anesthesia. After it was ascertained that a pleural symphysis existed, the abscess cavity was entered, preferably by cautery, with the objective of sealing the lung parenchyma and insuring against air embolism. If symphysis was missing, gauze packing was placed and the wound closed, in the hope that this foreign body would cause symphysis to occur and be strong enough to support a drainage tract when the procedure was attempted again some 2 weeks later. Drainage from such abscesses was often prolonged, although a number of successful results were reported.

Efforts to reduce the ravages of *tuberculosis* began with the realization that total body rest provided the best marshaling of the defenses against the disease. This collecting of patients in one area generally provided with abundant fresh air to which was added rest and nutritious food established the sanatorium regime. All this stimulated interest in the disease and segregated its victims, thereby reducing the contagiousness of the process. The debate that had raged over contagiousness in this disease had been solved by the work of Koch when he isolated the tubercle bacillus and demonstrated his postulates.

The observation that nature tended to immobilize and contract the chest in tuberculosis sparked the concept of achieving this as a therapeutic measure. Measures ranging from the placement of sandbags or having the patient lie on the affected side to intercostal neurectomy and scalenotomy were suggested as means of immobilizing the thoracic cage.

Introduction of air into the pleura-pneumothorax to directly rest the lung was apparently conceived by Carson about 1825, applied by Forlanini in Italy just before the turn of the century, and highly publicized by Murphy in 1898. Saugman added control to the process by introducing the manometer in 1904.

When visceroparietal adhesions prevented appropriate collapse by pneumothorax, these adhesions were divided by cautery under vision through a thoracoscope. This operation was referred to as "closed" pneumolysis and was developed by Jacobaeus in 1913. Rarely was an open approach for dividing such adhesions considered. Complications of pneumothorax were frequent and effusions of pyogenic or tuberculous etiology were common. Limitations in re-expansion were all too frequent after the requisite 4 to 6 years of collapse had transpired and were associated with a penalty in reduced pulmonary function. During the 1940s, intraperitoneal injection of air, producing *pneumoperitoneum,* was used to elevate the diaphragms and cause pulmonary collapse. Although less liable to complications, this approach was also less effective.

Phrenic nerve paralysis produced by crushing the nerve in the neck, introduced by Stuertz in 1911, enjoyed great popularity as a simple yet reversible (in 6 to 9 months) means of elevating the corresponding hemidiaphragm. Permanent paralysis by sectioning or avulsing the nerve had little usage.

The idea of resecting ribs to produce pulmonary collapse, *thoracoplasty,* probably originated with de Cerenville about 1885. The technique underwent many modifications contributed by Brauer, Friedrich, Boiffin, Gourdet, Wilms, and Sauerbruch. It finally became established as the most reliable of the collapse procedures. Its standard form required resection of long lengths of the upper seven ribs subperiosteally in three stages, including removal of the transverse processes of the corresponding vertebrae after the manner of Alexander and O'Brien of Detroit (Fig. 3). Further elective collapse could be provided by anterior stages if necessary. Freeing the apex of the lung in an attempt to bring an upper lobe cavity to a point for better collapse under the thoracoplasty, a procedure termed "apicolysis," was practiced by Semb of Norway in the late 1930s.

The era of chemotherapy began with the intro-

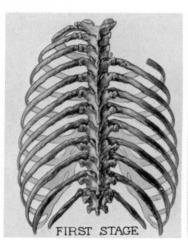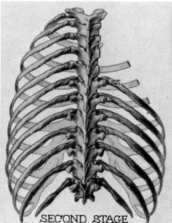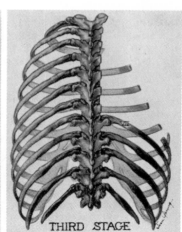

**Figure 3**   General schema for staged thoracoplasty as practiced by John Alexander. (From Alexander, J.: The Collapse Therapy of Pulmonary Tuberculosis. Springfield, Ill., Charles C Thomas, 1937.)

duction of streptomycin in 1944. In 1952, isoniazid was introduced and became the keystone of chemotherapeutic regimes. Prior to this time, resection had been infrequently employed in the treatment of pulmonary tuberculosis. It was found that patients with active pulmonary tuberculosis not brought under control by chemotherapy did poorly after these earlier resections. Insistence on conversion of sputum to negative and clearing of pneumonic areas of disease to a point of radiologic stability with drug therapy greatly improved the success of resection. The lesions that remained after these points had been reached by means of chemotherapeutic control became the targets of surgical resection. The efficacy of the new and improved drug regimens as well as the success of surgical programs has now greatly changed the prognosis of this disease.

## SELECTED REFERENCES

Alexander, J.: The Collapse Therapy of Pulmonary Tuberculosis. Springfield, Ill., Charles C Thomas, 1937.
*Afflicted by the very disease that led to his worldwide recognition, Alexander worked under the handicap of renal and osseous tuberculosis. This volume reflects the penchant for meticulous detail and completeness that characterized this highly disciplined man. It contains all that was of value in the management of pulmonary tuberculosis to the date of its publication in 1937. A medical counterpart, his long-time colleague, John B. Barnwell, was a contributor to the book.*

Brock, R. C.: The Anatomy of the Bronchial Tree with Special Reference to the Surgery of Lung Abscess. New York, Oxford University Press, 1946.
*This classic publication correlating an anatomic study of the bronchial tree with the clinical problem of lung abscess appeared at a time when antibiotics were changing surgical management in this disease from drainage to resection. It points up the relative scarcity of anatomic detail available from descriptive anatomists for the tracheobronchial tree.*

Craford, C.: On the technique of pneumonectomy in man. Acta Chir. Scand., Supp. 54, 81:1, 1938.
*This profusely illustrated monograph describes the experimental as well as the clinical experiences to that date. The author includes his own technique of anesthesia, thoracotomy, and management of the hilar structures.*

Delorme, E.: Précis de chirurgie de guerre. Paris, Masson et Cie, 1914, pp. 139–145.
*The very brief discussion of chest injuries in a monograph of at least quasiofficial stature from the pen of an eminent surgeon reflects the lack of insight into these problems during the early days of World War I (French).*

Eloesser, L.: Milestones in chest surgery. J. Thorac. Cardiovasc. Surg., 60:157, 1970.
*As invited speaker before the American Association for Thoracic Surgery in 1970, Eloesser, the oldest living member of that organization, recounted some of the milestones in thoracic surgery, to the delight of his audience.*

Graham, E. A., Singer, J. J., and Ballon, H. C.: Surgical Diseases of the chest. Philadelphia, Lea & Febiger, 1935.
*This volume is a repository for the ultimate views in thoracic surgery at the time of its publication (1935). The senior author, Graham, a giant among surgeons, a legend in his own time, pushed back many frontiers in surgical physiology. In the pages of this volume, the reader will find much that is basic to the development of thoracic surgery written while history was in the making.*

Hochberg, L. A.: Thoracic Surgery Before the 20th Century. New York, Vantage Press, 1960.
*This interesting book of considerable size brings together the nebulous background of fable and fantasy against which the halting yet firmer steps of the early 1900s laid the foundation for successful intrathoracic surgical maneuvers.*

Langston, H. T., and Tuttle, W. M.: The pathology of chronic traumatic hemothorax. J. Thorac. Surg., 16:99, 1947.

Samson, P. C., and Burford, T. H.: Total pulmonary decortication. Its evolution and present concepts of indications and operative technique. J. Thorac. Surg., 16:127, 1947.
*These two papers bring together the basic concepts evolved from the military experience of World War II concerning the fate of the blood in the pleura and what to do about it.*

Lilienthal, H.: Thoracic Surgery. Philadelphia, W. B. Saunders Company, 1925.
*This two-volume work is one of the comprehensive and early American texts on the subject. It represents the gleanings from a large surgical practice, described in voluminous detail, and includes many case histories that illustrate the opinions expressed. It appeared at a time when thoracic surgery was striving for stability as an emerging specialty, and clearly portrays the problems and conflicts of the era.*

Meade, R. H.: A History of Thoracic Surgery. Springfield, Ill., Charles C Thomas, 1961.
*This book culminates a lifelong interest in the history of surgery and specifically that dealing with the chest. It is exhaustive in scope, accurate in detail, and factual in its content. Above and beyond this, it contains much in the way of clinical assessment that lends flavor to the drier facts of history.*

Murphy, J. K.: Wounds of the Thorax in War. London, Oxford University Press, 1915.
*This monograph illustrates the imprecision of attitudes in management of chest injuries at the outset of World War I (British).*

Nissen, R., and Wilson, R. H. L.: Pages in the History of Chest Surgery. Springfield, Ill., Charles C Thomas, 1960.
*From the pen of the surgeon who first successfully removed an entire lung from a human being, this compendium is concise, accurate, modest, and entertaining. Profusely illustrated, it is a delight to read as it unfolds the story of thoracic surgery.*

Sauerbruch, F.: Die Chirurgie der Brustorgane. Berlin, J. Springer, 1920.
*This publication presents the output of the dynamic and imaginative service of the man who epitomized thoracic surgery in his time. His clinic attracted worldwide visitors interested in the infant specialty. The text is profusely illustrated by artists' drawings.*

Steele, J. D., ed.: The Surgical Management of Pulmonary Tuberculosis. Springfield, Ill., Charles C Thomas, 1957.
*This monograph, prepared by trainees of John Alexander and executed in his honor, brings together in contrast the two eras in pulmonary tuberculosis—that before and that after availability of effective chemotherapy.*

# II

# Anatomy

*Walter G. Wolfe, M.D.*

Marcello Malpighi in the seventeenth century demonstrated that the trachea terminated in dilated vesicles and not porous parenchyma. By inflating and then drying a lung, he demonstrated that membranous vesicles formed from the ends of the trachea which terminated "in spaces and unequal vesicles."[31] These observations made it clear for the first time that air passes from the trachea in and out of the sacs in the lung and provided the anatomic basis for true conception of the respiratory process. In 1880 Christoph Theodor Aeby published a treatise that was the first work of any consequence devoted to analysis of the branching of the bronchial tree.[5] Nine years later William Ewart, a pathologist, recognizing that the human lung must be divided into yet smaller regions than lobes, described nine bronchial distributions.[5]

In 1932 Kramer and Glass,[21] to better localize lung abscess, established smaller and more accurate units within the lobes which they named *bronchopulmonary segments*. Brock[7, 8] developed the clinical aspects of these segments and Churchill and Belsey[10] established the principle of the bronchopulmonary segments as surgical units. The importance of segmental anatomy was illustrated by Churchill and Belsey's observation that 80 per cent of patients with bronchiectasis in the left lower lobe also had involvement of the lower portion of the upper lobe. They named this segment the *lingula*. In 1943 the decisive studies of Jackson and Huber[16, 17] on the branching of the bronchopulmonary segments were reported and established the terminology accepted today.

While bronchial anatomy was of importance, development of microscopic anatomy led to the study of the lung as a physiologic unit. Malpighi described microscopic anatomy of the alveolus and used the terms "pulmonary artery" and "pulmonary vein." In 1733 Stephen Hales referred to the closed connections between artery and veins described by Malpighi as "capillary vessels."[31] The century-old question of whether alveoli of the mature lung were lined by continuous epithelium or whether the alveolar capillaries as viewed with the conventional light microscope were nakedly exposed to inspired air was resolved with electron microscopic studies of Low[25, 26] when he demonstrated a complete epithelial lining covering each alveolar surface. Electron microscopic study of the lung combined with physical and chemical studies of pulmonary tissue continues to complete and clarify the anatomy of the lung.

## EMBRYOLOGY

The primordia of the principal respiratory organs appear as a medial longitudinal groove in the ventral wall of the pharynx.[1, 12] The tube is lined with endoderm from which the epithelium of the respiratory tract develops. The cephalic part of the tube becomes the larynx, followed by the trachea, and from its caudal end, two lateral outgrowths arise, i.e., the left and right lung buds. From these, the bronchi and lungs develop. The right and left lung buds are initially symmetric. Their ends, however, soon become lobulated, three lobules appearing on the right and two on the left. During the course of development, the lungs migrate caudally so that by the time of birth, the bifurcation of the trachea is opposite the fourth thoracic vertebra. As the lungs grow, they project into that part of the coelom which ultimately forms the pleural cavities.

The pulmonary arteries form from the sixth arch.[1] Each pulmonary artery is closely related to the main stem bronchus and provides an arterial partner for each new bronchial ramification. As the airway-artery pairs enter first the lobe, then the segments, and finally lobules of developing lung tissue, they assume a central location in each and project branches toward the particular subdivision of the lung. As the veins develop, they receive tributaries from the pleura and the rich vascular networks developing about the growing tips of the respiratory tree. They arch across the base of the secondary lobules toward the periphery where they turn into the planes of connective tissue that separate adjacent pulmonary lobules. Interlobular veins unite to form and serve as tributaries to intersegmental veins, which, near the pulmonary hilus, combine in most cases into the superior and inferior pulmonary veins.

## ANATOMY

The respiratory system consists of the nose, nasal passages, nasopharynx, larynx, trachea, bronchi, and lungs. The respiratory tree functions proximate to the thorax and its bony and muscular components as well as to the pleura, pleural cavity, and mediastinum. The influence of pathologic changes in associated structures on the function of the respiratory system is important and one should be familiar with these anatomic relationships and the "topographical anatomy" of the thorax[12, 37] (Fig. 1). This chapter will consider only the tracheobronchial tree and the lungs.

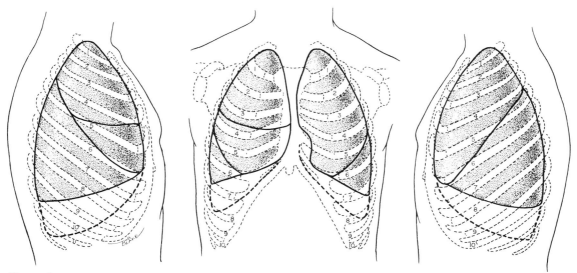

**Figure 1** The relationships of the pleural reflections and the lobes of the lung to the ribs. Topographic anatomy and the relationship of the fissures of the lobes to ribs in inspiration and expiration are important in evaluation of the routine PA and lateral chest film.

## TRACHEA

The entrance to the trachea is guarded by the larynx. It functions to prevent aspiration and as the organ of phonation and plays an important role in production of the cough. The mucous membrane lining the larynx is covered by ciliated epithelial cells and a few goblet cells. The epithelial surfaces in contact with food and pressure are covered by stratified squamous epithelium.[13] Except for the cricothyroid muscle, which is innervated by the external laryngeal branch of the superior laryngeal nerve, the larynx receives both motor and sensory innervation by way of the vagal accessory complex of nerve fibers. The intrinsic muscles of the larynx receive their motor innervation by way of the inferior laryngeal branch of the recurrent vagus nerve.[12]

The trachea is a fibromuscular tube 10 to 12 cm. in length and varying from 13 to 22 mm. in width, supported laterally and ventrally by approximately 20 U-shaped hyaline cartilages. The trachea originates at the level of the cricoid cartilage and descends through the superior aperture of the thorax and the superior mediastinum to its bifurcation at the level of the sternal angle (lower border of the fourth thoracic vertebra). Here it divides into the right and left primary bronchi. The spur formed at the point of bifurcation is called the carina. Half the trachea lies in the neck and the other half within the thorax.[12, 20]

The dimensions of the trachea are constantly changing with the movement of the head and neck. It is attached to a movable structure at both ends, namely, the larynx cranially and the pericardial sac and diaphragm caudally. During forced expira-

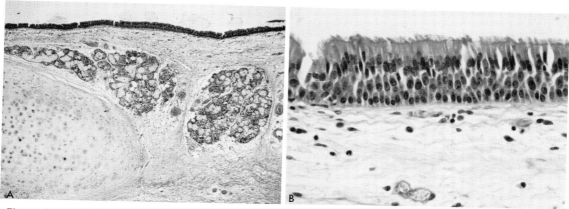

**Figure 2** *A,* Photomicrograph of human trachea demonstrating the relationship between epithelium, lamina propria, submucosa, and cartilage. × 45. *B,* Pseudostratified columnar ciliated epithelium containing goblet cells resting on an elastic lamina propria. × 400.

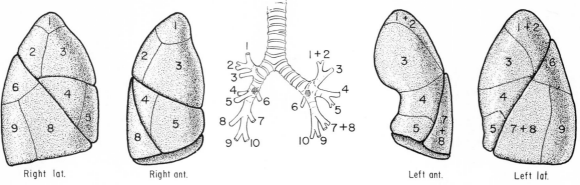

**Figure 3** Segments of the pulmonary lobes. (Modified from Jackson, C. L., and Huber, J. F.: Dis. Chest, *9*:319, 1943.)

tion, especially when the glottis is suddenly opened as in coughing, the trachea is markedly narrowed. In young subjects the lumen may be reduced to one-tenth its original size. Prior to cough, the bifurcation may ascend as much as 5 cm.[20]

The mucous membrane of the trachea rests on elastic lamina propria, beneath which is the sub-

mucosa. These layers are supported by another fibrous coat containing cartilage and smooth muscle. The dorsal membranous wall is fibromuscular. Smooth musculature elsewhere in the respiratory tree disposes in a helical arrangement about the airways; however, in the trachea it lies only in its dorsal wall. The submucosa varies in thickness with the thinnest portion on the inner surface of

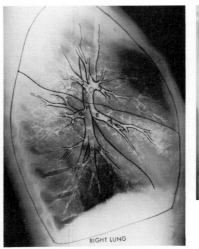
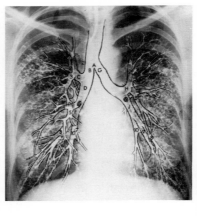
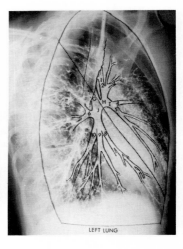

**Figure 4** Normal bronchogram. The major bronchi are indicated by the letters; segmental bronchi are numbered. Key for Figures 3 and 4

*Right*
1. Apical ⎤
2. Posterior ⎬ upper lobe
3. Anterior ⎦
4. Lateral ⎤ middle lobe
5. Medial ⎦
6. Superior ⎤
7. Medial (basal) RLL ⎥
8. Anterior basal ⎬ lower lobe
9. Lateral basal ⎥
10. Posterior basal ⎦

*Left*
1-2. Apical posterior ⎤
3. Anterior ⎬ upper lobe
4. Superior of lingula ⎥
5. Inferior of lingula ⎦
6. Superior ⎤
7. ⎥
8. Anterior-medial basal ⎬ lower lobe
9. Lateral basal ⎥
10. Posterior basal ⎦

A. Carina
B. R. main stem bronchus
C. RUL bronchus
D. Bronchus intermedius
E. RML bronchus

F. RLL bronchus
G. L main stem bronchus
H. LUL bronchus
I. Lingula bronchus
J. LLL bronchus

the cartilage and the thicker, more loosely organized portion being present on the muscular wall. In addition to blood vessels, nerves, and lymphatics, this layer contains the secretory portions of the mucous and serous glandular units. The trachea is lined with pseudostratified columnar ciliated epithelium containing goblet cells.[13] Near the basement membrane the formative cells may differentiate into new ciliated cells or goblet cells (Fig. 2).

## BRONCHI

At its termination, the trachea divides into the right and left principal bronchi. The right bronchus is 12 to 16 mm. in diameter and the left 10 to 14 mm. The combined cross-sectional area exceeds that of the trachea. The right main bronchus deviates less from the axis of the trachea than does the left; this explains why foreign objects entering the trachea more often lodge in the right bronchus or one of its branches.[12, 20]

Within a primary lobe, the secondary bronchus soon divides into tertiary branches which are remarkably constant in number and distribution. The segment of a lobe, aerated by a tertiary bronchus, is usually well delineated from adjoining segments by nearly complete planes of connective tissue. Knowledge of segmental anatomy is of great practical importance in radiology, bronchoscopy, and pulmonary surgery. Through painstaking anatomic studies of Jackson and Huber[16, 17] and others, the description of the segments of the pulmonary lobes has been completed (Fig. 3). Each segment is identified by its position in the lobe of the lung and the corresponding segmental bronchus is named for the segment it supplies (Fig. 4).

In the human lung, bronchial branches usually arise from bifurcations, and although the resulting branches are smaller than the parent stem, their total cross-sectional area is always greater by approximately six-fifths (Fig. 5). Structurally, large bronchi do not differ markedly from the trachea. Medium bronchi are distinguished by the large plates of cartilage, by the musculature, and by their relative abundance of glands (Fig. 6). The most peripheral airways containing cartilage are the terminal bronchi. The smaller bronchi have fewer glands, and are distinguished by rich venous plexuses between the muscular and cartilaginous fibrous layers. The effect of bronchial muscle contraction on venous and lymphatic channels probably plays an important role in propelling the vascular fluids toward the hilus of the lung. Also, these rich venous networks are thought to be an

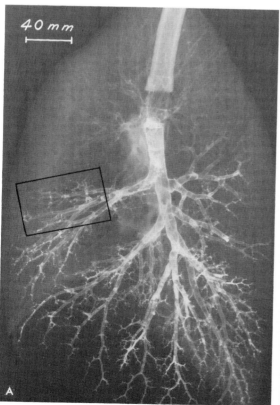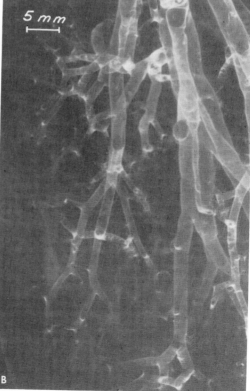

**Figure 5** The airways in a postmortem human lung outlined with powdered tantalum, demonstrating in fine detail the branching of the bronchi. (From Nadel, J. A., et al.: Invest. Radiol., 3:229, 1968.)

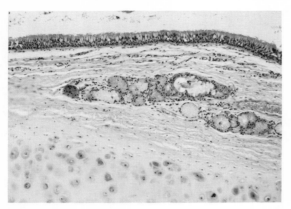

**Figure 6** Section through a bronchus. The relationship of the mucosa, glands, and cartilage is essentially the same as that seen in the trachea.

important factor in the warming of air en route to the pulmonary parenchyma[20] (Fig. 7).

The mucous membrane of the bronchial mucosa is made up of an epithelium, a basement membrane, and richly vascular and fibrous tunica propria. Like that of the trachea, the bronchial epithelium consists of pseudostratified ciliated and nonciliated cells, including goblet cells.[13] Peribronchial tissue consists of connective tissue that extends from the pulmonary hilus to the primary bronchioles. The peribronchium is continuous with the connective tissue investment of the arterial partners of the bronchi and the connective tissue sheath of the large veins. These connections form the basis for understanding the location and spread of certain types of edema and inflammation and the paths followed by air in and about the lung in interstitial emphysema. Interestingly, the peribronchium occupies a space in which subatmospheric pressure prevails. Von Hayek[14] feels that this subatmospheric pressure plays an important role in the flow of venous blood, lymph, and alveolar fluid as well as in migration of inhaled particulate matter.

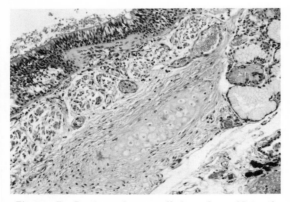

**Figure 7** Section of a small bronchus. Note the prominence of the muscle layer as compared to trachea and bronchi, and the rich vascular network between the muscular and cartilaginous fibrous layer. × 100.

## CILIATED, GOBLET, AND BRUSH CELLS

It has been demonstrated that each cilia-bearing cell has approximately 270 cilia. Each cilium originates in a basal corpuscle just beneath the cell surface and measures approximately 0.5 $\mu$ in length and 0.14 $\mu$ in diameter. The cilium is round on cross section and contains a pair of separate central filaments and a peripheral ring of nine paired, closely branched filaments. Cilia are phylogenetically ancient structures and all cilia, whether in the plant or animal kingdom, have the same basic structure.[18, 20, 36]

Although the cilia are borne by separate cells, these many thousands of cilia beat in an organized, coordinated manner. Studies have shown that they beat in a whiplike fashion, the cycle of activity being divided into a rapid forward propulsive stroke and a slower recovery stroke.[18, 20, 36] This propulsion is effective in moving a superimposed carpet of mucus along with a variable number of trapped particles and cells upward toward the larynx. The rate at which particulate matter is propelled by cilia varies according to species and that portion of the respiratory tree involved and has been recorded to be approximately 10 to 35 mm. per minute. The cilia do not beat within the viscous sheet of mucus but are bathed instead in fluid of considerably lower viscosity. The source of the fluid, factors controlling its viscosity, and rate of production are not known.[18, 27, 34] The ciliated cells disappear gradually as respiratory bronchioles are approached.

The nonciliated cells are the goblet and brush cells. Goblet cells occur singly and in groups between the ciliated epithelial cells. When filled with secretion, they are conspicuous by their bulging walls. In cases of chronic irritation of the tracheobronchial mucosa, there is marked increase in goblet cells at the expense of ciliated cells. It has been suggested that when mucus laden with particles of carcinogenic material has been carried to the branching point of an airway there may be a temporary stasis at that site owing to the local paucity of cilia.[20]

The brush cells are tall, standing from the basement membrane of the lumen of the airway. Electron photomicrographs demonstrate dovetailed cytoplastic processes rearing on their sides interlocking with neighboring goblet cells. This arrangement may serve to add mechanical stability to the epithelial sheet. Whether or not the brush cells are sustentacular in function or are the source of low-viscosity fluid that bathes the cilia is not known.[20, 35]

## BRONCHIOLES

Bronchioles are said to have a diameter of 1 mm. or less and to be devoid of cartilage support. Of all the airways, bronchioles have the highest proportion of smooth muscle in their walls relative to the diameter of the lumen. Since small bronchi are also without connective tissue sheaths, the fibrous

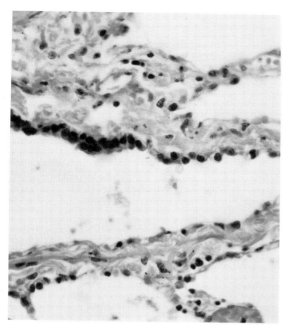

**Figure 8** Section of a terminal bronchus, demonstrating the cuboidal epithelium, which grades off into a flat epithelium near the alveolar entrances. Also, a large amount of smooth muscle is evident. × 400.

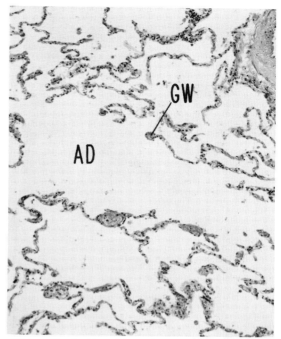

**Figure 10** Section of lung demonstrating an alveolar duct (AD) with its contiguous alveoli. Note that the alveolar duct is not a structural entity in and of itself. Its walls are, in fact, alveolar septa. GW is a cross section of a collagen bundle. These bundles are important in maintaining patency of the alveolar ducts and the openings into the alveoli. They are analogous to guy wires.

strands of the fibrocartilagines must extend peripherally into the mucous membrane of the bronchiole. The fibrous elements intermingle freely with the surrounding pulmonary parenchyma, exerting circumferential traction on the airway, maintaining its patency.

Bronchioles of the first order arise at the tip of the terminal bronchus and continue branching to produce three or four further divisions fully lined by cuboidal epithelium. The last to be lined is the terminal bronchiole. Estimates of the number of terminal bronchioles resulting from a single bronchus vary between 10 and 20 (Fig. 8).

A terminal bronchiole usually divides at an angle of 60 to 90 degrees into respiratory bronchioles, which in turn may give rise to further divisions. The branching of the terminal bronchiole is by no means uniform, as a single branch may be given off laterally and two or more may follow (Fig. 9). Respiratory bronchioles vary also in size (in man ranging from 1 through 3.5 mm. in length and approximately 1.5 mm. in diameter). The cuboidal epithelium stops abruptly at the entrance of the alveoli, which are lined by extremely thin squamous epithelium not revealed by conventional light microscopes. The last in a series of respiratory bronchioles usually bifurcate to produce the first in a series of alveolar ducts (Fig. 10).

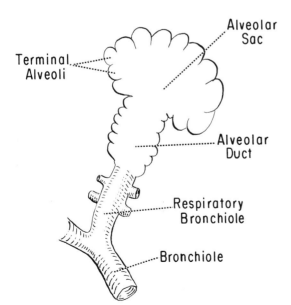

**Figure 9** The relationship of the airway in the periphery of the respiratory tree. Bronchioles lead to the respiratory bronchioles, which then terminate in the alveolar duct and the alveolar sac.

## ALVEOLI

The alveolar ducts terminate in one of several rotunda-like enclosures called alveolar sacs. The sacs bear a small and variable number of terminal alveoli. Like the alveolar ducts, the sacs lack

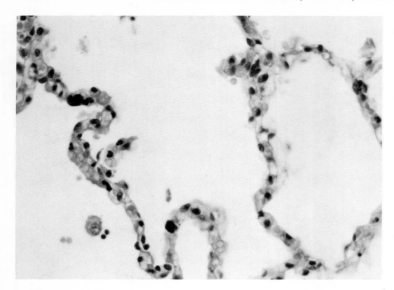

**Figure 11** Section through an alveolus. Light microscopy shows the blood-air interface as a simple thin line but when it is seen by electron microscopy (Fig. 12) it is a complex structure. Endothelial and epithelial nuclei are easily seen, but the cytoplasm of these cells cannot be resolved by light microscopy. × 400.

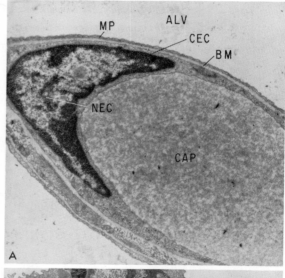

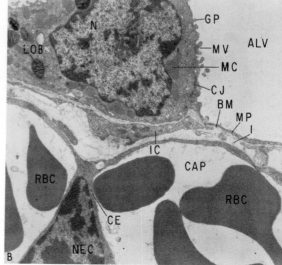

**Figure 12** *A,* Electron photomicrograph of an alveolus. This demonstrates the structure of the thinnest part of the blood-air interface. Note that the blood is separated from the alveolar air only by the attenuated cytoplasm of an endothelial cell and a membranous pneumocyte joined by a basement membrane. × 6700; print magnification 13,725. *B,* Note the relationship of the granular pneumocyte to the alveolar wall. The granular pneumocyte is an integral part of the alveolar lining. This cell has been referred to as "Type II cell," "great alveolar cell," and "alveolar phagocyte." It is thought to produce surfactant; the laminated osmiophilic bodies illustrated here may be surfactant or surfactant precursors. × 6700; print magnification 13,725. N, Nucleus of granular pneumocyte; LO, laminated osmiophilic body (these cells thought to be the site of surfactant production); GP, granular pneumocyte (sometimes called the alveolar Type II or the great alveolar cell); MV, microvilli; ALV, alveolus; MC, mitochondria; CJ, cell junction; BM, basement membrane; MP, membranous pneumocyte; I, interstitium; IC, interstitial cell; CAP, capillary; RBC, red blood cell; CE, capillary endothelium; NEC, nucleus of the endothelial cell; CEC, cytoplasm of the endothelial cell.

proper walls and open on all sides into alveoli. Each alveolus shares an entrance frame and a wall with its neighbor similar to two rooms being separated by a single wall. Because the alveoli surrounding an alveolar duct are an integral part of the pulmonary parenchyma, they are subjected to all of the stages of the respiratory cycle and to tractional forces which hold them open.

Pulmonary alveoli vary considerably in shape and size with the various mammalian species, corresponding in general to body size (Fig. 11). The factors determining the dimensions in given species are not clearly understood but probably relate to a combination of factors, including the metabolic rate of the animal and the number and size of red blood cells. In man, the alveoli are approximately 160 $\mu$ in size.[20]

## ALVEOLAR EPITHELIUM

The alveolar epithelial sheet rests on a basement membrane that lies on or near the basement membrane of the adjacent capillary. The structural layers composing the so-called air-blood barrier are the stratum of the alveolar epithelial cells, their basement membrane, the variable connective tissue layer, basement membrane of the capillary, and the cells of the capillary endothelium (Fig. 12).[2, 19, 25, 26, 32]

Knowledge of the structures separating the alveolar air and capillary blood is of importance. Alveolar epithelial cells are known to be sensitive to the noxious fumes and foreign particles that may be carried by the inspired air. Simple, rapid hypertrophy of the alveolar lining cell layer is possible and the cells are able to undergo metamorphosis into at least one type of alveolar phagocyte.[3, 14, 20, 29] The hypertrophy of the alveolar lining cells could provide the quantity of cells found in the pulmonary alveoli, in the alveolar cell carcinoma, and in the lung disease of sheep ("jagziekte").

There is evidence that some of the alveolar lining cells elaborate secretion products, one of importance being the surface-active fluid layer that lines pulmonary alveoli.[14, 20, 29]

## ALVEOLAR CAPILLARY NETWORK

Pulmonary capillary networks are the richest in the body, so dense that openings in them are frequently smaller than the diameter of the capillaries. Since the connective tissue fibers form the principal support of the capillary networks, any disease state, such as emphysema, in which there is destruction of the alveolar wall and supporting framework would permit stretching, attenuation, and destruction of the entire capillary bed.[23]

## PULMONARY AND BRONCHIAL VESSELS

The surgical anatomy of pulmonary arteries and veins, particularly their relation to each other and to other structures of the pulmonary hilus, is of obvious importance in pulmonary surgery. Knowledge of the "anatomy" of the normal pulmonary angiogram is critical so that pathologic conditions can be recognized (Fig. 13).[6, 12, 37] Pulmonary arteries and their ramifications are invested in connective tissue sleeves, permitting continuous spatial adjustments to changing positions and volumes of surrounding lung tissue. This permits marked dynamic changes in the arterial diameters while not imposing direct mechanical change on lung tissue.

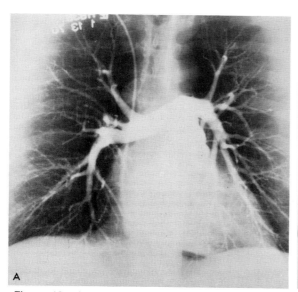
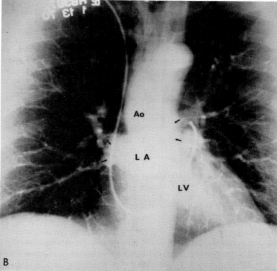

**Figure 13** *A,* Normal pulmonary angiogram illustrating the branching of the pulmonary arteries in the right and left lungs to their respective lobes. *B,* Venous phase of the same arteriogram demonstrating the superior and inferior pulmonary veins entering the left atrium (arrows). AO, Aorta; LA, left atrium; LV, left ventricle.

Pulmonary veins do not travel the same course as their arterial partners, a feature that is in marked contrast to the systemic circulation. They course along interlobular connective tissue planes and adapt longitudinally to surrounding parenchyma but cannot withdraw from it. The direct connection of vein to adjacent lung tissue by connective tissue fibers is the anatomic device that makes their diameter largely dependent on lung volume. This arrangement provides the mechanism for promoting venous return in the special situation of the low-pressure pulmonary circuit.

Although blood from the rich pulmonary capillaries undoubtedly supplies the metabolic needs of the pulmonary parenchyma, the many servant tissues (conducting airways, pulmonary vessels, lymphoid tissue, and so forth) require their own circulation supplied by vessels derived from the systemic circulation, the bronchial arteries. These originate either directly from the aorta or indirectly via the intercostals. Bronchial arteries accompany the bronchial ramifications and eventually lose their identity along the respiratory bronchioles where the capillaries that they supply drain into the alveolar capillary network and into the pulmonary veins. There is no bronchial vein corresponding to the bronchial artery; however, there is a rich peribronchial venous network that opens at many points into the pulmonary veins. Although the bronchial veins are described, their presence in normal persons has been questioned. They may, however, appear as sizable vessels in those with diseases such as pulmonary emphysema and mitral stenosis.[11, 23]

Literature on pulmonary vascular anastomoses covers more than two centuries of anatomic studies. Weibel's studies[41] have led him to conclude that pulmonary arteries and veins are end vessels and that there is no possibility for production of the collateral circulation. He found no precapillary arteriovenous pulmonary anastomosis that might permit blood to bypass the alveolar capillary net. Extensive studies of pulmonary vasculature and its anastomotic connection have been made by von Hayek.[14] He has described arterio-arterial communications between pulmonary arteries and bronchial arteries which are distinguishable by their remarkable thickness and unusual corkscrew course in addition to the abundant longitudinal musculature. Nothing is known at present about their importance in the regulation of vascular perfusion in the lung.

## PULMONARY LYMPHATICS

Pulmonary lymphatic vessels enter the hilar region in the second month of fetal life and continue to ramify and produce plexiform channels along the bronchi and pulmonary arteries and veins and in the subpleural connective tissue.[14, 20] According to Miller,[30] the lungs are more extensively supplied by lymphatics than the more metabolically active organs such as the liver and kidneys.

Studies of Tobin[38, 39] have demonstrated that pulmonary lymphatics do extend as far as alveoli. In most instances, the distance between the alveolus and the nearest lymphatic is extremely small. At the pulmonary hilus, the lymphatics, having gained both connective tissue and smooth muscle fibers, are relatively thick-walled and bear a histologic resemblance to the thoracic duct.

Collectively, the lymph nodes found along the lobar branches are called hilar nodes and are included in the great group of nodes about the root of the lung. The tracheobronchial nodes are usually larger on the right. On the left, one or more nodes are commonly related to the ligamentum arteriosum and thus to the recurrent branch of vagus nerve and to the vagal contributions to the anterior pulmonary plexus. Tracheal nodes form chains and are intimately related to the recurrent nerves.

## NERVE SUPPLY

Histologic studies and physiologic experiments have shown both afferent and efferent fibers present in the nerves that follow the vessels and airways to the lung.[12, 20] Right and left vagus nerves send one or more bronchial branches to the smaller anterior pulmonary plexus and many others to the rich posterior pulmonary plexus dorsal to the pulmonary hilus. A great many ganglion cells are found scattered along the cervical and thoracic portions of the vagus nerves. Those in the cervical vagus are thought to be sensory while the thoracic vagus is considered to be motor in function. Ganglion cells often lie adjacent to bronchial mucous glands and send short fibers with nonterminal twigs to the cells of glandular epithelium.

Sympathetic nerves arise from the second to fourth thoracic sympathetic ganglia and join the vagi in formation of the pulmonary plexus. The clinical and experimental evidence points to the presence of sympathetic bronchodilator fibers having cells or origin in spinal cord levels T2 to T4.

The phrenic nerve, in addition to the usual fibers of origin in the third to fifth cervical nerves, has been found to receive various contributions from the cervical sympathetics. A number of afferent fibers from the diaphragm as well as the mediastinum also appear to ascend in the phrenic nerve.

## COLLATERAL VENTILATION

In airways less than 1 mm. in diameter (bronchioles) reduction of normal traction forces in the lungs by infection, inflammation, fluid accumulation, or secretions singly or in combination may occlude the bronchial lumen. The consequences of such blockage may in some cases be offset by channels of collateral ventilation which form connections between well aerated alveoli and those normally supplied by the occluded small airway.

There are two principal mechanisms of collateral ventilation, interalveolar communications (pores of Kohn) and bronchial alveolar communications.

Alveolar pores are round to oval. Their shape and size are dictated by the delicate encirclements of elastic and other connective tissue fibers. As long as their fibrous framework is intact, the pores cannot enlarge beyond set limits. Alveolar pores may have the beneficial effect of preventing collapse of the lobules supplied by an occluded bronchiole. They may serve also as a temporary lodging place for alveolar phagocytes. Each communication may also provide pathways for the spread of fluid accumulations and for the transmission of bacteria between the communicating pulmonary lobules.[15, 29, 40]

In the past decade Lambert[22] described short, epithelial-like communications between distant bronchioles and neighboring alveoli. Such connections probably escaped discovery until recently because they are difficult or impossible to see in routine sections. They are approximately 30 $\mu$ in diameter, thus three or more times the diameter of most interalveolar pores. These communications are evidently able to remain open regardless of the degree of contraction of the bronchiolar smooth muscle. The benefit of pores may be shared only by the immediately adjacent alveoli while the bronchiole-alveolar communications provide means of aerating hundreds of alveoli. Recently, Chen[9] has demonstrated the dynamic nature of the collateral ventilatory channels.

## SELECTED REFERENCES

Boyden, E. A.: Segmental Anatomy of the Lungs, New York, McGraw-Hill Book Company, 1955.
*This excellent monograph not only reviews the historical development of the segmental anatomy of the lungs, but provides the groundwork for basic concepts of functional anatomy as it can be applied surgically and to the physiology of respiration.*

Hayek, H. von: The Human Lung. translated by V. E. Krahl. New York, Hafner Publishing Company, 1960.
*This monograph records the sophisticated anatomy of the respiratory system. It presents some of the newest concepts and findings in the functional anatomy of the lung and is one of the outstanding contributions to this field.*

Krahl, V. E.: Anatomy of the mammalian lung. In: American Physiological Society: Handbook of Physiology. Section 3, Respiration. Vol. I. Fenn, W. O., and Rahn, H., eds. Baltimore, Williams & Wilkins Company, 1964, p. 213.
*This chapter on the anatomy of the mammalian lung is one of the most complete treatises on the subject. It also contains more than 200 references, many of which are the original contributions that brought knowledge of the respiratory system to its present state.*

Perkins, J. F.: Historical development of respiratory physiology. In: American Physiological Society: Handbook of Physiology. Section 3, Respiration. Vol. I. Fenn, W. O., and Rahn, H., eds. Baltimore, Williams & Wilkins Company, 1964, p. 62.
*This chapter contains numerous pictures of original contributors to respiratory anatomy and physiology and also an extensive bibliography of the original works. It offers a complete review of the development and history of respiratory anatomy and physiology.*

## REFERENCES

1. Arey, L. B.: Developmental Anatomy. 7th ed. Philadelphia, W. B. Saunders Company, 1965.

2. Bertalanffy, F. D.: On the nomenclature of the cellular elements in respiratory tissue. Amer. Rev. Resp. Dis., 91:605, 1965.

3. Bertalanffy, F. D., and Leblond, C. P.: The continuous renewal of the two types of alveolar cells in the lung of the rat. Anat. Rec., 115:515, 1953.

4. Blumenthal, B. J., and Boren, H. G.: Lung structure in three dimensions after inflation and fume fixation. Amer. Rev. Tuberc., 79:764, 1959.

5. Boyden, E. A.: Segmental Anatomy of the Lungs. New York, McGraw-Hill Book Company, 1955.

6. Boyden, E. A.: The nomenclature of the bronchopulmonary segments and their blood supply. Dis. Chest, 39:1, 1961.

7. Brock, R. C.: The Anatomy of the Bronchial Tree with Special Reference to Surgery of Lung Abscess. 2nd ed. New York, Oxford University Press, 1954.

8. Brock, R. C.: The Anatomy of the Respiratory Tree. London, Oxford University Press, 1954.

9. Chen, C., Sealy, W. C., and Seaber, A. V.: The dynamic nature of collateral ventilation. J. Thorac. Cardiovasc. Surg., 59:518, 1970.

10. Churchill, E. D., and Belsey, R.: Segmental pneumonectomy in bronchiectasis. Ann. Surg., 109:481, 1939.

11. Ferguson, F. C., Kobilak, R. E., and Detrick, J. E.: Varices of bronchial veins as a source of hemoptysis in mitral stenosis. Amer. Heart J., 28:445, 1944.

12. Goss, C. M., ed.: Gray's Anatomy of the Human Body. 28th ed. Philadelphia, Lea & Febiger, 1966.

13. Ham, A. W., and Wilson, T. S.: The Respiratory System in Histology. 4th ed. Philadelphia, J. B. Lippincott Company, 1961, p. 663.

14. Hayek, H. von: The Human Lung. translated by V. E. Krahl. New York, Hafner Publishing Company, 1960.

15. Hesse, F. E., and Loosli, C. L.: The lining of the alveoli in mice, rats, dogs, and frogs following acute pulmonary edema produced by ANTU poisoning. Anat. Rec., 105:299, 1949.

16. Huber, J. F.: Practical correlative anatomy of the bronchial tree and lungs. J. Nat. Med. Ass., 41:49, 1949.

17. Jackson, C. L., and Huber, J. F.: Correlated applied anatomy of the bronchial tree and lungs with a system of nomenclature. Dis. Chest, 9:319, 1943.

18. Kilburn, K. H.: A hypothesis for pulmonary clearance and its implications. Amer. Rev. Resp. Dis., 98:449, 1968.

19. King, D. W., ed.: Ultrastructural Aspects of Disease. New York, Hoeber Medical Division, Harper & Row, 1966.

20. Krahl, V. E.: Anatomy of the mammalian lung. In: American Physiological Society: Handbook of Physiology. Section 3, Respiration. Vol. I. Fenn, W. O., and Rahn, H., eds. Baltimore, Williams & Wilkins Company, 1964, p. 213.

21. Kramer, R., and Glass, A.: Bronchoscopic localization of lung abscess. Ann. Otol., 41:1210, 1932.

22. Lambert, M. W.: Accessory bronchial alveolar channels. Anat. Rec., 127:472, 1957.

23. Liebow, A. A.: Pulmonary emphysema with special reference to vascular changes. Amer. Rev. Resp. Dis., 80:67, 1959.

24. Loosli, C. G.: Interalveolar communications in normal and in pathologic mammalian lungs. Arch. Path., 24:743, 1937.

25. Low, F. N.: Electron microscopy of the rat lung. Anat. Rec., 113:437, 1952.

26. Low, F. N.: The pulmonary alveolar epithelium of laboratory mammals and man. Anat. Rec., 117:241, 1953.

27. Luchsinger, P. C., LaGarde, B., and Kilfeather, J. E.: Particle clearance from the human tracheobronchial tree. Amer. Rev. Resp. Dis. 97:1046, 1968.

28. Macklin, C. C.: Alveolar pores and their significance in the human lung. Arch. Path., 21:202, 1936.

29. Macklin, C. C.: The alveoli of the mammalian lung. An anatomical study with clinical correlations. Proc. Inst. Med. Chicago, 18:78, 1950.

30. Miller, W. S.: The Lung. 2nd ed. Springfield, Ill., Charles C Thomas, 1947.

31. Perkins, J. F.: Historical development of respiratory physiology. In: American Physiological Society: Handbook of Physiology. Section 3, Respiration. Vol. I. Fenn, W. O., and Rahn, H., eds. Baltimore, Williams & Wilkins Company, 1964, p. 62.

32. Porter, K., and Bonneville, M. A.: Fine Structure of Cells and Tissues. Philadelphia, Lea & Febiger, 1968.

33. Pratt, P. C., and Klugh, G. A.: A technique for the study of

ventilatory capacity, compliance, and residual volume of excised lungs and for fixation, drying, and serial sectioning in the inflated state. Amer. Rev. Resp. Dis., *83*:690, 1961.

34. Quinlan, M. F., Salman, S. D., Swift, D. L., Wagner, H. N., Jr., and Proctor, D. F.: Measurement of mucociliary function in man. Amer. Rev. Resp. Dis., *99*:13, 1969.
35. Rhodin, J. A. G.: An Atlas of Ultrastructure. Philadelphia, W. B. Saunders Company, 1963.
36. Spock, A., Heick, H. M. C., Cress, H., and Logan, W. S.: Abnormal serum factor in patients with cystic fibrosis of the pancreas. Pediat. Res., *1*:173, 1967.

37. Thorek, P.: Anatomy in Surgery. Philadelphia, J. B. Lippincott Company, 1962.
38. Tobin, C. E.: Lymphatics of the pulmonary alveoli. Anat. Rec., *120*:625, 1954.
39. Tobin, C. E.: Pulmonary lymphatics with reference to emphysema. Amer. Rev. Resp. Dis., *80*:50, 1959.
40. Van Allen, C. M., and Lindskog, G. E.: Collateral respiration in the lung. Role in bronchial obstruction to prevent atelectasis and to restore patency. Surg. Gynec. Obstet., *53*:16, 1931.
41. Weibel, E. R., and Gomez, D. M.: Architecture of the human lung. Science, *137*:577, 1962.

# III

# Lung Function: Physiologic Considerations Applicable to Surgery

*Myron B. Laver, M.D., and W. Gerald Austen, M.D.*

*For it is much more high and philosophical to discover things a priori than a posteriori.*
— Robert Boyle, *Sceptical Chymist*, 1661

A significant advance in patient care has been achieved since we have recognized that acute respiratory failure is a likely complication in the critically ill patient and that successful prevention of pulmonary problems requires early and aggressive support of lung function. Both are particularly relevant when the surgery is extensive, when the patient has been the victim of severe body trauma, or when he has suffered the consequences of chronic lung disease.

Knowledge of the factors that control lung function will allow for early implementation of prophylactic measures or ventilator support and reduce significantly the morbidity and mortality associated with abnormal blood gas exchange.

The considerations to follow will be addressed to the following aspects of lung function: (1) mechanics of gas movement; (2) distribution of ventilation; (3) distribution of blood flow; (4) blood-gas exchange; (5) diffusion of gas between upper airway and pulmonary capillary blood; and (6) respiratory failure.

## MECHANICS OF GAS MOVEMENT

Ventilation is composed of three sequential phenomena: pressure change, followed by gas flow, and, finally, volume displacement. The lungs and chest wall (i.e., chest cage and diaphragm) exhibit changes in physical characteristics during the process of ventilation that can be subjected to mathematical formulations. Depending on body position, the abdominal contents may exert a highly restrictive effect on diaphragmatic motion and may in turn influence the effectiveness of pulmonary mechanics.

The action of the respiratory muscles is directed toward overcoming elastic recoil of the lung parenchyma and resistance to gas flow in the major airways, better known as flow resistivity. Deformation of the tissues involved, or viscous resistance, is also a component of flow resistivity, but the energy required to overcome it is small, and we usually consider flow resistivity as the work expended to achieve movement of gas.

The changes in volume, flow, and pressure characteristics for a single respiratory cycle are shown in Figure 1. This is all the information necessary for derivation of the formulas that define ventilatory mechanics.

Elastic recoil (elastance) is expressed as a relationship of change of pressure produced by a step change of volume:

$$\text{Elastance (cm. } H_2O/\text{ml.)} = \frac{\text{Pressure change (cm. } H_2O)}{\text{Volume change (ml.)}} \quad (1)$$

The reciprocal of elastance is called compliance (expressed as ml./cm. $H_2O$) and is preferred for a description of elastic property since the dynamic change we usually introduce is one of volume (V) for which a change in pressure (P) is recorded (i.e., pressure is the independent variable). The changes in volume and pressure seen during inspiration and expiration are shown in Figure 2 (P-V curve).

Compliance of the respiratory system (i.e., volume change per unit pressure) can be calculated by noting the change in volume and pressure

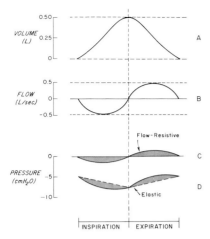

**Figure 1** Changes in volume, flow, and esophageal (pleural) pressure during a complete respiratory cycle. Zero flow is recorded at three points where the flow curve crosses the x-axis. At peak inspiration, the volume displaced is approximately 0.5 liter (curve $A$), while the change in pressure (between points of zero flow) is from $-5$ to $-8$ cm. $H_2O$ or 3 cm. $H_2O$ (curve $D$). Thus, lung compliance equals 0.5/3 or 0.167 liter/cm. $H_2O$.

The dashed line on curve $D$ was drawn between points of zero flow. The difference in pressure between dashed and solid lines on curve $D$, divided by the flow (curve $B$) recorded at the same point in the respiratory cycle, is equal to the resistance in cm. $H_2O$/liter/sec. Curve $C$ is the flow-resistive curve redrawn with the ordinate equal to the pressure differences obtained from curve $D$. The rate of change of elastic pressure (dashed line, curve $D$) is constant throughout inspiration and expiration (although not strictly true, it is a permissible assumption); rate of change of flow-resistive pressure varies as flow changes (solid line, curve $C$). (From Mead, J., and Martin, H.: Phys. Ther., $48$:478, 1968.)

on the appropriate curves shown in Figure 1. The change in pressure is required to overcome elastic recoil as well as resistance to flow. These two can be separated, and the pressure change necessary for overcoming elastic recoil can be assessed if we choose a point during the respiratory cycle when resistance to flow (i.e., flow-resistive pressure) is zero. According to Figure 1, we note that flow is equal to zero when inspiration is complete, immediately before expiration is initiated. At this point, no pressure change can be attributed to flow, and the relationship between increase in lung volume and change in pressure across the lung is equal to lung compliance. Reading from these curves, we have:

$$\text{Compliance} = \frac{0.5 \text{ liter}}{(8-5) \text{ cm. } H_2O} = 0.17 \text{ liter/cm. } H_2O$$
(2)

If we draw a straight line between points of zero flow (dashed line, curve $D$), we are implying that compliance, or volume change per unit pressure, remains constant throughout the respiratory cycle. Therefore, the pressure difference between the total pressure generated (solid line, curve $D$) and the pressure exerted to overcome elastic recoil

(dashed line, curve $D$) represents the pressure needed to overcome resistance to flow. This difference has been replotted for the entire respiratory cycle as curve $C$. The flow-resistive pressure curve generally has the same shape as curve $B$, the curve defining gas flow at the mouth, implying the need for greater pressure to overcome resistance to flow when the flow rate rises. Although a high flow rate results in turbulence and a corresponding increase in resistance to flow, it is *not* accompanied by a change in compliance (i.e., the area between the dashed and solid lines of curve $D$ may vary without changing the pressure coordinates at zero flow).

Figure 1 also allows calculation of resistance to flow by relating the flow-resistive pressure to the value for flow at any particular point:

$$R = \frac{P_{RES}}{V}$$
(3)

where

$R$ = resistance (cm. $H_2O$/liter/sec.)
$P_{RES}$ = flow-resistive pressure (cm. $H_2O$)
$V$ = gas flow (liter/sec.)

During normal tidal ventilation, expiration is a passive process. An increased resistance to expiratory flow may be caused by a narrowing of major airways secondary to edema, spasm, excessive secretions, or external pressure, so that an otherwise passive process may be transformed into one that requires active work and greater consumption of oxygen. Thus, we may be able to eliminate the need for inspiratory work, if the patient receives controlled mechanical ventilation during or after surgery, but without influencing the need for work on expiration. An overdistended lung, a narrowed or obstructed airway, and a high flow rate are factors that in combination lead to expiratory work. To ensure proper emptying of the lung, it is best to use slow frequencies during mechanical ventilation and insist on adequate preoperative preparation whenever pre-existing lung disease may increase the possibility of retained secretions during the postoperative period.

The work expended by the respiratory muscles during inspiration can be expressed as a product of the pressure generated and the volume of tidal ventilation. Inspiratory work is achieved to overcome elastic recoil and flow resistance. Reference to Figure 2 indicates how this work can be calculated. The elastic component of pressure ($P_{EL}$) is expressed by the straight line AC (slope equals change of volume divided by change of pressure and in turn equals compliance). Area ABC, which represents elastic work ($W_{EL}$), is simply:

$$W_{EL} = \frac{1}{2} P_{EL} \times V_T$$
(4)

Where $V_T$ = tidal volume (ml.)

However, $P_{EL}$ is related to compliance (C); therefore:

$$C = \frac{V_T}{P_{EL}} \quad \text{or} \quad P_{EL} = \frac{V_T}{C}$$
(5)

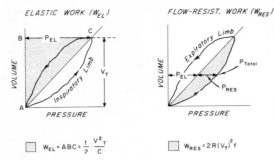

$$W_{EL} = ABC = \frac{1}{2} \cdot \frac{V_T^2}{C}$$

$$W_{RES} = 2R(V_T)^2 f$$

**Figure 2**  Calculation of the work of breathing ($W_{EL}$ + $W_{RES}$). Work of breathing (W) is the sum of work required to overcome elastic recoil ($W_{EL}$) and flow resistivity ($W_{RES}$). The sum of the two shaded areas represents the total work of breathing. Area at left ($W_{EL}$) is simply the area of the triangle ABC; area at right ($W_{RES}$) can be obtained directly by planimetry or by applying certain mathematical assumptions. The formula in the text for $W_{RES}$ is approximate at best and is given only to indicate relationships between work, tidal volume, and respiratory frequency. Note that work performed against elastic recoil is not frequency-dependent (f does not appear in the formula used to calculate area); on the other hand, work expended to overcome resistance to flow is frequency-dependent. Total pressure ($P_{TOTAL}$) developed during inspiration is the sum of elastic pressure ($P_{EL}$) and flow-resistive pressure ($P_{RES}$) as indicated in the right-hand loop. (From Mead, J., and Martin, H.: Phys. Ther., 48:478, 1968.)

Substituting for $P_{EL}$ in equation 4, we have:

$$W_{EL} = \frac{1}{2} \times \frac{V_T^2}{C} \qquad (6)$$

According to equation 6, a small rise in tidal volume will increase the work required to overcome elastic recoil more than a small fall in compliance. Consequently, if a patient has a low compliance, he will attempt to ventilate with smaller tidal volumes (and consequently more rapid frequencies) in order to minimize the work of breathing.

Work performed against resistance to flow is another component of the energy normally dissipated during respiration. This work is represented by the stippled area shown under the flow-resistive work curve in Figure 2. Inspection of this pressure-volume curve indicates that certain simplifying assumptions are necessary to facilitate calculation of the appropriate area. The detailed formulations are beyond the scope of this brief introduction, and the following expression is presented for descriptive purposes only. Details of its derivation are available by reference to the original literature.[1]

Thus:

$$W_{RES} = 2R \cdot (V_T)^2 \cdot f \qquad (7)$$

where  $W_{RES}$ = flow-resistive work
  R  = resistance to flow
  $V_T$  = tidal volume
  f  = frequency

Total work is equal to the sum of $W_{EL}$ + $W_{RES}$ (i.e., equations 6 and 7):

$$\text{Total work of breathing} = \frac{1}{2}\frac{V_T^2}{C} + 2R\,(V_T)^2\,f \qquad (8)$$

According to equation 8, an increase in tidal volume adds considerably more work to overcome resistance to flow than an increase in respiratory frequency.

The work expended for normal breathing at rest is approximately 6 kg.-m. or 3 ml. $O_2$/min. Oxygen consumed ($\dot{V}_{O_2}$) for the work of breathing at rest cannot be calculated directly. It can be estimated by measuring the change in body oxygen consumption achieved when a load (elastic or resistive) is

**TABLE 1**  EFFECT OF MODERATE AND HEAVY EXERCISE ON THE OXYGEN REQUIRED FOR BREATHING

Heavy exercise is accompanied by a 10-fold increase in oxygen consumption. The distribution of elastic and resistive work is reversed as compared with quiet breathing (elastic component falls from 66 to 39 per cent, and the resistive component rises from 33 to 61 per cent). A change from quiet breathing to heavy exercise is associated with a fivefold rise in tidal volume but only a threefold increase in respiratory frequency. See also equation 8 in the text. Maximal voluntary ventilation is achieved by a significantly greater increase in frequency than tidal volume as compared with heavy exercise. The elastic component is smaller and the resistive component higher than during heavy exercise. An increase in minute ventilation during the postoperative period is achieved by increasing work to overcome resistance to gas flow. Thus an increase in respiratory rate is indicative of inefficient respiration and incipient respiratory failure.

| Condition | External Work (kg.-m./ min.) | Tidal Vol. (ml.) | Resp. Rate (breaths/ min.) | Min. Vol. (L./min.) | $O_2$ Consumption (ml./min.) | Respiratory Work (kg.-m./ min.) | (% elastic) | (% resistive) | ($O_2$ cost ml./min.) |
|---|---|---|---|---|---|---|---|---|---|
| Quiet breathing | 0 | 500 | 15 | 7.5 | 300 | 0.3 | 66 | 33 | 3 |
| Moderate exercise | 620 | 1600 | 23 | 37.0 | 1500 | 5.2 | 57 | 43 | 52 |
| Heavy exercise | 1660 | 2400 | 48 | 115.0 | 3500 | 35.2 | 39 | 61 | 352 |
| Maximal voluntary ventilation | 0 | 1500 | 120 | 180 | — | 65.0 | 20 | 80+ | — |

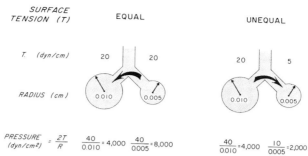

**Figure 3** Effect of distribution of airway diameter (R) and surface tension (T) on direction of gas flow between terminal airways. It is assumed that T remains constant during changes in volume (i.e., inspiration or expiration). At left, surface tension is equal in both alveoli; the transmural pressure for the individual gas spaces can be calculated from the Laplace expression: P = 2T/R. Since the alveolus at left is larger, its transmural pressure will be lower, and gas will flow from right to left as indicated by the arrow. If the distribution of surface tensions is unequal, then gas will flow in the reverse direction. Were this to occur in situ, then all gas spaces in the lung would empty into one alveolus and the lung would end up as a single giant balloon. Since the inhomogeneity of airway size persists in the normal lung, we must assume that changes in airway diameter (i.e., volume) are associated with continuous changes in surface tension. Thus the smallest alveoli must have the lowest surface tension in order to reaccommodate for the reduction in R. Considered in practical terms, a progressive reduction in T (as volume diminishes) serves as a protective mechanism against collapse whenever size is reduced toward a critical volume. Conversely, if surface tension is high because of pathologic changes within the lung, a large transmural pressure must be generated in order to prevent alveolar collapse. Some patients cannot achieve it in the postoperative period, and the elevated pressure can be provided only by a mechanical ventilator. (Redrawn from Nunn, J. F.: Applied Respiratory Physiology. New York, Appleton-Century-Crofts, 1969.)

added during the respiratory cycle. This allows us to plot the oxygen consumption for each increment of load and extrapolate the oxygen requirements under basal conditions, when no load is present.

The increase in ventilation following increasing levels of exercise leads to a disproportionate rise in oxygen consumption by the muscles of respiration (see Table 1). In fact, at the highest levels of exercise, the additional oxygen uptake achieved by the increase in ventilation is no longer adequate to provide the oxygen needed for the work of breathing, and the distribution of available oxygen becomes a limiting factor in performance.

We have noted earlier that the pressure-volume relationship of the lung is characterized by significant difference in the curves obtained during inspiration and during expiration (see Figs. 2 and 3). If one removes the lung from the chest cavity and fills the lung with liquid (e.g., saline), then the pressure-volume curves obtained during inspiration and expiration are superimposed. This difference between the gas-filled and liquid-filled lung is due to the presence of surface-active material ("surfactant"), which lines the terminal airways and maintains the geometric integrity of the lung. The interaction between transmural pressure, surface tension, and radius of the terminal airway is defined by the Laplace expression:

$$P = \frac{2T}{R} \tag{9}$$

where  P = transmural pressure (dynes/cm.²)
       T = surface tension (dynes/cm.)
       R = radius (cm.)

Pressure and radius fluctuate during the normal respiratory cycle. If surface tension (T) were to

remain constant throughout, then the regional differences in radii (R) would be accompanied by a greater discrepancy in regional pressure (P), and the lung would become sufficiently unstable for all high-pressure alveoli to empty into those with

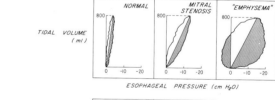

**Figure 4** Mechanics of breathing in patients with mitral stenosis and chronic obstructive lung disease ("emphysema"). Slope of the diagonal line that connects the extremes of the pressure-volume loop (change in volume/change in pressure) equals lung compliance in ml./cm. H₂O. A decrease in slope indicates a fall in compliance, and this is apparent in the presence of mitral stenosis or in "emphysema." Values for compliance are similar in these disorders; however, the work required to overcome resistance to flow is normal in patients with mitral valve disease but markedly increased (from 20 to 68 per cent of total work of breathing) in "emphysema." The pressure-volume loops are defined by the inspiratory limb (right of the diagonal) and an expiratory limb (left of the diagonal). During expiration, the line defining the pressure-volume relationship moves to the left of the y-axis in "emphysema," indicating the need for active work during the second half of expiration. End-expiration is at the origin. (From Turino, G. M., and Fishman, A. P.: J. Chron. Dis., 9:510, 1959.)

**TABLE 2**   WORK AND OXYGEN COST OF BREATHING IN MITRAL STENOSIS AND
CHRONIC OBSTRUCTIVE LUNG DISEASE ("EMPHYSEMA") AS
COMPARED WITH THE NORMAL INDIVIDUAL*

The increase in the oxygen cost of breathing due to a rise in minute ventilation differs little in the presence of mitral stenosis as compared with the normal person (threefold increase); however, in absolute values the rise is greater in mitral stenosis owing to elevated control values. In "emphysema," compliance decreases significantly as minute ventilation is increased, and the rise in ventilation is achieved with higher frequency and lower tidal volume than in mitral stenosis. This permits a lesser increase in the work of breathing necessary to overcome the abnormal resistance to gas flow (see equation 7). The increase in respiratory frequency requires an increase in work done against high air-flow resistance; accommodation is achieved by a reduction in tidal volume. Oxygen cost of breathing was calculated from the work of breathing on the assumption of a respiratory muscle efficiency of 5 per cent.

| Diagnosis, Age, Sex | Compliance (ml./cm. $H_2O$) | Respiratory Rate (per min.) | Tidal Volume (ml.) | Minute Ventilation (L./min.) | Work of Breathing (kg.-m./L. of expired tidal vol.) | Oxygen Cost of Breathing (ml./L. of expired tidal vol.) |
|---|---|---|---|---|---|---|
| Normal | 192 | 24 | 336 | 8.07 | 0.015 | 0.3 |
| 27, F. | 195 | 18 | 876 | 15.8 | 0.030 | 0.6 |
| | 160 | 43 | 438 | 18.8 | 0.026 | 0.5 |
| | 138 | 63 | 438 | 27.4 | 0.050 | 0.9 |
| Mitral stenosis | 61 | 25 | 418 | 10.6 | 0.045 | 0.8 |
| with severe | 63 | 18 | 811 | 14.7 | 0.070 | 1.2 |
| pulmonary | 50 | 44 | 581 | 24.3 | 0.107 | 1.9 |
| congestion | 43 | 67 | 551 | 36.7 | 0.133 | 2.4 |
| 30, F. | | | | | | |
| Pulmonary emphysema | 54 | 17 | 576 | 10.0 | 0.17 | 3.0 |
| with bronchial | 36 | 33 | 380 | 12.7 | 0.19 | 3.4 |
| obstruction, | 18 | 46 | 349 | 16.1 | 0.23 | 4.1 |
| severe | | | | | | |
| 55, M. | | | | | | |

*From Turino, G. M., and Fishman, A. P.: J. Chron. Dis., 9:510, 1959.

a low transmural pressure (see Fig. 3). This rather disadvantageous state of affairs is obviated by continuous fluctuation in regional surface tensions, and a low value is achieved at end-expiration, when alveoli are at their lowest radius. This fluctuation in surface forces serves as a protective mechanism and provides for optimal alveolar stability at low volumes. Cyclic changes in surface activity are probably the result of surfactant realignment as it folds and unfolds during alterations in alveolar size. A thorough discussion of the subject can be found in a recent monograph to which the interested reader is referred.[18]

Changes in lung structure, as in mitral stenosis or chronic obstructive lung disease, alter the compliance of the lung and the work needed to initiate gas flow. In Figure 4, lung mechanics of a normal individual are compared with the values obtained in mitral stenosis and in "emphysema." Compliance was found to be markedly decreased in the presence of both mitral stenosis and "emphysema," while the work required to overcome resistance to gas flow was normal in association with mitral valve disease but markedly elevated in "emphysema." In mitral stenosis, the work of breathing is increased only slightly above normal, as compared with the work increase seen in "emphysema." The expiratory limb of the pressure-volume loop in "emphysema" moves to the left of the y-axis, indicative of the work added to provide effective expiration. According to Table 2, both the work and oxygen cost of breathing rise significantly when respiratory frequency is elevated in the presence of mitral stenosis and chronic obstructive lung disease. However, the patient with

chronic lung disease ("emphysema") is unable to achieve a significant elevation of minute ventilation, because the oxygen cost of breathing is well above normal at rest.

This inability to respond appropriately to a necessary rise in ventilation should alert the physician to the potential need for prophylactic ventilator support following major abdominal or thoracic surgery. As noted in Table 2, a patient with normal lungs can increase the work of breathing and the attendant oxygen requirement several fold (0.3 to 0.9 ml. oxygen per liter of expired minute ventilation) and still keep this fraction at a small level of the total oxygen consumed. If the patient with abnormal lungs requires a greater effort for an added effective alveolar ventilation, then the work of breathing may represent a significant portion of the total oxygen consumption and place an important load on the heart to achieve greater oxygen uptake.

## DISTRIBUTION OF VENTILATION

Improved respiratory care has been achieved as a direct result of better understanding of the factors controlling distribution of ventilation and perfusion and of the manner in which the lung matches these two to achieve optimal gas exchange.[2, 23]

The discussion to follow relies heavily on studies performed in the isolated lung and intact man.[4, 5, 7, 8, 12] Although our knowledge of distribution of ventilation and perfusion in the patient with acute respiratory failure is incomplete, the

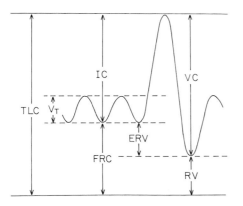

**Figure 5** Subdivisions of normal lung volumes.

TLC = total lung capacity
$V_T$ = tidal volume
IC = inspiratory capacity
FRC = functional residual capacity, i.e., lung volume at end-expiration
ERV = expiratory reserve volume
RV = residual volume, i.e., lung volume after forced expiration from FRC
VC = vital capacity, i.e., the maximal volume of gas inspired from RV

For normal values in the adult, see Table 3.

**Figure 6** *A*, Model of alveolar size distribution at end-expiration and following a maximal inspiration. Behavior of the lung is qualitatively similar to a steel spring hanging under its own weight. The situation at rest (end-expiration) is shown in the left-hand panel. The top portion of the spring (equivalent to the lung apex) is stretched (alveoli are largest), while the lower segments (lung base) are barely separated (alveoli are smallest). The effect of a deep inspiration is shown in the right-hand panel where the spring is stretched by pull applied to the lower end. Note that the maximal increase in the distance between turns occurs at the bottom of the spring (i.e., basal alveoli increase in size more than alveoli at the apex).

*B*, Effect of inspiration from different end-expiratory volumes on regional pressure-volume changes. In the normal upright lung, pleural pressure becomes less negative (i.e., approaches atmospheric pressure) as one moves down the upright lung. Thus, the transpulmonary pressure is less at the base than apex (airway pressure equals atmospheric when the upper airway is open and there is no gas flow). The two pressure-volume curves shown in the panels at left and right characterize the changes that occur during inspiration (lung volume rises) and expiration (lung volume falls). This lack of coincidence in the pressure-volume relationship between inspiration and expiration is known as hysteresis. It is due principally to the presence of surface-active material (surfactant), which normally lines the terminal lung units. These conclusions are drawn from the finding that hysteresis disappears if the pressure-volume measurements are made in a liquid-filled lung. Differences in transpulmonary pressure between top and bottom of the lung lead to differences in terminal lung unit volume (represented by dots on the inspiratory limb of the pressure-volume [P-V] curves). An inspiration taken from FRC will cause a change in transpulmonary pressure of equal magnitude at the apex and base of the lung (i.e., $\Delta P_{apex} = \Delta P_{base}$). However, owing to different positions of the respective alveoli on the P-V curve, the alveoli at the base will expand more ($\Delta V_{base}$) than those at the apex ($\Delta V_{apex}$). Similarly, the slope of the curve for basal alveoli (volume/pressure = compliance) is higher than for the apical region, and so inspired air will move preferentially to the dependent part of the lung. If the lung volume is reduced, or inspiration is initiated at residual volume, then alveoli at the base will require an initial change in transpulmonary pressure before they exhibit an increase in volume. Thus, more gas moves to the apex, and the sequence of gas distribution is reversed. (Redrawn from Bates, D. V., Macklem, P. T., and Christie, R. V.: Respiratory Function in Disease. 2nd ed. Philadelphia, W. B. Saunders Company, 1971.)

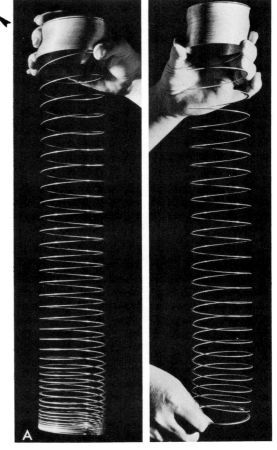

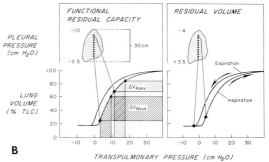

**TABLE 3**  PREDICTED VALUES FOR PULMONARY FUNCTION TESTS: PART A—MEN*

| 1 | 2 | 3 | 4 | 5 | 6 | 7 | 8 | 9 | 10 | 11 | 12 | 13 |
|---|---|---|---|---|---|---|---|---|---|---|---|---|
| Ht (cm) | Age (yrs) | VC | FRC | RV | TLC | $FEV_{0.75}$ × 40 (l/min) | $FEV_{1.0}$ liters | MMFR (l/sec) | $D_{Lco}SS_2$ | $\dfrac{F_{Ico}-F_{EXco}}{F_{Ico}}$ | $D_{Lco}SB$ | ME% |
| 155 | 20 | 3.97 | 2.72 | 1.13 | 5.10 | 136 | 3.6 | 4.3 | 23.8 | .56 | 26.7 | 70 |
|  | 30 | 3.65 | 2.72 | 1.30 | 4.95 | 121 | 3.3 | 3.9 | 21.0 | .52 | 23.7 | 65 |
|  | 40 | 3.35 | 2.72 | 1.45 | 4.80 | 106 | 3.0 | 3.5 | 18.2 | .49 | 20.7 | 60 |
|  | 50 | 3.04 | 2.72 | 1.61 | 4.65 | 91 | 2.7 | 3.1 | 15.4 | .45 | 17.7 | 55 |
|  | 60 | 2.73 | 2.72 | 1.77 | 4.50 | 76 | 2.4 | 2.7 | 12.6 | .42 | 14.7 | 50 |
|  | 70 | 2.42 | 2.72 | 1.91 | 4.35 | 61 | 2.1 | 2.3 | 9.8 | .39 | 11.7 | 45 |
| 160 | 20 | 4.30 | 2.98 | 1.27 | 5.57 | 141 | 3.8 | 4.4 | 24.1 | .55 | 29.0 | 70 |
|  | 30 | 4.00 | 2.98 | 1.42 | 5.42 | 126 | 3.5 | 4.0 | 21.3 | .52 | 26.0 | 65 |
|  | 40 | 3.70 | 2.98 | 1.57 | 5.27 | 111 | 3.2 | 3.6 | 18.6 | .48 | 23.0 | 60 |
|  | 50 | 3.40 | 2.98 | 1.72 | 5.12 | 96 | 2.8 | 3.2 | 15.8 | .45 | 20.0 | 55 |
|  | 60 | 3.10 | 2.98 | 1.87 | 4.97 | 81 | 2.5 | 2.8 | 13.0 | .41 | 17.0 | 50 |
|  | 70 | 2.80 | 2.98 | 2.02 | 4.82 | 65 | 2.2 | 2.4 | 10.1 | .39 | 14.0 | 45 |
| 165 | 20 | 4.62 | 3.23 | 1.42 | 6.04 | 145 | 3.9 | 4.5 | 24.5 | .55 | 31.3 | 70 |
|  | 30 | 4.32 | 3.23 | 1.57 | 5.89 | 130 | 3.7 | 4.1 | 21.7 | .52 | 28.3 | 65 |
|  | 40 | 4.02 | 3.23 | 1.72 | 5.74 | 115 | 3.3 | 3.7 | 18.9 | .48 | 25.3 | 60 |
|  | 50 | 3.72 | 3.23 | 1.87 | 5.59 | 100 | 3.0 | 3.3 | 16.1 | .44 | 22.3 | 55 |
|  | 60 | 3.42 | 3.23 | 2.02 | 5.44 | 85 | 2.7 | 2.9 | 13.3 | .42 | 19.3 | 50 |
|  | 70 | 3.12 | 3.23 | 2.17 | 5.29 | 70 | 2.4 | 2.5 | 10.6 | .38 | 16.3 | 45 |
| 170 | 20 | 4.94 | 3.48 | 1.57 | 6.51 | 150 | 4.1 | 4.6 | 24.9 | .54 | 33.6 | 70 |
|  | 30 | 4.64 | 3.48 | 1.72 | 6.36 | 135 | 3.8 | 4.2 | 22.1 | .50 | 30.6 | 65 |
|  | 40 | 4.35 | 3.48 | 1.86 | 6.21 | 120 | 3.5 | 3.8 | 19.3 | .47 | 27.6 | 60 |
|  | 50 | 4.05 | 3.48 | 2.01 | 6.06 | 105 | 3.2 | 3.4 | 16.5 | .43 | 24.6 | 55 |
|  | 60 | 3.74 | 3.48 | 2.17 | 5.91 | 90 | 2.9 | 3.0 | 13.7 | .40 | 21.6 | 50 |
|  | 70 | 3.44 | 3.48 | 2.32 | 5.76 | 75 | 2.6 | 2.6 | 10.9 | .37 | 18.6 | 45 |
| 175 | 20 | 5.26 | 3.74 | 1.72 | 6.98 | 155 | 4.3 | 4.7 | 25.2 | .53 | 35.8 | 70 |
|  | 30 | 4.96 | 3.74 | 1.87 | 6.83 | 140 | 4.0 | 4.3 | 22.4 | .50 | 32.8 | 65 |
|  | 40 | 4.66 | 3.74 | 2.02 | 6.68 | 124 | 3.7 | 3.9 | 19.6 | .47 | 29.9 | 60 |
|  | 50 | 4.36 | 3.74 | 2.17 | 6.53 | 110 | 3.4 | 3.5 | 16.9 | .43 | 26.9 | 55 |
|  | 60 | 4.06 | 3.74 | 2.32 | 6.38 | 94 | 3.1 | 3.1 | 14.1 | .39 | 23.9 | 50 |
|  | 70 | 3.76 | 3.74 | 2.47 | 6.23 | 79 | 2.8 | 2.7 | 11.3 | .36 | 20.9 | 45 |
| 180 | 20 | 5.58 | 3.99 | 1.87 | 7.45 | 159 | 4.5 | 4.8 | 25.6 | .52 | 38.1 | 70 |
|  | 30 | 5.28 | 3.99 | 2.02 | 7.30 | 145 | 4.2 | 4.4 | 22.8 | .49 | 35.1 | 65 |
|  | 40 | 4.98 | 3.99 | 2.17 | 7.15 | 129 | 3.9 | 4.0 | 20.0 | .46 | 32.1 | 60 |
|  | 50 | 4.68 | 3.99 | 2.32 | 7.00 | 114 | 3.6 | 3.6 | 17.2 | .42 | 29.2 | 55 |
|  | 60 | 4.38 | 3.99 | 2.47 | 6.85 | 99 | 3.3 | 3.2 | 14.2 | .39 | 26.2 | 50 |
|  | 70 | 4.08 | 3.99 | 2.62 | 6.70 | 83 | 2.9 | 2.8 | 11.6 | .35 | 23.2 | 45 |
| 185 | 20 | 5.90 | 4.25 | 2.02 | 7.92 | 163 | 4.7 | 4.9 | 25.9 | .53 | 40.4 | 70 |
|  | 30 | 5.60 | 4.25 | 2.17 | 7.77 | 148 | 4.3 | 4.5 | 23.2 | .48 | 37.4 | 65 |
|  | 40 | 5.30 | 4.25 | 2.32 | 7.62 | 133 | 4.1 | 4.1 | 20.4 | .46 | 34.4 | 60 |
|  | 50 | 5.00 | 4.25 | 2.47 | 7.47 | 118 | 3.7 | 3.7 | 17.6 | .42 | 31.4 | 55 |
|  | 60 | 4.70 | 4.25 | 2.62 | 7.32 | 103 | 3.5 | 3.3 | 14.8 | .38 | 28.4 | 50 |
|  | 70 | 4.40 | 4.25 | 2.77 | 7.17 | 88 | 3.1 | 2.9 | 12.0 | .35 | 25.5 | 45 |

*From Bates, D. V., Macklem, P. T., and Christy, R. V.: Respiratory Function in Disease. 2nd ed. Philadelphia, W. B. Saunders Company, 1971.

Subdivisions of lung volume measured in seated subjects.
Ventilatory tests performed with subjects standing.
Diffusing capacity tests performed on seated subjects.

MMFR = maximal mid-expiratory flow rate
$D_{Lco}SS$ = diffusion capacity; steady-state carbon monoxide uptake with alveolar carbon monoxide measured from an end-tidal sample of gas
VC = vital capacity
FRC = functional residual capacity
RV = residual volume
TLC = total lung capacity

$FEV_{0.75}$ = forced expiratory volume at 0.75 second (the $FEV_{0.75}$ multiplied by 40 gives an approximate indication of the maximal breathing capacity in liters/min.)
$FEV_{1.0}$ = forced expiratory volume at 1.0 second
$\dfrac{F_{Ico}-F_{EXco}}{F_{Ico}}$ = fractional uptake of carbon monoxide where $F_{Ico}$ equals the inspired and $F_{EXco}$ equals the expired fraction of carbon monoxide
$D_{Lco}SB$ = diffusion capacity; single-breath method using helium and carbon monoxide, modified Krogh technique
ME% = closed circuit helium index; measure of FRC

**TABLE 3** *Continued* PREDICTED VALUES FOR PULMONARY FUNCTION TESTS: PART B—WOMEN*

| 1 | 2 | 3 | 4 | 5 | 6 | 7 | 8 | 9 | 10 | 11 | 12 | 13 |
|---|---|---|---|---|---|---|---|---|---|---|---|---|
| Ht (cm) | Age (yrs) | VC | FRC | RV | TLC | $FEV_{0.75}$ ×40 (l/min) | $FEV_{1.0}$ liters | MMFR (l/sec) | $D_{Lco}SS_2$ | $\frac{F_{Ico} - F_{EXco}}{F_{Ico}}$ | $D_{Lco}SB$ | ME% |
| 145 | 20 | 2.81 | 1.96 | 1.00 | 3.81 | 88 | 2.6 | 3.6 | 20.7 | .58 | 19.5 | 70 |
|  | 30 | 2.63 | 1.96 | 1.08 | 3.71 | 80 | 2.4 | 3.3 | 18.2 | .55 | 16.9 | 65 |
|  | 40 | 2.45 | 1.96 | 1.16 | 3.61 | 72 | 2.1 | 2.9 | 15.7 | .51 | 14.2 | 60 |
|  | 50 | 2.27 | 1.96 | 1.24 | 3.51 | 64 | 1.9 | 2.5 | 13.2 | .48 | 11.7 | 55 |
|  | 60 | 2.09 | 1.96 | 1.32 | 3.41 | 56 | 1.5 | 2.2 | 10.7 | .44 | 9.0 | 50 |
|  | 70 | 1.91 | 1.96 | 1.40 | 3.31 | 48 | 1.4 | 1.8 | 8.2 | .41 | 6.4 | 45 |
| 150 | 20 | 3.08 | 2.20 | 1.05 | 4.13 | 92 | 2.7 | 3.7 | 21.1 | .57 | 21.7 | 70 |
|  | 30 | 2.89 | 2.20 | 1.14 | 4.03 | 84 | 2.5 | 3.3 | 18.6 | .54 | 19.1 | 65 |
|  | 40 | 2.71 | 2.20 | 1.22 | 3.93 | 76 | 2.2 | 3.0 | 16.0 | .51 | 16.4 | 60 |
|  | 50 | 2.53 | 2.20 | 1.30 | 3.83 | 67 | 2.0 | 2.6 | 13.5 | .47 | 13.7 | 55 |
|  | 60 | 2.35 | 2.20 | 1.38 | 3.73 | 60 | 1.6 | 2.3 | 11.0 | .43 | 11.1 | 50 |
|  | 70 | 2.17 | 2.20 | 1.46 | 3.63 | 52 | 1.5 | 1.9 | 8.5 | .40 | 8.5 | 45 |
| 155 | 20 | 3.34 | 2.43 | 1.19 | 4.53 | 95 | 2.8 | 3.8 | 21.5 | .56 | 23.9 | 70 |
|  | 30 | 3.15 | 2.43 | 1.28 | 4.43 | 88 | 2.6 | 3.4 | 18.9 | .52 | 21.2 | 65 |
|  | 40 | 2.97 | 2.43 | 1.36 | 4.33 | 79 | 2.4 | 3.1 | 16.4 | .49 | 18.5 | 60 |
|  | 50 | 2.79 | 2.43 | 1.44 | 4.23 | 71 | 2.1 | 2.7 | 13.9 | .45 | 15.8 | 55 |
|  | 60 | 2.61 | 2.43 | 1.52 | 4.13 | 63 | 1.7 | 2.3 | 11.4 | .42 | 13.1 | 50 |
|  | 70 | 2.43 | 2.43 | 1.60 | 4.03 | 55 | 1.6 | 2.0 | 8.9 | .39 | 10.5 | 45 |
| 160 | 20 | 3.60 | 2.67 | 1.32 | 4.92 | 99 | 2.9 | 3.9 | 21.9 | .55 | 26.0 | 70 |
|  | 30 | 3.41 | 2.67 | 1.41 | 4.82 | 91 | 2.7 | 3.5 | 19.4 | .52 | 23.3 | 65 |
|  | 40 | 3.22 | 2.67 | 1.50 | 4.72 | 83 | 2.5 | 3.2 | 16.8 | .48 | 20.6 | 60 |
|  | 50 | 3.05 | 2.67 | 1.57 | 4.62 | 75 | 2.2 | 2.8 | 14.3 | .45 | 17.9 | 55 |
|  | 60 | 2.87 | 2.67 | 1.65 | 4.52 | 67 | 1.8 | 2.4 | 11.8 | .41 | 15.2 | 50 |
|  | 70 | 2.69 | 2.67 | 1.73 | 4.42 | 59 | 1.7 | 2.1 | 9.2 | .39 | 12.5 | 45 |
| 165 | 20 | 3.88 | 2.90 | 1.44 | 5.32 | 103 | 3.1 | 4.0 | 22.2 | .55 | 28.1 | 70 |
|  | 30 | 3.68 | 2.90 | 1.54 | 5.22 | 95 | 2.8 | 3.6 | 19.7 | .52 | 25.4 | 65 |
|  | 40 | 3.50 | 2.90 | 1.62 | 5.12 | 87 | 2.6 | 3.3 | 17.2 | .48 | 22.7 | 60 |
|  | 50 | 3.32 | 2.90 | 1.70 | 5.02 | 79 | 2.3 | 2.9 | 14.6 | .44 | 20.0 | 55 |
|  | 60 | 3.14 | 2.90 | 1.78 | 4.92 | 71 | 1.9 | 2.5 | 12.1 | .42 | 17.3 | 50 |
|  | 70 | 2.96 | 2.90 | 1.86 | 4.82 | 63 | 1.8 | 2.2 | 9.6 | .38 | 14.6 | 45 |
| 170 | 20 | 4.13 | 3.14 | 1.58 | 1.58 | 107 | 3.2 | 4.1 | 22.6 | .54 | 30.3 | 70 |
|  | 30 | 3.94 | 3.14 | 1.67 | 5.61 | 99 | 2.9 | 3.7 | 20.1 | .50 | 27.6 | 65 |
|  | 40 | 3.76 | 3.14 | 1.75 | 5.51 | 90 | 2.7 | 3.3 | 17.5 | .47 | 24.9 | 60 |
|  | 50 | 3.58 | 3.14 | 1.83 | 5.41 | 82 | 2.4 | 3.0 | 15.0 | .43 | 22.2 | 55 |
|  | 60 | 3.40 | 3.14 | 1.91 | 5.31 | 74 | 2.0 | 2.6 | 12.5 | .40 | 19.5 | 50 |
|  | 70 | 3.22 | 3.14 | 1.99 | 5.21 | 66 | 1.9 | 2.3 | 9.9 | .37 | 16.8 | 45 |
| 175 | 20 | 4.38 | 3.37 | 1.80 | 6.18 | 111 | 3.3 | 4.1 | 22.7 | .53 | 32.3 | 70 |
|  | 30 | 4.20 | 3.37 | 1.90 | 6.10 | 102 | 3.0 | 3.8 | 20.0 | .50 | 29.6 | 65 |
|  | 40 | 4.02 | 3.37 | 2.00 | 6.02 | 94 | 2.8 | 3.4 | 17.7 | .47 | 26.9 | 60 |
|  | 50 | 3.84 | 3.37 | 2.10 | 5.94 | 86 | 2.5 | 3.1 | 15.2 | .43 | 24.2 | 55 |
|  | 60 | 3.66 | 3.37 | 2.20 | 5.86 | 78 | 2.1 | 2.7 | 12.7 | .38 | 21.5 | 50 |
|  | 70 | 3.38 | 3.37 | 2.40 | 5.78 | 70 | 2.0 | 2.3 | 10.2 | .36 | 18.8 | 45 |

*From Bates, D. V., Macklem, P. T., and Christy, R. V.: Respiratory Function in Disease. 2nd ed. Philadelphia, W. B. Saunders Company, 1971.
Subdivisions of lung volume measured in seated subjects.
Ventilatory tests performed with subjects standing.
Diffusing capacity tests performed on seated subjects.
For key, see Table 3, Part A.

therapeutic approach that has relied on data obtained in otherwise normal lungs has been remarkably successful. Further advance will be possible whenever the relevance of these principles to the patient with abnormal pulmonary function has been established.

The lung is subject to gravitational forces, partly as a function of its weight and partly because of the deforming tendencies of abdominal contents applied to the diaphragm. To understand function, we must appreciate the fact that the lung typifies inhomogeneity owing to regional variations in mechanical properties. We are all familiar with the classic subdivisions of lung volume shown in Figure 5, but this graph is hardly informative

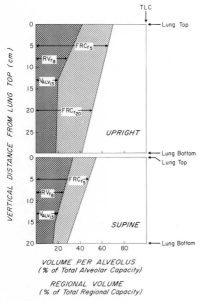

**Figure 7**  Regional distribution of lung volumes in the upright and supine lung. Full inspiration to total lung capacity (TLC) fills all alveoli (top to bottom of lung) to 100 per cent of their capacity. At end-expiration, the volume of gas remaining in the lung (FRC) will vary according to the level of the lung at which it is measured. For example, in the upright lung, a region 20 cm. from the top will contain 50 per cent of its total gas capacity ($FRC_{r20}$); a portion of the lung at 5 cm. from the top will contain 66 per cent of its total gas capacity for this level ($FRC_{r5}$). Thus, the distribution of gas volumes at end-expiration (FRC) is such that the dependent lung contains less gas than it can potentially accommodate as compared to the lung top. Conversely, the lung bottom expands more than the lung top on inspiration from FRC. The regional volume of gas per alveolus (at residual volume, or RV) 13 cm. from the lung top ($V_{ALV_{13}}$) is 20 per cent of the total alveolar capacity for this level. $RV_{r8}$ and $RV_{r25}$ represent the regional residual volumes expressed in per cent of total regional capacity at 8 and 25 cm. from the lung top. Note that FRC and RV are diminished in the supine as compared to the upright position. The reduction in lung volume, in part due to closure of terminal lung units, is caused by a reduction in FRC owing to push of abdominal contents and a decrease in RV because of increased pulmonary blood volume. (Redrawn from Bates, D. V., Macklem, P. T., and Christie, R. V.: Respiratory Function in Disease. 2nd ed. Philadelphia, W. B. Saunders Company, 1971.)

when it comes to an appreciation of regional variations. Part of the problem is detailed in Figures 6 and 7. Gravity produces a difference in transpulmonary pressure gradient that acts differently at the top and bottom of the lung. This is eminently obvious in the upright position when lung height may average 30 cm. in the normal adult. This difference in height has a significant effect on the change in size of regional terminal airways (or alveoli), in turn dependent on the lung volume from which gas movement is initiated.

A model of how the lung behaves in situ is shown in Figure 6A. If a flexible spring is allowed to hang under its own weight, the upper portion is distended more than the bottom. When the spring is stretched, major expansion is seen to take place among the turns least distended. If we apply these principles to the lung, an inspiration initiated from functional residual capacity (FRC) will find apical and basal alveoli on different parts of the pressure-volume curve (Fig. 6B), so that for a particular change in transpulmonary pressure ($\Delta P_{base}$), basal alveoli will exhibit a greater change in volume ($\Delta V_{base}$) than alveoli at the apex ($\Delta V_{apex}$). As already stated, this difference is due to the gradient in pleural pressures, since gravity tends to keep pleural pressure in the dependent part less negative than at the apex.* The regional differences in pleural pressure are determined by: (1) height of the lung; (2) position of the diaphragm; and (3) regional characteristics of compliance. The variations found among normal lungs are small and predictable, but the volume change may be significantly different in the patient with regional pathologic change.

If one starts inspiration from residual volume, then a considerable change in transpulmonary pressure will not be associated with a corresponding change in volume of basal alveoli (i.e., alveoli are on the flat portion of their pressure-volume curves), while a change in size will be evident for apical alveoli (see Fig. 6B). Thus the state of lung inflation at end-expiration is crucial in determining the distribution of change in lung volume during the ensuing tidal breath. Stated a little differently, the *distribution of ventilation* (i.e., how much gas will move to where) is critically dependent on the volume history of the previous exhalation. When lung volume is normal (at end-expiration, the inspired tidal volume), in a normal inspiration the air will distribute itself preferentially to the dependent lung region, where alveoli are smaller and more compliant because they are located on the steeper portion of the pressure-volume curve. If the depend-

---

*At end-expiration (i.e., at functional residual capacity), the chest wall tends to expand the lung, while the normal elastic recoil causes the lungs to retract. As a result, the pleural pressure is "negative" or several cm. $H_2O$ below atmospheric pressure. When the glottis is open, the chest wall is relaxed, and pressure throughout the gas phase of the lung is atmospheric. The transpulmonary pressure (TPP) is the arithmetic difference between the measured esophageal (or pleural) pressure and atmospheric pressure.

ent lung is collapsed, or if its compliance is very low (e.g., Fig. 6*B*, at residual volume), then the air inspired will move preferentially to the upper lobes. The significance of such distribution to the patient with acute respiratory failure should be obvious, and its practical implications will be apparent once we discuss its relationship to the distribution of blood flow.

The consequences of regional differences in mechanical properties on the distribution of lung (gas) volume at end-expiration are shown in Figure 7. These values differ depending on the position (upright or supine) in which the measurements are made. The data were accumulated from analyses of distribution of inhaled and intravenously administered radioactive xenon ($^{133}$Xe) with simultaneous recording of radioactivity over the chest surface or in expired gas or both. Referring to Figure 7, we note that in the upright position the lung top contains approximately 70 per cent of the volume it can achieve on inspiration to total lung capacity, while the lung base contains slightly over 40 per cent of its maximal volume. In the supine position, both apex and base contain significantly less than their maximal inspired volumes (approximately 55 per cent for the lung top and 28 per cent for the lung bottom), implying marked reduction in regional lung volumes due to change in body position. When the lung is affected by acute disease (e.g., infection or simply atelectasis), similar regional variations will occur and reduce FRC. Considered in a dynamic sense, as in Figure 8, we see that the rate of volume change will depend on whether we examine an upper (nondependent) or lower (dependent) lobe. In the normal lung, in which inspiration is initiated at FRC (Fig. 8), the differences in the slopes between upper, middle, and lower lung are not large and converge to the point of maximal inspiration. If the lung volume is diminished (as may happen in a patient with abdominal distention), then the end-expiratory position may shift close to residual volume (RV), a point normally reached after a maximal expiration from the end-expiratory position. As a consequence, an inspired breath will inflate initially the upper lobes (U) but achieve no expansion of the lower portions (L) until a critical opening pressure has been generated to cause these airways to increase in size. Figure 9 demonstrates how this phenomenon can be documented in terms of the radioactivity measured externally over the chest wall. At normal FRC, a bolus of radioactive xenon inhaled at the beginning of inspiration moves first to the lung base. If the bases are collapsed at end-expiration, then the distribution is reversed, and most of the inspired air moves to the apex. Thus, with basal collapse we face a double problem: absence of oxygenation of the blood flowing to the collapsed area during the expiratory pause, and reversal of flow during inspiration with a mismatch between normal ventilation and perfusion.

At this point we need to define the *airway closure* and *closing volume* concepts because they play an important role in understanding how acute

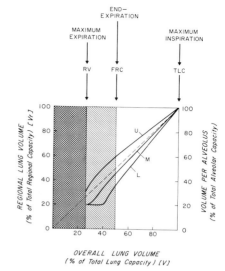

**Figure 8** Pattern of expansion of upper (U), middle (M), and lower (L) lung zones in a normal subject. The ratio $\Delta V_r/\Delta V$ is the rate of change of regional lung volume ($\Delta V_r$) as compared to the rate of change of overall lung volume ($\Delta V$) and defines the slopes for the lines marked U, M, and L. The lower lung zone (L) has the highest slope; i.e., the change of volume is maximal as one inspires from FRC. When FRC is reduced to less than 25 per cent of normal (as it may be in severe respiratory failure), tidal ventilation (initiated at RV) is distributed primarily to the upper zone (U), and the lower zone (L) does not begin to expand until lung volume has reached 40 per cent of TLC. The line marked L remains flat when a pressure change is initiated at RV, and regional lung volume for this zone begins to increase only when overall lung volume has reached approximately 40 per cent of TLC. This is the closing volume for the lung. The overall lung volume (per cent of TLC) at which L, M, and U have constant slopes is defined as "opening volume." It occurs at approximately 50 per cent of TLC. (Redrawn from Bates, D. V., Macklem, P. T., and Christie, R. V.: Respiratory Function in Disease. 2nd ed. Philadelphia, W. B. Saunders Company, 1971.)

disease and the patterns imposed by mechanical ventilation can affect gas exchange, particularly oxygenation. Reference to Figure 8, and the curve marked L, will be helpful. During expiration below FRC, a point is reached at which this curve becomes flat (horizontal), indicating no change in regional lung volume despite continued decrease of overall lung volume. This has been interpreted as indicative of *airway closure.** The volume at which it occurs (expressed as per cent of vital capacity) is called the closing volume, and normally it occurs at approximately 40 per cent of total lung capacity or 20 per cent of vital capacity (see Fig. 8).

---

*Evidence obtained in the isolated lung suggests that this is due to closure of conducting airways less than 1 mm. in diameter, with trapping of gas behind the closure.[9] Whether this also is true in acute respiratory failure is less clear. Limited data suggest that the criteria required for demonstrating airway closure have not been met in acute disease. The difference may be due to terminal airway collapse rather than gas trapping.

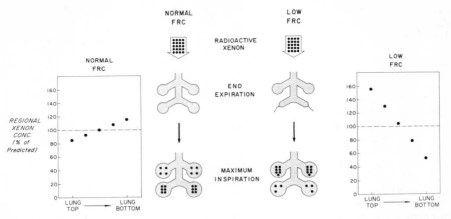

**Figure 9**   Effect of end-expiratory regional lung volume on distribution of an inspired breath. A bolus of radioactive xenon was injected at the beginning of inspiration, and regional radioactivity was measured with counters placed external to the chest at different lung levels. An inspiration taken from normal FRC is distributed preferentially to the dependent lung region (lung bottom). If these areas collapse on expiration, then the pattern of distribution is reversed, and the nondependent regions will receive a principal portion of the air inspired. Since perfusion of the dependent lung regions is higher than that at the apex, a marked mismatch will occur between ventilation and perfusion. Blood flowing past collapsed alveoli during the expiratory pause will not be oxygenated properly and this will contribute to the appearance of arterial hypoxemia. (From Pontoppidan, H., Laver, M. B., and Geffin, B.: Advances Surg., *4*:163, 1970. Copyright © 1970, Year Book Medical Publishers. Used by permission. Redrawn with permission from data of Milic-Emili, J., et al.: J. Appl. Physiol., *21*:744, 1966.)

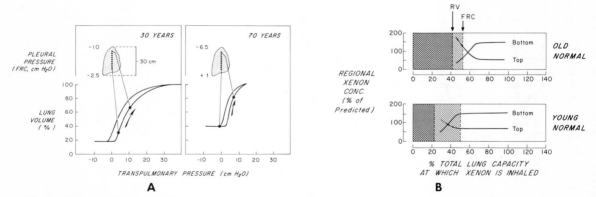

**Figure 10**   *A*, Effect of aging on regional compliance and distribution of ventilation. Owing to a diminution of lung recoil, transpulmonary pressure (TPP) is lower in the older lung. Basal alveoli lie on a portion of the P-V curve that is near or below their closing volume. When inspiration is started, the initial change in TPP is not associated with a change in volume of basal alveoli, and gas moves perferentially to the apex. Once the critical opening pressure of basal alveoli has been overcome, their volume will increase and proceed to move around the knee of the curve on the inspiratory limb, as shown in Figure 6*B*. (Redrawn from Bates, D. V., Macklem, P. T., and Christie, R. V.: Respiratory Function in Disease. 2nd ed. Philadelphia, W. B. Saunders Company, 1971.)

*B*, Effect of age on closing volume. Note that the older person has a significantly higher RV than the young adult, despite little difference in FRC. If a bolus of radioactive xenon is inhaled at FRC, regional distribution of radioactivity between top and bottom of the lung will be similar in young and old persons at total lung capacity. If the regional concentration is monitored during the ensuing expiration, little regional difference will be found in the young adult at FRC. When expiration is continued below this point, a volume is reached at which the concentration of radioactive xenon at the lung decreases while the apical xenon concentration rises.

The point (per cent of TLC) at which these concentrations begin to reverse is known as the closing volume. Note that these changes occur much earlier during expiration in the old adult, implying a higher closing volume. Advancing age is associated with a greater incidence of collapse above FRC during normal tidal ventilation. It should be possible (at least in theory) to prevent such collapse by preventing complete expiration. The practical aspects of this postulate become significant when one treats acute respiratory failure by ventilation with positive end-expiratory pressure (PEEP). (From Pontoppidan, H., Laver, M. B., and Geffin, B.: Advances Surg., *4*:163, 1970. Copyright © 1970, Year Book Medical Publishers. Used by permission. Redrawn with permission from Holland, J., et al.: J. Clin. Invest., *47*:81, 1968.)

The *opening volume* is defined as the lung volume above which regional gas distribution is independent of lung volume because all airways are open and the ratios of volume to pressure change are equal throughout. This is generally assumed to take place at 65 per cent of total lung capacity.

Two factors are important in determining the volume at which airway closure appears: body position and age. According to Figure 7, FRC is less in the supine than in the upright position, and the difference is due to a greater closing volume when a person is lying down. The effect of age is more complex but equally important, particularly in view of the high incidence of respiratory complications in the elderly patient. The transpulmonary pressures active at lung base and apex as well as closing volumes in young and old adults are compared in Figure 10. In Figure 10A, we note that the pleural pressure gradient from top to bottom of the lung is similar for the two age groups (i.e., $-10 - [-2.5] = -6.5 - [+1] = -7.5$ cm. $H_2O$). However, the absolute values of pleural pressure are slightly higher in the older person. This is reflected in altered degrees of expansion of the bases and apices for the same rise in transpulmonary pressure. In fact, as shown in the patient aged 70 years, advancing age is associated with a significant change in the distribution of ventilation. Basal alveoli, operating near the bottom of their pressure-volume curves, will change less in volume than their counterparts in the young adult, and tidal ventilation will take place near closing volume. Evidently, the increased propensity for postoperative respiratory failure in aged patients may be due to less than optimal distribution of ventilation. Figure 10B indicates that the older adult may reach closing volume at end-expiration and be particularly susceptible to hypoxemia (i.e., continued perfusion of nonventilated alveoli) consequent to minor alterations in mechanical performance. External restriction of the chest or abdominal wall produced by a tightly applied bandage can have a significant effect on vital capacity and, more important, on functional residual capacity. This is shown in Table 4. The fall in FRC with a reduction of chest or abdominal wall motion is due to airway collapse.

When invoking the "closing volume" concept, it is important to keep in mind that it has primarily functional rather than morphologic significance. Although the term does imply a reduction in the volume of terminal airways that participate in active gas exchange, the mode of alteration is far from established. We prefer to look upon "closing volume" as that lung volume at which the mechanical characteristics of the regional airways are altered abruptly, be this by actual collapse of terminal airways, closure of conducting airways with gas trapping, or narrowing with a marked increase in resistance to gas flow. Regardless of how one chooses to use the term, it is important to be aware of this change in the mechanical properties of the lung during normal ventilation, advancing age, or the mechanical limitations imposed by trauma, heart disease, or extensive surgery in order to provide a rational approach for respiratory therapy.

**TABLE 4** EFFECT OF STRAPPING THE THORACIC CAGE OR THE APPLICATION OF AN ABDOMINAL BINDER ON VITAL CAPACITY AND FRC*

Chest strapping caused a significant reduction in FRC, an increase of respiratory frequency, and a decrease in tidal volume, although minute volume of ventilation was not affected significantly. Following removal of the chest strap, FRC returned to normal after a deep breath. When the nitrogen concentration was monitored in expired air, the deep breath was associated with a sudden rise in $N_2$ concentration, suggesting that the drop in FRC was due to gas trapping.

| Vital Capacity (liters) | | Functional Residual Capacity (liters) |
|---|---|---|
| 4.99 | Control | 3.40 |
| 2.73 | Chest Restricted | 2.20 |
| 6.30 | Control | 3.28 |
| 5.17 | Abdomen Restricted | 2.33 |

*From Caro, C. G., Butler, J., and Dubois, A. B.: J. Clin. Invest., 39:573, 1960.

## DISTRIBUTION OF BLOOD FLOW

As with ventilation, gravitational forces and an interaction of vascular and airway pressures combine to give the lung great inhomogeneity in the distribution of blood flow. This inhomogeneity is characteristic for the normal lung and mandatory for optimal gas exchange. An understanding of this phenomenon is enhanced if we use a physical model as a starting point (Fig. 11). First, let us examine how vascular and airway (transpulmonary) pressures influence the distribution of blood flow. Regardless of position (upright, supine, or lateral), the lung is subject to the effects of gravity, modified primarily, but not exclusively, by the magnitude of both pulmonary arterial and venous pressures (see Fig. 11). In the upright lung, with the upper airway open and zero gas flow, alveolar pressure is the same throughout. A glance at Figure 11 indicates that a small portion of lung near the apex is not perfused, since pulmonary artery pressure (reflected by the height of the appropriate column) does not exceed alveolar pressure. Keep in mind that we are dealing with collapsible but nondistensible blood vessels at the alveolar level (better known in physiologic terminology as Starling resistors) and that left atrial pressure is considerably lower than pulmonary artery pressure. The ventilated but nonperfused alveolus constitutes a physiologic dead space ($V_D$), and the area of the lung where this situation prevails is defined arbitrarily as Zone I.[23] As we move from the apex to the base of the lung, the pressure within the pulmonary

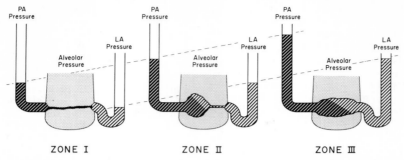

**Figure 11**   Effect of pulmonary artery, left atrial, and airway pressures on distribution of blood flow in the upright lung. At left, according to the model, pulmonary artery pressure is not high enough to overcome alveolar (transmural) pressure, and perfusion is nil. This is characteristic for the lung apex in the upright posture and is defined arbitrarily as Zone I.[23] Since gas movement continues during tidal ventilation while perfusion is absent, the effect is equivalent to the presence of dead space (i.e., alveolar dead space). As one moves down the lung, a level is reached where pulmonary artery pressure overcomes alveolar pressure and the inflow portion of the capillary opens. Since alveolar pressure is still higher than left atrial pressure, the effluent portion remains closed. Fluctuations in airway and vascular pressures during the breathing and cardiac cycles cause "fluttering", and blood flows intermittently. This middle portion of the lung, characterized by a pulmonary artery pressure ($P_{PA}$) higher than alveolar pressure ($P_{ALV}$), in turn higher than left atrial pressure ($P_{LA}$), is defined as Zone II. Zone III is the dependent part of the lung where left atrial pressure is higher than alveolar pressure and blood flows at all times. (From Laver, M. B., Hallowell, P., and Goldblatt, A.: Anesthesiology, *33*:161, 1970.)

artery will suddenly become high enough to overcome alveolar pressure and the collapsible tube (i.e., capillary) will open. Although the inflow portion is open, the effluent end is closed because alveolar pressure is higher than left atrial pressure. The portion of lung where this situation prevails is known as Zone II. Fluctuations in alveolar pressure during the respiratory cycle and in pulmonary artery pressure during the cardiac cycle are associated with intermittent patency of the effluent end of the capillary, and blood flow through this part of the lung is phasic in nature. *Velocity* of the fluid (cm./sec.) leaving the collapsible tube is determined by the difference between alveolar and left atrial pressures while *acceleration* is proportional to the square root of the pressure difference across the plane of constriction (Bernoulli's principle). *Flow* (ml./sec.), however, is independent of the difference between alveolar and left atrial pressures. This has been referred to as the waterfall phenomenon.*

In physical models similar to the one illustrated, flow through the distal portion of the collapsible tube (i.e., Zone II) is intermittent, and the tube is noted to "flutter."[17] If the effluent pressure is elevated (achieved by moving our level closer to the base of the lung), we note that the collapsible tube is distended maximally and flow is dependent on the difference between pulmonary artery and left atrial pressures. This is known as Zone III. Since the vessels in this zone are open at all times, resistance to flow is less than in Zone II, but still

dependent upon the diameter of the inflowing arterioles and effluent venules.

Under pathologic conditions, an increase in left atrial pressure will enhance fluid movement from the intravascular to the interstitial space. In fact, any body position that subjects a major portion of the lung to the pressure distribution characterized by Zone III will enhance the accumulation of interstitial fluid, particularly so when left atrial pressure is abnormally high. This situation is illustrated in detail in Figure 12. In the upright lung, when left ventricular failure is present, pulmonary congestion appears principally at the bases. The lateral position will compromise the dependent lung, while the supine position will jeopardize the posterior (dependent) portion of both lungs. In either case, prolonged immobilization is of little benefit for lung function, particularly in the presence of congestive heart failure. The head-down (or Trendelenburg) position carries an equally potent hazard. One need only to be reminded of the requirements for an abdominal hysterectomy (in which the head-down position is mandatory to facilitate exposure of the pelvic cavity) to appreciate the consequences if the patient is a female with long-standing mitral stenosis and a high left atrial pressure. The appearance of pulmonary edema during or after surgery should not come as a surprise under these circumstances.

All other factors remaining constant, a rise in pulmonary artery pressure will improve perfusion of the nondependent lung and reduce the physiologic dead space (see the next section, Blood Gas Exchange). It is not uncommon to find a reduction in physiologic dead space with the onset of congestive heart failure (left atrial and pulmonary artery pressures rise), only to see it return to control levels when pulmonary artery pressure re-

---

*The flow (ml./sec.) of water across the rim of a waterfall is independent of the height of the waterfall. Similarly, blood flow (ml./sec.) across Zone II is independent of the pressure gradient between alveolar and left atrial pressure.

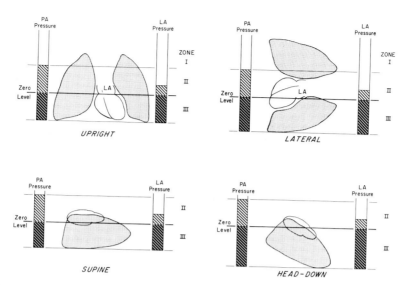

**Figure 12**  Effect of body position on the distribution of pulmonary perfusion. In the lateral position, all of the dependent (left) lung is Zone III. With the patient supine, the major portion of both lungs is Zone III. Pulmonary edema has a predilection for Zone III. Thus, in the lateral position, it will affect primarily the left lung; in the supine position, it will affect the posterior portion of both lungs from apex to base. The latter explains the "hypostatic pneumonia" known to appear in elderly bedridden patients. Finally, the head-down (Trendelenburg) position is the worst offender. Judging from its deleterious effects on lung function (effective left atrial pressure for the lung apex may exceed 30 cm. $H_2O$), there is little reason to justify its use in critically ill individuals. (From Laver, M. B., Hallowell, P., and Goldblatt, A.: Anesthesiology, 33:161, 1970.)

turns to normal. The onset of left ventricular failure and the increase in left atrial pressure will diminish the extent of zones I and II while increasing Zone III. More of the collapsible alveolar vessels will be open, and pulmonary vascular resistance will be reduced. Viewed as described in terms of changing pressures and their effects on

lung perfusion, most intraoperative and postoperative pulmonary problems seem less puzzling and definitely more amenable to therapy.

When the alveolar vessels are open at all times, flow rate will depend on the pressure gradient between pulmonary artery and left atrium. On the other hand, the rate at which water will move from

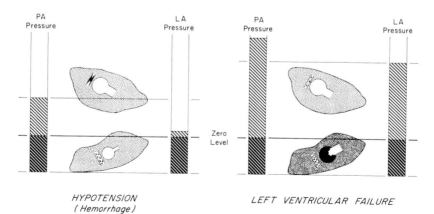

**Figure 13**  Effect of hypotension and left ventricular failure on the distribution of vascular pressures. The lungs were placed in the lateral position to emphasize the effect on blood gas exchange. Lowering of pulmonary artery pressure leads to cessation of blood flow in the upper (right) lung, while congestive heart failure improves perfusion of the nondependent (right) lung; however, edema formation in the dependent lung is enhanced because of the high "effective" left atrial pressure to which it is subjected. This "effective" pressure is the sum of the left atrial pressure measured at zero level (mitral anulus) plus the height of the hydrostatic column of blood below it. In the left-hand panel, the upper lung is shown to have an open, ventilated, but nonperfused alveolus. Pulmonary artery hypotension leads to an increase in physiologic dead space and a decreased efficiency of carbon dioxide removal. In the right-hand panel, the dependent lung is edematous, containing collapsed but perfused terminal airspaces. Since perfusion continues, arterial hypoxema must be present.

the intravascular to the extravascular space will depend largely on the pressure gradient between left atrium and alveolus (i.e., $P_{LA} - P_{ALV}$). A practical corollary to be drawn from these considerations concerns appropriate treatment of pulmonary edema. Diuresis and water restriction are im-

portant, but pulmonary edema cannot be relieved unless left atrial pressure is lowered.

Two common sources of abnormal pulmonary blood flow distribution are shown in Figure 13. Emphasis has been achieved by placing the patient in the lateral position. Hypotension, for what-

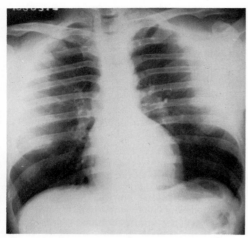

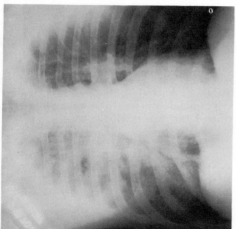

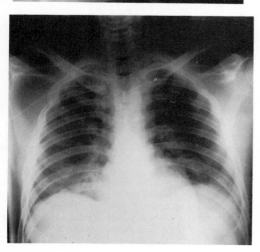

**Figure 14** The practical consequence of prolonged surgery in the lateral position in a patient with congestive heart failure. The operation, left hip arthroplasty, lasted 5 hours. One hour postoperatively the patient developed all the clinical signs of severe pulmonary edema. The chest film at the top was taken preoperatively; the film in the center (obtained with the patient upright, taken at the time of pulmonary edema (1 hour postoperatively), is placed on its side, similar to the position maintained by the patient during surgery. The film at the bottom was taken 48 hours later, after pulmonary edema had resolved. The most prominent congestive changes appeared in the dependent (right) lung.

ever reason, associated with a fall in pulmonary artery pressure will limit perfusion of the non-dependent lung, increase physiologic dead space, and limit carbon dioxide removal. Thus, more ventilation than normal (i.e., a higher tidal volume) is required to prevent arterial $P_{CO_2}$ from rising. Left ventricular failure will improve perfusion of the nondependent lung, but the high left atrial pressure will enhance pulmonary edema in the dependent lobes. As shown in Figure 14, this can happen in a patient with congestive heart failure whose operation requires immobilization in the right lateral decubitus position for several hours.

If we incorporate all the principles enunciated so far into our clinical thinking, we can outline some practical consequences to patient care that are particularly critical in the presence of acute respiratory failure. For example, what can we expect to happen to a patient with an extensive unilateral lung lesion containing a myriad of collapsed but perfused terminal air spaces who has been placed in the lateral position? Let us refer to Figure 15. In the normal lung, ventilation and perfusion are matched, both being distributed primarily to the dependent lung. When the diseased lung is uppermost, distribution of ventilation and perfusion are unchanged, and the degree of blood gas abnormality will be determined only by the extent of upper lung perfusion, i.e., the height of pulmonary artery pressure. If the collapsed lung is dependent, then its perfusion will be maximal, while ventilation will proceed preferentially to the nondependent lung (i.e., the lung with the higher compliance; see also Figure 9 for the redistribution of ventilation when inspiration is initiated in the presence of basal collapse). This mismatch will cause gross abnormalities in blood gas exchange, principally severe hypoxemia.

Extrinsic factors such as marked obesity may cause similar problems (Fig. 16). Excessive corpulence prevents proper expansion of dependent alveoli, which, in the upright position, receive the bulk of pulmonary blood flow. Again, a mismatch between ventilation and perfusion compromises gas exchange and explains why obesity is a significant contributor to postoperative respiratory failure.

This simplistic approach to the problem of distribution of pulmonary blood flow requires additional modification. Variations in blood vessel diameter are known to occur during the normal respiratory cycle. Several years ago, Macklin[11] noted that perfusion of the isolated lung from a reservoir containing liquids of different consistencies was associated with a contrasting response in liquid distribution during respiration. Thus, with saline as the perfusate, the fluid was pressed out of the lung during inflation; if a latex suspension was used instead, then inspiration was associated with an uptake of fluid by the lung. On the basis of this evidence, Macklin[11] concluded that the lung possesses a dual vasculature, which he divided into the intra-alveolar and extra-alveolar vessels, each affected differently during lung expansion.* The small, intra-alveolar capillaries perfused with saline bear the brunt of the rise in airway pressure during inspiration, and flow diminishes proportionally to the increase in transmural pressure. The extra-alveolar vessels, which include arteries and veins down to vessels

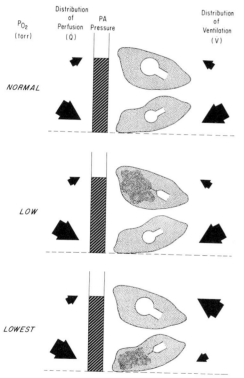

**Figure 15** Effect of body position and site of airway collapse on arterial oxygenation. Distribution of perfusion undergoes only minor alteration secondary to an acute change of airway geometry. Normally, the dependent lung receives the major portion of blood flow and ventilation (top). If the nondependent lung contains areas of nonventilation, distribution of ventilation and perfusion remain unchanged but moderate hypoxemia will be present, the degree depending on the pulmonary artery pressure and the amount of blood flow to the non-dependent lung (middle). If the lung containing non-ventilated alveoli is dependent and if its compliance is low preferential ventilation of the upper lung will occur; since distribution of perfusion remains unchanged, arterial hypoxemia will be severe (bottom). Arrow thickness reflects the relative magnitude of flow, be it blood or gas.

In the figure, the labels are: $P_{O_2}$ (torr); Distribution of Perfusion (Q); PA Pressure; Distribution of Ventilation (V); NORMAL; LOW; LOWEST.

*Saline fills all blood vessels including the intra-alveolar capillaries. The more viscous latex suspension fills only the larger blood vessels; a change in its volume of distribution is indicative only of the behavior of these larger or extra-alveolar vessels. The fact that saline is extruded during inspiration indicates the overall response of the lung with a normal FRC to a rise in mean airway pressure. If FRC is diminished by disease, then the overall response of flow to change in airway pressure may be dictated by the behavior of the extra-alveolar vessels.

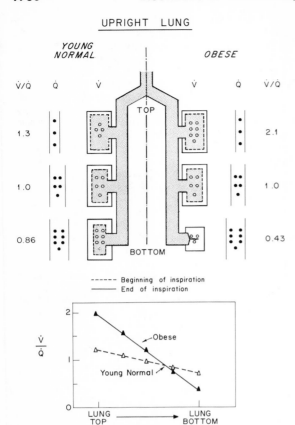

**Figure 16** Distribution of ventilation and perfusion in the presence of obesity, compared with that in the normal person. A marked increase in chest and abdominal wall weight leads to underventilation of the dependent lung regions, and the distribution of ventilation in the upright lung is reversed. Circles and solid dots represent units of ventilation and perfusion, respectively. In the normal lung, *apical* $\dot{V}/\dot{Q}$ is highest, although *basal* blood flow and ventilation are greater in absolute terms. The higher apical ratio is due to the rise of perfusion as one moves from apex to base. In the obese person, progression of the $\dot{V}/\dot{Q}$ ratio from top to bottom is steeper than normal (bottom graph) because of intermittent airway closure at the base and reversed $\dot{V}$ distribution of during inspiration. The obese patient comes to surgery with atelectasis built in. (From Pontoppidan, H., Laver, M. B., and Geffin, B.: Advances Surg., 4:163, 1970. Copyright © 1970, Year Book Medical Publishers. Used by permission. Redrawn with permission from Holland, J., et al.: J. Clin. Invest., 47:81, 1968.)

in alveolar septal junctions, are distended during lung expansion, and thereby their intraluminal diameter and volume are increased (Fig. 17). The tethering effect of an expanded airway may be considered as a supporting framework that keeps the vessel at its maximal diameter. This mechanism is probably of significance in controlling resistance to flow whenever lung volume is compromised by disease or extrinsic pressure. According to Figure 18, the relationship between measured pulmonary vascular resistance (PVR) and lung volume is

described by an inverted bell-shaped curve with minimal PVR achieved at normal FRC. An increase in lung volume above FRC (e.g., mechanical ventilation in the presence of normal lungs) will be reflected by an overwhelming effect on intra-alveolar vessels, and PVR will rise. In acute respiratory failure, when FRC may diminish to less than 50 per cent of normal, PVR is high because the tethering effect of the expanded alveolus has been lost and the extra-alveolar vessel diameter is small (see Fig. 17). Mechanical ventilation and the consequent increase in FRC will diminish resistance to flow, and perfusion of the lung may improve. Similarly, one may find a rise in cardiac output, when controlled ventilation is initiated in the face of respiratory failure, quite contrary to the response in the normal lung.

Changes in vessel diameter reponsive to altered airway geometry will help us understand variations in blood flow distribution that are at variance with the behavior of blood flow throughout Zone III described earlier in this section.[16] For instance,

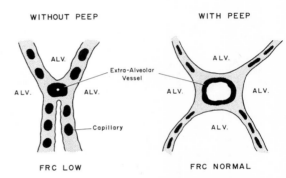

**Figure 17** Effect of lung expansion on the diameter of extra-alveolar vessels. When the lung is collapsed, the supporting effect of the alveolar surface is lost, and the lumen of the extra-alveolar vessel is small. Since pressure applied to the airway (P), surface tension (T), and radius (R) are related by the Laplace equation ($P = 2T/R$), an increase in R with T remaining constant can be achieved with lesser applied pressure. A reduction in pressure at the surface results in a commensurate reduction in the interstitial pressure, and the vascular transmural pressure (VTP) gradient rises; the result is an increase in vessel diameter. If the surface tension (T) is high (often the case with respiratory failure), then the pressure applied to the airway to keep the terminal airspace open must also be high. The effective pressure transmitted to the interstitium is always a function of P and T. Two important consequences arise from these considerations: (1) Collapse or diminution in airway size leads to a narrowing of extra-alveolar (resistance) vessels and an increase in vascular resistance; flow diminishes but does not cease; therefore, airway closure is associated with hypoxemia. (2) An increase in the VTP gradient enhances the movement of water from the intravascular to the extravascular space; this implies (but does not prove) that interstitial fluid accumulation (edema) is promoted by marked distention of the lung. PEEP = mechanical ventilation with positive end-expiratory pressure. The latter is used in order to increase FRC and improve arterial oxygenation during therapy for acute respiratory failure.

**Figure 18** Relationship between lung volume and pulmonary vascular resistance (PVR) in the isolated lung. Minimal resistance to blood flow is found at the normal end-expiratory position (FRC). With an increase in lung volume, pressure transmitted to the alveolar capillary has a significant effect on resistance to blood flow, which overrides the resistance-lowering effect of distending extra-alveolar vessels (shown in Fig. 17). Below FRC, collapse of terminal airways increases resistance in the extra-alveolar vessels (see Fig. 17), and overall PVR rises. (Redrawn from Thomas, L. J., Jr., Roos, A., and Griffo, Z. J.: J. Appl. Physiol., *16*:457, 1961.)

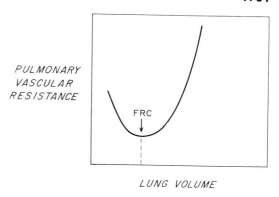

if one injects minute, isotope-containing spheres into the pulmonary artery and then counts radioactivity in lung slices at different levels of the lung, one finds that blood flow to the most dependent parts decreases to a volume only slightly higher than that at the apex. Thus, as one moves down the upright lung, blood flow rises as predicted by the model, until the lower third of the lung is reached. Below this point, blood flow is reduced. If we take into account the distribution of airway and vascular pressures, as well as regional differences in airspace size and its effect on extra-alveolar vessels, we can integrate this information into a picture of how the lung behaves in situ. According to Figure

19, basal airways are smaller in volume at end-expiration than their apical counterpart, with the result that basal extra-alveolar vessel diameters are reduced, vascular resistance is elevated, and blood flow is diminished. The pragmatic value of this arrangement is obvious. Blood flow past non-ventilated airways is tantamount to "luxury perfusion." The lung probably does not require it for nutritive purposes; it results only in the addition of mixed venous to oxygenated blood and arterial hypoxemia. Collapse of terminal airways or a marked reduction in size influences extra-alveolar (resistance) vessels sufficiently to reduce perfusion, but unfortunately not to stop it. If the latter

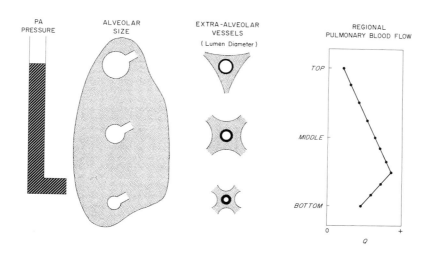

**Figure 19** Composite of factors influencing regional pulmonary blood flow in the upright lung. At the lung apex (top), the effect of pulmonary artery pressure is minimal, but mechanical factors promote maximal alveolar size and optimal diameter of extra-alveolar vessels. Blood flow is minimal. As one descends to lower portions of the lung, the influence of the pulmonary artery pressure increases but alveoli gradually diminish in size, as do the extra-alveolar vessels. As one moves down to a segment of lung below the middle, the rise in pulmonary artery pressure dominates, and flow rises to a maximum slightly above lung bottom. In the most dependent lung regions (bottom), alveolar size and extra-alveolar vessel diameter are sufficiently reduced to offset the effect of an increased pulmonary artery pressure, and blood flow is reduced. In vivo, changes in blood flow from middle to bottom of lung are less abrupt than shown in the graph at right.

were the case (i.e., acute cessation of flow to non-ventilated or hypoventilated areas), postoperative hypoxemia would be less of a clinical problem.

## BLOOD GAS EXCHANGE

Once the factors responsible for control of distribution of ventilation ($\dot{V}$) and perfusion ($\dot{Q}$) are defined, it is possible to consider how alterations in $\dot{V}/\dot{Q}$ will affect gas exchange, particularly oxygen uptake (i.e., arterial oxygenation) and carbon dioxide removal (i.e., arterial carbon dioxide levels).

### Oxygenation

In the awake person, normal oxygen uptake and carbon dioxide elimination are maintained by an exquisite balance between ventilation ($\dot{V}$)* and perfusion ($\dot{Q}$). The normal pattern and the common deviations seen during and after surgery are presented diagrammatically in Figure 20. Simplification has been achieved by assuming that the lung consists of a two-alveoli system (large square boxes), each with its appropriate blood flow. Under normal conditions at rest, as depicted in Figure 20, there is equal distribution of ventilation and perfusion to each lung. Possible sources of a deviation from normal in the arterial partial pressure of oxygen ($Pa_{O_2}$) are shown in part *II* of Figure 20; similarly, sources of abnormality in the arterial partial pressure of carbon dioxide ($Pa_{CO_2}$) are shown in part *III* of Figure 20.

Less than optimal oxygen exchange occurs as a consequence of airway collapse or marked hypoventilation (e.g., bronchial obstruction or mechanical compression of the lung), while perfusion of these airways continues. Normally, the difference between the alveolar partial pressure of oxygen ($P_{A_{O_2}}$) and arterial blood partial pressure of oxygen ($Pa_{O_2}$), i.e., the $P(A-aDO_2)$, is quite small. With alveolar collapse and continued perfusion, the $P(A-aDO_2)$ becomes large. The magnitude of this discrepancy in oxygenation can be analyzed readily during ventilation with 100 per cent oxygen because this maneuver simplifies calculation of $P_{A_{O_2}}$:

$$P_{A_{O_2}} = P_B - (P_{A_{CO_2}} - P_{H_2O}{}^T) \qquad (10)$$

where $P_B$      = barometric pressure
$P_{H_2O}{}^T$ = water vapor pressure at the patient's temperature (T)
$P_{A_{CO_2}} = Pa_{CO_2}$ = arterial partial pressure of carbon dioxide (it is assumed that arterial and alveolar $P_{CO_2}$ are equal; although this is not strictly true, the error involved is small)

All partial pressure measurements are expressed

in Torr rather than mm. Hg.* Thus, the alveolar-arterial oxygen tension gradient reflects the degree of "contamination" of well oxygenated with mixed venous blood. We say "reflects" because calculation of the right-to-left shunt must take into account the cardiac output, as we shall see.

First, keep in mind that the amount of oxygen carried in arterial blood per unit time is a product of the cardiac output ($\dot{Q}_T$ in ml./min.) and the arterial oxygen content ($Ca_{O_2}$ in ml./100 ml.), or $\dot{Q}_T \times Ca_{O_2}$. Within the lung, blood is partitioned into: (1) flow to capillaries supplying ventilated alveoli (here the amount of oxygen picked up is the product of flow [$\dot{Q}_C$] and the oxygen content of the pulmonary end-capillary blood [$C_{C_{O_2}}$], or $\dot{Q}_C \times C_{C_{O_2}}$); and (2) blood flow past nonventilated alveoli (oxygen contributed from these areas is expressed by the product of flow ($\dot{Q}_S$) and the oxygen content of mixed venous blood ($C_{\bar{V}_{O_2}}$) or $\dot{Q}_S \times C_{\bar{V}_{O_2}}$. Thus:

$$\dot{Q}_T \cdot Ca_{O_2} = (\dot{Q}_C \cdot C_{C_{O_2}}) + (\dot{Q}_S \cdot C_{\bar{V}_{O_2}}) \qquad (11)$$

Cardiac output ($\dot{Q}_T$) consists of flow to ventilated $\dot{Q}_C$ and nonventilated $\dot{Q}_S$ areas, or:

$$\dot{Q}_T = \dot{Q}_S + \dot{Q}_C \qquad (12)$$

Substituting for $\dot{Q}_C$ from equation 12 into equation 11 and rearranging, we obtain the "shunt equation," an expression devised to quantify the degree of venous admixture:

$$\frac{\dot{Q}_S}{\dot{Q}_T} = \frac{C_{C_{O_2}} - Ca_{O_2}}{C_{C_{O_2}} - C_{\bar{V}_{O_2}}} \qquad (13)$$

The oxygen content of end-capillary blood in ventilated alveoli ($C_{C_{O_2}}$) is not accessible for direct measurement, and certain assumptions are necessary to obtain a workable expression. When 100 per cent oxygen is breathed, alveolar $P_{O_2}$ is well above the value necessary to achieve full saturation of hemoglobin (calculable as $P_{A_{O_2}}$ in equation 10 when $P_B = 760$ Torr). This facilitates calculation of the oxygen content of pulmonary end-capillary blood, as follows:

$$C_{C_{O_2}} = \underbrace{[Hb \times 1.38]}_{\text{O}_2 \text{ bound by hemoglobin}} + \underbrace{[P_{A_{O_2}} \times 0.0031]}_{\text{O}_2 \text{ in solution}} \qquad (14)$$

---

*Symbols used throughout conform with established standards now in general use: see Pappenheimer, J. L.: Standardization of definitions and symbols in respiratory physiology. Fed. Proc., *9*:902, 1950. (For more details, see Appendix.)

*Pressure (mass per unit area) has usually been described in units of length, i.e., mm. Hg, an obvious error. To correct it, we have chosen to use the standards recommended by the International System of Units. Accordingly, partial pressure should be designated in bars (1 bar = $10^5$ newtons/M.², and 1 mm. Hg = 1.333 millibars). To avoid corrections of all pressure measurements from mm. Hg to millibars, it has been generally agreed to substitute the unit Torr for mm. Hg (1 Torr = 1 mm. Hg). Torr is taken from the name of Evangelista Torricelli, an Italian mathematician and physicist (died 1647), who was first to describe the effects of altitude on barometric pressure expressed as a length of a standard column of mercury. (See also Nahas, G. G., ed.: Current concepts of acid-base measurement. Ann. N.Y. Acad. Sci., *133*:1, 1966.)

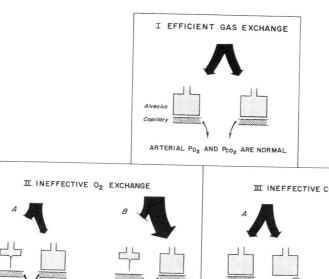

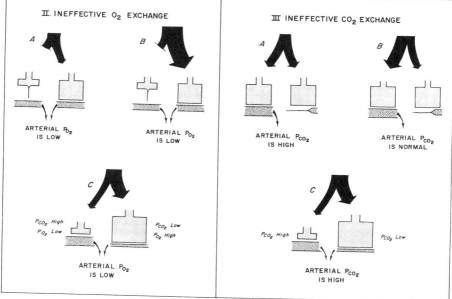

**Figure 20**   Effect of changes in ventilation and perfusion on arterial $P_{O_2}$ and $P_{CO_2}$. Solid black arrows represent tidal volume, and differences in thickness refer to changes in magnitude of the tidal volume.

*I,* The normal lung is assumed to consist of two alveoli, each perfused with one-half of the cardiac output.

*II, A* and *B,* Acute collapse of a terminal airspace is associated with continued perfusion. The addition of mixed venous to well oxygenated blood (intrapulmonary right-to-left shunt) results in arterial hypoxemia. The extent of hypoxemia depends on the percentage of cardiac output passing nonventilated alveoli and the inspired oxygen concentration. Despite an increase in tidal volume to the ventilated-perfused airspace, oxygenation is still deficient because of the "venous admixture" effect.

*II C,* Marked $\dot{V}/\dot{Q}$ maldistribution (e.g., collapse of terminal airways, hypoventilation) can also result in hypoxemia. The alveolus at left receives less ventilation but most of perfusion, and the blood moving past this area is incompletely oxygenated. The reverse occurs in the alveolus at right. Since the bulk of cardiac output is underoxygenated and underventilated, arterial $P_{O_2}$ will be low and $P_{CO_2}$ will be high.

*III A* and *B,* Flow has ceased to one ventilated airspace, and this has now assumed the role of a dead space. Since it is a "variable dead space" (i.e., its effectiveness in carbon dioxide removal is dependent on the degree of ventilation and perfusion, as compared to an anatomic dead space, where gas exchange does not take place), it can be designated as an alveolar dead space. The sum of the anatomic ($V_{D_{ANAT}}$) and the alveolar ($V_{D_{ALV}}$) dead spaces is called the physiologic ($V_{D_{PHYS}}$) dead space. Changes in alveolar dead space can be produced by complete cessation of blood flow (e.g., pulmonary embolism, fall in pulmonary artery pressure due to hypotension, hemorrhage). Lesser degrees of dead space change are produced by a marked imbalance between ventilation and perfusion, as in *III C.* The arterial $P_{CO_2}$ may be reduced to normal values if ventilation to the perfused alveolus is increased. Thus, when physiologic dead space is high, a corresponding elevation in tidal ventilation is required to maintain arterial $P_{CO_2}$ within normal limits. (From Laver, M. B., and Austen, W. G.: In: Gibbon, J. H., Jr., Sabiston, D. C., Jr., and Spencer, F. C., eds.: Surgery of the Chest. 2nd ed. Philadelphia, W. B. Saunders Company, 1969.)

where Hb = hemoglobin concentration in gm./100 ml.

1.38 = ml. oxygen bound per gram of hemoglobin (one gram molecular weight of oxygen is equivalent to 22,400 ml., and four molecules of oxygen react with one gram molecular weight of hemoglobin [i.e., 64,800 gm.]. Thus, each gram of hemoglobin binds $4 \times 22,400/64,800$, or 1.38 ml. of oxygen)

0.0031 = factor for converting partial pressure of oxygen to oxygen content (ml./100 ml.) at 37° C., i.e., $\alpha \cdot 100 \cdot 1/760$, where $\alpha$ = Bunsen solubility coefficient for oxygen at the specified temperature

Similar conditions apply to the arterial oxygen content, whenever hemoglobin is fully saturated:

$$Ca_{O_2} = [Hb \times 1.38] + [Pa_{O_2} \times 0.0031] \quad (15)$$

If we substitute equations 14 and 15 into equation 13, we obtain the modified shunt equation, which is considerably more useful:

$$\frac{\dot{Q}_S}{\dot{Q}_T} = \frac{0.0031\,(P_{A_{O_2}} - Pa_{O_2})}{[Ca_{O_2} - C\bar{v}_{O_2}] + 0.0031\,[P_{A_{O_2}} - Pa_{O_2}]} \quad (16)$$

All variables found in equation 16 are available for measurement. Mixed venous blood and its oxygen content ($C\bar{v}_{O_2}$) is not routinely available, but the recent introduction of a technique for floating a catheter into the pulmonary artery of critically ill patients has placed this measurement within our reach.[21]

In practice, equation 16, or the modified shunt equation, should be used only if $Pa_{O_2}$ is above 150 Torr. We have chosen this value arbitrarily on the assumption that at this $P_{O_2}$ incomplete saturation of hemoglobin with oxygen is small and introduces insignificant errors in the clinical setting. If $Pa_{O_2}$ is below 150 Torr and the patient is ventilated with 100 per cent oxygen, arterial oxygen content must be measured, and the calculation of $\dot{Q}_S/\dot{Q}_T$ must be performed according to equation 13. A less accurate approximation is obtained by calculation of the arterial and mixed venous contents from the measurement of oxyhemoglobin saturation and hemoglobin levels or the combination of $P_{O_2}$, pH, and hemoglobin with saturation calculated from a standard dissociation curve.[19]

$$Ca_{O_2} = \frac{Sa_{O_2}}{100} \cdot [Hb \times 1.38] + [Pa_{O_2} \times 0.0031] \quad (17)$$

where $Sa_{O_2}$ = oxyhemoglobin saturation in per cent

If a right ventricular or pulmonary artery blood sample is unavailable, its oxygen content can be calculated from the Fick equation when cardiac output and oxygen consumption are known:

Cardiac output (C.O.) =

$$\frac{O_2 \text{ consumption } (\dot{V}_{O_2})}{\text{Arterial minus mixed venous } O_2 \text{ content}} \quad (18)$$
$$\text{or } C\,(a-\bar{v}DO_2)$$

Monitoring changes in $P\,(A-aDO_2)$ while the patient is breathing 100 per cent oxygen is a useful

maneuver for approximating the inefficiency of oxygenation, provided we remember that the changes recorded are not always indicative of a changing shunt. Examination of equations 16 and 18 indicates that cardiac output and pulmonary right-to-left shunt are related (i.e., $Ca_{O_2} - C\bar{v}_{O_2}$, or $C[a-\bar{v}DO_2]$, appears in both). If oxygen consumption ($\dot{V}_{O_2}$) remains constant, changes in cardiac

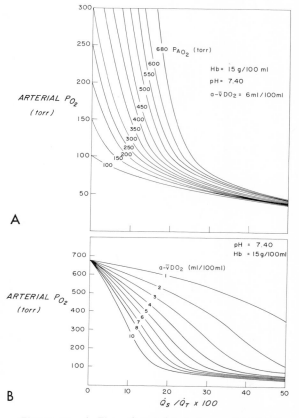

**Figure 21** *A*, The relationship between arterial $P_{O_2}$ ($Pa_{O_2}$) and intrapulmonary right-to-left shunt at different levels of alveolar $P_{O_2}$ ($P_{A_{O_2}}$) or arteriovenous $O_2$ content differences ($C[a-\bar{V}DO_2]$). $P_{A_{O_2}}$ varies according to the inspired oxygen concentration. The curves were calculated on the basis of a standard oxyhemoglobin dissociation curve (i.e., $P_{O_2}$ at 50 per cent saturation = 26.6 Torr), a pH of 7.4, and a hemoglobin concentration of 15 gm. per 100 ml. Note the convergences of arterial $P_{O_2}$ values as $\dot{Q}_S/\dot{Q}_T \times 100$ rises.

*B*, The effect of a change in the arterial minus mixed venous oxygen content ($C[a-\bar{V}DO_2]$) (secondary to an alteration in cardiac output or oxygen consumption) on arterial $P_{O_2}$. Note the marked rise in $Pa_{O_2}$ as $C[a-\bar{V}DO_2]$ falls at moderate levels of right-to-left shunt (i.e., $\dot{Q}_S/\dot{Q}_T \times 100$ range: 10 to 20 per cent). If $\dot{Q}_S/\dot{Q}_T \times 100 = 30$ and $C[a-\bar{V}DO_2] = 8$ ml. per 100 ml., then $Pa_{O_2}$ can be raised from approximately 80 Torr to 400 Torr by a fourfold rise in cardiac output. (From Pontoppidan, H., Laver, M. B., and Geffin, B.: Acute respiratory failure in the surgical patient. Advances Surg., 4:163, 1970. Copyright © 1970, Year Book Medical Publishers. Used by permission.)

output must be reflected by simultaneous changes in $C[a-\bar{V}DO_2]$, or changes in cardiac output must be reflected by changes in $P[A-aDO_2]$, whenever $\dot{Q}_S/\dot{Q}_T$ is constant. For example, if $Pa_{O_2} = 350$ Torr: (1) with a high cardiac output (i.e., $C[a-\bar{V}DO_2]$ = 3 ml./100 ml. and $Pa_{CO_2}$ = 40 Torr, according to equations 10 and 16, $\dot{Q}_S/\dot{Q}_T = 0.25$, i.e., 25 per cent of the cardiac output perfuses nonventilated areas; and (2) with a low cardiac output (i.e., $C[a-\bar{V}DO_2]$ = 8 ml./100 ml. and $Pa_{CO_2}$ = 40 Torr), $\dot{Q}_S/\dot{Q}_T = 0.11$, or 11 per cent of cardiac output perfuses nonventilated areas. Thus, despite a constant $Pa_{O_2}$, a twofold rise in cardiac output represents a proportionate rise in perfusion of nonventilated alveoli.

A graphic presentation of equation 13 or its modified form, equation 16, is given in Figure 21. The effect that a change in alveolar $P_{O_2}$ ($P_{A_{O_2}}$) will have on arterial $P_{O_2}$ ($Pa_{O_2}$) as the intrapulmonary right-to-left shunt rises up to 50 per cent of cardiac output is shown in Figure 21A. It is of interest that in the face of a high $\dot{Q}_S/\dot{Q}_T$ value, an increase in inspired oxygen concentration to 100 per cent ($F_{I_{O_2}} = 1$ and $P_{A_{O_2}} = 680$ Torr) produces a minimal rise in $Pa_{O_2}$ above that achieved on ventilation with ambient air (i.e., $F_{I_{O_2}} = 0.21$ and $P_{A_{O_2}} = 100$ Torr). This has important practical consequences. When the intrapulmonary right-to-left shunt is large and requires ventilation with a high concentration of oxygen, little will be gained by increasing the inspired oxygen concentration from 70 or 80 per cent to 100 per cent. Since prolonged ventilation with 100 per cent oxygen (24 hours or longer) is probably detrimental to the lung parenchyma, and since the presence of a nonabsorbable gas (nitrogen) assists in maintaining terminal airway integrity, little is to be gained by utilizing 100 per cent oxygen instead of a slightly lower concentration (e.g., 70 to 80 per cent) for prolonged ventilation. In critical cases it is recommended that $F_{I_{O_2}}$ be maintained in the 0.7 to 0.8 range, although higher concentrations should be used if hypoxemia is severe.

Examination of Figure 21 helps to clarify another source of confusion. It has been stated in the past that in the presence of an anatomic right-to-left shunt the diagnosis can be made from the lack of change in arterial oxygenation when the patient is given 100 per cent oxygen to breathe. This is false. Whether the change as it occurs is large enough to be interpreted as significant depends on the degree of right-to-left shunt. As shown in Figure 21, when $\dot{Q}_S/\dot{Q}_T \times 100$ is greater than 50 per cent of cardiac output, the resulting benefits are modest. When it is less than 50 per cent, the change can be substantial.

Figure 21B illustrates the effect of a change in cardiac output (or oxygen consumption) on arterial $P_{O_2}$ at different values for $\dot{Q}_S/\dot{Q}_T$. Note that arterial hypoxemia due to a large intrapulmonary right-to-left shunt ($\dot{Q}_S/\dot{Q}_T \times 100 = 50$) and a low cardiac output (i.e., $C[a-\bar{V}DO_2] = 10$) can be improved by an increase in cardiac output or a decrease in $C[a-\bar{V}DO_2]$. Obviously, when the right-to-left shunt is large, improvement in $Pa_{O_2}$ can be

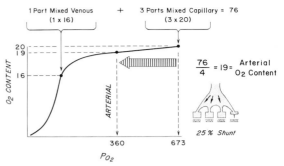

**Figure 22** Effect of an intrapulmonary right-to-left shunt on arterial $P_{O_2}$ and oxygen content during ventilation with 100 per cent oxygen. A 25 per cent right-to-left shunt is shown at right. Above full saturation of hemoglobin (i.e., $P_{O_2} = 150$ Torr), the relationship between oxygen content and $Pa_{O_2}$ is expressed by a straight line (top of curve). As the mixed venous point begins to move down to the steep portion of the curve, the arterial $P_{O_2}$ moves to the left. At this stage ($Pa_{O_2}$ less than 100 Torr), the drop in $P_{O_2}$ is small despite the increase in $\dot{Q}_S/\dot{Q}_T \times 100$. It is this gradual diminution in $P_{O_2}$ that leads to convergences of the lines at high $\dot{Q}_S/\dot{Q}_T$ in Figure 17. (From Laver, M. B., and Austen, W. G. In: Gibbon, J. H., Jr., Sabiston, D. C., Jr., and Spencer, F. C., eds.: Surgery of the Chest. 2nd ed. Philadelphia, W. B. Saunders Company, 1969.)

achieved only with a substantial rise in flow. However, the graph underscores the importance of cardiac output in determining the efficiency of arterial oxygenation in the critically ill patient. The same reasoning applies to changes in oxygen consumption.

**TABLE 5** FACTORS THAT INFLUENCE THE ALVEOLAR-ARTERIAL OXYGEN TENSION DIFFERENCE $|P(A-aDO_2)|^*$

1. Right to left shunt ($\dot{Q}_S/\dot{Q}_T \times 100$), i.e., per cent of cardiac output ($\dot{Q}_T$) flowing past nonventilated alveoli ($\dot{Q}_S$).
2. Arteriovenous oxygen content difference ($Ca_{O_2} - C_{\bar{V}_{O_2}}$, or $C[a-\bar{V}DO_2]$).
3. Oxygen consumption ($\dot{V}_{O_2}$) through its effect on mixed venous oxygen content ($C_{\bar{V}_{O_2}}$).
4. Cardiac output ($\dot{Q}_T$)
   A. Secondary to change in $C[a-\bar{V}DO_2]$ when oxygen consumption ($\dot{V}_{O_2}$) remains constant ($\dot{Q}_T = \dot{V}_{O_2}/C(a-\bar{V}DO_2)$).
   B. Secondary to redistribution of pulmonary blood flow.
5. Inspired-oxygen concentration (uneven distribution plays a greater role when less than 100 per cent oxygen is inspired).
6. Position of the hemoglobin-oxygen dissociation curve (pH, body temperature, red cell 2,3-diphosphoglyceric acid concentration).
7. Position of the arterial point ($Pa_{O_2}$ on the oxygen-hemoglobin dissociation curve, i.e., above or below full saturation).

*The list does not include the influence of a change in distribution of ventilation or body position as discussed in the text.

A rise in $\dot{V}_{O_2}$ is associated with an increase in $C[a - \overline{V}DO_2]$ and a deterioration of arterial oxygenation. The reader is encouraged to familiarize himself with the graphs shown in Figure 21, as they provide the essence for understanding the influence of different factors on arterial oxygenation. The alinearity shown in these graphs is caused by the specific shape of the oxyhemoglobin dissociation curve because the magnitude of arterial $P_{O_2}$ is a composite of oxygen contents taken from the linear part of the curve (ventilated and perfused airspaces, i.e., $C_{C_{O_2}}$) and its steeper, alinear portion (mixed venous blood, i.e., $C_{\overline{V}_{O_2}}$). An example is shown in Figure 22; Table 5 lists the factors that influence the magnitude of $P[A-aDO_2]$.

### Carbon Dioxide

As indicated in Figure 20, part *III*, *A*, *B*, and *C*, an imbalance between ventilation and perfusion may increase the inefficiency of carbon dioxide removal. Nonperfusion of a ventilated airspace represents the same obstacle to efficient carbon dioxide removal as the addition of a mechanical dead space. Bohr (1891) was first to suggest that the ratio between alveolar carbon dioxide concentration and that in mixed expired air is proportional to the dead space volume. To appreciate this concept, it is necessary to review the relationship between carbon dioxide output and tidal volume.

Total carbon dioxide expired per breath consists of carbon dioxide removal from ventilated, perfused alveoli, represented by the volume of gas from these alveoli ($V_A$) times its carbon dioxide concentration ($P_{ACO_2}$), or $V_A \cdot P_{ACO_2}$. However, expired air is a combination from both ventilated, perfused and ventilated, nonperfused alveoli. Thus, volume of gas contributed from dead space ($V_D$), per breath, times its carbon dioxide concentration ($P_{DCO_2}$) (i.e., $V_D \cdot P_{DCO_2}$) plus $V_A \cdot P_{ACO_2}$ equals expired tidal volume ($V_E$) times the mixed expired carbon dioxide concentration ($P_{ECO_2}$).*

$$V_A \cdot P_{ACO_2} = V_E \cdot P_{\overline{E}CO_2} + V_D \cdot P_{DCO_2} \quad (19)$$

A more practical equation is obtained with the following assumptions:

$$V_A = V_E - V_D; \; P_{DCO_2} = 0; \; P_{ACO_2} = Pa_{CO_2} \quad (20)$$

The assumption that $P_{DCO_2} = 0$ is not strictly true, since gas inspired into a nonperfused, ventilated alveolus is not free of carbon dioxide; for practical purposes, the error introduced by the assumption is small and may be ignored.

Substituting the assumptions from equation 20 into equation 19, we obtain:

$$V_T \cdot P_{\overline{E}CO_2} = (V_T - V_D) \, Pa_{CO_2} \quad (21)$$

According to equation 21 a rise in tidal volume ($V_T$) is necessary to keep alveolar tidal volume

---

*The quantity of carbon dioxide removed is obtained from a product of gas volume expired ($V_E$) and the fractional concentration of carbon dioxide in mixed expired air ($F_{E_{CO_2}}$); however, in the gas phase, fractional concentration and partial pressure are equivalent, but not equal ($P_{\overline{E}_{CO_2}} = F_{\overline{E}_{CO_2}} \cdot [P_B - P_{H_2O}^T]$).

($V_D-V_T$) constant when dead space ($V_D$) rises. Rearranging and dividing equation 21:

$$\frac{V_D}{V_T} = \frac{Pa_{CO_2} - P_{\overline{E}CO_2}}{Pa_{CO_2}} = 1 - \frac{P_{\overline{E}CO_2}}{Pa_{CO_2}} \quad (22)$$

The effects of an increase in physiologic dead space on the $V_D/V_T$ ratio are illustrated in Figures 23 and 24. A rise in this ratio implies decreased efficiency of carbon dioxide removal and requires an increase in tidal volume if $Pa_{CO_2}$ is to remain constant. Changes in carbon dioxide production ($\dot{V}_{CO_2}$) can also influence $Pa_{CO_2}$ if $V_D/V_T$ is unaltered. A rise in $V_{CO_2}$ (e.g., caused by a rise in temperature) will elevate $Pa_{CO_2}$ (if ventilation is unchanged), and the evaluation of arterial blood gases and lung function must take this into account.

Nonperfusion of ventilated alveoli is caused by

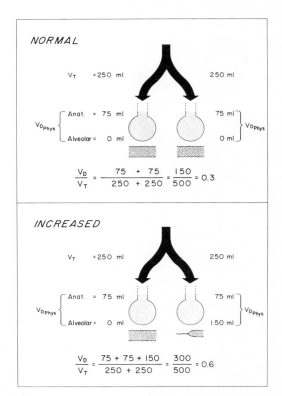

**Figure 23**   A schematic presentation of the influence of a rise in alveolar dead space on the $V_D/V_T$ ratio. Physiologic dead space ($V_{D_{PHYS}}$) is the sum of anatomic ($V_{D_{ANAT}}$) and alveolar ($V_{D_{ALV}}$) dead space. $V_{D_{ANAT}}$ in the adult is equal to body weight in pounds. Significant changes in $V_{D_{PHYS}}$ arise from changes in the ventilation-perfusion relationship. In the normal lung (top), $V_{D_{ALV}}$ is essentially zero, and the $V_{D_{PHYS}}/V_T$ ratio varies from 0.35 to 0.45. When perfusion to a major portion of the lung ceases (bottom), $V_{D_{PHYS}}$ rises and alveolar ventilation of the perfused airspace must be increased substantially if $Pa_{CO_2}$ is to be kept within normal limits. It is not unusual to find a $V_{D_{PHYS}}/V_T$ ratio as high as 0.85 in patients with acute respiratory failure. This means that minute ventilation delivered from a ventilator must be nearly twice the estimated normal to keep $P_{CO_2}$ at 40 Torr.

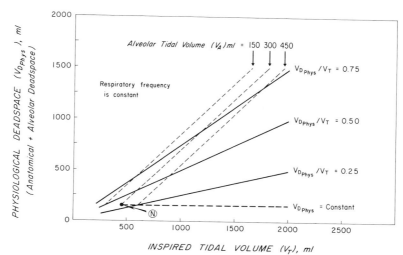

**Figure 24** Effect of tidal volume on alveolar ventilation at constant $V_{D_{PHYS}}/V_T$ ratios. If $V_{D_{PHYS}}/V_T = 0.75$ and an increase in alveolar tidal volume from 150 to 300 ml. is desired, then the inspired tidal volume must also be doubled (from 400 to approximately 800 ml.). Extensive experience with critically ill patients has shown that the average value for $V_D/V_T$ during moderate respiratory failure is 0.6. Proper ventilation is achieved by increasing tidal volume (recommended value: 15 ml. per kilogram body weight) while keeping frequency in the normal range of 10 to 14 breaths per minute. (Redrawn from Bendixen, H. H., Egbert, L. D., Hedley-Whyte, J., Laver, M. B., and Pontoppidan, H.: Respiratory Care. St. Louis, C. V. Mosby Company, 1965.)

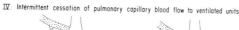

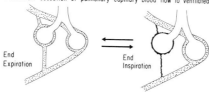

**Figure 25** Potential sources of an increased physiologic dead space during and after surgery. The problem in every case is due to a marked deviation of $\dot{V}/\dot{Q}$ from normal. *I*, Permanent cessation of pulmonary capillary blood flow arises as a result of embolism or pulmonary artery hypotension. *II*, Marked regional variation between $\dot{V}/\dot{Q}$ is conspicuous in chronic obstructive lung disease and during thoracotomy. *III*, Perfusion of a nonventilated unit leads to an increase in arterial $P_{CO_2}$ because mixed venous blood, with a high carbon dioxide content, raises the $P_{CO_2}$ of the oxygenated and ventilated blood ("pseudo-dead space effect"). *IV*, Intermittent cessation of pulmonary capillary blood flow is common in acute respiratory failure when major portions of the lung have a low compliance, and ventilation with a high airway pressure distends excessively the high-compliance airspaces.

**TABLE 6**   THE EFFECT OF AGE ON ARTERIAL $P_{O_2}$ AND $P_{CO_2}$ WHILE BREATHING AMBIENT AIR AT REST*

| Age Group (in Years) | No. Obs. | $Pa_{O_2}$ (Torr) Mean ± SD | $Pa_{CO_2}$ (Torr) Mean ± SD |
|---|---|---|---|
| <30 (median = 23) | 38 | 94.2   3.31 | 39.0   1.8 |
| 31–40 (median = 36) | 30 | 87.2   3.47 | 38.5   2.0 |
| 41–50 (median = 46) | 30 | 83.9   4.07 | 39.6   2.4 |
| 51–60 (median = 55) | 30 | 81.2   3.74 | 39.0   1.9 |
| >60 (median = 71) | 24 | 74.3   4.43 | 39.8   2.1 |

*From Sorbini, C. A., et al.: Respiration, *25*:3, 1968.

pulmonary emboli, hemorrhagic hypotension, a fall in cardiac output, or a pharmacologic lowering of mean pulmonary artery pressure. Except for embolism, all these factors are associated with an increase in the size of Zone I. Carbon dioxide retention in chronic obstructive lung disease arises from a marked discrepancy between $\dot{V}$ and $\dot{Q}$. Most of the lung is hypoventilated but overperfused, while a small portion is hyperventilated but underperfused; the coalescent flow is weighted by the bulk of the hypoventilated blood, and $Pa_{CO_2}$ remains high (Fig. 20, *III C*).

Increase in physiologic dead space secondary to or independent of a diminished cardiac output inevitably contributes to inadequate carbon dioxide removal during and after surgery, as well as in acute respiratory failure. Hypoventilation due to excessive narcotic medication or an improperly functioning ventilator is a preventable disorder and otherwise readily corrected.

Possible sources of an increased physiologic dead space are summarized in Figure 25.

We have discussed a host of variables that affect blood gas exchange in the patient subjected to surgery. All of these must be weighted vis-à-vis the patient's disease when evaluating arterial blood gases. However, one must not forget that age per se can have a definite effect on lung mechanics (see Distribution of Ventilation, earlier) and arterial oxygenation. Table 6 lists the values for arterial $P_{O_2}$ and $P_{CO_2}$ in adults from age 30 to above 60 years. Aging is associated with a progressive fall in $Pa_{O_2}$ but no change in $Pa_{CO_2}$ even in the absence of heart or lung disease. Although the source of the fall in $P_{O_2}$ is not immediately obvious, it has been attributed to the higher closing volume found in the old adult.[10] Intermittent airway closure lowers arterial $P_{O_2}$ because mixed venous blood perfuses collapsed areas during the expiratory pause and passes intermittently into the arterial side without being fully oxygenated.

## DIFFUSION OF GAS BETWEEN UPPER AIRWAY AND PULMONARY CAPILLARY BLOOD

Gas transport between upper and terminal airways is promoted by gas pressure gradients that arise from change in volume (ventilation) and oxygen uptake or carbon dioxide output at the alveolar-capillary boundary. The relative importance of ventilation vis-à-vis diffusion in the gas phase is illustrated by the arterial blood gas changes found in the absence of ventilatory movement. If a person is apneic while the endotracheal tube is attached to a reservoir containing oxygen, blood flowing through the lung will continue to take up oxygen, and arterial $P_{O_2}$ will remain high. The partial pressure gradient between upper and terminal airway will be large* and will promote rapid diffusion through the gas phase. On the other hand, the $P_{CO_2}$ gradient between alveolus and upper airway is small, and $P_{CO_2}$ will rise in proportion to the duration of apnea. If the endotracheal tube is attached to a reservoir of ambient air, arterial hypoxemia will ensue, the $P_{O_2}$ gradient being inadequate to promote its rapid diffusion.

With these comments out of the way, we can consider what diffusion-limiting influences reside within the lung, from the alveolar-capillary barrier down to the red cell interior and ending with the reaction rate between hemoglobin and oxygen. Diffusivity of gas through different layers of tissue is understood best if expressed as an electrical analogy. The lung contains two principal resistances to gas transfer, which may be considered to be in series. The first is a composite of several layers (membrane, M) including the alveolar lining cells, basal membrane, interstitium, capillary endothelium, the plasma layer, and finally the red cell membrane. The second resistance is the reaction rate between hemoglobin and carbon monoxide, a tracer gas commonly used for quantifying diffusion properties of the lung. Using the electrical analogy for summing resistance, we have:

$$\frac{1}{R_L} = \frac{1}{K \cdot \Theta} + \frac{1}{R_M} \qquad (23)$$

where $R_L$ = total resistance to gas transfer
$R_M$ = resistance to the different tissue layers to gas transfer
$\Theta$ = reaction rate between carbon monoxide and hemoglobin
$K$ = constant dependent on the amount of hemoglobin (i.e., red cells) in the pulmonary capillary bed

Substituting the symbol D for R in equation 23, we can write:

$$\frac{1}{D_L} = \frac{1}{V_C\Theta} + \frac{1}{D_M} \qquad (24)$$

where $D_L$ = diffusivity of lung to transfer of test gas (ml./min./Torr)

---

*$P_{O_2}$ in the reservoir is close to 1 atmosphere, while in mixed venous blood it is 40 to 70 Torr. The large gradient is sufficient to move oxygen almost as fast as it is removed by blood flow; $P_{CO_2}$ gradient is small (mixed venous $P_{CO_2}$ is 45 to 55 Torr and upper airway $P_{CO_2}$ near zero) and insufficient to allow for proper removal by gas diffusion alone.

$V_C$ = volume of red cells in pulmonary capillaries

$D_M$ = diffusivity of "membrane" component (ml./min./Torr)

$\Theta$ = reaction rate between the test gas (usually carbon monoxide) and hemoglobin (ml./min./Torr)

$\Theta$ is oxygen dependent. Thus, proper assessment of $D_L$ and $D_M$ can be made only by defining the quantity of carbon monoxide taken up per unit time at different alveolar oxygen concentrations. Equation 23 describes the straight line (Fig. 26):

$$y = mx + b \qquad (25)$$

Lung diffusion capacity, expressed on the ordinate as $\frac{1}{D_L}$, is measured at different concentrations of alveolar $P_{O_2}$ for which $\Theta$ (drawn on the abscissa) is known (Fig. 26). $\frac{1}{D_M}$ is obtained from the y-intercept of the straight line, while pulmonary capillary blood volume ($V_C$) is equal to the reciprocal of the slope.

This type of analysis has elucidated the contribution of the "membrane" component to the abnormalities of gas exchange seen with respiratory failure. Previously, conclusions on changes of diffusivity were based on a measurement of $D_L$ and on the assumption that $D_L$ equals $D_M$ without taking into account $V_C$ or $\Theta$. Thus, a rise of diffusivity was attributed glibly to an "alveolar-capillary block." A single measurement of diffusivity when ambient air is breathed (e.g., $P_{A_{O_2}} = 100$ mm. Hg) may result in an abnormally high value for $D_L$ due to a change in pulmonary capillary blood volume (slope equals $\frac{1}{V_C}$) while $D_M$ (the intercept) remains constant. According to recent studies,[2] the measured reduction of $D_M$ is not sufficient to account for the inadequate oxygenation seen to accompany respiratory failure. This is even less likely to be a factor when $P_{A_{O_2}}$ is elevated during therapy.

A decrease in lung diffusivity ($D_L$), i.e., greater resistance to gas transfer, can be detected in the presence of pulmonary vascular congestion owing to a slight decrease in $D_M$ and a rise in pulmonary capillary blood volume ($V_C$). Again, the change in $D_M$ is not sufficiently large to justify a diagnosis of "alveolar-capillary block" as a cause of hypoxemia.

Equation 24 defines the diffusivity of any gas from upper airway to the red cells. The test gas generally used is carbon monoxide. Diffusivity for oxygen can be calculated by combining the effects of (1) gas solubility on diffusivity with (2) Graham's law, which states that the ratio of diffusivity of two gases is inversely proportional to the square root of their molecular weights. Thus:

$$\frac{D_{L_{CO}}}{D_{L_{O_2}}} = \frac{\alpha CO}{\alpha O_2} \cdot \frac{\sqrt{\text{mol. wt. } O_2}}{\sqrt{\text{mol. wt. CO}}} = \frac{0.018}{0.024} \div \frac{\sqrt{32}}{\sqrt{28}} = 0.8$$

where $\alpha$ = Bunsen solubility for oxygen and carbon monoxide in water at 37° C.

A clinically significant increase in $D_M$ is seen in such disorders as pulmonary fibrosis, various "collagen" disorders, diffuse infiltration by lymphoma, and alveolar hemorrhage.

Consideration of diffusion has been exceedingly brief. However, this approach is prompted by the general belief that its role in the etiology and therapeutic considerations of acute respiratory failure is a minor one.

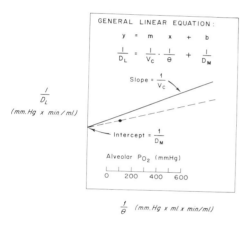

Figure 26 Effect of a change in alveolar $P_{O_2}$ on lung ($D_L$) and "membrane" ($D_M$) diffusion capacity. The lung diffusion capacity measured with carbon monoxide ($D_{L_{CO}}$) varies according to the diffusivity of the alveolar capillary membrane ($D_{M_{CO}}$), the pulmonary capillary blood volume ($V_c$), and the reaction rate between hemoglobin and carbon monoxide ($\theta$). Magnitude of the latter is dependent upon the alveolar $P_{O_2}$. The linear equation for diffusion shown at top can be solved for $D_{L_{CO}}$ if the measurements are carried out at different values for $P_{A_{O_2}}$. Values for $\theta$ are assumed from data obtained in vitro. If the gas transfer rate is diminished, then $D_L$ falls and $1/D_L$ rises. The solid circle on the dashed line represents the value for $D_L$ in a normal lung with membrane diffusivity ($D_M$) obtained from the y-intercept. If the pulmonary blood volume ($V_c$) falls, then $1/V_c$ (solid line) must rise, and a single measurement of $D_L$ while ambient air is breathed (i.e., alveolar $P_{O_2} = 100$ Torr) will indicate a fall in lung diffusivity ($1/D_L$ rises) without implying a change in membrane component; i.e., the $D_M$ intercept is constant. Comprehensive studies of diffusion have indicated that "alveolar-capillary block" is a minor contributor to hypoxemia in most disease states. (From Laver, M. B. and Austen, W. G. In: Gibbon, J. H., Jr., Sabiston, D. C., Jr., and Spencer, F. C., eds.: Surgery of the Chest. 2nd ed. Philadelphia, W. B. Saunders Company, 1969.)

## RESPIRATORY FAILURE

Prevention, recognition, and treatment of acute respiratory failure in the surgical patient cannot be discussed in detail within the confines of an introductory chapter on lung function. Several recent monographs and reviews have dealt with the subject at length and will serve as appropriate references for the interested reader.[2, 3, 13, 15]

The difficulty with providing guidelines for

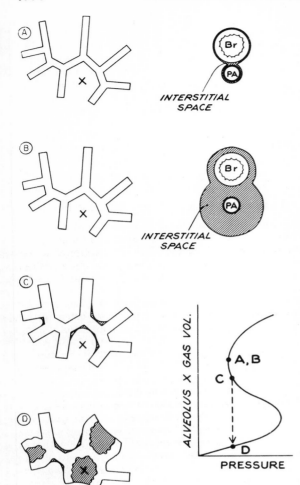

**Figure 27** Effect of pulmonary edema on alveolar geometry. Edema was produced in the experimental animal by fluid overload, epinephrine infusion, or toxic damage to capillary permeability; histologic sections were obtained from lungs frozen rapidly at constant pulmonary pressure after opening the thorax. The pattern of fluid accumulation was remarkably constant regardless of the etiology of pulmonary edema. *A* and *B*, The initial accumulation of fluid was found to progress around the bronchi (Br) and pulmonary artery (PA) complex ("perivascular cuffing"), without evidence of fluid present in or immediately adjacent to alveoli. *C*, Further increase in intrapulmonary fluid volume was associated with a "thickening" of the alveolar wall, consistent with increased interstitial edema and slight decrease in alveolar diameter. *D*, Progression of interstitial edema encroaches on alveolar geometry sufficiently to cause marked instability on the volume-pressure curve. Fluid accumulates rapidly within the alveolus (intra-alveolar edema) and gas exchange ceases but perfusion continues. Collapse of alveoli (i.e., apposition of alveolar walls, as noted in the unexpanded, gas-free lung of the neonate) is not evident. (From Staub, N. C., Nagano, H., and Pearce, M. B.: J. Appl. Physiol., *22*:227, 1967.)

treatment is based on our inability to establish an appropriate definition of the term "acute respiratory failure." Expressed in the most vague of terminologies, it is characterized by inadequate gas exchange. Unfortunately, the definition substitutes one vague term for another and fails to provide a foundation for early diagnosis.

The principal source of respiratory failure in the surgical patient is an acute diminution of functional residual capacity (FRC), associated with hypoxemia and decreased lung compliance. Changes in FRC are generally secondary to a marked increase in lung fluid, either interstitial or intra-alveolar, and an increase in surface activity. Both reduce the ability of terminal airways to maintain their stability, and closure or collapse ensues.

The effect of pulmonary edema on alveolar geometry is shown in Figure 27. When the duration of capillary nonperfusion is prolonged excessively (e.g., hemorrhage, pulmonary artery hypotension), loss of fluid into the extravascular space is prominent once circulation is re-estab-

lished. As with pulmonary edema of cardiac origin, the excess of interstitial fluid compromises alveolar stability, fluid fills the terminal airways, and hypoxemia appears owing to continued perfusion of these nonventilated airspaces (Fig. 28).

The following points will serve as a guideline for diagnosis and therapy. Although suggestive of dogma, they illustrate a philosophy proven successful in practice. Common sources of inadequate gas exchange are listed in Table 7, and the physiologic changes are illustrated in Figure 29.

1. In all critically ill patients arterial blood gases must be determined intermittently to ascertain the adequacy of blood gas exchange. We do not consider the timing of arterial blood gas analyses appropriate if performed only after respiratory insufficiency has set in. The recognition of incipient pulmonary failure can depend on no other tests.

2. Prophylactic ventilator therapy has proved more successful than therapy of established complications. Morbidity and mortality of this therapeutic mode, in experienced hands, has declined rapidly to a point where no patient should be

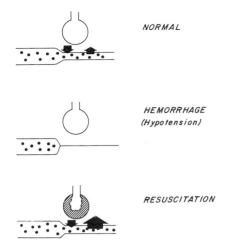

**Figure 28** Effect of an acute fall in pulmonary perfusion pressure and subsequent resuscitation on extraalveolar distribution of fluid. Depending on the duration of arrested flow, resuscitation and re-establishment of perfusion are associated with enhanced movement of fluid into the extravascular space, ultimately sufficient to compromise alveolar integrity, as shown in Figure 27. The etiology of these changes in vascular integrity is the subject of active investigation and debate.

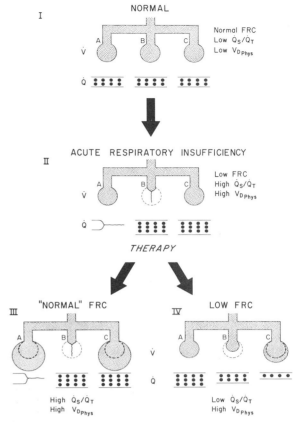

**Figure 29** Common changes in lung function that accompany respiratory failure, and their response to therapy.

*I* and *II*, Acute decompensation is characterized by a diminution of the functional residual capacity (FRC) and an increase in the intrapulmonary right-to-left shunt ($\dot{Q}_S/\dot{Q}_T$) as well as in the physiologic dead space ($V_{D_{PHYS}}$). The fall in FRC and rise in $\dot{Q}_S/\dot{Q}_T$ are associated with arterial hypoxemia, frequently relieved only by ventilator support, not simply by increasing the inspired oxygen concentration. The high physiologic dead space implies the need for an increase in tidal ventilation if arterial $P_{CO_2}$ is to remain within normal limits. The characteristic response to acute failure of lung function in a patient without previously demonstrable lung disease is hypoxemia associated with an increase in minute ventilation and a normal, or frequently low, arterial $P_{CO_2}$. Arterial $P_{CO_2}$ usually rises as a preterminal event.

*III* and *IV*, Changes in lung function following the onset of ventilator therapy. A higher than normal minute ventilation will be required in both *III* and *IV* to maintain $P_{CO_2}$ within normal limits; the $F_{I_{O_2}}$ necessary to maintain an adequate arterial $P_{O_2}$ will depend on the effect of therapy on $\dot{Q}_S/\dot{Q}_T$. Regardless of pattern, adequate therapy can be guided only by repeated measurement of arterial blood gases.

denied its benefits once the need has been established.

3. Regardless of etiology, ventilator support with an adequate inspired concentration of oxygen is mandatory. Treatment of abnormal gas exchange includes appropriate support of the circulation and kidney function. Like other organs, the lung responds similarly to different stimuli, but hypoxemia is a common response to all. Pragmatism is critical if the lessons learned from basic pulmonary physiology are to find rational application in the clinical setting.

4. Acute respiratory failure occurs with frightening frequency in patients who have had no previous history of lung disease. Prevention and properly timed therapy imply recognition of the risk. Most important, and often overlooked, acute hypoxemia may be tolerated well by a patient who is otherwise chronically hypoxemic (e.g., residence

**TABLE 7** COMMON CAUSES OF ACUTE RESPIRATORY FAILURE IN THE SURGICAL PATIENT

1. Trauma (crushed chest, extensive burn, etc.)
2. Massive blood transfusion (?vascular reaction to leukocytes, platelets)
3. Embolism (e.g., fat or blood clot)
4. Sepsis (intrapulmonary or extrapulmonary)
5. Aspiration (gastric contents, drowning, etc.)
6. Abdominal distention
7. Pulmonary edema (left ventricular failure, mitral stenosis, fluid overload)
8. Prolonged loss of consciousness (head injury, drug intoxication, etc.)

of high altitude, chronic obstructive lung disease, mitral valve disease with chronic pulmonary congestion) but may be disastrous in someone whose physiologic apparatus is unprepared for the challenge.

## APPENDIX: SYMBOLS FOR RESPIRATORY PHYSIOLOGY

### General Variables

| | |
|---|---|
| V | Gas volume in general. Pressure, temperature, and percentage saturation with water vapor must be stated |
| $\dot{V}$ | Volume flow of gas per unit time |
| P | Gas pressure in general |
| F | Fractional concentration in dry gas phase |
| $\dot{Q}$ | Volume flow of blood per unit time |
| C | Concentration in blood phase |
| f | Respiratory frequency |
| R | Respiratory exchange ratio in general (volume $CO_2$/volume $O_2$) |
| D | Diffusion capacity in general (volume per unit time per unit pressure difference) |

### Symbols for Gas Phase (Subscripts)

| | |
|---|---|
| I | Inspired gas |
| E | Expired gas |
| A | Alveolar gas |
| T | Tidal gas |
| D | Dead space gas |
| B | Barometric |

### Symbols for Blood Phase (Subscripts)

| | |
|---|---|
| b | Blood in general |
| a | Arterial |
| v | Venous |
| c | Capillary |

### Special Symbols and Abbreviations

| | |
|---|---|
| $\overline{X}$ | Dash above any symbol indicates a mean value |
| $\dot{X}$ | Dot above any symbol indicates a time derivative |
| s | Subscript to denote the steady state |
| STPD | Standard temperature, pressure, dry (0° C., 760 Torr) |
| BTPS | Body temperature, pressure, saturated with water |
| ATPD | Ambient temperature, pressure, dry |
| ATPS | Ambient temperature, pressure, saturated with water |

### Examples

| | |
|---|---|
| $V_{T_I}$ | = Tidal volume (inspired) (ml.) |
| $V_D$ | = Dead space volume (ml.) (second subscript identifies the specific dead space, e.g., $V_{D_{ANAT}}$ = anatomic dead space; $V_{D_{ALV}}$ = alveolar dead space; $V_{D_{PHYS}}$ = physiologic dead space). |
| $F_{I_{O_2}}$ | = Fractional concentration of oxygen in inspired gas |
| $\dot{V}_A$ | = Alveolar ventilation (liters/min.) |
| $\dot{V}_{O_2}$ | = Oxygen consumption (ml./min. — STPD) |

| | |
|---|---|
| $\dot{V}_{CO_2}$ | = Carbon dioxide production (ml./min. — STPD) |
| $\dot{Q}_T$ | = Cardiac output (liters/min.) |
| $\dot{Q}_S$ | = Blood flow through pulmonary capillaries exposed to nonventilated alveoli (liters/min.) |
| $\dot{Q}_C$ | = Blood flow through pulmonary capillaries exposed to ventilated alveoli (liters/min.) |
| $\dfrac{\dot{Q}_S}{\dot{Q}_T} \times 100$ | = Per cent of cardiac output perfusing nonventilated areas. This is a functional definition. In normal lungs, $\dot{Q}_S/\dot{Q}_T$ measured while 100 per cent oxygen is breathed defines what is probably an anatomic intrapulmonary right-to-left shunt |
| $\dfrac{V_{D_{PHYS}}}{V_T} \times 100$ | = Per cent of expired tidal volume distributed to physiologic dead space; $V_{D_{PHYS}}$ = sum of alveolar and anatomic dead spaces. $V_{D_{PHYS}}/V_T$ is a purely functional definition because it includes all areas that contribute to a $P_{CO_2}$ gradient (the test gas). Thus, areas with a low $\dot{V}/\dot{Q}$ ratio are included |
| $P\,(A\text{-a}DO_2)$ | = Alveolar to arterial gradient for $P_{O_2}$ (Torr) |
| $P\,(a\text{-}ADCO_2)$ | = Arterial to alveolar gradient for $P_{CO_2}$ (Torr) |
| $C\,(a\text{-}\overline{V}DO_2)$ | = Arterial to mixed venous oxygen content difference (ml./ml.) |
| $C\,(\overline{V}\text{-a}DCO_2)$ | = Mixed venous to arterial carbon dioxide content difference (ml./ml.) |

### SELECTED REFERENCES

American Physiological Society: Handbook of Physiology. Section 3, Respiration. Fenn, W . O., and Rahn, H., eds.: Baltimore, Williams & Wilkins Company, Vol. I, 1964; Vol. II, 1965.

*These volumes are a must for the serious student of respiratory physiology. The time, effort, and expense provided to publish this superb edition will not be duplicated for years to come.*

Bates, D. V., Macklem, P. T., and Christie, R. V.: Respiratory Function in Disease. An Introduction to the Integrated Study of the Lung. 2nd ed. Philadelphia, W. B. Saunders Company, 1971.

*This is the standard reference for lung disease with heavy emphasis on chronic disorders. The pioneering work performed by these authors in pulmonary physiology is reflected beautifully in their approach to the clinical problem.*

Bendixen, H. H., Egbert, L. D., Hedley-Whyte, J., Laver, M. B., and Pontoppidan, H.: Respiratory Care. St. Louis, C. V. Mosby Company, 1965.

*This monograph deals primarily with the clinical aspects of acute respiratory failure. Although it is still a valid position paper up to the time of publication, it is badly in need of revision.*

Campbell, E. J. M., Agostoni, E., and Davis, J. N.: The Respiratory Muscles: Mechanics and Neural Control. 2nd ed. Philadelphia, W. B. Saunders Company, 1970.

*The senior author has now expanded his original, slim monograph into a high-powered analysis of the subject. It does not read easily and requires the same care as one would accord a legal document. If one is interested in the mechanics of respiration, then this book is a must.*

Caro, C. G.: Advances in Respiratory Physiology. Baltimore, Williams & Wilkins Company, 1966.

*This monograph includes eight chapters, each written by an authority, on different aspects of respiratory physiology, ranging from CSF and Regulation of Respiration to Tissue Respiration. The discussion is detailed and at times complex. It is not a book for the beginner.*

Fishman, A. P., and Hecht, H. H.: The Pulmonary Circulation and Interstitial Space. Chicago, The University of Chicago Press, 1969.
*The proceedings of a satellite symposium on the pulmonary circulation sponsored by the 24th International Congress of Physiological Sciences consist of 27 individual papers and the ensuing discussion. The range of the contributors' interests is wide, and not all of the material is clinically relevant. The discussions and critiques of individual papers are particularly valuable.*

Moore, F. D., Lyons, J. H., Jr., Pierce, E. C., Jr., Morgan, A. P., Jr., Drinker, P. A., MacArthur, J. D., and Dammin, G. J.: Post-traumatic Pulmonary Insufficiency. Philadelphia, W. B. Saunders Company, 1969.
*An excellent presentation of the clinical problem. Particularly noteworthy is the definition of the syndrome of respiratory failure.*

Scarpelli, E. M.: The Surfactant System of the Lung. Philadelphia, Lea & Febiger, 1968.
*A basic, extensive, and critical review on surface active material; the chapters on pulmonary mechanics, morphology, and physiology are particularly valuable as an introduction to the subject.*

West, J. B.: Ventilation/Blood Flow and Gas Exchange. 2nd ed. Philadelphia, F. A. Davis Company, 1970.
*This book has been widely quoted and needs little or no introduction. Few changes characterize the second edition, but it continues with its high ratio of information per ounce book weight. One should begin here if interested to know more about lung function.*

## REFERENCES

Ths list has been biased toward an up-to-date overview of lung function most relevant to the management of respiratory failure. Although many of the articles are nonclinical, patience and careful reading will make one aware of how much of what is known awaits evaluation in the critically ill patient.

1. American Physiological Society: Handbook of Physiology. Section 3, Respiration. Fenn, W. O., and Rahn, H., eds. Baltimore, Williams & Wilkins Company, Vol. I, 1964; Vol. II, 1965.
2. Bates, D. V., Macklem, P. T., and Christy, R. V.: Respiratory Function in Disease. An Introduction to the Integrated Study of the Lung. 2nd ed. Philadelphia, W. B. Saunders Company, 1971.
3. Bendixen, H. H., Egbert, L. D., Hedley-Whyte, J., Laver, M. B., and Pontoppidan, H.: Respiratory Care. St. Louis, C. V. Mosby Company, 1965.
4. Dolfuss, R. E., Milic-Emili, J., and Bates, D. V.: Regional ventilation of the lung studied with boluses of xenon. Resp. Physiol., 2:234, 1967.
5. Glazier, J. B., Hughes, J. M. B., Maloney, J. E., and West, J. B.: Vertical gradient in alveolar size in lungs of dogs frozen intact. J. Appl. Physiol., 23:694, 1967.
6. Howell, J. B. L., Permut, S., Proctor, D. F., and Riley, R. L.: Effect of inflation of the lung on different parts of the pulmonary vascular bed. J. Appl. Physiol., 16:71, 1961.
7. Hughes, J. M. B., Glazier, J. B., Maloney, J. E., and West, J. B.: Effect of extra-alveolar vessels on distribution of blood flow in the dog lung. J. Appl. Physiol., 25:701, 1968.
8. Hughes, J. M. B., Glazier, J. B., Maloney, J. E., and West, J. B.: Effect of lung volume on the distribution of pulmonary blood flow in man. J. Appl. Physiol., 25:701, 1968.
9. Hughes, J. M. B., Rosenzweig, D. Y., and Kivitz, P. B.: Site of airway closure in excised dog lungs: histologic demonstration. J. Appl. Physiol., 29:340, 1970.
10. LeBlanc, P., Ruff, F., and Milic-Emili, J.: Effects of age and body position on "airway closure" in man. J. Appl. Physiol., 28:448, 1970.
11. Macklin, C. C.: Evidences of increase in the capacity of the pulmonary arteries and veins in dogs, cats and rabbits during inflation of the freshly excised lung. Rev. Canad. Biol., 5:199, 1946.
12. Milic-Emili, J., Henderson, A. M., Dolovich, M. B., Trop, D., and Kaneko, K.: Regional distribution of inspired gas in the lung. J. Appl. Physiol., 21:749, 1966.
13. Moore, F. D., Lyons, J. H., Jr., Pierce, E. C., Jr., Morgan, A. P., Jr., Drinker, P. A., MacArthur, J. D., and Dammin, G. J.: Post-traumatic Pulmonary Insufficiency. Philadelphia, W. B. Saunders Company, 1969.
14. Permutt, S., Bromberger-Barnea, B., and Bane, H. N.: Alveolar pressure, pulmonary venous pressure, and the vascular waterfall. Med. Thorac., 19:239, 1962.
15. Pontoppidan, H., Laver, M. B., and Geffin, B.: Acute respiratory failure in the surgical patient. Advances Surg., 4:163, 1970.
16. Reed, J. H., Jr., and Wood, E. H.: Effect of body position on vertical distribution of pulmonary blood flow. J. Appl. Physiol., 28:303, 1970.
17. Rodbard, S.: Flow through collapsible tubes: Augmented flow produced by resistance at the outlet. Circulation, 11:280, 1955.
18. Scarpelli, E. M.: The Surfactant System of the Lung. Philadelphia, Lea & Febiger, 1968.
19. Severinghaus, J. W.: Blood gas calculator. J. Appl. Physiol., 21:1108, 1966.
20. Staub, N. C., Nagano, H., and Pearce, M. L.: Acute pulmonary edema in dogs, especially the sequence of fluid accumulation in the lungs. J. Appl. Physiol., 22:227, 1967.
21. Swan, H. J. C., Ganz, W., Forrester, J., Marcus, H., Diamond, G., and Chonette, D.: Catheterization of the heart in man using a flow-directed balloon tipped catheter. New Eng. J. Med., 283:447, 1970.
22. Thomas, J. L., Jr., Roos, A., and Griffo, Z. J.: Relation between alveolar surface tension and pulmonary vascular resistance. J. Appl. Physiol., 16:457, 1961.
23. West, J. B.: Ventilation/Blood Flow and Gas Exchange. 2nd ed. Philadelphia, F. A. Davis Company, 1970.

# IV
# Bronchoscopy

*Robert W. Anderson, M.D.*

Since the time of its development, the bronchoscope has come to be regarded as an invaluable instrument for the diagnosis and treatment of thoracic disease. Bronchoscopy in conjunction with history and physical examination, x-rays, and laboratory examinations enables the physician, and most particularly the thoracic surgeon, to diagnose and treat conditions of a large portion of the respiratory tract with minimal discomfort and risk to the patient.

Although recent developments enable simultaneous visualization by two people during a bronchoscopic examination, clinical instruction in bronchoscopy has always been difficult by the very nature of the examination. In order to gain familiarity with the landmarks and anatomy of the tracheobronchial tree through a bronchoscope, the performance of examinations on an opened-chest cadaver is an excellent and worthwhile exercise.

## HISTORICAL ASPECTS

The inspection of body orifices and cavities beyond the region of the eye was hampered initially by lack of a proper light source. In 1806, Bozzini[1] reported the use of an endoscopic instrument with a wax candle as a light source to carry out examinations of the uterus and rectum. The invention of the electric light bulb by Edison in the United States began a new era in the development of endoscopy. Professor Gustav Killian[6] concluded in 1898 that it should be possible to introduce a lighted tube into the tracheobronchial tree with the use of topical cocaine anesthesia and that valuable information could be obtained from such an examination. Killian's early reports of foreign body extractions and endobronchial examinations mark him as the "Father of Bronchoscopy."

With the development of better techniques and instrumentation, bronchoscopy rapidly progressed from the art of looking into the air passages and removing foreign bodies to the science of bronchology, which is concerned with the visual examination and direct study of the anatomy, pathology, and physiology of, and also with the treatment of the diseases of, the tracheobronchial tree. The science of bronchoesophagology in America was developed by Chevalier Jackson and his associates at the Jackson Clinic in Philadelphia. For many years this group devoted themselves to the establishment and advancement of bronchoesophagology as a science, and their classic monograph

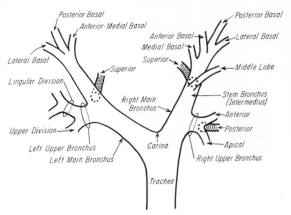

**Figure 1**   The inverted bronchial tree as visualized by the bronchoscopist. A rigid bronchoscope with forward-vision and right-angle telescopes allows visualization to the limits diagramed under optimal conditions.

on bronchoesophagology is recommended to anyone who is concerned with this field.[5]

## BRONCHOSCOPIC ANATOMY AND PHYSIOLOGY

The early development of bronchology was hampered by the bronchial anatomic classifications which were extremely confusing and complex. An accurate and simple nomenclature which was first outlined by Jackson and Huber[3] in 1943 now enables physicians in all fields to discuss pulmonary conditions with great accuracy. The terminology proposed by Jackson and Huber takes cognizance of the important fact that the bronchopulmonary segments are subdivisions of the lungs which function as individual units and are individually served by their own bronchus and arterial and venous blood supply. Since many disease processes are segmental in nature, it is essential that physicians diagnosing or treating chest diseases be familiar with bronchial anatomy from a radiologic, bronchographic, endoscopic, and surgical viewpoint.

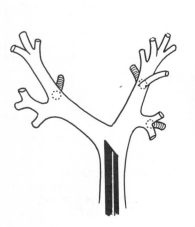

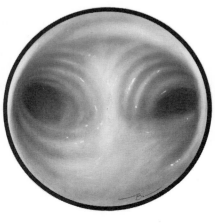

**Figure 2**   A normal, sharp-appearing carina during inspiration. During the expiratory phase of respiration there is some shortening and widening. Bronchial cartilage outlines are well seen and the mucosa is healthy.

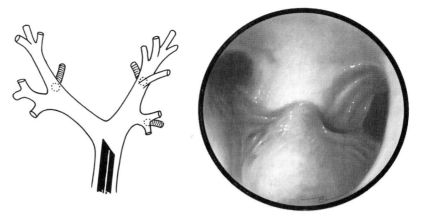

**Figure 3** Widened, abnormally fixed carina caused by subcarinal lymph node metastases. The diagnosis was made by a transcarinal needle biopsy and inoperability established.

An inverted schematic drawing showing the tracheobronchial tree and its bronchoscopically visible subdivisions as visualized by the endoscopist is shown in Figure 1. The trachea ends at the carina by dividing into the right and left main bronchi. The carina is an important landmark for the bronchoscopist; it should be nearly vertical and sharp if subcarinal lymphadenopathy or other distorting factors are not present (Figs. 2 and 3). The right main bronchus lies in almost the same axis as the trachea and extends for about 2 cm. before it divides into the laterally directed right upper lobe bronchus and the stem bronchus (bronchus intermedius), which is a continuation of the main bronchus. The right upper lobe bronchus commonly subdivides into three segmental branches (Fig. 4) and the bronchus intermedius divides into the anteriorly directed middle lobe bronchus and the lower lobe bronchus. The middle lobe bronchus divides into its two segmental branches while the lower lobe bronchus, after giving off the superior segmental branch, then subdivides into four basilar bronchi (Fig. 5). The left main bronchus makes a greater angle with the trachea and extends about twice as far as the right main bronchus before dividing into the upper and lower lobe bronchi. The upper lobe bronchus

subdivides into the upper division bronchus and the lingular bronchus, which then yields the superior and inferior segmental bronchi and is equivalent to the middle lobe bronchus on the right. The left lower lobe bronchus subdivides into the superior segmental bronchus and three basilar segmental bronchi.

This brief description outlines the usual pattern of the tracheobronchial tree, but anatomic variations are frequent and the presence of pathologic changes distorts normal anatomy and obscures sought-after landmarks.

The color of the bronchial mucosa, as it is visualized through a bronchoscope, depends upon the lighting source used, whether there has been trauma to the mucosa during instrumentation, and whether pathologic changes are present. A pale flesh-pink color is to be expected, but each endoscopist must become familiar with the standard of normality in his own clinic. Since many patients who undergo bronchoscopy suffer from chronic bronchitis, the distinct reddening and erythematous changes found in this disease must not be accepted as normal because of their frequent appearance. The trachea and main bronchi have a supporting framework of partially enclosing cartilaginous rings which diminish to

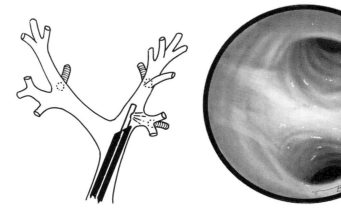

**Figure 4** Normal right upper lobe bronchial orifice as visualized through the right-angle telescopic lens. The usual division into anterior, posterior, and apical branches is well seen.

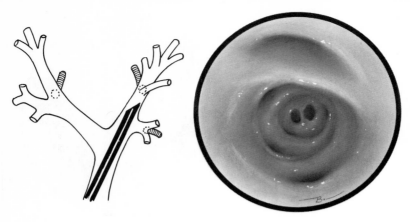

**Figure 5** Termination of the right main bronchus with the middle lobe orifice seen superiorly and the superior segmented bronchus posteriorly. Distally are the basilar bronchi with the posterior basilar bronchus and its subcarina appearing in the center of the field.

cartilaginous plaques in the more distal secondary bronchi and finally disappear in the bronchioles. Nowhere in the bronchial tree are these rings completely encircling or rigid, and for this reason there is normal mobility of the tracheobronchial tree during respiration which includes changes in both caliber and length of the airway. The loss of this mobility suggests fixation due to some disease process.

Physiologically, the tracheobronchial tree functions as a conduit system to conduct air from the upper airway to the alveoli, where gas exchange takes place. In addition to its mechanical function of conducting air, the tracheobronchial system also acts in concert with the upper airway as a heat exchanger and humidifier to prepare the air for delivery to the alveoli. The final physiologic function of the airways is to provide a drainage and cleansing system for the lungs by means of a protective layer of mucus and retrograde ciliary sweeping action which moves particulate matter and secretions upward. The expulsive forces and peristaltic activity of the airways caused by normal inspiration and expiration are aided by

forceful blasts of air during reflex-stimulated acts such as clearing of the throat or coughing.

In the normal tracheobronchial tree there are no visible secretions and their presence during a bronchoscopic examination represents an abnormality. Furthermore, the cleansing mechanisms of the airways are less efficient in protecting the alveoli against liquids than they are against particulate matter, and conditions such as bronchitis which are characterized by increased bronchial secretions result in distal airway changes as the defense mechanisms are overwhelmed.

## INSTRUMENTATION AND TECHNIQUE

The standard rigid bronchoscope is a hollow tube with a beveled tip which has a light source at the end. These bronchoscopes are available in a variety of sizes and the 7 × 40 mm. is most commonly employed in adults (Fig. 6). Broyles developed a series of telescopes which can be inserted through the lumen of the standard bronchoscope. The most useful are the forward-vision

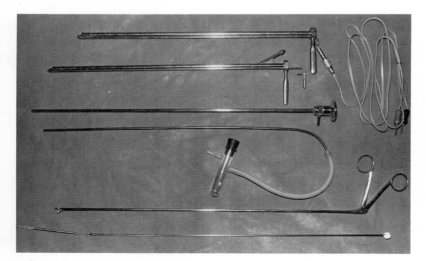

**Figure 6** The standard 7 × 40 mm. bronchoscope with carrier for the light source is seen at top. Below are a side-arm ventilating bronchoscope; right-angle Broyles telescope, which is passed through standard bronchoscope to visualize upper lobes; aspirating tube; biopsy forceps; and sponge carrier for removal of secretions and cytologic smears.

**Figure 7** The flexible fiber bronchoscope, which may be introduced perorally or through a rigid bronchoscope or tracheoscope. Light is introduced from an outside power source and travels via optic fibers to the flexible distal tip, which is operator-controlled by an angle lever located near the eyepiece. Cytologic specimens are obtained from the bronchi with a brush, curet, or biopsy forceps passed through a channel in the bronchofiberscope. (Courtesy of Olympus Corporation.)

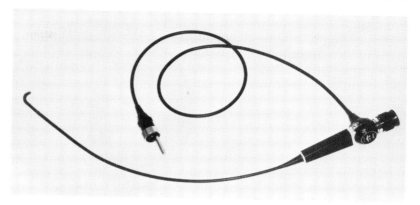

type which magnifies the lower lobe bronchi and the right-angled lens which provides a clear view of the upper lobe bronchi. The recent development of a flexible fiber bronchoscope extends the visual range of a bronchoscopic examination and should improve the diagnostic yield in more peripheral and earlier lung tumors. The fiberoptic bronchoscope has an operator-controlled, flexible distal tip and can be manipulated into the far reaches of the tracheobronchial tree where cytologic specimens can be obtained under direct visualization by the use of a brush (Figs. 7 and 8).

When general anesthesia is employed or the patient is in severe respiratory distress, a ventilating bronchoscope with side arm is utilized, so that insufflation of the lungs can be carried out during the course of the procedure. Ancillary equipment required for the bronchoscopic clinic includes an adjustable and reliable power source for the light employed, aspirating apparatus, biopsy and foreign body extraction forceps, sponge carriers,

a suitable examination table, cytologic brushes for excoriating suspicious areas for cells, and some type of shield or spectacles to protect the operator's eyes during the procedure. The technique of bronchoscopy is described in magnificent detail in the works of Stradling[8] and Jackson and Jackson.[5] Only the more salient features will be discussed here.

Although Jackson strongly advised the use of topical anesthesia for all endoscopic procedures, the development of safer anesthetic drugs and muscle relaxants has made general anesthesia safe for bronchscosopic examinations. It is most important to prepare the patient psychologically and pharmacologically for the procedure in order to allay his anxieties and fears. Topical anesthetics are applied to the oropharynx either by spray or swab and then dropped on the epiglottis and cords under mirror observation. While this is being accomplished, a thorough oral examination is carried out and vocal cord motion is evaluated.

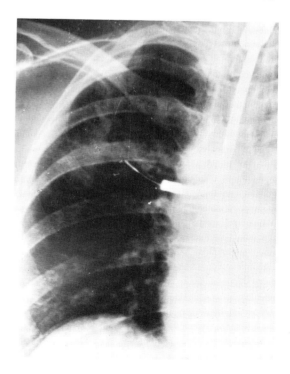

**Figure 8** Bronchofiberscope passed through rigid bronchoscope into anterior segmental bronchus of right upper lobe. A cytologic brush protrudes from the tip of the instrument into the mass in the lung which appeared malignant and was cytologically confirmed to be so. (Courtesy of Olympus Corporation.)

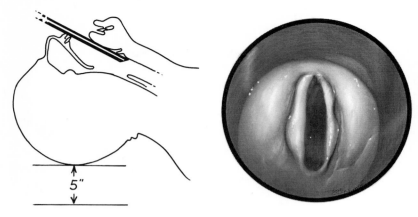

**Figure 9** With the head in proper position and the bronchoscope in the midline, the epiglottis has been displaced forward by the tip of the bronchoscope and the vocal cords are well seen. The instrument can now be gently passed through the cords and into the trachea.

Finally, the material is instilled into the trachea and bronchi by dripping it through the cords or by a transtracheal needle puncture.

After anesthesia is complete, the patient is properly positioned in the dorsal recumbent position with the shoulders flat, the head elevated about 5 inches, and the neck extended so that the chin points toward the ceiling (Fig. 9). While the patient's head is maintained in this position by an assistant, the bronchoscope is carefully insinuated through the cords until the trachea is identified. From this point, the examination must be methodically and gently performed and the bronchoscopist must look for details of anatomic form, mucosal coloration, nature and volume of secretions, and tracheobronchial motion. Suspicious areas should be noted during the initial examination and biopsied at the end of the procedure, since the bleeding which occurs following biopsy makes further evaluation difficult. Aspiration must be done atraumatically and small saline lavages utilized to aid in the removal of obscuring secretions and to help liquefy purulent material so that culture specimens can be obtained.

The complications associated with bronchoscopy are usually related to adverse reactions to the anesthesia utilized, cardiac problems secondary to vagal stimulation, and bleeding caused by biopsy or foreign body extraction. Particular care must be exercised in biopsying areas adjacent to major vessels.

## INDICATIONS AND CONTRAINDICATIONS

Bronchoscopy is both a diagnostic and therapeutic procedure and should be performed in the presence of pulmonary disease which is undiagnosed but presents as either unexplained symptoms, signs, or radiologic findings. Diagnosed chest lesions that fail to respond to medical therapy within a short period of time may be due to underlying processes (i.e., tumor, foreign body, stenosis, and so on) and bronchoscopy is therefore indicated. Bronchoscopy is specifically indicated when there is a chronic cough, signs or symptoms of bronchial obstruction,[2] or hemoptysis; as part of any work-up for suspected lung or esophageal cancer; whenever

foreign body aspiration is suspected; and in any patient for whom the inability to clear bronchial secretions is a problem. Patients being evaluated for pulmonary resection for tuberculosis or those who are found to have a positive sputum with no radiologically detectable abnormality require evaluation for endobronchial tuberculosis and this can be accomplished only by a bronchoscopic examination.

In suppurative disease, bronchoscopy is an invaluable aid toward restoring peroral drainage.[7] Thick secretions may be removed by aspiration in pneumonia, pulmonary abscess, persistent pneumothorax, bronchiectasis, or persistent atelectasis. Specimens for culture and cytologic evaluation are obtained while a search for tumors, foreign bodies, stenotic lesions, or other etiologic factors is conducted.

The contraindications to bronchoscopy are few and the recent introduction of the flexible fiberoptic bronchoscope makes examination feasible under almost any circumstance. Disease or injury of the cervical spine which makes hyperextension impossible or the presence of an aortic arch aneurysm contraindicates rigid tube bronchoscopy, but presents no problem when a flexible fiberoptic bronchoscope is used. Status asthmaticus, massive active pulmonary hemorrhage, and severe cardiac failure or arrhythmias are relative contraindications to bronchoscopy.

## TRACHEOBRONCHIAL PATHOLOGY

The pathologic changes observed in the tracheobronchial tree during a bronchoscopic examination fall into certain patterns which include inflammatory responses, bronchial distortion and displacement, new growths, and foreign bodies.

Inflammatory changes may be generalized as in bronchitis, in which the mucosa of the entire tracheobronchial tree appears reddened and hyperemic, with excessive secretions frequently noted. These secretions vary from thin mucoid material to thick purulent matter of high viscosity. The mucosa is often swollen and edematous in appearance, and normal sharp edges and contours may be obliterated by a thick enfolding carpet of swollen mucosa. Long-standing generalized bronchitis destroys the submucosal structures of the bronchial wall and the normal tone of the bronchus is lost. Areas of dilatation and puddling of secretions may occur as consequences of the loss of ciliary function and the milking action or "tussive squeeze"[4] of bronchial peristalsis during respirations. During forceful expiration, there may be complete collapse of the bronchial structures, since supporting tissue has been destroyed, and even the most vigorous expiratory efforts will fail to propel material past this obstruction.

The more common etiologic factors producing localized endobronchial inflammatory changes are pneumonia, lung abscess, bronchiectasis, foreign bodies, tuberculosis, mycotic diseases, and endobronchial tumors, particularly carcinoma. The changes noted in these conditions vary from localized mucosal erythema with purulent secretions issuing from a bronchial orifice in pneumonia or lung abscess, to granuloma formation or ulceration with scarring and stenosis in endobronchial tuberculosis or mycosis. Inert foreign bodies (i.e., metal) present for only a short time provoke only minimal local reaction, whereas long-standing irritants or vegetable matter (i.e., peanuts) may result in extensive changes with florid granulation tissue and edema. Any local inflammatory response must be explained, since a carcinoma in proximity may produce such changes although the tumor itself may not be visible through the bronchoscope.

Hemoptysis may occur as a result of friable vascular granulation tissue in any inflammatory process or may be the result of an ulcerating or eroding tumor. Bronchial adenomas and certain other rare tumors are extremely vascular and may present as severe hemoptysis. These tumors may bleed profusely if biopsied too deeply. Bronchoscopy is often best deferred in the face of large hemorrhages, since visibility is obscured.

Defining tracheal and bronchial distortion and displacement during a bronchoscopic examination provides valuable insight as to the nature and extent of the underlying disease process. Enlarged extrabronchial lymph nodes are the usual cause of these changes, but developmental anomalies; inflammatory scarring and contraction; radiation therapy sequelae; or extrinsic pressure secondary to effusions, cysts, tumor, or diaphragmatic elevation may also cause changes. Resection of pulmonary tissue with consequent rearrangement of lobes, kyphoscoliosis, or atelectasis may also produce very confusing pictures secondary to the attendant distortion of tracheobronchial anatomy.

In the evaluation of suspected lung cancer, bronchial distortion is carefully looked for at the sites of lymph node groups which may be involved by the tumor. Widening of the carina is produced by enlarged subcarinal nodes and may confirm inoperability. Enlarged paratracheal or parabronchial nodes may cause bronchial compression and fixation, and cautious biopsies may demonstrate invasion by tumor at these sites.

The great majority of bronchoscopically visible tumors are proved histologically to be bronchogenic carcinoma. However, the bronchoscopist's role is to define the anatomic and physiologic behavior of the tumor, since therapy is dictated by these observations as well as by the histologic identification which may result from a biopsy or cytologic study of bronchial secretions. Tumors may present as polypoid growths, as intraluminal masses which have eroded through the mucosa (Fig. 10), or as submucosal mural growths which may produce localized inflammatory changes with rigidity and partial stenosis. An unrushed and thorough examination is essential in any suspected lung tumor, and the diagnostic yield should be greater than 80 per cent if biopsies and washings for cytologic examination are judiciously performed.

## PEDIATRIC BRONCHOSCOPY

A bronchoscopic examination may be given to patients of any age, but bronchoscopy in infants should be limited to patients with suspected foreign body aspiration or evidence of bronchial

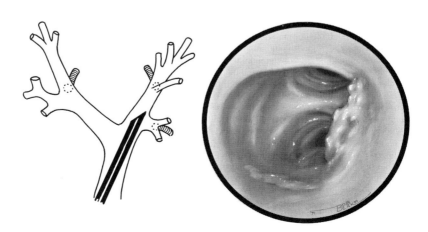

**Figure 10** A squamous carcinoma protruding into the bronchus intermedius just below the take-off of the right upper lobe bronchus. A biopsy was positive and there was no evidence of inoperability. A right pneumonectomy was performed.

obstruction. Small, delicate instruments are required, and the examination should be carried out gently and rapidly to keep laryngeal and bronchial edema at a minimum. In newborn infants and in most children below the age of 6, no anesthesia is employed for the procedure. Older children may be examined under general anesthesia or with topical anesthesia and mild sedation.

## SELECTED REFERENCES

Holinger, P., and Andrews, A. H.: Bronchial obstruction. Signs, symptoms and diagnosis. Amer. Surg., *54*:193, 1941.
*This article discusses the fundamental pathologic process of bronchial obstruction and the signs and symptoms it produces. The disease entities responsible for bronchial obstruction and the changes produced secondarily by obstruction are discussed in detail. The role of bronchoscopy in the diagnosis and treatment of bronchial obstruction is considered.*

Jackson, C., and Jackson, C. L.: Bronchoesophagology. Philadelphia, W. B. Saunders Company, 1950.
*In this monograph, the "Dean of American Bronchology" and his son summarize the extensive experience of the Jackson Clinic with endoscopic procedures. Recent advances in fiberoptic technology are not covered in this book, but it remains the standard work, and methodology is extensively discussed.*

Kassay, D.: Clinical Applications of Bronchology. New York, McGraw-Hill Book Company, 1960.
*A concise summary of the anatomy, physiology, and radiologic appearance of the tracheobronchial tree initiates this book.*

*The author then covers bronchoscopy and bronchography in relation to specific disease entities and includes an adequate list of selected references.*

Stradling, P.: Diagnostic Bronchoscopy. An Introduction. London, E. & S. Livingstone, 1968.
*This superb monograph provides an introduction to bronchoscopic technique and the anatomy of the tracheobronchial tree. Anyone preparing to carry out his first bronchoscopic examination will find this to be an invaluable guide. The color photographs are of the highest quality and the text is succinct and highly readable.*

## REFERENCES

1. Bozzini, P.: Lichtleiter, eine Erfindung zur Anschauung innerer Teile und Krankheiten nebst Abbildung. J. prakt. Heilunde, *24*:107, 1806.
2. Holinger, P., and Andrews, A. H.: Bronchial obstruction. Signs, symptoms and diagnosis. Amer. J. Surg., *54*:193, 1941.
3. Jackson, C. L., and Huber, J. F.: Correlated applied anatomy of the bronchial tree and lungs with a system of nomenclature. Dis. Chest, *9*:319, 1943.
4. Jackson, C., and Jackson, C. L.: Peroral pulmonary drainage—natural and therapeutic, with especial reference to the "tussive squeeze." Amer. J. Med. Sci., *186*:849, 1933.
5. Jackson, C., and Jackson, C. L.: Bronchoesophagology. Philadelphia, W. B. Saunders Company, 1950.
6. Killian, G.: Meeting of the Society of Physicians of Freiburg, Dec. 17, 1897. Munchen. Med. Wschr., *45*:378, 1898.
7. Peabody, J. W.: Bronchoscopic aids in medical conditions within the chest. Dis. Chest, *9*:307, 1943.
8. Stradling, P.: Diagnostic Bronchoscopy: An Introduction. London, E. & S. Livingstone, 1968.

# V

# Tracheostomy and Its Complications

*Hermes C. Grillo, M.D.*

Tracheostomy is one of the most ancient of operations and has long been used for the emergency management of upper airway obstruction. In the past two decades, tracheostomy has been increasingly employed to control secretions in severely ill patients. More recently, tracheostomy has provided a route for ventilatory support in respiratory insufficiency. This increased use of tracheostomy has reawakened appreciation of the large number of serious complications that may follow the procedure. A new spectrum of lesions, principally associated with its use for ventilatory support, has been identified.

## INDICATIONS FOR TRACHEOSTOMY

The occurrence of serious complications has caused critical reappraisal of the three classic indications for tracheostomy: (1) relief of upper airway obstruction, (2) control of secretions, and

(3) ventilatory support in respiratory failure. Tracheostomy often cannot be avoided in organic upper airway obstruction, although sometimes a tube may be slipped past an obstruction transiently until definitive treatment is provided. However, the accumulation of secretions has increasingly been controlled by adequate humidification and by intensive pulmonary physiotherapy, consisting of expert instruction and assistance in cough, positional drainage, and thoracic percussion. Tracheal suctioning is used in conjunction with these measures, and occasionally transcricoid instillation of saline has been of assistance. Bronchoscopy, formerly used so frequently, is rarely necessary.

Patients with respiratory insufficiency or impending failure are usually supported by respirator with an endotracheal tube for varying lengths of time. If it appears that more than a day or so of support will be required, a nasotracheal tube is generally preferred for patients' comfort.

Patients may thus be tided over a brief period of need for ventilatory support postoperatively without the need for tracheostomy. There is no firm rule about the length of time an endotracheal tube may be left in place. If it becomes clear that long-term support will be needed, a tracheostomy is usually done as an elective procedure within 5 to 7 days. Such a transfer becomes necessary because of the dangers of tube obstruction, the discomfort to the patient of a nasal or oral tube, and the considerable damage to the larynx that may result from prolonged intubation. This injury occurs especially in the posterior commissure, with damage to the arytenoid and interarytenoid area.[13]

## TECHNIQUE OF TRACHEOSTOMY

Tracheostomy is only rarely an emergency procedure. The safest way to establish an emergency airway is by insertion of an endotracheal tube or, failing that, introduction of a ventilating bronchoscope. Even obstructing lesions can often be bypassed in this way or enough ventilatory force applied past an obstruction through a tube so that a patient may be maintained until a more carefully considered procedure can be done. For this reason, the simplest emergency surgical airway,

an opening in the superficially located cricothyroid membrane, is rarely required. If this is done, it must be promptly followed by an elective tracheostomy in order to avoid irreversible damage to the larynx.

Tracheostomy may be done under local anesthesia, with the patient supine and the neck hyperextended. An anesthetist should be in attendance to maintain a clear airway, to adjust the positioning of the endotracheal tube during the procedure, and to supply oxygen or other support as needed. The procedure should be performed in the operating room, if only to maintain the most sterile conditions and to impress the operator with the need for meticulous technique. Blind tracheotomy procedures are unnecessary and are only to be condemned because of the high incidence of complications associated with them. The speedily made vertical cutaneous incision for emergency tracheostomy has been replaced by a carefully placed horizontal incision. This avoids the late tethering scars that may follow the vertical incision. Palpation of the extended neck always reveals the position of the cricothyroid membrane and the cricoid cartilage below this. The incision is placed at the level of the second tracheal cartilage and carried through the platysma (Fig. 1). The strap muscles are separated vertically in

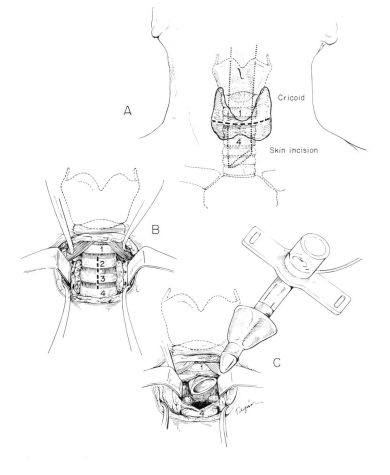

**Figure 1** Technique of tracheostomy. *A,* An endotracheal airway is in place. With the patient's neck extended and centered in the midline, a short horizontal incision is made over the second or third tracheal ring after the level of the cricoid cartilage has been carefully palpated. The first and fourth tracheal cartilages are numbered. *B,* Following horizontal division of the platysma, the strap muscles are separated in the midline, the cricoid is identified, and the thyroid isthmus usually is divided and sutured to allow easy access to the second and third tracheal rings. The second and third rings are incised vertically. Occasionally an additional partial incision of the fourth ring is necessary. *C,* Smooth thyroid pole retractors are used to spread the opening in the trachea. The endotracheal tube is withdrawn to a point just above the incision. The tracheostomy tube is introduced with a small amount of water-soluble lubricant and with its large-volume cuff collapsed. The endotracheal airway is not removed until it is demonstrated that the tracheostomy tube is properly seated and permits suitable air exchange. Closure is made with simple skin sutures. The flange of the tracheostomy tube is both sutured to the skin and tied with the usual tapes around the neck. On a rare occasion when an airway cannot be established from above, an emergency incision may be necessary over the cricothyroid membrane for rapid establishment of a temporary airway.

the midline with minimal bleeding. The lower border of the cricoid cartilage is clearly defined and the incision between the strap muscles and its subjacent fascia is carried down to a point below the thyroid isthmus. The isthmus is usually divided between hemostats after careful dissection beneath it in the pretracheal plane. The thyroid tissue on either side is controlled with mattress sutures. Exact levels of the cartilaginous rings must be determined. The first cartilage must be left intact, and the opening in the trachea must be placed so that there will be no tendency for the tube subsequently to erode the first ring or the adjacent cricoid cartilage by upward pressure. The second and third cartilages (and all or part of the fourth if necessary) are incised vertically in the midline to avoid the potential danger of upward pressure by the outside of the elbow of the tube. If there is any question, it is better to incise a lower cartilage than damage a higher cartilage. Even after centuries of tracheostomy, there is little controlled work to prove the superiority of the vertical incision over the cruciate or the horizontal incision, the excision of a disc or a segment of cartilage, or the turning of a Björk or other type of flap. The tracheal opening probably enlarges to the size of the tube in most cases after some days. The important point is not to make too large an opening in the tracheal wall, whether with a flap or not, since the flap may well be destroyed or deformed. Any opening heals by cicatrization, and the larger the opening, the greater is the chance for narrowing during stomal healing. If fine retractors are used in the open trachea, even tubes with a bulky low-pressure cuff may be inserted with ease with the assistance of a little water-soluble lubricant. With such an elective procedure, hemostasis should be precise throughout.

Hypoxia and subsequent cardiac arrest, which formerly occurred during emergency tracheostomy, should not occur with this technique, since an airway has already been established. Former texts indicated the site of tracheostomy to be the suprasternal notch in the extended neck. In many, such an approach selects a midtracheal location and places the point of potential damage from cuff injury low in the trachea. The trachea is also farthest away from the cervical skin surface at this level. Further, it tends to angulate the tube more. In children and in some adults, a low incision also places the inner side of the elbow of the tube close to a high innominate artery, with greater potential for later erosive major hemorrhage.

Once the tube has been securely seated and any attached cuff is functioning satisfactorily, the endotracheal tube is withdrawn and supportive oxygenation given through a light-weight connector attached to the tube or to its inner cannula if it is a two-part tube. The skin is loosely closed with vertical mattress sutures on either side of the tracheostomy tube. The loops of the sutures on either side are passed through the flanges of the tracheostomy tube, fixing it securely in place, in addition to the usual tracheostomy tapes. Such

fixation is particularly important in the first few days, especially when a vertical incision in the trachea has been used, so that displacement of the tube will not occur at a time when replacement may be difficult. Too long a tube should be avoided to prevent placement in the right main bronchus. Cuffs must be firmly fixed or cemented, if they are not an integral part of the tube, to prevent dislodgment or prolapse over the end of the tube. Suctioning during tracheostomy and immediately after its completion helps to avoid postoperative atelectasis. Prolonged suctioning, which may cause hypoxia, is avoided.

## COMPLICATIONS OF TRACHEOSTOMY

Conversion of tracheostomy to a carefully performed elective procedure has largely eliminated the immediate and early complications of the procedure.[8, 10, 14] The longer-term complications of tracheostomy present largely in three ways: (1) sepsis, (2) hemorrhage, or (3) obstruction of the airway. Additional complications are tracheoesophageal fistula and persistence of the stoma. In general, the longer a tracheostomy is in place (especially with an inflated cuff), the greater is the chance that complications will occur.

### Sepsis

All tracheostomies are clinically contaminated, and *Staphylococcus aureus* (often a resistant strain), *Pseudomonas aeruginosa*, and a variety of other bacteria such as *Escherichia coli* and streptococcus can be cultured. Despite this inevitability, sterile care and cleansing of the stoma and respiratory equipment must be maintained to minimize the possibility of invasive infection of the lower airway. Antibiotics are probably best reserved for use when there is evidence of tracheobronchitis, pneumonitis, or cellulitis, since their premature use will not sterilize the stoma but may merely permit other flora to establish themselves.

### Hemorrhage

It has been noted that the curve of the tube may erode the innominate artery and produce late hemorrhage, especially in children, in whom the trachea is small and the artery high. Massive hemorrhage also occurs from erosion by tracheostomy cuffs or even the tip of a tube through the trachea into the innominate artery as it passes obliquely over the trachea. Bleeding from granulations or more superficial tracheal erosions is less common and usually less massive. Only immediate tamponade of a major arterial leak with an inflated cuff and prompt surgical treatment can lead to salvage. Resection of the injured artery with suture of both ends is one of the few possibilities in such a contaminated field. In the small number of cases in which this has been done successfully, neurologic problems have not yet appeared. The tracheal injury must also be handled by resection and repair as will be discussed.

**Figure 2**  Obstructive lesions that may result from cuffed tracheostomy tubes. A conventional cuffed tube is in place at the left (*A*). Sagittal and cross-sectional (bronchoscopic) views of pathologic lesions are shown at the right (*B*). Anterolateral strictures are seen at the stoma (a) and granulomas also occur here (b). The lesions may occur concurrently. Circumferential stricture develops at the level of cuff injury (c). Between the stomal level and the cuff stricture, varying degrees of tracheal malacia may be seen; this leads to partial collapse during respiration (d). Granulomas may also occur at the level of the tip of the tube (e). (From Geffin, B., Grillo, H. C., Cooper, J. D., and Pontoppidan, H.: J.A.M.A., *216*:1984, 1971.)

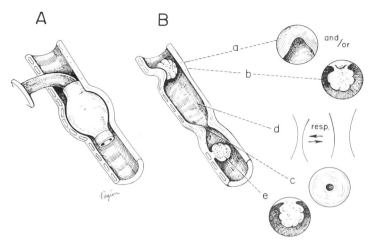

## Obstruction

Airway obstruction may occur while the tube is still in place. Cuff prolapse and its avoidance have been discussed. If a tube with an inner cannula is used, crusts may be easily cleaned. With proper humidification, obstruction of single-lumen tubes is less commonly seen. Occasionally, a valve type of crust may form at the tip of a tube so that a suction catheter may be easily passed without relieving the obstruction. If such is suspected, the only course is to change the tube. If the change is necessary early after tracheostomy, this should be done over a guiding catheter with adequate instruments and personnel available to reinsert an endotracheal tube or a bronchoscope from above in the event that the tube is not easily replaced. Occasionally, obstructive granulations also form at the tip of a tube that is still in place.

A major syndrome of postintubation airway obstruction has been recognized in the last decade[1, 6, 7] (Fig. 2). It is difficult to establish absolute incidence, but it may be that as many as 15 per cent of the survivors of prolonged ventilatory therapy have had such symptoms, as well as some patients who have had no ventilatory support but simply a cuffed tracheostomy tube that was placed to prevent aspiration. *Every patient with signs of upper airway obstruction—wheezing or stridor, dyspnea on effort, episodes of obstruction from secretions—who has been previously intubated with either an endotracheal tube or a tracheostomy tube must be considered to have organic obstruction until proved otherwise.* Unfortunately, many such patients who have been discharged from the hospital are treated for asthma to the point of death or subtotal obstruction before the lesion is recognized.

Obstructive *laryngeal lesions* from prolonged endotracheal intubation may occur at vocal cord level and consist of granulation tissue or cicatrix, particularly in the posterior commissure.[8, 13] *At*

**Figure 3**  Tracheal injury due to a cuffed tracheostomy tube. Autopsy specimen of larynx and trachea. *A*, A metal tracheostomy tube with rubber cuff inflated had been in place for 16 days. *B*, Cartilaginous rings are exposed and fragmented at the cuff site. The tracheal wall is thinned and distended. Similar injuries occur with plastic tubes and cuffs. (From Cooper, J. D., and Grillo, H. C.: Ann. Surg., *169*:334, 1969.)

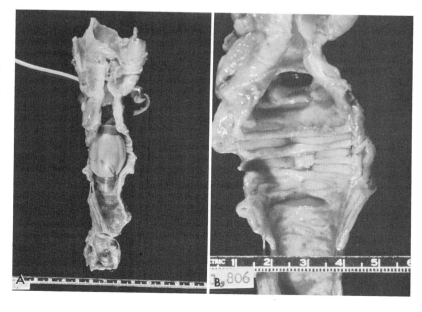

*the stomal level*, obstruction may be due to a polypoid granuloma that forms on the healing surface of the stomal site. Narrowing and indentation at the point of cicatrization of the stoma is often seen after tracheostomy. When the stoma is large—because of overgenerous initial surgery or erosion by local infection or, most commonly, by the prying action of heavy-weight equipment that connects the tracheostomy to the ventilator—healing may produce clinically obvious obstruction. Such stomal obstruction is usually three-sided, obstructing anteriorly and laterally, since the posterior wall is intact. Occasionally, some scarring occurs posteriorly as well. A combination of granuloma and stenosis may also produce obstruction. If the tracheostomy was placed too high, erosion of the cricoid cartilage may have occurred, with loss of substance and resultant subglottic stricture, one of the most difficult lesions to correct.

*At the cuff site*, pressure by the sealing cuff causes varying degrees of damage. Prior to the introduction of true large-volume, low-pressure cuffs, damage occurred in varying degrees in all patients in whom a cuff was inflated for more than 48 hours.[4] In the days and weeks following, erosion frequently bares numerous cartilages, leading to their fragmentation, and, eventually, total destruction (Fig. 3). Occasionally, the erosion progresses anteriorly, through the wall of the innominate artery, or posteriorly, to produce a tracheoesophageal fistula. With lesser degrees of damage, healing occurs with varying degrees of deformity and narrowing. If the tracheal wall has been deeply eroded circumferentially, a circumferential stricture results during healing (Fig. 4). This may become arrested with partial closure and produce only dyspnea on effort, or it may go on to complete closure with a fatal obstructive episode. The lengths of such strictures are extremely variable, extending from 0.5 cm. to 4 cm. Such lesions may occur with either endotracheal tubes or tracheostomy tubes since they are due to the cuff and not to the tube itself. A far greater number have resulted from cuffs on tracheostomy tubes since there is greater long-term exposure to them. Other factors have been implicated in the etiology of cuff strictures, including periods of hypotension, which make it easier to compress the mucosal vascular supply, bacterial infection, which is always present, and toxic products from various materials and from ethylene oxide sterilization with inadequate aeration. However, clinical, pathologic, and experimental evidence clearly demonstrates that the common denominator is pressure.[4, 5]

The tracheal cartilages *between the stoma and cuff level* are often thinned, presumably by inflammatory changes, and this segment may become malacic. With respiratory effort, the malacic segment tends to collapse, contributing to the obstructive picture. Granuloma may also form at a point of erosion by the *tip of the tracheostomy tube*. Children are more likely to show this lesion, since they are usually managed postoperatively without a cuff.

While most tracheostomies close spontaneously, a large and long *persistent stoma* will fail to close occasionally and require precise surgical repair.[12] This is apt to occur in aged or debilitated patients, in patients with metabolic disease, or in those who have been exposed to steroids.

Once a clinical diagnosis of obstruction is made, confirmation is easily obtained by simple radiologic studies (Fig. 5). Routine chest x-rays most frequently show clear lung fields. The unwary physician may treat the patient for adult-onset asthma or other vague diagnoses. Lateral neck roentgenograms will reveal tracheal deformities at the stomal level. Oblique views of the chest, which

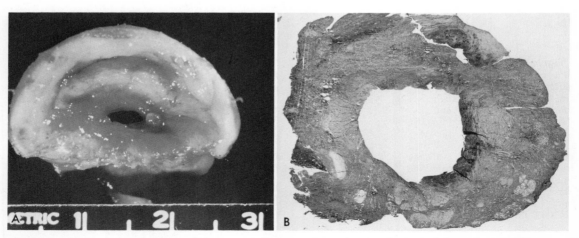

**Figure 4** Tracheal stenosis from cuff damage. *A*, Gross specimen showing the typical circumferential fibrous and inflammatory lesion. *B*, Photomicrograph showing that the stricture in a severe case is composed almost entirely of scar tissue; little normal tracheal architecture identifiable. Such strictures do not respond even to prolonged dilation or splinting. (From Grillo, H. C.: J. Thorac. Cardiovasc. Surg., *57*:52, 1969.)

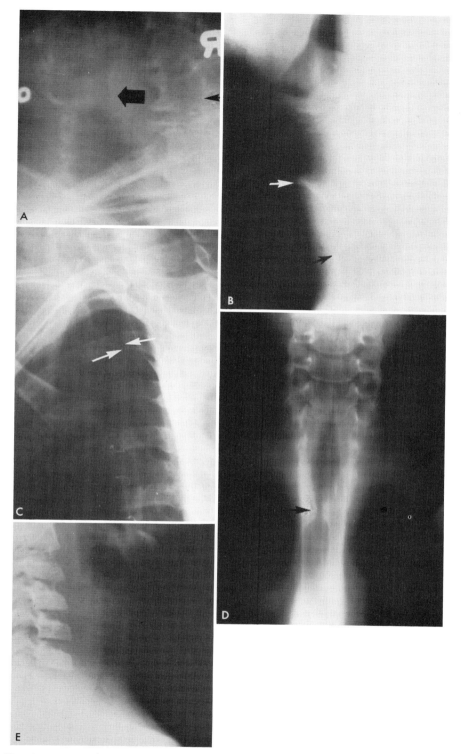

**Figure 5** Roentgenograms demonstrating tracheal lesions. *A*, Granuloma at stomal site. Circular radiopaque marker is on skin at site of prior stoma. Arrow points to partially narrowed air column with large anterior granuloma visible. *B*, Stricture at tracheostomy site, shown in detail of lateral neck view. Larynx is clearly seen above. Arrows mark longitudinal limits of anterior stricture. The posterior wall of trachea is not involved. *C*, Cuff-level stenosis is demonstrated on oblique view of chest, which rotates mediastinal structures away from the trachea and shows its full length. Arrows indicate the narrowness of the airway. The lesion is circumferential. *D*, Cuff stricture shown on laminagram. The exact length of the stenosis, degree of airway narrowing, and level of stricture in relation to larynx and carina are detailed. *E*, Granuloma at level of anterior erosion by tip of tracheostomy tube, shown in lateral neck roentgenogram. In this child, a cuff had not been used.

rotate the mediastinum to the side, reveal the entire trachea and demonstrate areas of narrowing at cuff level or elsewhere. A radiopaque marker taped to the skin at the site of an existing stoma or at the scar of such a stoma is helpful in pinpointing the level of a lesion. Fluoroscopy demonstrates the presence of malacia in the segment between the stoma and a cuff stricture. Tracheal laminagrams best define the character, the level, and the extent of a lesion, facts that are necessary to plan correction. Contrast medium produces a crisper picture but is not necessary. Insufflation of powdered tantalum avoids the possibility of obstruction that liquid media present in the tightest lesions.

**Treatment.** With the development of techniques of tracheal surgery that permit safe end-to-end anastomosis after resection of lengthy segments, the majority of these patients may be returned to normal function by surgical excision of the obstructing lesion and anatomic reconstruction of the upper airway.[7, 8, 15] If the patient is too ill for repair or has a disease that will soon require repeated tracheostomy, conservative management is recommended. This is possible in all but those cases in which the lesion is immediately above the carina, by reinstituting a tracheostomy, dilating the stricture and passing a fenestrated tube through it. In an occasional patient in whom the original damage was small in amount, repeated dilations or prolonged splinting with an inlying tube may produce a satisfactory airway over a long period of time. In most, however, conservative treatment will not succeed despite prolonged attempts, and a permanent tracheostomy tube is required.

In a series of 67 patients with *tracheal stenosis* seen between 1964 and 1971 at the Massachusetts General Hospital, 56 were submitted to surgical reconstruction. Ten were treated conservatively because their basic diseases did not suggest that a reconstruction would be tolerated or, more often, because they were likely to require tracheostomy again in the near future for diseases such as severe myasthenia gravis. One patient, early in the series, underwent exploration but died before resection could be done. Of the 57 surgical cases of stenosis, 54 followed intubation and three were post-traumatic. There were 13 postintubation lesions at the *stomal* level and 37 at the *cuff* level, three patients had stenoses at *both* levels, and in one the lesion was of uncertain origin. Two of the "cuff" stenoses were in patients who had had endotracheal intubation only, one for only 48 hours. Fifteen of the patients incurred their strictures at the Massachusetts General Hospital and the remaining 41 were referred.

The results of aggressive surgical treatment are good. Forty-six patients had good to excellent anatomic and functional results. Six had results that were clinically satisfactory although not ideal if the patients were to stress themselves physically. Three represented failures, one predictably in completely unfavorable circumstances in which the operation was forced because of the extremely low level of the stricture. The other two exhibited factors that were not fully appreciated early in our operative experience, namely, severe accompanying tracheomalacia and destruction of the cricoid cartilage. One patient in whom there was no alternative was operated upon as a desperate measure but required ventilatory support postoperatively, which led to erosion of the suture line. This was the sole fatality.

**Prevention.** Prevention of tracheal stenosis is of key importance. Diminution in the incidence of stomal strictures was noted at the Toronto General Hospital when heavy connecting tubing was abandoned for light-weight swivel connectors.[1]

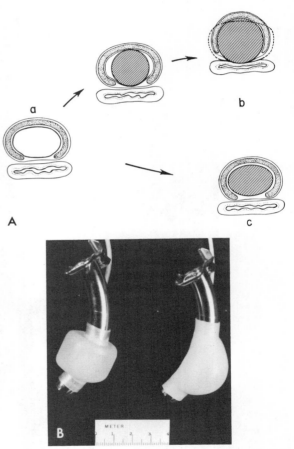

**Figure 6** *A,* Diagram of the mechanism of cuff injury to the trachea and its avoidance. Above, a conventional cuff must be inflated under high pressure to effect a seal of the irregular tracheal airway. It distorts the trachea and exerts great pressure on the mucosa. Below, a cuff with large resting volume fills the irregular tracheal lumen by conforming to its shape at low intracuff pressures, below the point of elastic distention of the cuff. *B,* The experimental cuff and a Rusch cuff mounted on standard Jackson tracheostomy tubes. The new cuff (left) is shown at its resting size. It must be collapsed with gentle syringe suction for insertion. The standard cuff (right) has been inflated with 8 cc. of air. It has a high intracuff pressure, is asymmetric, and is quite rigid. (From Grillo, H. C., Cooper, J. D., Geffin, B., and Pontoppidan, H.: J. Thorac. Cardiovasc. Surg., *62:*898, 1971.)

A relatively low incidence of stomal strictures in a corresponding period at the Massachusetts General Hospital, where light-weight connectors were in use, confirms this observation. Obviously, the surgical stoma should not be excessively large in the first place.

Strictures have been associated with tubes of every material and with cuffs of varying types of materials. At cuff level, the principal preventive factor is elimination of pressure necrosis.[3, 5, 9, 11] The large-volume, low-pressure cuffs, which occlude the irregularly shaped tracheal lumen by conforming to the shape of the trachea rather than by expanding to distend and so close the airway, seem to be accomplishing this end. Such a cuff was devised initially in animal experiments and then tested clinically in patients[5, 9] (Fig. 6).

Alternative methods of safeguarding the trachea have also been proposed or used. The most promising of these methods appears to be that of intermittent inflation of the cuff with the inspiratory phase of the respiratory cycle, thereby reducing the time of exposure of the trachea to a high-pressure cuff.[2] It is entirely possible that future advances in respiratory therapy will ultimately make tracheostomy unnecessary, but this era would appear to be far off.

## SELECTED REFERENCES

Andrews, M. J., and Pearson, F. G.: The incidence and pathogenesis of tracheal injury following cuffed tube tracheostomy with assisted ventilation: An analysis of a two-year prospective study. Ann. Surg., *173*:249, 1971.
*This excellent study correlates the factors attendant upon respiratory therapy, the gross pathologic observations per stomam at the time of extubation, and subsequent appearance of stenosis.*

Cooper, J. D., and Grillo, H. C.: The evolution of tracheal injury due to ventilatory assistance through cuffed tubes. A pathologic study. Ann. Surg., *169*:334, 1969.
*The pathogenesis of tracheal injuries is traced by means of study of autopsy specimens of tracheas from patients who died while in respiratory therapy and surgically resected specimens of fully developed strictures. Pressure necrosis is identified as the major etiologic factor.*

Grillo, H. C.: The management of tracheal stenosis following assisted respiration. J. Thorac. Cardiovasc. Surg., *57*:52, 1969.
*The failure of conservative management is emphasized, and the successful application of new techniques of surgical re-*

construction in the management of postintubation lesions is described.

Grillo, H. C.: Surgery of the trachea. Curr. Prob. Surg., July 1970.
*This brief monograph summarizes the literature on tracheal lesions and their management and presents the author's data and views on both inflammatory and neoplastic lesions of the trachea.*

Lindholm, C. E.: Prolonged endotracheal intubation. Acta Anaesth. Scand., Supp. 33, 1969.
*This exhaustive study of postintubation tracheal injury emphasizes the problems created by pressure of endotracheal tubes on the posterior commissural area of the larynx. It also describes post-tracheostomy injury.*

## REFERENCES

1. Andrews, M. J., and Pearson, F. G.: The incidence and pathogenesis of tracheal injury following cuffed tube tracheostomy with assisted ventilation: An analysis of a two-year prospective study. Ann. Surg., *173*:249, 1971.
2. Arens, J. F., Ochsner, J. L., and Gee, G.: Volume-limited intermittent cuff inflation for long-term respiratory assistance. J. Thorac. Cardiovasc. Surg., *58*:837, 1969.
3. Carroll, R., Hedden, M., and Safar, P.: Intratracheal cuffs: Performance characteristics. Anesthesiology, *31*:275, 1969.
4. Cooper, J. D., and Grillo, H. C.: The evolution of tracheal injury due to ventilatory assistance through cuffed tubes. A pathologic study. Ann. Surg., *169*:334, 1969.
5. Cooper, J. D., and Grillo, H. C.: Experimental production and prevention of injury due to cuffed tracheal tubes. Surg. Gynec. Obstet., *129*:1235, 1969.
6. Geffin, B., Grillo, H. C., Cooper, J. D., and Pontoppidan, H.: Stenosis following tracheostomy for respiratory care. J.A.M.A., *216*:1984, 1971.
7. Grillo, H. C.: The management of tracheal stenosis following assisted respiration. J. Thorac. Cardiovasc. Surg., *57*:52, 1969.
8. Grillo, H. C.: Surgery of the trachea. Curr. Probl. Surg., July 1970.
9. Grillo, H. C., Cooper, J. D., Geffin, B., and Pontoppidan, H.: A low pressure cuff for tracheostomy tubes to minimize tracheal injury: A comparative clinical trial. J. Thorac. Cardiovasc. Surg., *62*:898, 1971.
10. Head, J. M.: Tracheostomy in the management of respiratory problems. New Eng. J. Med., *264*:587, 1961.
11. Knowlson, G. T. G., and Bassett, H. F. M.: The pressures exerted on the trachea by endotracheal inflatable cuffs. Brit. J. Anaesth., *42*:834, 1970.
12. Lawson, D. W., and Grillo, H. C.: Closure of a persistent tracheal stoma. Surg. Gynec. Obstet., *130*:995, 1970.
13. Lindholm, C. E.: Prolonged endotracheal intubation. Acta Anaesth. Scand., Supp. 33, 1969.
14. Mulder, D. S., and Rubush, J. L.: Complications of tracheostomy: Relationship to long term ventilatory assistance. J. Trauma, *9*:389, 1969.
15. Pearson, F. G., and Andrews, M. J.: Detection and management of tracheal stenosis following cuffed tube tracheostomy. Ann. Thorac. Surg., *12*:359, 1971.

# VI

# Thoracic Trauma

## Paul A. Ebert, M.D.

Injuries of the chest occur with increased frequency, and they represent one of the most difficult and often most frustrating diagnostic complexes to the practicing physician. The thoracic cavity contains extremely vital organs, which can be injured without significant external evidence of trauma. Too often, the patient looks surprisingly well, and then suddenly shock, respiratory distress, and cardiac or respiratory arrest develop.

In patients with penetrating thoracic injuries,

the potential seriousness of the condition is usually immediately appreciated by the initial examiner. On the other hand, patients suffering from blunt thoracic trauma commonly have associated injuries that occupy the physician's attention, and often the extent and potential hazard of the intrathoracic injury are not appreciated until a catastrophic event occurs. Most blunt injuries to the chest result from automobile accidents, and the majority of these patients have associated injuries. The mortality from thoracic injuries increases markedly when associated injuries are present. This may simply be a reflection of the severity of the accident, or it may be due in part to the difficulties in managing patients with multiple injuries.

It has been estimated that as many as 20 per cent of deaths from trauma result primarily from chest injuries. Surprisingly, a very small percentage of hospital deaths can be attributed to the thoracic injury. For example, only approximately 20 per cent of patients with a ruptured thoracic aorta reach the hospital alive. In injuries of the chest, the most common cause of death between the site of accident and the emergency room is respiratory insufficiency. This may be due to simple obstruction of the airway in the mouth or throat, to development of tension pneumothorax, to a sucking chest wound, or to paradoxical movement of a fractured segment of the chest wall. Many of these conditions can be treated without elaborate equipment if the initial examining physician understands the urgency required in adequate management of respiratory difficulties.

Evaluation of ventilation should be one of the physician's first concerns. This can be accomplished by simply examining the patient and estimating the force of the respirations and the amount of air inspired and expired. Obviously, if the patient has multiple secretions or blood in the nasopharynx, these should be removed to assure an adequate airway. By palpating the pulse, one can determine whether it has respiratory variation; this would suggest hemopneumothorax or pericardial tamponade. The majority of patients in shock from blood loss alone, unless they also have a severe head injury or are in intense pain, will lie quietly and will not be restless or agitated. In a patient with thoracic injuries there may be both tension pneumothorax and loss of a large amount of blood into the thoracic cavity. The major sign of respiratory insufficiency is agitation and restlessness. Of course, if the patient also has a cerebral injury, signs of restlessness and agitation may be less meaningful.

An initial precursory examination should identify any obvious open wounds of the chest. Respiratory insufficiency from a flail chest may be apparent on inspection, but frequently in a large patient the amount of subcutaneous fluid or blood will conceal the extent of paradoxical movement and make the external appearance of the skin rather smooth and concentric. The presence of crepitus or actual free movement of ribs on palpation should suggest a possible flail segment. If respiratory efforts are adequate and the chest moves symmetrically but

ventilatory exchange is poor, some form of airway obstruction probably exists. The initial diagnosis of pneumothorax or hemothorax may be more difficult on physical examination than is often described. Often the involved hemithorax is diminished in volume, and there are poor respiratory excursions on the involved side. With the patient in the recumbent position, hemopneumothorax may be difficult to diagnose since blood will lie in the posterior aspect of the thorax, while the compressed lung will be near the anterior chest wall. Breath sounds may be normal over the anterior and lateral thorax; this makes the diagnosis by physical examination alone difficult.

The neck should be examined to determine the relative position of the trachea in the suprasternal notch. In tension pneumothorax or hemothorax, the trachea may be shifted away from the involved side, and this can be a useful clinical observation. Subcutaneous emphysema and crepitance may be present in the neck about the trachea. Neck veins may be distended if there is increased intrathoracic pressure or cardiac tamponade. If percussion can be performed far enough posteriorly, a large hemothorax will be associated with a dull percussion note, whereas pneumothorax will obviously be associated with a hyperresonant sound. The aforementioned important points for evaluation of thoracic injuries should accompany a complete, thorough physical examination to evaluate other areas of the body as well. It is important to emphasize that once obvious massive hemorrhage from open arteries has been controlled by pressure, tourniquet, or vascular clamp, the chest and respiratory system demand the most attention.

It is interesting to note certain overall mortality statistics of closed chest trauma. In a review of traffic fatalities with chest injury, Kemmerer[9] found rib fractures in 39 per cent, hemothorax in 28 per cent, lung lacerations in 10 per cent, and ruptured great vessels in 10 per cent. About 40 per cent of these victims were thought to have died as a result of their thoracic injuries. It is apparent that the extent of chest injuries often is not appreciated, and institution of proper treatment is unnecessarily delayed. Perry and Galway[14] reported that 21 per cent of patients with serious chest injury reaching the hospital alive died during the first 24 hours. Associated injuries have a great influence on survival after chest trauma. Schramel[16] observed a 42 per cent mortality in patients with a significant associated injury. When a cerebral injury significant enough to cause unconsciousness for 72 hours was associated with a major thoracic injury, a survival of only 12 per cent was observed. However, in isolated thoracic injuries alone, the survival is approximately 90 per cent.

## MECHANISMS OF INJURY

In the majority of incidences, it is difficult to isolate the exact mechanism of injury since several occur simultaneously. It is important, however, to attempt to divide the mechanisms of injury so that some understanding of the etiology of internal organ damage can be appreciated. Penetrating injuries, such as bullet or knife wounds, need little explanation since they cause injury by direct contact with the internal structure. Blunt thoracic trauma can be more complex, and the internal damage considerably more extensive than the external evidence of injury.

*Direct trauma* to the thoracic cage has always been a common form of injury. The victim is struck in the chest by a moving object; this may result in fractures of ribs or sternum over a localized area, but a major vascular or cardiac injury is rare. The lung may be contused by a fragment of rib driven inward, with pulmonary laceration or hemopneumothorax resulting. The majority of patients suffering direct local trauma survive, and associated injuries are uncommon. The area of the actual injury is usually clearly defined.

A *compression-type injury* of the thorax or upper abdomen may result in a specific type of damage. This is commonly seen in patients trapped in landslides, cave-ins, or building collapses. There may be direct local trauma to the thoracic cage, although in many instances no actual injury can be defined. Sustained thoracic compression causes traumatic asphyxia or cervicofacial static cyanosis. In this situation, the skin of the face, neck, and shoulders has a red to purple discoloration, and subconjunctival hemorrhages are usually present (Fig. 1). This results from blood being forced out of

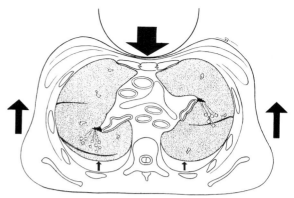

**Figure 2** Diagram of a sagittal section through the thorax, demonstrating the usual point of impact over the anterior chest. The bony thorax decelerates rapidly, while the internal structures may continue to move forward. The major attachment of the lung with the least elasticity is the bronchus, and the momentum of the lung may cause this structure to tear.

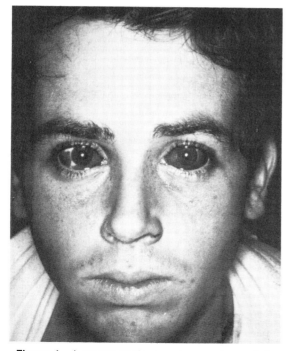

**Figure 1** A young workman who was trapped in a landslide and was subjected to thoracic compression for approximately 15 minutes. Note the marked bilateral subconjunctival hemorrhage. There was red to purple discoloration and multiple petechiae over the face, neck, and shoulder areas.

the thorax, with reflux cephalad through the venous system. Similar lesions can be produced experimentally by occluding the superior vena cava for approximately 10 minutes. These patients with vena caval occlusion are not asphyxiated in the usual meaning of the term, but suffer excessive oxygen removal in the capillary bed due to stasis. Compression injuries can rupture the diaphragm and contuse the lungs and the heart. In children, because of the marked pliability of the rib cage, severe thoracic compression can occur with minimal damage to the thoracic cage. Thoracic compression can result in the "crush syndrome," although it is not as common as in compression injuries of the extremities.

*Deceleration-type injuries* are usually classified under the broad headings of "impact" and "momentum," although most victims incur both concomitantly. Since most patients suffering blunt trauma to the chest are victims of automobile accidents, the effects of rapid deceleration are quite important. Impact injury results from direct contact of the thoracic cage with a hard object. The majority of force is dissipated against the bony thorax, with rib fractures and sternum fractures the result (Fig. 2). Contusion, laceration, and compression of soft tissues and internal organs occur. The fracture of ribs and the elasticity of the thoracic cage reduce the rate of deceleration and lessen the likelihood of a momentum-type injury occurring to internal organs. A momentum injury results from the rapid deceleration of the body with continued movement of the internal organ. For example, the heart is attached by the great arteries and veins, but the major mass is suspended in the pericardium. Patients sustaining a major fall have impact injury, but in addition the suspended heart continues to travel and one of its attachments tears. An aortic tear in the sinus of Valsalva is common in vertical deceleration, whereas tearing of the main bronchus results when the lung continues to move after rapid deceleration in a horizontal direction.

## PATHOPHYSIOLOGY

The most common thoracic injury is a simple fracture of ribs. Fracture of a rib in one place does not significantly alter the stability of the thoracic cage, but if the rib is fractured in two places, the segment between fracture sites has no stable attachment and is subject to movement related to changes in intrathoracic pressure. When several ribs are fractured in two sites, or in a single site in association with tearing of the anterior or posterior attachments, a large segment of chest wall becomes unstable, and so-called paradoxical movement of this area occurs. The loss of structural integrity of the thoracic cage reduces the efficiency of breathing, increases the work of respiration, and limits the volume of air moved with each breath. During inspiration, the flail segment moves inward, and during expiration it moves outward. For years the inadequacy of ventilation associated with a flail chest was attributed to a pendulum-like movement of air from one hemithorax to the other in association with paradoxical movement of the chest wall. Maloney[10] showed that this "pendelluft" effect did not occur and that the paradoxical movement of the chest wall simply limited the patient's ability to create adequate negative pressure to ventilate the lungs. Respiratory insufficiency may develop from mechanical instability of the chest wall, as a result of limited ventilation due to severe pain, and from alterations in ventilation and perfusion in the lungs secondary to trauma.

Most patients suffering a combination of impact and momentum injuries are subject to some pulmonary contusion. The initial response of the lung to trauma seems to be increased fluid production with retention of that fluid. This may be in the form of edema in the walls of the alveoli or frank outpouring of fluid into the alveolar spaces with development of pulmonary edema and pneumonitis. Comroe et al.[4] emphasized that there are changes in distribution of blood flow through the traumatized lung and alterations in ventilation within these traumatized segments. Thus, a degree of ventilation-perfusion inequality develops. This simply means that the relationship of ventilation and blood flow to the alveoli may not be uniform. One area of lung may be ventilated normally, while blood flow is decreased. In another or adjacent segment, blood flow may be increased, while ventilation is normal or decreased. Certainly, in normal man, blood flow to the capillary bed is not evenly distributed; in the erect position, gravitational force acting on blood in the longitudinal vessels causes an increase in blood flow to the base of the lungs. Some changes in vascular compliance of the pulmonary arteries may also be active and tend to make flow more nonuniform. The outpouring of fluid into lung parenchyma alters ventilation-perfusion relationships. Diffusion along the capillary membranes is altered in

areas of trauma, but the vast size of the pulmonary capillary bed usually permits adequate gas exchange. In some patients, the response to trauma is marked outpouring of fluid not isolated to the area of injury but involving the entire pulmonary tree. This finding has been commonly associated with severe head injury; the physiologic mechanism responsible is not well clarified, although it is thought to be related to an increase in intracranial pressure.

The physiologic shunt develops in the lung whenever blood flow through a segment of lung is greater than the ventilation to that segment. Thus, pulmonary venous blood draining the area will be incompletely oxygenated. Wilson[19] emphasized that physiologic shunting may be the earliest sign of impending respiratory failure. The ventilation-perfusion ratios are constantly changing in areas of injured lung, and the common physiologic disturbance is a reduction in oxygen content of the arterial blood. Since carbon dioxide diffusion across the alveolar membrane is approximately 20 times more efficient than oxygen transport, increased arterial carbon dioxide content is unusual. Oxygenation of the blood in capillaries is more time-consuming and is not completely accomplished in the injured lung. Increasing the oxygen content of inspired air will usually improve systemic arterial saturation. Thus, physiologic shunting can be decreased by raising the oxygen content of inspired air.

If arterial desaturation continues, some degree of tissue hypoxia occurs. The initial response is peripheral vasoconstriction, and the hypoxic tissue is thus further deprived of adequate oxygen. Patients usually become quite restless when peripheral tissue hypoxia occurs and often are quite hypertensive during this period unless associated major blood loss has occurred. There is usually an increase in the rate and depth of respiration, requiring additional work with increased oxygen consumption. Metabolic acidosis occurs, and the vicious cycle of tissue hypoxia is further amplified.

Following thoracic injury, ventilatory rate is usually increased and tidal volume is reduced. Thus, the calculated functional dead space is increased. Arterial carbon dioxide tension does not increase, although mild arterial hypoxemia has been noted when patients were breathing room air. Patients seem to be able to compensate for impaired ventilation for a period of time, but the added work of breathing to ensure adequate ventilation reduces arterial oxygen content and gradually results in accumulation of carbon dioxide, with the possibility of respiratory arrest. It is important that serial measurements of blood gases be done in any patient with evidence of arterial desaturation, since patients with flail chest injuries commonly do not show signs of respiratory insufficiency for 12 to 24 hours after admission to the hospital.

Impending respiratory failure should be appreciated before the arterial carbon dioxide level is elevated. Unless there is a major defect in diffusion

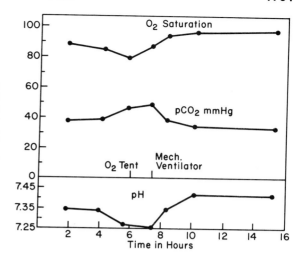

**Figure 3** Measurements of blood gases in a patient with a flail chest injury. Immediately after injury, there was a decrease in the arterial oxygen saturation. Placing the patient in an oxygen tent brought only slight improvement, and the arterial $pCO_2$ began to rise, suggesting further impairment in ventilation. Institution of positive-pressure ventilation with room air increased oxygen saturation, reduced the $pCO_2$, and raised the pH.

of gas from the alveoli to the pulmonary capillaries, arterial carbon dioxide does not become elevated until the tidal volume and dead space become nearly equal (Fig. 3). At this stage, arterial oxygen content is markedly reduced, and some type of ventilatory support is mandatory. There is only minimal reward in becoming expert in resuscitation after respiratory arrest, but great merit in recognizing and treating the early signs of respiratory insufficiency.

## FRACTURE OF THE RIBS

Simple fracture of the ribs resulting from blunt trauma to the chest is probably the most common injury encountered. Simple rib fracture can be lethal if the lung is lacerated and tension pneumothorax is produced. Tearing of an intercostal artery by the bony fragment may result in hemothorax and require thoracotomy for control of hemorrhage. In blunt injuries of the chest, the finding of subcutaneous emphysema over the site of the injury almost certainly indicates that the lung was torn and air escaped from the lung into the pleural space and then into the soft tissues.

Most of the time simple rib fracture does not result in internal injury to the lung, and the person complains only of a sharp, knifelike pain in the rib cage. This is accentuated by breathing or movement, and the patient attempts to splint the injured side. There is a tendency to underventilate the lung on the side of injury, and the possibilities of retention of secretions and atelectasis become a major problem.

In general, strapping of the hemithorax with tape should be discouraged since it further limits ventilatory excursion and enhances the possibility of atelectasis and pneumonitis. It is true that some relief of pain can be accomplished by strapping, but the overall benefits do not outweigh the disadvantages. Local anesthetic block of the intercostal nerves of the fractured rib and of the ribs above and below it provides considerable relief of pain. The anesthetic may last only 2 to 3 hours but often the pain is diminished because the patient breathes normally while the block is in effect. Administration of oral analgesics and expectorants is to be encouraged.

In all patients with suspected rib fractures, chest x-ray examination should be done to determine the presence or absence of pneumothorax. If a small pneumothorax is present, the physician should be alerted, as vigorous coughing and deep breathing by the patient may convert the simple pneumothorax into tension pneumothorax. If the pneumothorax is extensive, the insertion of an intercostal catheter with connection to an underwater seal is indicated. When pneumothorax alone is treated, the catheter is usually placed in the second intercostal space anteriorly. If considerable fluid or blood is present, the catheter may be inserted laterally through the sixth or seventh interspace.

## TENSION PNEUMOTHORAX

A small puncture wound in the lung may produce a ball valve action in the visceral pleura and allow air to enter the pleural cavity during inspiration but prevent its escape during expiration. The lung gradually collapses and the mediastinum shifts to the opposite side (Fig. 4). The patient becomes severely dyspneic from compression and inability to expand the opposite lung, and respiratory arrest may ensue. The patient will usually have pain on the side of the pneumothorax, and physical examination will confirm the diagnosis. Breath sounds will be diminished and the percussion note will be hyperresonant. A needle should immediately be inserted in the chest and air aspirated. Often air will be released under pressure, and continuing decompression of the hemithorax is necessary. A chest catheter should be inserted and connected to a closed drainage system. In patients in respiratory distress with the physical findings of tension pneumothorax, needle

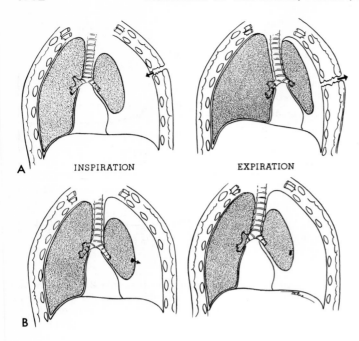

INSPIRATION        EXPIRATION

**Figure 4** *A,* Pleurocutaneous tract and movement of the mediastinum away from the site of injury during inspiration and toward the opening during expiration. *B,* In a tension pneumothorax, air leaves the lung during inspiration and cannot return through the small hole during expiration. The amount trapped in the pleural space increases, and the mediastinum shifts away from the involved side.

aspiration should be performed before a chest x-ray is obtained, as this is a life-threatening emergency.

## OPEN PLEUROCUTANEOUS TRACTS

A defect in the chest wall can be large enough that an open communication exists between the pleural space and the atmosphere. This is the so-called sucking-type chest wound. Often these wounds result from explosions or gunfire. The degree of respiratory distress will depend on the size of the opening. In large wounds, all air during inspiration passes through the pleurocutaneous wound rather than the trachea. This results in collapse of the lung and practically no intrapulmonary ventilation. The sound of air going through the defect is usually apparent. This rapid exchange of air through the chest wall defect results in inadequate ventilation because a positive intrathoracic pressure cannot be developed. The mediastinum shifts back and forth with each breath, and cardiac output is reduced. Immediate closure of the defect with mild external pressure will usually improve ventilation.

In most instances, an injury severe enough to cause an open thoracic wound will also injure the lung. When integrity of the chest wall is re-established by direct pressure or by a sealed dressing, the possibility of development of tension pneumothorax must be considered. In the emergency room it is best to pass a chest catheter through the wound and then restore integrity of the chest wall by applying a sealed dressing around the catheter. The catheter is attached to an underwater seal, and air leaking from the lung will be removed. If the wound is large, a urethral catheter with a 30 ml. inflatable balloon can be inserted, the balloon

inflated, and the wound sealed by gentle traction on the catheter. Surgical dressing of the defect can be accomplished, and a chest catheter can be inserted in another location to maintain expansion of the lung.

## FLAIL CHEST

Fractures of four or five ribs may result in paradoxical movement of a segment of chest wall. This reduces the efficiency of breathing and limits the ability of the patient to cough effectively. Frequently the paradoxical movement of the chest wall can easily be seen, but in some cases, soft tissue swelling and hematoma obscure the magnitude of the movement. Dyspnea and cyanosis may be present when the patient reaches the hospital, and in these situations treatment is quickly instituted. Too often, the patient looks well on admission, and the extent of the flail chest injury is thought not to justify corrective measures. Spencer[17] emphasized the potential seriousness of the flail chest, which is too often not appreciated on initial examination. These patients do well for several hours, but eventually accumulations of secretions, fatigue, bronchorrhea, and decrease in pulmonary compliance render them unable to continue adequate spontaneous respiration. Hypoxia becomes more severe, and eventually retention of carbon dioxide occurs.

Many methods of immobilization of the flail segment have been tried. In emergency situations, compression of the flail segment with a soft pressure bandage or application of a sandbag will suffice until definitive treatment is available. Strapping the flail segment with tape has the disadvantage of immobilizing normal chest wall, and further limiting respiratory function. External traction has been utilized to elevate the flail segment, stabilizing it in an outward position. Towel clip traction has been quite popular; this can be effected by placing a towel clip around one of the center ribs of the flail segment and applying outward traction, especially during inspiration. Many types of soft tissue traction, suction devices, and skeletal traction have been described. Most of these are very bulky and limit mobility of the patient. Open surgical pinning or wiring of fractures of the sternum has been quite satisfactory.

The copious secretions resulting from trauma to the lung remain a major problem. Patients with signs of respiratory insufficiency secondary to flail chest injuries should be managed by means of controlled positive-pressure ventilation. Mörch et al. in 1955 showed the value of this type of treatment, emphasizing that the flail segment can be stabilized by positive-pressure breathing and the problem of hypoxia can be eliminated.[12] If the patient is in severe respiratory distress, an endotracheal tube should be placed and positive-pressure ventilation instituted immediately. A tracheostomy is performed to facilitate use of the respirator and removal of secretions. The increase of mean intrathoracic pressure has not proved harmful, even in hypovolemic patients, in whom the circulatory reflexes are assumed to be retained. Respiration may be controlled by mild hyperventilation, which produces slight alkalosis and apnea. Other physicians prefer assistance of ventilation only, but this has the disadvantage of requiring the patient to initiate inspiration and thus continually move the flail segment of the chest. Positive-pressure ventilation is necessary until the chest wall stabilizes. This may require 3 to 4 weeks; too often a patient is removed from the respirator before the chest wall is stable, and paradoxical movement resumes. Both Border[2] and Rutherford[15] suggest that positive-pressure ventilation immediately after injury should be beneficial in re-expanding atelectactic lung, reducing edema, and decreasing pulmonary hemorrhage. Experimental work has shown that a delay of 24 hours allows a post-traumatic pulmonary lesion to be established, which is much more difficult to reverse. The appearance on chest x-ray has proved to be a poor index of the extent of pulmonary dysfunction. Arterial oxygen content or the alveolar-arterial oxygen tension difference is a much more reliable index.

Long-term management of patients with crushed-chest injuries requiring positive-pressure ventilation demands expert nursing care. Absolute sterile technique must be employed during suctioning and handling of the tracheostomy tube, which should be changed at least every 48 hours. Shortly after injury, endotracheal suctioning may have to be performed frequently to remove the copious secretions. The patients are routinely given antibiotics to reduce the possibility of infection in the traumatized lung. In some instances, positive-pressure ventilation is discontinued because of the fear that a lower respiratory tract infection will develop. Ebert[6] demonstrated that

pneumonitis develops in most patients with crushed-chest injuries, and positive cultures can be obtained from the trachea around the eighth to twelfth day. At this time, the general condition of the patient usually is such that proper antibiotics will control the infection (Fig. 5).

In any patient in whom positive-pressure ventilation is used, there is a risk that tension pneumothorax will develop, since the expanding lung may rub against a fragment of rib. The visceral pleura previously may have been perforated, and the fibrinous seal may be disrupted by administration of positive pressure. Thus, it is important that a routine chest x-ray be taken approximately 30 to 60 minutes after institution of positive-pressure ventilation, and the proper equipment for insertion of a chest catheter should be available.

Burford and Burbank in 1945 attributed the cause of traumatic wet lung to persistence of fluid, such as mucus, blood, or serum, in the lungs.[3] This condition lasted for several days after injury and patients were difficult to resuscitate from shock and were poor operative risks.

In patients suffering severe chest trauma, the amount of crystalloid fluid administered during the initial 48 hours after injury should be carefully calculated. The damaged capillary-alveolar membranes may leak fluid and cause increased respiratory difficulties. The lung reacts after trauma by producing an increased amount of interstitial and intra-alveolar fluid. Many patients have been made considerably worse by the injudicious use of large volumes of crystalloid fluid following trauma. In these circumstances, colloid osmotic pressure cannot hold a large volume of crystalloid fluid in the vascular space, and damaged capillaries in the lung increase the amount lost into the alveoli. There is considerable variance in the individual response to injury, in that the fluid produced by the lung may be so little that it is almost unrecognized or so great that it actually drowns the patient.

### Mechanical Ventilation

Whether a *volume-* or a *pressure-*regulated respirator should be used in management of flail chest injury is debated. The major advantage of the volume-regulated machine is the ability to control tidal volume and concentration of inspired oxygen. Most pressure-regulated respirators acquire their power from oxygen under pressure. If the ventilatory pressure increases, a greater concentration of oxygen is required to move the same volume of air. The problem is easily solved if compressed air is available to power the respirator.

Prolonged ventilation with high concentration of oxygen has been shown to produce changes in alveolar lining cells. These alterations are thought to be due to oxygen toxicity. Nash et al.[13] have divided these changes into two phases, an early exudative phase, with congestion, edema, hemorrhage, and fibrin, and a late proliferative phase, in which there is alveolar edema and fibroblastic proliferation with hyperplasia of the alveolar lining cells. The fundamental factors influencing oxygen toxicity are the oxygen concentration,

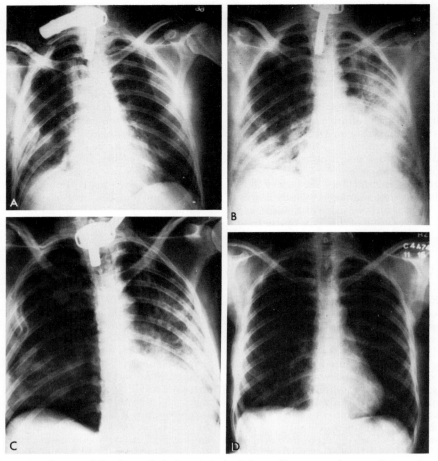

**Figure 5**   Sequence of x-rays following a flail chest injury. *A,* Immediate x-ray shows a chest catheter in the right thorax and a tracheostomy tube in place. The lung fields look reasonably clear. *B,* Twenty-four hours after injury, the extent of pulmonary contusion and fluid outpouring in the lung can be appreciated. *C,* Twelve days after injury, the right lung has cleared but residual pneumonitis is present on the left. *D,* Follow-up film 3 months after injury looks entirely normal.

susceptibility of the patient, and the length of exposure. In general, older patients are more susceptible than younger ones. The syndrome is progressive, and the changes are apparently irreversible. Prevention is the only known therapy, and there is no general agreement as to the length of time or concentration of oxygen required to produce alveolar changes. Prolonged ventilation with oxygen concentration no greater than 50 per cent seems to be tolerated without difficulty. However, if adequate arterial saturation cannot be accomplished with low oxygen concentrations, there is no choice but to increase the concentration of inspired oxygen. The possibility of toxic effects to the lung is realized, but the aim of treatment is maintenance until traumatized, nonfunctioning lung recovers. In all patients in whom positive-pressure ventilation is used, frequent measurements of arterial oxygen tension are necessary, and the level should be kept between 80 and 120 mm. Hg.

Prolonged use of mechanical ventilators has been incriminated as a cause of lung damage, and the term respirator lung or respirator pneumonitis has frequently appeared. Many patients who require assisted ventilation because of respiratory insufficiency have pre-existing pulmonary disease. Patients with mitral valve disease and secondary pulmonary changes often require prolonged ventilatory support after open heart surgery. Lungs from the patients, when seen at postmortem examination, often are congested, fluid-filled, and hepar-like, and unfortunately the term respirator lung was used to describe this appearance. More often, other factors such as prolonged administration of high concentrations of oxygen, infection, prior lung disease, and postperfusion pulmonary congestion syndrome were present and were primarily responsible for the pathologic findings. These changes are uncommon in patients suffering crushed-chest injury who had normal lungs before the accident, and it is known that a properly adjusted mechanical ventilation system can function for practically unlimited periods of time if tracheal, bronchial, and pulmonary infections are prevented.

## COSTOCHONDRAL OR STERNOCHONDRAL INJURIES

A direct blow over an anterior costal cartilage may result in severe pain at the point of impact, resulting from a separation or fracture of the cartilage at either a sternal or costal junction. These injuries are extremely painful and often disabling and frustrating to the patient. Complications are rare, and the diagnosis is based on the physical findings of pain and tenderness directly over the point of the chondral junction. These cartilaginous fractures heal slowly, and the period of discomfort may be prolonged. Treatment is usually with oral analgesics.

## FRACTURE OF THE STERNUM

In general, sternal fractures cause little disability except when associated with other major rib fractures. In severe flail chest injuries with associated sternal fractures, the sternum may have to be pinned or wired to provide stability of the thoracic cage. If the fracture is an isolated injury, relief of pain is the only treatment necessary.

## INJURIES TO TRACHEA OR MAIN BRONCHI

When blunt trauma to the chest causes a deceleration or momentum type of injury, the bronchus may be completely transected. Hemoptysis, pneumothorax, and subcutaneous emphysema usually occur, and the pneumothorax can quickly become a tension pneumothorax. Often subcutaneous emphysema of the neck appears early, and the trachea may be shifted to the opposite side (Fig. 6). Insertion of an intrathoracic tube to control the pneumothorax and air leak is important. If the patient will tolerate major surgery, direct anastomosis or bronchoplasty is recommended when the injury is recognized early. Often rupture of the bronchus is not immediately diagnosed, and it may be some time before development of pneumonitis or bronchial obstruction with distal pneumonia leads to its recognition. A ruptured bronchus heals with stenosis or occlusion. When stenosis is complete, the lung may be atelectatic and the diagnosis may remain obscure for years. If the stenosis is incomplete, air movement is partially obstructed, and coughing, due to blocking of the lumen by mucus, may occur. The likelihood of infection distal to the bronchial injury is greater when the obstruction is incomplete. Johnson[8] emphasized that patients with severe tracheal lacerations would be greatly improved by insertion of a tracheostomy tube. In these patients, massive air leaks usually develop, with extensive

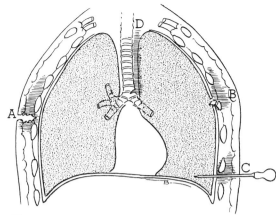

**Figure 6**  Possible causes of subcutaneous emphysema. *A,* Air may enter the soft tissues through external openings in the skin. *B,* A fractured rib may lacerate the parietal pleura and the lung; this results in a pneumothorax with escape of air through the parietal pleura into the subcutaneous tissue. *C,* A penetrating injury may result in subcutaneous emphysema from a combination of air entering from the outside and from a pneumothorax. *D,* A torn bronchus may cause mediastinal emphysema, which presents as subcutaneous air in the neck.

mediastinal emphysema. The tracheostomy tube lowers endotracheal pressure and decreases the amount of air escaping into the subcutaneous tissues. If the site of the laceration can be identified, it should be repaired at operation with interrupted nonabsorbable sutures (Fig. 7).

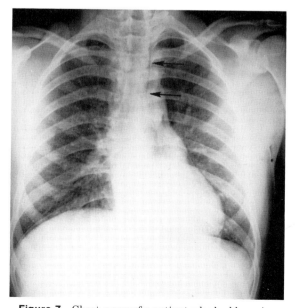

**Figure 7**  Chest x-ray of a patient who had been in an automobile accident with point of impact over the sternum. A small amount of subcutaneous emphysema was noted in the neck, and chest x-ray showed minimal mediastinal emphysema on the left. Bronchoscopy confirmed a tear in the left main stem bronchus, which was repaired at thoracotomy.

## INJURIES TO THE HEART

Blunt trauma to the chest can cause a wide variety of cardiac injuries. Bleeding in the pericardial sac with resultant tamponade may occur. A reliable central venous pressure measurement should be obtained before aspiration of the pericardial sac is attempted. If blood reaccumulates, open thoracotomy should be considered. Contusion of the heart or actual myocardial infarction probably occurs more frequently than is appreciated. Cardiac arrhythmias are common after chest injuries and are probably related to myocardial injury. Atrial fibrillation is often seen, and the rapid ventricular response may be controlled with digitalis. If electrocardiographic evidence of myocardial injury is observed, treatment for myocardial infarction should be instituted. The late development of ventricular aneurysm has been seen after blunt thoracic injury.

Injury to the heart should be suspected particularly after a steering column injury, since the broken end of the sternum or rib may be driven into the heart, with direct rupture of the heart wall. The heart may be so severely compressed between the sternum and the vertebrae that a laceration results. Signs of cardiac failure may occur and are treated with fluid restriction, diuretics, and digitalis. If ventricular irritability is evidenced by frequent premature ventricular beats, it probably is best managed by a continuous intravenous infusion of lidocaine. Persistent tachycardia is common after chest injury, and frequent x-rays should be obtained so that signs of cardiac dilatation or frank congestive heart failure may be detected.

## TRAUMATIC RUPTURE OF THE AORTA

It has been estimated that approximately 20 per cent of patients with rupture of the thoracic aorta reach the hospital alive. The majority die from exsanguination or pericardial tamponade. This subject is discussed in detail in another section.

## TRAUMATIC DIAPHRAGMATIC HERNIA

The diaphragm can be injured by direct penetration or as the result of blunt abdominal or thoracic trauma. Blunt injuries to the abdomen or chest produce a marked increase in intra-abdominal or

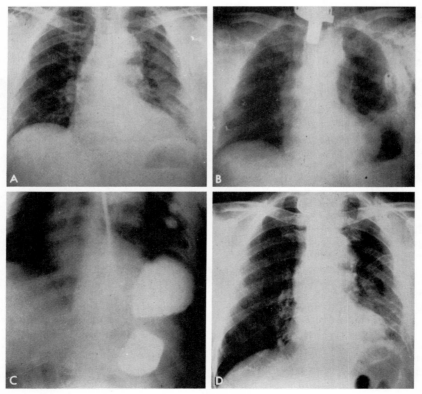

**Figure 8**   Sequence of chest x-rays of a patient with a left flail chest injury. *A,* The initial chest x-ray shows haziness in the left lower chest and contusion of the left lung. *B,* Two hours later, after institution of positive-pressure ventilation and tracheostomy. The suggestion of a left diaphragmatic hernia is now apparent. *C,* Radiopaque material given through the nasogastric tube confirms the presence of stomach in the left chest. *D,* Two days later, after left thoracotomy and repair of the diaphragmatic hernia.

intrathoracic pressure, usually resulting in a tear in the posterior central section of the diaphragm. Occasionally, the peripheral attachments of the diaphragm may be avulsed from the chest wall. Traumatic diaphragmatic hernias occur on the left side 98 per cent of the time; the liver apparently protects the right diaphragm. The defect is usually quite large, and abdominal viscera commonly herniate into the thorax. A high degree of suspicion is necessary when the possibility of diaphragmatic hernia exists, because often only a small portion of the stomach, spleen, or liver may be present in the left chest, producing only minimal changes on routine chest x-ray. Harrington has proposed that these tears in the diaphragm occur at the time of trauma but that often actual herniation of abdominal viscera into the chest occurs much later. Dyspnea, cyanosis, and restlessness in a patient with no evidence of actual pulmonary injury should suggest that the diaphragm is incompetent.

Operative repair is indicated as soon as the general condition of the patient permits. The preferred approach has been through a left posterior lateral thoracotomy or a thoracoabdominal incision. In many of these patients, the diaphragmatic rupture is associated with multiple rib fractures or other thoracic injuries (Fig. 8). Ebert et al.[6] showed that repair of the diaphragmatic hernia should be performed in patients with flail chest, and the usual methods of managing the unstable thoracic wall should be invoked in the postoperative period. Positive-pressure ventilation will be required and will be more easily managed after visceral organs have been returned to the abdominal cavity.

In small defects of the diaphragm, the possibility of strangulation of herniated viscera must be considered. Early surgical exploration will decrease the likelihood of this complication. In some instances, the diaphragmatic hernia will not be detected for many years, and a portion of lung will be collapsed because of the space occupied by abdominal viscera. Even when operation is performed late, results should be satisfactory, because re-expansion of the collapsed lung usually results in improved ventilatory function. The defect usually can be closed by direct suture, although in some instances of long-standing hernias some type of prosthetic material or cloth may be needed to bridge the defect. The operative results are excellent, with the main difficulty being in establishing the initial diagnosis.

## PENETRATING WOUNDS

Penetrating wounds of the chest are of serious concern because of the uncertainty as to whether major internal structures have been injured. One must consider the type of injury, and knowledge of the size or shape of the weapon can be extremely helpful. Unlike most abdominal wounds, which require an exploratory operation, many penetrating chest wounds do not require exploratory thoracotomy. However, a large number of these wounds are incurred in the lower left chest, and damage to the diaphragm or to intra-abdominal organs may occur, since the diaphragm lies at a much higher level than the lower limit of the rib cage. These injuries can be immediately life-threatening or, in many instances, seem highly insignificant, considering the mode of injury.

The major initial problem is that of hemopneumothorax, and most penetrating injuries of the chest require at least the insertion of an intercostal catheter connected to an underwater seal and suction. Bleeding from the lung is usually controlled by re-expansion of the lung, and thoracotomy usually is not necessary. In cardiac tamponade resulting from penetrating injuries, needle aspiration may initially provide relief but probably should be followed by exploratory thoracotomy. Wounds of the heart should be closed by direct suture, and evacuation of blood from the pericardium may reduce the possibility of subsequent constrictive pericarditis. It should be remembered that all penetrating injuries to the chest invariably contaminate the pleural space. Blood in the thorax is partially defibrinated by movement of the lung; this facilitates evacuation by chest catheter. Antibiotics are routinely administered because of intrapleural contamination. Elimination of the majority of blood in the pleural space decreases the possibility of subsequent pleuritis or empyema. Air leaks from the lung are usually controlled by maintaining adequate suction through the chest catheter.

Obviously, if blood continues to accumulate in the chest after insertion of a chest catheter, thoracotomy should be undertaken to control the hemorrhage. It is rare for significant bleeding to occur from the lung itself, but if major branches of the pulmonary artery or vein are injured, a lobectomy or even pneumonectomy may be necessary to control the hemorrhage. Intrapulmonary hematomas may develop after bullet or other penetrating injuries. These usually are asymptomatic and resolve spontaneously. Pulmonary lacerations may appear as cavitary lesions and contain a fluid level. This represents a tear in lung parenchyma, with leaking of air and fluid or blood into this space. These injuries are more common in young patients, and resolution is spontaneous, requiring an average of 6 to 10 weeks. Intrapulmonary hematomas discovered at the time of thoracotomy should be opened and the source of bleeding controlled by direct suture. The lung parenchyma is left exposed, with an intercostal catheter placed near the open area and connected to suction apparatus to maintain expansion of the lung. Development of lung abscesses in these intraparenchymal hematomas or cavities is uncommon.

## SELECTED REFERENCES

Moore, F. D., Lyons, J. H., Jr., Pierce, E. C., Jr., Morgan, A. P., Jr., Drinker, P. A., MacArthur, J. D., and Dammin, G. J.: Post-Traumatic Pulmonary Insufficiency. Philadelphia, W. B. Saunders Company, 1969.
*This excellent monograph considers pulmonary processes*

*associated with trauma or other illnesses that often are re-sponsible for respiratory insufficiency considered to be out of proportion to the primary disease. Respiratory difficulties associated with multiple fractures, sepsis, and shock are well defined. The pathophysiology of the pulmonary lesions is well illustrated, and the approach to management and pre-vention is emphasized. This presentation is easy to under-stand, and the clinical syndromes are separated by their physiologic consequences.*

Nealon, T. F., Jr.: Trauma to the chest. In: Gibbon, J. H., Jr., Sabiston, D. C., Jr., and Spencer, F. C., eds.: Surgery of the Chest. 2nd ed. Philadelphia, W. B. Saunders Company, 1969.

*This chapter provides an excellent overview of management and evaluation of patients suffering thoracic injuries. There are good series of chest x-rays demonstrating various conse-quences of trauma. Many specific areas such as wounds of the heart are well covered. Certain complications of thoracic injuries such as empyema or cardiac tamponade are dis-cussed in detail in other chapters.*

## REFERENCES

1. Battersby, J. S., and Kilman, J. W.: Traumatic injuries of the tracheobronchial tree. Arch. Surg., 88:644, 1964.
2. Border, J. R., Hopkinson, B. R., and Schenk, W. G., Jr.: Mechanisms of pulmonary trauma: an experimental study. J. Trauma, 8:47, 1968.
3. Burford, T. H., and Burbank, B.: Traumatic wet lung. J. Thorac. Surg., 14:415, 1945.
4. Comroe, J. H., Forster, R. E., Dubois, A. B., Briscoe, W. A., and Carlsen, E.: The Lung: Clinical Physiology and Pulmonary Function Tests. 2nd ed. Chicago, Year Book Medical Publishers, 1962, Chapter 4.
5. Conn, J. H., Hardy, J. D., Fain, W. R., and Netterville, R. E.: Thoracic trauma: analysis of 1022 cases. J. Trauma, 3:22, 1963.
6. Ebert, P. A.: Physiologic principles in the management of the crushed-chest syndrome. Monogr. Surg. Sci., 4:69, 1967.
7. Ebert, P. A., Gaertner, R. A., and Zuidema, G. D.: Traumatic diaphragmatic hernia. Surg. Gynec. Obstet., 125:59, 1967.
8. Johnson, J.: Battle wounds of the thoracic cavity. Ann. Surg., 123:321, 1946.
9. Kemmerer, W. T., Eckert, W. G., Gathright, J. B., Reemtsma, K., and Creech, O., Jr.: Patterns of thoracic injuries in fatal traffic accidents. J. Trauma, 1:595, 1961.
10. Maloney, J. V., Jr., Schmutzer, K. J., and Raschke, E.: Para-doxical respiration and "pendelluft." J. Thorac. Cardio-vasc. Surg., 41:291, 1961.
11. Martin, A. M., Simmons, R. L., and Heisterkamp, C. A., 3rd: Respiratory insufficiency in combat casualties. I. Pathologic changes in the lungs of patients dying of wounds. Ann. Surg., 170:30, 1969.
12. Mörch, E. T., Avery, E. E., and Benson, D. W.: Hyperventila-tion in the treatment of crushing injuries of the chest. Surg. Forum, 6:270, 1955.
13. Nash, G., Blennerhassett, J. B., and Pontoppidan, H.: Pul-monary lesions associated with oxygen therapy and artificial ventilation. New Eng. J. Med., 276:368, 1967.
14. Perry, J., and Galway, C. F.: Chest injury due to blunt trauma. J. Thorac. Cardiovasc. Surg., 49:684, 1965.
15. Rutherford, R. B., and Valenta, J.: An experimental study of "traumatic wet lung." J. Trauma, 11:146, 1971.
16. Schramel, R., Kellum, H., and Creech, O.: Analysis of factors affecting survival after chest injuries. J. Trauma, 1:600, 1961.
17. Spencer, F. C.: Treatment of chest injuries. Curr. Probl. Surg., Jan. 1964.
18. Whitwam, J. G., and Norman, J.: Hypoxaemia after crush injury of the chest. Brit. Med. J., 1:349, 1964.
19. Wilson, R. F., Larned, P. A., Corr, J. J., Sarver, E. J., and Barrett, D. M.: Physiologic shunting in the lung in critically ill or injured patients. J. Surg. Res., 10:571, 1970.

# VII

# Lung Abscess and Fungal Infections

*Timothy Takaro, M.D.*

## LUNG ABSCESS

A lung abscess is a localized area of suppuration and cavitation in the lung. This definition can en-compass such diverse conditions as tuberculous, mycotic, or parasitic cavitation; bronchiectasis; infected cyst; and even pulmonary infarction with abscess formation. Cavitation of a tumor may also occur. Most of these conditions are discussed in other chapters of the text. In this section, we are concerned first with primary pyogenic lung abscesses, and second with those which occur in association with other diseases or conditions re-sulting in the weakening of the natural defenses of the body to infection. The former are declining in incidence, while the latter have achieved in-creasing prominence in recent years.[20,36,54,61]

### Pathogenesis

Edentulous patients rarely have primary lung abscesses. Primary pyogenic lung abscesses usu-ally occur as a result of aspiration of a bit of septic debris from the oropharynx into the lung, in a patient with gingivodental disease or oral sepsis, during a period when the cough reflex is sup-pressed.[21] Dental or tonsillar operations also commonly precede the development of lung abscesses. Since these episodes occur during periods of unconsciousness from alcoholism or general anesthesia, epilepsy, cerebral vascular accident, or immersion, the victim is usually in a recumbent, and often a supine, position.[65] The most direct route for the airway embolus to travel is into the right main bronchus, and the first de-pendent bronchus in a supine patient is that to the superior division of the right lower lobe.[8] The posterior segment of the right upper lobe is also dependent and accessible. These two segments are therefore the most common sites of lodgment of septic emboli, and thus the commonest sites of primary lung abscesses. Esophageal disease that permits regurgitation and subsequent aspiration

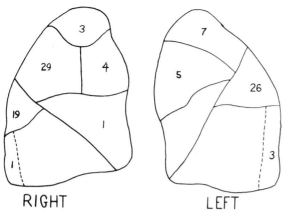

RIGHT          LEFT

**Figure 1** Diagram showing the segmental distribution in the two lungs of 98 lung abscesses due to aspiration. Note the predilection for three principal sites: the superior segment of the right lower lobe, the posterior segment of the right upper lobe, and the superior segment of the left lower lobe. (From Bernhard, W. F., Malcolm, J. A., and Wylie, R. H.: Dis. Chest, *43*:620, 1963.)

of esophageal contents into the lungs is another predisposing clinical setting. Rarely, an esophagobronchial fistula is the primary problem.[40]

Following the development of a severe pneumonitis in response to the embolus, liquefaction necrosis may occur. The microorganisms most commonly responsible for this chain of events are alpha and beta hemolytic streptococci, staphylococci, nonhemolytic streptococci, and *Escherichia coli*; other organisms are isolated less commonly. As the liquefied necrotic material empties through the draining bronchus, a necrotic cavity containing pus and air is formed. Typically, the patient presents with a history of upper respiratory infection and is febrile and often toxic. Chest pain is not uncommon.

Hemoptysis often heralds the evacuation of the necrotic contents of the abscess cavity, and expectoration of purulent and sometimes putrid sputum will commonly follow. This may be copious or scant, and green, brown, gray, or yellow in color. The expectoration of anchovy-sauce-type sputum is suggestive of an amebic lung abscess, a rather rare condition in the United States.[64, 70] Clubbing of the fingers can occur in as many as 20 per cent of cases.[61]

In the suppurative pneumonias of infancy due to staphylococci, clinical symptoms and signs of abscess may be overshadowed by those of toxemia, dyspnea, cyanosis, and septic shock. These may appear suddenly, or may be greatly intensified, if pyopneumothorax, due to rupture of the subpleural abscess, ensues.

The thoracic roentgenogram in lung abscess is not pathognomonic in the early stages prior to establishment of a communication between the abscess cavity and the draining bronchus. An area or areas of dense pneumonic consolidation precede the appearance of the characteristic cavitary

lesion. Multiple abscesses may form multiple cavities. A distinguishing roentgenographic feature of lung abscess, the air-fluid level, is seen only on thoracic roentgenograms exposed in the upright position (or lateral decubitus, in a very sick patient). Accompanying pleural thickening, pneumothorax, or atelectasis may obscure or confuse this picture. Staphylococcal pneumonia of infancy, which may lead to infected pneumoceles, differs in appearance from the classic lung abscess in that the lesions are characteristically thin-walled and cystlike, and are often accompanied by pleural

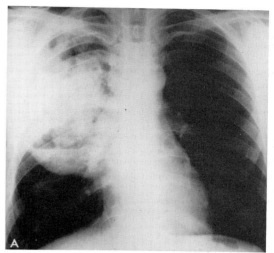

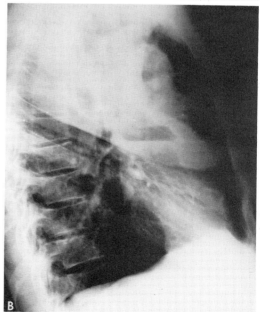

**Figure 2** *A*, Posteroanterior, and *B*, right lateral, thoracic roentgenograms of a patient with a pyogenic lung abscess, from which *Klebsiella pneumoniae* and alpha streptococci were cultured. After a month of intensive antimicrobial therapy, a residual dense, thick-walled cavitary mass, 4 cm. in diameter, was resected by right upper lobectomy.

effusion, empyema, or pyopneumothorax. Complete or partial opacification of the hemithorax may be the presenting roentgenographic picture under these circumstances. With adequate therapy, even the most dramatic roentgenographic features may disappear completely.

Because of the availability of effective broad-spectrum antibiotics such as penicillin, lung abscesses can often be aborted in the stage of pneumonitis; hence, the incidence of this type of abscess has sharply declined in recent years.[61] On the other hand, much more difficult clinical problems are presented by patients, often at the extremes of age, who have serious associated diseases ranging from prematurity to incurable malignant disease, in whom therapeutic efforts have allowed survival, but without the normal defense mechanisms to enable them to combat infections successfully.[36] In such patients, lung abscess may occur as a complication of a systemic disease. Prematurity, bronchopneumonia, congenital defects requiring surgical treatment, the postoperative state itself, and the presence of other infections, blood dyscrasias, or systemic diseases are common predisposing conditions in early infancy. Systemic diseases, malignant diseases (especially of the lung and oropharynx), prolonged use of corticosteroid, immunosuppressive, or radiation therapy, and the postoperative period constitute the common conditions of the older age group in which this type of lung abscess is seen.[42] Such conditions often give rise to multiple (rather than single) abscesses, and the majority of these infections are acquired in the hospital. Bacteriologically, also, these abscesses differ somewhat from classic aspiration-type abscesses. *Staphylococcus aureus* is a common causative organism, but alpha streptococci, *Neisseria catarrhalis*, pneumococci, Pseudomonas, Proteus, *Escherichia coli*, and Klebsiella are all recognized, and occasionally, after prolonged antibiotic treatment, rather unusual bacteria are all that remain to be cultured from the sputum. There is no predilection for particular sites for these abscesses—they can occur almost anywhere, except that the right lung is more commonly involved than the left.

### Treatment

The treatment of classic primary aspiration lung abscess is prolonged antimicrobial therapy.[20, 47, 78] An appropriate regimen, begun even before the results of sputum cultures are known, might be penicillin G in combination with streptomycin or kanamycin; other antibiotics are used as indicated by subsequent bacteriologic studies.[47] In Britain and Canada, more than in the United States, physical measures such as postural drainage and percussion are used and apparently found to be effective adjunctive measures. Bronchoscopy for diagnostic purposes, to remove a foreign body if one is present, and to provide drainage of the abscess by aspiration of the appropriate bronchus through the bronchoscope is also usually indicated. Surgical treatment is reserved for the compli-

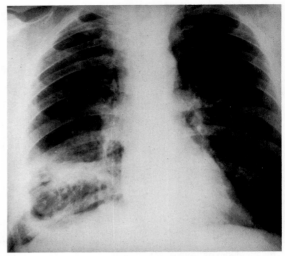

**Figure 3**　Thoracic roentgenogram of a patient with a huge lung abscess, right lower lobe, from which only the usually nonvirulent *Serratia marcescens* was cultured. This patient had had extensive corticosteroid therapy for severe asthma, and multiple broad-spectrum antibiotics for superimposed infection, prior to surgery. This type of abscess is currently being seen with greater frequency in similar clinical situations.

cated problems of massive hemoptysis,[73] lack of response to antibiotics, and presence of a cavity that is thick-walled or of large size (6 cm. or more).[2, 20] When a malignant lesion is suspected, or when empyema develops, surgery may also be appropriate. In most instances, resective surgery is performed—rarely is surgical drainage of lung abscesses indicated. The need for surgical resection for primary lung abscess has declined markedly in recent years, as the effectiveness of antibiotics has increased.

The complications of lung abscesses include the occurrence of empyema, septicemia, metastatic brain abscess,[58] and bronchogenic spread.[41] The commonest complication is the development of chronicity.[77] A bronchiectatic, often epithelialized residual cavity remains behind, if complete healing of the abscess has not taken place. Such a lesion is itself considered to be an indication for resection if it is symptomatic, or if infection recurs.

The mortality from primary aspiration-type lung abscess is emphatically different from that accompanying abscesses that occur as a complication of some other serious disease. The mortality from the former has declined from approximately 25 per cent, 10 to 15 years ago, to 5 per cent or less with prolonged and adequate antimicrobial therapy. On the other hand, 75 to 90 per cent of patients whose abscesses complicate some other systemic disease succumb—an appalling mortality, and a reflection of the gravity of the accompanying disease as well as of the prognostic significance of this complication.[36, 54] It is conceivable that prompt recognition and urgently applied and appropriate antibiotic therapy might in some measure alter this dismal picture.

**TABLE 1**  CURRENTLY AVAILABLE ANTIMYCOTIC ANTIBIOTICS*

| Mycosis | Antibiotic |
| --- | --- |
| Histoplasmosis | Amphotericin B; saramycetin |
| Coccidioidomycosis | Amphotericin B |
| North American blastomycosis | Amphotericin B; 2-hydroxystilbamidine |
| Cryptococcosis | Amphotericin B; 5-fluoro-cytosine |
| Aspergillosis | Amphotericin B |
| Nocardiosis | Sulfadiazine |
| Actinomycosis | Penicillin; erythromycin; broad-spectrum antibiotics |
| Candidiasis (moniliasis) | Amphotericin B; 5-fluoro-cytosine; nystatin† |
| Sporotrichosis | Iodides; amphotericin B; saramycetin |
| Phycomycosis (mucormycosis) | Amphotericin B; iodides |
| Monosporosis | None known |
| South American blastomycosis | Amphotericin B; sulfonamides |

*Adapted from Procknow, J. J.: Lab. Invest., *11*:1217, 1962; and American Thoracic Society: Amer. Rev. Resp. Dis., *100*:908, 1969; and Utz, J. P., Kravetz, H. M., Einstein, H. E., Campbell, G. D., and Buechner, H. A.: Chest, *60*:260, 1971.

†Topically only.

## FUNGUS INFECTION OF THE LUNGS

Attitudes concerning mycotic infections in general have changed considerably in recent years. While this section emphasizes fungus infections of the lungs, much of it is broadly applicable also to systemic infections of mycotic origin.

Formerly, blastomycosis, histoplasmosis, coccidioidomycosis, and cryptococcosis were considered to be rare, almost invariably fatal infections. Now it is recognized that benign, self-limited, and almost undetectable infections by all of these organisms are much more common. Millions of persons exhibit evidence of subclinical histoplasmosis and coccidioidomycosis, for instance, with spontaneous healing.

On the other hand, the widespread use of antimetabolites for neoplasms, of antibiotics for infections, and of steroids for a variety of conditions has given fungi such as Aspergillus, Candida, and Mucor the opportunity to invade the host and to cause disease. Thus, the formerly sharp line between so-called "pathogenic" and "nonpathogenic" fungi is blurred and no longer clear-cut. Both true pathogens and saprophytes *can* cause opportunistic infection—that is, invasion of the host when body defenses have been weakened or altered by drugs or disease. The surgeon must be aware of the variety of fungus infections that can beset his patient.[50, 69]

The surgeon is entirely dependent upon the pathologist for definitive diagnosis of these condi-

**Figure 4**  Map showing approximate areas in the United States recognized as endemic for North American blastomycosis, histoplasmosis, and coccidioidomycosis. (From Takaro, T. In: Lewis' Practice of Surgery. New York, Hoeber Medical Division, Harper & Row, 1968.)

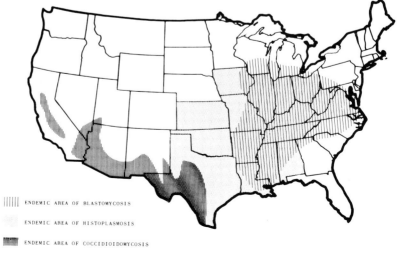

|||||| ENDEMIC AREA OF BLASTOMYCOSIS

ENDEMIC AREA OF HISTOPLASMOSIS

▓▓▓▓ ENDEMIC AREA OF COCCIDIOIDOMYCOSIS

tions, but the pathologist must rely upon the surgeon or physician to provide suspicion of fungus infection, and also to provide appropriate samples of sputum or tissue to make possible positive identification of the offending organism.[17, 60] This is important, because specific but rather toxic antimycotic drugs are now available for treatment (Table 1).[3, 63]

## Epidemiology

Many of the fungi causing human infection are inhabitants of the soil, and most infections are believed to be caused by direct inhalation of the organisms in contaminated dust. Thus, they are considered to be *exogenous* infections.

Three of these organisms are known to occur in the soil of specific and relatively delimited geographic areas in the United States. These are *Histoplasma capsulatum* (histoplasmosis), *Coccidioides immitis* (coccidioidomycosis), and *Blastomyces dermatitidis* (North American blastomycosis). A soil reservoir is fairly well accepted for Cryptococcus, Aspergillus, Nocardia, and Mucor. On the other hand, actinomycosis and candidiasis are considered *endogenous* infections, since these are part of the normal flora of human being and animals, and are not found free in nature.

## Histoplasmosis

Histoplasmosis is probably the most common of the fungus infections and occurs in the Mississippi Valley and its tributaries. The causative organism, *Histoplasma capsulatum*, is found in soil contaminated by pigeon, chicken, or bat droppings. Some 30 million persons are estimated to have been infected, judging from skin reactions to histoplasmin.[13]

The macropathology and micropathology resemble those of pulmonary tuberculosis, except for the finding of the tiny yeast cells of *H. capsulatum* in macrophages, or the capsules of nonviable organisms in the necrotic center of granulomas.

While most cases of infection are asymptomatic, acute pulmonic infection may be accompanied by diffuse pulmonary infiltration, or scattered nodular densities, and may be characterized by an acute febrile course. By far the commonest clinical presentation of histoplasmosis is as an asymptomatic chronic granuloma, appearing on a thoracic roentgenogram as a solitary pulmonary nodule of undiagnosed etiology.

Chronic cavitary histoplasmosis resembles pulmonary tuberculosis both symptomatically and roentgenographically, although it appears to progress somewhat more slowly. In a considerable percentage of cases, pulmonary tuberculosis has been found to coexist in such patients; in many others, a mistaken diagnosis of pulmonary tuberculosis, based on roentgenographic findings, has led to hospitalization in sanatoriums. Only in the past two decades has this error begun to be recognized.

The treatment of histoplasmosis depends upon the form of the disease that is encountered. For severe acute infections, therapy with amphotericin B, currently the only available effective drug, may be necessary. The solitary nodule may pose a problem in management. In a cooperative study of almost 1000 solitary pulmonary nodules resected in adult males, 53 per cent were found to be granulomas and 36 per cent malignant tumors.[67]

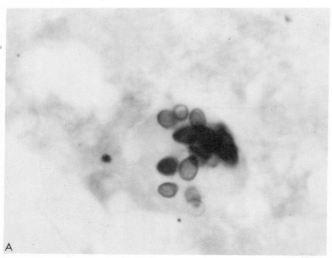

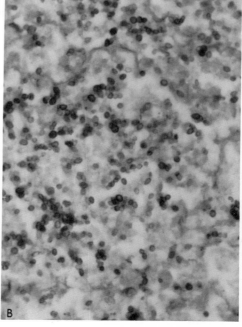

**Figure 5** Forms of *Histoplasma capsulatum* found in tissues. *A*, Intracellular viable organisms. H & E stain × 500. *B*, Nonviable capsules of *H. capsulatum* in necrotic center of a histoplasmoma. Gomori stain × 1000. (From Takaro, T. In: Lewis' Practice of Surgery. New York, Hoeber Medical Division, Harper & Row, 1968.)

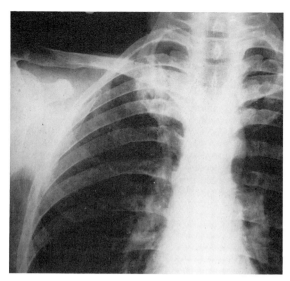

**Figure 6** Thoracic roentgenogram of patient with chronic cavitary histoplasmosis who underwent upper lobectomy prior to the availability of amphotericin B. (From Takaro, T. In: Lewis' Practice of Surgery. New York, Hoeber Medical Division, Harper & Row, 1968.)

Fungi, most commonly *H. capsulatum* or *Coccidioides immitis*, were isolated from the majority of these granulomas. However, since malignancy was found in such a high percentage of cases,

and since the presence of calcium in a nodule does not rule out carcinoma (unless perhaps calcification is concentric, dense, or unchanged for years), exploratory thoracotomy for the undiagnosed nodule will very often be indicated, especially in adult males. On the other hand, if the diagnosis can be made by transbronchial brushing of the lesion, neither thoracotomy nor drug therapy may be necessary. Cavitary histoplasmosis, proven by culturing the organism in the sputum, should be treated primarily with amphotericin B. Pulmonary resection for chronic cavitary pulmonary histoplasmosis has often been recommended in the past,[68] but in a cooperative study involving more than 400 patients, there was no evidence that this modality, even in conjunction with amphotericin B, resulted in a greater reduction in relapses and deaths than did use of the drug alone.[43] On the other hand, there is general agreement that if resectional surgery is undertaken, amphotericin B should be used, until a total dosage of at least 2 gm. is reached.[1, 48] This can be given over a period of a month before and a month after surgery if the diagnosis is established prior to surgery. If chronic cavitary histoplasmosis is diagnosed only after surgery, treatment with 2 gm. of amphotericin B is recommended to prevent recurrence and to lower the statistically higher death rate seen in patients who have not received the drug.

For disseminated forms of histoplasmosis, amphotericin B is urgently needed to prevent death.

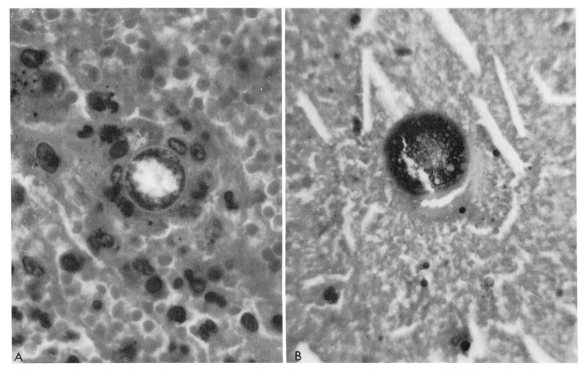

**Figure 7** Spherules of *Coccidioides immitis*, packed with endospores. *A*, In a giant cell. H & E × 500. *B*, In necrotic tissue. Gomori stain × 250. (From Takaro, T. In: Lewis' Practice of Surgery. New York, Hoeber Medical Division, Harper & Row, 1968.)

## Coccidioidomycosis

Coccidioidomycosis is caused by the dimorphic fungus *Coccidioides immitis*, which may occur in tissues in the form of large spherules packed with endospores, but also as individual small endospores (following rupture of a spherule) or as mycelial elements or hyphae (in cavities).[56]

Coccidioidomycosis is also an exogenous infection occurring in the area corresponding to the zone of mesquite, found in certain well defined regions of California, Nevada, Arizona, New Mexico, and Texas.[35] This is a region characterized by a dry, windy, dusty, hot climate. Modern irrigation has made this area a very important one from the agricultural standpoint and, therefore, also from the epidemiologic point of view, since population growth in this zone has been rapid in the past several decades. Extensive travel through the area has helped to spread coccidioidomycosis to every part of the United States as well as to other countries. Some 10 million people in the United States are estimated to have been infected at some time in their lives with *C. immitis.*

The gross and microscopic lesions of coccidioidomycosis strongly resemble those of pulmonary tuberculosis, but with two characteristic differences. These are the occurrence of thin-walled cavities and of suppuration in coccidioidomycosis. However, thick-walled cavities, and chronic granulomas appearing as solitary nodules, as in histoplasmosis, are also common. Finally, apical or subapical infiltrates or cavities or both, indistinguishable roentgenographically from either chronic pulmonary tuberculosis or chronic pulmonary histoplasmosis, are also seen.

A history of "valley fever" while residing in an endemic area is classically obtainable, but often no clinical evidence is available of the onset of the disease. With acute cavitation, hemoptysis is the commonest symptom; with chronic infection, cough, weight loss, fever, and chest pain are the presenting complaints. Skin tests and complement fixation tests are almost always positive in active cases.

The most effective specific therapy is amphotericin B, but many patients will require no treatment at all. The drug should be reserved for acutely ill patients and those with cavitary disease and sputum cultures positive for *C. immitis.*

The indications for resective surgery include enlarging, thick-walled, or ruptured cavities or abscesses, severe or recurrent hemoptysis, and the coexistence of pulmonary tuberculosis with coccidioidomycosis. Drug coverage with amphotericin B is recommended, but it is not clear that the use of amphotericin B has resulted in significantly fewer complications of bronchopleural fistula, empyema, and recurrent cavitation.[22, 26, 39, 59, 79] A program is proposed specifically for the troublesome problem of diagnostic confusion with pulmonary tuberculosis, or coexisting tuberculosis and coccidioidomycosis, in which one or both diseases are treated by appropriate drugs for 2 to 3 months prior to surgery.[39]

## North American Blastomycosis

North American blastomycosis, the third fungus infection endemic in a definable geographic area, largely east of the Mississippi River, is caused by *Blastomyces dermatitidis*, a round, thick-walled, single-budding yeast.[24, 76] The disease often occurs in a cutaneous form, with chronic, indolent, usually enlarging papulopustules with thick adherent crusts and purple raised edges.[80] Biopsy in these areas may show microabscesses containing the organism. This form, with no evidence of systemic (including pulmonary) involvement, is the most favorable form of the disease. Pulmonary symptoms may be nonspecific. On the thoracic roentgenogram, cavitary, nodular, fibrotic, or disseminated lesions may be observed; bronchogenic carcinoma may be mimicked.[80]

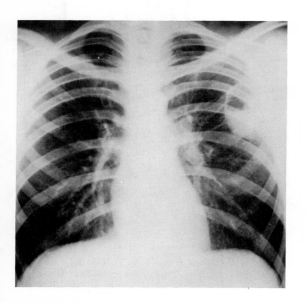

**Figure 8**  Cavitary lesion due to coccidioidomycosis, left lung. (From Hyde, L.: Dis. Chest, Supp. 1, *54*:213, 1968.)

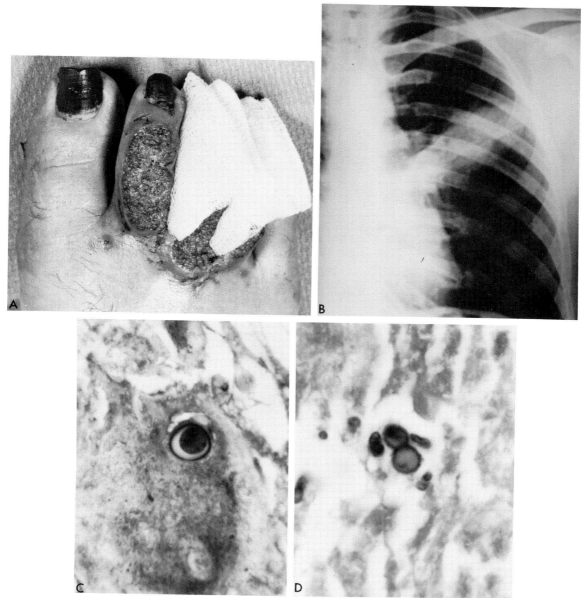

**Figure 9** *A*, Skin lesions of blastomycosis on the dorsum of the toes. Biopsy of the characteristic raised edges showed multiple microabscesses containing *Blastomyces dermatitidis. B*, Blastomycotic pneumonic lesion of the lung. *C* and *D*, Organisms of *B. dermatitidis* from resected lung tissue: Thick-walled yeast form with refractile cell wall on left; single budding yeast form on right. PAS stain × 1100. (From Takaro, T. In: Lewis' Practice of Surgery. New York, Hoeber Medical Division, Harper & Row, 1968.)

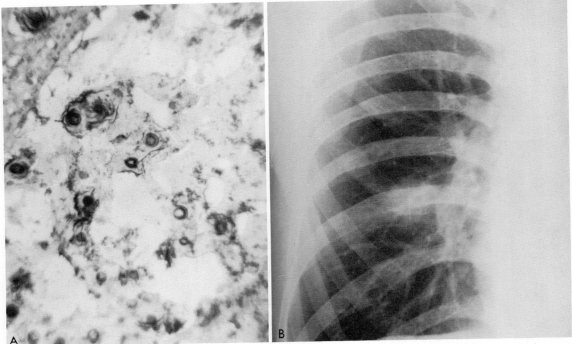

**Figure 10**   *A,* Organisms of *Cryptococcus neoformans* showing thick capsules. Mucicarmine × 950. *B,* Thoracic roentgenogram showing solitary cryptococcal granuloma. This was removed by wedge resection. (From Takaro, T. In: Lewis' Practice of Surgery. New York, Hoeber Medical Division, Harper & Row, 1968.)

The two drugs considered most useful for blastomycosis are 2-hydroxystilbamidine and amphotericin B. Because of its wider margin of safety, 2-hydroxystilbamidine should be considered the drug of first choice.[33] Amphotericin B should be held in reserve for treatment failures with 2-hydroxystilbamidine. Resectional surgery is only rarely needed except for diagnosis, especially in those in whom cancer is suspected. This disease is still a serious one, with a 5 year mortality of approximately 20 per cent. The prognosis is worsened if the disease coexists with pulmonary tuberculosis.[24, 71] Involvement of the genitourinary tract, the bones, and the nasal and oral mucosa is not uncommon.[80]

### Cryptococcosis

Cryptococcosis was earlier considered to be a rare and fatal disease, often accompanied by meningitis. Now, apparently benign and indeed subclinical bronchopulmonary infections are being recognized with increasing frequency. Even the dreaded meningeal form is controllable by drug therapy.[10, 16, 69]

*Cryptococcus neoformans* is found in nature in soil, dust, and pigeon dung. The organisms are round, budding yeast cells with thick gelatinous capsules. Opportunistic infection with Cryptococcus is frequently seen, especially in patients with lymphomas, collagen diseases, leukemias and other blood dyscrasias, diabetes, and sarcoidosis, especially after prolonged steroid or immunosuppressive drug therapy.

If cryptococci are cultured from sputum, with no demonstrable pulmonary lesion, or are isolated from lung tissue resected as an undiagnosed lesion, with no symptoms or signs of active disease, opinions differ regarding the need for antifungal therapy.[46, 72] Amphotericin B is not the only effective treatment at the moment, 5-fluoro-cytosine being recommended as preferable because of its lesser toxicity and oral route of administration.[74] Since the mere presence of cryptococci does not necessarily denote a pathogenic process, active treatment may not be necessary if there is no evidence of central nervous system involvement and no organisms are found in spinal fluid.[25]

On the other hand, if active cryptococcosis can be shown to be present by evidence of progression of a pulmonary lesion, and continued sputum positivity, or by evidence of meningeal involvement, treatment with 5-fluoro-cytosine or with amphotericin B is indicated and may be urgently needed.[46, 72, 74]

### Aspergillosis

Aspergillosis is usually caused by *Aspergillus fumigatus,* which presents in pathologic material as a filamentous organism with coarse, septate, fragmented hyphae.[69] Only rarely are characteristic vesicular spore heads identified. Of surgical interest is the tendency for this organism to invade pre-existing pulmonary cavities, there to

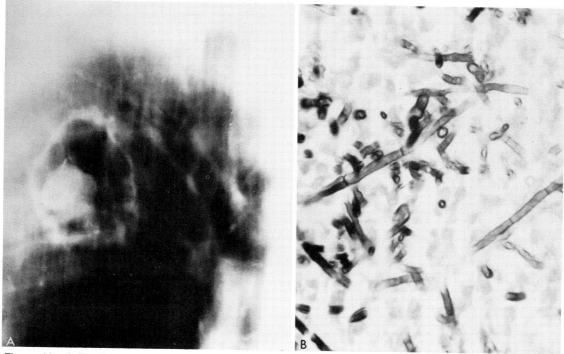

**Figure 11** *A*, Laminagram showing typical aspergilloma ("fungus ball") lying free in large cavitary lesion. This ball characteristically will alter its location as the patient changes position. (From Aslam, P. A., Larkin, J., Eastridge, C. A., and Hughes, F. A., Jr.: Chest, *57*:94, 1970.) *B*, Coarse, fragmented, septate mycelia of *Aspergillus fumigatus*. (From Takaro, T. In: Lewis' Practice of Surgery. New York, Hoeber Medical Division, Harper & Row, 1968.)

form a rounded necrotic mass of matted hyphae, fibrin, and inflammatory cells, called an aspergilloma or fungus ball.[12] This nondescript mass usually lies free in the cavity, and can change its location in the cavity as the patient changes his position from upright to recumbent. On the chest x-ray, a moon-shaped radiolucency adjacent to a rounded mass within a cavitary lesion is almost pathognomonic of an aspergilloma. Chronic cystic lesions of the upper lobes that remain as residua of pulmonary tuberculosis, sarcoidosis, lung cyst, or bronchiectasis commonly harbor such fungus balls; hemoptysis, occasionally severe, is the usual presenting symptom.[27]

The medical management of aspergillosis has been unsatisfactory. Iodides, nystatin, hydroxystilbamidine, and amphotericin B have all been used. Surgical excision of an aspergilloma is usually curative of symptoms of hemoptysis, and should be undertaken if the patient's condition permits and pre-existing disease has not produced generalized lung damage.[55] If excisional surgery is contraindicated, as it often is because of pulmonary fibrosis and respiratory insufficiency, endocavitary or endobronchial treatment with sodium iodide or amphotericin B may be helpful.[4] Aspergillus empyema is a serious complication, requiring drainage and local instillations of amphotericin B or nystatin for effective management.[31]

## Nocardiosis

Nocardiosis is occasionally classified as an infection by one of the higher bacteria; more usually, it is still considered a mycotic infection. It is caused by the aerobic actinomycete *Nocardia asteroides*; this organism has been isolated from the soil.[9, 45] It occurs in pathologic material in clumps or granules, made up of short or long branching filaments that are gram-positive and acid-fast. This property, as well as cultural and roentgenographic similarities, has led to confusion in the past with *Mycobacterium tuberculosis*.

Pulmonary nocardiosis may mimic pulmonary tuberculosis, pneumonia, or lung abscess, both clinically and roentgenographically. In the past decade, the majority of patients with nocardiosis have had some underlying disease, such as lymphoma, leukemia, other malignant diseases, or (surprisingly) alveolar proteinosis, or have received corticosteroid therapy.[57] Thus, nocardiosis is more often than not an opportunistic infection, and in these situations, the prognosis is grave, even with treatment. The treatment of choice is sulfadiazine, continued on a long-term basis— a minimum of 2 months after arrest of the disease. This method can be curative. On the other hand, if the disease is resectable, a cure rate of 100 per cent is reported. In many instances, the diagnosis

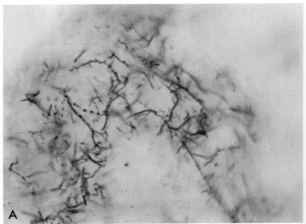

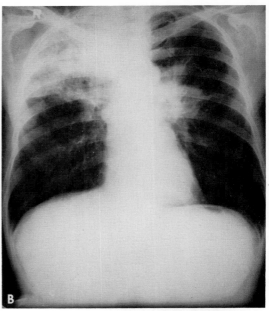

**Figure 12**   *A*, Organisms of *Nocardia asteroides*. Gram stain × 1000. These organisms have been mistaken for tubercle bacilli in the past, because of acid-fast staining characteristics. *B*, Roentgenogram of thorax showing pneumonic lesion of nocardiosis. (From Takaro, T. In: Lewis' Practice of Surgery. New York, Hoeber Medical Division, Harper & Row, 1968.)

has been made for the first time from the resected specimen.

### Actinomycosis

Actinomycosis is caused by the anaerobic actinomycete *Actinomyces israelii*, and is characterized by abscess and sinus formation, with dense scarring. It is the only fungus infection caused by an anaerobic or microaerophilic organism, and, therefore, special cultural techniques are required.[45, 69]

In pathologic material, organisms with branching filaments occur in clusters or microcolonies called granules. The much larger, yellow-brown granules in draining material from abscesses or sinuses are called "sulfur granules," and again are dense clusters of organisms.

Since *A. israelii* is a normal inhabitant of the oral cavity, one cannot make the diagnosis simply

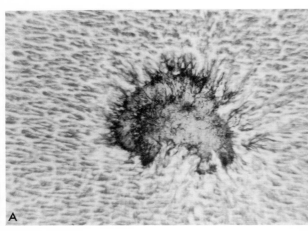

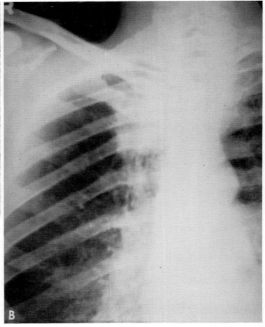

**Figure 13**   *A*, Actinomycotic granule showing branching filaments of a microscopic colony of *Actinomyces israelii*. Gomori stain × 250. *B*, Thoracic roentgenogram of a patient who subsequently underwent right upper lobectomy for a suspected malignant lesion. Actinomycosis was found in the resected specimen. (From Takaro, T. In: Lewis' Practice of Surgery. New York, Hoeber Medical Division, Harper & Row, 1968.)

by recovering the organism from sputum. It must be recovered from closed tissue spaces or draining sinuses or abscesses, or shown to be invasive in histopathologic sections.

Thoracic actinomycosis is most commonly due to bronchopulmonary invasion of infectious material from the oropharynx. The infection that results may be so indolent that symptoms may be few until pleural or chest wall involvement takes place.

Empyema and chronic draining chest wall sinuses are characteristic, but insidious, non-specific-appearing pulmonary infiltration, consolidation, or hilar mass strongly suggestive of bronchogenic carcinoma are also observed. This has been well shown by McQuarrie[38] and others.[75]

The drug of choice for actinomycosis is penicillin. Because of the dense, fibrous, avascular tissue surrounding the colonies of organisms and the concentration of organisms in dense clusters, high doses of drug must be used for long periods, and radical surgical excision should accompany antibiotic therapy, if possible. The difficulties of establishing a diagnosis in this disease also frequently result in surgical excision of the pulmonary lesions of actinomycosis, or of chest wall abscesses.[49] Empyema may require decortication or pleural drainage plus thoracoplasty.

### Fungal Endocarditis

Candidiasis is of special interest to cardiac surgeons because of the occurrence of Candida endocarditis in association with cardiac (usually valvular) lesions, 55 cases of which are already on record.[28] In a considerable number of patients, Candida endocarditis was diagnosed during or after prolonged and intensive antibiotic treatment for established subacute bacterial endocarditis. In another sizable group, fungal endocarditis (mostly due to Candida, but in some cases due to Aspergillus) has been reported following valve replacement.[14] Heart operations offer a portal of entry through indwelling catheters, a damaged endocardial surface, and prolonged parenteral and antibiotic therapy, all of which favor the growth of this organism.[15,18] The fungus is characterized by both budding yeast forms and mycelial ele-

ments. Candida infections of aortotomies have also been recorded twice.[37,51]

The clinical features of Candida endocarditis are almost indistinguishable from those of bacterial endocarditis, suspicion of and treatment for which may actually aggravate the fungal infection. The finding of sterile blood cultures in the face of a clinical picture of bacterial endocarditis should dictate a search for Candida; Candida species found on blood culture must not be taken as a laboratory contaminant, but as an indication of a potentially lethal infection. Distinguishing features of Candida endocarditis are embolic episodes to major vessels, owing to the unusually large size of the mycotic valvular vegetations. Potentially beneficial treatment in the form of amphotericin B (and more recently, 5-fluorocytosine) is available, but the number of cures is extremely small, the mortality being almost 90 per cent. Surgical excision of vegetations together with administration of amphotericin B has been the only method of treatment offering any real hope, three of four patients surviving following this modality.[28]

### Miscellaneous Fungal Infections

*Sporotrichosis* is caused by *Sporotrichum schenckii*, and pulmonary involvement is rare, the condition usually being encountered in its cutaneous or lymphatic manifestations. Agricultural workers and florists are especially susceptible. Localized cavitary pulmonary disease has been reported on a number of occasions recently.[6,62] Iodides are often effective in this disease, and surgical excision of localized disease with a successful outcome has been reported. If iodides are ineffective, a trial of amphotericin B, 2-hydroxystilbamidine, and saramycetin is recommended.

*Phycomycosis (mucormycosis)* is another rare and serious infection by any of the members of the order of fungi known as Phycomycetes.[5] The organisms are characterized by broad, nonseptate hyphae, and characteristically blood vessel invasion, thrombosis, and infarction of organs are seen. Extensive necrosis of face, lungs, or brain may occur. Debilitated persons and uncontrolled

**Figure 14** The organisms of *Candida albicans,* showing both mycelial and yeast forms. (From Takaro, T. In: Lewis' Practice of Surgery. New York, Hoeber Medical Division, Harper & Row, 1968.)

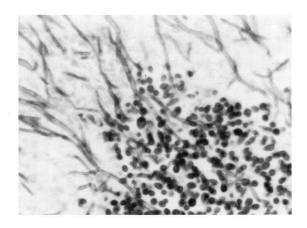

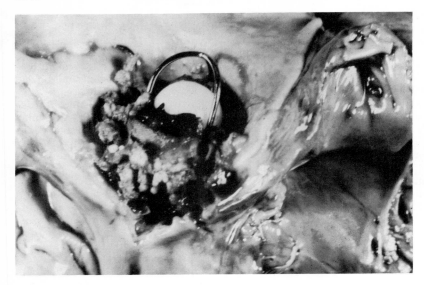

**Figure 15** Fungal endocarditis due to Aspergillus species, causing aortic prosthetic dehiscence due to perivalvular tissue necrosis. More commonly, *Candida albicans* has been the etiologic agent in opportunistic fungal infections following cardiac surgery. (From Ostermiller, W. E., and Weinberg, M.: J. Thorac. Cardiovasc. Surg., *61*: 670, 1970.)

diabetics seem to be especially prone to this infection. Control of the underlying disease, amphotericin B administration, and surgical excision of necrotic or infected tissue may prove to be helpful.[11, 19, 53]

*Pulmonary monosporosis* is a rare mycotic infection caused by *Monosporium apiospermum.* This inhabitant of soil appears to act as a secondary invader of previously damaged lung tissue, such as a cavity, cyst, or saccule. Sometimes (but not characteristically), a fungus ball is formed. Amphotericin B has not been reported used. Localized resections have been successful in two cases.[52]

*South American blastomycosis (paracoccidioidomycosis)* is a chronic granulomatous infection involving the skin, mucous membrane, lymph nodes, and visceral organs, including the lungs, that is caused by *Paracoccidioides brasiliensis,* presumably a soil saprophyte. It is endemic in South America, and perhaps also in Central America, but it has not been recognized outside these areas. The organisms resemble *Blastomyces dermatitidis* in tissues. Cavitary pulmonary disease occurs in about a third of cases. Treatment with sulfonamides is suppressive but not curative. Amphotericin B shows more promise. Surgery usually is not required.[34]

## SELECTED REFERENCES

American Thoracic Society: Treatment of fungal diseases. A statement by the committee on therapy. Amer. Rev. Resp. Dis., *100*:908, 1969.
*This is a brief but complete statement of the current consensus regarding optimal therapy for each of the mycotic infections.*

Busey, J. F.: Blastomycosis. I. A review of 198 collected cases in Veterans Administration Hospitals. Amer. Rev. Resp. Dis., *89*:659, 1964.
*This retrospective cooperative study makes available clinical data in a large number of patients, and covers the broad range of organ systems that may be involved in this disease.*

Emmons, C. W., Binford, C. H., and Utz, J. P.: Medical Mycology. Philadelphia, Lea & Febiger, 1963.
*This comprehensive textbook attempts to bridge the gap between mycology and its medical application, and does it very well.*

Goodwin, R. A., Snell, J. D., Hubbard, W. W., and Terry, R. T.: Early chronic pulmonary histoplasmosis. Amer. Rev. Resp. Dis., *93*:47, 1966.
*This in-depth analysis of one phase of the problem of histoplasmosis presents a balanced therapeutic approach.*

Hildick-Smith, G., Blank, H., and Sarkany, J.: Fungus diseases and their treatment. Boston, Little, Brown and Company, 1964.
*This beautifully illustrated textbook covers the entire field of mycology, especially its dermatologic aspects, and includes discussion of some of the rarer mycoses.*

Littman, M. L., and Walter, J. E.: Cryptococcosis: Current status. Amer. J. Med., *45*:922, 1968.
*This is a general review article, giving a broad exposition of the epidemiologic, diagnostic, therapeutic, and preventive aspects of cryptococcosis.*

Mark, P. H., and Turner, J. A. P.: Lung abscess in childhood. Thorax, 23:216, 1968.
*This review from Canada classifies abscesses in children into primary and secondary types; the emphasis is on conservative measures.*

McQuarrie, D. G., and Hall, W. H.: Actinomycosis of the lung and chest wall. Surgery, *64*:905, 1968.
*This excellent report, while focusing on the thoracic manifestations of actinomycosis, alludes also to the broader spectrum of the disease, its variable clinical presentation, and the problems of diagnosis and treatment.*

Perlman, L. V., Lerner, E., and D'Esopo, N.: Clinical classification and analysis of 97 cases of lung abscess. Amer. Rev. Resp. Dis., *99*:390, 1969.
*The sharp differentiation, based on clinical characteristics and on response to therapy, between primary (or simple) lung abscesses and those occurring in association with systemic disease, malignant or nonmalignant, in adults is emphasized in this review of 97 cases.*

Reed, W. A., and Allbritten, F. F.: The lungs: suppurative and fungal diseases. In: Gibbon, F. C., Jr., Sabiston, D. C., Jr., and Spencer, F. C., eds.: Surgery of the Chest. 2nd ed. Philadelphia, W. B. Saunders Company, 1969, pp. 349–356.
*This is a good general exposition of the subject of lung abscess.*

Schwarz, J., and Salfelder, K.: Diagnosis of surgical deep mycoses. Surg. Gynec. Obstet., *128*:259, 1969.
*This is a general exposition of the subject, with emphasis on the need for close cooperation between the surgeon and the bacteriologist for diagnostic accuracy.*

Steele, J. D., ed.: Treatment of Mycotic and Parasitic Diseases of the Chest. Springfield, Ill., Charles C Thomas, 1964.
*This is an excellent text, complete and clinically oriented.*

# REFERENCES

1. Ahn, C., Kilman, J. W., Vasko, J., and Andrews, N. C.: Therapy of cavitary pulmonary histoplasmosis. J. Thorac. Cardiovasc. Surg., 57:42, 1969.
2. Andersen, M. N., and McDonald, K. E.: Prognostic factors and results of treatment in pyogenic pulmonary abscess. J. Thorac. Cardiovasc. Surg., 39:573, 1960.
3. Andriole, V. T., and Kravetz, H. M.: Use of amphotericin B in man. J.A.M.A., 180:269, 1962.
4. Aslam, P. A., Larkin, J., Eastridge, C. E., and Hughes, F. A., Jr.: Endocavitary infusion through percutaneous endobronchial catheter. Chest, 57:94, 1970.
5. Baker, R. D.: Mucormycosis: A new disease? J.A.M.A., 163:805, 1957.
6. Baum, G. L., Donnerberg, R. L., Stewart, D., Mulligan, W. J., and Putman, L. R.: Pulmonary sporotrichosis. New Eng. J. Med., 280:410, 1969.
7. Baum, G. L., Larkin, J. C., Jr., and Sutliff, W. D.: Follow-up of patients with chronic pulmonary histoplasmosis treated with amphotericin B. Chest, 58:562, 1970.
8. Bernhard, W. F., Malcolm, J. A., and Wylie, R. H.: Lung abscess: A study of 148 cases due to aspiration. Dis. Chest, 43:620, 1963.
9. Buechner, H. A., Furcolow, M. L., Farness, O. J., Reagan, W. P., Saliba, N. A., and Abernathy, R.: Epidemiology of the pulmonary mycoses. Chest, 58:68, 1970.
10. Butler, W. T., Alling, D. W., Spickard, A., and Utz, J. P.: Diagnostic and prognostic value of clinical and laboratory findings in cryptococcal meningitis. New Eng. J. Med., 270:59, 1964.
11. Callard, G. M., Wright, C. B., Wray, R. C., and Minor, G. R.: False aneurysm due to Mucor following repair of coarctation with Dacron prosthesis. J. Thorac. Cardiovasc. Surg., 61:181, 1971.
12. Campbell, M. J., and Clayton, Y. M.: Bronchopulmonary aspergillosis: Correlation of the clinical and laboratory findings in 272 patients investigated for bronchopulmonary aspergillosis. Amer. Rev. Resp. Dis., 89:186, 1964.
13. Carr, D., and Sutliff, W. D.: Histoplasmosis. In: Steele, J. D., ed.: Treatment of Mycotic and Parasitic Diseases of the Chest. Springfield, Ill., Charles C Thomas, 1964, pp. 31–54.
14. Chaudhuri, M. R.: Fungal endocarditis after valve replacements. J. Thorac. Cardiovasc. Surg., 60:207, 1970.
15. Climie, A. R. W., and Rachmaninoff, N.: Fungal (Candida) endocarditis following open-heart surgery. J. Thorac. Cardiovasc. Surg., 50:431, 1965.
16. Cohen, A. A., Davis, A., and Finegold, S. M.: Chronic pulmonary cryptococcosis. Amer. Rev. Resp. Dis., 91:414, 1965.
17. Conant, N. F., Smith, D. T., Baker, R. D., Cellaway, J. L., and Martin, D. S.: Manual of Clinical Mycology. 2nd ed. Philadelphia, W. B. Saunders Company, 1954.
18. Dennis, D., Miller, M. J., and Peterson, C. G.: Candida septicemia. Surg. Gynec. Obstet., 119:520, 1964.
19. Dillon, M. L., Sealy, W. C., and Fetter, B. F.: Mucormycosis of the bronchus successfully treated by lobectomy. J. Thorac. Surg., 35:464, 1958.
20. Duffy, T. J., and Chofnas, I.: Primary lung abscess. Amer. J. Med. Sci., 243:269, 1962.
21. Flavell, G.: Respiratory tract disease: Lung abscess. Brit. Med. J., 1:1032, 1966.
22. Fosburg, R. G., Baisch, B. F., and Trummer, M. J.: Limited pulmonary resection for coccidioidomycosis. Ann. Thorac. Surg., 7:420, 1969.
23. Furcolow, M. L., Chick, E. W., Busey, J. F., and Menges, R. W.: Prevalence and incidence studies of human and canine blastomycosis. Amer. Rev. Resp. Dis., 102:60, 1970.
24. Furcolow, M. L., Watson, K. A., Tisdall, O. F., Julian, W. A., Saliba, N. A., and Ralows, A.: Some factors affecting survival in systemic blastomycosis. Dis. Chest, Supp. I, 54:285, 1968.
25. Geraci, J. E., Donoghue, F. E., Ellis, F. H., Jr., Witten, D. M., and Weed, L. A.: Focal pulmonary cryptococcosis: Evaluation of necessity of amphotericin B therapy. Mayo Clin. Proc., 40:552, 1965.
26. Hyde, L.: Coccidioidal pulmonary cavitation. Dis. Chest, Supp. I, 54:273, 1968.
27. Israel, H. L., and Ostrow, A.: Sarcoidosis and aspergilloma. Amer. J. Med., 47:243, 1969.
28. Kay, J. H., Bernstein, S., and Tsugi, H. K., et al.: Surgical treatment of Candida endocarditis. J.A.M.A., 203:621, 1968.
29. Khan, T. H., Kane, E. G., and Dean, D. C.: Aspergillus endocarditis of mitral prosthesis. Amer. J. Cardiol., 22:277, 1968.
30. Knudson, R. J., Burch, H. B., and Hatch, H. B.: Primary pulmonary cryptococcosis: Report of 3 cases and review of the literature. J. Thorac. Cardiovasc. Surg., 45:730, 1963.
31. Krakowka, P., Rowinska, E., and Halweg, H.: Infection of the pleura by Aspergillus fumigatus. Thorax, 25:245, 1970.
32. Leffert, R. L., and Hackett, R. L.: Aspergillus aortitis following replacement of aortic valve. J. Thorac. Cardiovasc. Surg., 53:866, 1967.
33. Lockwood, W. R., Busey, J. F., Batson, B. E., and Allison, F., Jr.: Experiences in the treatment of North American blastomycosis with 2-hydroxystilbamidine. Ann. Intern. Med., 57:553, 1962.
34. Machado Filho, J., and Lisboa Miranda, J.: Considerations concerning South American blastomycosis—localizations, initial symptoms, pathways of penetration and dissemination in 313 consecutive cases. Hospital (Rio), 58:99, 1960.
35. Maddy, K. T.: Geographic distribution of Coccidioides immitis and possible ecologic implications. Arizona Med., 15:178, 1958.
36. Mark, P. H., and Turner, J. A. P.: Lung abscess in childhood. Thorax, 23:216, 1968.
37. Marsten, J. L., Greenberg, J. J., Piccinini, J. C., and Rywlin, A. M.: Aortitis due to Candida stellatoidea developing in a supravalvular suture line. Ann. Thorac. Surg., 7:134, 1969.
38. McQuarrie, D. G., and Hall, W. H.: Actinomycosis of the lung and chest wall. Surgery, 64:905, 1968.
39. Melick, D. W., and Grant, A. R.: Surgery in primary pulmonary coccidioidomycosis and in the combined diseases of coccidioidomycosis and tuberculosis. Dis. Chest, Supp. I, 54:278, 1968.
40. Nelson, R. J., and Benfield, J. R.: Benign esophagobronchial fistula. A curable cause of adult pulmonary suppuration. Arch. Surg., 100:685, 1970.
41. Nicks, R.: Empyema and ruptured lung abscess in adults. Thorax, 19:492, 1964.
42. Pappas, G., Schröter, G., Brettschneider, L., Penn, I., and Starzl, T. E.: Pulmonary surgery in immunosuppressed patients. J. Thorac. Cardiovasc. Surg., 59:882, 1970.
43. Parker, J. D., Sarosi, G. A., Doto, I. L., Bailey, R. E., and Tosh, F. E.: Treatment of chronic pulmonary histoplasmosis. A National Communicable Disease Center Cooperative Mycoses Study. New Eng. J. Med., 283:225, 1970.
44. Parker, J. D., Sarosi, G. A., Doto, I. L., and Tosh, F. E.: Pulmonary aspergillosis in sanatoriums in the South Central United States. A National Communicable Disease Center Cooperative Mycoses Study. Amer. Rev. Dis., 101:551, 1970.
45. Peabody, J. W., Jr., Katz, S., Lyons, W. S., and Davis, E. W.: Actinomycosis, nocardiosis, and miscellaneous pulmonary mycoses. In: Steele, J. D., ed.: Treatment of Mycotic and Parasitic Diseases of the Chest. Springfield, Ill., Charles C Thomas, 1964, pp. 125–130.
46. Perkins, W.: Pulmonary cryptococcosis: Report on the treatment of nine cases. Dis. Chest, 56:389, 1969.
47. Petty, T. L., and Mitchell, R. S.: Suppurative lung disease. Med. Clin. N. Amer., 51:529, 1967.
48. Polk, J. W.: Treatment of pulmonary histoplasmosis. Dis. Chest, 56:149, 1969.
49. Prather, J. R., Eastridge, C. E., Hughes, F. A., Jr., and McCaughan, J. J., Jr.: Actinomycosis of the thorax: diagnosis and treatment. Ann. Thorac. Surg., 9:307, 1970.
50. Procknow, J. J.: Treatment of opportunistic infections. Lab. Invest., 11:1217, 1962.
51. Rainer, W. G., Liggett, M. S., Quianzon, E. P., and Dirks,

D. W.: Infected aortotomy due to Mucor following aortic valve replacement. J. Thorac. Cardiovasc. Surg., *59*: 781, 1970.

52. Reddy, P. C., Christianson, C. S., Gorelick, D. F., and Larsh, H. W.: Pulmonary monosporosis: An uncommon pulmonary mycotic infection. Thorax, *24*:722, 1969.

53. Reich, J., and Renzetti, A. D., Jr.: Pulmonary phycomycosis. Amer. Rev. Resp. Dis., *102*:959, 1970.

54. Sabiston, D. C., Jr., Hopkins, E. H., Cooke, R. E., and Bennett, I. L., Jr.: Surgical management of complications of staphylococcal pneumonia in infancy and childhood. J. Thorac. Cardiovasc. Surg., *38*:421, 1959.

55. Saliba, A., Pacini, L., and Beatty, O. A.: Intracavitary fungus balls in pulmonary aspergillosis. Brit. J. Dis. Chest, *55*:65, 1961.

56. Salkin, D., and Evans, B. H.: Coccidioidomycosis. In: Steele, J. D., ed.: The Treatment of Mycotic and Parasitic Diseases of the Chest. Springfield, Ill., Charles C Thomas, 1964, pp. 55–119.

57. Saltzman, H. A., Chick, E. W., Conant, N. F.: Nocardiosis as a complication of other diseases. Lab. Invest., *11*:1110, 1962.

58. Sandler, B. P.: Prevention of cerebral abscess secondary to pulmonary suppuration. Dis. Chest, *48*:32, 1965.

59. Sarosi, G. A., Parker, J. D., Doto, I. L., and Tosh, F. E.: Chronic pulmonary coccidioidomycosis. New Eng. J. Med., *283*:325, 1970.

60. Schwartz, J., and Salfelder, K.: Diagnosis of surgical deep Mycoses. Surg. Gynec. Obstet., *128*:259, 1969.

61. Schweppe, H. I., Knowles, J. H., and Kane, L.: Lung abscess: An analysis of Massachusetts General Hospital cases from 1943 through 1956. New Eng. J. Med., *265*:1039, 1961.

62. Scott, S. M., Peasley, E. D., and Crymes, T. P.: Pulmonary sporotrichosis: report of two cases with cavitation. New Eng. J. Med., *265*:453, 1961.

63. Seabury, J. H., Dascomb, H. E.: Results of treatment of systemic mycoses. J.A.M.A., *188*:509, 1964.

64. Sethi, J. P., Gupta, M. L., and Kasliwal, R. M.: Amebic pulmonary suppuration. Dis. Chest, *51*:148, 1967.

65. Shafron, R. D., and Tate, C. F., Jr.: Lung abscesses: A five year evaluation. Dis. Chest, *53*:12, 1968.

66. Siegrist, H. D., and Ferrington, E.: Primary pulmonary sporotrichosis. Southern Med. J., *58*:728, 1965.

67. Steele, J. D.: The Solitary Pulmonary Nodule. Springfield, Ill., Charles C Thomas, 1964.

68. Sutaria, M. K., Polk, J. W., Reddy, P., and Mohanty, S. K.: Surgical aspects of pulmonary histoplasmosis. Thorax, *25*:31, 1970.

69. Takaro, T.: Mycotic infections of interest to thoracic surgeons. Ann. Thorac. Surg., *3*:71, 1967.

70. Takaro, T., and Bond, W. M.: Pleuropulmonary, pericardial, and cerebral complications of amebiasis. Surg. Gynec. Obstet. (Int. Abstr.), *107*:209, 1958.

71. Takaro, T., Walkup, H. E., and Matthews, J. H.: The place of excisional surgery in the treatment of pulmonary mycotic infections. Dis. Chest, *36*:19, 1959.

72. Taylor, E. R.: Pulmonary cryptococcosis; an analysis of 15 cases from the Columbia area. Ann. Thorac. Surg., *10*:309, 1970.

73. Thoms, N. W., Puro, H. E., and Arbulu, A.: Significance of hemoptysis in lung abscess. J. Thorac. Cardiovasc. Surg., *59*:617, 1970.

74. Utz, J. P., Tynes, B. S., Shadomy, H. J., Duma, R. J., Kannan, M. M., and Mason, K. N.: 5-Fluoro-cytosine in human cryptococcosis. Antimicrob. Agents Chemother., *8*:344, 1968.

75. Villegas, A. H., and Sala, C. A.: Pulmonary actinomycosis of pseudotumoral form. J. Thorac. Cardiovasc. Surg., *49*:677, 1965.

76. Walkup, H. E., and Moore, J. A.: North American blastomycosis. In: Steele, J. D., ed.: The Treatment of Mycotic and Parasitic Diseases of the Chest. Springfield, Ill., Charles C Thomas, 1964, pp. 3–25.

77. Weiss, W.: Delayed cavity closure in acute nonspecific primary lung abscess. Amer. J. Med. Sci., *255*:313, 1968.

78. Weiss, W., and Flippin, H. F.: Treatment of acute nonspecific primary lung abscess: Use of orally administered penicillin G. Arch. Intern. Med., *120*:8, 1967.

79. Winn, W. A.: Long-term study of 300 patients with cavitary-abscess lesions of the lung of coccidioidal origin. Dis. Chest, Supp. 1, *54*:268, 1968.

80. Witorsch, P., and Utz, J. P.: North American blastomycosis: A study of 40 patients. Medicine, *47*:169, 1968.

# VIII

# The Pleura and Empyema

*Timothy Takaro, M.D.*

## THE PLEURA

The pleura is the serous membrane that invests the lungs and is reflected upon the walls of the thorax and on the diaphragm. In man, the pleura forms the lining of two complete and independent pleural sacs or potential cavities. Each extends into the neck, the retrosternal area, and the costophrenic sinuses, and also into the interlobar fissures. Familiarity with these ramifications of the pleural cavity can be extremely important since unwitting violation of the pleural space with its special anatomic and physiologic attributes may be followed by serious consequences. Thus, the earliest experiences of surgeons with wounds penetrating into the pleural cavities, or with

deliberate attempts to open them, often resulted in disaster, or near-disaster, from collapse of the lung, shift of the mediastinum, tension pneumothorax, and, later, infection.

A major surgical milestone was passed when the millimeter or two of potential space between the two layers of the pleural cavity could at last be crossed safely. This at first seemed to require that the whole operating team enter the area of negative pressure in the patient's pleural cavity, in order to operate within the thorax. Only the patient's head and neck remained outside, exposed to atmospheric pressure, when Sauerbruch's pioneering chamber was used at the turn of the century. This cumbersome arrangement was found to be unnecessary after Meltzer and Auer reported that positive-pressure insufflation of the lungs could sustain respirations, even with the chest open. The Empyema Commission's findings during World War I marked another milestone when it was understood that opening the pleural cavity to atmospheric pressure in order to drain an empyema prior to the development of adhesions limiting the extent of the infection could be catastrophic. In the years that followed World War I, intrathoracic surgery gradually evolved. Following World War II, this evolution progressed at a vastly accelerated pace, and the pleural cavities were regularly transgressed as a matter of course. These surgical developments added greatly to our knowledge of pleuropulmonary physiology and pathology.[8]

### Anatomic Features

Histologically, the pleural surface consists of a uniform layer of flattened mesothelial cells without a basement membrane, beneath which are layers of areolar connective tissue containing an abundance of blood vessels, nerves, and lymphatics. The visceral pleura is thinner, remarkably elastic, and intimately attached to the underlying lung by intrapulmonary fibrous prolongations of the deeper layer of connective tissue. The parietal pleura, on the other hand, is thicker, and easily separable from the thoracic wall because of the loose layer of areolar tissue separating it from the endothoracic fascia. It is supplied by the intercostal arteries. The visceral pleura is largely supplied by the bronchial arteries. Both are relatively insensitive and pain-free, parietal pleural pain fibers probably being present mostly in the endothoracic fascia.[62]

### Physiologic Characteristics

The two outstanding physiologic features of the pleural cavities are (1) the subatmospheric pressures in the normally nonexistent pleural space; and (2) the serous secreting and absorbing surface of the pleural membranes. These two characteristics seem to be interrelated. The natural elastic recoil of the lungs produces intrapleural negative pressures of −6 to −12 cm. $H_2O$ during inspiration, and −4 to −8 cm. during expiration. Extremes of +40 cm. $H_2O$ during the Valsalva maneuver or −40 cm. $H_2O$ during inspiratory effort against a closed glottis are also seen.

The secreting and absorbing properties of the pleura are substantial. With special techniques, a rate of formation of 600 to 1000 ml. of fluid per day has been observed in patients, and an equal volume has been noted to be reabsorbed by the pleural lymphatics.[65] Increased capillary hydrostatic pressure, or a greater negative intrapleural pressure, tends to increase transudation into the pleural cavities. Loss of intrapleural negative pressure diminishes transudation, while increased diaphragmatic and intercostal activity increases the absorption of transudate. Particulate matter such as red blood cells can also be absorbed directly by the normal pleura.[17] All these properties may be greatly altered by disease.[44]

## PLEURAL EFFUSIONS

While pleural effusions are almost invariably secondary to some primary condition, they often provide the first indication of that condition. Pleural effusions are always significant. Bloody effusions are ominous, for they may signify primary or secondary pleural tumor. Therefore, attempts to make a precise diagnosis of the cause of effusion should be intelligently and persistently pursued. The finding of the classic signs of fluid — flatness, absence of tactile and vocal fremitus, diminished breath sounds, and mediastinal displacement — depends upon the size of the fluid collection and on the care with which the signs are sought.

A pleural effusion of up to half a liter may not be apparent clinically or roentgenographically in the upright position in the adult, since it ordinarily gravitates into the costophrenic sinuses and is obscured by the diaphragm. Thus, when the characteristic appearance of a "small" effusion is noted on a thoracic roentgenogram, usually considerable fluid is already present and can be obtained by a carefully performed thoracentesis. On the other hand, fluid may collect almost anywhere from the apex to the base of the pleural cavity, in one or more loculated pockets, either in contact with the parietal pleura or in an interlobar fissure. Quite uncharacteristic and often bizarre roentgenographic pictures may then result, and needle aspiration may be necessary to establish the presence of a pleural effusion and thus to differentiate it from other thoracic conditions.[12]

The major causes of effusions and their differ-

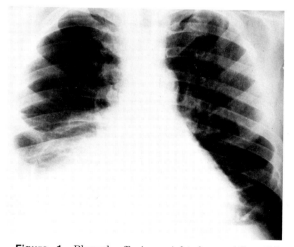

**Figure 1** Pleural effusion, right base. After this thoracic roentgenogram was taken, 1300 ml. of straw-colored fluid was aspirated at thoracentesis. Surprisingly large volumes of fluid may not be apparent clinically or roentgenographically when they gravitate into the costophrenic sinuses and are partially obscured by the diaphragm. A roentgenogram obtained in the lateral decubitus position may be more revealing.

**TABLE 1**   ETIOLOGIC CHARACTERISTICS OF PLEURAL EFFUSIONS

| | Tuberculosis | Malignancy | Congestive Failure | Pneumonia and Other Nontuberculous Infections | Rheumatoid Arthritis and Collagen Disease | Pulmonary Embolism | Fungal Infection | Trauma | Chylothorax |
|---|---|---|---|---|---|---|---|---|---|
| Clinical | Younger patient, exposure to tuberculosis, good health prior to effusion | Older patient, poor health prior to effusion | Signs and symptoms of congestive failure | Signs and symptoms of respiratory tract infection | History of joint involvement may or may not be present, subcutaneous nodules | Postoperative patient, immobilized patient, venous disease | Exposure in endemic area | History of trauma | History of trauma, known malignancy |
| Gross appearance | Usually serous, may be sanguineous | Often sanguineous | Serous | Serous | Turbid or yellow-green | Often sanguineous | Serous | Sanguineous | Chylous |
| Microscopic examination | Positive for acid-fast bacilli 30 to 70 per cent of cases, cholesterol crystals | Cytology positive in 50 per cent of cases | 0 | May or may not be positive for bacilli | 0 | 0 | May or may not be positive for fungi | 0 | Fat droplets |
| Cell count | 5 per cent over 10,000 erythrocytes; 75 per cent over 1000 leukocytes, mainly lymphocytes | 65 per cent bloody, 40 per cent over 1000 leukocytes, mainly lymphocytes | 10 per cent over 10,000 erythrocytes; 10 per cent over 1000 leukocytes | Polymorphonuclears predominate | Lymphocytes predominate | Erythrocytes predominate | 0 | Erythrocytes | 0 |
| Culture | 10 to 70 per cent pleural effusion positive; 10 to 15 per cent sputum or gastric positive | 0 | 0 | May or may not be positive | 0 | 0 | May or may not be positive | 0 | 0 |
| Specific gravity | 75 per cent over 1.016 | 75 per cent over 1.016 | 90 per cent under 1.016 (unless pulmonary embolism) | Over 1.016 | Over 1.016 | Over 1.016 | Over 1.016 | Over 1.016 | Over 1.016 |
| Protein | 90 per cent 3 g or more | 90 per cent 3 g or more | 75 per cent less than 3 g | 3.0 g or more | 3.0 g or more | 3.0 g or more | 3.0 g or more | 3.0 g or more | 0 |
| Sugar | 60 per cent less than 60 mg per cent | Less than 60 mg per cent rarely | 0 | Occasionally less than 60 mg per cent | 5–17 mg per cent; (only in rheumatoid arthritis) | 0 | 0 | 0 | 0 |
| Other | No mesothelial cells on cytology; will be the cause in 75 per cent of males under 25 years of age, 50 per cent of males 25 or over; tuberculin test usually positive | If hemorrhagic fluid, 65 per cent will be due to tumor; tends to continue to form after removed | Right-sided in 55 to 70 per cent | Associated with infiltrate on roentgenogram | Rapid clotting time; lupus erythematosus cell or rheumatoid factor may be present | Source of emboli may or may not be noted | Skin and serologic tests may be helpful | | |

*From Therapy of pleural effusion. A statement by the Committee on Therapy of the American Thoracic Society. Amer. Rev. Resp. Dis., 97:479, 1968.

entiation are outlined in Table 1. Infections (often tuberculous), tumor, and congestive failure account for at least 75 per cent of effusions in almost all types of patient populations. The problem of differential diagnosis often depends upon obtaining samples of either the fluid, the parietal pleura, or the lung and subjecting these to appropriate examinations. This does not always solve the problem, however.

Often a specific diagnosis cannot be made from pleural fluid alone, in spite of cultures and smears for pathogenic organisms and cell blocks for tumor cells.[4] Biopsy by needle or trephine may be expected to yield a specific diagnosis in less than half the cases in which it is attempted.[36, 56, 64] A small open thoracotomy may be necessary to make a definitive diagnosis, since this allows the surgeon to inspect both the visceral and the parietal pleura, as well as the lung, and to select the most promising areas for biopsy. Decortication of the lung, if indicated, may also be carried out after the incision has been enlarged. This approach is preferable to biopsies of the internal thoracic (mammary) lymph nodes, because the diagnostic yield in conditions other than tuberculosis is low.[11, 18] Thoracoscopy has rarely been used in recent years.

Pleural effusions may occur from subdiaphragmatic or intra-abdominal processes such as subphrenic or hepatic abscesses, cirrhosis of the liver, nephritis, pancreatitis,[35, 60] or ovarian fibroma.[50]

This last combination is called Meigs' syndrome. Whether passage of fluid from the peritoneal into the pleural cavities occurs through the lymphatics, or through recognized or unrecognized openings in the diaphragm, is a matter of debate.[54]

Thoracentesis is best done after careful localization of the effusion by roentgenograms in frontal, lateral, or oblique plane, or by the use of the fluoroscopic image intensifier. A syringe no larger than 20 ml., with a three-way stopcock interposed between needle and syringe, allows the most adequate control. After thorough infiltration of skin, intercostal muscle, and parietal pleura with a local anesthetic agent, the needle of appropriate caliber and length is directed just above the superior border of the lower rib of the appropriate interspace and allowed to penetrate the parietal pleura until fluid is reached, constant moderate negative pressure being applied to the syringe. When aspirating low in the costophrenic sinus, the needle tip should be directed cephalad to avoid puncturing the diaphragm. After the appropriate depth has been reached, a clamp may be placed on the needle at the level of the skin to prevent further penetration and thus to avoid injuring the lung. Removing all available fluid is usually not difficult unless a massive acute effusion is being completely evacuated. In some instances under these circumstances, pain, discomfort, and severe coughing may be initiated. Rarely, transient unilateral pulmonary edema may occur. Thus it may be wiser to evacuate no more than 1500 ml. of a massive effusion at the initial attempt.[72]

## "SPONTANEOUS" PNEUMOTHORAX

The accumulation of air in the pleural cavity without any apparent antecedent event – so-called spontaneous pneumothorax – is almost always due to rupture of a subpleural cyst, bleb, or bulla, often in an otherwise apparently normal lung in a young (20 to 40 year old) male cigarette smoker. It can occur, however, at any age, from the newborn, in whom vigorous resuscitative efforts may result in pneumothorax, to the elderly and emphysematous patient, in whom it may pose a very serious problem.[22] Rupture of a tuberculous focus as a cause is now quite uncommon. Occasionally, primary or metastatic tumor may be found in association with pneumothorax. Hemorrhage (hemopneumothorax) may accompany collapse of the lung due to a torn, vascular adhesion. Although this is uncommon, it may be severe enough to warrant emergency thoracotomy for control.

Symptoms depend upon the degree of collapse of the lung and on its previous condition. There may be no symptoms whatever, or severe dyspnea, hypoxemia, and even shock may be observed. Chest pain may be prominent or absent. Hyperresonance and absent or diminished breath sounds are the characteristic physical findings.

The diagnosis is usually apparent from the

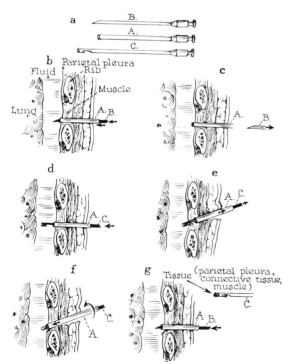

**Figure 2** Diagrams illustrating a method of obtaining a pleural biopsy using the Cope needle. (From Levine, H., and Cugell, D. W.: Arch. Intern. Med., *109*:516, 1962.)

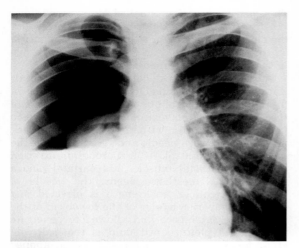

**Figure 3**   Thoracic roentgenogram illustrating spontaneous hemopneumothorax in a 22 year old male. This was treated by closed tube thoracostomy and responded with prompt and complete re-expansion of the lung. The etiology was undetermined.

In tension pneumothorax, intrapleural pressures on one or both sides may rise precipitately. This is due to a valvelike mechanism that allows air to enter the pleural spaces from the lung parenchyma or airways during brief episodes of markedly elevated intrabronchial or intra-alveolar pressure, as occurs during coughing. Because of collapse of the lung and shift of the mediastinum, severe and even life-threatening respiratory distress may develop, requiring emergency needle aspiration followed by tube thoracostomy drainage. Physical findings of hyperresonance, absent breath sounds, and mediastinal shift away from the involved side are diagnostic.

Spontaneous pneumothorax and especially roentgenogram of the chest. A film taken during expiration may help demonstrate a small pneumothorax more readily, while appropriate laminagrams of the lung may aid in the differentiation of localized pneumothorax from a large, thin-walled pulmonary cyst or pneumatocele.

Treatment depends upon a variety of factors. An initial, small (5 to 20 per cent), asymptomatic pneumothorax may safely be kept under observation. Intercostal rubber tube thoracostomy with a closed drainage system is adequate for the vast majority of patients with large pneumothoraces.[49] Prevention of recurrences is said to be favored by keeping the rubber (not plastic) tube in place for at least 4 days, to foster a sterile pleuritis. The rounded, closed-end, S-shaped needle introduced by Clagett is less traumatic and more convenient, but it lacks the desirable feature of acting as an irritant to the pleura.[22] Gentle suction on either catheter or S-needle facilitates expansion of the lung. If air leakage persists or is larger than can be handled by a high-volume vacuum system, if the episode is a recurrent one, or if obvious bullae or cysts are seen in the collapsed lung, open thoracotomy is advocated, with suturing, ligation, or excision of the ruptured bleb or bulla, and vigorous abrasion of especially the parietal, but also the visceral, pleura. This produces filmy adhesions and helps prevent recurrences. Excision of the parietal pleura is advocated by some observers, but the consensus is against its use, as being unnecessary, more traumatic, and associated with a higher complication rate.[13, 71, 79] Subsequent thoracotomy, if it should become necessary, is rendered more difficult also. Talc poudrage, or the use of other irritants to obtain pleurodesis, is not recommended.

Appropriate antimicrobial therapy is obviously indicated if an infectious process such as tuberculosis is present.

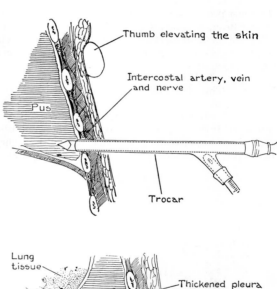

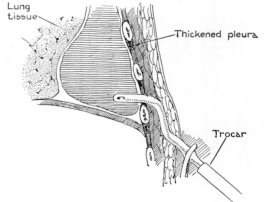

**Figure 4**   Diagrams illustrating a method of inserting an intercostal catheter for closed tube thoracostomy drainage. *A*, Step 1: Insertion of trocar into pleural space. (The patient's skin is being elevated by the surgeon's thumb to provide a flap valve effect for closure of the catheter tract following removal of the intercostal catheter.) *B*, Step 2: The intercostal catheter has been inserted through the trocar and into the pleural space. The trocar is being removed. (Note flap valve effect produced by Step 1.) (From Cutler, E. C., Elliott, C., and Zollinger, R. M.: Atlas of Surgical Operations. 2nd ed. New York, Macmillan, 1949.)

tension pneumothorax in the emphysematous patient with marginal respiratory function and cor pulmonale may present a grave and sometimes insurmountable problem of management. Monitoring of blood gases and of the electrocardiogram, assisted ventilation, tracheostomy, appropriate cardiac drugs, multiple closed thoracotomies, and open thoracotomy may all be necessary. In a recent series from the Mayo Clinic, 10 of 57 such patients died, 5 before adequate therapy could be instituted.[22] Two of eleven succumbed following thoracotomy. The prognosis in the average patient with pneumothorax, however, is very good, with few recurrences if a sterile pleuritis has been successfully produced by closed tube thoracostomy.

Rarely, as with pleural effusions, rapid re-expansion of a complete pneumothorax by means of high negative pressure can be followed by ipsilateral pulmonary edema. A slower decompression, using lesser negative pressure, might obviate this occurrence.[34]

Closed pleural drainage systems should be simple, but may be more complex, depending upon the particular clinical problem. Of primary importance is that the characteristics of the system used should be understood by both the responsible physician and the attending nursing staff. When little or no continuing air escape is expected, and only fluid drainage is required, simple, single-bottle, underwater-seal apparatus, or even a rubber flutter valve and plastic bag arrangement, is adequate.[5, 29] A two-bottle system, with a "dry trap" for the first bottle, provides a separate bottle for collection, in addition to the underwater seal, but adds to the volume of "dead space" between the pleural space and the water-seal surface. In small patients this may be of significance.[5] When air leaks are expected, more complicated systems, involving two or three bottles, with provision for active suction, are recommended.[5, 26, 58] The first bottle may be a collecting bottle, the second a water seal, and the third a vacuum regulator with a long tube open to air, and extending under water a determinate number of centimeters to correspond with the maximal negative suction in centimeters of water required (20 to 40 cm.). Very strong suction (−30 cm. Hg) has been advocated recently for patients who have had pulmonary resections.[67] Either a wall vacuum source or a high air flow capacity, electrically driven turbine type of pump is effective.[26] Pumps with a low air flow capacity should not be used when large air leaks, either continuous or intermittent (as during coughing), may be expected.[5] The drainage system should function to prevent ingress of air into the pleural cavity, even when the vacuum source fails. It is equally important that the system should allow egress of large volumes of air, suddenly, whether the vacuum source is functioning or not. Time spent in understanding the physiologic and physical principles of pleural drainage systems and communicating this understanding to attending nurses will be well spent.[26]

## HEMOTHORAX

An accumulation of blood in the pleural cavities (hemothorax) may result from trauma to the chest wall, the lung, the mediastinal structures, or the diaphragm. It can also be found with pulmonary infarction, with pleural or pulmonary neoplasm, or following tearing of a pleural adhesion, as with spontaneous pneumothorax. It can occur as a complication of anticoagulant therapy. Hemothorax following surgery on the heart or lungs is unfortunately all too common. Partial defibrination of the blood may occur, with deposition of fibrin on the pleural surface. However, a sterile hemothorax can be completely reabsorbed, leaving little or no residue.[17] An infected hemothorax, or hemothoracic empyema, on the other hand, can lead to the development of a fibrothorax, with serious compromise of pulmonary function.[10] This is more likely to occur after war wounds and gunshot wounds, with underlying lung damage; it is less likely to occur after a clean stab wound.[23] Hemopneumothorax is more likely to be followed by such a complication than hemothorax alone.

The management of hemothorax depends upon the rate of bleeding and the total volume bled, as well as the underlying cause. If the hemothorax is small, and bleeding has stopped, judging from clinical signs and serial roentgenograms, nothing need be done. For moderate amounts of estimated blood accumulation (500 ml. or more), a closed thoracostomy with intercostal tube drainage for complete evacuation of blood allows observation of its reaccumulation, plus re-expansion of the lung, and is preferable to needle aspiration. Continuing active bleeding, as judged from serial thoracic roentgenograms, clinical signs, or output from chest tubes, demands open thoracotomy for control of hemorrhage. It has often been observed that continuing postoperative bleeding will cease upon re-exploration and removal of blood clots, even if no active bleeding point is found.

In order to forestall the development of an imprisoning fibrothorax, and to gain re-expansion of lung compressed by blood, early decortication (within 3 weeks of the gunshot type of injury) is advocated. The fibrinous deposit will still peel off the visceral pleura readily, and pulmonary expansibility can be restored. On the other hand, one should not resort to decortication precipitately, since an uncomplicated hemothorax can be completely resorbed.

## CHYLOTHORAX

Chylothorax, that is, chyle in the pleural cavity, is most commonly due to trauma or tumor. The thin, fibromuscular thoracic duct that transports chyle along the length of the mediastinum from the cysterna chyli to the left subclavian vein may be ruptured anywhere along its course. Rupture above the fifth or sixth thoracic vertebra

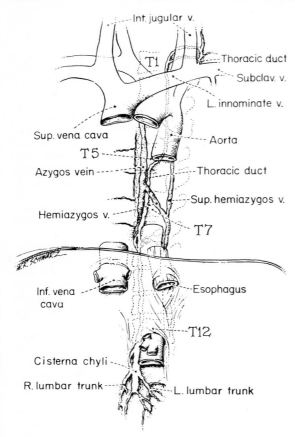

**Figure 5**    Diagram showing anatomic relationships of the thoracic duct. (From Williams, K. R., and Burford, T. H.: J. Trauma, 3:317, 1963.)

generally results in left-sided chylothorax; injury below that level often results in a right-sided collection. Because of excellent collateral pathways, the duct can be ligated with impunity.

Owing to the high fat and protein content of the milky white chyle, loss of this material into the pleural cavity can be a serious matter from the nutritional standpoint. The large volume of the effusion may also cause severe respiratory embarrassment.

Of traumatic cases, 80 per cent are the result of gunshot wounds, automobile accidents, stab wounds, and blunt trauma; and 20 per cent are iatrogenic, mostly postsurgical, usually following operations for congenital cardiovascular anomalies.[27, 32] Lymphosarcomas and metastatic carcinomas account for most cases due to tumor. Aspiration or closed intercostal drainage coupled with *increased* oral fat intake is often effective, if the patient's general condition permits persistence of such therapy for 3 to 4 weeks.[45] If not, and if conservative measures fail to control the leakage of chyle, or if it recurs, thoracotomy in 7 to 10 days is advocated to forestall severe nutritional depletion.[32] The ingestion of a fatty meal or

a quantity of a lipophilic dye just prior to surgery may aid in identifying the site of leakage.[37] Unless this leakage can be identified and controlled by suture ligation, ligation of the duct low in the mediastinum below the level of the eighth thoracic vertebra is the treatment of choice. It has been pointed out that in traumatic cases of chylothorax, surgery will usually be unnecessary, whereas in those cases due to malignant disease, it will rarely be effective.[77]

## PLEURAL TUMORS

These are classified as primary and secondary. Primary pleural tumors are mostly mesotheliomas, of which localized benign types and diffuse malignant types are recognized.[41, 53, 73] In both types, fibrous or fibrosarcomatous and epithelioid varieties are seen. Mixtures of the two histologic varieties also occur. Therefore, the pathologic classification of benign versus malignant and the

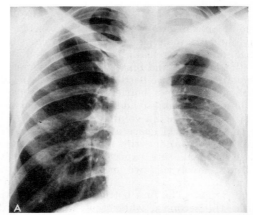

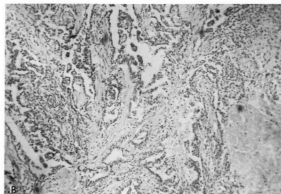

**Figure 6**    *A,* Thoracic roentgenogram showing marked pleural thickening around entire left lung, in an adult male. At open thoracotomy and biopsy, a pleural tumor was found which proved to be a diffuse malignant pleural mesothelioma. *B,* Reproduction of photomicrograph showing histologic pattern of pleural mesothelioma illustrated in *A.* This is only one of a variety of histologic patterns that can occur in this disease.

differentiation from carcinoma are sometimes difficult.

Patients with localized fibrous mesotheliomas may be asymptomatic, or they may complain of symptoms of arthralgia, clubbing of the fingers, or fever.[15, 33, 68] When the solitary, often encapsulated and pedunculated, usually easily removable tumor, arising ordinarily from the visceral pleura, is excised, the symptoms and signs of arthralgia and pulmonary osteoarthropathy disappear, and longevity seems to be unaffected. These tumors may range in size from a few to 20 cm. or more in diameter.

Diffuse or malignant mesotheliomas, on the other hand, cause chest pain and bloody pleural effusion containing malignant mesothelial cells.[30] These tumors are characterized by findings ranging from multiple papillary projections on both visceral and parietal pleurae to encasement of the entire lung in a thick rind of tumor, with similar findings on the parietal side. Part or all of the pleural space may be obliterated. Metastases are uncommon, except late in the disease, and are often limited to the regional lymph nodes. Extrathoracic metastases do occur, however. Death within 1 or 2 years is the rule in the majority of cases.[7]

At issue currently is the precise relationship between exposure to asbestos dust and the development of malignant mesotheliomas and, even more frequently, bronchogenic carcinoma. Circumstantial evidence for a causal relationship is strong and is based on experimental evidence[76] and on occupational exposure, with a high incidence of both pleural mesothelioma and bronchogenic carcinoma in asbestos workers or those exposed to asbestos.[20, 51] The identification of "asbestos bodies," the ferruginous or iron-staining foreign body capsules that coat the ultramicroscopic asbestos fibrils, in some patients with pleural mesotheliomas but also in random autopsies in 30 to 97 per cent of lungs weakens somewhat the chain of circumstantial evidence.[24]

Treatment of malignant mesothelioma has been unsatisfactory. There have been no cures. A small number of 4 to 7 year survivals have been achieved by "complete" pleurectomy or pleuropneumonectomy, but the great majority of patients have succumbed within 1 or 2 years of the diagnosis, regardless of the type of treatment used. Radiation is nevertheless recommended, if excisional surgery is impossible or incomplete.[41, 53]

Pleural involvement by metastatic disease is far more common than primary pleural tumor and is usually associated with implants involving the lung or with blockage of or interference with the lymphatic drainage of the visceral, parietal, diaphragmatic, or mediastinal pleura. The most common sites of primary tumor are the lung, breast, pancreas, and stomach. With direct involvement of the pleura by tumor implants, bloody fluid containing neoplastic cells can often be obtained. Various types of palliative treatment are advocated, depending upon the site of the primary tumor, the expansibility of the lung, the degree of disability from pleural effusion, and so forth. Hormonal therapy, radiation or radioisotope therapy, multiple aspirations of the chest, closed tube thoracostomy,[38] and the insufflation of talc[1, 52] or the instillation of chemotherapeutic agents[31] have all been reported, with varying degrees of palliation having been achieved.[40, 48]

## EMPYEMA

Pleural empyema is a collection of purulent fluid in the pleural space. It may be localized (encapsulated), or it may involve the entire pleural cavity. Empyema is classified by some authors as "acute" or "chronic," depending upon duration and pathologic reaction, but there is no sharp dividing line between the two types with respect to either time or pathologic response. A more informative but less popular differentiation between the stages of empyema might be that offered by the American Thoracic Society. *Exudative* empyema is characterized by thin fluid with low cellular content and by an underlying lung that will re-expand readily. *Fibrinopurulent* empyema is characterized by large numbers of polymorphonuclear leukocytes and by deposition of fibrin on both the visceral and parietal surfaces of the involved pleura. In this transitional phase between acute and chronic empyema, there is a progressive tendency toward loculation and delimitation of the extent of the empyema space, accompanied by beginning fixation of the lung. In *organizing* empyema, fibroblasts appear in the now heavier fibrin coating of the pleural membranes, and the exudate is quite thick. Over 75 to 80 per cent of the fluid consists of sediment, as is seen when the fluid is left standing.

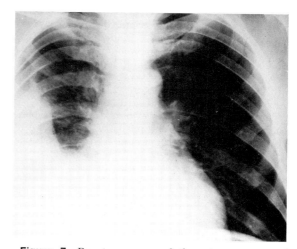

**Figure 7**  Roentgenogram of thoracic empyema of 2 months' duration, from which anaerobic streptococci and gram-negative bacteroides bacilli were isolated. This patient was treated by open drainage following resection of a 2 inch segment of the seventh rib. The right lung re-expanded completely and the empyema space was obliterated in approximately 2 weeks.

These distinctions are important, because therapy differs with each stage of the disease.

Both acute and chronic empyema in adults are relatively less common conditions in the present era of antibiotics than they were in the past.[42, 78] In spite of the antibiotics, however, there was an impressive increase in incidence of both staphylococcal pneumonia and empyema in children during the late 1950s.[57, 66] Such recrudescences of infections can surely be expected again. Today, because of the increasing age and debility of patients with empyema who have underlying serious illness, this disease may still pose serious problems of diagnosis and management.[75]

### Etiology

Acute empyema ordinarily results from a primary pathologic condition elsewhere. Most commonly, this condition is a pneumonic process in the underlying lung, such as lobar pneumonia, pneumonitis, or lung abscess.[42] This may extend to the pleura directly, by way of the lymphatics, by hematogenous spread, or by rupture of necrotic pulmonary parenchyma. The pneumonic process may itself be secondary to other conditions, such as bronchial obstruction due to bronchogenic carcinoma or a foreign body in the airway, or to bronchial infection, as seen in bronchiectasis. A ruptured emphysematous bleb with spontaneous pneumothorax may also occasionally result in empyema. Less commonly, the source of infection may be a mediastinal structure, such as the trachea or bronchi (bronchopleural fistula); the esophagus (perforation, leaking esophagogastric anastomosis);[63, 70] an abscessed lymph node; or osteomyelitis of the dorsal spine. Subphrenic or intrahepatic abscesses may spread via the rich lymphatics of the diaphragm and cause empyema. Finally, infection may be introduced into the pleural spaces from without by means of trauma, needle aspiration, or operation. Chronic empyema results from untreated or inadequately treated acute empyema. This development should be prevented if it is at all possible to do so. *Empyema necessitatis,* encapsulated empyema discharging into the subcutaneous tissues of the chest wall, is now rarely reported but still occurs.[46]

The most common bacteriologic agents responsible for empyema in the past—pneumococci and streptococci—have been displaced in importance and in frequency in recent years by *Staphylococcus aureus* and by a variety of gram-negative organisms: Pseudomonas, *Klebsiella pneumoniae, Escherichia coli, Aerobacter aerogenes,* Proteus, Bacteroides, and Salmonella. Tuberculous empyema is now uncommon. Empyema caused by fungi is discussed in the preceding section. Amebic empyema, now quite rare, occurs usually as the result of an amebic liver abscess, with rupture into the right pleural cavity.[69]

### Diagnosis

The diagnosis depends upon the detection of signs and symptoms of the underlying infectious

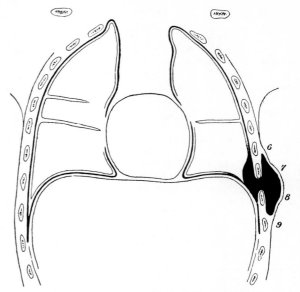

**Figure 8**    Diagram of empyema necessitatis showing its characteristic components: encapsulated pleural empyema, a narrow opening between the ribs through which the empyema has burrowed, and the externally presenting collection of pus in the subcutaneous tissues. (From Ashhurst, A. P. C.: Int. Clin., *4*:173, 1916.)

process and of the accumulation of purulent material in the pleural cavity. This is supported and localized by the clinical examination of the patient and the roentgenographic appearance of fluid, or fluid and air, or of a pleural or interlobar opacification compatible with fluid. It is confirmed by needle aspiration with the demonstration of pus. Bacteria may not be identified if intensive antibiotic therapy has been employed previously or if the etiologic agent is not bacterial.

### Treatment

The objectives of treatment for all stages of empyema are: (1) control of the primary infection and its secondary manifestation, empyema; (2) evacuation of the purulent contents of the empyema sac and eradication of the sac, to prevent chronicity; and (3) re-expansion of the underlying lung in order to restore function. The methods used to achieve these objectives depend upon the stage of empyema being treated and the nature of the primary infection or source of contamination. These objectives are realized by the use of appropriate antibiotic therapy, based upon the bacteriologic diagnosis, and by prompt and adequate drainage. *Needle aspiration* is sometimes adequate, but only in the exudative state with thin pus. Even in this stage, insertion of an intercostal tube for *continuous closed drainage* should not be delayed if the purulent fluid cannot be completely evacuated by thoracentesis, if the fluid reaccumulates, or if infection and toxicity are difficult to control. There is an increasing trend toward the early use of closed tube drainage for all acute empyemas.[6, 42, 74] For the fibrinopurulent stage, prompt use of closed tube drainage is indicated, especially if there is concern that open drainage would result in collapse of the lung. Negative pressure may have to be applied to hasten pulmonary expansion, especially in the presence of a bronchopleural fistula. The tube is usually inserted through a trocar; it should be of a caliber commensurate with the type of material being evacuated and should not be permitted to become plugged. It should be placed in the most dependent part of the empyema pocket, with care being exercised to avoid perforation of the diaphragm upon insertion of the trocar. Accurate localization is greatly facilitated by the use of biplane roentgenograms of the chest or a fluoroscopic intensifier. More than one tube may be necessary. Malecot or right-angle catheters that can be inserted directly through a stab incision and pulled flush with the parietal wall of the pleural cavity are preferred by some surgeons.[59]

*Open drainage* accompanied by resection of a short segment of rib is used if closed tube thoracostomy is ineffective, if the pus is too thick or is loculated in multiple pockets, or if the patient's toxic condition continues.[42, 43] At this stage, the empyema is localized by adherence of those parts of visceral and parietal pleura which are not involved in the empyema. In most instances, after the pus is evacuated, the obvious locules are broken up and the empyema cavity is washed, a wide-bore tube is left in place, open to atmospheric pressure. However, if it is found that the visceral pleural peel is still quite thin, and there is danger of pulmonary collapse or possible spread of empyema, the snug fit of an intercostal catheter can be duplicated by appropriate mechanical sealing of the wound around the tube and application of underwater-seal closed drainage or even negative pressure.[39, 59] Another variation, the Eloesser skin flap, originally designed for tuberculous empyema, combines some of the virtues of open and closed drainage and eliminates the need for wide-bore tubes open to air.[16, 25] With open drainage, the appropriate, most dependent site must be carefully localized roentgenographically or fluoroscopically and by repeated exploratory thoracenteses before the rib is resected. The drainage tube is removed only when the empyema sac has been eliminated, as determined by measurement of its capacity or radiographically, after introduction of contrast material.[3]

In some instances, *decortication* will achieve the goals of therapy more efficiently than open drainage. This is more likely to be true in managing infected or noninfected hemothorax, when the lung has become imprisoned by its nonelastic fibrinopurulent coat, but presumably remains expandible, and the patient is not in a toxic condition. Decortication may follow closed or open tube drainage.[9, 59] Although advocated by some as primary treatment for empyema,[47] decortication is not generally advocated as primary treatment, except in unusual circumstances in which there is major pulmonary collapse and an obvious, thick

visceral and parietal peel. Even here, closed drainage as a preliminary step to aid in cleansing the cavity contents and improving the patient's general condition may have a place. Infrequently, conventional *thoracoplasty* to obliterate the pleural space or Schede thoracoplasty to unroof an empyema pocket may be necessary. The use of skin flap open drainage,[59, 63] of pedicled muscle flaps as described by Maier, or of "thoracomediastinal plication" as described by Andrews[2] may be needed for complicated problems involving bronchopleural-cutaneous fistulas, if simple open drainage fails to obliterate empyema.

Treatment of empyema following pneumonectomy has changed in recent years with the observation that elimination of the empyema space is not necessary if it can be sterilized and if there is no underlying bronchopleural or esophagopleural fistula.[14] It can be accomplished in a variety of ways, involving instillation of a solution of antibiotics, with or without debridement of the lining of the empyema cavity.[19, 21, 55]

### Results of Treatment

The results of treatment of empyema depend upon the underlying condition, the age of the patient, and associated diseases. In Snider's series of 105 adult patients, there were 49 deaths. However, in only five patients was the empyema thought to be a significant factor. In one 30 year experience involving 138 children, mortality from postpneumonic empyema remained remarkably constant (9 to 14 per cent) in spite of the fact that the time span encompassed the preantibiotic and presulfonamide periods.[6] When empyema was secondary to surgical procedures or trauma, however, the mortality rate was in the range of 60 per cent.[6, 63] On the other hand, better results, with a 1.6 per cent mortality, have been reported when conservative measures were used, including methicillin and thoracentesis alone in most cases.[66] Thus some types of empyema remain a serious problem, requiring early diagnosis, accurate bacteriologic identification, and prompt and vigorous management.

### SELECTED REFERENCES

American Thoracic Society: Management of nontuberculous empyema. Amer. Rev. Resp. Dis., 85:935, 1962.
  *A statement of the Subcommittee on Surgery of the American Thoracic Society summarizing well a reasonable consensus regarding etiology, pathology, and appropriate therapy for the various phases of nontuberculous empyema.*

American Thoracic Society: Therapy of pleural effusion: a statement by the Committee on Therapy. Amer. Rev. Resp. Dis., 97:479, 1968.
  *A reasoned and detailed approach to the differential diagnosis and management of pleural effusions.*

Barrett, N. R.: The pleura—with special reference to fibrothorax. Thorax, 24:515, 1970.
  *The Tudor Edwards Memorial Lecture, 1970; thoughts, observations, and interpretations that present a fresh insight into the structure and function of the pleura in health and in disease.*

Eloesser, L.: Milestones in chest surgery. J. Thorac. Cardiovasc. Surg., 60:157, 1970.

*A brief but fascinating recapitulation of some of the major landmarks in the development of thoracic and cardiovascular surgery, from Sauerbruch's chamber to Gibbon's pumpoxygenator.*

Green, R. A.: Diseases of the pleura. In: Baum, G. L., ed.: Textbook of Pulmonary Diseases. Boston, Little, Brown and Company, 1965, pp. 655–707.
*An excellent exposition of many of the facets of pleural disease.*

Maier, H. C.: The pleura. In: Gibbon, J. H., Jr., Sabiston, D. C., Jr., and Spencer, F. C., eds.: Surgery of the Chest. 2nd ed. Philadelphia, W. B. Saunders Company, 1969, pp. 212–242.
*Recommended reading for a more complete exposition of this subject, including important details of surgical techniques.*

Ratzer, E. R., Pool, J. L., and Melamed, M. T.: Pleural mesotheliomas. Amer. J. Roentgen., 99:863, 1967.
*A well documented clinical and pathologic review of 37 patients seen at the Memorial and James Ewing Hospital in New York.*

Snider, G., and Saleh, S. S.: Empyema of the thorax in adults. Review of 105 cases. Dis. Chest., 54:410, 1968.
*A complete presentation of the subject, with specific details concerning antibiotic drug therapy.*

## REFERENCES

1. Adler, R. H., and Rappole, B. W.: Recurrent malignant pleural effusions and talc powder aerosol treatment. Surgery, 62:1000, 1967.
2. Andrews, N. C.: The surgical treatment of chronic empyema. Dis. Chest, 47:533, 1965.
3. Andrews, N. C., Ver Meulen, V. R., and Christoforidis, A. J.: Injection of contrast media in postresection pleural spaces; diagnostic, prognostic, and therapeutic value. Dis. Chest, 52:656, 1967.
4. Arrington, C. W., Hawkins, J. A., Rickert, J. H., and Hopeman, A. R.: Management of undiagnosed pleural effusions in positive tuberculin reactors. Amer. Rev. Resp. Dis., 93:587, 1966.
5. Batchelder, T. L., and Morris, K. A.: Critical factors in determining adequate pleural drainage in both the operated and non-operated chest. Amer. Surg., 28:296, 1962.
6. Bechamps, G. J., Lynn, H. B., and Wenzl, J. E.: Empyema in children. Mayo Clin. Proc., 45:43, 1970.
7. Borow, M., Conston, A., Livornese, L. L., and Schalet, N.: Mesothelioma and its association with asbestosis. J.A.M.A., 201:587, 1967.
8. Brock, L.: Evarts A. Graham: Recollections. Ann. Thorac. Surg., 9:272, 1970.
9. Bryant, L. R., Chicklo, J. M., Crutcher, R., Danielson, G. K., Malette, W. G., and Trinkle, J. K.: Management of thoracic empyema. J. Thorac. Cardiovasc. Surg., 55:850, 1968.
10. Burford, T. H.: Hemothorax and hemothoracic empyema. In Berry, B., ed.: Surgery in World War II: Thoracic Surgery. Vol. II. Washington, D.C., Office of the Surgeon General, Department of the Army, 1965, pp. 237–324.
11. Burke, H. E., and Wilson, J. A. S.: A new method for establishing the diagnosis of pleural disease—parasternal lymph node biopsy. Amer. Rev. Resp. Dis., 93:201, 1966.
12. Carr, D. T., Soule, E. H., and Ellis, F. H., Jr.: Management of pleural effusions. Med. Clin. N. Amer., 48:961, 1964.
13. Clagett, O. T.: The management of spontaneous pneumothorax. (Editorial.) J. Thorac. Cardiovasc. Surg., 55:761, 1968.
14. Clagett, O. T., and Geraci, J. E.: A procedure for the management of postpneumonectomy empyema. J. Thorac. Cardiovasc. Surg., 45:141, 1963.
15. Clagett, O. T., McDonald, J. R., and Schmidt, H. W.: Localized fibrous mesothelioma of pleura. J. Thorac. Surg., 24:213, 1952.
16. Cohn, L. H., and Blaisdall, E. W.: Surgical treatment of nontuberculous empyema. Arch. Surg., 100:376, 1970.
17. Condon, R. E.: Spontaneous resolution of experimental clotted hemothorax. Surg. Gynec. Obstet., 126:505, 1968.
18. Conklin, E. F., Yeoh, C. B., Jones, J. M., Malcolm, J. A., and Ford, J. M.: Internal–mammary–lymph–node

biopsy as a diagnostic aid in pleural effusion. New Eng. J. Med., 271:1346, 1964.
19. Conklin, W. S.: Post-pneumonectomy empyema. J. Thorac. Cardiovasc. Surg., 55:634, 1968.
20. Demy, N. G., and Adler, H.: Asbestosis and malignancy. Amer. J. Roentgen., 100:597, 1967.
21. Dieter, R. A., Pifarré, R., Neville, W. E., Magno, M., and Jasuja, M.: Empyema treated with neomycin irrigation and closed-chest drainage. J. Thorac. Cardiovasc. Surg., 59:496, 1970.
22. Dines, D. E., Clagett, O. T., and Payne, W. S.: Spontaneous pneumothorax in emphysema. Mayo Clin. Proc., 45:481, 1970.
23. Drummond, D. S., and Craig, R. H.: Traumatic hemothorax: complications and management. Amer. Surg., 33:403, 1967.
24. Editorial: Asbestos dust—a community hazard? J.A.M.A., 209:1216, 1969.
25. Eloesser, L.: Of an operation for tuberculous empyema. Ann. Thorac. Surg., 8:355, 1969.
26. Enerson, D. M., and McIntire, J.: A comparative study of the physiology and physics of pleural drainage systems. J. Thorac. Cardiovasc. Surg., 52:40, 1966.
27. Goorwitch, J.: Traumatic chylothorax and thoracic duct ligation. Case report and review of the literature. J. Thorac. Surg., 29:467, 1955.
28. Hamaker, W. R., Buchman, R. J., Cox, W. A., and Fisher, G. W.: Hemothorax: a complication of anticoagulant therapy. Ann. Thorac. Surg., 8:564, 1969.
29. Heimlich, H. J.: Valve drainage of the pleural cavity. Dis. Chest, 53:282, 1968.
30. Heller, R. M., Janower, M. L., Wever, A. L.: Radiological manifestations of malignant pleural mesothelioma. Amer. J. Roentgen., 108:53, 1970.
31. Hickman, J. A., and Jones, M. C.: Treatment of neoplastic pleural effusions with local instillations of quinacrine (mepacrine) hydrocloride. Thorax, 25:226, 1970.
32. Higgins, C. B., and Mulder, D. G.: Chylothorax after surgery for congenital heart disease. J. Thorac. Cardiovasc. Surg., 61:411, 1971.
33. Hudspeth, A. S.: Benign localized pleural mesotheliomas presenting as arthritis. Ann. Thorac. Surg., 2:691, 1966.
34. Humphreys, R. L., and Berne, A. S.: Rapid re-expansion of pneumothorax Radiology, 96:509, 1970.
35. Kaye, M. D.: Pleuropulmonary complications of pancreatitis. Thorax, 23:297, 1968.
36. Kettel, L. J., and Cugell, D. W.: Pleural biopsy. J.A.M.A., 200:317, 1967.
37. Klepser, R. G., and Berry, J. F.: Diagnosis and surgical management of chylothorax with the aid of lipophilic dyes. Dis. Chest, 25:409, 1954.
38. Lambert, C. J., Shah, M. H., Urschel, H. C., Jr., and Paulson, D. L.: Treatment of malignant pleural effusions by closed trocar tube drainage. Ann. Thorac. Surg., 3:1, 1967.
39. Langston, H. T.: Empyema thoracis. (Editorial.) Ann. Thorac. Surg., 2:766, 1966.
40. Leininger, B. J., Barker, W. L., and Langston, H. T.: A simplified method for management of malignant pleural effusion. J. Thorac. Cardiovasc. Surg., 58:758, 1969.
41. LeRoux, B. T.: Pleural tumors. Thorax, 17:111, 1962.
42. LeRoux, B. T.: Empyema thoracis. Brit. J. Surg., 52:89, 1965.
43. Levitsky, S., Annable, C. A., and Thomas, P. A.: Management of empyema after thoracic wounding. Observations on 25 Vietnam casualties. J. Thorac. Cardiovasc. Surg., 59:630, 1970.
44. Maier, H. C.: Pulmonary and pleural lymphatics: a challenge to the thoracic explorer. J. Thorac. Cardiovasc. Surg., 52:155, 1966.
45. Maloney, J. V., Jr., and Spencer, F. C.: Nonoperative treatment of traumatic chylothorax. Surgery, 40:121, 1956.
46. Marks, M. I., and Eickhoff, T. C.: Empyema necessitatis. Amer. Rev. Resp. Dis., 101:759, 1970.
47. Mayo, P., and McElvein, R. B.: Early thoracotomy for pyogenic empyema. Ann. Thorac. Surg., 2:649, 1966.
48. Meyer, P. C.: Metastatic carcinoma of the pleura. Thorax, 21:437, 1966.
49. Mills, M., and Baisch, B. F.: Spontaneous pneumothorax—A series of 400 cases. Ann. Thorac. Surg., 1:286, 1965.
50. Neustadt, J. E., and Levy, R. C.: Hemorrhagic pleural effusion in Meigs' syndrome. J.A.M.A., 204:81, 1968.

51. Newhouse, M. L., and Wagner, J. C.: Validation of death certificates in asbestos workers. Brit. J. Industr. Med., 26:302, 1969.
52. Pearson, F. G., and MacGregor, D. C.: Talc poudrage for malignant pleural effusion. J. Thorac. Cardiovasc. Surg., 51:732, 1966.
53. Porter, J. M., and Cheek, J. M.: Pleural mesothelioma. Review of tumor histogenesis and report of 12 cases. J. Thorac. Cardiovasc. Surg., 55:882, 1968.
54. Pratt, J. H., and Shamblin, W. R.: Spontaneous hemothorax as a direct complication of hemoperitoneum. Ann. Surg., 167:867, 1968.
55. Provan, J. L.: Management of postpneumonectomy empyema. J. Thorac. Cardiovasc. Surg., 61:107, 1971.
56. Rao, N. V., Jones, P. O., Greenberg, S. D., Bahar, D., Daysog, A. O., Jr., Schweppe, H. I., and Jenkins, D. E.: Needle biopsy of parietal pleura in 124 cases. Arch. Intern. Med., 115:34, 1965.
57. Ravitch, M. M., and Fein, R.: Changing picture of pneumonia and empyema in infants and children: review of the experience at the Harriet Lane Home from 1934 through 1958. J.A.M.A., 175:1039, 1961.
58. Roe, B. B.: Physiological principles of drainage of the pleural space. Amer. J. Surg., 96:246, 1958.
59. Samson, P. C.: Empyema thoracis—essentials of present-day management. Ann. Thorac. Surg., 11:210, 1971.
60. Shapiro, D. H., Anagnostopoulos, C. E., and Dineen, J. P.: Decortication and pleurectomy for the pleuropulmonary complications of pancreatitis. Ann. Thorac. Surg., 9:76, 1970.
61. Simon, H. B., Daggett, W. M., and DeSanctis, R. W.: Hemothorax as a complication of anticoagulant therapy in the presence of pulmonary infarction. J.A.M.A., 208:1830, 1969.
62. Spencer, H.: Pathology of the Lung, Excluding Pulmonary Tuberculosis. 2nd ed. Oxford, Pergamon Press, 1968.
63. Starkey, G. W. B., and Ullyot, D. J.: Pleural empyema—a grave surgical complication. Surg. Clin. N. Amer., 48:507, 1968.
64. Steel, S. J., and Winstanley, D. P.: Trephine biopsy of the lung and pleura. Thorax, 24:576, 1969.
65. Stewart, P. B.: The rate of formation and lymphatic removal of fluid in pleural effusions. J. Clin. Invest., 42:258, 1963.
66. Stiles, Q. R., Lindesmith, G. G., Tucker, B. L., Meyer, B. W., and Jones, J. C.: Pleural empyema in children. Ann. Thorac. Surg., 10:37, 1970.
67. Storey, C. F.: Intrapleural suction: Is it being used to best advantage. (Editorial.) Ann. Thorac. Surg., 6:196, 1968.
68. Stout, A. P., and Himadi, G. M.: Solitary (localized) mesothelioma of the pleura. Ann. Surg., 133:50, 1951.
69. Takaro, T., and Bond, W. M.: Pleuropulmonary, pericardial, and cerebral complications of amebiasis—a 20-year survey. Int. Abstr. Surg. (Surg. Gynec. Obstet.), 107:209, 1958.
70. Takaro, T., Walkup, H. E., and Okano, T.: Esophagopleural fistula as a complication of thoracic surgery. J. Thorac. Cardiovasc. Surg., 40:179, 1960.
71. Thomas, P. A., and Gebauer, P. W.: Results and complications of pleurectomy for bullous emphysema and recurrent pneumothorax. J. Thorac. Cardiovasc. Surg., 39:194, 1960.
72. Trapnell, D. H., and Thurston, J. G. B.: Unilateral pulmonary edema after pleural aspiration. Lancet, 1:1367, 1970.
73. Urschel, H. C., Jr., and Paulson, D. L.: Mesotheliomas of the pleura. Ann. Thorac. Surg., 1:559, 1965.
74. Van de Water, J. M.: Treatment of pleural effusion complicating pneumonia. Chest, 57:259, 1970.
75. Vianna, N. J.: Nontuberculous bacterial empyema in patients with and without underlying disease. J.A.M.A., 215:69, 1971.
76. Wagner, J. C., and Berry, G.: Mesotheliomas in rats following inoculation with asbestos. Brit. J. Cancer, 23:567, 1969.
77. Williams, K. R., and Burford, T. H.: Management of chylothorax. Ann. Surg., 160:131, 1964.
78. Yeh, T. J., Hall, D. P., and Ellison, R. G.: Empyema thoracis: a review of 110 cases. Amer. Rev. Resp. Dis., 88:785, 1963.
79. Youmans, C. R., Jr., Williams, R. D., McMinn, M. R., and Derrick, J. R.: Surgical management of spontaneous pneumothorax by bleb ligation and pleural dry sponge abrasion. Amer. J. Surg., 120:644, 1970.

# IX

# Bronchiectasis

*Gilbert S. Campbell, M.D.*

Bronchiectasis means dilatation of bronchi. René Laennec (1781–1826) was the first to give a clear description of this condition in 1819. However, the condition had first been observed by one of his pupils, Cayol, 11 years earlier.[11]

Debate still rages as to the etiology of bronchiectasis. In 1907, Carl Beck wrote, "Bronchiectasis is, as a rule, not a disease per se, but a consequence of various affections of the lungs or bronchi."[3]

Surgeons have been aggressive leaders in the crusade against bronchiectasis, and the development of pulmonary resection was stimulated by this disease. Resection of a lung lobe diseased with bronchiectasis was attempted periodically during the nineteenth century. Because of the high mortality and morbidity, lesser procedures were undertaken, such as cautery excision with diver-sion of the bronchial drainage to the outside through multiple fistulas. Surgical principles underlying one-stage lobectomy were proposed by Harold Brunn in 1929. He employed intrapleural suction drainage to remove fluid and air to augment expansion of the remaining lung lobes. Rudolph Nissen performed the first successful pneumonectomy in 1931 on a 12 year old girl with bronchiectasis. Two years later, Cameron Haight performed an identical procedure. Evarts Graham made a double advance in the third successful pneumonectomy in 1933, using a single-stage operation in a patient with bronchogenic carcinoma.[24]

Riggins stressed the morbidity in patients with advanced bronchiectasis and suppurative pneumonitis, "consisting of chronic invalidism, psychological changes varying from mild depressive states to psychopathic personalities, complete economic instability, a life alone, apart, helpless and hopeless."[27]

the respiratory tract as well as the pancreas produce a scanty, thick, and sticky secretion. Successful management of respiratory problems in these patients is extremely difficult.

## ETIOLOGY

Bronchial obstruction and infection beyond the bronchial obstruction are important precursors of bronchiectasis. The bronchial obstruction may result from a foreign body, plugs of tenacious mucopurulent material, tumors, and extrabronchial occlusion by lymph nodes. Mucopurulent material fills the bronchi beyond the obstruction, with subsequent infection of the bronchial wall and destruction of its muscle and elastic tissue. The diseased lung segments lose their normal cleansing power and are easy prey for further endogenous or exogenous infection. Bronchiectasis is a disease of the pulmonary parenchyma as well as of the bronchi. Pneumonitis with resultant pulmonary fibrosis may follow pertussis, measles, or other viral or bacterial infections. The theory that bronchiectasis is a result of scarring and contraction of lung tissue around bronchi was first proposed by Corrigan in 1838. He wrote, "If the fingers of the reader's hand, separated one from another, be supposed to represent a bunch of bronchial tubes, and at the intervals be supposed to be filled up with fibers undergoing a slow contraction, it is obvious that the first tendency of that contractile action will be to draw the sides of the fingers towards one another or if they were tubes to dilate them."[9]

Bronchiectasis may occur in association with situs inversus and sinusitis (Kartagener's syndrome), cystic fibrosis of the pancreas (mucoviscidosis), and agammaglobulinemia. True congenital bronchiectasis is rare. There was not a single case thought to be due to congenital malformation in a recent review of 100 cases of bronchiectasis in Alaskan native children.[17] Churchill reported that bronchiectasis in the Kartagener complex had the characteristics of acquired bronchiectasis and cited two patients with only two features of the triad (dextrocardia and absence of accessory nasal sinuses). Churchill described the moist bronchial secretion of these two patients, who were carefully treated with chemotherapy when respiratory infection occurred, in the hope that this treatment might prevent the development of bronchiectasis, which is probably acquired secondarily in Kartagener's syndrome and is not truly a congenital lung condition.[7] Culiner has suggested that congenital cystic bronchiectasis, intralobar bronchial cystic disease, and the "sequestration complex" are variants of a single primary complex of bronchovascular anomalies in otherwise normal lung parenchyma.[10] The incidence of "congenital" bronchiectasis has dropped sharply since antibiotics have become available to control acute pulmonary infections in the neonate. However, bronchiectasis is still a prominent feature of mucoviscidosis; the mucus-secreting glands of

## PATHOPHYSIOLOGY

As the bronchi enter the lung, they normally become smaller as they taper and divide, and the bronchial walls become correspondingly thinner. Normal bronchi telescope during the respiratory cycle—lengthening and widening during inspiration, shortening and contracting during expiration. There is a normal peristaltic muscular contractility that tends to keep the bronchial tubes clean by moving any intrabronchial material centrally where it can be coughed free from the respiratory tract. William Boyd has said the cough is the watchdog of the respiratory tract. Bronchiectasis damages or destroys these normal defense mechanisms.

Bronchiectasis may be classified anatomically as (1) cylindrical, (2) varicose, and (3) saccular.[26] Reid selected for study 45 cases of lobectomy with well preserved operative specimens and technically clear preoperative bronchograms. He counted the number of bronchial subdivisions in a single bronchopulmonary segment by examining the bronchograms, operative specimens, and microscopic serial sections. With cylindrical or tubular bronchiectasis, the bronchi do not taper in their normal way but usually end squarely and abruptly. Study of the operative specimens revealed a normal number of bronchial subdivisions, many of which did not fill on bronchography because they were filled with mucopurulent secretion. With saccular bronchiectasis, the dilated bronchi are usually subpleural, and for this reason "cystic" bronchiectasis has generally been considered to involve the terminal bronchioles. However, by counting the number of generations of the bronchial tree between the hilum and the cyst, Reid redemonstrated that saccular bronchiectasis usually involves proximal divisions of the segmental bronchi (Fig. 1).

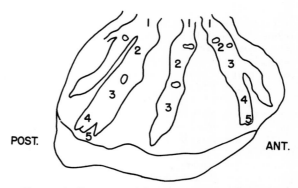

**Figure 1**  Diagram of lung segment with saccular bronchiectasis, showing involvement of proximal divisions of segmental bronchi. (From Reid, L. M.: Thorax, 5:233, 1950.)

Bronchi involved with bronchiectasis undergo destruction of elastic tissue and muscular coats of the bronchial walls, with replacement by fibrous tissue. Small branch bronchi may become fibrosed and cordlike. The ciliated columnar epithelial lining may show inflammatory change plus squamous metaplasia. Mucous gland hyperplasia and excess mucus production with stagnation occur and because of the impaired cleansing function of the lung, bacteria that lodge at these sites are not properly cleared.

Liebow and his associates have demonstrated extreme enlargement of the bronchial arteries and numerous anastomoses of these vessels with the pulmonary arteries in lung segments diseased by bronchiectasis.[22] Because of these rich bronchopulmonary anastomoses, bright red blood under systemic pressure may pour into the respiratory tree, with serious or even fatal consequences. In addition to being a troublesome source of hemoptysis, the expanded bronchial arterial supply to the diseased lung may impose an added circulatory burden on the heart, contributing to pulmonary hypertension and ultimately to the development of cor pulmonale. From the standpoint of respiratory gas exchange, the bronchial-pulmonary artery anastomoses may be beneficial, minimizing the ventilation-perfusion imbalance that would result from continued perfusion of the unventilated lung segments by pulmonary arterial blood. Advanced saccular bronchiectasis of the entire left lung may result in absence of uptake on a pulmonary scan (Fig. 2) and nonfilling of the left pulmonary artery on a pulmonary angiogram.[20] Dye injected into the descending aorta of such a patient showed marked tortuosity of the bronchial vessels and retrograde filling of the left pulmonary artery.[1, 20]

Bronchiectasis is usually located in the basal segments of the lower lobes and is associated with involvement of the corresponding middle lobe. Ordinarily the superior segments of the lower lobes are free of disease. The lingula is diseased in 60 to 80 per cent of patients with bronchiectasis of the left basilar segments.[8] Similarly, from 45 to 60 per cent of patients with bronchiectasis of the right basilar segments will have involvement of the right middle lobe. There is approximately a 40 per cent incidence of bilateral bronchiectasis. Involvement of the upper lobes is rare but may follow scarring of old tuberculosis; the disease here is a dry type of bronchiectasis.

Blades and Dugan documented that atypical pneumonia may produce temporary dilatations of the bronchi, and repeat bronchography a few weeks later shows complete return to normal of the bronchograms. This reversible type of bronchiectasis they termed pseudobronchiectasis.[4]

Lung function tests in patients with bronchiectasis show a reduced vital capacity and forced expiratory volume at 1 second.[6] Other authors have reported reduced ventilation, depressed ventilation-perfusion ratios, and decreased perfusion in lung regions involved by bronchiectasis. They suggested that radioactive xenon studies may be helpful for patients with bilateral disease and abnormal overall lung function in whom care must be taken to preserve a maximal amount of functional tissue.[2] Uneven ventilation and air trapping may occur in bronchiectasis. Pulmonary artery perfusion of poorly ventilated segments may result in decreased peripheral arterial oxygen saturation. Macklem et al. have stressed the obstruction in the small airways in patients with bronchiectasis; the contribution of disease in small airways to hypoxia and subsequent pulmonary hypertension is real.[23]

## DIAGNOSIS AND TREATMENT

Characteristically, bronchiectasis is a disease of young people—in 41 to 42 per cent onset occurs in the first decade, and in 64 to 69 per cent, before age 20.[25, 27] Since the bronchi of children are quite small, obstructive bronchitis develops readily during respiratory infections in infants and children. Some authors believe that the collateral air circulation through the pores of Kohn is not well developed in the youngster. Most cases of bronchiectasis were diagnosed as chronic bronchitis until 1922, when bronchography was introduced by Sicard and Forestier.[29] The left lung is more frequently involved in bronchiectasis than the right because (1) the right bronchus is really a continuation of the trachea and is more easily drained, (2) the left bronchus is somewhat constricted where the left pulmonary artery crosses it, and (3) the left bronchus is narrower and more easily compressed by the pulmonary artery in children.

A chronic, productive cough that persists in infants and children after an episode of measles, pertussis, or influenza may be due to secondary bronchiectasis. Septic pneumonitis and secondary

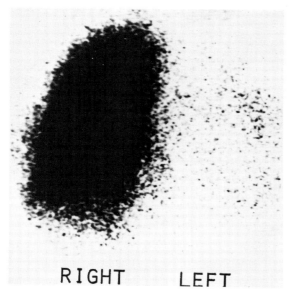

**Figure 2**  Lung scan from 9 year old boy with advanced saccular bronchiectasis of left lung.

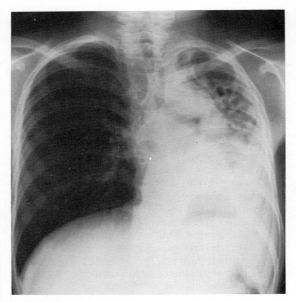

**Figure 3**    Chest film from same patient as in Figure 2.

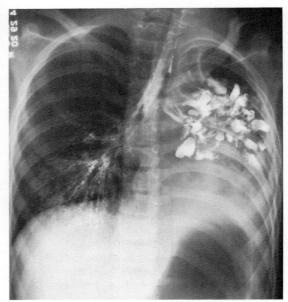

**Figure 4**    Preoperative bronchogram with nonfilling of left lower lobe because of impacted foreign body.

bronchiectasis may follow aspiration of foreign bodies into the bronchial tree. Cough with purulent expectoration, hemoptysis, and recurrent localized pneumonitis are important clinical manifestations of bronchiectasis. Auscultation over involved areas reveals depressed breath sounds and coarse rales. Digital clubbing is found in 25 per cent of patients.[21]

With cylindrical or tubular bronchiectasis, the x-ray film of the chest may be amazingly normal, but with saccular bronchiectasis, the diagnosis can sometimes be made on a plain chest film (Fig. 3).

Bronchoscopy is helpful in the diagnosis of bronchiectasis, enabling one to rule out foreign body, tumor, or stenosis. One can observe which bronchi are discharging pus and obtain uncontaminated material for culture.

Bronchography is the best means of demonstrating bronchiectasis. When bronchography is done for preoperative evaluation, every segment of both lungs must be visualized. Preliminary postural drainage is important prior to bronchography. The presence of thick sputum not only interferes with adherence of thick viscous iodized oil to the walls of bronchi, but is often the cause of severe coughing during the bronchographic examination, giving a faulty bronchogram.

In patients with septic bronchiectasis, appropriate sputum studies and sensitivity tests lead one to the optimal antimicrobial agent. In addition to antimicrobial drugs for septic exacerbation of bronchiectasis, other forms of medical treatment are postural drainage, expectorants, cessation of smoking, and treatment of any upper respiratory problem (such as sinusitis if this exists). Local complications of bronchiectasis are: recurrent pneumonia, lung abscess, empyema, and pyopneu-

mothorax. Other complications are cor pulmonale, brain abscess, and amyloid disease (rarely).

Field has made extensive follow-up studies on bronchiectasis in children.[12-16] She found that there was a trend for definite improvement in the second decade, which was maintained into the third and fourth decade. There was a sharp fall

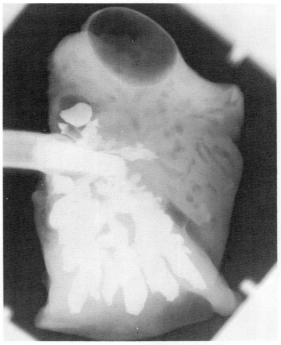

**Figure 5**    Selective bronchogram of left lower lobe of resected lung, showing extreme saccular bronchiectasis.

in incidence of cases of bronchiectasis between 1950 and 1960, at the time broad-spectrum antibiotics were introduced. Field recommended surgery for severe localized disease but suggested that diffuse bronchiectasis is best treated medically with postural drainage and antibiotics for exacerbations. With bilateral disease, the more involved lung should be operated upon first. Occasionally the relief of symptoms is so gratifying after an operation on one side that the remaining disease does not require resection.

Sealy, Bradham, and Young reported surgical treatment of multisegmental and localized bronchiectasis.[28] They performed pulmonary resections on 70 patients with localized disease, which they defined as bronchiectasis confined to a site distal to the bronchus of one lung, one lobe, or one segment. There were also 70 patients with generalized disease. Repeated respiratory infections were commoner in the multisegmental group. Eighty per cent of patients with localized bronchiectasis were relieved of all respiratory symptoms following surgery, whereas 36 per cent of patients with multisegmental disease were symptom-free after surgery. The right middle lobe was involved 22 times (16 per cent). During this same period, 41 patients with middle lobe syndrome[5] were operated upon, and 19 of these patients did not have true bronchiectasis.

Patients with multisegmental bronchiectasis have a tendency toward panrespiratory infections accentuated by prolonged periods of bronchial infections, suggesting an allergic background or lowered resistance or both. The disorder tends to develop in early life, and then for an unknown reason remains stabilized once the second decade is reached. Sealy et al. were impressed by the small percentage of asthmatics in the multisegmental group. In contrast to the findings of Ginsberg et al.[18] of recurrent or new bronchiectasis, there was only one patient in the Duke series in whom new disease developed postoperatively.

Modern surgical approach to bronchiectasis is based upon the principle of conservation of pulmonary tissue. Results of surgery are far better with localized than with multisegmental disease. Patients with diffuse bronchiectasis are not good candidates for surgical treatment as a general rule.

Surgical treatment of patients with localized bronchiectasis yields excellent results with a very low morbidity and mortality. Procrastination and prolongation of nonoperative therapy in this group of patients seem imprudent. Conversely, multiple pulmonary resections in patients with diffuse bronchiectasis seem impetuous.

## REFERENCES

1. Alley, R. D., Stranahan, A., Kausel, H., Formel, P., and Van Mierop, L. H. S.: Demonstration of bronchial-pulmonary artery reverse flow in suppurative pulmonary disease. Clin. Res., 6:41, 1958.
2. Bass, H., Henderson, J. A. M., Heckscher, T., Oriol, A., and Anthonisen, N. R.: Regional structure and function in bronchiectasis. A correlative study using bronchography and $^{133}$Xe. Amer. Rev. Resp. Dis., 97:598, 1968.
3. Beck, C.: Surgical Diseases of the Chest. Philadelphia, Blakiston, 1907, p. 213.
4. Blades, B., and Dugan, D. J.: Pseudobronchiectasis. J. Thorac. Surg., 13:40, 1944.
5. Brock, R. C.: Post-tuberculous broncho-stenosis and bronchiectasis of middle lobe. Thorax, 5:5, 1950.
6. Cherniack, N. S., and Carton, R. W.: Factors associated with respiratory insufficiency in bronchiectasis. Amer. J. Med., 41:562, 1966.
7. Churchill, E. D.: The segmental and lobular physiology and pathology of the lung. J. Thorac. Surg., 18:279, 1949.
8. Churchill, E. D., and Belsey, R.: Segmental pneumonectomy in bronchiectasis; the lingula segment of the left upper lobe. Ann. Surg., 109:481, 1939.
9. Corrigan, D. J.: On cirrhosis of the lung. Dublin J. Med. Sci., 13:266, 1838.
10. Culiner, M. M.: Intralobar bronchial cystic disease, the "sequestration complex" and cystic bronchiectasis. Dis. Chest, 53:462, 1968.
11. Duken, J., and Von den Steinen, R.: Das Krankheitsbild der Bronchiektasie im Kindesalter. Ergebn. Inn. Med. Kinderheilk., 34:457, 1928.
12. Field, C. E.: Bronchiectasis in childhood: clinical survey of 160 cases. Pediatrics, 4:21, 1949.
13. Field, C. E.: Bronchiectasis in childhood; etiology and pathogenesis, including survey of 272 cases of doubtful irreversible bronchiectasis. Pediatrics, 4:231, 1949.
14. Field, C. E.: Bronchiectasis in childhood; prophylaxis, treatment and progress with follow-up study of 202 cases of established bronchiectasis. Pediatrics, 4:355, 1949.
15. Field, C. E.: Bronchiectasis. A long-term follow-up of medical and surgical cases from childhood. Arch. Dis. Child., 36:587, 1961.
16. Field, C. E.: Bronchiectasis. Third report on a follow-up study of medical and surgical cases from childhood. Arch. Dis. Child., 44:551, 1969.
17. Fleshman, J. K., Wilson, J. F., and Cohen, J. J.: Bronchiectasis in Alaska native children. Arch. Environ. Health, 17:517, 1968.
18. Ginsberg, R. L., Cooley, J. C., Olsen, A. M., and Kirklin, J. W.: An analysis of unfavorable results in the surgical treatment of bronchiectasis. J. Thorac. Surg., 30:331, 1955.
19. Graham, E. A., Singer, J. J., and Ballon, H. C.: Surgical Diseases of the Chest. Philadelphia, Lea & Febiger, 1935, pp. 575–703.
20. Hutchin, P., Terzi, R. G., and Peters, R. M.: Bronchial-pulmonary artery reverse flow. Angiographic demonstration in bronchiectasis. Ann. Thorac. Surg., 4:391, 1967.
21. Laurenzi, G. A.: A critical reappraisal of bronchiectasis. Med. Times, 98:89, 1970.
22. Liebow, A. A., Hales, M. R., and Lindskog, G. E.: Enlargement of the bronchial arteries, and their anastomoses with the pulmonary arteries in bronchiectasis. Amer. J. Path., 25:211, 1949.
23. Macklem, P. T., Thurlbeck, W. M., and Fraser, R. G.: Chronic obstructive disease of small airways. Ann. Intern. Med., 74:167, 1971.
24. Nissen, R., and Wilson, R. H. L.: Pages in the History of Chest Surgery. Springfield, Ill., Charles C Thomas, 1960, pp. 35–45.
25. Perry, K. M. A., and King, D. S.: Bronchiectasis; a study of prognosis based on a follow-up of 400 patients. Amer. Rev. Tuberc., 41:531, 1940.
26. Reid, L. M.: Reduction in bronchial subdivision in bronchiectasis. Thorax, 5:233, 1950.
27. Riggins, H. M.: Bronchiectasis; morbidity and mortality of medically treated patients. Amer. J. Surg., 54:50, 1941.
28. Sealy, W. C., Bradham, R. R., and Young, W. G., Jr.: The surgical treatment of multisegmental and localized bronchiectasis. Surg. Gynec. Obstet., 123:80, 1966.
29. Sicard, J. A., and Forestier, J.: Méthode générale d'exploration radiologique par l'huile iodée. Bull. Soc. Med. Hop. Paris, 46:463, 1922.

# X

# The Surgical Treatment of Pulmonary Tuberculosis

*W. Glenn Young, Jr., M.D., and Gordon F. Moor, M.D.*

A study of the evolution of the surgical treatment of pulmonary tuberculosis is fundamental to an understanding of the entire field of current surgery of the chest. Just as the journals of the past 15 or 20 years picture the burgeoning field of cardiac surgery, the journals of the preceding 100 years or so are filled with the efforts, trials, frustrations, and successes of pioneer thoracic surgeons attempting to cope with suppurative disease of the chest, particularly tuberculosis.

Although the number of patients operated upon for tuberculosis has rapidly declined in the past few years, there are approximately 50,000 new cases of active tuberculosis being reported annually and, in addition, 6000 to 8000 patients who suffer clinical relapses each year. The number of patients presented for operation remains relatively constant, and is estimated to be from 5 to 15 per cent of those admitted. Thus, the topic remains pertinent and the need exists for surgeons to understand thoroughly the vagaries of the disease and the pitfalls in its treatment.

## HISTORICAL ASPECTS

The ancient Greeks recognized tuberculosis as a wasting disease and named it *phthisis,* meaning a wasting of the body, for its most conspicuous symptom. Hippocrates (470–376 B.C.) wrote the first elaborate description of the clinical disease, and apparently recognized an acute and chronic form. Hindu references to the disease were translated into Latin as consumption, from the consuming nature of the illness. The term tuberculosis was used in 1839 by Schönlein as a descriptive term for the nodule or tuber found in the lungs of patients so afflicted.

Pulmonary tuberculosis reached epidemic proportions in Europe in the eighteenth and nineteenth centuries, and one-seventh of all deaths in London at the time were believed to be due to consumption. Tuberculosis was long considered to be of many varieties and origins; the unity of the disease was first recognized by Laennec (1826). The correctness of his conceptions was disputed until 1882, when Koch isolated the specific organism and reproduced the disease experimentally.

## BACTERIOLOGY

Koch, in discovering the tubercle bacillus, not only identified the organism causing a disease that is still the number one infectious killer today, but also established the criteria that must be fulfilled before a particular microorganism can be accepted as the cause of a specific disease. Koch (1) found the bacillus associated constantly with the clinical disease, (2) collected it in pure culture, (3) reproduced the disease in guinea pigs and rabbits with the culture, and (4) recovered the bacillus in pure culture from the experimentally infected animals. These requirements, known as *Koch's postulates,* were introduced at a time when the infectious nature of many diseases was being recognized, and thereafter became the standard for bacteriologic research.

The avian type of bacillus was isolated in 1890 by Mafucci, and the bovine type in 1898 by Theobald Smith. The vast majority of human clinical disease is caused by the human strain (*Mycobacterium tuberculosis*).

### Skin Tests

Koch, in a search for a cure for tuberculosis, turned his attention to the investigation of injection of heat-killed or chemically destroyed tubercle bacilli subcutaneously. He found that in patients with the disease this resulted in a violent systemic reaction with a high fever. The point of injection became painful and red and occasionally sloughed. Although the injection of this *old tuberculin* did not prove valuable in treatment, it did lead to a useful diagnostic skin test. Seibert and Long[14] isolated the protein fraction from the bacillus in 1937 and called it PPD (purified protein derivative). This test reagent is used most commonly in this country now.

Patients become sensitized to the protein fraction from the tubercle bacillus 2 to 4 weeks after infection with the organism. This is a delayed hypersensitivity reaction and is manifested by an area of induration 48 to 72 hours after the intradermal injection of tuberculin. Patients critically ill with tuberculosis or other disease, and especially patients with tuberculous effusions of the pleura, pericardium, meninges, or peritoneum, may fail to react to tuberculin or may react only to the stronger doses. Steroids will also decrease reactivity to the test substance.

### Smear and Culture

The diagnosis of active pulmonary tuberculosis is made by identifying the tubercle bacillus in the sputum smear and is confirmed by isolating the organism in culture from sputum or gastric aspirate. A sputum specimen, preferably obtained as a fresh, early morning sample or from bronchial aspirate, is stained by the Ziehl-Neelsen method, which will identify the bacilli as brilliant red rods against a deep sky-blue background. It is sometimes necessary to examine multiple samples before a positive smear can be obtained. The human and bovine strains grow slowly, producing after 10 to 20 days small, dry, scaly colonies with corrugated surfaces. The niacin test for the human strain is based upon the findings that this bacillus is the only mycobacterium that can synthesize excess nicotinic acid.

### Atypical Acid-Fast Bacilli

Atypical acid-fast bacilli are often resistant to the standard chemotherapeutic agents. Since patients infected with these organisms present a particular problem in therapy, they are often seen by the surgeon early in the course of the disease. Since 1950 there has been a rapid increase in the number of reported cases of human disease caused by the atypical mycobacteria. Before then, there were only infrequent reports in which sufficient evidence was presented to justify implication of the atypical acid-fast bacilli as the probable cause of disease. Since these organisms, unlike *M. tuberculosis* and *M. bovis* often did not cause disease in guinea pigs, they were considered to be saprophytes and nonvirulent. Rather than there being a true increase in the incidence of atypical disease, it may be that we are today isolating and identifying the organisms more frequently.[6]

The various strains of mycobacteria differ from one another and are classified by differences in microscopic and cultural morphology, rate of growth, thermic requirements, ability to produce pigment, susceptibility to drugs, biologic activity in animal tissues, and ability to react to certain chemical and biologic tests. A wide variety of terms have been applied to the groups of acid-fast organisms that do not conform to characteristics of the classic species of *M. tuberculosis*. Runyon's classification is widely used[13] (Table 1).

It would appear from careful differential skin testing that the atypical organisms may actually

be more prevalent than the human strain.[15] While thus apparently being relatively nonvirulent, they do occasionally produce human pulmonary disease, which is characteristically slowly progressive, indolent, and difficult to treat with the standard chemotherapeutic agents.

## PATHOLOGY

The basic lesion in pulmonary tuberculosis follows inhalation of the tubercle bacilli and consists of a necrotizing reaction in the pneumonic process in the midlung fields and may proceed to resolution, organization and fibrosis, or caseous necrosis. The bacilli drain into the lymphatics and lodge in the hilar nodes to cause necrosis there or, in a small number of cases, may proceed to produce widespread systemic disease. The lesion in the periphery of the lung combined with hilar node involvement is called the "primary Ghon complex." This primary complex heals completely except in a few instances in which there is rapid pathologic progression. This progression may take the form of miliary tuberculosis by way of massive bloodstream infection and is often seen in early childhood, usually in the first 2 years of life.

Microscopically, the parenchymal lesion consists of a small central area of necrosis containing tubercle bacilli surrounded by a layer of epithelioid cells derived from mononuclear phagocytes. In this layer are also seen the characteristic multinuclear giant cells of the Langhans type.

Reinfection tuberculosis is almost exclusively a disease of the lungs. Chronic pulmonary tuberculosis may be the result of reactivation of an old focus in the lungs (endogenous) or may occur from reinfection (exogenous).[11, 16] It develops as a pneumonia in a segment or lobe and is usually located in the apical or posterior segment of the upper lobes or the superior segment of the lower lobes. Caseation necrosis may occur and result in liquefaction of pulmonary tissue. A cavity is formed if the necrotic process, which is surrounded by a fibrinous perifocal reaction, has involved an adjacent bronchus; this results in drainage and expectoration of the liquefied contents, which contain viable tuberculous organisms. The untreated disease process may then spread to other lobes, the contralateral lung, bronchi, the larynx, or the gastrointestinal tract.

Bronchiectatic changes occasionally accompany the destructive process of pulmonary tuberculosis, particularly in the area distal to a stenotic bronchus. This may be caused by a secondary nontuberculous infection or may occur in combination with true bronchiectasis. Caseous material may rupture into the pleural space, particularly if the lesion is near the pleural surface and has not drained into a bronchus; this results in a tuberculous or mixed tuberculous and bacterial empyema. A tuberculous pleural effusion may also be hematogenous in origin. Because of the intense perifocal reaction of pulmonary tuberculosis, fibrinous pleural adhesions frequently form between the visceral and parietal pleura and may obliterate

**TABLE 1**   CLASSIFICATION OF ATYPICAL MYCOBACTERIA (RUNYON)

| Group I | Photochromogens (*M. Kansasii*) (common in Southwest and upper Midwest) |
|---|---|
| Group II | Scotochromogens (frequent cause of cervical adenitis) |
| Group III | Nonphotochromogens (Battey-avian complex) (common in Southwest) |
| Group IV | Rapid growers (including *M. fortuitum*) |

the pleural space in an area adjacent to the disease process. The late stage of the disease is characterized by contraction of the lobe or lobes involved by fibrosis, with or without concomitant cavitation.

Endobronchial tuberculosis occurs as a result of infection of the bronchial mucosa by bacteria carried by liquefied necrotic material being discharged from the parenchymal lesion. The mucosa is thickened and congested and is occasionally ulcerated. Ulcerative endobronchial lesions may result in scarring and stenosis of the bronchus.

## COLLAPSE THERAPY

Prior to the advent of specific chemotherapy, the most successful type of surgery directed toward pulmonary tuberculosis evolved from the idea of putting the affected part at rest, allowing the lung to "relax or collapse." Open drainage of cavitary lesions by marsupialization or tube drainage (*cavernostomy*) was employed occasionally with success, but most such direct surgical approaches were followed by unacceptable complications.

### Artificial Pneumothorax

Hippocrates, using a pig's bladder and tube, introduced air into the pleural cavity to relieve the pain of pleurisy. The procedure received widespread popularity after the reporting of successful case series by Forlanini (1882, 1894) and John B. Murphy (1898).

Pneumothorax was employed in countless patients during the first 40 years of this century but often was unsuccessful in producing the desired collapse because of adhesions between the lung and chest wall, or was forcibly terminated by the appearance of pleural fluid not uncommonly infected by the acid-fast bacillus.

### Extrapleural Paravertebral Thoracoplasty

The direct surgical measures to relax or compress the tuberculous lung were introduced by master surgeons of continental Europe around the turn of the century. Their fascinating story was brought to this country by classic writings of John Alexander[1, 2] and is only briefly summarized here.

Estlander first used the term *thoracoplasty* in 1879 to denote removal of ribs so as to bring the chest wall down to the lung that would not expand after drainage of empyema. De Cerenville in 1885 first applied this operation to collapse the cavity in a tuberculous lung. An internist, Ludolph Brauer, emphasized that the thoracoplasty must collapse the diseased lung in order to be as effective as pneumothorax. Friedrich, following Brauer's suggestions, performed an operation in 1907 in which he resected all of the second through the ninth ribs. He resected the periosteum, intercostal muscle, and even the nerves as well as the ribs, and four out of his first seven patients survived. Brauer then suggested that subperiosteal resection of the ribs be carried out so that they might regenerate and stabilize the chest wall. Gourdet, Wilms, Sauerbruch, and others modified the very

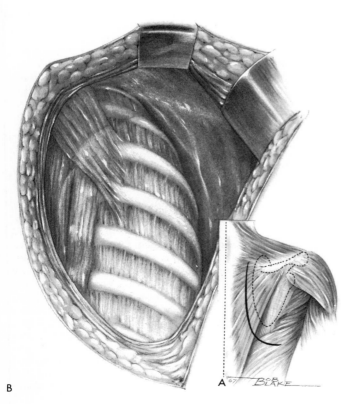

**Figure 1**  Technique of first-stage, standard thoracoplasty, showing incision (*A*) and exposure (*B*) following mobilization and retraction of scapula. (From Young, W. G., Jr., and Moor, G. F. In: Gibbon, J. H., Jr., et al.: Surgery of the Chest. 2nd ed. Philadelphia, W. B. Saunders Company, 1969.)

B

radical operation of Brauer and Friedrich. In addition to bringing the operation to this country, Alexander refined the "modern" operation of thoracoplasty. He carefully separated the procedure into stages and recognized the value of resection of the transverse processes in increasing the amount of collapse obtained. Alexander and Haight reported the results of paravertebral thoracoplasty from 1932 to 1934 in 119 patients. The mortality was 11 per cent, with cavity closure in 93 per cent of the survivors. In 1957, Strieder was able to report an operative mortality of 2 per cent in 99 consecutive cases.

The most important variation of the classic thoracoplasty is the so-called *plombage thoracoplasty*, a descendant of the old operation of extrapleural pneumonolysis which was introduced by Tuffier in 1891. In this version of the procedure, an extraperiosteal pocket is developed by denuding the ribs overlying the disease area to be collapsed and filling this pocket with a "plomb" such as polyethylene spheres enclosed in a polyethylene bag.

**Indications for Thoracoplasty.** During the past 10 to 15 years, the standard and plombage thoracoplasties have become rarely employed operations in the surgical clinics of the country. By far the majority of patients requiring surgery are successfully treated by resection. Thoracoplasty may still be justifiably considered in certain "salvage cases" in which extensive disease, highly productive of drug-resistant organisms, makes primary resection hazardous. It may also still be indicated in elderly patients as a compromise procedure.

Modified or "tailoring" thoracoplasty is used as a secondary procedure following resection when the primary operation is complicated by an infected residual space or bronchopleural fistula. In these cases, obliteration of the space can usually be accomplished in a single-stage operation without removal of the first rib or the transverse processes.

The general plan of the operation of thoracoplasty is to remove a sufficient portion of the bony chest wall to collapse the cavity-bearing portion of the lung. For the common upper lobe cavity, this usually involves removal of portions of the ribs down to the seventh or eighth (Fig. 1).

## CHEMOTHERAPY

Specific chemotherapeutic agents have been introduced in the treatment of pulmonary tuberculosis during the past 25 years and have had a profound effect on the course of the disease. Case fatality and overall mortality rates have dropped faster than new case rates. The length of hospital stay for patients has been significantly shortened, and, most important for the surgeon, the drugs have allowed resectional therapy to be accomplished with an acceptable morbidity and mortality.

The plan for initial treatment is a program of chemotherapy that is so effective that bacteriosta-

sis and conversion of sputum bacteriologic findings are achieved within 3 to 6 months, and the emergence of significant bacterial drug resistance is prevented. The treatment of patients with disease caused by drug-resistant bacilli frequently presents difficult problems. Drug sensitivity testing is helpful in selecting the most effective combination of chemotherapeutic agents.

Streptomycin (SM), isoniazid (INH), and para-aminosalicylic acid (PAS) are the major drugs used in treatment of pulmonary tuberculosis. The standard initial chemotherapy consists of a combination of INH-SM, INH-PAS, or INH-PAS-SM (triple therapy). Isoniazid is almost always included in any combination and SM-PAS is no longer recommended.

Organism resistance is a serious problem and may occur early if one drug is used alone. Drug-resistant bacteria are probably present in small numbers in all infections and multiply to become the predominant organism. The objective in chemotherapy is to allow healing to occur before the drug-resistant bacteria multiply to numbers sufficient to continue the disease process. When streptomycin became available in 1944, it was found that this drug halted the progress of the disease and brought about temporary improvement of the patient's condition; this state lasted 3 to 4 months, only to be followed by progression of the disease and recurrence of organisms in the sputum. With the beginning of use of para-aminosalicylic acid in combination with streptomycin in 1946, this situation was markedly changed. Isoniazid, the third and probably most valuable of the major drugs, became available in 1952. Since then many other drugs, such as viomycin, cycloserine, pyrazinamide, ethionamide, kanamycin, and others, have been found to be moderately effective. These agents are usually held in reserve because they are more toxic, more expensive, and less effective than the basic drugs. They are particularly useful when given as an *added drug* to increase antimicrobial coverage for resectional therapy. Their primary role is in the retreatment group of patients whose organisms are resistant to some or all of three major drugs.

### Isonicotinic Acid Hydrazide

Isoniazid is the most active antituberculous agent in a large family of synthetic pyridine-carboxylic acid compounds and was first synthesized in 1912. Its antituberculous activity was not recognized until 1951. The ease of administration and high efficacy were immediately demonstrated in man, but it soon became evident that the administration of isoniazid alone favored the development of bacterial resistance, just as in the case of streptomycin. In uncomplicated pulmonary tuberculosis, the average adult dose is 5 mg. per kilogram of body weight, and is usually given as 100 mg. orally three times a day. Children receive 10 to 15 mg. per kilogram of body weight for far advanced disease. The dosage may be increased to 10 to 20 mg. per kilogram in all age groups.

In the high dosage ranges, pyridoxine is added in doses of at least 10 mg. for each 100 mg. of INH. Rarely, allergic manifestations or toxicity prevents its use. Toxic reactions are usually related to the nervous system. Peripheral neuritis is the most common side effect and can be prevented or treated with pyridoxine.

### Para-aminosalicylic Acid

In 1941, Bernheim found that the sodium salts of benzoic and salicylic acid specifically stimulated the oxygen uptake of *Mycobacterium tuberculosis.* J. Lehman first used PAS clinically and announced his results in 1946. Para-aminosalicylic acid is a weakly tuberculostatic agent when used alone, but is very useful in delaying the emergence of resistant organisms when used in combination with other drugs, especially INH and SM. When it is used as a single drug, resistance usually develops in approximately 120 days. The chief disadvantage in the use of PAS is the frequency of side reactions. Such reactions are usually confined to the gastrointestinal tract, and include anorexia, nausea, vomiting, and diarrhea.

### Streptomycin

Streptomycin was discovered by Waksman and his colleagues in 1944, and was the first chemotherapeutic agent found to be effective against *M. tuberculosis.* It was soon found that streptomycin damaged the auditory portion of the eighth cranial nerve. When it was realized that smaller doses of streptomycin were effective, and when PAS became available 2 years later, effective chemotherapy was possible with less toxicity. The dosage of streptomycin varies, depending upon the combinations of drugs selected. When it is used as one of the primary drugs, 1.0 gm. (20 mg. per kilogram) per day is usually given initially, and later the dose is decreased to 1.0 gm. twice weekly.

The following drugs are second-choice agents and are used when patients do not tolerate the major drugs, when the organisms are resistant to the major drugs, or for added coverage for resection. As previously noted, these drugs are generally more toxic and less effective than the major drugs.

*Cycloserine* is an antibiotic and is a fairly effective "second-line" drug used in various combinations, probably best with INH. Its primary use is in retreatment chemotherapy. The commonly accepted dosage is 0.5 gm. (10 mg. per kilogram) per day, usually given in two divided doses. Up to 20 mg. per kilogram may be given if concomitant diphenylhydantoin (Dilantin) and phenobarbital sedation is administered. In doses over 20 mg. per kilogram per day, cycloserine is toxic for the central nervous system and may cause convulsions, psychoses, dizziness, personality changes, or somnolence.

*Pyrazinamide* (PZA) is structurally very similar to isoniazid and may be administered orally. This drug is very effective, especially for short-term use, and is particularly suited for additional coverage for resection. Resistance develops rapidly when this drug is used alone. The recommended dosage is 3 gm. per day (40 to 50 mg. per kilogram), given orally in three divided doses. In approximately 15 per cent of the patients receiving an oral dose of 3.0 gm. per day, liver toxicity will develop, with anorexia, nausea, malaise, liver tenderness with hepatomegaly, and abnormal liver function. Two to three per cent of patients may become jaundiced. Usually these toxic manifestations will subside after the dose is decreased or administration of the drug is stopped.

*Ethionamide* is a good "second-line" drug for combined therapy. High concentrations of this drug are bactericidal in vitro. Some of the photochromogenic bacteria, as well as *M. tuberculosis,* are fairly sensitive to this drug. The usual adult dose is 250 mg. given twice daily with meals, and may be gradually increased to 250 mg. three or four times a day with nourishment. The most frequent untoward reaction is that of gastrointestinal intolerance, which occurs in 50 per cent or more of patients.

*Ethambutal* is a promising antituberculous agent, which may be used in combination with any of the other drugs. The usual adult dose is 15 to 25 mg. per kilogram per day, most often given as a single oral dose. The toxic effects usually involve the optic nerve, but fortunately this is rare and the visual disturbances are usually reversible upon cessation of administration of the drug.

Other drugs used in difficult retreatment problems include viomycin, capreomycin, kanamycin, thiocarlide (Isoxyl), oxytetracycline, and antithiazane.

# RESECTION FOR PULMONARY TUBERCULOSIS

### Historical Aspects

Although the five patients operated upon by Block (1883), Kronlein (1884), and Ruggi (1885) died following attempted partial resection of the tuberculous lung, Tuffier successfully resected the apex of the right lung of a 25 year old man in 1891. He made an incision in the second interspace and separated the upper part of the lung in the extrapleural plane. He then passed a ligature around the lung and removed the involved area in the apex. His patient was alive 5 years later and was presented before the Surgical Conference in Paris. Subsequently, successful case reports were rare, and resection of tuberculous lung tissue was rightfully considered a dangerous mode of therapy.

Freedlander of Cleveland performed the first successful complete lobectomy for tuberculosis in 1934, and during the next several years enthusiasm was rekindled. The use of the individual ligation technique as proposed by Blades and Kent, Churchill, and others made pulmonary resection in general a safer procedure; however, in 1943 resections in tuberculous patients were still associated with a morbidity of 50 per cent or more and

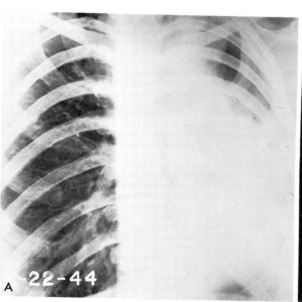
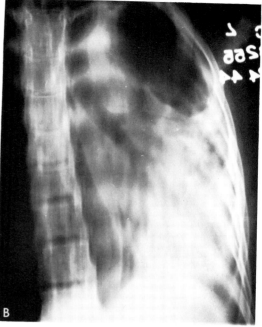

**Figure 2**  Plain x-ray and planigram illustrating destroyed left lung of a 33 year old female. Candidate for pneumonectomy. (From Young, W. G., Jr., and Moor, G. F. In: Gibbon, J. H., Jr., et al.: Surgery of the Chest. 2nd ed. Philadelphia, W. B. Saunders Company, 1969.)

a mortality in the range of 25 per cent.[8] It was not until after the discovery of streptomycin and PAS and particularly after the advent of isoniazid that selective resection of tuberculous lung tissue could be performed without the fear of catastrophic spread of the infection. Segmental resection, by which maximal preservation of functioning lung tissue could be accomplished, was introduced by Churchill and Belsey in 1939.[5] In 1953, Chamberlain and his associates[4] presented a series of 300 segmental resections for pulmonary tuberculosis. Ninety-three per cent of the patients were well, and the operative mortality was 3 per cent.

### Indications for Resection

The surgical approach to pulmonary tuberculosis is a valuable complement to medical therapy and when properly applied can result in a combined program that is nearly 100 per cent successful. The purpose of surgery is to remove or to assist in the healing or control of destructive residuals, which would otherwise contribute to failure of medical treatment or to reactivation of the disease process. Surgical assistance is required in a variable number of cases, depending upon selection, but the number may be as high as 20 per cent.[9] The indications for resection have become fairly well standardized:

1. An open cavity associated with positive sputum (so-called open positive) beyond 3 to 6 months after the initiation of chemotherapy. The need for surgery is increased if the organism is resistant to one or more of the major drugs.

2. Persistent positive sputum cultures after

adequate initial or retreatment programs in patients without demonstrable cavitation, but with pathologic residuals such as a destroyed lobe or lung (Fig. 2), localized bronchiectasis, bronchial stenosis with resultant atelectasis, or large residual nodular foci.

It is important that resection be performed in the first two groups before total bacterial resistance develops, and while an additional effective drug is available to increase antibacterial cover-

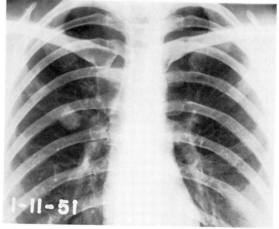

**Figure 3**  Solid lesion in superior segment, right lower lobe. Tuberculoma. (From Young, W. G., Jr., and Moor, G. F. In: Gibbon, J. H., Jr., et al.: Surgery of the Chest. 2nd ed. Philadelphia, W. B. Saunders Company, 1969.)

age for surgery. With increased coverage, fewer complications result.

3. Patients with negative sputum who have a residual destroyed segment, lobe, or lung; blocked cavities; tuberculomas; and significant fibrocaseous disease. In general, localized nodules larger than 2 cm. in diameter should be considered for resection (Figs. 3 and 4). Since antituberculous drugs may not penetrate dense fibrous tissue in sufficient concentration, sterilization of these lesions cannot be expected. In addition to the threat of reactivation of the tuberculous disease, the destroyed lobe may result in troublesome hemoptysis and bronchial obstruction with atelectasis and secondary infection.

4. The presence of localized infection with one of the atypical acid-fast organisms. This is an accepted indication for resection because of the organism's primary resistance to drugs and the tendency to progression or reactivation of the disease process. Therapy with INH-SM-PAS is given in spite of apparent resistance, and the decision for resection should be made early to take advan-

tage of the organism's temporary response to chemotherapy.

5. Tuberculous bronchiectasis most commonly occurs in the upper lobes, and because of free drainage afforded the affected areas in the upright position, resection is usually not required. Bronchiectasis of the middle and lower lobes, however, is quite apt to cause subsequent difficulty because of inadequate drainage, and resection of the involved segments is often indicated (Fig. 5).

6. Recent follow-up studies of patients with cavitary disease and negative sputum (so-called open negative) have shown that most of these patients do well with prolonged drug therapy. The trend in the treatment of these patients is toward the nonoperative approach. There are, however, a small number who will undergo reactivation with positive sputum and spread of their disease. Resection may be recommended in: (a) patients with thick-walled cavities; (b) patients who have responded slowly, as determined by sputum conversion and by lack of radiographic improvement; (c) patients who are likely to be unreliable in tak-

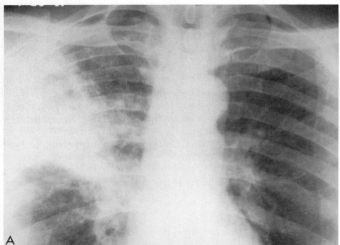

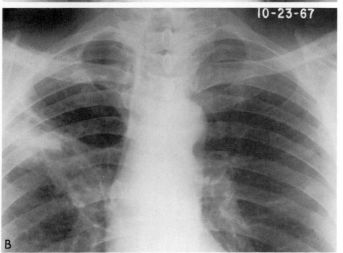

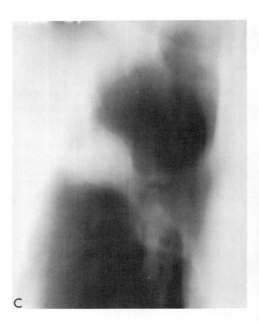

**Figure 4** Forty-nine year old male laborer with conversion of sputum after 3 months of chemotherapy but significant residual fibrocaseous disease at 6 months. Segmental resection performed. (From Young, W. G., Jr., and Moor, G. F. In: Gibbon, J. H., Jr., et al.: Surgery of the Chest. 2nd ed. Philadelphia, W. B. Saunders Company, 1969.)

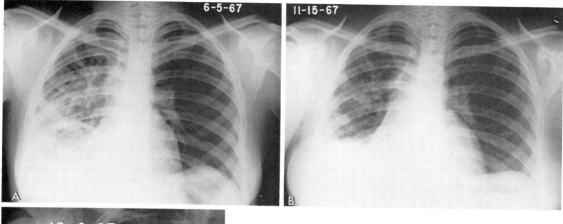

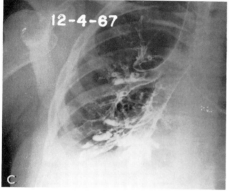

**Figure 5**   Lower and middle lobe tuberculosis in a 16 year old female with resultant "bronchiectasis" despite adequate response to chemotherapy and conversion of sputum. Bilobectomy performed. (From Young, W. G., Jr., and Moor, G. F. In: Gibbon, J. H., Jr., et al.: Surgery of the Chest. 2nd ed. Philadelphia, W. B. Saunders Company, 1969.)

ing medication or obtaining follow-up examination, such as alcoholics; and (d) those patients, men in particular, who for socioeconomic and educational reasons must perform strenuous labor for a livelihood.

7. Some tuberculous lesions will be removed because a neoplasm is suspected. In addition, concomitant tuberculosis and cancer, and the development of carcinoma in a site previously scarred by tuberculous infection, are entities that have assumed increasing importance in recent years. They require diligent observation and awareness on the part of the physician to prevent delay in the necessary resection.

8. Patients with recurrent or persistent hemoptysis, which is often the result of an open cavity (Fig. 6), bronchiectasis, or erosion of the bronchial wall by calcified hilar lymph nodes. Emergency resection may be life-saving in a patient with massive hemoptysis.

9. Patients with pleural empyema and encapsulated unexpandable lobe or lung may need a resection as well as decortication.

### Selection and Preoperative Preparation

The selection of patients for operation requires close cooperation between internist and surgeon. There is some variation of opinion regarding the timing of surgical intervention. In any event, the disease should appear stable or improving on serial x-rays. An effort should be made to convert the patient's sputum to negative before operation. This is not always possible, and undue delay carries the risk of the emergence of drug-resistant strains of bacteria. In a large number of cases, the optimal time is approximately 6 months after the institution of chemotherapy. After this period most of the reversible lesions have healed or resolved. In patients whose condition is optimal, early resectional surgery after 3 to 4 months of chemotherapy carries little more danger than postponement of operation and will decrease total hospital time.

Once it is seen that a patient will require surgery, a program of ambulation should be begun with improvement in general physical condition in mind. In addition to the standard preoperative evaluation, pulmonary function studies are helpful, particularly in the borderline case. Planigrams will demonstrate more clearly lesions that are to be resected. Occasionally, bronchograms are useful in demonstrating unsuspected bronchiectasis and in delineating the diseased segments. Bronchoscopy is called for in all patients to detect the unsuspected presence of bronchial stenosis, endobronchial tuberculosis, or other nontuberculous endobronchial lesions. It is wise to add a new chemotherapeutic agent to the ones already in use to protect the patient during and immediately following surgery. Pyrazinamide is an excellent drug in this context, since it is a potent although short-term drug.

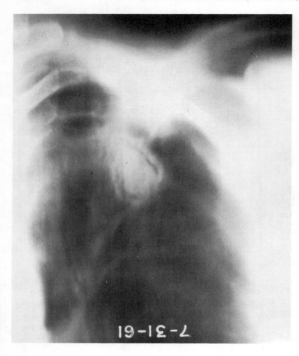

**Figure 6**   Residual cavitation associated with recurrent hemoptysis. The density within the cavity proved to be a "fungus ball" (aspergilloma). (From Young, W. G., Jr., and Moor, G. F. In: Gibbon, J. H., Jr., et al.: Surgery of the Chest. 2nd ed. Philadelphia, W. B. Saunders Company, 1969.)

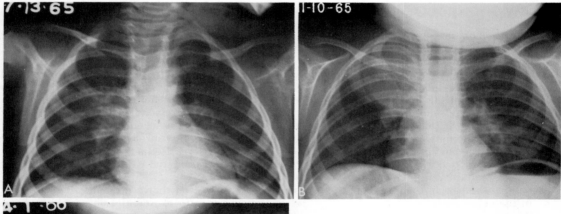

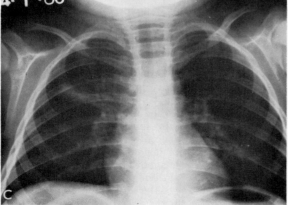

**Figure 7**   Pulmonary tuberculosis in a 2 year old infant with hilar adenopathy leading to right upper lobe atelectasis. Upper lobe re-expanded and asymptomatic after prolonged chemotherapy. (From Young, W. G., Jr., and Moor, G. F. In: Gibbon, J. H., Jr., et al.: Surgery of the Chest. 2nd ed. Philadelphia, W. B. Saunders Company, 1969.)

The type of resection depends upon the extent of disease, as determined by preoperative x-rays, including planigrams, and palpation at the time of surgery. Wedge resection is adequate for tuberculomas and for "coin lesions" removed for diagnosis and proved by frozen section to be granulomas. Segmental resection is ideal for localized residual cavities and fibrocaseous disease. Lobectomy is perhaps the procedure of choice when the patient has active disease with positive sputum and drug-resistant bacilli. Pneumonectomy should be reserved for the patient with a destroyed lung and persistently positive sputum, recurrent hemoptysis, or secondary infection.

### Resection for Childhood Tuberculosis

In the vast majority of children, standard long-term chemotherapy will cure pulmonary tuberculosis. Of almost 2000 children admitted to the Chicago Municipal Tuberculosis Sanatorium, Lees and associates[10] found that 101 (5.0 per cent) required surgery for the control of progressive pri-

mary disease or for excision of destructive residua of reinfection tuberculosis. There were two operative deaths, one late death, and no recurrence or reactivation of the disease in the 98 survivors.

The surgeon should be overly conservative, however, in advising excisional surgery for children with lobar atelectasis or obstructive emphysema accompanying the hilar adenopathy of primary tuberculosis. In the absence of secondary infection, these obstructed lobes will often return to normal as the lymph nodes regress with chemotherapy (Fig. 7), and functioning lung tissue will have been preserved.

### Decortication for Pleural Tuberculosis

Although pleural effusion is still a common first sign of pulmonary tuberculosis, purulent tuberculous empyema is now rarely encountered. By the time purulent empyema becomes evident, there is usually sufficient pleural thickening and "peel" formation to produce entrapment of the underlying lung. Simple thoracentesis or even tube

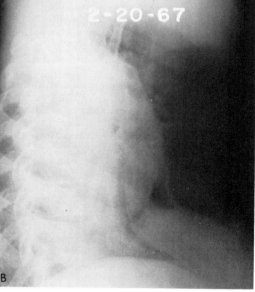
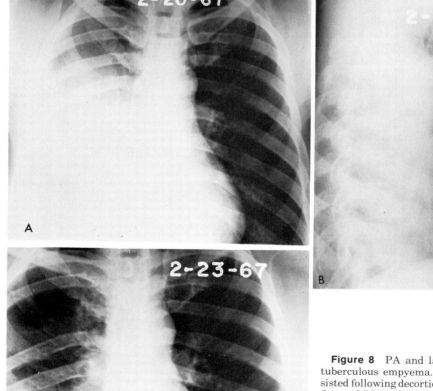

**Figure 8** PA and lateral x-rays showing pure tuberculous empyema. Re-expansion of lung persisted following decortication. (From Young, W. G., Jr., and Moor, G. F. In: Gibbon, J. H., Jr., et al.: Surgery of the Chest. 2nd ed. Philadelphia, W. B. Saunders Company, 1969.)

drainage and suction will not result in obliteration of the empyema space. For this reason, early decortication under drug coverage should be considered (Fig. 8). If complete and early re-expansion of the lung is obtained, an excellent result will ensue.

When the empyema is associated with pulmonary disease (cavitation or positive sputum or both), some form of concomitant resection will usually be required. In more complicated cases, empyema with bronchopleural fistula and secondary pyogenic infection will necessitate preliminary open drainage followed by decortication with resection (perhaps pleuropneumonectomy) and eventual thoracoplasty.

### Complcations of Resection

The three most important factors in the prevention of complications are: (1) the correct timing of the operative procedure and early recognition of an effective chemotherapeutic program; (2) meticulous surgical technique and rapid re-expansion of remaining lung tissue; and (3) careful postoperative care.

In addition to the usual complications of thoracotomy, two major specific complications occur in tuberculous patients. These are empyema, with or without bronchopleural fistula, and bronchogenic spread of the disease. The incidence of these complications is increased when the patient has positive sputum, when the bacteria are drug-resistant, and when extensive resection is necessary.

**Bronchopleural Fistula.**   A bronchopleural fistula is said to be present if there is air or an air-fluid level in the pleural cavity. It is also present if air continues to leak via the intercostal catheter for more than 10 to 14 days and if an increasing airspace develops when the intercostal tube is clamped or removed.

The incidence of this complication has been distinctly greater in tuberculous patients than in comparable patients in whom the indication for resection was not tuberculosis. It is often the result of unsuspected or occult tuberculous disease in the bronchial stump or the result of failure of the remaining lung to fill the hemithorax. The latter is often accompanied by small alveolar air leaks. With subsequent infection of the space with tuberculous organisms, the small fistula may persist and the sputum may become positive.

It is important to differentiate between simple postresectional space problems and true bronchopleural fistulas. An asymptomatic space that demonstrates a gradual decrease in size will rarely require tube drainage and obliteration by tailoring thoracoplasty.[3] Serial x-rays will show eventual complete closure, although several months may be required. Such a benign airspace may be seen in approximately 20 per cent of cases in a series of resections. Symptomatic bronchopleural fistula will occur in 5 to 10 per cent.

**Spread of Tuberculosis.**   This serious complication occurs in a small percentage of cases but is usually prevented by adequate added drug coverage. Spread of the disease rarely occurs if the patient's sputum is noninfectious at the time of the resection. A bronchopleural fistula, as already mentioned, may be responsible for the spread. Other factors such as techniques of anesthesia, positioning the patient, and inefficient clearing of pulmonary secretions in the postoperative period may contribute to disease spread.

### Mortality and Results

Operative mortality rates have continued to decrease during the past 15 years. In a combined study from the Veterans Administration–Armed Forces hospitals, 4126 pulmonary resections were performed between 1961 and 1966 with an overall mortality of 1.7 per cent.[12] Pneumonectomy carried a risk of 8.8 per cent (reported series vary between 2.5 and 12 per cent). The operative death rate following lobectomy was 2 per cent, segmentectomy 0.7 per cent, and subsegmental resection 0.3 per cent. It is interesting that in the Armed Forces hospitals participating in the study, 762 resections were performed with only four deaths, a mortality rate of 0.5 per cent. This would appear to represent the operative risk in a relatively young and otherwise healthy group of patients. The major fatal complications in the VA–Armed Forces study were pulmonary insufficiency or cor pulmonale and bronchopleural fistula and its sequelae.

The long-term prognosis for patients undergoing resectional therapy for pulmonary tuberculosis is excellent. A representative study, using the life table method of analyzing results, indicates that 90 to 96 per cent of such patients will be free of disease (as determined by sputum culture and x-ray examination) at the end of a 5 year period of follow-up.[7]

### SELECTED REFERENCES

*Historical Aspects*

Flick, L. F.: Development of Our Knowledge of Tuberculosis. Lancaster, Wickersham Printing Company, 1925.

Hochberg, L. A.: Thoracic Surgery Before the Twentieth Century. New York, Vantage Press, 1960.

*Chemotherapy*

Cohen, A. C.: Drug Treatment of Tuberculosis. Springfield, Ill., Charles C Thomas, 1966.

Mitchell, R. S.: Control of tuberculosis. New Eng. J. Med., 276:842, 905, 1967.

Newman, R., Doster, B., Murray, F. J., and Ferebee, S.: Rifampin in initial treatment of pulmonary tuberculosis. A U.S. Public Health Service tuberculosis therapy trial (early results with a new drug). Amer. Rev. Resp. Dis., 103:461, 1971.

*Surgical Treatment*

Alexander, J.: The Collapse Therapy of Pulmonary Tuberculosis. Springfield, Ill., Charles C Thomas, 1937.

Steele, J. D.,: Surgical Management of Tuberculosis. Springfield, Ill., Charles C Thomas, 1957.

### REFERENCES

1. Alexander, J.: The Surgery of Pulmonary Tuberculosis. New York, Lea & Febiger, 1925.
2. Alexander, J.: The Collapse Therapy of Pulmonary Tuberculosis. Springfield, Ill., Charles C Thomas, 1937.

 3. Barker, W. L., Langston, H. T., and Naffah, P.: Postresectional thoracic space. Ann. Thorac. Surg., 2:299, 1966.
 4. Chamberlain, J. M., Storey, C. F., Klopstock, R., and Daniels, C. F.: Segmental resection for pulmonary tuberculosis (300 cases). J. Thorac. Surg., 26:471, 1953.
 5. Churchill, E. D., and Belsey, R.: Segmental pneumonectomy in bronchiectasis. Ann. Surg., 109:481, 1939.
 6. Gentry, W. H.: Atypical mycobacterial infections. In: Tice-Harvey Practice of Medicine. Vol. III. Hagerstown, W. F. Prior Company, 1966.
 7. Johnson, G., Jr., and Peters, R. M.: Pulmonary resection for tuberculosis: Life table analysis of results. Ann. Thorac. Surg., 1:634, 1965.
 8. Jones, J. C.: Early experiences with resection in pulmonary tuberculosis. In: Steele, J. D., ed.: The Surgical Management of Pulmonary Tuberculosis. Springfield, Ill., Charles C Thomas, 1957.
 9. Langston, H. T., Barker, W. L., and Pyle, M. M.: Surgery in pulmonary tuberculosis: 11-year review of indications and results. Ann. Surg., 164:567, 1966.
10. Lees, W. M., Fox, R. T., and Shields, T. W.: Pulmonary sur-gery for tuberculosis in children. Ann. Thorac. Surg., 4:327, 1967.
11. Medlar, E. M.: The behavior of pulmonary tuberculosis lesions; a pathologic study. Amer. Rev. Tuberc., Vol. 71; part 2, 1955.
12. Mendenhall, J. T.: Report of Thoracic Surgery for Pulmonary Tuberculosis in VA-Armed Forces Study Unit Hospitals, July 1, 1965–June 30, 1966. Transactions of the 26th VA-Armed Forces Pulmonary Diseases Research Conference, Cleveland, 1967, p. 2.
13. Runyon, E. H.: Anonymous mycobacteria in pulmonary disease. Med. Clin. N. Amer., 43:273, 1959.
14. Seibert, F. B., and Long, E. R.: Further studies on purified protein derivative of tuberculin. Amer. Rev. Tuberc., 35:281, 1937.
15. Smith, D. T., and Johnston, W. W.: Single and multiple infections with typical and atypical mycobacteria. Amer. Rev. Resp. Dis., 90:899, 1964.
16. Stead, W. W.: Pathogenesis of the sporadic case of tuberculosis. New Eng. J. Med., 277:1008, 1967.

# XI

# Benign Tumors of the Trachea and Bronchi
*Marcus L. Dillon, M.D.*

Classification of benign tumors of the trachea and bronchi is fraught with several basic difficulties. First, many of these tumors have malignant neoplastic potential; second, they may be difficult to distinguish histologically from the malignant form; and third, some of the tumors are so rare that the natural history of significant numbers is unknown. In practice, the determination of whether a tumor arises from a bronchus or is malignant is frequently made after definitive removal. Peripheral lesions can seldom be differentiated radiologically from carcinoma of the lung and require removal for diagnosis. The endobronchial lesions not only may simulate carcinoma of the lung but also can be as deadly to the patient when they are associated with bronchial obstruction, distal infection, or hemorrhage. The frequency of destruction of lung tissue distal to an endobronchial lesion has led some to believe that resection of the lesion along with the distal tissue is preferable to segmental bronchial resection with anastomosis of the bronchus for benign lesions.

In the classification of tumors of the trachea and bronchi that follows, some of the tumors have considerable malignant potential, some have vascular or neurogenic origin, and some are so uncommon that the natural history is unknown, but all present clinically with features that simulate those of benign tumors of the trachea and bronchi. These lesions are listed more or less in order of frequency of occurrence.

1. Bronchial adenomas
   a. Carcinoid
   b. Salivary gland type
      1. Cylindroma (adenoid cystic)
      2. Mucoepidermoid
      3. Pleomorphic (mixed tumors)
2. Hamartoma
   a. Chondromatous hamartoma
   b. Congenital adenomatous malformation (diffuse hamartoma)
   c. Blastoma
3. Polyps
   a. Papillomatosis
   b. Inflammatory polyp
   c. Squamous papilloma
   d. Tumorlet
4. Vascular tumors
   a. Angiomas
      1. Hemangiomas
      2. Lymphangioma
      3. Hemangioendothelioma
   b. Pulmonary arteriovenous fistula
   c. Hemangiopericytoma
   d. Sclerosing hemangioma
5. Pseudotumors
   a. Tracheobronchopathia osteoplastica
   b. Amyloid
   c. Xanthoma
6. Granular cell myoblastoma
7. Lipomas
8. Leiomyoma

9. Fibroma
10. Chondroma
11. Neurogenic tumors
12. Myxoma
13. Plasmacytoma
14. Chemodectoma (nonchromaffin paraganglioma)
15. Clear cell tumor
16. Teratoma
17. Aberrant tissue
    a. Endometriosis
    b. Splenosis

## TRACHEAL TUMORS

Benign tumors of the trachea are uncommon, but their incidence is the same as that of malignant tracheal tumors in the adult; malignant tumors of the trachea are rare in children.[8] The predominant lesions are tracheopathia osteoplastica (adult), papilloma, fibroma, hemangioma (child), and bronchial adenoma.[4] Many of the rare bronchial tumors have also been found in the trachea. Tracheal tumors have the advantage of being accessible for bronchoscopic biopsy, and, if they do not involve the tracheal wall, may be removed endoscopically. Those localized tumors which involve the tracheal wall should be removed by tracheal resection. Some of the principles of this resection are shown in Figure 1. More than 2 cm. of tracheal resection requires extended mobilization of the remaining trachea, and as much as 6.6 cm. may be removed by freezing the right hilum and inferior pulmonary ligament, transplanting the left main bronchus into the bronchus intermedius, and maintaining the head in comfortable flexion of 15 to 35 degrees;[9] additional relaxation from the larynx can be obtained by dividing the sternohyoid and thyrohyoid muscles transversely. Prosthetic replacement has been unsatisfactory owing to infection, disruption, and stenosis. Successful resection of all but the distal 2 cm. of the trachea has been reported; the distal tracheal stump was sutured to the back of a hole made in the sternum, which was lined by a flap of skin.

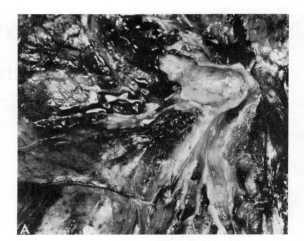

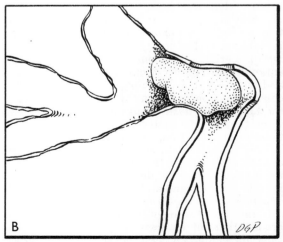

**Figure 1**   Diagram of a large lesion of the trachea and the extent of resection necessary for removal. Freeing of the larynx and division of the thyrohyoid and sternohyoid muscles are also represented, with displacement of the larynx inferiorly. The inset, *A,* illustrates the anastomosis of the right main bronchus, and the transposition of the left main bronchus to the bronchus intermedius.

**Figure 2**   *A,* Bronchial adenoma obstructing the right upper lobe bronchus, having caused bronchiectatic changes distally in the upper lobe. The mass impinges on the lumen of the lower lobe bronchus and has not yet produced such extensive changes. This adenoma is covered by bronchial mucosa and is almost entirely endobronchial. *B,* Diagrammatic representation of the bronchial changes and relationships to the tumor.

## BRONCHIAL TUMORS

Clinical symptomatology of the bronchial tumors varies from none (in peripherally located lesions) to cough, dyspnea, hemoptysis, and suffocation (in proximal endobronchial lesions). The mechanisms by which the endobronchial tumors produce symptoms and changes in the lung distal to the lesion are shown in Figures 2 and 3. A partially obstructing tumor may cause localized wheezing, whereas complete obstruction of a major bronchus will cause distal atelectasis. Partial obstruction prevents adequate cleansing and contributes to recurrent distal pneumonia with necrotizing bronchitis and subsequent bronchiectasis and lung abscess. Ball valve action of a tumor will allow filling of the lung with air on inspiration and trap the air in a lobe or segment on expiration. This can be seen radiographically as lobar or segmental emphysema (Fig. 3). Involvement of the bronchial wall is frequent with the most com-

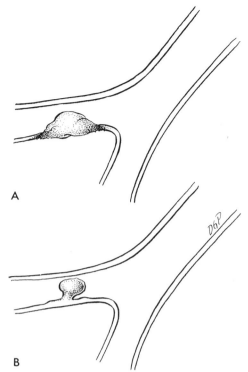

**Figure 4** *A,* Involvement of the bronchial wall, common with bronchial adenomas. Complete removal of this type of tumor by endoscopy is not feasible. Pedunculated tumors not involving the wall of the bronchus, as illustrated in *B,* can at times be completely removed endoscopically.

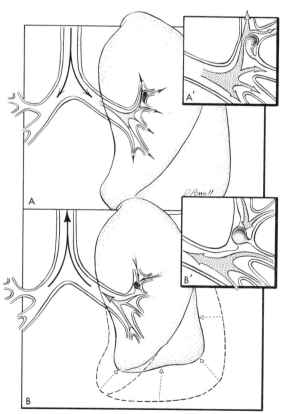

**Figure 3** *A,* Pedunculated endobronchial tumor in the bronchus to the apical posterior and anterior segments of the left upper lobe. In the position shown, all segments are allowed to fill on inspiration. This is emphasized in *A'. B,* On expiration, the tumor obstructs the apical posterior and anterior segmental bronchi and prevents the segments from decreasing in size; the expiratory contraction of the left lower lobe and lingula of the upper lobe is normal. The ball valve action of the pedunculated tumor in its closed position on expiration is emphasized in *B'.*

mon bronchial tumor, the bronchial adenoma. When there is bronchial wall involvement, removal of the tumor will create a defect that cannot be repaired bronchoscopically (Fig. 4). An endobronchial polypoid lesion that involves only the epithelium, as bronchial papilloma, can be removed bronchoscopically, and should be, because of the frequent recurrence in other areas (Fig. 4B).

## BRONCHIAL ADENOMAS

Although Müller first described a bronchial adenoma from an autopsy in 1882, Laennec had reported a vascular bronchial polyp in 1831 that probably represented the same entity. Langston, in a critical collective review of benign endobronchial tumors, found that prior collective reviews varied greatly in tabulation, and that reclassification of tumors was common.[14] He found, after critical appraisal of the literature (prior to 1950), that it was confused, laconic, and (at times) even possibly inaccurate. It was as recently as 1965 that the first two mixed tumors of the bronchus were described by Payne, Schier, and Woolner.[24] Bronchial adenoma is the most frequently encountered benign tumor, but is rare as compared to carcinoma of the lung, with a 1:50 ratio. The malignant potential is reported to be 10 per cent, as determined from lymph node metastases. Approximately 80 per cent of these tumors arise from the major bronchi, and between 55 and 70 per cent are associated with distal bronchiectasis.[6] These tumors arise from the epithelium of the ducts of the bronchial mucous glands, and the carcinoid type can arise from neurosecretory cells of both the mucous glands and bronchial epithelium.[29] Payne et al. reported the incidence of the various types of bronchial adenomas to be: carcinoid, 89 per cent; cylindromatous, 8 per cent; mucoepidermoid, 2 per cent; and mixed tumors, 1 per cent.[24]

*Carcinoid adenomas* have the characteristic histologic appearance of carcinoid tumors in other areas.[16] Some have been found to produce ACTH and MSH, with Cushing's syndrome resulting. Some are associated with other endocrine disorders. An insulin-secreting bronchial carcinoid tumor with immunoreactive insulin within the tumor has been reported. The "carcinoid syndrome," consisting of anxiety, tremulousness, temperature elevation, periorbital and facial edema, increased lacrimation and salivation, rhinorrhea, diaphoresis, explosive diarrhea, nausea and vomiting, hypotension, and oliguria, was originally attributed to the effects of serotonin produced by carcinoid tumors. As investigation continued, it was found that serotonin did not produce all of these changes, and additional factors not definitely identified, as kinins, catecholamines, histamines, substance P, components of complement, and prostaglandins, probably contribute to producing the syndrome.[21] Carcinoid adenomas are vascular and present the real possibility of severe hemorrhage on bronchoscopic biopsy. Degeneration of the vascular component can result in calcification and ossification, which can be seen radiographically but is not a common finding. Heimburger et al. reported that two separate tumors were present in one of five patients with peripheral carcinoid adenomas at their hospital.[10] They reviewed the eleven previously reported multiple adenomas and found that they were mostly of the carcinoid type (when classified) and frequently microscopic. Spencer believes that these lesions are occasionally confused with the epithelial proliferations associated with inflammation called tumorlets and that they can be differentiated by the absence of inflammatory lesions.[29] Planned, function-preserving surgical resection produces good immediate and long-term results.[1]

*Cylindromatous adenomas* make up only 8 per cent of the adenomas occurring in the bronchi, but they are the most common adenomas found in the trachea.[8] They frequently occur near the tracheal bifurcation and are vascular but seldom show necrosis or ossification. Markel and Abell (1964) described five patients with tracheal cylindroma.[20] Three were treated by partial endoscopic resection plus cobalt-60 radiation (6000 R), one had partial endoscopic resection, and one had complete endoscopic resection. Despite these inade-

quate resections, two of the patients were living at 8 years and 6.8 years, respectively, after operation. Three had died, one at 8 years, one at 12.5 years, and one at 13 years after treatment. Only one had distant pulmonary metastases. The authors predicted accurately that the future treatment of choice would be wide surgical excision. Cylindroma is a slow-growing, infiltrative carcinoma; however, as illustrated by this series, a 5 year survival is likely, even with less than optimal therapy, but cure cannot be expected. Cylindromas of the bronchi are best treated by resection with removal of the distal lung, which is frequently a site of infection and bronchiectasis.

*Mucoepidermoid adenomas* usually involve the major bronchi and frequently present as pedunculated endobronchial tumors. Reichle and Rosemond (1966)[25] reviewed the 29 reported cases and two of their own, and found no recurrences in those in whom complete resection was done. However, Welborn, Fahmy, and Gobbel (1969) report a 28 per cent incidence of high-grade malignancy among all reported cases, with metastasis frequently by all routes.[33] Of special interest was the finding in one of their cases of an elevated urine 5-HIAA level that fell after bronchoscopic removal of the tumor. This suggests a possible relationship between tumors of mucous gland origin and those of enterochromaffin origin (carcinoid adenoma). Liebow[16] gives credit to H. F. Smetana for separating this group of adenomas and calling them "mucoepidermoid tumors" in accordance with the mucoepidermoid tumors of the salivary gland described by Stewart, Foote, and Becker.[30] A pathologic malignant counterpart was also recognized by Dr. Smetana.

*Mixed tumors* are so rare and so recently identified that the natural history is unknown. They have been compared to mixed tumors of the salivary gland type elsewhere in the body, in which carcinomatous transformation does occur. One patient has been reported with recurrent tumor in the stump and in nodes about the stump of the bronchus intermedius 8 years after resection. The patient was doing well 3 years after discovery of recurrence.

## HAMARTOMA

This term was coined by Albrecht in 1904 (from the Greek words $\alpha\mu\alpha\rho\tau\iota\alpha$ = error and $\omega\mu\alpha$ = tumor)[29] to describe tumors resulting from errors in development.

*Chondromatous hamartoma* characteristically presents as an asymptomatic solitary pulmonary nodule and is rarely, if ever, malignant. This is not an uncommon tumor and makes up from 8 per cent to 14 per cent of reported solitary pulmonary nodules in large series. Bateson (1965) reported that, although 80.5 per cent present as peripherally localized parenchymal tumors and 19.5 per cent present as endobronchial lesions, there is good evidence that they are similar and that the peripheral tumors arise from peripheral bronchi.[3]

These tumors occur most commonly in persons between the ages of 50 to 60 years but have also been found in children. Tracheal hamartomas are rare but have been reported. Only once has malignant change been implied. The endobronchial lesions require removal for relief of obstructive and irritating symptoms and prevention of the inevitable distal lung destruction from infection. The peripheral lesions cannot be differentiated clinically from carcinoma of the lung and require removal for diagnosis.

*Diffuse hamartoma or congenital adenomatous malformation* of the lung rarely presents as a clinical problem, not only because it is rare, but also because it is usually found in premature or stillborn infants with other congenital pulmonary abnormalities. Usually a lobe or part of a lobe is involved, but it can be more extensive.[29] An adult patient with a small firm mass in the right upper lobe has been reported.

*Pulmonary blastoma* is a very rare tumor first described by Bernard in 1952, who believed it was benign because the patient was alive and well many years later. These tumors arise from embryonal lung tissue, and Spencer has found that they may ultimately metastasize by way of the bloodstream and lymphatics.[29]

## POLYPS

*Papillomatosis* is a common laryngeal tumor of infancy and childhood. There is distal spread in approximately 2 per cent of cases, usually only to the trachea; however, bronchial and alveolar papillomatosis does rarely occur. The sex incidence is equal, and the tumor rarely occurs in adults. The incidence of recurrence has been reported to be as high as 90 per cent. The tumors tend to transplant to adjoining structures and to regress spontaneously and disappear after puberty. Local treatment of laryngeal lesions with estrogenic hormones has caused regression. Lesions have disappeared with pregnancy and reappeared after pregnancy. They have been produced experimentally in animals by mechanical and chemical irritation of the larynx and trachea. There is frequent coexistence of papillomas and warts. Papillomas have been transferred by extract to the skin of humans and the vaginal mucosa of dogs. With extracts of papillomas, Ono et al. have produced patches of growth on chorioallantoic membranes, but were unable to produce serial transplants of the growth in chick eggs.[23] Autogenous vaccine preparations from tumor tissue have prevented recurrence during the period of vaccination, with rapid reappearance between courses.[27] Serum complement-fixing antibodies against autologous or homologous papilloma antigens have been demonstrated in patients.[13] An interesting aspect is the finding of low serum calcium and magnesium levels in patients with laryngeal papillomas. Shilovtseva has used calcium and magnesium in treatment of rabbits with tracheal and laryngeal papillomatosis and noted a reduction in the size of

papillomas.[28] In 1966, the seventh patient with bronchoalveolar papillomatosis associated with laryngeal papillomatosis was reported. Three of the seven patients have died as a consequence of their disease. Treatment of these patients may be frustrating because of the high incidence of recurrence, the frequent necessity of tracheotomy, and the need for multiple attempts at operative removal by bronchoscopy in an effort to maintain an adequate airway and prevent distal parenchymal infection over a period of many years.

*Inflammatory polyps* of the trachea and bronchi may be associated with laryngeal papillomatosis, chronic bronchitis, or allergic bronchitis and appear as single or multiple lesions. They are characterized by edema and inflammatory infiltration of the stalk with squamous metaplasia of the surface. Less common is the allergic-type polyp. In the absence of squamous metaplasia, the surface is covered with ciliated columnar epithelium. In inflammatory polyps (differentiated from papillomatosis), recurrence is not common. Conservative bronchoscopic removal is the treatment of choice. Mucous polyps of the upper air passage are thought to be of this type.

*Squamous papilloma* is pedunculated and is usually covered with stratified squamous epithelium, often with keratinization. It occurs most commonly in the fifth to seventh decade. It is not associated with prolonged respiratory infections. Inflammatory cells are absent; however, minimal inflammation occurs if the tumor has produced obstruction with distal infection. These lesions belong to the same class of tumors as pedunculated papillomas of the skin and mucous membrane, and are localized dysplasias rather than true neoplasms. These are rare lesions.

*Tumorlet* is a term coined by Whitwell (1955) to describe epithelial proliferative lesions associated with chronic inflammation that resemble oat cell carcinoma morphologically but behave as benign lesions. Small peripheral carcinoids have been confused with tumorlets and are differentiated by the absence of inflammation and lung damage. Inflammatory tumorlets have been produced in rabbits by tracheal instillation of 1 per cent nitric acid. In one reported patient from whom an endobronchial tumorlet had been removed bronchoscopically, there was no evidence of recurrence at autopsy 12 years later.

## VASCULAR TUMORS

**Angiomas.** *Hemangiomatous malformation* occurs in the subglottic area of the larynx and may extend into the trachea in infants. Because of the location, the consequences of these lesions can be sudden ventilatory obstruction. The lesions behave like hemangiomas of the skin in infants, with an increase in size after a month or more of life. Then, toward the later part of the first year of life, the lesions regress. The frequency of occurrence of this lesion is probably greatly underestimated, since croup is a common occurrence in infants, the engorged mass may collapse during examination and be completely missed, and, unless severe symptoms persist, examination is not done. Even at autopsy, unless they are engorged with blood they go unrecognized. Association with other vascular malformations occurs, encompassed by the term phlebarteriectasia (as telangiectases, port-wine stain, congenital arteriovenous malformations, capillary hemangiomas, and cavernous hemangiomas). Tracheotomy may be necessary to allow ventilation, along with repeated small doses of radiation to shrink the tumor. Hemangiomas may be multiple, extensive, or localized but fortunately rarely occur at the site of the usual tracheotomy.

*Lymphangiomatous malformations* usually present as cystic hygromas of the neck and axilla but may be associated with hemangiomas. They more frequently appear with venous hemangiomas as mixed lesions.

*Hemangioendothelioma* may present histologically as part of an angiomatous malformation that contains more of the endothelial component and grossly is a more solid tumor. Hemangioendothelioma has been reported as a polypoid lesion in the trachea, treated by local excision.

**Pulmonary Arteriovenous Fistula.** In 1897, Churton demonstrated the lungs from a 12 year old boy to the Leeds and West-Riding Medico-Chirurgical Society.[5] During life, the boy had a loud roaring pulmonary systolic bruit, a highly accentuated second sound, hemoptysis, epistaxis, and dropsy. Four blood-clot-filled aneurysms of the pulmonary artery in one lung and three in the other were described. The first clinical diagnosis of pulmonary arteriovenous fistula was reported in 1939, with the lesion demonstrated angiographically. The first resection was not reported until 1942, and the lesion was called a cavernous angioma. Pulsation of the whole lower lobe controlled by compression of the pulmonary artery was noted at operation. Stringer et al., in a comprehensive review, found reports of 148 patients by 1955 and emphasized that the pathologic physiology of pulmonary arteriovenous fistula is due to the shunt between pulmonary artery and vein.[32] The characteristic findings in these patients are telangiectasia, cyanosis, clubbing, exertional dyspnea, polycythemia, opacities seen in the chest x-ray, and a murmur heard over the lesion in the lung. Brain abscesses are frequent because the filtering action of the lung is bypassed. The treatment is conservative surgical excision since multiple lesions are common. The lesion is frequently found in patients with hereditary hemorrhagic telangiectasia.

**Hemangiopericytoma.** This is a rare lung tumor that was first described by Stout and Murray in 1942.[31] Only four tumors in the lung had been reported by 1964. The tumors are thought to originate from the pericytes (modified contractile smooth muscle cells) closely related to the capillary walls and may be benign or malignant. The diagnosis is made by removal, which also constitutes the treatment. Malignant hemangiopericytomas are somewhat radiosensitive.

**Sclerosing Hemangioma.** Sclerosing hemangiomas are unusual pulmonary tumors first described by Liebow and Hubbell in 1956.[17] They are benign tumors arising from alveolar capillary endothelial cells that do not usually involve bronchi, but do present as opacities in chest films and do cause hemoptysis as a frequent symptom. They may be multiple and may be associated with hereditary hemorrhagic telangiectasia. Localized xanthomas can be an end stage of sclerosing hemangioma.

## PSEUDOTUMORS

*Tracheobronchopathia osteoplastica* is the most common benign tumor occurring in the trachea of adults.[8] It is a process of cartilagenous growth from the ecchondrosis of the tracheal rings, which ossifies and lines the tracheal submucosa with nodular projections over the rings. This can extend into the bronchi and has caused death from stenosis with distal pneumonia. Reported cases frequently represent incidental findings at autopsy or are recognized in life from routine chest films followed by bronchoscopy.

*Amyloid deposits,* either focal or diffuse, beneath the tracheal and bronchial mucosa occur rarely and are not associated with other amyloid lesions.[4] Amyloid also is usually an incidental autopsy finding, but it may extend into the bronchi and produce stenosis and pneumonia. Localized lesions may be removed bronchoscopically, but when there is diffuse involvement resection is done only in those areas necessary to maintain the bronchial patency.

*Xanthoma* of the trachea and bronchus occurs rarely and is associated with lipoprotein disorders with fat deposits in the skin.[4] Xanthomas may arise from other pathologic processes as the end stage of sclerosing hemangioma or as maturation of a granuloma from an inflammatory process.

## GRANULAR CELL MYOBLASTOMA

Granular cell myoblastoma was first described in 1926 by Abrikossoff and usually arises in the tongue, skin, or subcutaneous tissue. Thirty-eight tumors have been reported in the lung, most in the large bronchi. They may be multiple and may occur in association with subcutaneous lesions. Local removal is adequate treatment, but because of its usual location in the large bronchi, the tumor may have caused distal pulmonary infection with destruction of the lung. Malignant forms are rare, but do occur.

## LIPOMA

Lipoma of the bronchus is an uncommon benign lesion. Only 33 had been reported in the English literature by 1968; five of them had been discovered at autopsy. Bronchial lipoma was first seen bronchoscopically and successfully removed through a bronchoscope in 1927.[12] The tumor may extend outside the bronchus and may require resection of distal lung because of bronchiectasis or pulmonary destruction from infection. Lipomas have also been reported to arise in the trachea.

## LEIOMYOMA

Leiomyoma of the trachea and bronchus is a rare tumor. Of 22 cases collected by 1969, the tumor had arisen within a major bronchus in only 9. Ten tracheal leiomyomas had been reported in the English literature through 1968. One was removed by tracheal resection. Bronchoscopic removal has been used in others, but is certainly not adequate for the malignant forms.

## FIBROMA

Fibromas of the trachea and bronchus are rare. Lieutaud described the first tracheal fibroma in 1767, and only 36 were reported during the next 200 years. In two cases, fibroma has been reported in the trachea in children. Local excision is adequate treatment. Intrapulmonary fibromas appear in x-rays as "coin lesions" and require removal for diagnosis.

## CHONDROMA

Chondroma of the bronchus is an extremely rare lesion, only four of which have been reported. It differs from a chondromatous hamartoma in that it consists of cartilage without glands or other tissue.

## NEUROGENIC TUMORS

Neurogenic tumors of the lung are rare. The first bronchial neurofibroma was described in 1940, and the first excision of a solitary primary neurogenic tumor of the lung was described by Bartlett and Adams in 1946.[2] By 1951, only two benign bronchial neurogenic tumors had been reported. Schwannomatous neurofibromatous lesions have been reported to erode a bronchus. Whether the neurofibroma lesions are benign or malignant can be difficult to determine from histologic examination.

## MYXOMA

Myxoma is a rare lesion described by Placitelli in 1953. Littlefield and Drash in 1959 described a patient in whom a myxoma presented as a "coin lesion" and who was doing well 26 months after wedge resection.[19]

## PLASMACYTOMA

In 1959, Kennedy and Kneafsey reported a tracheal plasmacytoma and a right main stem bronchial plasmacytoma, which were removed locally. There was no recurrence at 4 years and at 10 months, respectively.[11] However, plasmacytoma should be considered malignant, as a variant of multiple myeloma.

## CHEMODECTOMA

Chemodectomas are tumors of the chemoreceptor organs of the aorta, carotid, and jugular glomera. A glomus pulmonale has been located anatomically on the dorsal side of the main pulmonary artery. Minute, occasionally multiple glomus structures related to anastomosing pulmonary venules have been encountered in the periphery of the lung; however, their function as chemoreceptors has not been established. Of the 15 intrathoracic chemodectomas described through 1966, only one was present in the pulmonary parenchyma. These lesions may appear benign or malignant histologically, and none have been described with abnormal physiologic function.

## CLEAR CELL TUMOR

In 1963, Liebow and Castleman reported four examples of what they call benign clear cell tumors of the lung, which resemble metastases from renal carcinoma.[18] On the basis of a study of 13 patients, Morgan and Mackenzie believe these are adenocarcinomas of the lung.[22]

## TERATOMA

Of the 15 reported intrapulmonary teratomas, only one was endobronchial. In this patient, there was a mass in the left upper lobe surrounded by a crescent-shaped translucent area simulating a mycetoma. A left pneumonectomy was done, and the lesion was found to be an endobronchial teratoma with distal bronchiectasis.

## ABERRANT TISSUE

*Endometriosis* of the lung was first documented by Lattes et al. in 1956 in a 34 year old woman in whom a 1 cm. round mass developed in the right middle lobe with pregnancy.[15] She had undergone dilatation and curettage of the uterus twice in 1952, and hemoptysis with menses had followed. On removal, the mass was found to be pulmonary endometriosis with decidual tissue. The first case of endobronchial endometriosis was reported by Rodman and Jones in 1962 in a patient with an abnormal chest film and hemoptysis during menses and a normal chest film without hemoptysis between periods.[26] This lesion was in the bronchial wall with bronchial artery supply to it.

*Splenosis* in the bronchus has not been reported, but Davis et al. (1963) found autotransplantation to the pleural cavity in 3 of 36 reported cases. In one of their patients, an asymptomatic tumor could be seen in the left lung field on the chest film. At thoracotomy, six splenic implants were found and removed from the visceral pleura, parietal pleura, and left lung.[7] The mechanism of transplantation in splenosis is fragmentation of splenic tissue due to trauma, implantation at a foreign site, and development of a parasitic blood supply.

## SELECTED REFERENCES

Bateson, E. M.: Relationship between intrapulmonary and endobronchial cartilage-containing tumours (so-called hamartomata). Thorax, *20*:447, 1965.
*This article includes a rather extensive review of the literature and a detailed review of the relation of intrapulmonary and endobronchial hamartomas. It is well illustrated, and the author's argument—that they are similar lesions—is developed well.*

Caldarola, V. T., Harrison, E. G., Jr., Clagett, O. T., and Schmidt, H. W.: Benign tumors and tumor-like conditions of the trachea and bronchi. Ann. Otol., *73*:1042, 1964.
*This is a report of all benign tumors and tumor-like conditions of the trachea and bronchi encountered clinically (63 cases) at the Mayo Clinic from 1930 to 1960. It gives a thorough clinical discussion of these conditions and their frequency.*

Gilbert, J. G., Mazzarella, L. A., and Feit, L. J.: Primary tracheal tumors in the infant and adult. Arch. Otolaryng., *58*:1, 1953.
*This is a study of one of the largest collections of primary tracheal tumors in infants and adults and has been referred to by practically all authors writing on the subject.*

Grillo, H. C., Dignan, E. F., and Miura, T.: Extensive resection and reconstruction of mediastinal trachea without prosthesis or graft: an anatomical study in man. J. Thorac. Cardiovasc. Surg., *48*:741, 1964.
*This is a study done on human cadavers to establish the maximal amount of trachea that might be removed and still permit effective reconstruction. It is pertinent and informative.*

Liebow, A. A.: Tumors of the Respiratory Tract. Atlas of Tumor Pathology, Section 5, Fascicle 17. Washington, D.C., Armed Forces Institute of Pathology, 1952.
*This fascicle has served as a study reference for 19 years. It is beautifully illustrated with both black and white and color photographs of tumors of the lower respiratory tract.*

Melmon, K. L.: The endocrinologic manifestations of the carcinoid tumor. In: Williams, R. H., ed.: Textbook of Endocrinology. 4th ed. Philadelphia, W. B. Saunders Company, 1968, pp. 1161–1180.
*This is an excellent source giving the differences among functional carcinoid tumors in relation to their location, the biochemical substances involved, and their symptoms and treatment.*

Spencer, H.: Pathology of the Lung. 2nd ed. New York, Pergamon Press, 1968.
*This is a comprehensive reference text in the specialized study of the lung. It is especially useful as a source of both gross and microscopic pictures of all lesions of the lung except tuberculosis.*

Stewart, F. W., Foote, F. W., and Becker, W. F.: Muco-epidermoid tumors of salivary glands. Ann. Surg., *122*:820, 1945.
*This is an analysis of approximately 700 major and minor salivary gland tumors seen at the Memorial Hospital in New York between 1928 and 1943. The presentation of the material, utilizing color photomicrographs, is as impressive as the tabulated findings and the discussion of the various aspects of these tumors. The pathologic aspects are correlated with*

*the clinical behavior. An understanding of the salivary-gland-type bronchial adenoma can be gained from this evaluation of salivary gland tumors.*

## REFERENCES

1. Baldwin, J. N., and Grimes, O. F.: Bronchial adenomas. Surg. Gynec. Obstet., *124*:813, 1967.
2. Bartlett, J. P., and Adams, W. E.: Solitary primary neurogenic tumor of the lung. J. Thorac. Surg., *15*:251, 1946.
3. Bateson, E. M.: Relationship between intrapulmonary and endobronchial cartilage-containing tumours (so-called hamartomata). Thorax, *20*:447, 1965.
4. Caldarola, V. T., Harrison, E. G., Jr., Clagett, O. T., and Schmidt, H. W.: Benign tumors and tumor-like conditions of the trachea and bronchi. Ann. Otol., *73*:1042, 1964.
5. Churton, T.: Multiple aneurysms of pulmonary artery. Brit. Med. J., *1*:1223, 1897.
6. Condon, V. R., and Phillips, E. W.: Bronchial adenomas in children: A review of the literature and report of three cases. Amer. J. Roentgen., *88*:543, 1962.
7. Davis, C., Alexander, R. W., and DeYoung, H. D.: Splenosis: A sequel to traumatic rupture of the spleen. Arch. Surg., *86*:523, 1963.
8. Gilbert, J. G., Mazzarella, L. A., and Feit, L. J.: Primary tracheal tumors in the infant and adult. Arch. Otolaryng., *58*:1, 1953.
9. Grillo, H. C., Dignan, E. F., and Miura, T.: Extensive resection and reconstruction of mediastinal trachea without prosthesis or graft: an anatomical study in man. J. Thorac. Cardiovasc. Surg., *48*:741, 1964.
10. Heimburger, I. L., Kilman, J. W., and Battersby, J. S.: Peripheral bronchial adenomas. J. Thorac. Cardiovasc. Surg., *52*:542, 1966.
11. Kennedy, J. D., and Kneafsey, D. V.: Two cases of plasmacytoma of the lower respiratory tract. Thorax, *14*:353, 1959.
12. Kernan, J. D.: Three unusual endoscopic cases. Laryngoscope, *37*:62, 1927.
13. Klos, J., and Jezkova, Z.: A cytopathic agent in laryngeal papillomas of children. The relation of serum antibodies to the clinical course of laryngeal papillomatosis. Ann. Otol., *75*:225, 1966.
14. Langston, H. T.: Benign endobronchial tumors. Surg. Gynec. Obstet., *91*:521, 1950.
15. Lattes, R., Shepard, F., Tovell, H., and Wylie, R.: A clinical and pathologic study of endometriosis of the lung. Surg. Gynec. Obstet., *103*:552, 1956.
16. Liebow, A. A.: Tumors of the Respiratory Tract. Atlas of Tumor Pathology, Section 5, Fascicle 17. Washington, D.C., Armed Forces Institute of Pathology, 1952.
17. Liebow, A. A., and Hubbell, D. S.: Sclerosing hemangioma (histiocytoma, xanthoma) of lung. Cancer, *9*:53, 1956.
18. Liebow, A. A., and Castleman, B.: Benign "clear cell tumors" of the lung. Amer. J. Path., *43*:13a, 1963 (abstract).
19. Littlefield, J. B., and Drash, E. C.: Myxoma of the lung. J. Thorac. Surg., *37*:745, 1959.
20. Markel, S. F., and Abell, M. R.: Adenocystic basal cell carcinoma of the trachea. J. Thorac. Cardiovasc. Surg., *48*: 211, 1964.
21. Melmon, K. L.: The endocrinologic manifestations of the carcinoid tumor. In: Williams, R. H., ed.: Textbook of Endocrinology. 4th ed. Philadelphia, W. B. Saunders Company, 1968, pp. 1161–1180.
22. Morgan, A. D., and Mackenzie, D. H.: Clear-cell carcinoma of the lung. J. Path. Bact., *87*:25, 1964.
23. Ono, J., Saito, H., Igarashi, M., and Ito, M.: The etiology of papilloma of the larynx. Ann. Otol., *66*:119, 1957.
24. Payne, W. S., Schier, J., and Woolner, L. B.: Mixed tumors of the bronchus (salivary gland type). J. Thorac. Cardiovasc. Surg., *49*:663, 1965.
25. Reichle, F. A., and Rosemond, G. P.: Mucoepidermoid tumors of the bronchus. J. Thorac. Cardiovasc. Surg., *51*:443, 1966.
26. Rodman, M. H., and Jones, C. W.: Catamenial hemoptysis due to endobronchial endometriosis. New Eng. J. Med., *266*:805, 1962.
27. Rosenbaum, H. D., Alavi, S. M., and Bryant, L. R.: Pulmo-

nary parenchymal spread of juvenile laryngeal papillomatosis. Radiology, *90*:654, 1968.

28. Shilovtseva, A. S.: The complex treatment of patients affected with papillomatosis of the larynx and trachea. Arch. Otolaryng., *89*:552, 1969.

29. Spencer, H.: Pathology of the Lung. 2nd ed. New York, Pergamon Press, 1968.

30. Stewart, F. W., Foote, F. W., and Becker, W. F.: Muco-epidermoid tumors of salivary glands. Ann. Surg., *122*:820, 1945.

31. Stout, A. P., and Murray, M. R.: Hemangiopericytoma, vascular tumor featuring Zimmerman's pericytes. Ann. Surg., *116*:26, 1942.

32. Stringer, C. J., Stanley, A. L., Bates, R. C., and Summers, J. E.: Pulmonary arteriovenous fistula. Amer. J. Surg., *89*:1054, 1955.

33. Welborn, M. B., Fahmy, A., and Gobell, W. G.: Mucoepidermoid carcinoma of bronchus with chondroid metaplasia and elevated 5-hydroxyindoleacetic acid excretion. J. Thorac. Cardiovasc. Surg., *57*:618, 1969.

# XII

# Carcinoma of the Lung

*Will C. Sealy, M.D.*

In the past 35 years bronchogenic carcinoma has become a major surgical problem and in the opinion of some has assumed epidemic proportions. Any condition increasing in incidence and causing 65,000 deaths annually would be expected to be of concern, although there are two emotional reasons as well that account for some of this unusual attention. First, the cancer affects mostly men who are in their most influential period of life. Second, smoking, a minor vice and thus a natural subject for a crusade, has been related to the increased incidence of this cancer.

In the surgical treatment of cancer of the lung, the most important historical event was the first successful pneumonectomy, performed in 1933 on a physician by Dr. Everts Graham.[7] The patient was cured of squamous cell carcinoma of the lung. As happens with many successful therapeutic measures, widespread application of pneumonectomy had to await the development of a cluster of clinical procedures, and this occurred between 1933 and 1942. A major development was a practical clinical method of intratracheal anesthesia. Next came demonstration of means of acquiring and storing blood for transfusion. Later came the introduction of effective antibacterial agents for prevention and control of postoperative infections.

Other events of historical importance in the surgical treatment of carcinoma of the lung were grouped around the turn of the century. Diagnostic bronchoscopy was introduced by Kirstein and Killian and then applied widely by Chevalier Jackson. The use of x-ray in clinical medicine, advances in bacteriology, and the aggressive treatment of pulmonary tuberculosis were other notable developments that increased the role of the surgeon in the treatment of thoracic disease. The application of these principles by Alexander and Graham in the United States, Edwards in England, and Sauerbruch in Germany led to the development of the specialty of thoracic surgery, and to surgical treatment of carcinoma of the lung.

## PATHOLOGY OF BRONCHOGENIC CARCINOMA[11]

The morphology of bronchogenic carcinoma may be manifested in a variety of cell types, and because of this, it has been the subject of complicated classifications. From the surgeon's point of view, the simplest and most practical classification is: (1) squamous cell (or epidermoid) carcinoma; (2) undifferentiated carcinoma; (3) adenocarcinoma; and (4) alveolar or bronchiolar carcinoma. Difficulties in classification arise from the fact that one carcinoma may contain more than one cell type. The pathologist labels the cancer by the predominant cell noted. The clinician's interest is primarily in the degree of undifferentiation of the cancer.

Bronchial adenoma should be included among the bronchogenic malignant lesions despite the fact that its name implies that it is benign. It is not unexpected that other malignant tumors, such as lymphosarcomas, fibrosarcomas, and even melanosarcomas, occur in the lung.

*Squamous cell* (or epidermoid) carcinoma (Fig. 1), representing epithelial metaplasia, is the most common of the bronchogenic types, accounting for 40 to 50 per cent of cases in most series. In the majority of the patients, the cancer originates in the large bronchi. It is rare in females, in whom approximately 6 to 10 per cent of the reported cases occur. It is unusual to find this type of cancer in a patient who is not a cigarette smoker. The degree of differentiation varies considerably, ranging from pearl formation and intercellular bridges to areas that merge into the undifferentiated type. Because of the location, bronchial obstruction and infection are frequent. Like squamous cell carcinomas elsewhere, it spreads early by way of the lymphatics. However, it also has ready access to the systemic arterial system and therefore is disseminated in this manner as well.

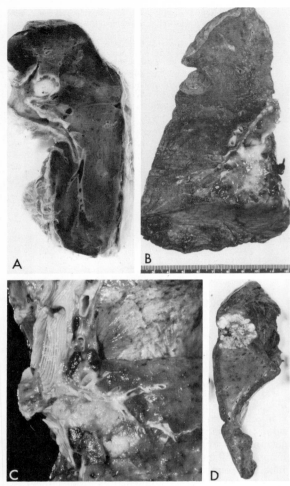

**Figure 1** *A*, Large bronchial adenoma obstructing the right upper lobe bronchus, causing marked cystic changes in the upper lobe. *B*, A large, undifferentiated carcinoma involving the lower lobe. *C*, A squamous cell carcinoma originating in a segmental branch of the upper lobe. This was just visible with a telescopic lens through the bronchoscope. *D*, A peripheral adenocarcinoma showing early necrosis in the central portion.

The second most common tumor is *undifferentiated* carcinoma, which includes small cell, large cell anaplastic, and oat cell carcinomas. Approximately 30 to 50 per cent of carcinomas seen are of this type, and many of its clinical features are similar to those seen in epidermoid cancer since it actually fuses with this group. The incidence of this tumor in women is approximately the same as that of epidermoid cancer. The larger bronchi are more commonly involved, and smoking is thought to be a factor in its development. This type spreads rapidly both by way of lymphatics and by early invasion of the pulmonary veins and subsequent metastasis via the systemic arterial system.

*Adenocarcinomas* are more frequently located peripherally, although they can occur anywhere,

for they are thought to originate both in the bronchial glands and from the surface epithelium. This variety makes up about 10 to 20 per cent of cancers of the lung. In some series, about 30 per cent of the cases are in women. Because of its peripheral location, an adenocarcinoma may not be symptomatic until late in its course. Therefore, it has frequently invaded the pulmonary veins by the time it is recognized.

*Alveolar* or *bronchiolar* carcinomas originate from the bronchiolar epithelium. They are occasionally multicentric in origin, although the multiple sites could result from bronchial spread. The tumor tends to follow the alveolar outlines and may be papillary in appearance. This carcinoma accounts for about 5 to 10 per cent of the cases in most series, although more and more it is being included in the adenocarcinoma group. It may occur in and about scars in the lung, as may squamous carcinomas. This variant has been called *scar cancer*. It occurs more frequently in men than in women, with about one-third of the cases occurring in the latter. Approximately a third of patients have a diffuse form, characterized by a pneumonic appearance on x-ray, that may involve an entire lung. Alveolar or bronchiolar cancer metastasizes by way of the bloodstream and the lymphatics.

*Bronchial adenoma* is another bronchogenic lesion. It almost always originates in the larger bronchi and trachea. There are two distinct tumors listed under this classification. The *cylindroma*, the much more malignant, originates in the mucous glands and is identical with adenoid cystic carcinoma of the salivary gland. This is a rare carcinoma, is locally invasive, and spreads by way of both the bloodstream and the lymphatics. About one-fifth of the bronchial adenomas are cylindromas. The *carcinoid* type of bronchial adenoma is the predominant form. It occurs about as frequently in women as it does in men and is distributed among all age groups. Its origin is from the argentaffin cells present in the bronchial mucous membrane. Histologically, it resembles similar tumors in the intestinal tract. In about 10 to 15 per cent of cases, it metastasizes to the regional nodes and by way of the bloodstream. Some carcinoids secrete serotonin.

*Fibrosarcomas* of the lung originate from the connective and fibrous tissue in the lung and behave as do similar lesions elsewhere in the body. *Lymphomas* of the lung may occur along with lymphosarcoma elsewhere or as isolated lesions. They are usually indistinct in outline and almost always occur in the peripheral portions of the lung. It may be difficult to separate a so-called pseudolymphoma from a truly malignant lesion. Other neoplasms rarely seen in the lung are melanosarcomas and myosarcomas.

Bronchogenic tumors spread by local extension to surrounding tissues and to lymphatics both by embolization and by permeation of the lymphatic system. The lymphatic supply of the lung is connected both superiorly with that of the cervical region and inferiorly with that of the abdomen.

Borrie made an excellent study of the lymphatic spread of carcinoma to the lymph nodes of the lung and mediastinum. He used the expression "sump drainage" to designate the main site of pulmonary lymph drainage. On the *right*, this is between the superior segment of the right lower lobe and the main bronchus and on the superior aspect of the right middle lobe bronchus where it joins the main bronchus. On the *left*, it is between the upper lobe bronchus and main bronchus and superior segment of the lower lobe bronchus and main bronchus. Although this study is of interest, there are only two differentiations that need be made. Carcinomas of the lung that spread by direct extension to the nodes about the bronchus of origin are usually amenable to curative surgical treatment. If there is spread to the mediastinal nodes, surgery is likely to be only palliative.

Cancers of the lung are particularly predisposed to dissemination through the systemic arterial system because of their frequent direct invasion of the pulmonary venous tree. Of the more malignant tumors, 60 per cent or more show vascular spread when first seen, as compared to 25 per cent of the more differentiated squamous cell ones. Aylwin was the first to emphasize the surgical significance of this mode of spread.

Speculation concerning the *etiology* of the bronchogenic carcinoma has attracted much attention. The lung and the stomach are two internal organs that are continuously exposed to the external environment. Thus, the chance of inoculation with a potential cancer-inducing agent is great in both. As an example, various mineral dusts have been indicated as agents causing lung cancer. It is of interest to note the rather marked change in incidence of both cancer of the lung and cancer of the stomach since 1930 (Fig. 2). No one has yet advanced a plausible theory for the marked diminution in the incidence of cancer of the stomach, while many have supported a direct cause-and-

effect relationship between smoking and cancer of the lung.

There are many facts that have been advanced to substantiate the cause and effect of the relationship between smoking and lung cancer. The incidence of lung cancer is much greater in cigarette smokers than in the users of pipes and cigars. The types of cancer usually associated with smoking are the ones that originate in the larger bronchi. Smoking is associated with bronchial epithelial alterations that might well be considered precancerous. From 1950 to 1964, the number of deaths from cancer of the lung in the United States increased from 18,313 to 45,838. The incidence of the disease rose from 12.2 to 24 per 100,000. For males this increase was more striking, being 19.4 to 41.4 per 100,000. In women, the incidence also increased, although it was only from 4.5 to 7.0 per 100,000. In select groups, such as men who have smoked more than 20 cigarettes per day, and inhaled, for 20 years or more, the incidence may be as high as 201 per 100,000, and in those of this group who are between the ages 65 and 79, the incidence is 262 per 100,000. In women, however, the incidence in the extreme select group is only about 35 per 100,000. It was estimated that in 1970 65,000 people would die from lung cancer.

Some counter arguments may be cited. Other areas of the respiratory tract, such as the nasopharynx, larynx, and trachea, are exposed to greater concentrations of tobacco smoke than the bronchi, yet the incidence of cancer in these areas has not markedly increased. Although the incidence of cancer in women, both smokers and nonsmokers, has increased slightly, it is still quite low.

## CLINICAL MANIFESTATIONS OF CARCINOMA OF THE LUNG[1, 6]

The clinical manifestations of carcinoma of the lung follow several different patterns that are related to the pathologic characteristics of the cancer, the manner in which it disseminates, and the peculiarities of the structures that surround it. Although the pattern may mimic almost any type of pulmonary inflammation, the experienced physician can usually make the clinical diagnosis from a careful history, physical examination, and x-ray studies. The classic symptoms of cough (40 per cent of patients), pain (20 per cent), and hemoptysis (15 per cent) are useful in suggesting the possibility of cancer.

### *Asymptomatic Carcinoma of the Lung*

In this form, the cancer is usually peripherally located and is frequently an adenocarcinoma, although it may be either squamous or bronchiolar (Figs. 3 and 4). This is frequently a scar cancer. When small, the tumors are sometimes called "coin lesions." The principal problem in differential diagnosis with this type of lesion is the separation of a cancerous lesion from an inflammatory one. A negative skin test for various fungi

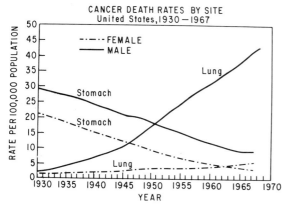

**Figure 2** Chart derived from statistics compiled by the American Cancer Society showing marked increase in the incidence of carcinoma of the lung and a decrease of the same magnitude in the incidence of carcinoma of the stomach.

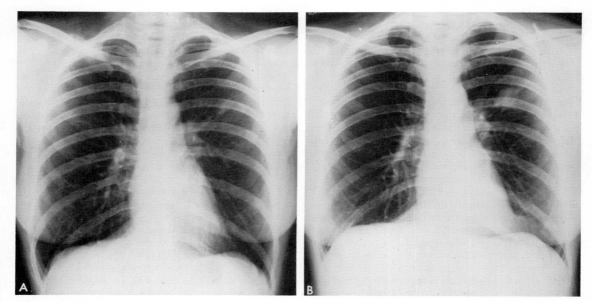

**Figure 3** *A,* The small shadow in the left upper lung showed very modest growth over a 5 year period *(B).* This carcinoma was treated by lobectomy, but the patient died 6 years later of recurrence in the lymphatics of the mediastinum.

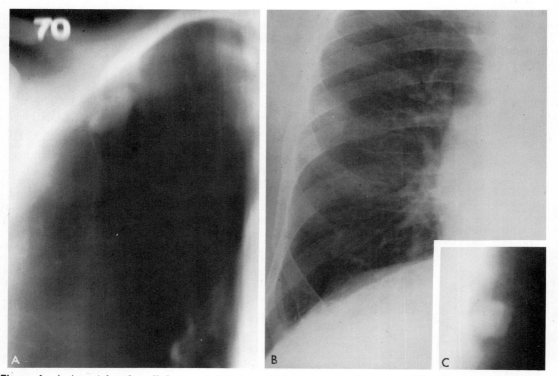

**Figure 4** *A,* A peripheral, well demarcated lesion, which was a granuloma caused by Cryptococcus. *B,* A round lesion, an adenocarcinoma, peripherally located, that is more clearly defined on the planigram shown in *C.* The differentiation of these two lesions by diagnostic measures, short of thoracotomy, is difficult.

and for tuberculin aids in exclusion of these lesions. Occasionally, planigrams demonstrate a large area of circular and laminated calcium in the center of the coin lesion; when this is seen, the lesion is likely to be inflammatory. Rarely, it may represent a *hamartoma*. A small fleck of calcium does not exclude the presence of a carcinoma. Rarely, a bronchial cyst may also have to be considered.

Occasionally, a solitary *metastatic* lesion may be a problem. This always poses the question of how extensive a search should be pursued when a solitary pulmonary nodule has been found. According to Steele,[10] experience has shown that extensive diagnostic tests may not be helpful in most patients. There are, however, certain areas where "silent cancers" occur and cause pulmonary metastases. These include the kidney, colon, stomach, and pancreas.

## Symptoms Due to Inflammation and Ulceration of the Bronchial Wall

The lesion that causes this syndrome is nearly always an undifferentiated or a squamous cell carcinoma located in the larger bronchi. Cancers are frequently associated with considerable inflammatory response in the bronchus around them. When ulcerated, these tumors bleed freely. The inflammation and infiltration may cause a particularly harassing nonproductive cough. The lesion usually can be seen with the bronchoscope, and it frequently exfoliates cells. X-rays of the chest may be normal or show only signs of partial bronchial obstruction on careful study. This symptom complex commonly melds with the next type.

## Obstructive Pneumonitis Due to Carcinoma of the Lung

The most common group of symptoms associated with carcinoma of the lung is that due to infection resulting from either complete or partial obstruction of the bronchus by the carcinoma (Fig. 5). Squamous cell and undifferentiated tumors are the usual cause of this syndrome. When drainage of the bronchus distal to the cancer becomes impeded, secondary infection occurs. The infection may cause cough, pleurisy, temperature elevation, and all the other symptoms associated with pneumonitis. If the bronchus is completely obstructed, atelectasis may occur first and then infection develops later.

On *physical examination* the important findings are associated with infection and atelectasis. If the obstruction is incomplete and the lung is even partially aerated distal to this point, an expiratory wheeze may be demonstrated.

The most common finding on x-ray is that of a pneumonitis associated with atelectasis. This may involve a segment, a lobe, or an entire lung. Atelectasis causes loss of lung volume, with mediastinal shift and a typical area of consolidation.

The infection may proceed to abscess formation unless antibiotics are administered. Fortunately, most patients receive antibiotic therapy before the surgeon is consulted, and the initial response is usually good, with correction of most of the patient's symptoms. The characteristic finding, however, is persistence of the x-ray changes. Most primary bacterial pneumonias tend to clear rapidly with antibiotic therapy, but viral pneu-

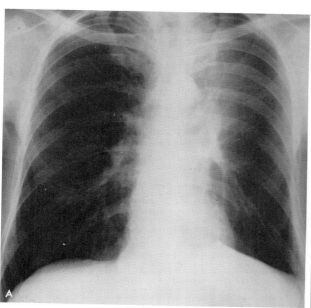
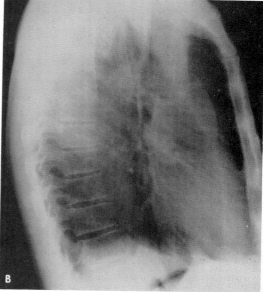

**Figure 5** Films from a patient with a squamous cell carcinoma of the lung causing collapse of the left upper lobe. This is seen high in the apex and quite far anteriorly (*B*). In *A*, the mediastinal shift is marked, the left diaphragm is high, the heart is shifted toward the left, and there is overdistension of the remaining left lower lobe.

monitis may respond more slowly, and this may provide a source of difficulty in differential diagnosis.

A subgroup under this heading includes cases in which infection accompanies necrosis of a large peripheral cancer, especially an epidermoid carcinoma. The necrotic lesions may drain into a bronchus, and infection may either precede or follow this event. On the x-ray, the shadow of the thick wall cavity with papillary projections into it is typical. Acute symptoms usually respond to antibiotics.

### Symptoms Due to Extension of the Carcinoma to Adjacent Areas

The initial finding in carcinoma of the lung may be evidence of local extension of the carcinoma into surrounding structures (Fig. 6). The symptoms can be divided into several syndromes. In the best known, the *Pancoast syndrome,* the tumors are almost always *squamous* or poorly *differentiated* lesions that originate in the apex of the lung and then spread to the adjacent chest wall, involving the cords of the brachial plexus or the upper one or two intercostal nerves. Later, involvement of the superior cervical ganglion causes *Horner's syndrome.* Eventually, the tumor invades the adjacent rib, transverse process, or vertebral body. Pain referral occurs at various times, over most of the distribution of the brachial plexus, giving pain in the arm, in the hand over the ulnar distribution to the fingers, the shoulder, the scapular region, the jaw, and the pectoral area. Characteristically, the pain is not very bothersome during the day but is quite difficult to control at night.

Physical examination may yield little information since neurologic signs may not be present.

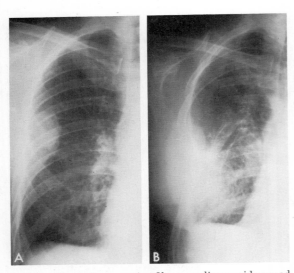

**Figure 6**  *A,* Preoperative film revealing a widespread squamous cell carcinoma originating in the peripheral portion of the right lung. This had involved the three ribs and the interspaces. It was removed by wide resection. The chest wall was reconstructed with a free rib graft and soft tissue, and no plastic material was needed (*B*).

X-ray studies are usually diagnostic, but often the lesion must be suspected before it is found on the x-ray film because it lies adjacent to dense shadows of the apex and of the mediastinum. Spot films over the ribs and spine as well as planigrams through the area may demonstrate the lesion more clearly and may also reveal unsuspected areas of bone erosion.

The *superior vena caval syndrome* may be caused by invasion of the lymph nodes around the vena cava or by extension of the carcinoma into the wall of the vena cava. The onset of venous occlusion is usually so acute that it is associated with alarming swelling and edema of the upper extremity, neck, and face and the prompt development of many superficial collateral veins about the chest. Laryngeal edema rarely occurs, although some patients may have cough syncope. Headaches are frequent. Since the lesion is close to the mediastinum, it may be difficult to detect on x-ray.

Carcinoma of the lung can directly invade the pericardium and may rarely cause cardiac tamponade requiring surgical intervention. It may extend the esophagus and cause a fistula or obstruction. Another common location of direct spread of lung cancer is the chest wall, and pain over the intercostal nerves may be the presenting symptom.

### Symptoms Due to Distant Metastasis from Carcinoma of the Lung

Carcinomas of the lung readily invade the pulmonary venous system and have direct access to the arterial system. Metastatic cancer from the lung frequently involves the liver. This may be shown by palpation, by radioisotope liver scan, and by liver function studies, and confirmed by needle biopsy. In autopsy series, the incidence of bone involvement is about 30 per cent. The most common site of lung cancer metastasis is the adrenal glands, although rarely does a recognizable clinical picture result. Manifestations of carcinoma of the lung due to unusual metastases are not infrequent. They may occur in the thumb, around the anal margin, and on the scalp. Involvement of the central nervous system, with signs of a space-consuming lesion, and spread to joints and peripheral nerves, causing severe pain, are frequent admission complaints. These manifestations are the reason for admission to the hospital in 15 to 20 per cent of cases of carcinoma of the lung.

### Symptoms Due to Extrapulmonary Nonmetastatic Manifestations of Carcinoma of the Lung

Since each cell in the body has the potential to perform the function of any other cell, it is not unexpected to find that the dedifferentiation occurs physiologically as well as morphologically in cancer of the lung (Fig. 7). Substances with an endocrine action and toxic substances have both been recognized as arising from lung cancer. In addition, an antigen may be elaborated that sensitizes the patient to his own tissue. Therefore, degenera-

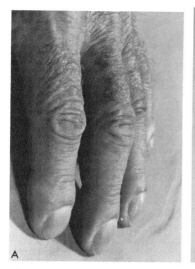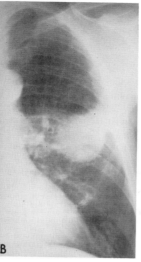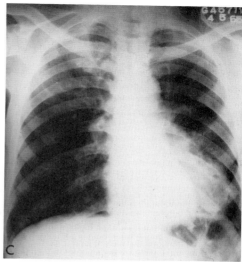

**Figure 7** *A*, Marked clubbing of fingers in a patient with a poorly differentiated carcinoma of the lung. *B*, Condition in a 65 year old male. *C*, Poorly differentiated carcinoma originating in the left lower lung that was associated with hypercalcemia. After surgical removal blood chemistry reverted to normal.

tive changes, particularly in the central nervous system, may follow.

The most common of these hormonal manifestations is a fulminant type of *Cushing's syndrome*, due to elaboration of an ACTH-like substance by the carcinoma (usually an oat cell type). Parathyroid hormone can also be elaborated by carcinomas of the lung (usually squamous cell type) and causes a rather rapid onset of symptoms, with a high calcium level and marked mental changes. Occasionally, a carcinoma of the lung elaborates *antidiuretic hormone.* A poorly differentiated cancer or an adenocarcinoma is most frequently responsible, and the principal clinical manifestation is mental confusion, as is also true in Cushing's syndrome and hyperparathyroidism associated with carcinoma of the lung. The serum sodium level may drop to 110 to 120 mEq. per liter. The only effective symptomatic treatment is reduction of fluid intake to as little as 800 ml. per day in order to maintain sodium levels high enough to correct systemic symptoms.

*Pulmonary osteoarthropathy* is the most common nonmetastatic extrapulmonary syndrome associated with carcinoma of the lung. The lesion in the lung may be a small, solitary, asymptomatic nodule. The *sudden* onset of clubbing of the fingers in an adult is highly suggestive of lung cancer, although it occurs in a variety of other pulmonary disorders. The clubbing is due to vascular proliferation in the bone at the tips of the fingers, and the classic sign of ballottement of the nail base, a raised, convex nail bed, and red hyperemic skin over terminal phalanges are seen. There may be edema and swelling of the small joints of the hand and ankles and the complaint of pain in the knees. X-ray examination reveals periosteal proliferation of the long bones, and the metacarpals and metatarsals may also be involved. Removal of the can-

cer is followed by almost immediate and dramatic relief of joint pains and rapid subsidence of clubbing.

Another bizarre manifestation of carcinoma of the lung is degeneration in the brain, principally the cerebellum. This is thought to be due to the elaboration of antibodies to brain tissue incited by an antigen derived from the carcinoma. A similar situation occurs in the posterior lateral columns of the spinal cord. Carcinoma of the lung may cause myasthenia, gynecomastia, and peripheral neuritis. Dermatomyositis as well as "toxic" dermatitis may also be found in patients with carcinoma of the lung.

## DIAGNOSIS OF CARCINOMA OF THE LUNG[1, 6]

Carcinoma of the lung with its varied manifestations may mimic most of the inflammatory diseases of the lung. The most reliable diagnostic maneuver is a careful history. Physical examination affords an opportunity to elicit signs of the primary lesion and to find evidence of spread to regional nodes, liver, skin, and bone. There may be evidence of consolidation of the lung, fluid in the thorax, or complete or partial bronchial obstruction. Unusual signs of extrapulmonary change such as clubbing of fingers, periarticular and joint changes, skin changes, and evidence of Cushing habitus may be present.

Radiologic changes are of prime importance. Careful study provides a unique opportunity to relate these changes to the history, physical, and operative findings. The usual posterior-anterior and lateral films, supplemented only when indicated with spot films and planigrams, usually suffice. With careful correlation of the physical examination, history and x-ray, it is possible to make the clinical diagnosis in most patients with lung cancer.

The more complicated and expensive diagnostic procedures for long cancer are indicated for two reasons: (1) to determine microscopically the presence of the cancer; and (2) to determine the extent of the cancer not evident by history, physical examination, or the x-ray study.

Examination of the sputum for malignant cells may be diagnostic in 60 to 80 per cent of patients with lung cancer, particularly if the small peripheral carcinomas are excluded. False-positive results are rare, but a negative result does not exclude a cancer.

Bronchoscopy is the next most important diagnostic measure employed to obtain a positive microscopic diagnosis and to determine the extent of the cancer. Lesions that originate in the larger bronchi (usually *squamous cell* or *undifferentiated* lesions) may be seen on bronchoscopic examination. A positive diagnosis is obtained in 30 to 40 per cent of patients. Occasionally, blind biopsy of the mucosa in areas close to the cancer may yield positive results. Bronchoscopy also affords an excellent opportunity to obtain washings of the bronchial system for cytologic study. A brush can be passed into the bronchus leading to the lesion to obtain appropriate material. Indirect signs of cancer such as fixation, blunting, and widening of the carina can be seen. Bronchial adenomas can be frequently visualized and have a typical appearance. They are notorious for brisk bleeding after biopsy.

Bronchography is sometimes employed in the diagnosis of carcinoma of the lung when there is either a deformity or complete obstruction of the bronchus. Bronchography is not particularly useful since the presence of bronchial secretions or blood clots can simulate bronchial obstruction and lead to uncertainty in interpretation. Bronchial brushing with fluoroscopic control may be helpful in obtaining a positive diagnosis of cancer and may demonstrate a specific organism causing an inflammatory nodule in the lung. A peripheral lesion may be approached externally with an aspirating needle, preferably with fluoroscopic guidance. There is danger of inducing pneumothorax, producing air emboli, implanting cells in the pleura and chest wall, and injuring a large blood vessel.

Scalene lymph node biopsy will occasionally demonstrate metastases even when nodes are not palpable. It has been accepted with considerable enthusiasm, and, unfortunately, has become in some instances a routine study in all patients suspected of having lung cancer. The scalenus anticus muscle is easily approached through a small anterior neck incision after the sternomastoid muscle is split. There is a fat pad located in this area which can easily be removed. The right scalene nodes tend to drain both the right lung and the left lower lobe, and when the lesion is on the left side both the right and left scalene areas should be examined. It has been optimistically estimated that in 10 to 15 per cent of cases node excision gives a positive diagnosis in the absence of palpable nodes. This procedure should not be employed as a routine diagnostic procedure but is indicated in: (1) patients with palpable lymph nodes in the low cervical area, (2) those with mediastinal lymph node enlargement, and (3) certain elderly patients in whom cytologic examination is negative and a microscopic diagnosis is needed to provide a firm basis for radiation therapy.

As an extension of scalene node biopsy, *mediastinoscopy* may be performed. This is essentially an exploration of the mediastinum with a laryngoscope, and it requires general anesthesia. A midline low neck incision is made, the pretracheal fascia is identified, and then a space beneath it is developed. Finally, an instrument similar to a laryngoscope is introduced into the developed space. On the right side, the dissection may be extended to the tracheal bifurcation and permits examination of the paratracheal nodes. On the left side, the extent of the exploration is limited because of the transverse aorta. It is obvious that such a procedure involves risk of complications, should be performed in the operating room, and requires the presence of an anesthesiologist. Similar information can be obtained at some risk by using the bed of the second costal cartilage to gain access to the mediastinum.

Exploratory thoracotomy is indicated in many patients for microscopic determination of extent of disease and is extended for surgical treatment when appropriate. A small chest incision can be made and extended as necessary if the lesion proves to be operable.

## TREATMENT OF CANCER OF THE LUNG

The surgeon must seek to answer two questions in planning treatment for carcinoma of the lung: (1) is the patient likely to be *cured*? and (2) if not, will surgery, radiation, or chemotherapy provide *palliation*? Evidence of distant metastases is easy to demonstrate in approximately a quarter of the patients with lung cancer. The usual sites are the central nervous system, bones, joints, liver, or pleura. Involvement of any of the areas rules out a cure and usually prohibits a palliative operation. Local invasion by the carcinoma may also be evident, although this may not always be a contraindication to curative surgery. *Superior sulcus tumors* have been successfully treated with a combination of radiation and wide excision of the involved chest wall. Occlusion of the superior vena cava may be evident and, except in rare instances, is a contraindication to surgery. Extension into the esophagus, causing obstructive symptoms, or into the pericardium, causing effusion, occasionally occurs. Either indicates that the cancer is incurable.

Pleural invasion from carcinoma of the lung by direct extension can cause multiple pleural implants and bloody effusion. When the pleura is involved by permeation of the lymphatics, the pleural fluid may be straw-colored. Rarely, pleural effusion is associated with obstructive pneumonitis secondary to carcinoma in the bronchus. Cytologic examination of the pleural fluid generally is more difficult, but cancer cells can usually be identified. Needle biopsy of the pleura should also be tried. When spread of the cancer to the pleura causes effusion, the cancer is not removable. *Paralysis* of the recurrent laryngeal nerve may occur from extension of the carcinoma. The left nerve is involved more frequently than the right. Recurrent nerve involvement is, without exception, an indication that the lung lesion is not removable. *Phrenic* nerve paralysis occurs from direct extension of the tumor into the phrenic nerve. Rarely, one may find a situation, when the extension is local, involving the nerve as it courses along the pericardium. Then the pericardium along with the tumor can be removed. Horner's syndrome indicates stellate ganglion invasion and irremovability.

Involvement of the scalene nodes and paratracheal nodes with carcinoma is a definite contraindication to direct surgical attack on the lesion. Involvement of the liver, a common site of metastasis, can be identified by physical examination and radioactive scan followed by needle biopsy. Then only symptomatic treatment is indicated.

After careful evaluation of the extent of the tumor, the total physical condition of the patient must be considered, particularly the state of the respiratory and cardiovascular systems. These two factors not only will limit the extent of resection but sometimes may contraindicate completely any type of surgical intervention. Pulmonary function must be evaluated carefully from the history and physical and x-ray findings as well as direct measurements of ventilatory and respiratory function. The latter include blood gas determinations and measurement of lung volumes and gas flow rates. For example, when one plans a pneumonectomy, provided the lesion does not greatly affect the function of the involved lung, the values for ventilatory function should be at least 75 per cent of normal. If the entire lung has been rendered functionless by the cancer, ventilatory function values of 50 per cent of normal would be sufficient. Certainly, when ventilatory measurements are below 50 per cent of normal and are associated with abnormal arterial $pO_2$ and $pCO_2$, great care should be exercised in considering removal of any functioning pulmonary tissue. The functional status of the cardiovascular system is almost as important as the functional status of the pulmonary system. The majority of patients with lung cancer are smokers and middle-aged or older, and thus have a high incidence of coronary artery disease. A history of myocardial infarction or angina pectoris may be a contraindication to pneumonectomy, from the point of view of both long-time function and immediate survival after operation. However, many patients will withstand lobectomy if proper measures are instituted to prevent shock and hypoxia during and immediately after surgery.

Throughout various accounts of experiences

with carcinoma of the lung, admonitions are found concerning the incurable nature of undifferentiated carcinoma, particularly of the oat cell type. It would be an exaggeration to imply that a poorly differentiated carcinoma, whether oat cell, small round cell, or large cell, is likely to be a curable lesion. However, any tumor that can be removed surgically with assurance that all of the local tumor has been excised should be treated, regardless of the diagnosis of cell type. When it is decided that the lesion is amenable to complete removal, the surgical procedure is removal of the primary site and the local extension. Evaluation of the results of treatment should be on this basis. Thus, a lobectomy that removes all the tumor and all the involved nodes should be as curative as a pneumonectomy that accomplishes this. In certain instances, a segmental resection or even wide local excision might well have the same result, provided it fulfills the principles given.

*Pneumonectomy* is indicated for all lesions that originate in the stem bronchi and the lobar branches, when the physiologic status of the patient permits. The technique of pneumonectomy consists of division of both pulmonary veins and the main pulmonary artery and transection of the bronchus as close to the trachea as feasible. The bronchus is best closed with nonabsorbable sutures. Prevention of bronchopleural fistulas is further enhanced if second layers of pleura or adjacent mediastinal tissue are provided. Some have advocated extending the scope of the pneumonectomy to what could be called a radical pneumonectomy by removal of all the lymph nodes that drain the lung, along with the lymphatics and fatty and areolar tissue. This means beginning just below the subclavian artery and extending the dissection in the anterior and posterior mediastinum downward to the hilum of the lung. The great vessels are then ligated within the pericardium. A portion of the pericardial sac may be removed. The dissection is extended inferiorly in order to remove all the lymphatics in the mediastinum. Unfortunately, there is no indication from reported results that this type of pneumonectomy gives any better result than the standard one. The mortality ranges from 5 to 20 per cent.

*Lobectomy* is indicated for peripheral carcinomas, that is, those in areas away from stem and lobar bronchi. When there are nodes at the hilum, cure by lobectomy is not probable. The bronchus should be amputated as high as possible and all lymphatics in the hilar area adjacent to the lobe should be removed. Occasionally, there may be direct extension of the carcinoma from one lobe to an adjacent one. If this is not extensive, wide local excision of the adjacent lobe in continuity with the lobe containing the tumor can be performed. The results insofar as cure is concerned are similar to those with pneumonectomy. The operative mortality is about 2 per cent as compared with 5 to 20 per cent with pneumonectomy. In some poor-risk patients, a segmental resection may occasionally result in cure.

Bronchial adenomas of the carcinoid type deserve special consideration. They are low-grade malignant tumors and thus particularly amenable to local excision and to "sleeve" resection. There are special surgical procedures that may be indicated in rare instances. Occasionally, operations for removal of tumors about the tracheal bifurcation, especially cylindromas, may require cardiopulmonary bypass. Chest wall infiltration with the cancer may sometimes be removed by block dissection together with lobectomy. Reconstitution of the chest wall can nearly always be achieved without using a prosthesis.

*Anesthesia* for pulmonary surgery for cancer deserves comment. Adequate ventilation is needed for prevention of hypoxia and hypercarbia, both of which are precursors of cardiac arrest. Bleeding from the chest wall has been easier to control since the introduction of nonexplosive agents has permitted the use of electrocautery. The use of the blocking agents at the myoneural junction has made both the problem of hemorrhage and the problem of intraoperative ventilation easier to deal with.

Postoperative care directed toward maintenance of the airway is particularly important since anesthetic agents, trauma to airways, hemorrhage in the lung, and postoperative pain all interfere with maintenance of its patency. Turning and encouraging of coughing are the most important preventive measures. Intratracheal suction is the most useful procedure for refractory situations, and only rarely is bronchoscopy necessary. In some poor-risk patients, postoperative respiratory assistance may be needed, first with a nasotracheal tube and later with tracheostomy. Drain-

age of the pleural cavity with underwater seal is indicated after all resection procedures except pneumonectomy.

As in other cancers within the body cavities, the use of radiation before and after surgery for lung cancer is recommended by some. Paulson and colleagues have reported excellent results with this combination in the treatment of cancers of the apex of the lung that have invaded the chest wall and neurovascular structures. In such instances, between 2500 and 3000 rads is usually employed, and the tumor is removed about 4 weeks later. The resection may be extensive, including ribs, transverse process, part of the vertebral bodies, and occasionally portions of the brachial plexus. If the dose of radiation is greater than that recommended, the bronchial stump may not heal and prevention of infection may be difficult. The use of this combination, particularly if larger doses of radiation are used, is associated with too many complications and has been abandoned.

The use of radiation after surgery is also advocated by many. It is again difficult to be certain whether or not this is beneficial. It is probably reasonable to use postoperative radiation in those patients in whom cancer-containing lymph nodes remain in the mediastinum or when the margin of the bronchial stump is close to or involved with cancer.

In patients with irremovable cancers (Fig. 8) and in those deemed poor surgical candidates because of the presence of severe cardiovascular or respiratory dysfunction, radiation therapy is an excellent means of palliation. When cobalt is given in two 5 day courses, 3 weeks apart (with a

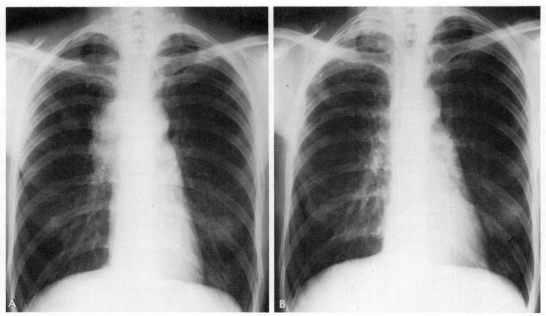

**Figure 8** *A*, Pretreatment film of a 45 year old woman with poorly differentiated carcinoma originating in the right upper lobe. There are metastases to the superior mediastinal lymph nodes. *B*, After a course of cobalt therapy (5000 rads given in two courses of 5 days each, 3 weeks apart), the upper lobe lesion and the metastases disappeared. The patient was symptom-free for 16 months, after treatment.

total of 5500 to 6000 rads delivered to the lesion), good palliation can be obtained with little morbidity. Enthusiasm for the use of chemotherapy in these patients waxes and wanes. Unfortunately, drugs are rarely effective in most carcinomas of the lung. Occasionally, a good response occurs in a patient with a very poorly differentiated cancer, particularly when the cancer has shown a rapid response to radiation therapy. Otherwise, chemotherapy may only aggravate the patient's terminal illness.

## Results of Treatment

Appraisals of the results of treatment of cancer of the lung frequently overemphasize the goal of 5 year survival and neglect the attainment of palliative results. The former can be easily expressed, but the latter is more difficult to evaluate. Careful application of surgery in some incurable cancers can reduce or eliminate the chances of repeated pulmonary infection, hemorrhage, and a harassing productive cough. In others, radiation will achieve the same result. Radiation is of great help in relieving pain from metastases to bone and soft tissue and occasionally other central nervous system symptoms. Unfortunately, neurosurgical procedures, such as root section and chordotomy, are only rarely helpful. Occasionally, craniotomy is needed to relieve increased intracranial pressure. In some, the nonmetastatic extrapulmonary symptoms of lung cancer can be effectively relieved by appropriate medical therapy. In terms of survival in the incurable group, there may be little or no difference between untreated patients and those treated with surgery, chemotherapy, or radiation, all surviving 6 to 8 months on the average. Rarely, survival will continue beyond 1 year.

The results of surgical treatment have changed little if any over the past 25 years. Surgical mortality has decreased, and there has been a trend away from pneumonectomy toward lobectomy. In about 50 per cent of the patients, the cancer is considered irremovable when the patient is first seen. Of those operated upon, approximately half have a removable lesion, 25 per cent of all patients. Of the ones with a removable lesion, about 35 per cent achieve a 5 year cure; *this represents a survival of about 8 per cent for the total sample for a period of 5 years.* Among patients with the more malignant cancers, such as oat cell carcinomas, there is only a rare 5 year survivor. Adenocarcinoma also has a poor prognosis. Bronchiolar carcinoma has a relatively good prognosis, almost as good as that of epidermoid cancer. In a series of 1205 patients from Memorial Hospital of New York admitted with squamous cell carcinomas (from a total of 2565 lung cancer patients), exploration was performed in 51 per cent but resection was done in only 24 per cent. Of those who underwent resection, 35 per cent survived 5 years. In other words, 17 per cent of the patients operated upon, or 9 per cent of those admitted, were alive at 5 years. In the Memorial Hospital experience with 368 patients with the most malignant of the un-

differentiated carcinomas (oat cell lesions), only 18 pneumonectomies, 6 lobectomies, and 3 subtotal resections were performed, and there were only *three* 5 year survivors.

Carcinoma of the lung is a major surgical problem because not only treatment but also diagnosis is nearly always obtained by surgery. The disorder is of great public interest because of the high incidence of the disease among smokers. In the 35 years since the operation became established, the results of surgical treatment have changed very little. This statement could be applied to the results of surgical treatment of most malignant tumors of epithelial origin.

## REFERENCES

1. Auerbach, O., Gere, J. B., Forman, J. B., Petrick, T. G., Smolin, H. J., Muehsam, G. E., Kassouny, D. Y., and Stout, A. P.: Changes in bronchial epithelium in relation to smoking and cancer of the lung: Report of progress. New Eng. J. Med., 250:97, 1957.
   The Health Consequences of Smoking: A Public Health Service Review: 1967. Washington, D.C., U.S. Department of Health, Education and Welfare, Public Health Service.
   Silverberg, E., and Holleb, A. I.: Cancer statistics, 1971. Cancer, 21:13, 1971.
   *These papers relate the statistical and clinical evidence of the possible relationship between smoking and cancer.*

2. Aylwin, J. A.: Avoidable vascular spread in resection for bronchial carcinoma. Thorax, 6:250, 1951.
   Baird, J. A.: The pathways of lymphatic spread of carcinoma of the lung. Brit. J. Surg., 52:868, 1965.
   Borrie, J.: Lung Cancer. New York, Appleton-Century-Crofts, 1965.
   *These works discuss the manner of spread of carcinoma of the lung.*

3. Berger, R. L., Boyd, T. F., and Strieder, J. W.: Complications of scalene lymph node biopsy. J. Thorac. Cardiovasc. Surg., 45:307, 1963.
   Carlens, E.: Mediastinoscopy: A method for inspection and tissue biopsy in the superior mediastinum. Dis. Chest, 36:343, 1959.
   Daniels, A. C.: A method of biopsy useful in diagnosing certain intra-thoracic disease. Dis. Chest, 16:360, 1949.
   Palva, T.: Mediastinoscopy. Chicago, Ill., Year Book Medical Publishers, 1964.
   *These articles give the rationale, technique, and results of three procedures designed for diagnosis and determination of the spread of carcinoma to lymphatics of mediastinum and cervical area.*

4. Clagett, O. T., Allen, T. H., Payne, W. S., and Woolner, L. B.: The surgical treatment of pulmonary neoplasms: A ten-year experience. J. Thorac. Cardiovasc. Surg., 48:391, 1964.
   *This paper describes the experience in an excellent clinic with a large series of patients.*

5. Fry, W. A., and Manalo-Estralla, P.: Bronchial brushing. Surg. Gynec. Obstet., 130:67, 1970.
   *Bronchial brushing is a standard diagnostic procedure for lung cancer. Not only does it afford an opportunity for direct biopsy, but it permits bronchial washings, sponging, and brushing.*

6. Galofre, M., Payne, W. S., Woolner, L. B., Clagett, O. T., and Gage, R. P.: Pathologic classification and surgical treatment of bronchogenic carcinoma. Surg. Gynec. Obstet., 119:51, 1964.
   Hyde, L., Yee, J., Wilson, R., and Patno, M. E.: Cell type and the natural history of lung cancer. J.A.M.A., 193:52, 1965.
   Storey, C. F., Knudtson, K. P., and Lawrence, B. J.: Bronchial (alveolar cell) cancer of the lung. J. Thorac. Surg., 26:331, 1953.
   *These references give descriptions of classification of bronchogenic cancer. Because of the varied morphology, considerable*

*effort is given to defining clearly boundaries that are in fact indistinct.*

7. Graham, E. A., and Singer, J. J.: Successful removal of an entire lung for carcinoma of the bronchus. J.A.M.A., *101:* 1371, 1933.
   *The first successful pneumonectomy for carcinoma is described in this paper. The patient, a physician, was cured and continued the practice of medicine until death from other causes many years later.*

8. Hughes, F. A., Higgins, G. A., and Beebe, G. W.: Present status of surgical adjuvant lung-cancer chemotherapy. J.A.M.A., *196:*343, 1966.
   *This paper describes attempts at palliation of carcinoma of the lung with nitrogen mustard.*

9. Sealy, W. C.: Non-metastatic extra pulmonary manifestations of bronchogenic carcinoma. Surgery, *68:*906, 1970.
   *This interesting clinical picture resulting from physiologic*

*aberrations of lung cancer is of importance from the point of view of both understanding the disease and planning palliative treatment of the patient.*

10. Steele, J. D.: The Solitary Pulmonary Nodule. Springfield, Ill., Charles C Thomas, 1964 (Also, J. Thorac. Cardiovasc. Surg., *46:*21, 1963.)
    *This is an excellent summary of the experience in treating the solitary pulmonary nodule in a large number of Veterans Administration Hospitals. Although most of the patients were men, the author's clear outline of the problems of management and their solutions is helpful.*

11. Watson, W. L.: Lung Cancer. St. Louis, C. V. Mosby Company, 1968.
    *This is an excellent review of the entire subject of lung cancer with abundant historical references concerning both anesthesia and the development of surgical approach to lung cancer.*

# XIII

# Thoracic Outlet Syndrome

## *Donald Silver, M.D.*

The thoracic outlet syndrome is the preferred term for those syndromes, e.g., the cervical rib syndrome, scalenus anticus syndrome, hyperabduction syndrome, costoclavicular syndrome, pectoralis minor syndrome, and the first thoracic rib syndrome, which result from compression of the neurovascular structures to the upper extremities. The thoracic outlet syndrome is a symptom complex consisting of either neural or vascular (arterial and/or venous) disorders, or both, of the upper extremities caused by compression of the brachial plexus or subclavian-axillary artery or vein in the region between the thoracic outlet and the insertion of the pectoralis minor onto the coracoid process. Symptoms may arise from neural, arterial, or venous compression, or any combination thereof.

### HISTORICAL ASPECTS

One of the earliest descriptions of the thoracic outlet syndrome appeared in 1860, when a Dr. Willshire reported a pulsating subclavian artery (possibly an aneurysm) that crossed a presumed cervical rib.[21] In 1861, Coote excised a cervical rib to relieve pressure on the axillary vessels and nerves.[4] Murphy in 1905[10] and Keen in 1907[8] emphasized the role of cervical ribs in the etiology of the neurovascular symptoms. In 1919, Stopford and Telford demonstrated that the brachial plexus and subclavian artery could be compressed by the thoracic rib and indicated that resection of the rib would relieve symptoms.[17]

In 1927, Adson and Coffey emphasized the role of the scalene muscles in the neurovascular com-

pression and popularized scalenotomy as a method of therapy.[2] Various operative maneuvers were tried with varying degrees of success until 1962, when the role of the first rib, and the ligamentous and muscular attachments to it, in the pathogenesis of the thoracic outlet syndrome was reemphasized.[3,6] Since then, the preferred form of operative therapy has been resection of the first rib with division of the pectoralis minor tendon if the symptoms are produced by hyperabduction.

### ANATOMY

An understanding of the spaces of potential pressure in the thoracic outlet region is necessary for proper evaluation and treatment of this syndrome. The anterior rami of five spinal nerves, C5, C6, C7, C8, and T1 (C4 and T2 may also contribute to the brachial plexus), exit through the intervertebral foramina and form trunks that pass through the scalene triangle and then divide behind the clavicle. The divisions of the trunks reunite to form cords that surround the axillary artery as it passes behind the pectoralis minor tendon. The motor and sensory branches of the brachial plexus are usually distal to the pectoralis minor tendon.

Rami from C8 and T1 form the lowest trunk, which lies on the first rib behind the subclavian artery and is responsible for the groove in the rib (which is often attributed to the artery). The peripheral distribution of C8 and T1 provides sensory reception from the fifth finger and medial half of the fourth finger and from the medial aspect of the forearm. The motor distribution of these rami controls flexion of the wrist and fingers and innervates the intrinsic muscles of the hand.

Both subclavian arteries exit from the thorax behind the sternoclavicular joints and pass over the first rib between the scalenus medius and scalenus anticus muscles. The arteries then course laterally behind the clavicles and become the axillary arteries. The axillary arteries pass posterior to the tendons of the pectoralis minor and become the brachial arteries.

The axillary veins pass behind the costocoracoid ligaments and pectoralis minor tendons. At the edge of the first rib, each axillary vein becomes a subclavian vein which passes over the first rib *anterior* to the scalenus anticus muscle to join the jugular vein at the base of the neck before it enters the thorax as the innominate vein. Each vein courses through a narrow area consisting of the first rib and the scalenus anticus muscle posteriorly, and the costocoracoid ligament, subclavian muscle, and clavicle anteriorly.

The arteries, veins, and components of the brachial plexus may be compressed in any of several areas as they pass from the neck or the thoracic outlet into the upper extremity. The sites of compression from medial to lateral include: (1) the interscalene triangle (arteries and nerves); (2) the space between the scalenus anticus muscle and the clavicle (vein); (3) the first rib, or between the first rib and clavicle (nerves, arteries, and veins); (4) the costocoracoid fascia (nerves, arteries, and veins); (5) the pectoralis minor tendon (nerves, arteries, and veins).

Other anatomic functional causes of compression of the neurovascular structures include:

1. Cervical ribs, which occur in approximately 1 per cent of the population and are bilateral in 80 per cent of the cases. Cervical ribs compress or irritate portions of the adjacent brachial plexus and compress or elevate the subclavian artery. However, less than 10 per cent of cervical ribs produce symptoms.

2. Long transverse processes of C7, which may function as cervical ribs.

3. Abnormal first thoracic ribs. These ribs frequently fail to reach the sternum, may be attached to the sternum or to the second rib by ligaments, and may cause distortion or compression of the lowest components of the brachial plexus.

4. Postural changes during which there is downward displacement of the upper extremity and shoulder girdle. Occupations that require carrying heavy loads or working in narrow quarters so that the upper extremities are drawn forward and down are frequently associated with thoracic outlet symptoms.

5. Occupations that require hyperabduction.

6. Acquired lesions such as fractures of the first rib or clavicle with deformity or callus formation.

## SYMPTOMS

The symptoms of the thoracic outlet syndrome vary, depending on the vessels or nerves compressed. The symptoms may be neurologic or vascular or both. The clinical manifestations rarely indicate the site of obstruction. Neurologic symptoms consist of pain, paresthesias, and numbness, usually in the fingers and hands. The symptoms usually occur in an ulnar distribution, but may occur anywhere in the upper extremity or shoulder girdle. Late neurologic defects include sensory loss, motor weakness, and atrophy.

Symptoms of arterial compression include ischemic pain, numbness, fatigue, paresthesias, coldness, and weakness in the arm or hand. These symptoms are accentuated by exercise and exposure to cold. Thromboses may occur in the compressed or poststenotic dilated areas of subclavian-axillary artery and produce distal ischemic changes. Distal embolization may also be part of the picture. The venous symptoms include pain, swelling, aching, distal edema, and cyanosis.

## DIAGNOSIS

A complete history and a thorough physical examination should establish the diagnosis in most cases. The symptom complexes plus a history of trauma with fracture(s) of the clavicle or ribs or both, a history of unusual exercise or occupation, poor posture, sagging bed, and so forth, should suggest the thoracic outlet syndrome. A careful history will also indicate whether or not the symptoms are part of a generalized process such as occurs with cord tumors, multiple peripheral embolizations, osteoarthritis, and collagen or metabolic disorders.

The physical examination should be thorough, with special emphasis given to detecting the neural, arterial, and venous signs. Neural signs include sensory deficits, weakness, and atrophy. Most often the sensory and motor deficits occur in the distribution of the ulnar nerve. Signs of arterial compression include weakened or absent brachial and radial pulses, a bruit in the supraclavicular or axillary space, delayed capillary blush, and occasional areas of distal gangrene. Signs of venous compression include distended veins, distal edema, and cyanosis.

The physical findings are not constant, and several examinations may be required before the thoracic outlet syndrome is suspected. The findings may vary according to the patient's position. Except when produced by hyperabduction, compression is rarely detected when patients are examined in the supine position, but is usually readily detected when the patient is sitting or standing. There are three specific diagnostic maneuvers for the thoracic outlet syndrome:

1. Adson or scalene maneuver.[1,2] While the physician monitors the radial pulse, the patient takes a deep breath, extends the neck, and turns the chin toward the side being examined. Disappearance or reduction of the radial pulse constitutes a positive finding. During a positive test a bruit frequently will become audible in the supraclavicular fossa, and the hand may become cool

and pale. The deep breath causes elevation of the first rib, and extending and turning the neck causes narrowing of the interscalene triangle. The symptoms are caused by compression of the subclavian artery and probably the brachial plexus by the first rib and scalene muscles. If the pulse is altered before the head is turned, one should suspect the presence of a cervical rib.

2. Costoclavicular compressive maneuver.[5] While the radial pulse is monitored, the patient throws his shoulders back and downward into an exaggerated military position. Disappearance or reduction of the radial pulse with the appearance of subclavian bruit constitutes a positive finding. The results are produced by compression of the subclavian artery (or vein, or brachial plexus) between the clavicle and first rib.

3. Hyperabduction maneuver.[20] The radial pulse is monitored while the arm is passively moved into a hyperabducted position. Reduction or cessation of the radial pulse and the appearance of an axillary bruit indicate arterial compression by the pectoralis minor tendon.

### Objective Examinations

Roentgenograms of the neck and chest may demonstrate cervical ribs, anomalous first ribs, prominent transverse processes, bony exostoses, calluses, abnormalities of the clavicle, and so forth. The roentgenograms also yield information about narrowing of the intervertebral foramina and tumors. Myelograms may be necessary to demonstrate a cervical disc or other causes of cervical cord compression. Arteriograms will demonstrate sites of partial or complete arterial occlusion. Arteriography should be performed with the patient's arms by his side and while he is performing the Adson, costoclavicular, and hyperabduction maneuvers. Occasionally, poststenotic dilatation or aneurysms of the subclavian artery distal to the site of compression will be demonstrated. Phlebograms are useful to demonstrate the sites of compression of the axillary or subclavian vein, and to indicate whether these veins are totally or partially occluded.

Plethysmography[15] has been used to document arterial compression. This technique[18] records changes in digit volume that occur with each heartbeat and can demonstrate obstruction to arterial flow. Electromyography is useful in detecting sites of compression of peripheral nerves by recording the altered response of the distal muscles to proximal electrical stimuli. Nerve conduction times between the thoracic outlet and elbow and wrist may be significantly prolonged. These conduction times return to normal range after surgical relief of the compression.[19]

## MANAGEMENT

For all patients, except those with complete vascular occlusion or poststenotic aneurysm, initial management should consist of a trial of weight reduction and an exercise program directed toward improving posture, strengthening the elevators of the shoulder girdle, and avoiding hyperabduction. These measures relieve symptoms in 50[19] to 70 per cent of patients.[7,11] Nonoperative management seems to be most successful in the obese, middle-aged female with poor posture.

Patients with major neurologic or vascular complications and those who do not respond to nonoperative management should be offered surgical intervention. A variety of only partially successful operative procedures have been devised for managing the thoracic outlet syndrome. The operative management has included excision of a cervical rib, division of the scalenus anticus muscle, resection of the clavicle, and division of the pectoralis minor tendon.[12,16] Falconer and Li,[6] Clagett,[3] and Roos[14] have emphasized that removal of the major portion of the first rib effectively decompresses the neurovascular structures. Removal of the first rib, and of a cervical rib if it is present, has become the preferred method of treatment for the thoracic outlet syndrome.

Clagett suggested that the rib be removed through a posterior incision identical to that used

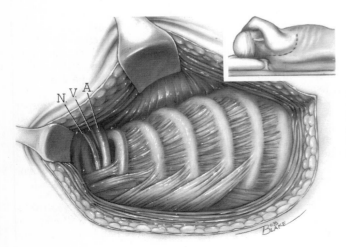

**Figure 1** Posterior approach to the first thoracic rib. The surgeon is behind the patient, who is in the left lateral decubitus position. Extension of the incision cephalad along the scapula provides exposure of the first rib, scalene muscles, brachial plexus (N.), and subclavian artery (A.) and vein (V.).

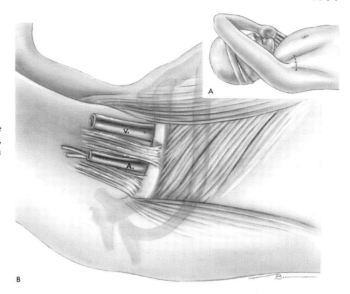

**Figure 2** The transaxillary approach to the first rib provides good exposure of the first rib, scalene muscles, brachial plexus, and subclavian artery (A.) and vein (V.).

for an upper thoracoplasty (Fig. 1). When the posterior approach is used, the subclavian vessels and brachial plexus are easily exposed and displaced anteriorly out of harm's way. Cervical ribs may also be easily excised through this approach, and it usually affords ample exposure for reconstructive vascular procedures when necessary.

Roos has popularized use of a transaxillary incision for removal of the rib (Fig. 2). The author prefers this incision, which is small and is readily hidden by the arm. The vessels and nerves are lifted off the first rib when the arm is hyperabducted during surgery. Of necessity, the scalene muscles are divided during removal of the rib. The disability is minimal and the postoperative course is usually uncomplicated. Most patients may be discharged by the third or fourth postoperative day and frequently return to work in 7 to 10 days. However, reconstructive vascular procedures are more difficult through this incision, and if reconstructive procedures are anticipated, the posterior approach is preferred.

Resection of the first thoracic rib, and of a cervical rib if it is present, effectively removes all the potential sites of neurovascular compression that produce the thoracic outlet syndrome save one. The neurovascular structures may be compressed by the pectoralis minor tendon when positions of hyperabduction are maintained. If, because of occupation or other reasons, the patient cannot avoid these positions, division of the tendon should be undertaken and can be performed through the posterior or transaxillary incision at the time the first rib is resected.

Nelson and Jenson[13] have employed an anterior extrapleural approach for excision of the first rib, and have found this incision to be cosmetically acceptable with a minimal complication rate. However, this approach is not suitable for removing cervical ribs or anomalous first ribs.

Although the limited operations often failed to relieve the symptoms of the thoracic outlet syndrome, resection of the first rib with an occasional division of the pectoralis minor tendon offers lasting relief to 90 per cent of the patients undergoing operation.

Mild poststenotic dilatation of the subclavian artery usually regresses once the compression is relieved. However, significant aneurysms of the artery should be excised and replaced with grafts, preferably vein grafts. Thrombosis of the subclavian artery should be treated by thromboendarterectomy or by replacement or bypass grafting of the involved segment. Thrombosis of the subclavian-axillary vein requires elimination of the causative factors and treatment with heparin, elevation, and an elastic sleeve until recanalization occurs. On rare occasions, a thrombectomy as suggested by Mahorner may be useful.[9]

## REFERENCES

1. Adson, A. W.: Surgical treatment for symptoms produced by cervical ribs and the scalenus anticus muscle. Surg. Gynec. Obstet., 85:687, 1947.
2. Adson, A. W., and Coffey, J. R.: Cervical rib: A method of anterior approach for relief of symptoms by division of scalenus anterior. Ann. Surg., 85:839, 1927.
3. Clagett, O. T.: Research and prosearch. Presidential Address. J. Thorac. Cardiovasc. Surg., 44:153, 1962.
4. Coote, H.: Pressure on the axillary vessels and nerve by the exostosis from a cervical rib: Interference with the circulation of the arm: Removal of the rib and exostosis: Recovery. Med. Times Gaz., 2:108, 1861; cited in Clagett.[3]
5. Falconer, M. A., and Li, F. W. P.: Resection of the first rib in costoclavicular compression of the brachial plexus. Lancet, 1:59, 1962.
6. Falconer, M. A., and Weddell, G.: Costoclavicular compression of the subclavian artery and vein: Relation to the scalenus anticus syndrome. Lancet, 2:539, 1943.
7. Haggart, G. E.: Value of conservative management in cervicobrachial pain. J.A.M.A., 137:508, 1948.
8. Keen, W.: The symptomatology, diagnosis, and surgical treatment of cervical ribs. Amer. J. Med. Sci., 133:173, 1907.
9. Mahorner, H., Castleberry, J. W., and Coleman, W. O.:

Attempts to restore function in major veins which are the site of massive thrombosis. Ann. Surg., *146*:510, 1957.

10. Murphy, J. B.: A case of cervical rib with symptoms resembling subclavian aneurysm. Ann. Surg., *41*:399, 1905.
11. Nelson, P. A.: Treatment of patients with cervicodorsal outlet syndrome. J.A.M.A., *163*:1570, 1957.
12. Nelson, R. M., and Davis, R. W.: Thoracic outlet compression syndrome. Ann. Thorac. Surg., *8*:437, 1969.
13. Nelson, R. M., and Jenson, C. B.: Anterior approach for excision of the first rib. Ann. Thorac. Surg., *9*:30, 1970.
14. Roos, D. B.: Transaxillary approach for first rib resection to relieve thoracic outlet syndrome. Ann. Surg., *163*:354, 1966.
15. Sanders, R. J., Monsour, J. W., and Baer, S. B.: Transaxillary first rib resection for the thoracic outlet syndrome. Arch. Surg., *97*:1014, 1968.
16. Silver, D.: The thoracic outlet syndrome. In: Lewis' Practice of Surgery. Vol. XI. New York, Harper & Row, 1968.

17. Stopford, J. S. B., and Telford, E. D.: Compression of the lower trunk of the brachial plexus by a first dorsal rib with a note on the surgical treatment. Brit. J. Surg., *7*:168, 1919.
18. Strandness, D. E., Jr., and Bell, J. W.: Peripheral vascular disease: Diagnosis and objective evaluation using a mercury strain gauge. Ann. Surg., Vol. 161, Supp. 4, 1965.
19. Urschel, H. C., Paulson, D. L., and McNamara, J. J.: Thoracic outlet syndrome. Ann. Thorac Surg., *6*:1, 1968.
20. Wright, I. S.: The neurovascular syndrome produced by hyperabduction of the arms: The immediate changes produced in 150 normal controls, and the effects on some persons of prolonged hyperabduction of the arms, as in sleeping, and in certain occupations. Amer. Heart J., *29*:1, 1945.
21. A mirror of the practice of medicine and surgery in the hospitals of London, clinical records, supernumerary first rib. Lancet, *2*:633, 1860.

# XIV

# Disorders of the Chest Wall

## *Mark M. Ravitch, M.D.*

## CONGENITAL MALFORMATIONS OF THE RIBS AND STERNUM

Deformities of the ribs and sternum are often sufficiently grotesque and obvious that one would expect them to have been recorded from ancient times. However, apart from descriptions of ectopia cordis in discussions of monsters, the congenital deformities of the type under discussion in this chapter received scant attention until the last half of the nineteenth century. The operative correction of these deformities has been largely a development of thoracic surgery since World War II. The depression deformity of the sternum, funnel chest or pectus excavatum, is by all odds the commonest. There were a few early successful operations for this, beginning with Sauerbruch's[16] in 1913 on a patient who was profoundly symptomatic and was improved. The operation for pectus excavatum was put in proper perspective by the classic paper of Ochsner and DeBakey[10] in 1939 and by the report of a series of patients presented by Lincoln Brown[3] of San Francisco in the following year. The publications of Sweet,[17] Lester,[7] and others[11] after World War II stimulated widespread interest and established the basic operative principles. The literature up to that time, and to some extent still, is replete with statements that these deformities are rare, that they are not amenable to satisfactory or lasting correction, and that in any case they cause no problems. As with most conditions, familiarity with these deformities and interest in their treatment have resulted in awareness that they occur relatively

frequently. The associated physiologic, orthopedic, social, and psychologic problems are well recognized, and satisfactory operative methods for the correction of these deformities have been devised.

The sternal deformities are of three principal types: (1) depression deformities (pectus excavatum or funnel chest); (2) protrusion deformities (pectus carinatum or pigeon or chicken breast); and (3) sternal clefts (cervicothoracic ectopia cordis and thoracoabdominal ectopia cordis).

### STERNAL DEFORMITIES

#### Depression Deformities (Pectus Excavatum, Funnel Chest, Trichterbrust, Schusterbrust)

**Appearance.** The deformity is marked by a sharp posterior concavity of the body of the sternum from above downward, deepest just above its junction with the xiphoid. The lower costal cartilages dip posteriorly to meet the depressed sternum so that there results a concavity from above downward and from side to side (Fig. 1). In some instances, the sternum itself is scaphoid. We recognize two principal types: (1) In the deep central deformity, in which there is a pocket that can literally hold a tennis ball or a fist, the manubrium is in proper position, and the chest on each side is well formed (Fig. 1A). This is the most striking-looking deformity, but because the remainder of the chest is properly formed, restitution to an almost normal chest wall after operation can be assured. (2) The broad, somewhat

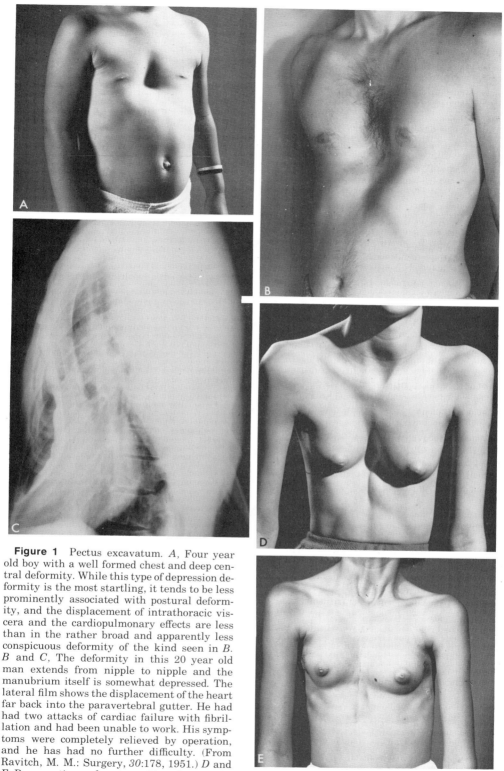

**Figure 1** Pectus excavatum. *A,* Four year old boy with a well formed chest and deep central deformity. While this type of depression deformity is the most startling, it tends to be less prominently associated with postural deformity, and the displacement of intrathoracic viscera and the cardiopulmonary effects are less than in the rather broad and apparently less conspicuous deformity of the kind seen in *B.* *B* and *C,* The deformity in this 20 year old man extends from nipple to nipple and the manubrium itself is somewhat depressed. The lateral film shows the displacement of the heart far back into the paravertebral gutter. He had had two attacks of cardiac failure with fibrillation and had been unable to work. His symptoms were completely relieved by operation, and he has had no further difficulty. (From Ravitch, M. M.: Surgery, *30:*178, 1951.) *D* and *E,* Preoperative and postoperative photographs of a girl with a severe funnel chest deformity as well as congenital agenesis of the left lung, the combination of which produced severe limitation of exercise tolerance and unrelieved tachycardia. Note the restitution of normal thoracic contour and the inconspicuous vertical scar. The right breast is seen to be less well developed than the left, as is often the case in pectus excavatum in females.

flatter deformity may go from nipple to nipple and may begin at the manubrium or may even involve a depression of the manubrium. In these patients, the chest is likely to have a narrow anteroposterior diameter on both sides lateral to the defect. The defect itself, being extremely broad, may seem not quite as impressive as the purely central defect; however, the cubic displacement of intrathoracic space is likely to be greater, and these deformities may in fact be the most significant physiologically (Fig. 1B and C). The children evidence a frequently striking paradoxical inward inspiratory motion of the sternum, a displacement of the heart invariably to the left, and frequently a forceful cardiac heave and thrust against the chest wall. In the more severe instances, with the hand placed around the left chest one can feel the imprisoned heart expanding the hemithorax with each impulse. The protuberant, potbellied abdomen is conspicuous, and as the children stand and walk the characteristic slumped shoulders, rounded back, and forward-thrust neck are noted.

**Etiology.** Funnel chest is a congenital deformity, most often sporadic, although familial incidence is common. We have, for instance, operated upon three children in one family whose three other siblings had varying degrees of the same deformity, operated on one father and daughter combination and seen others, and in numerous instances operated upon two siblings in a family. The deformity tends to be progressive from birth, and this, combined with the fact that it becomes more conspicuous as baby fat disappears, leads to the occasional statement that the child was perfectly normal at birth. The progression of the deformity is irregular and unpredictable. Sudden accentuation of the deformity is common during the adolescent growth spurt.

The deformity is, in general, unassociated with other congenital lesions, although it is one of the types of chest deformity that do occur in association with congenital cardiac deformities, and it is specifically associated with Marfan's disease (Ochsner and DeBakey's[10] patient had Marfan's disease). While attempts have been made to impute faulty development of the diaphragm, no developmental mechanism has been clearly demonstrated to be at fault. As reasonable as any is the suggestion that there occurs an overgrowth of costal cartilage that forces the sternum to either protrude or recede, and that under the influence of the diaphragm it is pulled posteriorly. Neither rickets nor any other disease of bone plays any part.

**Physiologic Effects.** Symptoms in infancy are few. We have seen one infant who was sufficiently difficult to feed that comment was made upon this before operation, and in whom the dysphagia was relieved after operation, and have treated a number of others in whom it was noted only after operation that the children now ate much more easily and rapidly. We and others have seen infants with severe stridor that was relieved by operative correction of the thoracic deformity. In childhood no

incapacity is generally recognized, but it is frequently pointed out after operation that children who had been quiet, well behaved, "good" youngsters became energetic, tireless, and quite different in their behavior and vigor. In adolescence it is not at all uncommon to have these children described as sedentary or to have it recognized that they are somewhat less energetic than their fellows and cannot sustain activity as long. In those who undertake athletics seriously, the disability is at times obvious and the improvement after operation measurable. Physiologic evaluation of the deficit in patients with sternal depressions has been undertaken by many.[1, 4, 5, 9, 19] Cardiac murmurs are common, particularly systolic murmurs to the left of the sternum, at the base of the heart. The heart is invariably displaced to the left and rotated, as demonstrated by physical examination, plain films, angiocardiography, and electrocardiography. A fair conclusion from the extensive studies of the electrocardiographic and vectorcardiographic[18] changes would be that most of the changes seen in the records can be attributed to the displacement and rotation of the heart and to the abnormal position of the chest leads on the malformed chest. Arrhythmias of several kinds have been observed, usually intermittent and relieved by correction of the deformity. Angiocardiography shows not only the displacement of the heart but in some instances deformity of the right ventricle or atrium. Although in our experience we have cited a number of diverse and striking patients with gross physiologic defects, even to cardiac failure and atrial fibrillation[12, 19] (Fig. 1B and C), in general, physiologic measurements of cardiac and pulmonary function have not yielded the kind of documentation one would like of a significant cardiopulmonary deficit. Most studies of cardiac output and respiratory function in these patients have shown results that fall within the rather broad limits of the normal range, if often at the lower limit of the range. We have long thought that the fault has lain in our inability to measure the subtle decrease in function which, to cite specific examples, accounts for the boy who can hike with his scout troop on the level but falls behind on a hill, the high school boy who can "fool around" on the basketball court, but not play a game, and the college man who can volley on the tennis court, but not play a set. We have reported an 11 year old girl with severe funnel chest and agenesis of the left lung[14] (Fig. 1D and E). She had progressively severe and disabling exertional dyspnea. A combination of two tolerable physiologic handicaps had produced an intolerable handicap. After operation she described, as a number of older patients have, a sense of freedom in inspiration, and returned to unrestricted activity; her pulmonary function tests, which had shown a restrictive respiratory defect, returned toward normal.

The literature on physiologic studies in patients with pectus excavatum is conflicting, depending to some extent upon the design of the physiologic studies. Fishman and associates[5] found no abnormalities in those respiratory functions they tested, but Weg[19] and associates, in 25 Air Force trainees with pectus excavatum and some exercise intolerance, found a decrease in the forced expiratory flow and a significant decrease in maximal voluntary ventilation. We and others have described a diastolic dip and plateau in the right ventricular pressure curve, similar to that seen in constrictive pericarditis, suggesting that the right ventricle is compressed between sternum and vertebral column, and in fact this can sometimes be seen by angiocardiography. Bevegard's[1] sophisticated studies of cardiac function yielded the information that the increase in the physical working capacity of the heart and the stroke volume was significantly less than in normal subjects in the sitting position on transition from rest to exercise, resulting in a higher pulse rate at a given oxygen uptake and explaining the lower physical working capacity. He attributes this to impaired ventricular filling.

**Indications for Operation.** We consider operation advisable to correct an existing defect, to prevent progression of the defect with the attendant hangdog posture (and hangdog self-image) and increasing probability of physiologic disadvantage, if not necessarily disability. While the structural and physiologic effects of the deformity are the principal basis for correction of the defect, it would be a mistake to minimize the social and psychologic significance of the deformity, and considerations on these scores would of themselves warrant operation. In infants and children we advise operation for deep or progressive deformities. We have not seen significant spontaneous recession of deformities, but on the other hand are not able to predict which will progress more extensively than others. Evidence of exercise intolerance and social embarrassment are added indications in later childhood and adolescence. In general, the adults upon whom we have operated have all been severely symptomatic. The younger the child at the time of operation, the less extensive need the operation be and the more likely is an optimal result.

**Technique of Operation.**[13] The operation (Fig. 2), which we have evolved in the course of 25 years and more than 300 operations, is based on the following considerations:

1. All of the deformed costal cartilages must be resected subperichondrially for the full extent of the deformity. The perichondrium will re-form new cartilage in the correct position.

2. The sternum must be separated from the xiphoid and from the intercostal bundles to release it for its new position.

3. A posterior sternal osteotomy above the beginning of the down curve of the deformity allows the sternum to be lifted forward in corrected position, and to be maintained there by a bone graft wedged into the osteotomy.

A great variety of other operations and techniques have been proposed, including reliance upon rigid temporary or permanent struts or upon external traction, excision and reversal of the

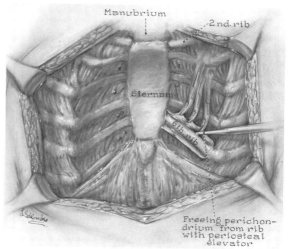

**Figure 2** The operation for pectus excavatum. The pectoral muscles have been stripped to either side. The costal cartilages will be removed subperichondrially for the full extent of the deformity, in this case the third, fourth, fifth, sixth, and seventh cartilages. The sternum will be divided from the xiphoid and the intercostal bundles divided from the sternum, so that the sternum is isolated as a peninsula. The second rib will be incised obliquely from medially and in front to laterally and behind, and the sternum elevated by a posterior osteotomy in the first interspace. This will allow a chock block of rib bone to be placed in the osteotomy, wedging it open. The medial stumps of the second costal cartilages will then lie on the lateral stumps and will be sutured there. The resulting three-point fixation provides a secure fixation of the sternum in overcorrected position. In rare instances, usually in adults with very large sternums, a Kirschner wire may be placed through the sternum and across the defect, to rest on the chest wall on either side, under the pectoral muscles.

sternum, multiple chondrotomies, and multiple sternotomies. We believe the operation described here to be the simplest and safest that will yield good results.

No mortality need be expected (the only death in our series was that of the second patient, 25 years ago). The operation can confidently be expected to relieve symptoms and prevent progression of the deformity. In the central deformities, the result is an essentially normal chest. In the wide deformities with a flat chest overall and sometimes with a depressed manubrium, improvement is dramatic, but parents should be forewarned that the general configuration of the chest, apart from the depressed sternum, limits the degree of restitution to a normal contour. Unsatisfactory results are likely to be due to inadequate mobilization of the sternum, insufficiently extensive resection of cartilages, or failure to devise a stable method of retaining the sternum in its new position. External traction, employed by some, is burdensome and unnecessary. In occasional adults or in very large adolescents, we employ internal Kirschner wire fixation.

Fascinatingly enough, the removal of large segments of five or six cartilages and fracture of the sternum does not cause any respiratory difficulty. We have never seen physiologic distress from the operation and have never had to use respirator support.

### Protrusion Deformities of the Sternum (Pigeon Breast, Chicken Breast, Pectus Carinatum)

**Clinical Manifestations.** This congenital deformity, occasionally familial, and occasionally associated with congenital heart disease, shows a much wider range of variation than is seen in pectus excavatum, although we recognize two typical varieties.[20-23]

1. In the chicken breast, or classic deformity (Fig. 3), the sternum appears prominently bowed forward but is in fact chiefly made to appear so because of the parallel vertical runnels of depressed cartilage on either side. These chests function as inefficiently in the mechanics of respiration as do funnel chests, and the impingement upon the proper intrathoracic space is significant.

2. Less common is what we have termed the pouter pigeon deformity, which is characterized by a forward tilt of the manubrium followed by a posterior angulation of the gladiolus and then a reverse anterior angulation of the distal portion of the sternum, so that a sagittal section of the sternum would be Z-shaped. The sternum tends to be broad, the xiphoid to be bifid, and the sternebrae to be prematurely fused.

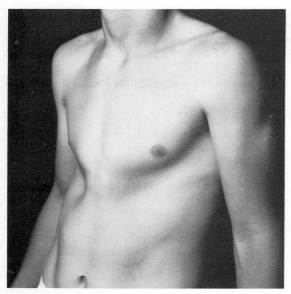

**Figure 3** Pectus carinatum of chicken breast type. A 16 year old boy referred because of a prominent sternum. In fact, it is the depression of the ribs on either side that causes the apparent prominence of the sternum. At operation, excision of four cartilages, subperichondrially, and reefing sutures in the now redundant perichondrium to provide a taut, straight course from the outer ends of the ribs to the sternum corrected the deformity very satisfactorily.

The grotesqueness of the various protrusion deformities in itself constitutes an adequate indication for operation, but we have been pleased to have our patients report substantially increased capacity for exercise after operation. Protrusion deformities are much less common than depression deformities, and physiologic studies of patients with protrusion deformities have been few.

**Treatment.** The variation from patient to patient in protrusion deformities invites the exercise of a good deal of surgical ingenuity in their correction, but the general experience with the correction of protrusion deformities has been extremely satisfactory.[23] In the commoner chicken breast, or true keeled-sternum variety of pectus carinatum, we have found that if we resect the depressed costal cartilages on either side, the lung with inspiration lifts forward the remaining perichondrium, which now, running a shorter course from the lateral limit of the rib resection to the sternum, has become redundant. If reefing sutures are taken in the perichondrium to stretch it tautly from rib to sternum, the cartilages as they regenerate provide an essentially normal thoracic contour. Ordinarily, nothing need be done to the sternum unless it is of unusual thickness or presents atypical bosses or angulations, which may be shaved away.

### Sternal Clefts

Sternal clefts were in the past reported as instances of ectopia cordis. In true ectopia cordis, the infant is born with the heart partially or entirely outside the thoracic cavity, covered, if at all, only by pericardium. This generally occurs in association with a distal sternal cleft. True ectopia cordis of this kind is invariably associated with an internal cardiac malformation that is incompatible with life and thus far insusceptible of correction. At least, no infant of this kind has survived.

The three principal types of sternal cleft are: (1) superior, usually involving the manubrium and the gladiolus to the third or fourth interspace but occasionally extending almost to the xiphoid; (2) distal, involving the distal half or third of the sternum and generally part of a complex syndrome; and (3) complete sternal cleft, the rarest of all.

**Superior Cervical Cleft (Cervicothoracic Ectopia Cordis).** The sternum develops from paired primordia, the lateral sternal bars, which properly fuse at the ninth week. The reasons for failure of fusion in the various types of sternal cleft can only be guessed at. In the case of the superior sternal cleft, the heart is covered only by skin and pericardium. It is not actually displaced cephalad, but its prominence and the soft midline, uncovered by manubrium, make it appear to be in the neck (Fig. 4A and B). There is ample experience now to state that in the first few weeks of life there is little difficulty in freeing up or wedging out the lower ends of the two sternal bars, and bringing the sternal halves together in the midline for a complete correction of the deformity. The heart is usually normal. Without operation, as weeks and

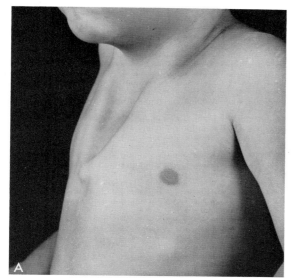

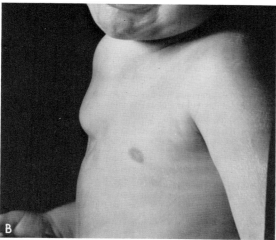

**Figure 4** Cleft sternum. *A*, At rest. *B*, During forced expiration. Superior clefts of the sternum are variously V- or U-shaped. The appearance of the child as he cries explains the term "ectopia cordis," although the heart is actually not misplaced. In the newborn, defects of this kind can be corrected by direct apposition of the sternal halves. In this child, closure of the defect was made possible by sliding chondrotomies on either side. (From Sabiston, D. C., Jr., J. Thorac. Surg., *35*:118, 1958.)

months pass, the weight of the shoulder girdle tends to hold the gap apart, and the increasing firmness of the chest wall makes approximation of the sternal halves in the midline difficult without additional procedures such as sliding chondrotomies. In still older children, even this does not avail and prosthetic reconstruction is required, with artificial materials and rib grafts, to eliminate the unsightly pulsating defect and to protect the heart and great vessels against injury. At times, a superior sternal cleft may extend almost to the xiphoid. The restitution to absolute normality of an infant with this striking deformity is accomplished with relative ease in early infancy.[26-28]

**Distal Sternal Defect (Thoracoabdominal Ectopia Cordis).** This is almost invariably a part of a pentalogy of defects.[25, 29, 30] (1) The distal portion of the sternum is cleft. (2) The epigastric midline is the seat of an omphalocele-like soft tissue defect or an actual omphalocele. (3) There is a ventral crescentic defect in the diaphragm. (4) The diaphragmatic pericardium is deficient as well, and the pericardium communicates with the peritoneal cavity. (5) There is an intrinsic cardiac defect, usually a ventricular septal defect, alone or as part of a complex deformity such as the tetralogy of Fallot. Occasionally there is a ventricular diverticulum.

Although the heart appears to be beating in the epigastrium, it is in fact not displaced. Operation in the first few months of life will make the midline somatic closure easiest. Closure of the diaphragm and pericardium poses no problems. The cardiac defect is treated at the time and manner determined by its nature. It has occasionally proved possible to repair the abdominal wall, the diaphragm, the chest wall, and the heart at one operation.[29, 30]

**Complete Sternal Cleft.** This is particularly uncommon. We have had experience with it in a single child,[31] who had also a ventral abdominal defect, a diaphragmatic defect, and a pericardial defect but no intracardiac defect. When he was first seen at the age of 1½ years, it was no longer possible to bring the lateral sternal bars together in the midline, but a reconstruction with prosthetic material (Teflon felt) and autogenous rib grafts has resulted in a normal-appearing and normally functioning chest, now 12 years later.

## RIB DEFORMITIES

A variety of bizarre deformities of the ribs occur, including missing ribs, fused ribs, and supernumerary ribs, often accompanied by other, distant, skeletal malformations as well. Each patient poses a separate problem. If there are large areas of paradoxical movement that cause respiratory embarrassment, or repeated pulmonary infections, some operative chest wall reconstruction may be considered. Most commonly, in association with these bizarre rib deformities one finds hemivertebrae, paravertebral bars of fused bone, and progressive scoliosis. It is the spinal deformity, with the possibility of progressive scoliosis, that is the serious problem and the one to which attention must usually be primarily directed, rather than to the ribs.[35, 36]

### Breast-Pectoral-Rib Syndrome

One anomaly of the ribs repeats itself with sufficient frequency to constitute a syndrome. This consists of absence of the costal cartilages and of portions of ribs, usually the second, third, and fourth, hypoplasia of nipple and breast, hypoplasia of subcutaneous fat, absence of the costal portion of the pectoralis major, and absence of the pectoralis minor.[36, 37] The area of absent cartilage, uncovered by muscle, and with unusually thin skin, presents a conspicuous deformity, an area of striking paradoxical motion of the chest wall and a "soft spot," which, particularly on the left side, is alarming. Failure to correct the deformity may lead to progressive increase in the deformity, as the cartilages above and below, unsupported and not connected to their mates, buckle and bulge. The deformity is unassociated with any visceral or distal skeletal malformations. As a substitute for the chest wall, and to provide some thickness to the tissues, we implant a sheet of prosthetic material (Teflon felt) stretched across the defect, supported by autogenous rib grafts for rigidity and some contour effect. This results in a stable chest wall, abolition of paradoxical movement, and protection of the subjacent viscera. In the absence of the pectoralis major and with deficient breast and subcutaneous tissue, the chest is still visibly asymmetric. In girls, after puberty, depending upon the degree of mammary development, prosthetic mammary augmentation may be worthwhile. This deformity is not to be confused with the much commoner absence of the costal portion of the pectoralis major, unassociated with rib or cartilage deformities but often associated with syndactylism or other deformity of the hand on the same side.[33, 34, 38] The muscular absence (as after radical mastectomy) does not constitute a significant functional handicap. All of our patients with the combined syndrome of rib, muscle, and breast deficiency have been females. All but one of our patients with pectoralis deficiency but normal ribs and cartilage have been boys. This sex difference has not been universally reported.

## ACQUIRED DEFORMITIES OF THE CHEST WALL

The physiologic cardiorespiratory embarrassment that may occur with extreme scoliosis or kyphoscoliosis is well known, and in the days when Pott's disease and grotesque hunchbacks were common, death from respiratory failure and from pulmonary hypertension with cardiac failure was well recognized. Lam[40] reported a remarkable improvement in a patient with severe "idiopathic" scoliosis in whom the progressive fatigue and dyspnea were strikingly relieved by decompression of the heart compressed by the deformed chest. We would expect that there would be patients with either scoliotic or kyphoscoliotic deformity in whom correction of a deep lateral incurvation on the concave side of the major curve might be possible, enlarging the hemithorax and permitting the lung to expand, but have never found such a patient. Block, Wexler, and McDonnell[39] demonstrated a remarkable increase in thoracic volume and pulmonary function in a 49 year old kyphoscoliotic by the application of halo-femoral traction to stretch the patient and decrease the scoliosis. While clearly it is preferable to prevent such severe deformities and their secondary cardiopulmonary complications by appropriate orthopedic

procedures early in life, it is worth bearing in mind that there may be instances in which, in addition to such measures as breathing exercises, bronchodilators, pulmonary toilet, and intermittent positive-pressure breathing that have been shown to be helpful, the basic mechanism of the disability might be attacked by procedures directed at correction of the thoracic deformity.

Fractured ribs have a remarkable capacity for springing back into shape, and deformity from this cause is uncommon. Even if double fractures of several ribs have produced a flail chest, the preferred treatment of prolonged respiratory support with a respirator maintains the segments in reasonably good position. In the rare patient in whom such segments heal in a depressed position, ultimate operative correction would be possible, although we have not ourselves seen a patient in whom this seemed advisable or justifiable.

## TUMORS OF THE RIBS AND STERNUM

Tumors of the ribs and sternum are relatively uncommon. Any of the structures in the soft tissues of the chest wall may be involved in all of the histologic types of connective tissue tumors, and these may secondarily involve the ribs or sternum. A soft tissue tumor that is hard, painful, fixed to the chest wall, or growing rapidly should be considered to be malignant. Benign tumors of soft tissues (as opposed to congenital malformations such as hemangiomas and lymphangiomas) are much less common in children than in adults, and any lump in the chest wall should be viewed with suspicion.

A soft tissue tumor, or a bony tumor for that matter, must be excised with a wide margin of normal tissues on all sides, and encapsulation, real or apparent, should be neither looked for nor trusted to. A soft tissue tumor involving the medial portion of the pectoralis major would therefore require resection of the chest wall to and including the pleura, whereas a tumor of similar size in the latissimus dorsi or trapezius might require only wide resection of soft tissue.

Tumors of the ribs and sternum are sufficiently uncommon that there are no large individual series, and the collected reports list scattered cases of every conceivable histologic type in all age groups. Vieta and Maier,[47] from 74 published reports on tumors of the sternum, found that the majority were malignant. Chondrosarcomas were the single commonest variety, and experience showed that pathologists had a tendency to "underdiagnose."

Chondrosarcoma was seen five to ten times more commonly arising from ribs than from sternum. The chondrosarcomas grow slowly, recur after long intervals, and cause distant metastases infrequently, death usually resulting from inoperable local extension. Plasmacytoma of the sternum, reticulum cell sarcoma of ribs and sternum, osteogenic sarcoma, Ewing's sarcoma, and other even rarer tumors occur. Results after resection and irradiation vary for each type.

Certain valid generalizations and particularizations may be made. Malignant tumors of the ribs and sternum are more common than benign tumors, and this is true in childhood and infancy as well. Again, at all ages, metastatic tumors to the chest wall are commoner than primary tumors. The discovery of a mass fixed to the chest wall requires a systematic investigation for a possible primary tumor, the lung, thyroid, breast, and kidney being the most likely sources apart from the lymphomas. If no primary tumor can be found, operation should be undertaken as if the chest wall tumor were malignant.[41] In general, biopsy is to be avoided because: (1) In the most common situation, chondrosarcoma, the histologic picture is notoriously treacherous and continues to seem benign even after the tumor has metastasized (quite the reverse of the situation with chondromas of the fingers, which look histologically malignant and are clinically benign). (2) If the skin is not attached to the tumor, it is desirable to plan the incision so that the ultimate suture line will be over intact chest wall, and this will not be possible if an incision is made directly over the tumor for biopsy. (3) Instances of seeding, even with the relatively benign chondrosarcoma, have been clearly documented.

The principles of resection of a chest wall tumor are straightforward.[42, 45, 46] (1) The incision should be designed so as to fall outside the ultimate defect in the chest wall. If the skin is involved or a biopsy has been performed, a wide margin should be given the tumor from the skin on down, and the original draping planned so that appropriate flaps can be swung. (2) The chest should be entered at least one interspace away from the tumor so that a finger may be inserted to determine the extent of any visceral involvement, usually an attachment to the lung. If the lung is involved, the contiguous portion, or the involved lobe, is resected. The problem of carcinoma of the lung extending into the chest wall is discussed in the section on carcinoma of the lung. (3) For lesions involving the ribs, one uninvolved rib above and below the lesion should be resected together with all the overlying muscle externally (and the skin as indicated) and the pleura internally, and a wide margin laterally and medially should be given to the apparent area of involvement. (4) For tumors of the sternum, a similarly wide margin is required, and full thickness of the sternum must be taken together with ample lengths of costal cartilages on either side of the involved portion of the sternum. The pericardium, if adherent, should be taken with the tumor, and the pleura with the attached costal cartilages.

Fortunately, very large portions of the sternum —in fact practically all of it if the upper border of the manubrium is left for attachment of the clavicles—can be removed without necessarily causing significant respiratory distress or paradoxical motion. If large areas of the costal portion of the chest wall are removed, significant paradoxical movement and respiratory embarrassment may occur. If skin has not had to be sacrificed, then for either a sternal or a costal defect we prefer a composite reconstruction, bridging the defect with autogenous rib grafts to support a tautly stretched prosthetic material such as Marlex or Teflon felt. If large areas of skin have had to be sacrificed, the cutaneous defect is best compensated for by rotation of a flap. In anterior chest wall defects in females, a flap composed of a breast, the substance of which has been split from its deep side so that it may be flattened out, will cover an enormous area at a considerable distance, if need be, from the original location of the breast. The abnormality of a misplaced breast is an acceptable price to pay for this readily available and thick covering for a chest wall defect. If heavy muscle flaps (e.g., latissimus dorsi) or a large breast or both are used to cover a defect, further reconstruction of the chest wall is often unnecessary.

Chondrosarcomas may reach enormous size and still be resectable and curable. We have had the experience of finding such a tumor invading the diaphragm, a portion of which had to be resected and the diaphragm then reattached to the reconstructed chest wall. The abdominal viscera may be involved by direct extension in large but resectable and potentially curable chest wall chondrosarcoma.[43]

The presence of a parasternal ulcerating lesion in a patient who has had a radical mastectomy for carcinoma of the breast presents both a diagnostic and a therapeutic problem. The lesion may be a chronic benign ulcer in ischemic scar tissue. It may be an irradiation ulcer. It may be squamous cell carcinoma in irradiated tissue. It may be the result of chondritis following irradiation or infection. It may be persistent carcinoma or a recurrence of carcinoma from the original lesion, or it may be the result of the extension through the chest wall of a metastatic deposit originating in the internal mammary chain. Since some of the possibilities represent benign lesions and others represent curable malignant lesions, no patient with such a lesion should be abandoned without careful biopsy and consideration as to whether a chest wall resection and reconstruction should be performed. Even if one gains only 6 months or a year of life in a patient with recurrent carcinoma of the breast, a period of that duration free from pain, ulceration, and discharge would justify the excision of the tumor and chest wall reconstruction. In these patients, who have had a radical mastectomy, chest wall resection inevitably requires migration of a flap, usually the entire opposite breast.

## INFECTIONS OF THE CHEST WALL

Subpectoral abscesses of remarkable size may be concealed by the pectoral muscle and breast over them. The subpectoral position of an abscess is demonstrated by the disappearance of bulge and fluctuation when the patient places his hands akimbo and tightens the pectoral muscle. The abscess may be pyogenic or tuberculous, originating from the pectoral lymph nodes, from infections of the ribs, or occasionally in communication with an empyema (empyema necessitatus). Evacuation of the abscess is performed through an incision below the pectoralis major, and appropriate therapy is directed to the underlying lesion.

Pyogenic infections of the ribs and sternum occur in association with disseminated infections. As with osteomyelitis elsewhere, the initial treatment is massive and prolonged administration of antibiotics. The thinness and softness of the cortical bone makes incision and drainage of an osteomyelitic focus even less urgent than in the long bones, and the anatomic situation is such as to allow wide decortication or resection of any affected portion of the ribs or sternum. Whereas pyogenically infected rib or sternum, once adequately exposed, will generally heal, cartilage will generally not heal once the perichondrium has been breached by infection, whether resulting from an infected traumatic or operative wound or some contiguous pyogenic process. After the period of active infection and systemic reaction has been passed, the area of involved cartilage should be cleanly resected, through its full thickness, by transection of the cartilage on either side with a sharp knife, with care to avoid elevation of the perichondrium over cartilage that is to remain. The relative avascularity of cartilage renders it extremely vulnerable.

### Specific Infections

Formerly, tuberculosis of the ribs, sternum, and cartilages created problems that are rarely seen in this country today. Tuberculous osteomyelitis of ribs or sternum generally perforates through the soft tissues and becomes secondarily infected. The earlier treatment of wide resection and secondary healing of the open wound has now been replaced by specific antimycobacterial therapy and expectant and limited operative treatment. A sinus or discharge a centimeter or two lateral to the sternum should be suspected of arising from the lymph nodes of the internal mammary chain; this is the route of infection that involves the costal cartilages in tuberculosis, or in the spread of cancer of the breast.

Actinomycosis of the chest wall is now similarly infrequently seen and responds to a combination of antibiotic therapy and such local operative therapy as general surgical principles dictate.

# REFERENCES

### Pectus Excavatum

1. Bevegard, S.: Postural circulatory changes after and during exercise in patients with a funnel chest, with special reference to factors affecting stroke volume. Acta Med. Scand., 171:695, 1962.
2. Brodkin, H. A.: Congenital chondrosternal depression (funnel chest): Its treatment by phrenosternolysis and chondrosternoplasty. Dis. Chest, 19:288, 1951.
3. Brown, A. L.: Pectus excavatum (funnel chest). J. Thorac. Surg., 9:164, 1939.
4. Diaz, F. V., Pelons, A. N., Valdis, F. G., Grandi, F. G. G., and Granados, A.: Pectus excavatum: Hemodynamic and electrocardiographic considerations. Amer. J. Cardiol., 10:272, 1962.
5. Fishman, A. P., Turino, G. M., and Bergofsky, E. H.: Disorders of the respiration and circulation in subjects with deformities of the thorax. Mod. Conc. Cardiovasc. Dis., 27:449, 1958.
6. Howard, R.: Funnel chest, its effect on cardiac function. Arch. Dis. Child., 34:5, 1958.
7. Lester, C. W.: Tissue replacement after subperichondrial resection of costal cartilage—two case reports. Plast. Reconstr. Surg., 23:49, 1959.
8. Lyons, H. A., Zuhdi, M. N., and Kelly, J. S., Jr.: Pectus excavatum ("funnel breast"): Cause of impaired ventricular distensibility as exhibited by right ventricular pressure pattern. Amer. Heart J., 50:921, 1955.
9. Mankin, H. J., Graham, J. F., and Schack, J.: Cardiopulmonary function in mild and moderate idiopathic scoliosis. J. Bone Joint Surg., 46-A:53, 1964.
10. Ochsner, A., and DeBakey, M.: Chone-Chondrosternon—Report of a case and review of the literature. J. Thorac. Surg., 8:469, 1939.
11. Ravitch, M. M.: The operative treatment of pectus excavatum. Ann. Surg., 128:429, 1949.
12. Ravitch, M. M.: Pectus excavatum and heart failure. Surgery, 30:178, 1951.
13. Ravitch, M. M.: The chest wall. In: Mustard, W. T., Ravitch, M. M., Snyder, W. H., Jr., Welch, C. E., and Benson, C. D.: Pediatric Surgery. 2nd ed. Chicago, Year Book Medical Publishers, 1969.
14. Ravitch, M. M., and Matzen, R. N.: Pulmonary insufficiency in pectus excavatum associated with left pulmonary agenesis, congenital clubbed feet and ectromelia. Dis. Chest, 54:58, 1968.
15. Reusch, C. S.: Hemodynamic studies in pectus excavatum. Circulation, 24:1143, 1961.
16. Sauerbruch, D. F.: Die Chirurgie der Brustorgane. 3rd ed. Berlin, G. Springer, 1928, pp. 735–741.
17. Sweet, R. H.: Pectus excavatum. Ann. Surg., 119:922, 1964.
18. Wachtel, F., Ravitch, M. M., and Grishman, A.: The relation of pectus excavatum to heart disease. Amer. Heart J., 52:121, 1956.
19. Weg, J. G., Krumholz, R. A., and Harkleroad, L. E.: Pulmonary dysfunction in pectus excavatum. Amer. Rev. Resp. Dis., 96:936, 1967.

### Pectus Carinatum

20. Howard, R.: Pigeon chest (protrusion deformity of the sternum). Med. J. Aust., 45:664, 1958.
21. Ravitch, M. M.: Unusual sternal deformity with cardiac symptoms. Operative correction. J. Thorac. Surg., 23:138, 1952.
22. Ravitch, M. M.: The operative correction of pectus carinatum (pigeon breast). Ann. Surg., 151:705, 1960.
23. Ravitch, M. M.: The chest wall. In: Mustard, W. T., Ravitch, M. M., Snyder, W. H., Jr., Welch, C. E., and Benson, C. D.: Pediatric Surgery. 2nd ed. Chicago, Year Book Medical Publishers, 1969.

### Sternal Clefts

24. Asp, K. A., and Sulamaa, M.: Ectopia cordis. Acta Chir. Scand., Supp. 283:52, 1961.
25. Cantrell, J. R., Haller, J. A., and Ravitch, M. M.: A syndrome of congenital defects involving the abdominal wall, sternum, diaphragm, pericardium and heart. Surg. Gynec. Obstet., 107:602, 1958.
26. Jewett, T. C., Jr., Hutsch, W. L., and Hug, H. R.: Congenital bifid sternum. Surgery, 52:932, 1962.
27. Longino, L. A., and Jewett, T. C., Jr.: Congenital bifid sternum. Surgery, 38:610, 1955.
28. Maier, H. G., and Bortone, F.: Complete failure of sternal fusion with herniation of pericardium. J. Thorac. Surg., 18:851, 1949.
29. Mulder, D. G., Crittenden, I. H., and Adams, F. H.: Complete repair of syndrome of congenital defects involving the abdominal wall, sternum, diaphragm, pericardium and heart: Excision of left ventricular diverticulum. Ann. Surg., 151:113, 1960.
30. Murphy, D. A., Aberdeen, E., Dobbs, R. H., and Waterston, D. J.: The surgical treatment of a syndrome consisting of

thoracoabdominal wall, diaphragmatic, pericardial, and ventricular septal defects, and a left ventricular diverticulum. Ann. Thorac. Surg., 6:528, 1969.

31. Ravitch, M. M.: Spectacular problems in surgery. Congenital absence of sternum. Surg. Gynec. Obstet., *116*: 1963.

32. Ravitch, M. M.: The chest wall. In: Mustard, W. T., Ravitch, M. M., Snyder, W. H., Jr., Welch, C. E., and Benson, C. D.: Pediatric Surgery. 2nd ed. Chicago, Year Book Medical Publishers, 1969.

### Rib Abnormalities

33. De Beneditti, M., and Chiapuzzo, A.: Malformazione Unilaterale dei Muscoli Pettorali. Arch. Ortop., *73*:408–417, 1960.

34. Epstein, L. I., and Bennett, J. W.: Syndactyly with ipsilateral chest deformity. Plast. Reconstr. Surg., *46*:236, 1970.

35. MacEwen, G. G., Conway, J. J., and Miller, W. T.: Congenital scoliosis with a unilateral bar. Radiology, *90*:711, 1968.

36. Ravitch, M. M.: Atypical deformities of the chest wall—absence and deformities of the ribs and costal cartilages. Surgery, *59*:438, 1966.

37. Sulamaa, M., and Asp, K.: Treatment of some thoracic deformities. Acta Chir. Scand., *122*:267, 1961.

38. Walker, J. C., Jr., Meijer, R., and Aranda, D.: Syndactylism with deformity of the pectoralis muscle—Poland's syndrome. J. Pediat. Surg. *4*:569, 1969.

### Acquired Deformities

39. Block, A. J., Wexler, J., and McDonnell, E. J.: Cardiopulmonary failure of the hunchback. J.A.M.A., *212*:1520, 1970.

40. Lam, C. R., and McClure, R. D.: Decompression of the heart in severe scoliosis. J. Thorac. Surg., *12*:517, 1943.

### Tumors

41. Brindley, G. V., Jr.: Primary malignant tumors of the chest wall (excluding primary cutaneous neoplasms). Ann. Surg., *153*:684, 1961.

42. Dineen, J. P., and Boltax, R. S.: Problems in the management of chest wall tumor. J. Thorac. Cardiovasc. Surg., *52*: 588, 1966.

43. Hull, D. A.: Massive chondrosarcoma of the rib with extension into the colon: Repair with tantalum mesh. Ann. Surg., *140*:886, 1954.

44. Kauffman, S. L., and Stout, A. P.: Extraskeletal osteogenic sarcomas and chondrosarcomas in children. Cancer, *16*: 432, 1963.

45. Maier, H. C.: Surgical management of large defects of the thoracic wall. Surgery, *22*:169, 1947.

46. Pickrell, K. L., Baker, H. M., and Collins, J. O.: Reconstructive surgery of the chest wall. Surg. Gynec. Obstet., *84*:465, 1947.

47. Vieta, J. O., and Maier, H. C.: Tumors of the sternum. Int. Abstr. Surg., *114*:513, 1962.

# 54

# THE MEDIASTINUM

*H. Newland Oldham, Jr., M.D., and David C. Sabiston, Jr., M.D.*

The mediastinum is an important subdivision of the thorax that is located between the pleural cavities. This space contains numerous organs and anatomic structures and is the site of a wide variety of primary and secondary disorders. The most important of these are infections, emphysema, and primary tumors and cysts. Other conditions such as esophageal and aortic lesions relate more appropriately to the specific organ system rather than to the mediastinum itself. The increasing use of chest roentgenography and the simultaneous advances in thoracic surgical techniques have emphasized the importance of accurate diagnosis and prompt surgical treatment of lesions of the mediastinum.

## HISTORICAL ASPECTS

Prior to the introduction of endotracheal anesthesia, few attempts were made to operate within the mediastinum because of the hazards of collapse of the lung following entry into the pleura. The Italian surgeon Bastianelli in 1893 performed one of the earliest successful operations, removing a dermoid cyst from the anterior mediastinum after resecting the manubrium.[1] An outstanding description of early mediastinal surgery was given by Milton in 1897.[27] Working first with cadavers and later with goats, he devised a sternal splitting approach to the mediastinum that avoided entrance into either pleural cavity. Using this technique, he operated on a patient with caseating tuberculous nodes in the mediastinum, leaving the sternum and the wound open at the end of the procedure. The patient did well, and 2 days later the incision was closed without difficulty. Milton was impressed with the access afforded by this incision, and after the operation he made the prediction that a sternal splitting approach to the mediastinum might be useful for operations on valvular lesions of the heart.

With the introduction of endotracheal anesthesia, which allowed the pleural cavities to be opened safely, major advances in surgery of the mediastinum rapidly followed. Although mediastinal lesions may occasionally be removed without entry into the pleura, thoracotomy with intrapleural dissection is the surgical approach most often employed. The most significant contributions leading to contemporary surgery of the mediastinum are found in the classic writings of Harrington,[16, 17] Blalock,[3] and Heuer and Andrus.[21]

## ANATOMY

The mediastinum is that portion of the thoracic cavity extending from the thoracic inlet superiorly to the diaphragms below. This space is bounded laterally by the mediastinal pleura, posteriorly by the vertebral column, and anteriorly by the sternum. Certain arbitrary divisions of the mediastinum have been made for convenience in localizing specific types of lesions. A plane extending from the lower manubrium to the fourth thoracic vertebra separates the superior from the inferior mediastinum. The inferior compartment is further subdivided by the pericardial sac into anterior, middle, and posterior compartments (Fig. 1). The superior mediastinum contains the upper trachea and esophagus, the thymus gland, and the aortic arch and its branches. Located in the anterior mediastinum are the thymus gland and adipose, lymphatic, and areolar tissues. The middle mediastinum contains the pericardium, heart, aorta, tracheal bifurcation and main bronchi, and the bronchial lymph nodes. The contents of the posterior mediastinum include the esophagus, descend-

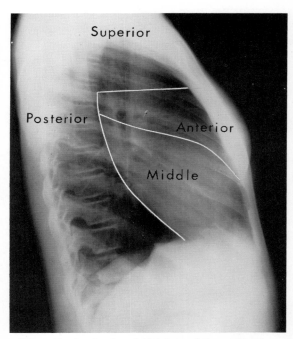

**Figure 1** Anatomic subdivisions of the mediastinum superimposed on a lateral chest film.

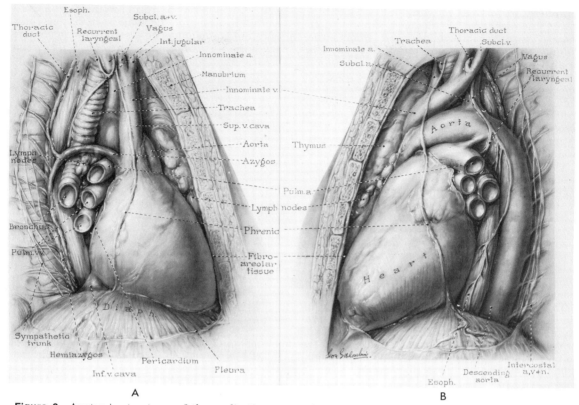

**Figure 2** Anatomic structures of the mediastinum seen from the right side (*A*) and the left side (*B*). (From Sabiston, D. C., Jr. In: Cooke, R. E., and Levin, S., eds.: Biologic Basis of Pediatric Practices. New York, McGraw-Hill Book Company, 1968.)

ing aorta, and sympathetic and peripheral nerves. The various structures present in the mediastinum are shown in Figure 2. Because many lesions in the superior mediastinum extend into the anterior or posterior compartment, it has been suggested that a more practical partition would consist of only three subdivisions: anterosuperior, posterior, and middle mediastinum.[5]

## INFECTIONS OF THE MEDIASTINUM

Acute mediastinitis is a serious condition that usually produces impressive clinical manifestations. The process is found in association with a variety of disorders, including perforation of the esophagus following trauma or esophagoscopy, penetrating wounds of the thorax, esophageal leaks following surgical anastomoses, and tracheobronchial perforation. The symptoms are usually quite dramatic and are characteristically of sudden onset. High fever, tachycardia, malaise, and leukocytosis are common. Severe pain in the neck or chest is usually present. If the mediastinitis is secondary to an esophageal perforation, the pain and discomfort are most often in the neck, since the perforation is usually at the level of the cricopharyngeal muscle. Subcutaneous emphysema producing cervical swelling is nearly always found.

The treatment of the mediastinitis is directed toward the inciting cause. Antimicrobial therapy

should be begun immediately as well as supportive treatment including sedation, oxygen, and careful observation. Although some patients may respond to nonoperative management alone, prompt surgical drainage is most often indicated as the safest and most certain means of controlling the infection.

Chronic mediastinitis is usually due to a granulomatous inflammatory process such as tuberculosis or one of the mycoses. Histoplasmosis commonly involves the lymph nodes of the mediastinum and has been identified as one of the agents associated with mediastinal fibrosis.[22] Antituberculosis or antifungal therapy is indicated in the presence of active infection. With progressive chronic infection, direct involvement or compression of a variety of structures adjacent to the mediastinal lymph nodes may occur. This may ultimately produce obstruction of the superior vena cava, the esophagus, the trachea, or a major bronchus.

## MEDIASTINAL EMPHYSEMA

The introduction of air into the mediastinum from numerous sources produces mediastinal emphysema or pneumomediastinum. The air may enter from the tracheobronchial tree, the esophagus, the neck, or the abdomen. Penetrating wounds and perforation of these structures are common causes of this condition. Blunt trauma with fracture of ribs or vertebrae is not infrequently accompanied by pneumomediastinum. Increased intrapulmonary pressure from either trauma or positive-pressure anesthesia may lead to alveolar rupture with subsequent dissection of air along the vascular structures of the lung into the hilum and then into the tissue planes of the mediastinum. In addition to these predisposing factors, "spontaneous mediastinal emphysema" is also a recognized entity.[15] In this condition mediastinal air is thought to follow interstitial emphysema of the lung, frequently occurring without specific known cause.

Mediastinal emphysema may make its clinical appearance in the deep and subcutaneous tissues of the neck and in the pleural cavity. It may also dissect into the retroperitoneal structures through the diaphragmatic hiatus. If the air within the mediastinum is under significant tension, the pressure may be sufficiently great to collapse the veins and interfere with venous return to the heart, and therefore produce clinical manifestations.

The symptoms of mediastinal emphysema include substernal pain and crepitus in the suprasternal notch and cervical region. With increasing pressure, the mediastinal air may spread to the soft tissues of the neck, chest, abdomen, and extremities. In spontaneous mediastinal emphysema, a characteristic crunching sound that is synchronous with systole is often heard over the precordium (Hamman's sign), and subcutaneous emphysema may be detectable in the cervical region. In this form of emphysema, this sign and precordial pain may be the only clinical manifestations and the disorder slowly subsides. In the more severe forms resulting from other causes, dyspnea, cyanosis, and prominence of the neck veins appear, especially if the air is under considerable tension. Rarely, circulatory failure may develop. The diagnosis is established by the clinical features as well as by roentgenography. Chest films show the presence of the air within the planes of the mediastinum dissecting also into the neck, pectoral muscles, and occasionally the extremities. The treatment of mediastinal emphysema is directed toward the inciting cause when such can be identified. The "spontaneous" form is apt to subside without producing significant sequelae. Careful observation of the patient is always indicated, so that the symptoms of increased tension and serious manifestations will be recognized promptly. Sedation and the administration of oxygen are important. Only rarely is surgical decompression necessary for the mediastinal emphysema itself, although it may be required for the underlying lesion.

# MEDIASTINAL COMPRESSION SYNDROMES

## Hemorrhage

Hemorrhage into the mediastinum may be due to a number of causes, but it is most commonly the result of trauma. Penetrating wounds often cause laceration of one of the major arteries or veins, and blunt trauma may be associated with transection of the aorta or other major vessels. Dissecting thoracic aneurysms are usually accompanied by significant bleeding into the mediastinum. Following cardiac surgery performed through a sternal splitting incision, especially when cardiopulmonary bypass is used, it is not uncommon to see a large accumulation of blood within the mediastinum. Less common causes of this condition are hemorrhagic diathesis, anticoagulation therapy, uremia, infection, and bleeding from a primary tumor or cyst of the mediastinum.[25] On rare occasions, superior mediastinal hemorrhage is seen in patients in whom no underlying cause can be established. This "spontaneous" form of bleeding sometimes follows episodes of violent coughing, and is presumably due to rupture of small mediastinal vessels during a period of markedly elevated intrathoracic pressure.[10] With progressive bleeding, mediastinal tamponade may occur, with hypotension, cyanosis, dyspnea, and venous distention, and ecchymoses extending into the neck. This syndrome is more insidious in onset than pericardial tamponade, as the mediastinum is capable of containing a large volume of blood before compression of its contents occurs. Surgical treatment may be urgently required to treat the underlying source of bleeding and to evacuate the blood causing compression.

## Superior Vena Caval Obstruction

Obstruction of the superior vena cava may result from a variety of benign and malignant lesions involving the mediastinum. As the primary process that obstructs the vena cava progresses, characteristic symptoms appear. The classic features of this syndrome include increased venous pressure; edema of the head, neck, and upper extremities; dilated venous collateral channels in the chest wall; and cyanosis. The venous distention is most apparent in the recumbent position, but in most instances the veins do not collapse in the normal manner with the patient upright. The pressure in the dilated veins ranges between 20 and 50 cm. of saline. In some instances, the superior vena cava becomes occluded quite slowly and the symptoms may be insidious in onset. When the occlusion is relatively rapid, all clinical manifestations are more prominent, and edema involving the eyelids and face as well as the arms and chest may be present. Moreoover, rapidly increasing venous pressure in the cerebral circulation leads to neurologic impairment.

The majority of patients with the superior vena caval syndrome have an underlying malignant tumor involving the mediastinum. The most common lesion is bronchogenic carcinoma of the right upper lobe. Other malignant tumors including those of the thymus and thyroid may also be responsible. In less than one-fourth of patients with superior vena caval obstruction, the syndrome is the result of a benign lesion. Causes of the latter include idiopathic mediastinal fibrosis,

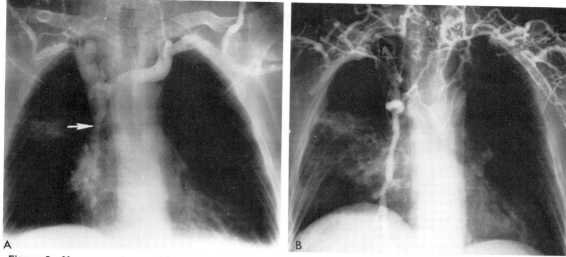

**Figure 3**   Venous angiogram illustrating narrowing of the superior vena cava (A). With later complete obstruction there are extensive channels bypassing the obstructed cava (B), and the azygos vein is noted as a prominent collateral pathway.

mediastinal granuloma (especially histoplasmosis), multinodular goiter, and pleural calcification.

The diagnosis of the superior vena caval syndrome is directed toward identification of the primary condition. Since more than three-fourths of these patients have a malignant tumor, a histologic diagnosis is usually possible and desirable. Venous angiography will demonstrate the site of obstruction of the superior vena cava and usually shows filling of extensive collateral vessels (Fig. 3). Surgical treatment is rarely indicated in this group, since the lesions are usually inoperable. Radiation therapy produces favorable symptomatic results in many instances. Although decompression of the superior vena caval system by use of various types of grafts has been tried frequently, it has usually been unsuccessful.[41] In patients with benign lesions, the course is usually one of spontaneous regression as collateral channels develop over the chest wall. Thus, with the passage of time marked symptomatic improvement occurs, and operation is rarely indicated.

## PRIMARY TUMORS AND CYSTS

A large number of histologically different tumors and cysts arise from the many anatomic structures located within the mediastinum. Since this area is also the site of numerous lymph nodes, metastases secondary to lesions in other parts of the body are also frequently found. Both benign and malignant lesions occur with considerable frequency, and a differential diagnosis is important whenever possible. Experience has shown that the majority of the primary lesions that occur in the

**TABLE 1**   INCIDENCE OF NEOPLASMS AND CYSTS OF THE MEDIASTINUM IN A COLLECTED SERIES OF 1000 PATIENTS*

| Type of Tumor or Cyst | Herlitzka and Gale, 1958[20] | Morrison, 1958[28] | Key, 1954[23] | Harrington, 1949[16] | Oldham and Sabiston, 1967[29] | Total | Per Cent |
|---|---|---|---|---|---|---|---|
| Neurogenic tumors | 35 | 101 | 10 | 51 | 43 | 240 | 24 |
| Cysts | | | | | | | |
|   Pericardial | 17 | 13 | 4 | 7 | 33 | 74 | 7.4 |
|   Bronchogenic | 24 | 23 | 3 | 10 | 27 | 87 | 8.7 |
|   Enteric | 2 | 6 | | 4 | 10 | 22 | 2.2 |
|   Nonspecific | 4 | 6 | | 8 | 13 | 31 | 3.1 |
| Teratodermoids | 26 | 36 | 31 | 40 | 36 | 169 | 17 |
| Thymomas | 14 | 47 | 4 | 8 | 52 | 125 | 12 |
| Lymphomas | 12 | 33 | 43 | | 38 | 126 | 13 |
| Other | 20 | 26 | 6 | 30 | 44 | 126 | 13 |
| Totals | 154 | 291 | 101 | 158 | 296 | 1000 | |

*Excluding primary carcinoma of the mediastinum and substernal extension of cervical goiter.

**TABLE 2**　USUAL LOCATION OF MEDIASTINAL TUMORS AND CYSTS

| Anterior Mediastinum | Superior Mediastinum | Posterior Mediastinum | Middle Mediastinum |
|---|---|---|---|
| Thymoma | Thymoma | Neurogenic tumor | Pericardial cyst |
| Teratodermoid | Lymphoma | Enteric cyst | Bronchogenic cyst |
| Carcinoma | Thyroid adenoma | | Lymphoma |
| Lymphangioma | Parathyroid adenoma | | |
| Hemangioma | | | |
| Lipoma | | | |

mediastinum can be cured by surgical means, and observation of mediastinal masses can only rarely be justified. Therefore, early diagnosis and definitive treatment are mandatory in the vast majority of patients with these disorders.

Primary lesions of the mediastinum are being recognized with increasing frequency, and in any large hospital population tumors and cysts of the mediastinum will be seen often enough to warrant a thorough understanding of their clinical characteristics. The relative incidence of the different types of mediastinal tumors and cysts in a collected series of 1000 patients is shown in Table 1. The incidence of the specific types is different in the various series, although definite tendencies for predominant lesions are apparent.[17, 20, 23, 28, 29] Thus, neurogenic tumors are the most frequent neoplasms of the mediastinum, followed by teratodermoids and lymphomas.

### Location

The division of the mediastinum into anatomic compartments as shown in Figure 1 is of value, since specific lesions characteristically arise in certain locations. The tumors and cysts most commonly occurring in each of the four compartments of the mediastinum are listed in Table 2. When a discrete mass is found in the superior mediastinum, the most likely diagnosis is thymoma or lymphoma, with tumors of the thyroid or parathyroid being less common possibilities. There are rare exceptions with each lesion, such as the occasional neurogenic tumor arising in the anterior mediastinum, or an ectopic thyroid located in the posterior mediastinum. As the tumor enlarges, it will occupy more than one compartment of the mediastinum, since there are no anatomic boundaries between them. It is not unusual to see a thymoma located in the superior mediastinum extending into the anterior mediastinum. A knowledge of the usual tumors and cysts located in each portion of the mediastinum is of help in planning the preoperative evaluation and operative procedure.

### Mediastinal Tumors

**Neurogenic Tumors.**　The most common mediastinal neoplasms in the majority of reported series are neurogenic tumors.[19, 28, 29, 38, 39] These tumors occur at any age and are most often benign, but when seen in children they have a somewhat greater tendency to be malignant. Several specific histologic types occur, including neurilemmoma, neurofibroma, neurosarcoma, ganglioneuroma, neuroblastoma, sympathicoblastoma, paraganglioma, and pheochromocytoma. The typical location is in the posterior mediastinum along the paravertebral gutter, with the tumor arising from either the intercostal nerves or the sympathetic chain. There are rare reported cases of neurogenic tumors occurring in the anterior mediastinum. Most neurogenic tumors produce few symptoms, and the diagnosis is often made from an incidental chest film. Symptoms of chest pain and cough may be present and are due to pressure on adjacent structures.

Recently it has been found that neurogenic tumors other than pheochromocytoma may exhibit hormonal activity.[14] This has been especially true of ganglioneuroma and neuroblastoma. Two syndromes have been seen: diarrhea and abdominal distention; and hypertension, flushing, and sweating. Elevated vanillylmandelic acid levels in the urine have been seen with ganglioneuroma, and the levels have returned to normal postoperatively.

*Neurofibromas* arise from nerve sheaths and nerve fibers of the posterior mediastinum (Fig. 4). Histologically, they are composed of a random arrangement of spindle-shaped cells lacking the uniform pattern usually seen in a neurilemmoma. Neurofibromas of the mediastinum may be seen in association with von Recklinghausen's disease, but a posterior mediastinal mass in a patient with this disease is not necessarily a neurofibroma, since meningiomas also occur with neurofibromatosis.[49] *Neurilemmomas* arise from the sheath of Schwann and microscopically show a regular pattern of elongated fusiform cells. They have been classified into several histologic types, but various theories concerning their histogenesis have produced many descriptions and names for these tumors. *Neurogenic sarcomas* (malignant schwannomas) originate by malignant degeneration from both neurilemmomas and neurofibromas. They occasionally are associated with hypoglycemia, and the blood sugar may return to normal levels after removal of the tumor. *Ganglioneuromas* originate from the sympathetic chain and contain ganglion cells and nerve fibers. These tumors occur more commonly in children than do other types of neurogenic tumors. A partially differentiated type of ganglioneuroma, or ganglioneuroblastoma, may occur, and contains immature cells of the sympathetic

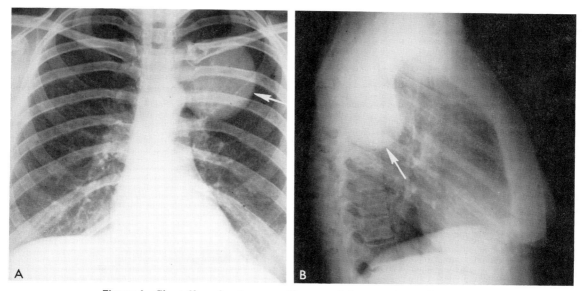

**Figure 4** Chest films showing neurofibromas of the posterior mediastinum.

nervous system mixed with mature ganglion cells. Ganglioneuroblastomas may behave in a benign fashion if completely excised, but they may present with widespread metastases and have the malignant potential of neuroblastomas. As many as 25 per cent of ganglioneuromas have been reported to contain immature elements with a malignant potential.

*Neuroblastoma* is the general term for malignant tumors of the sympathetic nervous system and includes sympathicogonioma and sympathicoblastoma. The various types are based on the histogenesis of the sympathetic nervous system. Neuroblastomas are highly invasive tumors that are most commonly seen in the retroperitoneal area in children, but also arise from any portion of the sympathetic nervous system. In spite of their very malignant nature, neuroblastomas are responsive to radiation therapy. Rare cases of spontaneous regression have been reported, and maturation from a malignant form to a benign form has also been documented. Immature neuroblastoma cells grown in tissue culture differentiate into mature ganglion cells.[12] Recently it has been shown that lymphocytes from children with neuroblastomas strongly inhibit the growth of neuroblastoma cells in tissue culture.[2] Histologically, neuroblastomas are composed of uni-

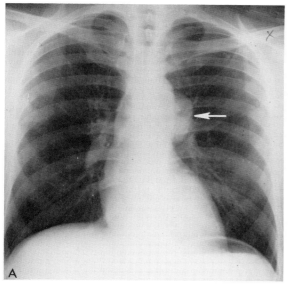
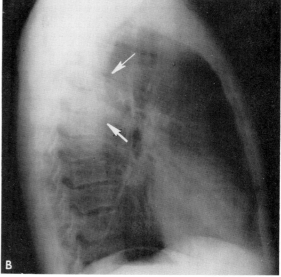

**Figure 5** Chest films showing pheochromocytoma of the mediastinum which was associated with episodic hypertension.

form sheets of small, round immature cells that may form pseudorosettes.

*Paragangliomas and pheochromocytomas* of the mediastinum originate from derivatives of the neural crest. They arise from any portion of the chemoreceptor apparatus and are similar to tumors of the carotid body, jugular glomus, and organ of Zuckerkandl. Usually the chromaffin-positive tumors or paragangliomas are hormonally inactive, but lack of correlation between the chromaffin reaction and hormonal activity does occur. Non chromaffin paragangliomas usually arise from the chemoreceptors and are located adjacent to the aortic arch, but they may also be found in the posterior mediastinum. Pheochromocytomas are almost always located posteriorly in the paravertebral region[9] (Fig. 5). By histologic criteria, the incidence of malignancy of paragangliomas and pheochromocytomas has been reported to be as high as 50 per cent. A more accurate index of the frequency of malignancy with these tumors is the gross appearance and presence of metastases. Based on these findings, the incidence of malignancy is probably less than 3 per cent. The hormonally active tumors present with persistent or episodic hypertension and may be diagnosed by measuring urinary catecholamine levels. Because of their location near the aorta and their extreme vascularity, these tumors may usually be visualized by means of thoracic aortography. The possibility of an associated mediastinal pheochromocytoma is an important consideration in evaluating a hypertensive patient who fails to become normotensive following resection of an abdominal pheochromocytoma.

**Teratodermoid Tumors.** Teratomas are tumors composed of multiple types of tissue foreign to the part in which they arise. Although the simplest form of teratoma, the dermoid cyst, appears to be different from the solid teratoma, careful microscopic examination usually reveals tissue from each germ layer rather than ectodermal tissue alone.[40, 48] Characteristically, mediastinal teratomas are located anteriorly, with only rare incidence in the posterior mediastinum (Fig. 6). Teratomas are usually first recognized in adult life and are rarely diagnosed in infancy. The gross appearance may vary from the smooth outline of the benign form to a lobulated, irregular surface in the malignant type, and on sectioning they may contain hair and teeth. Microscopically, the composition ranges from predominantly ectodermal tissues in the simple cystic type to a variety of tissues of endodermal, ectodermal, and mesodermal origin in the more complex solid types. Teratomas may present as very large tumors compressing the adjacent structures, and occasionally they may rupture into the pleural space, pericardium, aorta, or vena cava.

**Thymoma.** Thymic lesions represent one of the most common types of mediastinal tumors. Rare in childhood, they usually appear in adult life. These tumors are located in the superior and anterior mediastinum and vary in their appearance on chest roentgenogram from a small, circumscribed mass to an ill-defined, lobulated density (Fig. 7).

The association of thymoma with myasthenia gravis has been recognized for many years but remains incompletely defined.[7] The incidence of myasthenia gravis in patients with thymoma ranges from 10 to 50 per cent, whereas the incidence of thymoma in patients with myasthenia gravis ranges from 8 to 15 per cent.[47] The beneficial effects of thymectomy for myasthenia gravis are usually greatest in female patients without a thymoma and in whom the disease has been of

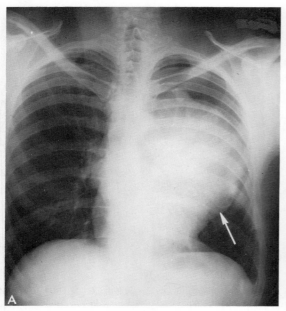 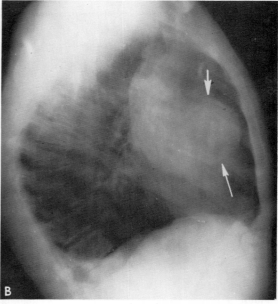

**Figure 6**   Chest films demonstrating teratoma of anterior mediastinum.

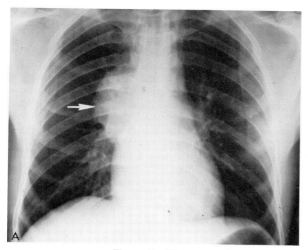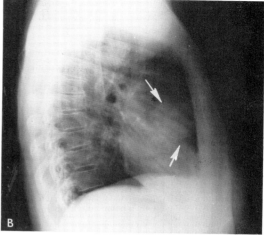

**Figure 7**  Thymoma of anterior mediastinum illustrated by chest films.

short duration. Patients with thymoma and myasthenia gravis in general have a much poorer prognosis than patients having a thymoma without myasthenia gravis.

One of the problems presented by tumors of the thymus is the difficulty in establishing a histologic diagnosis of malignancy. Usually, this diagnosis must be confirmed by the gross characteristics of the tumor as demonstrated by invasion into the lung, pericardium, or blood vessels.[7, 47] Distant metastases from malignant thymic tumors have been documented but are an unusual occurrence.

Thymomas have been associated with a wide variety of clinical conditions in addition to myasthenia gravis. There are reports of thymoma occurring with red blood cell aplasia, Cushing's syndrome, hypogammaglobulinemia, megaesophagus, and several collagen vascular disorders.[37] The exact incidence and etiology of these relationships is not well established. Cysts may occur in the thymus and may be inflammatory, neoplastic, or congenital. Of these, hemorrhagic cysts within a thymoma are the most common. True congenital thymic cysts are very rare and are thought to originate from the third branchial pouch remnant and to bear no relationship to thymoma.

**Lymphoma.**  The lymph nodes of the mediastinum are frequently involved with disseminated lymphoma. It is not unusual, however, for lymphoma to present primarily in the mediastinum without evidence of spread to other parts of the body. Hodgkin's disease, lymphosarcoma, reticulum cell sarcoma, and lymphoblastoma may present as primary mediastinal tumors. These tumors are characteristically situated in the anterior mediastinum, although they may involve lymph nodes elsewhere, especially around the bronchi. By definition, all these lesions are malignant. Surgical excision is indicated in those patients in whom the lesion is localized, especially in Hodgkin's disease.[4] Radiation therapy should be employed for most patients with these conditions.

**Carcinoma.**  Carcinoma arising within the mediastinum in the absence of any other primary source has been reported to account for 3 to 11 per cent of primary mediastinal lesions. The origin of these lesions is unclear. Since they occur most frequently in males and the most common lesion is squamous cell carcinoma, it is likely that the primary source is in the lung in many of these patients, although such an origin cannot be confirmed. It is also possible that these carcinomas may arise in previously benign cysts. The prognosis is very poor, and although radiation is usually employed, the benefits in most instances are not striking and the disease progresses rapidly.

**Other Tumors.**  *Thyroid tumors* within the mediastinum occur quite rarely. True intrathoracic thyroid tissue or ectopic mediastinal thyroid is not to be confused with the more common mediastinal extensions of cervical goiter. Patients with mediastinal thyroid tissue are usually asymptomatic, but they may have symptoms of compression or rarely may be hyperthyroid. The diagnosis may be made with radioactive iodine scanning.[26] The vascular supply of intrathoracic goiters is usually thoracic rather than cervical, and these lesions may be visualized by thoracic angiography. The usual histologic diagnosis is thyroid adenoma. These tumors are located in the anterior mediastinum with rare exceptions.

*Parathyroid adenomas* occur in the anterior and superior mediastinum in 10 per cent of patients and are often embedded in thymic tissue. Rarely, an adenoma may be located in the posterior mediastinum. Most mediastinal parathyroid tumors are hormonally active, and the diagnosis is usually made after mediastinal exploration in a patient with clinical and laboratory evidence of hyperparathyroidism. Diagnostic techniques utilized in evaluating patients suspected of having a mediastinal parathyroid adenoma include the routine chest film, barium swallow, inferior thyroid artery angiography, and radioactive selenium scanning.[18, 43] Recent advances in radioimmuno-assay for parathyroid hormone have been helpful, and parathyroid adenomas have been localized to the mediastinum preoperatively by selective venous catheterization combined with radioimmuno-assay.[36] Although very rare, carcinoma of the parathyroid gland may occur in the mediastinum.

*Mesenchymal tumors* found in the mediastinum include lipomas, liposarcomas, fibrosarcomas, myxomas, tumors of muscle origin (leiomyosarcomas), and mesotheliomas.[31] All are uncommon in the mediastinum when compared to their incidence in other portions of the body. Their behavior in the mediastinum is generally no different from that in other locations. It is not unusual for soft tissue tumors to contain elements of more than one tissue type; this makes their classification difficult and accounts for the variety of descriptive names. Treatment of these tumors is surgical excision, with the malignant lesions showing little response to radiation or chemotherapy. Mesotheliomas are listed as mesenchymal tumors, although there has been some speculation concerning their exact origin. The classification as a primary tumor has even been questioned, but studies with tissue culture, histochemical techniques, and special stains have helped clarify its histogenesis.[35] It is generally thought that these tumors arise from mesothelial cells and have the potential of developing both a fibroblastic and an epithelial counterpart. They may arise from the pleura or pericardium, or may appear as a solitary mediastinal mass without an obvious attachment to a mesothelial structure. The diagnosis of benign mesothelioma must be viewed with caution, since the biologic behavior of these tumors is very unpredictable, and distant metastases may occur many years after resection of a localized lesion.[46]

*Vascular and lymphatic tumors* are extremely common in other parts of the body but are distinctly uncommon within the mediastinum.[32] These tumors may be seen in all age groups and are found in all portions of the mediastinum but are most characteristically located in the anterior mediastinum. The histologic types include hemangioma, hemangioendothelioma, hemangiopericytoma, lymphangioma, and lymphangiomyoma. The histologic classification depends on the morphologic structure and the relative number of endothelial cells, smooth muscle cells, and pericytes. These tumors often grow to large proportions before they are diagnosed and produce symptoms by compressing adjacent structures. Included with vascular tumors is the rare occurrence of intrathoracic extramedullary hematopoiesis. This unusual tumor is composed of hematopoietic tissue and is seen in association with spherocytic anemia and other disorders affecting the bone marrow. The mass is characteristically located in the posterior mediastinum and may be interpreted as a neurogenic tumor because of this location. This disorder may be diagnosed by scanning after injection of radioactive gold.[34]

*Seminomas* are germinal tumors occurring as primary tumors of the mediastinum. In spite of the close histologic similarity between these tumors and the testicular seminomas, multiple sections of the testes have shown that the mediastinal tumors are not metastatic lesions.[24] Clinically, seminomas occur in men in the third and fourth decades of life, with no diagnostic symptoms or specific radiologic findings. The rare choriocarcinomas, as opposed to seminomas, are hormonally active, causing elevation of urinary gonadotropin levels, and frequently are associated with gynecomastia. Choriocarcinomas are rapidly metastasizing, usually fatal tumors. Seminomas, however, behave like testicular seminomas, and both the primary tumors and metastatic lesions are sensitive to irradiation.

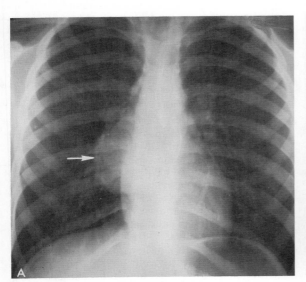 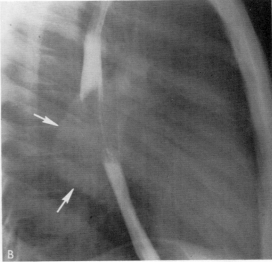

**Figure 8** Chest films of bronchogenic cyst.

## Cysts of the Mediastinum

The various cysts that arise in the mediastinum form a significant portion of the primary lesions. The cysts may originate in the pericardium, bronchi, trachea, esophagus, and thymus gland.

**Bronchogenic Cysts.** These cysts originate from the ventral foregut that forms the respiratory system and may occur in the mediastinum or in the lung. In the mediastinum they are usually located close to the trachea or main stem bronchi, most often immediately posterior to the carina (Fig. 8). A communication may exist with the tracheal lumen, but usually the cysts are adjacent to the trachea or connected to it by a cartilaginous tract. Histologically they are composed of ciliated respiratory epithelium, cartilage, smooth muscle, fibrous tissue, and mucous glands. Bronchogenic cysts are uncommon in infancy, but when they occur in this age group they may cause severe respiratory distress by compressing the trachea or bronchus.[11] In the older child, symptoms of cough, dyspnea, and stridor are not unusual. The roentgenogram shows a smooth density at the carinal level that may be seen to compress the esophagus on barium swallow. In the rare patient in whom the cyst communicates with the trachea, an air-fluid level may be seen within the cyst. Malignant degeneration has not been seen within a mediastinal bronchogenic cyst, but a bronchial adenoma has been found within the wall of a bronchogenic cyst.[13]

**Enteric Cysts.** Also called enterogenous cysts, reduplication cysts, inclusion cysts, or gastric cysts, these cysts of the mediastinum originate from the dorsal division of the foregut that develops into the gastrointestinal tract.[42] Duplications of the gut may be found at any level in the posterior mediastinum adjacent to the esophagus (Fig. 9). The cysts are smooth-walled and are composed of a muscular coat and a mucosa that may resemble that of the esophagus, stomach, or small intestine, though it is usually ciliated. They are usually attached to the wall of the esophagus but occasionally may be completely embedded within the muscularis of the esophagus. Symptoms due to pressure on the esophagus or tracheobronchial tree are common and typically occur at an early age. Since many of these cysts are lined with gastric mucosa, acid secretion with peptic ulceration, perforation, and bleeding are recognized complications.

Enteric cysts are occasionally associated with vertebral anomalies, and may be attached to the meninges or spinal cord by a tract containing neural elements. This tract may be patent and may be shown by myelography to communicate with the spinal cord. Rarely, mediastinal enteric cysts may be multiple or may be associated with duplications of abdominal portions of the gastrointestinal tract, with a communication through the diaphragm between the thoracic and abdominal portions of the duplication.

**Pericardial Cysts.** These cysts are rather common mediastinal lesions, usually occurring at the cardiophrenic angles, especially on the right side (Fig. 10). They are thought to originate either from a failure of fusion of the primitive pericardial lacunae or from abnormal folds in the embryonic pleura.[8] The cysts either may be separate from the pericardial cavity or, more rarely, may communicate with it. The radiologic appearance of these lesions is frequently characteristic. These cysts are benign and only occasionally produce symptoms. Surgical excision is indicated, primarily for diagnosis.

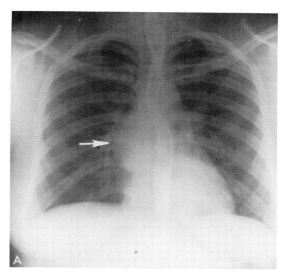 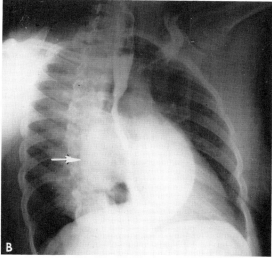

**Figure 9** Chest films illustrating enteric cyst of posterior mediastinum. (From Sabiston, D. C., Jr., and Oldham, H. N., Jr. In: Gibbon, J. H., Jr., et al.: Surgery of the Chest. 2nd ed. Philadelphia, W. B. Saunders Company, 1969.)

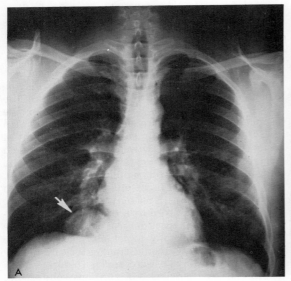
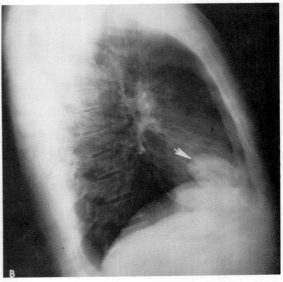

**Figure 10**   Chest films showing typical location of pericardial cyst in the right cardiophrenic angle. (From Sabiston, D. C., Jr., and Oldham, H. N., Jr. In: Gibbon, J. H., Jr., et al.: Surgery of the Chest. 2nd ed. Philadelphia, W. B. Saunders Company, 1969.)

### Symptoms

The presenting symptoms in patients with primary tumors and cysts of the mediastinum are diverse. Although a number of lesions are found initially on routine chest films, approximately two-thirds of patients have specific symptoms. The most common complaints include chest pain, cough, and dyspnea. The presence of symptoms in a patient with a mediastinal mass is of some significance, since such symptoms correlate with the incidence of malignancy (Table 3). The lesion is benign in 95 per cent of the patients in whom diagnosis is made from a routine chest film. In the group of patients who are symptomatic, half the lesions are benign and half are malignant.[29]

Symptoms that suggest direct invasion of nerves, such as hoarseness, Horner's syndrome, and severe pain, are generally associated with a poor prognosis. Similarly, evidence of major vascular obstruction such as the superior vena caval syndrome is also an unfavorable sign.

It is recognized that specific syndromes are often associated with primary lesions of the mediastinum. For example, myasthenia gravis is known to occur more frequently in the presence of a thymoma. Thymomas have also been reported in association with hypogammaglobulinemia, Whipple's disease, red blood cell aplasia, and Cushing's disease. Hypoglycemia is found with mesotheliomas, teratomas, and fibrosarcomas. Hypertension occurs in association with mediastinal pheochromocytomas and ganglioneuromas, and diarrhea may also be associated with these lesions. Neurofibromas accompany von Recklinghausen's disease, and vertebral anomalies are common with enteric cysts of the mediastinum. Malignant tumors of the mediastinum may produce chylothorax, and neurogenic tumors that press on the spinal cord may produce neurologic symptoms, including hemiplegia. A positive relationship between hypertrophic osteoarthropathy and neurogenic tumors has been established. Finally, many mediastinal tumors, especially those which are malignant, are associated with fever. One of the more classic types is the intermittent fever (Pel-Ebstein) characteristic of Hodgkin's disease.

### Diagnosis

A careful evaluation of the history and symptoms is of much aid in localizing the mediastinal lesion and suggesting a possible diagnosis. Specific symptoms such as hoarseness and Horner's syndrome suggest pressure on the recurrent laryngeal nerve and the cervical-thoracic sympathetic chain. Back pain suggests a posterior mediastinal lesion, especially one of the neurogenic lesions arising from the intercostal nerves.

Roentgenographic studies remain the most helpful diagnostic tools.[5] The standard chest film usu-

**TABLE 3**   SIGNIFICANCE OF SYMPTOMS IN 164 CONSECUTIVE PATIENTS WITH MEDIASTINAL TUMOR OR CYST*

|  | Total | Benign | Malignant |
|---|---|---|---|
| Asymptomatic† | 57 | 54 (95%) | 3 (5%) |
| Symptomatic | 107 | 57 (53%) | 50 (47%) |

*At the Duke University Medical Center.
†Lesion found on routine chest film.

ally will show the anatomic location of the mass and will allow a description of its size, its relationship to adjacent structures, and its relative density, cystic or solid. Further information concerning the location and character of the mass may be obtained by fluoroscopy, barium swallow, and laminagraphy. Methods of inclined frontal laminagraphy and horizontal laminagraphy have been reported to allow a more precise localization of mediastinal masses. Carbon dioxide pneumo-mediastinography has also been described for evaluation of mediastinal tumors.

The recent advances in radioisotope scanning have been applied to lesions of the mediastinum. The use of radioactive iodine for the evaluation of superior mediastinal masses is occasionally very helpful, since there have been rare instances in which the ectopic mediastinal thyroid was the only functioning thyroid tissue present. Techniques currently are being reported for the scanning of radioisotopes localized in the thymic tissue, parathyroid tissue, and heterotopic marrow.[34, 18, 45] Conceivably, these and other more refined procedures will soon allow precise diagnosis of a variety of mediastinal tumors. The use of selective venous catheterization and radioimmunoassay for parathyroid hormone is a significant advance in the preoperative localization of parathyroid adenoma in the mediastinum.[36]

Various methods of obtaining tissue from the mediastinum have been described, including needle biopsy, needle aspiration of cystic lesions, anterior mediastinal exploration, and mediastinoscopy.[6, 33, 44] Of these, mediastinoscopy has been the most widely used.[30] In properly selected patients, this technique will often give both a tissue diagnosis and an indication of resectability.

A wide variety of both intrathoracic and extrathoracic lesions may resemble primary mediastinal tumors and cysts. Mediastinal masses may resemble cardiovascular abnormalities, and angiocardiography may be necessary to make the proper differentiation.[30] Cardiovascular abnormalities such as aneurysms of the heart or great vessels can also resemble primary mediastinal lesions, and angiography may also be required for a proper diagnosis. Abnormalities of the vertebral column, spinal cord, or meninges may exist in the posterior mediastinum and be confused with primary mediastinal tumors. Other disease processes such as achalasia, hiatal hernia, coarctation of the aorta, mediastinitis, and many more may initially resemble tumors and cysts of the mediastinum. The experienced use of the many diagnostic tests available and the proper evaluation of the clinical presentation should in most cases lead to the proper differentiation between these abnormalities and primary tumors and cysts of the mediastinum.

### Treatment

An accurate assessment of the patient's symptoms, chest film, and special diagnostic tests will lead to the proper preoperative diagnosis. The precise histologic diagnosis, however, is rarely made prior to operation. Since the incidence of malignancy is quite high, thoracotomy is usually indicated. This allows both objective diagnosis and definitive treatment. Moreover, early diagnosis and treatment are accompanied by the most favorable prognosis in those patients with malignant tumors. It is also important to emphasize that a number of benign tumors of the mediastinum may ultimately become malignant unless resection is performed. The mortality accompanying operation is quite low, and in a consecutive group of 164 patients there was no operative mortality.[29] In this series there were three postoperative deaths (1.8 per cent), and in two of the patients, who had myasthenia gravis, death followed severe respiratory complications. Of 53 patients in this series with malignant tumors, 37 required postoperative irradiation or chemotherapy for advanced lesions. Of these, 36 per cent survived 5 years or more, demonstrating the importance of obtaining an objective diagnosis and of instituting proper therapy.

It is recommended that all patients diagnosed as having a primary tumor or cyst of the mediastinum receive the benefit of expeditious preoperative evaluation followed by a thoracotomy for excision or biopsy of the lesion, with appropriate supportive chemotherapy and irradiation when indicated. The mortality and morbidity from this approach are negligible, and the relief of symptoms in patients with benign lesions and the survival rate in patients with malignant lesions are significant.

## SELECTED REFERENCES

Castleman, B.: Tumors of the thymus gland. In: Atlas of Tumor Pathology, Section 5, Fascicle 19. Washington, D.C., Armed Forces Institute of Pathology, 1955.

Schlumberger, H. G.: Tumors of the mediastinum. In: Atlas of Tumor Pathology, Section 5, Fascicle 18. Washington, D.C., Armed Forces Institute of Pathology, 1951.

Willis, R. A.: Teratomas. In: Atlas of Tumor Pathology, Section 3, Fascicle 9. Washington, D.C., Armed Forces Institute of Pathology, 1951.
*These three volumes of the* Atlas of Tumor Pathology *from the Armed Forces Institute of Pathology are a fundamental reference for those interested in a detailed description of the gross and microscopic characteristics of mediastinal tumors. Each volume is prepared by an authority on the subject. The various histologic patterns of each type of tumor are clearly illustrated with excellent photomicrographs.*

Blalock, A., Mason, M. F., Morgan, H. J., and Riven, S. S.: Myasthenia gravis and tumors of the thymic region: Report of a case in which tumor was removed. Ann. Surg., *110:*544, 1939.
*This classic paper describes the first successful removal of a thymic tumor associated with myasthenia gravis with subsequent symptomatic remission. The author presented 53 instances from the literature showing an association of myasthenia gravis with abnormalities of the thymus gland. This review was responsible for establishing surgical removal as the treatment for patients with myasthenia gravis and a thymic tumor.*

Burkell, C. C., Cross, J. M., Kent, H. P., and Nanson, E. M.: Mass Lesions of the Mediastinum. Chicago, Year Book Medical Publishers, 1969.

*This recent monograph presents the authors' experience in the diagnostic evaluation and treatment of patients with primary lesions of the mediastinum. Emphasis is placed on the proper use of the diagnostic tests available and on the use of radiotherapy both as an adjunct to surgery and as a palliative measure. Clinical management of patients with a mediastinal mass is illustrated by case histories of patients with each of the various disorders. This work is a concise summary of current information concerning mediastinal lesions.*

Greenfield, L. J., and Shelley, W. M.: The spectrum of neurogenic tumors of the sympathetic nervous system: Maturation and adrenergic function. J. Nat. Cancer Inst., 35:215, 1965.
*The authors present a careful analysis of the pathologic findings in 66 patients with ganglioneuroma or neuroblastoma. They report complete maturation of a fully malignant neuroblastoma to a benign ganglioneuroma in 11 patients, and partial maturation in 19 patients. The secretion of catecholamines was demonstrated in 10 of these patients and was associated with symptoms of hypertension or diarrhea. This study emphasizes the correlation between maturation of the tumor and the results of surgery, and also documents the secretion of catecholamines by neurogenic tumors other than pheochromocytoma.*

Harrington, S. W.: Intrathoracic tumors. Arch. Surg., 19:1679, 1929.
*This article presents one of the earlier series of patients with primary tumors and cysts of the mediastinum. The excellent results obtained with surgical treatment documented the feasibility of excision of these lesions and was responsible for subsequent advances in mediastinal surgery.*

Leigh, T. F., and Weens, H. S.: The Mediastinum. Springfield, Ill., Charles C Thomas, 1959.
*This monograph describes a wide variety of conditions within the mediastinum, including infections, emphysema, tumors, and cysts. A thorough description is given of the anatomy of the mediastinum, including the patterns of lymphatic drainage. The indications for and uses of the various radiographic tests available are presented. The excellent reproduction of roentgenograms adds to the value of this work.*

Palva, T.: Mediastinoscopy. Chicago, Year Book Medical Publishers, 1964.
*This monograph thoroughly presents the indications and techniques of mediastinoscopy as first described by Carlens. The various pathologic diagnoses obtained in this series of 295 patients demonstrate the usefulness of this procedure in a number of clinical situations. The detailed description of the anatomy of the mediastinum and the excellent color photographs of views through the mediastinoscope add to the quality of this book.*

# REFERENCES

1. Bastianelli, R. Quoted by Meade, R. H.: A History of Thoracic Surgery. Springfield, Ill., Charles C Thomas, 1961.
2. Bill, A. H.: The implications of immune reactions to neuroblastoma. Surgery, 66:415, 1969.
3. Blalock, A., Mason, M. F., Morgan, H. J., and Riven, S. S.: Myasthenia gravis and tumors of the thymic region: Report of a case in which tumor was removed. Ann. Surg., 110:544, 1939.
4. Burk, W. A., Burford, T. H., and Dorfman, R. F.: Hodgkin's disease of the mediastinum. Ann. Thorac. Surg., 3:287, 1967.
5. Burkell, C. C., Cross, J. M., Kent, H. P., and Nanson, E. M.: Mass Lesion of the Mediastinum. Chicago, Year Book Medical Publishers, 1969.
6. Carlens, E.: Mediastinoscopy. Dis. Chest, 36:343, 1959.
7. Castleman, B.: Tumors of the thymus gland. In: Atlas of Tumor Pathology, Section 5, Fascicle 19. Washington, D.C., Armed Forces Institute of Pathology, 1955.
8. Drash, E. C., and Hyer, H. J.: Mesothelial mediastinal cysts. J. Thorac. Surg., 19:755, 1950.
9. Edmunds, L. H.: Mediastinal pheochromocytoma. Ann. Thorac. Surg., 2:743, 1966.
10. Epstein, A. M., and Klassen, K. P.: Spontaneous superior mediastinal hemorrhage. J. Thorac. Cardiovasc. Surg., 39:740, 1960.
11. Gerami, S., Richardson, R., Harrington, B., and Pate, J. W.: Obstructive emphysema due to mediastinal bronchogenic cysts in infancy. J. Thorac. Cardiovasc. Surg., 58:432, 1969.
12. Goldstein, M., Burdman, J. A., and Journey, L. J.: Long term tissue culture of neuroblastomas. J. Nat. Cancer Inst., 32:165, 1964.
13. Greenfield, L. J., and Howe, J. S.: Bronchial adenoma within the wall of a bronchogenic cyst. J. Thorac. Cardiovasc. Surg., 49:398, 1965.
14. Greenfield, L. J., and Shelley, W. M.: The spectrum of neurogenic tumors of the sympathetic nervous system: Maturation and adrenergic function. J. Nat. Cancer Inst., 35:215, 1965.
15. Hamman, L.: Spontaneous mediastinal emphysema. Bull. Johns Hopkins Hosp., 64:1, 1939.
16. Harrington, S. W.: Intrathoracic tumors. Arch. Surg., 19:1679, 1929.
17. Harrington, S. W.: Intrathoracic extrapulmonary tumors: Diagnosis and treatment. Postgrad. Med., 6:6, 1949.
18. Haynie, T. P., Otte, W. K., and Wright, J. C.: Visualization of hyperfunctioning parathyroid adenoma using Se75 selenomethionine and the photoscanner. J. Nucl. Med., 5:710, 1964.
19. Heimburger, I. L., Battersby, J. S., and Vellios, F.: Primary neoplasms of the mediastinum. Arch. Surg., 86:978, 1963.
20. Herlitzka, A. J., and Gale, J. W.: Tumors and cysts of the mediastinum. Arch. Surg., 76:697, 1958.
21. Heuer, G. J., and Andrus, W. O.: The surgery of mediastinal tumors. Amer. J. Surg., 50:146, 1940.
22. Hewlett, T. H., Steer, A., and Thomas, D. E.: Progressive fibrosing mediastinitis. Ann. Thorac. Surg., 2:345, 1966.
23. Key, J. A.: Mediastinal tumors. Surg. Clin. N. Amer., 34: 959, 1954.
24. Koyntz, S. L., Connolly, J. E., and Cohn, R.: Seminoma-like (or seminomatous) tumors of the anterior mediastinum. J. Thorac. Cardiovasc. Surg., 45:289, 1963.
25. Leigh, T. F., and Weens, H. S.: The Mediastinum. Springfield, Ill., Charles C Thomas, 1959.
26. Lindskog, B. I., and Malin, A.: Diagnostic and surgical considerations in mediastinal (intrathoracic) goiter. Dis. Chest, 47:201, 1965.
27. Milton, H.: Mediastinal surgery. Lancet, 1:872, 1897.
28. Morrison, I. M.: Tumors and cysts of the mediastinum. Thorax, 13:294, 1958.
29. Oldham, H. N., Jr., and Sabiston, D. C., Jr.: Primary tumors and cysts of the mediastinum. Monogr. Surg. Sci., 4:243, 1967.
30. Oldham, H. N., Jr., and Sabiston, D. C., Jr.: Primary tumors and cysts of the mediastinum presenting as cardiovascular abnormalities. Arch. Surg., 96:71, 1968.
31. Pachter, M. R., and Lattes, R.: Mesenchymal tumors of the mediastinum. I. Tumors of fibrous tissue, adipose tissue, smooth muscle, and striated muscle. Cancer, 16:74, 1963.
32. Pachter, M. R., and Lattes, R.: Mesenchymal tumors of the mediastinum. III. Tumors of lymphvascular origin. Cancer, 16:108, 1963.
33. Palva, T.: Mediastinoscopy. Chicago, Year Book Medical Publishers, 1964.
34. Papavasiliou, C. G.: Tumors stimulating intrathoracic extramedullary hematopoiesis: Clinical and roentgenologic considerations. Amer. J. Roentgen., 93:695, 1965.
35. Porter, J. M., and Cheek, J. M.: Pleural mesothelioma: Review of tumor histogenesis and report of 12 cases. J. Thorac. Cardiovasc. Surg., 55:882, 1968.
36. Reitz, R. E., Pollard, J. J., Wang, C., Fleischli, D. J., Cope, O., Murray, T. M., Deftos, L. J., and Potts, J. T.: Localization parathyroid adenomas by selective venous catheterization and radioimmunoassay. New Eng. J. Med., 281:348, 1969.
37. Rubin, M., Stravo, B., and Allen, L.: Clinical disorders associated with thymic tumors. Arch. Intern. Med., 114:389, 1964.
38. Sabiston, D. C., Jr.: The digestive system: Esophagus and mediastinum. In: Cooke, R. E., and Levin, S., eds.:

Biologic Basis of Pediatric Practices. New York, Mc-Graw-Hill Book Company, 1968.

39. Sabiston, D. C., Jr., and Scott, H. W.: Primary neoplasms and cysts of the mediastinum. Ann. Surg., 136:777, 1952.

40. Schlumberger, H. G.: Tumors of the mediastinum. In: Atlas of Tumor Pathology, Section 5, Fascicle 18. Washington, D.C., Armed Forces Institute of Pathology, 1951.

41. Skinner, D. B., and Salzman, E. W.: The challenge of superior vena caval obstruction. J. Thorac. Cardiovasc. Surg., 49:824, 1965.

42. Spock, A., Schneider, S., and Baylin, C. J.: Mediastinal gastric cysts: A case report and review of English literature. Amer. Rev. Resp. Dis., 94:97, 1966.

43. Steiner, R. E., Fraser, R., and Aird, I.: Operative parathyroid arteriography for location of parathyroid tumor. Brit. Med. J., 2:400, 1956.

44. Stemmer, E. A., Calvin, J. W., Chandor, S. B., and Connolly, J. E.: Mediastinal biopsy for indeterminate pulmonary and mediastinal lesions. J. Thorac. Cardiovasc. Surg., 49:405, 1965.

45. Tool, J. F., and Witcofski, R.: Selenomethionine Se$^{75}$ scan for thymoma. J.A.M.A., 198:1219, 1966.

46. Urschel, H. C., and Paulson, D. C.: Mesotheliomas of the pleura. Ann. Thorac. Surg., 1:559, 1965.

47. Wilkins, E. W., Edmunds, L. H., and Castleman, B.: Cases of thymomas at the Massachusetts General Hospital. J. Thorac. Cardiovasc. Surg., 52:322, 1966.

48. Willis, R. A.: Teratomas. In: Atlas of Tumor Pathology, Section 3, Fascicle 9. Washington, D.C., Armed Forces Institute of Pathology, 1951.

49. YaDeau, R. E., Clagett, O. T., and Divertie, M. B.: Intrathoracic meningocele. J. Thorac. Cardiovasc. Surg., 49:202, 1965.

# 55

# THE PERICARDIUM

*Paul A. Ebert, M.D.*

## HISTORICAL ASPECTS

Hippocrates in 460 B.C. described the pericardium as a smooth tunic that enveloped the heart and contained a small amount of fluid resembling urine. Lower, in the seventeenth century, described the pericardial effusion that compressed the walls of the heart and could result in death. Lancisi in 1728 elucidated the clinical and necropsy findings of constrictive pericarditis. In 1761 Morgagni recognized the danger of cardiac compression and described constrictive pericarditis of such a degree that the heart could not receive a proper quantity of blood.[20] Romero in 1819 incised the pericardium in three patients, two of whom survived.[23] Schuh and Karanaeff (1840) performed pericardicenteses for relief of massive pericardial effusion. In 1842 Chevers presented the first clear clinical picture of the development of constrictive pericarditis.[3] Kussmaul (1873) described the paradoxical pulse and rise in venous pressure on inspiration in patients with constrictive pericarditis.[15]

Resection of the pericardium was performed independently by Rehn and by Sauerbruch in 1913. Churchill in 1929 performed the first successful pericardiectomy for constrictive pericarditis in the United States. Parsons and Holman (1951, 1955)[21] and Isaacs et al. (1952)[10] reported classic experimental studies clarifying the physiologic effects of segmental compression of the heart. Many surgeons have emphasized the necessity of performing radical pericardiectomy to prevent recurrences of pericardial constriction requiring secondary operations.

## FUNCTIONS OF THE PERICARDIUM

The pericardium provides a smooth serous sac that allows the heart a frictionless chamber in which to function. It is a strong fibrous material with a restraining influence against overdilatation of the heart. The pericardium may be stretched over a period of time by cardiac enlargement, but sudden changes in heart size are restricted. The pericardium may protect the heart from extension of infection from the chest, lungs, mediastinum, esophagus, and infradiaphragmatic areas.

Congenital absence of the entire pericardium is extremely rare. More commonly, small segments may be missing, and absence of small portions of the pericardium on the left side is most common. No clinical symptoms are known to result from congenital absence of the pericardium. It has been shown experimentally that without the pericardium the heart ruptures at a lower intracardiac pressure.

## PERICARDIAL CYSTS

The pericardium forms from a series of disconnected lacunae, and for a brief period during developmental stages these lacunae remain as individual spaces. Occasionally, the communication with the pericardium in such lacunae persists and is called a diverticulum. If one of these lacunar cavities fails to fuse, it may remain and form a pericardial cyst or may simply atrophy. Cysts in general do not cause symptoms and are usually discovered on routine chest x-ray. The classic description of such cysts as given by radiologists is a mass lying anteriorly in the chest in either cardiophrenic sulcus. These masses may be confused with lung tumors, thymomas, and other mediastinal lesions. Cysts may become of such size that they can be incapacitating and life-threatening because of their space-occupying characteristics. (See Chapter 54, The Mediastinum.)

Pericardial diverticula are simply described as protrusions of the pericardial sac at points of weakness. These vary greatly in size, from 0.5 to 12.0 cm. They are usually more frequent on the right side and can be confused with aneurysms of the ascending aorta or with mediastinal tumors. The diverticula are rarely symptomatic, and excision is advised to establish a definitive diagnosis.

## NEOPLASMS

Neoplasms arising in the pericardium are extremely rare. Such benign tumors as lipomas, lobulated fibrous polyps, and hemangiomas have been reported. Primary mesotheliomas arising from the lining endothelium have been described. Sarcomas and teratomas occasionally arise from the pericardium, and the pericardium is commonly infiltrated by primary myocardial tumors or infiltrating lung cancers.

Precordial or pleuritic pain in the left chest associated with a soft tissue mass that cannot be distinguished from the heart on chest x-ray is the usual description of acute necrosis of pericardial fat. Necrosis is thought to be due to a vascular accident with extravasation of blood and the formation of a hematoma. Hydropneumopericardium has been reported and is a rare lesion in which the clinical signs are precordial tympany and metallic splashing sounds that can be quite loud. Chest film showing air in the pericardium is conclusive. An infection may be present, and if improvement is not prompt, pericardiotomy is indicated. Air in the pericardium is also common after severe chest trauma.

## PERICARDITIS

Pericarditis may occur as a primary disease process or as a secondary manifestation of a systemic disease. In its simplest form, pericarditis is an acute self-limiting inflammation most likely caused by a virus. The disease may be preceded by an upper respiratory tract infection, and symptoms vary considerably. Usually, fever is present, with the temperature around 101° F. but sometimes as high as 104 to 105° F. There is substernal or precordial pain, and a pericardial friction rub is usually heard. All degrees of severity are observed; the disease may be minimal, lasting only a few days, or symptoms may persist for weeks. Shortness of breath, shallow grunting respirations, cough, and orthopnea with a tendency to lean forward are characteristic symptoms. The pain may be sharp or dull and is usually accentuated by coughing, respiration, or activity. Commonly it is relieved by sitting up and aggravated by lying down. Leukocytosis with a predominant increase in lymphocytes is usually noted, and chest x-ray may show mild cardiac enlargement due to pericardial effusion. ST segment elevation on the electrocardiogram with absent Q waves in the presence of a pericardial friction rub is strongly suggestive of pericarditis. Pleuritis and pleural effusion may also be present.

The disease process is usually self-limiting, and complications are rare. There are isolated reports of constrictive pericarditis developing after supposedly viral pericarditis, but this is unusual. Atrial fibrillation commonly occurs, and signs of cardiac failure secondary to rhythm disturbance may be noted.

Treatment usually consists of bed rest and analgesics. Salicylates have been successful in relieving pain. If the patient does not respond to supportive treatment, steroids may be beneficial. Routine use of steroids is not encouraged, since the disease may recur when the steroids are withdrawn. Remissions are not uncommon, with pain, fever, friction rub, and even pericardial effusion frequently receding, only to recur a short time later. Heart failure is infrequent and usually can be controlled with digitalis.

Pericarditis often accompanies systemic diseases such as scleroderma, rheumatic fever, and lupus erythematosus. Sarcoidosis may involve the pericardium and heart but is rarely responsible for pericarditis. Such hypersensitivity states as serum sickness, autoimmune reactions, and various drug reactions may result in pericarditis or effusion. In cholesterol pericarditis, the pericardial fluid has a characteristic gold-paint color. The diagnosis is confirmed by pericardial aspiration and identification of cholesterol crystals. Hypothyroidism is commonly present, and pericarditis may disappear with thyroid replacement.

Acute pyogenic pericarditis may occur as a result of direct contamination of the pericardium or from septicemia or pyemia. Abscesses from below the diaphragm may rupture into the pericardial sac, or pyogenic pericarditis may result as a complication from operations on the heart, lungs, or esophagus. Severe chest pain and fever are the usual clinical signs. In the early stages, it is difficult to differentiate pyogenic pericarditis from the more common benign form. Pericardial effusion can occur more rapidly and cardiac tamponade must be expected. Tamponade may develop under these circumstances with the presence of as little as 100 ml. of fluid or pus. The electrocardiogram shows low voltage in the QRS and inverted T waves. Venous pressure is usually elevated, and a paradoxical pulse may be felt. The diagnosis is confirmed by pericardial aspiration, and repeated pericardicenteses may be necessary to evacuate accumulated fluid and pus. In most instances, resection of a costal cartilage and direct drainage of the pericardium should be performed. Very rapid forms of constrictive pericarditis have been identified, with the interval between injury and actual constriction as short as 11 weeks. Pericardial constriction occurs after cardiac surgery, but the incidence seems to be quite low.

## TUBERCULOUS PERICARDITIS

Tuberculous pericarditis is thought to be secondary to tuberculosis elsewhere, with the disease spreading to the pericardial sac by direct extension from the pleura or lung, by way of lymph nodes, or through the vascular system. The onset of symptoms is usually insidious, and most often the patient is not known to have pulmonary tuberculosis.

Symptoms may be very nonspecific and include malaise, fever, sweats, pleural pain, cough, and a pericardial friction rub. In some instances, a slowly developing pericardial effusion occurs in which the fluid may be clear, straw-colored, or sanguineous. Early pericardicenteses may establish the diagnosis with the finding of acid-fast bacilli in the fluid. In many instances the skin test for tuberculosis will be negative, since a large reservoir of antibody has reacted against the massive amount of antigen in the pericardial sac. In these instances it may be several weeks after institution of treatment before an actual positive skin test will develop. Untreated patients may show progressive emaciation, toxemia, and subsequent death. The patient may die of cardiac failure, but the most common cause of death is widespread tuberculosis.

There appears to be a direct relationship between pericardial constriction and the length of time the disease is present prior to institution of treatment. Wood (1956) emphasized that pericardial constriction was a rule if treatment was delayed more than 4 months. The fibrotic process of healing, which is beneficial in pulmonary tuberculosis, is associated with a threat of pericardial contracture and constriction.

Treatment with antituberculous drugs should be started as soon as the diagnosis is established. In some cases confirmation of the diagnosis may be time-consuming; therefore, if the clinical picture is convincing, it is probably better to administer antituberculous therapy before confirmation. Single drug therapy is ineffectual, and the combination most frequently used is isoniazid and para-aminosalicylic acid. Clinical signs of improvement usually appear within 2 to 3 weeks. Heart size, elevated venous pressure, and amount of effusion disappear more slowly. There does not seem to be any benefit in administering corticosteroids to minimize effusions and scarring.

A significant number of patients with tuberculous pericarditis will suffer the effects of pericardial constriction. As the fluid is absorbed, it becomes more viscid and more irritating to the surrounding structures. It has been postulated that the fluid then gravitates toward the diaphragmatic pericardium and that this area is subject to a longer period of irritation and thus to a greater deposition of fibrous tissue. When tuberculosis is established as a cause of effusion, drug therapy should be instituted for a period of 6 to 8 weeks. If the effusion disappears and signs of constriction occur within a short period of time, pericardiectomy is indicated. Likewise, if the effusion recurs after repeated pericardicenteses, pericardiectomy should be performed. Excellent results have been obtained when resection has been performed during the effusion stage, since the pericardium can be removed with ease. Holman and Willett[9] have emphasized that at this stage of the disease atrophy of the myocardium, fibrous infiltration, and calcification are usually not present.

Obviously it is futile to operate on febrile patients with acute toxicity and active tuberculous pericarditis. However, it is equally unwise to await a period of relative inactivity, by which time constriction and calcification have occurred. The optimal time for operation appears to be the period in the early healing phase when the patient is clinically well, aside from early signs of constriction. Constrictive pericarditis is a mechanical limitation of ventricular filling, which operative removal of the scarred pericardium will relieve. Surgical results must be evaluated in reference to the period of time during which the operation was performed. In earlier stages of thoracic surgery, the pericardium was removed only from the anterior and lateral surfaces of the heart, and recurrences were common. Shumacker and Roshe[27] have emphasized the necessity of performing a radical pericardiectomy, which includes removing the pericardium from both the anterior and posterior surfaces of the heart. When this procedure has been followed, operative results have been extremely good and recurrences uncommon.

## CARDIAC TAMPONADE

Fluid or blood in the pericardial space may limit filling of the heart during diastole. This is due to the increased pressure from within the pericardium, and systolic contraction is rarely limited, whereas filling the ventricles requires a greater venous pressure. Tamponade commonly occurs after penetrating injuries to the heart in which blood escapes into the pericardial sac. The blood or fluid cannot escape through the laceration in the pericardium, and tamponade may follow. A very small amount of blood, 150 to 200 cc., may be sufficient to cause tamponade, whereas in chronic effusion the pericardium stretches over a period of time and has the capacity to contain considerably more fluid with minimal cardiac effect. In cardiac tamponade a critical point exists prior to which cardiac output is only minimally reduced. But when this critical point is reached, accumulation of a very small additional volume may reduce cardiac output, and death ensues. The treatment can be equally dramatic when removal of blood or fluid results in the quick return of blood pressure and cardiac output to near normal.

In cardiac tamponade, diastolic filling pressure rises and the amount of blood pumped per beat is reduced. Sympathetic activity increases in an attempt to maintain a normal arterial pressure, and the result is vasoconstriction. Heart rate increases and systolic ejection may become more vigorous. Venous pressure rises owing to compression of the heart during diastole, and no gradients have been demonstrated between the great veins and the right atrium during experimental cardiac tamponade. Coronary blood flow may be reduced, and myocardial failure may result from inadequate coronary perfusion.

Clinically, the patient appears to be in shock at a time when venous distention is present. Cyanosis due to marked venous stasis may be noted, and the venous pressure rather than the arterial pressure should be used as a guide to treatment, since the latter may be artificially maintained by an elevated peripheral resistance.

Treatment must not be delayed, since this is an emergency situation. Venous pressure should be obtained, and pericardial aspiration should be performed with an electrocardiogram lead attached to the needle to identify contact with the heart surface (Fig. 1). The blood or fluid can be aspirated, and a fall in venous pressure should be noted. If venous pressure rises, additional pericardicenteses should be performed. In some cases

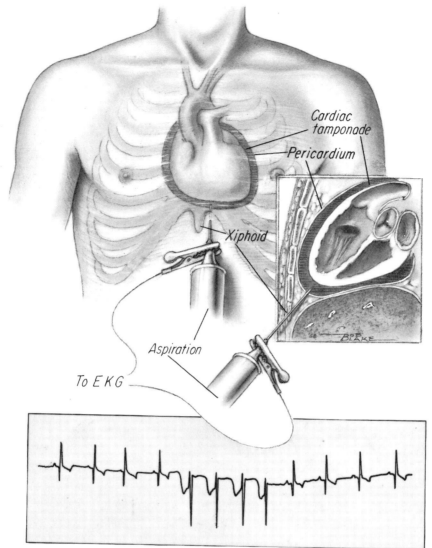

Cardiac tamponade
Pericardium
Xiphoid
Aspiration
To EKG

**Figure 1**   The technique for pericardicentesis for relief of cardiac tamponade. The needle with an electrocardio-graphic lead attached is introduced beneath the xiphoid. Contact with the epicardial surface of the heart produces a marked change in the electrocardiogram. The needle is withdrawn until the electrocardiogram reverts to normal. The needle may also be inserted just to the left of the sternum through the fourth intercostal space. (From Ebert, P. A. In: Gibbon, J. H., Jr., Sabiston, D. C., Jr., and Spencer, F. C., eds.: Surgery of the Chest. 2nd ed. Philadelphia, W. B. Saunders Company, 1969.)

of chronic effusion, a small plastic catheter may be passed percutaneously into the pericardial sac and left in place for continual decompression. Pericardiotomy should be considered as an emergency procedure if repeated aspirations do not relieve tamponade. Pericardicenteses occasionally may result in sudden death due to laceration of a coronary artery or to ventricular fibrillation. The procedure must be considered to be serious and must be performed with care. The use of the electrocardiogram to detect contact with the heart reduces the chance of myocardial or coronary artery injury.

## CHRONIC PERICARDIAL EFFUSION

In most cases, pericardial effusion develops over a period of time, and the heart shadow is usually markedly enlarged. The differential diagnosis is usually between pericardial effusion and marked cardiomegaly due to heart failure. In effusion, the heart sounds are usually distant, there is absence of murmurs, and shifting intensity of heart sounds is more likely to be seen. A pericardial splash or friction rub is rarely heard. Electrocardiogram usually shows low voltage, ST segment elevation, and electrical alternans of the

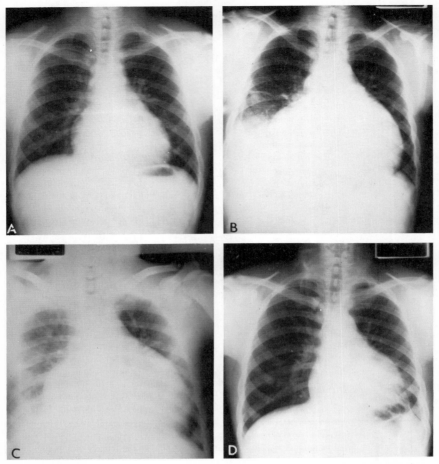

**Figure 2** A sequence of chest x-rays from a patient with pericardial effusion. *A*, Minimal cardiac enlargement when the patient presented with malaise and night sweats. *B*, Two weeks later there is marked pericardial effusion. *C*, Repeated pericardicenteses were temporarily effective, but fluid accumulated again and the cardiac silhouette enlarged. *D*, Pericardiectomy was performed and 3 weeks later the chest x-ray was nearly normal.

QRS complex. In this situation the QRS complexes are regular in time but alternate in height or direction of the major deflection. ST segment elevation may be seen in acute tamponade resulting from compression of the heart and myocardial ischemia.

Numerous diagnostic techniques have been used in attempts to differentiate effusion from cardiomegaly. Echocardiography, injection of intravenous carbon dioxide, with the patient lying on his left side in order to differentiate the right atrial wall from the pericardium, and routine angiocardiography outline the heart in reference to the cardiac silhouette. Pericardicentesis is probably the most direct means of confirming the diagnosis of effusion. Repeated pericardicenteses may provide temporary relief, but surgical therapy offers the best prognosis. The creation of a window between the pericardial sac and the pleural space to drain the fluid for absorption has produced good results. Resection of the pericardium is a more definitive form of treatment (Fig. 2). Recur-

rences are extremely uncommon after pericardiectomy. Pericardial resection also eliminates the possibility of the development of subsequent constrictive pericarditis. Operative resection is usually fairly easy at this stage, since the pericardium is not attached to the heart. The remnant can drain into either pleural space, and excellent results have been reported.

## CHRONIC CONSTRICTIVE PERICARDITIS

Constrictive pericarditis results from a chronic inflammatory process producing a fibrous thickened pericardium that surrounds the heart and limits diastolic ventricular filling. As the scar continues to shrink, further compression of the heart limits stroke volume and decreases cardiac output. In the late stages, this thickened and scarred pericardium, which becomes densely adherent to the heart, limits systolic ejection as well as restricting diastolic filling. In contrast to cardiac tamponade resulting from fluid accumulation around the heart, furthur elevation of venous pressure by infusion of blood or plasma results in no change in cardiac output. This reflects the severe restriction of diastolic filling imposed by the fibrous calcified pericardium.

Reduction in cardiac output means less effective perfusion to the liver, kidneys, and other tissues. Salt and water accumulation occurs; this further expands blood volume and increases venous pressure. In theory, the function of the kidney actually worsens the condition, since increases in venous pressure and blood volume will not increase cardiac output. Diuretics are of value, since patients may undergo diuresis with the reduction of venous pressure and diastolic pressure in both the left and right heart without significant decrease in cardiac output. Lange (1956) showed that ganglionic blocking agents may reduce venous pressure without changing cardiac output.

Symptoms are usually those of heart failure, with weakness, easy fatigability, and shortness of breath. Ascites formation without peripheral edema is common. Syncopal attacks may occur with activity and are thought to be due to the inability of the heart to increase its output. Liver engorgement may cause abdominal pain.

In the late stages, the physical findings are classic; the patient's face is puffy and his abdomen is protuberant. The heart is quiet and the apex beat may or may not be felt. Sometimes a distinct diastolic shock may be palpated at the time of rapid ventricular filling. Murmurs are usually absent. Generally the liver is enlarged and ascites may be present. Peripheral edema is usually not marked. Approximately one-third of the patients present with atrial fibrillation, and the peripheral pulse may be paradoxical, disappearing completely during inspiration. The arterial blood pressure is usually low, with a very narrow pulse pressure.

On chest x-ray the heart is usually normal or only moderately enlarged. Calcium deposits are commonly seen on the lateral films, and the superior vena cava may be prominent (Fig. 3). Electrocardiogram shows low voltage in the QRS complexes, and T waves are often flat and inverted. A bifid P wave may be present, with the second wave taller than the first. Serum proteins are usually low, owing to loss through the gastrointestinal tract. Increased portal pressure causes increased lymph production and increased rate of thoracic duct flow. Chylous effusions may occur in the chest and abdomen. Intestinal lymphangiectasia results from increased pressure in the capillaries and lymphatics. This congestion of the intestinal wall mucosal surface results in diminished absorption of ingested protein accompanied by an actual loss of protein from the congested lymphatics. Thoracic duct lymph will show a very low protein content, even though fluid production is increased. Fat transport is also reduced after ingestion.

The diagnosis of constrictive pericarditis is not always easy, since it can easily be confused with various forms of familial and acquired myocardiopathies. Cardiac catheterization has been the best technique in differentiating myocardial and pericardial disease. In constrictive pericarditis, the diastolic pressure in the right ventricle shows a rapid rise during early filling, with a plateau effect and a very small A wave. The systolic pulmonary artery pressure is rarely ever above 45 mm. Hg, and the right atrial pressure is always elevated. Left ventricular end-diastolic pressure is usually normal, whereas in myocardiopathies it is usually much greater, with an average as high as 15 to 18 mm. Hg. Angiocardiography is helpful in outlining the thickness of the atrial wall and the stiffness of the atrium. In a certain number of cases, the diagnosis remains uncertain and can be accurately defined only by pericardial biopsy. This is usually performed

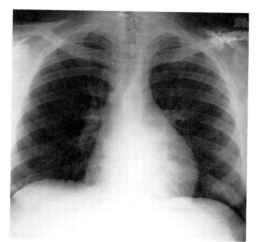
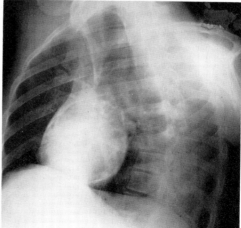

**Figure 3**   Posteroanterior and oblique chest x-rays from a 46 year old male with calcific constrictive pericarditis secondary to tuberculosis. The heart size and lung markings are normal on the posteroanterior film, and calcification is not apparent. On the oblique projection, a ring of calcium almost completely encircles the heart.

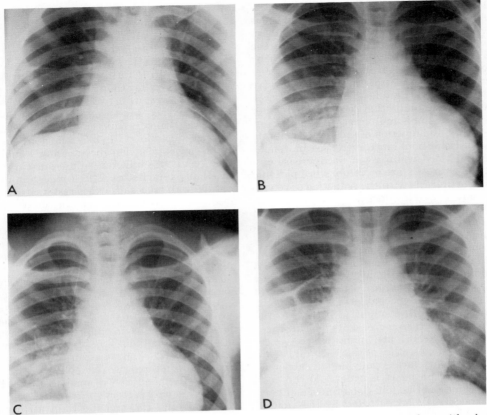

**Figure 4**  Sequence of chest x-rays from an 18 year old male stabbed in the left anterior chest with a knife. *A*, On admission the cardiac silhouette was enlarged. Blood was aspirated from the pericardial sac and the patient hospitalized 8 days. *B*, Four weeks later the cardiac silhouette was larger. There was a slight haziness in the right lower lung field and the patient remained asymptomatic. *C*, At 11 weeks symptoms of constrictive pericarditis developed, with a smaller heart but marked exercise limitation and venous stasis. *D*, Pericardiectomy was performed and the postoperative x-ray showed the heart to be smaller, with residual pleural reaction in the right chest.

through a small incision, with resection of the fourth or fifth costal cartilage. If the diagnosis of constrictive pericarditis is confirmed, a formal thoracotomy should be performed.

Pericardial constriction often follows suppurative forms of pericarditis, a common cause of which has been tuberculosis. Simple penetrating injuries of the heart result in hemopericardium, but this has been a rare cause of chronic pericardial constriction (Fig. 4). Blunt trauma to the chest may cause hemopericardium and precipitate scarring. In some instances the time interval between injury and pericardial constriction is considerable.

# PERICARDIECTOMY

## Preoperative Preparation

Patients are usually hospitalized and brought to an optimal nutritional and cardiovascular state. Vigorous efforts to relieve ascites and cardiac failure should be made by salt restriction, control of arrhythmias, adequate digitalization, and use of diuretics. Antituberculous therapy

should consist of two drugs, with the possible addition of a third drug 10 days prior to operation.

## Operative Technique

Adequate exposure of the heart is necessary to remove the pericardium from the anterior and posterior surfaces. A sternal splitting incision is commonly employed, although a left anterior thoracotomy with extension across the sternum into the right chest has also been advocated. The extent of pericardial resection should be determined by the operative findings; most errors have been the result of removal of an insufficient amount of the pericardium. The myocardium may be quite thinned and atrophic because of the long period of compression by the pericardium, and care must be taken when removing the pericardium from the thin-walled right ventricle. Injury to the coronary vessels must be carefully avoided, and bleeding areas from the heart surface must be controlled by finely placed sutures. The phrenic nerves should be mobilized away from the pericardium to avoid damage to them and to allow resection of the pericardium posterior to the nerve.

Small pockets of localized fluid or pus may be encountered between the epicardium and the thickened pericardium, and the epicardial lining of such pockets should be removed to lessen the chance of subsequent scarring. Oozing from the heart surface usually ceases with gentle pressure, and the pleura is opened widely on both sides. Intercostal catheters are placed in each chest for drainage.

### Postoperative Care

The main concern of the postoperative period is fluid overload. Venous pressure usually falls after the constricted pericardium is removed, and intravenous fluid or blood must be administered conservatively to avoid overloading the heart or lungs. A mild cardiac stimulant may be needed if cardiac contractility decreases. Usually a slow infusion of dilute isoproterenol will improve cardiac function. Antibiotics are usually administered for 8 to 10 days, and tuberculous chemotherapy is continued for 3 to 6 months depending upon culture reports of pericardial material. In proved cases of tuberculosis, antituberculous therapy should be continued for a minimum of 6 months, and many advise treatment for 1 year.

Salt restriction is usually necessary; however, if a profound diuresis occurs after operation, salt replacement may be indicated. Electrolytes must be closely observed, and digitalis administration usually is continued. Ambulation and exercise are gradually encouraged, since ascites and edema usually subside soon after operation.

It has been emphasized that the pericardium must be removed from the caval orifices to the right atrium to be certain of relieving ascites. In experiments in animals, Isaacs et al.[10] showed that removal of the pericardium from the right heart resulted in a decrease in central venous pressure, but the animals expired from pulmonary congestion. In other instances, removal of the pericardium from the left heart alone had no effect on venous pressure or ascites.

# POSTPERICARDIOTOMY SYNDROME

Postpericardiotomy syndrome is an unusual syndrome typically characterized by fever, pericardial pain, pleural pain, pulmonary infiltrates, arthralgias, dyspnea, pericardial effusion, pleural effusion, pericardial friction rub, or any combination of these signs and symptoms. Symptoms suggesting the postpericardiotomy syndrome have been noted in 10 to 40 per cent of patients undergoing cardiac surgery, and the actual incidence may be higher, since mild cases may remain unrecognized. The sedimentation rate is elevated, and leukocytosis with an increase in lymphocytes is usually present. The electrocardiogram may show changes of pericarditis.

Cox[5] and Koucky and Milles[14] initially referred to this syndrome as polyserositis occurring after wounds of the heart. It was called postcommissur-otomy syndrome because of its frequency of occurrence after mitral commissurotomy and was thought at one time to be due to reactivation of rheumatic fever. Dresdale et al.[6] observed similar symptoms after a pericardiotomy and termed the syndrome postpericardiotomy syndrome. It has been seen to occur after such minor violations of the pericardium as percutaneous left ventricular punctures.

The etiology of postpericardiotomy syndrome has received considerable speculation. It was originally thought that the syndrome represented an exacerbation of rheumatic fever, but the occurrence of the syndrome in persons without evidence of rheumatic heart disease seems to rule out this possibility. Bacterial infection was considered, but repeated cultures of pericardium or pericardial fluid in patients suffering from the syndrome did not reveal any pathogenic organism. Cohen et al.[4] noticed that there were periods of increased incidence of the syndrome with seasonal variation. This suggested the possibility of a virus infection being activated by operation and causing symptoms. Kahn and co-workers[11] in 1967 reported the isolation of parainfluenza virus from a group of patients with postpericardiotomy syndrome; this suggests that a virus infection may be responsible in some cases at least.

The possibility that the syndrome represents an autoimmune response has been suggested, the symptoms resulting from a delayed hypersensitivity reaction to damaged tissues in the pericardial cavity. The pertinent structural alterations render tissue somewhat foreign to the host, and this induces the production of autoantibody. It has been suggested that the myocardium, red blood cells, and pericardial tissue may be the organs against which the antibodies react. Van der Geld[30] detected antiheart antibodies in 21 of 29 patients with postpericardiotomy syndrome. The severity of symptoms could be correlated with falling or rising titers of circulating antibodies.

Aronstam and Cox[1] described low serum albumin associated with poor nutrition in patients with symptoms of postpericardiotomy syndrome. Reversal of negative nitrogen balance by administration of intravenous albumin resulted in clinical improvement. If collections of fluid persisted, pericardicentesis or thoracentesis was done. No evidence of the syndrome appeared in any patient showing normal blood protein levels in the postoperative period.

The syndrome is generally self-limiting and benign. The illness may last from 1 to 6 weeks, and recurrences are possible. Chronic pericardial effusion and constrictive pericarditis have not been reported to occur after postpericardiotomy syndrome. The diagnosis is based primarily on the clinical findings. Treatment is generally symptomatic, with the patient being made as comfortable as possible. Physical activity is restricted, and fever and pain are controlled by appropriate medications. Salicylates have been effective in lowering temperature and relieving pain. Stronger analgesics may be required in more severe cases.

Steroid therapy may cause dramatic relief of symptoms, with temperature returning to normal. In some cases the symptoms linger and low doses of steroids are necessary for a considerable period of time. Steroid therapy is generally not recommended for the milder cases, since recurrences are common when the steroids are withdrawn.

The main complications of this syndrome are misdiagnosis resulting in failure to treat a specific infection, delay in recuperation with prolongation of hospitalization, and recurrences. Postpericardiotomy syndrome usually does not play a role in the ultimate prognosis of the patient, even though convalescence can be prolonged.

## SELECTED REFERENCES

Ebert, P. A.: The pericardium. In: Gibbon, J. H., Jr., Sabiston, D. C., Jr., and Spencer, F. C., eds.: Surgery of the Chest. 2nd ed. Philadelphia, W. B. Saunders Company, 1969.
*In this detailed account of diseases of the pericardium, the techniques of pericardial aspiration are discussed, and the potential problems associated with various methods are analyzed. The pathophysiology of pericardial tamponade is presented and the clinical course discussed. The operative technique of pericardiectomy is well illustrated, and the importance of performing a radical pericardiectomy is emphasized.*

Kirsh, M. M., McIntosh, K., Kahn, D. R., and Sloan, H.: Postpericardiotomy syndromes. Ann. Thorac. Surg., 9:158, 1970.
*This review article gives an excellent résumé of the current concepts of the rather vague syndromes seen after operations on the heart. A good review of possible etiologies of the postpericardiotomy and postperfusion syndromes, such as autoimmune states, virus infection, and protein deficiencies, is presented. Treatment is outlined and the usual benign course of these syndromes emphasized.*

## REFERENCES

1. Aronstam, E. M., and Cox, W. A.: A new concept of the pleuropericardial syndrome. Postpericardiotomy or postcardiotomy syndrome. J. Thorac. Cardiovasc. Surg., 51:341, 1966.
2. Brawley, R. K., Vasko, J. S., and Morrow, A. G.: Cholesterol pericarditis. Amer. J. Med., 41:235, 1966.
3. Chevers, N.: Observations on the disease of the orifice and valves of the aorta. Guy's Hosp. Rep., 7:387, 1842.
4. Cohen, G., Dardick, I., and Greenblatt, J.: Pleurisy and pericarditis complicating myocardial infarction: The so-called post myocardial infarction syndrome. Canad. Med. Ass. J., 82:123, 1960.
5. Cox, W. M.: Wounds of the heart. Arch. Surg., 17:484, 1928.
6. Dresdale, D. T., Ropstein, C. B., Gusman, S. J., and Greene, M. A.: Postpericardiotomy syndrome in patients with rheumatic heart disease. Amer. J. Med., 21:57, 1956.
7. Holman, C. W., and Steinberg, I.: The role of angiocardiography in the surgical treatment of massive pericardial effusions. Surg. Gynec. Obstet., 107:639, 1958.
8. Holman, E., and Willett, F.: Treatment of active tuberculous pericarditis by pericardiectomy. J.A.M.A., 146:1, 1951.
9. Holman, E., and Willett, F.: Results of radical pericardiectomy for constrictive pericarditis. J.A.M.A., 157:789, 1955.
10. Isaacs, J. P., Carter, B. N., II, and Haller, J. A., Jr.: Pathologic physiology of constrictive pericarditis. Bull. Johns Hopkins Hosp., 90:259, 1952.
11. Kahn, D. R., Ertel, P. Y., Murphy, W. H., Kirsh, M. M., Vathayanon, S., Stern, A. M., and Sloan, H.: Pathogenesis of the postpericardiotomy syndrome. J. Thorac. Cardiovasc. Surg., 54:682, 1967.
12. Kaplan, M. H.: The concept of autoantibodies in rheumatic fever and in the postcommissurotomy state. Ann. N.Y. Acad. Sci., 86:974, 1960.
13. Karanaeff: Paracentese des Brustkastens und des Pericardiums. Med. Ztg., 9:251, 1840.
14. Koucky, J. D., and Milles, G.: Stab wounds of the heart. Arch. Intern. Med., 56:281, 1935.
15. Kussmaul, A.: Ueber schwielige Mediastino-Perikarditis und den paradoxen Puls. Berlin. Klin. Wschr., 10:433, 461, 1873.
16. Lower, R.: Tractatus de Corde. London, 1669. (Cited in Major, R. H.: Classic Descriptions of Disease. Springfield, Ill., Charles C Thomas, 1932, p. 630.)
17. Martin, A.: Acute non-specific pericarditis. A description of nineteen cases. Brit. Med. J., 2:279, 1966.
18. Martin, J. W., and Schenk, W. G., Jr.: Pericardial tamponade; newer dynamic concepts. Amer. J. Surg., 99:782, 1960.
19. McKusick, V. A., Kay, J. H., and Isaacs, J. P.: Constrictive pericarditis following traumatic hemopericardium. Ann. Surg., 142:97, 1955.
20. Morgagni, G. B.: De Sedibus et Causis Morborum per Anatomen Indagatis. Venetiis, Typ. Remondiniana, 1761.
21. Parsons, H. G., and Holman, E.: Experimental segmental pericarditis. Arch. Surg., 70:479, 1955.
22. Rehn, L.: Zur experimentellen Pathologie des Herzbeutels. Ver. Deutsch. Ges. Chir., 42:339, 1913.
23. Romero, cited by Baizeau: Mémoire sur le ponction du péricarde au point de vue chirurgical. Gaz. Med. Chir., 1868, p. 565.
24. Roshe, J., and Shumacker, H. B., Jr.: Pericardiectomy for chronic cardiac tamponade in children. Surgery, 46:1152, 1959.
25. Sauerbruch, F.: Die Chirurgie der Brustorgane. Vol. II. Berlin, 1925.
26. Sellors, T. H.: General observations on constricitive pericarditis with special reference to results of surgery. Minerva Cardioangiol. Europ., 4:489, 1956.
27. Shumacker, H. B., Jr., and Roshe, J.: Pericardiectomy. J. Cardiovasc. Surg., 1:65, 1960.
28. Soulen, R. L., Lapayowker, M. S., and Gimenz, J. L.: Echocardiography in the diagnosis of pericardial effusion. Radiology, 86:1047, 1966.
29. Turner, A. F., Meyers, H. L., Jacobson, G., and Lo, W.: Carbon dioxide cineangiocardiography in the diagnosis of pericardial disease. Amer. J. Roentgen., 97:342, 1966.
30. Van der Geld, H.: Anti-heart antibodies in the postpericardiotomy and the postmyocardial-infarction syndromes. Lancet, 2:617, 1964.
31. Vieussens, R.: Traité nouveau de la structure et des causes du mouvement naturel de coeur. Toulouse, J. Guillemette, 1715.
32. White, P.: Chronic constrictive pericarditis. (Pick's disease) treated by pericardial resection. Lancet, 2:597, 1935.
33. Wood, P.: Diagnosis of pericardial effusion by means of cardiac catheterization. Brit. Heart J., 13:574, 1951.

# 56

# THE HEART

I

## Cardiac Catheterization

*Erwin Robin, M.D., Sunilendu N. Ganguly, M.D.,*
*and Richard J. Bing, M.D.*

### HISTORICAL ASPECTS

In 1861, Chaveau and Marey performed cardiac catheterization in animals. In 1905, Fritz Bleichroeder had a ureteral catheter placed in his axillary vein from the arm and in his inferior vena cava from the thigh. Forssman, in 1929, under fluoroscopic control, catheterized his right atrium from a left antecubital vein. Right heart catheterization was introduced clinically in 1941 by Cournand and Ranges and was further developed by Richards, Bing, and Dexter. Since that time, rapid advances have been made with the introduction of new methods, such as indicator dilution methods, left heart catheterization, and selective angiography.

### INDICATIONS

There are no absolute contraindications to cardiac catheterization. From a clinical viewpoint, it is indicated whenever it is necessary to establish a precise and definite diagnosis. This has become increasingly important as surgical techniques have been devised for correction of more and more cardiac lesions.

### PREPARATION OF THE PATIENT

The patient should be psychologically prepared. This is best accomplished by explaining the procedure and its goal, and thus gaining his confidence.

General anesthesia is neither necessary nor desirable. In adults, small amounts of a narcotic or barbiturate may be used. In children, intramuscular injection of a combination of 6.25 mg. promethezine (Phenergan), 6.25 mg. chlorpromazine (Thorazine), and 25 mg. meperidine hydrochloride (Demerol) per cubic centimeter of mixture provides good sedation. The dose varies according to the age, weight, and condition of the patient. Noncyanotic children receive 1 ml. per 20 pounds of body weight. Cyanotic children should receive a smaller dose. Newborns rarely need sedation. However, if it is needed, oral chloral hydrate may be administered in a dose of 10 to 15 mg. per pound of body weight.

The patient should fast for 3 to 6 hours prior to the study. Sedation is given 30 to 60 minutes before catheterization. Cyanotic children, because of the high viscosity of their blood, are permitted to receive fluids 2 to 3 hours prior to the procedure. As a rule, prophylactic antibiotics are not necessary.

### CHOICE OF CATHETERS

Catheters are available in a variety of models and sizes (Fig. 1). Pressures are best recorded with open-end catheters. During the performance of angiocardiography, closed-end catheters are used to prevent recoil and intramural injection of contrast material.

### RIGHT HEART CATHETERIZATION

Under sterile conditions and fluoroscopic control, a radiopaque catheter is inserted percutaneously or via a cutdown into a peripheral vein and passed into the right atrium, right ventricle, and pulmonary arterial vessels. In newborns, the superficial femoral or umbilical vein is used. In infants and small children, the superficial saphenous vein is usually used (Fig. 2*A*). In older children and adults, an antecubital vein is preferred (Fig. 2*B*).

#### Recording of Pressures

Normal values of pressures obtained during right cardiac catheterization are shown in Table 1. **Pulmonary Capillary Pressure.** The pulmonary

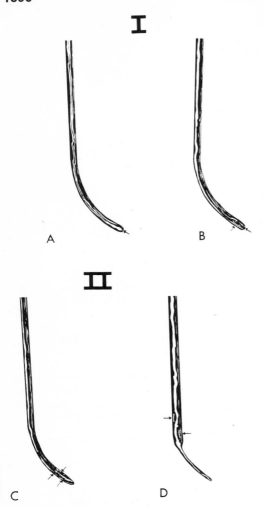

**Figure 1** Catheters used during cardiac catheterization. *I,* Open-end catheter tips: A, Cournand catheter tip; B, Birdseye catheter tip with two laterally opposed eyes close to the distal tip. *II,* Closed-end catheter tips: C, NIH catheter tip with six round openings arranged in three laterally opposed pairs within 1 cm. of the tip; D, Lehman ventriculography catheter tip with four eyes arranged in two laterally opposed pairs within 4 cm. of the distal tip. (Arrows point toward openings.)

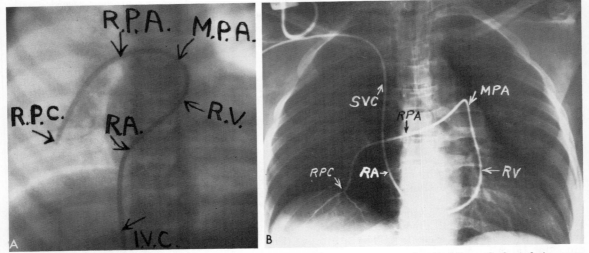

**Figure 2** *A,* A catheter has been introduced into the right saphenous vein and guided through the inferior vena cava (I.V.C.), right atrium (R.A.), right ventricle (R.V.), main pulmonary artery (M.P.A.), and right pulmonary artery (R.P.A.) to the right pulmonary capillary position (R.P.C.). *B,* A catheter has been introduced into a right antecubital vein and passed through the superior vena cava (S.V.C.), right atrium (R.A.), right ventricle (R.V.), main pulmonary artery (M.P.A.), right pulmonary artery (R.P.A.), and right pulmonary capillary position (R.P.C.).

**TABLE 1**  NORMAL PRESSURES OBTAINED BY
RIGHT HEART CATHETERIZATION*

| | Pressure (mm. Hg) | | |
| --- | --- | --- | --- |
| | *Systolic* | *Diastolic* | *Mean* |
| Right atrium | 5 to 7 | −2 to 2 | −2 to 7 |
| Right ventricle | 15 to 30 | 0 to 7 | |
| Pulmonary artery | 15 to 30 | 5 to 15 | 10 to 20 |
| Pulmonary capillary | | | 5 to 12 |

*Modified from Robin, E., et al. In: Gibbon, J. H., Jr., Sabiston, D. C., Jr., and Spencer, F. C., eds.: Surgery of the Chest. 2nd ed. Philadelphia, W. B. Saunders Company, 1969.

capillary pressure (also referred to as wedge pressure) resembles the left atrial pressure (Fig. 3). This is due to the fact that there are no valves between the left atrium and pulmonary veins and capillaries. Incomplete wedging or wedging of the catheter tip into the wall of a tortuous pulmonary artery is a common cause of a distorted pulmonary capillary pressure tracing.

**Pulmonary Artery Pressure.** The pulmonary artery pressure ranges from 15 to 30 mm. Hg systolic, and 5 to 15 mm. Hg diastolic, with a mean of 10 to 20 mm. Hg.

Pulmonary hypertension is classified into hyperkinetic and obstructive types. The former type is due to a marked increase in pulmonary flow from a left-to-right shunt. During childhood and adolescence, pulmonary hypertension is more common in cases of ventricular septal defect and patent ductus arteriosus than in those of atrial septal defect.

Obstructive pulmonary hypertension may be the end result of the hyperkinetic type. In this case, the pulmonary blood flow can be normal or even decreased. Other causes are chronic pulmonary parenchymal diseases, multiple pulmonary emboli, chronic left heart failure, mitral valve disease, and pulmonary vasculitis.

**Right Ventricular Pressure.** A maximal systolic gradient of 10 mm. Hg between the main pulmonary artery and the right ventricle is considered normal. In pulmonic valvular stenosis, the systolic gradient between the main pulmonary trunk and the outflow tract of the right ventricle is abrupt

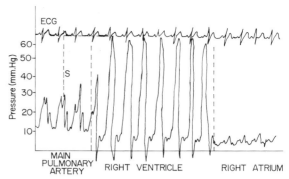

**Figure 4**  Pulmonic valvular stenosis: There is an abrupt systolic gradient (S) of 40 mm. Hg between the main pulmonary trunk and the outflow tract of the right ventricle at the level of the pulmonic valve. (From Robin, E., et al. In: Gibbon, J. H., Jr., Sabiston, D. C., Jr., and Spencer, F. C., eds.: Surgery of the Chest. 2nd ed. Philadelphia, W. B. Saunders Company, 1969.)

(Fig. 4); in infundibular stenosis, on the other hand, progressive gradients are found between the main pulmonary artery, the infundibular chamber, and the right ventricle (Fig. 5).

In 90 per cent of cases of isolated pulmonic stenosis, the lesion is at the level of the pulmonic valve. In tetralogy of Fallot, infundibular pulmonic stenosis is present in 40 per cent, valvular stenosis in 35 per cent, and combined valvular and infundibular stenosis in 25 per cent of cases. Isolated infundibular stenosis can develop late in the course of large ventricular septal defects.

**Right Atrial Pressure.** The right atrial pressure curve consists of three waves, "a," "c," and "v," each of which is followed by a descent "x," "x'," and "y." The "a" wave is produced by atrial systole, the "c" wave by transmission of the right ventricular systole through the closed tricuspid valve, and the "v" wave by the inflow of blood into the right atrium during atrial diastole.

In tricuspid atresia and stenosis, in the absence of atrial fibrillation, there is a tall "a" wave; if the

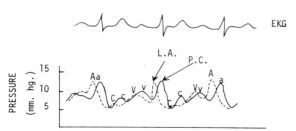

**Figure 3**  Simultaneous left atrial (L.A.) and pulmonary capillary (P.C.) pressures: The left atrial pressure was obtained by means of the transseptal technique. Both curves are similar in their contour and magnitude. The pulmonary capillary pressure is slightly delayed.

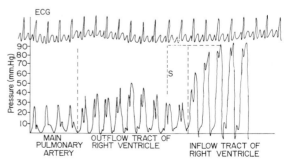

**Figure 5**  Pulmonic infundibular stenosis: There is a systolic gradient (S) of 40 mm. Hg between the outflow and inflow tracts of the right ventricle below the pulmonic valve. (From Robin, E., et al. In: Gibbon, J. H., Jr., Sabiston, D. C., Jr., and Spencer, F. C., eds.: Surgery of the Chest. 2nd ed. Philadelphia, W. B. Saunders Company, 1969.)

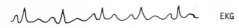

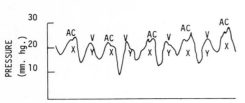

PRESSURE (mm. hg.)

**Figure 6** Right atrial pressure in a case of constrictive pericarditis: The pressure curve has an M or W shape because of the prominent and steep "x" and "y" descents.

| | O$_2$ Saturation Difference (%) | O$_2$ Content Difference (Vol. %) | Type of Defect |
|---|---|---|---|
| SVC-RA | 9.0 | 2.0 | ASD |
| RA-RV | 5.0 | 1.0 | VSD |
| RV-PA | 3.0 | 0.5 | PDA |

**TABLE 2** SIGNIFICANT DIFFERENCES IN OXYGEN SATURATION AND CONTENT*

*Modified from Robin, E., et al. In: Gibbon, J. H., Jr., Sabiston, D. C., Jr., and Spencer, F. C., eds.: Surgery of the Chest. 2nd ed. Philadelphia, W. B. Saunders Company, 1969.

valve is incompetent, the "v" wave is prominent. An increase in right atrial pressure occurs in right heart failure. In constrictive pericarditis, the mean right atrial pressure is elevated, and the pressure curve assumes a distinctive pattern (Fig. 6).

### Sampling of Blood for Oxygen Determination and Calculation of Flow

The most commonly used method of identifying, localizing, and quantifying shunts involves the analysis of oxygen in blood drawn from the heart and the great veins and arteries. Normally, there is great variability in the oxygen in blood withdrawn from the right atrium because of laminar flow from the superior and inferior venae cavae and coronary sinus. Truly mixed venous blood is found only in the pulmonary artery.

Multiple samples of blood should be obtained in rapid succession, beginning at the pulmonary artery and ending at the venae cavae. At least two samples should be obtained in the right ventricle: one in the outflow tract and the other in the main cavity. In the right atrium, at least three samples should be drawn: one near the inferior vena cava, one in the middle of the atrium near the lateral wall, and the third just below the superior vena cava.

Flows are calculated according to the Fick principle (see Equations 1 and 2 at bottom of page).

If pulmonary flow is more than systemic flow, there is a left-to-right shunt. If the systemic flow is greater than the pulmonary flow, there is a right-to-left shunt.

If bidirectional shunting is present, the "effective pulmonary blood flow" must be calculated first. The "effective pulmonary blood flow" is the volume of mixed blood that, after returning to the right atrium, is aerated in the pulmonary capillaries (see Equation 3 at bottom of page).

At the level of a left-to-right shunt and downstream from it, the oxygen saturation of blood is higher than in the chamber immediately upstream. The pulmonary flow also exceeds the systemic flow. In contrast, in the right-to-left shunts the pulmonary flow is less than the systemic flow; the oxygen saturation is normal in the pulmonary veins and decreased in the peripheral arterial blood. In many cases, a bidirectional shunt is present. This results in a left-to-right shunt and a diminished oxygen saturation in the peripheral arterial blood.

Significant differences in oxygen saturation and content are summarized in Table 2. Left-to-right shunts that are less than 20 per cent of the pul-

---

1. Systemic flow (S.F.) (liters/min.) $= \dfrac{O_2 \text{ consumption (ml./min.)}}{\text{Systemic A-V difference} \times 10}$  where A (vol. %) = peripheral arterial blood
   V (vol. %) = mixed venous blood

2. Pulmonary flow (P.F.) (liters/min.) $= \dfrac{O_2 \text{ consumption (ml./min.)}}{\text{Pulmonary A-V difference} \times 10}$  where A (vol.%) = pulmonary vein blood
   V (vol.%) = pulmonary artery blood

3. Effective pulmonary flow (E.F.) =

   $$\dfrac{O_2 \text{ consumption (ml./min.)}}{\text{Pulmonary venous } O_2 \text{ content (vol. \%)} - \text{mixed venous } O_2 \text{ content (vol. \%)} \times 10}$$

   Then: a. left-to-right shunt = P.F. − E.F.
   (liters/min.)
   b. right-to-left shunt = S.F. − E.F.
   (liters/min.)

monary flow are not detectable by the conventional blood oxygen saturation methods.

### Oxygen Analysis

Oxygen content determination can be accomplished by the manometric method of Van Slyke and Neill or by spectrophotometry. These methods are time-consuming, and in infants multiple sampling may constitute a considerable loss of blood. By use of either transmission or reflection methods, direct analysis of blood oxygen content can be obtained rapidly by flow through cuvettes connected directly to a catheter. Oxygen tension ($pO_2$) may be monitored continually by means of a platinum electrode. A fiberoptic catheter incorporates instantaneous and continuous measurement of oxygen saturation without withdrawal of blood samples. The same instrument can also be used in the determination of cardiac output.

### Observation of the Position of the Catheter

The position of the catheter is important in the recognition of abnormal communications between the cardiac chambers and the great vessels. If abnormal channels are encountered, serial blood samples should be drawn, and continuous pressures should be recorded.

The tip of the catheter may pass over the left side of the heart through a patent foramen ovale or atrial or ventricular septal defect. In endocardial cushion defects, either partial or complete, the position of the catheter is lower than in septum secundum defects. If the tip of the catheter is manipulated into the left ventricle, one may obtain, on withdrawal, an abrupt pressure change from the left ventricular to the right atrial form.

If an anomalous draining pulmonary vein is intubated, the shaft of the catheter will take an abnormal position in relation to the cardiac silhouette. However, distinction between an atrial septal defect and an anomalous pulmonary vein cannot be made from the position of the catheter alone.

Often the catheter may be threaded through the patent ductus arteriosus into the descending aorta. In the tetralogy of Fallot, aortic transposition, or ventricular defects in the membranous part of the septum, the ascending aorta may be intubated directly from the right ventricle.

## LEFT HEART CATHETERIZATION

The development of left heart catheterization has made it possible to assess more accurately the size and location of left-to-right shunts and to evaluate lesions of the mitral and aortic valves. Selective angiocardiography of the left heart chambers, aorta, and coronary arteries can be performed, and postoperative results can be evaluated.

The normal pressures observed during left heart catheterization are summarized in Table 3.

**TABLE 3** NORMAL PRESSURES RECORDED DURING LEFT HEART CATHETERIZATION*

| | Pressures (mm. Hg) | | |
| | Systolic | Diastolic | Mean |
| --- | --- | --- | --- |
| Left atrium | | | 4 to 12 |
| Left ventricle | 100 to 140 | 4 to 12 | |
| Aorta | 100 to 140 | 60 to 90 | 70 to 90 |

*From Robin, E., et al. In: Gibbon, J. H., Jr., Sabiston, D. C., Jr., and Spencer, F. C., eds.: Surgery of the Chest. 2nd ed. Philadelphia, W. B. Saunders Company, 1969.

### Pressure Relationships of the Left Heart

The diagnostic value of left heart catheterization is to a large extent based on the pressure relationships between the left atrium, the left ventricle, and the aorta (Fig. 7). The components of the normal left atrial pressure are diagramed in Figure 8.

The "v" wave ranges normally between 5 and 15 mm. Hg, and the "a" wave between 3 and 7 mm. Hg. In auricular fibrillation, the "a" wave is absent, whereas in atrioventricular block, giant "a" waves may be present. In heart failure or valvular disease, normal pressure tracings are modified by changes in contour or height. In congestive heart failure, there is an elevation of the left ventricular end-diastolic and left atrial pressures. In mitral stenosis, there is usually an increase in the left atrial pressure and a prolongation of the "y" descent, indicating resistance to flow across the mitral valve (Fig. 9).

Although pressure contours are of value in the evaluation of patients with mitral disease, the most important criterion of the severity of mitral stenosis is the left atrioventricular diastolic pressure gradient across the mitral valve at rest and during exercise. Normally this gradient is 1 mm. or less, whereas in mitral stenosis gradients of 5 to 30 mm. Hg at rest have been found. The gradient rises significantly with exercise. Following suc-

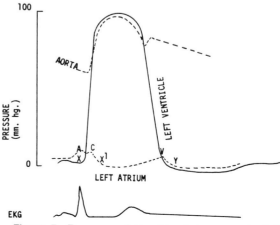

**Figure 7** Pressure relationships between aorta, left ventricle, and left atrium.

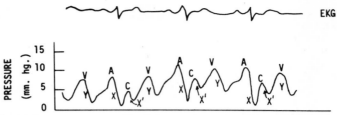

**Figure 8**   Normal left atrial pressure curve: The "a" wave is produced by atrial systole, the "c" wave by transmission of the rising pressure in the left ventricle through the closed mitral valve during ventricular systole, and the "v" wave by the inflow of blood into the left atrium during atrial diastole. Each wave is followed by a descent; the "v" wave is followed by the "x" descent, the "c" wave by the "x'" descent, and the "v" wave by the "y" descent. (The right atrial curve has a similar contour.)

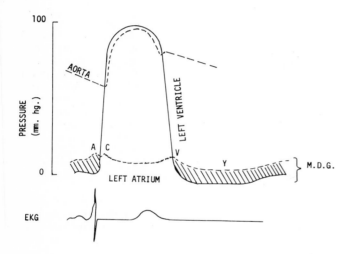

**Figure 9**   Mitral stenosis: There is a diastolic gradient (M.D.G.) between the left atrium and left ventricle. The "y" descent is prolonged because of the resistance to flow across the mitral valve.

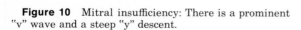

**Figure 10**   Mitral insufficiency: There is a prominent "v" wave and a steep "y" descent.

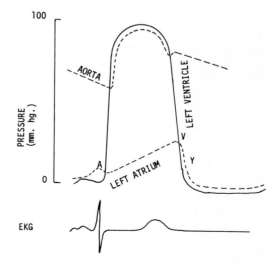

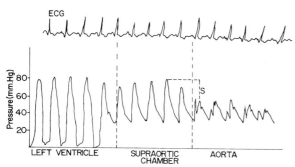

**Figure 11** Supravalvular aortic stenosis: There is a systolic gradient (S) of 20 mm. Hg within the ascending aorta above the aortic valve. (From Robin, E., et al. In: Gibbon, J. H., Jr., Sabiston, D. C., Jr., and Spencer, F. C., eds.: Surgery of the Chest. 2nd ed. Philadelphia, W. B. Saunders Company, 1969.)

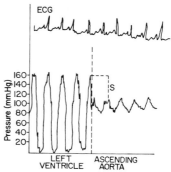

**Figure 12** Aortic valvular stenosis: There is a systolic gradient (S) of 45 mm. Hg between the ascending aorta and left ventricle at the level of the aortic valve. (From Robin, E., et al. In: Gibbon, J. H., Jr., Sabiston, D. C., Jr., and Spencer, F. C., eds.: Surgery of the Chest. 2nd ed. Philadelphia, W. B. Saunders Company, 1969.)

cessful mitral commissurotomy, a marked reduction or abolition of the mitral gradient is observed.

A mitral diastolic gradient does not always indicate mitral stenosis. It may result from obstructive hypertrophy of the anterior papillary muscles, myxoma of the left atrium, anomalous myocardial hypertrophy adjacent to the mitral valve, or generalized obstructive left ventricular hypertrophy.

In mitral insufficiency, the characteristic features are a tall "v" wave (the so-called regurgitant wave) and a steep "y" descent, indicating little or no resistance to flow across the valve (Fig. 10). In combined lesions of the mitral valve, the pressure tracing reveals a combination of the findings described in mitral insufficiency and stenosis, the gradations depending on the severity of each.

The normal left ventricular pressure in man is 120 mm. Hg (100 to 140) systolic and 4 to 12 mm. Hg diastolic. In infants, the systemic arterial pressure averages 60 to 70 mm. Hg. There is a difference of 10 to 15 mm. Hg between the central systolic aortic pressure and the peripheral systolic pressure, the latter being higher. Supravalvular aortic stenosis is characterized by an abrupt fall in

pressure as the catheter passes the site of a narrowing above the aortic valve (Fig. 11). In congenital or acquired valvular aortic stenosis, the systolic gradient between the aorta and the left ventricle is sudden (Fig. 12). In discrete subaortic stenosis, the systolic pressure gradient shows a progressive fall between the left ventricle and the aorta similar to that described in isolated pulmonic infundibular stenosis (Fig. 13). In idiopathic hypertrophic subaortic stenosis, the site of obstruction has been localized to the left ventricular outflow tract. The ascending limb of the left ventricular pressure tracing, recorded proximally to the obstruction, generally exhibits a notch at a level that corresponds to the peak pressure distal to the obstruction (Fig. 13). Administration of digitalis, amyl nitrite, nitroglycerin, and isoproterenol or a Valsalva maneuver increases the systolic gradient (Figs. 14 and 15), whereas methoxamine and beta-adrenergic blocking agents, such as propranolol, tend to decrease the systolic gradient (Fig. 16). There is a fall in the peripheral pulse pressure following the normal beat that succeeds a ventricular premature con-

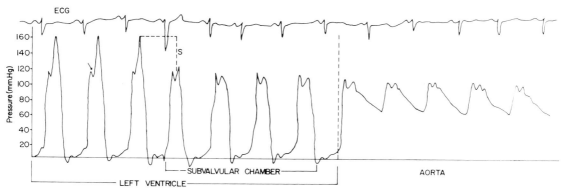

**Figure 13** Subaortic hypertrophic stenosis: There is a systolic gradient (S) of 45 mm. Hg below the aortic valve within the left ventricle. The arrow denotes the notch on the ascending limb of the left ventricular pressure curve that corresponds to the peak systolic pressure distal to the obstruction. (From Robin, E., et al. In: Gibbon, J. H., Jr., Sabiston, D. C., Jr., and Spencer, F. C., eds.: Surgery of the Chest. 2nd ed. Philadelphia, W. B. Saunders Company, 1969.)

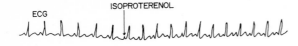

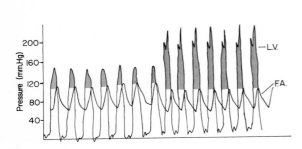

**Figure 14**  Effect of intravenous isoproterenol on the systolic gradient (shaded area) between left ventricle (L.V.) and femoral artery (F.A.) in subaortic hypertrophic stenosis: The baseline systolic gradient (shaded area) is about 40 mm. Hg. During infusion of isoproterenol it increases to 90 mm. Hg (shaded area). (From Robin, E., et al. In: Gibbon, J. H., Jr., Sabiston, D. C., Jr., and Spencer, F. C., eds.: Surgery of the Chest. 2nd ed. Philadelphia, W. B. Saunders Company, 1969.)

**Figure 15**  Effect of Valsalva maneuver on the systolic gradient (shaded area) between left ventricle (L.V.) and femoral artery (F.A.) in subaortic hypertrophic stenosis: The baseline systolic gradient (shaded area) is about 60 mm. Hg. During the maneuver it is increased to 110 mm. Hg (shaded area). (From Robin, E., et al. In: Gibbon, J. H., Jr., Sabiston, D. C., Jr., and Spencer, F. C., eds.: Surgery of the Chest. 2nd ed. Philadelphia, W. B. Saunders Company, 1969.)

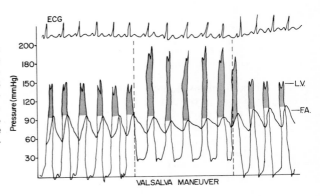

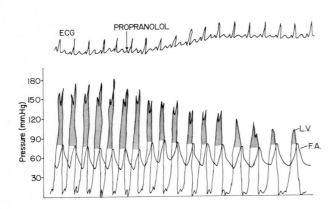

**Figure 16**  Effect of a beta-adrenergic blocking agent (propranolol) on the systolic gradient (shaded area) between left ventricle (L.V.) and femoral artery (F.A.) in subaortic hypertrophic stenosis: The baseline systolic gradient (shaded area) is about 80 mm. Hg. During infusion of propranolol it decreases to about 20 mm. Hg (shaded area). (From Robin, E., et al. In: Gibbon, J. H., Jr., Sabiston, D. C., Jr., and Spencer, F. C., eds.: Surgery of the Chest. 2nd ed. Philadelphia, W. B. Saunders Company, 1969.)

**Figure 17**  Effect of a post-premature contraction on pulse pressure of the femoral artery (F.A.) in subaortic hypertrophic stenosis: The baseline pulse pressure (P) in the femoral artery (F.A.) is about 35 mm. Hg. During the post-premature contraction, pulse pressure (P$_1$) in the femoral artery (F.A.) is about 25 mm. Hg. Shaded area represents the systolic gradient between the left ventricle (L.V.) and the femoral artery (F.A.). (From Robin, E., et al. In: Gibbon, J. H., Jr., Sabiston, D. C., Jr., and Spencer, F. C., eds.: Surgery of the Chest. 2nd ed. Philadelphia, W. B. Saunders Company, 1969.)

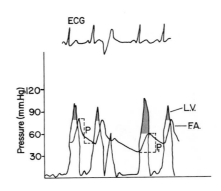

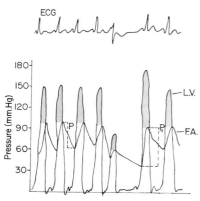

**Figure 18** Effect of a post-premature contraction on pulse pressure of the femoral artery (F.A.) in valvular aortic stenosis: The baseline pulse pressure (P) of the femoral artery (F.A.) is about 35 mm. Hg. During post-premature contraction, pulse pressure (P₁) of the femoral artery (F.A.) is about 55 mm. Hg. Shaded area represents the systolic gradient between the left ventricle (L.V.) and the femoral artery (F.A.). (From Robin, E., et al. In: Gibbon, J. H., Jr., Sabiston, D. C., Jr., and Spencer, F. C., eds.: Surgery of the Chest. 2nd ed. Philadelphia, W. B. Saunders Company, 1969.)

traction (Fig. 17). In contrast, in patients with discrete supravalvular, valvular, or subvalvular stenosis, a widened pulse pressure occurs after the first normal beat following a premature ventricular contraction (Fig. 18).

In aortic insufficiency, left ventricular diastolic pressure exceeds left atrial pressure in mid-diastole and continues to rise so that the aortic and ventricular diastolic pressures are about equal at the onset of systole. The aortic pressure contour also exhibits a low diastolic pressure and a wide pulse pressure. In patients with aortic insufficiency and aortic stenosis, a combination of these signs is seen, and the brachial artery pulse pressure exhibits the so-called pulsus bisferiens.

### Methods of Left Heart Catheterization

During the last 15 years, numerous methods of catheterizing the left heart have been employed clinically. These have included the transbronchial technique, the posterior percutaneous left atrial puncture technique, the suprasternal left atrial puncture technique, and the anterior left ventricular approach technique.

In recent years, these methods have been completely replaced by the transseptal left heart and retrograde aortic left heart catheterization techniques. The latter method is by far the more popular because of its relative ease and low morbidity. It can be performed percutaneously through the femoral artery or through the brachial artery via a cutdown. With either approach, the aorta, left ventricle, and coronary vascular bed can be selectively visualized. In addition, with the transbrachial route, the left atrium can be intubated from the left ventricle.

## COMPLICATIONS OF CARDIAC CATHETERIZATION

Transient arrhythmias occur during every procedure. Conduction defects, knotted catheters, pyrogenic reactions, air emboli, venous or arterial spasm, thrombophlebitis, and perforation of the atria, ventricles, and coronary sinus with subsequent hemopericardium and cardiac tamponade have been reported. An increased risk is expected in cyanotic children and in patients with severe pulmonary hypertension. (See also the discussion of contrast materials under the heading Angiocardiography.)

## INDICATOR DILUTION TECHNIQUES

### Dye Dilution Method

The direct recording of the peripheral arterial dye dilution curve yields much information about the circulation in a relatively short time. Thus, it is possible to estimate the cardiac output and to determine the presence of shunts or valvular insufficiency. The usefulness of the technique is increased when it is employed in conjunction with right and left heart catheterization. Selective injection and selective sampling have made possible the localization of the sites of intracardiac and extracardiac shunts as well as the establishment of the direction of shunts. Methods for localizing incompetent valves and estimating the degree of regurgitant flow have also been described. The residual volume of the right and left ventricles can be estimated by injection of dye in the respective ventricle.

The indicator dilution techniques, helpful as they are as diagnostic aids, have definite limita-

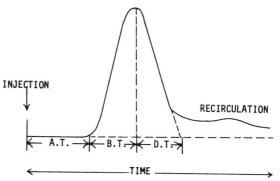

**Figure 19** Diagrammatic representation of a normal indicator dilution curve: The appearance time (A.T.) represents the interval between the injection of the indicator and the appearance of the indicator at the site of sampling. The buildup time (B.T.) represents the interval between the appearance time and the time of peak indicator concentration. The disappearance time (D.T.) is represented by the downslope of the curve. To exclude any recirculating indicator, the concentration is plotted logarithmically against time (dashed segment of the downslope).

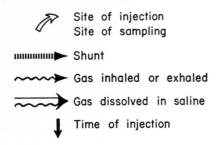

Site of injection
Site of sampling

Shunt

Gas inhaled or exhaled

Gas dissolved in saline

Time of injection

**Figure 20**   Symbols used in Figures 21 to 32.

**Figure 21**  The altered dye curve produced by dilution of the dye by an increased central blood volume (b). The appearance time is delayed, the peak concentration is reduced, and the disappearance time is prolonged when compared to a normal dye dilution curve (a).

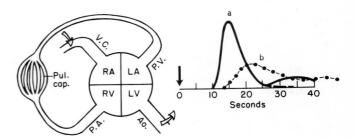

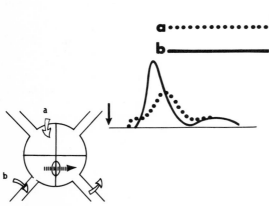

**Figure 22**   a, Ventricular septal defect with a right-to-left shunt. Diagrammatic representation of the dye curve showing the early appearance time of the shunted dye, which modifies the upslope of the curve. This modified upslope is produced by the portion of the dye that circulates through the abnormal pathway. b, When dye is injected downstream from the right-to-left shunt, a normal curve is produced.

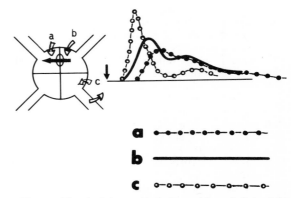

**Figure 23**  Atrial septal defect with a left-to-right shunt: a, The downslope of the dye curve is altered by the recirculation through the lungs of left-to-right shunted dye. The appearance time is normal and the peak concentration of the dye is decreased. b, Injection proximal to or at the site of the left-to-right shunt causes an altered downslope. The appearance time is early and the peak concentration of dye is decreased. c, Injection of dye downstream from the shunt results in a curve of normal contour with an early appearance time.

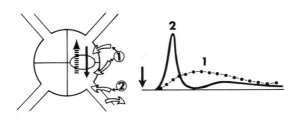

**Figure 24**  Mitral insufficiency: 1, Dye injected either in the left atrium or left ventricle in the presence of mitral insufficiency is diluted in increasing volumes of blood as the dye is washed back and forth through the incompetent valve. The upslope and downslope of the curve are prolonged, the appearance time is normal, and the peak concentration of dye is decreased. 2, Injection of dye at the root of the aorta results in a normal curve.

tions, particularly when they are used for quantitative studies. This is especially true at very low flows because of the large area under the curve and its prolonged downslope. This applies also to measurements of central volume when that volume is greatly increased. Equally important, the presence of high flow may lead to a considerable error because of the small area under the curve. At high flows, an error can be introduced because of the lag of the recording system; under these conditions, the peak of the dye concentration is often obscured. When a continuously recording densitometer is used, the flow through the sampling system must be controlled critically to avoid distortion. In the interpretation of dye dilution curves, adequate mixing of the indicator with the blood is assumed; mixing may be inadequate, however, particularly when injection and sampling sites are too close together. It is important to keep the limitations of this technique in mind when interpreting quantitative results obtained with this method.

**Dye Dilution Curves.** The concentration of dye in the blood is measured by recording the change in optical density of the blood by photoelectric means (decrease in the transmission of light) as the blood is drawn through a cuvette at a constant rate. Arterial sampling after rapid injection of a known amount of nondiffusible dye into the venous side of the circulation (i.e., pulmonary artery, left ventricle or atrium, or any vein) reveals a sudden appearance of the dye a few seconds after the injection. The concentration of the dye rises rapidly to a peak and then falls to a point above the baseline. A smaller, blunter peak of recirculating dye is recorded. The final dye concentration represents a state of equilibrium of dye concentration in the vascular system (Fig. 19).

The time course of the downstream concentration of an injected indicator is related to the flow of the volume of blood that diluted it. When the downslope of the initial appearance curve is replotted on semilogarithmic paper, it assumes a straight line. The extrapolation of that line to zero (or nearly zero, since the zero point is approached asymptotically) separates the area under the curve due to the first circulation of the indicator from the area due to recirculation.

The cardiac output is determined from the Stewart-Hamilton formula:

$$F = \frac{60\ I}{CT}$$

where F = cardiac output in liters per minute, I = the amount of dye injected expressed in milligrams, 60 = number of seconds per minute, C = mean concentration of dye in milligrams per liter, and T = time in seconds from the first appearance of the dye to the theoretic disappearance.

The contour of the normal dye dilution curve is modified by: (1) increased central blood volume (Fig. 21b); (2) right-to-left shunts (Fig. 22); (3) left-to-right shunts (Fig. 23a); and (4) valvular insufficiency (Fig. 24).

**Localization of Left-to-Right Shunts.** The indicator dilution method can be utilized to locate left-to-right shunts. This is accomplished by several techniques:

1. Injection of dye in the left atrium, left ventricle, or aorta and sampling from a peripheral artery (Figs. 23b and 23c).

2. Injection of dye into the left atrium, left ventricle, or aorta and sampling from the right atrium, right ventricle, or pulmonary artery (Fig. 25).

3. Peripheral venous injection of dye with sampling from the right atrium or ventricle (Fig. 26).

4. Injection of dye into a branch of the main pulmonary artery and sampling from the right atrium, right ventricle, or main pulmonary artery (Fig. 27).

### Other Methods for the Diagnosis and Localization of Shunts

Included among the substances that may be used as indicators for the detection of shunts are nitrous oxide, hydrogen, sodium ascorbate, krypton-85, and iodine-131-tagged albumin. Except for [131]I-tagged albumin, most of these substances are not true indicators, such as tricarbocyanine (Cardio-Green), since they diffuse freely into the extracellular and often the intracellular spaces. Also, the gaseous substances are exhaled by the lung.

**The Nitrous Oxide Technique.** This test is based

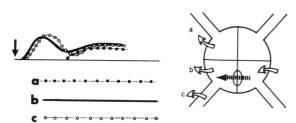

**Figure 25** Ventricular septal defect with left-to-right shunt: Injection of dye into the left ventricle results in early appearance of dye in the right ventricle (b) and in the pulmonary artery (c) but not in the right atrium (a). The shunt is thus located at the ventricular level.

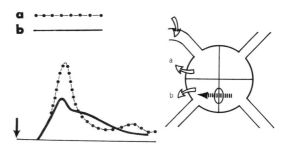

**Figure 26** Ventricular septal defect with left-to-right shunt: Peripheral venous injection of dye with sample upstream from (a) or at the site of a left-to-right shunt localizes the shunt to the chamber in which an altered downslope first appears (b).

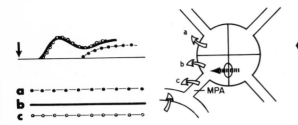

**Figure 27** Ventricular septal defect with left-to-right shunt: Dye injected into a distal branch of the main pulmonary artery appears early in the right ventricle (b) and in the main pulmonary artery (c) and late in the right atrium (a).

**Figure 28** Ventricular septal defect with left-to-right shunt: When nitrous oxide is inhaled, there is normally a wide arteriovenous difference in the first half minute. $\frac{N_2O_{RA}}{N_2O_A} \times 100 = \frac{0.3}{2.7} = 11\%$ (less than 15%: shunt at the atrial level). However, $\frac{N_2O_{RV}}{N_2O_A} \times 100 = \frac{0.9}{2.7} \times 100 = 33\%$ (greater than 20%: left-to-right shunt at the ventricular level). The ratio of pulmonary to systemic flow = $\frac{100\% - 11\%}{100\% - \dfrac{N_2O_{RV}}{N_2O_A}} \times 100 = \frac{89}{67} = 1.33$.

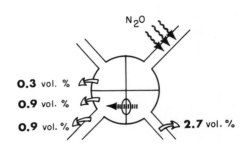

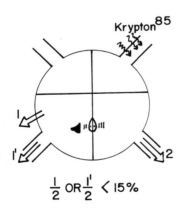

**Figure 29** Localization of ventricular septal defect with left-to-right shunt with krypton-85. Inhaled [85]Kr appears rapidly in the left cardiac chambers. It diffuses freely in the interstitial and cellular compartments, and so its concentration in venous blood returning to the heart is low. Thus, in the presence of a left-to-right shunt at the ventricular level there will be an increase in the concentration of [85]Kr in the right ventricle and the pulmonary artery. As a result, the ratio of the concentration of the gas in the right heart to systemic arterial blood is increased. Normally, this ratio is less than 15 per cent. (From Robin, E., et al. In: Gibbon, J. H., Jr., Sabiston, D. C., Jr., and Spencer, F. C., eds.: Surgery of the Chest. 2nd ed. Philadelphia, W. B. Saunders Company, 1969.)

**Figure 30** Atrial septal defect with left-to-right shunt: A rapid appearance time of [85]Kr in the expired air after a solution of the gas is injected in the left atrium indicates the presence of a left-to-right shunt at the atrial level (a). If the solution of gas is injected in the left ventricle, the appearance time will be delayed (b).

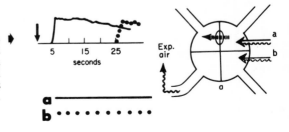

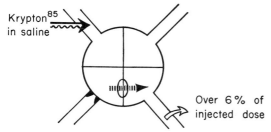

**Figure 31** Ventricular septal defect with right-to-left shunt with [85]Kr: Since 95 per cent of the [85]Kr injected into the venous side of the circulation is excreted by the lungs during its first passage through the pulmonary circulation, the finding of a significant amount of radioactivity in the blood sampled from a peripheral artery indicates a right-to-left shunt. (From Robin, E., et al. In: Gibbon, J. H., Jr., Sabiston, D. C., Jr., and Spencer, F. C., eds.: Surgery of the Chest. 2nd ed. Philadelphia, W. B. Saunders Company, 1969.)

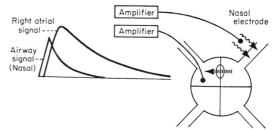

**Figure 32** Atrial septal defect with a left-to-right shunt with hydrogen: The early appearance in the right atrium of a change in potential caused by inhaled hydrogen indicates the presence of an interatrial septal defect with a left-to-right shunt. The inhalation of hydrogen is timed by an electrode placed in the nose as shown in the diagram. (From Robin, E., et al. In: Gibbon, J. H., Jr., Sabiston, D. C., Jr., and Spencer, F. C., eds.: Surgery of the Chest. 2nd ed. Philadelphia, W. B. Saunders Company, 1969.)

on the fact that during the first minute of inhalation of nitrous oxide, the arteriovenous difference is relatively large owing to the avid tissue uptake of the gas. The patient breathes a mixture of 50 per cent nitrous oxide with 21 per cent oxygen for a period of 30 seconds. From the tenth to the thirtieth seconds, integrated simultaneous samples are drawn from a peripheral artery and from the pulmonary artery, the right ventricle, or the right atrium. The nitrous oxide content of the blood is analyzed in a Van Slyke manometric apparatus, and an arbitrary ratio between the nitrous oxide content of the right heart blood and that of the arterial blood is determined. A value of 15 per cent or less demonstrates the absence of a shunt, while a value over 20 per cent is diagnostic of a left-to-right shunt. The tests may be repeated several times during a catheterization to permit selective sampling. The relative flow of the shunt may be quantified (Fig. 28).

The quantification, as given, also applies to the use of [85]Kr to be described for left-to-right shunts. The chief advantages of the nitrous oxide test are simplicity and accuracy in localizing the site of the shunt. The chief disadvantage is that the results of the tests are not immediately available to the operator because of time-consuming analysis.

**The Use of Radioactive Krypton.** Krypton-85 also may be used for the detection of shunts. It can be inhaled (Fig. 29) or dissolved in saline and injected into the left or right circulation (Figs. 30 and 31). These tests are technically simple, and the results are immediately available. They are more sensitive in the detection of small left-to-right shunts than in the analysis of the oxygen content of blood, and they can be used in locating the site of entry of a shunt.

**The Hydrogen Ion Electrode.** The presence of dissolved hydrogen in the blood changes the potential difference between a platinized electrode in the blood and a silver reference electrode placed on the skin with suitable contact. The electrodes are connected directly to the D.C. input of a recording amplifier. One silver reference electrode may be used with several platinum electrodes.

For the detection of left-to-right shunts, the patient is given a breath of hydrogen, the timing of the breath being recorded from a platinum electrode at the tip of a nasal catheter. A left-to-right shunt results in an early deflection recorded by a suitably placed right heart electrode (Fig. 32). For the detection of right-to-left shunts, an arterial electrode is used. Hydrogen, dissolved in saline by being bubbled through the solution, is injected into a peripheral vein. Since the hydrogen is exhaled almost completely by the lungs during its first circulation, the appearance of a deflection on the left side of the circulation indicates a right-to-left shunt. Blood sampling is not necessary, and multiple simultaneous recordings from different sites can be obtained easily. However, hydrogen is an explosive gas; furthermore, quantification of shunts has not yet been achieved.

Sodium ascorbate also produces a potential in the presence of a platinum electrode and is used to test the electrode in situ before hydrogen is administered. Thus, sodium ascorbate is of value in the detection of shunts without blood sampling.

## INTRACARDIAC PHONOCARDIOGRAPHY

The first and second sounds are recorded throughout the heart, but the first sound reaches its maximal intensity in the ventricles and the second sound in the pulmonary artery and aorta. If a third heart sound is present, its greatest intensity is in the ventricles. The fourth heart sound is present in all patients with normal sinus rhythm; it is best recorded from the atria.

In patent ductus arteriosus, the murmur is localized to the pulmonary artery, and in pulmonic stenosis, to the pulmonary artery just downstream from the valve. In ventricular septal defect with a left-to-right shunt, the murmur is recorded in the right ventricle. In atrial septal defects, the systolic murmur is found to arise in the pulmonary artery.

Left-sided sounds and murmurs can be studied

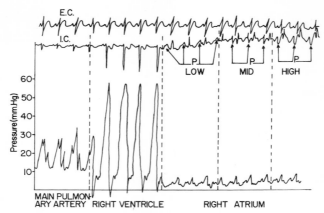

**Figure 33**   Intracardiac electrocardiography: Tracings from pulmonary artery to right atrium obtained from a patient with pulmonic valvular stenosis. E.C. = external electrocardiogram; I.C. = intracardiac electrocardiogram. The superior vena cava and atrial electrocardiograms consist of relatively large P waves, generally inverted in the superior vena cava and high in the right atrium, diphasic in midatrium, and positive in the lower portion of the atrium. In contrast to the large P waves, the QRS voltage within the superior vena cava and right atrium is small. The ventricular electrocardiogram demonstrates isoelectric or relatively small P waves, while the QRS complex is large. The electrocardiogram recorded from the pulmonary artery resembles the atrial electrocardiogram in that the QRS voltage is small, but differs in that the P waves are of similar magnitude to those observed within the ventricle. (From Robin, E., et al. In: Gibbon, J. H., Jr., Sabiston, D. C., Jr., and Spencer, F. C., eds.: Surgery of the Chest. 2nd ed. Philadelphia, W. B. Saunders Company, 1969.)

by retrograde or by transseptal left heart techniques.

The murmur of aortic stenosis originates at the level of the valve and travels distally, diminishing in intensity as the catheter is passed into the left ventricle. In aortic insufficiency, the murmur appears in the left ventricular cavity and radiates toward the apex.

The murmur of mitral stenosis is best recorded in the inflow tract of the left ventricle, and that of mitral insufficiency in the left atrium.

## INTRACARDIAC ELECTROCARDIOGRAPHY

Intracardiac electrocardiography is the study of electrical potentials as obtained from the endo-

cardial surface of the heart. During the performance of cardiac catheterization, a small electrode attached to the catheter serves as the exploring electrode.

Intracardiac electrocardiography has been useful for the following reasons: (1) better understanding of the genesis of the electrocardiogram; (2) precise location of the various cardiac chambers and vessels in complicated malformations; this is accomplished by the analysis of the shape and voltage of the P waves and QRS complexes as recorded in the cardiac chambers and vessels (Fig. 33); (3) diagnosis of Ebstein's anomaly; this is accomplished by recording simultaneously intracavitary pressures and electrocardiographic patterns proximal to the tricuspid valve (Fig. 34); and (4) improved definition of atrial activity in cases of arrhythmias.

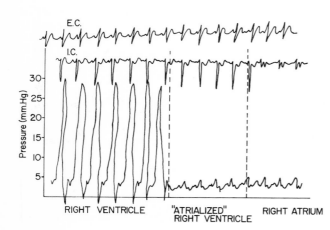

**Figure 34**   Intracardiac electrocardiography: Tracings obtained during pullback from right ventricle to right atrium in a patient with Ebstein's anomaly. E.C. = external electrocardiogram. There is a change from right ventricular to atrial pressure, but the intracardiac electrocardiogram (I.C.) maintains its right ventricular morphology. (From Robin, E., et al. In: Gibbon, J. H., Jr., Sabiston, D. C., Jr., and Spencer, F. C., eds.: Surgery of the Chest. 2nd ed. Philadelphia, W. B. Saunders Company, 1969.)

# CALCULATION OF VALVE AREAS

In order to calculate the surface area of the valves, the following general equation is used:

$$A = \frac{F}{C \times 44.5 \sqrt{P_1 - P_2}}$$

where A (cm.²)          = orifice area
F (ml./sec.)          = flow through orifice
44.5          = constant related to gravity acceleration
$P_1 - P_2$ (mm. Hg) = pressure gradient across the orifice
$P_1$          = pressure proximal to orifice
$P_2$          = pressure distal to orifice

## Mitral Valve Area

With the foregoing formula, the mitral valve area can be calculated as follows:

$$MVA = \frac{MVF = \dfrac{CO}{DFP}}{31 \sqrt{LAm - LVmd}}$$

where MVA (cm.²)      = mitral valve area
MVF (ml./sec.)   = mitral valve flow
CO (ml./min.)    = cardiac output
DFP (sec./min.) = diastolic filling time
LAm (mm. Hg)    = left atrial mean pressure
LVmd (mm. Hg)  = left ventricular mean diastolic pressure (This may be assumed to be 5 mm. Hg in most cases.)

Although in the majority of cases there is a good correlation between the calculated and the actually measured surface area of the mitral valve, the following factors may introduce errors in the calculations: (1) the presence of mitral insufficiency; (2) small pressure gradients across the mitral valve; (3) left ventricular failure; and (4) changes in flow and in pressure gradients between measurements.

The average effective surface area of the normal mitral valve is about 4 to 5 cm.². The surface area of the mitral valve can be narrowed down to 2.5 cm.² without the presence of significant symptoms. Between 2.5 cm.² and 2.0 cm.², the narrowing produces symptoms on severe exertion only. Between 2.0 cm.² and 1.5 cm.², symptoms are present with moderate exertion. Below 1.5 cm.², minimal exercise may provoke severe symptoms.

## Aortic Valve Area

The formula used to calculate the effective aortic valve surface area is:

$$AVA = AVF = \frac{\dfrac{CO}{SEP}}{C \times 44.5 \sqrt{LVsm - Asm}}$$

where AVA (cm.²)        = aortic valve area
AVF (ml./sec.)     = aortic valve flow
CO (ml./min.)     = cardiac output
SEP (sec./min.)   = systolic ejection period
C          = empirical constant = 1.0
44.5          = gravity acceleration factor
LVsm (mm. Hg) = left ventricular mean systolic pressure
Asm (mm. Hg)   = aortic mean systolic pressure

Calculations of the aortic valve surface area are not accurate in the presence of aortic insufficiency. The normal effective surface area of the aortic valve is about 3 to 4 cm.². Usually the symptoms of angina and syncope do not appear until the aortic valve area measures between 0.5 to 0.7 cm.².

# CALCULATION OF RESISTANCE

Vascular resistance can be defined as an impedance to blood flow. This can be translated in a simplified form of Poiseuille's equation:

$$\text{Resistance (R)} = \frac{\text{pressure gradient}}{\text{flow}}$$

The result can be expressed in simple units (R). However, one can express resistance in fundamental units of force as follows (see equation at bottom of page).

Each unit of resistance (R) can be converted into dynes-sec./cm.⁵ by multiplying by 80.* In order to compare data obtained from infants, children and adults, resistance should be related to flow index (liters/min./m.²). Thus, the formula for systemic resistance is as follows:

$$SVR = \frac{Aom - RAm \times 80}{SBF}$$

where SVR (dynes-sec./cm.⁵) = systemic vascular resistance
Aom (mm. Hg) = mean aortic pressure
RAm (mm. Hg) = mean right atrial pressure
SBF (liters/min. or liters/min./m.²) = systemic blood flow

*$\dfrac{1332 \text{ dynes/cm.}^2 \times 60 \text{ sec.}}{1000 \text{ cm.}^3}$

---

$$\text{Resistance (dynes-sec./cm.}^5) = \frac{\text{pressure gradient (mm. Hg)} \times 1332 \text{ dynes/cm.}^2}{\text{blood flow (cm.}^3\text{/sec.)}}$$

Pulmonary vascular resistance can be calculated as follows:

$$PVR = \frac{PAm - LAm \times 80}{PBF}$$

where PVR (dynes-sec./cm.⁵) = pulmonary vascular resistance

PAm (mm. Hg) = mean pulmonary artery pressure

LAm (mm. Hg) = mean left atrial pressure

PBF (liters/min. or liters/min./m.²) = pulmonary blood flow

The normal values for pulmonary vascular resistance are one to three units (80 to 240 dynes-sec./cm.⁵).

As described previously (see Pulmonary Artery Pressure, p. 1897, pulmonary hypertension can be classified in hyperkinetic and obstructive types. In the hyperkinetic type, the pulmonary artery pressure may be high in spite of a normal and fixed pulmonary arterial resistance. In contrast, in the obstructive type, the pulmonary arterial resistance is usually elevated.

## ANGIOCARDIOGRAPHY

### Contrast Materials

The most commonly used preparations are: sodium and methylglucamine diatrizoate (Hypaque 75 per cent or 90 per cent, Renovist 69 per cent, Renografin 60 and 76 per cent), sodium acetrizoate (Urokon 70 per cent), sodium iothalamate (Angio-Conray 80 per cent), iodopyracet (Diodrast 70 per cent), and sodium iodomethamate (Neo-Iopax 75 per cent).

Because of their hypertonicity (greater than 1500 mOsm./liter), injection of large quantities of contrast medium has been shown to cause a temporary increase in cardiac output, blood volume, and left ventricular end-diastolic and pulmonary artery pressures. In addition, an increase in heart rate and a decrease in systemic arterial pressure have been observed. In normal patients and in patients with mitral valve disease, there is a rise in left atrial pressure, the increase being more marked in the latter group.

All iodinated contrast substances are capable of producing reactions. A previous allergic history or pre-existing cerebral and renal disease should prompt careful evaluation of the indications to perform angiocardiography. Reactions are also related to the quantity, concentration, and duration of action of the material used. Because of systemic arterial vasodilation, a feeling of heat and a flushing of the skin are almost universal. Osmotic red cell agglutination can occur in cyanotic children.

Electrocardiographic changes are frequently noted. They may consist of premature auricular, nodal, and ventricular systoles. Occasionally these arrhythmias may persist for a long period of time. T waves may become flat or even inverted. The occurrence of arrhythmias may lead to temporary mitral insufficiency. A diagnosis of true mitral insufficiency is justified only if the contrast material appears in the left atrium in the absence of bradycardia or ventricular arrhythmias. The same reservations also must be made in the case of aortic insufficiency.

### Selective Angiocardiography

Until 1947 peripheral intravenous angiocardiography was the most commonly used method. This technique afforded good visualization of the right heart chambers. However, a considerable degree of dilution occurred in the pulmonary vascular bed. As a result, the left cardiac chambers and aorta were ill defined.

The advantages of selective angiocardiography include: (1) the injection of small quantities of less diluted radiopaque materials, (2) the injection of a radiopaque medium in the chamber of interest so that surrounding structures do not superimpose each other, and (3) the detection of shunts by a sensitive and precise method.

Delivery of contrast material should be as rapid as possible. This is accomplished by choosing a catheter with a large lumen. Because of the possibility of recoil, the catheter should have a closed end with laterally placed holes. Injection of radiopaque material is performed either by hand or by a power injector, the latter being five times more efficient.

To study anatomic or physiologic changes, films must be taken in rapid sequence. This is made possible by rapid film changers or by image intensifiers with cine-camera attachments. Single or biplane rapid film changers can take from one to four frames per second. These machines use either precut film loaded in a cassette or roll films. This technique provides excellent anatomic details. However, the amount of radiation used is high, and the injection of contrast material cannot be monitored.

Cineangiocardiography permits recording of the passage of contrast medium by means of x-ray motion picture photography. This has been made possible by the development of amplification and intensification fluoroscopy, whereby the ordinary fluoroscopic image is converted into an electron image. The electron image is then reconverted into a light image of much increased brightness, which can be viewed by mirror optics, photographed by a cine-camera, or monitored by television. The signal can also be relayed to a video recorder for immediate replay. This method permites motion pictures from 7½ to 60 frames per second with a 16 or 35 mm. movie camera. Thus, cardiac anatomy, as well as the direction of blood flow, can be studied while keeping the dose of radiation low.

Complications occurring during the course of angiocardiography are related to the radiopaque media and to the pressure generated by the injector. Before pressure injection, the tip of the catheter should be free in the cardiac chamber,

**TABLE 4** SELECTIVE ANGIOCARDIOGRAPHY*

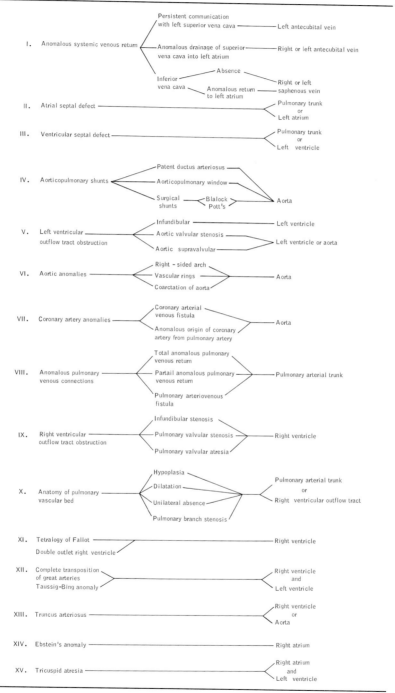

*From Robin, E., et al. In: Gibbon, J. H., Jr., Sabiston,
D. C., Jr., and Spencer, F. C., eds.: Surgery of the Chest.
2nd ed. Philadelphia, W. B. Saunders Company, 1969.

**TABLE 5**   SELECTIVE ANGIOCARDIOGRAPHY*

| | | |
|---|---|---|
| I. | Pericardial disease — Effusion / Scar — | Right atrium |
| II. | Pulmonary embolism ——————— | Main pulmonary trunk |
| III. | Mitral stenosis ——————— | Left atrium or Left ventricle |
| IV. | Mitral insufficiency ——————— | Left ventricle |
| V. | Aortic stenosis ——————— | Left ventricle or Aorta |
| VI. | Aortic insufficiency ——————— | Aorta |
| VII. | Aortic aneurysm ——————— | Aorta or Left ventricle |

*From Robin, E., et al. In: Gibbon, J. H., Jr., Sabiston, D. C., Jr., and Spencer, F. C., eds.: Surgery of the Chest. 2nd ed. Philadelphia, W. B. Saunders Company, 1969.

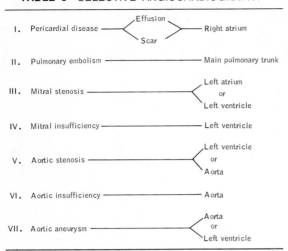

**Figure 35**   Catheter tips used during the performance of selective coronary angiography: *A*, Sones catheter tip; *B*, femoro-right coronary artery catheter tip; *C*, femoro-left coronary artery catheter tip. (Arrows point toward openings.)

away from the myocardial wall. The position of the catheter tip can be ascertained by the injection of small quantities of contrast material under low pressure. Myocardial extravasation of radiopaque medium occurs in about 5 per cent of cases, but the majority of cases are asymptomatic. Occasionally, perforation of the atria or ventricles occurs, resulting in cardiac tamponade. Myocardial infarction and ventricular fibrillation have also been observed. Some of the types of congenital and acquired cardiac anomalies that can be identified by the selective injection of contrast medium are summarized in Tables 4 and 5.

The indications for angiocardiography depend upon the nature of the malformation. The need for it is particularly great in complicated anomalies, since data obtained from cardiac catheterization may be misleading. Anatomic demonstration of a defect by properly obtained selective angiograms is superior to or at least complementary to results obtained from catheterization.

With selective angiocardiography, the following can be accomplished: (1) assessment of the position and size of the cardiac chambers in relation to each other and the great veins and arteries; (2) precise localization of intracardiac and extracardiac defects, including shunts; (3) assessment of the location, anatomy, and motion of the cardiac valves; (4) rough estimation of the degree of valvular insufficiency; and (5) visualization of the coronary vascular tree.

### Coronary Arteriography

Until the late 1950s, opacification of the coronary arteries was achieved indirectly by such methods as: (1) random injection of contrast material at the root of the ascending aorta; (2) phasic injection of contrast medium at the aortic root during ventricular diastole; (3) injection of con-

trast material medium at the aortic root during ventricular asystole produced by acetylcholine; (4) temporary occlusion of the ascending aorta by means of a balloon catheter and injection of contrast medium above the aortic valve; and (5) differential opacification of the aortic root by means of a preformed, spiral-shaped catheter.

In 1959, Sones described a technique of *direct, selective* coronary arteriography using the transbrachial approach and a special catheter with a flexible tip (Fig. 35A). In 1962, Ricketts and Abrams introduced two catheters with tips formed in a way that facilitates their entrance into either the right or left coronary artery (Figs. 35B and 35C). Both catheters are introduced in succession in the aorta with the percutaneous transfemoral approach. In recent years the Ricketts-Abrams method, with some modifications, has gained wide recognition following the reports of Judkins.

**Indications.**   Coronary arteriography is indicated: (1) in a patient whose symptoms, clinical course, and electrocardiographic changes are so atypical as to raise doubt regarding the diagnosis of coronary arteriosclerosis; (2) in a patient with intractable angina pectoris or heart failure in spite of adequate medical treatment and in whom coronary artery surgery is considered; (3) in the evaluation of coronary artery and myocardial revascularization surgical procedures; and (4) in a patient with suspected congenital anomalies of his coronary arterial system.

The right and left coronary arterial patterns are shown in Figures 36 and 37.

**Complications.**   The mortality rate attributed to coronary arteriography is less than 0.5 per cent. Ventricular fibrillation occurs in 1 to 2 per cent of patients studied. Other uncommon complications are myocardial infarction and dissection of the coronary arteries.

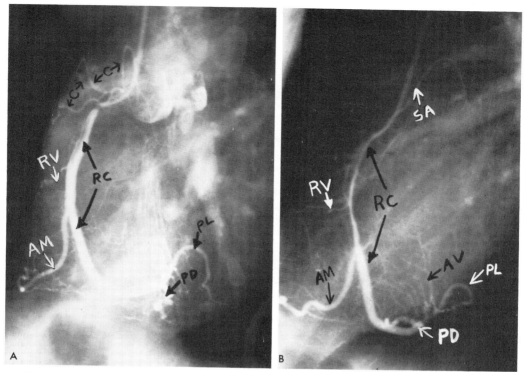

**Figure 36** *A,* Selective right coronary angiogram in the left anterior oblique projection: RC = right coronary artery; C = conal branches; RV = right ventricular artery; AM = acute marginal artery; PD = posterior descending artery; PL = posterior lateral artery. *B,* Later phase in the same patient showing the sinus node (SA) and atrioventricular (AV) arteries.

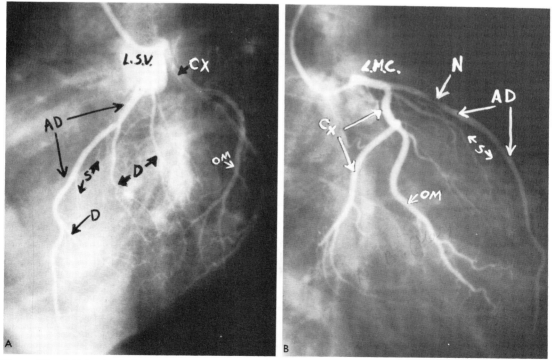

**Figure 37** *A,* Selective left coronary angiogram in the left anterior oblique projection: L.S.V. = contrast material in left sinus of Valsalva; AD = anterior descending artery; CX = circumflex artery; OM = obtuse marginal artery; S = septal branches; D = diagonal branches. *B,* Selective left coronary angiogram in right anterior oblique projection: L.M.C. = left main coronary artery; N = severe narrowing involving the proximal segment of anterior descending artery (AD).

## CORONARY BLOOD FLOW IN MAN—
## ITS CLINICAL IMPORTANCE

Coronary angiocardiography provides a study of the anatomy and direction of blood flow in the larger vessels. It does not give any information about the physiologic status of the coronary circulation. For this purpose, several methods have been devised (Table 6).

Our interest has centered on the development of the coincidence counting technique, using a positron emitter, rubidium-84, to measure coronary blood flow.

The dynamics of $^{84}$Rb in the fluid compartments of the body are similar to those of potassium. The half-life of $^{84}$Rb is 33 days. It decays by positron emission 19 per cent of the time. The positron travels a few millimeters inside the body before annihilation with a negative electron, thereby producing two gamma photons of 0.51 million electron volts (MEV) directed 180 degrees apart (Fig. 38A). Coronary blood flow in patients is measured by a specially designed instrument, which consists of two pairs of coincidence detectors provided with two 4 inch diameter crystals

**TABLE 6** METHODS USED IN THE MEASUREMENT OF CORONARY BLOOD FLOW*

| Substance | Method |
| --- | --- |
| Nitrous oxide | Inhalation-coronary sinus intubation |
| Krypton-85 | Inhalation-coronary sinus intubation |
| | Left ventricular injection-coronary sinus intubation |
| | Coronary artery injection-precordial counting |
| Xenon-133 | Coronary artery injection-precordial counting |
| Iodine-131 iodoantipyrine | Intravenous injection-coronary sinus intubation |
| Sodium-131 | Intramyocardial injection-precordial counting |
| Potassium-42–Rubidium-84 | Intravenous injection-precordial counting |
| Rubidium-84 | Intravenous injection-coincidence counting |

*Modified from Robin, E., et al. In: Gibbon, J. H., Jr., Sabiston, D. C., Jr., and Spencer, F. C., eds.: Surgery of the Chest. 2nd ed. Philadelphia, W. B. Saunders Company, 1969.

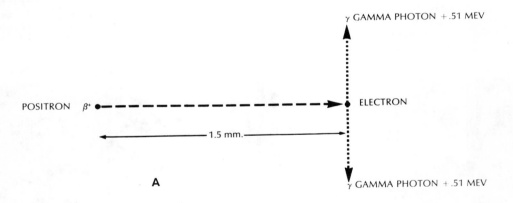

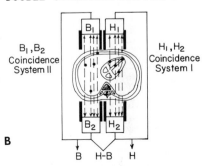

**Figure 38** *A*, Rubidium-84 decays by positron emission 19 per cent of the time. The positron travels about 1.5 mm. inside the body before annihilation with a negative electron, thereby producing two gamma photons of 0.51 million electron volts directed 180 degrees apart. Only events resulting from simultaneous detection of the photons are recorded. *B*, Schematic representation of the double coincidence counting system. One pair of detectors (H$_1$ and H$_2$) is located in front and back of the left chest. The other pair (B$_1$ and B$_2$) is located over the right side of the chest. All detectors are shielded with half-inch lead. The apparatus subtracts electronically the precordial counts (H) from the chest background (B), and this difference expresses the myocardial uptake of $^{84}$Rb (H − B). (From Robin, E., et al. In: Gibbon, J. H., Jr., Sabiston, D. C., Jr., and Spencer, F. C., eds.: Surgery of the Chest. 2nd ed. Philadelphia, W. B. Saunders Company, 1969.)

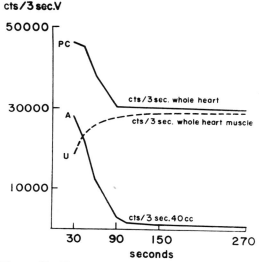

cts/3 sec.V

**Figure 39** Time concentration curves 30 to 270 seconds after an intravenous bolus injection of [84]Rb: PC = the curve monitored by the external counters over the heart; A = radioactivity of arterial blood as measured in the well-counter; U = net counting rate of myocardial [84]Rb uptake (determined by graphic subtraction PC − A). Note that from 90 to 270 seconds following injection of [84]Rb the precordial counting rate is stable and is closely related to the myocardial uptake of the isotope as the arterial concentration remains low.

over and behind the left precordium (coincidence system I), and two 2 inch diameter crystals over and behind the right chest (coincidence system II) (Fig. 38B), and a conventional well-counter for continuously monitoring arterial specific activity. The counting rates of the precordial coincidence pair ($H_1$, $H_2$) and of the background (right chest) coincidence pair ($B_1$, $B_2$), the difference between the two (H − B), and the rate measured in the well-counter (A) are registered on a fast recorder every 3 seconds. Only events resulting from the simultaneous detection of gamma photons originating 180 degrees apart from collision of a positron and an electron are counted (Fig. 38). The difference in transmission between the two sides of the chest introduced by differences in density is corrected by counting the emissions of a [84]Rb source of known dilution in saline placed in succession on both sides of the chest. Once the projections of the heart and domes of the diaphragm are determined on the chest wall by fluoroscopy and roentgenography, each pair of detectors is aligned in such a manner that the upper shields touch the chest, while the pair of lower detectors is separated from it by the table.

The main advantages of the coincidence counting technique using [84]Rb are that there is no need to intubate the coronary sinus, coronary arteries, or left ventricle; background counting rates, natural radioactivity, and cosmic rays are eliminated; the radioactivity of the heart muscle can be separated from that of surrounding structures; and the activity of rubidium in the blood of the cardiac chambers is not "seen" by the detectors.

The concentration of the activity of [84]Rb in arterial blood and its uptake by the heart following a single rapid injection of the isotope are shown in Figure 39.

It is possible with the coincidence counting technique, combined with a bolus injection of [84]Rb, to measure total coronary and nutritional blood flows, the latter being the circulation that is involved in the metabolic exchange with the tissues. With this method, it was found that isoproterenol increases total and nutritional coronary blood flow in equal proportion. In contrast, after norepinephrine administration, total coronary blood flow increases to a greater extent than nutritional coronary flow. Sublingual nitroglycerin increases nutritional coronary blood flow in normal subjects and in patients with coronary artery disease. This effect is still noticeable 90 seconds after administration of the drug.

In addition to the evaluation of drugs upon coronary arterial circulation, the coincidence counting technique may be of value in the assessment of coronary blood flow prior to and following coronary artery surgery and myocardial revascularization procedures.

## SELECTED REFERENCES

Beckmann, C. H., and Dooley, B.: Complications of left heart angiography, a study of 1,000 consecutive cases. Circulation, 41:825, 1970.
*A study of 1000 consecutive left heart cineangiocardiograms is presented. Major problems were associated with the procedure in 3.1 per cent of the cases. Most cardiac complications resulted from open-end catheter angiography, especially through transseptal catheters.*

Braunwald, E., Lambrew, C. T., Morrow, A. G., Pierce, G. E., Rockoff, S. D., and Ross, J., Jr.: Idiopathic hypertrophic subaortic stenosis. Circulation, Vol. 30, Supp. IV, 1964.
*This classic monograph represents the prime source of information about this most fascinating disease.*

Braunwald, E., Moscovitz, H. L., Amram, S. S., Lasser, R. P., Sapin, S. O., Himmelstein, A., Ravitch, M. M., and Gordon, A. J.: The hemodynamics of the left side of the heart as studied by simultaneous left atrial, left ventricular and aortic pressure. Particular reference to left mitral stenosis. Circulation, 12:69, 1955.
*In six patients without mitral stenosis and in patients with mitral stenosis the hemodynamics of the left heart were studied at operation by means of simultaneous needle puncture of the left atrium, left ventricle, and aorta.*

Braunwald, E., and Swan, H. J. C., eds.: Cooperative study on cardiac catheterization. Circulation, Vol. 37, Supp. III, 1968.
*This monograph is the latest study in the assessment of the risks of various cardiac catheterization methods in a total of 12,367 procedures carried out over a period of 2 years.*

Brock, R.: The surgical treatment of pulmonary stenosis. Brit. Heart J., 23:337, 1961.
*This excellent presentation of the problem of congenital pulmonic stenosis is based on data obtained from 198 patients. A survey of the incidence, morbid anatomy, and clinical significance of this condition is presented. Indications and results of closed and open valvotomy are discussed.*

Brockenbrough, E. C., Braunwald, E., and Ross, J., Jr.: Transseptal left heart catheterization—a review of 450 studies and description of an improved technic. Circulation, 25:15, 1962.
*The technique of transseptal left heart catheterization is described. This method was applied in 450 studies. The left atrium was intubated in all but two patients. The left ventricle was entered in 95 per cent of the cases. The only serious complication was accidental puncture of the aorta in three patients.*

Hildner, F. J., Drake, E. H., Gale, H. H., and Ormond, R. S.: Transbrachial retrograde left heart catheterization. Evaluation of 600 consecutive cases in adults. Amer. J. Cardiol., 18:52, 1966.
*The transbrachial retrograde arterial approach was used in 600 consecutive adult cases. The left ventricle was intubated in 96 per cent of the cases. The failure rate of 4 per cent was due to tortuous or aberrant great arteries, tortuous aortas, calcified valves, and local arteriospasm. In 216 cases of significant aortic stenosis, the left ventricle was entered in 98 per cent of cases.*

Judkins, M. P.: Percutaneous transfemoral selective coronary arteriography. Radiol. Clin. N. Amer., 6:467, 1968.
*The technique of coronary angiography using the percutaneous transfemoral approach and especially designed catheters is described. Results obtained in 500 patients are discussed. Reproductions of coronary angiograms are excellent.*

Leonard, J. J., and Kroetz, F. W.: Lessons learned through intracardiac phonocardiography. Mod. Conc. Cardiovasc. Dis., 35:69, 1966.
*A summary of the current concepts of the origin of cardiac sounds and murmurs as obtained by intracardiac phonocardiography is presented. Sounds and murmurs related to congenital anomalies such as atrial and ventricular septal defects, patent ductus arteriosus, pulmonic stenosis, and acquired defects of the mitral, aortic, and tricuspid valves are discussed.*

Ross, R. J., and Friesinger, G. C.: Anatomic and physiologic considerations in measurements of myocardial blood flow. Circulation, 32:630, 1965.
*The different techniques for measuring coronary blood flow are discussed. It has not been possible to separate normal persons from patients with coronary artery disease on the basis of myocardial blood flow measurements. However, they have been useful in the study of exercise or the acute administration of drugs.*

Rudolph, A. M., and Cayler, G. G.: Cardiac catheterization in infants and children. Pediat. Clin. N. Amer., 5:907, 1958.
*An excellent and concise report on the different cardiac catheterization techniques and their application to the evaluation of heart disease in infants and children.*

Shirey, E. K., and Sones, F. M., Jr.: Retrograde transaortic and mitral valve catheterization. Physiologic and morphologic evaluation of aortic and mitral valve lesions. Amer. J. Cardiol., 18:745, 1966.
*The retrograde method of left atrial catheterization using the right brachial arterial approach is discussed. This technique was used in 310 patients for a total of 315 studies. The left atrium was intubated in 285 studies. In 84 per cent of cases of mitral stenosis, the left atrium was successfully catheterized. Ventricular fibrillation occurred in five cases.*

Sones, F. M., Jr.: Cine coronary arteriography. In: Hurst, J. W., and Logue, R. B., eds.: Heart. 2nd ed. New York, McGraw-Hill Book Company, 1970, pp. 377–385.
*The technique of coronary cineangiography using the right retrograde transbrachial route is described by the man who was the first to introduce and develop the technique of direct, selective coronary arteriography. His experience with the procedure in more than 15,000 patients is discussed.*

# REFERENCES

1. Abrams, H. L.: Radiologic aspects of operable heart disease. III. The hazards of retrograde aortography: A survey. Radiology, 68:812, 1957.
2. Androuny, Z. A., Southerland, D. W., Griswold, H. E., and Ritzman, L. W.: Complications with transseptal left heart catheterization. Amer. Heart J., 65:327, 1963.
3. Arcilla, R. A., Agutsson, M. M., Bicoff, J. P., Lynfeld, J., Weinberg, M., Jr., Fell, H. G., and Gasul, B. M.: Further observations on the natural history of isolated ventricular septal defect in infancy and childhood. Circulation, 28:560, 1963.
4. Bagger, M., et al.: On methods and complications in catheterization of heart and large vessels with and without contrast injection. Amer. Heart J., 54:767, 1957.
5. Bargeron, L., Clark, L. C., and Lyons, C.: Use of an electrode for continuously recording intracardiac $PO_2$

changes in cardiac catheterizations. Circulation, 24:881, 1961.
6. Battro, A., and Bidoggia, H.: Endocardial electrocardiogram obtained by heart catheterization in man. Amer. Heart J., 33:604, 1947.
7. Beckmann, C. H., and Dooley, B.: Complications of left heart angiography, a study of 1,000 consecutive cases. Circulation, 41:825, 1970.
8. Bedford, D. E., and Sellors, T. H.: Atrial septal defects. In: Modern Trends in Cardiology. London, Butterworth and Company, 1960, p. 138.
9. Bell, L. A. L., Haynes, W. F., Jr., Shimomura, S., and Dallas, D. P.: Influence of catheter tip position on pulmonary wedge pressures. Circ. Res., 10:215, 1962.
10. Beuren, A. J., and Apitz, J.: Left ventricular angiography by transseptal puncture of the left atrium. Circulation, 28:209, 1963.
11. Bing, R. J., Bennish, A., Bluemchen, G., Cohen, A., Gallagher, J. P., and Zaleski, E. J.: The determination of coronary flow equivalent with coincidence counting technic. Circulation, 29:833, 1964.
12. Bing, R. J., Heimbecker, R., and Falholt, W.: An estimation of the residual volume of blood in the right ventricle of normal and diseased human hearts in vivo. Amer. Heart J., 42:483, 1951.
13. Bing, R. J., Vandam, L. D., and Gray, F. D., Jr.: Physiological studies in congenital heart disease: Results of preoperative studies in patients with tetralogy of Fallot. Bull. Johns Hopkins Hosp., 80:121, 1947.
14. Bing, R. J., Vandam, L. D., and Gray, F. D., Jr.: Physiological studies in congenital heart disease: Procedures. Bull. Johns Hopkins Hosp., 80:107, 1947.
15. Björk, V. O., and Loden, H.: Left heart catheterization with selective left atrial and ventricular angiocardiography in the diagnosis of mitral and aortic valvular disease. Progr. Cardiovasc. Dis., 2:116, 1959.
16. Björk, V. O., and Loden, H.: Evaluation of mitral stenosis with selective left ventricular angiocardiography. J. Thorac. Cardiovasc. Surg., 40:17, 1960.
17. Björk, V. O., Loden, H., and Malers, E.: The evaluation of the degree of mitral insufficiency by selective left ventricular angiocardiography. Amer. Heart J., 60:691, 1960.
18. Björk, V. O., Malmström, G., and Uggla, L. G.: Left auricular pressure measurements in man. Ann. Surg., 138:718, 1953.
19. Bleichroeder, F.: Intra arterielle Therapie. Berlin. Klin. Wschr., 2:1503, 1912.
20. Bookstein, J. J., and Sigmann, J. M.: Intramural deposition of contrast agent during selective angiography. Radiology, 81:932, 1963.
21. Braunwald, E., Brockenbrough, E. C., Talbert, J. L., Folse, J. R., and Rockoff, S. D.: Selective left heart angiography by the transseptal route. Amer. J. Med., 33:213, 1962.
22. Braunwald, E., Goldblatt, A., Long, R. T. L., and Morrow, A. G.: The krypton inhalation test for the detection of left-to-right shunts. Brit. Heart J., 24:47, 1962.
23. Braunwald, E., Lambrew, C. T., Morrow, A. G., Pierce, G. E., Rockoff, S. D., and Ross, J., Jr.: Idiopathic hypertrophic subaortic stenosis. Circulation, Vol. 30, Supp. IV, 1964.
24. Braunwald, E., Morrow, A. G., Cornell, W. P., Augen, M. M., and Hilbish, T.: Idiopathic hypertrophic subaortic stenosis. Clinical hemodynamic and angiographic manifestations. Amer. J. Med., 29:940, 1960.
25. Braunwald, E., Moscovitz, H. L., Amram, S. S., Lasser, R. P., Sapin, S. O., Himmelstein, A., Ravitch, M. M., and Gordon, A. J.: The hemodynamics of the left side of the heart as studied by simultaneous left atrial, left ventricular, and aortic pressures: Particular reference to mitral stenosis. Circulation, 12:69, 1955.
26. Braunwald, E., Pfaff, W. W., Long, R. T. L., and Morrow, A. G.: A simplified indicator-dilution technique for the localization of left-to-right circulatory shunts. An experimental and clinical study of intravenous injection and right heart sampling. Circulation, 20:875, 1959.
27. Braunwald, E., and Swan, H. J. C., eds.: Cooperative study on cardiac catheterization. Circulation, Vol. 37, Supp. III, 1968.
28. Braunwald, E., Tanenbaum, H. L., and Morrow, A. G.: Dye-

dilution curves from left heart and aorta for localization of left-to-right shunts and detection of valvular insufficiency. Proc. Soc. Exp. Biol. Med., 94:510, 1957.

29. Brock, R.: Anatomy of Congenital Pulmonic Stenosis. New York, Paul B. Hoeber, 1957.

30. Brock, R.: The surgical treatment of pulmonary stenosis. Brit. Heart J., 23:337, 1961.

31. Brock, R., Milstein, B. B., and Ross, D. N.: Percutaneous left ventricular puncture in the assessment of aortic stenosis. Thorax, 11:163, 1956.

32. Brockenbrough, E. C., and Braunwald, E.: A new technique for left ventricular angiocardiography and transseptal left heart catheterization. Amer. J. Cardiol., 6:1062, 1960.

33. Brockenbrough, E. C., Braunwald, E., and Morrow, A. G.: A hemodynamic technique for the detection of hypertrophic subaortic stenosis. Circulation, 23:189, 1961.

34. Brockenbrough, E. C., Braunwald, E., and Ross, J., Jr.: Transseptal left heart catheterization—a review of 450 studies and description of an improved technic. Circulation, 25:15, 1962.

35. Brown, R., Rahimtoola, S. H., Davis, G. D., and Swan, H. J. C.: The effect of angiographic contrast medium on circulatory dynamics in man. Cardiac output during angiocardiography. Circulation, 31:234, 1965.

36. Calazel, P., Gerard, R., Daley, R., Draper, A., Foster, J., and Bing, R. J.: Physiological studies in congenital heart disease. XI. A comparison of the right and left auricular, capillary and pulmonary artery pressures in nine patients with auricular septal defect. Bull. Johns Hopkins Hosp., 88:20, 1951.

37. Campbell, J. A., Klatte, E. C., and Shalkowski, R. A.: Factors influencing image quality in cineroentgenography. Amer. J. Roentgen., 83:345, 1960.

38. Chavez, I., Dorbecker, N., and Celis, A.: Direct intracardial angiocardiography; its diagnostic value. Amer. Heart J., 33:560, 1947.

39. Cheng, T. O.: Myocardial infarction following transmural extravasation of contrast medium during left ventricular cineangiography. Circulation, 28:105, 1963.

40. Clark, L. C., and Bargeron, L. M., Jr.: Detection and direct recording of left-to-right shunts with the hydrogen electrode catheter. Surgery, 46:797, 1959.

41. Clark, L. C., Bargeron, L. M., Jr., Lyons, C., Bradely, M. N., and McArthur, K. T.: Detection of right-to-left shunts with an arterial potentiometric electrode. Circulation, 22:949, 1960.

42. Clark, L. C., Kaplan, S., Matthews, E. C., Edwards, F. K., and Helmworth, J. A.: Monitor and control of blood oxygen tension and pH during total body perfusions. J. Thorac. Surg., 36:488, 1958.

43. Cohen, L. S., Elliott, W. C., and Gorlin, R.: Measurement of myocardial blood flow using krypton[85]. Amer. J. Physiol., 206:997, 1964.

44. Connolly, D. C., Kirklin, J. W., and Wood, E. H.: The relationship between pulmonary artery wedge pressure and left atrial pressure in man. Circ. Res., 2:434, 1954.

45. Cope, C.: Technique for transseptal catheterization of left atrium. Preliminary report. J. Thorac. Surg., 37:482, 1959.

46. Cope, C.: Intravascular breakage of Seldinger spring guide wires. J.A.M.A., 180:1061, 1962.

47. Cournand, A., Bing, R. J., Dexter, L., and Dotter, C.: Report of the Committee on Cardiac Catheterization and Angiocardiography. Circulation, 7:769, 1953.

48. Cournand, A., Motley, H. L., Himmelstein, A., Dresdale, D., and Baldwin, J.: Recording of blood pressure from the left auricle and the pulmonary veins in human subjects with interauricular septal defect. Amer. J. Physiol., 150:267, 1947.

49. Cournand, A., and Ranges, H. A.: Catheterization of the right auricle in man. Proc. Soc. Exp. Biol. Med., 46:462, 1941.

50. Cournand, A., Riley, R. L., Breed, E. S., Baldwin, E. de F. and Richards, D. W., Jr.: Measurement of cardiac output in man using the technique of catheterization of the right auricle or ventricle. J. Clin. Invest., 24:106, 1945.

51. Cowan, C., Duran, P. M. V., Corsini, G., Goldschlager, N., and Bing, R. J.: The effects of nitroglycerin on myocardial blood flow in man measured by coincidence

counting and bolus injections of [84]rubidium. Amer. J. Cardiol., 24:154, 1969.

52. Davis, F. W., Jr., and Andrus, E. C.: Mitral stenosis in facsimile. New Eng. J. Med., 251:297, 1954.

53. Dexter, L., Haynes, F. W., Burwell, C. S., Eppinger, E. C., Siebel, R. E., and Evans, J. M.: Studies of congenital heart disease. I. Technique of venous catheterization as a diagnostic procedure. J. Clin. Invest., 26:547, 1947.

54. Dexter, L., Haynes, F. W., Burwell, C. S., Eppinger, E. C., Sogerson, R. P., and Evans, J. M.: Studies of congenital heart disease. II. The pressure and oxygen content of blood in the right auricle, right ventricle and pulmonary artery in control patients with observation on the oxygen saturation and source of pulmonary "capillary" blood. J. Clin. Invest., 26:554, 1947.

55. Donato, L., Bartolomei, G., and Giordani, R.: Evaluation of myocardial perfusion in man with radioactive potassium or rubidium and precordial counting. Circulation, 29:195, 1964.

56. Dotter, C. T.: Left ventricle and systemic arterial catheterization: A simple percutaneous method using a spring guide. Amer. J. Roentgen., 6:969, 1960.

57. Dow, P.: Dimensional relationships in dye-dilution curves from humans and dogs, with an empirical formula for certain troublesome curves. J. Appl. Physiol., 7:399, 1955.

58. Dow, P.: Estimations of cardiac output and central blood volume by dye-dilution. Physiol. Rev., 36:77, 1956.

59. Duchosal, P. W., Ferrero, C., Doret, J. P., Andereggen, P., and Rilliet, B.: Les potentiels intra-cardiaques récueillis par cathétérisme chez l'homme. Cardiologia, 13:113, 1948.

60. Eckenhoff, J. E., Hafkenschiel, J. H., Harmel, M. H., Goodale, W. T., Lubin, M., Bing, R. J., and Kety, S. S.: Measurement of coronary blood flow by the nitrous oxide method. Amer. J. Physiol., 152:356, 1948.

61. Edwards, E. A., and Biguria, F. A.: A comparison of Skiodan and Diodrast as vasographic media: with special reference to their effect on blood pressure. New Eng. J. Med., 211:589, 1934.

62. Enson, Y., Briscoe, W. A., Polanyi, M. L., and Cournand, A.: In vivo studies with an intravascular and intracardiac reflection oximeter. J. Appl. Physiol., 17:552, 1962.

63. Facquet, J., Lemoine, J. M., Alhomme, P., and Lefebvre, J.: La mesure de la pression auriculaire gauche par voie transbronchique. Arch. Mal. Coeur, 45:741, 1952.

64. Feruglio, G. A.: Intracardiac phonocardiography: A valuable diagnostic technique in congenital and acquired heart disease. Amer. Heart J., 58:827, 1959.

65. Fisher, D. L.: The use of pressure recordings obtained at transthoracic left heart catheterization in the diagnosis of valvular heart disease. J. Thorac. Surg., 30:379, 1955.

66. Fleming, H. A., Hancock, E. W., Milstein, B. B., and Ross, D. H.: Percutaneous left ventricular puncture with catheterization of aorta. Thorax, 13:97, 1958.

67. Fleming, P., and Gibson, R.: Percutaneous left ventricular puncture in the assessment of aortic stenosis. Thorax, 12:37, 1957.

68. Forman, J., Laurens, P., and Serville, M.: Catheterization of the left cavities with micromanometry by transseptal route. Arch. Mal. Coeur, 55:601, 1962.

69. Forssmann, W.: Die Sondierung des rechten Herzens. Klin. Wschr., 8:2085, 1929.

70. Fox, I. J., and Wood, E. H.: Applications of dilution curves recorded from the right side of the heart or venous circulation with the aid of a new indicator dye. Proc. Mayo Clin., 32:541, 1957.

71. Fox, S. M.: Pretracheal left heart catheterization: Difficult technique with some advantages. Circulation, 20:696, 1959.

72. Freis, E. D., Rivara, G. L., and Gilmore, B. L.: Estimation of residual and end-diastolic volumes of the right ventricle of men without heart disease, using the dye-dilution method. Amer. Heart. J., 60:898, 1960.

73. Friedlich, A., Heimbecker, R., and Bing, R. J.: A device for continuous recording of concentration of Evans blue dye in whole blood and its application to determination of cardiac output. J. Appl. Physiol., 3:12, 1950.

74. Gasul, B. M., Dillon, R. J., Vrla, V., and Hart, G.: Ventric-

ular septal defects. Their natural transformation in those with infundibular stenosis or with the cyanotic or non-cyanotic type of tetralogy of Fallot. J.A.M.A., *164*:847, 1957.

75. Gilford, S. R., Gregg, D. E., Shadle, O. W., Ferguson, T. B., and Marzetta, L. A.: An improved cuvette densitometer for cardiac output determination by the dye-dilution method. Rev. Sci. Instrum., *24*:696, 1953.

76. Gorlin, R., and Gorlin, S. G.: Hydraulic formula for calculations of the area of the stenotic mitral valve, other cardiac valves and central circulatory shunts. Amer. Heart J., *41*:1, 1951.

77. Gorlin, R., Lewis, B. M., Haynes, F. W., and Dexter, L.: Studies of the circulatory dynamics at rest in mitral valvular regurgitation with and without stenosis. Amer. Heart J., *43*:357, 1952.

78. Grundemann, A. M., Bosch, C., Schwantje, E. J. M., Reijns, G. A., and Verheught, A. P. M.: Retrograde catheterization of the left ventricle in aortic stenosis. Amer. J. Cardiol., *6*:915, 1960.

79. Hallermann, F. J., Rostelle, G. C., and Swan, H. J. E.: Comparison of left ventricular volumes by dye-dilution and angiographic methods in the dog. Amer. J. Physiol., *204*:446, 1963.

80. Hamilton, W. F., Moore, J. W., Kinsman, J. M., and Spurling, R. G.: Studies on the circulation. IV. Further analysis of the injection method, and of changes in hemodynamics under physiological and pathological conditions. Amer. J. Physiol., *99*:534, 1932.

81. Hansen, A. T., Haxholdt, B. F., Husfeldt, E., Lassen, N. A., Munck, O., Sorenson, H. R., and Winkler, K.: Measurement of coronary blood flow and cardiac efficiency in hypothermia by use of radioactive krypton[85]. Scand. J. Clin. Lab. Invest., *8*:182, 1956.

82. Harned, H. S., Lurie, P. R., Croethers, C. H., and Whittmore, R.: Use of the whole blood oximeter during cardiac catheterization. J. Lab. Clin. Med., *40*:445, 1952.

83. Hecht, H. H.: Potential variations of the right auricular and ventricular cavities in man. Amer. Heart J., *32*:39, 1946.

84. Herd, J. A., Hollenberg, M., Thorburn, G. D., Kopald, H. H., and Barger, A. C.: Myocardial blood flow determined by krypton[85] in unanesthetized dogs. Amer. J. Physiol., *203*:122, 1962.

85. Hernandez, F. A., Rockkind, R., and Cooper, H. R.: The intracavitary electrocardiogram in the diagnosis of Ebstein's anomaly. Amer. J. Cardiol., *1*:181, 1958.

86. Hickam, J. B., and Frazer, R.: Spectrophotometric determination of blood oxygen. J. Biol. Chem., *180*:457, 1949.

87. Hilder, F. J., Drake, E. H., Gale, H. H., and Ormond, R. S.: Transbrachial retrograde left heart catheterization. Evaluation of 600 consecutive cases in adults. Amer. J. Cardiol., *18*:52, 1966.

88. Hollander, W., Madoff, I. M., and Chobanian, A. V.: Local myocardial blood flow as indicated by the disappearance of Na-I-131 from the heart muscle: Studies at rest during exercise and following nitrite administration. J. Pharmacol. Exp. Ther., *139*:53, 1963.

89. Holling, H. E., MacDonald, I., O'Holloran, J. A., and Venner, A.: Reliability of a spectrophotometric method of estimating blood oxygen. J. Appl. Physiol., *8*:249, 1955.

90. Horger, E. L., Dotter, C. T., and Steinberg, E.: Electrocardiographic changes during angiocardiography. Amer. Heart J., *41*:651, 1951.

91. Hugenholtz, P. G., Gamble, W. J., Monroe, R. G., and Polanyi, M.: The use of fiberoptics in clinical cardiac catheterization. II. In vivo dye-dilution curves. Circulation, *31*:344, 1965.

92. Judkins, M. P.: Percutaneous transfemoral selective coronary arteriography. Radiol. Clin. N. Amer., *6*:467, 1968.

93. Kent, E. M., Ford, W. B., Fisher, D. L., and Childs, T. B.: The estimation of the severity of mitral regurgitation. Ann. Surg., *141*:47, 1955.

94. Kidd, L.: The hemodynamics in ventricular septal defect in childhood. Amer. Heart. J., *70*:732, 1965.

95. Kinsman, J. M., Moore, J. W., and Hamilton, W. F.: Studies on the circulation. I. Injection method: Physical and mathematical considerations. Amer. J. Physiol., *89*: 322, 1929.

96. Klatte, E. C., Campbell, J. A., and Lurie, P. R.: Technical factors in selective cinecardioangiography. Radiology, *73*:539, 1959.

97. Kossman, C. E., Berger, A. R., Rader, B., Brumlik, J., Briller, S. A., and Donnolly, J. H.: Intracardiac and intravascular potentials resulting from electrical activity of the normal human heart. Circulation, *2*:10, 1950.

98. Krasnow, N., Levine, H. J., Wagman, R. J., and Gorlin, R.: Coronary blood flow measured by I-131 iodo-antipyrinine. Circ. Res., *12*:58, 1963.

99. Leb, G., Derntl, F., Goldschlager, N., Cowan, C., and Bing, R. J.: Determination of effective and total coronary blood flow using Rb[84]. Amer. J. Med. Sci., *257*:203, 1969.

100. Lenegre, J., and Maurice, P.: De quelques résultats obtenus par la dérivation directe intracavitaire des courants électriques de l'oreillette et du ventricule droits. Arch. Mal. Coeur, *38*:298, 1945.

101. Leonard, J. J., and Kreutz, F. W.: Lessons learned through intracardial phonocardiography. Mod. Conc. Cardiovasc. Dis., *35*:69, 1966.

102. Levin, A. R., Spach, M. S., Anderson, P. A. W., and Capp, M. P.: Cardiac perforation following left ventricular cineangiocardiography. Circulation, *32*:593, 1965.

103. Levine, H. D., Hellems, H. K., Dexter, L., and Tucker, A. S.: Studies in intracardiac electrocardiography in man. II. The potential variations in the right ventricle. Amer. Heart J., *37*:64, 1949.

104. Levine, H. D., Hellems, H. K., Wittenberg, M. H., and Dexter. L.: Studies in intracardiac electrocardiography in man. I. The potential variations in the right atrium. Amer. Heart J., *37*:46, 1949.

105. Lewis, D. H., Deitz, G. W., Wallace, J. D., and Brown, J. R., Jr.: Intracardiac phonocardiography. Progr. Cardiovasc. Dis., *2*:85, 1959.

106. Lewis, D. H., Ertugrul, A. E., Deitz, G. W., Wallace, J. D., Brown, J. R., Jr., and Moghadam, A. N.: Intracardiac phonocardiography in the diagnosis of congenital heart disease. Pediatrics, *23*:837, 1959.

107. Lind, J., Boesen, I. B., and Wegelius, C.: Selective angiocardiography in congenital heart disease. Progr. Cardiovasc. Dis., *2*:293, 1959.

108. Litwak, R. S., Bernstein, W. H., and Samet, P.: Problems in the interpretation of left atrial, left ventricular, and mean diastolic gradients. Amer. J. Cardiol., *6*:1023, 1960.

109. Long, R. T. L., Braunwald, E., and Morrow, A. G.: Intracardiac injection of radioactive krypton[85]. Clinical applications of new methods for characterization of circulatory shunts. Circulation, *21*:1126, 1960.

110. Lucas, R. V., Jr., Adams, P., Jr., Anderson, R. C., Meyne, N. G., Lillihei, C. W., and Varco, R. L.: The natural history of isolated ventricular septal defect. A serial physiological study. Circulation, *24*:1372, 1961.

111. Luchsinger, P. C., Seipp, H. W., Jr., and Patel, D. J.: Relationship of pulmonary artery wedge pressures to left atrial pressures in man. Circ. Res., *11*:315, 1962.

112. Lurie, P. R., Shumacker, H. B., Jr., Schulz, D. M., Klatte, E. C., and Grajo, M. Z.: Obstructive hypertrophy in congenital heart disease: Definition, classification, and surgical importance. Circulation, *20*:732, 1959.

113. McMichael, J., and Mounsey, J. P.: Complication following coronary sinus and cardiac vein catheterization in man. Brit. Heart J., *13*:397, 1951.

114. Moffit, E. A., Dawson, B., and O'Neill, N. C.: Anesthesia for pediatric cardiac catheterization and angiography. Anesth. Analg., *40*:483, 1961.

115. Moore, J. W., Kinsman, J. M., Hamilton, W. F., and Spurling, R. G.: Studies on the circulation. II. Cardiac output determinations; comparison of the injection method with the direct Fick procedure. Amer. J. Physiol., *89*:331, 1929.

116. Morrow, A. G., Braunwald, E., Haller, J. A., Jr., and Sharp, E. H.: Left heart catheterization by the transbronchial route: Technique and applications in physiologic and diagnostic investigations. Circulation, *16*:1033, 1957.

117. Morrow, A. G., Braunwald, E., and Ross, J., Jr.: Left heart catheterization. An appraisal of techniques and their

applications in cardiovascular disease. Arch. Intern. Med., *105*:645, 1960.

118. Morrow, A. G., Sanders, R. J., and Breaunwald, E.: The nitrous oxide test. An improved method for the detection of left-to-right shunts. Circulation, *17*:284, 1958.

119. Morrow, A. G., Sharp, E. H., and Braunwald, E.: Congenital aortic stenosis: Clinical and hemodynamic findings, surgical technique, and results of operation. Circulation, *18*:1091, 1958.

120. Morrow, A. G., Waldhausen, J. A., Peters, R. L., Bloodwell, R. D., and Braunwald, E.: Supravalvular aortic stenosis, clinical hemodynamics and pathological observations. Circulation, *20*:1003, 1959.

121. Moscovitz, H. L., Donoso, E., and Gelb, I. J.: The demonstration of flow murmurs by intracardiac phonocardiography. Clin. Res. Proc., *5*:162, 1957.

122. Nadas, A. S., Rudolph, A. M., and Gross, R. E.: Pulmonary hypertension in congenital heart disease. Circulation, *22*:1041, 1960.

123. Nicholson, J. W., III, and Wood, E. H.: Estimation of cardiac output and blood volume by continuous recording of Evans blue time-concentration curves in man employing an oximeter. Amer. J. Physiol., *163*:738, 1950 (abstract).

124. Nunez, V. B., and Ponsdomenech, E. R.: Heart puncture cardioangiography: Clinical and electrocardiographic results. Amer. Heart J., *41*:855, 1951.

125. Nutter, D. O., and Kelser, G. A.: The percutaneous intracavitary electrocardiogram in the diagnosis of arrhythmias. Ann. Intern. Med., *62*:706, 1965.

126. Owen, S. G., and Wood, P.: A new method of determining the degree or absence of mitral obstruction: An analysis of the diastolic part of indirect left atrial pressure tracings. Brit. Heart J., *17*:41, 1955.

127. Polanyi, M. L., and Hehir, R. M.: New reflection oximeter. Rev. Instrum., *31*:401, 1960.

128. Popper, R. W., Schumacher, D., and Quinn, C. H.: Cardiac tamponade due to hypertonic contrast medium in the pericardial sac following cineangiography. Circulation, *35*:933, 1967.

129. Priotin, J. B., Thévenet, A., Pelissier, M., Puech, P., Latous, H., and Pourquier, J.: Cardiographie ventriculaire gauche par cathétérisme retrograde percutane fémoral. Presse Méd., *65*:1948, 1957.

130. Radner, S.: Extended suprasternal puncture technique. Acta Med. Scand., *151*:223, 1955.

131. Rahimtoola, S. H., Duffy, J. P., and Swan, H. J. C.: Hemodynamic changes associated with injection of angiographic contrast medium in assessment of valvular lesions. Circulation, *22*:52, 1966.

132. Read, J. L., Bong, E. G., and Porter, R. R.: The hazard of unrecognized catheterization of the coronary sinus. Arch. Intern. Med., *96*:176, 1955.

133. Read, R. C.: Cause of death in cardioangiography. J. Thorac. Cardiovasc. Surg., *38*:685, 1959.

134. Richards, D. W., Jr.: Cardiac output by catheterization technique in various clinical conditions. Fed. Proc., *4*:215, 1945.

135. Ricketts, J. H., and Abrams, H. L.: Percutaneous selective coronary cinearteriography. J.A.M.A., *181*:620, 1962.

136. Rodrigo, J. A.: Determination of the oxygen saturation of blood in vitro by using reflected light. Amer. Heart J., *45*:809, 1953.

137. Rodriguez-Alvarez, A., and Martinez de Rodriguez, G.: Studies in angiocardiography. The problems involved in the rapid, selective and safe injections of radiopaque materials. Development of a special catheter for selective angiocardiography. Amer. Heart J., *53*:841, 1957.

138. Ross, J., Jr.: Transseptal left heart catheterization: A new method of left atrial puncture. Ann. Surg., *37*:482, 1959.

139. Ross, J., Jr.: Considerations regarding the technique for transseptal left heart catheterization. Circulation, *34*:391, 1966.

140. Ross, J., Jr., Braunwald, E., and Morrow, A. G.: Transseptal left atrium puncture: New technique for measurement of left atrial pressure in man. Amer. J. Cardiol., *3*:653, 1959.

141. Ross, J., Jr., Braunwald, E., and Morrow, A. G.: Left heart catheterization by the transseptal route. A description

of the technique and its applications. Circulation, *22*: 927, 1960.

142. Ross, R. S., Ueda, K., Lichtlen, P. R., and Rees, J. R.: The measurement of myocardial blood flow in animals and man by selective injection of radioactive inert gas into the coronary arteries. Circ. Res., *15*:28, 1964.

143. Rowe, G. G., and Zarnstorff, W. C.: Ventricular fibrillation during selective angiocardiography. J.A.M.A., *192*:105, 1965.

144. Rudolph, A. M., and Cayler, G. G.: Cardiac catheterization in infants and children. Pediat. Clin. N. Amer., *5*:907, 1958.

145. Russell, R. O., Caroll, J. F., and Hood, W. G., Jr.: Cardiac tamponade. A complication of the transseptal technique of left heart catheterization resulting in a fatality. Amer. J. Cardiol., *13*:558, 1964.

146. Sanders, R. J., and Morrow, A. G.: The diagnosis of circulatory shunts by the nitrous oxide test. Improvements in technique and methods for quantification of shunts. Circulation, *18*:856, 1958.

147. Sanders, R. J., and Morrow, A. G.: The identification and quantification of left-to-right circulation shunts. A new diagnostic method utilizing the inhalation of a radioactive gas, Kr[85]. Amer. J. Med., *26*:508, 1959.

148. Schafer, H., Blain, J. M., Ceballos, R., and Bing, R. J.: Essential pulmonary hypertension. A report of clinical physiologic studies in three patients with death following catherization of the heart. Ann. Intern. Med., *44*:505, 1956.

149. Scott, S. M., Fish, R. G., and Takaro, T.: A double needle technique for transbronchial left heart catheterization. Circulation, *22*:976, 1960.

150. Scott, W. G., and Moore, S.: Rapid serialization of x-ray exposures by the radiography utilizing roll of film nine and one-half inches wide. Radiology, *53*:846, 1949.

151. Scott, W. G., and Moore, S.: The development of the tautography and the advantages of automatization in cardiovascular angiography. Amer. J. Roentgen., *62*:33, 1949.

152. Segal, B. L., Novack, P., and Kasparian, H.: Intracardiac phonocardiography. Amer. J. Cardiol., *13*:188, 1964.

153. Seldinger, S. L.: Catheter replacement of the needle in percutaneous arteriography: New technique. Acta Radiol., *39*:368, 1953.

154. Shaffer, A. B., and Silber, E. N.: Factors influencing the character of the pulmonary arterial wedge pressure. Amer. Heart J., *5*:522, 1956.

155. Shirey, E. K., and Sones, F. M., Jr.: Retrograde transaortic and mitral valve catheterization. Physiologic and morphologic evaluation of aortic and mitral valve lesions. Amer. J. Cardiol., *18*:745, 1966.

156. Singleton, R. T., Dembo, D. H., and Scherlis, L.: Krypton[85] in the detection of intracardiac left-to-right shunts. Circulation, *32*:134, 1965.

157. Smith, C., Rowe, R. D., and Vlad, P.: Sedation of children for cardiac catheterization with an ataractic mixture. Canad. Anaesth. Soc. J., *5*:35, 1958.

158. Sodi Pallares, D., Vizcaino, M., Soberon, J., and Cabrera Cosio, E.: Comparative study of the intracavitary potential in man and in dog. Amer. Heart J., *33*:819, 1947.

159. Sones, F. M., Jr.: Cine coronary arteriography. In: Hurst, J. W., and Logue, R. B.: Heart. 2nd ed. New York, McGraw-Hill Book Company, 1970, pp. 377–385.

160. Sones, F. M., Jr., and Shirey, E. K.: Cine coronary arteriography. Mod. Conc. Cardiovasc. Dis., *31*:735, 1962.

161. Soulie, P., Laurens, P., Bouchard, F., Cornu, C., and Brial, E.: Enregistrement des pressions et des bruits intracardiaques à l'aide d'un micromanomètre. Bull. Soc. Med. Hop. Paris, *22*:713, 1957.

162. Stern, T. N., Tacket, H. S., and Zachary, E. G.: Penetration into pericardial cavity during cardiac catheterization. Amer. Heart J., *44*:448, 1952.

163. Stewart, G. N.: Researches on the circulation time and on the influences which affect it. IV. The output of the heart. J. Physiol., *22*:11, 1897.

164. Swan, H. J. C., Burchell, H. B., Linder, E., Birkhead, N. C., and Wood, E. H.: Symposium on diagnostic applications of indicator-dilution curves recorded from left and right sides of the heart. Part II. Proc. Mayo Clin., *33*:581, 1958.

165. Van Slyke, D. D., and Neill, J. M.: Determination of gases in blood and other solutions by vacuum extraction and manometric measurement. J. Biol. Chem., *61*:523, 1924.

166. Vogel, J. H. K., Tabari, K., Averill, K. H., and Blount, S. G., Jr.: A simple technique for identifying P waves in complex arrhythmias. Amer. Heart J., *67*:158, 1964.

167. Wallace, J. O., Brown, J. R., Lewis, D. H., and Deitz, G. W.: Acoustic mapping within the heart. J. Acoust. Soc. Amer., *29*:9, 1957.

168. Watson, H.: Electrode catheters and the diagnostic application of intracardiac electrography in small children. Circulation, *29*:284, 1964.

169. Wood, E. H., Swan, H. J. C., Fox, I. J., et al.: Symposium on diagnostic applications of indicator-dilution techniques. Proc. Mayo Clin., *32*:463, 1957.

170. Wright, J. L., Toscano-Barboza, E., and Brandenburg, R. O.: Left ventricular and aortic pressure pulses in aortic valvular disease. Proc. Mayo Clin., *31*:120, 1956.

171. Yamakawa, K., Shionoya, Y., Kitamura, K., Nagai, T., Yamomoto, T., and Ohta, S.: Intracardiac phonocardiography. Amer. Heart J., *47*:424, 1954.

172. Zimmerman, H. A., and Hellerstein, H. K.: Cavity potentials of the human ventricles. Circulation, *3*:95, 1951.

173. Zimmerman, H. A., Scott, R. W., and Becker, N. O.: Catheterization of the left side of the heart in man. Circulation, *1*:357, 1950.

174. Zinn, W. J., Levinson, D. C., Johns, V., and Griffith, J. C.: The effect of angiocardiography on the heart as measured by electrocardiographic alterations. Circulation, *3*:658, 1951.

# II

# Cardiac Arrest

*James R. Jude, M.D.*

Cardiac arrest in the narrow surgical sense is sudden cessation of effective cardiac action. Modern concepts of this problem and its prevention and therapy require a broader definition. In the operating room, if cardiac arrest occurs, pulmonary ventilation is generally under control, and consideration need be directed to the heart and circulation only. Treatable cardiac arrest more frequently occurs outside the operating theater and is often preceded or followed by respiratory arrest. Consequently, cardiopulmonary arrest is a more appropriate term, and it can be defined as the sudden and unexpected cessation of ventilation or functional circulation or both. While spontaneous ventilation may cease suddenly, the subsequent occurrence of circulatory and cardiac arrest will depend on whether poor ventilation is recognized and treated. Primary circulatory and cardiac arrest will always be followed immediately by spontaneous respiratory ventilatory arrest.

## DEATH

Death, while inevitably the natural conclusion of life, may occur prematurely and suddenly. It can be thwarted before irreversible final biologic cellular alterations occur. The definition of death is currently undergoing evaluation and change and must be related to the entire organism. A single organ system may be dead and yet the overall organism may survive, at least temporarily. Organ death refers to irreversible cellular, biochemical, microscopic, and enzymatic changes in an organ that render it incapable of functioning to a degree compatible with its purpose correlative with other organ systems and the entire organism. Thus, an embolism to the superior mesenteric artery may cause gangrene of the entire small bowel with subsequent organism death. A less necessary organ such as a leg may be lost without loss of the entire organism. In the case of central nervous system death, the organism may exist at least temporarily in a comatose, nonreactive, vegetative state, with survival not independent but contingent upon external assistance with respect to nutrition, mobility, and so forth. We see, therefore, that death must be considered in terms of the relationship of the various body organs to each other and the entire organism.

With untreated respiratory and circulatory arrest, death of the entire organism is immediate and obvious to all, even nonmedical people. With central nervous system death, the human organism as we know it is just as dead in regard to autonomic and vegetative functions, but death is not so obvious to the nonphysician.

We must consider cardiopulmonary resuscitation from the point of view of prevention of the situation of central nervous system death, the central nervous tissue being the first to sustain the irreversible biologic cellular changes, only 4 to 6 minutes after cerebral circulation ceases. Even though the cerebral circulation may again be returned to normal, if such time periods are exceeded cellular changes of swelling, pyknosis, and lysosome and nucleus degeneration occur. The heart may go without circulation for as long as 45 to 60 minutes, as may renal tissue, and skeletal muscle may survive with a functional potential for up to 6 to 8 hours of ischemia.

## RESUSCITATION

The term resuscitation is being employed frequently to indicate the therapy directed at returning a patient to a stable state. Burn resuscitation includes correction of fluid and electrolyte balance and treatment of toxemic shock in order to stabilize the hemodynamic response; resuscitation of a patient with severe body trauma indicates stabilization of the respiratory dynamics and prevention and replacement of blood loss. The more specific and common definition of resuscitation is the restoration to life and consciousness of one apparently dead. Concisely stated for our purposes, cardiopulmonary resuscitation is the therapy directed at sustaining circulation and ventilation while efforts are made to correct the cause of the sudden and unexpected cessation of spontaneous ventilation or circulation, or both, so that these may again regain their automaticity.

## HISTORICAL ASPECTS

Surgeons have long been involved in prevention and therapy of sudden death largely because the treatable occurrence was first seen in patients undergoing general anesthesia, and also because the available effective mode of therapy required the surgical procedure of open-chest cardiac massage. The first described cardiac arrest occurred in 1848 and was secondary to chloroform anesthesia.[2] Resuscitation by closed-chest cardiac resuscitation was first successfully accomplished about 1883,[23] and by open-chest cardiac resuscitation in 1901.[17, 22] Schiff was the real pioneer of cardiac resuscitation by the open-chest method.[41] In 1874 he stated, ". . . if the thorax is opened and at the same time air is insufflated into the lungs, by rhythmical compression of the heart with the hands (care being taken in so doing not to interfere with the coronary circulation) and continuous pressure of the abdominal aorta so as to bring the blood in greater quantity towards the head, it is possible to re-establish the heartbeat even up to a period of eleven and one-half minutes after the stoppage of that organ." The pioneer of the closed-chest cardiac resuscitation method was Boehm, who in 1878 resuscitated cats asphyxiated with chloroform to cardiac asystole by an external cardiac compression method.

The internal cardiac defibrillator was developed by Kouwenhoven and associates[15] following earlier work by Prevost and Batelli.[35] Beck accomplished the first successful human heart defibrillation in 1946, using the internal-type, alternating current defibrillator.[1, 25] Zoll was the first to apply the external defibrillator successfully to the human.[43] The direct current defibrillator now in common use was originally conceived by Peleska.[26, 33]

Drug therapy in cardiopulmonary resuscitation began with the use of epinephrine by Crile in 1904.[6] The present techniques of total cardiopulmonary resuscitation have evolved over the past 10 years, proceeding from the rediscovery of closed-chest cardiac massage by Kouwenhoven and associates at Johns Hopkins in 1958.[10, 20, 24, 40] Multiple advances in pharmacologic therapy and electrical defibrillation as well as a better understanding of the physiology of sudden death have opened a new era in the treatment of cardiac arrest.

## OBJECTIVES OF THERAPY

Knowledge of the basic physiology of cardiopulmonary arrest should lead to the prevention of the majority of sudden death situations in the preoperative, intraoperative, and postoperative periods. When unexpected sudden death does occur, immediate recognition leads to a high likelihood of successful return to the original basal state. Resuscitative therapy is directed to provision of oxygenated blood circulation specifically to the central nervous system and myocardium, thereby to prevent central nervous system damage and to stimulate the return of effective cardiac action. Ancillary treatment consists of determination of the type of cardiac electrical activity and employment of pharmacologic agents and defibrillation as needed; these are directed also to early return of effective cardiac function. Postresuscitation therapy has as its aim prevention of recurrence of the circulatory arrest and correction of the inciting cause. Finally, evaluation is made in an attempt to prevent a similar occurrence in another patient in the future.

## ETIOLOGY AND INCIDENCE

The incidence of cardiac arrest in the operating room has long been reported to be between 1 in 900 and 1 in 2000 procedures using general and epidural anesthesia.[42] Recent studies confirm that this incidence remains approximately the same, although cardiac arrest is less likely during uncomplicated nonemergent operations. Jude et al. found an incidence of 1 in 1216 operations involving general and epidural anesthesia.[18] Fifty-eight per cent of the cases occurred during emergency procedures. Cardiac arrest is most likely to occur during anesthesia induction, during the actual operation procedure, and during transfer to or in the recovery or intensive care room.

The etiology of cardiac arrest in these circumstances is related to myocardial depression or irritability. Myocardial depression may be secondary to anoxia, anesthesia sensitivity or overdose, hyperkalemia, hypercarbia, low blood pressure, blood loss with decreased coronary perfusion, or vagovagal sensitization. Myocardial irritability may result from systemic acidosis, hypokalemia, anesthesia idiosyncrasy, decreased coronary perfusion, or myocardial infarction.

In surgical wards the incidence of cardiac arrest

is similar to that in the general hospital population. The causes are also similar, and are related largely to metabolic imbalances, especially hypokalemia or hyperkalemia, digitalis toxicity, myocardial ischemia or infarction, and pulmonary embolism. Patients with borderline cardiac function with or without large fluid losses are especially prone to cardiac arrhythmias and cardiac arrest.

Cardiac arrest is a rather common occurrence in the emergency room. Blood loss from trauma with secondary hypoperfusion, myocardial depression, respiratory insufficiency of whatever cause (usually trauma) with hypoxic myocardial depression, and myocardial infarction are the common causes.

Sudden cardiac arrest may occur anywhere else in the hospital,[29] e.g., the x-ray department during contrast radiographic procedures, or in the cardiac catheterization laboratory; the etiology and therapy are similar to those of cardiac arrest occurring elsewhere.

## PREVENTION

Proper preoperative preparation of the patient is vital to the prevention of sudden cardiac arrest. Blood volume, hematocrit, and serum electrolytes should be as near normal as compatible with the patient's basic disease. The status of the myocardium as evaluated by electrocardiography or more elaborate study should be known. If the adequacy of pulmonary function is in doubt after history and physical examination, pulmonary function studies should be done. Blood gas determinations might be indicated. Preoperative medication with parasympatholytic drugs generally will prevent vagovagal arrest. The anesthesiologist's knowledge of the toxic effects of the anesthetic agent to be employed will generally prevent idiosyncratic or overdose effect, but any history of allergy will necessitate great care in employment of agents with a high sensitization factor.

In most cases, cardiac arrest during the surgical procedure is caused by direct interference with cardiovascular or respiratory dynamics. Obviously, good ventilation and adequate objective blood replacement should be maintained at all times. Myocardial irritability and myocardial infarction are most commonly associated with inadequacy in these respects. In all patients if possible, and certainly in those with a history of cardiovascular or pulmonary difficulty, those with massive blood loss, those with extrinsic operative procedures, and the elderly, the vital signs should be monitored by a cardiac monitor during operation, and in some cases an intra-arterial pressure line may be necessary.

In the postoperative period, sudden cardiopulmonary collapse most commonly is secondary to asphyxia and its consequences or myocardial depression or myocardial ischemia secondary to acute coronary occlusion. Ventilatory exchange should be closely observed. Tracheal detubation should be delayed until tidal volume is adequate and the patient is wide awake. In some patients muscle relaxants cause a delayed reaction, with development of shallow inefficient ventilatory exchange that may lead to hypoxia and hypercarbia. Hypotension secondary to excess analgesia or reflex vasodilation may trigger decreased coronary perfusion, which in the presence of coronary arteriosclerosis causes subendocardial ischemia or transmural myocardial infarction.

Patients with a higher likelihood of perfusion problems, e.g., the elderly, patients who have undergone massive general, cardiac, or thoracic surgical procedures, and those in whom intraoperative difficulties or large blood loss have occurred, require postoperative monitoring of intra-arterial blood pressure and electrocardiogram, frequent blood gas analyses, measurement of cardiac output, and hourly urinary output measurement.

## RECOGNITION

Being alert to the ever present danger of sudden cardiac arrest is of greatest importance (Fig. 1). The proper monitoring of vital signs *and* electrocardiogram in the higher-risk patients will tell of the sudden onset of loss of effective cardiac action. There may be no premonitory sign of any type, although to the trained and perceiving eye this is usually not the case. During surgery the anesthesiologist is usually the first to recognize the absence of pulse or electrocardiographic change or both. One must remember that the QRS electrical activity of the heart shown by the electrocardiogram may not reflect underlying ineffective cardiac action. The pupils of the eyes will begin to dilate 30 to 40 seconds after cardiac arrest and will be fully dilated in 90 to 120 seconds. In the absence of mydriatic drugs, pupil dilation indicates almost certain circulatory arrest. Absence of capillary bleeding is an important sign, although the surgeon, with his interest centered on details of the operative procedure, may not notice it immediately. The surgeon must always be sensitive to the appearance of the operative field, i.e., the amount of blood and the presence or absence of capillary pulsation. Quick palpation of an available artery, e.g., abdominal aorta or femoral artery, will indicate the state of the blood pressure. The surgeon should become accustomed to the feel of normal aortic pulsation by palpating the aorta deliberately during the course of a laparotomy so that he will always be ready to make a mental comparison in the emergency situation. Outside the operating room, e.g., in the recovery room, sudden cardiac arrest is evidenced by respiratory arrest, absence of major pulses, and, in 90 to 120 seconds, full dilation of the pupils. Obviously, resuscitation should not be delayed until the pupillary change has occurred. A check of blood pressure is not usually necessary.

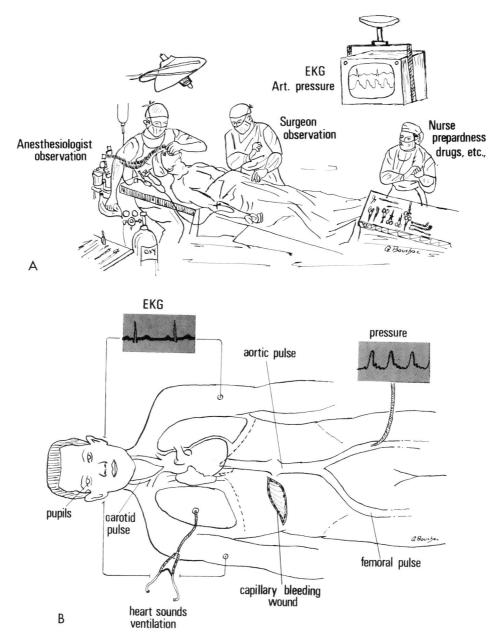

**Figure 1** *A*, Prevention of cardiopulmonary arrest. Proper monitoring of the electrocardiogram (and arterial pressure in selected cases) with close observation by the anesthesiologist and surgeon will prevent most cases of unexpected circulatory arrest. Preparedness by the nurse will allow immediate proper drug therapy in those few cases that do occur. *B*, Diagnostic points. All team personnel must be attuned to the possibility of sudden cardiac arrest. The absence of capillary bleeding, for example, should be checked immediately by palpating for the carotid, femoral, or aortic pulse. Pupil dilation is a late and inexact sign.

## TREATMENT

Therapy in cardiopulmonary arrest can be divided into three major categories:[19, 21] (1) emergency care (to sustain circulation of oxygenated blood and prevent irreversible cellular change); (2) definitive therapy (to reinstitute spontaneous respiratory and cardiac function; and (3) postresuscitative care (to correct the cause of the cardiopulmonary arrest and treat complications resulting from the circulatory cessation).

### Emergency Care

An acute time limit exists in therapy because of the risk of irreversible cellular alterations in the central nervous system within 4 to 6 minutes of circulation cessation. Thus, cardiopulmonary arrest is a true emergency of the highest order; no time is available for consultation or calling other assistance or obtaining mechanical aids or tools. Artificial ventilation and artificial circulation must be provided *immediately*. Adequate effective ventilation can be obtained in the operating room by controlled positive-pressure respiration with 100 per cent oxygen. Since in most patients tracheal intubation has already been established, this is no problem. If this is not the case, then a tight-fitting face mask will suffice. Outside the operating room, expired-air (mouth-to-mouth) artificial respiration can be performed, and, when it becomes available, a self-inflating bag and mask with 100 per cent oxygen to a reservoir tube inlet may be substituted. Ultimately, tracheal intubation can be accomplished. Expired-air ventilation

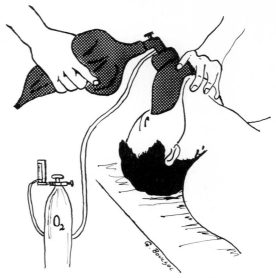

**Figure 3** The use of a self-inflating bag and mask, if available, is more acceptable on aesthetic grounds. The surgeon should be experienced in their use.

provides sufficient oxygen concentration (16 to 18 vol. %) to the victim's lungs if capillary-alveolar block is not present.

**Technique of Expired-Air Ventilation (Mouth-to-Mouth) (Fig. 2).** The resuscitator hyperextends the head of the patient by lifting behind the neck with one hand and pushing backward on the forehead with the palm of the other. This causes the patient's mouth to gape open. The resuscitator takes a deep breath, places his wide-open mouth over the patient's, occluding the nostrils with his cheek, and blows (huffs) air in until the chest expands. Then, maintaining the patient's head in the hyperextended position, the resuscitator removes his mouth from the patient's, to allow passive expiration. Alternatively, the resuscitator places one hand behind the patient's neck, grasps and occludes the nostrils between the thumb and index finger of the other hand, and pulls upward and cephalad to hyperextend the head and open the mouth. Insufflation proceeds as described.

In the mouth-to-nose variation (needed in case of spasm of the masseter muscles), the resuscitator places one hand under the patient's mandible and holds the head hyperextended and the mouth closed. He then applies his open mouth over the nostrils, making a seal, and begins insufflation.

The self-inflating bag and mask can also be employed (Fig. 3). An airway should be inserted over the tongue. The resuscitator holds the mask in place over the patient's nose and mouth and with the same hand maintains the head in hyperextension. With his other hand he squeezes the bag. Some experience is necessary to do this well. The inlet to the bag should if possible be a 3 foot tube reservoir into which flows 100 per cent oxygen.

The respiratory rate is 12 to 16 per minute no matter what technique is used.

When circulatory arrest is present, cardiac massage must be instituted immediately. Either the closed-chest or open-chest technique may be employed. In the operating theater, closed-chest cardiac compression can be carried out through the sterilely draped field.[30] This technique is

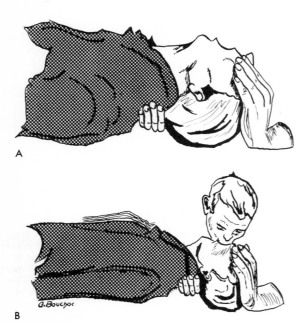

**Figure 2** Mouth-to-mouth artificial respiration. *A*, The patient's head is held hyperextended to open the airway. This can be done as shown by grasping the nose and pulling cephalad and posteriorly. *B*, Air should be huffed in until the chest is seen to expand.

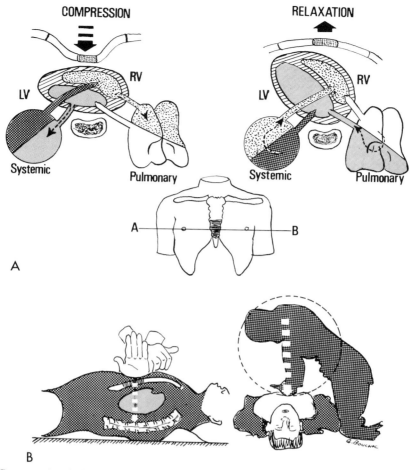

**Figure 4** *A*, Cross-sectional illustration (diagrammatic) at cut A–B. With compression (at left), blood forced is from the ventricles into the lungs (pulmonary artery) and body (aorta). With relaxation, the sternum recoils and, by negative pressure and venous pressure, venous blood is drawn into the ventricles from the pulmonary veins and venae cavae. *B*, On left, sagittal illustration of proper external cardiac compression. On right is cephalad view of hand position.

thus especially valuable in preventing contamination of the primary operative field. Outside the operating theater, the necessary adjuncts for open cardiac massage are not always readily available, and so closed-chest compression is the only approach immediately possible.

**Technique of Closed-Chest Cardiac Compression (Fig. 4).** The anatomic basis of the closed method of cardiac massage is that the heart, a centrally located organ enclosed in the pericardium, almost completely fills the space between the lower half of the sternum anteriorly and the thoracic vertebral spine posteriorly. Depression of the sternum compresses the heart against the vertebral column, and blood is forced out of the right and left ventricles into the pulmonary and systemic circulations. During relaxation of the sternal pressure, blood is returned passively and actively into the heart from the systemic and pulmonary venous circulations. The patient should be supine on a firm surface. The operating table is very appropriate. The base of the resuscitator's hand, between the thenar and hypothenar eminences,

is placed longitudinally on the lower one-half of the sternum. The other hand is placed on top of the first, and pressure is exerted directly posteriorly toward the vertebral column. The resuscitator should be slightly higher than the patient and he should hold his elbows straight in order to utilize the body weight effectively in delivery of the pressure. The downward pressure should depress the sternum 1$\frac{1}{2}$ to 2 inches in the adult and is held for $\frac{1}{2}$ second and then rapidly released for $\frac{1}{2}$ second. The cycle is repeated at a rate of 60 to 80 times per minute. Care should be taken not to exert pressure on ribs either to the right or left or on the epigastrium. A palpable pulse should be present with each compression. Movement of an aneroid barometer needle can even indicate the approximate systolic arterial pressure delivered.[13]

**Technique of Open-Chest Cardiac Massage (Internal Cardiac Massage)**[14] **(Fig. 5).** In the emergency situation, with or without brief antiseptic preparation of the chest, a scalpel is obtained, an intercostal incision is made anteriorly below the left nipple, and the chest is entered in the fifth intercostal space. When available, a rib

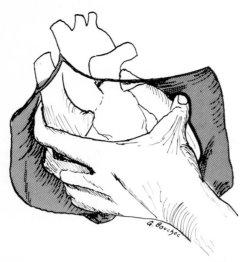

**Figure 5** Placement of hand in left-hand direct cardiac massage. Location of incision is shown in Figure 6. The pericardium is opened anterior to the phrenic nerve. Care must be taken to avoid traumatizing the myocardium excessively.

spreader is inserted. The heart is initially compressed through the pericardium either with the left hand grasping it with the fingers and palm over the right ventricle and the thumb over the left ventricle, or with the hand behind the heart compressing it anteriorly against the posterior sternum. If cardiac action does not immediately resume with good forceful beats and arterial pressure, the pericardium is opened longitudinally anterior to the phrenic nerve and the heart is compressed directly; a better effect can usually be obtained with this method. The compression should be held for approximately ½ second and then released completely for ½ second to enable the heart to fill passively with systemic or pulmonary venous blood. Drugs may be injected directly into the blood inside the left ventricle. Defibrillation can be carried out with the electrode paddles directly in contact with the myocardium. As soon as effective cardiac action resumes, the patient is taken to the operating room, where the chest wall is sterilized and draped properly. The pericardium and left pleural space are then irrigated voluminously with saline and the pericardium is closed loosely with interrupted catgut sutures. A single intercostal chest tube is generally left in place. The ribs are approximated with catgut and the wound is closed in layers, also with catgut. The skin is generally closed but may be left open if the contamination was severe. Generally 1 gm. of cephalothin is left in the left pleural space. Empyema or wound infection is not commonly a problem, even if the procedure is initially performed without any sterile preparation.

**Technique of Transdiaphragmatic Cardiac Massage.** If the abdomen is already open, the heart can be compressed through the diaphragm by pressure against the diaphragmatic portion of the left ventricle, compressing the heart against the posterior sternum. This technique is very inefficient and should not be pursued beyond a few compressions unless cardiac action begins to resume. A better technique is to make an incision in the dome of the left diaphragm and to insert the hand into the left chest and directly squeeze the heart through the pericardium, grasping the heart in the right hand with the thumb over the right ventricle and the palm and fingers over the left ventricle. Direct electric defibrilla-

tion is not possible through this approach, but if the heart is in ventricular fibrillation, and if adequate circulation is being given by this technique, *external* defibrillation of the heart can be done to reverse the ventricular fibrillation.

**Indications for the Various Types of Cardiac Massage.**[7, 16, 36] In most situations when resuscitation is possible, external cardiac compression will suffice. The cardiac output that can be obtained by this method varies from 30 to 40 per cent of normal. With internal direct cardiac compression, cardiac outputs of 40 to 60 per cent of normal may be possible. Open-chest direct cardiac massage is indicated in cases of penetrating injury to the chest, when there is possible associated cardiac tamponade, in cases of suspected tension pneumothorax, when crush injury to the chest is associated with cardiac arrest, and in all those cases in which, because of rigid thorax anatomy or other reasons, external cardiac compression does not seem to be producing adequate circulation.

With the employment of acceptable and effective respiratory and cardiac emergency measures, the patient is essentially sustained on a plateau, and the sinking into irreversible biologic death is totally reversed or slowed. Efforts can now be more coherently directed toward reinstituting spontaneity of respiratory action and cardiac function.

### Definitive therapy

Definitive therapy consists of methods directed at regaining spontaneous effective ventilatory activity and cardiac output. It employs pharmacologic agents, diagnostic determination of the type of cardiac rhythm, and electrical defibrillation as needed.

**Pharmacologic Adjuncts (Table 1).**[12, 27, 38] The purpose of employment of vasoactive agents in cardiac resuscitation is essentially to provide a pharmacologic "tourniquet" to direct the limited cardiac output produced by cardiac massage to the central nervous system and to the heart itself. Inotropic drugs are used to stimulate contraction of the myocardium. Antacids reverse the metabolic acidosis incumbent upon the low cardiac output produced by the artificial circulation of internal or external cardiac massage. Other pharmacologic agents are used to decrease myo-

**TABLE 1** DRUG THERAPY IN CARDIOPULMONARY ARREST

A. Cardiotonic and vasopressor
   Epinephrine, 0.5 to 1.0 mg. I.V. or I.C. every 3 to 5 min.

B. Antacid
   Sodium bicarbonate, 44 mEq. I.V. every 5 to 10 min.

C. Cardiotonic
   Calcium chloride or lactate, 0.5 to 1.0 gm. I.V. or I.C. every 5 min.

D. Antiarrhythmic
   Lidocaine hydrochloride, 25 to 75 mg. I.V. p.r.n.

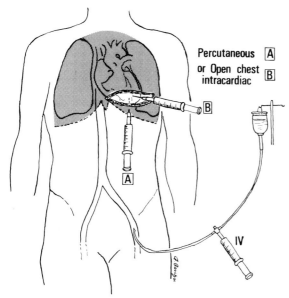

**Figure 6** Intracardiac administration of cardiotonic-vasopressor agents by direct left ventricular puncture through a thoracotomy incision or percutaneously via the substernal route. Intravenous administration may be started by cutdown or puncture of the saphenous vein at the ankle or femoral vein in the groin.

cardial irritability, which may cause persistence of ventricular tachycardia or fibrillation, and additional agents are used to sustain or maintain adequate arterial pressure. All are given directly into the bloodstream (Fig. 6).

Epinephrine is employed both as a vasoconstrictor ("tourniquet") and as an inotropic agent. Because of this alpha and beta effect, it is especially valuable. As soon as epinephrine becomes available, it is given into the blood by the intracardiac or intravenous route in 0.5 to 1 mg. aliquots every 4 to 5 minutes. Other drugs such as isoproterenol may be employed for the inotropic effect but must be accompanied by an alpha stimulator such as phenylephrine hydrochloride.

The exact amount of antacid needed can be determined from arterial or venous blood gases if time is available for this.[9, 11] In most situations, there is not time, and the amount must be estimated. Sodium bicarbonate as a 5 or 7.5 per cent solution may be employed. An empirical dosage of 3.75 gm. (44.2 mEq.) every 5 to 10 minutes generally will maintain arterial pH close to normal during the resuscitation period. Following resuscitation, acidosis may increase as the retained anaerobic metabolic products are released from the previously underperfused periphery.

Calcium chloride and gluconate are additional inotropic agents commonly employed when only weak cardiac action resumes or when there is coordinated electrical activity of the myocardium but inadequate cardiac output. Generally, 0.5 to 1 gm. every 5 minutes is appropriate as long as

adequate circulation is not present. The effectiveness of the calcium lies in its ability to counteract the hyperkalemia occurring in the hypoxic myocardium.

**Cardiac Rhythm.** Cardiac arrest may exist as (1) asystole, (2) ventricular fibrillation, and (3) what is called profound cardiovascular collapse (Fig. 7). When the heart is observed directly, with the chest open, asystole is evidenced by totally inactive cardiac ventricles. In ventricular fibrillation, the ventricular muscle is very active but the movement is totally chaotic and disorganized, and the muscle feels like a "bag of worms" to the grasp. In profound cardiovascular collapse, there is very slight, nonproductive, but coordinated contraction of the heart. If closed-chest cardiac compression is being employed, the exact type of electrical activity of the myocardium can be determined only by electrocardiography. Any lead is satisfactory, such as lead II. Asystole produces a straight line on the electrocardiogram; ventricular fibrillation is characterized by totally chaotic and erratic activity without any QRS complexes; and in profound cardiovascular collapse there are coordinated QRS complexes but the pacing origin may be displaced downward. Asystole is generally caused by anoxia or massive vagovagal stimulation. It may be the end result of severe, diffuse myocardial ischemia. Ventricular fibrillation is generally due to some irritable focus in the ventricle that causes a discharge stimulus with re-entry, so that a "circus" movement results. The various segments or cells of the myocardium are contracting totally independently of one another, without any coordinated rhythm. In profound cardiovascular collapse, electrical activity of the myocardium is coordinated, and there may be some muscular action but this is totally ineffective in producing circulation and would soon lead to complete cardiac asystole or possibly ventricular fibrillation.

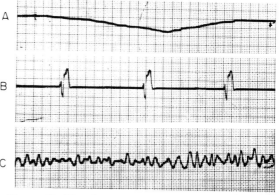

**Figure 7** The three types of electrical patterns in cardiac (circulatory) arrest. When closed-chest cardiac compression is used, an electrocardiogram must be taken, as ventricular fibrillation requires specific therapy (electrical defibrillation). A, Asystole; B, profound cardiovascular collapse; C, ventricular fibrillation.

Knowledge of the exact type of cardiac rhythm is important in determining the type of therapy needed. If asystole or profound cardiovascular collapse is present, therapy with inotropic, vasoconstrictor, and antacid agents must continue. Calcium chloride or gluconate may be especially valuable in this group of patients. If ventricular fibrillation is present, inotropic agents are necessary to improve the quality of the fibrillatory activity and to prod the heart back to spontaneity of activity; myocardial depressants are also necessary to depress irritable foci that may make defibrillation difficult or may cause recurrent ventricular tachycardia or fibrillation. Lidocaine hydrochloride in 25 to 75 mg. aliquots should be given until the irritable focus is permanently brought under control.

**Defibrillation.**[37] This may be carried out either internally or externally. Defibrillation will be successful only if the quality and amplitude of myocardial fibrillations indicate a well oxygenated myocardium. The purpose of defibrillation is complete depolarization, by a massive, overpowering discharge stimulus, of all myocardial segments, allowing essentially simultaneous repolarization and then, it is hoped, a coordinated discharge. If irritable foci remain, additional depressing agents such as lidocaine may be necessary. In some situations, intravenous administration of propranolol in 2 to 3 mg. doses may be tried. External defibrillation is carried out by placing the large paddle electrodes at the base of the heart, on the right second intercostal space parasternally, and over the apex of the heart, in the left fifth intercostal space in the midclavicular line. The direct current defibrillator is the one most commonly employed and is extremely effective. A total of 200 to 400 watt-seconds is delivered in a brief, 2 to 4 millisecond shock. Repeated shocks are frequently required. Internal defibrillation is accomplished by opening the pericardium and placing the spoon-shaped paddles over the left ventricle and the right atrium and discharging between 40 and 60 watt-seconds of current between the electrodes.

## Postresuscitation Care

Once resuscitation has been accomplished, therapy is aimed at determining the exact etiology of the cardiac arrest, preventing recurrence, and treating any complications resulting from the period of circulatory arrest.

Central nervous system damage may occur even though there were not prolonged periods of total absence of cerebral circulation.[3] Cardiac output may have been inadequate or the circulation directed to the brain insufficient. If the patient does not awaken immediately, one must consider that there has been some central nervous system damage. Since the damage may be marginal, cerebral function may recover completely if additional damage is prevented. Every effort should be made, therefore, to prevent further central nervous system insult. Since organ damage will

result in cellular edema which in turn will cause compression and damage to the brain, efforts should be directed at preventing this edema. This can be done by the use of diuretics such as mannitol, urea, or ethacrynic acid (Edecrin). Total body temperature and the temperature of the brain may be lowered to 32 to 34° C. and maintained there for up to 96 hours in an effort to decrease cerebral edema. Corticoids may also be employed to decrease cerebral edema.

Respiratory assistance is frequently necessary, and a pressure or volume respirator may be used. The endotracheal tube may be left in place for up to 72 hours and then replaced with a tracheostomy if indicated. Blood gases should be followed carefully and the patient maintained on as low an oxygen concentration as will provide adequate arterial $pO_2$. Acidosis should be corrected.

A full 12-lead electrocardiogram should be taken to determine if there is any evidence of subendocardial or transmural myocardial ischemia or infarction. This information must be known, especially if reoperation is considered. Also, further therapy to prevent recurrent arrhythmias and cardiac arrest may be indicated. In most situations, the exact cause of the cardiac arrest cannot be determined. Close observation of the patient must be maintained by monitoring of arterial pressure, electrocardiogram, and urine output during the early postrecovery phase. Oral and parenteral fluids are restricted for 1 to 2 days to a maximum of 800 cc. daily. Antibiotics are administered if open-chest cardiac massage was performed under unsterile conditions.

## Results of Application[4, 8, 28, 31, 34, 39]

When intraoperative cardiac arrest occurs, it must be decided whether to continue the operation or to terminate it as soon as possible. In most situations cardiac function returns immediately, and when there is no electrocardiographic evidence of ischemia of the myocardium, the operative procedure can be completed in its normal course. If, however, there is persistent myocardial irritability or a prolonged period of time (more than 10 minutes) passes before spontaneous cardiac function returns, then the operation should be terminated as soon as possible even though the surgeon will have to reoperate later. The operation can be completed as soon as the patient recovers completely from the cardiac arrest, with both cardiac and central nervous system function returned to normal. If there is evidence after resuscitation of myocardial ischemia or transmural myocardial infarction, then the operation should be delayed until complete healing and recovery have occurred; this may take 8 to 12 weeks.

The faults in previous techniques in cardiopulmonary resuscitation have been largely in the area of procrastination rather than in lack of effectiveness. The open-chest method of cardiac massage is totally satisfactory as far as production of cardiac output is concerned, but it requires thoracotomy and special equipment. Because of the magnitude of this procedure, procrastination is common, and this delay results in a higher incidence of central nervous system damage. On the other hand, external cardiac massage can be carried out immediately when the cardiac arrest is first suspected, even though the diagnosis is wrong or there may be weak cardiac action. External cardiac massage can be administered to the fully draped patient so that there is no disruption of the sterility of the operative field. Checking or contemplating whether or not cardiac arrest is actually present can be done by a second person, and there is absolutely no delay or procrastination in initiation of circulation. The reported effectiveness of cardiac resuscitation is extremely variable, by whatever technique employed. It would seem that there is generally much wider application of cardiac resuscitation by the closed-chest technique, with results superior to those of the open method. This is thought to be due largely to the ease and speed of application.

## ADJUNCTS IN CARDIOPULMONARY RESUSCITATION

Many different techniques and methods of applying both internal and external cardiac compression have been offered over the years. In the 1930s, a mechanical internal cardiac massage machine was developed but never received extensive application. The logistics of application are so difficult that the large majority of patients who might be saved have already been saved by time a machine is set up. Similarly, mechanical devices have been proposed and employed for external cardiac compression. These do not have any general application in the operating room but occasionally could be employed for recurrent cardiac arrest in the recovery or intensive care areas. Any dependence upon such devices as a primary approach to resuscitative therapy would immediately cause a delay that would be extremely detrimental to success of the resuscitation efforts.

Respirators can be employed during the resuscitation but must be of the volume-controlled rather than the pressure-controlled variety. Since the anesthesiologist in surgery will provide a combination of both methods, this is not the problem it might be in the intensive care unit or in the surgical wards, where if a pressure-sensitive type of respirator is employed it would be triggered with every precordial cardiac compression and ventilation of the lungs would be prevented altogether.

In selected cases, when resuscitation is initiated immediately and there is evidence of good central nervous system function, use of temporary complete cardiopulmonary bypass in an effort to obtain return of spontaneous cardiac activity might be considered. There have been numerous reports of such successful application, sometimes extremely dramatic. The possibility of this application should always be kept in mind.

## PERSPECTIVE

Life and death are a heartbeat apart. During elective surgery, when the patient is in the operating room for a nonemergent problem, cardiac arrest is generally a severe tragedy. Preventing cardiac arrest, and, when it occurs, treating it appropriately, will eliminate the majority of such tragic episodes. Only in the emergency situation, when the cause is beyond the control of anyone, should we see failures of treatment.

Cardiac and pulmonary resuscitation is but a very small part of the large medical picture, but it is the most urgent of all problems with respect to both diagnosis and therapy. The primary disease problem is of little concern if resuscitation is not successful. Everyone should therefore understand completely the biophysical characteristics of sudden death as opposed to the normal exit of life and be ready to direct efforts toward re-establishing the normal circulatory and respiratory processes. Controversy about the definition of death — that is, between central nervous system and cardiac and a combination of both, and between cellular and organismal — can only complicate the realization of the value of resuscitation efforts. Principles can be learned but are of little value unless properly applied in the practical situation.

## SELECTED REFERENCES

Dupont, B., Flensted-Jensen, E., and Sandoe, E.: The long-term prognosis for patients resuscitated after cardiac arrest. A follow-up study. Amer. Heart J., 78:444, 1969.
*The authors review the short- and long-term results in the management of cardiac arrest in 161 patients, 95 of whom had acute myocardial infarction. Included are the initial and discharge survival incidence, the relationship of duration of cardiac arrest to long-term survival, and the incidence of psychiatric complications. The statistics are quite typical of results of present-day resuscitation techniques and substantiate their use.*

Jude, J. R., and Nagel, E.: Cardiopulmonary resuscitation— 1970. Mod. Conc. Cardiovasc. Dis., 39:133, 1970.
*The authors, as representatives of the American Heart Association's Committee on the title subject, give a brief review of the first 10 years of closed-chest cardiopulmonary resuscitation and present concisely the current status of resuscitation procedures. This paper provides an excellent review of current methods, drugs, and equipment.*

Kouwenhoven, W. B., Jude, J. R., and Knickerbocker, G. G.: Closed chest cardiac massage. J.A.M.A., 173:1064, 1960.
*This brief article was the introduction to the modern era of resuscitation by its new presentation of nonoperative resuscitation techniques. It is historically significant.*

Stephenson, H. E.: Cardiac Arrest and Resuscitation. 3rd ed. St. Louis, C. V. Mosby Company, 1969.
*The monograph of cardiopulmonary resuscitation contains a very complete bibliography, is well indexed, and serves as a good reference when in-depth treatment of the subject is desired.*

## REFERENCES

1. Beck, C. S., Pritchard, W. H., and Feil, H. S.: Ventricular fibrillation abolished by electric shock. J.A.M.A., 135: 985, 1947.
2. Beecher, H. K.: The first anesthesia death, with some remarks suggested by it on the fields of the laboratory

and the clinic in the appraisal of new anesthetic agents. Anesthesiology, 2:443, 1941.

3. Bengtsson, M., Holmberg, S., and Jansson, B.: A psychiatric-psychological investigation of patients who had survived circulatory arrest Acta Psychiat. Scand., 45:327, 1969.

4. Benson, D. W., Williams, G. R., Spencer, F. C., and Yates, A. J.: The use of hypothermia after cardiac arrest. Anesth. Analg., (Cleveland), 38:423, 1959.

5. Boehm, R. V.: Arbeiten aus dem pharmakologischen Institut der Universitat Dorpat XIII. Uber Weiderbelebung nach Vergifungen und Asphyxie. Arch. Exp. Path., 8:68, 1878.

6. Crile, G. W.: The resuscitation of the apparently dead and a demonstration of the pneumatic rubber suit as a means of controlling the blood pressure. Trans. Southern Surg. Gynec. Ass., 16:362, 1904.

7. Del Guercio, L. R. M., Coomaraswamy, R. P., and State, D.: Cardiac output and other hemodynamic variables during external cardiac massage in man. New Eng. J. Med., 269:1398, 1963.

8. Dupont, B., Flensted-Jensen, E., and Sandoe, E.: The long-term prognosis for patients resuscitated after cardiac arrest. A follow up study. Amer. Heart J., 78:444, 1969.

9. Edmonds-Seal, J.: Acid-base studies after cardiac arrest. A report on 64 cases. Acta Anaesth. Scand., Supp. 23:235, 1966.

10. Elam, J. O., Brown, E. S., and Elder, J. D., Jr.: Artificial respiration by mouth-to-mask method; a study of the respiratory gas exchange of paralyzed patients ventilated by operator's expired air. New Eng. J. Med., 250:749, 1954.

11. Fillmore, S. J., Shapiro, M., and Killip, T.: Serial blood gas studies during cardiopulmonary resuscitation. Ann. Intern. Med., 72:465, 1970.

12. Flensted-Jensen, E., and Sandoe, E.: Lidocaine as an antiarrhythmic. Acta Med. Scand., 185:297, 1969.

13. Fletcher, G. F.: Hazardous complications of "closed chest" cardiopulmonary resuscitation. Amer. Heart J., 77:431, 1969.

14. Foley, W. J.: Open cardiac massage. Surg. Gynec. Obstet., 128:827, 1969.

15. Hooker, D. R., Kouwenhaven, W. B., and Langworthy, O. R.: The effect of alternating electric currents on the heart. Amer. J. Physiol., 103:444, 1933.

16. Hugin, W.: A comparison of closed and open chest cardiac massage. Acta Anaesth. Scand., Supp. 9:122, 1961.

17. Igelsrud, K.: Tromso, Norway, 1901; first successful case. Reported by Keen.[22]

18. Jude, J. R., Bolooki, H., and Nagel, E.: Cardiac resuscitation in the operating room — current status. Ann. Surg., 171:948, 1970.

19. Jude, J. R., and Elam, J. O.: Fundamentals of cardiopulmonary resuscitation. Philadelphia, F. A. Davis Company, 1965.

20. Jude, J. R., Kouwenhoven, W. B., and Knickerbocker, G. G.: External cardiac resuscitation. Monog. Surg. Sci., 1:59, 117, 1964.

21. Jude, J. R., and Nagel, E.: Cardiopulmonary resuscitation, 1970. Mod. Con. Cardiovasc. Dis., 39:133, 1970.

22. Keen, W. W.: Case of total laryngectomy (unsuccessful) and a case of abdominal hysterectomy (successful) in both of which massage of the heart for chloroform collapse was employed, with notes of 25 other cases of cardiac massage. Ther. Gaz., 28:217, 1904.

23. Koenig, F.: Lehrbuch allgemeinen Chirurgie. Gottingen, 1883, pp. 60–61.

24. Kouwenhoven, W. B., Jude, J. R., and Knickerbocker, G. G.: Closed chest cardiac massage. J.A.M.A., 173:1064, 1960.

25. Kouwenhoven, W. B., and Kay, J. H.: A simple electrical apparatus for clinical treatment of ventricular fibrillation. Surgery, 30:781, 1951.

26. Kouwenhoven, W. B., and Milnor, W. R.: Treatment of ventricular fibrillation using a capacitor discharge. J. Appl. Physiol., 7:283, 1954.

27. Malm, O. J.: Treatment of acidosis and electrolyte disturbances in asphyxia and cardiac arrest. Acta Anaesth. Scand., Supp. 29:165, 1968.

28. Minuck, M., and Perkins, R.: Long-term study of patients successfully resuscitated following cardiac arrest. Anesth. Analg. (Cleveland), 49:115, 1970.

29. Moss, A. J., Osborne, R. K., Baue, A. E., Lees, R. S., Jamison, R. L., and Spann, J.: Closed chest cardiac massage in the treatment of ventricular fibrillation complicating acute myocardial infarction. New Eng. J. Med., 267:679, 1962.

30. Nixon, P. G.: The arterial pulse in successful closed-chest cardiac massage. Lancet, 2:844, 1961.

31. Norris, R. M.: Long-term survival after cardiac arrest. New Zeal. Med. J., 69:144, 1969.

32. Pearson, J. W., and Redding, J. S.: The role of epinephrine in cardiac resuscitation. Anesth. Analg. (Cleveland), 42:599, 1963.

33. Peleska, B.: Transthoracic and direct defibrillation., Rozhl. Chir. 26:731, 1957.

34. Peschin, A., and Coakley, C. S.: A five year review of 734 cardiopulmonary arrests. Southern Med. J., 63:506, 1970.

35. Prevost, J. L., and Batelli, F.: La mort des courants électriques — courants alternatifs à haute tension. J. Physiol. Path. Gen., 1:427, 1899.

36. Redding, J. S., and Cozine, R. A.: A comparison of open-chest and closed-chest cardiac massage in dogs. Anesthesiology, 22:280, 1961.

37. Redding, J. S., and Pearson, J. W.: Resuscitation from ventricular fibrillation drug therapy. J.A.M.A., 203:255, 1968.

38. Rothwell-Jackson, R. L.: The adjuvant use of pressor amines during cardiac massage. Brit. J. Surg., 55:545, 1968.

39. Russell, E. S.: Cardiac arrest. A. Survival after 2½ hours' open chest cardiac massage. B. Survival after closed chest cardiac massage. Canad. Med. Ass. J., 87:512, 1962.

40. Safar, P., Escarrage, L., and Elam, J.: A comparison of the mouth-to-mouth and mouth-to-airway methods of artificial respiration with the chest-pressure air-lift methods. New Eng. J. Med., 259:671, 1958.

41. Schiff, M.: Uber directke Reizung der Herzoberflache. Arch Ges. Physiol., 28:200, 1882.

42. Stephenson, H. E.: Cardiac Arrest and Resuscitation. 3rd ed. St. Louis, C. V. Mosby Company, 1969.

43. Zoll, P. M., Limenthal, A. J., Gibson, W., Paul, M. H., and Norman, L. R.: Termination of ventricular fibrillation in man by externally applied electric countershock. New Eng. J. Med., 254:727, 1956.

# III

# Patent Ductus Arteriosus, Coarctation of the Aorta, and Anomalies of the Aortic Arch

*Henry T. Bahnson, M.D.*

## HISTORICAL ASPECTS

The history of these three conditions, generally included in classifications of congenital heart disease, centers on the contributions of Robert E. Gross, who in 1938 first successfully ligated a patent ductus arteriosus and thus introduced the use of surgical treatment for congenital heart disease. In 1944, Blalock and Park described experimental methods for treatment of coarctation of the aorta by anastomosis of the left subclavian artery to the distal aorta. In the following year (1945), Gross and Craoord and Nylin independently described excision of the coarctation and primary anastomosis of the aorta, the method preferred today. Gross and his associates in 1949 used aortic homografts to replace deficiencies following excision of coarctation of the aorta, reviving a technique that had been described by Carrel and Guthrie in 1906. Gross and Ware were the first to recognize that anomalies of the aortic arch caused tracheal or esophageal obstruction that was amenable to surgical treatment and described this in 1946. In the two to three decades that have followed these milestones, numerous contributions have further clarified the pathophysiology and the diagnostic and therapeutic variations of these defects, and all can now be satisfactorily treated surgically.

## PATENT DUCTUS ARTERIOSUS

Treatment of the patent ductus arteriosus is representative of the rapid advances made in thoracic surgery in the last 30 years. Less than three decades ago ligation of a ductus arteriosus was a "pièce de résistance" performed by a few surgeons in the country. Now, interruption is done by most thoracic surgeons, and it is considered one of the simplest operations, often performed incidentally at the time of open repair of intracardiac defects. Interruption of a ductus can be accomplished with little risk and is one of the most satisfactory and curative operations in the field of surgery of the heart and great vessels.

### Pathologic Anatomy

In the majority of typical cases the only discernible abnormality is the presence of the duct joining the main, or left, pulmonary artery with the lesser curvature of the aortic arch opposite the left subclavian artery, and the channel thus conducts an aortic-pulmonary shunt of blood. The diameter may vary from several millimeters to 1 or 2 cm. It is variable in length, some of the large ductus being almost flush aortic-pulmonary connections. Aberrant positions of the ductus do occur but are rare; it is almost always on the left, even in the presence of a right aortic arch, when it joins the pulmonary artery and distal left innominate artery. The ductus, a structure present during fetal life, normally closes soon after birth. Christie (1930)[6] studied 558 infants and found that the ductus was open 2 weeks after birth in 65 per cent but that this number rapidly decreased, and only 2 per cent were open after 32 weeks and 1 per cent at 1 year. Many of these were small openings and functionally unimportant.

In most cases of patent ductus arteriosus there are no secondary changes, but in those patients with pulmonary hypertension there may be marked intimal proliferation of the medium and small pulmonary arteries, muscular hypertrophy of these vessels, and organizing or organized thrombi in the pulmonary arteries.[8] Somewhat similar pathologic findings are noted in the lungs of normal infants, but these changes regress with age and with lowering of the pulmonary arterial pressure.[9] Whether the pulmonary vascular changes are present at birth and never regress in patients with patent ductus and pulmonary hypertension, or whether they regress and then re-form with the continued high pulmonary flow, has not been conclusively demonstrated. It is unlikely that this will be proved in the future, since, in view of the low operative risk, the condition will not be allowed to follow its natural course without treatment.

### Clinical Manifestations

The symptoms of patients with patent ductus arteriosus vary widely from none to severe cardiac failure, the variation depending upon age, the size of the aortic-pulmonary shunt, and undetermined factors. Some children grow normally, have no shortness of breath or other limitation of activity, and lead fairly normal lives. A significant number of children are retarded in physical growth, in some instances strikingly. In many cases, particularly if the ductus is a moderately large one, the additional burden on the heart becomes apparent as the patient ages, as evidenced by loss of energy, shortness of breath, and fatigue. A typical ductus not accompanied by superimposed pulmonary hypertension or an additional cardiac defect rarely causes cardiac failure, but failure may be a problem, particularly in infants with a large ductus in whom there is pulmonary hypertension and often a high pulmonary blood flow.

Subacute bacterial endarteritis at the site of the ductus is a less frequent problem now than it was prior to the use of antibiotics. Endarteritis occurs most commonly in young adults but rather infrequently in children and is manifested by fever, weight loss, anemia, and positive blood cultures.

That the typical patent ductus arteriosus appears to be an innocuous lesion in many children may lead to the assumption that the condition is compatible with a long life and little or no disability, but such is not usually the case. Keys and Shapiro (1943) found that those who are alive at 17 years of age with a patent ductus arteriosus have a subsequent life expectancy about one-half that of the normal population. Campbell[4] has concluded, on the basis of review of his own large experience and others' reported experiences, that by age 45, 42 per cent of patients with a patent ductus arteriosus will have died. Although his data also showed that spontaneous closure of the ductus may occur even later in life, this occurs too infrequently to justify it as a hoped-for solution to the problem.

The heart is usually normal in size or only slightly enlarged. In the presence of a large ductus it may be overactive. There may be a normal systolic blood pressure with a low diastolic level because of the run-off into the pulmonary circuit, and this may be accompanied by peripheral signs similar to those of aortic insufficiency. The murmur is a characteristic one and allows an accurate diagnosis of the condition in about 95 per cent of cases. In the typical case, it is a continuous murmur, often rumbling in systole, sometimes obscuring the pulmonary second sound, is heard most prominently in the right second to third intercostal space, and is frequently associated with a thrill. The pulmonary second sound may be accentuated. The rumbling systolic phase, the banging second sound, and the continuous murmur give the impression of machinery, the name usually applied to it. Transmission of the murmur depends largely on its intensity, the systolic phase usually being transmitted more widely than the diastolic. If the channel is small, only a systolic murmur may be heard, although the flow and turbulence are probably continuous. If the shunt of blood through the ductus is extremely large, there may be a rumbling diastolic murmur at the apex of the heart suggestive of relative mitral stenosis; there may be other murmurs due to a large blood flow through the active heart. When heart failure occurs with pulmonary hypertension, the murmur may be obscured or otherwise altered. Other variations in the murmur will be mentioned in connection with the atypical ductus.

Roentgenologic studies show the heart to be of normal size or slightly enlarged. When enlargement is significant, it is apt to be predominantly of the left atrium and left ventricle. The region of the left pulmonary artery is often full along the upper left contour of the heart. The lung fields show increased vascularity, and there may be a hilar dance, although this is not so striking in patients with a ductus as in those with a left-to-right intracardiac shunt. These changes are not specific for the patent ductus, since the picture may be similar to that of other shunts, notably a ventricular septal defect. Although it often cannot be determined by routine radiologic methods, the ascending aorta characteristically is larger in the patient with a patent ductus (by virtue of the flow through it) than in one with a ventricular septal defect.

**Atypical Patent Ductus Arteriosus.** When significant pulmonary hypertension exists, the patient does not present a typical picture. This may be the case in infants with an otherwise ordinary ductus. At birth the pulmonary artery pressure is elevated, but it normally falls rapidly in the first few months. Because of the reduced pressure gradient between the aorta and the pulmonary artery in neonatal life, blood does not flow continuously, and only a systolic murmur may be heard. As the child becomes older, the typical, continuous murmur appears.

On the other hand, there is a group of patients in whom moderate to severe distress is caused by a ductus and pulmonary hypertension. Dammann and Sell[8] and Ziegler[28] focused attention upon the ductus as a cause of disability and of cardiac failure in this group of infants and young children. The atypical ductus is seen most frequently in infants and young children and again in young adults, with a paucity of cases in the intermediate age. In almost all instances the ductus proves to be a large one. Infants and young children frequently are scrawny, underdeveloped, and subject to colds and infection, with dyspnea, some cardiac enlargement, and often signs of cardiac failure. The precordium is active. The murmur is usually a systolic one or one with a short diastolic element, often separated by a pause, indicating the lack of a continuous aortic-pulmonary pressure gradient. The pulmonary second sound is characteristically loud, indicative of hypertension. Radiologically the lung fields are vascular, both from increased flow and from congestive changes.

In infants and many children there is apt to be a high pulmonary blood flow with only a moderate increase in pulmonary vascular resistance. In some children and in most adults with pulmonary hypertension and an atypical ductus, there is a tendency toward lower pulmonary blood flow and high pulmonary vascular resistance. In such instances, the heart is less active and not so large. In its extreme, the atypical ductus is associated with a reverse flow, pulmonary blood entering the aorta and causing cyanosis of the toes in contrast to fingers of normal color. This late and probably irreversible stage is rarely seen in children, a fact that lends support to the concept that the pulmonary vascular changes are progressive.

## Diagnosis

In 95 per cent of cases the diagnosis can be made easily and simply, largely on the basis of the characteristic continuous murmur. The murmur may be simulated by a venous hum, although a hum is usually more prominent over the right upper chest, is less intense with the patient supine, and may be obliterated by compression of the jugular vein in the neck. Arteriovenous fistulas of the lung cause a similar murmur, although this type is usually high-pitched and is transmitted more widely for its intensity, and the lesion frequently can be seen in the lung field on a plain roentgenogram.

In three conditions, the initial differential diagnosis may be extremely difficult: ventricular septal defect, possibly with associated aortic insufficiency; aorticopulmonary window; and patent ductus arteriosus with pulmonary valvular insufficiency. All may present an almost identical clinical picture. Although sampling of blood for oxygen content may give similar findings in these three conditions, appropriate injections and selective angiocardiography will usually establish the diagnosis prior to operation. In some instances, exploration for a patent ductus or for correction of either of the other two lesions with cardiopulmonary bypass may be necessary to establish the diagnosis.

### Selection of Patients for Operation

A difficult problem arises in treating the patient, usually an adult, with pulmonary hypertension and a reverse ductus. When pulmonary hypertension is striking and in the presence of a reversed shunt, there may be such severe pulmonary vascular resistance that the patient will not tolerate the stresses of the postoperative period. Cyanosis of the toes or evidence of significant right ventricular hypertrophy as seen electrocardiographically suggests that an irreversible condition has developed. Ellis et al.[11] presented a good analysis of the problem and concluded that if the shunt is predominantly left to right but nearly balanced, operation is probably indicated but involves considerable risk. Indications are clearer for operation when the shunt is only left to right without right to left, since several studies have shown a decrease in pulmonary artery pressure and pulmonary vascular resistance after interruption of a ductus with pulmonary hypertension. The condition is more apt to be reversible in young children than in adults. When flow is predominantly right to left, there is great operative risk and little chance of benefit from the operative closure.

In some cases, as in the tetralogy of Fallot, the ductus is a compensating structure. The ductus must not be interrupted in such cases unless the condition for which it is compensating can be corrected.

Clatworthy and McDonald[7] pointed out that the operative morbidity in infants and young children is no greater than that seen in older children and advocated operation in children with symptoms when the diagnosis is established or in asymptomatic patients before the age of 5. They saw little advantage in postponing operation. Trusler et al.[25] advocate closure before age 2 years to avoid the greater psychologic trauma between ages 2 and 4. The operative risk is small; the only deaths were in infants in failure less than 6 months old. At present a new indication for ductal obliteration is in some premature infants with the respiratory distress syndrome who show signs of increased pulmonary blood flow. Interruption in some infants weighing 1 to 2 kg. has strikingly changed the course of their illness.

### Operative Technique

Whether the ductus is surgically exposed from an anterolateral or posterolateral incision is largely a matter of personal preference. Mobilization of the aorta may be accomplished more easily through a posterolateral fourth interspace incision. However, exposure is more time-consuming and the position increases ventilatory embarrassment; we have used this approach only for the uncommon patient with a mycotic aneurysm involving the ductus or for the patient with an extremely large main pulmonary artery, which might obscure the exposure of the ductus anteriorly.

We prefer to make an incision through the third interspace, going below the breast in females (Fig. 1). The incision must extend well around laterally, with division of almost the entire intercostal muscle bundle, separating the serratus and dividing the anterior edge of the latissimus dorsi, so that one obtains good exposure well up into the axilla. In our experience this has given wide and ample exposure of the ductus, adjacent aorta, and pulmonary artery. An incision is made overlying the pulmonary artery between the phrenic and vagus nerves. If the ductus is not readily seen, it may be found by tracing the recurrent branch of the vagus nerve around the ductus and the aorta. There is usually a small lappet of pericardium extending over the ductus that should be elevated, and the ductus should be bared of its adventitia and freed of attachments.

Sharp dissection around the great vessels under direct vision is preferable to blunt, tearing dissection. The angle between the distal pulmonary artery and the ductus is particularly susceptible to injury. Attachments between the pericardium, pulmonary artery, and lesser curvature of the aortic arch should be exposed and divided. After the ductus is mobilized as much as possible and the adjacent pulmonary artery and aorta freed, a right-angle clamp may be placed around the ductus and umbilical tape passed. This clamp is probably more safely passed behind the ductus from the caudal, distal, aortic side. In order to obtain additional length slight traction may be applied on the tape and the ductus can be freed posteriorly.

There is room for personal preference also in the method of interruption of the ductus.[10] Most would agree that, theoretically, closure of any large artery can best be accomplished by division of the artery. In actual practice, however, multiple-suture ligation of the ductus with occlusion over the entire length of the ductus has given excellent results (Scott, 1950). Ligation with multiple transfixing sutures was championed by Blalock[2] (1946) at a time when division was associated with considerably greater risk than it is at present. The method is safe and satisfactory. If ligation is to be done, purse-string sutures are placed at the aortic and pulmonary ends and tied snugly, so that the flow through the ductus is nearly obliterated (Fig. 1). Two mattress sutures are then placed between these, and the ductus is obliterated over a length of 1 cm. or more.

Increased experience with the great vessels and particularly the development of finer clamps for occluding vessels have greatly reduced the risk of division of the ductus. This procedure is probably now practiced more widely than ligation. After the ductus is mobilized as much as possible, fine vascular clamps, such as the multitooth Potts ductus clamp, are placed on the aortic and pulmonary ends with sufficient room in between for division and closure (Fig. 2). When the ductus is divided, the occluding clamps must be held against the pulmonary artery and the aorta; this lessens the danger of their being pulled off and at the same time gives greater exposure for suture closure. A satisfactory method is to

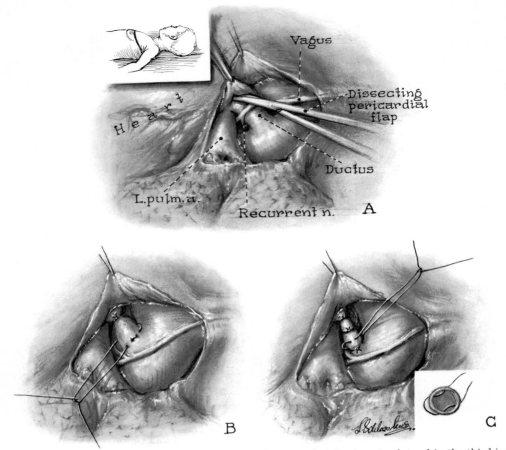

**Figure 1** Operative treatment of ductus arteriosus by ligation. Incision is anterolateral in the third interspace. In females the incision circles beneath the breast. Elevation of pericardial lappet exposes the ductus. A purse-string suture, which does not enter the lumen, is placed at each end, and perforating mattress sutures are placed in between. The ductus should be obliterated over an 8 to 10 mm. distance. (From Bahnson, H. T. In: Gibbon, J. H., Jr., Sabiston, D. C., Jr., and Spencer, F. C., eds.: Surgery of the Chest. 2nd ed. Philadelphia, W. B. Saunders Company, 1969.)

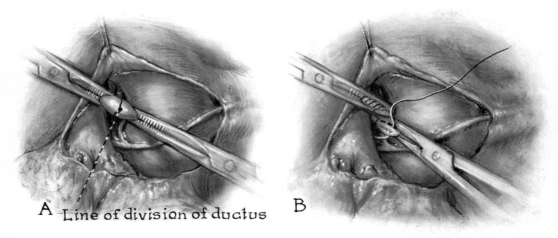

**Figure 2** Treatment of ductus arteriosus by division. Anterolateral third interspace incision is used with exposure as for ligation. A thin occluding clamp is placed at each end and the ductus is divided. Pressing the clamp against the pulmonary artery or aorta after division reduces likelihood of slipping. Suture of ductus is by a continuous mattress suture adjacent to clamp, followed by whip stitch back up over the free edge. Suture of the pulmonary artery end is easier when done from the patient's right side. (From Bahnson, H. T. In: Gibbon, J. H., Jr., Sabiston, D. C., Jr., and Spencer, F. C., eds.: Surgery of the Chest. 2nd ed. Philadelphia, W. B. Saunders Company, 1969.)

suture adjacent to the clamp with a mattress suture and continue back over the free edge with an over-and-over whip suture. After both openings are sutured, a sponge is held in the area for compression while the occluding vascular clamps are removed. An additional suture occasionally may be necessary to control bleeding. Suturing the lappet of pericardium across the pulmonary end of the divided ductus to tissue posterior, between the pulmonary artery and aorta, separates the two ends more completely.

If the ductus is unusually large, greater than 1.5 cm. in diameter, simple ligation is dangerous because of the possibility of the suture's tearing through the wall. Division of the ductus is advocated in such patients. When the ductus is extremely short and large, one can gain added length for closure by clamping the ductus at the pulmonary end and then cross-clamping the aorta just above and below the ductus. The ductus is then divided with sufficient cuff on the pulmonary end for closure, and the tangential opening in the aorta is closed while the aorta is collapsed. The safe occlusion time of the aorta is unknown and unpredictable,[15] but 15 minutes' occlusion is probably safe, and this should be ample to allow closure.

Convalescence should be uneventful in the patient with the typical ductus. When cardiac failure, pulmonary hypertension, or endarteritis of the ductus is present, the convalescence may be correspondingly less smooth.

### Results of Operation

Few operations in cardiac surgery are more satisfyingly curative than that for patent ductus arteriosus. The work of the heart is immediately lowered as the burden of the excessive shunt is removed. In 689 cases of all types at the Johns Hopkins Hospital, both typical and atypical, with and without cardiac failure, and with additional defects in a number of cases, the mortality was 2.6 per cent. Gross[13] reported that in his experience in patients who had no failure or infection prior to operation the mortality was less than 0.5 per cent. In a collective review of 3986 cases, the operative mortality was 2.0 per cent with ligation and 2.1 per cent with division in children, and 4.3 and 5.2 per cent, respectively, in adults.[27]

Although patients usually are clinically entirely well after interruption of a patent ductus arteriosus, Lueker et al.[17] have demonstrated evidence of residual pulmonary vascular hyperactivity with exercise and hypoxemia. This is in keeping with other studies following operative treatment of congenital left-to-right shunt with pulmonary hypertension, showing that increased pulmonary resistance diminishes little after operation even though pressure may significantly fall with the decrease in pulmonary blood flow.

Long-term evaluation of patients who have been operated upon clearly demonstrates the value of occlusion of the ductus. In view of the low risk, prophylactic occlusion seems indicated in all children and young adults, even in the absence of symptoms. There is even greater reason for operation in most of the patients who are symptomatic. The low operative risk when balanced against the likelihood of complications and a shortened life expectancy indicates to most cardi-ologists and surgeons that the ductus should be interrupted in asymptomatic children and young adults. In symptomatic patients the interruption may be urgent and necessary for the control of cardiac failure.

## AORTICOPULMONARY WINDOW

Aorticopulmonary window (or aorticopulmonary fenestration, fistula, or septal defect) resembles patent ductus arteriosus in its functional and clinical manifestations. In fact, differential diagnosis is difficult, and many cases have been discovered at the time of operation for patent ductus arteriosus or ventricular septal defect, the two commonly confused conditions.

### Pathologic Anatomy

Between the fifth and eighth weeks of fetal life the aortic septum divides the truncus arteriosus into the aorta and the pulmonary artery. At the same time, the cardiac chambers are developing. The bulbus cordis connects the right ventricle to the pulmonary artery, and the ventricular septum separates the left ventricle and permits its attachment to the aorta. Ultimately the aortic septum from above fuses with the ventricular septum from below. Failure of development of the various septa may result in an aorticopulmonary window, a ventricular septal defect, or (if there is complete failure in development) a truncus arteriosus.

The typical fistula is anatomically located just above the aortic valve (Fig. 3) and varies in size from a few millimeters to several centimeters. Although in many instances the aorta and pulmonary artery are separate between the heart and the region of the window, in some instances the defect is located immediately adjacent to the coronary arteries and valves, and the condition may be indistinguishable externally from a truncus arteriosus in which the aortic and pulmonary valves are part of a single opening.

### Clinical Manifestations

The clinical manifestations of this condition are practically indistinguishable from those of a large patent ductus. Cardiac enlargement is almost always present, along with physical underdevelopment. The murmur produced varies from a continuous to a soft systolic one, and in some instances there is no murmur at all. The murmur has been described as more superficial than that of patent ductus and may be loudest along the left sternal border in the third and fourth interspaces. As in patent ductus arteriosus with pulmonary hypertension, the pressure in the two vessels may be essentially equal, so that there is not a continuous murmur. The pulmonary second sound is usually loud, and there may be a diastolic murmur of pulmonary insufficiency. A wide pulse pressure may be noted. Increased pulmonary vascularity, often with dilatation of the main pulmonary artery, is similar to that seen roent-

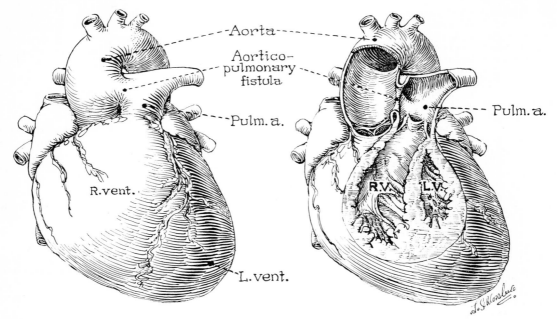

**Figure 3** Aorticopulmonary window similar to that shown treated in Figure 4. Size of the fistula and its relation to the semilunar valves are variable. (From Scott, H. W., Jr., and Sabiston, D. C., Jr.: J. Thorac. Surg., 25:26, 1953.)

genologically in patent ductus arteriosus, as is the electrocardiographic evidence of left ventricular hypertrophy or both left and right hypertrophy in the presence of pulmonary hypertension.

Cardiac catheterization and, more specifically, selective cineangiocardiography make possible an accurate preoperative diagnosis in most instances.

These studies are usually reserved for the patient without the typical clinical picture, however, and without a certain preoperative diagnosis one must be prepared to encounter the unusual lesion. Similarly, when operating for a patent ductus arteriosus the clinical findings should fit the size of the ductus, and if one encounters a small ductus

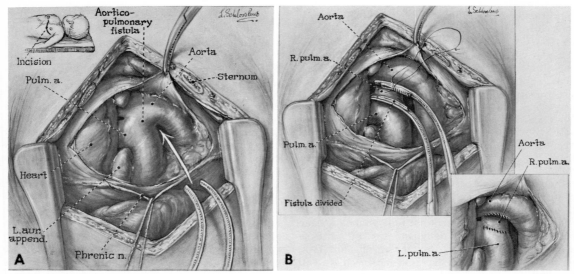

**Figure 4** Closure of aorticopulmonary window during cardiopulmonary bypass. *A*, The aorta is occluded while the fistula is divided and the aortic end closed. The cannula in the left atrium through the appendage helps keep the operative area free of blood; this is clamped as closure of the aortic opening is completed and air is evacuated from the left side. *B*, The aorta is unclamped and coronary circulation restored while the pulmonary opening is closed. (From Bahnson, H. T. In: Gibbon, J. H., Jr., Sabiston, D. C., Jr., and Spencer, F. C., eds.: Surgery of the Chest. 2nd ed. Philadelphia, W. B. Saunders Company, 1969.)

in the presence of bounding pulses and a hyperactive heart, he should suspect and look for an aorticopulmonary window.

### Operative Technique

Aorticopulmonary windows have been treated by ligation, by simple clamping and division, and by division and suture during caval occlusion with hypothermia or cardiopulmonary bypass. In cases in which the defect is small or in which there is no significant pulmonary hypertension and there is sufficient room between the defect and the cardiac valves to allow mobilization, clamping and division may be used. In most cases, however, the conditions are not favorable for clamping. The vessels are large and tense with pulmonary hypertension; the right pulmonary artery seems to arise almost from the back wall of the fistula; and the vessels are easily torn during mobilization or attempted occlusion. In such instances the use of cardiopulmonary bypass converts a difficult and hazardous procedure into a relatively straightforward and easy one (Fig. 4).

### Results of Operation

The condition is not a common one. Pulmonary hypertension has been present in almost all instances. Decrease in heart size and relief of cardiac failure are usually impressive. In most instances the pulmonary arterial pressure falls and approaches the normal level. Whether the pulmonary vascular bed will return to normal in the majority of cases is not known, but at least the cause of the increased pulmonary flow and pulmonary hypertension can be removed so that the pulmonary hypertension is no longer progressive.

# COARCTATION OF THE AORTA

Coarctation of the aorta is an important congenital cardiovascular defect that occurs in a significant number of persons. It shortens life if untreated, but it can be corrected to render the patient functionally normal.

### Pathologic Anatomy

Coarctation most commonly occurs in the region of the aortic isthmus just distal to the left subclavian artery. It occurs less frequently in the aortic arch itself, and in occasional cases the constriction is in the midthoracic aorta at the level of the diaphragm or below in the region of the renal arteries.[1] In rare instances the coarctation may be multiple.

Formerly, the condition was classified as infantile or adult, depending primarily upon the duration of life. The terms are misnomers, since the two types overlap, and, moreover, the terms are not accurately descriptive. From an anatomic point of view, the infantile type can more properly be called preductal coarctation and the adult type postductal (Fig. 5). In the former condition, the pulmonary artery communicates through a large ductus with the distal aorta, and there are usually additional major intracardiac defects, most commonly a ventricular septal defect but in a significant number of cases transposition of the great vessels, atrial septal defect, and other anomalies. The coarctation then separates the flow from the left ventricle to the head and arms and the flow from the pulmonary artery and right ventricle to the caudal half of the body through the ductus. This type of coarctation often involves the distal aortic arch along with the isthmus and tends to be more elongated or diffuse. It is generally discovered in infancy because of the striking disturbance of the circulation by the aortic obstruction in addition to the cardiac defect. Cardiac failure usually occurs, is intractable, and results in death unless correction is possible.

Interrupted aorta, or aortic atresia, is a severe form of coarctation of aorta, usually but not always associated with persistence of the ductus arteriosus. Although most cases have been found at autopsy in newborn infants, a few patients have survived to reach adulthood.

In the typical, uncomplicated, postductal type occurring in the adult, there is a localized constriction just distal to the ductus or ligamentum arteriosum. The aortic valve is bicuspid in 25 to 40 per cent of cases, but other cardiac defects are uncommon. Most patients with this type of anomaly survive to adult life. Although the typical postductal coarctation is usually localized to the region of the ligamentum arteriosum, it may involve the mouth of the left subclavian artery, may be more elongated and diffuse, or may be associated with a hypoplastic distal aortic arch.

POSTDUCTAL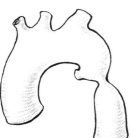

PREDUCTAL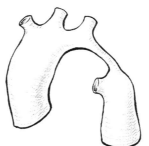

INTERRUPTED AORTA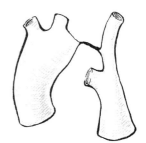

**Figure 5**  Sketches of representative types of coarctation.

In patients who survive beyond infancy, a number of additional features are often noted, the most striking being development of collateral circulation, as was well demonstrated by Bramwell and Jones (1941). Arteries connecting the upper and lower parts of the body, notably the internal mammary, subscapular, and lateral thoracic arteries, become dilated. These communicate with the intercostal arteries, which may be greatly dilated, thin-walled, friable, and subject to dangerous aneurysm formation. Immediately distal to the coarctation there is often poststenotic dilatation of the thoracic aorta, which has the appearance as much of a congenital dilation as of a functional one caused by flow through the stenotic area. There is an increased incidence of cystic medial necrosis of the ascending aorta in association with coarctation.

The etiology is unknown, although the most widely mentioned cause is in connection with the obliterative process, which causes disappearance of the aortic arches and possibly closure of the ductus arteriosus. In the unusual type of coarctation that occurs in the midthoracic aorta, there appears to be a more diffuse inflammatory process, also of unknown etiology.

### Clinical Manifestations

Most children with coarctation are asymptomatic, and their condition is discovered because of a murmur or the presence of arterial hypertension discovered during a routine examination. Symptoms are more common in the adult. Headache, dyspnea, palpitation, vertigo, throbbing in the head, visual troubles, precordial pain, or symptoms of cardiac decompensation—all related to hypertension of the upper part of the body—may drive the patient to seek medical aid. General weakness is a common complaint. In a number of instances weakness and fatigue of the legs and even intermittent claudication are present, but conversely it is striking how many patients have no difficulty with the lower extremities, some even being unusually athletic before the condition is recognized.

Diagnosis is made simply and easily in almost all cases by finding a difference in arterial pulsations and blood pressure in the upper and lower extremities. A comparison of radial and femoral pulsations should be part of every complete physical examination and of course is essential in any patient with hypertension or in one who has complaints such as those just listed. Normally the pulses in the radial and the femoral arteries are synchronous, but in the presence of coarctation there is a noticeable delay in the femoral pulse. Blood pressures and pulses in both upper extremities should be compared with the same measurements in the legs, because, in rare cases, the orifice of one subclavian, usually the left, may be involved in the coarctation, giving rise to a low blood pressure in that arm. Indeed, either subclavian artery may arise below the coarctation. One case has been described in which both subclavian arteries arose from the region of the coarctation and were hypoplastic. Consequently there was no brachial hypertension. In such patients, observation of collateral circulation is most important in the diagnosis.

In addition to the pathognomonic pulse and pressure gradient, there are often pulsations in the neck and supraclavicular areas due to hypertension. A systolic murmur is often heard over the base of the heart or in the midback around the sixth or seventh dorsal vertebra. Diastolic murmurs may be heard in either place. A posterior diastolic murmur probably represents flow through the narrowed area or through the dilated intercostal arteries. Wells, Rappaport, and Sprague (1949) found posterior diastolic sounds in all 15 patients with coarctation of the aorta examined by phonocardiography. These sounds were a continuation of those noted during systole. An anterior diastolic murmur should also be carefully sought, since its presence may indicate a patent ductus arteriosus or aortic regurgitation due to a bicuspid aortic valve or dilatation of the proximal aorta.

Except in young children, enlarged collateral vessels may often be felt over the back, adjacent to the scapula, and in some cases a murmur may even be heard over these vessels. Sir Thomas Lewis in 1933 pointed out that, in the proper light, pulsations can be seen in these vessels, and he carefully mapped the circulation in this condition. The subscapular artery is often enlarged also and can be felt by compressing the subscapular tissue between the thumb and index finger. Collateral circulation should always be looked for, because the disparity of pressure and pulse characteristic of coarctation may also be caused by the Leriche syndrome and terminal aortic thrombosis.

The heart may show some increase in size, particularly of the left ventricle, but when it is unduly large, other anomalies must be considered. The upper mediastinum is often widened because of the enlarged left subclavian artery. Prominence of the left subclavian artery and the proximal and distal aorta is responsible for a characteristic notch in the upper left mediastinal shadow on the roentgenogram, giving the appearance of the number 3; the upper convexity is the proximal aorta, the notch is the coarctation, and the lower convexity is the poststenotic dilatation (Fig. 6). Notching of the ribs, as first noted by Railsbach and Dock (1929), remains one of the most characteristic radiologic features and is caused by dilatation, elongation, and tortuosity of the intercostal vessels that serve as collaterals between the subclavian arteries above and the aorta below the narrowing (Fig. 6). When present in the uncomplicated case, notching is most noticeable in the third to the seventh ribs and is bilaterally symmetric. If the distribution is more prominent in other areas or is asymmetric, one must consider an atypical coarctation or involvement of the mouth of the subclavian artery. When a subclavian artery arises from the aorta below the coarctation,

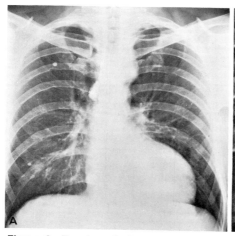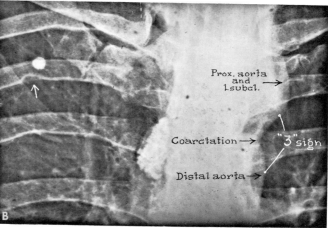

**Figure 6**   Roentgenologic signs, which are diagnostic but not always present in coarctation, include notching of the ribs and the "3" sign caused by the dilated proximal segment and left subclavian artery, by the constricted area, and by poststenotic dilatation. *A*, Note rounded lower left cardiac border, indicating left ventricular enlargement. *B*, Enlargement from *(A)* showing notching of rib (adjacent to calcified lesion) and "3" sign. (From Bahnson, H. T. In: Gibbon, J. H., Jr., Sabiston, D. C., Jr., and Spencer, F. C., eds.: Surgery of the Chest. 2nd ed. Philadelphia, W. B. Saunders Company, 1969.)

notching will be present only on the contralateral side.

The electrocardiogram may vary from normal to that of a striking left ventricular hypertrophy, depending upon the severity of the coarctation and the degree of hypertension. This examination is especially important in older patients in whom changes associated with myocardial damage presage a greater operative risk.

All the signs mentioned point to an obstruction to blood flow in the aorta between the origin of the vessels to the head and arms and the origin of those to the lower extremities. In the majority of cases beyond infancy, one would be correct in assuming that the coarctation is at the junction of the arch and the descending aorta. There is an occasional patient, however, with constriction distal to the usual site. It is important to identify these cases prior to thoracotomy, since successful treatment of such a lesion often requires an aortic replacement and the area may not be readily accessible with the usual thoracotomy incision.

A satisfactory aortogram will demonstrate the lesion in the unusual site, but this examination is unnecessary in most instances of typical coarctation. If one is aware of the possibility of the unusual coarctation, there are several features that suggest the use of aortography. A diffuse murmur heard low in the back is unusual in the typical case and suggests an atypical site in the back or abdomen. Notching that is most prominent in the lower ribs or the absence of notching in patients with other signs of significant aortic obstruction, such as definite hypertension or the brachial-femoral pressure gradient, is suggestive. When the coarctation is in the abdominal aorta, pulsations in the upper abdominal aorta may be palpable. If the possibility is kept in mind, one may

safely reserve aortography for patients presenting any or all of the atypical signs mentioned.

Coarctation is an important cause of cardiac failure in infants, in either the preductal or the postductal site. Such children with failure are irritable and dyspneic, fail to grow and eat normally, and may have cyanosis. The baby may look quite sick, with tachypnea, tachycardia, rales over the lungs, hepatomegaly, and an overactive heart. The diagnosis may be difficult to make in sick infants, and the discrepancy in the pulses of the upper and lower extremities may not be readily apparent. Examination should be repeated until the diagnosis is clarified, although in doubtful cases aortography may be used to demonstrate the coarctation.

### Prognosis

In a review of 108 infants with coarctation by Glass et al.,[12] 90 per cent of the fatalities in those under 1 year of age were due to preductal coarctation, usually in association with cardiac defects. Many infants with postductal coarctation can tolerate the failure when given nonoperative treatment and can improve, presumably as the collateral channels develop.[13] In others this is not possible and surgical relief is necessary.

Adults with typical postductal coarctation have an abbreviated life expectancy. Campbell[5] found the mean age at death to be 34 years, less than half the normal life expectancy. Reifenstein et al. (1947) reviewed a large group of patients and found that 61 per cent died in or before the fortieth year. About one-fourth of the patients lived far into adult life with no incapacity; about one-fourth died of bacterial endocarditis or aortitis; about one-fourth died suddenly of rupture of the aorta (the aorta is susceptible to rupture both proximal and distal to the coarctation); and about one-fourth died of cardiac failure or cerebral hemorrhage resulting from the hypertensive state. It is evident that, although some subjects may live a normal life and be unhindered by coarctation, the defect is in most instances a hazardous one.

### Pathologic Physiology

Physiologic studies have been concerned primarily with the cause of hypertension above coarctation of the aorta. Whether peripheral resistance of the coarctation and collateral vessels per se is sufficient cause, or whether a renal mechanism is involved, remains a controversial issue. Bing and co-workers (1948) observed no evidence of generalized increase in peripheral resistance and from their data demonstrated that the coarctation and collateral vessels alone produce sufficient increase in peripheral resistance to cause elevated pressure. On the other hand, Scott and Bahnson[22] produced coarctation experimentally in dogs, with a resultant discrepancy in femoral and carotid arterial pressures similar to that seen in clinical cases. In such animals, transplantation of a kidney to the neck and removal of the contralateral kidney caused a prompt fall in carotid pressure, although the gradient between carotid and femoral pressures remained. Perhaps there is truth in both concepts and there are some cases of coarctation of the aorta in which the resistance of the coarctation and collateral vessels alone causes hypertension and others in which there is an additional renal factor.

### Selection of Patients for Operation

Almost all patients with coarctation of the aorta should be operated on at an appropriate time unless there are significant contraindications. There are degrees of coarctation, and in some patients in whom only a slight discrepancy in pressure exists between the upper and lower extremities, suggesting less total obstruction, it may be difficult to be sure that the obstruction is not more complete and that it is not simply compensated by adequate collateral circulation.

Probably the most satisfactory age for operation is between 6 and 16 years. Although technically easy in younger children, the operation is apt to be more permanently beneficial if the aorta is allowed to approach its adult size. With increasing age beyond the optimum, the operation is of greater magnitude; the aorta is more sclerotic, less elastic, and more difficult to approximate and suture, and aneurysms of the intercostal arteries are found more frequently. Hypertension also is more apt to be of a fixed nature and responds less satisfactorily to the relief of the aortic obstruction.

Operation is clearly indicated in some patients above and below the optimal age. As Gross[13] has emphasized, during the first few months of life many babies have cardiac embarrassment from uncomplicated coarctation of the aorta, but the majority of them can be supported by nonoperative means. Once compensation is gained, they often survive to later childhood without difficulty. On the other hand, there are a significant number of infants who will not survive unless surgical help can be given. In such infants the operative risk is undoubtedly high. However, Glass et al.[12] recommended that babies with symptoms in the first month of life be operated upon promptly unless they show dramatic response during a 12 hour trial of treatment with digitalis, and that babies over 1 month of age who respond to digitalis be kept on this medication until adequate compensation has taken place and operation can be performed at the optimal age.

At the other end of the age scale, some persons are unaware of coarctation of the aorta until well into adult life. Beyond the age of 30 there is some increase in the operative risk, and although statistics are not available, this almost surely rises with increased age. Of 51 patients older than 30 years treated by Dr. Blalock and his staff, there was a 10 per cent hospital mortality as compared to a 7 per cent risk for patients in the 4 to 15 year age group. It should be emphasized, however, that there is no more specific treatment for arterial hypertension than excision of a coarctation of the aorta, and the operation should be seriously considered at any age. Successful results have been obtained in the fifth and sixth decades.

Certain conditions greatly increase the operative risk.[21] Mild to moderate aortic insufficiency may be present, caused by either rheumatic heart disease or a congenitally bicuspid valve. In a few instances the valve as well as the coarctation has been surgically treated. The risk is greater when there are significant cardiac abnormalities: mitral disease from rheumatic fever, septal defects, or myocardial damage. In almost all such cases the burden on the heart would be decreased if the hypertension due to coarctation could be relieved, but the risk may be prohibitive and operation inadvisable.

### Operative Technique

Blalock and Park (1944) reported an experimental operation designed to bypass coarctation of the aorta by anastomosing the left subclavian artery to the distal aorta. This method was not attempted on a patient until Crafoord and Nylin (1945) and Gross and Hufnagel (1945) did so independently, resecting the involved area and performing end-to-end anastomosis of the divided aorta. Theoretically and actually, such an operation is more desirable when possible, and the use of the subclavian is rarely advisable. The subclavian artery is usually of large size, but a large number of collaterals must be severed when the artery is divided.

The operation is performed with the patient in the lateral position (Fig. 7). Almost the entire length of the fifth rib is removed, as suggested by Crafoord, and the chest is entered through the bed of this rib. If the entire rib from neck to cartilage is removed, good exposure can be obtained and the removal of segments of other ribs is not necessary. In infants, incision in the fourth interspace is satisfactory. The coarctation and the arrangement of the aorta and the vessels should be inspected before the pleura is opened, because often a good view is obtained before the tissues are stained. A long incision

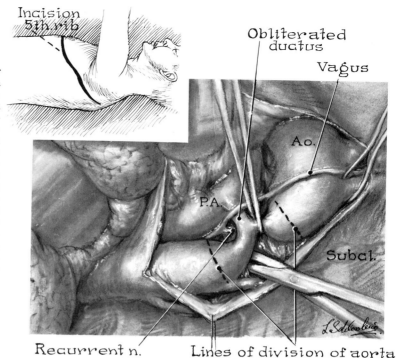

**Figure 7** Operative exposure for resection of coarctation of the aorta is through the bed of the fifth rib. The entire rib is removed from neck to cartilage. The constricted segment is usually held medially by an obliterated ductus, division of which allows considerable mobility. The coarctation is held forward to facilitate dissection posteriorly. Large intercostal arteries must be carefully avoided. Division of the aorta should be through a point of normal diameter. (From Bahnson, H. T. In: Gibbon, J. H., Jr., Sabiston, D. C., Jr., and Spencer, F. C., eds.: Surgery of the Chest. 2nd ed. Philadelphia, W. B. Saunders Company, 1969.)

is made in the pleura over the coarctation, the adjacent subclavian above, and the aorta below, and the pleural flaps are held back with sutures. The easier dissection is done first, namely, mobilizing the left subclavian and the adjacent aorta, the coarctation, and the ligamentum arteriosum or the ductus. Considerable mobility of the aorta is often obtained when the ductus or ligament is divided, so that division of this as soon as possible is helpful. If there are large intercostal arteries adjacent to the coarctation, mobilization of the aorta a short distance below may help to avoid injury to these thin-walled and sometimes troublesome collaterals.

Once this area is mobilized, the intercostals can be visualized from both sides and isolated more carefully. Great care must be exercised in dissection around the intercostal arteries, since they are friable and easily torn from the wall of the aorta. This portion of the operation for coarctation is a perfect example of a situation in which it is easier to avoid difficulty than it is to solve problems once they occur. It is preferable to divide none of these collateral vessels, but although this is often feasible, one or two of the upper ones must usually be severed. As soon as tapes can be placed around the aorta, it can be pulled up slightly away from the vertebral column and better visualization of the posterior aspect can be obtained.

In most patients with an uncomplicated postductal coarctation, the constricted segment is short, but in some instances there is a narrow proximal aortic segment and in others a long area of marked constriction. It must be emphasized that in order to obtain relief of hypertension all of the coarctation must be removed. It is tempting to remove only a short segment and thus avoid tension in the anastomosis. If in doing this an anastomosis smaller than the diameter of the distal aortic arch is obtained, or if the ends cannot be approximated because sufficient length has been removed to relieve the constriction, some form of aortoplasty or of aortic replace-

ment must be used.[21] Such procedures have been used in 2 to 40 per cent of cases, depending on inclination of the surgeon and the age range of his patients. Less elasticity of the aorta and greater frequency of aneurysms and atherosclerotic lesions in the adult require more frequent use of complicated reconstruction.

Various types of anastomoses may be performed. We prefer a single row of continuous 4-0 silk or synthetic sutures in adults (5-0 in young children) through all layers, the intima being everted with a mattress suture (Fig. 8). In the usual case this gives a smooth approximation of the intima of the two vessels. An overhand, noneverting suture works satisfactorily, particularly if the anastomosis is begun with eversion and efforts are made to continue the everting. In view of experimental work showing that a continuous suture may prevent growth of the anastomosis,[20] we interrupt the suture frequently on the anterior row, or, especially in children when growth is important, we use interrupted sutures for the entire anterior portion. It is often helpful to place much of the posterior row of an everting mattress suture before the vessels are closely approximated and the posterior suture line pulled up, as described by Blalock[2] (Fig. 8).

Following completion of the anastomosis, the distal clamp is removed and any necessary sutures are placed in order to obtain a tight anastomosis. The proximal clamp should be released slowly and blood given intravenously during this time. In some patients, too rapid a release of the clamp may lead to profound hypotension.

The infant with coarctation requires careful operative technique and conscientious postoperative care. Interruption of the aorta between the great vessels in the aortic arch is especially hazardous, and only a few survivors have been reported. Tyson et al.[26] advised temporary and then permanent banding of the pulmonary artery to reduce the left-to-right shunt during and after operation, and thus reduce the load on the left

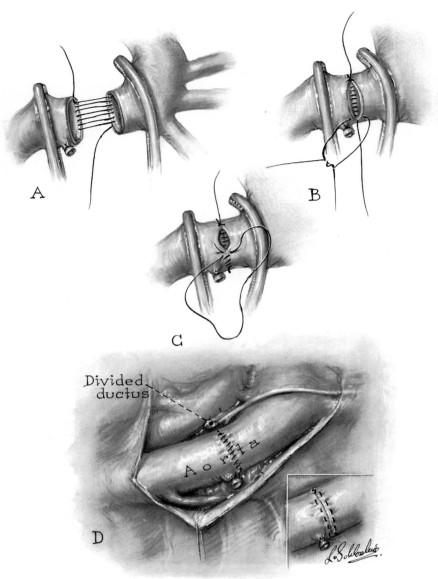

A

B

C

Divided ductus

Aorta

D

**Figure 8**  Anastomosis following excision of coarctation. An everting mattress suture is placed over about one-third of the posterior row before the vessels are approximated and the suture is pulled up. The anastomosis is completed with continuous over-and-over suture. Inset in *D* shows the everting mattress suture sometimes used. In children, interrupted mattress sutures are used for the entire anterior row. (From Bahnson, H. T. In: Gibbon, J. H., Jr., Sabiston, D. C., Jr., and Spencer, F. C., eds.: Surgery of the Chest. 2nd ed. Philadelphia, W. B. Saunders Company, 1969.)

ventricle. Their unique success in repair of the interrupted aorta in the newborn supports this admonition.

### Results of Operation

In 1601 cases collected from around the world, the average mortality was 8.6 per cent.[19] It was 6.8 per cent in patients between the ages of 4 and 15 years and significantly higher in those below age 3 or over age 30. Heart failure and pulmonary edema, often related to associated defects, and disruption of the anastomosis, probably most often due to infection, were the most common causes

of death and in conjunction with cardiac arrest or fibrillation and operative hemorrhage accounted for 72.9 per cent of the deaths.

Among the patients who survived, satisfactory relief of hypertension was obtained in 95.2 per cent, and entirely normal readings were present in 72.0 per cent. The incidence of persistent hypertension increased progressively with the age of the patient. For unknown reasons, the blood pressure does not always reach its final level immediately after operation. In the majority of patients, the pressure is normal at the time of discharge from the hospital, but it usually remains elevated for 10 to 14 days and occasionally for several months.

One complication, which appears to be an unfortunate byproduct of the relief of hypertension, has been *necrotizing arteritis*. Although rare, this condition has occasionally been fatal. Examination shows the arteritis to be limited to the lower part of the body. Most of the clinical manifestations have been in the abdomen, causing abdominal pain and in some instances resulting in gangrene of the intestine. In about one-third of young patients operated upon with resection of the coarctation, blood pressure may rise to a higher level after operation than before—a "paradoxical hypertension." Abdominal symptoms are usually confined to this group of patients and occur in one-fourth to one-half of them (Tawes et al., 1970). Sympatholytic drugs are indicated in such cases.[24] The cause of this complication is unknown, although it is recognized that there is increased sympathetic nerve activity following resection of coarctation (Goodall and Sealy, 1969).

A rare but distressing complication has been paraplegia or weakness of the lower part of the body after operation. This appears to result from inadequate circulation through the anterior spinal artery, possibly owing to interruption of important intercostal arteries or collateral vessels; again, this emphasizes the desirability of preserving, if not all, as many collaterals as possible.

In the late 1960s several reports of recoarctation appeared, possibly reflecting the greater use of operation in infants earlier in the decade.[15] Restenosis has been due to insufficient resection, residual ductal or fibrous tissue, thrombosis, or failure to grow because of a constricting continuous suture.[16]

The ultimate long-term results of the treatment of coarctation are unknown, since the longest follow-up extends only to 1944, but it is evident that surgery rests on a firm basis and has a great deal to offer most of these patients.

# ANOMALIES OF THE AORTIC ARCH

Constriction by an abnormality of the aortic arch must be considered in patients, especially infants, who present evidence of tracheal or esophageal obstruction. Many anomalies of the aortic arch, of its branches, and of the great veins in the superior mediastinum are of no clinical significance, and in fact most of the reported cases were discovered incidentally. Gross and Ware in 1946, however, clearly demonstrated that embarrassing and sometimes fatal obstruction of the trachea and esophagus may arise from a double aortic arch; a right aortic arch with a ligamentum arteriosum completing a ring about the trachea; or an anomalous innominate, left common carotid, or subclavian artery.[13, 14]

## Embryology

In order to understand the variations that might be encountered, it is helpful to review the embryology of the aortic arch system.[1] During the first 3 weeks of embryonic life, six aortic arches join the ventral aortic sac and the dorsal paired aortas around the interposed pharynx. The aortas caudal to the branchial arches become fused as an unpaired dorsal aorta. Figure 9A shows diagrammatically the approximate configuration of the aortic arches in the 12 mm. embryo. The embryonic subclavian artery is the seventh cervical segmental artery, which supplies the limb bud. As the heart and aortic sac move caudad and the cranial portion of the embryo elongates, the subclavian artery moves craniad on the aorta. Normally the most caudal segment of the right fourth arch becomes obliterated as the left fourth arch takes over the majority of the cardiac output. The right third arch persists as the proximal part of the carotid artery. It ultimately arises from the fourth arch, which persists as the innominate and subclavian arteries. The left fourth arch persists as the definitive aorta, and the carotid and subclavian arteries arise independently. In rare instances the left subclavian artery may ascend to the third arch, and a left innominate artery results. If the right aortic arch persists and the left arch becomes obliterated, the mirror image of the arrangement just described may occur.

If the proximal rather than the distal part of the right fourth arch becomes obliterated, the right subclavian artery arises from the unpaired aorta and courses behind the esophagus to reach the right arm. In rare instances the vessel may go between the trachea and the esophagus or anterior to the trachea. A short segment of the distal end of the right fourth arch may persist as an aortic diverticulum from which the subclavian arises. The ductus arteriosus usually connects the main or the left pulmonary artery (derived from the sixth arch) with the left aortic arch. When the proximal left fourth arch becomes obliterated, the ductus arteriosus is connected with the most distal portion of the left dorsal aorta along with the subclavian artery (Fig. 9C). If the arch becomes obliterated distal to the ductus arteriosus, this relationship is lost. When both aortic arches persist, a complete aortic ring is formed around the trachea and esophagus (Fig. 9B). In such instances the brachiocephalic vessels usually arise from the arches independently, although double aortic arches with an innominate artery have been described.

## Pathologic Anatomy

A vascular ring around the trachea and esophagus may be composed of any of the several remnants of the aortic arch system. A double aortic arch results when neither of the aortic arches regresses. In such cases the ascending aorta bifurcates, one branch going to the right and behind the trachea and esophagus, and the other to the left in front of the trachea. Both limbs join behind to complete a ring around the trachea and esophagus (Fig. 10). In most instances the descending aorta is on the left side, although a right descending aorta may occur, with the aorta lying to the right of the vertebral column. Regardless of the side of the descending aorta, the smaller of the two arches is usually to the left and anterior, an important consideration in selecting the side of surgical approach.

If the left fourth aortic arch, rather than the right, disappears in the embryo, the subject is born with a right aortic arch, which ascends,

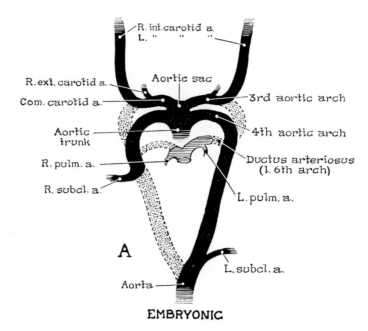

EMBRYONIC

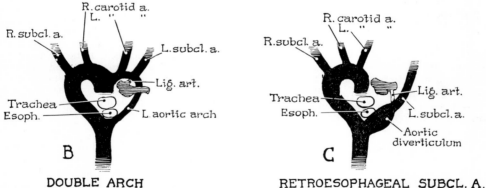

B
DOUBLE ARCH

C
RETROESOPHAGEAL SUBCL. A.
WITH LIG. ARTERIOSUM

**Figure 9** Development of aortic arch and anomalies. The stippled areas normally disappear. Normally only the left fourth arch persists in its entirety. Both fourth arches persist in the double aortic arch. When the right fourth arch persists and the left fourth arch disappears, the left subclavian artery is retroesophageal. A ligamentum arteriosum may join this to the pulmonary artery and complete the ring. (From Bahnson, H. T., and Blalock, A.: Ann. Surg., *131*:356, 1950.)

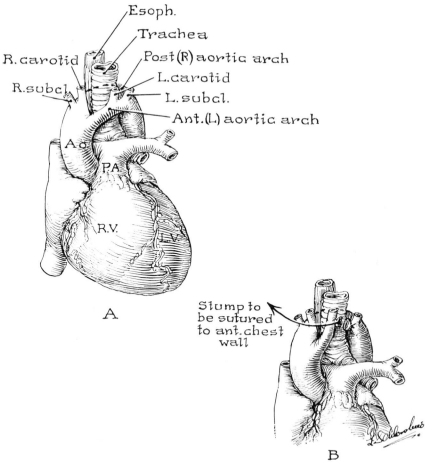

**Figure 10**  Double aortic arch. *A*, The larger channel is usually the posterior one and on the right. Branches of the arch arise independently. In almost all instances the descending thoracic aortic is on the left as shown. *B*, Point of division of the smaller arch is selected to preserve circulation to the branches. The left common carotid artery is then tacked to the anterior chest wall to further relieve tracheal compression. (From Bahnson, H. T. In: Gibbon, J. H., Jr., Sabiston, D. C., Jr., and Spencer, F. C., eds.: Surgery of the Chest. 2nd ed. Philadelphia, W. B. Saunders Company, 1969.)

passes to the right of the trachea and esophagus, and descends usually on the left, but occasionally on the right, of the vertebral column. Such an arch in itself rarely causes symptoms, although there may be some tracheal or right bronchial compression. In many such cases the ligamentum arteriosum courses from the pulmonary artery and joins the innominate artery* at its bifurcation into the carotid and subclavian. In some instances, however, the ligamentum passes from the pulmonary artery to the left of the trachea and esophagus and to the distal end of the right aortic arch, thus completing a ring around the trachea and esophagus (Fig. 11). This ring may be small enough to compress and interfere with the function of the trachea and esophagus.

Of the anomalies of the branches of the aortic arch, that of the right subclavian is the most easily recognized and understood. If in the development of the aortic arch system the proximal portion of the right fourth arch disappears instead of the distal portion, the right subclavian artery will arise as the last branch of the aortic arch and course behind the esophagus (or in rare instances between the esophagus and trachea or in front of the trachea) to supply the right arm. This anomaly was clearly recognized by Bayford in 1794 and has long been known to cause "dysphagia lusoria."

Although the innominate artery normally arises to the left of the trachea, in some instances it arises farther along the arch than normal and must wind across the trachea in reaching the apex of the right chest. If the vessel is lax, no symptoms are caused, but when it is tight there may be constriction of the trachea. Similarly, if the left common carotid branches from the aortic

---

*The innominate artery arises as the first vessel branching off the aortic arch, regardless of the side of the arch, and, hence, in this case supplies the left arm and left common carotid.

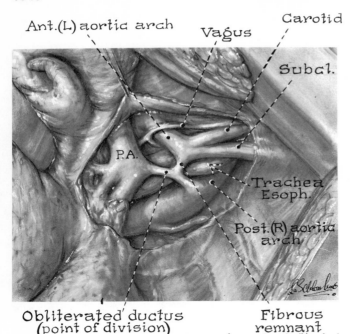

Ant.(L) aortic arch　　Vagus　　Carotid

Subcl.

P.A.

Trachea
Esoph.

Post.(R) aortic
arch

Obliterated ductus
(point of division)

Fibrous
remnant
(point of division)

**Figure 11** Operative view of tracheal ring completed by obliterated remnant of distal left arch and ligamentum arteriosum. After complete exposure of the vascular components, the proper point of division of the ligaments can easily be determined. (From Bahnson, H. T. In: Gibbon, J. H., Jr., Sabiston, D. C., Jr., and Spencer, F. C., eds.: Surgery of the Chest. 2nd ed. Philadelphia, W. B. Saunders Company, 1969.)

arch farther to the right than usual, it may wind across the anterior surface of the trachea as it courses upward and to the left and may cause tracheal compression.

Of the 160 babies operated upon by Gross,[14] 40 per cent had a double arch, 25 per cent had a right arch and left ligamentum arteriosum, 12 per cent had an anomalous innominate or carotid artery, 10 per cent had an aberrant right subclavian artery, and 13 per cent had miscellaneous other anomalies.

### Clinical Manifestations

Why some children with anomalies of the aortic arch remain asymptomatic and others are severely bothered is an unanswered question. Symptoms are those of tracheal obstruction, often with stridor and even a crowing type of respiration, frequent respiratory infections with secretions that cannot adequately be cleared, and a wheeze that often may be heard without a stethoscope. There may be difficulty in swallowing, and in some instances this is the complaint that brings the patient to the physician. Respiratory distress is frequently worse after eating or drinking, and aspiration pneumonia is often seen because of esophageal obstruction. The infant appears to obtain some relief by lying in a position of hyperextension, and this is frequently the preferred position. Respiratory obstruction may be exaggerated if the neck is flexed forcibly.

Symptoms may be alarming with any of the compressing anomalies, but they are usually more prominent with the double aortic arch or a right arch with a ring completed by the liga-

mentum arteriosum. When difficulty occurs, it is almost always evident in infancy or early childhood, many patients being under 6 months of age. Few older patients have symptoms or require treatment. The anomalous right subclavian causes difficulty principally in swallowing, there usually being little or no respiratory distress except that occasioned by dysphagia and aspiration after eating. Conversely, pressure from an aberrant innominate or carotid artery on the trachea causes predominantly respiratory symptoms.

### Diagnosis

Consideration of the possibility of an aortic arch anomaly is the most important step in diagnosing the condition. Roentgenograms may show pneumonitis and in some instances the outline of the trachea and its compression. Barium swallow shows the posterior compression of the esophagus (Fig. 12), and by careful examination of the films and the direction and level of the compression, the exact anomaly can often be determined.[18] The combination of anterior tracheal compression and posterior esophageal compression justifies an almost certain diagnosis of a vascular ring. The relative sizes of the right and left arches can be determined by the size of the indentation on barium swallow. Angiocardiography may demonstrate the anomaly but is rarely necessary. A tracheogram with Lipiodol instillation may clearly identify the tracheal compression. The level and obliquity of the tracheal and esophageal compression usually allow identification of the type of vessel when obstruction is due to anomalous arteries from the aortic arch.

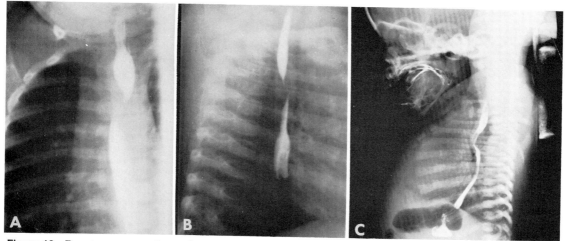

**Figure 12**   Roentgenograms of vascular ring. *A* and *B*, Double aortic arch. The location and direction of esophageal compression suggest a larger posterior arch coursing from above downward but with anterior compression also. *C*, Obstruction from remnant of left fourth arch and obliterated ductus as shown in Figure 11. The large posterior arch is pulled forward and compresses the trachea and esophagus. (From Bahnson, H. T. In: Gibbon, J. H., Jr., Sabiston, D. C., Jr., and Spencer, F. C., eds.: Surgery of the Chest. 2nd ed. Philadelphia, W. B. Saunders Company, 1969.)

## Operative Technique

Division of the constricting ring or displacement of an aberrant vessel has much to offer these patients in providing more room for the trachea and esophagus and in relieving their obstruction. Adequate exposure is an absolute necessity, and this usually is obtained through the left chest. The arch and the vessels arising from it, the ductus, and the fibrous tissue attached to the vascular ring must be clearly exposed. Removal of the thymus often helps.

Once adequate exposure is obtained, selection of the proper component for division is usually not difficult. In the case of the right aortic arch with a ligamentum arteriosum completing the vascular ring, simple division of the ligamentum arteriosum and mobilization of the arch should relieve the constriction. When a double arch is present, the side and position of the smaller arch must be determined. The smaller arch, usually anterior and on the left, is divided in a manner that does not interfere with circulation to the common carotid arteries. This usually means division of the arch between the left common carotid and the left subclavian arteries. The adjacent and possibly constricting fibrous tissue must be divided, and, if the divided arch and carotid in any way compress the trachea, the arch should be tacked with multiple stitches through the adventitia to the posterior surface of the sternum or chest wall in order to hold the vessel away from the trachea. Gross[14] advocates leaving the adhesions between arch and trachea, so that tacking the arch to the sternum will pull the anterior wall of the trachea forward. Although theoretically the smaller arch can be divided at any site and circulation will continue into the branches through the distal or proximal opening, in some instances the distal end of the smaller arch is narrowed and circulation to the carotid through this opening may be curtailed.

The subclavian artery, if it is causing compression, arises as the last branch of the aortic arch; by dissecting in the posterior mediastinum, it can be mobilized behind the aorta. It can be divided with impunity, and in cases of the aberrant retroesophageal left subclavian artery, freeing of the artery from its bed and doubly ligating and dividing it is all that is required. Sufficient collateral circulation is available through the second and third portions of the subclavian artery to maintain adequate circulation to the arm. In cases of compression by an anomalous innominate or carotid artery, the continuity of the artery must be maintained. Hence, proper treatment consists of complete mobilization of the artery, division of any constricting fibrous tissue around it, and suture of the vessel away from the trachea and against the back wall of the sternum with multiple fine sutures through the adventitia.

After operation in patients in whom there has been some tracheal compression, particular care must be taken to provide an atmosphere with high humidity; there must also be close supervision of tracheobronchial secretions. Persistent tracheal obstruction may be caused by tracheomalacia or by tracheal hypoplasia resulting from tracheal pressure and narrowing present since early fetal life. Not infrequently, because of the tracheal manipulation and pre-existing obstruction, there may be respiratory obstruction and even stridor for the first few postoperative days. In rare cases this has persisted for months.[3]

## Results of Treatment

Relief of the tracheal and esophageal obstruction is usually associated with dramatic clinical improvement, often evident immediately after operation. In some instances there is deformity of the trachea, which may persist. No long-term follow-up of such cases is yet available, but it is likely that relief of the compression will allow the trachea to grow in a normal fashion. Persisting deformity of the tracheal cartilage is more common in patients with a double arch or a right arch with a ligamentum arteriosum.

There were 5 deaths among the 57 patients of all types treated by Gross,[13] and all 5 were among the 21 patients with double aortic arch. The ages of the 57 patients ranged from 3 weeks to 12 years, the majority being under 2 years of age.

## SELECTED REFERENCES

Gross, R. E.: The Surgery of Infancy and Childhood, Its Principles and Practice. Philadelphia, W. B. Saunders Company, 1953.
*This is the classic text on children's surgery by the author who figured prominently in the development of surgical treatment for all the conditions discussed in this chapter.*

Gross, R. E.: An Atlas of Children's Surgery. Philadelphia, W. B. Saunders Company, 1970.
*This altas is a companion piece to the textbook by the same author and shows the pathologic anatomy and operative treatment of many conditions encountered in pediatric surgery. Results of the long experience with pediatric surgery for many of the conditions are given.*

Schumacker, H. B., Jr., King, H., Nahrwald, D. L., and Waldhausen, J. A.: Coarctation of the aorta. Curr. Probl. Surg., Feb. 1968.
*This is a comprehensive review of the condition, including all but the most recent references.*

## REFERENCES

1. Bahnson, H. T.: Coarctation of the aorta and anomalies of the aortic arch. Surg. Clin. N. Amer., 32:1313, 1952.
2. Blalock, A.: The technique of creation of artificial ductus arteriosus in the treatment of pulmonic stenosis. J. Thorac. Surg., 16:244, 1947.
3. Bradham, R. R., Sealy, W. C., and Young, W. G.: Respiratory distress associated with anomalies of the aortic arch. Surg. Gynec. Obstet., 126:9, 1968.
4. Campbell, M.: Natural history of patent ductus arteriosus. Brit. Heart J., 30:4, 1968.
5. Campbell, M.: Natural history of coarctation of the aorta. Brit. Heart J., 32:633, 1970.
6. Christie, A.: Normal closing time of the foramen ovale and the ductus arteriosus: Anatomical and statistical study. Amer. J. Dis. Child., 40:323, 1930.
7. Clatworthy, H. W., Jr., and McDonald, V. G., Jr.: Optimum age for surgical closure of patent ductus arteriosus. J.A.M.A., 167:444, 1958.
8. Dammann, J. F., Jr., and Sell, C. G. R.: Patent ductus arteriosus in the absence of a continuous murmur. Circulation, 6:110, 1952.
9. Edwards, J. E.: Structural changes of the pulmonary vascular bed and their functional significance in congenital cardiac disease. Proc. Inst. Med. Chicago, 18:134, 1950.
10. Ekstrom, G.: The surgical treatment of patent ductus arteriosus. A clinical study of 290 cases. Acta Chir. Scand., Supp. 169, 1952.
11. Ellis, F. H., Jr., Kirklin, J. W., Callahan, J. A., and Wood, E. H.: Patent ductus with pulmonary hypertension. J. Thorac. Surg., 31:268, 1956.
12. Glass, I. H., Mustard, W. T., and Keith, J. D.: Coarctation

of the aorta in infants. A review of twelve years' experience. Pediatrics, 26:109, 1960.
13. Gross, R. E.: The Surgery of Infancy and Childhood, Its Principles and Practice. Philadelphia, W. B. Saunders Company, 1953.
14. Gross, R. E.: An Atlas of Children's Surgery. Philadelphia, W. B. Saunders Company, 1970.
15. Hartmann, A. F., Jr., Goldring, D., Hernandez, A., Behrer, M. R., Schad, N., Ferguson, T., and Burford, T.: Recurrent coarctation of the aorta after successful repair in infancy. Amer. J. Cardiol., 25:405, 1970.
16. Iberra-Perez, C., Castaneda, A. R., Varco, R. L., and Lillehei, C. W.: Recoarctation of the aorta. Nineteen year clinical experience. Amer. J. Cardiol., 23:778, 1969.
17. Lueker, R. D., Vogel, J. N. K., and Blount, S. G., Jr.: Cardiovascular abnormality following surgery for left to right shunts. Observations in atrial septal defect, ventricular septal defect and patent ductus arteriosus. Circulation, 40:783, 1969.
18. Neuhauser, E. B. D.: The roentgen diagnosis of double aortic arch and other anomalies of the great vessels. Amer. J. Roentgen., 56:1, 1946.
19. Rumel, W. R., Bailey, C. P., Samson, P. C., Waterman, D. H., and Bing, R. J.: Surgical treatment of coarctation of aorta. Report of the Section on Cardiovascular Surgery, American College of Chest Physicians. J.A.M.A., 164:5. 1957.
20. Sauvage, L. R., and Harkins, H. N.: Growth of vascular anastomoses: An experimental study of the influence of suture type and suture method with a note on certain mechanical factors involved. Bull. Johns Hopkins Hosp., 91:276, 1952.
21. Schumacker, H. B., Jr., King, H., Nahrwald, D. L., and Waldhausen, J. A.: Coarctation of the aorta. Curr. Probl. Surg., Feb. 1968.
22. Scott, H. W., Jr., and Bahnson, H. T.: Evidence for a renal factor in the hypertension of experimental coarctation of the aorta. Surgery, 30:206, 1951.
23. Scott, H. W., Jr., and Sabiston, D. C., Jr.: Surgical treatment for congenital aorticopulmonary fistula. Experimental and clinical aspects. J. Thorac. Surg., 25:26, 1953.
24. Sealy, W. C., Harris, J. S., Young, W. G., Jr., and Callaway, H. A., Jr.: Paradoxical hypertension following resection of coarctation of the aorta. Surgery, 42:135, 1957.
25. Trusler, G. A., Arayangkoon, P., and Mustard, W. T.: Operative closure of isolated patent ductus arteriosus in the first two years of life. Canad. Med. Ass. J., 99:879, 1968.
26. Tyson, K. R., Harris, L. S., and Nghiem, Q. X.: Repair of aortic arch interruption in the neonate. Surgery, 67:1006, 1970.
27. Waterman, D. H., Samson, P. C., and Bailey, C. P.: The surgery of patent ductus arteriosus. A report of the Section on Cardiovascular Surgery. Dis. Chest, 29:102, 1956.
28. Ziegler, R. F.: The importance of patent ductus arteriosus in infants. Amer. Heart J., 43:553, 1952.

# IV

# Atrial Septal Defects, Ostium Primum Defects, and Atrioventricular Canals

*John A. Waldhausen, M.D., and G. Frank O. Tyers, M.D., F.R.C.S.(C.)*

## HISTORICAL ASPECTS

The clinical features and pathophysiology of atrial septal defects have been studied for the past 150 years, and the first true anatomic description of septal defects was published by Rokitansky[58] in 1875. The first operation for atrial septal defect in man was reported in 1948.[48] The blind external techniques of invaginating the atrial wall into the defect[16] and of ligating the defect[48] resulted in some successful results.[2] However, incomplete closures and direction of a portion of the systemic venous return into the left atrium often followed these procedures. The blind internal technique described by Gross et al.[33] used a rubber well sewn into the atrial opening and allowed suturing inside the heart without direct vision.[34] Results were surprisingly good, but the technique was of limited value for complex defects.

Combination of moderate hypothermia with temporary occlusion of the systemic venous return permitted accurate closure of atrial septal defects under direct vision,[43] but even with multiple periods of venous occlusion, operating time was limited and complex defects could not be repaired.[44] In 1953, Gibbon, after 20 years of laboratory work, first used mechanical cardiopulmonary bypass successfully for an operation on the human heart—closure of an atrial septal defect.[30] This is now the method of choice.

## INCIDENCE

*Atrial septal defect* is the fifth most common congenital cardiac abnormality, occurring in one in 13,500 children under 14 years of age.[40] In the early years of cardiac surgery, atrial septal defects seemed to be the most common congenital cardiac defect, because its relatively benign early course without treatment had permitted accumulation of a large number of patients. This also explains its low incidence, only 3 per cent, in Abbott's[1] postmortem series. It is still the most

common congenital cardiac defect detected in persons over 20 years of age, but in children the incidence has stabilized at approximately 7 per cent. Atrial septal defects occur three times as frequently in females as in males.

The incidence of *ostium primum* compared to that of other atrial defects can be seen in Table 1. Weidman and DuShane[73] cite a similar incidence. In contrast to ostium secundum defects, the sex distribution of ostium primum defects is equal.

At birth, persistent *common atrioventricular canal* defects are more prevalent than ostium primum defects, but since the life span with this defect is significantly curtailed, the lesion is less common in older children and adolescents. It made up only 2 per cent of the congenital cardiac lesions in the series reported by Keith and his associates.[40] However, it represented 20 per cent of all atrial defects (Table 1). The sex incidence is equal. Down's syndrome has been reported in 37 per cent of patients with the complete form of atrioventricular canal,[40] and in a series of 55 cases, Rogers and Edwards[57] showed an incidence of mongolism of 30 per cent. Six patients had other major associated anomalies, and 19 had minor associated defects.

## ETIOLOGY

That atrial septal defect may result from genetic abnormalities is evidenced by its increased incidence in patients with such hereditary disorders as mongolism,[9] Turner's syndrome,[54] Ellis–van Creveld syndrome,[31] Marfan's syndrome, and the Ehler-Danlos syndrome.[74] The atrial septal defect in these disorders may be of the simple secundum variety, but more frequently single atrium (cor triloculare) or complex endocardial cusion defects are present. A familial incidence of atrial septal defect has been reported,[76] and the inheritance of the defects in these cases is best explained on the basis of a dominant autosomal gene with incomplete penetrance. In another study, the risk to offspring of parents with atrial septal defects was 21 times greater than average.[52]

Undetermined environmental influences are thought to cause the majority of atrial septal defects, however. This impression is based on the lack of association of most septal defects with known hereditary abnormalities, the high incidence of associated nongenetic abnormalities of other structures, and the lack of concordance of cardiac defects in identical twins.[41, 72] Two environmental influences known to produce septal defects are maternal rubella infection[66] and the ingestion of thalidomide during the first trimester of pregnancy.

**TABLE 1**  ATRIAL SEPTAL DEFECTS, INCIDENCE OF SUBGROUPS, HOSPITAL FOR SICK CHILDREN, TORONTO*

| Defect | Number of Cases | Per Cent of Total |
|---|---|---|
| Ostium secundum | 307 | 68 |
| Ostium primum | 58 | 12 |
| Atrioventricularis communis | 87 | 20 |
| Total | 452 | 100 |
| Ostium secundum | 307 cases | |
| Isolated form | | 68.4 |
| With pulmonary stenosis | | 10 |
| With partial anomalous pulmonary vein drainage | | 7 |
| With mitral stenosis | | 1 |
| With rheumatic mitral insufficiency | | 0.3 |
| With ventricular septal defect | | 5.0 |
| With patent ductus | | 3.0 |
| With coarctation of the aorta | | 0.3 |
| | Total | 95 |

*From Keith, J. D., Rowe, R. D., and Vlad, P.: Heart Disease in Infancy and Childhood. New York, Macmillan Company, 1958.

## EMBRYOLOGY

By the fourth week of embryonic life, the venous end of the heart is composed of the sinus venosus, receiving two superior and two inferior venous channels; the primi-

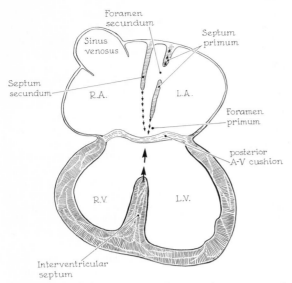

**Figure 1**  Embryology of the atrial septum and endocardial cushion. Arrows show direction of growth or regression of septal structures.

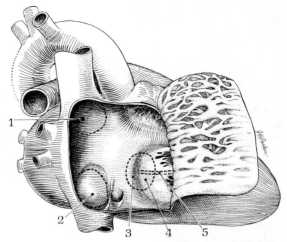

**Figure 2**  The different types of atrial septal defects. 1, Sinus venosus defect. 2, Ostium secundum defect. 3, Ostium primum defect. 4, Ventricular septal defect of a complete atrioventricular canal. 5, Cleft septal leaflet of mitral valve. 3, 4, and 5, Complete atrioventricular canal.

tive common atrium; and the atrioventricular canal.[22] During the fourth week, the septum primum begins to grow down from the posterior-superior aspect of the common atrium toward the endocardial cushions (Fig. 1). Its growth is temporarily arrested, and a crescentic inferior defect—ostium primum—is left just above the endocardial cushions. During the fifth and sixth weeks, growth of the septum primum resumes and the foramen primum is obliterated by union of the free edge of the septum primum with the fusing posterior and anterior endocardial cushions. The atrioventricular valves differentiate from the endocardial cushions, and the interventricular foramen is closed by proliferating tissue from the fused endocardial cushions and the bulbar ridges. Prior to obliteration of the foramen primum a second oval defect—the foramen secundum—is formed by cephalic degeneration of the septum primum. Later, a second septum—septum secundum—grows down from the right of the superior attachment of the septum primum between the septum primum and the left valve of the sinus venosus. It envelops the foramen secundum to form a unidirectional valve that allows passage of venous blood from the lower portion of the embryo and the placenta into the left atrium.

During the development of the interatrial septum, the sinus venosus is gradually absorbed into the atrium, and part of it eventually fuses with the posterior-superior portion of the interatrial septum. The right superior venous channel becomes the superior vena cava; the left superior venous channel becomes the coronary sinus, and the inferior venous channels become the inferior vena cava.

## PATHOLOGIC ANATOMY

The morphology of interatrial defects is best understood when related to the previous section on embryology. Figure 2 shows the typical atrial septal and atrioventricular canal (endocardial cushion) defects superimposed on the normal right atrial anatomy.

### Sinus Venosus and Secundum Defects

Failure of fusion of the left valve of the sinus venosus with the posterior-superior portion of the interatrial septum results in a high defect overlying the superior vena cava. This is frequently associated with absorption of a portion of the venous drainage of the right upper and middle lobes into what becomes the superior vena cava and the right atrium. As the sinus venosus defect or superior caval defect underlies the superior caval orifice, this channel opens into both atria; there is no upper margin, and often the posterior margin is incomplete. The right upper pulmonary veins open into the superior vena cava, the middle vein opens into either atrium, and the lower pulmonary vein drains normally.[6]

Ostium secundum defects in the lower midportion of the interatrial septum result from failure of the septum secundum to close the ostium secundum. At times the defect may extend down to the inferior vena cava, leaving no atrial margin at the inferior border of the defect. If the degenerative process that produces the ostium secundum is excessive, multiple secundum defects result, or almost total lack of the interatrial septum can occur. Secundum defects are less frequently associated with venous drainage from the right lung into the right atrium, but if the defect is low, the right lower lobe may drain into what becomes the inferior vena cava. Probe patency (patent foramen ovale) of the ostium secundum occurs in approximately 30 per cent of adults[70] but is seldom of pathologic significance. There is a greater than expected incidence of mitral stenosis of rheumatic origin[20] associated with secundum defects (Lutembacher's syndrome). Other associated congenital cardiac anomalies include pulmonary stenosis, mitral valve disease, and ventricular septal defects[27] (see Table 1).

## Endocardial Cushion Defects

When the septum primum fails to resume its downward growth, an ostium primum defect with a crescentic upper border centered over the junction of the atrioventricular valve annuli occurs. This has also been referred to a partial persistent common atrioventricular canal. This usually is associated with a cleft in the septal leaflets of the mitral and tricuspid valves and some abnormality of the chordae tendineae. There may be narrowing of the aortic outflow tract, resulting in the characteristic "gooseneck" deformity on cineangiocardiography.[3] An ostium primum defect can occur either alone, with a mitral valve cleft, or with both a mitral and tricuspid valve cleft (Fig. 3). The isolated form is uncommon (Table 2). When an ostium primum defect is associated with persistence of a high ventricular septal defect, it is known as a persistent common atrioventricular canal. Rarely the atrial portion is closed and only the valve leaflet clefts occur in association with a ventricular septal defect. An isolated mitral valve cleft or an isolated ventricular septal defect may also occur and represent a form of endocardial cushion defect.[50] However, in the usual persistent common atrioventricular canal, the ostium primum is associated with a single atrioventricular valve with common anterior and posterior leaflets and a large interventricular septal defect, which may be almost complete.[55]

**TABLE 2** INCIDENCE OF ASSOCIATED ABNORMALITIES IN FIFTY PATIENTS WITH OSTIUM PRIMUM DEFECTS OF THE ATRIAL SEPTUM*

| Type of Lesion | No. of Patients |
|---|---|
| Isolated ostium primum atrial septal defect | 3+ |
| Primum atrial septal defect with cleft mitral valve | 15 |
| Primum atrial septal defect with cleft mitral and tricuspid valves | 6 |
| Common atrium with cleft mitral valve | 3 |
| Common atrioventricular canal | 23 |
| Total | 50 |

*From Evans, J. R., Rowe, R. D., and Keith, J. D.: Amer. J. Med., *30*:345, 1961.

†One patient had, in addition, a secundum atrial septal defect and pulmonary stenosis.

Rastelli et al.[55] observed three forms of complete atrioventricular canal.

Type I. Here the common anterior leaflet is divided into two distinct portions, one relating to the entrance into the left ventricle and one to that into the right ventricle (Fig. 4). Both portions are attached medially to the ventricular septum, while laterally they are attached to normally placed papillary muscles. The posterior leaflet is single and may or may not be attached to the septum. The membranous septum is intact.

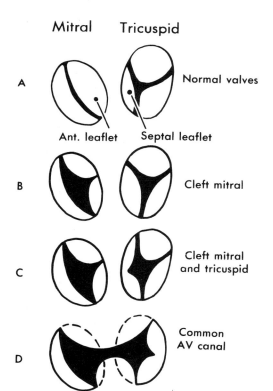

**Figure 3** The mitral and tricuspid valve abnormalities seen in endocardial cushion defects. (Modified from Bedford, D. E., et al.: Lancet, *1*:1255, 1957.)

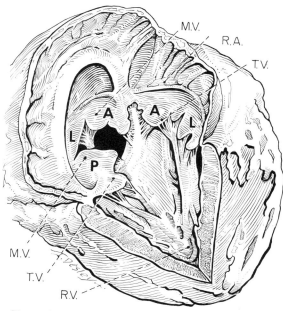

**Figure 4** Most common type of complete form of atrioventricular canal as viewed from the right atrium and right ventricle. The anterior leaflet is divided into two distinct portions, both attached medially to the ventricular septum. A and P indicate common anterior and posterior leaflets of this single atrioventricular valve. L indicates a lateral leaflet. M.V. and T.V. indicate mitral and tricuspid portions of leaflets; R.A. and R.V. indicate right atrium and right ventricle. (From McGoon, D. C. In: Cooper, P.: The Craft of Surgery. Vol. 1. 2nd ed. Boston, Little, Brown and Company, 1971.)

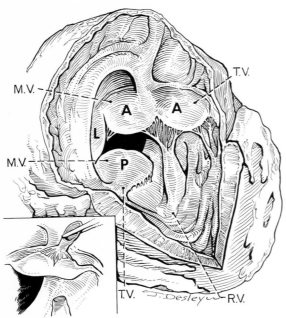

**Figure 5**   Complete form of atrioventricular canal in which the anterior leaflet is divided, and the medial aspect of each portion (A) is attached by chordae to a papillary muscle in the right ventricle (R.V.). P indicates common posterior leaflet, L indicates lateral leaflet, and M.V. and T.V. indicate mitral and tricuspid portions of leaflets. (From McGoon, D. C. In: Cooper, P.: The Craft of Surgery. Vol. 1. 2nd ed. Boston, Little, Brown and Company, 1971.)

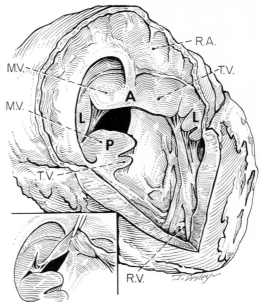

**Figure 6**   Complete form of common atrioventricular canal most commonly associated with other major cardiac anomalies. The undivided anterior leaflet is unattached to the ventricular septum (inset). A and P are common anterior and posterior leaflets of single, atrioventricular valve, L and L are lateral leaflets, M.V. and T.V. are mitral and tricuspid portions of common valve, and R.A. and R.V. are right atrium and right ventricle. (From McGoon, D. C. In: Cooper, P.: The Craft of Surgery. Vol. 1. 2nd ed. Boston, Little, Brown and Company, 1971.)

Type II. This lesion differs from Type I in that the medial portion of each of the two distinct parts of the anterior leaflet is attached by chordae to an anomalous papillary muscle in the right ventricle (Fig. 5). The membranous portion of the septum is incompletely developed, with a defect subjacent to the aortic valve.

Type III. In this form of atrioventricular canal, the anterior leaflet is undivided and there are no attachments to the ventricular septum (Fig. 6). The membranous septum is also deficient, and an interventricular communication beneath the aortic valve results.

Type I is by far the most common (70 per cent) form of persistent atrioventricular canal if only minor associated cardiac defects are present. However, Types II and III are most common when major cardiac malformations are associated. Posterior displacement and elongation of the bundle of His associated with this defect render the conduction system very susceptible to injury. Pulmonary vascular changes associated with pulmonary hypertension are also frequent.

Complete absence of the atrial septum, or cor triloculare, also occurs and probably results from failure of multiple embryologic processes during the development of the heart. It is usually associated with other severe congenital defects.[25]

The distribution of the various forms of endocardial cushion defects can be seen in Table 2.[27] Another lesion described in association is pul-

monic stenosis, which may be valvular or combined valvular and infundibular.[59]

## SECUNDUM AND SINUS VENOSUS DEFECTS OF THE ATRIUM

### Physiology

In the normal heart, there is a positive pressure difference between the left and right atrium that is responsible for keeping the foramen ovale closed. This pressure gradient is reduced in small atrial septal defects but still contributes to the left-to-right shunt. Correlation of instantaneous pressure differences across the defect with the direction of flow, as seen by cineangiocardiography, showed the onset of flow across the defect to occur 50 to 75 milliseconds after the onset of the gradient. The major left-to-right shunt and pressure gradient occurred over an interval encompassing ventricular systole and early diastole (Fig. 7).[42] Also, there was augmentation of the left-to-right shunt during atrial contraction. In large atrial septal defects, this gradient is abolished. Direction of shunt flow then is determined to a large extent by the compliance of the right and left ventricles.[11] In infancy, the ventricles are of nearly equal thickness and compliance, but as the pressure in the pulmonary artery falls, the right ventricular muscle mass decreases, with a resultant increase in compliance. This causes more blood from the

**Figure 7** Intracardiac pressure dynamics in secundum atrial septum defects. The tracings were obtained with simultaneous monitoring of right and left ventricular pressures by means of Statham SF-1 pressure-tipped transducer catheters. The catheters were subsequently withdrawn to record both atrial pressures. There was no change in rate (R-R interval remained constant). All data were recorded simultaneously with the lead II electrocardiogram and the phonocardiogram in the second left interspace. A composite was made by direct overlay tracings to produce the time-aligned data as indicated.

The predominant left-to-right gradient occurred over an interval extending from midventricular systole into early diastole. The peak of the left atrial v wave was coincident with the interval of the second sound. The fluctuations in left atrial pressure can be seen to be more prominent than those of the right atrium. The transient right-to-left gradient occurred coincident with the onset of ventricular contraction. (From Levin, A. R., et al.: Circulation, 37:476, 1968. By permission of the American Heart Association, Inc.)

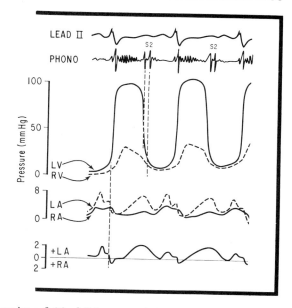

"common" atrium to enter the right ventricle and results in a gradually enlarging left-to-right shunt. As pulmonary hypertension develops later in life, hypertrophy of the right ventricle results in decreased compliance. The left-to-right shunt diminishes or even reverses and becomes a right-to-left shunt.

Even in the absence of pulmonary hypertension, some right-to-left shunting can be demonstrated in most atrial septal defects. It is due in part to streaming of blood from the inferior vena cava across the defect because of some overriding of the cava by the defect and the flap action of the eustachian valve. This small right-to-left shunt is not sufficient to cause cyanosis and usually can be detected only by dye dilution curves with injection into the inferior vena cava and sampling from the aorta or its branches.[67] However, right-to-left shunting does permit emboli from the peripheral veins and the right side of the heart to enter the systemic circulation (paradoxical embolism).[70] Pulmonary embolism (non-paradoxical embolism) is frequently associated. The paradoxical emboli usually lodge in the middle cerebral artery or one of its branches and cause stroke and occasionally brain abscess. The kidney and other viscera are less frequently involved.

Because of the proximity of the right pulmonary vein orifices to the atrial defect, there is preferential left-to-right shunting of blood from the right lung.[68] Studies of patients with atrial septal defects during exercise show that pulmonary blood flow increases in proportion to systemic blood flow in those with small left-to-right shunts. However, in patients with large shunts, pulmonary blood flow either stays the same or occasionally falls slightly;[51] this suggests that maximal output from the right ventricle has become the limiting factor.

The left-to-right shunt may be quite large and result in a pulmonary blood flow three to four times systemic blood flow ($Q_p:Q_s$ = 3 to 4:1). In a

series of 26 children aged 3 to 14, Levin et al.[42] found the mean left-to-right shunt to be 65 per cent (range, 59 to 74 per cent) of total pulmonary blood flow. At operation the atrial septal defects varied from 1.5 to 3 cm. in diameter. Systemic blood flow is usually normal. In spite of this large pulmonary blood flow, pulmonary hypertension is rare in children and begins to appear only in adulthood, in the second or third decade of life. Pulmonary arteries may show medial hypertrophy and intimal proliferation. The changes are rarely greater than grade 2 (Heath and Edwards classification).[39] Pulmonary diffusing capacity, as measured by $D_{L_{CO}}$, in patients with atrial septal defects is increased compared to that in normal subjects and increases in the same proportion during exercise.[5]

The large flow across the pulmonary outflow tract often results in a right ventricular pulmonary artery gradient as high as 40 mm. Hg. The pulmonary valve is normal, and after repair the flow gradient is abolished.

The physiologic changes in patients with sinus venosus defects and partial anomalous venous return are not significantly different from those in patients with ostium secundum defects.

### Clinical Manifestations

Children with moderate shunts usually have few if any symptoms, and therefore the diagnosis is often made during a routine preschool physical examination. Patients with large shunts may have symptoms of fatigue, exertional dyspnea, and at times frank congestive heart failure. Similarly, patients with pulmonary hypertension will have exertional dyspnea and possibly cyanosis. Significant disease may, however, exist without symptoms.[73]

On physical examination, the findings are dependent upon the presence or absence of pulmonary hypertension. The typical child with a sinus venosus or secundum defect looks healthy. A right ventricular lift is palpable. The first heart sound is often accentuated, while the second is almost always split in all phases of respiration, in part as a result of delayed right ventricular emptying.[27] The second sound is often slightly increased in intensity, even in the absence of pulmonary hypertension.

Because of the increased pulmonary blood flow, there is usually a pulmonary ejection-type systolic murmur audible along the left sternal border in the second and third intercostal spaces. The large flow across the tricuspid valve results in an early diastolic murmur along the lower left sternal border.[49]

With the development of pulmonary hypertension, the pulmonary second sound increases while the systolic ejection murmur decreases and the diastolic murmur is no longer audible.

On phonocardiography the peaked jugular "v" wave exceeded the "A" wave in approximately 40 per cent of patients with atrial septal defect.[69]

### Electrocardiographic Features

The electrocardiogram usually shows some variant of incomplete right bundle branch block in the first precordial lead. The mean axis of the QRS complex lies between +60 and −150 degrees, although in most patients the axis will be between +90 and +150. Prominent P waves may suggest atrial enlargement.

The vectorcardiogram shows a clockwise loop directed inferiorly and to the right in the frontal projection (Fig. 8).[27]

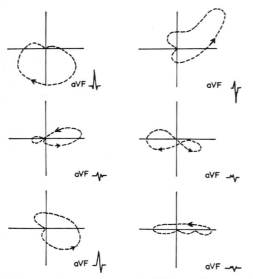

**Figure 8**   Frontal vector of the QRS complex computed from the electrocardiogram of six patients showing clockwise loop usually seen with secundum defects and counterclockwise loop above the horizontal plane typical of ostium primum defects. Vectors with a figure-of-eight pattern of flat loop closely applied to the horizontal axis may be seen with either secundum or primum defects. The configuration of the QRS complex in lead aVF is shown alongside the vector loop. (From Evans, J. R., et al.: Amer. J. Med., *30*:345, 1961.)

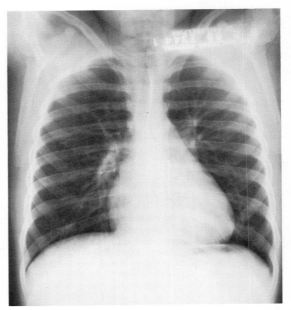

**Figure 9**   Chest roentgenogram of a 9 year old child with ostium secundum defect.

### Radiologic Features

Slight to moderate cardiac enlargement is common (Fig. 9). Chamber analysis usually shows enlargement of the right atrium and ventricle and main pulmonary artery. Pulmonary vascular markings are increased. The left ventricle and aorta are either normal or slightly small.

### Cardiac Catheterization and Angiocardiography

Cardiac catheterization and oxygen measurements show a step-up in oxygen saturation in the right atrium when compared to the superior and inferior venae cavae. (Measurement of such a step-up may be inaccurate because of streaming and catheter tip location.) Partial anomalous venous return may produce similar findings, and it may be possible to differentiate it by inserting the catheter into the abnormally located orifice of the pulmonary vein. Injection of contrast medium into the left atrium during cineangiography will show the left-to-right shunt as well as the pulmonary recirculation. Injection of contrast medium into the left ventricle will help rule out an ostium primum defect with mitral incompetence. A systolic flow gradient as high as 40 mm. Hg may be detected across the pulmonary outflow tract. Accurate diagnosis of an atrial septal defect can usually be made from the clinical findings, the results of cardiac catheterization and cineangiocardiography, and the electrocardiogram.[23]

### Natural History

Prognosis is based on shunt size, but a simple atrial defect is compatible with a longer life than a ventricular septal defect. Reports of patients living into the seventh and eighth decades are not

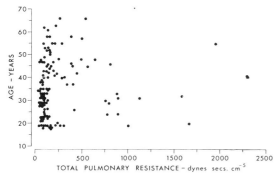

**Figure 10** Relationship between patients' ages at the time of cardiac catheterization and the total pulmonary vascular resistance. (From Craig, R. J., and Selzer, A.: Circulation, 37:805, 1968. By permission of the American Heart Association, Inc.)

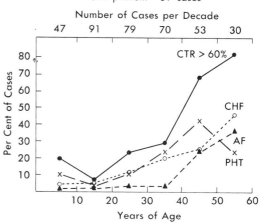

**Figure 11** Complications in 440 patients with atrial septal defects, chiefly ostium secundum. CTR, cardiothoracic ratio; CHF, congestive heart failure; AF, atrial fibrillation; PHT, pulmonary hypertension. After the age of 40 years these complications increase significantly. (From Bedford, D. E., and Besterman, E. M. M. In: Keith, J. D., et al.: Heart Disease in Infancy and Childhood. 2nd ed. New York, The Macmillan Company, 1967.)

uncommon. Life expectancy in two series of untreated patients was 42 and 38 years, respectively.[7, 17]

The majority of patients have few symptoms in infancy and childhood. Nevertheless, on rare occasions congestive failure in infancy does occur in association with very large shunts and requires an aggressive therapeutic approach.[12, 36] Spontaneous closure has been reported in infancy but is a rare occurrence.[15, 35]

The development of pulmonary hypertension is a serious prognostic finding and usually occurs in adult life (Fig. 10).[20] Gault et al.[29] studied 62 patients who were 40 years of age or older. Forty-five per cent were in functional class III or IV. Sixty-nine per cent had pulmonary artery hypertension, and in 28 per cent it was severe.

In other adults with moderate shunts, without significant pulmonary hypertension, symptoms develop after the onset of coronary artery disease. The decreased myocardial oxygenation and the persistent overload of the right ventricle result in congestive heart failure. Cardiac arrhythmias such as atrial flutter or fibrillation are common in patients over 40 years old, although they may occur at any age.[60] A composite graphic presentation of the principal factors influencing the course of patients with atrial septal defects is shown in Figure 11.[40] Patients living at lower altitudes have less severe pulmonary hypertension than those at high elevations. The average mean pulmonary artery pressure in a group of patients under 20 years old living below 2000 ft. was 18.7 mm. Hg, whereas in a comparable group living at 4000 ft. the mean pressure was 30.4 mm. Hg.[21] Bacterial endocarditis is rare in patients with ostium secundum defects. When it does occur, it usually involves the pulmonary valve and right ventricular outflow tract; in patients without septal defects, it is more likely to involve the tricuspid valve.[32]

### Indications for Operation

Indication for operation is the presence of a shunt resulting in a pulmonary blood flow at least 1.5 times systemic flow ($Q_p:Q_s > 1.5$, where $Q_p$ equals pulmonary flow and $Q_s$ equals systemic flow) without severe pulmonary vascular disease ($R_p:R_s > 0.7$, where $R_p$ equals pulmonary vascular resistance and $R_s$ equals systemic resistance). The optimal time for repair is between 5 and 8 years of age even if the patient is asymptomatic. Repair at any age thereafter is also indicated but less desirable in view of such diverse factors as family responsibilities of the patient, emotional stability, pulmonary hypertension, and coronary artery disease.

### Treatment

Cardiopulmonary bypass should be used in operations for closure of sinus venosus and secundum defects. This allows for precise closure as well as insertion of a patch in large defects. Furthermore, failure to recognize partial anomalous pulmonary venous drainage at the time of catheterization is of little significance since the repair is not very difficult when cardiopulmonary bypass is used. The use of hypothermia and venous inflow occlusion has as its main virtue simplicity and the lack of need for blood to prime the extracorporeal circuit. However, the time available for intracardiac repair is limited and is insufficient for accurate repair of unforeseen complicating defects.

Normothermic cardiopulmonary bypass is usually preferred, and left ventricular drainage may be employed to avoid air embolism. Others have temporarily induced ventricular fibrillation to prevent the left ventricle from ejecting air into the systemic circulation while the right atrium is

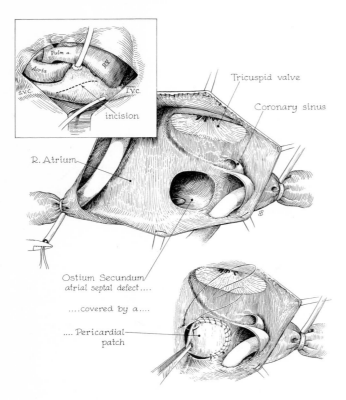

Tricuspid valve

Coronary sinus

R. Atrium

incision

Pulm. a.

Aorta

S.V.C.

I.V.C.

**Figure 12**  Repair of ostium secundum type atrial septal defect.

Ostium Secundum
atrial septal defect....

....covered by a....

.... Pericardial
patch

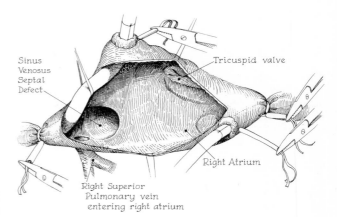

Sinus
Venosus
Septal
Defect

Tricuspid valve

Right Atrium

Right Superior
Pulmonary vein
entering right atrium

**Figure 13**  Repair of sinus venosus type atrial septal defect with anomalous return of right upper lobe veins.

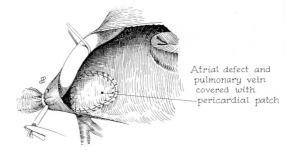

Atrial defect and
pulmonary vein
covered with
pericardial patch

open. Through an atrial incision, the atrial septum is visualized (Fig. 12). Small defects can readily be closed with a continuous suture, but larger defects should be closed with a patch.[47] It has been shown that postoperative residual defects are common in those patients with large defects closed without a patch. Although Dacron or Teflon is quite satisfactory, we prefer to use the patient's own pericardium since it is autogenous tissue. In the rare instances of postoperative bacterial endocarditis, bloodstream sterilization can be achieved in patients who have pericardial patches but not in those in whom synthetic material was used.[53]

Operative mortality in patients without pulmonary artery hypertension is quite low, less than 2 per cent in most series.[46] Sellers et al.[61] reported a 1.8 per cent hospital mortality and no late deaths in 225 operations for ostium secundum defects with normal pulmonary artery pressure. Even in older patients, mortality has been quite low, and age per se should not be a contraindication to operation.[24] In patients with pulmonary artery hypertension, mortality will increase in direct proportion to the degree of hypertension, but results are still acceptable if the ratio of pulmonary vascular resistance to systemic resistance is below 0.7. Beck et al.[4] showed that in 9 of 11 patients the pulmonary vascular resistance fell from a preoperative average of 510 dynes/sec./cm.$^{-5}$ to 230 dynes/sec./cm.$^{-5}$ postoperatively. Attempts to close defects in patients in whom pulmonary vascular resistance approaches systemic resistance have been fatal or have not produced a significant fall in pulmonary artery pressure. Closure of ostium secundum defects by means of a perforated prosthesis that eventually closed completely appeared to improve survival in these very ill patients but did not alter the course of the patients' pulmonary hypertension.[13]

Repair of sinus venosus defects usually requires a patch to divert the anomalous pulmonary venous drainage through the atrial septal defect into the left atrium (Fig. 13). Results are quite good and comparable to those of repair of ostium secundum defects.[19]

Thromboembolism postoperatively following closure of an atrial septal defect is well documented and occurred in 35 of 546 patients traced 2 to 15 years after closure of an uncomplicated defect. Eleven of the 35 patients succumbed to the embolism. This complication is more common in older patients and those with atrial fibrillation.[37]

## OSTIUM PRIMUM DEFECT

### Physiology

As in secundum defects, the left-to-right shunt is usually large and dependent upon the size of the defect as well as upon ventricular compliance. Isolated ostium primum defects differ little physiologically from ostium secundum defects. However, a cleft mitral valve with mitral insufficiency may result in a greater left-to-right shunt. Often the regurgitant jet is ejected almost directly into the right atrium through the large septal defect. There is also volume overloading of the left ventricle. A large degree of mitral insufficiency associated with a large left-to-right shunt results in more pronounced symptoms and earlier onset of pulmonary artery hypertension than in the usual atrial septal defect.

### Clinical Manifestations

The lesion is commonly discovered in infancy because of the mitral insufficiency murmur. Dyspnea and fatigue, failure to gain weight, and frequent respiratory infections are common. Congestive heart failure is not uncommon. These findings are dependent upon the degree of mitral insufficiency. The clinical features in patients with ostium primum defects without mitral regurgitation are similar to those in patients with ostium secundum defects.[27] Involvement of the tricuspid valve leads to an increased incidence and earlier onset of congestive heart failure and pulmonary hypertension.[75]

On physical examination, bulging of the left anterior chest wall and both right and left ventricular lifts are found. The pulmonary ejection murmur is more prominent than in an ostium secundum defect. The most characteristic finding is the murmur of mitral regurgitation at the apex extending out to the axilla. A mid-diastolic flow murmur across the tricuspid valve may be audible along the lower left sternal border. The second heart sound is widely split and possibly accentuated, depending upon the degree of pulmonary artery hypertension.

### Electrocardiographic Features

The electrocardiogram is diagnostic and shows left axis deviation. The P waves show changes indicating atrial enlargement. The vector loop shows a counterclockwise rotation to the left and superiorly in all cases (see Fig. 8).[40, 71, 27] In most cases, the frontal plane loop lies above the isoelectric line. Delay in right ventricular activation due to volume overload is constant, while left ventricular overload is seen in those with marked mitral insufficiency.

### Radiologic Features

Cardiac enlargement and increased pulmonary vascularity are more prominent than in patients with ostium secundum defects but differentiation between the two lesions on a chest roentgenogram may be difficult (Fig. 14).

### Cardiac Catheterization and Angiocardiography

A large left-to-right shunt can be demonstrated by a step-up in the oxygen saturation from the venae cavae to the right atrium. Often this step-up is low near the tricuspid valve, and at times, because of streaming, the increase may be detected only after entrance of the catheter through the tricuspid valve into right ventricular inflow tract; this may falsely suggest a ventricular septal de-

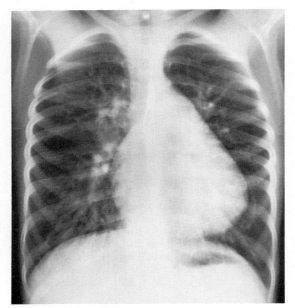

**Figure 14**   Chest roentgenogram of an 11 year old boy with an ostium primum defect with a cleft mitral valve and mitral incompetence.

fect. The left ventricular angiogram is quite diagnostic, showing the gooseneck deformity of the outflow tract as well as mitral regurgitation (Fig. 15). The gooseneck deformity is due to the abnormal mitral valve.[3]

### Natural History

In a series of 122 patients ranging in age from 11 days to 69 years reviewed by Somerville,[64] death occurred at all ages, from 2 weeks to 56 years. Heath[38] reported a patient who died at 69 years of age and at autopsy was found to have an ostium primum defect. The median age at death was 23 years in 18 cases collected from the literature by Fontana and Edwards.[28] The development of dysrhythmia was relatively common, occurring in 20 per cent of patients. It was a poor prognostic sign and was more common after the age of 30[27] (see Fig. 11). The arrhythmias were usually atrial fibrillation, nodal rhythm, ventricular tachycardia, or complete heart block.

Another complication is congestive heart failure, which was most common in infancy and childhood but was seen at all ages in Fontana and Edwards' series.[28] Pulmonary hypertension was more common than in ostium secundum defects, but in Somerville's review[64] only four such patients were identified and only two died of pulmonary hypertension. In the series of Ellis et al.,[26] 16 of 48 patients with ostium primum defects had significant pulmonary hypertension although all were less than 16 years old.

Mitral regurgitation appears to be a major determining factor in the ultimate prognosis of a patient with an ostium primum defect. Although

most patients with primum defects have a shorter life expectancy, this is especially true when the lesion is associated with severe mitral regurgitation. Significant tricuspid regurgitation also worsens the prognosis.

### Indications for Operation

In view of the relatively poor prognosis, virtually all patients with ostium primum defects should have repair. Shunts almost never are so small that repair is not indicated.[75] More complex is the question of mitral valve repair. Injudicious suture of a competent although cleft valve may lead to severe distortion and regurgitation or stenosis. Aortic obstruction has also been seen.[45] Clearly, all valves showing significant regurgitation during left ventricular angiography should be repaired. To omit this part of the operation can be most serious since repair of the atrial defect destroys the "blowoff" effect through the atrial defect. It has been our practice to assess the competence of the valve carefully with cineangiography and at operation. With careful placement of sutures, valve distortion occurred in only one patient in a series of 25 ostium primum repairs. This patient had a marked valve

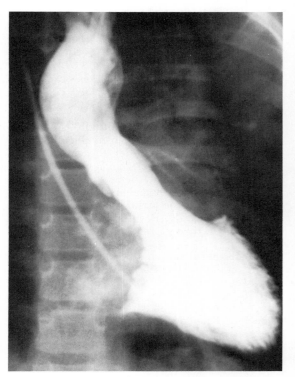

**Figure 15**   Frontal left ventriculogram in systole in a case of ostium primum defect. Note the elongation and narrowing of the left ventricular outflow tract. The right outline of the ventricular silhouette is scalloped and shows a deep, nonopaque indentation in the area where the two segments of the divided anterior mitral leaflet coapt. (From Moss, A. J., and Adams, F. H.: Heart Disease in Infants, Children and Adolescents. Baltimore, Williams & Wilkins Company, 1968.)

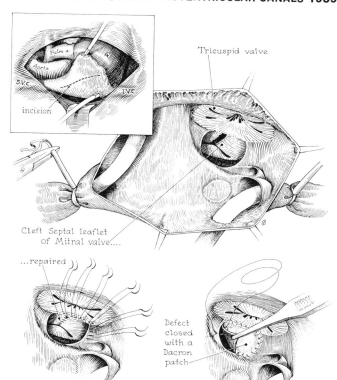

**Figure 16** Repair of an ostium primum defect with cleft mitral valve.

leaflet deficiency and ultimately required a mitral valve prosthesis.

The optimal age for repair is somewhere between 5 and 8 years, but at times earlier repair, because of cardiac failure, or later repair, because of lack of recognition, will be required.

### Treatment

Defects are repaired with the patient supported by cardiopulmonary bypass. Through the right atrium, the interatrial septum is visualized and the defect inspected (Fig. 16). The characteristic low location of the defect and the lack of atrial tissue between the valve annulus and the defect make the nature of the anomaly apparent. Inspection of the septal leaflet of the mitral valve usually shows the cleft. This leaflet is carefully elevated out of the ventricle with nerve hooks. Proper anatomic approximation of the leaflet halves can then readily be accomplished with interrupted sutures.

The septal defect is closed with a patch of either pericardium or synthetic material such as Dacron. Interrupted sutures are carefully placed superficially at the inferior margin of the defect in order to avoid damage to the conduction system and complete heart block. A running suture is then used to sew the patch to the remaining atrial wall. In addition, there may be an ostium secundum defect requiring separate closure. Inspection of the tricuspid valve may also show a cleft in the septal leaflet, but repair is generally not required.

Postoperative care is not unusual save for the management of arrhythmias. Complete heart block requires the use of cardiac pacing, and pacing wires should be attached to the ventricle. However, surgically produced permanent third-degree heart block is exceedingly rare. If it is acquired, a permanent pacemaker should be implanted since all patients with postsurgical heart block are in danger of sudden death. In some patients, preoperative heart block exists and may require permanent pacing if the ventricular rate is below 60 beats per minute.

Results have been excellent and operative mortality is quite low.[18, 26, 63] A residual murmur of mitral insufficiency is quite common but is usually of little hemodynamic significance.

A serious complication of repair of this lesion has been the development of hemolytic anemia that is difficult to control medically. At times there is hemoglobinuria. Hemolysis results when a regurgitant jet through an incompetent, inadequately repaired mitral valve strikes the septal Teflon prosthesis, which acts like a "washboard." Repair of the valve or, at times, valve replacement may be required.[62] Replacement of the Teflon patch by pericardium may further improve the condition.

## COMMON ATRIUM

This uncommon lesion represents a form of partial atrioventricular canal with absence of the entire atrial septum. The septal leaflet of the mitral valve is usually cleft, and the septal leaflet of the tricuspid valve may also be involved (see Table 2). Patients with this condition usually show symptoms of decreased exercise tolerance, fatigue, and dyspnea. Cyanosis may be noted on exercise. Symptoms may occur in infancy. Physical findings include a hyperactive heart, a widely split second heart sound, and a loud systolic ejection murmur at the left upper sternal border. The characteristic high-pitched holosystolic murmur due to mitral insufficiency can be heard at the apex with transmission to the axilla. The electrocardiogram is similar to that seen in patients with atrioventricular canal, while the roentgenogram shows marked cardiomegaly with increased pulmonary vascular markings owing to the large pulmonary blood flow. Cardiac catheterization shows almost complete mixing of the pulmonary and systemic venous blood, resulting in nearly equal oxygen saturation in the pulmonary artery and aortic blood. Indicator dilution curves may be of some help in demonstrating the lesion.[25] Angiocardiography shows simultaneous filling of both atria. Differentiation from total anomalous pulmonary venous return may be difficult, but many patients with this defect have an anomalous left vertical vein, and its absence lends support to a diagnosis of common atrium. Most patients require operative treatment. Contraindication to operation is primarily the severe pulmonary vascular disease, and the guidelines are similar to those for other atrial defects ($R_p:R_s > 0.7$). The large atrial defect is closed with a Dacron prosthesis. Mitral valve repair should be performed as in the more common ostium primum defects.

## PERSISTENT COMMON ATRIOVENTRICULAR CANAL

### Physiology

The degree of pathophysiologic change is determined by several factors: (1) size of the ventricular septal defect; (2) degree of atrioventricular valve insufficiency; (3) degree of pulmonary hypertension; and (4) size of the atrial septal defect. Associated defects such as pulmonic stenosis or patent ductus may also significantly affect hemodynamics.

In many patients with persistent common atrioventricular canal the ventricular septal defect is large and contributes to a large left-to-right shunt. Because of the increased pulmonary blood flow and the direct pressure transmission from the left ventricle to the pulmonary artery, patients with an atrioventricular canal frequently have pulmonary hypertension. This is further aggravated by atrioventricular valve insufficiency. Indeed, right ventricular blood may eject through the incompetent common atrioventricular valve into the left atrium. This results in pressure elevation in the left atrium (in addition to the usual pressure elevation in the right atrium) and cyanosis. This cyanosis is not dependent on high pulmonary vascular re-

sistance and therefore is not necessarily a sign of inoperability.

### Clinical Manifestations

Most patients have severe symptoms early in life, and heart failure is common. Cyanosis is present in approximately 15 per cent and may be severe if there is associated pulmonary stenosis. Failure to thrive and repeated respiratory infections are common.

On physical examination, these patients are often found to be dyspneic, underdeveloped, thin infants or children with marked precordial activity and a precordial bulge. A thrill may be palpable. On auscultation the first heart sound is accentuated, and the second heart sound is split and accentuated because of pulmonary hypertension. A loud holosystolic murmur from the ventricular septal defect is heard along the lower left sternal border, and is often transmitted to the back. A high-pitched murmur due to mitral insufficiency may be heard at the apex radiating into the axilla. A pulmonic ejection murmur may also be audible, as well as a mid-diastolic flow murmur across the common atrioventricular valve.

### Electrocardiographic Features

These are quite characteristic.[14] The mean electric axis of the QRS lies above the isoelectric line, and the vector loop in the frontal plane is directed counterclockwise. In all cases there is scalar electrocardiographic and vectorcardiographic evidence of right ventricular hypertrophy.

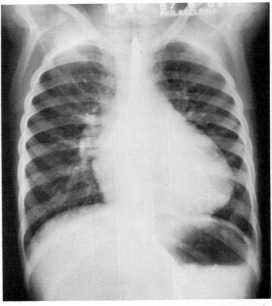

**Figure 17** Preoperative chest roentgenogram of a 6 year old girl with a complete atrioventricular canal and pulmonary hypertension in whom total correction was successful.

### Radiologic Features

The heart is always enlarged (average cardio-thoracic ratio, 0.62), and all four chambers are usually involved. The pulmonary artery is prominent, and the pulmonary vascular markings are increased (Fig. 17).

### Cardiac Catheterization and Angiocardiography

Cardiac catheterization shows an oxygen step-up in both the right atrium and the right ventricle. Pulmonary artery pressure may be quite high, while pulmonary to systemic flow ratios will usually be above 2. The majority of patients have severe pulmonary hypertension ($>75$ per cent of systolic systemic pressure $- R_p:R_s > 0.75$).

The frontal ventricular angiocardiogram demonstrates a characteristic picture. There is a long, narrow outflow tract with a scalloped right margin. A notch in the mitral valve can frequently be seen (Fig. 18). A similar left ventriculogram may be seen in patients with the partial form of persistent atrioventricular canal, as well as in those with a common atrium. If the anterior leaflet is not divided and attached to the septum, the usual picture may not be present. There may be a right-angled appearance of the right border of the left ventricle (Fig. 19). The angle s horizontal component is formed by the undivided anterior common leaflet, and the vertical side is formed by contrast medium trapped under the lateral "mitral" leaflet.

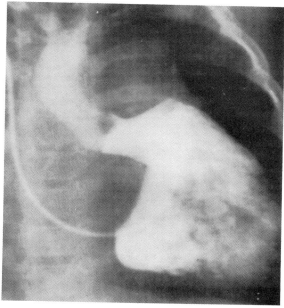

**Figure 19** Frontal left ventriculogram in a case of complete atrioventricular canal with anterior common leaflet not divided and not attached to the septum. Note the right-angle appearance of the right border of the ventricle. The angle's horizontal component is formed by the undivided anterior common leaflet, and the vertical side is formed by contrast medium trapped under the lateral "mitral" leaflet. (From Moss, A. J., and Adams, F. H.: Heart Disease in Infants, Children and Adolescents. Baltimore, The Williams & Wilkins Company, 1968.)

### Natural History and Indications for Operation

These patients have a short life span and often die in the first or second year of life. The median age at death is 2 years, but if there are associated defects the median age is only 4 months. The cause of death in infancy is usually congestive heart failure and pneumonia. Thereafter, irreversible pulmonary vascular changes rapidly render the outlook hopeless.

### Treatment

Initial attempts to repair this defect often failed because of lack of understanding of the complex anatomy. Persistent atrioventricular valve insufficiency and inadequate closure of ventricular septal defects were common. Surgically produced heart block was frequent, and the postoperative mortality was between 60 and 75 per cent.

With better understanding of the anatomy,[55] a new repair was developed that has proved satisfactory.[56] Since these patients often are in serious difficulty in infancy, and because of the complexity of total operative correction, palliation by pulmonary artery banding may be indicated. Somerville et al.[65] were able to provide palliation for 66 per cent of infants with a complete atrioventricular canal in whom congestive heart failure was present. Although the mortality rate is still quite high, especially when compared to that of operations for

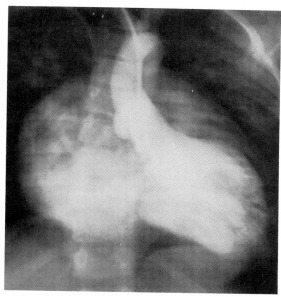

**Figure 18** Frontal left ventriculogram in early systole in a case of complete atrioventricular canal with anterior common leaflet divided and attached medially to the ventricular septum. Note elongation and narrowing of the left ventricular outflow tract, with scalloping of the right border of the ventricle and a notch from which region a jet originates. (From Moss, A. J., and Adams, F. H.: Heart Disease in Infants, Children, and Adolescents. Baltimore, The Williams & Wilkins Company, 1968.)

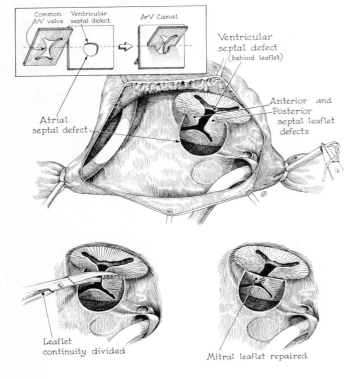

**Figure 20**  Repair of a complete atrioventricular canal. The anterior and posterior leaflets are divided. The mitral leaflet is repaired.

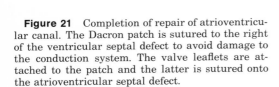

**Figure 21**  Completion of repair of atrioventricular canal. The Dacron patch is sutured to the right of the ventricular septal defect to avoid damage to the conduction system. The valve leaflets are attached to the patch and the latter is sutured onto the atrioventricular septal defect.

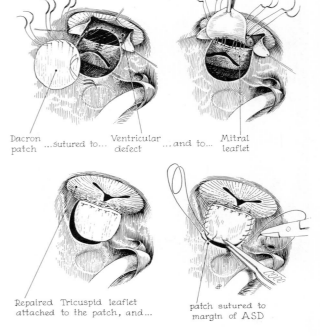

isolated ventricular septal defect in infants,[10] this operative procedure may offer the only hope for a desperately ill infant with persistent atrioventricular canal. Subsequent repair can be carried out at an age when this complex operation is feasible. The increased mortality with pulmonary artery banding in infants with persistent atrioventricular canals is related to the atrioventricular valve insufficiency and the advanced pulmonary vascular disease.

Total correction of persistent common atrioventricular canal is shown in Figures 20 and 21. Cardiopulmonary bypass is used. The right atrium is opened widely, and the details of the defect are assessed. In the most common form, there is a common posterior leaflet with or without attachments to the ventricular septum, the anterior leaflet is subdivided and attached to the ventricular septum, and the membranous septum is closed (see Fig. 4). During correction, division of the posterior leaflet is done slightly to the right side. The "mitral" portions of the anterior and posterior leaflets are approximated with sutures, to close the "cleft" mitral valve. The defect is repaired by suturing a Dacron prosthesis to the right side of the ventricular septum. The medial portion of the mitral leaflet is then attached to the appropriate level of the patch. The cleft in the tricuspid valve is repaired and the septal leaflet attached to the right side of the patch. The patch is then sutured into the atrial portion of the defect.

In the less common form of persistent atrioventricular canal (see Fig. 6), the common anterior leaflet also will require division, but the repair is similar to that just described. In addition, the membranous ventricular septum is absent and will require closure with the patch. In the least common form of this defect (see Fig. 5), the common anterior leaflet is attached to an anomalous papillary muscle in the right ventricle, and the membranous septum is absent; repair is similar to that for the second type of persistent atrioventricular canal.

The most frequent complication of total correction is complete heart block. This can usually be avoided, at the expense of a small residual shunt, if the division of the leaflet is kept well to the right side of the septum and if the patch is sutured posteriorly to the divided common posterior leaflet (especially in the common form of persistent common atrioventricular canal). With this repair, the mortality has been reduced to 20 per cent. Surviving patients have done well, although most have mild to moderate mitral valve incompetence.

## SELECTED REFERENCES

Cooley, D. A., and Hallman, G. L.: Surgical Treatment of Congenital Heart Disease. Philadelphia, Lea & Febiger, 1966.
*This monograph details the experience of a group that has managed a large number of infants and children with congenital heart disease. The book is well illustrated and adequately covers the basic operations and their results.*

Gould, S. E.: Pathology of the Heart and Blood Vessels. Springfield, Ill., Charles C Thomas, 1968.

*This textbook written by a number of authors clearly details the embryology and pathologic anatomy of the various defects of the heart. It has excellent references and is of special help to the student who desires more detailed information about the morbid anatomy of the heart and great vessels.*

Keith, J. D., Rowe, R. D., and Vlad, P.: Heart Disease in Infancy and Childhood. 2nd ed. New York, Macmillan Company, 1967.
*This textbook of pediatric cardiology is based largely on the personal experience of the authors in one of the major pediatric centers of the world. The medical and diagnostic aspects of congenital heart disease are given particular attention.*

Johnson, J., MacVaugh, H., III, and Waldhausen, J. A.: Surgery of the Chest. 4th ed. Chicago, Year Book Medical Publishers, 1970.
*This monograph describes the steps in the operative procedures of cardiothoracic surgery and is especially helpful to students and house officers who desire better understanding of the operations.*

Moss, A. J., and Adams, F. H., eds.: Heart Disease in Infants. Baltimore, Williams & Wilkins Company, 1968.
*A large number of authors contributed to this textbook of cardiology. The chapters are encyclopedic, particularly in regard to pathologic, medical, and diagnostic aspects of pediatric cardiology.*

## REFERENCES

1. Abbott, M. E.: Atlas of Congenital Heart Diseases. New York, American Heart Association, 1936.
2. Bailey, C. P.: Congenital interatrial connections: clinical and surgical considerations with a description of a new surgical technique—atrioseptopexy. Ann. Int. Med., 37:888, 1952.
3. Baron, M. G., Wolf, B. S., Steinfeld, L., and Van Mierop, L. M. S.: Endocardial cushion defects: specific diagnosis by angiocardiography. Amer. J. Cardiol., 13:162, 1964.
4. Beck, W., Swan, H. J. C., Burchell, H. B., and Kirklin, J. W.: Pulmonary vascular resistance after repair of atrial septal defects in patients with pulmonary hypertension. Circulation, 22:938, 1960.
5. Bedell, G. N., and Adams, R. W.: Pulmonary diffusing capacity during rest and exercise. A study of normal persons and persons with atrial septal defect, pregnancy and pulmonary disease. J. Clin. Invest., 41:1908, 1962.
6. Bedford, D. E.: The anatomical types of atrial septal defect. Amer. J. Cardiol., 6:568, 1960.
7. Bedford, D. E., Papp, C., and Parkinson, J.: Atrial septal defect. Brit. Heart J., 3:37, 1941.
8. Bedford, D. E., Sellors, T. H., Somerville, W., Belcher, J. R., and Besterman, E. M. M.: Atrial septal defect and its surgical treatment. Lancet, 1:1255, 1957.
9. Berg, J. M., Crome, L., and France, N. E.: Congenital cardiac malformations in mongolism. Brit. Heart J., 22:331, 1960.
10. Boruchow, I., Waldhausen, J. A., Miller, W. W., Rashkind, W. J., and Friedman, S.: Pulmonary artery hypertension in infants with congenital heart disease. Palliative management by pulmonary artery binding. Arch. Surg., 99:716, 1969.
11. Brannon, E. S., Weens, H. S., and Warren, J. V.: Atrial septal defect; study of hemodynamics by technique of right heart catheterization. Amer. J. Med. Sci., 210:480, 1945.
12. Braudo, J. L., Nadas, A. S., Rudolph, A. M., and Neuhauser, E. B. D.: Atrial septal defects in children. Pediatrics, 14:618, 1954.
13. Braunwald, N. S., and Morrow, A. C.: The delayed closure of atrial septal defects with perforated prostheses. Surg. Gynec. Obstet., 116:579, 1963.
14. Burchell, H. B., DuShane, J. W., and Brandenburg, R. O.: The electrocardiogram of patients with atrioventricular cushion defects (defects of the atrioventricular canal). Amer. J. Cardiol., 6:575, 1960.
15. Cayler, G. G.: Spontaneous functional closure of symptomatic atrial septal defects. New Eng. Med., 276:65, 1967.
16. Cohn, R.: An experimental method for the closure of interauricular septal defects in dogs. Amer. Heart J., 33:453, 1947.

17. Colmers, R. A.: Atrial septal defects in elderly patients: report of three patients aged 68, 72, and 78. Amer. J. Cardiol., 1:768, 1958.

18. Cooley, D. A.: Results of surgical treatment of atrial septal defects. Amer. J. Cardiol., 6:605, 1960.

19. Cooley, D. A., Ellis, P. R., Jr., and Bellizzi, M. E.: Atrial septal defects of the sinus venosus type: surgical considerations. Dis. Chest, 39:185, 1961.

20. Craig, R. J., and Selzer, A.: Natural history and prognosis of atrial septal defect. Circulation, 37:805, 1968.

21. Dalen, J. E., Bruce, R. A., and Cobb, L. A.: Interaction of chronic hypoxia of moderate altitude on pulmonary hypertension complicating defect of the atrial septum. New Eng. J. Med., 266:272, 1962.

22. Davis, C. L.: Development of the human heart from its first appearance to the stage found in embryos of 20 paired somites. Contrib. Embryol., 19:245, 1927.

23. DuShane, J. W., Weidman, W. H., Brandenburg, R. O., and Kirklin, J. W.: Differentiation of interatrial communications by clinical methods: ostium secundum, ostium primum, common atrium and total anomalous pulmonary venous connection. Circulation, 21:363, 1960.

24. Ellis, F. H., Jr., Brandenburg, R. O., and Swan, H. J. C.: Defect of the atrial septum in the elderly. Report of successful correction in five patients sixty years of age or older. New Eng. J. Med., 262:219, 1960.

25. Ellis, F. H., Jr., Kirklin, J. W., Swan, H. J. C., DuShane, J. W., and Edwards, J. R.: Diagnosis and surgical treatment of common atrium. Surgery, 45:160, 1959.

26. Ellis, F. H., Jr., McGoon, D. C., and Kirklin, J. W.: Surgical management of persistent common atrioventricular canal. Amer. J. Cardiol., 6:598, 1960.

27. Evans, J. R., Rowe, R. D., and Keith, J. D.: The clinical diagnosis of atrial septal defect in children. Amer. J. Med., 30:345, 1961.

28. Fontana, R. S., and Edwards, J. E.: Congenital Cardiac Disease: A Review of 357 Cases Studied Pathologically. Philadelphia, W. B. Saunders Company, 1962.

29. Gault, J. H., Morrow, A. G., Gay, W. A., Jr., and Ross, J., Jr.: Atrial septal defect in patients over the age of forty years. Circulation, 37:261, 1968.

30. Gibbon, J. H., Jr.: Application of a mechanical heart and lung apparatus to cardiac surgery. Minn. Med., 37:171, 1954.

31. Giknis, F. L.: Single atrium and the Ellis-van Creveld syndrome. J. Pediat., 62:558, 1963.

32. Griffiths, S. P.: Bacterial endocarditis associated with atrial septal defect of the ostium secundum type. Amer. Heart J., 61:543, 1961.

33. Gross, R. E., Pomeranz, A. A., Watkins, E., Jr., and Goldsmith, E. I.: Surgical closure of defects of the interauricular septum by use of an atrial well. New Eng. J. Med., 247:455, 1952.

34. Gross, R. E., Watkins, E., Jr., Pomeranz, A. A., and Goldsmith, E. I.: A method for surgical closure of interauricular septal defects. Surg. Gynec. Obstet., 96:1, 1953.

35. Hartmann, A. F., and Elliott, L. P.: Spontaneous physiologic closure of an atrial septal defect after infancy. Amer. J. Cardiol., 19:290, 1967.

36. Hastreiter, A. R., Wennemark, S. R., Miller, R. A., and Paul, M. H.: Secundum atrial septal defects with congestive heart failure during infancy and early childhood. Amer. Heart J., 64:467, 1962.

37. Hawe, A., Rastelli, G. C., Brandenburg, R. O., and McGoon, D. C.: Embolic complications following repair of atrial septal defects. Circulation, Supp. 39:185, 1969.

38. Heath, D.: Long survival in partial persistent common atrioventricular canal. Brit. J. Dis. Chest, 62:207, 1968.

39. Heath, D., and Edwards, J. E.: The pathology of hypertensive pulmonary vascular disease: a description of six grades of structural changes in the pulmonary arteries with special reference to congenital cardiac septal defects. Circulation, 18:533, 1958.

40. Keith, J. D., Rowe, R. D., and Vlad, P.: Heart Disease in Infancy and Childhood. New York, Macmillan Company, 1958.

41. Lamy, M., de Grouchy, D., and Schweisguth, O.: Genetic and nongenetic factors in the etiology of congenital heart disease: study of 1188 cases. Amer. J. Hum. Genet., 9:17, 1957.

42. Levin, A. R., Spach, M. S., Boineau, J. P., Canent, R. V., Jr.,

Capp, M. P., and Jewett, P. H.: Atrial pressure-flow dynamics in atrial septal defects (secundum type). Circulation, 37:476, 1968.

43. Lewis, F. J., and Tauffic, M.: Closure of atrial septal defects with aid of hypothermia: experimental accomplishments and report of one successful case. Surgery, 33:52, 1952.

44. Lewis, F. J., Tauffic, M., Varco, R. L., and Niazi, S.: The surgical anatomy of atrial septal defects: experiences with repair under direct vision. Ann. Surg., 142:401, 1955.

45. Lillehei, C. W., Anderson, R. C., Ferlic, R. M., and Bonnabeau, R. C., Jr.: Persistent common atrioventricular canal. J. Thorac. Cardiovasc. Surg., 57:83, 1969.

46. McGoon, D. C., DuShane, J. W., and Kirklin, J. W.: Surgical treatment of atrial septal defect in children. Pediatrics, 24:992, 1959.

47. Morrow, A. G., Gilbert, J. W., Baker, R. R., and Collins, N. P.: The closure of atrial septal defects utilizing general hypothermia. J. Thorac. Cardiovasc. Surg., 40:776, 1960.

48. Murray, G.: Closure of defects in cardiac septa. Ann. Surg., 128:843, 1948.

49. Nadas, A. S., and Ellison, R. C.: Phonocardiographic analysis of diastolic flow murmurs in secundum atrial septal defect and ventricular septal defect. Brit. Heart J., 29:684, 1967.

50. Neufeld, H. N., Titus, J. L., DuShane, J. W., Burchell, H. B., and Edwards, J. E.: Isolated ventricular septal defect of the persistent common atrioventricular canal type. Circulation, 23:685, 1961.

51. Nielsen, J. S., and Fabricius, J.: The effect of exercise on the size of the shunt in patients with atrial septal defects. Acta Med. Scand., 183:91, 1968.

52. Nora, J. J., Dodd, P. F., McNamara, D. G., Hattwick, M. A. W., Leachman, R. D., and Cooley, D. A.: Risk to offspring of parents with congenital heart defects. J.A.M.A., 209:2052, 1969.

53. Pierce, W. S., Peckham, G. J., Johnson, J., and Waldhausen, J. A.: Gram-negative sepsis following operation for congenital heart disease: diagnosis, management, and results. Arch. Surg., 101:698, 1970.

54. Rainier-Pope, C. R., Cunningham, R. D., Nadas, A. S., and Crigler, J. F.: Cardiovascular malformation in Turner's syndrome. Peidatrics, 33:919, 1964.

55. Rastelli, G. C., Kirklin, J. W., and Titus, J. L.: Anatomic observations on complete form of persistent common atrioventricular canal with special reference to atrioventricular valves. Mayo Clin. Proc., 41:296, 1966.

56. Rastelli, G. C., Ongley, P. A., Kirklin, J. W., and McGoon, D. C.: Surgical repair of the complete form of persistent common atrioventricular canal. J. Thorac. Cardiovasc. Surg., 55:299, 1968.

57. Rogers, H. M., and Edwards, J. E.: Incomplete division of the atrioventricular canal with patent interatrial foramen primum. Report of five cases and review of the literature. Amer. Heart J., 36:28, 1948.

58. Rokitansky, C. F.: Die Defekte der Scheidewände des Herzens. Vienna, Bräumuller, 1875.

59. Scott, L. B., Hauck, A. J., and Nadas, A. S.: Endocardial cushion defect with pulmonic stenosis. Circulation, 25:653, 1962.

60. Sealy, W. C., Farmer, J. C., Young, W. G., Jr., and Brown, I. W.: Atrial dysrhythmia and atrial secondum defects. J. Thorac. Cardiovasc. Surg., 57:245, 1969.

61. Sellers, R. D., Ferlic, R. M., Sterns, L. P., and Lillehei, C. W.: Secundum type atrial septal defects: early and late results of surgical repair using extracorporeal circulation in 275 patients. Surgery, 59:155, 1966.

62. Shumacker, H. B., Jr., and Herendeen, T. L.: Hemolytic anemia after repair of ostium primum septal defect and cleft mitral valve: surgical correction. J. Thorac. Cardiovasc. Surg., 55:489, 1968.

63. Shumacker, H. B., Jr., and King, H.: Septum primum atrial septal defects. J. Thorac. Cardiovasc. Surg., 43:366, 1962.

64. Somerville, J.: Ostium primum defect: factors causing deterioration in the natural history. Brit. Heart J., 27:413, 1965.

65. Somerville, J., Agnew, T., Stark, J., Waterston, D. J., Aberdeen, E., Carter, R. E. B., and Waich, S.: Banding of the pulmonary artery for common atrioventricular canal. Brit. Heart J., 29:816, 1967.

66. Swan, C., Tostevin, A. L., Mayo, H., and Black, G. H. B.:

Further observation on congenital defects in infants following infectious diseases during pregnancy with special reference to rubella. Med. J. Aust., 1:409, 1944.

67. Swan, H. J. C., Burchell, H. B., and Wood, E. H.: The presence of venoarterial shunts in patients with interatrial communications. Circulation, 10:705, 1954.

68. Swan, H. J. C., Hetzel, R. S., Burchell, B. H., and Wood, E. H.: Relative contribution of blood from each lung to the left-to-right shunt in atrial septal defect: demonstration by indicator-dilution techniques. Circulation, 14:200, 1956.

69. Tavel, M. E., Bard, R. A., Franks, L. C., Feigenbaum, H., and Fisch, C.: The jugular venous pulse in atrial septal defect. Arch. Intern. Med., 121:524, 1968.

70. Thompson, T., and Evans, W.: Paradoxical embolism. Quart. J. Med., 23:135, 1930.

71. Toscano-Barbosa, E., Brandenburg, R. O., and Burchell, H. B.: Symposium on persistent common atrioventricular canal: electrocardiographic studies of cases with intra-cardiac malformations of atrioventricular canal. Proc. Mayo Clin., 31:513, 1956.

72. Uchida, I. A., and Rowe, R. D.: Discordant heart anomalies in twins. Amer. J. Hum. Genet., 9:133, 1957.

73. Weidman, W. H., and DuShane, J. W.: Defects of the atrial septum and endocardial cushion. In: Moss, A. J., and Adams, F. H., eds.: Heart Disease in Infants, Children and Adolescents. Baltimore, Williams & Wilkins Company, 1968.

74. Wendet, V. E., Keech, M. K., Read, R. C., Bistue, A. R., and Bianchi, F. A.: Cardiovascular features of Marfan's syndrome: family studies. Circulation, Supp. 2, 32:218, 1965.

75. Weyn, A. S., Bartle, S. H., Nolan, T. B., and Dammann, J. F.: Atrial septal defect – primum type. Circulation, Supp. 3, 32:13, 1965.

76. Zuckerman, H. S., Zuckerman, G. H., Mammen, R. E., and Wassermil, M.: Atrial septal defect. Amer. J. Cardiol., 9:515, 1962.

V

# Disorders of Pulmonary Venous Return

*Dev R. Manhas, M.D., M.S., and*

*K. Alvin Merendino, M.D., Ph.D.*

Abnormalities of the pulmonary veins are uncommon. These anomalies can be divided in two groups: (1) anomalous connection of the pulmonary veins, so that the pulmonary venous return enters the right instead of the left atrium; and (2) obstruction of blood flow into the left atrium due to stenosis or atresia of the pulmonary veins or cor triatriatum.[32] Abnormalities in the latter group are rare and beyond the scope of this chapter.

## TOTAL ANOMALOUS PULMONARY VENOUS CONNECTION (TAPVC)

In this congenital abnormality, all pulmonary veins from both lungs fail to join the left atrium. Pulmonary venous blood instead goes to the right atrium either directly or through one of its tributaries. TAPVC constitutes about 1.6 to 2 per cent of all congenital heart anomalies.[11, 14] In the absence of pulmonary venous obstruction, TAPVC is distributed equally in both sexes; however, there is marked male preponderance if pulmonary venous obstruction is present.[21, 27]

### HISTORICAL ASPECTS

Wilson in 1798 was the first to describe TAPVC.[5] In 1942, Brody[5] stimulated interest in this disease with an excellent review of the literature; he found 37 autopsied cases of this anomaly. Muller[30] in 1951 reported partial surgical correction by anastomosis of the end of the left atrial appendix to the side of the common pulmonary trunk. Lewis and Varco[26] in 1956 achieved the first successful open heart correction of the cardiac type of TAPVC under direct vision using hypothermia and inflow occlusion; a few months later Burroughs and Kirklin[8] successfully employed extracorporeal circulation for repair of a similar defect. Senning[34] in 1956 performed total correction of a supracardiac TAPVC in a 21 year old patient. Cooley and Oschner,[10] through a transatrial approach, anastomosed the posterior wall of the left atrium to the common pulmonary trunk in an infant with supracardiac TAPVC in 1957. The first successful surgical correction of infradiaphragmatic type of TAPVC was reported by Sloan and associates[35] in 1962. In 1965, Dillard et al.[12] used surface induced deep hypothermia with total circulatory arrest for total surgical correction of TAPVC in infancy. Several reviews of surgical experience have been reported in recent years.[9, 18, 19, 31, 39-41]

### ANATOMIC AND HISTOLOGIC ASPECTS

#### Embryology

Primordia of the lungs develop from the foregut;[1, 15, 20] the pulmonary vascular network, formed early in the development of the lungs, initially drains into the cardinal and the umbilicovitelline system of veins. The common pulmonary vein sprouts as a small endothelial bud from the middle of the posterior aspect of the still undivided atrium. It divides into two branches, each of which further subdivides into two. Gradually, by process of differential growth, the dilated common pulmonary vein is absorbed into the enlarging left atrium up to its four subdivisions so that each subdivision becomes a pulmonary vein and opens separately into the left atrium. The pulmonary venous network in each lung establishes communication with the tributaries of the pulmonary veins and thereafter loses its connection with the cardinal and umbilicovitelline venous systems. If the common pulmonary vein persists but loses its connection with the left atrium in the early stage of embryonic life when the communication with the cardinal and the umbilicovitelline veins is still present, the latter will become the collateral channels of circulation, and various types of anomalous pulmonary venous connections will result. The most frequently used channel is the left anterior cardinal vein, which drains into the left innominate vein or the coronary sinus.[3, 7, 17]

### Anatomy

The pulmonary veins may open directly into the right atrium or, more often, unite with each to form a common venous pool behind the heart.[32] This venous pool has been called by various names, such as the common pulmonary trunk and horizontal anomalous vein. From the common pulmonary trunk arises one vein, which may join the left innominate vein or any other systemic vein in the thorax or abdomen.

There is a wide spectrum of anomalous pulmonary venous connection. Blake and associates[2] reviewed 113 cases from Brook General Hospital, Walter Reed General Hospital, and the Armed Forces Institute of Pathology and reported 27 different patterns of anomalous pulmonary venous connection. Snellen and associates[37] introduced an elaborate but useful code to describe the anatomic complexes briefly and accurately. Although there are various classifications of TAPVC, one suggested by Darling et al.[11] is very popular. According to this, there are four types of TAPVC:

1. *Supracardiac type.* This is the commonest type.[3, 7] Here the central connection is to the left innominate vein via an anomalous vertical vein. Infrequently the common pulmonary trunk may drain into the superior vena cava at or below the

level of the azygous vein. In this situation, the lower end of the superior vena cava is dilated, and the associated atrial septal defect is high.

The anomalous vertical vein on its way to join the left innominate vein usually passes in front of the left pulmonary artery. However, it may pass between the left main bronchus and the left pulmonary artery and be compressed between these two structures; this results in pulmonary venous obstruction.[16, 23]

2. *Cardiac type.* This is the second commonest in frequency.[3, 7] The common pulmonary trunk is connected to the coronary sinus (less often to the right atrium) through a vascular channel.

3. *Infracardiac type.* This should preferably be called the infradiaphragmatic type. A descending vein arises from the inferior portion of the common pulmonary trunk and runs downward in front of the esophagus, passes through the diaphragm at the esophageal hiatus, and joins the portal vein, ductus venosus, or rarely the inferior vena cava.[21]

4. *Mixed type.* The pulmonary veins from each lung and even from various lobes of the same lung have a different central connection in this type.

The most frequent sites of the central connection are the left innominate vein and the coronary sinus.[3, 7, 17] The incidence of various central connections is shown in Table 1.

The majority of patients with TAPVC do not have associated major cardiac defects.[3, 17] An interatrial communication is invariably present and is not considered a major cardiac defect for it is essential to life in this condition. This communication is usually a patent foramen ovale but may be a secundum atrial septal defect. The size of the interatrial communication is one of the factors that affect the natural history of uncomplicated TAPVC;[6] patients who survive beyond the first year of life without corrective surgery have a secundum atrial septal defect.[3] Irrespective of the type of TAPVC, the heart shows some common features on gross examination. The right atrium and ventricle are usually hypertrophied and dilated; the left cardiac chambers are comparatively small but in most cases normal or only

**TABLE 1** SITE OF THE CENTRAL CONNECTION IN TOTAL ANOMALOUS PULMONARY VENOUS CONNECTION UNASSOCIATED WITH MAJOR CARDIAC DEFECTS

| Authors | Total Number of Patients | Left Innominate Vein | Coronary Sinus | Right Atrium | Superior Vena Cava | Portal Vein | Multiple Sites | Others |
|---|---|---|---|---|---|---|---|---|
| Burroughs and Edwards (1960)[7] | 113 | 41 | 18 | 17 | 12 | 7 | 8 | 10 |
| Cooley et al. (1966)[9] | 62 | 28 | 12 | 8 | 7 | 2 | 4 | 1 |
| Bonham Carter et al. (1969)[3] | 58 | 30 | 16 | 2 | 3 | 3 | 2 | 2 |
| Gathman and Nadas (1970)[17] | 75 | 26 | 14 | 3 | 8 | 13 | 8 | 3 |
| Gomes et al. (1970)[18] | 59 | 32 | 10 | 11 | 5 | — | 1 | — |
| Total | 367 | 157 | 70 | 41 | 35 | 25 | 23 | 16 |

slightly hypoplastic. Microscopically, persistence of fetal pulmonary vascular pattern has been reported on histologic study of the lungs.[10]

## BIOLOGIC ASPECTS

In the fetus, because the lungs are not expanded, an increased pulmonic vascular resistance exists. Consequently, most of the blood from the right heart is shunted to the descending aorta via the patent ductus arteriosus. As the requirements for survival in utero require mainly an effective pump, TAPVC causes no disturbances. After birth, with the first breath the lung expands, the pulmonic vascular resistance falls, pulmonary circulation is established, and the need for a dual (pulmonic and systemic) circulation is necessary. In TAPVC, pulmonary venous blood empties into the right atrium or one of its tributaries, and a left-to-right shunt is created. In the absence of any communication between the right and left sides of the heart, the infant will die soon after birth. An interatrial communication, as already mentioned, is invariably present, and so a part of the mixture of the pulmonary and systemic venous blood goes to the left atrium, and thence to the systemic circulation. The amount of blood flow across the interatrial communication is directly related to its size.[6, 14, 38] If the interatrial communication is large, the volume of flow to the two ventricles will depend on the pressure and distensibility of each ventricle.[7] In the absence of pulmonary artery hypertension, the right ventricle exhibits a lower pressure and greater distensibility than the left ventricle; therefore, there is more flow across the tricuspid valve than the mitral valve. As pulmonary flow is greater than systemic flow, the oxygen saturation of pulmonary venous and systemic venous blood mixture in the right atrium is very near normal and therefore cyanosis is not apparent. On the other hand, in TAPVC with marked pulmonary artery hypertension (due to pulmonary venous obstruction or increased pulmonary vascular resistance), the right ventricle becomes hypertrophied and less distensible, and the pulmonary flow is diminished. The pulmonary venous blood available for mixing is decreased, and systemic arterial oxygen saturation falls. Cyanosis is therefore encountered more often when there is marked pulmonary artery hypertension.[21]

From the foregoing it is apparent that pulmonary venous obstruction plays a significant role in the pathophysiology and the natural history of TAPVC. It is invariably present in the infradiaphragmatic type, and there are a number of reasons for this:[21] (1) the descending channel may be intrinsically narrow or may be compressed at the level of the diaphragm; (2) the hepatic vascular bed presents obstruction to a large flow; and (3) the thoracoabdominal pressure changes during respiration are yet another factor. In the supradiaphragmatic types of TAPVC, the pulmonary venous obstruction may be the result of an unusual course of the anomalous vertical vein, which passes between

the left pulmonary artery and the left bronchus and is compressed at this point.[16, 23] Another site of obstruction may be a stenosis at the junction of the anomalous channel with the systemic vein. As mentioned earlier, owing to the development of pulmonary artery hypertension, cyanosis is usually present in patients with pulmonary venous obstruction, and congestive heart failure develops very early because of excessive right heart strain.[21] If compression between the left pulmonary artery and the left bronchus is the cause of obstruction, this is abetted by pulmonary artery hypertension and associated pulmonary artery dilatation. The vicious cycle thus created has been described by Elliot and Edwards[16] as a "hemodynamic vise."

## CLINICAL FEATURES

### Symptoms

The signs and symptoms of TAPVC are dependent upon the presence or absence of pulmonary venous obstruction. Infants without pulmonary venous obstruction may be asymptomatic at birth.[11] The earliest problem is tachypnea, which is especially noticeable during feeding. Cyanosis may be absent or so slight that it is unnoticed by parents.[3] With the passage of time, tachypnea becomes more prominent and feeding difficulties appear. The infant suffers frequent respiratory infections and fails to thrive, and congestive heart failure usually develops by the time the baby is 6 months of age.[29] Seventy-five to eighty per cent of these infants die by the age of 1 year;[3, 7] however, an occasional patient may reach adulthood.[7, 11, 20]

The clinical picture of TAPVC with severe pulmonary venous obstruction varies markedly from that of the unobstructed form. Symptoms appear at birth or soon thereafter and include tachypnea and feeding difficulties.[21] Cyanosis is apparent at birth and cardiac decompensation appears very early. In the infradiaphragmatic type of TAPVC, cyanosis and dyspnea are aggravated by crying, straining, and so forth, owing to impediment of the flow through the anomalous channel by increased intra-abdominal pressure or the diaphragm. These infants die within a few days to a few weeks after birth.[21, 27]

### Signs

**TAPVC without Pulmonary Venous Obstruction.** The birth weight of these infants is usually on the low side, and most gain little weight. The infants have been described as scrawny and irritable. Tachypnea and tachycardia are invariably present. Cyanosis is usually mild and may be difficult to detect clinically.[3] It may be delayed or intermittent and appear only during exertion.[14, 27] Clubbing is absent initially but may be seen in older patients.

In cardiac failure, hepatomegaly is a consistent finding; distention of neck veins, peripheral edema, and pulmonary rales also may be present. Right ventricular heave can be seen in most patients. The first heart sound is distinct and loud, while the second heart sound is usually widely split and does not vary with respiration. A soft systolic murmur is heard over the pulmonic area in 75 per cent of patients;[14, 21] a mid-diastolic flow murmur of relative tricuspid stenosis may be heard along the lower left sternal border.[24] Right ventricular failure is accompanied by a prominent third sound[14] and a holosystolic murmur of tricuspid regurgitation.[24]

**TAPVC with Pulmonary Venous Obstruction.** These infants are moderately cyanotic and show signs of cardiac decompensation such as hepatomegaly, dilated neck veins, and peripheral edema. The precordium is quiet and the heart is not enlarged.[21, 22] The pulmonic component of the second heart sound is accentuated, and splitting is decreased and may be heard only in inspiration. A soft ejection systolic murmur is heard along the upper left sternal border in 50 per cent of patients.[21] A continuous murmur may be audible along the upper left sternal border in the supracardiac type.[3, 14, 21] When heard, it usually indicates obstruction to the anomalous vertical vein,[3] although it may be occasionally heard in patients without venous obstruction.

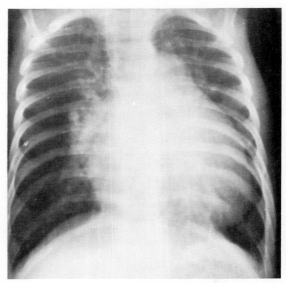

**Figure 1**   Chest roentgenogram of a mildly cyanotic 3 month old male with TAPVC to the coronary sinus. Note increased pulmonary vascular markings, cardiac enlargement, and prominent main pulmonary artery.

## DIAGNOSTIC STUDIES

### Electrocardiogram

Right axis deviation and right ventricular hypertrophy are invariably present. The P wave is tall and peaked; this indicates right atrial enlargement. Conduction defects are uncommon.[17] The presence of a Q wave used to be considered diagnostic of TAPVC, but is not thought so now.[29]

### Roentgenogram

In TAPVC without pulmonary venous obstruction, the heart is usually enlarged; this enlargement involves the right side of the heart. With a barium-filled esophagus, the left atrium is not enlarged; when the central connection is to the coronary sinus, the latter is dilated and may indent the esophagus and wrongly suggest left atrial enlargement. The pulmonary artery segment is prominent and the pulmonary vascular markings are accentuated; the aortic arch is small (Fig. 1). Classic "figure-of-eight"[36] or "snowman" configuration is seen only in TAPVC to the left innominate vein (Fig. 2).

In the presence of pulmonary venous obstruction, the heart is usually normal in size and configuration. The lung fields show a mottled, reticulated, or ground-glass appearance and prominent

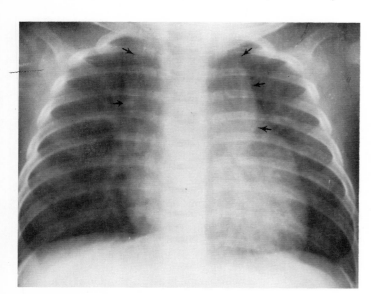

**Figure 2**   Roentgenogram of chest from a 5½ month old female with TAPVC to the left innominate vein. A well defined structure is seen both to the right and to the left of the midline which is neither thymus nor aorta. It is formed by the anomalous vertical vein, left innominate vein, and dilated superior vena cava; this imparts a "figure-of-eight" or "snowman" appearance to the cardiomediastinal silhouette.

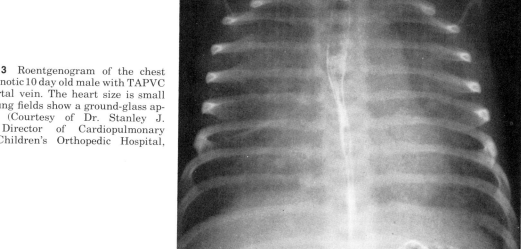

**Figure 3** Roentgenogram of the chest from a cyanotic 10 day old male with TAPVC to the portal vein. The heart size is small and the lung fields show a ground-glass appearance. (Courtesy of Dr. Stanley J. Stamm, Director of Cardiopulmonary Center, Children's Orthopedic Hospital, Seattle.)

septal lines suggestive of pulmonary venous congestion and pulmonary edema.[21] This appearance of the lung field with a small heart is characteristic of the infradiaphragmatic type of TAPVC, although an identical appearance is seen in other types with marked pulmonary venous obstruction (Fig. 3).

### Cardiac Catheterization

**Oxygen Saturation.** A step-up in oxygen saturation occurs where the pulmonary venous blood joins the systemic venous blood. When the anomalous connection is to the right atrium, oxygen step-up is seen at the right atrial level, and the oxygen saturation of blood in the four chambers of the heart, as well as in the pulmonary artery and the aorta, is equal. In the supracardiac type, the pulmonary artery blood has a higher oxygen saturation than systemic arterial blood, because the inferior vena cava blood shunts preferentially across the interatrial communication, while the superior vena cava blood streams into the right ventricle.[38] By the same token, the oxygen saturation of the pulmonary arterial blood is less than the systemic arterial blood in the infradiaphragmatic type.[17] In the presence of a large atrial septal defect, preferential flow occurs to a lesser degree.

**Pressures.** The right atrial pressure may be normal or higher than normal. There is a small mean gradient, in the range of 0 to 2 mm. Hg between the right and left atria.[17] The pressure in the right ventricle and pulmonary artery is usually normal. However, in patients with pulmonary venous obstruction, the right ventricular and pulmonary artery pressure is markedly elevated and may be equal to or more than systemic pressure.[21, 22] Also, the pulmonary wedge pressure is elevated, and there is a pronounced gradient between the mean pulmonary wedge pressure and the mean right atrial pressure.[21]

Accurate measurements of pulmonary and systemic flow ratios as well as measurement of resistance are difficult in TAPVC because of difficulty in obtaining a proper mixed-venous sample.[17] In general, the estimated pulmonary blood flow is

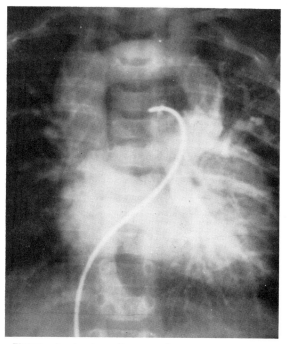

**Figure 4** Angiocardiogram from a patient with TAPVC to the left innominate vein (whose x-ray chest is seen in Figure 2). The contrast material was injected through a catheter into the main pulmonary artery. The pulmonary veins from both lungs unite to form a horizontal venous confluence behind the heart from which arises a vertical anomalous vein that joins the left innominate vein.

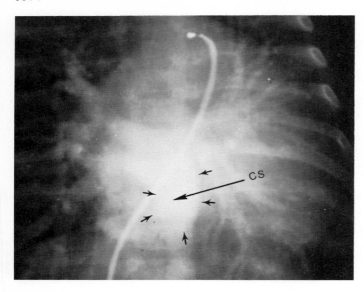

**Figure 5**　Angiocardiogram from a patient with TAPVC to the coronary sinus (Figure 1 shows x-ray chest of the same patient). A main pulmonary artery injection was made. The contrast material opacifies the pulmonary veins, which open into the dilated coronary sinus (CS).

moderately increased in patients without pulmonary venous obstruction, and is nearly normal in the presence of obstruction.

**Angiocardiography.** Injection of contrast medium in the pulmonary artery enables one to visualize the point of entry of the anomalous pulmonary venous trunk; other associated cardiac anomalies, which are sometimes present, can also be diagnosed (Figs. 4 and 5). The mixed type of TAPVC can be better seen by selective injection of contrast medium in the right and left pulmonary artery (Fig. 6).

## TREATMENT

If the defect is not corrected, 75 to 80 per cent of patients with TAPVC die within the first year of life.[7, 18] Gathman and Nadas[17] found that only 8 per cent of their patients survived up to 1 year without significant signs and symptoms. The prognosis is particularly poor in patients with pulmonary artery hypertension.[17, 18] The commonest cause of death is congestive heart failure. This natural history demands an aggressive approach in diagnosis and management.

Basically, the aims of surgical correction are: (1) to direct the pulmonary venous blood into the left atrium; (2) to interrupt the connection with the systemic veins; and (3) to repair the atrial septal defect. These aims can be achieved by total repair in one stage or by multistage procedures. Most workers recommend complete repair in one stage.[9, 12, 18, 39] Total correction can be done with the aid of cardiopulmonary bypass or during deep hypothermia with total circulatory arrest.[12, 13] The optimal age for total correction in a relatively asymptomatic patient is 3 to 5 years; however, surgery should be considered earlier if symptoms develop. Patients with pulmonary hypertension and pulmonary venous obstruction need total correction urgently.[17]

### Supracardiac Type

Pulmonary venous blood is directed into the left atrium through a large side-to-side anastomosis between the horizontal common pulmonary venous trunk and the posterior wall of the left atrium. This can be done by rotating the apex of the heart

**Figure 6**　Angiocardiogram from a patient with mixed type of TAPVC. Selective right and left pulmonary artery injections were made. The upper lobe veins including the lingular segment drain into an anomalous vertical vein that empties into the left innominate vein. The pulmonary venous return from the right lung and left lower lobe drains into the coronary sinus.

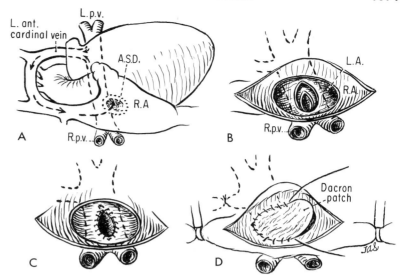

**Figure 7** Operative steps for transatrial correction of the supracardiac TAPVC. *A,* Schematic representation of the anomaly. *B* and *C,* The interatrial communication is enlarged, an incision is made in posterior wall of the left atrium and anterior wall of the common pulmonary trunk, and an anastomosis is created between the two. *D,* The interatrial defect is closed with a Dacron patch and the anomalous vertical vein (left anterior cardinal vein) is ligated. R.A., right atrium; L.A., left atrium; R.p.v., right pulmonary veins; L.p.v., left pulmonary veins; A.S.D., atrial septal defect.

up and performing the anastomosis posteriorly from outside, or it can be done transatrially. The most important point is the necessity of creating as large an anastomosis as possible. A small anastomosis usually produces pulmonary venous obstruction or relative obstruction aggravated by exercise. The interatrial communication is repaired, and the connection with the left innominate vein is ligated. If the anomalous connection is to the superior vena cava, a similar anastomosis is performed and the anomalous channel going to the superior vena cava is ligated (Fig. 7).

### Cardiac Type

When the anomalous connection is to the coronary sinus, the foramen ovale is enlarged and the common wall between the posterior left atrium and the coronary sinus is incised or excised. Because the incision proximally frequently extends into the free pericardial sac, a continuous suture uniting the posterior atrial wall and coronary sinus for the entire length of the incision is necessary. Otherwise a serious leak posteriorly may be difficult to repair when it becomes apparent later

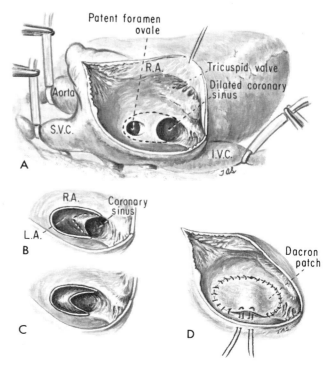

**Figure 8** Operative steps for correction of TAPVC to the coronary sinus. *A* and *B,* Through a right atriotomy, the foramen ovale is enlarged and the common wall between the left atrium and the coronary sinus is excised. *C* and *D,* The resultant defect is roofed with a Dacron patch. R.A., right atrium; L.A., left atrium; S.V.C., superior vena cava; I.V.C., inferior vena cava. (From Dillard, D. H., et al.: Circulation, Supp. 1, *35*:105, 1967. By permission of American Heart Association, Inc.)

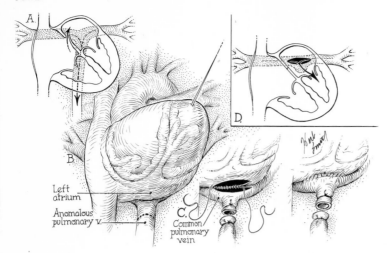

**Figure 9** Operative steps for correction of infradiaphragmatic TAPVC. *A,* Schematic representation of the anomaly. *B* and *C,* Anastomosis of the posterior wall of the left atrium with the common pulmonary trunk and ligation of the descending anomalous vein. *D,* Pattern of flow after the repair. (From Cooley, D. A., et al.: J. Thorac. Cardiovasc. Surg., *51*:88, 1966.)

in the procedure. This resultant defect is roofed with a Dacron patch so that all the pulmonary venous blood together with coronary sinus blood is directed into the left atrium (Fig. 8). Drainage of desaturated coronary sinus blood into the left atrium results in a right-to-left shunt without any obvious evidence of systemic desaturation or adverse effects. If the anomalous connection is to the right atrium, it can be managed in similar fashion. In repair of this type one must be careful to avoid injury to the atrioventricular node and to the conduction bundle of His, which lie below and in front of the coronary sinus opening. Likelihood of injury to the conduction bundle is less when the repair is done on a beating heart.

### Infradiaphragmatic Type

Here the common pulmonary trunk is anastomosed to the posterior wall of the left atrium by an extracardiac approach in a manner similar to that used for the supracardiac type (Fig. 9). The atrial septal defect is closed and the descending anomalous vein is ligated. An end-to-side anastomosis between the descending vein and the left atrium is not recommended because of the danger of kinking and stenosis.[9]

### Mixed Type

A combination of the aforementioned procedures is necessary, the choice depending on the pathologic anatomy. Because of the complicated nature of the anomaly, chances of obtaining a complete anatomic repair are not good.[9]

**Multistage Correction.** A large atrial septal defect allows good interchange of blood between the two atria and prolongs life in patients with TAPVC.[6] It would appear, therefore, that creation of a large atrial septal defect should provide palliation for moribund infants. When this was done surgically, results were disappointing.[31] The technique of balloon septostomy developed by Rashkind and Miller[33] looks promising as a palliative procedure. Good results have been reported after balloon atrial septostomy in TAPVC with

congestive heart failure but without pulmonary vascular obstruction.[28] It should be done at the time of initial catheterization if the interatrial communication seems small. If the patient improves after the septostomy, corrective surgery can be postponed until the child is old enough to tolerate surgical correction; if no improvement is seen following septostomy, however, immediate total correction should be considered. Mustard and associates[31] recommend leaving the anomalous channel open after anastomosis in the supracardiac type, so that it may decompress the left heart if necessary. It is ligated at a subsequent operation a few years later. Staged surgical procedures seem to have theoretical advantages; however, in actual practice the infant mortality has not been reduced, and a second operation with its inherent risk is necessary.

Acute pulmonary edema has been a common and serious postoperative complication occurring within the first 12 hours.[9, 31] Various explanations have been given for this. Some believe that the left ventricle is hypoplastic and cannot handle the circulatory load after total correction, and recommend leaving the vertical channel or the interatrial communication open to act as a safety valve for left heart decompression. The ligation of the former and closure of the latter may be done at a subsequent operation a few years later. This explanation seems unlikely, because prior to correction in most instances of uncomplicated TAPVC the left ventricle is maintaining an adequate pressure and output. Others[24] believe that the small left atrium predisposes to pulmonary edema after total correction. However, when one realizes that the capacious pulmonary venous bed distal to the pulmonary capillaries is in a sense an extension of the left atrium, it is difficult to accept this hypothesis. Probably the most important factor is related to the size of the common vein–atrial anastomosis and the possible presence of torsion when the heart is once again distended and in circuit. Obviously, narrowing for any reason would have the same pulmonic effects as mitral stenosis. As in the

TABLE 2 OPERATIVE MORTALITY ACCORDING TO AGE IN TOTAL ANOMALOUS PULMONARY VENOUS CONNECTION

| Authors | Less Than 1 Year in Age | | | More Than 1 Year in Age | | | Total | | |
|---|---|---|---|---|---|---|---|---|---|
| | Number of Patients | Number of Deaths | % | Number of Patients | Number of Deaths | % | Number of Patients | Number of Deaths | % |
| Cooley et al. (1966)[9] | 35 | 19 | 54 | 27 | 5 | 18.5 | 62 | 24 | 39 |
| Mustard et al. (1968)[31] | 45 | 38 | 84 | 26 | 7 | 26 | 71 | 45 | 64 |
| Gomes et al. (1970)[18] | 15 | 7 | 47 | 44 | 3 | 7 | 59 | 10 | 17 |

patient with pure mitral stenosis, whose symptoms increase as the size of the valve orifice decreases below 1.5 sq. cm., a large anastomosis between the common vein and atrium is necessary in order to avoid an increased pulmonary venous pressure and possibly acute pulmonary edema. Another contributing factor has been proposed by Gomes et al.,[18] who think that intraoperative maneuvers that raise the pulmonary venous pressure, such as temporary occlusion of the pulmonary veins, are important factors in the production of pulmonary edema. This complication was uncommon in their experience because they avoid temporary occlusion of the pulmonary veins, and recommend opening the horizontal common vein immediately after institution of bypass and occlusion of the anomalous communicating vein.

## RESULTS OF TREATMENT

The results after total correction of TAPVC are summarized in Table 2. The following factors play an important role in the results after total surgical correction of TAPVC. (1) *Age.* Hospital mortality is closely related to the age of the patient. Approximately 90 per cent of patients under 6 months of age died after surgery in one series.[31] The hospital mortality was about 50 per cent in children less than 1 year of age.[9, 18] Mortality progressively decreased when surgery was undertaken after 1 year of age.[9, 31] (2) *Type of anomaly.* The cardiac type of TAPVC is comparatively easy to correct and results are comparatively better;[39] results have been poor in the mixed variety.[9] (3) *Pulmonary hypertension.* Markedly elevated pulmonary artery pressure adversely influences the natural course of this disease and increases the operative mortality. Gomes et al.[18] reported that 5 of 11 patients with pulmonary artery pressures of more than 75 mm. Hg died after total correction. Pulmonary hypertension is particularly serious in patients less than 1 year of age and carries a very high operative mortality. (4) *Cyanosis.* Hospital mortality seems to be directly proportional to the degree of cyanosis. In patients with systemic arterial oxygen saturations of 80 to 85 per cent or less, mortality of 53 to 62 per cent has been reported.[9, 18] (5) *Size of atrial septal defect.* The presence of a large atrial septal defect appears to have a favorable influence on the course of this disease and also improves the

chance of survival after total surgical correction.[31] On the other hand, when the interatrial communication was 6 mm. or less, 8 of 11 patients died after total correction in one series.[18] (6) *Deep hypothermia versus cardiopulmonary bypass.* Open heart surgery with the aid of total cardiopulmonary bypass has generally carried a prohibitive mortality when used in total correction of TAPVC in infancy. However, recently some encouraging reports have come from some centers using cardiopulmonary bypass technique.[4, 25] At the University of Washington, deep hypothermia with total circulatory arrest has been used for correction of various congenital anomalies, including TAPVC in infancy, with gratifying results.[13] The authors believe that these infants tolerate deep hypothermia better than total cardiopulmonary bypass (with the present perfusion techniques), and that use of this method will be an important factor in reducing the mortality rate.

## SELECTED REFERENCES

Burroughs, J. T., and Edwards, J. E.: Total anomalous pulmonary venous connection. Amer. Heart J., 59:913, 1960.
*This review article is based on reports of 188 patients in the literature proved to have TAPVC at autopsy or operation or both. One hundred nineteen cases had no other associated cardiac defects except an interatrial communication while 66 patients had associated major cardiac abnormalities. Various anatomic and pathophysiologic patterns are described. Seventy-five per cent of patients died in infancy or early childhood; in the presence of short anomalous route and large interatrial communication the patients survived for a longer period of time. A detailed bibliography containing 120 references is included.*

Cooley, D. A., and Hallman, G. L.: Surgical Treatment of Congenital Heart Disease. Philadelphia, Lea & Febiger, 1966.
*In this monograph, history, embryology, clinical features, and diagnosis of various congenital heart diseases are presented in a clear and concise manner. The book includes a number of illustrations that simplify the understanding of these anomalies. The technique of operative correction of TAPVC (and other congenital defects) is very well illustrated with stepwise drawings.*

Gathman, G. E., and Nadas, A. S.: Total anomalous pulmonary venous connection. Circulation, 42:143, 1970.
*An excellent retrospective study based on 75 proved cases of TAPVC without other significant cardiac defects. Clinical, anatomic, and physiologic data are reviewed in detail. Guidelines are given for management of these patients. Early total surgical correction is recommended in the presence of pulmonary vascular obstruction; if pulmonary hypertension is absent and there is a significant gradient across the right ventricular outflow tract, the operation can be postponed to a later date, preferably after 4 years of age.*

Hastreiter, A. R., Paul, M. H., Malthan, M. E., and Miller, R. A.: Total anomalous pulmonary venous connection with severe pulmonary venous obstruction. A clinical entity. Circulation, 25:916, 1962.

*This paper deals with various aspects of TAPVC with pulmonary venous obstruction. The clinical picture is remarkably uniform and characteristic no matter what the site of pulmonary venous obstruction. The clinical presentation and hemodynamic data that help to differentiate it from TAPVC without obstruction are tabulated.*

## REFERENCES

1. Auer, J.: The development of the human pulmonary vein and its major variations. Anat. Rec., 101:581, 1948.
2. Blake, H. A., Hall, R. J., and Mannion, W. C.: Anomalous pulmonary venous return. Circulation, 32:406, 1965.
3. Bonham Carter, R. E., Caprils, M., and Noe, Y.: Total anomalous pulmonary venous drainage. A clinical and anatomical study of 75 children. Brit. Heart J., 31:45, 1969.
4. Bowman, F. O.: Personal communication.
5. Brody, H.: Drainage of the pulmonary vein into the right side of the heart. Arch. Path., 33:221, 1942.
6. Burchell, H. B.: Total anomalous pulmonary drainage and physiologic patterns. Proc. Mayo Clin., 31:161, 1956.
7. Burroughs, J. T., and Edwards, J. E.: Total anomalous pulmonary venous connection. Amer. Heart J., 59:913, 1960.
8. Burroughs, J. T., and Kirklin, J. W.: Complete surgical correction of total anomalous pulmonary venous connection. Report of three cases. Proc. Mayo Clin., 131:182, 1956.
9. Cooley, D. A., Hallman, G. L., and Leachman, R. D.: Total anomalous pulmonary venous drainage: Correction with the use of cardiopulmonary bypass in 62 cases. J. Thorac. Cardiovasc. Surg., 51:88, 1966.
10. Cooley, D. A., and Ochsner, A., Jr.: Correction of total anomalous pulmonary venous drainage. Surgery, 42:1014, 1957.
11. Darling, R. C., Rothney, W. B., and Craig, J. M.: Total pulmonary venous drainage into the right side of the heart: Report of 17 autopsied cases not associated with other major cardiovascular anomalies. Lab. Invest., 6:44, 1957.
12. Dillard, D. H., Mohri, H., Hessel, E. A., Anderson, H. N., Nelson, R. J., Crawford, E. W., Morgan, B. C., Winterscheid, L. C., and Merendino, K. A.: Correction of total anomalous pulmonary venous drainage in infancy utilizing deep hypothermia with total circulatory arrest. Circulation, Supp. 1, 35:105, 1967.
13. Dillard, D. H., Mohri, H., and Merendino, K. A.: Correction of heart disease in infancy utilizing deep hypothermia and total circulatory arrest. J. Thorac. Cardiovasc. Surg., 61:69, 1971.
14. DuShane, J. W.: Total anomalous pulmonary venous connection: Clinical aspects. Proc. Mayo Clin., 31:167, 1956.
15. Edwards, J. E.: Pathologic and developmental considerations in anomalous pulmonary venous connection. Proc. Mayo Clin., 28:441, 1953.
16. Elliot, L. P., and Edwards, J. E.: The problems of pulmonary venous obstruction in total anomalous pulmonary venous connection to the left innominate vein. Circulation, 25:913, 1962.
17. Gathman, G. E., and Nadas, A. S.: Total anomalous pulmonary venous connection. Circulation, 42:143, 1970.
18. Gomes, M. M. R., Feldt, R. H., McGoon, D. C., and Danielson, G. K.: Total anomalous pulmonary venous connection: Surgical considerations and results of operation. J. Thorac. Cardiovasc. Surg., 60:116, 1970.
19. Gomes, M. M. R., Feldt, R. H., McGoon, D. C., and Danielson, G. K.: Long-term results following correction of total

anomalous pulmonary venous connection. J. Thorac. Cardiovasc. Surg., 61:253, 1971.
20. Gott, V. L., Lester, R. G., Lillehei, C. W., and Varco, R. L.: Total anomalous pulmonary return: An analysis of thirty cases. Circulation, 13:543, 1956.
21. Hastreiter, A. R., Paul, M. H., Malthan, M. E., and Miller, R. A.: Total anomalous pulmonary venous connection with severe pulmonary venous obstruction. A clinical entity. Circulation, 25:916, 1962.
22. Hauck, A. J., Rudolph, A. M., and Nadas, A. S.: Pulmonary venous obstruction in infants with anomalous pulmonary venous drainage (abstract). Amer. J. Dis. Child., 100:744, 1960.
23. Kaufman, S. L., Ores, C. N., and Andersen, D. H.: Two cases of total anomalous pulmonary venous return of the supracardiac type with stenosis simulating infradiaphragmatic drainage. Circulation, 25:376, 1962.
24. Keither, J. D., Rowe, R. D., Vlad, P., and O'Hanley, J. H.: Complete anomalous pulmonary venous drainage. Amer. J. Med., 16:23, 1954.
25. Kirklin, J. W.: Personal communication.
26. Lewis, F. J., Varco, R. L., Taufic, M., and Niazi, S.: Direct vision repair of triatrial heart and total anomalous pulmonary venous drainage. Surg. Gynec. Obstet., 102:713, 1956.
27. Lucas, R. V., Jr., Adams, P., Jr., Anderson, R. C., Varco, R. L., Edwards, J. E., and Lester, R. G.: Total anomalous pulmonary venous connection to the portal venous system: A case of pulmonary venous obstruction. Amer. J. Roentgen., 86:561, 1961.
28. Miller, W. W., Rashkind, W. J., Miller, R. A., Hastreiter, A. R., Green, E. W., Golinko, R. J., and Young, D.: Total anomalous pulmonary venous return: Effective palliation of critically ill infants by balloon atrial septostomy (abstract). Circulation, Supp. 2, 36:189, 1967.
29. Moss, A. J., and Adams, F. H.: Heart Disease in Infants, Children and Adolescents. Baltimore, Williams & Wilkins Company, 1968, p. 672.
30. Muller, W. H., Jr.: The surgical treatment of transposition of the pulmonary veins. Amer. Surg., 134:683, 1951.
31. Mustard, W. T., Keon, W. J., and Trusler, G. A.: II. Transposition of the lesser veins (total anomalous pulmonary venous drainage). Progr. Cardiovasc. Dis., 11:145, 1968.
32. Nakib, A., Muller, J. H., Kanjub, V. I., and Edwards, J. E.: Anomalies of the pulmonary veins. Amer. J. Cardiol., 20:77, 1967.
33. Rashkind, W. J., and Miller, W. W.: Creation of an atrial septal defect without thoracotomy: A palliative approach to complete transposition of the great arteries. J.A.M.A., 196:991, 1966.
34. Senning, A.: Complete correction of total anomalous pulmonary venous return. Ann. Surg., 148:99, 1958.
35. Sloan, H. J., Mackenzie, J., Morris, J. D., Stern, A., and Sigmann, J.: Open-heart surgery in infancy. J. Thorac. Cardiovasc. Surg., 44:459, 1962.
36. Snellen, H. A., and Albers, F. H.: The clinical diagnosis of anomalous pulmonary venous drainage. Circulation, 6:801, 1952.
37. Snellen, H. A., Van Ingen, H. C., and Hoefsmit, E. C. M.: Patterns of anomalous pulmonary venous drainage. Circulation, 38:45, 1968.
38. Swan, H. J. C., Toscano-Barboza, E., and Wood, E. H.: Hemodynamic findings in total anomalous pulmonary venous drainage. Proc. Mayo Clin., 31:177, 1956.
39. Vetto, R. R., Dillard, D. H., Jones, T. W., Winterscheid, L. C., and Merendino, K. A.: The surgical therapy of extracardiac anomalous pulmonary drainage. Circulation, 23:907, 1961.
40. Williams, G. R., Thompson, W. M., Garrett, D. H., and Greenfield, L. J.: Surgical management of total anomalous pulmonary venous drainage via left vertical anomalous trunk. J. Cardiovasc. Surg., 9:470, 1968.
41. Zubiate, P., and Kay, J. H.: Surgical correction of anomalous pulmonary venous connection. Ann. Surg., 156:234, 1962.

# VI

# Ventricular Septal Defects

*Nicholas T. Kouchoukos, M.D., and John W. Kirklin, M.D.*

Isolated ventricular septal defect is the most common congenital cardiac lesion, accounting for 30 to 40 per cent of all congenital heart disease at birth.[8] The clinical signs of ventricular septal defect and the underlying pathological condition were described by Roger in 1879. By 1950 precise delineation of the hemodynamic alterations produced by such defects resulted from the use of cardiac catheterization. The first attempt at surgical management of a patient with ventricular septal defect was performed by Muller and Dammann,[23] who banded the pulmonary artery to reduce pressure in the pulmonary vascular system and thus the likelihood of development of irreversible pulmonary hypertension. The first successful repair of a ventricular septal defect with the use of controlled cross circulation was performed in 1954 by Lillehei et al.[19] The development of improved surgical techniques and the use of pump-oxygenators in the operation[15, 20] increased the safety with which closure of such defects could be performed. Increasing knowledge of the life history of patients with ventricular septal defects[8] and of the results of operation in various types of patients resulted in the present patient management programs for ventricular septal defect.

## ANATOMY

Ventricular septal defects that occur in patients (without transposition of the great arteries, inversion of the ventricles or corrected transposition, tetralogy of Fallot, or the complete form of common atrioventricular canal) can be divided generally into four anatomic groups[2, 16] (Fig. 1). The largest number are the so-called *high ventricular septal defects*. Viewed from the left ventricle,

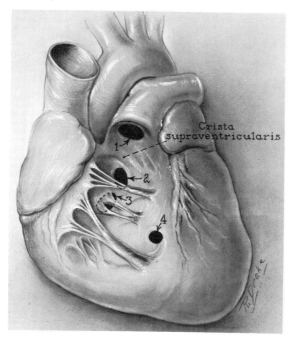

**Figure 1** Schematic representation of some of the common locations of isolated ventricular septal defects: (1) the so-called supracristal defect, immediately upstream to the pulmonary valve, but from the right ventricular aspect still under the aortic valve; (2) the most common type, the typical high defect that from the left ventricular aspect is immediately under the aortic valve; (3) the so-called atrioventricular canal type of ventricular septal defect; and (4) one of the common locations of defects of the muscular portion of the septum. (From Kirklin, J. W., Harshbarger, H. G., Donald, D. E., and Edwards, J. E.: J. Thorac. Surg., *33:*45, 1957.)

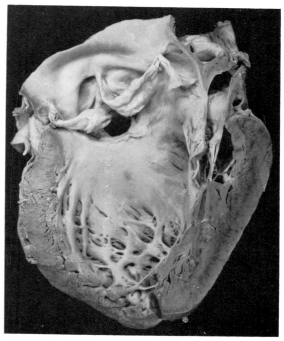

**Figure 2** A high ventricular septal defect viewed from the left ventricular side. Note that it is immediately under the commissure between the right and noncoronary cusps of the aortic valve. (From Kirklin, J. W., Harshbarger, H. G., Donald, D. E., and Edwards, J. E.: J. Thorac. Surg., *33:*45, 1957.)

they are located immediately upstream to (or under) the aortic valve, and they most commonly lie beneath the commissure between the noncoronary and right coronary cusps (Fig. 2). Viewed from the right ventricle, these defects appear to be in the region of the membranous septum. Often, however, they are slightly ventral, or anterior, to it. They are located in the inflow portion of the right ventricle, beneath the crista supraventricularis (infracristal in location) and in the portion of the septum adjacent to the junction of the septal and anterior leaflets of the tricuspid valve.

Some defects, when viewed from the left ventricle, are "high" defects but lie beneath the central portion of the right coronary cusp and that part of the right cusp adjacent to the commissure between it and the left coronary cusp. Viewed from the right ventricle, they are seen to be *supracristal ventricular septal defects*. They are located in the outflow portion, or infundibulum, of the right ventricle and lie immediately beneath the pulmonary valve (Fig. 3).

A third group of defects is located beneath the septal leaflet of the tricuspid valve, further removed from the aortic valve. There is no muscular tissue between these defects and the tricuspid valve. They are triangular in shape and are termed *defects of the atrioventricular canal type* because of their similarity to the defects observed in the complete form of common atrioventricular canal.

*Muscular ventricular septal defects* are located in the ventricular septum in the inflow portion of the right ventricle, in areas other than those described previously (Fig. 4). They may be multiple and can occur with the other types of defects as well.

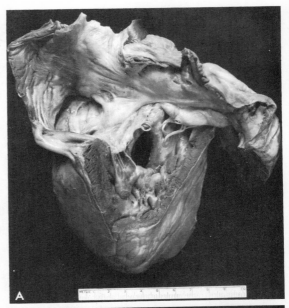

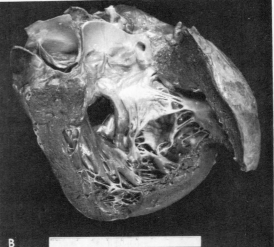

**Figure 4**   Muscular ventricular septal defects. *A,* The defect is near the tricuspid valve but is completely surrounded by ventricular septal muscle. *B,* This muscular ventricular septal defect, viewed from the left ventricular side, is low in the muscular septum. (From Kirklin, J. W., Harshbarger, H. G., Donald, D. E., and Edwards, J. E.: J. Thorac. Surg., *33:*45, 1957.)

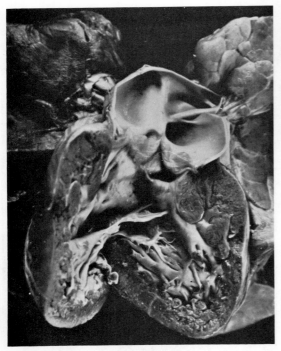

**Figure 3**   Supracristal ventricular septal defect viewed from the right ventricular side. Note that it is immediately beneath the pulmonary valve. (From Becu, L. M., Fontana, R. S., DuShane, J. W., Kirklin, J. W., Burchell, H. B., and Edwards, J. E.: Circulation, *14:*349, 1956. By permission of the American Heart Association, Inc.)

The location of the bundle of His with respect to ventricular septal defects must be understood when surgical repair is undertaken, in order to avoid producing heart block. In high ventricular septal defects, the bundle of His is located along the posterior and inferior margins of the defect (Fig. 5). The relations of the bundle of His to the margins of defects of the atrioventricular canal type are not so constant, but presumably here also the bundle is located along the edge of the ventricular component of the defect from its midportion to that extremity of the ventricular septal edge of the defect near the coronary sinus. The bundle of His is generally not in danger of being damaged when supracristal or muscular defects are closed.

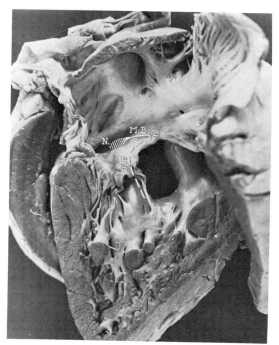

**Figure 5** In this specimen, the right ventricle and right atrium have been opened. The pulmonary valve and pulmonary artery are superior and to the right. The relations of the bundle of His (M.B.B.) are illustrated. The bundle lies not in the tricuspid valve tissue but in that part of the septum immediately beneath it. One cannot be certain that the main bundle has become the right bundle (R.B.) until one reaches the level of the papillary muscle of the conus. Stitches must not be placed in these areas when repairing the defect. (From Kirklin, J. W., Karp, R., B., and Bargeron, L. M., Jr. Surgical Treatment of Ventricular Septal Defect. In: Gibbon, J. H., Jr., Sabiston, D. C., Jr., and Spencer, F. C., eds.: Surgery of the Chest. 2nd ed. Philadelphia, W. B. Saunders Company, 1969.)

## ASSOCIATED LESIONS

In some patients with supracristal ventricular septal defects, aortic valvular incompetence develops presumably as a result of progressive prolapse of the right aortic cusp through the defect.[24,29] Abnormalities in the development of the aortic root may also contribute to the development of aortic incompetence. Peak pressure gradients between the inflow portion of the right ventricle and the outflow portion of the pulmonary artery are present in approximately one-half of the patients with ventricular septal defects and aortic valve incompetence as a result of associated displacement and hypertrophy of the crista supraventricularis and its bands.[13] The prolapsed aortic leaflet may contribute to the obstruction.[27]

Occasionally patients with ventricular septal defects have associated mild or moderate degrees of infundibular pulmonary stenosis. Less commonly, there is associated valvular pulmonary stenosis. These lesions should be recognized and treated appropriately when repair of ventricular septal defect is carried out. These lesions are different morphologically from the tetralogy of Fallot, which is discussed elsewhere in this text.

Other lesions that occur with ventricular septal defect include patent ductus arteriosus, atrial septal defect, coarctation of the aorta, congenital mitral stenosis or insufficiency, and persistent left superior vena cava. These lesions are of importance when decisions are made regarding therapy and in the conduct of the operation.

## PATHOPHYSIOLOGY

### Hemodynamics

The direction and magnitude of the shunt in patients with ventricular septal defect depends upon the size of the defect and the differences in pressure between the ventricles during systole and diastole. When the ventricular septal defect is small, it offers resistance to flow and only a relatively large pressure difference between the two ventricles, such as occurs during mid and late systole, results in significant flow across the defect. Since under these circumstances pressure is higher in the left than in the right ventricle, the shunt is left-to-right. When the defect is large, it offers little resistance to flow, and small pressure differences between the right and left ventricle then result in shunting.[11,18] The pressure differences between the two ventricles and the resultant shunting during mid and late systole, when most of the shunting occurs, are related primarily to the relative resistance to ejection in the systemic and pulmonary vasculature. In diastole and early systole, a number of other factors appear to influence the magnitude and direction of the gradients and the resultant shunting, including the relative compliances of the ventricles, their diastolic pressures, and the presence of asynchronous contraction of the two ventricles.[18] The size of the ventricular septal defect may vary during various phases of the cardiac cycle and may also influence the degree of shunting.

When a left-to-right shunt is present, pulmonary blood flow is increased relative to normal and to systemic blood flow. Flow through the left atrium and mitral valve orifice is similarly increased and thus greater work (pressure × flow) is performed by both the left and the right ventricles. Both ventricles enlarge when this work load is significantly increased by a large left-to-right shunt. The pressure and size of the left atrium increase to a degree corresponding to the magnitude of increase in pulmonary blood flow. In patients with severe pulmonary hypertension, severe elevation of pulmonary vascular resistance, and bidirectional shunting, pulmonary blood flow is about normal, left atrial and mitral valve flow are about normal, and the left ventricle and atrium are consequently not enlarged. The right ventricle is hypertrophied.

### Effects on the Pulmonary Vasculature

Patients with small ventricular septal defects (area < 1 cm.$^2$ per square meter body surface area) generally have normal right ventricular and pulmonary arterial pressure, slightly elevated pulmonary blood flow relative to systemic flow, and no pulmonary vascular disease as evidenced

**TABLE 1** A WAY OF CATEGORIZING PATIENTS WITH VENTRICULAR SEPTAL DEFECTS*

| Size of Defect | Pulmonary Arterial Hypertension | | Pulmonary Blood Flow | | Pulmonary Vascular Disease | |
| --- | --- | --- | --- | --- | --- | --- |
| | Degree | $P_p/P_s$† | Magnitude of Increase | $Q_p/Q_s$‡ | Severity | $R_p/R_s$§ |
| Small | None | <0.25 | Mild | <1.4 | None | <0.25 |
| | None | <0.25 | Moderate | 1.4–1.8 | None | <0.25 |
| Large | Mild | 0.25–0.45 | Large | >1.8 | Mild | <0.25 |
| | Moderate | 0.45–0.75 | Large | >1.8 | Mild | <0.25 |
| | Severe | >0.75 | Large | >1.8 | Mild | 0.25–0.45 |
| | | | Moderate | 1.4–1.8 | Moderate | 0.45–0.75 |
| | | | Small | <1.4 | Severe | >0.75 |

*From Kirklin, J. W., Karp, R. B., and Bargeron, L. M., Jr. In: Gibbon, J. H., Jr., Sabiston, D. C., Jr., and Spencer, F. C., eds.: Surgery of the Chest. 2nd ed. Philadelphia, W. B. Saunders Company, 1969.

†$P_p/P_s$ refers to the ratio between peak pressure in the pulmonary artery and that in a systemic artery (ratio between mean pressures is more commonly used, and is similar).

‡$Q_p/Q_s$ refers to ratio between pulmonary and systemic blood flow.

§$R_p/R_s$ refers to ratio between pulmonary and systemic vascular resistance.

histologically or by the measurement of pulmonary vascular resistance (Table 1).

The hemodynamic state in patients with large ventricular septal defects is determined largely by the pulmonary vascular resistance, which in these patients may be mildly, moderately, or severely elevated because of varying degrees of hypertensive pulmonary vascular disease. The pulmonary vascular disease develops as a result of the large ventricular septal defect. The pulmonary vascular resistance is expressed numerically in resistance units, normalized as to body surface area (BSA):

$$\frac{\text{Mean pulmonary artery pressure} - \text{Mean left atrial pressure}}{\text{Cardiac output /BSA}}$$

The absolute value for pulmonary vascular resistance is important, but so also is the relation between pulmonary and systemic vascular resistance, although the variability of the latter in a given patient dictates the use of caution in interpreting this ratio. In any event, some patients with large ventricular septal defects have a low pulmonary/systemic resistance ratio (less than 0.45) and a large pulmonary blood flow relative to systemic flow. This has been termed the hyperdynamic type of pulmonary hypertension. When the pulmonary/systemic resistance ratio is between 0.45 and 0.75, indicating significant pulmonary vascular disease (see later discussion), pulmonary blood flow is only moderately elevated relative to systemic flow. When the resistance ratio is greater than 0.75, the flow across the defect is bidirectional or right-to-left and the pulmonary blood flow is similar to or less than systemic blood flow.

In normal persons, a fourfold increase in pulmonary blood flow, as occurs with exercise, can be accommodated without an increase in pulmonary artery pressure; this indicates an actual decrease in pulmonary vascular resistance under these circumstances. In patients with ventricular septal defects and moderate or severe pulmonary vascular disease, the pulmonary vasculature usually loses the ability to accommodate increases in pulmonary blood flow caused by physiologic stresses such as exercise by a decline in pulmonary vascular resistance. In this case, closure of the ventricular septal defect is hazardous, since pulmonary, and thus systemic, blood flow cannot increase during exercise. With the defect open, systemic blood flow and oxygen consumption can increase, albeit by the mechanism of increased right-to-left shunting.

The elevations of pulmonary vascular resistance in patients with ventricular septal defects are associated with anatomic changes in the small arteries of the lungs.[6, 7, 30] The changes result from a decrease in the ratio between the diameter of the lumen and the total diameter of the small muscular pulmonary arteries and arterioles. In patients with moderately elevated pulmonary vascular resistance, the increase in vessel wall thickness is primarily due to increased thickness of the muscle of the media and to intimal fibrosis with actual occlusion of some of the vessels. In patients with severe elevation of pulmonary vascular resistance, the intimal proliferation is more pronounced, with widespread occlusion of the muscular pulmonary arteries and arterioles and plexiform dilatation of many of the remaining vessels.[6]

## NATURAL HISTORY

Many patients with ventricular septal defects have small defects and few or no symptoms, since the left-to-right shunt is small and pulmonary hypertension and vascular disease do not develop. It is estimated that only 10 to 20 per cent of patients have large defects and incur serious difficulties.[9]

Infants born with large ventricular septal defects also have moderate elevation of pulmonary vascular resistance, owing to persistence of the medial thickening of the small pulmonary arteries present in the normal fetus. As the pulmonary vessels mature, pulmonary resistance declines in the first few weeks of life and the magnitude of the left-to-right shunt across the defect increases and symptoms develop. Such infants may die of severe congestive heart failure during this period.[22] If they survive and the hemodynamic state stabilizes, the small systemic blood flow and breathlessness, which entails a large caloric expenditure and interferes with eating, can result in growth failure. If operation is not performed, death can occur during this period, usually from congestive failure or pneumonia, and usually in the first year of life.[9]

In a small number of infants with large ventricular septal defects who survive the neonatal period, severe pulmonary vascular disease and a significant increase in pulmonary vascular resistance begin to develop by the age of 6 to 12 months. If operation is not performed and this condition progresses over the ensuing months or years until it becomes severe, these patients can no longer be considered candidates for operation because of the severity of the pulmonary vascular changes. When the shunting becomes dominantly right-to-left across the defect as a result of the hypertensive pulmonary vascular disease, the patients become cyanotic and can be considered to have Eisenmenger's complex. Operation is then contraindicated.

Another group of infants with large defects have only mild elevation in pulmonary vascular resistance in the first few years of life, although significant pulmonary hypertension and a large pulmonary blood flow are present. These children are usually of small stature and have significantly impaired exercise tolerance. If the defect is still open or unrepaired by the time the patient is about 10 years old, the pulmonary vascular disease usually begins to progress, and at the age of 15 to 20 years these patients have Eisenmenger's complex with severe elevation of the pulmonary vascular resistance, and predominant right-to-left shunting occurs across the defect. Occasionally, severe pulmonary vascular disease does not develop, and heart failure may occur in the second or third decade of life. Those patients with Eisenmenger's complex become polycythemic and they eventually succumb to the complications of hypoxia and polycythemia, usually at the age of 25 to 30 years.

In some infants, the ventricular septal defect becomes smaller in size relative to the size of the heart as time passes. Pulmonary blood flow decreases because of the resistance to flow offered by the smaller defect, and pulmonary artery pressure also decreases. Although a left-to-right shunt is still present, severe pulmonary vascular disease does not develop. The growth and development of these children is quite normal. In a few of these patients bacterial endocarditis develops.[25]

Spontaneous complete closure of ventricular septal defects has been estimated to occur in 25 to 50 per cent of patients during childhood.[9] Even large defects may close in this way. Closure most commonly occurs before the age of 3 years and only occasionally after the early teen years. The mechanism of closure is usually related to ingrowth of fibrous tissue from the margins of the defect or adherence of the septal leaflet of the tricuspid valve to the margins of the defect.[9]

## DIAGNOSIS

### History

Infants with large ventricular septal defects do not usually have symptoms until they reach the age of 6 weeks to 3 months. At this time the pulmonary vascular resistance has fallen from the elevated levels present at birth, and this results in maximal left-to-right shunting of blood across the defect and a marked increase in pulmonary blood flow. Tachypnea, growth failure, pneumonia, and possibly severe cardiac failure then develop.

Many patients with ventricular septal defects are asymptomatic. Generally these are patients whose defects are small in size. Children with moderate-sized or large septal defects may demonstrate growth failure and have limitations in exercise tolerance. The growth failure is related to the size of the defect and the magnitude of the left-to-right shunt.

Patients with markedly elevated pulmonary vascular resistance and predominant right-to-left shunting across the septal defect (Eisenmenger's complex) are cyanosed, polycythemic, and severely limited in their activities.

### Examination

The infant with a large ventricular septal defect and increased pulmonary blood flow characteristically presents with tachypnea and marked subcostal retraction. Severe growth failure and a lack of subcutaneous tissue are often evident. The complexion may be waxen, and evidence of profuse sweating, such as damp or matted hair, may be noted. The jugular venous pulses are prominent even when the infant is held erect. On palpation, there is often a precordial bulge, and the heart is overactive with a rapid rate. A thrill is present in the third to fifth left intercostal spaces. A loud systolic murmur is also present in this same area. The second sound at the base is usually loud and may be split. The liver and spleen are usually enlarged, and the peripheral pulses are weak.

In older children with large ventricular septal defects, a protruding sternum or pigeon breast deformity is frequently present. Presumably this results from the enlarged right ventricle pushing the sternum anteriorly during the period of growth. The heart is hyperactive, there is a right ventricular lift, and the left ventricle is found to be enlarged on palpation. A systolic thrill is often present over the left precordium. The characteristic murmur is harsh and pansystolic and is heard best in the left fourth interspace along the sternal border. If pulmonary blood flow is large, there may be a superimposed midsystolic ejection murmur in the area of the pulmonary valve.[17] A mid-diastolic murmur is present at the apex and indicates a large flow across the mitral valve. The first sound at the base is normal. The second sound is characterized by an abnormally wide split in expiration, and the splitting is accentuated in inspiration.[17]

Patients with small defects and small left-to-right shunts have only a systolic murmur. The heart is not hyperactive, and there is no enlargement of the left ventricle or right ventricular lift. In patients with large defects and high pulmonary vascular resistance resulting in only small net left-to-right shunts or in bidirectional shunts of equal magnitude, the systolic murmur is soft and short or may be absent. There is no apical diastolic rumble and the second sound is markedly accentuated. There is no left ventricular enlargement and a right ventricular lift is prominent. When in addition the patient is cyanotic, pulmonary vascular disease is severe and the shunt is dominantly right-to-left.

### Chest Roentgenograms

As already emphasized, this and all other parts of the clinical and hemodynamic state are deter-

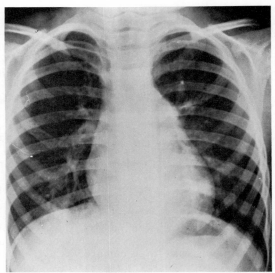

**Figure 7**   This chest roentgenogram is in contrast to that shown in Figure 6. The heart is not enlarged overall. The main pulmonary artery is enlarged; there is no evidence of increased pulmonary blood flow. This patient has a large ventricular septal defect, pulmonary hypertension, severe elevation of pulmonary vascular resistance, and pulmonary blood flow that is less than systemic blood flow. The condition is inoperable. (From DuShane, J. W., and Kirklin, J. W.: Circulation, *21*:13, 1960. By permission of the American Heart Association, Inc.)

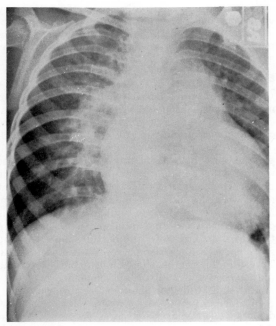

**Figure 6**   Chest roentgenogram of a child with a large ventricular septal defect, large pulmonary blood flow, and pulmonary hypertension, but only mild elevation of pulmonary vascular resistance. This is reflected in the evidence of left and right ventricular enlargement, enlargement of the main pulmonary artery, and marked increase in pulmonary blood flow. (From Kirklin, J. W., Karp, R. B., and Bargeron, L. M., Jr. In: Gibbon, J. H., Jr., Sabiston, D. C., Jr., and Spencer, F. C., eds.: Surgery of the Chest. 2nd ed. Philadelphia, W. B. Saunders Company, 1969.)

mined by the size of the defect and the degree of pulmonary vascular resistance.

In patients with small ventricular septal defects and small left-to-right shunts, chest roentgenograms are usually normal. Patients with large ventricular septal defects, mild elevation of pulmonary vascular resistance, and large left-to-right shunts have large pulmonary arteries, both centrally and peripherally, and therefore a large pulmonary blood flow (Fig. 6). The right ventricle and the left ventricle are enlarged, as is the left atrium. When marked enlargement of the left atrium is present in a patient suspected of having a ventricular septal defect, the presence of coexisting mitral valvular regurgitation should be considered.

In patients with large ventricular septal defects and severe elevation of the pulmonary vascular resistance, the chest roentgenogram is quite different (Fig. 7). The central pulmonary arteries appear normal in size or are enlarged, but the peripheral pulmonary arteries appear normal; this suggests a normal or decreased pulmonary blood flow. The right ventricle appears somewhat enlarged, but there is no evidence of significant left atrial or left ventricular enlargement. Aside from the enlarged central pulmonary arteries, the cardiac silhouette may appear normal.

### Electrocardiogram

The electrocardiographic findings, in the absence of a conduction defect, are likewise determined by the size of the defect and the pulmonary vascular resistance.

In patients with small ventricular septal defects, the electrocardiogram may be normal. When the defect and shunt are slightly larger ($Q_p/Q_s >$ about 1.8), the increase in left ventricular work from the large left ventricular stroke volume is evidenced by increased R wave voltage and tall peaked T waves from the left precordial leads. When the shunt is still larger, a pattern of mild right ventricular overload may be present as suggested by an RSR' pattern in the $V_1$ lead.

If the ventricular septal defect is large, and the left-to-right shunt is large ($Q_p/Q_s > 2$), but the pulmonary vascular resistance is significantly less than the systemic vascular resistance ($R_p/R_s < 0.75$), there is evidence of increased work of both ventricles. The R wave from the right precordial leads is tall, and when the right ventricular peak pressure is similar to the left ventricular peak pressure, it is notched on the upstroke. The left precordial leads in this situation have the pattern of left ventricular overload previously described, although there may be a deeper S wave.

When the ventricular septal defect is large and the pulmonary vascular resistance is equal to or greater than the systemic resistance, right axis deviation is usually present in the limb leads. The right precordial leads show the typical large, usually notched R waves of right ventricular hypertrophy while the left precordial leads no longer show left ventricular overload. The Q wave usually disappears in the left precordial leads, the R wave voltage is below normal, and a deep S wave appears.

In many patients with ventricular septal defect and large pulmonary blood flow, evidence of left atrial hypertrophy is seen in the broadened and even notched P waves present primarily in the left precordial leads.

The electrocardiogram then supplements the physical findings and chest roentgenogram. Taken together, they usually provide a useful categorization of patients as to the size of the ventricular septal defect, the size of the shunt, and the magnitude of the pulmonary vascular resistance.

### Cardiac Catheterization

Cardiac catheterization is indicated in patients in whom clinical assessment suggests elevated pulmonary vascular resistance. The physical findings, chest roentgenogram, and electrocardiogram do not by themselves allow accurate categorization of patients whose pulmonary/systemic resistance ratio is greater than about 0.5. The measurement of pulmonary and systemic flows and pressures and the calculation of pulmonary and systemic vascular resistance at rest, and whenever possible during exercise, are important in such patients in assessing the operability of the condition.

Measurement of the magnitude of the left-to-right shunt is helpful in deciding whether surgical intervention is necessary in patients with small ventricular septal defects. Cardiac catheterization

is also indicated when the clinical findings are atypical or when the presence of associated cardiac defects is suspected.

### Angiocardiography

Injection of radiopaque contrast material into the left ventricle at the time of catheterization will demonstrate the size and location of the ventricular septal defect. This study is not necessary in most patients with ventricular septal defects. However, when repair of ventricular septal defect is contemplated in infants, angiocardiography is useful, since preoperative information regarding the location and number of ventricular septal defects is of great assistance when one is planning the technical details of the operation. In those patients suspected of having associated defects, such as aortic valvular incompetence or pulmonary infundibular or valvular stenosis, angiocardiographic studies are indicated.

## INDICATIONS FOR OPERATION

The decision to recommend operation for an individual patient is made on the basis of knowledge of the natural history of similar untreated patients and of the results of surgical correction. Important considerations are the possibility of spontaneous closure of the defect on the one hand and of the development of severe pulmonary vascular disease on the other, along with the possible presence of congestive heart failure and growth failure.

In infants under 6 months of age operation is occasionally indicated because of severe cardiac failure from a large defect and a large shunt, which does not respond to medical treatment. Banding of the main pulmonary artery with deferral of intracardiac repair until the age of about 3 years has been recommended by many in the past. Banding increases right ventricular outflow resistance and thereby decreases pulmonary blood flow and prevents the development of pulmonary vascular disease.[10, 28] However, the morbidity and mortality with the procedure is 10 to 20 per cent and some increased risk is involved in later intracardiac repair. Therefore, although it remains controversial, we and others now perform primary intracardiac repair in infants less than 6 months of age when operation is indicated.[1, 4, 26]

Intracardiac repair is indicated in infants between 6 and 24 months of age with large defects and large shunts and pulmonary hypertension who present with persisting left ventricular failure, recurrent pulmonary infections, severe growth failure, or evidence of increasing pulmonary vascular disease. In patients between 2 and 5 years of age, repair is indicated if there is persisting left ventricular failure, growth failure, or evidence of progressing pulmonary vascular disease.

If the ventricular septal defect is large when a child is between 5 and 10 years of age, the likelihood of spontaneous closure still exists but is probably small, and usually some degree of pulmonary vascular disease and growth failure exists. Defects in patients in this group should be surgically corrected. If the defect is small or of moderate size, the possibility of spontaneous closure and the general well-being of the patient support a decision to defer operation. If such defects remain patent in patients who reach the age of 10 to 12 years, the likelihood of spontaneous closure is probably smaller, and surgical repair at that time is usually recommended.

At any age, the presence of pulmonary vascular disease so severe that the pulmonary/systemic resistance ratio is greater than 0.9 is considered a contraindication to operation. If the pulmonary/systemic resistance ratio is between 0.75 and 0.90, operation is generally advised but with the full knowledge of the possibility of an unsatisfactory long-term result.[3] The presence of severe pulmonary hypertension itself is not a contraindication to operation if the pulmonary/systemic resistance ratio is less than 0.75. However, the operation is, in fact, usually not truly curative in older patients with established pulmonary vascular disease.

When aortic valvular incompetence begins to develop in a child with a ventricular septal defect, closure of the defect should be undertaken to prevent further prolapse of the aortic cusps and progression of the aortic incompetence. When coexisting pulmonary infundibular or valvular stenosis is present, the ventricular septal defect is generally large and if the stenosis is severe, right-to-left shunting may be present. In these situations operation is advisable. Mild or moderate mitral incompetence in association with ventricular septal defect is not a contraindication to repair of the defect.

## SURGICAL TREATMENT

### Intracardiac Repair

A midline sternal splitting incision is used, and the pericardium is opened vertically to the level of the left innominate vein. Careful exploration of the pericardial cavity should be performed to determine the presence of a patent ductus arteriosus, a left superior vena cava, and any anomalous pulmonary venous connections. The sizes of the various cardiac chambers are estimated, and the peak systolic pressures in the right and left ventricles and in the pulmonary artery are measured. Prior to insertion of the superior caval cannula through the atrial appendage, the right atrium is digitally examined under tourniquet control (Fig. 8). The presence or absence of an atrial septal defect is noted, and the size and location of the ventricular septal defect are assessed by palpation through the tricuspid valve. The decision for use of an atrial or ventricular approach is made at this time. Generally, an atrial approach is preferred unless the following conditions prevail: the patient is an infant; the ventricular septal defect is felt to be inaccessible through the tricuspid valve; or pulmonary valvular or infundibular stenoses are present that will require correction.

Cardiopulmonary bypass is instituted (32° C.)

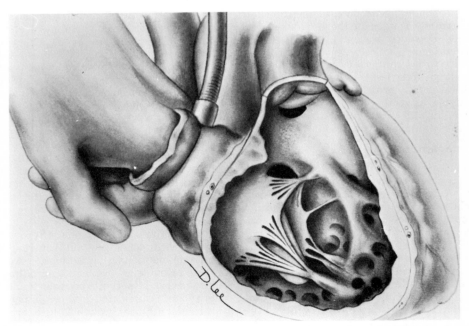

**Figure 8** Before the venous cannula is placed through the right atrial appendage, the left index finger is used to examine the interior of the right atrium and right ventricle. Generally, if the ventricular septal defect can be felt and seems reasonably accessible, the atrial approach is chosen. (From Kirklin, J. W., Karp, R. B., and Bargeron, L. M., Jr. In: Gibbon, J. H. Jr., Sabiston, D. C., Jr., and Spencer, F. C., eds.: Surgery of the Chest. 2nd ed. Philadelphia, W. B. Saunders Company, 1969.)

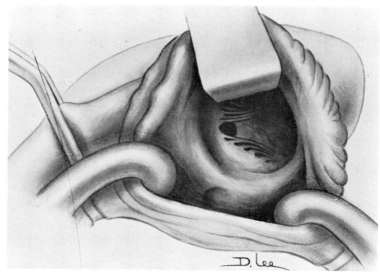

**Figure 9** The atrial approach, illustrated here, allows good exposure for most high ventricular septal defects, muscular defects, and defects of the atrioventricular canal type. Note that the tricuspid valve is not incised to obtain exposure. (From Cartmill, T. B., DuShane, J. W., McGoon, D. C., and Kirklin, J. W.: J. Thorac. Cardiovasc. Surg., 52:486, 1966.)

using two venous cannulas, one in each vena cava, and a catheter in the ascending aorta for arterial return from the pump-oxygenator (see later discussion for the technique in infants). Tapes previously placed around the superior and inferior venae cavae are then secured tightly around the cannulas. For the right atrial approach, the right atrium is opened obliquely between the caval catheters, and a vent is passed across the foramen ovale into the left atrium. The ventricular septal defect is then exposed by retracting the leaflets of the tricuspid valve (Fig. 9). It is not necessary to incise or disconnect the tricuspid valve leaflets. The relations of the defect to the tricuspid valve, to the area of the ventricular septum occupied by the bundle of His, and to the aortic and pulmonary valve cusps are carefully noted. The ventricular septum should be carefully visualized to determine the presence of multiple defects. Repair of the defect is carried out while the aorta is clamped intermittently for 10 to 15 minute intervals, with release of the clamp for 3 minute periods to allow perfusion of the coronary arteries.

Small defects are generally closed by direct suture and large defects are repaired with a patch of Dacron or Teflon cloth. When a patch is to be used, the first stitch is placed between the patch and the edge of the defect at the position most distant from the surgeon. The edge of the patch is sutured to the anterior rim of the ventricular septal defect with continuous sutures. The posterior half of the patch is then sutured to the inferior and posterior edges of the ventricular septal defect. It is in this area that the bundle of His is located. The stitches in the ventricular septum are therefore placed 3 to 4 mm. away from the edge of the defect in order to avoid injury to the conduction system. As the suture line is carried dorsally, the region of the tricuspid anulus is approached. In this area a transition stitch is placed between the septum, the base of the septal leaflet of the tricus-

pid valve, and the patch. Closure of the defect is then completed by suturing the patch to the base of the septal leaflet of the tricuspid valve and extending this suture line superiorly (to the surgeon's left) until the previously placed sutures on the anterior border of the defect are reached (Fig. 10).

When the defect is approached through the right ventricle, a transverse ventriculotomy is made in the location shown in Figure 11a after a vent has been inserted into the left ventricle through the apex. Repair of a high septal defect is similar to that just described except that the first stitch is placed through the posterior portion of the inferior margin of the defect, the base of the septal leaflet of the tricuspid valve, and then through the patch. The repair is carried anteriorly along the inferior border of the defect, the patch being sutured to the ventricular septum and the bites placed 3 to 4 mm. away from the edge of the defect. The repair is completed posteriorly by suturing the edge of the patch to the base of the septal leaflet of the tricuspid valve. Stitches are then placed between the patch and the superior margin of the defect with care to avoid injury to the aortic cusp, which lies beneath.

When the defect is of the supracristal type and lies immediately beneath the pulmonary valve, it is generally oval or triangular in shape and sometimes can be closed by direct suture. There is little danger of damage to the tricuspid valve or the bundle of His in this area. Care must be taken, however, to avoid injury to the aortic and pulmonary valve cusps.

Defects of the atrioventricular canal type, located beneath the septal leaflet of the tricuspid valve, are triangular in shape and must usually be closed with a patch. The patch is sewn into place with continuous sutures that secure it to the base of septal leaflet of the tricuspid valve along one side and to the margins of the ventricular

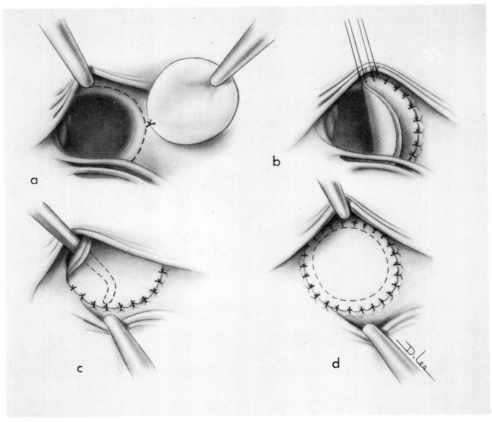

**Figure 10**   Steps in the repair of a large ventricular septal defect through the right atrium. The leaflets and chordae are retracted to provide visualization. Before the suture line is completed, a fine probe is used to detect any residual apertures, and any found are closed with additional sutures. (From Cartmill, T. B., DuShane, J. W., McGoon, D. C., and Kirklin, J. W.: J. Thorac. Cardiovasc. Surg., *52*:486, 1966.)

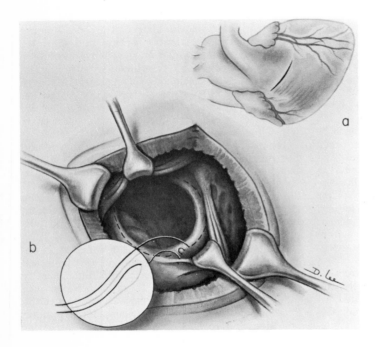

**Figure 11**   In infants, the right ventricular approach is usually employed for high defects; the transverse right ventriculotomy incision is illustrated (*a*). In *b*, the first stitch for the repair has been placed. This stitch is carried anteriorly along the dotted line and then to the left and anteriorly along the dotted line to the other side to complete the repair. (From Cartmill, T. B., DuShane, J. W., McGoon, D. C., and Kirklin, J. W.: J. Thorac. Cardiovasc. Surg., *52*:486, 1966.)

septal defect along the other two sides. When the patch is sutured to the posterior margin, the stitches should be placed well away from the edge of the defect to avoid injury to the conduction system. The cardiac rhythm must be carefully monitored during repair of this type of defect, since the location of the bundle of His is not as consistent in relation to the margins of the defect as it is with the high ventricular septal defect.

Defects in the muscular portion of the septum can usually be closed by direct suture. If these defects lie far anteriorly, it is best to place the sutures from outside the right ventricle, grasping the edges of the defect and bringing the stitch again outside the heart to be tied on the surface.

If pulmonary infundibular or valvular stenosis exists with the ventricular septal defect, valvotomy and resection of the infundibular muscle are performed prior to repair of the defect. If aortic incompetence exists in association with a ventricular septal defect and is severe enough to require replacement of the valve, the operation is performed through an incision in the proximal ascending aorta that extends into the noncoronary sinus of the aortic valve. The aortic valve leaflets are then excised and cannulas are inserted into the coronary ostia for their continuous perfusion. The ventricular septal defect can generally be closed with interrupted sutures, although occasionally a patch may be required. Care must be taken to avoid injury to the conduction system, which may lie in close proximity to the edges of the defect. After the defect has been closed, the aortic valve is replaced with an aortic allograft, by means of a standard technique.[5, 12]

Intracardiac repair of ventricular septal defects in infants less than 1 year old presents special problems because of the small size of the structures and because of the tendency to postoperative pulmonary complications. More or less standard perfusion techniques are used with satisfaction by some surgeons in this special situation,[26] but recently a combination of surface cooling, total circulatory arrest during the repair, and rewarming with cardiopulmonary bypass has been popularized for intracardiac surgery in infants.[1] At present we employ this technique for repair of ventricular septal defects in infants less than 1 year of age, primarily because the perfusion time is short and the technical aspects of the repair are facilitated by the superb exposure during total circulatory arrest.

### Pulmonary Arterial Banding

Although at present we rarely use the technique of banding of the pulmonary artery, it is employed still by some groups in managing infants with severe heart failure from ventricular septal defect.

A left anterolateral thoracotomy incision in the third intercostal space is employed. The pericardium overlying the pulmonary artery is incised longitudinally, and a plane is developed between the pulmonary artery and the aorta. A band of synthetic cloth (Dacron or Teflon) is passed through the aperture behind the pulmonary artery. The ends of the band are then placed in a right-angle clamp anteriorly and traction is placed on the band to produce the desired amount of constriction of the pulmonary artery. In such infants an indwelling arterial needle is helpful. As the band is tightened, the arterial blood pressure rises; but when the band is too tight, bradycardia and cardiac dilation occur. In addition, a fall in peripheral arterial oxygen saturation occurs as a result of the production of some right-to-left shunting as the pulmonary artery is constricted. Ideally, a pulmonary artery pressure of 30 to 50 mm. Hg distal to the band with an adequate systemic pressure is optimal. Once the desired level of constriction of the artery has been achieved by the right-angle clamp, the clamp is released slightly and horizontal mattress sutures are placed through the edges of the band to secure it at the desired level. The edges of the pericardium are then approximated and the thoracotomy incision is closed in the usual fashion. One small tube is left in the pleural cavity for drainage.

## POSTOPERATIVE CARE

Although the outcome of operation for closure of the ventricular septal defect is determined largely by events in the operating room and by proper preoperative selection of patients, the postoperative care is also of importance, particularly in infants.

Optimal cardiac performance is obtained by avoiding excessive trauma to the heart during operation and by maintaining adequate ventricular end-diastolic pressure and blood volume early after operation. Fine polyvinyl catheters in the left and right atria are used to monitor atrial pressures for the first 24 hours after operation. If the cardiac output is greater than about 3.0 liters per minute per square meter (by measurement or clinical estimate), the left atrial pressure should be kept low (6 to 10 mm. Hg). If the cardiac output is less, maintenance of left atrial pressure at 10 to 15 mm. Hg by infusion of blood will often improve cardiac output by increasing preload (the stretch of the sarcomeres at end-diastole). If blood infusion does not produce the desired effect, if the presence of cardiac tamponade can be excluded, and if the reduction in cardiac output is not severe (cardiac index > 2.2 and < 3.0), administration of digitalis is indicated. Digoxin is the drug of choice, since it can be given intravenously, intramuscularly, or orally and its onset of action and rate of elimination are reasonably rapid. In situations in which there is acute and severe depression of cardiac output, isoproterenol or epinephrine should be administered intravenously to improve myocardial contractility.

Ventilation is usually assisted for a few hours after operation with a positive-pressure ventilator and an endotracheal tube. In most patients, this can be discontinued within a few hours after operation. If the cardiac output is low or pulmonary dysfunction is present, ventilatory assistance via the endotracheal tube is continued for 24 to 36 hours. Infants require particular care of the respiratory subsystem in the early postoperative period, for success or failure in that group of patients is largely dependent upon the skill in managing assisted ventilation and clearing of the airway.

Urine flow is usually adequate after operation, particularly when some degree of hemodilution of the perfusate has been employed. In those unusual situations in which cardiac output is low and oliguria is present, an infusion of mannitol is indicated. If this does not produce the desired increase in urine output, infusion of a potent diuretic such as ethacrynic acid should be considered.

Excessive postoperative bleeding following surgical treatment of ventricular septal defect is quite unusual. When drainage from the chest tubes in the early postoperative period is excessive, reoperation is indicated. Generally, no specific bleeding point is found, but the evacuation of clotted blood is advantageous. With very small children and infants, reoperation would be indicated after smaller amounts of chest drainage.

## RESULTS OF SURGICAL TREATMENT

### Hospital Mortality

Hospital mortality rates and complications are directly related to the preoperative condition of the patient and to the conduct of the operative procedure (Table 2). At the present time, the risk for repair of small or moderate-sized ventricular septal defects and of large ventricular septal defects with mild pulmonary vascular disease is approximately 1 per cent. Properly selected patients with moderate or severe pulmonary vascular disease can be operated upon with a risk of less than 10 per cent.

In the past, operative mortality has been high following complete repair of ventricular septal de-

**TABLE 2**  HOSPITAL MORTALITY AFTER REPAIR OF VENTRICULAR SEPTAL DEFECT IN PATIENTS MORE THAN 6 MONTHS OF AGE*

| Category | Patients | Hospital Deaths No. | % |
|---|---|---|---|
| $P_p/P_s$ <0.45 | 108 | 0 | 0 |
| $P_p/P_s$  0.45–0.75 | 40 | 0 | 0 |
| $P_p/P_s$ > 0.75 | | | |
| $R_p/R_s$ < 0.45 | 50 | 3 | 6 |
| $R_p/R_s$  0.45–0.75 | 39 | 2 | 5 |
| $R_p/R_s$ > 0.75 | 6 | 1 | 17 |
| $P_p$ < 40 mm. Hg. | 13 | 0 | 0 |
| $P_{rv}/P_{lv}$ > 0.75 | | | |
| Totals | 256 | 6 | 2 |

*1962 through 1965. From Cartmill, T. B., DuShane, J. W., McGoon, D. C., and Kirklin, J. W.: J. Thorac. Cardiovasc. Surg., 52:486, 1966.

fects in infants less than 6 months of age. Recent experiences suggest that a low mortality rate (perhaps 10 per cent) can be achieved even in these sick small babies.[1] Mortality rates in older infants have been low for some years now, being approximately 5 per cent in children between 6 months and 2 years of age.[14, 21]

### Heart Block

Although permanent heart block occurred in a large percentage of patients after repair of ventricular septal defect in the early years when the operation was performed, this complication is quite unusual at present. In one group of 256 patients in whom closure of ventricular septal defects was performed between 1962 and 1965, permanent heart block did not occur in a single instance.[3] If heart block should occur at the time of operation, temporary ventricular pacing wires should be placed and connected to an external pacing unit. If heart block persists in the postoperative period, a permanent pacing unit can then be inserted when the patient has sufficiently recovered from the initial operative procedure.

### Incomplete Repair

With standardization of the operative technique, and with the use of synthetic patch material to close moderate-sized or large ventricular septal defects, the incidence of persistent or recurrent shunts approximates 10 per cent or less.[3]

### Resolution of Pulmonary Vascular Disease

The late results of the surgical treatment of ventricular septal defects in patients with abnormally elevated pulmonary vascular resistance are dependent not only upon the closure of the ventricular septal defect but also upon the behavior of the pulmonary vasculature.[3, 21]

Patients with mild elevation of pulmonary vascular resistance (pulmonary to systemic resistance ratios of less than 0.45) have for the most part shown a decline or no increase in the pulmonary vascular resistance after operation. About one-third of the patients over 2 years of age at the time of operation with moderate pulmonary vascular disease (pulmonary to systemic resistance ratios between 0.45 and 0.75) have no change in pulmonary vascular resistance 2 to 5 years after operation. Unfortunately, about one-third of patients with moderate elevation of pulmonary vascular resistance preoperatively have a progressive increase in pulmonary vascular resistance late in the postoperative period. These patients and approximately two-thirds of those patients with severe pulmonary vascular disease preoperatively (pulmonary to systemic resistance ratios of greater than 0.75) do not have a satisfactory long-term prognosis because of the severity of the pulmonary hypertension at rest and the pulmonary vascular disease. With exercise, such patients have a restriction of cardiac output because of the obstructive pulmonary vascular disease. If these patients

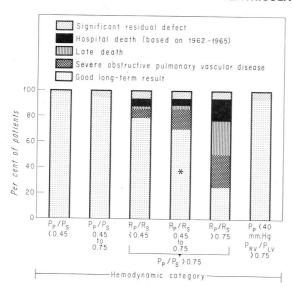

**Figure 12** Composite results of repair of ventricular septal defect in patients more than 6 months of age. (From Cartmill, T. B., DuShane, J. W., McGoon, D. C., and Kirklin, J. W.: J. Thorac. Cardiovasc. Surg., 52:486, 1966.)

could be identified with certainty preoperatively, it would be preferable to avoid operating on them.

Progression of pulmonary vascular disease seems to be uncommon when the ventricular septal defect is repaired before the age of 2 years.[4] This is one of the reasons for advising closure of ventricular septal defects in infants less than 2 years of age when there is increasing elevation of pulmonary vascular resistance.

### Overall Results

The overall results of the surgical treatment of patients with ventricular septal defects in the various categories outlined previously are indicated in Figure 12. The results are excellent in most patients with small or moderate-sized ventricular septal defects and in patients with ventricular septal defects and pulmonary stenosis. Satisfactory results have also been obtained in patients with ventricular septal defects and aortic valve incompetence in which the aortic valve is replaced with an aortic allograft.[5, 27] Nearly all patients with large ventricular septal defects and mild elevation of pulmonary vascular resistance have an excellent prognosis. Patients with large ventricular septal defects and moderate elevation of pulmonary vascular resistance may have an excellent long-term prognosis, but progressively more severe pulmonary vascular disease develops in about one-third of those over 2 years of age at the time of operation. Those patients who preoperatively have severe elevation of pulmonary vascular resistance have a high incidence of unsatisfactory results.

The results appear to be particularly favorable when the ventricular septal defect is repaired during the first 2 years of life.

## SELECTED REFERENCES

Becu, L. M., Fontana, R. S., DuShane, J. W., Kirklin, J. W., Burchell, H. B., and Edwards, J. E.: Anatomic and pathologic studies in ventricular septal defect. Circulation, 14:349, 1956.
*This paper analyzes in detail the anatomic features of ventricular septal defects in 50 hearts examined at autopsy. The precise anatomic relationships of the various types of septal defects to adjacent structures are outlined, and the defects are divided into two major groups according to their location, either in the inflow or the outflow portion of the right ventricle. In addition, the coexisting congenital anomalies of the cardiovascular system are tabulated. Although a subsequent classification (see text) has proved more useful from the surgical standpoint, the relationships of the various types of septal defects to the surrounding structures described in this paper are important to surgeons in particular.*

Cartmill, T. B., DuShane, J. W., McGoon, D. C., and Kirklin, J. W.: Results of repair of ventricular septal defect. J. Thorac. Cardiovasc. Surg., 52:486, 1966.
*This is a review of 447 patients having complete repair of ventricular septal defect during a 5 year period (1960 to 1965) at one institution. The patients are categorized according to the severity of the preoperative pulmonary hypertension and the pulmonary vascular resistance as compared to the systemic vascular resistance. In addition, particular emphasis is placed on the changes in pulmonary vascular resistance that occur as a result of surgical closure of the defects. The studies indicate that in some patients with only mild increase in pulmonary vascular resistance preoperatively, severe obstructive pulmonary vascular disease developed after operation. In 20 per cent of the patients with moderate elevations in pulmonary to systemic resistance, increased pulmonary vascular disease developed after operation. With these findings as the basis, specific indications for operative intervention in patients with ventricular septal defects are outlined.*

Hoffman, J. I. E., and Rudolph, A. M.: The natural history of isolated ventricular septal defect with special reference to selection of patients for surgery. Advances Pediat., 17:57, 1970.
*This excellent article contains an enormous amount of information regarding the natural history of patients with isolated ventricular septal defect. It deals extensively with the problems related to the severity of the disease, the frequency and the time course of spontaneous closure of ventricular septal defects, the incidence and importance of pulmonary vascular disease, and the changes in pulmonary vascular resistance that occur after surgical closure. In addition, a program is outlined for the management of patients with ventricular septal defect, particularly infants, and the indications for operative intervention are given.*

Leatham, A., and Segal, B.: Auscultatory and phonocardiographic signs of ventricular septal defect with left to right shunt. Circulation, 25:318, 1962.
*The auscultatory and phonocardiographic signs of ventricular septal defects in 23 patients with left-to-right shunts and normal or slightly elevated pulmonary vascular resistance were carefully correlated in this study. The origin of the systolic murmurs in such patients is discussed, and a mechanism for the widely split second heart sound present in the majority of the patients is proposed.*

Levin, A. R., Spach, M. S., Canent, R. V., Jr., Boineau, J. P., Capp, M. P., Jain, V., and Barr, R. C.: Intracardiac pressure-flow dynamics in isolated ventricular septal defects. Circulation, 35:430, 1967.
*This study characterizes the nature of intracardiac shunting in 50 children between the ages of 3 and 15 years with isolated ventricular septal defects. Intraventricular pressure measurements and biplane cineangiocardiography were utilized to study the timing and the direction of flow across the defects during the cardiac cycle. Patients with moderately elevated right ventricular pressures demonstrated left-to-right shunting across the defect throughout the cardiac cycle. When pressure in the right ventricle approximated that in the left, left-to-right shunting occurred across the defect into the left ventricle during isovolumic relaxation. All patients showed a predominant left-to-right pressure gradient and shunt across the defect into the right ventricle during diastole*

*and increase of the left-to-right pressure gradient with resultant increase of the shunt into the right ventricle during isovolumic contraction immediately before the aortic valve opened. During ventricular ejection and isovolumic relaxation, the pressure-flow relationships are affected significantly by the size of the defect and the ratio of the pulmonary to systemic vascular resistance.*

Wagenvoort, C. A., Neufeld, H. N., DuShane, J. W., and Edwards, J. E.: The pulmonary arterial tree in ventricular septal defect. A quantitative study of anatomic features in fetuses, infants and children. Circulation, 23:740, 1961.

*This paper is an anatomic study of the pulmonary arterial tree of 50 fetuses, infants, and children with uncomplicated ventricular septal defect. A detailed analysis of the pulmonary arterial medial thickness and the index of medial surface area (the ratio of medial tissue to pulmonary parenchyma) was carried out. During the fetal and newborn period, both the thickness and the index of surface area of the media were generally within normal limits. The subjects between 1 and 5 weeks of age had a medial thickness and an index of medial surface area that were lower than the average values at the time of birth. In this regard, the pulmonary arterial tree in cases of ventricular septal defect was similar to that from normal newborn infants. Soon after this period, however, and particularly from 8 weeks of age on, the subjects with ventricular septal defects showed a pronounced rise both in the medial thickness and in the index of medial surface area, indicating the presence of considerable medial hypertrophy. These findings correlate closely with the development of pulmonary hypertension and with the clinical findings in patients with ventricular septal defects.*

## REFERENCES

1. Barratt-Boyes, B. G., Simpson, M., and Neutze, J. M.: Intracardiac surgery in neonates and infants using deep hypothermia and limited cardiopulmonary bypass. Circulation, Supp. 1, 43:25, 1970.
2. Becu, L. M., Fontana, R. S., DuShane, J. W., Kirklin, J. W., Burchell, H. B., and Edwards, J. E.: Anatomic and pathologic studies in ventricular septal defect. Circulation, 14:349, 1956.
3. Cartmill, T. B., DuShane, J. W., McGoon, D. C., and Kirklin, J. W.: Results of repair of ventricular septal defect. J. Thorac. Cardiovasc. Surg., 52:486, 1966.
4. Ching, E., DuShane, J. W., McGoon, D. C., and Danielson, G. K.: Total correction of ventricular septal defect in infancy using extracorporeal circulation. Ann. Thorac. Surg., 12:1, 1971.
5. Gonzalez-Lavin, L., and Barratt-Boyes, B. G.: Surgical considerations in the treatment of ventricular septal defect associated with aortic valvular incompetence. J. Thorac. Cardiovasc. Surg., 57:422, 1969.
6. Heath, D., and Edwards, J. E.: The pathology of hypertensive pulmonary vascular disease. A description of six grades of structural changes in the pulmonary arteries with special reference to congenital cardiac septal defects. Circulation, 18:533, 1958.
7. Heath, D., Helmholz, H. F., Jr., Burchell, H. B., DuShane, J. W., and Edwards, J. E.: Graded pulmonary vascular changes and hemodynamic findings in cases of atrial and ventricular septal defect and patent ductus arteriosus. Circulation, 18:1155, 1958.
8. Hoffman, J. I. E.: Natural history of congenital heart disease: Problems in its assessment with special reference to ventricular septal defect. Circulation, 37:97, 1968.
9. Hoffman, J. I. E., and Rudolph, A. M.: The natural history of isolated ventricular septal defect with special reference to selection of patients for surgery. Advances Pediat., 17:57, 1970.
10. Hunt, C. E., Formanek, G., Levine, M. A., Castenada, A., and Moller, J. A.: Banding of the pulmonary artery. Results in 111 children. Circulation, 43:395, 1971.
11. Jarmakani, M. M., Edwards, S. B., Spach, M. S., Canent, R. V., Jr., Capp, M. P., Hagan, M. J., Barr, R. C., and Jain, V.: Left ventricular pressure-volume characteristics in congenital heart disease. Circulation, 37:879, 1968.
12. Karp, R. B., and Kirklin, J. W.: Replacement of diseased aortic valves with homografts. Ann. Surg., 169:921, 1969.
13. Keck, E. W. O., Ongley, P. A., Kincaid, O. W., and Swan, H. J. C.: Ventricular septal defect with aortic insufficiency. A clinical and hemodynamic study of 18 proved cases. Circulation, 27:203, 1963.
14. Kirklin, J. W., and DuShane, J. W.: Repair of ventricular septal defect in infancy. Pediatrics, 27:961, 1961.
15. Kirklin, J. W., DuShane, J. W., Patrick, R. T., Donald, D. E., Hetzel, P. S., Harshbarger, H. G., and Wood, E. H.: Intracardiac surgery with the aid of a mechanical pump-oxygenator system (Gibbon type): Report of eight cases. Proc. Mayo Clin., 30:201, 1955.
16. Kirklin, J. W., Harshbarger, H. G., Donald, D. E., and Edwards, J. E.: Surgical correction of ventricular septal defect: Anatomic and technical considerations. J. Thorac. Surg., 33:45, 1957.
17. Leatham, A., and Segal, B.: Auscultatory and phonocardiographic signs of ventricular septal defect with left to right shunt. Circulation, 25:318, 1962.
18. Levin, A. R., Spach, M. S., Canent, R. V., Jr., Boineau, J. P., Capp, M. P., Jain, V., and Barr, R. C.: Intracardiac pressure-flow dynamics in isolated ventricular septal defects. Circulation, 35:430, 1967.
19. Lillehei, C. W., Cohen, M., Warden, H. E., Ziegler, N., and Varco, R. L.: The results of direct vision closure of ventricular septal defects in eight patients by means of controlled cross circulation. Surg. Gynec. Obstet., 101:446, 1955.
20. Lillehei, C. W., DeWall, R. A., Read, R. C., Warden, H. E., and Varco, R. L.: Direct vision intracardiac surgery in man using a simple disposable artificial oxygenator. Dis. Chest, 29:1, 1956.
21. Lillehei, C. W., Levy, M. J., Adams, P., and Anderson, R. C.: High-pressure ventricular septal defects. J.A.M.A., 188:949, 1964.
22. Morgan, B. C., Griffiths, S. P., and Blumenthal, S.: Ventricular septal defect. I. Congestive heart failure in infancy. Pediatrics, 25:54, 1960.
23. Muller, W. H., Jr., and Dammann, J. F., Jr.: The treatment of certain congenital malformations of the heart by the creation of pulmonic stenosis to reduce pulmonary hypertension and excessive pulmonary flow. A preliminary report. Surg. Gynec. Obstet., 95:213, 1952.
24. Nadas, A. S., Thilenius, O. G., La Farge, C. G., and Hauck, A. J.: Ventricular septal defect with aortic regurgitation. Medical and pathologic aspects. Circulation, 29:862, 1964.
25. Shah, P., Singh, W. S. A., Rose, V., and Keith, J.: Incidence of bacterial endocarditis in ventricular septal defects. Circulation, 34:127, 1966.
26. Sigmann, J. M., Stern, A. M., and Sloan, H. E.: Early surgical correction of large ventricular septal defects. Pediatrics, 39:1, 1967.
27. Somerville, J., Brandao, A., and Ross, D. N.: Aortic regurgitation with ventricular septal defect. Surgical management and clinical features. Circulation, 41:317, 1970.
28. Stark, J., Aberdeen, E., Waterston, D. J., Bonham-Carter, R. E., and Tynan, M.: Pulmonary artery constriction (banding): A report of 146 cases. Surgery, 65:808, 1969.
29. Van Praagh, R., McNamara, J. J., and Gross, R. E.: Anatomic types of ventricular septal defect with aortic insufficiency. Circulation, Supp. 2, 36:256, 1967.
30. Wagenvoort, C. A., Neufeld, H. N., DuShane, J. W., and Edwards, J. E.: The pulmonary arterial tree in ventricular septal defect. A quantitative study of anatomic features in fetuses, infants and children. Circulation, 23:740, 1961.

# VII

# The Tetralogy of Fallot

*David C. Sabiston, Jr., M.D.*

The tetralogy of Fallot is one of the most frequent of the serious congenital cardiac malformations commonly accompanied by cyanosis. Of further significance is the fact that it was among the first of the congenital heart lesions to yield to a highly successful palliative operation. A landmark in cardiac surgery was established in 1944 by Blalock and Taussig when the first successful systemic-pulmonary artery anastomosis was performed. Since then a corrective procedure employing extracorporeal circulation has been developed, and the surgical treatment of tetralogy of Fallot is now one of the most satisfactory in cardiac surgery.

## HISTORICAL ASPECTS

There are a number of early descriptions of the tetralogy of Fallot, including those of Stensen (1672),[53] Sandifort (1777),[51] John Hunter (1783),[32] William Hunter (1784),[33] Farre (1814),[19] Gintrac (1824),[21] Hope (1839),[31] and Peacock (1866).[44] However, the most notable contribution was that of Étienne-Louis Arthur Fallot of Marseille, who in 1888 clearly described the clinical and pathological aspects. In these communications, Fallot referred to previously reported cases but emphasized the clinical manifestations of the malformation *during life*. His original communications appeared under the title "Contribution à l'anatomie pathologique de la maladie bleue (cyanose cardiaque)."[18] In translation, the following is Fallot's own description of the now famous *tetralogy*:

"This malformation consists of a true anatomopathological type represented by the following tetralogy: (1) stenosis of the pulmonary artery; (2) interventricular communication; (3) deviation of the origin of the aorta to the right; (4) hypertrophy, almost always concentric, of the right ventricle. Failure of obliteration of the foramen ovale may occasionally be added in a wholly accessory manner."

In his descriptions, Fallot reported 55 cases of congenital heart disease of which 74 per cent were of the tetralogy type. It is remarkable that such a large number of cases could have been reported by a single author at that time.

In 1944, Blalock operated upon a severely ill infant with tetralogy of Fallot and established a subclavian-pulmonary anastomosis.[6] The child greatly benefited from the procedure and this operation heralded the onset of a wide variety of additional cardiac procedures that were to follow. The first open correction of the tetralogy of Fallot was performed by Scott (1954), employing arrested circulation with hypothermia;[52] following the advent of extracorporeal circulation, the scope of intercardiac surgery advanced greatly. Open correction using cardiopulmonary bypass was first performed by Lillehei in 1955.[38] Although the mortality was originally quite high, it has progressively diminished.

## ANATOMY

In the original description, Fallot emphasized *four* primary anatomic points, including pulmonary stenosis, ventricular septal defect, dextroposition of the aorta, hypertrophy of the right ventricle. However, it is now recognized by most that the two most *important* features of the tetralogy of Fallot are (1) the right ventricular outflow tract obstruction (infundibular), and (2) the ventricular septal defect. The overriding of the aorta is related to the location of the ventricular septal defect, and the right ventricular hypertrophy is a secondary phenomenon due to the outflow tract obstruction of the right ventricle. Emphasis should be placed upon the fact that there is a wide variation in the spectrum of the severity of the anatomic malformations in the tetralogy of Fallot.[34] The wide differences in the severity of these components have led some to urge discontinuance of the term "tetralogy of Fallot." However, from the view of both diagnosis and surgical management, the term continues to have sufficient usefulness to justify its retention. In general, a working definition of the tetralogy includes the basic principle that it is a congenital cardiac malformation with a ventricular septal defect, the size of which approximates the aortic orifice, and with pulmonary stenosis of such a degree that approximately equal pressures result in both ventricles. In addition, there are varying degrees of dextroposition (or overriding) of the aorta. Moreover, the degree and nature of the infundibular pulmonary stenosis may be quite variable. Several types of infundibular chambers have been described, depending mostly upon the size of the chamber.[9,10] Thus, the infundibular chamber may be quite small when the outflow tract obstruction is near the pulmonary valve. At the opposite extreme, the muscular obstruction in the outflow tract may be quite proximally situated, resulting in a large infundibular chamber sometimes called a "third ventricle." Moreover, *stenosis* of the pulmonary valve is common, occurring in as many as one-third of patients with tetralogy of Fallot in addition to infundibular stenosis. Occasionally, the stenosis is confined solely to the pulmonary valve without the presence of infundibular obstruction.

It becomes apparent that from the physiologic point of view the majority of patients with tetralogy of Fallot exhibit a high resistance to right ventricular emptying owing to pulmonary stenosis. Therefore, the predominant shunt is from right-to-left, with flow across the ventricular defect into the aorta. This produces cyanosis and results in elevation of the hematocrit. In those instances in which the pulmonary stenosis is less severe, bidirectional shunting may occur. In some patients, the infundibular stenosis is minimal, and the predominant shunt is left-to-right, producing what is termed clinically "the pink tetralogy." Although such patients may not appear cyanotic, they may have slight oxygen desaturation in the systemic arterial blood.

Occasionally, no communication exists between the right ventricle and the pulmonary artery. In these patients, the outflow tract of the right ventricle or the pulmonary valve is *atretic*. The pulmonary valve ring and main pulmonary artery are often quite small, although the left and right branches may be of significant size. Such infants exhibit severe symptoms and usually require operation early in life. It has also been recognized that some patients with a previous systemic-pulmonary anastomosis may experience a progression of the outflow tract obstruction in the right ventricle. Thus, the infundibular stenosis or valvar stenosis may become more severe and can become total, representing an *acquired* lesion. Under these circumstances, life is maintained solely by a previous systemic-pulmonary shunt with additional help from collateral bronchial arterial circulation.[50]

# DIAGNOSIS

## Clinical Manifestations

Experience has shown that the clinical manifestations of the tetralogy of Fallot vary with the severity of the anatomic malformation. Infants with pulmonary atresia manifest distress shortly after birth and usually succumb unless operation is performed. Cyanosis is common, especially with crying. In most children, cyanosis is *not* present *at birth*, probably because of a persistent ductus arteriosus. As the child grows older, dyspnea on exertion usually follows, and a characteristic position *(squatting)* is assumed by the great majority of these patients to relieve fatigue. This position has diagnostic significance and is highly characteristic of the tetralogy of Fallot. It usually produces an increase in systemic arterial oxygen saturation.

Some patients with pulmonary atresia may present desperate problems in infancy. At the opposite end of the spectrum, rare instances of longevity with a reasonably normal life have been reported. One interesting example is that of an American composer, Gilbert, who lived to the age of 60 with tetralogy of Fallot and who led a relatively productive life without surgery.[58] Such a history is obviously rare. Statistics show that of the entire group of patients with tetralogy of Fallot half reach the age of 7, one-fifth reach age 14, and not more than one-tenth survive to age 21 in the absence of operative intervention.[11]

## Physical Examination

Cyanosis of the lips and nail beds is usually apparent, and the patient may appear to be smaller than expected for his or her age. The fingers and toes usually show clubbing (hypertrophic pulmonary osteoarthropathy). On palpation of the chest, a thrill is usually present anteriorly. A harsh systolic murmur is audible over the pulmonary area and along the left sternal border. Absence of a murmur in a patient suspected of having the tetralogy is suggestive of pulmonary atresia.

## Roentgenograms

The chest film in the tetralogy of Fallot usually shows diminished vascularity in the lungs and

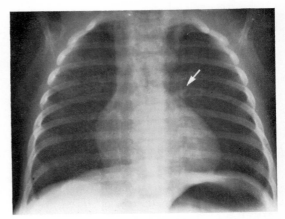

**Figure 1**   Chest film of infant with tetralogy of Fallot. Note diminished vascular markings in the lungs and reduced prominence of the pulmonary artery shadow. (From Sabiston, D. C., Jr. In: Gibbon, J. H., Jr., Sabiston, D. C., Jr., and Spencer, F. C., eds.: Surgery of the Chest. 2nd ed. Philadelphia, W. B. Saunders Company, 1969.)

absence of prominence of the pulmonary artery. In the early stages, the chest film may be entirely normal. The shadow of the great vessels in the superior mediastinum is narrow, owing to the diminished caliber of the pulmonary artery. If cyanosis and dyspnea are quite prominent, the pulmonary vascular markings are usually markedly diminished. Later, the classic boot-shaped heart (coeur en sabot) may develop and is recognized as a hallmark of the tetralogy of Fallot (Fig. 1). Diminution or absence of pulsations in the pulmonary arteries can be demonstrated by fluoroscopy. Right ventricular enlargement is present and is best demonstrated in the left anterior oblique position. The barium swallow provides evidence of the side on which the aortic arch descends. This is of considerable importance, since approximately one-fourth of the patients with tetralogy of Fallot have a *right* aortic arch. In fact, the presence of a right aortic arch with cyanosis is strong evidence that the malformation is indeed tetralogy of Fallot.

## Blood Studies

An elevation in the hemoglobin, hematocrit, and erythrocyte count is usually present. The magnitude of hemoconcentration is directly proportional to the cyanosis. Hematocrit values may vary from normal to as high as 90 per cent, the majority being between 50 and 70 per cent. The erythrocyte count varies between normal and a high of 12,000,000. Similarly, the oxygen saturation in the systemic arterial blood is variable, usually between 65 and 70 per cent. However, in severe forms of the malformation, the arterial oxygen saturation during exercise may fall as low as 25 per cent. It has been recognized that a bleeding tendency is present in many patients with the tetralogy of Fallot, especially those in whom cyanosis is intense. In the various studies that have been performed on these patients, the usual finding is a diminution in a variety of the factors responsible for blood coagulation, but none of the factors are reduced to critical levels. The platelet count and total blood fibrinogen are frequently slightly diminished, and clot retraction is sometimes poor and associated with prolonged prothrombin and coagulation times. Despite the defects in the clotting mechanism in some patients, the changes are usually insufficient to explain the hemorrhagic tendency noted at the time of operation.[29, 45]

### Electrocardiogram

The electrocardiogram usually shows right ventricular hypertrophy. This is usually apparent in the standard leads and is most consistently found in the unipolar leads. The more commonly encountered findings include tall and peaked T waves, reversal of the RS ratio, and a normal PR interval and QRS duration. It is to be emphasized that if right ventricular hypertrophy is absent, the diagnosis of tetralogy of Fallot should be seriously doubted.

### Angiocardiograms

The angiocardiogram is of great importance in establishing the diagnosis. Moreover, it demonstrates objectively the magnitude of pulmonary stenosis and the size of the pulmonary arteries (Fig. 2). The ventricular septal defect and overriding of the aorta are also shown (Fig. 3). An atrial septal defect may also be present. Occasionally, only one pulmonary artery is present, and in nearly all patients with a single artery, it is the left one that is absent.

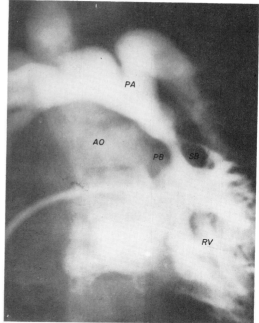

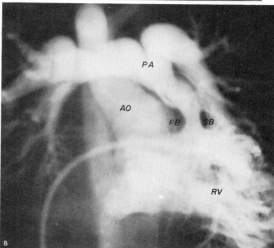

Figure 3  Obstruction in the region of the infundibulum. *A*, Frame made in systole. *B*, Frame made in diastole. The negative shadows of the hypertrophied parietal (PB) and septal (SB) bands are particularly well demonstrated. The pulmonary valve appears domed, and at operation was bicuspid, but not stenotic. The aorta (AO) is opacified by this right ventricular injection and its diameter is three times that of the pulmonary artery. The underdevelopment of the infundibulum of the right ventricle, a basic characteristic of the tetralogy of Fallot, is apparent in this angiocardiogram. RV = right ventricle; PA = pulmonary artery. (From Kirklin, J. W., and Karp, R. B.: The Tetralogy of Fallot from a Surgical Viewpoint. Philadelphia, W. B. Saunders Company, 1970.)

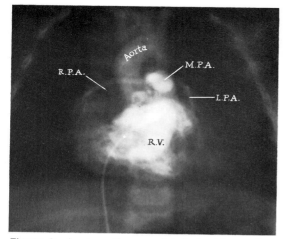

Figure 2  Angiocardiogram of infant with tetralogy of Fallot in whom pulmonary arteries are very small. An ascending aorta–right pulmonary artery anastomosis (Waterston) was performed because of serious symptoms. The infant greatly benefited from the procedure. (From Sabiston, D. C., Jr. In: Gibbon, J. H., Jr., Sabiston, D. C., Jr., and Spencer, F. C., eds.: Surgery of the Chest. 2nd ed. Philadelphia, W. B. Saunders Company, 1969.)

### Cardiac Catheterization

Much valuable information is provided by cardiac catheterization (Fig. 4). The presence of equal pressures in both ventricles distinguishes the con-

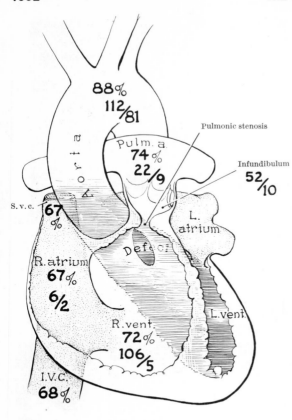

Pulmonic stenosis

Infundibulum

**Figure 4**  Diagram of results obtained at cardiac catheterization in patient with tetralogy of Fallot. This patient has a relatively high arterial oxygen saturation and represents one of the less severe anatomic types. Values for oxygen are expressed as percentage saturation. The pressures are given in millimeters of mercury. (From Sabiston, D. C., Jr., and Blalock, A. In: Derra, E., ed.: Encyclopedia of Thoracic Surgery. Heidelberg, Springer-Verlag, 1959.)

dition from isolated valvar pulmonary stenosis, in which the pressures in the right ventricle may be considerably greater than those in the left ventricle. Tracings also establish the level of right ventricular outflow tract obstruction and the presence of valvar stenosis.

## INDICATIONS FOR OPERATION

Nearly all patients with tetralogy of Fallot should be considered candidates for surgical correction. Since wide variations occur in the clinical manifestations, management must be individualized, especially the timing of operation. If surgery is indicated during the first 2 years of life, most recommend a systemic-pulmonary anastomosis, although corrective procedures have been performed during this period.[4] For patients between the ages of 3 and 5, the choice of operation is more debatable. Some recommend open correction, and acceptable morbidity and mortality results are available to support this position.[14] Many continue to perform systemic-pulmonary anastomoses in patients up to age 5. In older children, open correction is advised for nearly all those requiring surgical treatment.

## SURGICAL TECHNIQUE

The most versatile and frequently employed of the *shunt* operations is systemic-pulmonary anastomosis. This procedure has its maximal usefulness in the patient requiring operation between the ages of 2 and 5 years (Blalock and Taussig;[6] Blalock[5]). The result is an increase in blood flow to the lungs. An alternate technique is an anastomosis between the descending aorta and the left pulmonary artery (Potts operation),[47] a procedure used infrequently today, since enlargement of the anastomosis is more likely, producing an excessive shunt with pulmonary hypertension and aneurysm formation.[48,54] Moreover, a Potts anastomosis is more difficult to close at the time of subsequent correction. The use of an ascending aorta–right pulmonary artery anastomosis (Waterston) is usually recommended in young infants who require operation during the first several months of life.[57]

For a *subclavian-pulmonary anastomosis (Blalock-Taussig)*, the incision is generally made on the side opposite that on which the aorta descends (Fig. 5). In the majority of patients, the incision is made on the right side, since the aorta most often descends on the left. When the aorta descends on the right (20 to 25 per cent), the incision is made on the left. Ideally the subclavian branch of the innominate artery is used for the anastomosis because the angle produced at its origin from its parent vessel is better than that formed when the subclavian artery is used, as shown in Figure 6.[49] The latter arises directly from the aorta and is apt to kink at its origin when deflected inferiorly for anastomosis to the pulmonary artery. Experimental studies have shown that approximately three-fourths of the blood passing

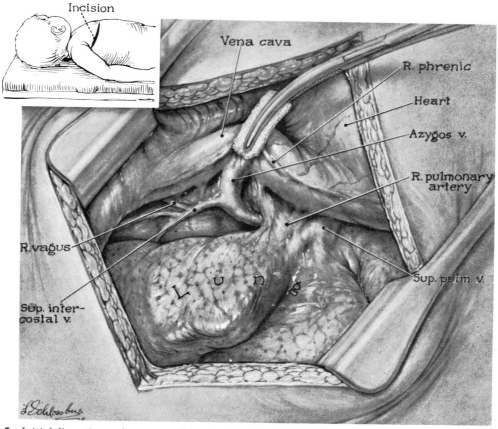

**Figure 5** Initial dissection and exposure of the pulmonary artery for construction of a right subclavian–pulmonary artery anastomosis. The insert at the top shows the position of the patient on the operating table. The entry into the pleural cavity is through the second intercostal space. (From Blalock, A.: Surg. Gynec. Obstet., 87:385, 1948.)

through a subclavian-pulmonary shunt is directed to the lung on the side of the anastomosis.[20]

Much attention must be paid to detail in performing the Blalock shunt, especially in the construction of the anastomosis itself. Every effort must be made to prevent constriction of the anastomosis; meticulous technique is essential (Fig. 7). Whereas the posterior row of sutures may be continuous, it is important to construct the anterior row with interrupted sutures. Use of the subclavian branch of the innominate is more difficult in patients over the age of 12, and generally the subclavian branch of the aorta is preferable.

Vascular anomalies are encountered frequently with the tetralogy of Fallot. For example, a right aortic arch

**Figure 6** Completed anastomosis. Note that the subclavian artery at its origin from the innominate artery is circular. When the anastomosis is performed between the subclavian branch of the aorta and the pulmonary artery, there is usually a kink (oval shape) of the left subclavian artery at its origin; this diminishes the blood flow through the anastomosis. (From Blalock, A.: Surg. Gynec. Obstet., 87:385, 1948.)

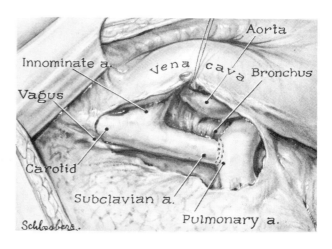

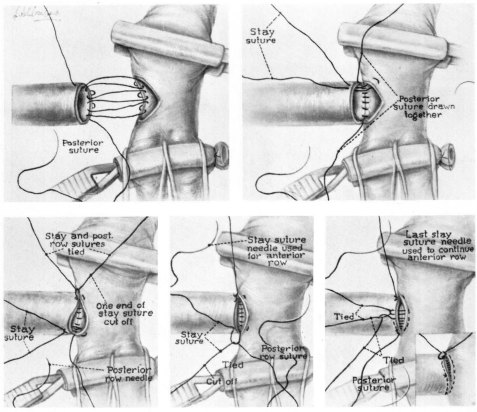

**Figure 7** Technique of anastomosis of the end of the subclavian artery to the side of the pulmonary artery. The suture is an everting and continuous one for the posterior row; 5–0 or 6–0 silk is used. The anterior row is constructed by interrupted mattress sutures. The space separating each "bite" in the vessel is approximately 1 mm. (From Blalock, A.: Surg. Gynec. Obstet., *87*:385, 1948.)

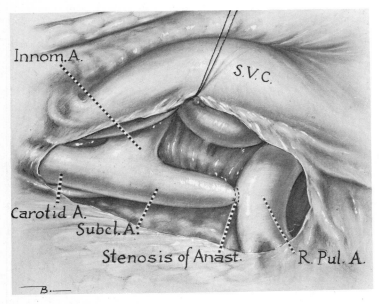

**Figure 8** Illustration of late stenosis of subclavian-pulmonary artery anastomosis at site of anastomosis. This is the usual site at which the constriction occurs, and diminished systemic-pulmonary blood flow results. This situation is frequently encountered at the time of open correction when the subclavian-pulmonary anastomosis is dissected in preparation for ligation of the subclavian artery. (From Sabiston, D. C., Jr., In: Gibbon, J. H., Jr., Sabiston, D. C., Jr., and Spencer, F. C., eds.: Surgery of the Chest. 2nd ed. Philadelphia, W. B. Saunders Company, 1969.)

is quite common, and a single pulmonary artery is occasionally seen. A retroesophageal subclavian artery occurs in approximately 5 per cent of patients and may involve either the right or left vessel. A persistent left superior vena cava occurs with about the same incidence.[43] It is quite *rare* for the retroesophageal subclavian vessels to cause dysphagia. In fact, it is usually not necessary to alter the retroesophageal relationship of the vessel in order to perform a proper anastomosis. Peripheral pulmonary arterial stenosis of the main artery or of branches has also been described.[25] In a number of patients in whom return of symptoms indicates inadequate blood flow because of stenosis of the anastomosis (Fig. 8) or because of occlusion, a second subclavian-pulmonary anastomosis may be performed with benefit.[26] However, in most instances open correction is indicated if a second operation is performed.

The *ascending aorta–pulmonary anastomosis* was originally described by Waterston and has since been emphasized by several others.[13,15] The procedure is performed through a right anterior thoracotomy entering the pleural cavity through the third intercostal space. The pericardium is opened anterior to the phrenic nerve, with exposure of the ascending aorta. The right pulmonary artery is then dissected as it passes beneath the ascending aorta. The vena cava is retracted laterally and a vascular clamp is placed so that one blade is beneath the pulmonary artery and the other anterior to the ascending aorta. Thus, it is possible to occlude both the right pulmonary artery and a portion of the ascending aorta with the same clamp (Fig. 9). An incision is then made in the anterior wall of the right pulmonary artery and a similar one on the lateral and slightly posterior aspect of the ascending aorta. An anastomosis approximately 4 to 5 mm. in diameter is then made between the

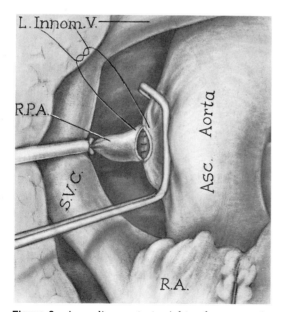

**Figure 9** Ascending aorta to right pulmonary artery anastomosis (Waterston). The anastomosis has a diameter of 4 to 5 mm., and care is taken to prevent its being larger. The clamp only partially occludes the aorta, whereas it totally occludes the right pulmonary artery. (From Sabiston, D. C., Jr. In: Gibbon, J. H., Jr., Sabiston, D. C., Jr., and Spencer, F. C., eds.: Surgery of the Chest. 2nd ed. Philadelphia, W. B. Saunders Company, 1969.)

ascending aorta and the right pulmonary artery. It has proved quite satisfactory and is the preferred procedure when systemic-pulmonary anastomosis is needed within the first several months of life. This procedure has the distinct advantage of being easily corrected at the time of open correction.

Rarely, *anastomosis of the superior vena cava to the right pulmonary artery (Glenn operation)* has been advocated in the treatment of tetralogy of Fallot.[3,23] In this procedure, the systemic venous blood from the superior vena cava passes directly into the pulmonary circulation, thus bypassing the right heart. Although the procedure has produced good results with respect to symptoms in some, more difficulty is experienced in the subsequent total correction. It is rarely employed in the treatment of the tetralogy of Fallot. A method for subsequent correction of the ventricular septal defect and relief of the right ventricular outflow obstruction following a superior vena cava to right pulmonary artery anastomosis has been described.[12]

### Open Correction

Open correction is the ideal operation for the tetralogy of Fallot and is accomplished with extracorporeal circulation. Through a median sternotomy, the pericardium is opened. Major branches of the right coronary artery may pass across the outflow tract to supply the left ventricle; occasionally, the anterior descending coronary artery arises from the right coronary artery and should be avoided. A careful estimate is made of the size of the main pulmonary artery as well as of the possible presence of valvar stenosis. The inferior and superior venae cavae are dissected, in preparation for insertion of venous cannulas into the right atrium. The left heart is vented through a catheter passed either through the right superior pulmonary vein, through the left atrial appendage, or through the left ventricular apex. A transverse or longitudinal ventriculotomy is then made in the outflow tract of the right ventricle (Fig. 10A). If valvar pulmonary stenosis is present, it is relieved by commissural incisions. The infundibular stenosis is carefully resected, with removal of all obstructing muscle (Fig. 10B). The ventricular septal defect is then identified. It is usually large and requires a plastic prosthesis for closure (Fig. 10C and D). Extreme care is devoted to the placement of the sutures, and it is important that the electrocardiogram and the atrial and ventricular contractions be monitored while these sutures are being placed. Should a pattern of heart block occur, the suture should be removed and reinserted. Intermittent occlusion of the ascending aorta is helpful when retraction and exposure of the defect produce aortic insufficiency and obscure the field. Air emboli in the coronary circulation must be prevented on reopening of the aorta by the passage of a clamp to render the aortic valve completely insufficient as the aortic clamp is released. Following closure of the interventricular septal defect, the right ventricle may be closed primarily or may require a patch. When feasible, primary closure is desirable; but if primary closure produces excessive obstruction, right ventricular hypertension and a low cardiac output syndrome will ensue. If the pulmonary artery or the valvar annulus is small, it may be necessary to extend the patch across the valve ring to the proximal portion of the pulmonary artery (Fig. 11). This produces pulmonary insufficiency, but it may be unavoidable and is apt to cause few problems. Residual right ventricular pulmonary artery gradients above 50 mm. Hg can be tolerated, although if this level is to be exceeded judicious assessment of the situation is required. The operation for correction is more difficult for patients with a previous left pulmonary artery-

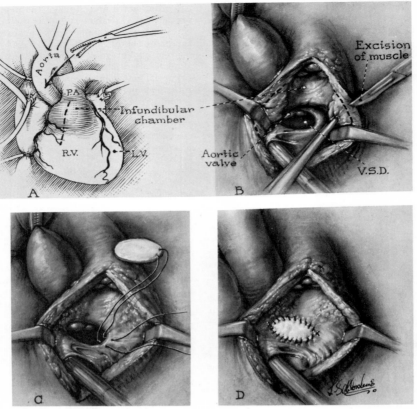

**Figure 10** Steps in the total correction of the tetralogy of Fallot. *A*, Note infundibular chamber and normal distribution of coronary vessels. The superior and inferior venae cavae are separately cannulated. The left atrium is decompressed by a catheter in the left atrial appendage. *B*, Marked infundibular stenosis is present in the outflow tract of the right ventricle. The pulmonary valve is normal. The interventricular defect is of the standard type. Through the defect, the cusps of the aortic valve are easily visualized. The aorta is temporarily occluded to prevent reflux of blood that would obscure the operative field in the region of the ventricular septal defect. *C*, The placement of the initial suture in the ventricular septal defect border. Intermittent aortic occlusion is employed. *D*, Completion of placement of ventricular prosthesis. (From Sabiston, D. C., Jr. In: Gibbon, J. H., Jr., Sabiston, D. C., Jr., and Spencer, F. C., eds.: Surgery of the Chest. 2nd ed. Philadelphia, W. B. Saunders Company, 1969.)

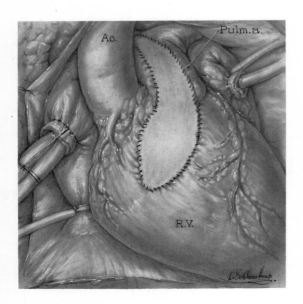

**Figure 11** In this patient with atresia of the pulmonary valve ring a large plastic prosthesis was required from the bifurcation of the pulmonary artery in order to decompress the right ventricle adequately. (From Sabiston, D. C., Jr. In: Gibbon, J. H., Sabiston, D. C., Jr., and Spencer, F. C., eds.: Surgery of the Chest. 2nd ed. Philadelphia, W. B. Saunders Company, 1969.)

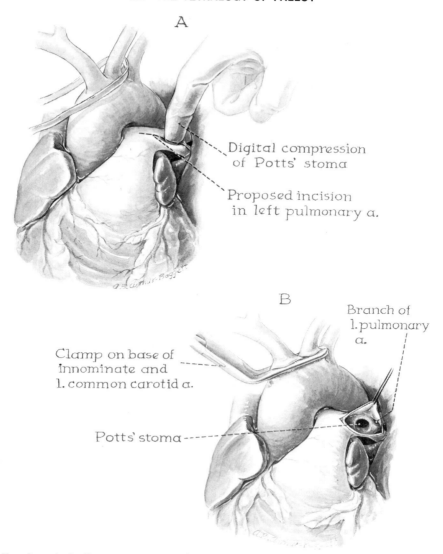

A

Digital compression
of Potts' stoma

Proposed incision
in left pulmonary a.

B

Branch of
l. pulmonary
a.

Clamp on base of
innominate and
l. common carotid a.

Potts' stoma

**Figure 12** For closure of a Potts anastomosis, the head vessels are clamped at their origin, circulatory arrest is established, and the stoma is visualized through an incision in the left pulmonary artery. (From Kirklin, J. W., and Karp, R. B.: The Tetralogy of Fallot from a Surgical Viewpoint. Philadelphia, W. B. Saunders Company, 1970.)

descending aorta anastomosis (Potts). The technique described by Kirklin is a very satisfactory one (Fig. 12).[36]

## RESULTS

The tetralogy of Fallot is now being corrected frequently and with an ever diminishing mortality. The results with open correction during the recent past have been impressive. The mortality in most series is now between 3 and 10 per cent.[2,37,41] In the majority of patients, the clinical and physiologic status is greatly improved, and good to excellent results have been reported in up to 90 per cent.[41] Some of the rarer and more severe anatomic malformations respond less well, but even these lesions are now yielding to surgery

with improved results.[1,27,55] Following open correction, the chest film usually shows slight enlargement of the heart, and murmurs of pulmonary insufficiency may be present. In early experience with the technique of open correction, left-to-right shunts through a ventricular septal defect or reopening of the defect occurred with some frequency but these are now uncommon.

## POSTOPERATIVE MANAGEMENT

Following operation, a number of variables must be followed carefully. Adequate *pulmonary function* is maintained by the use of an endotracheal tube, generally for the first 24 hours. This permits the maintenance of relatively normal values for the arterial $pO_2$, $pCO_2$ and pH. Whenever possible, the percentage of oxygen in the inspired air is maintained between 40 and 50 per cent, with attempts made not to exceed 60 per cent to prevent oxygen toxicity. Maintenance of an adequate *cardiac output* is also of crucial importance. It is appropriate to obtain dye dilution determinations of cardiac output when indicated. In general, the cardiac output can be increased by increasing the ventricular end-diastolic pressure, as accomplished by administration of blood or fluids. The atrial pressure can be raised should this be necessary. However, if evidence of *low* cardiac output persists, a search should be conducted for other primary causes. *Cardiac tamponade* is a recognized cause of the low output syndrome and may be present. If tamponade is not present, efforts should be made to improve the contractility of the cardiac muscle; this can be accomplished by the use of digitalis if the situation is not acute, and with inotropic agents such as isoproterenol if the clinical manifestations are more serious. If isoproterenol is ineffective, epinephrine or norepinephrine may be employed. Maintenance of *renal* function is also of critical importance. The urethral catheter is left in place with a desired output of at least 20 ml. per hour. It is generally necessary to limit fluid intake, especially during the first 24 hours following operation. This is due to the tendency to development of fluid retention of patients after repair of tetralogy of Fallot. On the first day, approximately 500 ml. of water per square meter of body surface should be administered. After the second postoperative day, the patient is allowed fluids by mouth but is placed on a low sodium diet (500 mg. daily). Following this, fluid intake may be regulated by total body weight examinations. Chlorothiazide (Diuril) may be used to counteract fluid retention. To prevent infection, especially when prosthetic materials have been used, antibiotics are given routinely. Arrhythmia, especially atrioventricular dissociation, is a serious postoperative complication. If this pattern is noted during operation or any suspicion of its occurrence exists, a myocardial wire for a pacemaker should be implanted. If this pattern develops postoperatively, a wire can be passed through a needle by the subxiphoid route. Following this, a pacing catheter can be inserted transvenously into the right ventricle. If atrial fibrillation develops, rapid digitalization is indicated. In the presence of *ventricular ectopic* beats, potassium chloride is employed (3 to 5 mEq. per 10 per cent solution).

## PULMONARY STENOSIS WITH INTACT VENTRICULAR SEPTUM

Pulmonary valvar stenosis with intact ventricular septum is one of the most favorable congenital cardiac lesions from the point of view of treatment. The symptoms are generally less pronounced than with the tetralogy of Fallot, although there are numerous examples of infants with extremely severe pulmonary stenosis that produces congestive heart failure. Some infants require immediate valvotomy as an *emergency* procedure, but in the majority of patients symptoms develop more slowly. In approximately three-fourths of this group, the foramen ovale is patent, and with development of increased pressure in the right atrium, blood is shunted to the left atrium and cyanosis is produced. Clubbing of the fingers may appear later. Characteristically, the pulmonary valvar commissures are fused into a dome-shaped structure with a small central lumen. A *jet* of blood that is forced through the aperture under great pressure from the right ventricle into the pulmonary artery creates eddy currents and a prominent thrill. Poststenotic dilatation of the main pulmonary artery ensues. In rare instances, *infundibular* stenosis may be associated with valvar stenosis and an intact ventricular septum. Moreover, frank atrial septal defects are also encountered, the latter combination being termed the *trilogy of Fallot.* The clinical findings are dependent upon the severity of the valvar pulmonary stenosis and the patency of the foramen ovale.[17] Dyspnea on exertion is the most common complaint, and cyanosis is usually present in those patients with a patent foramen ovale or an atrial septal defect. A harsh systolic murmur and thrill are present over the pulmonary area; the thrill can be palpated in the suprasternal notch. The pulmonary second sound is characteristically weak or absent. The chest film is often typical, demonstrating prominence of the pulmonary artery due to poststenotic dilatation (Fig. 13). The angiocardiogram is also helpful in demonstrating the classic dome-shaped pulmonary valve with small aperture and poststenotic dilatation, or an atrial septal defect and infundibular stenosis combined

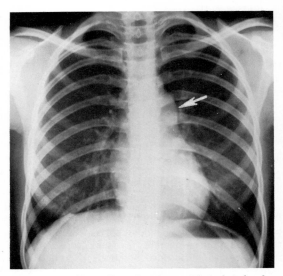

**Figure 13** Chest film of patient with isolated valvar pulmonary stenosis, demonstrating typical appearance of dilatation of the pulmonary artery. (From Sabiston, D. C., Jr. In: Gibbon, J. H., Jr., Sabiston, D. C., Jr., and Spencer, F. C., eds.: Surgery of the Chest. 2nd ed. Philadelphia, W. B. Saunders Company, 1969.)

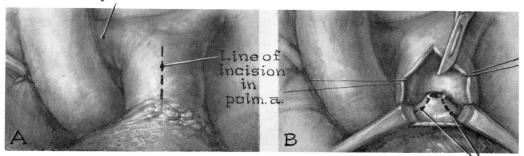

R. pulm. a.

Line of
incision
in
pulm. a.

A

B

Incisions

**Figure 14** Illustration of open correction of pulmonary valvar stenosis employing extracorporeal circulation. An incision is made in the main pulmonary artery, exposing the dome-shaped pulmonary valve. Radial incisions are made in each of the fused commissures, with complete opening of the valve. (From Sabiston, D. C., Jr. In: Gibbon, J. H., Jr., Sabiston, D. C., Jr., and Spencer, F. C., eds.: Surgery of the Chest. 2nd ed. Philadelphia, W. B. Saunders Company, 1969.)

with valvar stenosis. Cardiac catheterization demonstrates a gradient between the right ventricle and the pulmonary artery *without* evidence of a shunt at the ventricular level. In severe forms, the pressure gradient between the pulmonary artery and the right ventricle may exceed 200 mm. Hg.

### Treatment

The original treatment of valvar pulmonary stenosis was introduced by Brock[8] and consisted of transventricular valvotomy. A valvulotome was passed through the wall of the right ventricle into the pulmonary artery to open the stenotic valve. Later, an improved valvulotome was designed for transventricular use.[46] For a number of years this approach was used with moderate success and was associated with both clinical and hemodynamic improvement.[30] Nevertheless, closed valvotomy has definite disadvantages,[40] and it is now agreed that open repair of the valvar stenosis under direct vision produces the best results.[7] The use of extracorporeal circulation permits simultaneous correction of coexisting atrial septal defects and of infundibular stenosis when present.[42] Thus, the open approach to the correction of pulmonary valvar stenosis is most often indicated (Fig. 14). There is one exception that bears emphasis, namely, *valvar stenosis in infancy.* This situation is apt to lead to severe congestive heart failure and death unless the stenosis is relieved. Under these circumstances, transventricular division of the valve with a valvulotome is expeditious, safe, and quite effective.

Open correction of pulmonary valvar stenosis yields excellent results and recurrence of the condition is rare. Moreover, the compensatory infundibular hypertrophy that frequently accompanies the valvar stenosis usually regresses with time. Although the gradient between the right ventricle and the pulmonary artery may not be totally abolished immediately after operation, regression of the secondary hypertrophy of the right ventricular outflow tract occurs and repeat

catheterization later shows a marked reduction in the gradient.[16]

In addition to valvar pulmonary stenosis, *isolated infundibular stenosis* of the right ventricle may also occur as a congenital anomaly. The symptoms are quite similar to those of valvar stenosis, although the murmur may be located somewhat lower in the precordium. The angiocardiogram demonstrates the lesion with precision, and cardiac catheterization demonstrates two gradients: (1) between the pulmonary artery and the infundibulum, and (2) between the infundibulum and the right ventricle. Management of these cases is resection of the infundibular stenosis in the open heart employing extracorporeal circulation. The results are excellent.

## TRICUSPID ATRESIA

In this malformation, the primary lesion is *atresia* of the tricuspid valve, usually associated with *defective development of the right ventricle.* The latter is usually a rudimentary chamber or may be absent. Another prominent feature of this defect is the presence of an interatrial communication that allows the blood to pass from the right atrium to the left heart and thence into the aorta. A small ventricular septal defect passing into the rudimentary right ventricle is usually present, and *pulmonary stenosis* is a frequent associated finding. Transposition of the great vessels may also occur with this disorder.

The most common anatomic form is tricuspid atresia associated with subpulmonary stenosis. A small opening is present between the left ventricle and the infundibulum of the right ventricle, and a stenotic pulmonary artery arises from a rudimentary right ventricle. The size of the interatrial communication is of importance in that it determines the amount of blood allowed to pass from the right to the left side of the heart.

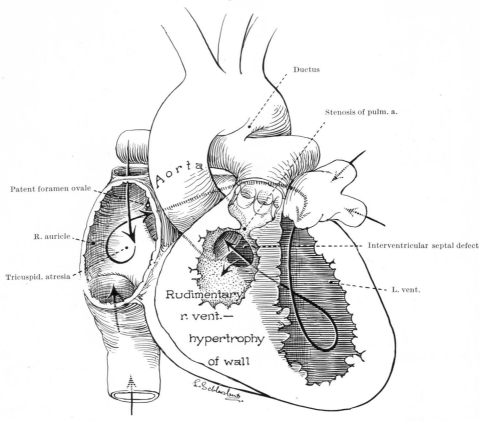

**Figure 15**  Diagram of tricuspid atresia with rudimentary right ventricle, patent foramen ovale, small ventricular septal defect, pulmonary stenosis, and patent ductus arteriosus. (From Sabiston, D. C., Jr., and Blalock, A. In: Derra, E., ed.: Encyclopedia of Thoracic Surgery. Heidelberg, Springer-Verlag, 1959.)

The *diagnosis* is usually made in a patient with cyanosis and dyspnea. An enlarged, pulsating liver may be palpable, and may suggest that the interatrial communication is a small one. The chest film often shows absence or diminution of the right ventricle, particularly in the left anterior oblique position. The most helpful diagnostic aid is the electrocardiogram, which nearly always shows a left axis deviation, unlike the case in most other types of congenital cyanotic heart disease. A firm diagnosis can be established by the angiocardiogram and cardiac catheterization, with demonstration of the characteristic features of the anatomy (Fig. 15).

The treatment of tricuspid atresia is most satisfactory in those patients with pulmonary stenosis, in whom surgical creation of a systemic-pulmonary shunt (Blalock) is done. When the interatrial communication is small, the creation of a larger interatrial defect often proves beneficial. Occasionally, a superior vena cava to right pulmonary artery anastomosis has been advocated for this condition.[22] If surgery is indicated in those patients with transposition of the great vessels without pulmonary stenosis, the operation is directed toward banding of the pulmonary artery to reduce pulmonary blood flow.

## DOUBLE-OUTLET RIGHT VENTRICLE (ORIGIN OF AORTA AND PULMONARY ARTERY FROM THE RIGHT VENTRICLE)

There are two major types of this condition: (1) with pulmonary stenosis, and (2) without pulmonary stenosis. The patients with pulmonary stenosis resemble those with the tetralogy of Fallot and are usually cyanotic. Those *without* pulmonary stenosis can be subdivided into two groups: (1) those with an interventricular defect located posterior and inferior to the crista supraventricularis, and (2) those in which the ventricular septal defect lies anterior and superior to the crista and in close proximity to the pulmonary valve (Taussig-Bing complex). In the latter group, associated cardiac malformation such as an atrioventricular canal, aortic arch hyperplasia, or coarctation of the aorta may be present.

In patients without pulmonary stenosis, the clinical manifestations and course resemble those of a patient with a large ventricular septal defect and excessive pulmonary blood flow. In the Taussig-Bing complex, left ventricular flow is primarily into the pulmonary artery, whereas the blood in the right ventricle flows primarily to the aorta and cyanosis results. Angiocardiography may reveal evidence that the pulmonary valve and aortic valve are approximately in the same plane, whereas in the tetralogy of Fallot the aortic valve is usually at a lower position than the pulmonary valve. The treatment consists of open correction of the defect with cardiopulmonary bypass, with closure of the ventricular septal defect and excision of the pulmonary stenosis when these conditions are present.[24, 35]

## TRUNCUS ARTERIOSUS (PERSISTENT TRUNCUS ARTERIOSUS COMMUNIS)

This is a rare congenital cardiac malformation in which a single artery arises from the base of the heart instead of the normal aorta and pulmonary artery. The primary anatomic features of this defect include (1) a single artery called the *persistent truncus arteriosus* originating from the base of both ventricles; (2) a valve between the heart and the truncus, with the number of cusps varying from two to six; (3) a high ventricular septal defect immediately below the single valve; and (4) origin of the pulmonary arteries directly from the truncus arteriosus.

Since the malformation is a severe one, prominent symptoms are usually apparent at birth, and death frequently occurs during the first year of life, although prolonged survival does occur. The clinical manifestations resemble those of a large left-to-right shunt such as in ventricular septal defect with pulmonary hypertension. With the pulmonary arteries arising directly from the aorta, cyanosis may be minimal or absent. The systolic pressures at cardiac catheterization are essentially identical in both ventricles, in the truncus, and in the pulmonary arteries that arise from the truncus. The *diagnosis* is further established by angiocardiography, which demonstrates the ventricular defect, the common vessel arising from the base of the heart (truncus), and the origin of the pulmonary arteries.

The treatment for this serious malformation is open correction with correction of the ventricular septal defect and construction of a pulmonary artery placed from the right ventricle to the arteries supplying the lungs by means of an aortic homograft.[56]

The term *pseudotruncus arteriosus* is applied to a congenital malformation in which there is absence of the pulmonary valve and of the main pulmonary artery. In this defect, the only vessel leaving the base of the heart is the aorta, but it does not give rise to pulmonary arteries. The blood supply to the lung is from a ductus arteriosus that is connected to the pulmonary arteries but does not communicate with the heart, since the main pulmonary artery is atretic. Enlarged bronchial arteries may also supply blood to the lungs. This malformation is much like a severe form of tetralogy of Fallot and is treated accordingly.

## EBSTEIN'S DISEASE

This malformation consists primarily of (1) downward displacement of the tricuspid valve into the right ventricle, and (2) origin of a septal leaflet (and frequently the posterior leaflet) from the wall of the right ventricle instead of the normal annulus fibrosus. The anterior leaflet arises normally from the ring, but the valve leaflets are frequently deformed. It is apparent that a large portion of the right ventricle then becomes "atrialized" and is actually a part of the right atrium. This produces gross right atrial enlargement. In most instances, an interatrial septal defect is present that permits a shunt of varying degree directly to the left side of the heart. A ventricular septal defect, and at times pulmonary stenosis, may also be present. The primary problem is ineffective pumping of the right ventricle due to its atrialization. The tricuspid valve is usually insufficient and occasionally stenotic as a result of the malformation.

The clinical manifestations are usually dyspnea and cyanosis, although the latter may be delayed in appearance. Sudden death, probably due to paroxysmal arrhythmias, is well recognized. Occasionally, longevity has been reported with this malformation. Physical examination usually reveals cyanosis, clubbing of the fingers, and a holosystolic murmur. The latter is apt to represent tricuspid insufficiency or the presence of a ventricular septal defect. Additional findings include cardiac enlargement, especially of the right atrium. The electrocardiogram characteristically demonstrates right bundle branch block and a prolonged PR interval. The P waves are tall and frequently of increased duration in leads II and III. The primary findings on angiocardiography are enlargement of the right atrium, downward displacement of the tricuspid valves, and the demonstration of possible atrial or ventricular septal defects. These findings are confirmed on cardiac catheterization. Although the clinical course with Ebstein's disease is variable, congestive heart failure usually occurs in childhood or early adult life. Occasionally, prolonged survival with signs of cardiac insufficiency and arrhythmia occurs.

The treatment of Ebstein's disease is not totally satisfactory, although plication of the tricuspid valve by direct suture may be helpful.[28] In other instances, excision and prosthetic replacement of the tricuspid valve has led to improvement.[39]

## SELECTED REFERENCES

Blalock, A., and Taussig, H. B.: Surgical treatment of malformations of the heart in which there is pulmonary stenosis or pulmonary atresia. J.A.M.A., *128*:189, 1945.
*In this paper, Dr. Blalock's first three operations for creation of a systemic-pulmonary artery anastomosis are reported. The first patient, a 15 month old infant with severe cyanosis, had a history of multiple episodes of loss of consciousness. An anastomosis of the left subclavian artery to the left pulmonary artery was made, and the clinical improvement was striking. Two additional patients with successful results are also described. It is of interest that Dr. Blalock refers to earlier experimental work in which subclavian-pulmonary*

*anastomoses were performed in the dog in an effort to produce pulmonary hypertension. Although these experiments did not succeed in producing an elevated pulmonary arterial pressure, the operation was subsequently used for an entirely different purpose. This procedure was the first of many additional cardiac surgical advances.*

Kirklin, J. W., and Karp, R. B.: Tetralogy of Fallot from a Surgical Viewpoint. Philadelphia, W. B. Saunders Company, 1970.

*This is a superb monograph with excellent presentations of the anatomy, natural history, hemodynamics, clinical features, and diagnosis of the tetralogy of Fallot. The techniques of palliative and open corrective surgery are superbly described and illustrated. A detailed account of the results is provided and ranks among the best in the world literature. This monograph is highly recommended for a complete analysis of the entire subject.*

Lillehei, C. W., Cohen, M., Warden, H. E., Read, R. C., Aust, J. B., DeWall, R. A., and Varco, R.: Vision intracardiac surgical correction of the tetralogy of Fallot, pentalogy of Fallot, and pulmonary atresia defects. Ann. Surg., 142:418, 1955.

*In this paper the original descriptions for surgical correction of the tetralogy of Fallot are provided. The paper is a classic one in the development of surgical techniques for complete correction of this malformation.*

Sabiston, D. C., Jr., Cornell, W. P., Criley, J. M., Neill, C. A., Ross, R. S., and Bahnson, H. T.: The diagnosis and surgical correction of total obstruction of the right ventricle. J. Thorac. Cardiovasc. Surg., 48:577, 1964.

*In this paper, the most severe of the forms of tetralogy of Fallot, those with complete obliteration of the outflow tract of the right ventricle and its communication with the pulmonary artery, are described together with the details of operative correction and results. It is interesting that in these patients who have no communication between the right ventricle and pulmonary artery and, following correction, have total pulmonary insufficiency, the subsequent course is generally surprisingly good. In other words, pulmonary valvar insufficiency can be well tolerated.*

Taussig, H. B.: Tetralogy of Fallot. In: Congenital Malformations of the Heart. 2nd ed. Cambridge, Harvard University Press, 1960.

*This chapter in an outstanding text of pediatric cardiology is an excellent resource for the descriptions of the clinical manifestations, physical findings, laboratory studies, and ultimate results in patients with the tetralogy of Fallot. Its author has probably examined and followed more patients with this condition than anyone else in the world.*

## REFERENCES

1. Allison, P. R., Gunning, A. J., Hamill, J., and Mody, S. M.: Fallot's tetralogy. A postoperative study. Circulation, 28:525, 1963.
2. Bahnson, H. T.: Discussion of Malm, J. R., Blumenthal, S., Bowman, F. O., Jr., Ellis, K., Jameson, A. G., Jesse, M. J., and Yeoh, C. B.: Factors that modify hemodynamic results in total correction of tetralogy of Fallot. J. Thorac. Cardiovasc. Surg., 52:502, 1966.
3. Bakulev, A. N., and Kolesnikov, S. A.: Anastomosis of the superior vena cava and pulmonary artery in the surgical treatment of certain congenital defects of the heart. J. Thorac. Surg., 37:693, 1959.
4. Barratt-Boyes, B. G., Simpson, M., and Neutze, J. M.: Intracardiac surgery in neonates and infants using deep hypothermia with surface cooling and limited cardiopulmonary bypass. Circulation, Suppl. 1, 43:1, 1971.
5. Blalock, A.: Surgical procedures employed and anatomical variations encountered in the treatment of congenital pulmonic stenosis. Surg. Gynec. Obstet., 87:385, 1948.
6. Blalock, A., and Taussig, H. B.: The surgical treatment of malformation of the heart in which there is pulmonary stenosis or pulmonary atresia. J.A.M.A., 128:189, 1945.
7. Blount, S. G., Jr., McCord, M. C., Mueller, H., and Swan, H.: Isolated valvular pulmonic stenosis; clinical and physiologic response to open valvuloplasty. Circulation, 10:161, 1954.
8. Brock, R. C.: Pulmonary valvulotomy for the relief of congenital pulmonary stenosis; report of 3 cases. Brit. Med. J., 1:1121, 1948.
9. Brock, R. C.: Congenital pulmonary stenosis. Amer. J. Med., 12:706, 1952.
10. Brock, R. C., and Campbell, M.: Infundibular resection for pulmonic stenosis. Brit. Heart J., 12:403, 1950.
11. Campbell, M., and Deuchar, D. C.: Results of the Blalock-Taussig operation in 200 cases of morbus caeruleus. Brit. Med. J., 1:349, 1953.
12. Claxton, C. P., Jr., and Sabiston, D. C., Jr.: Correction of tetralogy of Fallot following superior vena cava to pulmonary artery shunt. J. Thorac. Cardiovasc. Surg., 57:475, 1969.
13. Cooley, D. A., and Hallman, G. L.: Intrapericardial aortic-right pulmonary arterial anastomosis. Surg. Gynec. Obstet., 122:1084, 1966.
14. Dobell, A. R. C., Charrette, E. P., and Chughtai, M. S.: Correction of tetralogy in the young child. J. Thorac. Cardiovasc. Surg., 55:70, 1968.
15. Edwards, W. S., Mohtashemi, M., and Holdefer, W. F., Jr.: Ascending aorta to right pulmonary artery shunt for infants with tetralogy of Fallot. Surgery, 59:316, 1966.
16. Engle, M. A., Holswade, G. R., Goldberg, H. P., Lukas, D. S., and Glenn, F.: Regression after open valvotomy of infundibular stenosis accompanying severe valvular pulmonic stenosis. Circulation, 17:862, 1958.
17. Engle, M. A., and Taussig, H. B.: Valvular pulmonic stenosis with intact ventricular septum and patent foramen ovale: Report of illustrative cases and analysis of clinical syndrome. Circulation, 2:481, 1950.
18. Fallot, E. A. L.: Contribution à l'anatomie pathologique de la maladie bleue (cyanose cardiaque). Marseille Med., 25, 77, 138, 207, 270, 341, 403, 1888.
19. Farre, J. R.: Pathological Researches. Essay I. On Malformation of the Human Heart. London, 1814.
20. Fort, L., III, Morrow, A. G., Pierce, G. E., Saigusa, M., and McLaughlin, J. S.: The distribution of pulmonary blood flow after subclavian-pulmonary anastomosis: An experimental study. J. Thorac. Cardiovasc. Surg., 50:671, 1965.
21. Gintrac, E.: Observations et recherches sur la cyanose, ou maladie bleue. Paris, J. Pinard, 1824.
22. Glenn, W. W. L., Ordway, N. K., Talner, N. S., and Call, E. P.: Circulatory bypass of the right side of the heart. VI. Shunt between superior vena cava and distal right pulmonary artery. Report of clinical application in 38 cases. Circulation, 31:172, 1965.
23. Glenn, W. W. L., and Patino, J. F.: Circulatory bypass of the right heart. I. Preliminary observation on direct delivery of vena caval blood into pulmonary arterial circulation. Azygos vein–pulmonary artery shunt. Yale J. Biol. Med., 27:147, 1954.
24. Gomes, M. M. R., Weidman, W. H., McGoon, D. C., and Danielson, G. K.: Double-outlet right ventricle without pulmonary stenosis: Surgical considerations and results of operation. Circulation, Supp. 1, 43:31, 1971.
25. Gregoratos, G., Jones, R. C., and Jahnke, E. J., Jr.: Unilateral peripheral pulmonic stenosis complicating tetralogy of Fallot. J. Thorac. Cardiovasc. Surg., 50:202, 1965.
26. Haller, J. A., Jr.: Second shunting operations for pulmonary stenosis with cyanosis following failure of original systemic-pulmonary anastomoses. Surgery, 44:919, 1958.
27. Hallidie-Smith, K. A., Dulake, M., Wong, M., Oakley, C. M., and Goodwin, J. F.: Ventricular structure and function after radical correction of the tetralogy of Fallot. Brit. Heart J., 29:533, 1967.
28. Hardy, K. L., and Roe, B. R.: Ebstein's anomaly: Further experience with definitive repair. J. Thorac. Cardiovas. Surg., 58:553, 1969.
29. Hartmann, R. C.: A hemorrhagic disorder occurring in patients with cyanotic congenital heart disease. Bull. Johns Hopkins Hosp., 91:49, 1952.
30. Himmelstein, A., Jameson, A. G., Fishman, A. P., and Humphreys, G. H., II.: Closed transventricular valvulotomy for pulmonic stenosis. Surgery, 42:121, 1957.
31. Hope, J.: A Treatise on Disease of the Heart and Great Vessels and on the Affections which may be Mistaken for Them. London, J. & A. Churchill, 1839.
32. Hunter, J.: Medical Observations and Inquiries by a Society of Physicians of London. London, 1757–1784.

33. Hunter, W.: Three cases of malformation of the heart. Case II. Medical Observations and Inquiries by a Society of Physicians in London, 6:291, 1784.
34. Johns, T. N. P., Williams, G. R., and Blalock, A.: The anatomy of pulmonary stenosis and atresia with comments on surgical therapy. Surgery, 33:161, 1953.
35. Kirklin, J. W., Harp, R. A., and McGoon, D. C.: Surgical treatment of origin of both vessels from right ventricle, including cases of pulmonary stenosis. J. Thorac. Cardiovasc. Surg., 48:1026, 1964.
36. Kirklin, J. W., and Karp, R. B.: The Tetralogy of Fallot from a Surgical Viewpoint. Philadelphia, W. B. Saunders Company, 1970.
37. Kirklin, J. W., Wallace, R. B., McGoon, D. C., and DuShane, J. W.: Early and late results after intracardiac repair of tetralogy of Fallot. Trans. Amer. Surg. Ass., 83:258, 1965.
38. Lillehei, C. W., Cohen, M., Warden, H. E., Read, R. C., Aust, J. B., DeWall, R. A., and Varco, R. L.: Vision intracardiac surgical correction of the tetralogy of Fallot, pentalogy of Fallot, and pulmonary atresia defects. Ann. Surg., 142:418, 1955.
39. Lillehei, C. W., Kalke, B. R., and Carlson, R. G.: Evolution of corrective surgery for Ebstein's anomaly. Circulation, Supp. 1, 35:1, 1967.
40. Lillehei, C. W., Winchell, P., Adams, P., Baronofsky, I., Adams, F., and Varco, R. L.: Pulmonary valvular stenosis with intact ventricular septum. Amer. J. Med., 5:756, 1956.
41. Malm, J. R., Blumenthal, S., Bowman, F. O., Jr., Ellis, K., Jameson, A. G., Jesse, M. J., and Yeoh, C. B.: Factors that modify hemodynamic results in total correction of tetralogy of Fallot. J. Thorac. Cardiovasc. Surg., 52:502, 1966.
42. McGoon, D. C., and Kirklin, J. W.: Pulmonic stenosis with intact ventricular septum. Treatment utilizing extracorporeal circulation. Circulation, 17:180, 1958.
43. Nagao, G. I., Daoud, G. I., McAdams, A. J., Schwartz, D. C., and Kaplan, S.: Cardiovascular anomalies associated with tetralogy of Fallot. Amer. J. Cardiol., 20:206, 1967.
44. Peacock, T. B.: Malformations of the Human Heart. London, J. & A. Churchill, 1866.
45. Porter, J. M., and Silver, D.: Alterations in fibrinolysis and coagulation associated with cardiopulmonary bypass. J. Thorac. Cardiovasc. Surg., 56:869, 1968.
46. Potts, W. J., Gibson, S., Riker, W. L., and Leninger, C. R.: Congenital pulmonary stenosis with intact ventricular septum. J.A.M.A., 144:8, 1950.
47. Potts, W. J., Smith, S., and Gibson, S.: Anastomosis of the aorta to a pulmonary artery for certain types of congenital heart disease. J.A.M.A., 132:629, 1946.
48. Ross, R. S., Taussig, H. B., and Evans, M. H.: Late hemodynamic complications of anastomotic surgery for treatment of the tetralogy of Fallot. Circulation, 18:553, 1958.
49. Sabiston, D. C., Jr., and Blalock, A.: The tetralogy of Fallot, tricuspid atresia, transposition of the great vessels and associated disorders. In: Encyclopedia of Thoracic Surgery. Heidelberg, Springer-Verlag, 1959, Vol. 2, p. 697.
50. Sabiston, D. C., Jr., Cornell, W. P., Criley, J. M., Neill, C. A., Ross, R. S., and Bahnson, H. T.: The diagnosis and surgical correction of total obstruction of the right ventricle: An acquired condition developing after systemic artery–pulmonary artery anastomosis for tetralogy of Fallot. J. Thorac. Surg., 48:577, 1964.
51. Sandifort, E.: Observations Anatomico-Pathologicae. Ludg. Bat P.v.d. Eyk et D. Vygh, 1777, Chapter 1, Figure 1.
52. Scott, H. W., Collins, H. A., and Foster, J. H.: Hypothermia as an adjuvant in cardiovascular surgery. Experimental and clinical observations. Amer. Surg., 20:799, 1954.
53. Stensen, Hiels (Nicholaus Steno): In: Thomas Bartholin, Acta Medica et Philosophica Hafnienca, 1671/72, Vol. I, p. 302. Reprinted in Nicolae Stenosis: Opera Philosophica. Copenhagen, Vilhelm Maar, 1910, Vol. 2, pp. 49–53.
54. Stephens, H. B.: Aneurysm of the pulmonary artery following a Potts' shunt operation. J. Thorac. Cardiovasc. Surg., 53:642, 1967.
55. Theye, R. A., and Kirklin, J. W.: Physiologic studies early after repair of tetralogy of Fallot. Circulation, 28:42, 1963.
56. Wallace, R. B., Rastelli, G. C., Ongley, P. A., Titus, J. L., and McGoon, D. C.: Complete repair of truncus arteriosus defects. J. Thorac. Cardiovasc. Surg., 57:95, 1969.
57. Waterston, D. J.: Treatment of Fallot's tetralogy in children under 1 year of age. Rozhl. Chir., 41:181, 1962.
58. White, P. D., and Sprague, H. B.: The tetralogy of Fallot. Report of a case in a noted musician who lived to his sixtieth year. J.A.M.A., 92:787, 1929.

# VIII

# Transposition of the Great Vessels

*Paul A. Ebert, M.D.*

## HISTORICAL ASPECTS

Anatomic observation of transpositions of the great vessels was reported as early as 1672 by Steno, and by Morgani in 1761 and Bailey in 1779. Even in these early reports, variations in the anatomic configurations of the transposition malformation were described. Von Rokitansky[45] (1875) reported analysis of the pathogenesis of transposition and attempted to classify the various types. The clinical recognition of this anomaly during life was emphasized by Fanconi[12] in 1932. Taussig[40] in 1938 described not only the clinical manifestations of this anomaly during life but also the pathologic anatomy and hemodynamic manifestations of the disorder.

The era of surgery for transposition of the great arteries began in 1950 when Blalock and Hanlon[6] reported an ingenious method of creating an atrial septal defect to increase mixing between the two circulations. Although the mortality with this operation was extremely high in the early years of its use, the marked improvement observed in the survivors created considerable enthusiasm. In 1952, Mustard[31] attempted to reverse the transposed great arteries directly, and in the same year Bailey[4] also reversed the aorta and pulmonary artery, but neither patient survived. In 1952,

Lillehei and Varco[28] transferred the right pulmonary veins to the right atrium and the inferior vena cava to the left atrium to partially correct the circulation. In 1954, Glenn and Patino[15] anastomosed the right pulmonary artery to the superior vena cava in patients with transposition of the great vessels and pulmonary stenosis. Baffes[3] in 1956 successfully transferred the right pulmonary veins to the right atrium and grafted the right inferior vena cava to the left atrium. Kay and Cross[23] (1955) and Merendino[29] (1957) attempted intra-atrial diversionary procedures to redirect venous flow into the respective ventricles. In 1959, Senning[38] reported success in transposing the atria in a young boy. Barnard[5] in 1961 excised the atrial septum and inserted a plastic prosthesis around the orifices of the pulmonary veins, connecting the other end to the orifice of the systemic or right ventricle. Considerable enthusiasm for the management of transposition of the great vessels followed Mustard's[30] report in 1964 of an operation in which he excised the entire atrial septum and positioned a pericardial baffle in the atrium to redirect all the caval blood to the pulmonary ventricle and allow the oxygenated blood returning by pulmonary veins to enter the systemic ventricle. This procedure has received universal acceptance and has produced excellent results.

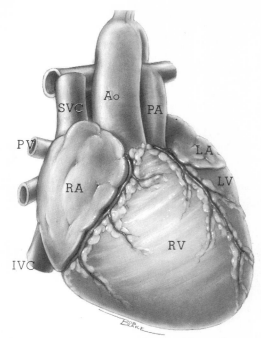

**Figure 1**   External view of the usual form of transposition of the great vessels. The aorta arises anteriorly from the right ventricle, and there is minimal if any rotation to the great vessels. The pulmonary valve lies almost directly posterior to the aortic valve. The left and right ventricles have a nearly normal relationship.

## ANATOMIC ASPECTS

Transposition of the great arteries accounts for approximately 9 per cent of cases of cyanotic congenital heart disease. This lesion represents approximately 15 per cent of congenital cardiac anomalies seen at autopsy in infants less than 1 month of age. Transposition is the leading cause of death due to congenital heart lesions in the first 2 months of life. There is a definite male preponderance, the ratio being between 2.3 and 3:1.

Complete transposition of the great vessels essentially means that the aorta and pulmonary artery are misplaced across the ventricular septum. The aorta usually arises anteriorly from trabeculated right ventricle that receives desaturated venous blood from the right atrium (Fig. 1). The pulmonary artery most commonly lies posterior to and to the left of the aorta and receives oxygenated blood from a smooth-walled left ventricle. There are many possible combinations of great vessel and chamber arrangements in transposition of the great vessels, depending on rotation of the heart and the side-to-side relationships of the ventricles. Paul[33] reported that complete transposition occurred as a relatively isolated anomaly 65 per cent of the time, with only simple associated lesions such as atrial septal defect, ventricular septal defect, patent ductus arteriosus, or these in combination. When transposition occurred with situs inversus (3 per cent of cases) or asplenia (6 per cent), associated complex intracardiac anomalies also were noted.

In the normal heart, the aortic valve is inferior to and in direct continuity with the mitral valve, while in transposition it lies superior, atop the subaortic conus. Many theories of morphogenesis have been proposed but the differential conal growth hypothesis[17] has been favored. It is postulated that in the normal heart, the subaortic segment of the conus does not grow and that dominant growth of the left-sided subpulmonary conus forces the pulmonary valve anteriorly and superiorly to the left, whereas in ordinary forms of transposition, growth of the subaortic part of the conus pushes the aorta anteriorly and disrupts aortic-mitral valve continuity. Failure of the subpulmonary portion of the conus to develop maintains posterior location of the pulmonary artery and pulmonary-mitral valve continuity.

Development of the conus determines truncal rotation, and the relationship of the great arteries proximally at the semilunar valves is similar to that at the arch. There is no twist in the great arteries simply because the aorta is anterior. In less common types of transposition, development of both right and left parts of the conus thrusts both the aortic and pulmonary valves forward. If growth of the two segments is approximately equal, the valves will lie side by side at about the same height. Bilateral conus development is more common in transposition associated with malposition of the heart.

## PATHOPHYSIOLOGY

The basic physiologic abnormality in complete transposition of the great vessels is that venous blood is pumped directly into the aorta while oxygenated blood is returned to the pulmonary artery. Thus, there are two separate circulations in parallel instead of in series. Oxygenated pulmonary venous blood enters the circulation only by way of intracirculatory shunts (Fig. 2). Thus, the greater the number of simple associated anomalies such as atrial septal defect, ventricular septal defect, and patent ductus arteriosus, the greater the opportunity for intracirculatory mixing of venous and oxygenated blood. Infants with these associated lesions are usually less cyanotic. When intracirculatory shunting is limited, the infant is extremely cyanotic because of recirculation of the systemic venous blood. Pulmonary flow is usually excessive, and often the pulmonary artery pressure is elevated. Heart work is increased, and the myocardium must sustain this load with marginal coronary oxygenation.

The degree of intracirculatory shunting that occurs appears to be related to simple pressure gradients present at the site of the communication. Most infants with transposition have an increased pulmonary blood flow and pulmonary venous return. As the left atrium enlarges, the foramen ovale is stretched, and this results in oxygenated blood being shunted into the right atrium and systemic circulation. A systemic-to-pulmonary shunt exists through the bronchial vessels and also through a ventricular septal defect or patent ductus arteriosus if either is present. Bidirectional shunting can usually be demonstrated across the atrial septum, but the amount of systemic blood entering the pulmonary circuit is usually related to the size of the atrial septal defect.

The pulmonary vascular resistance is usually normal or only mildly elevated in infants with transposition of the great vessels with or without an associated ventricular septal defect. Ferencz[13] observed advanced histologic changes in the lungs of children over 2 years of age, and intimal fibrosis was noted as early as 1 month of life. These changes seem to be present in most children with transposition of the great vessels and suggest that this malformation may be associated with a more advanced and malignant form of pulmonary vascular disease than ventricular septal defect with normal relationship of the great vessels. Whether the advanced changes are related to perfusion of the pulmonary arterial tree with oxygenated blood in association with systemic desaturation is not clear. Severe pulmonary vascular changes are present in most older children with transposition of the great vessels with associated moderate to large ventricular septal defects. Hemodynamic measurements do not completely agree with the histologic findings in children with intact ventricular septum or small ventricular septal defects, however, since the majority do not have physiologic evidence of increased pulmonary vascular resistance. It has been postulated that systemic hypoxia stimulates sympathetic activity, with a resultant increase in tone of pulmonary arterioles. Thus, after complete correction, a decrease in pulmonary vascular resistance might be anticipated in many cases.

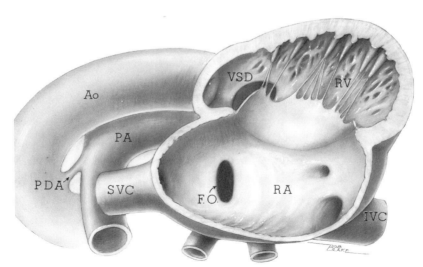

**Figure 2** The common anomalies associated with transposition of the great vessels are patent ductus arteriosus (PDA), ventricular septal defect (VSD), and patent foramen ovale (FO). These intracirculatory communications facilitate mixing of arterial and venous blood between the parallel circulations. The size and number of these associated anomalies determine the degree of cyanosis.

## CLINICAL FEATURES

Cyanosis and congestive heart failure are the common findings in infants with complete transposition of the great vessels. The cyanosis is usually observed by 1 week of age and is more pronounced when the ventricular septum is intact. When cyanosis appears later, there is usually significant intracirculatory shunting through a large ventricular septal defect or patent ductus arteriosus. Differential cyanosis, with the upper extremities more blue than the lower part of the body, indicates a large patent ductus and increased pulmonary vascular resistance, with pulmonary-to-systemic shunting through the ductus. Clubbing of the digits is rare before 6 months of age but may progress rapidly in the older infant. Squatting, which is so characteristic in children with tetralogy of Fallot, is rarely seen with transposition.

Birth weight is usually normal or above normal. Growth and physical development are always retarded. Anoxic spells are usually characterized by prolonged, labored breathing with increased cyanosis. The infant usually remains conscious and rarely has convulsions. These spells are due to hypoxemia from inadequate intracirculatory shunting, and metabolic acidosis results. Congestive heart failure is a common clinical finding, with dyspnea, cardiac enlargement, hepatomegaly, pulmonary rales, and occasionally peripheral edema. Symptoms of heart failure are present within the first week of life in about 10 per cent of patients but more commonly appear at about 1 month. Seventy-five per cent of these infants will have a systolic murmur even though the ventricular septum is intact. The second heart sound is single and loud because of the close proximity of the aorta to the chest wall. An apical diastolic gallop is commonly heard, and a mild diastolic apical murmur may be noted in those with an associated ventricular septal defect. The degree of pulmonary vascular obstruction cannot be assessed by auscultation since the second sound is usually loud and single. Pulmonary valvular or subvalvular stenosis is characteristically associated with a long crescendo-decrescendo systolic murmur along the left sternal border transmitted to the right clavicular area.

The common electrocardiographic findings are right atrial hypertrophy, right or combined ventricular hypertrophy, and right axis deviation. In early infancy the electrocardiogram may appear normal for age since the newborn characteristically has right ventricular hypertrophy. These findings vary, depending on age, presence or absence of ventricular septal defect, presence or absence of pulmonary valve or subvalvular stenosis, and the pulmonary vascular resistance. Right axis deviation is usually associated with an intact ventricular septum, whereas in approximately 40 per cent of patients with a moderate-sized ventricular septal defect the axis will be normal.

The routine chest x-ray is frequently diagnostic. The important factors are: progressive cardiomegaly in early infancy, an oval or egg-shaped cardiac configuration, a narrow superior mediastinum, and increased pulmonary vascular markings (Fig. 3). Characteristically, the heart is normal in size during the first 1 or 2 weeks of life, but then cardiac enlargement is observed in almost all infants with transposition of the great vessels and increased pulmonary blood flow. The pulmonary markings are prominent, and even pulmonary stenosis, unless unusually severe, does not significantly reduce the prominence of the pulmonary vasculature.

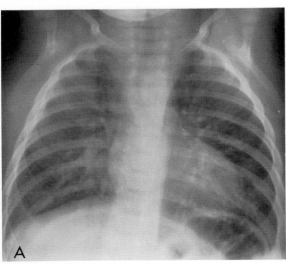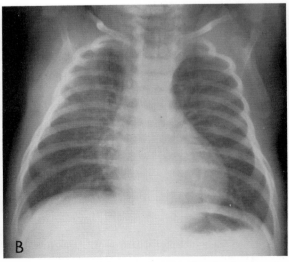

**Figure 3**  *A,* Typical chest x-ray of a 2 month old infant with transposition of the great vessels, showing hyperemic lung fields, narrow heart base, and the globular-shaped cardiac silhouette. *B,* Chest x-ray 3 weeks later, after creation of an atrial septal defect by the Blalock-Hanlon technique. Heart size is smaller and the lung fields are less plethoric.

## MANAGEMENT

Since most infants with transposition of the great vessels are cyanotic within the first week of life and the mortality is so high within the first 2 months, the majority usually are brought for treatment at a very early age. Cardiac catheterization should be undertaken to substantiate the diagnosis and confirm the position of intracardiac chambers. In most cases, the left atrial pressure will be greater than the right atrial pressure, and the pressure in the posterior or left ventricle will depend on the presence or absence of ventricular septal defect or pulmonary valvular or subvalvular stenosis as well as the state of the peripheral pulmonary vasculature. Catheterization must be performed in an expedient manner, as any stress in these severely ill infants increases metabolic requirements and the marked degree of cyanosis quickly results in systemic acidosis with marked reduction in arterial pH.

Once the diagnosis is confirmed in the newborn period, a balloon septostomy, performed as described by Rashkin and Miller in 1966,[34] is indicated in most of these infants. A balloon-tipped catheter is placed in a systemic vein and advanced into the right atrium and through the foramen ovale into the left atrium. The balloon is inflated with 1 to 3 ml. of contrast material so it can be visualized on the image intensifier, and then it is pulled vigorously across the atrial septum to enlarge or tear the foramen ovale (Fig. 4). This increases mixing of venous and oxygenated blood at the atrial level and has proved to be an excellent means of palliation in the very small infant. The balloon septostomy procedure can be repeated at subsequent dates if cyanosis becomes unmanageable. It is important that vigorous efforts at palliation in early infancy be undertaken since the more severely cyanotic infants are usually those with an intact ventricular septum and are therefore the best candidates for subsequent total correction.

### Palliative Operations

Since the advent of the balloon septostomy, the necessity of performing palliative operative procedures during the first month of life has been reduced. Approximately 70 per cent of infants with transposition of the great vessels and intact ventricular septum if left untreated will not survive the first month of life. It is currently recognized that these patients represent the most favorable group for subsequent total correction, and it is most imperative that successful palliation be accomplished. The technique in general use is the closed method of Blalock and Hanlon[6] by which the right pulmonary veins and a segment of right atrium are incorporated in a partial occluding clamp so that a segment of the atrial septum included within this clamp can be excised (Fig. 5). This procedure has certain advantages in that it removes the interatrial groove on the right side and allows enlargement of the right and left atria as a common chamber, which facilitates subsequent total correction.

The creation of an atrial septal defect under direct vision by inflow occlusion as recommended by Trusler in 1964[42] has generally carried a higher mortality than the closed procedure. The possibility of an air embolus entering the systemic circulation at the time the right atrium is opened is a serious complication of this technique. Palliative surgical procedures during the first month of life have been associated with a mortality of 40 to 50 per cent, which is reduced to 10 to 20 per cent if the operation is performed after the first month. The mortality with balloon septostomy during the first month of life has been less than 10 per cent, and this procedure has permitted many infants to undergo subsequent palliative operations at an age when the surgical procedure is much better tolerated.

### Ventricular Septal Defect

The presence of a small ventricular septal defect and only moderate elevation of pressure in the left ventricle should not cause major concern since irreversible pulmonary vascular disease is not likely to develop. Infants with large ventricular septal defects and systemic pressure in the left ventricle present one of the most difficult problems. These infants generally are not severely cyanotic, but irreversible vascular changes in the lungs develop at an early age if some type of pro-

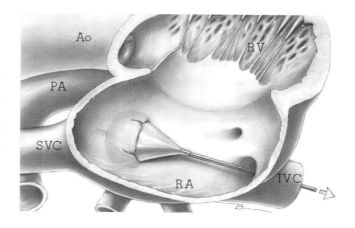

**Figure 4** The size of the interatrial communication is enlarged by passing a balloon-tipped catheter through the foramen ovale, inflating the balloon, and forcefully pulling it back into the right atrium. The atrial septum is torn and the patent foramen enlarged; this facilitates increased mixing of arterial and venous blood.

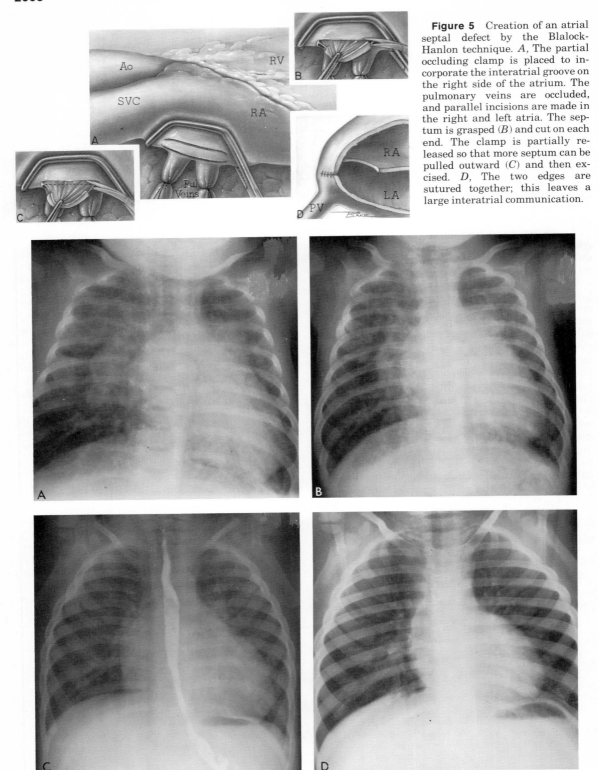

**Figure 5** Creation of an atrial septal defect by the Blalock-Hanlon technique. *A,* The partial occluding clamp is placed to incorporate the interatrial groove on the right side of the atrium. The pulmonary veins are occluded, and parallel incisions are made in the right and left atria. The septum is grasped (*B*) and cut on each end. The clamp is partially released so that more septum can be pulled outward (*C*) and then excised. *D,* The two edges are sutured together; this leaves a large interatrial communication.

**Figure 6** Sequence of chest x-rays showing: *A,* Age 3 weeks: Infant with transposition of the great vessels and a large ventricular septal defect in marked congestive heart failure. *B,* Age 5 weeks: Ten days after banding of the pulmonary artery the lung fields are less congested and heart failure is controlled. *C,* Age 3 months: Two weeks after creation of an atrial septal defect the lungs are even less congested and the heart size is smaller. *D,* Age 2½ years: Chest x-ray 6 months after removal of the pulmonary band, closure of the ventricular septal defect, and placement of an intra-atrial baffle for total correction. Heart size is reduced and lung markings are normal.

tection is not afforded. Banding of the pulmonary artery is a very delicate procedure in transposition of the great arteries. If the band is too tight, pulmonary flow is reduced too much and systemic hypoxia and metabolic acidosis ensue. On the other hand, if the band is too loose, flow to the lungs will not be significantly impeded and respiratory failure or pulmonary vascular changes will occur. If a patent ductus is present, it should be closed at the time of banding. In most instances, banding alone should not be considered but should be accompanied by some type of palliative procedure to improve mixing at the atrial level. This can be either open creation of an atrial septal defect, closed creation by the Blalock-Hanlon technique, or transposition of the atrial septum as recommended by Edwards and Bargeron in 1965[10] (Fig. 6). In general, if pulmonary flow is to be reduced by banding of the pulmonary artery to protect the pulmonary vasculature, improved mixing must be provided at the atrial level to prevent cyanosis from being too severe. It is *imperative* that a high pulmonary artery pressure not be allowed to persist beyond the first months of life, as irreversible pulmonary vascular changes are certain to develop.

### Left Ventricular Outflow Obstruction

This group of infants has proved to pose most perplexing problems as regards subsequent total correction. Palliative procedures probably should be designed so that subsequent total correction can be accomplished if the outflow obstruction can be relieved successfully. Many of these infants have an associated ventricular septal defect. Since the pressure in the pulmonary artery is quite low because of the outflow obstruction, anastomosis of the superior vena cava to the right pulmonary artery has been an attractive solution and has offered good palliation in children who do not have severe symptoms during the first 2 to 3 years of life. Subsequent total correction is not precluded by this procedure, but late studies of children in whom superior vena cava to right pulmonary artery shunts have been created have shown a progressive decrease in the amount of blood going to the right lung. If vascular resistance increases in the right lung or if pressure rises in the pulmonary venous system, more blood will be diverted away from the right lung through systemic venous collaterals and will return to the heart via the inferior vena cava. If total correction is attempted, the superior vena cava to right pulmonary artery anastomosis is usually left intact, and the inferior vena cava return is diverted to the posterior atrium. In most instances, pulmonary flow is reduced and must be increased in order to relieve cyanosis. Because of the anatomic relationship of the main pulmonary artery to the aorta, it is difficult to create a satisfactory Waterston-type shunt between the right pulmonary artery and the ascending aorta. In the infant, the best solution is probably a systemic-to-pulmonary shunt between the descending aorta and left pulmonary artery, accompanied by either balloon septostomy or crea-

tion of an atrial septal defect as a subsequent separate procedure. A direct anastomosis between the main pulmonary artery and ascending aorta also can be considered. If the child is above 1 year of age, a subclavian artery to pulmonary artery anastomosis can be accomplished. Fortunately, infants with outflow obstruction represent only a small minority of patients with transposition of the great vessels, and this type of palliation is seldom required.

### Reduced Pulmonary Flow

A small percentage of infants with transposition of the great vessels have diminished pulmonary markings, and usually an intact ventricular septum, and fail to thrive after creation of an atrial septal defect either by balloon septostomy or by operation. Whether in these infants there is some difference in compliance between the right and left ventricles that causes filling of the pulmonary ventricle to be inadequate to propel blood into the lungs has not been determined. However, some type of systemic-to-pulmonary shunting procedure often is required, and it may be that for these infants total correction during the first year of life should be considered. Dillard et al.[8] (1969) have had success in total correction in small infants, using deep hypothermia and total circulatory arrest for the time of intraoperative correction. Clark and Barrett-Boyes[7] (1967) reported similar success with the technique of deep hypothermia and circulatory arrest except that they employed a pump-oxygenator system during the rewarming phase.

### Total Correction

Correction of complete transposition of the great vessels by repositioning the transposed arteries over their appropriate ventricles has not been clinically successful. A major difficulty with this technique is that if the repositioning were accomplished above the orifice of the coronary arteries, coronary flow would come from the pulmonary artery and the heart would receive desaturated blood. Diversion of the venous inflow at the atrial level has appeared more appealing, and Senning in 1959[38] created two large interatrial channels for crossing the systemic and pulmonary venous circulations. This was accomplished by incising, realigning, and suturing interatrial septal tissue and the right atrial free wall in order to create these separate channels. This procedure was difficult to perform, and in the small infant it was practically impossible to obtain channels of adequate size. Mustard[32] in 1964 described an operation for total correction of transposition of the great vessels, based on principles proposed by Albert,[2] that provides an intra-atrial baffle, made of pericardial tissue, to direct the systemic venous return to the posterior ventricle and allow the pulmonary venous return to enter the systemic ventricle. Surgical success with this operation has been reported to be in the range of 80 to 90 per cent, and at present this technique certainly represents the best approach to total correction.[22]

If successful palliation has been provided in early infancy by balloon septostomy or a palliative operation, or both, elective total correction is usually undertaken when the child is between 18 and 36 months of age. It may be advisable to lower this elective age to 8 to 14 months in order to reduce the possibility of cerebral thrombosis or emboli, which are common in children with transposition. Although excision of a portion of the atrial septum and interatrial groove by the Blalock-Hanlon technique allows the two atria to enlarge in a spherical form and thus facilitates total correction, the operation described by Mustard has been performed with satisfactory results in children who have had only balloon septostomy.

The operative approach is through a median sternotomy incision. A large piece of anterior pericardium is excised, the pericardium is cleaned of as much scar or fibrous tissue and fat as possible,

and the venae cavae are mobilized for about 1 to 2 cm. into the pericardial orifices to facilitate cannulation. A purse-string suture is placed on the right lateral side of the atriocaval junction, and care is taken in placement of the superior vena cava catheter to avoid injury in the area of the sinus node. Total cardiopulmonary bypass is established, and the heart is electrically fibrillated to reduce the possibility of air emboli when the systemic atrium is opened (Fig. 7). The right atrium may be opened in either a longitudinal or transverse fashion. The ventricular septal defect, if present, is repaired by retraction of the leaflets of the tricuspid valve. If adequate exposure cannot be accomplished with retraction, the septal leaflet may be partially incised to facilitate visualization of the defect. The ventricular septal defects usually have a muscular rim owing to development of the subaortic conus. The defects are usually located

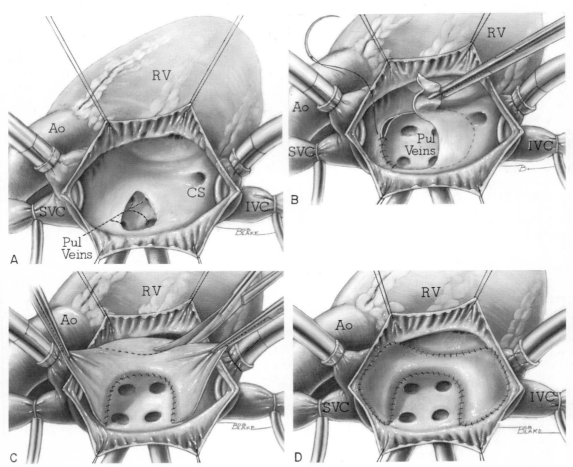

**Figure 7**   Total correction of transposition of the great vessels by intra-atrial diversion. *A*, The right atrium is opened, so that the atrial septum, coronary sinus, and atrial septal defect are exposed. *B*, The atrial septum is excised. If the excision extends outside the heart in the interatrial groove, it is repaired by direct suture. *C*, The pericardial or prosthetic patch is fashioned around the pulmonary veins and trimmed to fit the atrium. *D*, To complete repair, the baffle is sutured around the caval orifices and to the remnant of tissue across the top of the ventricular septum. Caval blood is now diverted posteriorly into the left ventricle, while pulmonary venous blood enters the right ventricle and then the aorta.

just below the posterior aspect of the aortic conus, and the conduction bundle passes along the superior aspect of the lower rim of the defect. Good exposure can be accomplished and closure is rarely a significant problem. In most instances, a patch should be used for closure of the ventricular septal defect.

The atrial septum is then completely excised; care must be taken to excise completely the interatrial groove in the cephalad area between the superior vena cava and the top of the ventricular septum. The incision may extend outside the heart and require suturing of the endocardial surfaces. If the rim of atrial septum is not completely removed between the medial junction of the superior cava and the superior border of the ventricular septum, this ridge may be too close to the pericardial baffle and obstruct flow from the superior cava. In some cases, it may be necessary to extend this incision superiorly along the medial side of the atriocaval junction and enlarge the area with a patch. A small rim is left attached to the top of the muscular ventricular septum between the tricuspid and mitral valves. This minimizes the possibility of damaging the conduction bundles when the baffle is sutured in place. The coronary sinus can be generously opened posteriorly into the left atrium to allow drainage into the venous circulation. The edges of the sinus are oversewn to ensure endothelialization. The baffle is tailored so that the center portion is somewhat narrower than the ends, and the center section is sutured to a position between the left pulmonary veins. The baffle is then sutured around the lateral orifice of the left pulmonary veins, and this suture line must be fairly close to the veins in order to allow adequate systemic venous return into the posterior ventricle. The suture line continues to the right across the floor of the left atrium onto the right lateral wall. Excess pericardium is removed since redundancy of the baffle may have a tendency to block the orifice of the mitral valve, or, if systemic venous pressure is elevated, bulging of the baffle into the right atrium may limit the volume of this chamber and result in pulmonary edema. The baffle extends over the orifices of the vena cava so that the venous catheters enter into the venous atrium. If a previous Blalock-Hanlon procedure has been performed and the interatrial septum has been removed on the right side, it is unusual to have to enlarge the systemic atrium (Fig. 8). If only a balloon septostomy has been performed, a pericardial patch is usually necessary to enlarge the left atrium by incorporating it in the closure of the atrium. The heart is allowed to fill with blood and care is taken to eliminate all air from the systemic ventricle. As closure of the atriotomy is accomplished and the heart is filled with blood, electrical fibrillation is discontinued and spontaneous defibrillation usually occurs. Usually, the superior vena caval catheter is removed before cardiopulmonary bypass is terminated.

One of the major complications of this operation has been associated tachycardia from an atrial origin or the creation of nodal rhythm. It seems

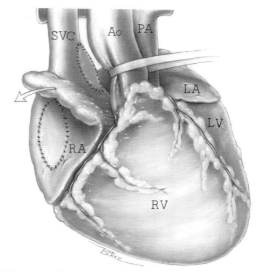

**Figure 8**   The atrium may require enlargement at two sites during complete correction. The right atrium may require an external patch over the lateral wall to enlarge the size of the chamber receiving blood from the pulmonary veins. In some cases, when the pulmonary veins arise more superiorly than usual, an external patch along the medial aspect of the superior caval-atrial junction is necessary to prevent obstruction of flow from the superior cava into the posterior atrium.

reasonable that when such large portions of the atrium have been excised and several incisions have been made in the walls of the atrium conduction from the sinus node to the atrioventricular node may be impaired or the scarring process about sutures may be responsible for ectopic atrial activity. The incidence of atrial flutter or supraventricular tachycardia has been high in the postoperative period, and both can be difficult to control. Definite care should be taken to preserve the sinus node, and positioning of the intra-atrial baffle in regard to the coronary sinus has been of concern. If the baffle is placed too near the atrioventricular node, it is possible that the atrioventricular node may be injured directly by suture, by scarring and fibrosis, or by ischemia produced by interruption of coronary vascular supply to the node. Thus, the suture line passing from the septal remnant between the atrioventricular orifices to the area of the coronary sinus should lie as far inside the anterior limit of the coronary sinus as possible. An alternative has been to eliminate the incision into the coronary sinus and extend the anterior suture line below the coronary sinus; this permits the coronary sinus to drain into the pulmonary atrium and assumes that the small right-to-left shunt will be of no significance. At present, the answer to the problem of how to avoid atrial rhythm disturbance has not been clearly defined. In the area between the ventricular septum and the inferior vena cava along the anterior suture line, meticulous care should be taken to keep the sutures as superficial as possible and to position the suture line inside the superior rim of the orifice of the coronary sinus.

The presence of pulmonary stenosis has been a most difficult problem to manage in the child with transposition of the great vessels. In most cases, this is a subvalvular stenosis that incorporates a portion of the mitral valve into the stenotic fibrotic band. Because of the posterior location of the pulmonary outflow tract and the presence of a major coronary vessel overlying the tract, it has not been possible to patch the outflow tract, as is commonly done in repair of tetralogy of Fallot. Excision or cutting of the fibromuscular components with a

rongeur through a pulmonary arteriotomy has been satisfactory in some children but complete relief of the stenosis may not be possible. If the child can be maintained to an older age, approximately 8 years, the procedure described by Rastelli[35] can be utilized. This technique is applicable in the presence of pulmonary stenosis and a large ventricular septal defect (Fig. 9). The pulmonary artery is simply divided and the end exiting from the heart sutured closed. A ventriculotomy is then performed between the aortic outflow and the ventricular septum, and an interventricular patch is positioned to divert the posterior ventricle efflux

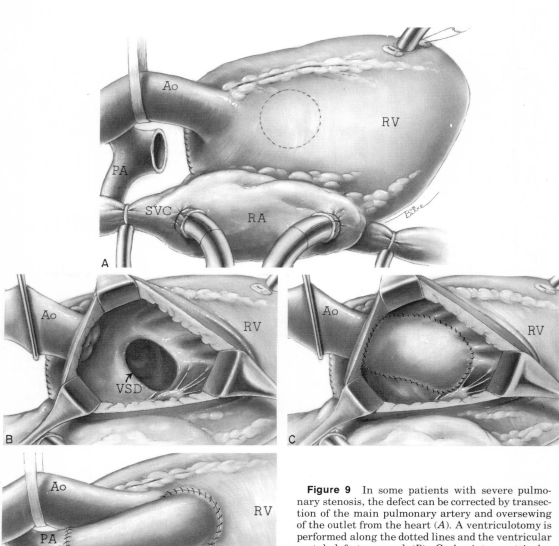

**Figure 9** In some patients with severe pulmonary stenosis, the defect can be corrected by transection of the main pulmonary artery and oversewing of the outlet from the heart (*A*). A ventriculotomy is performed along the dotted lines and the ventricular septal defect exposed (*B*). *C*, An intraventricular baffle is sutured so that flow from the posterior ventricle is directed out through the aorta. *D*, Venous blood reaches the lungs through an aortic root homograft connected to the ventriculotomy and the distal pulmonary artery.

through the ventricular septal defect and out through the aorta. An aortic homograft is then placed over the ventriculotomy and connected to the pulmonary artery to carry the systemic venous blood into the lungs. If a palliative atrial septal defect has previously been created, it is closed through a separate atriotomy.

If the pulmonary stenosis is mild, then direct surgical relief through the pulmonary artery should be adequate. It must be remembered that there usually is direct continuity between the pulmonary annulus and mitral annulus in the standard form of transposition, and good visualization must be accomplished to avoid damage to the mitral valve. The ventricular septal defect is closed in the usual fashion through the tricuspid valve and a routine intra-atrial baffle procedure is performed. Although this problem affects a very small percentage of infants with transposition of the great vessels, it certainly is the most challenging and difficult aspect of the anomaly to correct.

## OPERATIVE COMPLICATIONS

In any operative procedure when the systemic atrium and ventricles are open, air embolus must be prevented. Fibrillation of the heart during intracardiac repair and until the entire vascular system is refilled with blood has been a useful technique. The caval tapes should be released prior to defibrillation so that the surgeon can check for any leaks around the baffle and also detect any hemorrhage in areas where sutures may have torn the atrial wall during placement of the baffle. Blood will then pass through the lungs and any air trapped in the pulmonary veins should exit through the systemic atrium. Immediately before defibrillation, a small catheter is placed through the tricuspid valve to ensure that the ventricle is free of air.

The mediastinum must be drained well, because after correction of transposition the heart seems especially sensitive to any space-occupying lesions in the mediastinum. We have seen marked impairment of cardiac output caused by postoperative hemorrhage in the thymus. Clark and Barratt-Boyes[7] described two cases in which postoperative pulmonary edema was relieved by reoperation and removal of a clot positioned between the right pericardium and the right atrial wall. This extreme sensitivity of these children to mild postoperative mediastinal clot may be related to the anterior position of the systemic atrium and to its somewhat small size after the intra-atrial baffle procedure. The slightest compression of the right anterior atrial wall may impair filling of the systemic ventricle and result in low cardiac output and elevated pulmonary venous pressure. Partial obstruction of the superior vena cava by the baffle may occur since the pulmonary veins are located in the more superior aspect of the atrium, much nearer the superior vena cava orifice than the inferior vena cava orifice. Usually, partial obstruction of the superior cava will not be of clinical

significance, as venous collaterals easily divert the return to the lower part of the body and into the inferior vena cava. Redundancy of the baffle may partially obstruct the mitral orifice, or if the venous pressure is too high the baffle may bulge into the systemic atrium and cause pulmonary edema.

Rhythm disturbance following total correction of transposition of the great vessels has been quite common. Nodal rhythm will be present in a large percentage of these children in the postoperative period, and often a small amount of isoproterenol will be required to increase heart rate. Adjustment to a nodal rate of 80 to 90 per minute usually occurs after the first 4 to 5 days, but the use of a cardiotonic agent is most helpful during this time. Complete heart block is not common but certainly carries the same grave prognosis as when it occurs after surgical repair of other congenital heart defects. Atrial flutter with a rapid ventricular response has been a complication in the later postoperative period, and this can be extremely difficult to control with medications. In these children, it has proved difficult to block the atrioventricular node with digitalis, and antiarrhythmic agents such as quinidine have not been especially helpful in controlling the atrial disturbance. We have seen foci of atrial activity in the left atrium and in the coronary sinus as the source of atrial tachycardia or flutter. In one patient, propranolol proved effective in controlling these episodes. In most cases, these episodes are intermittent, usually self-terminating, and, in many instances, accentuated by sympathetic activity, as when the child is excited or frightened. These disturbances in rhythm have been less common in children with nodal rhythm in the postoperative period as compared to those with some type of conducted rhythm of atrial origin whether it be from the sinus node or other areas of the atrium.

Some degree of cardiac failure may be present in the immediate postoperative period and is usually manifested as mild pulmonary congestion and occasional accumulation of fluid in the pleural cavity. Since most of these children have a strong left ventricle, it is probably not advisable to elevate venous pressure above 8 to 10 cm. $H_2O$. A high venous pressure can cause bulging of the baffle into the right atrium and impede pulmonary venous return by diminishing the size of the atrium. This, of course, increases pulmonary congestion and compounds the problem if the pressure in the pulmonary artery is low and the left ventricle responds to a rise in central venous pressure. Tracheostomy has usually not been necessary, but the majority of children have required the use of an endotracheal tube and positive-pressure ventilation for 24 to 72 hours. Obviously, if the pulmonary vascular resistance is elevated or mild pulmonary stenosis remains, it may be necessary to increase venous pressure to improve the function of the left ventricle and elevate cardiac output. The hourly urine output has proved to be the best index of cardiac output, and we commonly use minute amounts of isoproterenol to improve cardiac function whenever urine output decreases, even though other measurements and clinical signs remain unchanged. Mild congestive heart failure may persist for several weeks or months but responds to proper medication, such as digitalis and diuretics, and appears to be self-limiting.

## RESULTS OF OPERATION

In transposition of the great vessels with intact atrial septum, total correction has been most gratifying, with operative survival between 80 and 90 per cent (Fig. 10). The presence of a small associated ventricular septal defect without evidence of pulmonary hypertension has also been associated with a high success rate. The majority of these children have been between the ages of 18 and 36 months at the time of correction, and obviously successful palliation in early infancy by balloon septostomy or operative creation of an atrial septal defect is most important in order to allow the majority of these infants to reach the age for definitive correction. The clinical responses have been excellent, with normal oxygen saturation and relatively unlimited activity. The pulmonary markings on chest x-ray decrease over 6 to 12 months, and progressive pulmonary hypertension has not been observed. Cardiac catheterization performed 1 to 3 years after operation has not demonstrated tricuspid insufficiency to be a major early complication, although the ability of the tricuspid valve to remain competent at systemic pressures continues to be a major unanswered question and ultimate success will depend greatly on this factor.

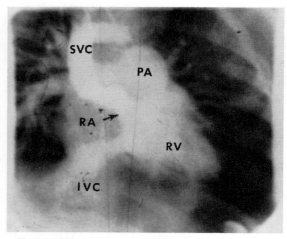

**Figure 10**　Postoperative cineangiocardiogram following total correction using an intra-atrial baffle. The arrow points to the baffle. Note that the blood flow from the venae cavae is directed posterior and to the left. The pulmonary venous return enters the right atrium, which is of adequate size.

## SELECTED REFERENCES

Aberdeen, E., and Carr, I.: Modern Trends in Cardiac Surgery. New York, Appleton-Century-Crofts, 1968.
*This monograph gives an excellent appraisal of the results of surgical treatment for transposition of the great vessels. It represents a review of the pertinent literature and presents a very large personal experience of the authors. The postoperative management and complications associated with total correction of transposition of the great vessels are well outlined.*

Blalock, A., and Hanlon, C. R.: The surgical treatment of complete transposition of the aorta and pulmonary artery. Surg. Gynec. Obstet., 90:1, 1950.
*This original article opened the era of surgical treatment of transposition of the great vessels. The illustrations and text emphasize to the student the necessity of complete understanding of the anatomic relationships necessary for the planning of a successful palliative procedure. The clinical histories relate the difficulties encountered in the preoperative and postoperative management of these severely ill infants.*

Mustard, W. T., Keith, J. D., Trusler, G. A., Fowler, R., and Kidd, L.: The surgical management of transposition of the great vessels. J. Thorac. Cardiovasc. Surg., 48:953, 1964.
*This excellent work describes the intra-atrial baffle procedure for total correction of transposition of the great vessels. The important details of the operative procedure are well defined, and many subtle points are emphasized to allow a better understanding of the complexity of this procedure. This paper was responsible for a complete change in thinking regarding the outlook for children with transposition of the great vessels.*

Paul, M. H.: Transposition of the great arteries. In: Moss, A. J., and Adams, F. H.: Heart Disease in Infants, Children, and Adolescents. Baltimore, Williams & Wilkins Company, 1968.
*This chapter clearly outlines the anatomic and embryologic development of transposition of the great vessels. Descriptions of the various types and possible positions of the great arteries and ventricles are presented. The basic pathophysiology of the circulatory anomaly is fully explained.*

## REFERENCES

1. Aberdeen, E., and Carr, I.: Modern Trends in Cardiac Surgery. New York, Appleton-Century-Crofts, 1968.
2. Albert, H. M.: Surgical correction of transposition of the great vessels. Surg. Forum, 5:74, 1955.
3. Baffes, T. G.: A new method for surgical correction of transposition of the aorta and pulmonary artery. Surg. Gynec. Obstet., 102:227, 1956.
4. Bailey, C. P.: Surgery of the Heart. Philadelphia, Lea & Febiger, 1955.
5. Barnard, C. N., Schrire, V., and Beck, W.: Complete transposition of the great vessels: A successful complete correction. J. Thorac. Cardiovasc. Surg., 43:768, 1962.
6. Blalock, A., and Hanlon, C. R.: The surgical treatment of complete transposition of the aorta and pulmonary artery. Surg. Gynec. Obstet., 90:1, 1950.
7. Clarke, C. P., and Barratt-Boyes, B. G.: The cause and treatment of pulmonary edema after the Mustard operation for correction of complete transposition of the great vessels. J. Thorac. Cardiovasc. Surg., 54:9, 1967.
8. Dillard, D. T., Mohri, H., Merendino, K. A., Morgan, B. C., Baum, D., and Crawford, E. W.: Total surgical correction of transposition of the great arteries in children less than six months of age. Surg. Gynec. Obstet., 129:1258, 1969.
9. Ebert, P. A., and Canent, R. V., Jr.: Corrective surgery for complete transposition of the great vessels. Amer. Surg., 36:28, 1970.
10. Edwards, W. S., and Bargeron, L. M., Jr.: More effective palliation of transposition of the great vessels. J. Thorac. Cardiovasc. Surg., 49:790, 1965.
11. Elliott, L. P., Anderson, R. C., Tuna, N., Adams, P., Jr., and Neufeld, H. N.: Complete transposition of the great vessels. I. An anatomic study of sixty cases. Circulation, 27:1105, 1963.
12. Fanconi, G.: Die Transposition der grossen Gefasse (das charakteristische Rontgenbild). Arch. Kinderheilk., 95:202, 1932.

13. Ferencz, C.: Transposition of the great vessels. Pathophysiologic considerations based upon a study of the lungs. Circulation, 33:232, 1966.
14. Ferguson, D. J., Adams, P., and Watson, D.: Pulmonary arteriosclerosis in transposition of the great vessels. Amer. J. Dis. Child., 99:653, 1960.
15. Glenn, W. W. L., and Patino, J. F.: Circulatory bypass of the right heart. I. Preliminary observations on the direct delivery of vena caval blood into the pulmonary arterial circulation. Azygos vein-pulmonary artery shunt. Yale J. Biol. Med., 27:147, 1954.
16. Glotzer, P., Young, D., and Bloomberg, A.: Sequential banding of the creation of atrial septal defect for transposition of the great vessels. J. Thorac. Cardiovasc. Surg., 46:104, 1963.
17. Grant, R. P.: The morphogenesis of transposition of the great vessels. Circulation, 26:819, 1962.
18. Hallman, G. L., and Cooley, D. A.: Complete transposition of great vessels: results of surgical treatment. Arch. Surg., 89:891, 1964.
19. Hanlon, C. R., and Blalock, A.: Complete transposition of the aorta and the pulmonary artery. Experimental observations on venous shunts as corrective procedures. Ann. Surg., 127:385, 1948.
20. Harris, J. S., and Farber, S.: Transposition of the great cardiac vessels with special reference to the phylogenetic theory of Spitzer. Arch. Path., 28:427, 1939.
21. Hightower, B. M., Weidman, W. H., and Kirklin, J. W.: Open intracardiac repair for complete transposition of the great arteries. Circulation, Supp. 1, 33:19, 1966.
22. Indeglia, R. A., Moller, J. H., Lucas, R. V., Jr., and Castaneda, A. R.: Treatment of transposition of the great vessels with an intra-atrial baffle (Mustard procedure). Arch. Surg., 101:797, 1970.
23. Kay, E. B., and Cross, F. S.: Transposition of the great vessels corrected by means of atrial transposition. Surgery, 41:938, 1957.
24. Keith, J. D., Neill, C. A., Vlad, P., Rowe, R. D., and Chute, A. L.: Transposition of the great vessels. Circulation, 7:830, 1953.
25. Kirklin, J. W., Devlon, R. A., and Weidman, W. H.: Open intracardiac repair of transposition of great vessels: 11 cases. Surgery, 50:58, 1961.
26. Lev, M., and Saphir, O.: A theory of transposition of the arterial trunks based on the phylogenetic and ontogenetic developments of the heart. Arch. Path., 39:172, 1945.
27. Liebman, J., Cullum, L., and Belloc, N. R.: Natural history of transposition of the great arteries. Circulation, 40: 237, 1969.
28. Lillehei, C. W., and Varco, R. L.: Certain physiologic, pathologic, and surgical features of complete transposition of the vessels. Surgery, 34:376, 1953.
29. Merendino, K. A., Jesseph, J. E., and Herron, P. W.: Interatrial venous transposition, a one stage intracardiac operation for the conversion of complete transposition of the aorta and pulmonary artery to corrected transposition: Theory and clinical experience. Surgery, 42:898, 1957.
30. Mustard, W. T.: Successful two-stage correction of transposition of the great vessels. Surgery, 55:469, 1964.
31. Mustard, W. T., Chute, A. L., Keith, J. D., Sirek, A., Rowe, R. D., and Vlad, P.: A surgical approach to transposition of the great vessels with extracorporeal circuit. Surgery, 36:39, 1954.
32. Mustard, W. T., Keith, J. D., Trusler, G. A., Fowler, R., and Kidd, L.: The surgical management of transposition of the great vessels. J. Thorac. Cardiovasc. Surg., 48:953, 1964.
33. Paul, M. H.: Transposition of the great arteries. In: Moss, A. J., and Adams, F. H.: Heart Disease in Infants, Children and Adolescents. Baltimore, Williams & Wilkins Company, 1968, p. 527.
34. Rashkind, W. J., and Miller, W. W.: Transposition of the great arteries: Results of palliation by balloon atrioseptotomy in 31 patients. Circulation, 38:453, 1968.
35. Rastelli, G. C., Wallace, R. B., and Ongley, P. A.: Complete repair of transposition of the great arteries with pulmonary stenosis: A review and report of a case corrected by using a new surgical technique. Circulation, 39:83, 1969.
36. Reed, W. A., Lauer, R. M., and Diehl, A. M.: Staged correction of total transposition of the great vessels. Circulation, Supp. 1, 33:13, 1966.
37. Rowlatt, U. F.: Coronary artery distribution in a complete transposition. J.A.M.A., 179:269, 1962.
38. Senning, A.: Surgical correction of transposition of the great vessels. Surgery, 45:966, 1959.
39. Shaher, R. M., and Kidd, L.: The hemodynamics of complete transposition of the great vessels before and after the creation of an atrial septal defect. Circulation, Supp. 1, 33:3, 1966.
40. Taussig, H. B.: Complete transposition of the great vessels. Amer. Heart J., 16:728, 1938.
41. Taussig, H. B.: Congenital Malformations of the Heart. 2nd ed. Cambridge, Mass., Harvard University Press, 1960.
42. Trusler, G. A., Mustard, W. T., and Fowler, R. S.: Role of surgery in the treatment of transposition of the great vessels. Canad. Med. Ass. J., 91:1096, 1964.
43. Van Mierop, L. H. S., and Wiglesworth, F. W.: Pathogenesis of transposition complexes. III. True transposition of the great vessels. Amer. J. Cardiol., 12:233, 1963.
44. Van Praagh, R., and Vlad, P.: Transposition of the great arteries. In: Keith, J. D., Rowe, R. D., and Vlad, P., eds.: Heart Disease in Infancy and Childhood. 2nd ed. New York, Macmillan Company, 1967.
45. Von Rokitansky, C.: Die Defekte der Scheidewände der Herzens. Vienna, Bräumuller, 1875.
46. Waldhausen, J. A., Pierce, W. S., Rashkind, W. J., et al.: Total correction of transposition of the great arteries following balloon atrioseptotomy. Circulation, Supp. 2, 41:123, 1970.

# IX

# Congenital Aortic Stenosis

*H. Newland Oldham, Jr., M.D.*

Congenital aortic stenosis is produced by a group of malformations that cause obstruction to the flow of blood from the left ventricle into the central aorta. This obstruction may be located at, above, or below the level of the aortic valve. These lesions are not uncommon and account for 5 to 10 per cent of all congenital heart defects.[22] Current information indicates that an abnormality of the aortic valve, although not always hemodynamically significant, is the single most common congenital cardiac defect encountered.[38] It is also now recognized that there is evidence of a pre-existing congenital valvular deformity in at least one-half of adult patients with isolated aortic valve lesions.[37]

There are no known etiologic or genetic factors associated with either valvular or discrete subvalvular aortic stenosis, although supravalvular stenosis may occur with derangements in vitamin D metabolism and infantile hypercalcemia. Both the aortic lesions and the associated craniofacial abnormalities seen with this type of stenosis may be induced experimentally by administration of large doses of vitamin D.[10] A genetic factor is present in patients with hypertrophic muscular subaortic stenosis, since this lesion occurs in a familial form in about one-third of patients.[3]

## HISTORICAL ASPECTS

Early descriptions of aortic valve disease such as that given by Riverius in 1646 primarily concerned calcific aortic stenosis in the adult.[36] In 1844 Paget described the tendency of congenitally bicuspid aortic valves to cause obstruction, and in 1886 Osler reported the occurrence of endocarditis with bicuspid aortic valves.[30,31] The association of arrhythmias and sudden death with aortic stenosis was recognized by Cowper in 1705 in a young adult, and Thursfield in 1913 called attention to sudden death in a child with subaortic stenosis.[8,43] Tuffier in 1913 successfully dilated a calcific aortic valve, but no further advances were made until 1950 when Bailey successfully performed a closed dilation of the aortic valve.[1,44] In 1955 Swan and Lewis independently performed valvulotomies using hypothermia.[20,42] With the development of extracorporeal circulation, techniques for accurate relief of various forms of congenital aortic stenosis were successfully introduced.

## PATHOLOGIC ANATOMY

The four types of obstruction that occur between the left ventricle and the aorta are valvular, discrete subvalvular, supravalvular, and hypertrophic muscular subaortic stenosis (Fig. 1). The stenosis is usually limited to one of these four types, but combinations of lesions may occur together in the same patient.[41] Between 20 and 25

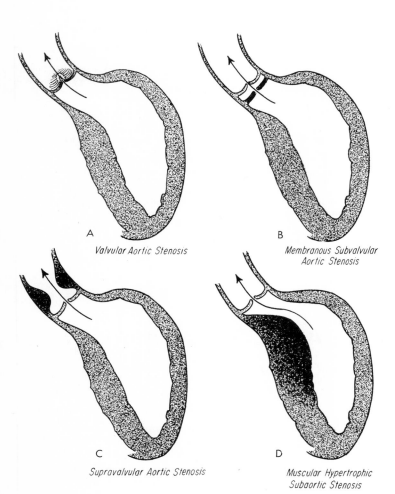

A  *Valvular Aortic Stenosis*

B  *Membranous Subvalvular Aortic Stenosis*

C  *Supravalvular Aortic Stenosis*

D  *Muscular Hypertrophic Subaortic Stenosis*

**Figure 1**  Diagrammatic representation of the types of congenital obstruction between the left ventricle and central aorta.

per cent of these patients have other associated cardiovascular defects, most commonly coarctation of the aorta, patent ductus arteriosus, ventricular septal defect, or pulmonary stenosis.

The type of obstruction in more than half the patients is isolated valvular aortic stenosis. The basic malformation is a thickening of the valve leaflets associated with varying degrees of fusion of the commissure. The annulus is usually not affected, although occasionally it is hypoplastic. The valve may be tricuspid, with partial fusion of each commissure producing a central stenotic orifice. Fusion of the commissure between the right and the left coronary cusps, producing a bicuspid valve with an eccentric narrowed opening, occurs in 60 to 80 per cent of patients with valvular stenosis.[9, 23] Less common types encountered are valves with four cusps or valves with only a single supporting commissure that functions as a monocusp.[25, 38] Histologically, the valves demonstrate fibrosis and a persistence of embryonic connective tissue.[40] Infants with critical stenosis may have fibrosis of the myocardium, necrosis of the papillary muscles, and fibroelastosis.[5, 24, 40] Calcification of a deformed aortic valve is quite common in patients over age 30 but is extremely rare during childhood.

Discrete subaortic stenosis is the second most common type of obstruction encountered and consists of a thin ring of fibrous tissue located 10 to 15 mm. below the aortic valve. This may form a concentric diaphragm with a central stenotic opening, but often the membrane is more prominent over the anterior portion of the left ventricular outflow tract and fuses at each end with the aortic leaflet of the mitral valve. The aortic valve in this situation is not stenotic, but the leaflets may be thickened, in which case mild aortic insufficiency is produced. This thickening may be due to the turbulence produced by blood ejected through the stenotic subvalvular membrane and may cause the valve to be more susceptible to bacterial endocarditis.[9, 27]

Supravalvular aortic stenosis occurs in several anatomic forms, ranging from localized narrowing just above the valve commissures to diffuse hypoplasia of the aortic annulus and ascending aorta.[7, 35] The outer diameter of the aorta is usually normal, but may be reduced at the site of localized obstruction. The obstructing ridge is composed of fibrous tissue and elastic fibers extending from the tunica media, and it may cover the sinuses of Valsalva and produce obstruction of the coronary artery ostia. Supravalvular aortic stenosis is commonly associated with peripheral pulmonary stenosis, abnormalities of the aortic valve leaflets, coronary artery abnormalities, and craniofacial deformities.[9, 10, 35, 46]

Muscular subaortic stenosis is a diffuse abnormality of the cardiac muscle with a broad area of hypertrophied tissue located several centimeters below the aortic valve. This type of obstruction may occur as a secondary phenomenon with other forms of aortic stenosis, or it may be a primary disorder with no other associated malformations.

Microscopically, the tissue is composed of muscle fibers arranged in whorl-like masses.

## PHYSIOLOGY

The basic hemodynamic alteration produced by obstruction of left ventricular outflow is an increase in left ventricular pressure. All four types of aortic stenosis result in a pressure gradient between the left ventricle and the aorta during the systolic ejection period. The degree of stenosis determines the pressure gradient at any given flow rate, but as cardiac output increases, the pressure gradient increases in proportion to the square of the flow rate.[14] Normal flow can be maintained through an abnormal valve at the expense of a sustained elevation of left ventricular pressure. With exercise, a doubling of cardiac output produces a fourfold increase in ventricular pressure. Both the increase in ventricular wall tension and the increased duration of tension due to increased systolic ejection time are associated with an increase in myocardial oxygen consumption. The ventricle adapts to this prolonged pressure overload by an increase in muscle mass and a subsequent decrease in left ventricular cavity size.[15] The increased systolic ejection period results in a decrease in the length of diastole and therefore reduces coronary perfusion. Increased myocardial energy requirements coupled with a relative decrease in coronary flow ultimately result in left ventricular failure or ischemia. With left ventricular failure there is a reduction in cardiac output and an increase in left ventricular end-diastolic, left atrial, and pulmonary artery pressures.

The resting cardiac output and stroke volume are usually within normal limits in children with congenital aortic stenosis. If the resting pressure gradient between the left ventricle and the aorta is less than 50 mm. Hg, or if the calculated aortic orifice size is greater than 0.7 sq. cm. per square meter of body surface area, the heart usually responds to the demands of exertion without failing. In the majority of patients with a greater degree of stenosis, manifested by a higher pressure gradient and a smaller effective valve area, cardiac output cannot be elevated by means of exercise.

The two most important sequelae of severe obstruction to left ventricular ejection are clearly increased stress on the myocardium and inability of the left ventricle to increase forward flow in response to exertion. These limitations explain the frequent occurrence of left ventricular strain, angina, and exertional syncope in children with congenital aortic stenosis.

These considerations are particularly applicable to congenital valvular, supravalvular, and discrete subaortic stenosis, all of which have a fixed area of obstruction. Hypertrophic muscular subaortic stenosis differs in that the severity of the obstruction varies, depending on the contractile state of the myocardium and left ventricular end-systolic volume. In this condition the pressure gradient is increased by infusion of inotropic drugs such as isoproterenol, by decreasing blood volume, and by the Valsalva maneuver. The obstruction is reduced by maneuvers such as increasing blood volume, general anesthesia, and administration of propranolol, an adrenergic blocking agent. A clear understanding of the effects of these influences on myocardial contraction and ventricular volume has helped to explain the different gradients measured by catheterization during varying physiologic states.[3, 4, 33, 45]

## CLINICAL FEATURES

Congenital aortic stenosis is three to four times more common in males than in females. The clinical presentation is essentially identical for each type of obstruction and the distinguishing factor is the capacity of the left ventricle to compensate for its pressure overload both at rest and during exercise. Even in the presence of significant stenosis, most patients are asymptomatic during early childhood and show normal growth and development. During later childhood, symptoms of exertional dyspnea and fatigue are common. It should be emphasized, however, that it is not unusual for children with critical stenosis to remain entirely free of symptoms, whereas others with minimal obstruction may have prominent symptoms. When the cardiac output is insufficient to meet the demands of the systemic or coronary circulation, symptoms of exertional syncope, angina, and congestive heart failure occur. These findings usually indicate a severe degree of stenosis. Left ventricular failure occurring in infancy is particularly ominous and is usually fatal if untreated.[5, 32]

Physical examination demonstrates a characteristic harsh systolic murmur, most prominent over the second right interspace and usually associated with a thrill. A diastolic murmur of mild aortic insufficiency is heard in one-fourth of patients with congenital aortic stenosis and is more common with discrete subvalvular stenosis. Phonocardiography characterizes the systolic murmur as the ejection type, beginning shortly after the

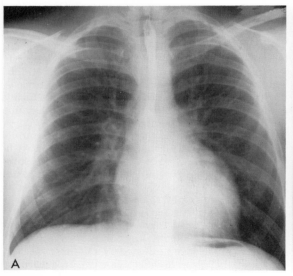

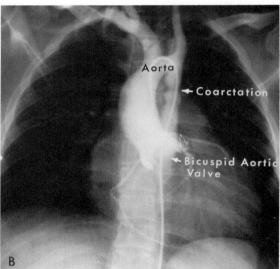

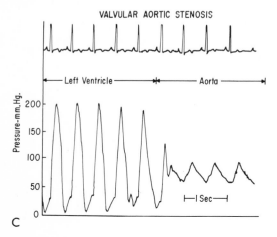

**Figure 2** Valvular aortic stenosis. *A*, Chest film demonstrating slight prominence of the left ventricle. *B*, Aortogram showing a bicuspid aortic valve, poststenotic dilatation of the ascending aorta, and associated coarctation of the descending thoracic aorta. *C*, Pressure tracing during withdrawal of a catheter from the left ventricle into the aorta, localizing the change in pressure to the level of the aortic valve.

first heart sound and ending just before the second heart sound. The second heart sound may be paradoxically split as a result of the increased duration of systolic ejection. On percussion, the heart is not found to be enlarged, but a prominent left ventricular lift is often present. The carotid pulse has a palpable slow upstroke, except with hypertrophic muscular subaortic stenosis, in which the upstroke is normal or rapid. The remainder of the physical examination is not remarkable, with the exception of the findings associated with supravalvular aortic stenosis. In this disorder a characteristic facies is frequently present, and the systolic blood pressure in the right arm is often higher than that in the left.[7,35,46]

The chest roentgenogram demonstrates little overall cardiomegaly, but 70 to 80 per cent of patients have evidence of left ventricular enlargement.[23,34] Unfortunately, the degree of enlargement does not correlate well with the severity of the stenosis, and severe obstruction may be present in children with a normal chest film. Poststenotic dilatation of the ascending aorta is present in approximately one-half of patients with moder-

ate to severe stenosis and occurs more commonly with valvular stenosis than with the other forms of obstruction (Fig. 2). Active pulsation of the ascending aorta is seen with fluoroscopy. Calcification is rarely present in children, but its presence in a young adult is evidence that the obstruction is valvular.

The electrocardiogram has been extensively used to judge the degree of obstruction in congenital aortic stenosis. It is now realized that the electrocardiographic findings do not correlate well with the magnitude of the pressure gradient. Stenosis that is severe enough to cause sudden death has been documented in children without any electrocardiographic abnormalities. In most patients with a pressure gradient of greater than 50 mm. Hg, changes of left ventricular hypertrophy and left ventricular strain are present. There is a much better correlation between these findings and the degree of stenosis in patients under 10 years of age.[2] The vectorcardiogram at times may demonstrate evidence of severe aortic stenosis despite a normal electrocardiogram.[12,17] Because of the difficulties in relating electrocardi-

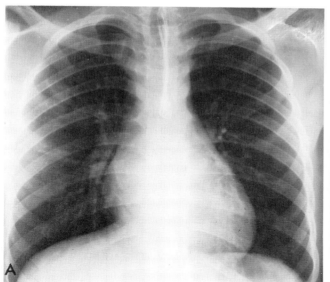
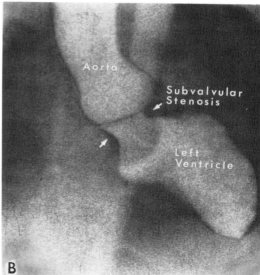
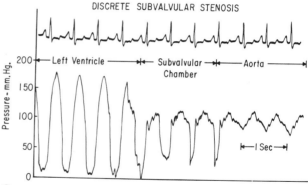

**Figure 3** Discrete subvalvular aortic stenosis. *A*, Chest film. *B*, Cineangiogram during left ventricular injection, demonstrating a subvalvular membrane. *C*, Pull-back pressure tracing showing systemic systolic pressure in the subvalvular chamber.

ographic findings to the presence of left ventricular overload in any individual patient, caution should be exercised in the use of these results in determining patient management.

## CARDIAC CATHETERIZATION

Congenital aortic stenosis may be diagnosed accurately on the basis of clinical findings, the chest roentgenogram, and the electrocardiogram without benefit of cardiac catheterization, but in order to determine the type and the degree of stenosis, and to eliminate the possibility of other associated defects, catheterization is essential. Combined right and left heart catheterization and selective angiocardiography are necessary to obtain this information. Catheterization of the right side of the heart will demonstrate any other lesions, such as a ventricular septal defect or pulmonary stenosis, that may be present, and it will also determine the presence or absence of pulmonary hypertension. Left heart catheterization is performed by either the transseptal or retrograde arterial approach. From the measurements of cardiac output and of the systolic pressure gradi-

ent between the left ventricle and the central aorta, it is possible to calculate the functional orifice area of the stenosis.[14] Selective left ventricular angiocardiography permits visualization of the level of obstruction and also allows assessment of left ventricular cavity size, ventricular wall thickness, and competency of the mitral valve (Figs. 2 to 5). If hypertrophic muscular subaortic stenosis is suspected, measurement of the pressure gradient is indicated during infusion of drugs that change peripheral vascular resistance or the inotropic state of the myocardium.[3]

## NATURAL HISTORY AND OPERATIVE INDICATIONS

Careful studies of the natural history of patients with congenital aortic stenosis have been limited by the development of surgical treatment of this condition. The finding of congenitally deformed valves in most adults with isolated calcific aortic stenosis indicates the progressive nature of the obstruction over a prolonged period of time.[37] The clinical course is quite variable, with a normal life expectancy in some patients and overt cardiac

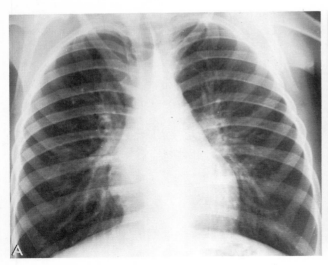

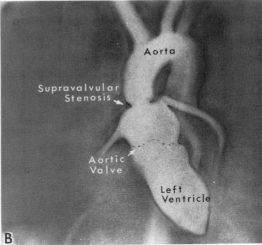

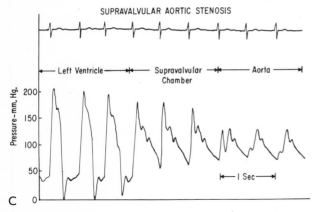

**Figure 4** Supravalvular aortic stenosis. *A*, Chest film. *B*, Cineangiogram illustrating an obstructing ridge just above the origin of the coronary arteries. *C*, Pressure recording demonstrating a supravalvular zone of elevated pressure.

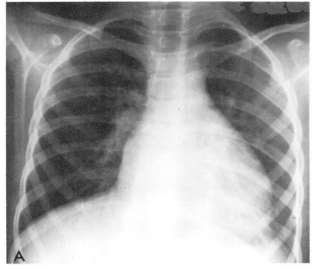

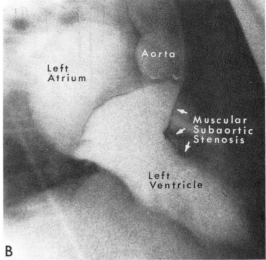

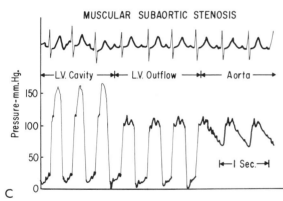

**Figure 5** Hypertrophic muscular subaortic stenosis. *A*, Chest film showing considerable enlargement of the left ventricle. *B*, Left ventricular cineangiogram illustrating a broad area of muscular obstruction. The left atrium is opacified as a result of associated mitral insufficiency. *C*, Pressure tracing showing an area of systemic pressure within the left ventricular outflow tract.

decompensation or sudden death in others. Severe aortic stenosis occurring in infancy is accompanied by a high incidence of associated malformations and often causes cardiac failure and death.[16] Older children who become symptomatic usually have a moderate to severe degree of stenosis. Evaluation of initially asymptomatic children by serial cardiac catheterization showed that severe obstruction developed in more than half over a period of several years. The majority of these patients who acquired significant gradients showed no progression of symptoms or electrocardiographic findings suggesting severe obstruction.[11] Sudden death is reported to occur in 1 to 19 per cent of children with aortic stenosis.[6,13] This phenomenon, probably related to arrhythmias, is seen in most patients only after development of serious symptoms and electrocardiographic changes of left ventricular strain. It should be emphasized, however, that patients with none of these abnormal signs or symptoms have experienced sudden death.[19]

Operative treatment is recommended in a child with severe obstruction, indicated by a systolic pressure gradient greater than 50 mm. Hg or by a calculated area of stenosis less than 0.5 sq. cm. per square meter of body surface area. It is advisable, if possible, to delay operation until the child is older, because surgical exposure and techniques are easier when the structures are larger. Since as many as one-fourth of infants with severe obstruction die during the first year of life, operative treatment may be indicated at this early age in spite of the increased operative risk.[5,6,18]

## SURGICAL TREATMENT AND RESULTS

Operative procedures are currently available for correction or palliation of all forms of left ventricular outflow obstruction. The general approach of the various types is the same, but specific methods for relief of the stenosis are quite different. With rare exceptions, all operations are performed with cardiopulmonary bypass, which allows ample time and exposure for complete assessment of the defect and utilization of precise surgical techniques. The heart is exposed through a median sternotomy. Venous drainage is provided by a catheter inserted into the right atrium, and arterial inflow is directed into the femoral artery

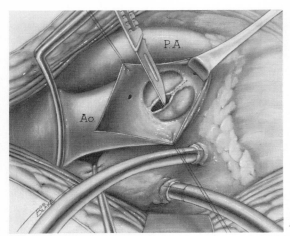

**Figure 6**  Valvular aortic stenosis. A longitudinal incision is made in the ascending aorta to expose the bicuspid aortic valve. The valve is incised along the line of fusion of the commissures to relieve the stenosis.

or the ascending aorta. The left ventricle is cannulated through its apex or the right superior pulmonary vein to produce a bloodless field. After the ascending aorta is clamped, a vertical aortotomy is made into the noncoronary sinus of Valsalva. Protection against myocardial ischemia is achieved by mild hypothermia and individual perfusion of the coronary arteries. At this point, careful evaluation of the anatomy is undertaken, with the realization that additional sites of obstruction may be present. Only after the exact nature of the lesion is established can specific methods for its correction be employed.

Valvular stenosis is corrected by incision of the fused commissures. If the valve is tricuspid, each of the three commissures is divided to within 1 mm. of the aortic annulus. With the more common

bicuspid valve, the two lines of fusion are carefully separated (Fig. 6). The incomplete commissure in the left half of the bicuspid valve representing the fusion point of the right and left coronary cusps should not be incised, since this destroys the support of that portion of the valve and produces significant aortic regurgitation. It is advisable to perform a limited valvulotomy, and leave a residual gradient, rather than to abolish the gradient completely at the expense of aortic insufficiency.[28] In the rare circumstance when a unicusp valve is encountered, extreme care must be exercised, since it may be impossible to enlarge the valve orifice safely.

Exposure of discrete subvalvular stenosis is obtained by retracting the aortic valve leaflets (Fig. 7). The fibrous membrane is partially removed in the safe portion of its circumference beneath each side of the commissure between the right and left leaflets. Extensive removal of the membrane in other areas can produce damage to the underlying structures and result in mitral insufficiency, ventricular septal defect, or third-degree heart block. The aortic valve leaflets are often thickened and may cause mild aortic insufficiency, but no attempt should be made to correct hemodynamically insignificant regurgitation.

When supravalvular stenosis is caused by diffuse hypoplasia of the ascending aorta, surgical procedures such as endarterectomy or enlarging the aorta by a long prosthetic patch may occasionally be successful, but in general the results of these maneuvers have not been satisfactory. The localized type of supravalvular stenosis is much more amenable to surgical correction. The deformed area is usually just above the commissures, so total excision of the tissue as a form of treatment is not possible. Partial excision of the intraluminal ridge is indicated if there is obstruction of the coronary ostia. Effective relief of the obstruction is achieved by suturing a patch of plastic

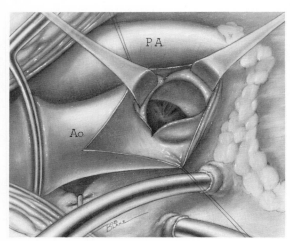

**Figure 7**  Discrete subvalvular aortic stenosis. The aortic valve leaflets are retracted to expose the subvalvular membrane. Partial excision of this membrane elminates the obstruction.

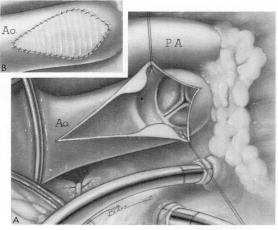

**Figure 8**  Supravalvular aortic stenosis. A, The aortotomy is performed through the ridge of obstructing tissue located just above the coronary ostia. B, A patch of plastic material is inserted into the aortic incision to enlarge the narrowed segment.

material to each side of a generous aortotomy and extending it through the constricting segment (Fig. 8).

Muscular subaortic stenosis is now recognized as a diffuse disorder of the left ventricular musculature. Pharmacologic alteration of the process by adrenergic blocking agents is occasionally helpful; however, in those patients with severe gradients, relief of the obstruction by surgical means is preferable. Numerous approaches for resection of a portion of the muscle mass have been advocated, but the transaortic route has been successfully used in most instances.[26, 29] After the aortic valve leaflets have been retracted, the diffuse area of hypertrophy is defined by palpation through the valve. Parallel incisions are made into the muscle and a strip of tissue is excised between these cuts for a considerable distance into the ventricle (Fig. 9). The incision must be properly placed to avoid perforation of the septum or injury to the conduction system.

At the conclusion of the operative procedure for the various types of aortic stenosis, simultaneous pressures should be recorded from the left ventricle and the ascending aorta to measure any residual gradient. It is preferable to accept a gradient of 30 mm. Hg or less rather than extend the opening and risk the production of aortic insufficiency or damage to adjacent structures. There is good correlation between the gradient recorded at the end of the procedure and measurements obtained during postoperative catheterization. In some patients with adequate correction of valvular stenosis, a gradient remains because of secondary muscular hypertrophy, but this usually resolves during the postoperative period.[9]

The risks of surgical correction of all types of aortic stenosis are small, and the postoperative results are generally good. The long-term results following relief of supravalvular, muscular subaortic, and discrete subaortic stenosis justify an aggressive surgical approach to these disorders.[21, 26, 35] The ultimate outcome following operation for congenital valvular stenosis is not as clearly established. At the present time it is not known whether opening a deformed valve during childhood will prevent the progression of subsequent stenosis and calcification during adult life. It is probable that a second operative procedure will be necessary in some of these patients, and insertion of a prosthetic valve may be required. Until these questions are answered, it seems wise to limit operative treatment for congenital valvular aortic stenosis to those patients with a significant pressure gradient or clinical findings of left ventricular compromise.

## SELECTED REFERENCES

Braunwald, E., Goldblatt, A., Aygen, M. M., Rockoff, S. D., and Morrow, A. G.: Congenital aortic stenosis. I. Clinical and hemodynamic findings in 100 patients. Circulation, 27:426, 1963.

Morrow, A. G., Goldblatt, A., and Braunwald, E.: Congenital aortic stenosis. II. Surgical treatment and results of operation. Circulation, 27:450, 1963.
*These companion papers represent excellent examples of the critical use of hemodynamic measurements in evaluating both the preoperative severity of congenital aortic stenosis and the results of operative intervention. A thorough analysis of the clinical findings, electrocardiographic patterns, and cardiac catheterization data from 100 children is presented. The surgical procedures used in 44 of these patients are clearly described and illustrated. Complete postoperative cardiac catheterization studies were performed in 33 patients, and the findings document the effectiveness of the methods of treatment utilized.*

Friedman, W. F., Modlinger, J., and Morgan, J. R.: Serial hemodynamic observation in asymptomatic children with valvar aortic stenosis. Circulation, 43:91, 1971.
*This evaluation of initially asymptomatic children by serial cardiac catheterizations demonstrated that severe obstruction developed in more than half over an average follow-up period of 6.8 years. In the majority of these patients, symptoms, electrocardiograms, and chest roentgenograms did not correlate well with the development of a significant transvalvular pressure gradient. The authors conclude that serial hemodynamic studies should be a routine part of the evaluation of asymptomatic children with aortic stenosis in order to determine properly the advisability of surgical treatment.*

McGoon, D. C., Geha, A. S., Scofield, E. L., and DuShane, J. W.: Surgical treatment of congenital aortic stenosis. Dis. Chest, 55:388, 1969.
*Extensive experience with the surgical treatment of the various forms of congenital aortic stenosis in 169 patients is presented. This is the largest series currently available for review. The operative mortality of only 3.5 per cent and the significant improvement achieved in these patients are commendable. The authors stress the fact that operative treatment for congenital valvular aortic stenosis is palliative rather than curative, since many of these children have a residual transvalvular pressure gradient at the completion of the procedure.*

Morrow, A. G.: Hypertrophic subaortic stenosis: Some physiologic concepts and the role of operative treatment. Arch. Surg., 99:677, 1969.
*The author presents an experience over a 10 year period in characterizing the physiologic basis for this form of aortic stenosis, and in developing a successful method of surgical treatment. A concise hemodynamic explanation for the changing nature of this type of obstruction is given. The results obtained with a transaortic resection of hypertrophied muscle in 34 patients clearly document the effectiveness of this approach in relieving the obstruction.*

Rastelli, G. C., McGoon, D. C., Ongley, P. A., Mankin, H. T., and Kirklin, J. W.: Surgical treatment of supravalvular aortic stenosis. J. Thorac. Cardiovasc. Surg., 51:873, 1966.

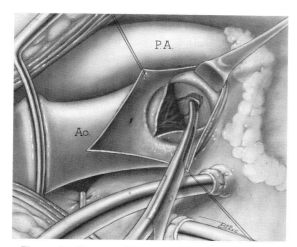

**Figure 9** Hypertrophic muscular subaortic stenosis. After retraction of the aortic valve leaflets, a portion of the hypertrophied tissue is removed with a rongeur to widen the left ventricular outflow tract.

*Surgical experience with 16 patients with congenital supravalvular aortic stenosis is presented in this article, and the literature on this unusual lesion is reviewed. The various types of supravalvular obstruction are described, and the surgical procedures recommended are clearly presented.*

Roberts, W. C.: The congenitally bicuspid aortic valve. Amer. J. Cardiol., 26:72, 1970.
*The author gives a detailed analysis of the postmortem examination of 105 adult patients with isolated aortic valve stenosis. Sixty-seven of these patients were found to have congenitally deformed valves, and in 54 the valve was bicuspid. This paper establishes the bicuspid aortic valve as the most common congenital malformation of the heart, and supports the concept that these valves progressively stenose and finally produce the adult form of calcific aortic stenosis. This is an excellent presentation of the pathologic anatomy and the ultimate fate of the congenitally bicuspid aortic valve.*

# REFERENCES

1. Bailey, C. P., Glover, R. P., O'Neill, T. J. E., and Redondo-Ramirez, H. P.: Surgical relief of aortic stenosis. J. Thorac. Surg., 20:516, 1950.
2. Braunwald, E., Goldblatt, A., Aygen, M. M., Rockoff, S. D., and Morrow, A. G.: Congenital aortic stenosis. I. Clinical and hemodynamic findings in 100 patients. Circulation, 27:426, 1963.
3. Braunwald, E., Lambrew, C. T., Rockoff, S. D., Ross, J., Jr., and Morrow, A. G.: Idiopathic hypertrophic subaortic stenosis. I. A description of the disease based upon an analysis of 64 patients. Circulation. Supp. IV, 30:3, 1964.
4. Braunwald, E., Oldham, H. N., Jr., Ross, J., Jr., Linhart, J. W., Mason, D. T., and Fort, L., III: The circulatory response of patients with idiopathic hypertrophic subaortic stenosis to nitroglycerin and to the Valsalva maneuver. Circulation, 29:422, 1964.
5. Burnell, R. H., Ghadiali, P. E., Joseph, M. C., and Paneth, M.: Management of critical valvular outflow obstruction in neonates. Thorax, 25:116, 1970.
6. Campbell, M.: The natural history of congenital aortic stenosis. Brit. Heart J., 30:514, 1968.
7. Cornell, W. P., Elkins, R. C., Criley, J. M., and Sabiston, D. C., Jr.: Supravalvular aortic stenosis. J. Thorac. Cardiovasc. Surg., 51:484, 1966.
8. Cowper, W.: Of ossification or petrifactions in the coats of arteries, particularly in the valves of the great artery. Trans. Phil. Tr. Roy. Soc. London, 5:215, 1703–1712.
9. Fisher, R. D., Mason, D. T., and Morrow, A. G.: Results of operative treatment in congenital aortic stenosis. J. Thorac. Cardiovasc. Surg., 59:218, 1970.
10. Friedman, W. F., and Mills, L. F.: The relationship between vitamin D and the craniofacial and dental anomalies of the supravalvular aortic stenosis syndrome. Pediatrics, 43:12, 1969.
11. Friedman, W. F., Modlinger, J., and Morgan, J. R.: Serial hemodynamic observations in asymptomatic children with valvar aortic stenosis. Circulation, 43:91, 1971.
12. Gamboa, R., Hugenholtz, P. G., and Nadas, A. S.: Comparison of electrocardiograms and vectorcardiograms in congenital aortic stenosis. Brit. Heart J., 27:344, 1965.
13. Glew, R. H., Varghese, P. J., Krovetz, L. J., Dorst, J. P., and Rowe, R. D.: Sudden death in congenital aortic stenosis: A review of eight cases with an evaluation of premonitory clinical features. Amer. Heart J., 78:615, 1969.
14. Gorlin, R., and Gorlin, S. G.: Hydraulic formula for calculation of area of stenotic mitral valve, other cardiac valves, and central circulatory shunts. Amer. Heart J., 41:1, 1951.
15. Graham, T. P., Jr., Lewis, B. W., Jarmakani, M. M., Canent, R. V., and Capp, M. P.: Left heart volume and mass quantification in children with left ventricular pressure overload. Circulation, 41:203, 1970.
16. Hoffman, J. I. E.: The natural history of congenital isolated pulmonic and aortic stenosis. Ann. Rev. Med., 20:15, 1969.
17. Hugenholtz, P. G., and Gamboa, R.: Effect of chronically increased ventricular pressure on electrical forces of the heart. Circulation, 30:511, 1964.
18. Idress, F. S., Dieter, R., Riker, W. L., and Paul, M. H.: Left ventricular outflow obstruction in infancy and childhood. Arch. Surg., 99:257, 1969.
19. Jones, R. C., Walker, W. J., Jahnke, E. J., and Winn, D. F.: Congenital aortic stenosis: Correlation of clinical severity with hemodynamic and surgical findings in 43 cases. Ann. Intern. Med., 58:486, 1963.
20. Lewis, F. J.: Aortic valvulotomy under direct vision during hypothermia. J. Thorac. Surg., 32:481, 1956.
21. Lillehei, C. W., Bonnabeau, R. C., Jr., and Sellers, R. D.: Subaortic stenosis: Diagnostic criteria, surgical approach, and late follow-up in 25 patients. J. Thorac. Cardiovasc. Surg., 55:94, 1968.
22. Mitchell, S. C., Korones, S. B., and Berendes, H. W.: Congenital heart disease in 56,109 births. Circulation, 43:323, 1971.
23. McGoon, D. C., Geha, A. S., Scofield, E. L., and DuShane, J. W.: Surgical treatment of congenital aortic stenosis. Dis. Chest, 55:388, 1969.
24. Moller, J. H., Nakib, A., and Edwards, J. E.: Infarction of papillary muscles and mitral insufficiency associated with congenital aortic stenosis. Circulation, 34:87, 1966.
25. Moller, J. H., Nakib, A., Eliot, R. S., and Edwards, J. E.: Symptomatic congenital aortic stenosis in the first year of life. J. Pediat., 69:728, 1966.
26. Morrow, A. G.: Hypertrophic subaortic stenosis. Arch. Surg., 99:677, 1969.
27. Morrow, A. G., Fort, L., III, Roberts, W. C., and Braunwald, E.: Discrete subaortic stenosis complicated by aortic valvular regurgitation: Clinical, hemodynamic, and pathologic studies and the results of operative treatment. Circulation, 31:163, 1965.
28. Morrow, A. G., Goldblatt, A., and Braunwald, E.: Congenital aortic stenosis. II. Surgical treatment and the results of operation. Circulation, 27:426, 1963.
29. Morrow, A. G., Lambrew, C. T., and Braunwald, E.: Idiopathic hypertrophic subaortic stenosis. II. Operative treatment and the results of pre- and postoperative hemodynamic evaluations. Circulation, Supp. IV, 30:120, 1964.
30. Osler, W.: The bicuspid condition of the aortic valves. Trans. Ass. Amer. Physicians, 2:185, 1886.
31. Paget, J.: On obstructions of the branches of the pulmonary artery. Med. Chir. Trans., 27:162, 1844.
32. Peckham, G. B., Keith, J. D., and Evans, J. R.: Congenital aortic stenosis: Some observations on the natural history and the clinical assessment. Canad. Med. Ass. J., 91:639, 1964.
33. Pierce, G. E., Morrow, A. G., and Braunwald, E.: Idiopathic hypertrophic subaortic stenosis. III. Intraoperative studies of the mechanism of obstruction and its hemodynamic consequences. Circulation. Supp. IV, 30:152, 1964.
34. Putnam, T. C., Harris, P. D., Bernhard, W. F., and Gross, R. E.: The surgical management of congenital aortic stenosis. J. Thorac. Cardiovasc. Surg., 48:540, 1964.
35. Rastelli, G. C., McGoon, D. C., Ongley, P. A., Mankin, H. T., and Kirklin, J. W.: Surgical treatment of supravalvular aortic stenosis: Report of 16 cases and review of literature. J. Thorac. Cardiovasc. Surg., 51:873, 1966.
36. Riverius, L.: Observations medical et curatives insignes, quebus accesserunt observations an Alles communicatae. M. Flesher, London, 1646.
37. Roberts, W. C.: The structure of the aortic valve in clinically isolated aortic stenosis. Circulation, 42:91, 1970.
38. Roberts, W. C.: The congenitally bicuspid aortic valve: A study of 85 autopsy cases. Amer. J. Cardiol., 26:72, 1970.
39. Robicsek, F., Sanger, P. W., Daugherty, H. K., and Montgomery, C. C.: Congenital quadricuspid aortic valve with displacement of the left coronary orifice. Amer. J. Cardiol., 23:288, 1969.
40. Serck-Hanssen, A.: Congenital valvular aortic stenosis: Histological changes in the valves and myocardium in 3 cases. Acta Path. Microbiol. Scand., 72:465, 1968.
41. Shumacker, H. B., and Nahrwold, D. L.: Associated subvalvular and supravalvular aortic stenosis with aortic valve anomaly. Ann. Thorac. Surg., 9:356, 1970.

42. Swan, H., Wilkenson, R. H., and Blount, S. G., Jr.: Visual repair of congenital aortic stenosis during hypothermia. J. Thorac. Surg., 35:139, 1958.

43. Thursfield, H., and Scott, H. W.: Sub-aortic stenosis. Brit. J. Child. Dis., 10:104, 1913.

44. Tuffier, T.: Etat actuel de la chirurgie intrathoracique. Trans. Int. Cong. Med., London, 1914.

45. Whalen, R. E., Cohen, A. I., Sumner, R. G., and McIntosh, H. D.: Demonstration of the dynamic nature of idiopathic hypertrophic subaortic stenosis. Amer. J. Cardiol., 11:8, 1963.

46. Williams, J. C. P., Barratt-Boyes, B. G., and Lowe, J. D.: Supravalvular aortic stenosis. Circulation, 24:1311, 1961.

# X

# The Coronary Circulation

## David C. Sabiston, Jr., M.D.

The coronary arteries provide the blood to the heart, the organ essential for maintenance of the circulation. A variety of distinct pathologic disorders may reduce blood flow to the myocardium and produce a serious threat to life. By far the most common cause of myocardial ischemia is coronary *atherosclerosis,* and this disorder is the greatest single cause of death among Americans today. Although the symptoms of *angina pectoris* have been known since Heberden's classic description in 1768,[29] and *acute myocardial infarction* has been recognized since the report by Herrick in 1912,[30] only in recent years has the *epidemic* nature of coronary disease been appreciated. The presence of extensive coronary atherosclerosis in otherwise healthy young males was emphasized in World War II by the incidence of fatal myocardial infarction occurring in soldiers. It was also shown in *routine* autopsies on young military casualties in the Korean conflict that 77 per cent had *gross* evidence of coronary atherosclerosis and 10 per cent showed *advanced* disease, with 70 per cent or greater occlusion of one of more major coronary arteries.[19] In a community study, it was found that coronary atherosclerosis (from 25 per cent to complete occlusion of one or more major arteries) was present in three-fourths of the entire population.[52] These figures indicate the extreme prevalence of the disorder, but unfortunately its presence is usually not made manifest until serious symptoms appear.

The advances that have been made in coronary arteriography and evaluation of ventricular function have been of great significance in the objective diagnosis of coronary occlusion and myocardial ischemia. In the recent past, the direct approach for myocardial revascularization by anastomosis of venous autografts from the aorta to the coronary arteries has assumed a primary position in the field of cardiovascular surgery.

### ANATOMY OF THE CORONARY ARTERIES

The right and left coronary arteries are the first branches of the aorta and arise from the sinuses of Valsalva. The right coronary artery passes deep in the right atrial ventricular groove and proceeds over the anterior surface of the heart. At the superior end of the acute margin of the heart on the right, the vessel turns posteriorly toward the crux of the heart and usually terminates as the *posterior descending* coronary artery as it passes forward on the diaphragmatic surface of the heart in the posterior interventricular groove. The right coronary artery initially branches into a number of small vessels, which anastomose on the anterior ventricle in the pulmonary conus region with corresponding branches from the left coronary artery (the arterial circle of Vieussens). It next supplies multiple ventricular branches and the sinus node artery (the latter *may* arise from the left circumflex artery). Along the acute right border of the heart, the right *marginal* artery takes origin. The right coronary artery terminates in the posterior descending artery and by an extension to the crux, and branches into an atrial ventricular nodal artery and several terminal left ventricular branches supplying the posterior surface of the left ventricle. A diagrammatic illustration of the right coronary artery and its branches is shown in Figure 1.[57]

The *left* coronary is usually about 1 cm. in length and gives rise to the *anterior descending* and *circumflex* arteries. The anterior descending gives branches to the arterial circle of Vieussens, and several *diagonal* branches to the left ventricular surface, and as it proceeds inferiorly, gives origin to a number of anterior penetrating branches to the interventricular septum. This artery terminates at the apex of the heart, usually anastomosing with the *posterior descending* artery. The anterior descending coronary artery supplies (1) the anterior left margin of the right ventricle, (2) the free wall of the left ventricle, (3) the apex of the heart, and (4) the principal blood supply of the interventricular septum.

The left *circumflex* artery lies in the atrioventricular groove on the left and proceeds inferiorly and posteriorly to pass around the obtuse margin of the heart, terminating in the left marginal artery or communicating via the crux with the posterior descending coronary artery. The first branch of the circumflex artery is usually the auricular anastomotic artery (Kugel's artery). A diagrammatic illustration of the left coronary artery and its anterior descending and circumflex branches is shown in Figure 2.[57]

The *venous drainage* of the heart is via *superficial* and deep circuits. The superficial veins conduct most of the venous blood and accompany the respective coronary

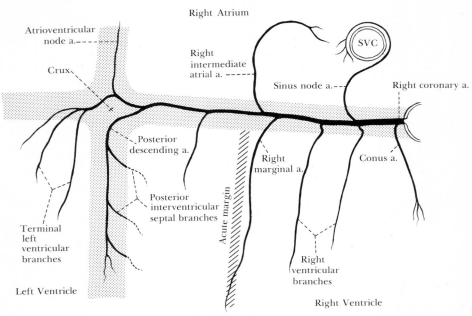

**Figure 1**    A schematic drawing of the right coronary artery, showing its usual branches and the common point of termination between the crux and obtuse margin of the heart. (From Winterscheid, L. C.: In: Strandness, D. E., Jr., ed.: Collateral Circulation in Clinical Surgery. Philadelphia, W. B. Saunders Company, 1969.)

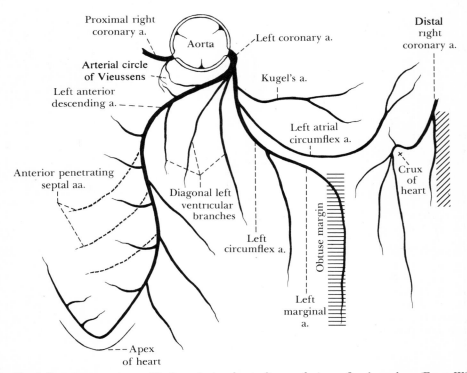

**Figure 2**    The left coronary artery with its anterior descending and circumflex branches. (From Winterscheid, L. C. In: Strandness, D. E., Jr., ed.: Collateral Circulation in Clinical Surgery. Philadelphia, W. B. Saunders Company, 1969.)

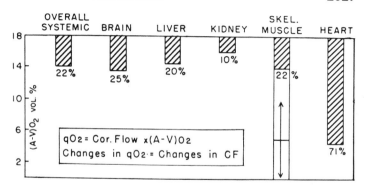

**Figure 3** Systemic and regional arteriovenous oxygen extraction. $qO_2$ = oxygen consumption per minute. Exercising skeletal muscle extracts an increasing but varying amount of oxygen during effort (arrow). Oxygen extraction by cardiac muscle remains relatively constant and exceeds that of other organs. (From Gorlin, R.: Brit. Heart J., Supp. 9, 33:1, 1971.)

arteries and empty either into the *coronary sinus* (which drains into the right atrium) or into the anterior cardiac veins, the latter emptying individually into the right atrium. The deep veins communicate with both the atrial and ventricular cavities via thebesian and sinusoidal channels.

## PHYSIOLOGIC DETERMINANTS OF CORONARY BLOOD FLOW

In normal man, the average coronary blood flow has been calculated to be approximately 80 ml. per 100 gm. per minute (range, 66 to 93 ml. per 100 gm. per minute).[44] Compared with other organs, the oxygen extraction is quite high (Fig. 3),[25] and the average coronary arteriovenous oxygen difference is approximately 11 ml. per 100 ml. of blood (range, 10.3 to 12.5).[44] The coronary venous $pO_2$ is in the range of 20 mm. Hg. These data emphasize the high oxygen *utilization* of the myocardium, which is approximately 10 ml. per 100 gm. of car-

diac muscle per minute. The arterial pressure is an important determinant of flow, and generally follows an essentially linear relationship in physiologic ranges. It is somewhat paradoxical that during *ventricular systole* coronary blood flow decreases because of the increased resistance as the cardiac muscle contracts. Conversely, there is an augmentation of coronary flow during *diastole* as the ventricles relax and resistance diminishes. Thus, the heart is the only organ in the body that consistently has a greater arterial blood flow in diastole than in systole. A sequential moment-to-moment flow through the coronary circulation is illustrated in Figure 4.[27]

The most powerful *vasodilator* of the coronary circulation is hypoxemia. As the oxygen content of arterial blood is reduced, or with reduction in coronary blood flow, impressive increases in coronary blood flow occur without an increase in perfusion pressure, a phenomenon termed *reactive hyperemia*. A composite diagram illustrating the factors regulating coronary blood flow is shown in Figure 5.[25]

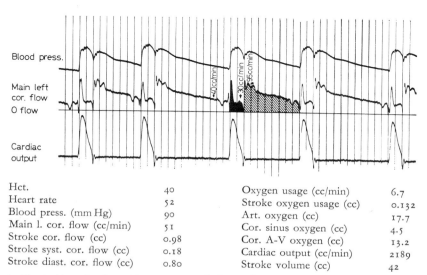

| | | | | |
|---|---|---|---|---|
| Hct. | 40 | Oxygen usage (cc/min) | 6.7 |
| Heart rate | 52 | Stroke oxygen usage (cc) | 0.132 |
| Blood press. (mm Hg) | 90 | Art. oxygen (cc) | 17.7 |
| Main l. cor. flow (cc/min) | 51 | Cor. sinus oxygen (cc) | 4.5 |
| Stroke cor. flow (cc) | 0.98 | Cor. A-V oxygen (cc) | 13.2 |
| Stroke syst. cor. flow (cc) | 0.18 | Cardiac output (cc/min) | 2189 |
| Stroke diast. cor. flow (cc) | 0.80 | Stroke volume (cc) | 42 |

**Figure 4** Data illustrating phasic aortic pressure and phasic flow in the left main coronary artery and ascending aorta obtained by means of a chronically implanted strain gauge and electromagnetic flowmeter in a dog at rest. (From Gregg, D. E. In: Marchetti, G., and Taccardi, B., eds.: Coronary Circulation and Energetics of the Myocardium. Basel, S. Karger, 1967.)

FACTORS REGULATING CORONARY FLOW

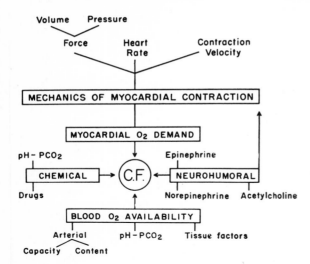

**Figure 5** Factors regulating coronary flow (C.F.). These factors can be subdivided into those affecting myocardial oxygen requirements (above), those affecting oxygen availability per unit flow (below), and those acting directly on the arteriole. Neurohumoral factors can affect coronary flow not only through primary vasomotion but also through altered oxygen demand. Likewise, pH can affect both arteriolar resistance and oxygen availability. (From Gorlin, R.: Brit. Heart J., Supp. 9, *33*:1, 1971.)

## MYOCARDIAL METABOLISM

The primary problem in myocardial ischemia is the reduction in oxygen available for myocardial metabolism. Normally, the heart extracts approximately 75 per cent of the oxygen present in the arterial blood, leaving little additional to be removed during stressful situations. The added oxygen required for the heart during exercise or emotional stress is normally provided by an appropriate *increase* in coronary flow. This is made difficult if not impossible in the presence of significant arterial obstruction. The basic substrates utilized in myocardial metabolism are glucose, fatty acids, and lactate. In the presence of adequate oxygen, glucose is converted to pyruvate with production of ATP (adenosine triphosphate) in the Krebs cycle. Lactate is also converted to pyruvate. Oxidative phosphorylation of pyruvate is greatly slowed with reduction or absence of oxygen, and the lactate-pyruvate reaction may be reversed, with production of lactate in the heart. *Anaerobic* metabolism is inefficient in the heart, and although glucose is degraded, much less energy is provided. The clinical manifestations of significant myocardial hypoxemia include (1) anginal pain; (2) cardiac arrhythmias (ventricular premature systoles, ventricular tachycardia, and ventricular fibrillation) and electrocardiographic abnormalities (inversion of T waves and ST segment depression, especially with exercise); and (3) signs of cardiac failure.

## PATHOLOGIC ASPECTS

Coronary atherosclerosis is a progressive disease, the earliest microscopic changes of which have been described in the newborn infant. The infantile lesions consist of rupture, degeneration, and regeneration of the internal elastic membrane, together with deposits of mucopolysaccharide and proliferation of endothelial cells and fibroblasts.[39] At this early stage in life, it is obvious that such lesions are quite minimal and are solely microscopic. However, *gross* lesions subsequently appear within a few years in the form of small yellow deposits of lipoid material visible beneath the intima. These lesions are present in half the hearts examined at autopsy during the second decade of life.[58] Careful pathologic studies have been done by a number of observers to assess the incidence and degree of atherosclerosis in *each* of the major coronary ateries. Nearly all of the studies have shown that the anterior descending coronary artery is the most frequently involved, followed in incidence by the right coronary, the left circumflex, the left main, and, least frequently of all, the right posterior descending coronary artery (Table 1).[4, 8, 12, 56]

It has also been noted that the more severe changes occur in the *proximal third* or *half* of the

**TABLE 1** FREQUENCY OF OBSTRUCTIVE LESIONS IN THE CORONARY ARTERIES DUE TO ATHEROSCLEROSIS AS FOUND IN A SERIES OF 300 CONSECUTIVE PATIENTS WITH CORONARY ATHEROSCLEROSIS*

| Coronary Artery | No. of Cases | — |
|---|---|---|
| Right | 165 | 28.4 |
| Left main | 26 | 4.5 |
| Left anterior descending | 251 | 43.4 |
| Left circumflex | 134 | 23.7 |
| Totals | 576 | 100.0 |

*From Berger, R. L., and Stary, H. C.: New Eng. J. Med., 285:248, 1971.

**TABLE 2** OPERABILITY IN 300 HEARTS WITH ATHEROSCLEROSIS STUDIED AT POSTMORTEM EXAMINATION (THE RELATIONSHIP OF OPERABILITY TO THE NUMBER OF VESSELS OBSTRUCTED— ANTERIOR DESCENDING, RIGHT, CIRCUMFLEX, AND LEFT CORONARY ARTERIES)*

| No. of Vessels Obstructed | Total Cases | No. of Operable Vessels | | | | | | Summary of Operability | | | | | |
|---|---|---|---|---|---|---|---|---|---|---|---|---|---|
| | | *1* | | *2* | | *3* | | Complete Repair | | Partial Repair | | Stenosis Inoperable | |
| | | *No. of Cases* | *%* | *No. of Cases* | *%* | *No. of Cases* | *%* | *No.* | *%* | *No.* | *%* | *No.* | *%* |
| One | 117 | 100 | 85.5 | | | | | 100 | 85.5 | | | 17 | 14.5 |
| Two | 99 | 28 | 28.3 | 63 | 63.6 | | | 63 | 63.6 | 28 | 28.3 | 8 | 8.1 |
| Three | 75 | 18 | 24 | 30 | 40 | 19 | 25.4 | 19 | 25.4 | 48 | 64 | 8 | 10.6 |
| Four | 9 | 1 | 11.1 | 4 | 44.5 | 3 | 33.3 | 3 | 33.3 | 5 | 55.6 | 1 | 11.1 |

*From Berger, R. L., and Stary, H. C.: New Eng. J. Med., *285*:248, 1971.

coronary arteries. In a thorough study of some 400 hearts, Schlesinger and Zoll[48] concluded that most occlusions were less than 5 mm. in length and that the majority were in the proximal third of the vessel. In a recent review of atherosclerotic lesions in 300 hearts studied primarily for an assessment of *operability* by direct bypass graft, a definite anatomic pattern was identified.[8] The usual pattern is one of *multifocal* lesions characteristically involving more than one major trunk in the same heart. The stenoses tend to be short but are contiguous with other areas of less severe coronary atherosclerosis. In general, lesions in the branches of the left coronary artery are usually proximal and originate at the bifurcation of the anterior descending and circumflex branches. However, there are appreciable numbers of distal lesions in these vessels. In the right coronary artery, the disease is more diffuse and involves primarily the proximal and middle portions of the artery. In this study, it was noted that 88 per cent of hearts with coronary atherosclerosis were anatomically suitable for a graft distal to the obstructing lesion. Further analysis indicated that bypass in *all* obstructed coronary arteries was achievable in 62 per cent of hearts, whereas of those with multiple lesions, only 27 per cent were suitable for surgical repair of *each* of the involved vessels (Table 2).[8] The site of obstruction for each of the three major coronary vessels in this study is shown in Figure 6.[8]

## CLINICAL MANIFESTATIONS OF ISCHEMIC HEART DISEASE

The symptoms associated with significant coronary atherosclerosis are those produced by a reduction in coronary blood flow. While coronary atherosclerosis is clearly the most common cause of myocardial ischemia, angina pectoris may also be associated with other lesions that cause a reduced coronary flow and enter the differential diagnosis. These include aortic stenosis, aortic insufficiency, syphilitic coronary ostial stenosis, hypertension, other forms of arteritis, embolism, and congenital malformations of the coronary arteries (Fig. 7).[11]

The *clinical syndrome* of angina pectoris was first described by Heberden in 1768. His original account is worth citing, since most believe that it has never been improved upon:

There is a disorder of the breast marked with strong and peculiar symptoms, considerable for the kind of danger belonging to it, and not extremely rare, which deserves to be mentioned more at length. The seat of it, and sense of strangling, and anxiety with which it is attended, may make it not improperly be called angina pectoris.

They who are afflicted with it, are seized while they are walking, (more especially if it be up hill, and soon after eating), with a painful and most disagreeable sensation in the breast, which seems as if it would extinguish life, if it were to increase or continue; but the moment they stand still, all this uneasiness vanishes.

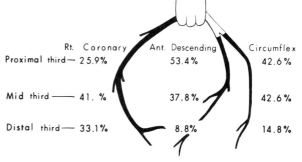

**Figure 6** Localization of the stenotic lesion in the three major coronary trunks. Each coronary artery is divided into three equal segments and the percentage of the total number of lesions in each third is noted. In the anterior descending circumflex arteries, the obstructions tend to be in the proximal half, whereas the primary involvement is in the distal half of the right coronary artery. (From Berger, R. L., and Stary, H. C.: New Eng. J. Med., *285*:248, 1971.)

Rt. Coronary | Ant. Descending | Circumflex
Proximal third— 25.9% | 53.4% | 42.6%
Mid third —— 41.% | 37.8% | 42.6%
Distal third— 33.1% | 8.8% | 14.8%

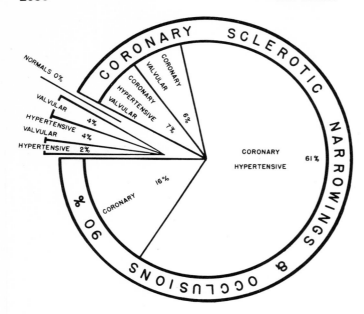

**Figure 7** The etiologic basis of angina pectoris based on studies in 177 patients. (From Blumgart, H. L., Pitt, B., Zoll, P. M., and Freiman, D. G. In: James, T. N., and Keyes, J. W., eds.: The Etiology of Myocardial Infarction, Boston, Little, Brown and Co., 1963.)

In all other respects, the patients are, at the beginning of this disorder, perfectly well, and in particular have no shortness of breath from which it is totally different. The pain is sometimes situated in the upper part, sometimes in the middle, sometimes at the bottom of the os sterni, and often more inclined to the left than to the right side. It likewise very frequently extends from the breast to the middle of the left arm. The pulse is, at least sometimes, not disturbed by this pain, as I have had opportunities of observing by feeling the pulse during the paroxysm. Males are most liable to that disease, especially such as have passed their fiftieth year.

After it has continued a year or more, it will not cease so instantaneously upon standing still; and it will come on not only when the persons are walking, but when they are lying down, especially if they lie on their left side, and oblige them to rise up out of their beds. In some inveterate cases it has been brought on by the motion of a horse, or a carriage, and even by swallowing, coughing, going to stool, or speaking, or any disturbance of the mind. . . .

The termination of the angina pectoris is remarkable. For, if no accidents intervene, but the disease go on to its height, the patients all suddenly fall down, and perish almost immediately. Of which indeed their frequent faintness, and sensations as if all the powers of life were failing, afford no obscure intimation.

The discomfort is generally substernal in location and is described by the patient as "a pressure, choking sensation or tightness which is quite discomforting." A variety of factors, primarily exercise and emotional stress, can initiate the symptoms. Occasionally angina occurs at rest and in the recumbent position and is termed *angina decubitus.* The pain frequently radiates down the left arm and into the left neck and occasionally to the right arm.

The physical examination is frequently not remarkable in the patient with angina pectoris. Occasionally the fourth heart sound can be heard on auscultation; it has been interpreted as an in-

crease in the amplitude of presystolic enlargement of the left ventricle.

The plain chest film is normal in the majority of patients, although cardiac enlargement may be present in those with more serious disease, especially those with heart failure. Left ventricular aneurysms of varying size may also be present. The electrocardiogram can be of substantial aid in the diagnosis of angina pectoris, although in at least half the patients it is within normal limits. Myocardial ischemia may be evidenced by the presence of inverted T waves, and especially ST segment and T wave changes, which occur during the course of an anginal episode. ST segment depression is an especially reliable sign and, if not present at rest, can often be elicited by an exercise stress test.

## CORONARY ARTERIOGRAPHY

Coronary arteriograms are essential for the *objective* diagnosis of angina pectoris caused by coronary atherosclerosis. The *selective* technique with placement of a tapered catheter *directly* into the coronary artery has been widely employed.[2] Since selective coronary arteriography was first performed by Sones in 1958, he and his associates have performed more than 20,000 of these examinations, with 19 fatalities or approximately one death per 1000.[50] A diagram of the arteriographic pattern is shown in Figure 8.[2] An example of the normal anatomy of the right and left coronary arteries is shown in Figure 9.[50] Obstructions are well demonstrated, together with the collateral vessels (Fig. 10).[50] For all patients being considered for surgery, coronary arteriography is essential.

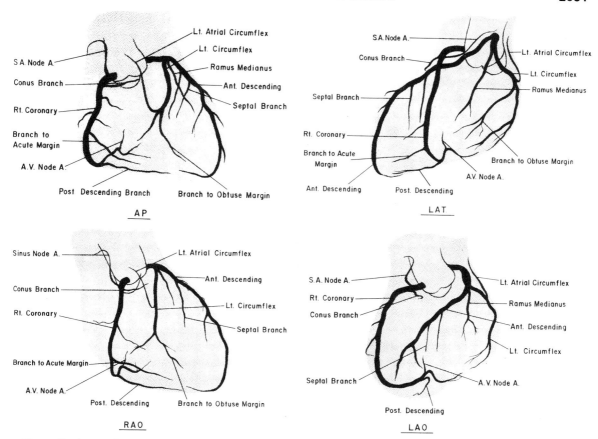

**Figure 8**   Anatomic representation of the coronary arteries. These vessels are represented as they would be seen on the angiogram. No attempt to convey the third dimension has been made. Careful study of the changes in position of the various branches with rotation of the heart is essential to intelligent interpretation of arteriograms. The combination of the left anterior oblique (LAO), lateral (LAT), and right anterior oblique (RAO) positions usually demonstrates all branches in profile. (From Abrams, H. L., and Adams, D. F.: New Eng. J. Med., *281*:1276, 1969.)

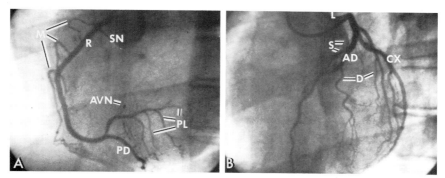

**Figure 9**   *A,* Right coronary arteriogram, left anterior oblique position. The right main trunk (R) supplies a series of marginal branches (M) to the right ventricle, as well as an atrial branch from which the artery to the sinus node arises (SN). After its major bifurcation and the origin of the posterior descending (PD) branch, the right coronary artery continues across the crux of the heart, giving rise to a branch to the atrioventricular node (AVN) and branches to the posterolateral aspect of the left ventricle (PL). *B,* Left coronary arteriogram, left anterior oblique projection. The main trunk of the left coronary artery (L) divides into its major anterior descending (AD) and circumflex (CX) divisions. The anterior descending division provides one or more branches to the interventricular septum (S), and a series of diagonal (D) branches to the anterolateral aspect of the left ventricle. The circumflex division contributes a series of branches distributed to the anterolateral, lateral, and posterolateral areas of the left ventricle. (From Sheldon, W. C.: Surg. Clin. N. Amer., *51*:1015, 1971.)

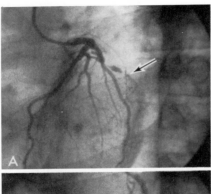
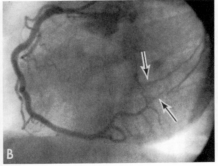
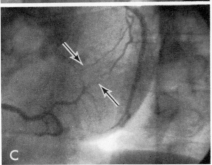

**Figure 10** *A,* Left coronary arteriogram, left anterior oblique (LAO) position, demonstrating total obstruction of the proximal left circumflex coronary artery (arrow). *B* and *C,* Right coronary arteriogram demonstrating retrograde perfusion of the obstructed left circumflex branches via intercoronary collateral anastomoses with distal right coronary branches (arrows). (From Sheldon, W. C.: Surg. Clin. N. Amer., *51*:1015, 1971.)

## MEDICAL MANAGEMENT

The medical management of coronary atherosclerosis and angina pectoris is both general and specific. If obesity and hypertension are present, both should be controlled. Smoking should be avoided, since the vasoconstrictive effects of nicotine and its influence upon the coronary circulation are well established. The presence of abnormal lipoproteins in the blood should be determined (Fredrickson types) and treated appropriately. Often it is necessary to adjust the patient's life style to reduce the likelihood of anginal attacks, especially if associated with myocardial irritability.

### Drug Therapy

The primary basis of medical therapy is the use of agents found to be successful in controlling the pain of angina pectoris. The majority of patients obtain relief with sublingual nitroglycerin (0.4 to 0.6 mg.), and results are usually quite prompt. Many patients anticipate attacks of pain, especially with exercise or emotional stress, and can prevent them by prophylactic use of nitroglycerin. Several long-acting coronary vasodilators are available but produce variable results. The use of beta-adrenergic blocking agents such as *propranolol* is frequently effective. The pharmacologic effects of propranolol are a reduction in cardiac output, lowering of the pulse rate, and decrease in the force of ventricular contraction. Since it reduces the work load, it may produce substantial relief when administered regularly. Although much has been written concerning the use of anticoagulants in the treatment of angina pectoris and coronary atherosclerosis, there is little definitive

evidence to support their use. Exercise has been advocated to aid in the development of coronary collateral circulation, and its beneficial effect has been shown both in the experimental animal[17] and in man.[38]

## SURGICAL MANAGEMENT

It has now been more than 50 years since the first surgical procedure was performed for the relief of angina pectoris. Although interest has remained high in the surgical attack on this serious problem, most of the procedures previously advocated have yielded in the recent past to the use of direct grafts from the aorta to the coronary arteries distal to the obstruction. This procedure has been supported widely by both cardiologists and surgeons, and the initial results are encouraging. Nevertheless, a cautious attitude remains appropriate until long-term assessment of this procedure is available. A number of distinct questions await answers that only appropriate observation will provide.

### Historical Aspects

A surgical approach for relief of angina pectoris was first suggested in 1899 by a professor of physiology in Paris, François-Franck.[23] He believed that section of the cervical sympathetics might interrupt the pain fibers to the heart and ameliorate the symptoms. This procedure was first employed in 1916 by Jonnesco[33] and produced symptomatic relief in the patient. The subsequent recognition that angina pectoris was usually accompanied by a reduction in arterial blood supply to the heart led to the development of a number of surgical procedures designed to improve coronary blood flow.

*Epicardial abrasion* was advocated by Beck[7] in 1935 to

stimulate the development of intramyocardial arterial collaterals. A number of tissues have been applied directly to the surface of the heart (omentum, pectoral muscle, pericardial fat pad, the spleen, and so forth) to promote the ingrowth of new arterial vessels to anastomose with the coronary circulation.[53] A procedure used in a large number of patients was that devised by Vineberg[54] in 1946 of *internal mammary artery implantation* into a tunnel in the left ventricle. From the implant a system of arterial communications with the intramyocardial vessels developed. Such arterial implants were demonstrated to remain patent, although the amount of blood flow that passed through them remained quite controversial. In 1957 Bailey[6] introduced coronary *endarterectomy,* a technique that was substantially modified by Longmire the following year.[36] This technique was applied primarily to proximally located lesions and was suitable for only a small number of patients, generally less than 10 per cent of the total.

The more recent and notable contributions of Johnson[32] and of Favaloro[20] and their associates have led to an extensive reappraisal of the surgical approach to ischemic myocardial heart disease. To these workers much credit is due for placing emphasis upon the basic principle that *coronary arteries of extremely small caliber may be successfully anastomosed to a venous autograft from the aorta.* It has since been demonstrated by these workers and others that coronary arteries as small as 1 mm. in diameter may be joined by a suture anastomosis with prolonged patency demonstrated by subsequent coronary arteriograms.

### Indications for Operation

The primary indications for a surgical approach in patients with angina pectoris are (1) for relief of severe and unresponsive anginal pain, (2) to improve the manifestations of congestive heart failure, and (3) to reduce the likelihood of subsequent myocardial infarction, especially in those patients with previous infarction and with extensive coronary lesions.

Most surgeons agree that in 80 to 90 per cent of patients with occlusive coronary artery disease the anatomy is appropriate for direct aortic-coronary grafts, provided the necessary indications for the procedure are also present. The majority of patients are likely to have more than one occlusion, and an appreciable number have three or more significant obstructing lesions, each potentially correctable by a graft. It is essential that the lesions be demonstrated accurately by coronary arteriography prior to operation. Moreover, in most instances at least 75 per cent occlusion of one or more vessels will be apparent in patients with angina pectoris. In some, especially those with evidence of congestive heart failure, a *dyskinetic* area is apt to be found in the left ventricle, with poor or paradoxical contraction. In a more severe form, these areas are actually *aneurysms* of the ventricular wall that bulge during systolic

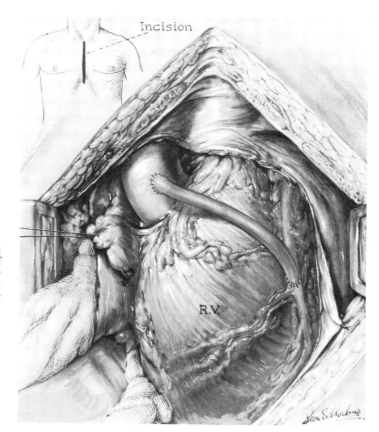

**Figure 11** Illustration of anastomosis of saphenous vein autograft from side of ascending aorta to side of left anterior descending coronary artery distal to an obstruction in the anterior descending coronary artery.

contraction. These aneurysms may contain thrombus, which may potentially embolize the systemic arteries. The dyskinetic areas may be suitable for plication or excision, depending upon their characteristics. Emergency aortocoronary bypass has been used in patients with impending or extending myocardial infarction with good results.[31] Patients with acute myocardial infarction and "power failure" (intractable shock) have also been treated successfully by direct grafts, with or without aneurysm resection.[41]

Cardiac catheterization studies have been quite helpful in documenting objective evidence of left ventricular function. In general, cardiomegaly, low ejection fractions from the left ventricle (especially below 25 per cent), increased left ventricular volume, and wide coronary arteriovenous differences (greater than 6 vol. per cent) all are associated with increased morbidity and mortality. To a lesser extent, an elevated end-diastolic pressure in the left ventricle may increase risk. However, the presence of any one of these variables does not necessarily preclude a successful surgical result. In addition, preoperative assessment and evaluation of dyskinesia, aneurysms, associated valvar disease, and diffuse myocardial damage with poor function are required in consideration of the advisability and extent of the operation planned.

### Surgical Procedures

The vast majority of patients with obstructive disease of the coronary circulation who are candidates for surgery are treated with grafts of autogenous veins anastomosed between the aorta and the coronary arteries. The saphenous vein is usually chosen, and the vessel is reversed so that blood may flow in the direction of the valves. The procedure is conducted with extracorporeal circulation, although the aortic anastomosis can usually be accomplished without the use of bypass since the aorta is relatively still and this anastomosis can be easily accomplished (Fig. 11). For the coronary artery anastomosis, bypass is instituted with cannulation of the left ventricle for continuous decompression. Ventricular fibrillation is usually induced to insure a quiet heart and thus permit a technically superior anastomosis to the coronary artery, which is usually 1 to 2.5 mm. in diameter. The body temperature is lowered to 30° C. and the anastomosis is performed in a quiet and nonbeating heart. Meticulous attention to surgical detail is mandatory, and the anastomosis is accomplished with very fine sutures (7–0) (Figs. 12 and 13).[20] Some advocate the use of interrupted sutures, whereas others employ a continuous suture. It is essential that the anastomosis be performed distal to the obstruction and preferably in a site in which there is little involvement of the wall with atherosclerotic change. The use of magnifying glasses has been found helpful.[51] After reconstruction, electromagnetic flowmeter determinations of volume of blood flow have shown average flows for right coronary grafts of 60 ml. per minute (range, 28 to 150 ml.); of the anterior descending, 80 ml. per minute (range, 20 to 160 ml.); and of the circumflex, 75 ml. per minute (range, 60 to 90 ml.).[40]

Areas of dyskinesia or aneurysm formation may require direct correction. Occasionally mitral insufficiency results from infarction of the papillary muscles and if severe may require replacement with a prosthetic valve. A direct anastomosis of the internal mammary artery to the coronary artery has also been recommended in preference to using a venous autograft.[26]

### Postoperative Management

The postoperative management of patients following revascularization procedures is of prime importance. The endotracheal tube is generally left in place for the first day, to permit adequate

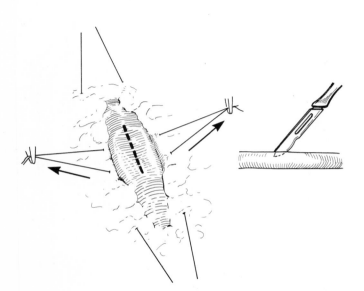

**Figure 12** Dissection of the coronary artery is avoided in the left coronary artery and its divisions, except when the anastomosis is performed on the main circumflex coronary artery. A No. 15 bistoury blade is utilized to open the artery layer by layer from outside. (From Favaloro, R. G.: Surg. Clin. N. Amer., *51*:1035, 1971.)

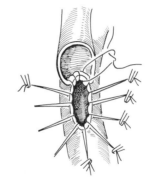
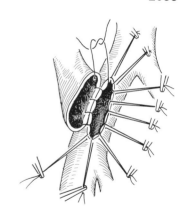

**Figure 13** The anastomosis starts at the proximal end of the arteriotomy (*left*) except for the proximal segment of the anterior descending and circumflex coronary arteries. To avoid kinking of the graft, the anastomosis should start in the middle of the medial side of the arteriotomy (*right*). (From Favaloro, R. G.: Surg. Clin. N. Amer., *51*:1035, 1971.)

ventilation by a respirator. It should remain in place until satisfactory ventilation can be assured, as shown by blood gas measurements of $pO_2$ and $pCO_2$. The cardiac output is maintained by attention to the central venous pressure, which is kept as high as 150 to 200 mm. of saline (10 to 15 mm. Hg) if necessary. The use of isoproterenol may be indicated to improve the *low output syndrome*. Similarly, various arrhythmias may develop and require the use of digitalis, procaine amide, xylocaine, potassium, or electrical cardioversion.

### Results

In most of the large series the mortality has been less than 10 per cent,[40, 45, 51] and in some, as low as 4 per cent.[20] The results in most series demonstrate an excellent symptomatic response, and improvement is noted in approximately 90 per cent of patients. In approximately 65 per cent, relief is complete, with no further symptoms, and distinct improvement occurs in an additional 25 per cent.[45] However, it is clear that changes in the grafts and in the coronary arteries themselves occur after revascularization. It has been demonstrated that the original stenosis present in the coronary artery may progress to complete occlusion after a bypass graft is placed distally.[5] In addition, progressive and late obstruction of the aortocoronary venous bypass graft has been demonstrated. The early patency rate during the first year after operation approximates 90 per cent in the grafts, although with the passage of time an *intimal fibrosis* may occur in the vein graft and cause obstruction (Figs. 14 and 15).[28, 55] In some instances, thrombi have also been noted. A distinctive *fibrous endarteritis* that occludes the grafts has been described in detail by Edwards.[18]

Despite the encouraging results currently reported, an objective attitude is essential relative to the late results of these procedures. A critique of direct surgery of the coronary circulation for atherosclerotic obstruction would include (1) the ultimate patency rates of the grafts, (2) the development of atherosclerosis in the venous grafts, (3) aneurysmal dilatation, fibrosis, or thrombosis of the graft, (4) progression of the previously existing coronary artery disease, (5) the ultimate amount of blood flow through the venous graft, (6) effect of the venous graft on prevention of subsequent myocardial infarction, and (7) the extension of the life span in those patients undergoing operation as compared to survival without operation. The answers to these important points will add much to the elucidation of the ultimate appraisal of the surgical management of coronary atherosclerosis.

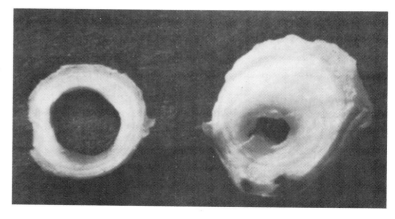

**Figure 14** Segments of the vein graft showing marked narrowing of the lumen in the first portion of the graft (*right*) in comparison to the "normal" lumen-wall ratio of the distal segment of the vein graft (*left*). (From Grondin, C. M., Meere, C., Castonguay, Y., Lepage, G., and Grondin, P.: Circulation, *43*:698, 1971. By permission of the American Heart Association, Inc.)

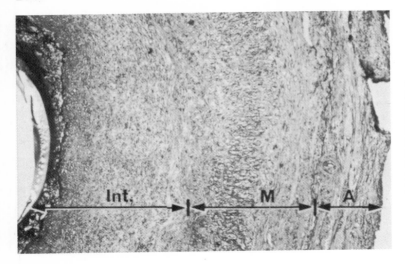

**Figure 15** Histologic section of the vein graft in the area of stenosis, showing marked fibrosis of all layers, but predominantly of the intimal layer (Int.). M = media; A = adventitia. Hematoxylin and eosin, × 65. (From Grondin, C. M., Meere, C., Castonguay, Y., Lepage, G., and Grondin, P.: Circulation, *43*:698, 1971. By permission of the American Heart Association, Inc.)

## VENTRICULAR ANEURYSMS

Ventricular aneurysms most commonly result from myocardial infarction but rarely may be the result of trauma, bacterial endocarditis, or congenital malformations. More than 95 per cent occur in the *left* ventricle. Formerly they were thought to occur in as few as 3 per cent of patients with myocardial infarction, but more recent studies with improved diagnostic methods indicate the incidence to be 12 to 15 per cent.[1] In a collected series, the site of the aneurysm formation in the left ventricle was found to be at the apex in 42 per cent of cases, the anterior wall in 16 per cent, the posterior basal wall in 26 per cent, and the interventricular septum in 12 per cent; the site was in the right ventricle in 4 per cent.[49]

After myocardial infarction, the fibrotic area that results from necrosis of muscular tissue may bulge with ventricular systole. Thus, when the ventricular myocardium contracts to pump blood into the aorta, the aneurysm distends, and this *paradoxical* behavior causes reduction of cardiac output. The left ventricular volume and frequently the left ventricular end-diastolic pressure are increased. The chest film usually demonstrates the aneurysm in the ventricular wall, usually best visualized in the oblique positions. Fluoroscopic examination is quite helpful, and *ventriculography* together with cardiac catheterization function studies confirms the diagnosis. Frequently patients with ventricular aneurysm also have symptoms of angina pectoris and exertional dyspnea. Others show frank manifestations of congestive heart failure and may have peripheral arterial emboli from thrombus arising in the aneurysm. The clinical manifestations observed in 100 consecutive patients with coronary disease are listed in Table 3.[14]

Surgical correction of ventricular aneurysms is indicated (1) when congestive heart failure is present, (2) in association with grafting operations for angina pectoris, and (3) when there are thromboembolic complications. In one large series of 301 patients treated surgically, 76 per cent underwent aneurysmectomy alone, although more recently revascularization procedures have been included in 56 per cent of operations. The mortality is approximately 10 per cent.[37] Ventricular aneurysms are excised through a median sternotomy, generally with the use of extracorporeal circulation. The aneurysmal sac is excised and the edges of the ventricle are resutured with two or three layers of sutures (Fig. 16).[37] Ventricular aneurysmectomy is designed to achieve several major objectives, including elimination of the *paradoxical* sac, removal of an actual or potential source of systemic emboli, and reduction in the left ventricular volume and end-diastolic pressure with corresponding improvement in cardiac function.

## VENTRICULAR SEPTAL DEFECT FOLLOWING MYOCARDIAL INFARCTION

Data obtained from postmortem studies indicate that 8 to 10 per cent of fatal cases of myocardial infarction are due to *rupture* of the heart.[42] In addition, infarction of the interventricular septum with subsequent formation of a ventricular septal

**TABLE 3** CLINICAL MANIFESTATIONS IN 100 PATIENTS*

| Presenting Symptoms | Coronary Artery Disease | Ventricular Aneurysm |
|---|---|---|
| Angina pectoris | 72 | 23 |
| Exertional dyspnea | 16 | 7 |
| Congestive heart failure | 5 | 3 |
| Previous myocardial infarcts | 5 | 1 |
| Recent myocardial infarction | 2 | 1 |
| Thromboembolism | 1† | 1† |
| Totals | 100 | 35 |

*From Cheng, T. O.: Amer. J. Med., *50*:340, 1971.
†One of those with congestive heart failure.

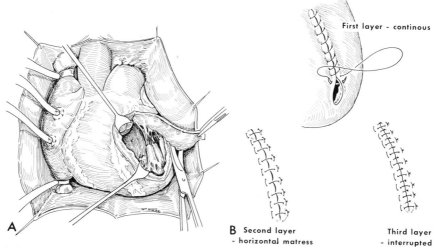

**Figure 16** *A,* Line drawing depicting a sizable ventricular scar in the typical location. The margins of the aneurysm are usually well defined. *B,* The ventricular wall is reconstructed with three separate layers of 0 and 2–0 mersilene. (From Loop, F. D.: Surg. Clin. N. Amer., *51:*1071, 1971.)

defect causes death in 1 to 2 per cent of cases of acute myocardial infarction. The usual interval between the acute infarct and rupture is 4 to 12 days; this correlates well with histologic findings of maximal cardiac muscle degeneration. Once rupture has occurred, the prognosis is poor, as demonstrated in one series of 157 patients of whom 24 per cent died on the first day after rupture, 65 per cent had died by the end of 2 weeks, and 81 per cent by 2 months. Only 7 per cent survived for a year after the development of a ventricular septal defect.[43]

This condition develops classically in a patient with myocardial infarction in whom shock or congestive heart failure appears. A loud, holosystolic murmur is usually heard over the apex, and two-thirds of the patients demonstrate a palpable thrill. The differential diagnosis includes papillary muscle dysfunction, rupture of a papillary muscle with acute mitral insufficiency, rupture of chordae tendineae, mitral insufficiency due to left ventricular failure, and a pericardial friction rub secondary to myocardial infarction. Although clinical findings may be highly suggestive, the definitive diagnosis is made by catheterization. The data demonstrate a left-to-right shunt at the ventricular level.

Since the natural history of the disease without surgical closure is dismal, surgical correction is indicated in nearly all patients. Whenever possible, it is preferable to allow the infarct to heal, with operation deferred for 6 to 8 weeks. However, the condition of the patient may not permit delay, and early operation may be a necessity. Since currently available figures indicate that some three-fourths of untreated patients will not survive for 2 months, it is recommended that surgery be considered before 6 weeks in any patient who no longer responds to vigorous medical management.

The first correction of a postinfarction ventricular defect was by Cooley in 1957.[15] These defects are usually in the apical septum and are most often associated with occlusion of the anterior descending coronary artery since it supplies the anterior two-thirds of the septum. *Multiple* defects are present in approximately one-third of patients. The operation is performed with the use of extracorporeal circulation. An incision is made in the right ventricle for exposure of the defect. If the infarct has healed (usually 6 or more weeks after onset), a fibrous rim may be present. If operation is done earlier, before complete healing, it may be necessary to remove a portion of the necrotic edges of the defect and to insert a plastic prosthesis for closure. Approximately two-thirds of reported patients have survived the operative procedure.

## OTHER COMPLICATIONS OF ACUTE MYOCARDIAL INFARCTION REQUIRING SURGICAL MANAGEMENT

In addition to the development of ventricular aneurysms and perforation of the interventricular septum, acute myocardial infarction may produce other specific complications that require surgical management. These include *heart block, peripheral arterial emboli, rupture of a papillary muscle, pulmonary embolism, and rupture of the ventricle.* Successful management of cardiac rupture has been reported.[22] The other complications listed are discussed in appropriate sections.

## CONGENITAL ORIGIN OF CORONARY ARTERY FROM THE PULMONARY ARTERY

A number of congenital anomalies of the coronary arteries have been reported, but the vast

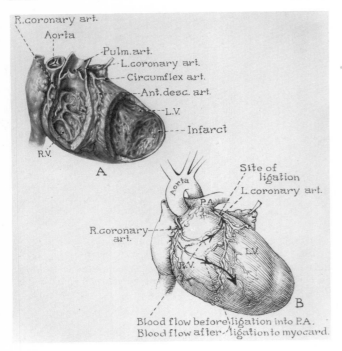

Figure 17    *A,* Specimen obtained at the time of postmortem examination. The left coronary artery arises anomalously from the pulmonary artery. The dilated left ventricle with aneurysmal area of infarction is seen. *B,* Diagrammatic illustration of blood flow in the anomalous left coronary artery before and after ligation at its origin. Prior to ligation the blood flowed from the aorta under systemic arterial pressure (with complete oxygen saturation) into the right coronary artery and through collateral vessels into the left coronary artery, with ultimate drainage into the pulmonary artery in a *retrograde* manner. Following ligation of the anomalous left coronary at its origin, the arterial blood from the right coronary artery is directed peripherally into the branches of the left coronary artery, where it reaches the myocardial vascular bed. (From Sabiston, D. C., Jr., et al.: J. Thorac. Cardiovasc. Surg., *40:*321, 1960.)

majority do not seriously affect coronary blood flow. For example, abnormal origin of the arteries from the aorta, single coronary arteries, and an abnormal course of distribution are all known to occur. Either the left or right coronary artery may arise from the pulmonary artery. It is of interest that when the *right* coronary artery arises from the pulmonary artery, few, if any, symptoms ensue and the lesion is usually discovered for the first time at postmortem examination. However, in those patients in whom the *left* coronary artery arises from the pulmonary artery, serious symptoms usually become manifest within the first months of life.

### Pathologic Features

The right coronary artery arises normally from the right sinus of Valsalva and is usually considerably larger than normal. It is distributed to the right ventricle, with many greatly enlarged collaterals anastomosing with the branches of the left coronary artery (Fig. 17).[47] The left ventricular wall is characteristically dilated and thin. The left coronary artery is generally larger than normal, quite tortuous, and thin-walled. Microscopic section of the ventricle frequently shows scarring with varying amounts of subendocardial fibrosis. Calcification is often present in the areas of fibrosis. The infarction pattern of the ventricle may extend into the ventricular septum, leading to infarction of the papillary muscle, which produces mitral insufficiency, especially in association with an enlarged left ventricular cavity, which may also stretch the mitral ring, preventing normal coaptation of the valve leaflets.

The first description of a left coronary artery arising from the pulmonary artery was published in 1911 by Abrikossoff.[3] The patient was a 5 month old infant who died of congestive heart failure with aneurysm formation in the left ventricle. Little attention was given this condition until 1933 when Bland, White, and Garland[10] described the electrocardiographic changes diagnostic of this malformation in early life. It has since become apparent that the vast majority of patients with this disorder become symptomatic in infancy generally within the first few months of life, but a smaller number survive to later life. Rarely, the condition is associated with minimal symptoms for many years.

### Clinical Manifestations

Keith[34] has estimated that 95 per cent of patients with this malformation have clinical symptoms during the first year of life. However, at birth the infant is usually normal, probably be-

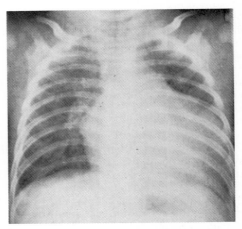

Figure 18    Chest film of infant with anomalous origin of left coronary artery from pulmonary artery, demonstrating marked cardiomegaly, primarily of the left ventricle. (From Sabiston, D. C., Jr., et al.: J. Thorac. Cardiovasc. Surg., *40:*321, 1960.)

cause elevation of the pulmonary arterial pressure at this stage allows perfusion of the left coronary artery from the pulmonary artery. Symptoms usually appear during the first several months of life and include tachypnea, dyspnea, coughing, wheezing, and cyanosis. Of interest is the fact that the infants may cry after feeding; this has been termed "angina of feeding." Later, frank congestive heart failure may appear. On physical examination, marked cardiomegaly is present. Early in the course, no murmurs are heard, although later the systolic murmur of relative mitral insufficiency may develop. The liver is often enlarged and, less often, the spleen is palpable.

The chest film shows evidence of cardiomegaly, especially of the left ventricle (Fig. 18).[47] Fluoroscopic examination may show poor motion of the left ventricle with aneurysmal dilatation. The electrocardiogram characteristically demonstrates inverted T waves in the standard leads. The ST segment in lead 1 may be slightly raised, the T waves in the precordial leads (especially $V_5$ and $V_6$) are usually inverted, and deep Q waves are present.

Angiocardiography demonstrates a normal right heart and pulmonary arteries. It is rare for the left coronary artery to fill from the pulmonary artery, and this probably occurs only in the presence of pulmonary hypertension. The left ventricle is shown to have a greatly enlarged cavity with associated thin wall, and frequently paradoxical activity of the ventricular myocardium is apparent. Arteriography shows the right coronary artery arising from the aorta but not the left coronary artery. Since the collaterals are markedly dilated, they fill the left coronary artery, and dye may be seen actually entering the pulmonary artery by *retrograde* flow (Fig. 19).[46] It is this examination that is the most definitive, as it clearly establishes the diagnosis. Cardiac catheterization is usually of little aid, although a left-to-right shunt at the pulmonary artery level from the retrograde flow through the left coronary artery can sometimes be demonstrated by dye dilution techniques.

### Management

Since the prognosis of origin of the left coronary artery from the pulmonary artery is quite poor once symptoms appear, a surgical approach is generally indicated. It has been established that the blood flow in the left coronary artery is *retrograde,* and the flow of fully oxygenated blood in the left coronary artery into the pulmonary artery should be prevented. In infants and young children, this is probably best accomplished by *ligation* of the artery at its origin from the pulmonary artery, thus forcing the blood in the left coronary artery into the capillary bed of the left ventricle where it is needed. In older children and adults, the preferred operation is anastomosis of a venous autograft from the aorta to the left coronary artery, with closure of the entry of the left coronary artery into the pulmonary artery.[46]

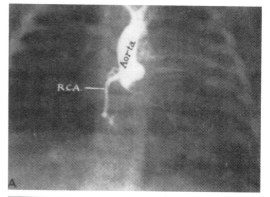
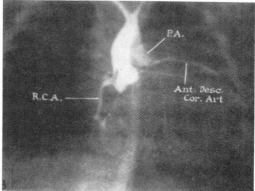
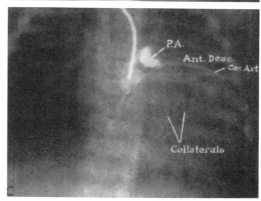

**Figure 19** Several cine frames taken from a series illustrating coronary arterial filling during aortography. *A,* Filling of the right coronary artery as it arises normally from the aorta. Note that its size is somewhat greater than normal. *B,* Filling of the branches of the left coronary artery through collaterals from the right coronary artery. *C,* Filling of the pulmonary artery by *retrograde* flow from the left coronary artery. (From Sabiston, D. C., Jr., and Orme, S. K.: J. Cardiovasc. Surg., 9:543, 1968.)

## CORONARY ARTERIOVENOUS FISTULA

In 1865, Krause described the first coronary arteriovenous fistula,[35] and since then numerous examples have been reported. Not until 1947 was it recognized that such lesions could be corrected surgically. Bjork and Crafoord,[9] in an operation on a patient with a preoperative diagnosis of a patent ductus arteriosus, did not find a ductus, but on further examination discovered a coronary arteriovenous fistula, which they closed.

The majority of patients with coronary arteriovenous fistulas are asymptomatic and have a murmur that is discovered on routine physical examination. The murmur is frequently continuous, and is heard best near the site of the fistula. However, definite complications do occur, including cardiac enlargement, high output cardiac failure, aneurysm formation, and bacterial endocarditis. These lesions are accurately localized by selective arteriography. Communications between a coronary artery and the right atrium, right ventricle, left atrium, left ventricle, pulmonary artery, coronary sinus, and great coronary vein, in order of incidence, have been described. The right coronary artery is most commonly involved with a fistula draining into the right ventricle.

### Clinical Manifestations

At the time of discovery the majority of coronary arteriovenous fistulas are *asymptomatic*. Detection of a continuous murmur is often the first sign and is often initially regarded as the murmur of a patent ductus arteriosus. Other conditions that must be differentiated include aorticopulmonary window, sinus of Valsalva fistula, ventricular septal defect with aortic insufficiency, arteriovenous fistula of the lung, and fistulas of the subclavian or internal mammary vessels. The site of the left-to-right shunt can usually be identified by cardiac catheterization. In some instances, the flow is massive and may exceed the cardiac output.

### Surgical Management

Following selective arteriography and localization of the site of the fistula, surgical correction is indicated. Since the complications produced by these lesions are appreciable, it is usually recommended that asymptomatic fistulas be closed. It is important to close the fistulas without interfering with the coronary arterial circulation distal to the lesion. In most instances this can be accomplished without cardiopulmonary bypass, although at times it is necessary. The results of surgical closure have been excellent.

## CONGENITAL ANEURYSMS OF THE CORONARY ARTERIES

The first report of an aneurysm of the coronary artery was made by Bougon in 1812.[13] By 1957, 68 cases had been reported in the literature,[24] and additional ones have been added.[16] The etiology of these aneurysms includes congenital, atherosclerotic, mycotic, syphilitic and rheumatic types. The complications that may occur include rupture, thrombosis, and infarction of the myocardium due to embolism.

In the past, the majority of aneurysms of the coronary arteries have been associated with arteriovenous fistulas. However, in the future it is likely that more isolated aneurysms of coronary arteries will be discovered with the increasing use of selective coronary arteriography. Treatment of these lesions is indicated if they are symptomatic, especially if there is evidence that emboli from the lesions are occluding the coronary arteries distally, producing myocardial ischemia.

### SELECTED REFERENCES

Abrams, H. L., and Adams, D. F.: The coronary arteriogram. Structural and functional aspects. New Eng. J. Med., *281*: 1276, 1969.
*This review of coronary arteriography is well done and includes a presentation of the anatomy, technique of arteriography, and indications for the procedure.*

Abrikossoff, A.: Aneurysma des linken Herzventrikels mit abnormer Abgangsstelle der linken Koronararterie von der Pulmonalis bei einem funfmonatlichen Kinde. Virchow's Arch. Path. Anat. Physiol. Med., 203:413, 1911.
*This is the first description of anomalous origin of the left coronary artery from the pulmonary artery. Both the gross and microscopic illustrations are excellent. The author describes in detail the clinical manifestations and postmortem findings.*

Baroldi, G., and Scomazzoni, G.: Coronary Circulation in the Normal and the Pathologic Heart. Washington, D.C., Office of the Surgeon General, Department of the Army, 1967.
*This monograph is an exhaustive study of numerous specimens of the normal heart and those with atherosclerotic occlusive disease. It is the most detailed of the studies of the anatomy and pathology of coronary atherosclerosis and is a classic.*

Daniel, T. M., Graham, T. P., and Sabiston, D. C., Jr.: Coronary artery–right ventricular fistula with congestive heart failure: Surgical correction in the neonatal period. Surgery, 67:985, 1970.
*Nearly 200 cases of coronary arteriovenous fistula are reviewed. The incidence of congestive heart failure was 14 per cent. Approximately half of all patients with isolated arteriovenous fistulas were symptomatic. The age of onset of dyspnea, congestive heart failure, bacterial endocarditis, and angina pectoris is reviewed.*

Favaloro, R. G., Effler, D. B., Groves, L. K., Sheldon, W. C., Shirey, E. K., and Sones, F. M., Jr.: Severe segmental obstruction of the left main coronary artery and its divisions: Surgical treatment by the saphenous vein graft technique. J. Thorac. Cardiovasc. Surg., 60:469, 1970.
*In this paper, pioneers in the establishment of aortic-coronary bypass surgery describe their experience; their series constitutes the largest group of patients managed surgically. The indications, operative technique, and results are emphasized.*

Gorlin, R.: Regulation of coronary blood flow. Brit. Heart J., Vol. 33, Supp. 9, 1971.
*This paper describes the various factors that regulate coronary blood flow. It is concise and well presented.*

James, T. N.: Anatomy of the Coronary Arteries. New York, Paul B. Hoeber, 1961.
*This monograph is the definitive source describing the anatomy of the coronary circulation. The work is superbly documented with numerous dissections and injections of specimens, which are carefully reproduced. This monograph is highly recommended.*

Johnson, W. D., Flemma, R. J., Lepley, D., Jr., and Ellison, E. H.: Extended treatment of severe coronary artery disease: A total surgical approach. Ann. Surg., 170:460, 1969.
*This paper represents the early experience of the group who deserve primary credit for the introduction of the aortic-venous bypass graft for myocardial revascularization.*

Marchetti, G., and Taccardi, B., eds.: Coronary Circulation and Energetics of the Myocardium. Basel, S. Karger, 1967.
*This monograph records the presentations made at an International Symposium on the Coronary Circulation and Myocardial Energetics. World leaders in this field partici-*

*pated, and these papers form the best single source of physiology and metabolism of the coronary circulation currently available. The illustrations are excellent.*

Sabiston, D. C., Jr., and Orme, S. K.: Congenital origin of the left coronary artery from the pulmonary artery. J. Cardiovasc. Surg., 9:543, 1968.

*The authors describe 23 patients, ranging in age from 1 day to 31 years, with this disorder. The natural history, clinical findings, laboratory data, and ultimate course are presented.*

Vlodaver, Z., and Edwards, J. E.: Pathologic changes in aortic-coronary arterial saphenous vein grafts. Circulation, 44:719, 1971.

*This is an excellent pathologic study of segments of saphenous vein used as grafts between the aorta and coronary artery. The earliest lesions were noted at 1 month and consisted primarily of intimal fibrotic proliferative lesions and organized thrombi. It is thought that the intimal fibrous proliferative lesion is primarily a response to arterial pressure within the segment of vein.*

# REFERENCES

1. Abrams, D. L., Edelist, A., Luria, M. H., and Miller, A. J.: Ventricular aneurysm. A reappraisal based on a study of 65 consecutive autopsy cases. Circulation, 24:164, 1963.
2. Abrams, H. L., and Adams, D. F.: The coronary arteriogram. Structural and functional aspects. New Eng. J. Med., 281:1276, 1969.
3. Abrikossoff, A.: Aneurysma des linken Herzventrikels mit abnormer Abgangsstelle der linken Koronararterie von der Pulmonalis bei einem funfmonatlichen Kinde. Virchow's Arch. Path. Anat. Physiol. Med., 203:413, 1911.
4. Ackerman, R. F., Dry, T. J., and Edwards, J. E.: Relationship of various factors to the degree of coronary atherosclerosis in women. Circulation, 1:1345, 1950.
5. Aldridge, H. E., and Trimble, A. S.: Progression of proximal coronary artery lesions to total occlusion after aorta-coronary saphenous vein bypass grafting. J. Thorac. Cardiovasc. Surg., 62:7, 1971.
6. Bailey, C. P., May, A., and Lemmon, W. M.: Survival after coronary endarterectomy in man. J.A.M.A., 164:641, 1957.
7. Beck, C. S.: The development of a new blood supply to the heart by operation. Ann. Surg., 102:801, 1935.
8. Berger, R. L., and Stary, H. C.: Anatomic assessment of operability by the saphenous-vein bypass operation in coronary-artery disease. New Eng. J. Med., 285:248, 1971.
9. Bjork, G., and Crafoord, G.: Arteriovenous aneurysm on the pulmonary artery simulating patent ductus arteriosus Botalli. Thorax, 2:65, 1947.
10. Bland, E. F., White, P. D., and Garland, J.: Congenital anomalies of coronary arteries: Report of an unusual case associated with cardiac hypertrophy. Amer. Heart J., 8:787, 1933.
11. Blumgart, H. L., Pitt, B., Zoll, P. M., and Freiman, D. G.: Anatomic factors influencing the locations of coronary occlusions and development of collateral coronary circulation (Henry Ford Hospital International Symposium). In: James, T. N., and Keyes, J. W., eds.: The Etiology of Myocardial Infarction. Boston, Little, Brown and Company, 1963.
12. Blumgart, H. L., Schlesinger, M. J., and Davis, D.: Studies on the relation of clinical manifestations of angina pectoris, coronary thrombosis and myocardial infarction to the pathologic findings with particular reference to significance of collateral circulation. Amer. Heart J., 19:1, 1940.
13. Bougon: Bibl. Med., 37:183, 1912; cited by Packard, M., and Wechsler, H. F.: Aneurysm of the coronary arteries. Arch. Intern. Med., 43:1, 1929.
14. Cheng, T. O.: Incidence of ventricular aneurysm in coronary artery disease. An angiographic appraisal. Amer. J. Med., 50:340, 1971.
15. Cooley, D. A., Belmonte, B. A., Zeis, L. B., and Schnur, S.:

Surgical repair of ruptured interventricular septum following acute myocardial infarction. Surgery, 41:930, 1957.
16. Ebert, P. A., Peter, R. H., Gunnells, J. C., and Sabiston, D. C., Jr.: Resecting and grafting of coronary artery aneurysm. Circulation, 43:593, 1971.
17. Eckstein, R. W.: Effect of exercise and coronary artery narrowing on coronary collateral circulation. Circ. Res., 5:230, 1957.
18. Edwards, J. E., et al.: Occlusion of saphenous vein autografts. Circulation, 1972, in press.
19. Enos, W. F., Holmes, R. H., and Beyer, J.: Coronary disease among United States soldiers killed in action in Korea. Preliminary report. J.A.M.A., 152:1090, 1953.
20. Favaloro, R. G.: Direct Myocardial Revascularization. Surg. Clin. N. Amer., 51:1035, 1971.
21. Favaloro, R. G., Effler, D. B., and Groves, L. K.: Severe segmental obstruction of the left main coronary artery and its divisions: Surgical treatment by the saphenous vein graft technic. J. Thorac. Cardiovasc. Surg., 60:469, 1970.
22. FitzGibbon, G. M., Hooper, G. D., and Heggtveit, H. A.: Successful surgical treatment of post-infarction external cardiac rupture. J. Thorac. Cardiovasc. Surg., 63:622, 1972.
23. François-Franck, C. A.: Signification physiologique de la résection du sympathique dans la maladie de Basedow, l'épilepsie, l'idiotie et le glaucome. Bull. Acad. Nat. Med., 41:565, 1899; cited by White, J. C.: Cardiac pain—anatomic pathways and physiologic mechanisms. Circulation, 16:644, 1957.
24. Gore, I., Smith, J., and Clancy, R.: Congenital aneurysms of the coronary arteries with report of a case. Circulation, 19:221, 1959.
25. Gorlin, R.: Regulation of coronary blood flow. Brit. Heart J., Vol. 33, Supp. 9, 1971.
26. Green, G. E., Stertzer, S. H., Gordon, R. B., and Tice, D. A.: Anastomosis of the internal mammary artery to the distal left anterior descending coronary artery. Circulation, Supp. 2, 41:79, 1970.
27. Gregg, D. E.: The coronary circulation in the unanesthetized dog. In: Marchetti, G., and Taccardi, B., eds.: Coronary Circulation and Energetics of the Myocardium. Basel, S. Karger, 1967.
28. Grondin, C. M., Meere C., Castonguay, Y., Lepage, G., and Grondin, P.: Progressive and late obstruction of an aortocoronary venous bypass graft. Circulation, 43:698, 1971.
29. Herberden, W.: Commentaries on the History and Cure of Diseases. Boston, Wells and Lilly, 1818, p. 292.
30. Herrick, J. B.: Clinical features of sudden obstruction of the coronary arteries. J.A.M.A., 59:2015, 1912.
31. Hill, J. D., Kerth, W. J., Kelly, J. J., Selzer, A., Armstrong, W., Popper, R. W., Langston, M., and Cohn, K. E.: Emergency aortocoronary bypass for impending or extending myocardial infarction. Circulation, Supp. 1, 43:105, 1971.
32. Johnson, W. D., Flemma, R. J., Lepley, D., Jr., and Ellison, E. H.: Extended treatment of severe coronary artery disease: A total surgical approach. Ann. Surg., 170:460, 1969.
33. Jonnesco, T.: Angine de poitrine guérie par la résection du sympathique cervico-thoracique. Bull. Acad. Med., 84:93, 1920.
34. Keith, J. D.: The anomalous origin of the left coronary artery from the pulmonary artery. Brit. Heart J., 21:149, 1959.
35. Krause, W.: Z. Rat. Med., 24, 1865.
36. Longmire, W. P., Jr., Cannon, J. A., and Kattus, A. A.: Direct-vision coronary endarterectomy for angina pectoris. New Eng. J. Med., 259:993, 1958.
37. Loop, F. D.: Ventricular aneurysmectomy. Surg. Clin. N. Amer., 51:1071, 1971.
38. Mann, G. V., Garrett, H. L., Farhi, A., Murray, H., and Billings, F. T.: Exercise to prevent coronary heart disease. Amer. J. Med., 46:12, 1969.
39. Moon, H. D.: Coronary arteries in infants and juveniles. Circulation, 16:263, 1957.
40. Morris, G. C., Jr., Howell, J. F., Crawford, E. S., Reul, G. J., Chapman, D. W., Beazley, H. L., Winters, W. L., and Peterson, P. K.: The distal coronary bypass. Ann. Surg., 172:652, 1970.
41. Mundth, E. D., Buckley, M. J., Leinbach, R. C., DeSanctis,

R. W., Sanders, C. A., Kantrowitz, A., and Austen, W. G.: Myocardial revascularization for the treatment of cardiogenic shock complicating acute myocardial infarction. Surgery, 70:78, 1971.

42. Oldham, H. N., Scott, S. M., Dart, C. H., Fish, R. G., Claxton, C. P., Dillon, M. L., and Sabiston, D. C., Jr.: Surgical correction of ventricular septal defect following acute myocardial infarction. Ann. Thorac. Surg., 7:193, 1969.

43. Oyamadi, A., and Queen, F. V.: Spontaneous rupture of the interventricular septum following acute myocardial infarction with some clinico-pathological observations on survival in 5 cases. Presented at Pan Pacific Pathology Congress, Tripler U. S. Army Hospital, 1961.

44. Rowe, G. G., Castillo, C. A., Maxwell, G. M., and Crumpton, C. W.: Comparison of systemic and coronary hemodynamics in the normal human male and female. Circ. Res., 7:728, 1959.

45. Sabiston, D. C., Jr.: Direct revascularization procedure in the management of myocardial ischemia. Circulation, 43:175, 1971.

46. Sabiston, D. C., Jr., and Orme, S. K.: Congenital origin of the left coronary artery from the pulmonary artery. J. Cardiovasc. Surg., 9:543, 1968.

47. Sabiston, D. C., Jr., Pelargonio, S., and Taussig, H. B.: Myocardial infarction in infancy. J. Thorac. Cardiovasc. Surg., 40:321, 1960.

48. Schlesinger, M. J., and Zoll, P. M.: Incidence and localization of coronary artery occlusions. Arch. Path., 32:178, 1941.

49. Schlichter, J., Hellerstein, H. K., and Katz, L. N.: Aneurysm of the heart. Medicine, 33:43, 1954.

50. Sheldon, W. C.: Cine coronary arteriography. Surg. Clin. N. Amer., 51:1015, 1971.

51. Spencer, F. C.: Bypass grafting for occlusive disease of the coronary arteries. Maryland Med. J., 20:2, 1971.

52. Spiekerman, R. E., Brandenburg, J. T., Achor, R. W. P., and Edwards, J. E.: The spectrum of coronary artery disease in a community of 30,000. A clinico-pathologic study. Circulation, 25:57, 1962.

53. Vansant, J. H., and Muller, W. H., Jr.: Surgical procedures to revascularize the heart: Review of the literature. Amer. J. Surg., 100:572, 1960.

54. Vineberg, A. M.: Development of an anastomosis between the coronary vessels and a transplanted internal mammary artery. Canad. Med. Ass. J., 55:117, 1946.

55. Vlodaver, Z., and Edwards, J. E.: Pathologic changes in aortic-coronary arterial saphenous vein grafts. Circulation, 44:719, 1971.

56. White, N. K., Edwards, J. E., and Dry, T. J.: The relationship of the degree of coronary atherosclerosis with age in men. Circulation 1:645, 1950.

57. Winterscheid, L. C.: Collateral circulation of the heart. In: Strandness, D. E., Jr., ed.: Collateral Circulation in Clinical Surgery. Philadelphia, W. B. Saunders Company, 1969.

58. Wolkoff, K.: Ueber die Atherosklerose der Koronararterien des Herzens. Beitr. Path. Anat., 82:55, 1929.

# XI

# Acquired Disorders of the Aortic Valve

*William H. Muller, Jr., M.D., and Stanton P. Nolan, M.D.*

## ANATOMY AND FUNCTION OF THE AORTIC VALVE

The normal aortic valve is tricuspid, and each leaflet forms a truncated parabola. The uppermost attachment of the commissures defines the distal limits of the sinuses of Valsalva, with the coronary arteries usually arising in the upper one-third. Pulse duplicator studies of valvular motion indicate a rapid retraction of all three cusps at the beginning of ejection to form a triangular orifice. A slow, wavelike motion of the free edge and billowing of the base of each cusp are caused by eddy currents within the sinuses of Valsalva. Occlusion of the coronary ostia by the leaflets is thus prevented, and a position is maintained that allows slight reversal of flow to result in immediate closure without regurgitation.[13] Only 20 per cent of total coronary blood flow occurs during systole.[8] Therefore, diastolic coronary blood flow is enhanced by the aortic pressure and decreased intramural pressure of the ventricles and retarded by increased right atrial and intraventricular pressures. Left ventricular ejection occurs when left ventricular pressure exceeds aortic pressure. The forward pressure gradient ceases during the first one-half of systole, and thereafter forward flow is maintained by a mass-acceleration effect. Closure of the normal aortic valve is accomplished by reversal of the flow rather than by reversal of the pressure gradient.[10]

## PATHOLOGY AND ETIOLOGY

### Rheumatic Fever

This process begins as myocarditis invading the aortic valve through the valvular ring. In the acute stage, there is edema, inflammation, formation of granulation tissue, and scarring, often resulting in thickened, scarred, contracted leaflets with rolled edges. The valvular ring frequently dilates because of destruction of its fibrous tissue. In addition, the tissues are more susceptible to degenerative alterations and may undergo atheromatous changes and calcium deposition (Fig. 1). Dilatation of the annulus may produce insufficiency with shortening or stiffening of the cusps, or stenosis may occur as a result of fusion of the commissures and agglutination of the leaflet borders.

### Syphilis

Syphilitic valvular disease, now seldom seen in the United States, begins in the aorta around the vasa vasorum. Initially, there is perivascular

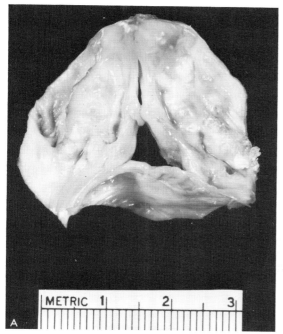
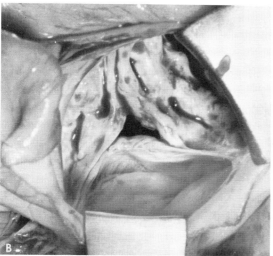

**Figure 1** *A*, Photograph of the excised valve, showing dense calcification of two leaflets. *B*, Operative view of a calcified stenotic aortic valve.

cellular infiltration that compromises the nutrient vessels, producing destruction of the muscular and elastic layers of the tunica media as well as associated elevation and roughening of the intima. Valvular dysfunction occurs when the process affects the aortic root, producing dilatation of the valvular ring and widening of the commissures. The cusps are rarely involved except for secondary stretching and patulence, and consequently pure aortic insufficiency most commonly results. A recent review of 258 autopsy reports of aortic regurgitation[1] indicated that syphilis now accounts for less than 5 per cent of the cases. Since the coronary ostia are involved, and coronary insufficiency occurs in most of these patients, it is possible that sudden death occurs and that this accounts for the relatively few patients referred for surgical consideration.

### Bacterial Endocarditis

Subacute bacterial endocarditis is characterized by the deposition of bacterial vegetations and thrombus formation on the valvular leaflets. These lesions induce inflammation and scarring or may progress to erosion and valvular perforation. The process usually occurs on a congenitally deformed valve or one damaged by rheumatic valvulitis. Either *insufficiency* or *stenosis* may result, the former being by far the more frequent lesion. Autopsy studies indicate that the inflammatory process subsides slowly over a period of several months following sterilization of the bloodstream.

### Traumatic Aortic Insufficiency

Traumatic rupture of the aortic valve is rare; it most frequently occurs in a previously diseased valve and usually follows extreme muscular exertion. Blunt trauma to the chest may also cause rupture of a diseased valve, and if it is severe enough it may affect similarly a normal valve. A linear tear through a single cusp or avulsion of a commissure from the aortic wall is generally found.

### Marfan's Syndrome

Marfan's syndrome is a heritable, generalized, systemic disease of connective tissue. Aortic insufficiency results when cystic medial necrosis of the aorta produces dilatation of the aortic ring and aneurysm formation. Sudden insufficiency often develops when spontaneous intimal rupture and retrograde dissection releases the commissural attachments of the valve, so that it partially invaginates into the left ventricle during diastole.[9]

### Congenital Valvular Disease

Acquired disease of the aortic valve may result from a congenital deformity. Although a congenitally deformed valve may remain asymptomatic for many years, it is more susceptible to bacterial endocarditis, rheumatic fever, or, particularly, calcification and may become stenotic or insufficient. Of 162 patients over the age of 15 years dying of aortic stenosis, Roberts found that 52 per cent had congenital deformities of the valve.[11]

## PATHOLOGIC PHYSIOLOGY

### Aortic Insufficiency

The hemodynamic changes in aortic insufficiency result from the reflux of a significant amount of blood into the left ventricle during diastole. What constitutes a "significant" volume of reflux in the human is difficult to define. Measurements performed in the operating room prior to valvular replacement and studies from the animal laboratory indicate that greater than 50 per cent of the left ventricular ejection must regurgitate into the left ventricle before symptoms of heart failure are produced.[7]

When significant aortic insufficiency alone is present, the pulse pressure is always increased, and there is an exaggeration of the normal elevation of peripheral over central systolic pressure. Mean systemic pressure generally remains in a normal range owing to a proportional increase in systolic pressure. There is much controversy concerning the left ventricular end-diastolic pressure in this disease. However, it probably remains normal until the onset of either cardiac failure or myocardial fibrosis.

Cardiac compensation is achieved by hypertrophy and dilatation of the left ventricle. Thus, addition of the volume of reflux to the normal left atrial inflow produces an increase in the initial intraventricular tension and results in a more forceful and rapid ejection. Additional compensation is achieved by the decrease in aortic diastolic pressure, which allows an abridgment of the isometric contraction phase and prolongation of the systolic ejection time. Experimentally, it has been shown that the normal phasic pattern of coronary arterial flow persists in aortic insufficiency, and that the major portion of coronary perfusion occurs during diastole.[10] Although there may be an increase in the absolute coronary flow in aortic insufficiency, in some patients relative coronary insufficiency will develop because of cardiac hypertrophy secondary to increased myocardial oxygen consumption and a shorter diastolic coronary perfusion time.

Symptoms are rare in uncomplicated, compensated aortic insufficiency. Occasionally, patients complain of nocturnal angina pectoris;[6] however, it is difficult to delineate the role played by the valvular disease from that of underlying coronary artery disease. Cardiac compensation may last for years, and the first indications of the progression of the disease are signs and symptoms of left ventricular failure.

### Aortic Stenosis

The systolic pressure gradient across the aortic valve is increased by left ventricular outflow obstruction. Experimental studies indicate that diminution of the cross-sectional area of the valve orifice to one-fourth its normal size must occur before a significant decrease in resting cardiac output or increase in pressure gradient is evident.

Systemic blood pressure is usually normal, although the pulse pressure is often decreased and the peripheral pulses diminished. Left ventricular aortic systolic gradients may range as high as 150 mm. Hg (Fig. 2). The resting cardiac output is normal unless failure is present; however, cardiac output does not increase with exercise in the presence of severe stenosis. Left ventricular hypertrophy and increased left ventricular diastolic volume act as compensatory mechanisms to maintain cardiac output. Prolongation of the isometric contraction phase, as well as the systolic ejection

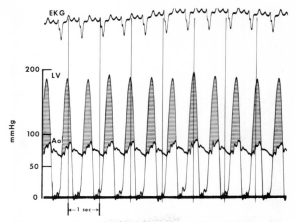

**Figure 2** Simultaneous recording of the electrocardiogram (EKG), left ventricular pressure (LV), and aortic pressure (Ao) obtained at cardiac catheterization in a patient with aortic stenosis. The shaded areas indicate the pressure gradient across the aortic valve. The LV-Ao peak systolic pressure gradient is 95 mm. Hg.

time, allows a longer period for emptying of the ventricle and compensation for the lower flow rate. These mechanisms allow maintenance of an adequate cardiac output but interfere with myocardial perfusion because the proportion of the cardiac cycle devoted to isometric contraction and systolic ejection is markedly lengthened, and the period of elevated intramural tension is increased. Thus, the duration of diastolic coronary perfusion is decreased. Coronary insufficiency in the absence of primary coronary artery disease may ensue, causing electrocardiographic changes consistent with myocardial ischemia and the symptoms of angina pectoris. The frequent occurrence of sudden death in aortic stenosis is probably due to sudden ventricular arrhythmias secondary to inadequate coronary blood flow.

## CRITERIA FOR SURGERY

The selection of patients for aortic valvular surgery is often difficult. Ideally, all patients with aortic valvular disease should undergo operation prior to the onset of *irreversible* myocardial changes. Unfortunately, there is no certain method of recognizing this state; thus, the surgeon is left with the decision to operate upon relatively asymptomatic patients whose prognosis with medical management may be good, or upon those with myocardial damage whose mortality will be higher and in whom the results will be less than satisfactory.

In general, surgery is contraindicated in anyone with active rheumatic heart disease. In those with bacterial endocarditis, surgery should be postponed, if possible, for approximately 3 months after blood cultures are negative. If one is forced to operate earlier, adequate antibiotics must be given with full knowledge that the results will not be as good. The degree of pulmonary fibrosis or emphysema, or both, if present, must be carefully determined before the decision to operate is made. Primary coronary artery disease, if recognized, requires consideration of the expected results in comparison to the increased operative risks.

### Aortic Insufficiency

The lack of a method for quantitating the degree of aortic insufficiency results in the selection of operative candidates primarily on the basis of clinical progression of signs and symptoms. The development of angina or congestive failure indicates subsequent progressive deterioration. Cineangiocardiography may be of help in estimating the degree of insufficiency but is of limited practical aid in selecting candidates for operation. Cardiac catheterization may be helpful in patients with an elevated left ventricular end-diastolic pressure prior to the recognition of overt heart failure and may provide additional evidence of dysfunction of other cardiac valves.

Any patient with advanced aortic insufficiency should be considered a candidate for surgery. Usually, there is a history of congestive heart failure, progressive electrocardiographic changes, and radiographic evidence of progressive cardiomegaly (Fig. 3).

### Aortic Stenosis

Aortic stenosis often produces no symptoms for 10 to 30 years. Once symptoms develop, however, the patient's condition is precarious, and the average life expectancy is 2 years.[12] Therefore, patients with symptomatic aortic stenosis should undergo cardiac catheterization. If electrocardio-

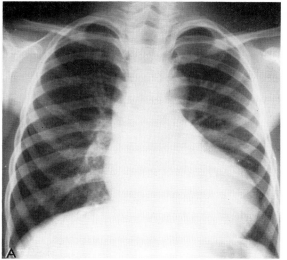
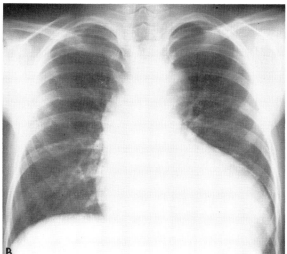
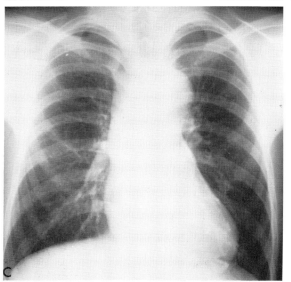

**Figure 3** Serial roentgenograms of a patient with aortic insufficiency, demonstrating changes in cardiac size. A, Five years before operation, patient asymptomatic. B, Immediate preoperative view, poorly controlled congestive heart failure for 6 months. C, Six months after aortic valvular replacement, patient asymptomatic.

graphic signs of coronary insufficiency are present, or if the history suggests such a condition, coronary angiography should be performed simultaneously in order to evaluate the coronary circulation, so that a more objective candidate selection may be made. In the symptomatic patient, the demonstration of a systolic gradient across the valve of more than 50 mm. Hg is sufficient to justify operative intervention. Serial x-ray evidence of rapid cardiac enlargement is an ominous sign and an urgent indication for operation.

## OPERATIVE TREATMENT

Operations on the aortic valve are performed through a median sternotomy. Cardiopulmonary bypass is achieved by cannulating the right atrium or the superior and inferior venae cavae and the ascending aorta or femoral artery. The aorta is occluded proximally, and the valve is exposed through a transverse or curved aortotomy. Exposure is facilitated by sump suction through the apex of the left ventricle. Coronary artery perfusion with a cannula in each coronary orifice is preferred, especially perfusion of the left coronary artery.

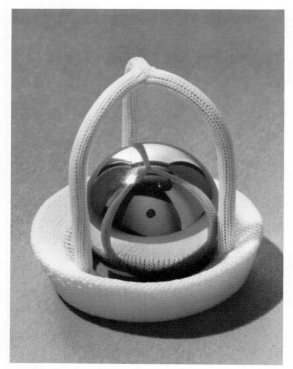

**Figure 4**  Starr-Edwards aortic ball valve prosthesis with plastic cover and metal ball. (Courtesy of Edwards Laboratories.)

Occasionally, valvular function can be restored by excising small amounts of calcium from the leaflets and incising the commissures to the annulus. Rarely, a valvuloplasty may restore competence. However, in the majority of adults with acquired aortic valve disease, the entire valve must be excised and replaced.

Although many devices have been employed for aortic valve replacement, none is ideal. The most widely used are prosthetic valves, which are usually composed of a metal frame exposed or covered with cloth and containing a moving obturator. The obturator may be a sphere, disc, toroid, or hinged flap fabricated from plastic or metal[3] (Fig. 4). Tissue valves are composed of human or animal tissues appropriately sterilized and preserved. Homografts excised at autopsy with their aortic attachments may be sutured directly to the patient's annulus. Homografts and heterografts are frequently presutured to a metal and fabric stent before insertion. Fascia lata excised from the patient's thigh, tailored, and sutured to a stent to form a trileaflet valve has been used for replacement.[5]

Prosthetic valves, especially if relatively small, may result in a moderate left ventricular–aortic pressure gradient. The majority carry some risk of thromboembolism, although many of the prostheses have been modified or redesigned in an effort to prevent this complication. Most surgeons advocate postoperative anticoagulants indefinitely. Homograft valves rarely cause thrombosis or embolism; however, they may be subject to fatigue and late calcification. The results are encouraging in several series of patients followed for more than 5 years.[2] At the present time, the long-term fate of heterograft valves is unknown.

## RESULTS OF SURGERY OF THE AORTIC VALVE

The results of aortic valvular surgery must be evaluated from several points of view: (1) the prognosis of patients with untreated aortic valvular disease; (2) the risk of operation; (3) the risk of complications secondary to the device used for valvular replacement; (4) the percentage of patients alive several years after operation; and (5) the percentage of patients living and functionally improved.

Duvoisin and McGoon[4] have reported results over a 6 year period in 550 patients undergoing insertion of an aortic ball valve prosthesis. Six per cent of their patients died in the first 30 days. At the end of 6 years, 66 per cent were alive, and 60 per cent had a good result. There was correlation between long-term survival and results and the presence or absence of preoperative heart failure and the preoperative New York Heart Association functional classification. Of patients without failure or those who were classified as functional Class II, 75 to 80 per cent had a good result 6 years after operation. Emboli occurred in 22 per cent of the survivors, but the embolization rate was reduced with adequate anticoagulation.

Homograft aortic valves were placed in 101 patients and followed for 5 years by Barratt-Boyes.[2] Six per cent of the patients died in the first month. After 5 years, 70 per cent were still alive; however, only 50 per cent were asymptomatic. Twelve per cent of the patients required another aortic valve operation.

# IDIOPATHIC HYPERTROPHIC SUBAORTIC STENOSIS (IHSS)

## Gross Pathology

IHSS is a syndrome consisting of eccentric hypertrophy of the left ventricle and particularly the outflow tract, producing severe subvalvular stenosis. Patients dying of this disease have large hearts in which the thickened left ventricular muscle encroaches on the ventricular cavity, thus narrowing the volume. There are two general types: by far the most common is asymmetric hypertrophy involving the outflow portion of the ventricular myocardium, usually including the ventricular septum; the second is a more or less symmetric diffuse hypertrophy of the entire ventricle and ventricular septum. There is often enlargement of the papillary muscles and trabeculae carneae, thickening and opacity of the endocardium, particularly in the outflow tract, and thickening of the anterior mitral leaflet. In some hearts, the texture of the hypertrophied muscle is coarser than that of adjacent, more normal-appearing muscle.

## Histopathology

The histopathologic appearance varies. There is a generalized increase in the amount of interstitial connective tissue. The muscle bundles are separated by this tissue and assume a bizarre arrangement. In some instances there are endothelial-lined channels between the muscle bundles opening into the ventricular cavities. Electron microscopic examination indicates not only thickening of the fibers but shortening as well. There is an increase in the size and number of nerve fibrils, elastic tissue, and mitochondria. Pearse[13] noted that hypertrophied myofibrils were being replaced by mitrochondria, and so myofibril bands were shortened. The similarity between these fibers and normal sinoauricular nodal cells and atrial muscle suggested to him that IHSS might be the result of displacement of atrial muscle or abnormal proliferation of cardiac sympathetic nerves.

## Clinical and Accessory Clinical Findings

Males are affected twice as frequently as females. In 64 patients reported by Braunwald and Morrow,[3] the ages ranged from 6 to 56 years of age. All patients had systolic murmurs, and 48 of them had complaints that were believed to be related to their disease. A heart murmur was most often the first clinical manifestation of disease. Dyspnea, angina, and dizzy spells were the most common symptoms, and syncope occurred not infrequently. The heart was usually enlarged, and a systolic thrill, best felt over the lower precordium on the left, was present in about half the patients. A systolic murmur along the lower left sternal border or at the apex was present in nearly all instances. Electrocardiographic abnormalities were present in virtually all patients. Roentgenologic examination showed an increased cardiothoracic ratio in more than 50 per cent. Angiocardiography demonstrated a smaller than normal left ventricular cavity during diastole and one that appeared to be almost entirely obliterated during systole. The left ventricular wall was generally much thicker than normal and often thicker than that found in patients with valvular or membranous subvalvular aortic stenosis.

## Hemodynamics

Hemodynamically, the most prominent feature is the variability of the obstruction. The pressure

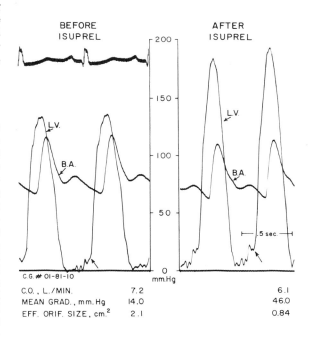

| | BEFORE ISUPREL | AFTER ISUPREL |
|---|---|---|
| C.O., L./MIN. | 7.2 | 6.1 |
| MEAN GRAD., mm.Hg | 14.0 | 46.0 |
| EFF. ORIF. SIZE, cm.² | 2.1 | 0.84 |

**Figure 5** Simultaneous left ventricular (LV) and brachial artery (BA) pressure recordings from a patient with IHSS made before and after the intravenous infusion of isoproterenol. The inotropic effect of this pharmacologic agent caused the pressure gradient to increase from 14 to 46 mm. Hg, while the effective aortic orifice area decreased from 2.1 to 0.8 cm.²

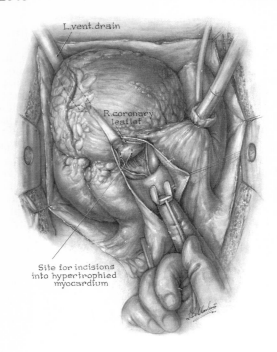

L.vent.drain

R.coronary
leaflet

Site for incisions
into hypertrophied
myocardium

**Figure 6**   Technique of ventriculomyotomy combined with resection. The aortic valve is retracted, and parallel superficial incisions are made about 1 cm. apart over the muscle mass. The incisions are usually oriented to the commissure between the left and right coronary leaflets of the aortic valve and may be made individually or with the double-bladed knife shown. The aortic leaflet of the mitral valve is shown posteriorly. (From Morrow, A. G.: Circulation, Supp. 29, Nov. 1964. By permission of the American Heart Association, Inc.)

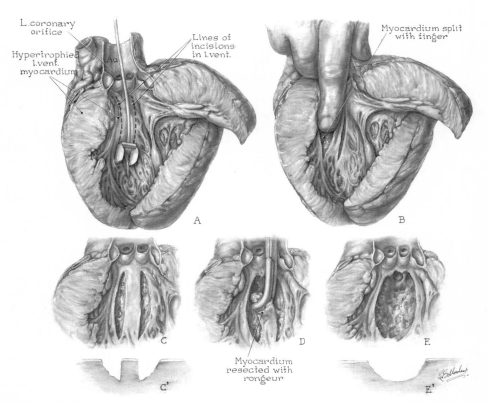

L.coronary
orifice

Hypertrophied
l.vent.
myocardium

Ao

Lines of
incisions
in l.vent.

Myocardium split
with finger

A

B

C

D

E

Myocardium
resected with
rongeur

C'

E'

**Figure 7**   Technique of ventriculomyotomy combined with resection. Two parallel incisions are made as shown in *A*, and the muscle beneath each of them is then split by digital pressure to a depth of 2 to 3 cm. (*B*). The ridge of endocardium and muscle between the incisions is then resected with an angled rongeur passed from the aortic incision (*C, D, E*). (From Morrow, A. G., Circulation, Supp. 29, Nov. 1964. By permission of the American Heart Association, Inc.)

gradient may vary tremendously during a single study, at times increasing severalfold, diminishing significantly, disappearing entirely, or appearing when none was present initially. This is explained by the fact that the obstruction is produced by the myocardial contractions and is subject to the same regulatory influences that control the contractile state of the entire myocardium. A number of factors can be introduced to influence the degree of stenosis and are based primarily upon whether or not the ventricular volume is diminished or increased. Those factors which reduce ventricular volume will increase the obstruction and include a decreased venous return produced by bleeding or by maneuvers to increase the intrapleural pressure, certain drugs with a positive inotropic effect on the myocardium (Fig. 5), and decreased afterloading. Conversely, those factors which increase ventricular volume reduce or alleviate the obstruction. These include an increased venous return, a negative inotropic effect on the myocardium, an increased afterload, and operations to relieve the obstruction.

### Operative Treatment and Results

A number of operations have been devised to treat this disease and are directed primarily toward relieving the outflow obstruction. The most effective and frequently employed operation is that devised by Morrow (Figs. 6 and 7), which consists of approaching the hypertrophied myocardium through an aortotomy and making two parallel incisions longitudinally through the muscle mass in the outflow tract.[8] These incisions are then increased in depth by digital pressure, and the mass of tissue between them is excised. At times, a rongeur passed through an apical incision may be necessary to reach the more distal part of the muscle mass.

The operative mortality is approximately 10 per cent. Symptomatic as well as hemodynamic results are excellent. There is no peak gradient at rest when the operation is properly executed. Maneuvers to decrease left ventricular volume and thereby increase outflow obstruction are effective only to a minimal degree in some patients. The end-diastolic pressure is reduced, and associated mitral insufficiency, when present before operation, is usually corrected.

### SELECTED REFERENCES

Barratt-Boyes, B. G., et al.: Aortic homograft valve replacement. Circulation, *40*:763, 1969.
*This article is a review of 101 patients undergoing homograft aortic valve replacement and followed from 4 to 6 years postoperatively. The problems and complications associated with homograft valves are evaluated and discussed.*

Duvoisin, G. E., and McGoon, D. C.: Aortic valve replacement with a ball-valve prosthesis. Arch. Surg., *99*:684, 1969.
*This report on 548 operations for replacement of the aortic valve with an aortic ball valve prosthesis includes an evaluation of the effects of many factors on early and late results. The authors urge the reporting of late results of operations for cardiac disease by means of time-oriented data such as actuarial curves in order to provide a true perspective for comparison to other studies.*

Morrow, A. G., Brawley, R. K., and Braunwald, E.: Effects of aortic regurgitation on left ventricular performance: Direct determinations of aortic blood flow before and after valve replacement. Circulation, Supp. 1, *31*:80, 1965.
*An operative study of instantaneous flows and pressures in patients with aortic valvular disease is presented. It provides valuable information concerning the effects of aortic valvular disease on left ventricular function in man and documents the favorable changes in flow, pressure, and left ventricular work that immediately follow aortic valvular replacement.*

Zimmerman, J.: The functional and surgical anatomy of the aortic valve. Fourth Asian-Pacific Congress of Cardiology, *5*:862, 1969.
*An excellent description and graphic representation of the dynamic behavior of the normal aortic valve is presented. The surgical implications of the normal anatomy as it relates to operative technique and prosthetic valve design are discussed.*

### REFERENCES

1. Barondess, J. A., and Sande, M.: Some changing aspects of aortic regurgitation. Arch. Inter. Med., *124*:600, 1969.
2. Barratt-Boyes, B. G., et al.: Aortic homograft valve replacement. Circulation, *40*:763, 1969.
3. Braunwald, E., Lambrew, C. T., Rockoff, S. D., Ross, J. Jr., and Morrow, A. G.: Idiopathic hypertrophic subaortic stenosis. Circulation, Supp. 4, *30*:3, 1964.
4. Brewer, L. A., III, ed.: Prosthetic Heart Valves. Springfield, Ill., Charles C Thomas, 1969.
5. Duvoisin, G. E., and McGoon, D. C.: Aortic valve replacement with a ball-valve prosthesis. Arch. Surg., *99*:684, 1969.
6. Ionescu, M. Z., et al.: Heart valve replacement with autologous fascia lata. J. Thorac. Cardiovasc. Surg., *60*:331, 1970.
7. Levinson, G. E., Frank, M., and Schwartz, C. J.: The effect of rest and physical effort on the left ventricular burden in mitral and aortic regurgitation. Amer. Heart J., *80*:791, 1970.
8. Morrow, A. G.: Hypertrophic subaortic stenosis. Arch. Surg., *99*:677, 1969.
9. Morrow, A. G., Brawley, R. K., and Braunwald, E.: Effects of aortic regurgitation on left ventricular performance: Direct determinations of aortic blood flow before and after valve replacement. Circulation, Supp. 1, *31*:80, 1965.
10. Muller, W. H., Jr., Dammann, J. F., Jr., and Warren, W. D.: Surgical correction of cardiovascular deformities in Marfan's syndrome. Ann. Surg., *152*:506, 1960.
11. Nolan, S. P., and Muller, W. H., Jr.: Instantaneous coronary artery blood flow in aortic insufficiency. Surg. Forum, *14*:251, 1963.
12. Nolan, S. P., and Muller, W. H., Jr.: The aortic valve. Ann. Rev. Med., *16*:33, 1965.
13. Pearse, A. G. E.: The histochemistry and electron microscopy of obstructive cardiomyopathy. In: Ciba Foundation Symposium on Cardiomyopathies. Boston, Little, Brown and Company, 1965.
14. Roberts, W. C.: The structure of the aortic valve in clinically isolated aortic stenosis: An autopsy study of 162 patients over 15 years of age. Circulation, *42*:91, 1970.
15. Ross, J., Jr., and Braunwald, E.: Aortic stenosis. Circulation, Supp. 5, *38*:61, 1968.
16. Zimmerman, J.: The functional and surgical anatomy of the aortic valve. Fourth Asian-Pacific Congress of Cardiology, *5*:862, 1969.

# Acquired Mitral and Tricuspid Valvular Disease

## W. Gerald Austen, M.D., and Adolph M. Hutter, Jr., M.D.

Mitral and tricuspid valvar diseases are most often acquired disorders and are usually the result of rheumatic fever. Within the past 25 years the prognosis for these lesions has changed as a result of remarkable advances in diagnostic techniques and cardiac surgery.

## HISTORICAL ASPECTS

Surgical correction of *mitral stenosis* was first suggested in 1902 by Brunton[23] and first attempted in 1923 by Cutler and Levine.[29] The result was unsatisfactory because partial resection of the stenosed valve resulted in severe mitral regurgitation. In 1925, Souttar[131] performed a digital commissurotomy in a single case but no significant progress was made over the next two decades. During this period, the technique of cardiac catheterization was developed and it added immensely to the understanding of valvular heart disease. Forssmann, a urologist, presented the first radiographic evidence of right atrial catheterization in man in an operation he performed on himself in 1929.[39] In 1941 Cournand and Ranges[28] established right cardiac catherization as a useful tool. In the late 1940s, Harken et al.,[54] Bailey,[7] and Brock,[21] independently, successfully accomplished closed digital commissurotomy for mitral stenosis, and thus made this procedure a practical reality. The addition of techniques employing various knives or *transatrial* valvulotomes did not result in significant improvement in results. However, the subsequent development of the Tubbs *transventricular* dilator in 1959 allowed a considerably more effective commissurotomy.

Effective surgical treatment of *mitral regurgitation* had to await development of cardiopulmonary bypass techniques, beginning in the early 1950s.[46] Various forms of open annuloplasty were subsequently employed, with variable results. The introduction of the rigid-ring, ball valve prosthesis by Starr and Edwards in 1961[133] provided a consistently successful surgical procedure for patients with mitral valvular heart disease (both regurgitation and stenosis), even in the presence of extensive valvular damage. Both the success and the complications of the early models have been taken into account in the subsequent modifications[58, 59, 132] and improvements of the Starr-Edwards prosthesis, and a number of other types of prostheses have been designed and clinically tested.[11, 15, 36, 60, 71, 84] Homograft, heterograft, and fascia lata valves have also been employed.[10, 24, 65, 66, 116]

Only recently has it become apparent that a significant number of patients have severe *tricuspid valvular disease* that can seriously affect the operative result following mitral or aortic valve surgery.[8, 97, 135, 139] Open valvulotomy has been shown to be helpful in patients with acquired tricuspid stenosis,[123] and annuloplasty may occasionally be of value in patients with tricuspid regurgitation. Frequently, however, valve replacement is necessary in patients with severe acquired or functional tricuspid disease.[135]

## MITRAL STENOSIS

### ETIOLOGY AND PATHOLOGY

Mitral stenosis is far more frequent in women than in men, the ratio being 2 or 3 to 1. Although a definite history of rheumatic fever is evident in only approximately one-half of patients with mitral stenosis, pathologic evidence reveals that rheumatic heart disease is the usual etiology. A history of Sydenham's chorea is particularly significant; rheumatic heart disease (usually mitral stenosis) will develop in up to 30 per cent of these patients, without apparent initial carditis, over the subsequent 30 years.[4] *Congenital* mitral stenosis is quite rare.

A number of pathologic changes contribute to narrowing of the mitral orifice secondary to rheumatic inflammation. The process is progressive, with pathologic changes occurring over a number of years after the initial attack of rheumatic carditis. The ingrowth of fibrous tissue results in a thickened, rigid leaflet. Concurrently, retraction develops, and fusion of the leaflets at the commissures produces narrowing of the orifice. Concomitantly, the chordae may become thickened, retracted, and fused, pulling the valve down into the left ventricle. In some cases, later calcification adds to the rigidity of the valve. These combined processes result in a rigid, narrowed, funnel-shaped orifice with the apex projecting into the left ventricle (Fig. 1). The inflammatory process usually involves the myocardium and pericardium, and direct myocardial injury may occasionally produce clinical manifestations. The extent of pathologic changes is an important determinant in the choice of surgical therapy. Pliable, nonregurgitant leaflets that are stenotic primarily because of fusion respond well to commissurotomy. On the other hand, extensive fibrosis and retraction of the leaflets, heavy calcification, marked shortening of the chordae tendineae with fusion of the leaflets to the underlying papillary muscles, or significant regurgitation requires mitral valve replacement for restoration of good valve function. *Restenosis* after mitral valvulotomy is very common but, in

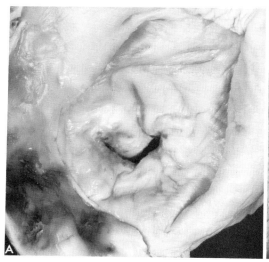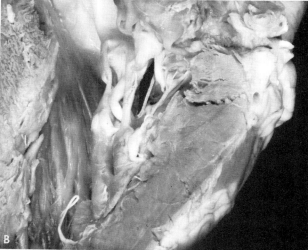

**Figure 1**  Typical pathologic changes in mitral stenosis: *A*, The mitral valve viewed from the atrial side. The leaflets are thickened and adherent. *B*, Left ventricular view. The thickened, fused, and retracted chordae tendineae are seen. The leaflet-chordal complex forms a funnel-shaped structure with the narrowed apex in the left ventricle. (From Eliot, R. S., and Edwards, J. E. In: Hurst, J. W., and Logue, R. B.: The Heart. 2nd ed. Copyright 1970, McGraw-Hill Book Company. Used with permission of McGraw-Hill Book Company.)

properly selected cases, usually does not occur for at least 5 to 10 years. Factors that predispose to early restenosis following commissurotomy are calcification of the valve leaflets and shortening of chordae, both of which tend to leave the leaflets immobile, favoring refusion and further stiffening of the leaflets.

## PHYSIOLOGY

The cross-sectional area of a normal mitral valve measures 4 to 6 sq. cm. Gorlin and Gorlin[50] have devised a formula that includes the relationship of valve area, blood flow, and the pressure gradient across the valve and allows a reliable approximation of the area of a nonregurgitant valve from data obtained at cardiac catheterization. As mentioned previously, it is probable that the mitral valve becomes progressively more narrowed over subsequent years after the initial attack of rheumatic carditis. Recurrent attacks of rheumatic fever hasten the process—hence the value of penicillin prophylaxis. Symptoms may appear early, but more often their appearance is delayed 20 to 30 years or more. Significant narrowing of the mitral valve is required before symptoms appear. When the valve area is 2.1 to 2.5 sq. cm., symptoms usually occur only with extreme exertion.[83] Moderate exertion may produce symptoms when the valve area is 1.6 to 2.0 sq. cm. When the valve area approaches 1.0 sq. cm., even normal activity may produce symptoms. A valve area of 1.0 sq. cm. is considered "critical stenosis," because when the valve is that small the left atrial pressure and hence pulmonary capillary pressure is usually about 25 to 30 mm. Hg at rest, i.e., about the level of oncotic pressure.[50, 83] Consequently,

with this degree of stenosis, the heart is unable to increase forward flow by elevations of the pressure gradient across the mitral valve without precipitating early pulmonary edema.[51, 83] The limitation of forward flow by the narrowed valve may also result in a low cardiac output. A valve area of approximately 0.4 sq. cm. is the minimal orifice size compatible with life.

The constant elevation of pulmonary capillary pressure results in vasoconstriction[68, 83] and, later, structural changes in the pulmonary arterioles resulting in pulmonary artery hypertension.[49, 61, 68, 140, 142] In a sense, pulmonary hypertension "protects" the pulmonary capillaries from sudden increases in right ventricular output and consequently lessens the occurrence of pulmonary congestion.[33, 83, 140] The price paid is right ventricular hypertrophy and eventual failure with secondary or "functional" tricuspid regurgitation.[83, 142] The pulmonary arterioles may become a second area of obstruction to flow, further contributing to low cardiac output.[83] Fortunately, even severe pulmonary artery hypertension in time usually recedes after effective mitral valve surgery.[19] The length of time required appears to be related to the relative contributions to the pulmonary hypertension of *vasoconstriction* and *structural changes*. On occasion, the pulmonary hypertension secondary to structural changes will take a number of months to decrease and may never return to normal.

The chronic left atrial hypertension produces left atrial enlargement and structural changes in the left atrial wall that eventually result in *atrial fibrillation*. The onset of atrial fibrillation frequently precipitates pulmonary congestion because the rapid rate shortens diastolic filling time with resultant increase in left atrial pressure. Rate control by digitalis may yield dramatic results. The loss of the "atrial kick" may also be important in decreasing cardiac efficiency. The combination of atrial fibrillation and mitral stenosis results in stasis of blood in the left atrium, a condition that greatly increases the risk of left atrial clot and subsequent systemic embolization.[30, 143]

## CLINICAL FEATURES

The patient is often a woman in the thirties who complains of dyspnea on exertion, fatigue, or palpitation. These symptoms may be precipitated by pregnancy or atrial fibrillation. The early course is usually dominated by manifestations of pulmonary congestion—dyspnea, orthopnea, paroxysmal nocturnal dyspnea, and a nocturnal cough.[83, 142] The latter three symptoms result from a return of fluids to the lungs from dependent portions of the body in the supine position. Mild bronchitis and coughing may result in hemoptysis from engorged pulmonary veins. On occasion, gross hemoptysis can be quite frightening.[88] The fear-induced tachycardia with its attendant rise in left atrial pressure only complicates the situation. As pulmonary artery hypertension develops, the patient notes fewer congestive symptoms and may believe she is "better." Left-sided failure is then replaced by right-sided failure, with peripheral edema and an elevated jugular venous pressure. An engorged liver may present as right upper quadrant pain; splanchnic congestion, as nausea, diarrhea, or protein-losing enteropathy.[136] Occasionally, hoarseness may develop from encroachment of a dilated left pulmonary artery on the left recurrent nerve (Ortner's syndrome).[37] Encroachment of the enlarged left atrium on the esophagus may give rise to dysphagia. At any time throughout this progression, the symptoms of a "low output state" may be dominant. Easy fatigability and weakness are the major early clues, and weight loss is a later sign. One is frequently amazed at the advanced state of incapacity a patient can reach without realizing it, because of the gradual adjustments in daily activities she has made to accommodate her disability. Precise questioning regarding the necessity of resting after minimal housework or similar activity often reveals a marked limitation of activity.

On *physical examination,* the patient may appear relatively normal. Patients with advanced disease may be thin and frail owing to long-

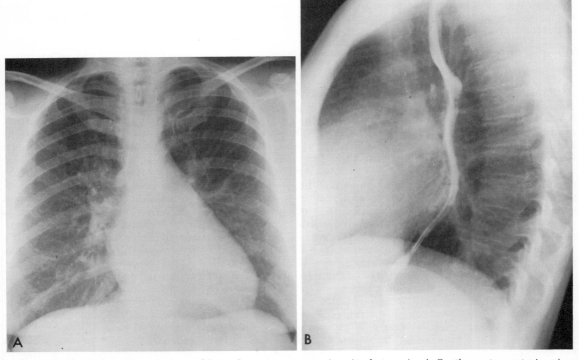

**Figure 2**  Typical posteroanterior and lateral roentgenograms in mitral stenosis: *A,* On the posteroanterior view, left atrial enlargement is evidenced by a double contour on the right, an elevated left main stem bronchus, and straightening of the mid left heart border. Distention of the upper lobe pulmonary veins results from pulmonary venous hypertension, and dilatation of the central pulmonary artery reflects pulmonary artery hypertension. *B,* On the lateral view, the enlarged left atrium displaces the barium-filled esophagus. The left ventricle is not enlarged, but the right ventricle is, and this is best seen as filling of the retrosternal space on the lateral view. (Courtesy of Dr. Robert E. Dinsmore.)

standing low cardiac output. Ruddiness of the cheeks with mild cyanosis of the lips, fingers, and toes may be present, probably the result of peripheral oxygen desaturation in the low output state. There may be basilar rales, or the lungs may be clear, even in severe stenosis. The heart size is usually normal. Careful assessment of the cardiac impulse yields much information. In pure mitral stenosis, the left ventricular impulse is often normal. A sustained or diffuse impulse suggests additional aortic valve disease or mitral regurgitation. A palpable pulmonic closure sound and right ventricular lift over the parasternal area indicate pulmonary hypertension and right ventricular hypertrophy. Right-sided failure is manifested by distended neck veins, an enlarged liver, and peripheral edema. Predominant systolic venous waves and a pulsatile liver indicate tricuspid regurgitation, usually secondary to pulmonary hypertension and right ventricular dilatation.

The primary *auscultatory* features are a loud first heart sound, an opening snap, and a low-pitched diastolic rumbling murmur heard at the apex.[80, 142] The pulmonic closure sound is accentuated if pulmonary hypertension is present. The diastolic rumble is best heard at the apex with the patient in the left lateral decubitus position. It is often well localized and may be inaudible even an inch away. In some patients, a murmur may be heard only after exercise; in others, it may be loud enough to produce a palpable thrill. The loudness of the murmur, however, does not correlate well with the severity of the stenosis.[48]

The earliest *radiologic* finding in mitral stenosis is left atrial enlargement. This is first evidenced by posterior displacement of the middle third of the barium-filled esophagus on the lateral view (Fig. 2).[3] In the posteroanterior view, the esophagus may be displaced to the right. When the atrium is larger, the left main stem bronchus may be elevated and may appear as an increased density extending to the right side within the cardiac shadow (double density). The overall cardiac size is often normal. Enlargement of the pulmonary artery and left atrial appendage characteristically obliterates the normal concavity in the upper and middle left heart border, producing a straightened or convex border. Right ventricular enlargement is revealed by anterior encroachment on the retrosternal space in the lateral view. Calcification of the mitral valve is rare in patients under 30.[86] When mild, it may be detected only by fluoroscopy with image amplification. Heavier calcification may be visualized on an overpenetrated film. Calcification of the left atrial wall may also be seen and indicates a higher incidence of mural thrombi and potential technical difficulties at surgery.[56] The lung fields initially reveal only distention of the upper pulmonary veins, a reflection of pulmonary venous hypertension.[79] Later, distended pulmonary lymphatics present as horizontal linear densities termed "Kerley's B lines,"[130] best seen just above the costophrenic angle on the right side. Pulmonary congestion or even frank pulmonary edema may be present.

The classic *electrocardiographic* pattern demonstrates left atrial enlargement with right ventricular hypertrophy. The former is reflected by a broad, double-humped P wave in lead II (P mitrale), or by a broad, deep, negative deflection in the terminal part of the P wave in lead $V_1$.[95] The most sensitive indication of right ventricular hypertrophy is right axis deviation. With more severe pulmonary hypertension and right ventricular hypertrophy, a high R/S ratio in $V_1$ and a clockwise rotation may appear. Any evidence of left ventricular hypertrophy should prompt a search for concomitant disease, such as aortic valve disease or mitral regurgitation. Atrial fibrillation is frequently seen and often marked by relatively coarse fibrillation waves.[110] Unfortunately, the electrocardiogram is not a reliable guide to the severity of mitral stenosis and may occasionally be completely normal even in cases of relatively severe mitral stenosis complicated by moderate pulmonary hypertension.[128, 142]

In most patients with pure mitral stenosis, the diagnosis and estimation of severity can be made from clinical findings. When quantitation is needed in unclear cases, most of the pertinent information can be obtained by right heart *catheterization*. Pulmonary capillary wedge pressure (which closely reflects the left atrial pressure), the pulmonary artery pressure, and the cardiac output can be measured. The stress of exercise is often helpful in detecting significant disease by precipitating a markedly abnormal rise in a near-normal resting "wedge" pressure, or by revealing an inability to appropriately elevate the cardiac index (cardiac output per square meter of body surface). Prominent "V" waves in the "wedge" pressure may indicate significant mitral regurgitation. A proper evaluation of aortic valve disease, mitral regurgitation, or left ventricular function requires left heart catheterization, usually by retrograde passage of a catheter across the aortic valve. This also allows precise measurement of the diastolic gradient across the mitral valve (Fig. 3), which, combined with the cardiac index and the length of diastole, permits calculation of the valve area by the formula of Gorlin and Gorlin.[50] The pulmonary wedge pressure may be substituted for the left atrial pressure if a left atrial pressure is not obtained. The mean diastolic gradient in significant mitral stenosis is usually 10 mm. Hg or more, depending on the cardiac output. A smaller gradient may be significant with low cardiac output. Left ventricular angiography is the best way to quantitate mitral regurgitation (the height of the "V" wave in the left atrium or on the pulmonary capillary wedge trace may also be helpful), and an aortic root angiogram provides the best quantification of aortic regurgitation. The presence of angina is usually an indication for coronary arteriography. The amount of valvular calcification is noted on fluoroscopy. Significant mitral regurgitation, or heavy calcification, indicates that mitral valve replacement will probably be necessary rather than a commissurotomy. The assessment of aortic and tricuspid valvular dis-

R.M.

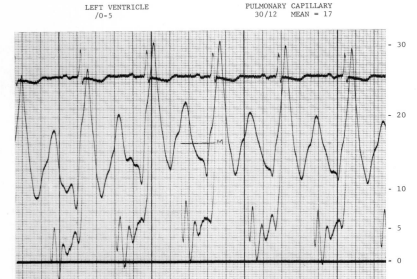

LEFT VENTRICLE /0-5

PULMONARY CAPILLARY 30/12   MEAN = 17

**Figure 3**  Typical cardiac catheterization findings in mitral stenosis: Simultaneous pulmonary capillary "wedge" and left ventricular pressure tracings. There is a delay in inscription of the wedge pressure which represents the transmission time from the left atrium to the right heart catheter tip. The "A" wave on the wedge tracing is predominant, rising to 30 mm. Hg. A mean diastolic gradient of about 12 mm. Hg is present across the mitral valve. (Courtesy of Dr. Charles A. Sanders.)

ease may be important in planning surgical correction. If any hint of aortic or tricuspid valve disease is present on clinical evaluation, catheterization may be indicated because the determination of relative severity of the different valvular lesions may be difficult on clinical grounds alone when multiple valves are diseased. If circumstances preclude catheterization, the state of the aortic and tricuspid valves should be carefully assessed at the time of surgery.

## INDICATIONS FOR SURGERY

In general, mitral valve surgery is indicated for any patient with significant limitation from the disease despite an appropriate medical regimen. Obviously, the definition of significant limitation depends on the patient and circumstances related to his disease. One would decide upon surgery earlier for a patient without mitral regurgitation or calcification in whom a commissurotomy appears feasible. Contrariwise, in patients with a clear-cut need for mitral valve replacement, a greater degree of disability (Class III*) would usually be required to justify surgery. It is important to emphasize, however, that the risk of surgery is considerably higher if symptoms are allowed to progress to a far advanced stage. Surgery should be advised before this occurs. One factor that may prompt surgery even in mildly symptomatic pa-

---

*New York Heart Association Functional Classification:

Class   I — No symptoms on ordinary physical activity.
Class  II — Symptoms on ordinary physical activity.
Class III — Symptoms on less than ordinary physical activity.
Class IV — Symptoms on any physical activity, usually at rest.

tients is evidence of pulmonary vascular disease with increased pulmonary arteriolar resistance. Fortunately, excellent results may be achieved even when marked pulmonary hypertension and markedly elevated pulmonary arteriolar resistance are present, although the risk of surgery is greater than for patients without pulmonary hypertension. No patient should be refused surgery because of the severity of pulmonary hypertension or congestive failure, as the prognosis for such patients with medical therapy alone is poor.

## SURGICAL THERAPY

### Closed Valvulotomy and Open Valvuloplasty

There has been considerable discussion during the past few years regarding the open versus the closed approach in the treatment of mitral stenosis.[44, 99, 102, 107] Some groups prefer the open technique for all cases; others feel that certain patients can be best managed with a closed operation. *Open* mitral valvuloplasty is usually accomplished by way of a median sternotomy or right anterolateral thoracotomy. After institution of cardiopulmonary bypass, the left atrium is incised and the valve inspected. Any thrombus in the atrium is removed. If the mitral valve is primarily stenotic and calcification is not severe enough to affect leaflet flexibility, the commissures are opened under direct vision, usually with a knife. Any subvalvular chordal fusion should be released, if possible, usually by finger dilation or knife incision or both. The advantages of this approach include a lessening of thrombotic or calcific embolic problems, the avoidance of hemorrhagic catastrophes from left atrial tears, and, on occasion, a more complete commissurotomy. Complications include the usual risks associated with open heart surgery, particularly the occasional cannulation problems and clotting difficulties. Great care must be taken to avoid peripheral arterial embolization of valvular debris or air trapped in the left heart. At the completion of the procedure (after cardiopulmonary bypass has been discontinued), the surgeon's finger should be inserted via a purse-string suture into the left atrium for estimation of the operative result in the functioning heart. If possible, left atrial and left ventricular pressures should also be measured, when the patient's cardiac output is satisfactory, in order to detect the presence of a significant diastolic gradient across the mitral valve or large "V" waves in the left atrium, suggesting significant mitral regurgitation. If adequate valvular function has not resulted, mitral valve replacement should be undertaken.

We prefer a *closed* commissurotomy in patients with relatively pure mitral stenosis and moderate to no valvular calcification as determined by fluoroscopic study. The procedure is best performed through a left posterolateral thoracotomy. We prefer to remove the fifth rib to provide adequate exposure for an open or closed operation; a fourth or fifth interspace incision can also be employed, with transection of a rib if necessary. Some prefer an anterolateral thoracotomy in the fourth interspace. The left groin is positioned in such a way that cannulation of the femoral vessels can be accomplished if necessary. The operation should be performed in an operating room equipped for open heart procedures with the pump-oxygenator assembled and ready for use ("pump standby"). Sufficient blood should be available in case cardiopulmonary bypass is required. The left atrium is carefully inspected visually for lack of motion suggesting thrombus. Careful external digital examination of the left atrial appendage for thrombus may be done. We believe that if thrombus is pres-

ent the closed operation should be converted to an open one; the clot can then be safely removed under direct vision, and this operation can be followed by the valvulotomy. If there is no evidence of atrial thrombus, a purse-string suture is placed in the atrial appendage, the appendage is incised, and a small amount of blood (and perhaps any thrombus) is permitted to flow from the incision. Then the surgeon's finger is inserted through the atrial incision into the atrial cavity. The purse-string suture may require tightening to prevent bleeding around the surgeon's finger. The surgeon should digitally examine the atrium for thrombus or calcification and then should assess the state of the mitral valve. Particularly important points to be considered include the amount of mitral regurgitation, the amount of valvular calcification, the extent of subvalvular fusion, and an estimation of the likelihood of calcium particles being dislodged from the valve during a closed valvulotomy. If thrombotic or calcific emboli from the valve or atrial wall appear to be a distinct possibility, the procedure should be converted to an open one. Some groups have employed temporary bilateral carotid occlusion during initial insertion of the surgeon's finger into the left atrium and at the time of valvulotomy. It was hoped that this maneuver would lessen the risk of cerebral emboli; however, we have not found this technique of significant value. If it appears that a satisfactory closed valvulotomy can be carried out (when predominant mitral stenosis with moderate to no valvular calcification exists), this is performed. Some prefer digital pressure to open the fused commissures gradually. Many groups, including our own, prefer use of the transventricular dilator[6, 45, 87] as the primary procedure (Fig. 4). A purse-string suture is placed in a relatively avascular area at the tip of the left ventricle. An incision is made in the epicardium and a tunnel is created in the left

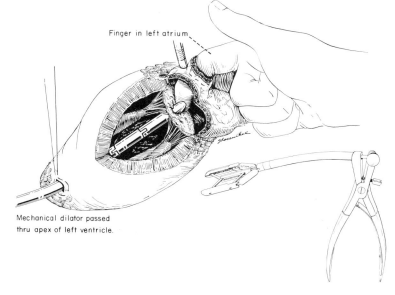

**Figure 4**   Illustration of the use of the transventricular mitral dilator for mitral stenosis: The dilator, with the blades closed, is inserted through a purse-string suture in the tip of the left ventricle and passed through the mitral valve. Then the blades are opened (inset) to accomplish valvulotomy.

Finger in left atrium

Mechanical dilator passed thru apex of left ventricle.

ventricular muscle by a clamp or scissors. The closed dilator is inserted and guided through the mitral valve. In order to lessen the risk of mitral regurgitation, it is essential that the dilator not be enmeshed in the chordae and that it be opened only when its tip is in the left atrium. Therefore, the dilator should be positioned to traverse the subvalvular area easily, and the surgeon's finger should palpate the tip of the dilator in the left atrium. It seems reasonable that the blades of the dilator should be opened against the valve leaflets,[6] but this is probably not crucial. The dilator should initially be opened only to 3.0 to 3.5 cm. and then gradually expanded further. Finger dilation may also be helpful in association with the dilator. No matter what technique is employed, the surgeon, with his finger in the left atrium, should intermittently assess the degree of relief of stenosis and the presence and amount of mitral regurgitation. In addition, subvalvular stenosis should be relieved by finger fracture, if possible. At the end of the procedure and at a time when the cardiac output is satisfactory, an attempt should be made to measure left atrial and left ventricular pressures. Minimal mitral regurgitation and small (3 or 4 mm. Hg) gradients across the mitral valve are acceptable. The advantages of a closed approach over open operation are: (1) it is simpler; (2) the operating time is shorter; (3) less blood is required; and (4) it permits assessment of valvular function in the working heart during the course of the operation. Operative complications particularly associated with closed mitral valvulotomy include systemic emboli, the creation of significant mitral regurgitation, inadequate relief of mitral stenosis, and hemorrhage from a tear in the left atrial wall secondary to the insertion of the surgeon's finger into the left atrium.

If adequate mitral valve function cannot be achieved by these closed techniques, cardiopul-monary bypass should be instituted, and an open valvuloplasty or valve replacement performed. Arterial cannulation for cardiopulmonary bypass with a left thoracotomy can be accomplished with femoral arterial cannulation or direct cannulation of the descending thoracic aorta via a purse-string suture. Venous return can sometimes be accomplished with femoral venous cannulation alone. As an alternative, a venous cannula can be inserted in the right ventricle directly or via the pulmonary artery, with or without femoral venous cannulation.

### Mitral Valve Replacement

If open mitral valvuloplasty or mitral valve replacement is definitely planned preoperatively, a median sternotomy or right anterolateral thoracotomy is usually employed. Arterial cannulation can be accomplished via the femoral artery or via a purse-string suture in the ascending aorta. Femoral arterial cannulation has the advantage of keeping the arterial cannulation out of the main operative field, and, if femoral venous cannulation is employed, early partial cardiopulmonary bypass is readily available to extremely ill patients. Femoral arterial cannulation does require an additional operative incision, and, particularly in patients with peripheral vascular disease, there is a significant incidence of arterial dissection from the trauma of the catheter tip and the retrograde arterial perfusion. Venous cannulation is usually accomplished by the insertion of catheters via the right atrium into the superior and inferior venae cavae. The left atrium is better visualized if the right atrium is mobilized and the intra-atrial groove is exposed. Perfusion flow depends on the temperature of the patient; the temperature is usually lowered to approximately 32° C., at which level a flow rate of 50 to 60 cc. per

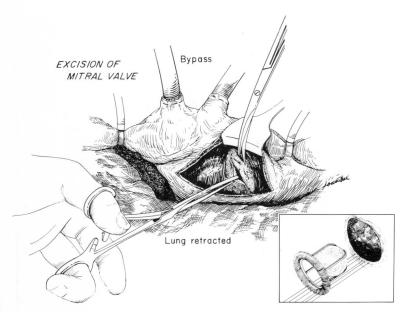

EXCISION OF MITRAL VALVE

Bypass

Lung retracted

**Figure 5** Schematic representation of mitral valve replacement: The deformed mitral valve is excised and (inset) a Starr-Edwards prosthetic valve is inserted by means of multiple sutures to the mitral annulus.

kilogram is satisfactory. The left atrium is usually incised parallel to the intra-atrial groove (Fig. 5), and the mitral valve is exposed by appropriate retraction. On occasion, because of a small atrium and consequent poor visualization, exposure of the mitral valve may be accomplished transseptally by incising both atria and the interatrial septum.

As mentioned previously, one of the major risks of open mitral surgery is air embolism. Many surgeons cross-clamp the aorta temporarily during valve replacement to avoid inadvertent ejection of air by the left ventricle. This also eliminates the possibility of any aortic regurgitation blood in the operative field, but on the other hand prevents coronary perfusion. Because of the anoxic effects on the heart, we usually do not cross-clamp the aorta unless there is significant aortic regurgitation. If the aorta is not cross-clamped, it is important to render the mitral valve regurgitant as soon as it is visualized. This can be accomplished by inserting a clamp or catheter through the valve. At the end of the procedure, before left ventricular ejection is allowed, the left ventricle should be aspirated with a needle and syringe. A needle should also be inserted into the upper aspect of the ascending aorta to allow air removal.

Valve replacement is usually performed if there is significant mitral regurgitation or if the valve is so stiff and calcified that relatively long-term relief of obstruction cannot be satisfactorily achieved. The diseased valve can be brought into better view if it is pulled toward the surgeon with a hook or clamp (Fig. 5). The valve is incised circumferentially on the inner margins of the annulus. Care must be taken to keep the incision well to the inside because of the close proximity of the atrioventricular node and the circumflex coronary artery. In addition, overly generous removal, particularly posteriorly, can result in a tear in the left ventricular wall at the annular level, with resultant hemorrhage.[90] While there has been some disagreement as to whether the papillary muscles and the attached chordae should be left intact,[85] most surgeons completely remove all chordae and transect the papillary muscles at a convenient point near the left ventricular wall. Any remaining detached chordae must be removed because they can become enmeshed in the prosthetic valve and cause dysfunction.

The technique of suture of the valve replacement is very important. Most surgeons employ multiple interrupted sutures, either "figure-of-eight" or mattress. If the annular tissue is soft, a buttress of Teflon felt may be helpful. Paravalvular leak, usually resulting from circumferential tearing of the patient's tissue or from cutting through of the tissues by the sutures, is an important complication.[1, 141] The resultant regurgitant flow, particularly in association with prosthetic valves such as the Starr-Edwards type, may lead to significant traumatic hemolysis. With proper technique, paravalvular leak should be a rare occurrence.

If the left ventricular cavity is of reasonable size, a Starr-Edwards prosthesis can be employed. It is important, however, not to use a prosthesis that is too large, because if the cage impinges upon the left ventricular endocardium ventricular irritability will result. The ball and cage can also cause left ventricular outflow obstruction. If the left ventricle is very small, it is probably wise to

**Figure 6** *A*, Earlier type Starr-Edwards valve (Model 6000) with a Silastic ball and a base with a large area of exposed metal. This prosthesis was removed at postmortem examination and the sewing ring is abnormally roughened and darkened. *B*, Starr-Edwards valve introduced in 1966 (Model 6120) with a Silastic ball and an extended Teflon cloth sewing ring. *C*, Newest type Starr-Edwards valve (Model 6320) with a hollow metal ball and a completely cloth-covered prosthesis with metal studs for seating. *D*, Smeloff-Cutter valve. Note descent of the ball below the sewing ring, resulting in minimal regurgitation.

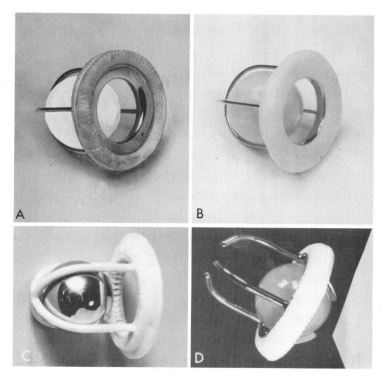

employ a low-profile prosthesis or some other valve substitute.

There are a large number of different types of artificial valves available. Of the prosthetic valves, certainly the Starr-Edwards prosthesis has been most commonly employed and most extensively evaluated by clinical follow-up.[1, 58, 59, 74, 132, 135] In the early type of Starr-Edwards prosthesis (Model 6000), a considerable amount of metal was exposed on the under surface of the valve (Fig. 6A), and embolization rates ranged between 20 and 40 per cent over a few years of follow-up.[1] Ball *variance* (swelling and surface irregularity) of the Silastic ball has been uncommon in the mitral position in contrast to the high incidence with the earlier Starr-Edwards models in the aortic position. The Model 6120 Starr-Edwards mitral valve (Fig. 6B) incorporates an extended Teflon cloth sewing ring to decrease the amount of exposed metal. Tissue ingrowth, which occurs in a matter of months, covers this Teflon cloth, and the incidence of embolization has been reduced markedly.[132] Valvular gradients have not usually been significant, although gradients of a few millimeters of mercury are common. With the first completely covered Starr-Edwards valve (Model 6300), in which both ring and struts were covered, significant valvular gradients occurred because of valve design, the thick cloth, and tissue ingrowth. With Model 6310,

there have not been significant gradient problems, but cloth wear on the struts and valvular thrombosis have caused difficulties. The most recent model (6320 series) Starr-Edwards mitral valve is completely covered except for multiple small metal studs for seating. The covering is two-ply, with an inner coat of Teflon and an outer coat of polypropylene. The ball is hollow metal (Fig. 6C).[58] In early studies of the 6320 Model, no wear or thrombosis problems have been found, and valvular gradients have been insignificant. Initial clinical evaluation has indicated a very low incidence of embolization, and this prosthesis appears quite promising.[58] However, this model has not been in use long enough for evaluation regarding late problems of wear and tissue ingrowth.

The Smeloff-Cutter mitral valve (Fig. 6D) has some similarities to the Starr-Edwards prosthesis. However, the ball descends below the sewing ring into the atrium; this results in minimal regurgitation and a smaller prosthetic ball with a larger diastolic orifice size. This variation of hemodynamics as well as other aspects of design has resulted in minimal valvular gradients and a relatively low embolization rate.[36]

Some surgeons have employed a low-profile, floating-disc type of prosthesis. Notable examples include the Beall valve (Fig. 7A),[11] the Kay-Shiley valve (Fig. 7B),[71] and the Starr-Edwards valve

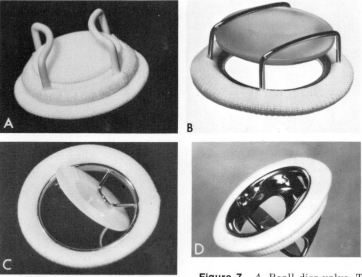

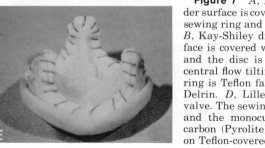

**Figure 7** *A,* Beall disc valve. The under surface is covered with a Dacron velour sewing ring and the disc is made of Teflon. *B,* Kay-Shiley disc valve. The under surface is covered with a Teflon sewing ring and the disc is Silastic. *C,* Bjork-Shiley central flow tilting disc valve. The sewing ring is Teflon fabric and the monocusp is Delrin. *D,* Lillehei-Kaster pivoting disc valve. The sewing ring is Teflon or Dacron and the monocusp is made of pyrolytic carbon (Pyrolite). *E,* Homograft mounted on Teflon-covered stent.

with a metal disc and Teflon-covered ring.[60] It is true that less inertial force is required to move the disc as compared to the ball, but there have been late problems with wear and a relatively high embolization rate in some early series. The newer models have a cloth-covered base to minimize the amount of exposed metal, with resultant reduction in embolization rates.

Another interesting type of prosthetic valve design is the hingeless eccentric monocusp. Examples include the Bjork-Shiley tilting disc valve (Fig. 7C)[15] and the Lillehei-Kaster pivoting disc valve (Fig. 7D).[84] The flow characteristics of these types of valves are very promising, but they have not been in use long enough for adequate clinical follow-up. With earlier types of hingeless monocusp valves, there were significant wear problems.[138]

The use of a homologous cadaver aortic valve for human valve substitute was suggested by Murray in 1955.[98] He inserted fresh aortic homografts into the descending thoracic aorta of patients with aortic regurgitation, and some of these grafts are still functioning. In 1964, Ross[116] and Barratt-Boyes[10] published their experience with the use of aortic homografts in the subcoronary position. The advantages of homografts (Fig. 7E) include: freedom from thromboembolic problems, relatively normal hemodynamic characteristics with central flow and no early gradients across the valves, no inherent defects such as ball variance, a very low incidence of hemolysis, and absence of abnormal valve sounds. Disadvantages include a somewhat greater complexity involved in insertion, problems of procurement and preservation, and relatively high incidence of infection, valvular regurgitation, and late failures. When used in the mitral position, the aortic homograft, sutured to a Teflon-covered metal stent of appropriate size, is inserted in the same way as a prosthetic valve. Initially, the grafts were excised and preserved by betapropiolactone or freeze-drying.[10, 116] Evidence suggested that these valves tended to fail because of shrinking after a number of years.[77] Now valves are usually used fresh,[77] or sterilized with irradiation and stored at −70° C.[91]

Heterografts (usually pig aortic valves on stents) have also been employed,[24, 66, 105, 106] but the incidence of valve shrinkage and disruption has been sufficiently high to discourage many. The method of preservation may have an important influence on the results.[105, 106]

Another type of valve replacement involves the use of autogenous fascia lata sutured as three leaflets onto a mitral valve stent.[65] The use of this readily available autogenous living graft material as a valvular substitute was first reported in 1964.[129] Initial clinical results with aortic valve replacement were encouraging, but more extensive experience has suggested a high late failure rate when these grafts are used in the mitral and tricuspid positions.[117]

Our own preference at present in mitral valve replacement continues to be the Starr-Edwards ball valve. We usually employ the 6120 Model, but we are also carefully evaluating Model 6320. We certainly recognize that other mitral valve substitutes may be equally satisfactory and that sufficient study and follow-up may show them to be superior.

## EARLY POSTOPERATIVE PROBLEMS

The primary early postoperative problems after mitral valve surgery, in addition to those already mentioned, are similar to the complications following other major heart procedures. They include low cardiac output or cardiac failure, cardiac arrhythmias, bleeding, respiratory failure, renal failure, the postpericardiotomy and the postperfusion syndromes, valvular infections, peripheral emboli, and psychologic problems.

*Low cardiac output* and *cardiac failure* are moderately common following mitral valve surgery. These clinical features usually occur in association with long-standing mitral valve disease with significant pulmonary hypertension, but they may occasionally be associated with unsatisfactory valvular repair or intraoperative myocardial damage. Cardiac failure is usually right ventricular in mitral stenosis and may be right ventricular or left ventricular or both in mitral regurgitation. Proper management of the low cardiac output syndrome or cardiac failure requires definition of its etiology. Central venous pressure and left atrial pressure measurements are very helpful. Central venous pressure levels of 15 mm. Hg or higher[89] may be required, and similar pressures may be required in the left atrium.[38] If the patient is hypovolemic, infusion of blood or other colloid may reverse the low output state. Care must be taken to avoid overinfusion, as reflected in pulmonary congestion, and, more sensitively, a lowered arterial $pO_2$ owing to increased pulmonary arteriovenous shunting. Acidosis, hypocalcemia, hyperkalemia, hypokalemia, and severe hyponatremia may have an adverse effect upon myocardial function and, if present, require therapy. Thus, frequent determinations of electrolytes and blood gases are essential to proper management. The digitalis glycosides should be appropriately used, with care to avoid digitalis toxicity, especially if hypokalemia is present. In the patient with volume overload, or congestion, the potent diuretics such as furosemide or ethacrynic acid are very helpful. The low output state frequently requires the use of inotropic agents such as isoproterenol and epinephrine. Heart rate augmentation by atrial pacing (or ventricular pacing in patients with atrial fibrillation or atrioventricular block) may greatly improve cardiac output in patients with relatively slow ventricular rates. Atrioventricular sequential pacing may sometimes be effectively used to preserve the contribution of the atrial "kick." There has been some use of peripheral vasodilation in these patients with low output to decrease left ventricular work and oxygen consumption.[34] Vasodilating agents include phenoxybenzamine and corticosteroids. With vasodilation, volume replacement must be simultaneously accomplished to maintain adequate cardiac filling pressures and cardiac output. Partial circulatory support may be of value in a limited number of patients with refractory, but potentially reversible, low cardiac output.[122]

Virtually any *cardiac arrhythmia* may occur following mitral valve surgery, with a frequency much higher than that associated with the standard general surgical procedures. In addition, these arrhythmias may have more serious consequences because they are occurring in a heart that is unable to perform at normal efficiency. Constant electrocardiographic monitoring during surgery and in the first few days following operation is essential. In patients without atrial fibrillation, both temporary atrial and ventricular pacing wires are inserted. In patients with atrial fibrillation, only ventricular pacing wires are inserted. The atrial wires may be used as sensing electrodes in diagnosing complicated arrhythmias.[32] In addition to rate augmentation for improved cardiac output as already mentioned, atrial or ventricular pacing may be effectively used for rate-overdrive suppression of ventricular arrhythmias, allowing a reduced dependence on antiarrhythmic agents.[12] Ventricular pacing is vital in heart block. Ventricular premature beats, especially if more than five or six occur per minute, require treatment either by rate-overdrive suppression or by antiarrhythmic agents. Intravenous lidocaine is probably the safest drug to use for ventricular irritability in the early postoperative state. Intramuscular procaine amide is very effective but depresses the myocardium when given in high doses.[55, 75] Diphenylhydantoin is useful, especially if the ventricular irritability is due to digitalis toxicity.[14, 69] Propranolol may also be used in this situation. Parenteral bretylium may be helpful in otherwise refractory ventricular arrhythmias, but it must be used with care because of its peripheral vasodilatory and hence hypotensive effects. Long-term suppressive therapy may be achieved by the use of quinidine, procaine amide, or diphenylhydantoin, or combinations of them. Accelerated junctional rhythms ("nodal") are not infrequently seen after mitral valve surgery and probably reflect transient inflammation of the atrioventricular junctional tissue adjacent to the mitral annulus. This rhythm is difficult to suppress pharmacologically, but it is usually benign and, therefore, requires no specific therapy. It almost always disappears with time. Atrial premature beats are frequent and do not themselves require suppression. However, they often presage atrial fibrillation, and their appearance might prompt one to start quinidine or digitalis administration in an attempt to "stabilize" the atrium and "prevent" atrial fibrillation. Atrial flutter may cause considerable difficulty because of a rapid ventricular rate that is difficult to control with digitalis. Digitalization may convert the rhythm to atrial fibrillation or, occasionally, to normal sinus rhythm. Intravenous propranolol can be quite effective in atrial flutter both for rate control and for conversion to normal sinus rhythm. Because rate control in flutter is difficult to achieve with drugs, electrical cardioversion is usually done early, either by rapid atrial pacing to "capture" the atrium or by external electrical countershock. Atrial fibrillation is very commonly present preoperatively, and operative countershock cardioversion is unlikely to be successful for a prolonged period. In general, we perform cardioversion 6 weeks to 3 months after surgery, usually in patients in whom atrial fibrillation has only recently begun. The incidence of long-term maintenance of normal sinus rhythm following cardioversion in this group is quite high.[127] In a sizable number of patients, with normal sinus rhythm preoperatively, atrial fibrillation occurs during the first week or so following surgery. In general, the treatment should be control of the ventricular rate with digitalis compounds. Many patients will revert to normal sinus rhythm spontaneously. Occasionally, rapid atrial fibrillation with significant hemodynamic depression requires early electrical cardioversion. Proper electrolyte balance, particularly the avoidance of hypokalemia and hyperkalemia, is essential to decrease of incidence of serious arrhythmias. Digitalis compounds must be given carefully to avoid toxicity.

Postoperative *bleeding problems* are much less common now than a few years ago and are almost exclusively associated with open rather than closed mitral procedures. A number of alterations in the hemostatic mechanism may occur following cardiopulmonary bypass, the two most important being circulating heparin and thrombocytopenia.[119] Protamine is usually employed to reverse the heparin effect following bypass. The protamine should be given slowly intravenously to avoid significant hypotension; on occasion vasopressors may be required. Usually 1 to 3 mg. of protamine for each milligram of heparin is required. Excessive amounts of protamine have a mild anticoagulant effect. The partial thromboplastin time may be used as an indication of the adequacy of neutralization of heparin. If after the standard amount of protamine is given the partial thromboplastin time is still prolonged, it is helpful to obtain a protamine titration test as an indication of the degree of heparin neutralization. A significant platelet deficiency may be present following cardiopulmonary bypass. Usually, nothing need be done. Occasionally, platelet-rich fresh blood or platelet concentrates may be required. Other less common problems in hemostasis include intravascular coagulation, fibrinolysis, and problems of hemostasis related to liver disease.[43] Certainly the most important measure that the cardiac surgeon can take is to obtain adequate mechanical hemostasis. It is essential to monitor the chest tube drainage carefully after operation, to obtain periodic chest x-rays, and to observe the patient carefully for signs suggestive of cardiac tamponade. If no coagulation defect can be elicited and bleeding continues for more than 4 to 6 hours at high rates (150 to 200 cc. per hour), re-exploration should be undertaken.

*Respiratory problems* represent one of the major

complications of mitral valve surgery. Prior to surgery, all patients should be taught respiratory exercises and be educated regarding their use in the postoperative period. Elective postoperative ventilatory support should be employed in the immediate postoperative period to insure adequate oxygenation. The length of respiratory support depends on the mitral procedure performed and on the state of the lungs. In patients with straightforward mitral stenosis, without significant pulmonary hypertension or other pulmonary problems, who undergo a closed mitral valvulotomy, respiratory support can be stopped in a few hours when they are awake. In the patient with mitral valve replacement, respiratory support can usually be withdrawn the day after surgery. On the other hand, patients with severe, long-standing mitral valve disease with significant pulmonary hypertension are likely to require respiratory support for at least 2 days and sometimes longer. Measurements of arterial gases are very helpful in safely weaning patients from the respirator.[13] In the rare instance when respiratory support is required for more than 3 or 4 days, tracheostomy should usually be performed.

*Renal failure* may occur following mitral valve surgery.[52] It is usually associated with operative or postoperative hypotension with secondary acute tubular necrosis.[144] Hemoglobinuria, from prolonged cardiopulmonary bypass, or renal arterial embolus, from left atrial clot or mitral valvular debris, may occasionally play a role. Oliguria is the usual manifestation. Acute tubular necrosis must be differentiated from prerenal azotemia and oliguria secondary to hypovolemia or poor cardiac function. An adequate blood volume should be achieved, and the most effective cardiac action should be maintained. Occasionally, severe vasoconstriction, secondary to the stress of surgery (catecholamines) and to hypothermia with resultant decreased renal perfusion, may be present. Maintaining a normal or slightly elevated body temperature plus the administration of modest amounts of a vasodilator drug such as chlorpromazine may improve urine output. If the patient has an adequate blood volume and there is a satisfactory degree of hydration and vasomotor tone, then a trial with diuretics such as furosemide or mannitol is reasonable. If renal failure is indeed present, the patient must be appropriately treated with fluid restriction and careful monitoring of electrolytes. Hyperkalemia should be managed with ion exchange resin enemas (Kayexalate) and, if necessary, intravenous glucose and insulin and sodium bicarbonate. Peritoneal dialysis, or hemodialysis, may be required.[104]

A frequent complication of mitral valve surgery, occurring in perhaps a third of the patients, is the *postcardiotomy syndrome.* The postcardiotomy syndrome[42] usually consists of abrupt development of fever, pericarditis, pleurisy, and pleural effusion. The white blood count may be normal or elevated; rarely, a few atypical lymphocytes may be noted. The postcardiotomy syndrome usually appears 2 to 4 weeks after cardiac surgery but

may occasionally be seen as early as 1 week following surgery or as late as 3 months. The etiology is not known, but an autoimmune phenomenon is thought most likely. Once other causes of fever are ruled out, treatment consists of administration of salicylates, indomethacin, or, in severe refractory cases, corticosteroids. Treatment should usually continue for a week or more. Relapses may occur. The less common *postperfusion syndrome*[41] consists of fever, malaise, splenomegaly, and a low white blood cell count with a high level of atypical lymphocytes, occurring in a patient who has undergone cardiopulmonary bypass and transfusions. Additional findings may include a maculopapular rash, hepatomegaly, lymphadenopathy, and hemolysis. Cytomegalic inclusion virus has been implicated in some cases.[78] Treatment is similar to that of the postcardiotomy syndrome. Again, relapses may occur.

Postoperative *valvular infection* following mitral valve surgery is, fortunately, an uncommon problem. When it does occur, it is a very serious matter, particularly if a mitral prosthesis is present.[2] Most surgeons employ high doses of antibiotics[100] that cover the gram-positive organisms (primarily staphylococcus), such as staphcillin or oxicillin. Antibiotic administration should be started preoperatively so that an adequate blood level will be reached by the time of surgery; it is usually continued for 3 to 5 days postoperatively. If an intracardiac infection occurs, aggressive antibiotic therapy is necessary. The patient should be treated with high doses of the appropriate antibiotic as determined by the sensitivity studies. Ideally, treatment should be continued for approximately 6 weeks and then stopped, with careful observation of the patient to determine whether the infection has been eradicated. In patients with mitral valve replacement, the infection is very difficult to eradicate, but occasionally antibiotics alone will be successful. Commonly, the infection causes disruption of the sutures and consequent mitral regurgitation. If the regurgitation becomes significant, or if antibiotics fail to clear the infection, reoperation is required, with removal of the previous valve replacement and any adjacent infected tissue, followed by the insertion of a new mitral valve.[16]

Peripheral *arterial emboli* have already been mentioned as a significant problem in association with mitral valve surgery. Peripheral pulses should be carefully checked after mitral surgery. Signs or symptoms of cerebral, mesenteric, or renal emboli should also be carefully sought. Operative intervention for mesenteric, renal, or peripheral emboli may be necessary. After prosthetic mitral valve replacement, warfarin therapy is usually begun 2 or 3 days postoperatively and continued indefinitely.[1] The prothrombin time should be maintained approximately twice normal. The incidence of emboli appears to be lessened significantly with warfarin therapy. Other agents that effect platelet adhesiveness, such as dipyridamole or aspirin, may be valuable in preventing emboli as well.[137]

*Psychologic problems* occur quite commonly following mitral valve surgery. They are most common in patients who are quite ill and require prolonged intensive care. Depression, agitation, disorientation, delusions, and hallucinations may occur. Treatment of such symptoms usually consists of mild sedation and gentle reassurance, and removal of the patient from the intensive care situation as soon as considered safe. These psychologic problems are transitory and almost always resolve in a short time.

## GENERAL POSTOPERATIVE CONSIDERATIONS

Because of the tendency to retain salt and water in the postoperative state, the average patient is initially limited to 500 mg. sodium and 1500 cc. fluid per day for a few days, and then this is progressively liberalized. Following mitral valve surgery the patient is usually discharged on a low sodium diet, but many patients can take a regular diet within a few months. Digitalis glycosides and diuretics are usually required in the early postoperative period, but are not necessarily still required by the time the patient is ready for discharge. The amount of activity advised depends on the degree of cardiac impairment. The patient usually is permitted to dangle his feet on the second postoperative day and is allowed out of bed on the second or third postoperative day. Activity is gradually increased to ambulation around the ward prior to discharge. Full activity may be possible 2 or 3 months after valvulotomy but may take longer after valve replacement. Patients with mild hemolytic anemia (particularly those with prosthetic mitral valves) should receive an iron supplement and folic acid.

Patients who have undergone mitral valvulotomy or mitral valve replacement should subsequently be given appropriate prophylactic antibiotic therapy to avoid bacteremia and valvular infection. They require antibiotics in association with surgery, dental extractions, and severe respiratory or other infections. In addition to bacterial endocarditis prophylaxis, young patients with rheumatic heart disease should also receive daily antibiotic prophylaxis for *rheumatic fever* (penicillin in the nonallergic patient).

## OPERATIVE RESULTS

The operative risk of mitral surgery depends primarily on the severity of the patient's disease. In appropriately selected patients, the mortality associated with closed mitral valvulotomy should not exceed 1 or 2 per cent.[72] With open valvuloplasty in comparable patients, the results are similar. Usually, however, patients undergoing open valvuloplasty have more complicated problems, and the operative mortality is in the range of 5 per cent. Symptomatic improvement following closed mitral valvulotomy or open mitral valvuloplasty has been excellent. However, in 20 to 50 per cent of these patients, hemodynamically significant *recurrent* mitral disease occurs in 5 to 10 years.[72]

The operative mortality with mitral valve replacement is in the range of 10 per cent. Again, this is related to the severity of the mitral disease and to secondary myocardial and pulmonary effects. Long-term results depend on these factors as well as on the type of valve replacement employed (Fig. 8A). Most surviving patients are essentially asymptomatic, but approximately one-fourth have slight to moderate limitation of activity.[96, 135] A small percentage of patients have quite significant limitation of activity. The late death rate over 3 or 4 years postoperatively with the newer, improved prostheses should be 10 per cent or less. (Fig. 8B). Problems with emboli in

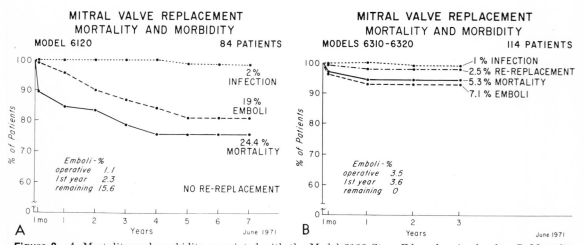

**Figure 8** *A*, Mortality and morbidity associated with the Model 6120 Starr-Edwards mitral valve. *B*, Mortality and morbidity associated with the Model 6320 Starr-Edwards mitral valve. (From Starr, A.: Outline of lectures in Cardiovascular Post-graduate Course of American College of Surgeons, 1971, p. 29.)

patients with prosthetic valves and concerns about late failure with other valve substitutes require further study.

## MITRAL REGURGITATION

### ETIOLOGY AND PATHOLOGY

In contrast to the etiology of mitral stenosis, that of mitral regurgitation is varied. The most common cause of mitral regurgitation requiring surgery is rheumatic valvulitis. Rupture of the chordae tendineae is also quite common. Other less frequent etiologic factors in mitral regurgitation requiring surgery include papillary muscle dysfunction or rupture, the "floppy valve syndrome," and bacterial endocarditis. Females are more commonly affected by rheumatic mitral regurgitation than males, although the ratio is not as high as that in mitral stenosis. Papillary muscle dysfunction, on the other hand, occurs more frequently in men because of the higher incidence of coronary artery disease in males.

In rheumatic mitral regurgitation, the pathologic process is similar to that in mitral stenosis, but the end result favors regurgitation, probably because of a preponderance of contraction of the leaflets and chordae tendineae. Immobility of the leaflets, particularly if they are calcified, contributes to the retention of the valve in an "open" position. Why the rheumatic process produces mitral regurgitation in one patient and mitral stenosis in another is not known. As one might expect, a variable component of mitral obstruction often accompanies regurgitation in rheumatic heart disease.

Perhaps the most common cause of mitral regurgitation is papillary muscle dysfunction,[22, 25, 57, 82, 101, 111, 120] but only a minority of these patients require mitral valve surgery. Three types of papillary muscle dysfunction may be considered:[120] (1) The first is due to alteration of spatial relationships between the papillary muscles and mitral leaflets, which causes loss of their normal parallel alignment. Abnormalities of this relationship may result from left ventricular dilatation from any cause[82] and may also be an important factor in the mitral regurgitation seen with idiopathic hypertrophic subaortic stenosis.[35] (2) Intrinsic papillary muscle dysfunction due to ischemia or infarction from coronary artery disease is the most common cause of papillary muscle dysfunction.[25, 27, 31, 120] The *posteromedial* papillary muscle is most prone to abnormalities in this situation,[27, 31, 57, 120] for its major nutrient vessel, the descending branch of the dominant coronary artery, has little collateral support.[67] In contrast, the blood supply to the anterolateral papillary muscle is rich in collaterals. (3) Actual rupture of the papillary muscle occurs uncommonly, but, when it does, it is usually in the setting of myocardial infarction.[31, 120, 125] Again, the posteromedial muscle appears more susceptible.[31, 125]

Rupture of the chordae tendineae may cause mitral regurgitation to a degree that is either acute and severe or insidious and chronic, depending on the number of chordae ruptured.[124, 126] Although the most common cause in the preantibiotic era was bacterial endocarditis, it is now apparent that some cases occur as a complication of rheumatic valvulitis. An increasing number of cases appear to occur as isolated spontaneous ruptures without evident pre-existing lesions;[121, 126] pathologic examination has revealed areas of lysis of elastin and collagen in these chordae.[26] Isolated spontaneous chordal rupture tends to occur in middle-aged or elderly males and usually involves the posterior leaflet.[9]

Recently, a number of patients have been described in whom prolapse (billowing) of one or both mitral leaflets is associated with mitral regurgitation ("floppy valve syndrome").[9, 53] This phenomenon may be associated with a variety of other cardiac abnormalities, or may occur as an isolated abnormality. Pathologically, the leaflets and chordae are thin and redundant and may show myxomatous degeneration. Other causes of mitral regurgitation include trauma,[94] active bacterial endocarditis, and massive calcification of the mitral annulus.[76]

### PHYSIOLOGY

In mitral regurgitation, a variable amount of left ventricular output is directed back to the left atrium; this causes a systolic rise in left atrial pressure represented as a "V" wave on a left atrial or pulmonary wedge pressure tracing. The extra blood is then returned as an added volume load to the left ventricle in diastole. Fortunately, the heart is capable of adapting to even large increments in volume work without great reduction in systemic blood flow. The stroke volume can be doubled without significant change in oxygen consumption, probably because the extra work is performed at low pressure.[18] This adaptive ability most likely accounts for the fact that some patients may do quite well for long periods of time despite severe mitral regurgitation. The volume of mitral regurgitation tends to rise in proportion to the increasing cardiac output with exercise, and it also reduces rapidly with a decline in cardiac output during rest.[88]

The physiologic and hence clinical consequences of mitral regurgitation are different in the acute and chronic forms. In acute regurgitation, the left atrium is usually small, and the rhythm is normal sinus. Thus, the high-pressure jet from the vigorous left ventricle is immediately transmitted back to the lungs, and a huge "V" wave and marked pulmonary hypertension result (Fig. 9).[112, 121] Since left ventricular function is often quite good, exercise increases cardiac output and hence mitral regurgitation, with resultant precipitous rises in left atrial pressure. Consequently, these patients have progressive exertional dyspnea marked by frequent episodes of pulmonary edema in the

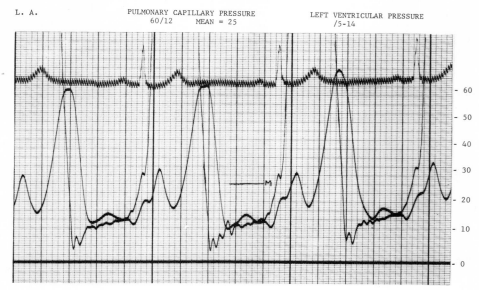

L. A.                     PULMONARY CAPILLARY PRESSURE                    LEFT VENTRICULAR PRESSURE
                              60/12        MEAN = 25                              /5-14

**Figure 9**  Typical cardiac catheterization findings in acute mitral regurgitation: Simultaneous pulmonary capillary "wedge" and left ventricular pressure tracings. There is normal sinus rhythm. The mean wedge pressure is elevated to 25 mm. Hg. A large "V" wave rises to over 60 mm. Hg without end-diastolic gradient across the mitral valve. (From Sanders, C. A., Scannell, J. G., Harthorne, J. W., and Austen, W. G.: Circulation, *31*:506, 1965. By permission of the American Heart Association, Inc.)

presence of a good forward output. At the other extreme, chronic mitral regurgitation is usually associated with a large left atrium that is often fibrillating. The combination of a dilated, more compliant atrium and often a poorly functioning left ventricle results in a low fixed cardiac output, small left atrial "V" waves, and lower pulmonary capillary pressure. In such patients, easy fatigability and weakness predominate, and acute episodes of pulmonary edema occur far less frequently.

An increase in pulmonary arteriolar resistance occurs more slowly and less frequently than in mitral stenosis, probably because the left atrial pressure is elevated only intermittently, i.e., only during systole. Furthermore, owing to the absence of stasis in the left atrium, the incidence of left atrial clot is much lower than in mitral stenosis.

## CLINICAL FEATURES

The major symptoms in mitral regurgitation are usually dyspnea on exertion, easy fatigability, and sometimes palpitation. Pulmonary hypertension and right ventricular failure are relatively infrequent until late in the course of the disease. In acute mitral regurgitation, pulmonary congestion dominates the picture. The sudden worsening of a patient's chronic course, especially with the appearance of marked pulmonary congestion, should alert the physician to the possibility of bacterial endocarditis or ruptured chordae tendineae.

The key *physical* finding is an apical systolic murmur, which is holosystolic. This occurs with fixed regurgitation, as in rheumatic heart lesions, ruptured papillary muscle, or ruptured chordae tendineae. The murmur of papillary muscle dysfunction may be variable in timing during systole.[27] The murmur of a prolapsed mitral leaflet ("floppy valve syndrome") is usually late systolic and is often accompanied by a midsystolic click[9, 53] or, occasionally, an early systolic click.[64] The murmur in all types of mitral regurgitation is usually best heard at the apex and radiates toward the axilla. With posterior leaflet chordal rupture, radiation to the left sternal border is likely. The first heart sound is frequently difficult to hear because it merges with the onset of the murmur. The second heart sound may be widely split owing to shortening of left ventricular systole. An opening snap may be heard in 10 per cent of patients with severe rheumatic mitral regurgitation and, when present, indicates a movable and pliable anterior mitral leaflet.[103] In diastole, a loud and palpable $S_3$ gallop represents the rapid filling of the left ventricle with the large volume of blood from the left atrium. A short filling rumble may follow the gallop. In acute mitral regurgitation with normal sinus rhythm, the small left atrium generates a loud $S_4$ gallop. In all types of mitral regurgitation, the left ventricular impulse is abnormally wide, hyperdynamic, and of normal duration. In chronic mitral regurgitation with left ventricular enlargement, the impulse is displaced downward and to the left. Occasionally, systolic expansion of the enlarged left atrium can be perceived as a late systolic parasternal impulse giving a rocking sensation to the precordium. This may be mistaken for the impulse of right ventricular hypertrophy.[92]

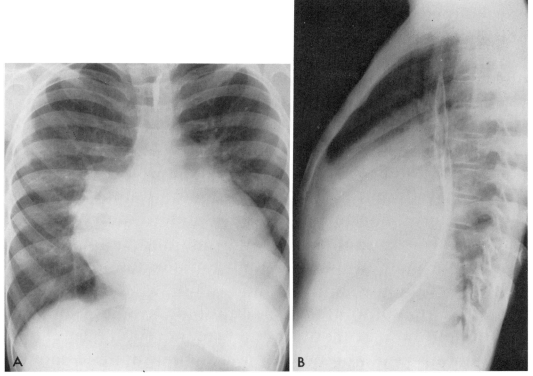

**Figure 10**   Typical posteroanterior and lateral roentgenograms in chronic mitral regurgitation: The chronicity of this patient's mitral regurgitation is suggested by a very large left atrium. In addition, there is left ventricular enlargement. (Courtesy of Dr. Robert E. Dinsmore.)

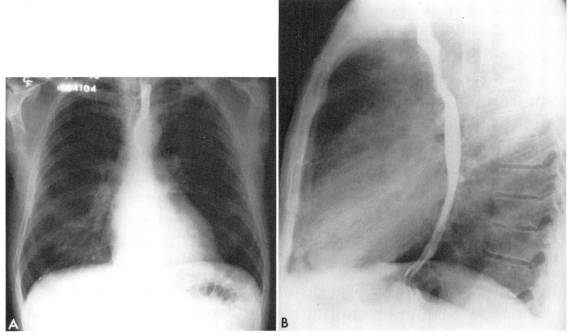

**Figure 11**   Typical posteroanterior and lateral roentgenograms in acute mitral regurgitation: The combination of a relatively small left atrium and marked pulmonary congestion in a patient with a loud apical holosystolic murmur suggests acute mitral regurgitation. In this patient, ruptured chordae tendineae with severe mitral regurgitation were found. (Courtesy of Dr. Robert E. Dinsmore.)

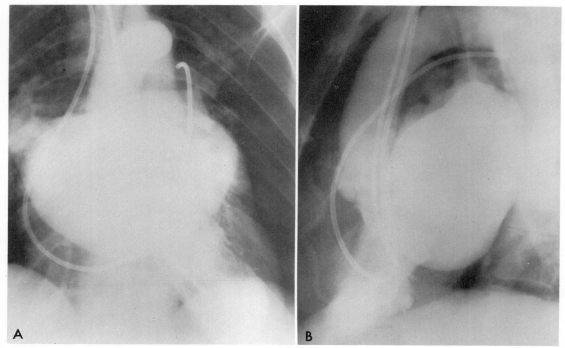

**Figure 12**  Biplane left ventricular angiogram of a patient with mitral regurgitation: Note the dense opacification of the left atrium by contrast medium injected into the left ventricle through a catheter passed retrograde across the aortic valve. A right heart catheter is also present with its tip in the pulmonary artery.

The *chest x-ray* in chronic mitral regurgitation reveals an enlarged left atrium (Fig. 10), which sometimes reaches gigantic proportions, and usually left ventricular dilatation. In spite of considerable cardiomegaly, the pulmonary vasculature may be unremarkable. Significant calcification of the mitral valve is unusual in pure mitral regurgitation. Acute mitral regurgitation in the absence of pre-existing heart disease presents a distinctive radiologic appearance of a relatively small heart with a disproportionate amount of pulmonary vascular congestion. Left atrial size will be normal or only moderately increased (Fig. 11).[121]

The *electrocardiogram* is of only modest help. One may see left ventricular hypertrophy and left atrial enlargement with normal sinus rhythm. Atrial fibrillation is frequent in long-standing cases. Right ventricular hypertrophy may appear in later stages of the disease.

Frequently, accurate quantitation of the severity of mitral regurgitation and the functional impairment of the patient can be made clinically, without *catheterization*. However, mitral regurgitation can best be quantitated by left ventricular angiography via a catheter passed retrograde across the aortic valve (Fig. 12). This study will also give important information about left ventricular size and the adequacy of left ventricular contraction. Left atrial or pulmonary capillary "wedge" pressure tracings may reveal an elevated mean pressure with tall "V" waves (see Fig. 9). A high left ventricular end-diastolic pressure may indicate left ventricular failure. In more severe cases, the cardiac index may be low at rest and unable to rise appropriately with exercise. Pulmonary hypertension may be present. The preoperative assessment, when indicated, of concomitant aortic or tricuspid valve disease or of significant coronary artery disease by catheterization is as important in patients with mitral regurgitation as it is in those with mitral stenosis.

## INDICATIONS FOR SURGERY

Since patients with significant mitral regurgitation can function very well for years with limitation of physical activity and medical management, and since mitral valve replacement, with its attendant risks and complications, is usually required for surgical correction, probably only patients of Class III status or worse, in spite of appropriate medical treatment, should be considered for surgery. As in mitral stenosis, surgery should not be delayed until the patient reaches Class IV, because of the considerable increase in the risk of surgery in such patients. Contrariwise, although the risk of surgery in Class IV patients is high, dramatic clinical improvement can be accomplished by operation.

## SURGICAL THERAPY

The operative repair of mitral regurgitation requires open heart techniques and cardiopulmonary bypass. The usual approach is via a median sternotomy or a right anterolateral thoracotomy. If significant mitral regurgitation is created or unexpectedly found during the performance of a closed mitral valvulotomy, cardiopulmonary bypass can be instituted through a left lateral thoracotomy.

### Mitral Valve Replacement

The standard procedure for the treatment of mitral regurgitation under most circumstances is mitral valve replacement. Many surgeons use *only* mitral valve replacement. The technical considerations, types of valve substitutes, and operative and postoperative problems are identical to those in mitral valve replacement for mitral stenosis and have already been discussed.

We currently employ the Starr-Edwards ball prosthesis for the surgical treatment of essentially all types of significant mitral regurgitation. In patients with mitral regurgitation, the left ventricle is usually large enough that problems of left ventricular endocardial irritation or outflow obstruction from the ball and cage are unlikely (if the proper-sized prosthesis is selected).

### Mitral Annuloplasty

In a small percentage of patients, who have relatively mobile leaflets and a dilated valve annulus, mitral annuloplasty, with cardiopulmonary bypass, may be considered for the treatment of mitral regurgitation. Any commissural fusion is incised, and the mitral annulus is narrowed with mattress sutures (usually with Teflon-felt buttressing) placed in the annulus, usually at one or both commissures.[70] In the process of improving the mitral regurgitation, this technique does decrease the mitral orifice size; an adequate mitral valve orifice of approximately 3 sq. cm. should be maintained if possible. At the completion of the procedure, with cardiopulmonary bypass discontinued, the function of the mitral valve and degree of mitral regurgitation or stenosis should be assessed by insertion of the surgeon's finger into the left atrium and also by simultaneous measurement of left atrial and left ventricular pressures. If adequate valve function has not been achieved, valve replacement should be carried out.

### Mitral Valvuloplasty

A number of different types of valvuloplasty, in addition to annuloplasty, have been suggested in the treatment of mitral regurgitation. Most have now been discarded in favor of valve replacement. When the regurgitation is due to loss of leaflet substance (particularly the mural leaflet), the leaflet area can be extended and increased by the insertion of pericardium or prosthetic material; this may be carried out in association with an annuloplasty as well.

When ruptured chordae are the cause of the mitral regurgitation, plication of the flail leaflet may be possible[70, 93] if the number of ruptured chordae is not too great and their location is appropriate. Mitral annuloplasty may also be necessary. Again, it should be stated that the function of the mitral valve must be checked after bypass is discontinued, and if function is not adequate, valve replacement should be carried out.

## EARLY POSTOPERATIVE PROBLEMS AND GENERAL POSTOPERATIVE CONSIDERATIONS

The postoperative problems and general postoperative considerations associated with the operative treatment of mitral regurgitation are similar to those for the open operative treatment of mitral stenosis and have already been discussed. Early valvular disruption and inadequate valvular function are additional concerns in patients who have undergone annuloplasty or other types of valvuloplasty.

## OPERATIVE RESULTS

The operative results of mitral valve replacement for mitral regurgitation are similar to those for mitral stenosis (operative mortality of approximately 10 per cent). The operative mortality depends in large part on the severity and duration of the mitral regurgitation and the secondary myocardial and pulmonary effects. Symptomatic improvement has been very satisfactory, again quite similar to that in the mitral stenosis group. Late mortality in 3 or 4 years of follow-up is in the range of 10 per cent or less.

Significant late recurrence of valvular dysfunction has been associated with annuloplasty and other types of valvuloplasty. Restenosis or regurgitation occurs in significant numbers of patients in whom leaflet extension procedures have been done. Regurgitation may occur after plication for ruptured chordae. In one well conducted series of annuloplasty operations, significant mitral regurgitation was found in approximately 10 per cent of patients.[113]

## TRICUSPID VALVULAR DISEASE

### ETIOLOGY AND PATHOLOGY

*Tricuspid stenosis* is most commonly due to rheumatic heart disease. It occurs as a clinically significant lesion in 3 to 5 per cent of rheumatic patients.[5, 73] Women are affected four to five times more frequently than men, a female preponderance exceeding that of mitral stenosis. Patients are usually between 25 and 40 years of age. Rheumatic tricuspid stenosis is essentially always associated with rheumatic mitral valve disease, generally with severe mitral stenosis.[47, 123] The pathologic changes seen in the tricuspid valve are quite similar to those found in the mitral valve in rheumatic stenosis. Valve leaflets are thickened, fused, and rigid; chordae tendineae are shortened and fused. Obstructing vegetations of bacterial endocarditis occasionally cause tricuspid stenosis. The endocardial thickenings seen with carcinoid may result in either tricuspid stenosis or tricuspid regurgitation.[115]

In contrast, *tricuspid regurgitation* is much more likely to be functional. Normal tricuspid leaflets are barely large enough to effect valve closure. Muscular contraction of the tricuspid ring in systole is thus an important adjunct in complete closure of the valve. Consequently, right ventricular dilatation, from any cause, may easily result in displacement of papillary muscles and dilatation of the tricuspid ring, leading to regurgitation. Organic tricuspid regurgitation may result from rheumatic retraction of the leaflets or chordae tendineae, bacterial endocarditis, carcinoid,[115] or trauma.[108]

## PHYSIOLOGY

The hemodynamic effects of both tricuspid stenosis and tricuspid regurgitation result in an increased systemic venous pressure and a reduced right ventricular output. The former is manifested by right atrial enlargement, distended neck veins, hepatic engorgement, and peripheral edema. In rheumatic heart disease, the low output of the right ventricle may have the effect of "protecting" the patient from paroxysms of pulmonary congestion by preventing abrupt increases in blood flow into the pulmonary circulation. The tricuspid lesions may also significantly contribute to the systemic manifestations of low cardiac output, i.e., easy fatigability, weight loss, and hypotension. Thus, the recognition, quantitation, and appropriate correction of tricuspid valve disease is important in the attainment of satisfactory hemodynamic results from surgery for other valvular lesions.

## CLINICAL FEATURES

The clinical manifestations are determined by the coexisting mitral or aortic valvular disease. Organic tricuspid disease should be suspected, however, in a female with severe disease of the mitral or aortic valve who presents with long-standing venous stasis and yet has been relatively spared from frequent pulmonary symptoms such as orthopnea and paroxysmal nocturnal dyspnea.[118] Gastrointestinal symptoms including anorexia, nausea, eructations, vomiting, and right upper quadrant pain result from splanchnic congestion and hepatic engorgement. Cardiac cachexia may be present.

The *physical findings* are frequently missed unless specifically searched for. Of great importance is the examination of the neck veins. In normal sinus rhythm, tricuspid stenosis may cause prominent presystolic "A" waves in the jugular venous pulse. They are more significant if seen in the absence of manifestations of pulmonary hypertension and right ventricular hypertrophy, which also can result in large "A" waves. The "V" wave occurring around the end of systole is not as prominent as the "A" wave, but the "Y" descent following it may be slow; this indicates obstruction to right atrial emptying. In addition to peripheral edema, elevated systemic venous pressure leads to hepatomegaly and may eventually result in cardiac cirrhosis with secondary ascites and splenomegaly. A protein-losing enteropathy with low albumin and globulin levels as well as a decreased number of circulating lymphocytes may be seen.[136] On auscultation, a diastolic murmur, often higher-pitched than the rumble of mitral stenosis,[17] may be heard at the left lower sternal border. Sometimes only a presystolic murmur is heard.[109] Augmentation by inspiration (Carvallo's sign) is an important feature, but sometimes is not present.[109] An opening snap may be heard but it may not be easily distinguished from that of mitral stenosis.[109] In the presence of atrial fibrillation, the diagnosis of tricuspid stenosis may be very difficult owing to loss of the "A" wave and changes in the murmur.[123]

In tricuspid regurgitation, a large systolic wave merging with a tall "V" wave in the jugular venous pulse is a key feature. A rapid collapsing venous pulse (sharp "Y" descent) following the systolic wave argues against concomitant tricuspid stenosis, especially if the collapse is followed by a brisk rebound.[109] The systolic expansion may move the ear lobe and cause the liver to pulsate. The murmur of tricuspid regurgitation is a high-pitched, usually holosystolic murmur heard at the left lower sternal border and often increased by inspiration. The intensity of the murmur is probably better correlated with right ventricular pressure than with the amount of regurgitation.[63] Presumably, the high pressure causes a higher velocity of flow and hence a more prominent murmur. In contrast, the murmur in severe tricuspid regurgitation with a normal right ventricular pressure, as might occur with traumatic etiology, is often very soft or may be absent.[108]

The major clue to tricuspid valvular disease on the *chest x-ray* is enlargement of the right atrium (Fig. 13). With significant right atrial enlargement, the right lower cardiac contour bulges to the right, and its convexity is increased in the frontal view. In the right anterior oblique projection, there is a local prominence posteriorly just above the diaphragm. The superior vena cava may be widened and may be seen to pulsate on fluoroscopy.

On the *electrocardiogram*, right atrial enlargement, characterized by tall peaked P waves in leads II, III, aVF, and VI, is the best clue to tricuspid valvular disease. Usually, however, the electrocardiographic pattern is determined by the associated mitral or aortic valve disease.

*Cardiac catheterization* is indicated in all patients suspected of having tricuspid valvular disease who are about to have other valvular surgery. Clinical assessment alone is often inaccurate. In

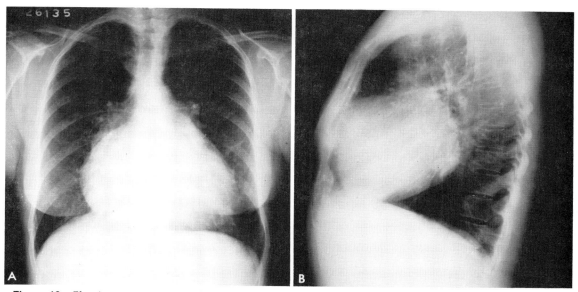

**Figure 13**  Classic roentgenograms of a patient with tricuspid valvular disease. Right atrial enlargement is indicated by the bulge of the entire right heart contour extending to the diaphragm on the posteroanterior view (*A*). This finding superimposed on the changes of mitral stenosis, as indicated by evidence of pulmonary venous hypertension and left atrial enlargement (double contour on the right and elevation of the left main stem bronchus), indicates tricuspid valvular disease. The sharply angulated bulge into the retrosternal space on the lateral view (*B*) is probably the large right atrial appendage.

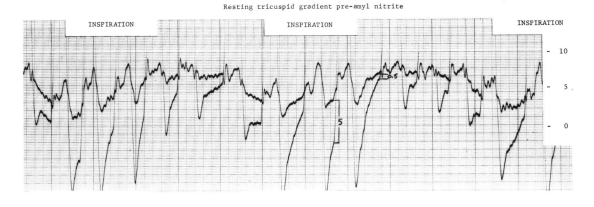

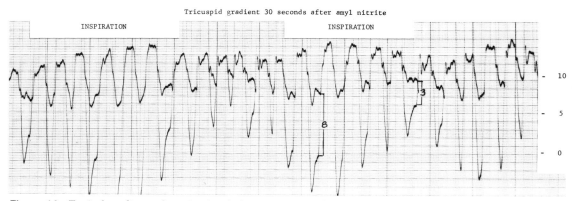

**Figure 14**  Typical cardiac catheterization findings in tricuspid stenosis: Simultaneous right atrial and right ventricular pressure tracings recorded through a double-lumen catheter. Inspiration and amyl nitrite increase the gradient by increasing venous return and hence flow across the tricuspid valve. (From Sanders, C. A., Harthorne, J. W., DeSanctis, R. W., and Austen, W. G.: Circulation, *33*:26, 1966. By permission of the American Heart Association, Inc.)

one series,[134] significant tricuspid valvular disease was unsuspected preoperatively in one-third of the patients who subsequently had an operative procedure on the tricuspid valve. Atrial fibrillation makes the clinical diagnosis of tricuspid stenosis even more difficult, and in 80 per cent of patients in another series,[123] diagnosis was not made until catheterization. At catheterization, the relatively low right-sided pressures permit quite a low gradient across the tricuspid valve, even with moderately severe stenosis. Thus, the double-lumen catheter, which allows simultaneous right atrial and right ventricular pressure tracings, is necessary[123] (Fig. 14); pullback tracings are not adequate. Right ventricular angiography to detect tricuspid regurgitation may yield many false-positive studies but very few false-negative ones.[134] A prominent right atrial "V" wave may indicate tricuspid regurgitation. A normal or only slightly elevated pulmonary artery pressure is helpful in differentiating organic from functional tricuspid regurgitation, for the latter is very unlikely if the pulmonary artery pressure is not significantly elevated.

## INDICATIONS FOR SURGERY

The decision to correct significant tricuspid regurgitation is best made after correction of the left-sided lesions at the time of surgery. Most surgeons would agree that tricuspid valve surgery can be lifesaving in a patient with severe tricuspid regurgitation who is unable to maintain an adequate circulation without the pump-oxygenator. On the other hand, how often functional tricuspid regurgitation of moderately severe degree requires correction is debated.[20, 134]

For tricuspid stenosis, it seems reasonable to correct significant tricuspid narrowing at the time of surgery for associated mitral or aortic valvular disease.

## SURGICAL TREATMENT

Tricuspid valve surgery requires open techniques and cardiopulmonary bypass. Usually, a median sternotomy incision is used because this allows the best exposure of the aortic, mitral, and tricuspid valves. If only the mitral and tricuspid valves are involved, a right anterolateral thoracotomy may occasionally be employed. Cannulation and the other aspects of cardiopulmonary bypass have already been discussed. The tricuspid valve should be palpated through a right atrial purse-string suture before cardiopulmonary bypass is instituted to determine the degree of stenosis or regurgitation. The left-sided valvular lesions are corrected first. If the tricuspid problem is functional regurgitation, cardiopulmonary bypass should usually be discontinued and the surgeon's finger should again be inserted into the right

atrium. We believe that if severe tricuspid regurgitation is still present repair is required. Significant organic tricuspid stenosis or regurgitation is also an indication for tricuspid surgery.

### Tricuspid Valve Replacement

In addition to the debate regarding the indications for corrective tricuspid valve surgery, there is argument concerning valve replacement versus annuloplasty or other valvuloplasty procedures. In general, in patients with significant tricuspid malfunction, we have felt that valve replacement is usually preferable.[134] The right atrium is incised and the tricuspid valve with its papillary muscle and chordae is removed. Because the bundle of His runs in close proximity to the septal leaflet, a rim of septal leaflet is preserved. Multiple interrupted mattress or figure-of-eight sutures, with Teflon-felt buttressing if necessary, are placed around the circumference of the annulus and septal leaflet and then in the ring of the valve substitute.

At present, we prefer the Starr-Edwards ball prosthesis, but other types may be equally satisfactory. In employing the Starr-Edwards ball valve, it is important to choose one that is not too large for the right ventricular cavity. Septal irritation and injury can occur if the prosthesis is too large. If a smaller valve is required, a low-profile disc, eccentric monocusp, or stented homograft valve should be employed. Some prefer a low-profile disc, eccentric monocusp, or stented homograft valve for all tricuspid valve replacements, in part because of the low pressures in the right heart and the decreased inertia required for these valves to function.

### Tricuspid Valvuloplasty

Various types of tricuspid valvuloplasty have been employed with varying success. In the rare patient with relatively pure tricuspid stenosis, open valvuloplasty with incision of the fused commissures may be performed.[123] It is difficult to be sure of the exact location of all the commissures, and, to avoid regurgitation, it is usually best to incise just one or two commissures. In the average-sized patients, an orifice size of greater than 3 sq. cm. is probably satisfactory.

In patients with mixed organic disease or severe functional regurgitation, an annuloplasty may be considered (in addition to incision of the commissures, if stenosis is also present). This procedure is difficult to perform and enthusiasm for it is variable. Multiple mattress sutures are usually placed in the annulus at one or two commissures, to decrease the annular size and make the valve more competent. It is important that the annuloplasty not narrow the orifice too much, or significant stenosis may result. At the completion of the procedure, with cardiopulmonary bypass discontinued, the surgeon should feel the valve with his finger through the right atrial wall. If there is significant tricuspid stenosis or regurgitation, valve replacement should be performed.

## EARLY POSTOPERATIVE COMPLICATIONS AND GENERAL POSTOPERATIVE CONSIDERATIONS

The postoperative problems and other considerations following tricuspid valve surgery are similar to those already discussed in association with mitral surgery. Patients with tricuspid valve disease are usually sicker and, of course, undergo a more complicated operation involving repair of more than one valve. The most troublesome group are the patients with pulmonary hypertension and severe functional tricuspid regurgitation. In addition to the problems already discussed in other sections of this chapter, patients undergoing tricuspid valve surgery may show evidence of postoperative liver failure because of long-standing high venous pressure secondary to the tricuspid valve disease. Because of the high incidence of pulmonary hypertension and because most of these patients have very severe, long-standing cardiac difficulties, prolonged respiratory support is usually required, and many patients will require tracheostomy. Low cardiac output states and cardiac failure are common, most particularly if significant tricuspid valve malfunction is still present in the postoperative period, but also frequently when the tricuspid valve is functioning well. Cardiac arrhythmias and renal failure occur in a relatively high proportion of cases.

## OPERATIVE RESULTS

The operative results depend on the other associated valve problems, the type of tricuspid valve disease, and the degree of myocardial damage and secondary pulmonary effects. In patients with organic tricuspid valve disease who undergo a satisfactory valvuloplasty or valve replacement, the operative mortality is only slightly higher than that related to the operative procedure for the associated left-sided valvular problems (usually in the range of 5 to 15 per cent). In patients with significant functional tricuspid regurgitation, the long-standing severe cardiac disease and pulmonary hypertension result in a relatively higher operative mortality (in the range of 20 to 25 per cent). Recurrence of tricuspid dysfunction may follow tricuspid valvuloplasty. Rarely, in patients with prosthetic valves, thrombosis of the prosthesis and pulmonary emboli may develop. In general, surviving patients do well, with marked improvement in symptoms. Because of the multiple valve problems and secondary myocardial and pulmonary effects, the late mortality in this group of patients is somewhat higher than in patients with single mitral valve replacement.

## REFERENCES

1. Akbarian, M., Austen, W. G., Yurchak, P. M., and Scannell, J. G.: Thromboembolic complications of prosthetic cardiac valves. Circulation, 37;826, 1968.
2. Amoury, R. A., Bowman, F. O., and Malm, J. R.: Endocarditis associated with intracardiac prostheses. Diagnosis, management and prophylaxis. J. Thorac. Cardiovasc. Surg., 51:36, 1966.
3. Amplatz, K.: The roentgenographic diagnosis of mitral and aortic valvular disease. Amer. Heart J., 64:556, 1962.
4. Aron, A. M., Freeman, J. M., and Carter, S.: The natural history of Sydenham's chorea: Review of the literature and long-term evaluation with emphasis on cardiac sequelae. Amer. J. Med., 38:83, 1965.
5. Auger, P., and Wigle, E. D.: Coarctation of the aorta associated with severe mitral insufficiency. Amer. J. Cardiol., 21:190, 1968.
6. Austen, W. G., and Wooler, G. H.: The surgical treatment of mitral stenosis by the transventricular approach employing a mechanical dilator. New Eng. J. Med., 263:661, 1960.
7. Bailey, C. P.: The surgical treatment of mitral stenosis (mitral commissurotomy). Dis. Chest, 15:377, 1949.
8. Bailey, C. P.: Surgery of the Heart. Philadelphia, Lea & Febiger, 1955.
9. Barlow, J. B., Bosman, C. K., Pocock, W. A., and Marchand, P.: Late systolic murmurs and non-ejection ("mid-late") systolic clicks: An analysis of 90 patients. Brit. Heart J., 30:203, 1968.
10. Barratt-Boyes, B. G.: Homograft aortic valve replacement in aortic incompetence and stenosis. Thorax, 19:131, 1964.
11. Beall, A. C., Jr., Bloodwell, R. D., Liotta, D., Cooley, D. A., and DeBakey, M. E.: Clinical experience with Dacron velour covered Teflon disc mitral prostheses. Ann. Thorac. Surg., 5:402, 1968.
12. Beller, B. M., Frates, R. W. M., and Wulfsohn, N.: Cardiac pacemaking in the management of postoperative arrhythmias. Ann. Thorac. Surg., 6:68, 1968.
13. Bendixen, H. H., Egbert, L. D., Hedley-Whyte, J., Laver, M. B., and Pontoppidan, H.: Respiratory Care. St. Louis, C. V. Mosby Company, 1965.
14. Biggers, J. T., Schmidt, D. H., and Kutt, H.: Relationship between the plasma level of diphenylhydantoin sodium and its cardiac antiarrhythmic effects. Circulation, 38:363, 1968.
15. Björk, V. O.: A new tilting disc valve prosthesis. Scand. J. Thorac. Cardiovasc. Surg., 3:1, 1969.
16. Block, P. C., DeSanctis, R. W., Weinberg, A. N., and Austen, W. G.: Prosthetic valve endocarditis. J. Thorac. Cardiovasc. Surg., 60:540, 1970.
17. Bousvaros, G. A., and Stubington, D.: Some auscultatory and phonocardiographic features of tricuspid stenosis. Circulation, 29:26, 1964.
18. Braunwald, E.: Mitral regurgitation: Physiologic, clinical and surgical considerations. New Eng. J. Med., 281:425, 1969.
19. Braunwald, E., Braunwald, N., Ross, J., Jr., and Morrow, A. G.: Effects of mitral valve replacement on the pulmonary vascular dynamics of patients with pulmonary hypertension. New Eng. J. Med., 273:509, 1965.
20. Braunwald, N. S., Ross, J., Jr., and Morrow, A. G.: Conservative management of tricuspid regurgitation in patients undergoing mitral valve replacement. Circulation, Supp. 1, 35:63, 1967.
21. Brock, R. C., and Campbell, M.: Discussion on surgery of the heart and great vessels. Proc. Roy. Soc. Med., 44:995, 1951.
22. Brody, W., and Criley, J. M.: Intermittent severe mitral regurgitation. New Eng. J. Med., 283:673, 1970.
23. Brunton, L.: Preliminary note on the possibility of treating mitral stenosis by surgical methods. Lancet, 1:352, 1902; Surgical operation for mitral stenosis. Lancet, 1:547, 1902.
24. Buch, W. S., Kosek, J. C., Angell, W. W., et al.: Deterioration of formalin-treated aortic valve heterografts. J. Thorac. Cardiovasc. Surg., 60:673, 1970.
25. Burch, G. E., DePasquale, N. P., and Phillips, J. H.: The syndrome of papillary muscle dysfunction. Amer. Heart J., 75:399, 1968.
26. Caulfield, J. B., Page, D. L., Kastor, J. A., and Sanders, C. A.: Dissolution of connective tissue in ruptured chordae tendineae. Circulation, Supp., 40:111, 1969.
27. Cheng, T. O.: Some new observations on the syndrome of papillary muscle dysfunction. Amer. J. Med., 47:924, 1969.
28. Cournand, A., and Ranges, H. A.: Catheterization of right

auricle in man. Proc. Soc. Exp. Biol. Med., *46*:462, 1941.

29. Cutler, E. C., and Levine, S. A.: Cardiotomy and valvulotomy for mitral stenosis. Boston Med. Surg. J., *188*: 1023, 1923.

30. Daley, R., Mattingly, T. W., Holt, C. L., Bland, E. F., and White, P. D.: Systemic arterial embolism in rheumatic heart disease. Amer. Heart J., *42*:566, 1951.

31. DeBusk, R. F., and Harrison, D. C.: The clinical spectrum of papillary muscle disease. New Eng. J. Med., *281*:1458, 1969.

32. Delman, A. J., Robinson, G., Stein, E., Yahr, W., and Lister, J. W.: Precise determination of cardiac arrhythmias during open heart surgery by monitoring of myocardial electrograms. Amer. J. Cardiol., *21*:714, 1968.

33. Dexter, C., Dow, J. W., Haynes, F. W., Whittenberger, J. L., Ferris, B. G., Goodale, W. T., and Hellems, H. K.: Studies of the pulmonary circulation at rest. Normal variations and the interrelations between increased pulmonary blood flow, elevated pulmonary arterial pressure and high pulmonary "capillary" pressure. J. Clin. Invest., *29*:602, 1950.

34. Dietzman, R. H., Motsay, G. J., and Lillehei, R. C.: Drugs in the treatment of shock. Pharmacol. Physicians, *4*:1, 1970.

35. Dinsmore, R. E., Sanders, C. A., and Harthorne, J. W.: Mitral regurgitation in idiopathic hypertrophic subaortic stenosis. New Eng. J. Med., *275*:1225, 1966.

36. Duvoisin, G. E., Brandenburg, R. O., and Ellis, F. H., Jr.: Mitral valve replacement with a full-orifice ball valve: Experience with 108 operations. In: Brewer, L. A., III, ed.: Prosthetic Heart Valves. Springfield, Ill., Charles C Thomas, 1969, p. 541.

37. Fetterolf, G., and Norris, G. W.: The anatomical explanation of the paralysis of the left recurrent laryngeal nerve found in certain cases of mitral stenosis. Amer. J. Med. Sci., *141*:625, 1911.

38. Fishman, N. H., Hutchinson, J. C., and Roe, B. B.: Controlled atrial hypertension: A method for supporting cardiac output following open heart surgery. J. Thorac. Cardiovasc. Surg., *52*:777, 1966.

39. Forssmann, W.: Ueber Kontrastdarstellung der Höhlen des labenden richten Herzens und der Lungen schlagader. Munchen. Med. Wschr., *78*:489, 1931.

40. Friedberg, C. K.: Acute pericarditis. In: Diseases of the Heart. 3rd ed. Philadelphia, W. B. Saunders Company, 1966, p. 933.

41. Friedberg, C. K.: Tricuspid and pulmonic valvular disease. In: Diseases of the Heart. 3rd ed. Philadelphia, W. B. Saunders Company, 1966, p. 1162.

42. Friedberg, C. K.: Surgical procedures in the cardiac patient. In: Diseases of the Heart. 3rd ed. Philadelphia, W. B. Saunders Company, 1966, p. 1746.

43. Gans, H., and Krivit, W.: Problems in hemostasis during open heart surgery. III. Epsilon amino caproic acid as an inhibitor of plasminogen activator activity. Ann. Surg., *155*:268, 1962.

44. Gerami, S., Messmer, B. J., Hallman, G. L., and Cooley, D. A.: Open mitral commissurotomy: Results of 100 consecutive cases. J. Thorac. Cardiovasc. Surg., *62*:366, 1971.

45. Gerbode, F.: Transventricular mitral valvulotomy. Circulation, *21*:563, 1960.

46. Gibbon, J. H., Jr.: Application of mechanical heart and lung apparatus to cardiac surgery. Minnesota Med., *37*:171, 185, 1954.

47. Gibson, R., and Wood, P.: The diagnosis of tricuspid stenosis. Brit. Heart J., *17*:552, 1955.

48. Goodwin, J. F.: Diagnosis of left atrial myxoma. Lancet, *1*:464, 1963.

49. Goodwin, J. F., Hunter, J. D., Cleland, W. P., Davis, L. G., and Steiner, R. E.: Mitral valve disease and mitral valvotomy. Brit. Med. J., *2*:573, 1955.

50. Gorlin, R., and Gorlin, S. G.: Hydraulic formula for calculation of the area of the stenotic mitral valve, other cardiac valves, and central circulatory shunts. Amer. Heart J., *41*:1, 1951.

51. Gorlin, R., Lewis, B. M., Haynes, F. W., Spiegl, R. J., and Dexter, L.: Factors regulating pulmonary "capillary" pressure in mitral stenosis. Amer. Heart J., *41*:834, 1951.

52. Grismer, J. T., Levy, M. J., Lillehei, R. C., Indeglia, R., and Lillehei, C. W.: Renal function in acquired valvular heart disease and effects of extracorporeal circulation. Surgery, *55*:24, 1964.

53. Hancock, E. W., and Cohn, K.: The syndrome associated with mid-systolic click and late systolic murmur. Amer. J. Med., *41*:183, 1966.

54. Harken, D. E., Ellis, L. B., Ware, P. F., and Norman, L. R.: The surgical treatment of mitral stenosis. New Eng. J. Med., *239*:802, 1948.

55. Harrison, D. C., Sprouse, J. H., and Morrow, A. G.: The antiarrhythmic properties of lidocaine and procaine amide. Circulation, *28*:486, 1963.

56. Harthorne, J. W., Seltzer, R. A., and Austen, W. G.: Left atrial calcification: Review of the literature and proposed management. Circulation, *34*:198, 1966.

57. Heikkila, J.: Mitral incompetence as a complication of acute myocardial infarction. Acta Med. Scand., Supp., 475, 1967.

58. Hodam, R., Anderson, R., Starr, A., Wood, J., Dobbs, J., and Raible, D.: Further evaluation of the composite seat cloth-covered aortic prosthesis. Presented at the Society of Thoracic Surgeons, Dallas, Texas, 1971.

59. Hodam, R., Starr, A., Herr, R., et al.: Early clinical experience with cloth-covered valvular prostheses. Ann. Surg., *170*:471, 1969.

60. Horsley, H. T., Jr., Rappoport, W. J., Vigoda, P. S., and Vogel, J. H. K.: Fatal malfunction of Edwards low-profile mitral valve. Circulation, Supp., *40*:111, 1969.

61. Hugenholtz, P. G., Ryan, T. H., Stein, S. W., and Abelman, W. H.: The spectrum of pure mitral stenosis: Hemodynamic studies in relation to clinical disability. Amer. J. Cardiol., *10*:773, 1962.

62. Hurst, J. W., and Logue, R. B.: Common diseases of the heart: Systemic tension in the heart. In: The Heart. 2nd ed. New York, McGraw-Hill Book Company, 1970, p. 773.

63. Hurst, J. W., and Logue, R. B.: Less common diseases of the heart. In: The Heart. 2nd ed. New York, McGraw-Hill Book Company, 1970, p. 863.

64. Hutter, A. M., Jr., Dinsmore, R. E., Willerson, J. T., and DeSanctis, R. W.: Early systolic clicks due to mitral valve prolapse. Circulation, *44*:516, 1971.

65. Ionescu, M. I., and Ross, D. N.: Heart-valve replacement with autologous fascia lata. Lancet, *1*:355, 1969.

66. Ionescu, M. I., Wooler, G. H., Smith, D. R., and Grimshaw, V. A.: Mitral valve replacement with aortic heterografts in humans. Thorax, *22*:305, 1967.

67. James, T. N.: Anatomy of coronary arteries in health and disease. Circulation, *32*:1020, 1965.

68. Jordan, S. C.: Development of pulmonary hypertension in mitral stenosis. Lancet, *2*:322, 1965.

69. Karliner, J. S.: Intravenous diphenylhydantoin sodium (Dilantin) in cardiac arrhythmias. Dis. Chest, *51*:256, 1967.

70. Kay, J. H., and Egerton, W. S.: The repair of mitral insufficiency associated with ruptured chordae tendineae. Ann. Surg., *157*:351, 1963.

71. Kay, J. H., Tsuji, H. K., Redington, J. V., Mendes, A., Saji, K., Kamata, K., Yokoyama, T., Magidson, O., and Krohn, B.: Experiences with the Kay-Shiley disc valve. In: Brewer, L. A., III, ed.: Prosthetic Heart Valves. Springfield, Ill., Charles C Thomas, 1969, p. 609.

72. Kiser, I. O., Hoeksema, T. D., Connolly, D. C., and Ellis, F. H., Jr.: Long-term results of closed mitral commissurotomy. J. Cardiovasc. Surg., *8*:263, 1967.

73. Kitchin, A., and Turner, R.: Diagnosis and treatment of tricuspid stenosis. Brit. Heart J., *26*:354, 1964.

74. Kloster, F. E., Herr, R. H., Starr, A., et al.: Hemodynamic evaluation of a cloth-covered Starr-Edwards valve prosthesis. Circulation, Supp. 1, *39*:119, 1969.

75. Koch-Weser, J., Klein, S. W., Foo-Cantu, L., Kastor, J. A., and DeSanctis, R. W.: Antiarrhythmic prophylaxis with procainamide in acute myocardial infarction. New Eng. J. Med., *281*:1253, 1969.

76. Korn, D., DeSanctis, R. W., and Sell, S.: Massive calcification of the mitral annulus: A clinicopathological study of fourteen cases. New Eng. J. Med., *267*:900, 1962.

77. Kosek, J. C., Iben, A. B., Shumway, N. E., and Angell,

W. W.: Morphology of fresh heart valve homografts. Surgery, 66:269, 1969.

78. Lang, D. L., Scolnick, E. M., and Willerson, J. T.: Association of cytomegalovirus infection with the postperfusion syndrome. New Eng. J. Med., 278:1147, 1968.

79. Lavender, J. P., Doppman, J., Shawdon, H., and Steiner, R. E.: Pulmonary veins in left ventricular failure and mitral stenosis. Brit. J. Radiol., 35:293, 1962.

80. Leatham, A.: Auscultation of the heart. Lancet, 2:703, 757, 1958.

81. Levinson, G. E., Schwartz, C. J., and Frank, M. J.: The effect of rest on the volume burden of mitral and aortic regurgitation. Clin. Res., 16:238, 1968.

82. Levy, M., and Edwards, J.: Anatomy of mitral insufficiency. Progr. Cardiovasc. Dis., 5:119, 1962.

83. Lewis, B. M., Gorlin, R., Houssay, H. E. J., Haynes, F. W., and Dexter, L.: Clinical and physiological correlations in patients with mitral stenosis. Amer. Heart J., 43:2, 1952.

84. Lillehei, C. W., Kaster, R. L., Starek, P. J., Block, J. H., and Rees, J. R.: A new central flow pivoting disc aortic and mitral prosthesis: Initial clinical experience. Amer. J. Cardiol., 26:688, 1970.

85. Lillehei, C. W., Levy, M. J., and Bonnabeau, R. C., Jr.: Mitral valve replacement with preservation of papillary muscles and chordae tendineae. J. Thorac. Cardiovasc. Surg., 47:532, 1964.

86. Links, E., and Sysimetsa, E.: Clinical and radiological aspects of calcification of the mitral valve. Brit. Heart J., 20:329, 1958.

87. Logan, A., and Turner, R.: Surgical treatment of mitral stenosis with particular reference to the transventricular approach with a mechanical dilator. Lancet, 2:874, 1959.

88. Lunger, M., Abelson, D. S., Elkind, A. H., and Kantrowitz, A.: Massive hemoptysis in mitral stenosis: Control by emergency commissurotomy. New Eng. J. Med., 261:393, 1959.

89. MacLean, L. D.: Venous pressure versus blood volume. Surg. Gynec. Obstet., 118:594, 1964.

90. MacVaugh, H., III, Joyner, C. R., and Johnson, J.: Unusual complications during mitral valve replacement in presence of calcification of the annulus. Ann. Thorac. Surg., 11:336, 1971.

91. Malm, J. R., Bowman, F. O., Jr., Harris, P. D., and Kowalik, A. T. W.: Evaluation of aortic valve homografts sterilized by electron beam energy. J. Thorac. Cardiovasc. Surg., 54:471, 1967.

92. Manchester, G. H., Block, P., and Gorlin, R.: Misleading signs in mitral insufficiency. J.A.M.A., 191:87, 1965.

93. McGoon, D. C.: Repair of mitral insufficiency due to ruptured chordae tendineae. J. Thorac. Surg., 39:357, 1960.

94. McLaughlin, J. S., Cowley, R. A., Smith, G., and Matheson, N. A.: Mitral valve disease from blunt trauma. J. Thorac. Cardiovasc. Surg., 48:261, 1964.

95. Morris, J. J., Jr., Estes, E. H., Whalen, R. E., Thompson, H. K., Jr., and McIntosh, H. D.: P-wave analysis in valvular heart disease. Circulation, 29:242, 1964.

96. Morrow, A. G., Oldham, H. N., Elkins, R. C., and Braunwald, E.: Prosthetic replacement of the mitral valve. Preoperative and postoperative clinical and hemodynamic assessments in 100 patients. Circulation, 35:962, 1967.

97. Mounsey, P.: Tricuspid incompetence following successful mitral valvulotomy. Brit. Heart J., 21:123, 1959.

98. Murray, G.: Homologous aortic valve segment transplants as surgical treatment for aortic and mitral insufficiency. Angiology, 7:446, 1956.

99. Nathaniels, E. K., Moncure, A. C., and Scannell, J. G.: A fifteen-year follow-up study of closed mitral valvuloplasty. Ann. Thorac. Surg., 10:27, 1970.

100. Nelson, R. M., Jenson, C. B., Peterson, C. A., and Sanders, B. C.: Effective use of prophylactic antibiotics in open heart surgery. Arch. Surg., 90:731, 1965.

101. Nexlin, V. E., and Shamesova, L. C.: Infarction of papillary muscles: Clinical and anatomico-pathologic observations. (In Russian.) Klin. Med. (Moskva), 29:51, 1951.

102. Nichols, H. T., Blanco, G., Morse, D. P., Adam, A., and Baltazar, N.: Open mitral commissurotomy: Experience with 200 consecutive cases. J.A.M.A., 182:268, 1962.

103. Nixon, P. G. F., Wooler, G. H., and Radigan, L. R.: Mitral incompetence caused by lesions of the mural cusp. Circulation, 19:839, 1959.

104. Norman, J. C., McDonald, H. P., and Sloan, J.: The early and aggressive treatment of acute renal failure following cardiopulmonary bypass with continuous peritoneal dialysis. Surgery, 56:1, 1964.

105. O'Brien, M. F., and Clarebrough, J. K.: Heterograft aortic valves for human valve disease. Amer. Heart J., 74:135, 1967.

106. O'Brien, M. F., Clarebrough, J. K., McDonald, I. G., Hale, G. S., Bray, H. S., and Cade, J. I.: Heterograft aortic valve replacement. Mitral follow-up studies. Thorax, 22:387, 1967.

107. Olinger, G. N., Rio, F. W., and Maloney, J. V., Jr.: Closed valvulotomy for calcific mitral stenosis. J. Thorac. Cardiovasc. Surg., 62:357, 1971.

108. Osborn, J. R., Jones, R. C., and Jahnke, E. J., Jr.: Traumatic tricuspid insufficiency. Hemodynamic data and surgical treatment. Circulation, 30:217, 1964.

109. Perloff, J. K., and Harvey, W. P.: Clinical recognition of tricuspid stenosis. Circulation, 22:346, 1960.

110. Peter, R. H., Gracey, J. G., and Beach, T. B.: Significance of fibrillatory waves and the P terminal force in idiopathic atrial fibrillation. Ann. Intern. Med., 68:1296, 1968.

111. Phillips, J. H., Burch, G. E., and DePasquale, N. P.: The syndrome of papillary muscle dysfunction. Ann. Intern. Med., 59:508, 1963.

112. Raftery, E. B., Oakley, C. M., and Goodwin, J. F.: Acute subvalvular mitral incompetence. Lancet, 2:360, 1966.

113. Reed, G. E., Clauss, R. H., and Spencer, F. C.: Controversy between replacement and repair of the mitral valve. In: Symposium on Prosthetic Valves, 1968. In press.

114. Roberts, W. C., Braunwald, E., and Morrow, A. G.: Acute severe mitral regurgitation secondary to ruptured chordae tendineae: Clinical hemodynamic and pathologic considerations. Circulation, 33:58, 1966.

115. Roberts, W. C., and Sjoerdsma, A.: The cardiac disease associated with the carcinoid syndrome (carcinoid heart disease). Amer. J. Med., 36:5, 1964.

116. Ross, D. N.: Homotransplantation of the aortic valve in the sub-coronary position. J. Thorac. Surg., 47:713, 1964.

117. Ross, D. N., Gonzalez-Lavin, L., and Dalichau, H.: A two-year experience with supporting autologous fascia lata for heart valve replacement. In press.

118. Salazar, E., and Levine, H. D.: Rheumatic tricuspid regurgitation. The clinical spectrum. Amer. J. Med., 33:111, 1962.

119. Salzman, E. W., and Britten, A.: Hemorrhage and Thrombosis. Boston, Little, Brown and Company, 1965.

120. Sanders, C. A., Armstrong, P. W., Willerson, J. T., and Dinsmore, R. E.: The etiology and differential diagnosis of acute mitral regurgitation. Progr. Cardiovasc. Dis., 14:129, 1971.

121. Sanders, C. A., Austen, W. G., Harthorne, J. W., Dinsmore, R. E., and Scannell, J. G.: Diagnosis and surgical treatment of mitral regurgitation secondary to ruptured chordae tendineae. New Eng. J. Med., 276:943, 1967.

122. Sanders, C. A., Buckley, M. J., Leinbach, R. C., Mundth, E. D., and Austen, W. G.: Mechanical circulatory assistance: Current status and experience with combining circulatory assistance, emergency coronary angiography and acute myocardial revascularization. Circulation, in press.

123. Sanders, C. A., Harthorne, J. W., DeSanctis, R. W., and Austen, W. G.: Tricuspid stenosis: A difficult diagnosis in the presence of atrial fibrillation. Circulation, 33:26, 1966.

124. Sanders, C. A., Scannell, J. G., Harthorne, J. W., and Austen, W. G.: Severe mitral regurgitation secondary to ruptured chordae tendineae. Circulation, 31:506, 1965.

125. Sanders, R. J., and Neuberger, K. T.: Rupture of the papillary muscles. Occurrence of rupture of the posterior muscle in posterior myocardial infarction. Dis. Chest, 31:316, 1957.

126. Selzer, A., Kelly, J. J., Jr., Vannitamby, M., Walker, P.,

Gerbode, F., and Kerth, W. J.: The syndrome of mitral insufficiency due to isolated rupture of the chordae tendineae. Amer. J. Med., *43*:822, 1967.

127. Semer, H., Hultgren, H., Kleiger, R., and Braniff, B.: Cardioversion following prosthetic mitral valve replacement. Circulation, *35*:523, 1967.

128. Semler, H. J., and Pruett, R. D.: An electrocardiographic estimation of pulmonary vascular obstruction in 80 patients with mitral stenosis. Amer. Heart J., *59*:541, 1960.

129. Senning, A.: Fascia lata replacement of aortic valves. J. Thorac. Cardiovasc. Surg., *48*:346, 1964.

130. Shanks, S. C., and Kerley, P.: A Text-book of X-ray Diagnosis. 3rd ed. Vol. 2. Philadelphia, W. B. Saunders Company, 1962.

131. Souttar, H. S.: Surgical treatment of mitral stenosis. Brit. Med. J., *2*:603, 1925.

132. Starr, A.: Mitral valve replacement with ball valve prostheses. Brit. Heart J., Supp. 33, 1971, p. 47.

133. Starr, A., and Edwards, M. L.: Mitral replacement: Clinical experience with a ball-valve prosthesis. Ann. Surg., *154*:726, 1961.

134. Starr, A., Herr, R., and Wood, J.: Tricuspid valve replacement for acquired valve disease. Surg. Gynec. Obstet., *122*:1295, 1966.

135. Starr, A., Herr, R. W., and Wood, J. A.: Mitral replacement: Review of six years' experience. J. Thorac. Cardiovasc. Surg., *54*:333, 1967.

136. Strober, W., Cohen, L. S., Waldman, T. A., and Braunwald,

E.: Tricuspid regurgitation: A newly recognized cause of protein-losing enteropathy, lymphocytopenia, and immunologic deficiency. Amer. J. Med., *44*:842, 1968.

137. Sullivan, J. M., Harkins, D. E., and Gorlin, R.: Pharmacologic control of thrombo-embolic complications of cardiac valve replacement. New Eng. J. Med., *284*:1391, 1971.

138. Wada, J.: Knotless suture method and Wada hingeless valve. Jap. J. Thorac. Surg., *15*:88, 1966.

139. Watson, H. L.: Severe tricuspid stenosis revealed after aortic valvulotomy. Brit. Heart J., *24*:241, 1962.

140. West, J. B., Doller, C. T., and Heard, B. E.: Increased pulmonary vascular resistance in the dependent zone of isolated dog lung caused by perivascular edema. Circ. Res., *17*:191, 1965.

141. Willerson, J. T., Kastor, J. A., Dinsmore, R. E., Mundth, E. D., Buckley, M. J., Austen, W. G., and Sanders, C. A.: Phonocardiographic and hemodynamic assessment of mitral paravalvular and intravalvular regurgitation. Brit. Heart J., Supp. 42, 1970, p. 32.

142. Wood, P.: An appreciation of mitral stenosis: I. Clinical features; II. Investigations and results. Brit. Med. J., *1*:1051, 1113, 1954.

143. Wood, P.: Systemic embolism. Brit. Med. J., *1*:1056, 1954.

144. Yeh, T. J., Brachney, E. L., Hall, D. P., and Ellison, R. G.: Renal complications of open heart surgery: Predisposing factors, prevention and management. J. Thorac. Cardiovasc. Surg., *47*:79, 1964.

# XIII

# Cardiac Neoplasms

*Brack G. Hattler, Jr., M.D., and David C. Sabiston, Jr., M.D.*

Cardiac tumors have been recognized since the mid-sixteenth century. In 1559, Columbus[5] recorded the first known report of a cardiac neoplasm, and in the ensuing centuries these lesions continued to remain largely autopsy curiosities. Barnes[2] in 1934 reported the first clinical diagnosis of a cardiac tumor, in a patient who later died of a primary sarcoma of the heart. The true impetus to the premortem discovery of these tumors, however, came with the development of cardiac surgery and refinements in angiocardiographic techniques. Prior to the development of extracorporeal circulation in the performance of open heart surgery, Steinberg[21] reported in 1953 an *unsuccessful* attempt to excise an atrial myxoma diagnosed by angiocardiography. The following year, Crafoord[6] performed the first successful removal of a cardiac neoplasm—an atrial myxoma—utilizing extracorporeal circulation. Since then cardiac tumors have been diagnosed and successfully excised from all chambers of the heart, a fact that is all the more important because of the frequently excellent prognosis with certain types of neoplasms. Of the cardiac tumors, metastatic lesions are most frequent, followed by primary benign lesions, and least common are primary malignant neoplasms.[19, 23]

Cardiac tumors, whether benign, malignant, or metastatic, produce clinical manifestations that vary with the location and size of the tumor and depend particularly upon whether or not cardiac function is compromised. In addition, intracavitary tumors produce bizarre symptoms mimicking a systemic illness. On occasion, these tumors are manifested initially by a peripheral arterial embolus or possibly an *immune reaction* to the tumor itself. Apart from this, cardiac tumors may continue to grow undetected, and it is interesting that more than 80 per cent of these neoplasms are first discovered at autopsy.[17] It is imperative, therefore, that the clinician be fully aware of the various presenting clinical manifestations.

## METASTATIC NEOPLASMS

The most frequent cardiac tumors are of *metastatic* origin. Metastases to the heart may occur with all types of malignant diseases and spread is by direct extension or hematogenous or lymphatic routes.[9, 15] Melanomas have a definite propensity for vascular spread to the myocardium, where they may appear as tumor implants in as many as 50 per cent of cases.[17] In spite of limited cardiac lymphatic connections,[19] lymphatic spread of bronchogenic and mammary carcinoma to the heart has been reported in over 25 per cent of cases in which dissemination has occurred. The spread within cardiac lymphatic channels is often retrograde. Metastatic infiltrates within the myocardium occur in over 15 per cent of cases of lymphoma and leukemia.[17] Direct cardiac extension of tumors from mediastinal structures or the surrounding lung also occurs. The pericardium is usually involved, and manifestations of acute pericarditis may appear. Associated pericardial friction rubs, hemorrhagic effusions with possible tamponade, and, on electrocardiogram, elevated ST segments and decreased voltage may be seen.

Metastatic tumor to the heart should be suspected in any patient with a known malignant neoplasm in whom signs of cardiac irregularity, electrocardiographic changes, or heart failure develops. Lack of cardiac dysfunction does not exclude cardiac metastasis, however. Relatively small tumors may produce complete heart block if they involve the atrioventricular node, and yet metastatic tumors may become quite large without producing signs or symptoms. Thus, the heart may compensate for a purely space-occupying lesion if critical areas are not compromised. Bisel[3] has reported a 21 per cent incidence of cardiac metastasis in patients dying of malignant disease, but only approximately 10 per cent of affected patients have symptoms.[17] Diagnosis may be facilitated by careful examination of pericardial fluid cell buttons, by pneumopericardiography following carbon dioxide injection into the pericardial space, or by direct biopsy of the lesion.

For metastatic tumors of the heart, treatment is palliative. Chemotherapy and irradiation have been tried with little benefit. Pericardicentesis for accumulated fluid provides temporary relief with improved cardiac filling. Rarely, pericardiectomy is indicated for treatment of metastatic pericarditis.

In addition to abnormalities due to direct involvement of the heart by metastasis, malignant carcinoids may affect the heart without actual mechanical invasion.[8] The overall manifestations of this endocrine-secreting tumor are discussed in detail elsewhere. Cardiac effects are of interest, however, because of their association with collections of fibrous tissue seen in the valvular cusps and endocardium, predominantly on the right side of the heart. Although the tumor actively produces serotonin (5-hydroxytryptophan), there is no evidence that the cardiac lesions are directly related to the production of this agent. Metastatic involvement of the liver is almost always encountered in patients with related cardiac abnormalities. Cardiac disturbances secondary to pulmonic stenosis or tricuspid insufficiency predispose to the development of right-sided heart failure. Because of the advanced state of the tumor when cardiac symptoms become manifest, chemotherapy directed at the carcinoid is of questionable benefit in alleviating the effects of the malignant neoplasm on the heart.

## BENIGN NEOPLASMS

Benign tumors constitute 70 per cent of primary neoplasms of the heart; approximately half of them are myxomas. Lipomas, angiomas, teratomas, fibromas, hemartomas, and leiomyomas are rare benign cardiac neoplasms seen usually as incidental findings at autopsy.[14] Death from complete heart block or cardiac compression, however, has been reported with these tumors.[4,13]

*Rhabdomyoma* is the most common cardiac tumor seen in infancy and childhood. More than 50 per cent of cases occur in association with tuberous sclerosis.[12] The tumor may be seen as single or multiple, ill defined, grayish nodules within the myocardium. It is thought to be the result of a disturbance in glycogen metabolism leading to a glycogenic infiltration of the myofibrils. Characteristically, the nodules appear on histologic examination as areas of myofibril degeneration, with a prominent vacuolated cytoplasm surrounding the centrally placed nucleus. Rather than a true tumor of the heart, it is considered more a form of isolated glycogen storage disease. Death, frequently of undetermined cause, is seen in over 50 per cent of cases during the first year of life. The diagnosis of this histologically benign tumor should be suspected in infants with tuberous sclerosis in whom cardiac symptoms develop. With no specific therapy available, treatment in these cases is symptomatic.

Clinically, *myxomas* constitute the most significant of all cardiac neoplasms.[16] Not only are they the most common intracavitary tumor but also, once they are diagnosed, the probability of surgical cure is excellent. Although approximately 75 per cent originate in the left atrium and some 20 per cent in the right atrium, myxomas have been successfully removed from all chambers of the heart. Myxomas are more commonly found in females and have been diagnosed in all age groups. A familial tendency has recently been noted.[18]

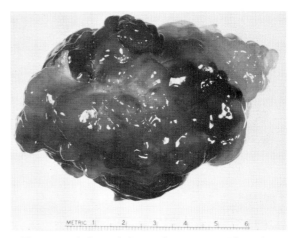

**Figure 1** A large left atrial myxoma with an irregular, glistening contour. A histologic section of this myxoma is shown in Figure 3.

Myxomas characteristically arise from a portion of the interatrial septum on a rim of the fossa ovalis. The tumors are usually situated on a pedicle and may vary in size from less than 0.5 cm. to more than 10 cm. in diameter (Fig. 1). Although at one time thought to represent an organized atrial thrombus, myxomas are now considered to be true neoplasms. Grossly, they appear as a pale, gelatinous, extremely friable mass throughout which areas of calcification may be seen. Microscopically, the tumor is composed of fibroblasts scattered within a loose connective tissue stroma. Plasma cells and lymphocytes may be seen in all areas, and hemosiderin-laden macrophages are regularly found. Endothelium lines the outermost edges of the neoplasm. Glycoproteins and mucopolysaccharides form the main constituents of the tumor. Biologically, the tumor is benign, lacking the ability both to invade locally and to metastasize. It may thus grow slowly over a period of years without producing symptoms or may cause intermittent symptoms that are sometimes difficult to interpret. With left atrial tumors, especially the larger pedunculated ones, symptoms of left atrial obstruction may occur and may be erroneously attributed to mitral stenosis (Fig. 2). Recurrent pulmonary edema may be noted and is resistant to treatment. Murmurs of mitral stenosis or insufficiency may be heard, and a "tumor plop" sometimes confused with an open-

ing snap has been described coinciding with movement of the pedunculated mass within the atrium or across the semilunar valves. These findings may vary with positional change. Right atrial myxomas producing atrioventricular valvular obstruction are most often confused with constrictive pericarditis, tricuspid stenosis, or Ebstein's anomaly. Hepatic enlargement, mild to severe peripheral edema, and varying tricuspid murmurs have been demonstrated in this setting. Acute circulatory failure may result from sudden blockage of the tricuspid or mitral valve.

Small tumors frequently remain asymptomatic unless they embolize or produce systemic symptoms. In any large series of myxomas, a small percentage of patients present with initial symptoms of peripheral embolization. The diagnosis of myxoma is made on pathologic examination of the specimen at thrombectomy (Fig. 3). Systemic symptoms including recurrent fever, weight loss, arthralgia, and anemia may be encountered in these patients and suggest an inflammatory illness such as collagen-vascular disease, myocarditis, subacute bacterial endocarditis, or even acute rheumatic fever. Blood cultures, however, are usually negative, and the time course, intermittent symptomatology, and past history may help to differentiate the myxoma from a lesion of inflammatory etiology.

Patients with atrial myxomas may thus present

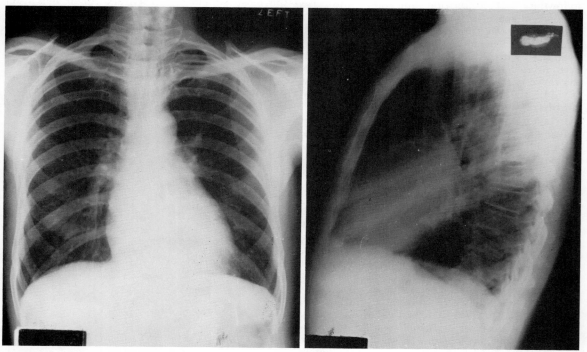

**Figure 2**　The calcified left atrial myxoma seen in the left lateral chest film was mistaken for the mitral valve. A roentgenogram of the removed myxoma is superimposed in the upper right corner. Although no calcium was present in the mitral valve, severe insufficiency was demonstrated. At the time of myxoma removal, the mitral valve was replaced with a ball valve prosthesis. The patient had had rheumatic fever as a young adult. (From Hattler, B. G., Jr., et al.: Ann. Thorac. Surg., *10*:65, 1970.)

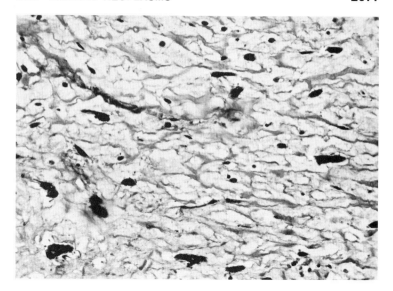

**Figure 3** A section of myxomatous material from a saddle embolus. × 150. The patient presented with an acute obstruction of the right femoral artery. Histologic examination of the embolized material established the diagnosis. A left atrial myxoma was successfully removed. (From Hattler, B. G., Jr., et al.: Ann. Thorac. Surg., *10*:65, 1970.)

with symptoms of peripheral embolization, atrioventricular valvular obstruction, or a systemic illness. In a consecutive series of 13 such patients, zone electrophoresis of serum proteins demonstrated elevated total globulin levels with prominent alpha-2, beta-1, or heterogeneous gamma globulin peaks. Immunoelectrophoresis localized the elevated globulins to either the IgM or IgA fractions. The levels return to normal with removal of the tumor (Fig. 4). Elevated erythrocyte sedimentation rates are usually seen. The electro-

cardiographic findings are usually nonspecific, although large right atrial P waves are sometimes seen in patients with right atrial tumors. Chest roentgenograms may be inconsistent, with a normal-sized heart evident in the presence of severe pulmonary venous and arterial congestion. Hemodynamic findings on cardiac catheterization and the analysis of pressure tracings are best correlated with the degree of atrioventricular valvular obstruction. Their value lies mainly in localizing the site of the disorder. The definitive method

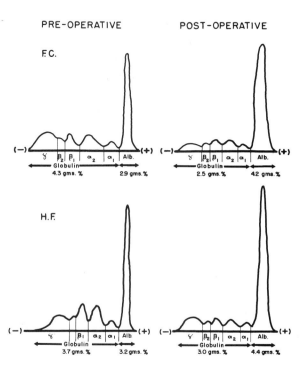

**Figure 4** Serum protein electrophoresis demonstrating prominent alpha-2, beta-1, and heterogeneous gamma globulin peaks in the preoperative specimens. Reversion to normal is demonstrated postoperatively. Both patients presented initially with recurrent fever, weight loss, and arthralgias, which cleared following tumor removal. (From Hattler, B. G., Jr., et al.: Ann. Thorac. Surg., *10*:65, 1970.)

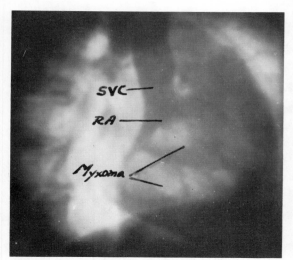

**Figure 5** Angiocardiogram following injection of contract medium into the superior vena cava (SVC). A large filling defect in the right atrium (RA) is demonstrated. A myxoma was removed the following day. (From Hattler, B. G., Jr., et al.: Ann. Thorac. Surg., *10*:65, 1970.)

of diagnosis is selective angiocardiography. In the series of cases of atrial myxoma mentioned earlier, angiocardiograms were diagnostic in all patients on whom the study was performed (Fig. 5), while cardiac catheterization without angiography was unsuccessful in establishing a diagnosis in two patients. Radioactive precordial scans utilizing radioiodinated serum albumin may demonstrate defects in the area of the myxoma.

## Management

Following diagnosis, all tumors should be surgically excised under direct vision with use of extracorporeal circulation. Operation should be performed promptly because of the constant threat of sudden death following any prolonged obstruction of the atrioventricular valve and the possibility of embolization. A right anterolateral incision provides ready access for incision into either the left or right atrium. During manipulation of these tumors, prophylaxis against embolization is accomplished by induction of ventricular fibrillation or temporary occlusion of the ascending aorta or both. Lavage of the atrium and ventricle aids in the removal of loose tumor fragments. Because invasion of the interatrial septum cannot be demonstrated at the point of origin of the myxoma, simple excision of the tumor base with only a superficial layer of the septum is generally performed, although recent reports describing recurrence of myxomas following simple excision imply that removal of an adjacent core of interatrial septum may be preferable.[1,10] Prognosis with surgery is excellent, and regression of all preoperative symptoms for follow-up periods of up to 10 years has been reported.

## MALIGNANT NEOPLASMS

The vast majority of primary malignant tumors of the heart are *sarcomas*.[22] With the exception of infants and children, in whom they are rarely found, these tumors are seen in persons of all ages and constitute approximately 20 per cent of primary cardiac neoplasms.[7] They originate most frequently from the endocardium or pericardium on the right side of the heart, occurring with equal frequency in the atrium and ventricle.[19] Grossly, neoplasms originating in the pericardium infiltrate diffusely, eventually obscuring the cardiac contour. Although an infiltrative lesion is commonly seen with tumors originating in the epicardium, intracavitary protrusions may also occur with more sessile forms of this neoplasm. Histologically, a wide range of sarcomatous tumors have been reported, with round cell and spindle cell sarcomas and angiosarcomas being most frequent. Metastatic spread is encountered in over 25 per cent of cases, with involvement of the mediastinum, lung, and pleura. More rarely, hematogenous spread to abdominal organs including the liver, kidney, and adrenals has been noted.[19]

Clinically, patients with primary sarcomas of the heart have progressive heart failure that generally is unresponsive to medical therapy. Because of preponderant involvement of the right side of the heart, symptoms of tricuspid valve or superior vena caval obstruction may predominate. Invasion of the conduction system produces arrhythmias or may result in complete heart block. With epicardial and pericardial extensions, a picture of bizarre, irregular cardiac enlargement is seen on chest roentgenograms or by pneumopericardiography in association with hemopericardium. In contrast to benign myxomas, in which angiocardiograms are diagnostic, intracavitary sarcomas are only occasionally revealed by angiocardiography. This may be attributed to the morphologic arrangement of the tumor, which is usually not pedunculated and has little or no free movement within the atrial or ventricular cavities.

A special malignant pericardial tumor is the *mesothelioma*.[20] It arises from the serous surface of the pericardium and is difficult to classify histologically. Both epithelial and connective tissue tumor components are seen microscopically with a frequently sarcomatous appearance intermingling in other areas with glandlike spaces or channels. Mesothelioma appears grossly as a flattened, nodular tumor mass spreading over the pericardium and resulting in voluminous hemorrhagic effusions. The clinical findings are those of pericarditis and tamponade. These highly malignant tumors grow rapidly and invade the surrounding myocardium. Distant metastases are commonly found.

Diagnosis of primary malignant cardiac tumors may be made from cytologic examination of pericardial fluid, but thoracotomy and direct biopsy may be required. With the exception of isolated reports, definitive therapy at the time of surgery is usually not possible. Symptomatic temporary relief can follow the removal of pericardial fluid or the excision of large space-occupying lesions. Further palliation may be obtained with drug and radiation therapy.[11] Death usually occurs within the first year following the onset of symptoms.

## SELECTED REFERENCES

Freiman, A. H.: Cardiovascular disturbances associated with cancer. Med. Clin. N. Amer., 50:733, 1966.
*This article considers in a concise fashion cardiac abnormalities that may arise as a result of either direct involvement of the heart by metastatic tumor or secondary mechanisms associated with cancer that alter the function of the heart. It emphasizes the various clinical manifestations the clinician may encounter and the pitfalls to be avoided.*

Gerbode, F., Keith, J. W., and Hill, J. D.: Surgical management of tumors of the heart. Surgery, 61:94, 1967.
*This concise, well illustrated article describes the technical aspects and surgical management of 10 patients with tumors of the heart. Eight myxomas, one teratoma, and one fibroma were surgically excised. Recurrence of myxoma was noted in one case 4 years after simple excision. The recurrent tumor was removed along with a portion of atrial septum; the authors now recommend this procedure to insure against recurrence.*

Hattler, B. G., Jr., Fuchs, J. C. A., Cosson, R., and Sabiston, D. C., Jr.: Atrial myxoma: an evaluation of clinical and laboratory manifestations. Ann. Thorac. Surg., 10:65, 1970.
*The diagnosis and management of 13 cases of atrial myxoma are reviewed. Emphasis is placed on the varied clinical manifestations these tumors may produce. Changes in the electrophoretic pattern of the serum proteins, with elevation in gamma globulins, are features of diagnostic importance that return to normal after excision of the myxoma. In 11 of the 13 patients the tumor was diagnosed correctly and managed by surgical excision.*

Prichard, R. W.: Tumors of the heart: review of the subject and report of one hundred and fifty cases. A.M.A. Arch. Path., 51:98, 1951.
*The article presents a general discussion of tumors of the heart, together with a report of 146 secondary and four primary cardiac neoplasms. Each type of tumor is reviewed at least briefly, and abundant gross and microscopic illustrations are included. The compilation of data and the references to works published up to that time make this paper a ready source of information.*

Whorton, C. M.: Primary malignant tumors of the heart. Cancer, 2:245, 1949.
*The paper presents a review of 100 cases of primary sarcomatous tumors of the heart. Discussion of their localization, histology, and metastatic spread is amplified by a table concisely listing each case with its salient features and literature references.*

## REFERENCES

1. Bahl, O. P., Oliver, C. G., Ferguson, T. B., Schod, N., and Parker, B. M.: Recurrent left atrial myxoma: report of a case. Circulation, 40:673, 1969.
2. Barnes, A. R., Beaver, D. C., and Snell, A. M.: Primary sarcoma of the heart: report of a case with electrocardiographic and pathological studies. Amer. Heart J., 9:480, 1934.
3. Bisel, H. F., Wroblewski, F., and La Due, J. S.: Incidence and clinical manifestations of cardiac metastases. J.A.M.A., 153:712, 1953.
4. Brandes, W. W., Gray, J. A. C., and MacLeod, N. W.: Leiomyoma of the pericardium: report of a case. Amer. Heart J., 23:426, 1942.
5. Columbus, M. R.: De Re Anatomica. Paris, 1562, Libri XV, p. 482.
6. Crafoord, C.: Case report. In: International Symposium Cardiovascular Surgery. Detroit, Henry Ford Hospital, 1955, p. 202.
7. Dong, E., Hurley, E. J., and Shumway, N. E.: Primary cardiac sarcoma. Amer. J. Cardiol., 10:871, 1962.
8. Freiman, A. H.: Cardiovascular disturbances associated with cancer. Med. Clin. N. Amer., 50:733, 1966.
9. Gassman, H. S., Meadows, R., Jr., and Baker, L. A.: Metastatic tumors of the heart. Amer. J. Med., 19:357, 1955.
10. Gerbode, F., Keith, J. W., and Hill, J. D.: Surgical management of tumors of the heart. Surgery, 61:94, 1967.
11. Goldstein, S., and Mahoney, E. B.: Right ventricular fibrosarcoma causing pulmonic stenosis. Amer. J. Cardiol., 17:570, 1966.
12. Goyer, R. A., and Bowden, D. H.: Endocardial fibroelastosis associated with glycogen tumors of the heart and tuberous sclerosis. Amer. Heart J., 64:539, 1962.
13. Grant, R. T., and Camp, P. D.: A case of complete heart block due to an arterial angioma. Heart, 16:137, 1932.
14. Griffiths, G. C.: Primary tumors of the heart. Clin. Radiol., 13:183, 1962.
15. Hanbury, W. J.: Secondary tumors of the heart. Brit. J. Cancer, 14:23, 1960.
16. Hattler, B. G., Jr., Fuchs, J. C. A., Cosson, R., and Sabiston, D. C., Jr.: Atrial myxoma: an evaluation of clinical and laboratory manifestations. Ann. Thorac. Surg., 10:65, 1970.
17. Hurst, J. W., and Cooper, H. R.: Neoplastic disease of the heart. Amer. Heart J., 50:782, 1955.
18. Magovern, G. J.: Discussion of Hattler, B. G., Jr., Fuchs, J. C. A., Cosson, R., and Sabiston, D. C., Jr.: Atrial myxoma: an evaluation of clinical and laboratory manifestations. Amer. Thorac. Surg., 10:65, 1970.
19. Prichard, R. W.: Tumors of the heart: review of the subject and report of one hundred and fifty cases. A.M.A. Arch. Path., 51:98, 1951.
20. Reals, W. J., Russman, B. C., and Walsh, E. M.: Primary mesothelioma of the pericardium. A.M.A. Arch. Path., 44:380, 1947.
21. Steinberg, I., Dotter, C. T., and Glenn, F.: Myxoma of the heart: roentgen diagnosis during life in three cases. Dis. Chest, 24:509, 1953.
22. Whorton, C. M.: Primary malignant tumors of the heart. Cancer, 2:245, 1949.
23. Yater, W. M.: Tumors of the heart and pericardium. Arch. Intern. Med., 48:627, 1931.

# XIV

# Cardiac Pacemakers

*William M. Chardack, M.D.*

Some accounts of the use of electrical currents to elicit contraction of the heart muscle date back to the eighteenth century, but the era of modern pacemaking began in 1932 when Hyman established the concept of pacing,[12] that is, the repetitive delivery of an electrical impulse that depolarizes only cardiac tissue adjacent to the electrode. The remainder of the myocardium is then acti-

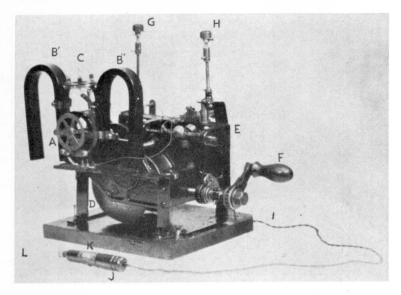

**Figure 1**  Artificial pacemaker consisting of a hand-operated magnetogenerator (A) and an electrode needle (L). (From Hyman, A. S.: Arch. Intern. Med., *50*:289, 1932.)

vated by a propagated action potential. The pulse generator and needle electrode developed by him (Fig. 1) were cumbersome but adequate for clinical use, which he thought of as being in the domain of resuscitation from cardiac arrest. At that time, the serious nature of heart block complicated by asystole had been known for more than a century, but another 20 years elapsed before Zoll, in 1952, successfully treated the condition by repetitive electrical stimuli applied to the chest wall.[27] External pacemakers operating through surface electrodes gained immediate acceptance, but the painful side effects of the high voltages required by this technique made it difficult to use on a long-term basis.

With the development of open heart surgery in the early 1950s, control of the heart rate became of great interest to surgeons because the inadvertent induction of heart block during the repair of intracardiac defects was then a not infrequent and often lethal complication; cardioaccelerating drugs were unsatisfactory, but the management of this complication was dramatically improved by the introduction of myocardial wires sutured to the myocardium and brought out through the chest wall at the time of operation.[26] The currents required to pacemake through such wires are below the threshold of sensation.

This approach stimulated the development of small battery-powered external pacemakers and of silicone rubber-insulated bipolar electrodes[11] and the application of pacing techniques to patients with other types of chronic heart block. About the same time, early clinical trials with pacing via transvenously placed endocardial electrodes were reported.[8] However, long-term pacemaking with electrodes traversing the skin had limitations because of the risk of infection and accidental disconnection and the inconvenience of an externally worn apparatus. Two solutions to these problems were developed.

Partially implanted pacemaker systems were introduced in 1959, consisting of an externally worn pulse generator coupled by radio-frequency waves[1,9] or by induction through the intact skin to an implanted receiver and electrode system. Other investigators pursued the concept of a completely implanted system, and the first successful long-term clinical use of a self-contained pacemaker carrying its own power supply was reported in 1960.[4] Since then, this approach has become the treatment of choice for chronic heart block.

In the ensuing decade, increasingly sophisticated instrumentation has been developed. Implanted pacemaker systems operating through transvenously placed endocardial electrodes became popular in 1963,[24] and soon thereafter implantable devices were introduced, the output of which was programed from spontaneous atrial[20] or ventricular electrical activity.[22] A recent report of the clinical use of a nuclear energy-powered pacemaker marked the introduction of an implantable power source with an extremely long life.[15]

Temporary and permanent pacing techniques are now frequently used to treat arrhythmias other than block, and temporary pacing has become an important tool in the postoperative care of cardiac and other surgical patients.

The surgeon is most commonly involved in the management of chronic atrioventricular block by implantation of a pacemaker system and this topic will be discussed first.

## ETIOLOGY AND CLINICAL FEATURES OF ACQUIRED CHRONIC HEART BLOCK

Most patients with this disease are elderly; about two-thirds are over 70 years old, and the ratio of males to females is 2:1. The incidence of the disorder has been estimated at 6.3 patients per 100,000 population per year, or about 13,000 new cases per year in the United States. Increasing longevity of the population and greater diagnostic awareness of the problem suggest a higher incidence in the future.

The etiology of chronic heart block is still the subject of controversy. Histologic findings suggest that about 40 to 50 per cent of cases are caused by degenerative fibrous and calcific changes—probably related to the aging process—either of the conduction system itself or in the closely adjacent fibrous cardiac skeleton.[16,17] There is convincing evidence linking the entity of chronic atrioventricular block in the elderly to bilateral bundle branch block, the so-called "hemiblocks," and "trifascicular blocks." Several of these entities, caused by various combinations of block in the distal branches of the bundle of His, are known to be precursors of complete block.[14] Recent techniques of recording an endocardiac electrogram (through a transvenously placed electrode) from various portions of the conduction system make it possible to localize accurately the site of the block.[19] They may also lead to a more precise classification of block than that based on the conventional electrocardiogram, which distinguishes between: (1) first degree block (prolongation of the atrioventricular conduction time); (2) second degree block (occasional dropped beats; higher grade block with 2:1, 3:1 atrioventricular conduction); and (3) complete block (atrial and ventricular activity are independent).

The role of coronary artery disease in the genesis of heart block is changing. Autopsy data reported in the past have shown only inconspicuous involvement of the coronary arterial tree, but current clinical experience reveals an increase in the number of patients in whom permanent block is a direct sequela of an acute myocardial infarction. Heart block complicates about 8 per cent of acute infarctions, and in only a few of these does it become a permanent residual, but because of the high incidence of acute myocardial infarction, it may cause as many as 5000 cases of block per year in the United States. This estimate may be low because improvements in coronary care by monitoring and pacing techniques are beginning to improve the chances for survival of patients in whom block complicates an acute infarction.

Chronic block can also be caused by focal and diffuse lesions observed in a wide variety of diseases—rheumatic heart disease, myopathies, and bacterial and parasitic infections, to list but a few.

Atrioventricular block may be permanent or intermittent; episodes of complete or higher degrees of block can alternate with periods of normal conduction or lesser degrees of block. The features of the disease are caused by bradycardia (a slow subsidiary pacemaker substitutes for the sinus node), which is compensated for by an increase of the stroke volume, leading to dilatation and hypertrophy of the heart. When the rate falls to below 40 beats per minute, stroke volume approaches its maximum and cardiac output be-

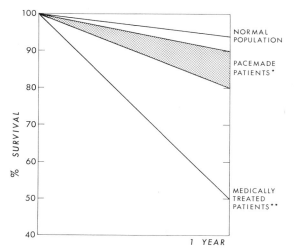

**Figure 2** Comparison of per cent survival at the 1 year point in chronic acquired heart block. The asterisk indicates range of percentages from several large series. The double asterisk indicates average of percentages in several series of medically treated patients. (From Chardack, W. M. In: Gibbon, J. H., Jr., Sabiston, D. C., Jr., and Spencer, F. C., eds.: Surgery of the Chest. 2nd ed. Philadelphia, W. B. Saunders Company, 1969.)

comes entirely rate-dependent. Decompensation occurs, first under the stress of physical activity and then at rest. Cardiac output is then subnormal, the arterial pulse pressure and the arteriovenous oxygen difference are high, and secondary renal and cerebral manifestations make their appearance.

The occurrence of syncopal attacks (Adams-Stokes or Morgagni-Adams-Stokes syndrome) is the cardinal feature of the disease. Syncope is caused by the sudden reduction of cardiac output and cerebral blood flow. The underlying mechanism may be bradycardia, asystole, ventricular tachycardia, or ventricular fibrillation, and one or more of these may be observed in any one patient. Normal conduction may prevail between syncopal episodes. Tachyarrhythmias not caused by block also may produce syncope, and syncopal attacks unrelated to cardiac disease may occur in patients with low-degree block and erroneously be ascribed to the latter. Continuous recording of the electrocardiogram may be required to establish the cause of syncope.

The natural course of chronic acquired heart block is unpredictable. Drug therapy has been unsatisfactory, and the ominous prognosis of the condition is well known. Without pacemaking, the mortality rate at the end of the first year following appearance of symptoms requiring treatment is between 50 and 60 per cent[3] (Fig. 2).

## OPERATIVE INSTALLATION OF AN IMPLANTED PACEMAKER SYSTEM

Implantable pacemaker systems consist of a pulse generator and the electrode(s) (Figs. 3 to 8).

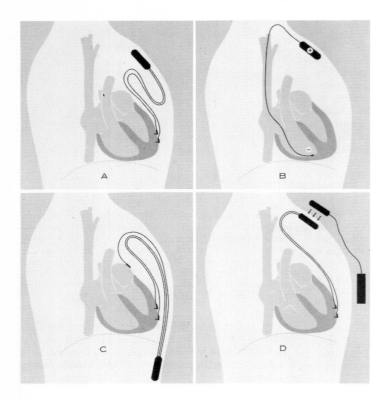

**Figure 3** Diagram of pacemaker systems. *A*, Bipolar myocardial electrodes. Pulse generator in subcutaneous tissues of chest wall. *B*, Unipolar endocardiac electrode. Pulse generator in subcutaneous tissues of chest wall. *C*, Synchronous (atrial-programed) pulse generator. Note sensing electrode on left atrium. *D*, Partially implanted system. Note external transmitting coil placed over implanted receiver.

**Figure 4** Patient with implanted myocardial-electrode pacemaker system. Pulse generator is in the subcutaneous tissues beneath the lateral margin of the pectoralis major muscle. (From Chardack, W. M. In: Gibbon, J. H., Jr., Sabiston, D. C., Jr., and Spencer, F. C., eds.: Surgery of the Chest. 2nd ed. Philadelphia, W. B. Saunders Company, 1969.)

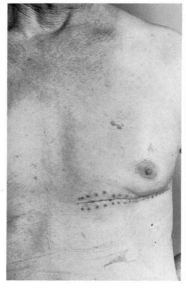
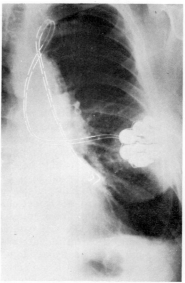

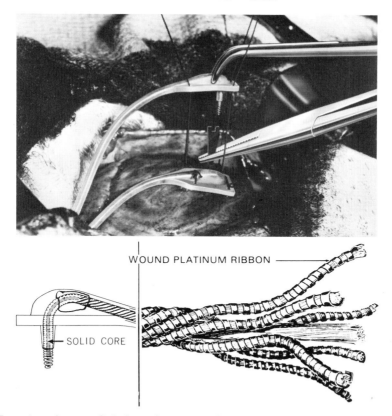

WOUND PLATINUM RIBBON

SOLID CORE

**Figure 5**  *Top,* Insertion of myocardial electrode (retouched). A stab wound is made on a bare area of the myocardium, the electrode point is advanced into the myocardium, and sutures are tied down. (From Chardack, W. M. In: Gibbon, J. H., Jr., Sabiston, D. C., Jr., and Spencer, F. C., eds.: Surgery of the Chest. 2nd ed. Philadelphia, W. B. Saunders Company, 1969.) *Bottom,* Details of electrode construction showing a solid platinum core, which strengthens platinum-iridium spring tip. Electrode lead consists of six intertwined platinum ribbons wound around Dacron cores.

Virtually all pulse generators currently in use are powered by zinc-mercuric oxide batteries. A transistorized electronic circuit regulates the emission of the electrical impulses. The components are encapsulated in various materials compatible with body tissue. The electrical pulse, roughly rectangular, ranging between 4 and 7 volts and lasting about 1 millisecond, is transmitted to the myocardium by either a myocardial or an endocardiac electrode (Figs. 3 to 8). This may be a single electrode structure (unipolar), which is used as the cathode (Fig. 3B) and the electrical circuit is completed either by a metal plate on the pulse generator or by the metallic housing of the pulse generator itself (anode) (Fig. 8), or a bipolar electrode, with both anode and cathode terminals on or in the heart (Figs. 5 and 7).

Implantation of pacemaker systems operating through myocardial electrodes requires thoracotomy or an extrapleural approach, usually with general anesthesia. Installation of a transvenously placed endocardiac electrode attached to a subcutaneously placed pulse generator can be carried out under local anesthesia. A variety of pulse generators are now available for use in combination with different electrode systems, and typical instrumentation is summarized in Table 1 and shown in Figures 3 to 8.*

The indications for installation of a permanent pacemaking system for acquired chronic block are: (1) permanent block, complete or incomplete, with syncope or congestive failure or both; (2) symptomatic intermittent block; (3) permanent postsurgical block, symptomatic or not; and (4) acquired heart block with low rates but apparently symptomatic. The last indication is controversial, but in practice only an exceptional patient with a very slow rate is truly asymptomatic. Pacemaking prolongs survival, and once heart block is present symptoms soon appear and sudden death often occurs. The indications for implantation of a pacemaker therefore should be liberal.

---

*The instrumentation used in these illustrations is the one in the development of which the author has participated and which is manufactured by Medtronic, Inc., Minneapolis, Minnesota. Other United States manufacturers of pacemaker systems are: Cordis, Inc., Miami, Florida; General Electric Company, Milwaukee, Wisconsin; Electrodyne, Inc., Boston, Massachusetts; American Optical Company, Boston, Massachusetts; among others.

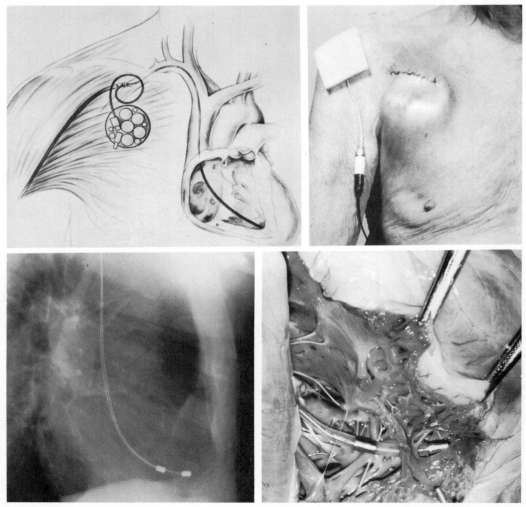

**Figure 6** *Top left,* Schematic drawing of endocardiac approach. Electrode is inserted through right cephalic vein found in deltopectoral groove. (From Furman, S.: Ann. Surg., *164:*465, 1966.) *Top right,* Photograph of patient shortly after operation. Monitoring electrode is taped to right shoulder. *Bottom left,* X-ray showing anterior direction of endocardiac electrode. *Bottom right,* Interior of right ventricular cavity showing electrode wedged into trabeculations. Electrode was inserted for demonstration purposes only in the course of an autopsy on a patient who had no heart block. (From Chardack, W. M., et al.: Progr. Cardiovasc. Dis., *9:*105, 1966. Reprinted by permission.)

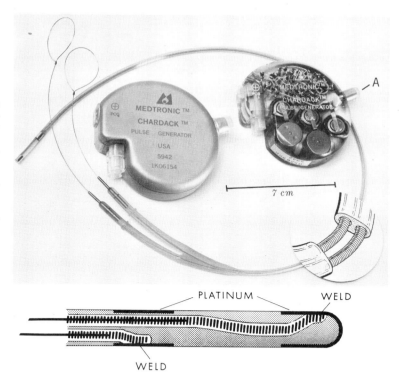

**Figure 7** Implantable demand pulse generator in titanium housing, which shields against radiated external electromagnetic fields (*left*). Circuitry and batteries are encapsulated in epoxy (*right*). Protuberance (A) contains a potentiometer, which controls the rate of stimulation. It can be adjusted by percutaneously inserting a needle of triangular cross section into this control. The electrode shown is a bipolar endocardial electrode. Stylets are removed after positioning of the electrode.

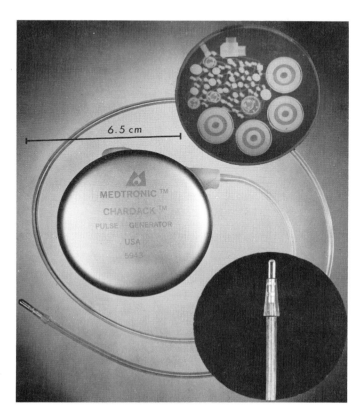

**Figure 8** Implantable demand pulse generator with monopolar electrode. Titanium housing serves as anode. X-ray shows that details of batteries are still discernible. Changes in their cross-sectional appearance permit a rough estimate of remaining capacity. Electrode tip is made of platinum and has a silicone rubber flange to facilitate retention of position.

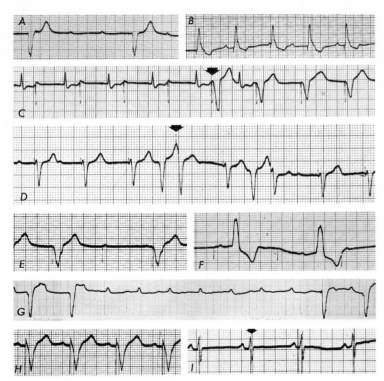

**Figure 9** Commonly encountered electrocardiographic patterns in heart block and pacing. *A,* Complete heart block. *B,* Asynchronous pacing (stimulus has no relationship with P wave.) *C,* Competitive rhythm. Runs of conducted depolarizations (first five on left) alternate with runs of pacemade beats (last three on right). The arrow shows a pacemade beat interspersed between two conducted depolarizations, leading to a summation of rate. *D,* Competitive rhythm caused by extrasystoles. First three complexes on left are pacemade, the fourth is an extrasystole, and the next pacemaker stimulus (arrow) falls into the vulnerable period after extrasystole. In this particular patient, this phenomenon was innocuous for many years. Extrasystoles during the postoperative period should be suppressed. *E,* Intermittent pacing. Second stimulus from left fails to depolarize. In this case, intermittency was caused by perforation, *F,* Complete failure to pace. None of the three stimuli depolarize. This may be because of inadequate pulse generator output, electrode displacement, or perforation. *G,* Long period of asystole during interruption of pacing. Note that this occurred even though the driving rate of the pacemaker was slightly below 60. *H,* Complete heart block corrected by synchronous pacemaking. Note constant time relationship between stimulus and preceding P wave. *I,* Resumption of normal conduction during synchronous pacemaking. Pacemaker stimulus (arrow) falls into absolute refractory period. (From Chardack, W. M. In: Gibbon, J. H., Jr., Sabiston, D. C., Jr., and Spencer, F. C., eds.: Surgery of the Chest. 2nd ed. Philadelphia, W. B. Saunders Company, 1969.)

**TABLE 1** FULLY IMPLANTED PACEMAKER SYSTEMS

1. *Electrodes*
   Endocardiac  ⎫
   Myocardial   ⎬ Unipolar or bipolar configuration
2. *Pulse generators*
   A. Asynchronous (independent of atrial and ventricular rate)
      Fixed-rate (although rate may be adjustable)
   B. Programed
      (1) Atrial-programed
          (P-wave synchronous, programed from atrial potentials)
      (2) Ventricular-programed
          (a) Ventricular-suppressed (true demand pacemaker)
              Detects spontaneous QRS, which suppresses output of pulse generator (does not fire during normal sinus rhythm)
          (b) Ventricular-triggered
              Spontaneous QRS triggers pulse generator and stimulus falls into absolute refractory period (fires during normal sinus rhythm)

## THORACOTOMY AND INSTALLATION OF A MYOCARDIAL-ELECTRODE PACEMAKER SYSTEM

Under general anesthesia, a left anterolateral thoracotomy is performed through the fifth intercostal space or through the bed of the resected fifth rib. The pericardium is incised anterior to the left phrenic nerve. The electrode(s) is affixed to a bare area of the left ventricular myocardium as shown in Figure 5. The pericardium is closed over the electrode leads with a small aperture left for drainage and with care to keep the phrenic nerve out of the immediate vicinity of the electrode. The pulse generator is then attached and placed subcutaneously either into a subcostal or more commonly now into a retropectoral position (Fig. 4). The chest is drained for 24 hours.

## Important Considerations in the Management of Patients Treated by Thoracotomy

Preoperative pacing by a temporary endocardiac electrode should always be used. It permits correction of congestive failure and electrolyte imbalance and an operation on a well prepared patient. The temporary electrode also provides a high stimulation rate during certain phases of the operative procedure. Stimulation at a rate of about 100 beats per minute, suddenly interrupted, is followed by a controllable period of asystole which facilitates the installation of the electrode (Fig. 9G). This structure is subject to flex stresses at a rate of 80,000 to 100,000 duty cycles per 24 hours, and attention to details of placement and fixation is essential.

If a bipolar electrode system is used, the terminals are placed side by side on an avascular area of the left ventricle. The distance between the two electrode pins is not critical. An avascular area can usually be found near the apex of the left ventricle (Fig. 5).

The subcutaneous pocket for the pulse generator should be tight enough to avoid rotation of the apparatus and should be drained for 24 hours by a catheter brought out through a separate stab wound. Prophylactic antibiotic therapy is advisable to protect against infection, especially that caused by coagulase-positive staphylococci.

Several modifications of operative techniques have been devised to avoid entrance into the pleural cavity by either an upper abdominal or a subcostal transdiaphragmatic approach.

## Management of Postoperative Complications

The pleural, pulmonary, and pericardial complications incident to a thoracotomy and pericardiotomy may have to be managed. Persistence of congestive failure may require drug therapy and a faster stimulation rate if the pulse generator allows adjustment of the rate. An important complication is the occurrence of runs of premature ventricular extrasystoles and multifocal ectopic activity (Fig. 10A and B). Myocardial injury and irritability, advanced dilatation and failure, and digitalis intoxication compounded by a low serum potassium concentration may play a part in the genesis of this complication. It should be treated immediately and aggressively by antiarrhythmic agents, restoration of a normal electrolyte pattern, and, if needed, an increase in the pacing rate (Fig. 10C).

Early infection around the implanted system is rare and usually caused by a coagulase-positive staphylococcus. It leads to an increase of the pacing threshold, often beyond the capabilities of the pulse generator. Aspiration and local and systemic administration of antibiotics is rarely successful. Exteriorization of the pulse generator is indicated, followed by implantation of a new permanent system at a different site.

Stimulation of the phrenic nerve(s), manifested by twitching of the upper abdomen and lower chest, is caused by too close a proximity of the nerve to the electrode current field. It may subside but if persistent and symptomatic it can be corrected by crushing or transposition of the nerve.

In the past, the most common complication was

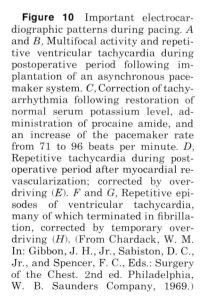

**Figure 10** Important electrocardiographic patterns during pacing. *A* and *B*, Multifocal activity and repetitive ventricular tachycardia during postoperative period following implantation of an asynchronous pacemaker system. *C*, Correction of tachyarrhythmia following restoration of normal serum potassium level, administration of procaine amide, and an increase of the pacemaker rate from 71 to 96 beats per minute. *D*, Repetitive tachycardia during postoperative period after myocardial revascularization; corrected by overdriving (*E*). *F* and *G*, Repetitive episodes of ventricular tachycardia, many of which terminated in fibrillation, corrected by temporary overdriving (*H*). (From Chardack, W. M. In: Gibbon, J. H., Jr., Sabiston, D. C., Jr., and Spencer, F. C., Eds.: Surgery of the Chest. 2nd ed. Philadelphia, W. B. Saunders Company, 1969.)

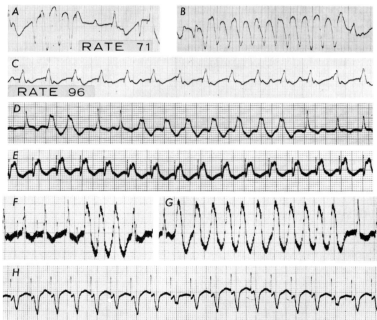

breakage of the electrode. If only one lead of a bipolar system was affected, the complication could be corrected by transforming the broken lead into an indifferent subcutaneous electrode. Currently available electrodes have a flex resistance far in excess of requirements, and disruption of an electrode lead should be exceptional.

The pulse generator requires periodic replacement under local anesthesia when the batteries are near the end of their life. Infection may follow such secondary operation. The electrode leads are by then firmly encapsulated by a tight sleeve of fibrous tissue, and extension proximally of the infection and loss of pacing are infrequent. The pulse generator should be exteriorized and worn as an external apparatus as long as the electrode leads remain intact (applicable only to bipolar systems).

## INSTALLATION OF AN IMPLANTED ENDOCARDIAC-ELECTRODE PACEMAKER SYSTEM

The technique and instrumentation for this approach are illustrated in Figures 3 and 6 to 8. Installation can be performed under local anesthesia. The electrical conductors of the electrode leads are one or two coils of a corrosion- and flex-resistant nickel or similar alloy. They terminate in a platinum ring and tip (bipolar) or in a tip only (unipolar). Stiffness and curvature required for insertion of the electrode are provided by removable stylets (Figs. 7 and 8).

For patients with a clearly established indication, installation of a permanent endocardiac system can be the first therapeutic step since it carries the same risk as the insertion of a temporary electrode. Support of the heart rate during insertion of the electrode is required rarely, usually only for a few minutes, and can be accomplished with an intravenous solution of isoproterenol (1 mg. in 500 ml. of 5 per cent dextrose). The rate of administration must be carefully titrated to avoid myocardial irritability. An intravenous solution of procaine amide (1 gm. in 250 to 500 ml. of normal saline) should be readily available. Positioning of the electrode requires an image intensifier, and in many centers the entire procedure is performed in the cardiac catheterization unit. Facilities must be available for monitoring the electrocardiogram and for defibrillation.

The right or left cephalic vein is now most commonly used, since this approach requires only one incision (Fig. 6). If this vein is inadequate in size, either the left or right external jugular vein can be used. If an internal jugular vein must be used, it should not be ligated, and the electrode entrance should be closed by a purse-string suture. The electrode with its stylets in place is guided into the right ventricle and advanced into the trabeculations of the apex. Accurate wedging of the electrode tip into the trabeculae of the right ventricular apex is essential (Fig. 6). Contact between the electrode terminals and the endocardium is critical and must be demonstrated not only by a satisfactory position of the electrode but also by the presence of appropriately low stimulation thresholds. An endocardiac electrogram recorded from the electrode may be helpful. Placement into the coronary sinus should be avoided unless specifically intended for atrial stimulation. To rule out a position in the coronary sinus, fluoroscopy in the lateral position and an endocardiac electrogram may be required. After placement of the electrode, the stylets are removed and the pulse generator is attached to the electrode terminal(s) and placed in a subcutaneous or retropectoral pocket. The pocket should be drained for 24 hours, and prophylactic antibiotics are recommended. Anticoagulants are not required.

### Complications of the Endocardiac-Electrode Pulse-Generator System

Because of the elimination of thoracotomy and general anesthesia, the endocardiac technique has a low postoperative mortality rate; however, it has its own characteristic complications:

1. Only a few instances of septicemia and mycotic infections have been reported, even though part of the system resides in the bloodstream.

2. Disruption of the electrode leads is also rare. The flex stresses on the endocardiac electrode are less severe than those on a myocardial electrode.

3. Perforation of the right ventricular myocardium or the interventricular septum can be caused by manipulation at insertion or later by erosion, resulting in one or more of the following: loss of pacing, pericardiac rub, diaphragmatic contractions, and electrocardiographic patterns indicating left ventricular activation. None of these are pathognomonic, and their presence will depend upon the position of the electrode terminals in relation to myocardium. Tamponade following perforation has been exceptional, but it can be acute and require decompression by pericardiocentesis or thoracotomy. In most cases, the complication can be corrected by withdrawal of the electrode after its entrance site into the vein in the neck has been exposed.

4. Air embolism has occurred during insertion of an endocardiac electrode. In the reported cases, the complication remained harmless, but it should be kept in mind for prophylaxis and therapy.

5. Thromboembolic phenomena were conspicuously absent in early reports covering large series,[3] although prophylactic anticoagulants had not been used. More recently, thrombosis of the right atrium, the superior vena caval system, and the axillary and jugular veins and pulmonary embolizations have been observed. In some cases, congestive failure may have been a contributory cause. These complications have been rare, but they should be kept in mind because angiography can help with an early diagnosis, and surgical intervention may be warranted. Also, embolization may occur when an endocardiac electrode is withdrawn.

It is likely that thrombi form around most, if not all, endovascular and endocardiac electrodes, as can be demonstrated by venograms. As time goes by, organization of the thrombus occurs, resulting in a fibrous sheath around the electrode and incorporation of the latter into the endothelium and endocardium. This sheath is covered by an outer endothelial layer which may be important in preventing thrombosis and embolization in the majority of cases.[3]

6. The most common complication of the endocardiac approach is dislodgment of the electrode followed by loss of pacing. This has been reported in most series, with an incidence of 10 to 18 per cent. Usually dislodgment occurs in the early days or weeks following operation, and the electrocardiogram should be continuously monitored for a few days and longer if this can be done by telemetering techniques that do not interfere with mobilization of the patient. Displacement can often be corrected by repositioning of the electrode under local anesthesia. Late displacement of the electrode is uncommon, probably because of the firm attachment between the electrode and the endocardium.

It is held by some that the incidence of electrode dislocation can be decreased by increasing proficiency of the operator; others believe that these complications must be considered an inherent and, at least with currently available electrodes, unavoidable feature of the endocardiac approach.

## TRANSVENOUS ENDOCARDIAC VERSUS MYOCARDIAL ELECTRODES (THORACOTOMY)

Some authors recommend the exclusive use of the endocardiac-electrode system, whereas others prefer thoracotomy for all patients. The author's own position is intermediate and can be summarized as follows: the endocardiac system, installed under local anesthesia, has a low initial mortality rate which makes it ideal for the very elderly, that is, for a considerable number of those who require treatment. Reported hospital mortality has varied from 0 to 3 per cent. Thoracotomy, on the other hand, has an overall mortality rate of 7.5 per cent.[24] The endocardiac approach is obviously indicated for patients in whom a thoracotomy would carry a high risk for reasons other than age or when thoracotomy is precluded because a previously installed myocardial system has become infected.

The complications of the endocardiac approach are usually correctable under local anesthesia by repositioning of the electrode or by replacement of the entire system. The potential risk associated with the long-term presence of an endovenous and endocardiac structure remains unknown. Tricuspid valvular disease is certainly a contraindication. Major thromboembolism has been rare, but the absence of microembolization over long periods of time has yet to be demonstrated. The endocardiac approach should therefore be avoided in children and in adults with a relatively long life expectancy,

and one must remember that the most common complications of the endocardiac system—albeit correctable under local anesthesia—are a potential hazard to life because of the associated cessation of pacing. Small as the risk may be, it should not be imposed upon patients in whom thoracotomy can be carried out with negligible risk. Where the line should be drawn in terms of chronologic and physiologic age must be determined by clinical judgment and cannot be specified by a rule of thumb.

## INSTALLATION OF SYNCHRONOUS AND PARTIALLY IMPLANTED PACEMAKER SYSTEMS

A synchronous pacemaking system is programed from atrial activity and requires an additional electrode to sense the atrial potential (Fig. 3C). The most commonly practiced surgical approach consists of a left anterolateral thoracotomy and fixation of the sensing electrode to the atrium. Because of the popularity of the endocardiac electrode, synchronous pacemaking systems have also been installed by a transvenously placed atrial electrode and a second ventricular endocardiac electrode. Curved and hooked atrial electrodes have been devised for placement into the atrial appendage, and a sensing electrode placed close to the atrium by mediastinoscopy has also been used. The long-term reliability of these techniques remains to be demonstrated.

Partially implanted systems transmit electrical energy through the intact skin by radio-frequency waves or induction coupling.[1, 9] The receiver is implanted (Fig. 3D) and may be a myocardial electrode, an endocardiac electrode, or a miniaturized receiver with prongs directly attached to the myocardium. The advantage of a partially implanted system is that replacement of the pulse generator does not entail another operation, but the patient must wear an external appliance, the transmitting coil of which must remain secured to the skin in proximity to the implanted receiver. This requires constant watching, and rehabilitation is incomplete. For this reason, partially implanted systems have seen much less clinical application than fully implanted devices.

## PERMANENT PACING FOR CONGENITAL AND SURGICALLY INDUCED HEART BLOCK

Congenital block has been thought to occur mostly in association with congenital cardiac defects, but now it is known that it is an isolated entity more often than was suspected. In congenital block, the QRS is often narrow; this indicates a high location of the subsidiary pacemaker. The rate is relatively high (40 to 60 beats per minute) and increases during exercise. Physical work capacity can be close to normal, and the prognosis is said to be good. This classic picture does not always obtain, and congenital block can produce congestive failure, Stokes-Adams attacks, tachyarrhythmia, and death, particularly in the neonatal period or under the stress of exercise and intercurrent disease. A number of young children with congenital block, some in the neonatal period, have been treated with implanted pacemakers. This therapy should be considered if there is a history of syncope, especially in the very young child, if the QRS is wide (low idioventricular pacemaker), or if the block is diagnosed in utero.

With better knowledge of the anatomy of the conduction system, the incidence of block following repair of cardiac defects has been reduced (to about 1 per cent) but it remains high (about 13 per cent) following operations on the aortic valve. The immediate management of this complication is pacemaking through myocardial wires. In about two-thirds of the cases, return of conduction can be expected to occur within several weeks because the block is caused by hemorrhage, edema, and ischemia rather than by severance of the conduction bundle.

The outlook for survival is poor when a surgically induced heart block remains a permanent sequela, and implantation of a pacemaker is indicated whether or not symptoms are present.

## PERMANENT PACING FOR SINUS ARREST, SINOATRIAL BLOCK, AND SINUS DISEASE

These entities may produce symptoms because of slow or arrested impulse formation in the sinoatrial node, blocked conduction from the node to the atrium, or episodes of bradycardia alternating with tachycardia. Correction by an implanted pacemaker system is then indicated. In some patients, an atrial driving site has been used to preserve atrioventricular synchrony. Before selecting an atrial driving site, one must remember that sinus disease is frequently associated with or followed by atrioventricular conduction disturbances. These can be brought to light by preliminary atrial pacing[13] and by His bundle electrograms.[19] The use of ventricular-programed demand pacemakers is advantageous in such patients since the pulse generator is suppressed during periods of adequate sinus impulse formation.

## PERMANENT PACING FOR TACHYARRHYTHMIAS NOT ASSOCIATED WITH BLOCK

Temporary pacing alone or in combination with antiarrhythmic or beta-adrenergic blocking drugs has been shown to be effective in suppressing a variety of ventricular and supraventricular tachyarrhythmias not associated with block (Fig. 10D to G), and therefore implanted systems have been used in patients in whom such rhythm disturbances were uncontrollable by medication

alone.[3, 7, 24] Maintenance of a moderately rapid rate ("overdriving"), faster than the normal sinus rate but slower than the rate during the episodes of tachycardia, suppresses the emergence of ectopic foci. In patients in whom atrioventricular conduction is normal, pacing from an atrial site is preferable. A few cases of uncontrollable supraventricular tachycardia have been managed by surgical division of the conduction bundle and installation of a pacemaking system.

## CLINICAL RESULTS

There is agreement that long-term pacing prevents Stokes-Adams attacks regardless of the mechanism of their genesis. Pacing relieves, or palliates, congestive failure and the cerebral and renal symptoms induced by bradycardia. Opinion remains divided as to the degree of restoration of normal hemodynamics in these patients. Improvement is striking in many patients, but the gains are questionable in others, depending upon age and the degree of coexistent impairment of myocardial infarction. Data extending now over a period of more than a decade support the conclusion that, in addition to palliation, pacing significantly increases survival (Fig. 2).[3]

## INSTRUMENTATION FOR LONG-TERM PACING

### ELECTRODES FOR LONG-TERM PACING

A limited increase (after initial installation) in the threshold current required to initiate depolarization has been observed with every type of electrode. This is due to scar tissue around the electrode (and some degree of displacement in the case of an endocardiac electrode). The result is an increase in the distance between electrode and responsive myocardium and a corresponding decrease in current density at the latter. In the presence of infection, fluid accumulation around the electrode results in a greater separation between it and myocardium. A high current threshold is then observed. The absolute values of voltage or current required to set off a propagated action potential late in diastole (aside from the properties of myocardium) depend upon electrode surface, polarity, and metal and duration of the stimulus. In regard to conservation of battery life (while maintaining an adequate margin of pulse-generator output over threshold requirement), a pulse duration of approximately 0.8 millisecond appears to be most useful.

The respective advantages of unipolar and bipolar electrode configurations have been the subject of much discussion. Unipolar cathodal threshold voltages are slightly lower than those of bipolar electrodes. The advantages of a bipolar configuration are redundancy, two opportunities instead of one to find a lower threshold (important mainly for endocardiac electrodes), and their lesser sensitivity to external electrical fields. Since pulse generators now are shielded against interference and electrode fracture is rare, there is little to choose between unipolar and bipolar electrode configurations.

Polarization and electrolytic corrosion effects on electrode metal are important considerations and support the choice of biphasic pulses and of platinum terminals for bipolar configurations. In unipolar configurations, the anodal surface should be large and the active cathode in the myocardium be made of platinum since polarization is reduced (efficiency increased) and electrical thresholds with this material have been shown to be stable over periods in excess of 10 years.

## PULSE GENERATORS

### Asynchronous Pulse Generators

Asynchronous pulse generators, the first to be developed, supply electrical stimuli at a fixed rate independent of the atrial and ventricular activity. Although the rate is fixed, in some pulse generators it may be adjustable by a switch actuated by an external magnet, providing a low and a high stimulation frequency. Others incorporate a control permitting adjustment of the rate by puncture with a percutaneous needle (Fig. 7). The ability to increase the pacing rate may be desirable in a few patients in whom one wishes to suppress ectopic activity or to increase cardiac output in the presence of myocardial failure. The circuitry of asynchronous pacemakers is the simplest one, and their current consumption is lower than that of the more sophisticated types of pulse generators.

### Programed Pulse Generators

**Atrial-Programed Pulse Generators ("P wave synchronous").**\* These require an additional electrode (Fig. 3C) to sense the atrial potential, which, amplified, triggers the pulse generator to deliver a stimulus to the ventricle after a set PR interval. To prevent tachycardia triggered from the atrium, a blocking circuit with a 2:1 reduction slows the rate of stimulation when the atrial signals occur at frequencies above 120 beats per minute. If the atrial potentials are inadequate, or if the atrial impulse formation is abnormally slow, the pulse generator reverts to a fixed rate of about 60 to 70 stimuli per minute.

**Ventricular-Programed Pacemakers.** Ventricular-programed pacemakers respond to any spontaneous QRS potential appearing at the electrode. The same electrode is used to carry the output stimulus from the pulse generator. Two types of ventricular-programed pulse generators are in clinical use.

VENTRICULAR-SUPPRESSED (TRUE DEMAND) PULSE GENERATORS. Any spontaneous QRS potential appearing at the electrode resets the tim-

ing circuit of the pulse generator; for instance, if the device is set to a stimulation frequency of 60 pulses per minute, it will emit pulses at 1 second intervals as long as there is no spontaneous ventricular activity. However, if a depolarization, ectopic or conducted, occurs before the end of the 1 second escape interval, it recycles the pulse generator and suppresses the output for another cycle of 1 second duration. Therefore, as long as spontaneous depolarizations occur at a beat-to-beat rate in excess of 60 per minute, the pulse generator remains quiescent. If none occur before the end of a 1 millisecond cycle, the pulse generator will escape, emit a stimulus, and continue to do so in the absence of further spontaneous ventricular electrical activity (Fig. 11 A to C).

The purpose of ventricular-programed pacemaker systems is to preclude competitive rhythms from either conducted or ectopic depolarizations, a phenomenon that can occur with asynchronous pacemakers (Fig. 8C and D). The ventricular-suppressed pulse generator precludes delivery of a stimulus into the vulnerable period (following a spontaneous depolarization) and avoids the hemodynamic consequences of competitive rhythms. During periods of normal conduction, its output is suppressed; this reduces current drain. In order to demonstrate that the pulse generator is operational during these periods, an external magnet is applied that switches the device into fixed-rate operation (Fig. 11C).

VENTRICULAR-TRIGGERED PACEMAKERS. Ventricular-triggered pacemakers differ from true demand pacemakers in that the R wave triggers emission of a stimulus following a short delay so that it falls into the absolute refractory period. If there is no spontaneous ventricular activity within a preset interval, the pulse generator escapes and produces a stimulus. In ventricular-triggered pacemakers during normal sinus rhythm, the stimulus artifact can be seen in the absolute refractory period on the electrocardiogram (this makes interpretation difficult; Fig. 11D), but this does not insure that the stimulus is adequate to elicit depolarization were it needed. The current drain of ventricular-triggered pulse generators is high since they emit a pulse even during periods of normal sinus rhythm, and they require protection, by a refractory period, against external electrical signals, which could accelerate the stimulation rate of these devices to a dangerous level.

A discussion of the respective merits of various types of pacemakers hinges upon the consideration of the hemodynamics during artificial pacing and the risks entailed by the pacing stimulus itself (see later).

### Reliability of Pulse Generators

During the first years after the development of implanted pacemaker systems, electrode failure was the predominant cause of system malfunction. As this problem was eliminated, the pulse-generator power supply became the factor limiting the life of the system. Development of a better

---

\*Model Atricor, manufactured in the United States by Cordis, Inc., Miami, Florida.

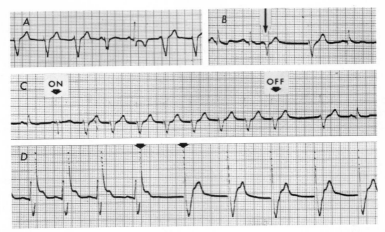

**Figure 11** Electrocardiographic patterns with ventricular-programed pacemakers. *A*, Three pacemade beats on left followed by a fusion beat and a conducted depolarization. The latter suppresses output of pacemaker, which does not appear until present interval has elapsed. *B*, Normal sinus rhythm—first two complexes on left. At the arrow, a ventricular extrasystole occurs and is followed by a pause that exceeds the programed cycle of the demand pulse generator. The next depolarization is pacemade, and the last (right) is again a normally conducted beat that suppresses pacemaker output. *C*, Normal sinus rhythm, pacemaker output suppressed, first complex on left. Between arrows, external magnet is applied and device functions as a fixed-rate pulse generator. All depolarizations are pacemade, and when the external control is turned off (arrow, right), a preautomatic pause follows, exceeding the standby interval. The next depolarization is therefore pacemade, and then the normal sinus rhythm (last complex on right) suppresses pacemaker output again. *D*, Ventricular-triggered standby pacemaker. First four depolarizations (left) are conducted, and pacemaker pulse is directed into the absolute refractory period. Pressure is then applied to the carotid sinus, cardiac rate falls below the standby cycle, and the five depolarizations (beginning at second arrow) are pacemade. (From Chardack, W. M. In: Gibbon, J. H., Jr., Sabiston, D. C., Jr., and Spencer, F. C., eds.: Surgery of the Chest. 2nd ed. Philadelphia, W. B. Saunders Company, 1969.)

power source remains the most pressing problem. Virtually all commercially available pulse generators are powered by mercuric oxide-zinc batteries.* At body temperature, the chemical processes in the batteries are accelerated, and internal losses occur that reduce the net capacity available to the pulse generator. Up to now, fixed-rate pacemakers had to be replaced at the end of approximately 30 months, and most programed pulse generators had an "end-of-life" failure after 22 to 24 months. Some of the causes leading to the premature end of life of the batteries have been identified, and the cells now in use should yield a longer life, albeit one that still falls short of the initial expectations of 4 to 5 years.

Because of the disappointing performance of the batteries, efforts have been made to predict impending failure of the pulse generator by oscillographic evaluation of the pacemaker stimulus potential as it appears on the surface of the body or by a measurement of the relative margin of pacemaker output over threshold requirement.[7, 21, 23–25] Specialized pacemaker clinics and the telephone transmission of the electrocardiogram or the pacemaker potential, or both, have been used to follow patients with implanted devices.[7, 21, 24, 25] Up to now the most important parameter in the follow-up has been the rate, since most pulse generators are programed for a decrease in the stimulation rate as the battery voltage drops. Recently, emphasis has been placed on an increase of pulse

width as battery voltage drops. The purpose of this is to provide an additional end-of-battery-life indicator and to compensate for decreasing pulse amplitude by an increase in pulse duration, thus maintaining capture as the battery nears exhaustion (Fig. 15). The author's practice has been oriented toward periodic prophylactic replacement of pulse generators based on performance data obtained from clinical experience and by placing representative numbers of pulse generators into a saline solution at body temperature. The various follow-up methods should be facilitated by the adoption of the pulse-width increase compensating for beginning battery depletion.

In addition to "end-of-life" failure of the pulse generator, malfunction due to component failure can occur. This is rare and mostly has led to intermittency or cessation of pacing and the resumption of an idioventricular rhythm. There have been instances in which the mode of failure was an inordinate increase in the rate, leading to tachycardia and in some cases to ventricular fibrillation. It must be emphasized that in all currently available circuitry, the failure of certain components can lead to an inordinate increase of the stimulation rate. The "runaway" pacemaker constitutes an acute emergency requiring immediate disabling of the malfunctioning unit and provision for resumption of pacing promptly.

In summary, the reliability and longevity of pulse generators has been improved, but their performance still falls short of initial expectations. Rechargeable batteries and bioelectric and piezo electric power sources are under experimental

---

*Mallory RM-1 cell, manufactured by Mallory Company, Tarrytown, New York.

evaluation, and nuclear energy-powered pulse generators are under initial clinical trial.[15]

## TEMPORARY PACEMAKING SYSTEMS

Instrumentation and techniques for temporary pacemaking of the heart have been summarized in Table 2. Selection of a technique should be based on the circumstances in a given case. If ample time is available, introduction of an endocardiac electrode either under fluoroscopy or by monitoring its position by the intracardiac electrogram should be considered. In an acute emergency, repetitive blows on the chest may be effective, and the percutaneous insertion of myocardial wires should be considered. This requires only a few seconds and materials, suture wires and a spinal needle, that are readily available in a hospital environment.

Temporary pacing techniques are important in the preoperative and operative management of patients with block who require installation or repair of a permanent pacemaking system. They have also been applied to conduction and other rhythm disturbances complicating acute myocardial infarction.

Temporary pacing is also used either to increase an inadequate cardiac rate and output or to suppress tachyarrhythmias in postoperative states following cardiac and general surgery[10] (Fig. 10D to H). In patients with normal atrioventricular conduction, an atrial stimulation site should be used. Temporary ventricular and atrial pacing by single or repetitive stimuli (alone or in combination with drugs) has been employed to control a variety of ventricular and supraventricular tachycardias.[7, 24] Controlled hypotension during surgical procedures can be induced by rapid packing, and atrial pacing at high rates has been used as a diagnostic procedure to bring to light latent disturbances of the atrioventricular conduction system.[13] Myocardial performance and the appearance of angina can be evaluated by electrically induced tachycardia.[24]

Pacing with paired electrical stimuli can slow the effective mechanical rate of the heart and induces postsystolic potentiation of cardiac contractility. The technique introduces a premature extrasystole into each cycle and creates a bigeminal rhythm in which mechanical ineffective beats alternate with potentiated effective contractions.

**TABLE 2** INSTRUMENTATION FOR TEMPORARY PACEMAKING

*External Electrodes*
  Painful, resuscitation only

*Endocardiac Electrodes*
  Repositioned by fluoroscopy or by following intracardiac electrogram

*Electrode Wires*
  Installed at time of cardiac operation.
  Introduced percutaneously through lumen of needle, advanced into right ventricle

The technique remains experimental, although the number of reported successful clinical trials is beginning to increase.[6]

## ELECTRICAL HAZARDS OF PACEMAKING

The potential hazards of electrical stimulation of the heart involve three mechanisms: (1) leakage of 60 cycle current from line-powered instruments connected to pacing electrodes; (2) potential hazards of the pacemaker stimulus; and (3) the effects of external electromagnetic fields on implanted devices.

### Leakage of Currents from Line-Powered Instruments

Pacing electrodes are low-resistant current pathways to the myocardium, and minute currents, of the order of 100 microamperes, can induce ventricular fibrillation. This danger is present when line-powered instruments are connected to an electrode, and if at the same time the patient is connected to a second line-powered instrument or in good contact with ground, such as through an x-ray table or an electrically powered bed. A case in point would be a patient paced with a line-powered pulse generator who then is connected to an electrocardiograph.

Only battery-driven devices should be connected to cardiac electrodes, and their terminals and connections to the electrodes should be protected against contact with potential sources of line current leakage. If a line-powered instrument must be used on a cardiac electrode (to obtain an endocardiac electrogram, for instance), it should be the only one in contact with the patient, and even then the hazard of ventricular fibrillation constantly must be kept in mind.

The dangers of line current leakage are always present with temporary electrodes traversing the skin and with permanent electrodes when they are being installed or exteriorized in the course of a pulse-generator exchange. With completely implanted devices, it is safe to use line-powered instruments, such as electrocardiographs and monitors.

### Hazards Arising from Pacemaker Stimulus

Ever since cardiac pacing was introduced, concern has been expressed about the risk of inducing ventricular fibrillation by the pacemaking stimulus itself. This possibility does not exist as long as the cardiac rhythm is dominated by the artificial pacemaker, because all stimuli are delivered in late diastole beyond the confines of the "vulnerable zone," which approximately coincides with the apex of the T wave. When there is competition between the artificial pacemaker and conducted or ectopic ventricular depolarizations, stimuli can fall into the vulnerable period following such an event (Fig. 9C and D). Extrasystoles and intermittent resumption of normal conduction commonly occur in pacemade patients.

Experimental data show that in the animal with

a presumably normal myocardium, fibrillation can be initiated by brief pacing stimuli falling into the vulnerable period, but high currents are required to produce this effect. The threshold of fibrillation exceeds the threshold of stimulation (late in diastole) by a factor of about 20.[5] In general, the currents required for fibrillation are beyond the output capabilities of implantable pulse generators. However, physiologic and pharmacologic interventions can reduce the margin between fibrillatory and stimulating pulses. Fibrillation is facilitated by large electrode surfaces, stimuli of long duration, alterations in electrolyte composition, acidosis, hypoxia, and adrenergic and other agents commonly administered to cardiac patients, such as large doses of digitalis. The fibrillatory threshold also drops sharply following ligation of a coronary artery that supplies a myocardial electrode site. However, the threshold of stimulation also increases considerably in the ischemic area.[5]

The margin of safety between the amplitude of a pacemaker stimulus and that required to provoke ventricular fibrillation varies with the time that has lapsed since implantation of the electrode. At installation, the threshold for stimulation is low and then rises (over 2 to 3 weeks) as the electrode matures. The output of the pulse generator must be set to anticipate this increase as well as fluctuations of the stimulation threshold related to physiologic and pharmacologic causes.[23] Immediately after implantation, it exceeds the stimulation threshold by a considerable margin, which then decreases.

A review of the reported clinical experience[5] leads to the conclusion that electrical parasystole can be dangerous either during temporary pacing for block complicating an acute myocardial infarction or in the early postoperative period following installation of a permanent pacemaking system. Under the latter circumstances, a high ratio between stimulus and threshold is present, and myocardial irritability may be high, especially in the presence of digitalis intoxication and a low serum potassium concentration. In most observations (linking ventricular fibrillation to pacing), competition was the result of premature ventricular extrasystoles and multifocal ectopic activity. This type of arrhythmia (Fig. 10A and B) is intrinsically dangerous (whether electrical stimuli are administered or not) and must be treated aggressively even when a demand pacemaker is used. Furthermore, the insertion of an electrode causes some injury to myocardial fibers in its vicinity, and the risk may be compounded when the procedure is performed in the presence of an unsuspected infarction or when a coronary occlusion supervenes as a postoperative complication.

The danger of electrical parasystole is remote in patients in whom the electrode has matured and the stimulation threshold has increased. Temporary return to normal sinus rhythm has been observed in 20 to 50 per cent of patients with implanted pacemakers, and the real incidence may well be greater since competitive rhythms are likely to escape documentation. Many thousands of patients with implanted fixed-rate pacemakers have now been observed for periods up to a decade, and uncountable stimuli have been delivered into the vulernable period. There is abundant evidence that such electrical parasystole is harmless in most cases. Pacemaker stimuli can be hazardous when the fibrillatory threshold decreases or the ratio between pacemaker stimulus and threshold is high. Because these circumstances are likely to be present in the postoperative period, ectopic ventricular activity and competitive rhythms should then be aggressively suppressed.

Pacemaker stimuli are also hazardous in the presence of an acute myocardial infarction when freshly placed electrodes are located in ischemic myocardium. Only demand pacemakers should be used in such patients, and excessive pulse amplitudes above threshold should be avoided.

### Hazards Arising from External Electrical Fields

There is considerable electrical and electromagnetic noise in the modern environment, and the effect of these fields on implanted pulse generators has been extensively studied. They vary with the source of interference and the type of pulse generator. Asynchronous pulse generators are insensitive to most environmental electrical fields. Ventricular-programed pacemakers, since they must respond to QRS potentials of a few millivolts, are more sensitive to external electrical fields, and interference with their output has been observed when patients were exposed to radiated electromagnetic energy, such as radio and television transmitters, microwave ovens, diathermy, automobile ignitions, electric razors, and fluorescent lights. These fields penetrate the implanted pulse generator. Ventricular-programed pacemakers can also be interfered with by conducted electricity, such as 60 cycle A.C. leakage current (below the level of sensory perception) from a faulty household appliance; these currents are sensed by the electrode. Protection of ventricular-programed pulse generators of current manufacture against radiated fields is obtained through shielding by the metal housing. In the presence of strong conducted currents, they will revert to fixed-rate operation.

In a medical environment, the electrical equipment that is most likely to produce interference with implanted pulse generators is electrosurgical and diathermy apparatus. To begin with, the latter should never be used on body areas overlying any implanted pulse generator because of the heating effect on the metallic components. Electrosurgical currents should not be used within 2 inches of even asynchronous and shielded programed pulse generators. Application in more distant areas may suppress the output of unshielded programed pulse generators of older manufacture. Patients still wearing devices of earlier types should be alerted to the hazards mentioned here.

## HEMODYNAMICS IN HEART BLOCK AND DURING ARTIFICIAL PACING

Oxygen demands of the body above the resting level are satisfied by an increase of cardiac output and of oxygen extraction from the blood. Cardiac output can be raised by an increase in the rate and the stroke volume. With maximal workloads, all three mechanisms—increasing rate, stroke volume, and oxygen consumption—come into play. In untrained man, adjustment to mild to moderate exercise is mediated chiefly by an increase in heart rate, but in the presence of a heart rate that is fixed or held constant, cardiac output can increase solely by a higher stroke volume.

In the experimental animal in which heart block has been induced, pacing at increasing rates shows that cardiac output is relatively constant except at the very low and very high rates. While cardiac output remains relatively constant over this range of rates, myocardial oxygen consumption increases as the rate goes up and efficiency decreases.[3]

Many studies have dealt with the hemodynamics in patients with pacemakers. In evaluating the results, one should keep in mind that cardiac output decreases and arteriovenous difference increases in the aged, whose exercise performance is often limited before the cardiorespiratory system is maximally stressed, and one must differentiate between the response observed following an abrupt change of the rate or the mode of pacing (atrial to ventricular, for instance) and that seen if such interventions are permitted to reach a steady or chronic stage. In many patients, some myocardial insufficiency is present, and therefore the reported observations show some variations.

In many studies made at rest and during exercise, increases in cardiac output were observed as the rate was raised by pacing. This increase occurred as the rate was raised from the slow idioventricular level to about 60 beats per minute, and, in general, cardiac output remained fairly constant from 60 to 110 beats, exhibiting a typical plateau type of curve. In other observations, cardiac output peaked between 70 and 90 beats and then decreased, and exercise produced only a negligible increment[3, 18, 24] (Fig. 12).

In regard to the energetics of the heart, an increase of cardiac output mediated by an increase in the stroke volume requires only a small increment of coronary blood flow and oxygen consumption, whereas increase of the output mediated by an increase of the rate requires large increments of these parameters. At slow rates, coronary arterial inflow is facilitated because of the long diastolic filling time. These considerations may be unimportant in regard to patients with block and relatively normal coronary arteries, but they are quite relevant to patients who have coexisting coronary artery disease. Patients with angina are known to tolerate poorly the higher driving rates that are produced by atrial-triggered pulse generators.[7]

In general, fixed-rate pacemaking at about 70 beats per minute has been satisfactory and has produced a reasonable exercise tolerance. With pacing, cardiac size and volume decrease and cardiac reserve is restored, since now stroke volume can be increased again as a response to stress. A rate of 70 per minute is usually more than adequate to suppress multifocal ectopic activity and runs of ventricular tachycardia and fibrillation that are associated with very slow idioventricular rates. There are occasional patients in whom such tachyarrhythmias (similar to those observed in patients without block—Fig. 10D to H) require higher driving rates in combination with drugs, and in a few patients with refractory competitive failure a faster rate may be of help.

## ASYNCHRONOUS VERSUS SYNCHRONOUS PACEMAKERS

With fixed-rate pacemakers, there is a limit to which cardiac output can increase in response to high workloads, but maximal performance is of little consequence in a group of patients of a mean age of 70 years. A fixed heart rate compels cardiac output to increase by augmenting stroke volume, which is less costly in energy than a rise in rate. Also, it has not been established that the rate response of the atrium by definition is an optimal response; in fact, it can be inappropriately high in many elderly patients and the "wisdom" of the node has been questioned.[7]

**Figure 12**   Cardiac output with increasing pacing rates. A, Peak response. B, Typical plateau (see text). (From McNally, E., and Benchimol, A.: Amer. Heart J., 75:380, 679, 1968.)

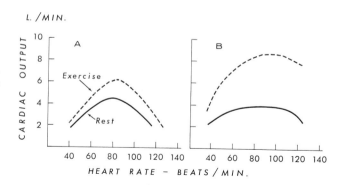

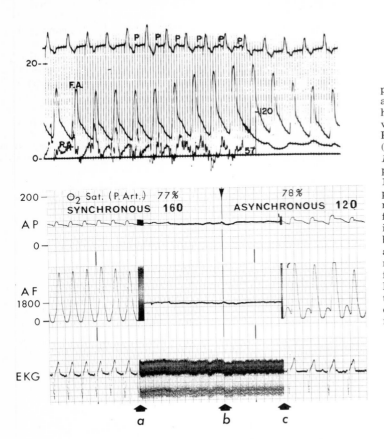

2/8/62

**Figure 13** *Top,* Electrocardiogram and pressures of femoral artery and right auricle during asynchronous pacing. Note higher pressure during cycles in which the ventricular stimulus happens to follow a P wave with an appropriate delay (P). (From Samet, P., et al.: Amer. J. Cardiol., *11*:594, 1963.) *Bottom,* Experimental comparison of synchronous pacing at rate of 160 beats per minute with asynchronous pacing at the slower rate of 120 beats per minute. Arterial pressure (AP), aortic flow (AF), and electrocardiogram recorded in an experimental animal with induced block. At *a,* slow paper speed is started and pressure and flow are recorded as mean values; at *b,* pacing is switched from synchronous to asynchronous mode. Paper speed increased again at *c.* Note that switch from synchronous to asynchronous mode has no significant influence on mean aortic pressure and flow.

**Figure 14** Diagram showing progression of conduction in the heart and the relationship between anatomic structures and the events observed in limb electrocardiogram and in an electrogram recorded from a transvenously inserted bipolar electrode positioned close to the conduction bundle (see text, page 2081, and references 14 and 19). SAN = Sinoatrial node, AVN = Atrioventricular node, BH = His bundle, RB = Right bundle branch, LB = Left bundle branch, (PD = posterior division; AD = anterior division).

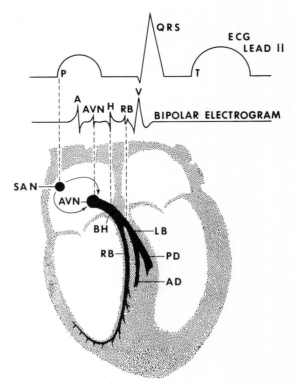

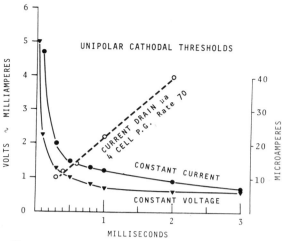

**Figure 15** Strength duration curve showing relationship between pulse duration and stimulus voltage (or current) required to depolarize from a myocardial electrode several months after implantation. Note that increasing pulse duration beyond 2 milliseconds does not lower threshold appreciably. Current drain on batteries increases linearly with pulse duration. Pulse generator functions with optimal efficiency at pulse durations from 0.5 to 0.8 millisecond (see text, page 2091).

In most experimental and clinical studies made to assess the contribution of atrioventricular synchronization to cardiac output, the performance parameters of a single ventricular contraction preceded by an appropriately timed atrial contraction are compared with a ventricular contraction that is out of phase with the preceding atrial event. Under these circumstances, a contraction with a normal atrioventricular timing always produces a higher output, and if the driving rate is close to the atrial rate, cyclic variations occur in pressure and cardiac output (Fig. 13). When one compares mean cardiac output and pressure during synchronous and those obtained with asynchronous driving at a slightly lower rate, the fluctuations become negligible, especially if the experiment is carried out long enough to allow physiologic feedback mechanisms to come into play (Fig. 13).[4]

Most studies show a difference in cardiac output between synchronous and asynchronous pacemaking of the order of 10 to 20 per cent related to the loss of atrioventricular synchrony and the dyssynergia of abnormal ventricular activation. Even if synchronous pacing could produce a small increase of cardiac output of the order of 10 per cent, this would not matter except at the uppermost and lowermost limits of the range of cardiac outputs. In younger patients with good myocardial function, a fixed rate of 70 is well tolerated, and in many patients with congenital heart block, even rates around 50 are adequate for a normal work capacity. It seems fair to conclude that both the loss of atrioventricular synchrony and dyssynergia produce experimentally demonstrable but limited reductions in cardiac output, which, in most patients, are of little clinical significance. They may be of importance in the presence of myocardial insufficiency.[2] Synchronous pacing or sequential pacing (delivering appropriately timed stimuli to the atrium and ventricle) may also be of value when temporary stimulation is required in the treatment of acute myocardial infarction complicated by block or tachyarrhythmia or both, especially when high driving rates are used, since atrioventricular coordination becomes more significant as the rate increases.

Synchronous pulse generators require instrumentation of greater complexity and, in order to protect against atrial-triggered tachycardias, they must provide for an automatic cutoff of the rate once a preset atrial rate is reached. This cutoff point varies between 120 and 150 beats, and it is questionable whether a sudden decrease of the heart rate during physical or emotional stress is always well tolerated. Synchronous pacing is contraindicated when there is an increase or a decrease in the frequency of atrial pulse formation and in the presence of angina.

It seems reasonable to conclude that although a pacemaker system programed from the atrium seems, at first glance, ideal because it accomplishes restoration of a normal physiologic state, in practice the gains have been more theoretical than practical, and for the majority of patients they do not warrant the increased complexity of the system and of its installation.

## THE PLACE OF VENTRICULAR-PROGRAMED PACEMAKERS

Pulse generators that are programed from ventricular activity are now used by many groups to the exclusion of other types. The purpose of ventricular-programed pacemaker systems is to preclude the delivery of a pacemaker stimulus into the vulnerable period as well as the hemodynamic consequences and the reduced efficiency inherent in a competitive rhythm. In regard to the risk of electrical parasystole, it is clear that external demand pacemaker systems should be the only ones used for temporary pacing for block complicating an acute myocardial infarction and in the suppression of various tachyarrhythmias when used in combination with otherwise dangerously high dosages of drugs.[5, 7] In regard to implanted pacemaker systems, the available evidence indicates that there is no significant hazard associated with electrical parasystole in patients with fixed-rate pulse generators. Long-term follow-up studies show that the life expectancy of patients with pacemakers approaches that of a comparable normal population. Since competitive rhythms are common in these patients, a substantial unexplained mortality rate should now be clearly evident if electrical parasystole were a substantial hazard. In the author's experience, there has been no significant difference in the incidence of sudden or unexplained deaths (which conceivably could have been caused by ventricular fibrillation) in patients with implanted fixed-rate pacemakers and those with implanted demand pulse generators in whom electrical parasystole is precluded.

In regard to the hemodynamic consequences of a competitive rhythm, they are tolerated well by most patients with pacemakers, although there are a few who exhibit symptoms probably because of a borderline functional cardiac competence. On the other hand, however negligible the risk and the loss of efficiency associated with electrical parasystole may be, it is clear that the principle of eliminating electrical stimulation when it is not needed is obviously sound, provided that the instrumentation required to do so does not introduce new hazards and failure mechanisms. The drawbacks formerly associated with demand systems, related to their sensitivity to external electrical fields, have now been virtually eliminated by the introduction of shielding. However, the circuitry of programed pulse generators requires a larger number of components than that for synchronous pacemakers, and their service life, at least up to now, has been shorter than that of asynchronous pulse generators. There is a clear-cut indication for demand systems for patients in whom sinus rhythm predominates and who experience only intermittent episodes of block. A demand pulse generator should also be used for the correction of intermittent sinus arrest, bradycardia, and sinoatrial block and for patients who have returned to a normal sinus rhythm following installation of a fixed-rate system and who either are symptomatic because of competition or require a change of their pulse generator. On the other hand, many elderly patients in apparently fixed chronic block can be satisfactorily and safely managed with asynchronous pulse generators.

## ACKNOWLEDGMENT

The clinical data used in this manuscript represent the combined experience of my associates and myself. I am indebted to Andrew A. Gage, M.D., Anthony J. Federico, M.D., and George Schimert, M.D., for their permission to include this material, and I am grateful to Miss Lillian R. Klinko for the technical assistance in the preparation of this text and to Mr. Harold C. Baitz, Chief, Medical Illustration Service, Veterans Administration Hospital, Buffalo, New York, for his assistance in the preparation of the illustrations.

## SELECTED REFERENCES

*Cardiac pacemakers have now been in clinical use for about a decade. The entire field of electrical control of cardiac activity is still under constant change and it involves the disciplines of surgery, cardiology, electrophysiology, and engineering. For a general review of the developments in this field, the reader is referred to:* Cardiac Pacemakers. Ann. N. Y. Acad. Sci., Volume 111, Number 3, June 1967; *and* Advances in Cardiac Pacemakers Ann. N. Y. Acad. Sci., Volume 167, Number 2, Oct. 1969. *These monographs contain numerous papers covering most aspects of pacing.*

*The views of the author have been set forth in greater detail in:* Cardiac pacemakers and heart block. In: Gibbon, J. H., Jr., Sabiston, D. C., Jr., and Spencer, F. C., eds.: Surgery of the Chest. 2nd ed. Philadelphia, W. B. Saunders Company, 1969. *The bibliography was up to date until 1969 and provides documentation of the views presented in this chapter.*

*Those who wish to study the subject in greater detail should consult:* Siddons H., and Sowton, E.: Cardiac Pacemakers, Springfield, Ill., Charles C Thomas, 1967; *and* Furman, S., and Escher, D. J. W.: Principles and Techniques of Cardiac Pacing. New York, Harper & Row, 1970.

*The reader interested in the electrocardiographic manifestations of pacing and their interpretation should review:* Kaster, J. A., and Leinbach, R. C.: Pacemakers and their arrhythmias. Progr. Cardiovasc. Dis., 13:3, 1970.

## REFERENCES

1. Abrams, L. D., Hudson, W. A., and Lightwood, R.: A surgical approach to the management of heart block using an inductive coupled artificial cardiac pacemaker. Lancet, 1:1372, 1960.
2. Braunwald, E.: Symposium on cardiac arrhythmias with comments on the hemodynamic significance of atrial systole. Amer. J. Med., 37:655, 1964.
3. Chardack, W. M.: Cardiac pacemakers and heart block. In: Gibbon, J. H., Jr., Sabiston, D. C., Jr., and Spencer, F. C., eds.: Surgery of the Chest. 2nd ed. Philadelphia, W. B. Saunders Company, 1969.
4. Chardack, W. M., Gage, A. A., and Greatbatch, W.: A transistorized, self-contained, implantable pacemaker for the long-term correction of complete heart block. Surgery, 48:643, 1960.
5. Chardack, W. M., Ishikawa, H., Fochler, F. J., Souther, S., and Gage, A. A.: Pacing and ventricular fibrillation. Ann. N. Y. Acad. Sci., 167:919, 1969.
6. Cranefield, P. F.: Paired pulse stimulation and postextrasystolic potentiation of the heart. Progr. Cardiovasc. Dis., 8:446, 1966.
7. Furman, S., and Escher, D. J. W.: Principles and Techniques of Cardiac Pacing. New York, Harper & Row, 1970.
8. Furman, S., and Robinson, G.: Stimulation of the ventricular endocardial surface in control of complete heart block. Ann. Surg., 159:841, 1959.
9. Glenn, W. W. L., Mauro, A., Longo, E., Lavietes, P. H., and Mackay, F.: Remote stimulation of the heart by radiofrequency transmission. New Eng. J. Med., 261:948, 1959.
10. Hodam, R. P., and Starr, F.: Temporary postoperative epicardial pacing electrodes—their value and management after open heart surgery. Ann. Thorac. Surg., 8:506, 1969.
11. Hunter, S. W., Roth, N. A., Bernardez, D., and Noble, J. L.: A bipolar myocardial electrode for complete heart block. J. Lancet, 79:506, 1959.
12. Hyman, A. S.: Resuscitation of the stopped heart by intracardiac therapy. II. Experimental use of an artificial pacemaker. Arch. Intern. Med., 50:283, 1932.
13. Imparato, A., Reppert, E., and Spencer, F.: Rapid atrial pacing to produce transient heart block: a preliminary report. Surgery, 63:198, 1968.
14. Lasser, R. P., Haft, J. I., and Friedberg, C. K.: Relationship of right bundle branch block and marked left axis deviation to complete heart block and syncope. Circulation, 37:429, 1968.
15. Laurens, P., and Piwnica, A.: Stimulateur cardiaque isotopique, recherche sur la sécurité et la fiabilité à long terme. Communication à la Société Française de Cardiologie, May 10, 1970. Arch. Mal. Coeur, 63:906, 1970.
16. Lenegre, J.: Etiology and pathology of the bundle branch block in relation to complete heart block. Progr. Cardiovasc. Dis., 6:409, 1964.
17. Lev, M.: The pathology of complete atrioventricular block. Progr. Cardiovasc. Dis., 6:317, 1964.
18. McNally, E., and Benchimol, A.: Medical and physiological considerations in the use of artificial cardiac pacing. Amer. Heart J., 75:380, 679, 1968.
19. Narula, O. S., Scherlag, B. J., Samet, P., and Javier, R. P.: Atrioventricular block—localization and classification by His bundle recordings. Amer. J. Med., 50:146, 1970.
20. Nathan, D. A., Center, S., Wu, C.-Y., and Keller, W.: An im-

plantable synchronous pacemaker for the long-term correction of complete heart block. Amer. J. Cardiol., 11:362, 1963.
21. Parsonnet, V., Myers, G. H., Gilbert, L., and Zucker, I. R.: Prediction of impending pacemaker failure in a pacemaker clinic. Amer. J. Cardiol., 25:311, 1970.
22. Parsonnet, V., Zucker, I. R., Gilbert, L., and Myers, G. H.: Clinical use of an implantable standby pacemaker. J.A.M.A., 196:104, 1966.
23. Preston, T., Fletcher, R., Lucchesi, B., and Judge, R.: Changes in myocardial threshold. Physiologic and pharmacologic factors in patients with implanted pacemaker. Amer. Heart J., 74:235, 1967.

24. Siddons, H., and Sowton, E.: Cardiac Pacemakers. Springfield, Ill., Charles C Thomas, 1967.
25. Thalen, H. J., van den Berg, J. S., van der Heide, J. H. N., and Nieveen, J.: The Artificial Cardiac Pacemaker—Its History, Development and Clinical Application. Springfield, Ill., Charles C Thomas, 1969.
26. Wierich, W. L., Gott, V. L., and Lillehei, C. W.: Treatment of complete heart block by combined use of myocardial electrode and artificial pacemaker. Surg. Forum, 8:360, 1957.
27. Zoll, P. M.: Resuscitation of the heart in ventricular standstill by external electric stimulation. New Eng. J. Med., 274:768, 1952.

# XV

# Surgical Pharmacology of the Cardiovascular System

*W. John Powell, Jr., M.D., and Willard M. Daggett, M.D.*

In this section, the pharmacology of low cardiac output states, cardiogenic shock, congestive heart failure, cardiac arrhythmias, and hypertension will be described. Discussions of the pharmacologic agents that act on the cardiovascular system can be found throughout other chapters within the context of the disease process described. This chapter is not intended to cover all aspects of cardiovascular pharmacology pertinent to the surgeon but rather emphasizes the treatment of pathophysiologic states commonly seen in patients with heart disease both before and after corrective cardiac surgical procedures.

left and right sides of the heart when assessing a patient with inadequate perfusion. This knowledge of intracardiac pressures is imperative to the selection of appropriate pharmacologic therapy. The recently developed Swan-Ganz flow-directed balloon catheter[30] has facilitated the continuous measurement of pulmonary capillary wedge pressure as an indirect index of left ventricular filling pressure. The measurement of central venous pressure as an index of right ventricular filling pressure is readily accomplished with an indwelling central venous cannula.

## LOW CARDIAC OUTPUT STATES

Inadequate cardiac output from a variety of causes may follow any cardiac surgical procedure. The first problem the surgeon faces in assessing this clinical situation is to determine the cause of inadequate peripheral perfusion. Measurement of cardiac performance is important in order to determine whether the low cardiac output has a myocardial basis or results from some other cause. In such patients with low cardiac output it is not uncommon to observe a discrepancy between left and right ventricular filling pressures, depending on which ventricle is more severely affected by the basic cardiac disorder. For example, in patients with coronary artery disease, left atrial pressure is frequently higher than right atrial pressure (Fig. 1). Conversely, in a patient with mitral valve disease and elevated pulmonary vascular resistance, the right-sided filling pressure frequently exceeds measured left atrial pressure. Thus, it is important to monitor filling pressures on both the

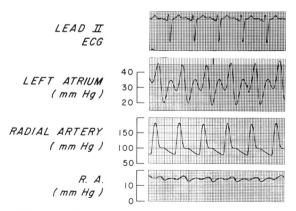

**Figure 1** Pressures recorded in a 52 year old male under anesthesia immediately after coronary artery bypass grafting. Mean left atrial pressure exceeds 30 mm. Hg, while right atrial (R.A.) pressure has a mean value of approximately 15 mm. Hg. This type of discrepancy between right-sided and left-sided filling pressures, depending on the basic cardiac disorder, underscores the need for measuring left- and right-sided filling pressures in critically ill postoperative patients.

Careful assessment of the state of ventricular filling provides a rational basis for treatment of inadequate cardiac output. The baseline requirement for the treatment of the low cardiac output syndrome is adequate intravascular volume. Such patients may require much higher ventricular filling pressures than would ordinarily be expected. It is not uncommon to observe improvement in cardiac output measured by the dye dilution technique following elevation of left atrial pressure to 20 mm. Hg by expansion of intravascular volume.[14] Similarly, in those instances in which right ventricular failure is very prominent, a central venous pressure of 20 to 30 cm. H₂O may be necessary for adequate cardiac output.

It is important to determine the arterial blood gas levels (pH, the pO₂, and the pCO₂) and to correct them if they are deranged. If the pH is low, this state should be corrected with the use of intravenous sodium bicarbonate, even if the amount of sodium that must be administered causes a slight volume overload of the circulation. Both a low pH and a low pO₂ substantially depress left ventricular function.

It is also important to monitor cardiac rhythm and to maintain heart rate within an optimal range (approximately 80 to 120 beats per minute). If a sinus bradycardia or atrioventricular block exists and the ventricular rate is slow, it is advisable to increase the ventricular rate through the use of ventricular pacing. If there is a supraventricular tachyarrhythmia, it is advisable to convert the tachyarrhythmia to sinus rhythm or to slow the ventricular rate response by appropriate therapy. Whenever possible, the sequence of an atrial contraction followed closely by a ventricular contraction should be maintained. The hemodynamic importance of an appropriately placed atrial contraction in increasing cardiac output in the acutely ill patient has been well documented.[16]

Sepsis must always be considered in a patient with poor perfusion, since this is an important potential cause of low cardiac output.

In severe low cardiac output states, inotropic support of the myocardium is usually required. Since the classification of catecholamine action by Ahlquist,[1] much insight has been gained into the mechanism of action of the various endogenous and synthetic sympathomimetic agents.[20] Ahlquist classified catecholamines according to their capability to act on the cardiovascular system at hypothetical sites known as *beta-adrenergic receptors* and *alpha-adrenergic receptors*. This concept provides a convenient way of classifying catecholamines according to their biologic effects (Table 1). Agents that act on beta-adrenergic receptors increase heart rate, increase strength of myocardial contraction (increase contractility), and dilate arteries. Catecholamines that act solely upon alpha-adrenergic receptors do not influence directly either heart rate or strength of myocardial contraction. The primary action of such agents is constriction of peripheral arteries and veins. Thus, all naturally occurring and synthetic catecholamines can be classified according to beta- or

**TABLE 1** CARDIOVASCULAR EFFECTS OF SELECTIVE ADRENERGIC RECEPTOR STIMULATION

|  | Alpha | Beta |
|---|---|---|
| Cardiac: |  | ↑ Heart rate |
|  |  | ↑ Contractility |
|  |  | ↑ Conduction velocity |
|  |  | ↑ Automaticity |
|  |  | ↑ Excitability |
| Vascular resistance: |  |  |
|   Coronary | ↑ | ↓ |
|   Skeletal muscle | ↑ | ↓ |
|   Abdominal viscera (excluding liver) | ↑ | ↓ |

alpha-adrenergic receptor stimulation or both. (See Table 2 for listing of catecholamines according to receptor site of action.)

In patients with the low cardiac output syndrome, intensive peripheral vasoconstriction may be counteracted (and peripheral blood flow thereby improved) by the administration of isoproterenol (Isuprel) by intravenous drip. This synthetic catecholamine, an essentially pure beta-adrenergic receptor stimulator, causes active vasodilation of systemic arterioles and pulmonary arterioles as well. In addition, the basic cause of peripheral vasoconstriction may be ameliorated by improvement in cardiac output secondary to enhancement of heart rate and myocardial contractile force by isoproterenol administration.[2] The substantial vasodilation produced by this drug frequently results in a translocation of blood volume peripherally and a decreased diastolic arterial pressure.[4] Therefore, following initiation of treatment with isoproterenol it is often necessary to reassess the status of ventricular filling and to increase central blood volume with blood, plasma, or albumin. Limitations to the amount of isoproterenol that can be delivered are related to its electrophysiologic effects. Isoproterenol increases rhythmicity, lowers threshold for pacemaker tissue, increases conduction velocity in Purkinje tissue,[9] and enhances excitability. Thus, marked increases in heart rate may attend higher doses of isoproterenol in association with either sinus tachycardia or a rapid ventricular response to atrial fibrillation owing to facilitation by this agent of atrioventricular con-

**TABLE 2** CLASSIFICATION OF CATECHOLAMINES ACCORDING TO ADRENERGIC RECEPTOR ACTIVITY

| Drug | Cardiac Effect | Peripheral Effect |
|---|---|---|
| Isoproterenol | Beta | Beta |
| Epinephrine | Beta | Beta – low dose / Alpha – high dose |
| Norepinephrine | Beta | Alpha |
| Metaraminol (Aramine) | Beta | Alpha |
| Phenylephrine (Neo-synephrine) | Alpha | Alpha |
| Methoxamine (Vasoxyl) | Alpha | Alpha |

| | Systemic Blood Pressure mm. Hg | Cardiac Output L./min. |
|---|---|---|
| 1. E − 2 μg./min. I − 0.8 μg./min. | 96 | 2.25 |
| 2. E − 4 μg./min. I − 0.8 μg./min. | 110 | 2.50 |
| 3. E − 2 μg./min. I − 8 μg./min. | 100 | 3.25 |

**Figure 2**  These data were obtained from a 48 year old woman 24 hours after mitral valve replacement. A severe low cardiac output state was present and the patient was oliguric and obtunded. The data clearly indicate the optimal dosage combination of epinephrine (E) and isoproterenol (I). The third combination, that is, 2 μg. epinephrine per minute and 8 μg. Isuprel per minute, led to a measurable improvement in cardiac output and marked improvement in the patient's clinical status. Inotropic support was continued for approximately 48 hours, after which it was gradually discontinued. Thereafter the patient recovered without incident. These types of data document the need for measurement of the hemodynamic effects of pressor agents or combinations thereof in any given patient.

duction across the atrioventricular node. The enhancement of excitability may lead to ventricular irritability at the higher doses. In patients with regional myocardial ischemia, ventricular irritability may be manifest at lower doses. Therapy with isoproterenol should be initiated at a dose of 1 to 2 μg. per minute delivered intravenously (1 to 2 mg. of isoproterenol in 250 cc. of dextrose and water).

Epinephrine is an endogenous catecholamine with mixed alpha- and beta-adrenergic stimulating effects.[26] This agent differs from isoproterenol in that, in addition to its capability for increasing strength of myocardial contraction and heart rate, it causes peripheral arterial and venous constriction at higher doses. Thus, arterial diastolic pressure is increased and peripheral vascular capacitance is decreased by high doses of epinephrine. The effect of epinephrine on heart rate is generally an increase, but may vary as a result of reflex vagal enhancement secondary to an increase in arterial pressure. Epinephrine, like isoproterenol, increases rhythmicity, lowers threshold, and enhances excitability. This agent also facilitates atrioventricular conduction. Ventricular irritability may complicate high-dose therapy with epinephrine but usually in a lesser degree than with isoproterenol. Therapy with epinephrine should be initiated at a dose of 1 to 2 μg. per minute delivered intravenously through a central venous cannula.

Although the vasodilatory capability of isoproterenol makes this agent the rational choice for treatment of low cardiac output, not all patients will respond favorably to this drug when it is used alone. The limitations of tachycardia, ventricular irritability, and decrease in coronary filling due to lower diastolic pressure limit the overall effectiveness of the agent. In many patients with low cardiac output, combinations of isoproterenol and epinephrine are required for an optimal balance

among cardiac output, peripheral blood flow, and perfusion pressure (Fig. 2). Underlying disease states often modify catecholamine requirements. Patients with chronic hypertension or arteriosclerosis may require higher perfusion pressures for adequate cerebral and renal blood flow. Patients with chronic congestive heart failure may require higher doses of catecholamines because of depletion of endogenous stores.[7]

Peripheral vasoconstriction in the presence of inadequate cardiac output may be so intense that additional specific pharmacologic agents are required. The catastrophic circle of events initiated by inadequate cardiac output and compounded by peripheral vasoconstriction often requires vigorous vasodilator therapy to break the chain of deterioration. Morphine given intravenously in increments of 5 to 10 mg.[17] may be of considerable aid in this regard, because of its effect on arterial smooth muscle.[18] Use of this agent in large doses will ordinarily require tracheal intubation and mechanical ventilation because of the resulting respiratory depression. Chlorpromazine, a direct alpha-adrenergic receptor blocking agent, has also been found to be particularly effective when arterial constriction is most intense. In such patients, chlorpromazine should be given in very small doses initially (1 mg. intravenously), since its effect is proportional to the degree of peripheral sympathetic activity present at the time the drug is administered. When sympathetic constriction is prominent, substantial decreases in arterial pressure may follow the administration of vasodilator agents in general, and alpha-adrenergic blocking agents, such as chlorpromazine, in particular. Thus, the administration of these agents should be initiated cautiously, with plasma expanders readily available to counteract a sudden increase in vascular capacitance due to the action of the drug.

Lillehei has presented data indicating that massive doses of steroids ( 1 gm. methylprednisolone or its equivalent) may have a favorable effect in the low cardiac output syndrome,[11] but the use of corticosteroids in these doses must be considered developmental rather than established conventional therapy.

Mannitol, a hyperosmotic agent, may be particularly helpful, when given as a test bolus of 12.5 gm. intravenously, in assessing the underlying cause of oliguria in the patient with inadequate cardiac output. This agent increases intravascular volume almost immediately, and thus may be used to determine whether hypovolemia is the cause of inadequate cardiac output from which oliguria results. For this type of situation, mannitol, given as a bolus, offers unique advantages as both a diagnostic and therapeutic agent.[3]

## CARDIOGENIC SHOCK

Cardiogenic shock may be defined as severe hypotension with inadequate perfusion of peripheral organs secondary to myocardial failure. It is accompanied by a vicious cycle of ischemia or necrosis of the myocardium leading to a decrease in systemic arterial pressure, which leads to a decrease in coronary perfusion pressure and to a further reduction in myocardial oxygen delivery; this in turn results in further ischemia or necrosis of the myocardium.

Cardiogenic shock occurs after acute myocardial infarction in approximately 10 per cent of patients. Although the treatment of myocardial infarction was formerly the province of the internist or cardiologist, the advent of the surgical treatment of coronary artery disease makes adequate understanding of the treatment of acute myocardial infarction and its hemodynamic complications of the utmost importance to the surgeon. The therapy of cardiogenic shock is based on sound physiologic rationale. First, as in all instances in which cardiac output is inadequate, it is necessary to be certain that there is adequate intravascular volume and oxygenation and to correct any disorder of acid-base balance. Cardiac rhythm must be closely monitored and arrhythmias treated appropriately.

Under conditions of severe hypotension, coronary blood flow varies directly with changes in systemic perfusion pressure. In these situations isoproterenol not only may increase the oxidative demands of the heart through its positive inotropic action, but also may lower systemic blood pressure through its peripheral vasodilatory effect. When this occurs, the demand for oxygen by the heart may outstrip the supply, and further ischemia and necrosis may ensue.[19] The importance of achieving an adequate systemic blood pressure in order to maintain coronary perfusion in severe hypotension bears emphasis. Norepinephrine, which increases peripheral vascular resistance, may be very helpful. Norepinephrine has a beta-adrenergic effect on the heart that is quantitatively equal to that of epinephrine and is the drug of choice for treatment of the rare patient in cardiogenic shock with low peripheral vascular resistance.

Calcium, delivered as a chloride or glucoheptonate salt, should be considered an important complementary agent for support of the injured or failing myocardium. The chloride delivers a much greater amount of ionized calcium. Confusion concerning which preparation is being used may lead to an overdose if the chloride is administered, or inadequate therapy may ensue if glucoheptonate is given. Calcium administered by intravenous drip is particularly helpful when large volumes of blood are being given rapidly, to counteract loss of ionized calcium due to binding with citrate.[6] Intravenous calcium should be administered only when there is a firm cardiovascular indication for its use, such as hypotension in the presence of an elevated left atrial pressure or electrocardiographic evidence of hypocalcemia. As calcium augments the arrhythmogenic effects of digitalis glycosides, the two agents should be given together only with great caution, to avoid ventricular irritability.

When cardiogenic shock is refractory to these therapeutic measures, it is probable that severe injury to the left ventricle has occurred. Page, Caulfield, and their co-workers have shown that in death due to cardiogenic shock 40 per cent or more of the left ventricular myocardium has been lost.[23] If cardiogenic shock is refractory and resistant to pharmacologic therapy, mechanical circulatory assistance should be instituted in an attempt to stop the progression of extensive myocardial necrosis. Of the various means available, counterpulsation by means of intra-aortic balloon pumping[24] appears to have greatest clinical promise.[5] Patients who require mechanical circulatory assistance may, in addition, require emergency coronary revascularization[22] or infarct resection[8] or both for survival.

## CONGESTIVE HEART FAILURE

The treatment of *congestive heart failure* in the surgical patient requires, in addition to the administration of cardiac glycosides and diuretic agents, treatment of the underlying cause. In patients undergoing cardiac surgical procedures, congestive heart failure may be temporarily aggravated by the stress of surgery and require vigorous treatment until the benefits of the operation are manifest. Since congestive heart failure in the surgical patient is often the result of fluid shifts that occur intraoperatively or postoperatively, the judicious use of diuretic agents assumes great importance. Because of the critical status of the patient, it is important to use a diuretic agent that is potent, rapid-acting, and parenterally administered.

*Ethacrynic acid* and *furosemide* are the two most potent diuretics available. Diuresis produced by these agents is associated with a urinary loss of sodium, chloride, potassium, and ammonium ions. This pattern is similar to that produced by the thiazide diuretics and must be kept in mind to ensure proper replacement of these electrolytes, particularly potassium and chloride. The indiscriminate use of these agents for the treatment of transient oliguria is to be discouraged, since large doses of either can produce irreversible auditory nerve damage. Rather, the cause of the oliguria should be sought and treated appropriately. If congestive heart failure is deemed the cause, then diuresis is appropriate. Since patients have been shown to tolerate sodium and water loading poorly after cardiac surgery, a central feature of prevention and treatment of congestive heart failure is stringent restriction of fluid and sodium intake.

Although the use of digitalis glycosides is important in the treatment of congestive heart failure in most clinical situations, the critically ill surgical patient presents special problems that dictate certain modifications in the use of glycosides. First, *long-acting* digitalis preparations are inappropriate for the treatment of the critically ill patient, since the usual signs of digitalis excess may be difficult to assess and a rapid-acting and rapidly excreted preparation is required. Digoxin is generally the preparation of choice for treatment of the hospitalized patient. The onset of inotropy after the intravenous administration of 0.5 mg. of digoxin occurs in approximately 30 to 60 minutes, and the half-life of this substance in the patient, assuming normal renal function, is 33 to 40 hours. Because of the arrhythmogenic effect of digitalis, significant impairment of renal function dictates a reduction of dosage. In the patient not treated with digitalis previously and with normal kidney function, 0.5 to 0.75 mg. intravenously can be given initially, followed by 0.25 mg. intravenously at 3 to 4 hour intervals over approximately 9 to 12 hours. During this time one should watch carefully for the onset of digitalis-induced arrhythmias, primarily *ventricular premature beats.* Other important signs of digitalis excess in the critically ill patient are the appearance of *paroxysmal atrial tachycardia with block* (see later discussion) and regularization of the ventricular response to *atrial fibrillation.* Gastrointestinal and visual signs are rarely of help in the severely ill patient. The recently developed technique of measuring glycoside blood levels by radioimmunoassay[28] adds significantly to the safe conduct of digitalis therapy.

The most important function of digitalis in the cardiac surgical patient is the control of the ventricular rate response to rapid atrial arrhythmias, such as atrial fibrillation, and flutter, by induction of a graded degree of atrioventricular block. Although digitalis strengthens myocardial contraction significantly, it is no substitute for catecholamine pressor agents in the treatment of hypotension.

Digitalis increases strength of contraction in the normal heart,[10] but it is of the greatest aid in situations in which severe congestive heart failure accompanies enlargement of the left ventricle. By improving contractility of the heart, digitalis may not only increase cardiac output but also decrease the end-diastolic volume. Since lowering of the end-diastolic volume is associated with a decrease in wall tension, myocardial oxygen consumption should be reduced. Thus, an increase in myocardial efficiency may be achieved by use of the cardiac glycosides in congestive heart failure.

It is important to remember that the hypoxic or ischemic myocardium may be more susceptible to the arrhythmogenic effects of digitalis than the normal well oxygenated heart. Similarly, serum potassium must be monitored closely and deficits must be corrected, since hypokalemia significantly enhances the likelihood of a digitalis-induced arrhythmia for any given blood level of the glycoside.

## CARDIAC ARRHYTHMIAS

### Atrial Arrhythmias

Of atrial arrhythmias, *atrial premature beats* are usually benign; however, if they are frequent and multifocal or if they are bigeminal in pattern, they may herald the onset of a more serious atrial tachyarrhythmia such as *atrial fibrillation.* Quinidine sulfate in a dose of 200 to 400 mg. every 4 to 6 hours orally (or quinidine lactate intramuscularly) is the drug of choice for treatment of atrial pre-

mature beats if it is deemed necessary to suppress them. If the patient cannot tolerate quinidine, procaine amide (250 to 500 mg. every 4 hours)[15] may be used. The treatment of *sinus tachycardia,* during which the pulse rate is usually between 100 and 160 beats per minute, is usually directed at the underlying cause of the sinus tachycardia, which may be anxiety, congestive heart failure, hypovolemia, or a hypermetabolic state, such as hyperthyroidism or sepsis.

*Paroxysmal atrial tachycardia* is an ectopic atrial arrhythmia with an atrial rate between 150 and 250 beats per minute. Usually, each atrial complex is conducted to the ventricle. If atrioventricular block exists, underlying digitalis toxicity should be suspected. Carotid sinus pressure or the Valsalva maneuver will often abruptly convert the arrhythmia to normal sinus rhythm. The right carotid sinus should be massaged first for no longer than 5 to 10 seconds with continuous electrocardiographic monitoring. If this is ineffective, the left carotid sinus should be massaged. Simultaneous massage of both carotid sinuses should never be done, because of the possibility of resultant asystole or cerebral ischemia. If these maneuvers fail to convert the arrhythmia, edrophonium chloride (Tensilon) may be given intravenously in a dose of 5 to 10 mg. If the paroxysmal atrial tachycardia is well tolerated by the patient, as shown by a well maintained systemic blood pressure, then rapid digitalization with intravenous digoxin is likely to convert the arrhythmia to sinus rhythm. Electrical cardioversion may be required if these techniques fail to convert the arrhythmia, particularly in a patient who is hypotensive.

*Atrial flutter* is a rapid ectopic atrial tachyarrhythmia with an atrial rate between 250 and 350 beats per minute. The ventricular rate depends on the degree of atrioventricular block, which is usually either 2:1 or 3:1. In many patients, digitalization will convert this arrhythmia to sinus rhythm or, short of conversion, induce a stable degree of atrioventricular block leading to an acceptable ventricular rate. If this is not successful, cardioversion is the treatment of choice, particularly in a patient who is not tolerating the arrhythmia. If cardioversion is ineffective, digitalization followed by the administration of quinidine is the next treatment of choice. Prevention of recurrent attacks is best achieved by the oral administration of quinidine sulfate in a dose of 200 to 400 mg. every 4 to 6 hours. Atrial flutter is a common arrhythmia following cardiac surgery. If the patient has not had recent cardiac surgery, an underlying cause such as pulmonary embolism should be considered. A point of practical importance is the fact that atrial flutter can be resistant to digitalis therapy; larger than usual doses may be required either to convert flutter to sinus rhythm or to induce an acceptable stable degree of atrioventricular block. Consideration must be given to the need for ultimate cardioversion in a given patient, lest the digoxin dose be pushed to toxicity level without success in treating the arrhythmia. The risk of ventricular fibrillation with cardioversion at this point is greater than it would have been had cardioversion been undertaken prior to the "digitalis push."

*Atrial fibrillation* is characterized by a rapid chaotic atrial rhythm at an atrial rate greater than 350 beats per minute. Digoxin is the drug of choice for controlling the ventricular rate. Digitalization should be continued until the ventricular rate is decreased to an acceptable range. In the acutely ill patient with chronic long-standing atrial fibrillation, attempts to convert the rhythm may not be successful or even hemodynamically useful. In such patients, satisfactory hemodynamics may be achieved merely by adequate ventricular rate control with digoxin. In the immediate postoperative period, attempts to reduce the ventricular rate below 100 with increments of digoxin should probably be avoided. Increased metabolic demands following surgery and augmented adrenergic activity, by facilitation of atrioventricular conduction, normally increase the heart rate. Thus, attempts to reduce the heart rate below this level with digoxin may lead to ventricular irritability without inducing block.

In a patient in whom digoxin therapy does not produce adequate rate control, propranolol in small doses (0.5 to 1.0 mg. intravenously as a single test dose, or 10 mg. orally 4 times a day) may be tried, assuming that the patient has basically good myocardial function. Use of this agent in this situation requires careful consideration, and the administration of propranolol to a patient with advanced myocardial disease is not recommended.

During digitalization, conversion to normal sinus rhythm may occur. If, however, neither conversion nor adequate rate control results from drug therapy, electrical cardioversion should be undertaken. Attempted conversion of atrial fibrillation with orally administered quinidine has little application in the acutely ill postoperative patient. If quinidine is given, full digitalization should be achieved prior to the administration of quinidine, because this drug is vagolytic and may increase the ventricular response to the atrial fibrillation. Moreover, if atrial flutter develops, a 1:1 conduction to the ventricle with resultant hypotension or congestive heart failure or both may ensue.

As with atrial flutter, forethought is advisable concerning the need for cardioversion, which should be undertaken before digitalis therapy approaches toxicity level. When atrial fibrillation develops abruptly with a rapid ventricular rate response (160 to 170 beats per minute), increments of digoxin are likely to be successful, particularly if administration of the drug was discontinued for several days previously. However, when the onset of atrial fibrillation is accompanied by a lower ventricular rate (120 to 130 per minute) and the patient's response to the arrhythmia is poor, digoxin therapy is less likely to help, and immediate cardioversion is indicated.

*Multifocal atrial tachycardia*[27] is a rapid ectopic atrial rhythm involving at least several different atrial foci with a ventricular response of greater than 100 beats per minute. Patients with this arrhythmia frequently have accompanying lung disease (acute or chronic), with arterial hypoxia. Treatment is aimed primarily at correction of the arterial blood gas levels. In the patient not previously given digitalis therapy, digitalization may assist in slowing the ventricular response to the atrial tachycardia, but further increments of digitalis are not of benefit and may actually contribute to the patient's deterioration. This is a complex, life-threatening arrhythmia that is often resistant to pharmacologic therapy.

### Nodal or Atrioventricular Junctional Rhythms

These arrhythmias may occur at any rate and are characterized electrocardiographically by relatively unchanged QRS complexes when compared to beats of supraventricular origin. However, an appropriately timed P wave does not appear before each QRS complex. From a hemodynamic standpoint, a nodal rhythm results in loss of an appropriately timed atrial systole prior to ventricular systole. This ectopic rhythm, if it occurs at a slow rate, as an "escape" rhythm, may be overcome by atrial pacing. Nodal tachycardia is a much more difficult problem, however, often indicating injury to or disease of the myocardium or digitalis excess. In the presence of nodal tachycardia, metabolic disorders such as acidosis, hypoxia, and hypokalemia must be corrected so that they can be excluded as possible etiologic factors. Diphenylhydantoin, procaine amide, lidocaine (Xylocaine), or propranolol may be used successfully on occasion, but nodal tachycardia is notoriously resistant to drug therapy. Resistant nodal tachycardia may respond to cardioversion, but if the arrhythmia is thought to be due to digitalis excess, cardioversion is most hazardous and drug treatment is far preferable. In the case of a refractory nodal tachycardia in a patient who cannot tolerate the arrhythmia hemodynamically, capture of the atrium by rapid atrial pacing and then gradual slowing of the atrial pacing rate to an acceptable level may suppress the nodal ectopic pacemaker.

### Ventricular Arrhythmias

*Ventricular premature beats* are the most common ventricular arrhythmias. Indications for treatment include the following: the occurrence of more than three or four ventricular premature beats per minute, ventricular premature beats that are multifocal in origin, those that occur in salvos of two or three or more, and those that occur near the peak of the T waves of the preceding QRS complexes. The latter type is likely to initiate ventricular tachycardia. In the early postoperative period, ventricular premature beats should be suppressed vigorously with appropriate therapy, unless the patient has been known to have longstanding, singly occurring ventricular premature beats prior to operation.

There are many potential causes for ventricular irritability in the form of ventricular premature beats in the patient who has had cardiac surgery. Among these are digitalis excess, systemic hypoxia, regional myocardial injury or ischemia, acidosis, and hypokalemia. These defects, if present, must be quickly corrected when possible, and at the same time the ventricular irritability should be appropriately suppressed. It is always helpful to recognize that although digitalis may aggravate ventricular irritability (particularly in the presence of hypokalemia), when ventricular premature beats occur in the presence of congestive heart failure, they may be eliminated by digitalis in a patient who has not received this agent previously.

The usual treatment for ventricular premature beats after cardiac surgery is lidocaine delivered intravenously at a rate of 1 to 2 mg. per minute (1 gm. lidocaine in 250 cc. of 5 per cent dextrose in water). Continuing ventricular irritability may require additional intravenous boluses (50 mg.) of lidocaine. If lidocaine does not adequately suppress the ventricular premature beats, procaine amide (250 to 500 mg. intramuscularly or orally every 4 hours) or quinidine (200 to 400 mg. of the sulfate orally or of the lactate intramuscularly) may be used to complement lidocaine therapy. In the patient with severe and threatening ventricular irritability but basically sound myocardial dynamics, propranolol (0.5 mg. to 1 mg. intravenously) may be used when other safer methods fail.

For ventricular irritability thought to be caused by digitalis excess, an intravenous potassium chloride infusion to replenish intracellular potassium losses may be effective. Diphenylhydantoin (100 mg. intravenously, intramuscularly, or orally every 6 to 8 hours) is particularly effective in the treatment of irritability due to digitalis excess.

*Ventricular tachycardia* should be treated immediately either with lidocaine by intravenous bolus (as described earlier) or, particularly if there is coexistent hypotension, with immediate electrical cardioversion. If immediate cardioversion is not successful with restoration of an acceptable systemic blood pressure (peak systolic pressure of 90 mm. Hg or greater), cardiopulmonary resuscitative efforts must be undertaken immediately. These include tracheal intubation, mechanical ventilation with 100 per cent oxygen, external cardiac massage, intravenous injection of sodium bicarbonate for acidosis, intravenous administration of 50 to 100 mg. lidocaine (once it has been established by electrocardiogram that the mode of the patient's cardiac arrest is not asystole), and repeated attempts at electrical defibrillation.[29] The intravenous administration of either norepinephrine or epinephrine may be indicated during and following the immediate period of cardiac "arrest" to effect an adequate coronary perfusion pressure initially.

The occurrence of *ventricular fibrillation* necessitates immediate electrical cardioversion. As with refractory ventricular tachycardia, failure to respond to electrical cardioversion should be treated with resuscitative maneuvers. If the condition is refractory to defibrillation, treatment should consist of intravenous administration of glucose (25 gm. in a 50 per cent solution) and crystalline zinc insulin (20 units), with or without 1 gm. of cal-

cium chloride,[13] to correct probable hyperkalemia due to circulatory stasis.

Cardiac arrest in patients in whom the underlying rhythm disturbance is not readily discernible should be treated with electrical defibrillation immediately, since in the majority of these patients underlying *ventricular fibrillation* is the basis for cardiac arrest.

## HYPERTENSION

Management of *hypertension* in the surgical patient is of importance in three distinct circumstances: (1) the routine management of the patient who is already hypertensive prior to surgery; (2) the antihypertensive treatment of the patient with an acute dissecting aneurysm of the aorta; and (3) severe paradoxical hypertension developing during or following surgery, as may occur after the repair of coarctation of the aorta or during or immediately following surgery in a patient with pheochromocytoma.

For patients receiving antihypertensive medications preoperatively, it is appropriate to stop administration of these agents at least 1 day before surgery. Usually patients with even moderately severe hypertension prior to surgery will be normotensive during the administration of anesthesia. It is important that both the surgeon and the anesthesiologist know which antihypertensive agents were used. Although it was formerly thought that some drugs such as reserpine should be withdrawn several weeks prior to surgery to allow repletion of catecholamine stores, it has now become apparent that this agent may be given almost until the time of surgery and that depleted catecholamine stores may be replaced with intravenous norepinephrine if required.

Although the majority of patients with dissecting aneurysm of the aorta are best managed by surgical repair, some very high-risk patients may be appropriately treated by means of a nonoperative antihypertensive program (see Chapter 52). Even the patient who has undergone operation will require pharmacologic control of blood pressure preoperatively and postoperatively to forestall further dissection. In addition to the usual antihypertensive agents, propranolol, a beta-adrenergic receptor blocking agent, may be of special benefit, since this drug lowers the rate of increase in pressure in the aorta with each ventricular systole and thereby decreases the tendency toward extension of the dissection.[32]

The third group of patients are those with severe paradoxical hypertension. Removal of pheochromocytomas is sometimes accompanied by a sharp increase in systemic blood pressure. This is particularly likely to occur at the time of manipulation of the tumor and is thought to represent a sudden release of catecholamines from the lesion. Prior treatment of these patients with phenoxybenzamine can substantially decrease the incidence of hypertension during and immediately following surgery (see Chapter 25).

Following surgical correction of coarctation of the aorta, paradoxical elevation of the blood pressure may occur. In some instances the extent of hypertension in this situation may be impressive. The exact mechanism of this change in blood pressure is not understood, but it is probably caused by neural release of catecholamines;[31] it can and should be treated, however, with the agents to be discussed in the succeeding paragraphs.

Diuretics such as chlorothiazide and spironolactone are mild antihypertensive agents that are commonly used, although their mechanism of action is not well understood. Either 500 mg. per day of chlorothiazide given orally or 100 mg. per day of spironolactone given orally (in four divided doses) or both, when not used in conjunction with other agents, may have a mild antihypertensive effect.[33] When used in conjunction with more potent antihypertensive agents, these drugs appear to potentiate the effect of the stronger medications. An advantage of using spironolactone, in contrast to other diuretics, is that potassium is conserved by this agent.

A second group of antihypertensive agents includes the rauwolfia alkaloids, of which reserpine is an example. These drugs act by inhibiting the binding of norepinephrine and epinephrine in the peripheral sympathetic nervous system. The usual oral dose of reserpine is in the range of 0.75 to 1 mg. per day in three or four equally divided doses. Reserpine can be administered intramuscularly to patients with severe hypertension in single injections of 0.5 to 1 mg., but there appears to be little added advantage to increasing the daily dose of parenteral reserpine above 8 mg. Depression and peptic ulceration are important side effects of these agents.

Hydralazine, a drug that acts directly on vascular smooth muscle to promote arteriolar relaxation, is useful in patients whose hypertension is accompanied by renal failure. The drug does not adversely affect renal function and is not dependent upon the kidneys for inactivation. The usual dose is 75 to 100 mg. per day in three or four divided doses. Side effects include associated beta-adrenergic receptor stimulation with an increase in heart rate and in cardiac output. This effect may be detrimental to patients with angina or dissecting aneurysm. A collagen vascular disease resembling lupus erythematosus develops in a small percentage of patients receiving high doses of hydralazine over prolonged periods (usually longer than 6 months). The clinical manifestations of this disease appear to be reversible when the drug is discontinued.

Alpha-methyldopa (Aldomet) is metabolized into alpha-methylnorepinephrine, a less potent pressor agent than norepinephrine. This metabolite displaces stored norepinephrine at nerve endings. The usual dose of Aldomet is 1 to 2 gm. per day orally or intravenously in divided doses. Side effects include postural hypotension and somnolence; in 10 to 15 per cent of patients receiving Aldomet a Coombs test produces positive results, which appear to be dose-related.

Guanethidine, a drug that is similar to Aldomet in its antihypertensive potential, probably acts by preventing the release of norepinephrine at myoneural junctions and by depleting peripheral stores of norepinephrine. Side effects include postural hypotension, which may become severe even when the drug is given in low therapeutic doses.

Diazoxide, a new agent that is structurally similar to chlorothiazide and is still under investigation, holds great promise as a therapeutic agent for the treatment of both malignant hypertension and chronic severe hypertension.[12, 21] Diazoxide appears to act directly on vascular smooth muscle to promote a lowering of vascular resistance.[25] The usual dose in acute severe or malignant hypertension is 300 mg. intravenously every 6 to 8 hours. Hypotension as a result of the use of this agent is unusual in a patient who is not being given other antihypertensive agents. Because of a lack of untoward side effects and because this agent increases renal blood flow, diazoxide may become an important agent in the treatment of hypertension.

Ganglionic blocking agents such as pentolinium tartrate (Ansolysen) and mecamylamine hydrochloride (Inversine) block both sympathetic and parasympathetic ganglia. These agents are indicated only for patients with severe hypertension. As might be anticipated, postural hypotension is a frequent complication of their use. Other side effects are attributable to blockade of the parasympathetic nervous system and include severe constipation and occasionally paralytic ileus.

All the antihypertensive drugs mentioned here, with the exception of diazoxide, can be administered orally. Trimethaphan camsylate (Arfonad) and nitroprusside are potent antihypertensive agents that are administered solely by the intravenous route. The delivery of both these agents must be titrated continuously with the patient's blood pressure. Failure to monitor continuously the rate of delivery of these drugs can result in severe hypotension and death. These drugs are indicated for treatment of severe hypertension refractory to other agents and for control of hypertension in situations in which the blood pressure must be rapidly controlled, as in acute dissecting aneurysm. The use of Arfonad or nitroprusside is best undertaken with continuous oscilloscopic display of the arterial blood pressure measured through an arterial catheter, since slight changes in rate of drug delivery may lead to precipitous changes in the blood pressure.

## REFERENCES

1. Ahlquist, R. P.: Adrenergic drugs. In: Drill, V. A., ed.: Pharmacology in Medicine. 2nd ed. New York, McGraw-Hill Book Company, 1958.
2. Armstrong, P. W., Gold, H. K., Buckley, M. J., Willerson, J. T., and Sanders, C. A.: A hemodynamic evaluation of rate augmentation produced by atrial pacing and isoproterenol in the early postoperative phase of cardiac surgery. Circulation, 44:649, 1971.
3. Barry, K. G., and Berman, A. R.: Mannitol infusion: The acute effect of intravenous infusion of mannitol on blood

and plasma volumes. New Eng. J. Med., *264*:1985, 1961.

4. Bendixen, H. H., Osgood, P. F., Hall, K. V., and Laver, M. B.: Dose dependent difference in catecholamine action on heart and periphery. J. Pharmacol. Exp. Ther., *145*:299, 1964.

5. Buckley, M. J., Mundth, E. D., Daggett, W. M., DeSanctis, R. W., Sanders, C. A., and Austen, W. G.: Surgical therapy for early complications of myocardial infarction. Surgery, *70*:814, 1971.

6. Bunker, J. P.: Metabolic effects of blood transfusion. Anesthesiology, *27*:446, 1966.

7. Chidsey, C. A., Braunwald, E., Morrow, A. G., and Mason, D. T.: Myocardial norepinephrine concentration in man: effects of reserpine and of congestive heart failure. New Eng. J. Med., *269*:653, 1963.

8. Daggett, W. M., Buckley, M. J., Mundth, E. D., Sanders, C. A., and Austen, W. G.: The role of infarctectomy in the surgical treatment of myocardial infarction. Amer. Heart J., in press.

9. Daggett, W. M., and Wallace, A. G.: Vagal and sympathetic influences on ectopic impulse formation. In: Dreifus, L., Likoff, W., and Moyer, J. H., eds.: Mechanisms and Therapy of Cardiac Arrhythmias. New York, Grune & Stratton, 1966, p. 64.

10. Daggett, W. M., and Weisfeldt, M. L.: Influence of the sympathetic nervous system on the response of the normal heart to digitalis. Amer. J. Cardiol., *16*:394, 1965.

11. Dietzman, R. H., Castaneda, A. R., Lillehei, C. W., Ersek, R. A., Motsay, G. J., and Lillehei, R. C.: Corticosteroids as effective vasodilators in the treatment of low output syndrome. Chest, *57*:440, 1970.

12. Finnerty, F. A., Jr., Davidov, M., and Kakaviatos, N.: Hypertensive vascular disease: the long term effect of rapid repeated reductions of arterial pressure with diazoxide. Amer. J. Cardiol., *19*:377, 1967.

13. Gilmore, J. P., Daggett, W. M., McDonald, R. H., and Sarnoff, S. J.: Influence of calcium on myocardial potassium balance, oxygen consumption, and performance. Amer. Heart J., *75*:215, 1968.

14. Kirklin, J. W.: Circulation and cardiac failure. In: American College of Surgeons, Committee on Pre and Postoperative Care: Manual of Preoperative and Postoperative Care. 2nd ed. Philadelphia, W. B. Saunders Company, 1971, pp. 195–210.

15. Koch-Weser, J., Klein, S. W., Foo-Canto, L. L., Kastor, J. A., and DeSanctis, R. W.: Anti-arrhythmic prophylaxis with procainamide in acute myocardial infarction. New Eng. J. Med., *281*:1253, 1969.

16. Leinbach, R. C., Chamberlain, D. A., Kastor, J. A., Harthorne, J. W., and Sanders, C. A.: A comparison of the hemodynamic effects of ventricular and sequential A-V pacing in patients with heart block. Amer. Heart J., *78*:502, 1969.

17. Lowenstein, E., Hallowell, P., Levine, F. H., Daggett, W. M., Austen, W. G., and Laver, M. B.: Cardiovascular response to large doses of intravenous morphine in man. New Eng. J. Med., *281*:1389, 1969.

18. Lowenstein, E., Whiting, R. B., Bittar, D. A., Sanders, C. A., and Powell, W. J., Jr.: Local and neurally mediated effects of morphine on skeletal muscle vascular resistance. J. Pharmacol. Exp. Ther., *180*:359, 1971.

19. Maroko, P. R., Kjekshus, J. K., Sobel, B. E., Watanabe, T., Covell, J. W., Ross, J., Jr., and Braunwald, E.: Factors influencing infarct size following experimental coronary artery occlusions. Circulation, *43*:67, 1971.

20. Moran, N. C.: Adrenergic receptors within the cardiovascular system. Circulation, *28*:987, 1963.

21. Mroczek, W. J., Liebel, B. A., Davidov, M., and Finnerty, F. A., Jr.: Rapid administration of diazoxide in accelerated hypertension. New Eng. J. Med., *285*:603, 1971.

22. Mundth, E. D., Buckley, M. J., Daggett, W. M., Sanders, C. A., and Austen, W. G.: Surgery for complications of acute myocardial infarction. Circulation, in press.

23. Page, D. L., Caulfield, J. B., Kastor, J. A., DeSanctis, R. W., and Sanders, C. A.: Myocardial changes associated with cardiogenic shock. New Eng. J. Med., *285*:133, 1971.

24. Powell, W. J., Jr., Daggett, W. M., Magro, A. E., Bianco, J. A., Buckley, M. J., Sanders, C. A., Kantrowitz, A. R., and Austen, W. G.: Effects of intra-aortic balloon counterpulsation on cardiac performance, oxygen consumption and coronary blood flow in dogs. Circ. Res., *26*:753, 1970.

25. Powell, W. J., Jr., Green, R. M., Whiting, R. B., and Sanders, C. A.: Action of diazoxide on skeletal muscle vascular resistance. Circ. Res., *28*:167, 1971.

26. Powell, W. J., Jr., and Skinner, N. S., Jr.: Effect of the catecholamines on ionic balance and vascular resistance in skeletal muscle. Amer. J. Cardiol., *18*:73, 1966.

27. Shine, K. I., Kastor, J. A., and Yurchak, P. M.: Multifocal atrial tachycardia: clinical and electrocardiographic features in 32 patients. New Eng. J. Med., *279*:344, 1968.

28. Smith, T. W., and Haber, E.: Digoxin intoxication: the relationship of clinical presentation to serum digoxin concentration. J. Clin. Invest., *49*:2377, 1970.

29. Stephenson, H. E.: Cardiac Arrest and Resuscitation. St. Louis, C. V. Mosby Company, 1969.

30. Swan, H. J. C., Ganz, W., Forrester, J., Marcus, H., Diamond, G., and Chonette, D.: Catheterization of the heart in man with use of a flow-directed balloon-tipped catheter. New Eng. J. Med., *283*:447, 1970.

31. Verska, J. J., DeQuattro, V., and Woolley, M. M.: Coarctation of the aorta: the abdominal pain syndrome and paradoxical hypertension. J. Thorac. Cardiovasc. Surg., *58*:746, 1969.

32. Wheat, M. W., Jr., Palmer, R. F., Bartley, T. D. and Seelman, R. C.: Treatment of dissecting aneurysms of the aorta without surgery. J. Thorac. Cardiovasc. Surg., *50*:364, 1965.

33. Wolf, R. L., Mendlowitz, M., Roboz, J., Styan, G. P. H., Kornfeld, P., and Weigl, A.: Treatment of hypertension with spironolactone. J.A.M.A., *198*:1143, 1966.

# XVI

# Extracorporeal Circulation

*Marvin Pomerantz, M.D.*

## HISTORICAL ASPECTS

Legallois[22] is credited with first suggesting the concept of artificial perfusion with oxygenated blood in 1813, and the discovery of heparin by Howell and Holt[16] in 1918 made this concept an achievable goal. The development of a clinically applicable heart-lung machine, however, awaited the contributions of Gibbon, who began work in this field in 1934. Gibbon made the following statement regarding the initiation of this research: "The idea of a heart-lung machine came to me while watching a patient die with a massive pulmonary embolus at the Massachusetts General Hospital in 1931. It occurred to me that it might be possible to help keep such a patient alive until the

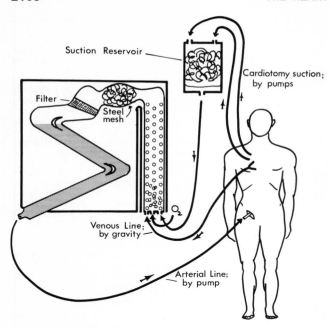

Suction Reservoir

Cardiotomy suction;
by pumps

Filter

Steel
mesh

Venous Line;
by gravity

$O_2$

Arterial Line;
by pump

CIRCUIT FOR BAG OXYGENATOR

**Figure 1** Diagrammatic illustration of an extracorporeal circuit. (From Paton, B. C.: J. Roy. Coll. Surg. Edinb., 8:301, 1963.)

embolus could be surgically removed if we could do a part of the work of the heart and lungs by continually removing systemic venous blood, adding oxygen to it, and getting rid of carbon dioxide and then continuously reinjecting the blood into a systemic artery."[25] In 1939, he commented as follows: "For example if the flow of blood through the heart and lungs could be safely stopped for 30 minutes, it is conceivable that a new field of cardiac surgery might be developed."[12] During the next decade, extracorporeal circulation was limited to laboratory experimentation as satisfactory pumps and oxygenators were developed. Dennis and associates[8] in 1951 first employed extracorporeal circulation in an attempt to close a large atrial septal defect in a 6 year old girl with massive cardiomegaly and congestive heart failure. Unfortunately, the patient did not survive the 40 minute bypass. The first successful open heart operation using extracorporeal circulation was performed by Gibbon on May 6, 1953.[13] An atrial septal defect in an 18 year old female was closed by direct suture. This patient had a 6 month history of heart failure and had been hospitalized three times during that period. The bypass lasted 45 minutes, with complete cardiopulmonary function being taken over by the heart-lung machine for 26 minutes. Cardiac catheterization performed in July, 1953, showed the defect to be closed, and at that time she was in good health. Following this monumental achievement, extracorporeal circulation and cardiac surgery developed rapidly as improvements in pumps, oxygenators, priming solutions, and technical aspects were forthcoming. A typical circuit is shown in Figure 1.

## PUMPS

The ideal blood pump should be able to pump at least 5 liters per minute, be easy to dismantle, clean, and sterilize, be easily calibrated, be automatic but with manual controls in case of power failure, have adjustable stroke volume and rate, have an output linear to pulse rate and independent of resistance, and produce minimal damage to blood elements. A pump with each of these ideal features has yet to be designed.

The *roller* pump originally described by De-Bakey in 1934[7] is the most commonly used (Fig. 2). This pump uses a progression of rollers along a flexible tube filled with blood to provide the pumping force and direction to flow. This pump requires an occlusive setting requiring exact adjustment of compression of the tubing to prevent excessive blood trauma. The rate of pumping is dependent upon the speed of rotation of the arm and the diam-

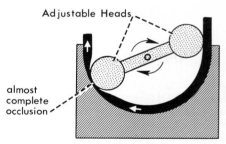

Adjustable Heads

almost
complete
occlusion

**Figure 2** Diagrammatic illustration of a roller pump.

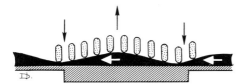

**Figure 3**    Diagrammatic illustration of a finger pump.

eter of the tubing employed. The advantages of the roller pump are its simplicity of design, accurate perfusion rate, and durability. However, as with all occlusive pumps, prohibitive degrees of blood trauma may occur unless the pump is carefully adjusted.[10]

Multiple *finger* pumps (sigmamotor pumps) were used initially in open heart surgery, but are now rarely employed (Fig. 3). These pumps propel fluid along a tube by creating progressive occlusion from metal phalanges. The pumps are durable and effective but, because of their size, trauma to blood, noisy operation, have been largely supplanted by the quieter, more compact roller pump.[27] Diaphragm pumps (Fig. 4), ventricle pumps, and piston pumps have been of little use in heart-lung machines.

Recently, Trinkle and associates[33] have constructed a pulsatile pump that may yield superior results as compared with nonpulsatile flow. With the pulsatile pump, less hemolysis, lower transfusion volume, lower vascular resistance, higher unbuffered arterial pH and $pO_2$, lower arterial lactate, less defibrination and a smaller decline in hematocrit and platelet count were found. As better pulsatile pumps are developed, it is possible that they may replace the standard roller pump for arterial perfusion.

## OXYGENATORS

Gas exchange is dependent upon the equilibration between blood and a gas mixture that usually flows counter to the blood. In 1952 Wesolowski and Welch[34] used homologous dog lungs as oxygenators. Lillehei[24] in 1955 used a human donor to serve as the pump and oxygenator in controlled cross-circulation as means to supply oxygenated blood to patients undergoing open heart surgery. These techniques are of historical interest only. Ideally,

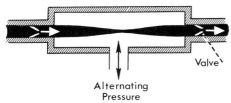

**Figure 4**    Diagrammatic illustration of a diaphragm pump.

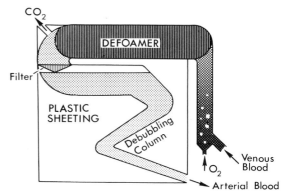

**Figure 5**    Diagrammatic illustration of a bubble oxygenator.

an oxygenator should be able to introduce adequate oxygenation of the blood, have a low priming volume, have little resistance to flow, and cause minimal damage to the blood elements.

There are three types of oxygenators of clinical use today: (1) bubble oxygenators, (2) film oxygenators, and (3) membrane oxygenators.

### Bubble Oxygenators

Blood can be oxygenated by the passage of bubbles through it (Fig. 5). The use of bubble oxygenators became practical with the introduction of antifoam by Clark and associates in 1950.[3] This substance alters the surface tension of the bubbles, allowing them to break. After the oxygen containing bubbles comes in contact with blood, foam is produced and intimate mixing of blood and oxygen occurs. Once this is completed, coalescence of foam and removal of bubbles are carried out by the action of surface-active agents by settling trapping, filtration, or centrifugation of the bubbles or by a combination of these means.[10]

Small bubbles are better for oxygenation and poorer for removal of carbon dioxide than large bubbles. Small bubbles furthermore may cause hemolysis by their jet action; therefore, there is usually a compromise in size of bubbles with most bubble oxygenators. Bubble oxygenators have a tendency to produce hemolysis if the rate of oxygen flow is too great and are more likely to produce protein denaturation than other oxygenators. However, for perfusions less than 2 hours, they are quite acceptable.

### Film Oxygenators

These oxygenators function by spreading out into a thin film a rapidly moving stream of blood. Gas exchange is then facilitated by exposing the blood film to oxygen. Inherent in these oxygenators for increased efficiency of gas transfer is the presence of turbulence to prevent layering of the blood. Of the various types of film oxygenators, the screen and rotating disc have received much popularity. Other oxygenators of the film type are the sponge, rotating spiral, and rotating cylinder.[10]

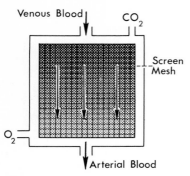

**Figure 6** Diagrammatic illustration of a screen oxygenator.

Gibbon and associates[14] were responsible for the development of the *screen* oxygenator (Fig. 6). In this apparatus, blood is spread over thin stainless steel screens where it is exposed to oxygen. The rotating *disc* oxygenator was popularized by Kay and Cross[17] (Fig. 7). In this oxygenator, venous blood is introduced at one end and oxygenated as the thin blood film is dispersed over the disc and exposed to oxygen. Optimal oxygenation depends upon the speed of disc rotation, distance between the discs, and depth of immersion of discs into blood.[10] The rotating disc yields a large surface of gas exchange per unit of time in a comparatively small apparatus. However, these oxygenators produce considerable blood trauma, which increases as the speed of disc rotation increases.

### Membrane Oxygenators

The first membrane oxygenator practical for human perfusion was an outgrowth of the multi-layered lung described by Clowes et al.[5] in 1956. Membrane oxygenators differ from other oxygenators in that there is no direct contact between blood and gas. All other oxygenators function by exposing blood in one phase to gas in another. In the membrane oxygenator, oxygen is separated from blood by a semipermeable membrane (Fig. 8). Gas transfer across the membrane depends upon the nature, thickness, surface, and degree of hydration of the membrane as well as the partial pressure differences of diffusing gases on opposite sides of the membrane.[10] At present, two materials are used in membrane oxygenators: Teflon and silicone. Of these, Teflon is cheaper, but silicone effects better gas exchange. The transfer of car-

bon dioxide is primarily limited by the membrane barrier, while oxygen transfer is controlled by the blood thickness. The main advantage of membrane oxygenators is minimal trauma to blood.[30]

## BLOOD AND OTHER PRIMING FLUIDS

Originally most pump-oxygenator systems were primed with whole blood, since it was assumed that this would most closely match the normal physiologic needs of the body. It was felt necessary to use blood, particularly with early oxygenators, to maintain sufficient oxygen-carrying capacity. Several problems were soon apparent with whole blood primes. The quantities of cross-matched heparinized blood required for the large priming volumes of some pump-oxygenator systems were sometimes difficult to obtain. Furthermore, the heparinized blood could at the time be stored safely for only 24 hours. Another problem concerned the fact that the greater the number of blood units used, the greater the chance for minor mismatches and serum hepatitis. For these reasons, attention was directed toward other solutions alone or in combination with blood for priming pump-oxygenator systems.

Dextrose 5 per cent in water, dextrose 5 per cent in saline, Ringer's solution, lactated Ringer's solution, and low molecular weight dextran as well as various crystalloid and blood combinations have been used to prime pump systems. In general, hemodilution has the following advantages: decreased renal damage, decreased hemolysis, increased postoperative urine output, and reduction of peripheral vasoconstriction, cyanosis, and metabolic acidosis.

Although Cooley and associates[6] report excellent results with the use of 5 per cent dextrose in water, others report postoperative dilution of serum electrolytes and hemolysis when this prime is used.[26, 27] The use of low molecular weight dextran in the priming fluid has resulted in good perfusion and excellent urine output, but in some cases it may produce an increase in postoperative bleeding and acid-base imbalance during perfusion. Neville[27] and Paton[26] advocate the use of a balanced salt solution or buffered Ringer's lactate as a priming fluid to reduce the severity of such complications as metabolic acidosis, postoperative electrolyte imbalance, and increased postoperative bleeding and to produce high flow rates and good output of urine. The contents of the extracorporeal

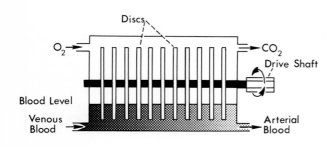

**Figure 7** Diagrammatic illustration of a disc oxygenator.

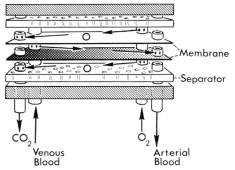

**Figure 8** Diagrammatic illustration of a membrane oxygenator.

unit may be infused at the completion of bypass to restore red cell mass. This is usually well tolerated, and the additional fluid load is probably partly responsible for the increased postoperative diuresis seen with hemodilution.

The availability of the various crystalloid solutions as well as the advantages of hemodilution already mentioned makes hemodilution a method of choice for priming pump-oxygenator systems.

## HEAT EXCHANGERS

Heat exchangers are incorporated into the extracorporeal circuit either to maintain body temperature within normal physiologic range during perfusion or to lower body temperature and thus metabolic demand during intracardiac procedures. Brown[2] and Sealy[32] early advocated the use of hypothermia with extracorporeal circulation, and this technique is frequently employed. Most heat exchangers can decrease esophageal temperatures 1 to 3° C. at flow rates of 1 to 4 liters per minute.[10] Rewarming is slower (0.5 to 1.0° C. per minute) because of the limit to which the temperature in the heat exchanger can be raised. If the rewarming temperature exceeds 40 to 41° C., red cells may be damaged or proteins may be coagulated.[15]

## PERFUSION

Arterial perfusion is accomplished by cannulation of either the ascending aorta or femoral artery. Cannulation of the ascending aorta avoids a second incision and shortens operative time. Cannulation of the femoral artery has the advantage of removing the cannula and tubing from the operative field. Both techniques are used, the choice depending upon the individual situation.

Flow rates are usually in the range of 2.4 liters per square meter of body surface area. Even with the addition of hypothermia, high flow rates are preferable. Longer perfusions (more than 2 hours) have been associated with increased mortality. This is probably due to the degree of difficulty of the procedure as well as the increased damage to blood elements by the extracorporeal system.

## METABOLISM

An ideal perfusion provides all body tissue with the oxygen needed for optimal metabolism and prevents abnormalities in acid-base balance; electrolyte abnormalities must be rigidly controlled if perfusion is to maintain normal homeostatic mechanisms.

*Oxygen* requirements are determined by the pre-existing metabolic rate, nature and depth of anesthetic agent, and body temperature.[4] Kirklin[19] has indicated that this value varies between 100 and 125 ml. per square meter per minute, while Clowes states that the basal metabolic rate of oxygen usage varies from 120 to 150 ml. per square meter per minute. The latter author states that anesthesia causes a reduction of oxygen consumption of 10 to 25 per cent. Lowering body temperature to 30° C. decreases the oxygen requirement by approximately 50 per cent.[15] Originally it was thought that hypothermia would permit use of low flow rates without the development of an oxygen debt. However, it has been shown that excess lactate, a measurement of tissue underperfusion, develops when low flow rates are maintained in combination with hypothermia.[27] The tremendous reduction in oxygen consumption, even with deep hypothermia, does not apparently prevent an oxygen debt in the presence of low flow rates. The use of hemodilution produces an improvement in oxygen consumption if the temperature is below 20° C., but a debt is paid during normothermic perfusion.[4] The shift of the oxyhemoglobin dissociation curve as the blood is cooled and the Bohr effect in the presence of respiratory alkalosis may also contribute to a decrease in oxygen delivery during hypothermia or hemodilution.[4]

The common denominator for disturbances of *acid-base metabolism* brought about by extracorporeal circulation is metabolic acidosis. It has been established that the acidosis associated with extracorporeal circulation develops as a result of insufficient oxygenation of the tissues, and that the accumulation of lactic acid during perfusion is inversely proportional to the flow rate.[27] It has also been demonstrated that with acute hypocarbia and respiratory alkalosis during bypass lactic acid concentrations increase and potassium levels decrease.[1] The addition of carbon dioxide (3 per cent) to the oxygenating gas has been found to prevent these changes. In addition to cellular hypoxia from inadequate perfusion and the hypocarbia of bypass, Galletti[10] cites the following factors as also contributing to the metabolic acidosis: anesthesia and thoracotomy as such, and accumulation of acid metabolites in the priming blood.

Although 5 per cent dextrose and water has been used extensively to prime oxygenators,[6] others have found this solution to produce a dilution of the serum *electrolytes*.[29] Clowes[4] states that the usual electrolyte pattern seen with extracorporeal circulation is more like that encountered in alkalosis. The most striking alteration is the decline in serum potassium by 1 to 2 mEq. per liter. This decline in serum potassium is particularly noted with hemodilution, and is accompanied by a rise in intracellular potassium.[27] Other electrolyte shifts include a modest decline in sodium and a fall of calcium. With high-flow perfusions producing little tissue hypoxia and less acidosis, there are fewer postperfusion electrolyte disturbances. With almost all perfusions there is a positive fluid balance at the end of perfusion, which may produce either dilutional electrolyte changes or edema. In view of this, fluid and electrolyte replacement should be used sparingly in the immediate postoperative period.

## COMPLICATIONS

Complications of extracorporeal circulation may be either mechanical or related to alterations in the circulating blood elements and their effect upon the body. *Mechanical* problems associated with extracorporeal circulation include aortic dissection from the arterial cannula, air embolism, and arterial thrombosis when the femoral artery is used. The mechanical complications are rarely seen. With proper venting, aortic cross-clamping, and elective cardiac arrest or fibrillation, air embolism seldom occurs.

Some of the problems such as bleeding, hemolysis, cerebral abnormalities, and "pump lung" are probably related to damage to blood elements by pumps, oxygenators, or suction devices and the effects of these damaged cells on the body. Destruction of red cells, denaturation of proteins, release of vasoactive substances, and intravascular coagulation can all lead to postperfusion abnormalities.

Lee[20, 21] reported evidence that plasma proteins are denatured by disc, bubble, and screen oxygenators. These oxygenators have in common a *blood-gas interface,* and it is at this interface that the plasma proteins are denatured by the stress of intermolecular forces. This denaturation of plasma proteins results in an increase in viscosity of plasma, release of free lipids, which can produce fat emboli, and intravascular hemagglutination, which can plug arterioles, venules, and capillaries. Plasma that is oxygenated by disc, bubble, or screen oxygenators and later infused into dogs may produce delayed anesthetic recovery, signs of decerebration, prolonged hypotension, and death. Comparison of the *membrane* oxygenator to these other oxygenators with regard to these parameters showed it to be superior, since there is no interface between blood and gas where plasma proteins can be denatured. With the membrane oxygenator there was less increase in viscosity, less protein denaturation, less turbidity, no chylomicron aggregation, less capillary sludging, and no shock, decerebration, or death.

It has been emphasized by Kessler[18] that microemboli are produced by various types of oxygenators. Osborn, Swank, and associates[28] have emphasized the deleterious effects of embolization on the perfused patient. With addition of a Dacron wool filter to the extracorporeal system, there was a significant decrease of microemboli returned to the perfused patient. Early clinical reports[28] indicate that with the use of the filter patients were more alert, more interested, and less confused following bypass. At postmortem fewer nonfat emboli were found in patients who had undergone bypass with a filter incorporated into the extracorporeal system than in those who had had bypass without filters.

Cardiopulmonary bypass may be followed by severe changes in the lungs characterized by congestion, hemorrhage, and consolidation, resulting in pulmonary insufficiency (*postperfusion lung syndrome, pump lung,* and so forth).[23] In the various explanations for this syndrome, the changes are attributed to the effects of denatured proteins, microemboli, or hypothermia.[23] It is probable that postperfusion lung is due to a combination of these factors, including the postoperative state itself, especially low cardiac output syndrome. Until a system devoid of these complications is developed, the use of mechanical respirators in the immediate postoperative period to maintain normal arterial blood gases and reduce the work of breathing is often indicated. A secondary effect of reducing the work of breathing may be an improvement of the patient's cardiovascular status.

Postperfusion cerebral dysfunction is a problem that appears to be decreasing in frequency. Various factors such as hypoxia due to poor perfusion, respiratory alkalosis, and embolization have been incriminated as causes of this dysfunction. Better physiologic perfusion and reduction of emboli associated with improved systems are undoubtedly responsible for the lowered incidence of postperfusion cerebral problems.

## TECHNIQUE AND MANAGEMENT OF EXTRACORPOREAL CIRCULATION

While many open heart procedures may be performed through right or left thoracotomy, the majority of operations employing extracorporeal circulation are now performed through a sternal splitting incision. After the pericardium is opened, the venae cavae, the ascending aorta, and occasionally the pulmonary artery are encircled with tapes. If perfusion is to be carried out via a femoral artery catheter, a groin incision is also made and the femoral artery isolated.

Heparinization is withheld until the dissection is complete and hemostasis has been obtained. Heparin, a sulfated mucopolysaccharide, acts as an anticoagulant by interfering with the conversion of fibrinogen to fibrin. It is administered intravenously in doses of 200 to 400 units (2 to 4 mg.) per kilogram of body weight. Since the in vivo disappearance of heparin is approximately 57 per cent per hour,[4] additional heparin is administered intravenously if perfusion extends beyond 1 hour.

Cannulation is accomplished with either thin-walled plastic or metal cannulas. It is wise to perform arterial cannulation before venous cannulation so that bypass can be instituted rapidly if bleeding or arrest occurs during cardiac manipulation. Arterial cannulation most commonly is performed via either the femoral artery or ascending aorta. Venous drainage is obtained by the insertion of catheters into the venae cavae through purse string sutures placed on the right atrium. Occasionally, for left-sided heart operations, a single right atrial catheter is inserted. Coronary perfusion is provided by specially designed catheters placed directly into the coronary ostia via an opening in the aorta, with the aorta clamped above, after perfusion has begun.

Venous blood is collected by either gravity drainage or mild negative suction from the caval catheters or the right heart. This blood flows either directly into an oxygenator or first into a reservoir and then into an oxygenator. The venous blood is oxygenated by contact with an oxygen-containing gas mixture within the oxygenator. Oxygenated blood is then pumped into the arterial system after it passes through a heat exchanger, bubble trap, and, in many perfusion systems, a filter. After bypass is begun and while blood is still perfusing the pulmonary circuit (partial bypass), the anesthesiologist must continue ventilation of the patient. To establish complete bypass, blood is prevented from flowing through the pulmonary artery by tightening of the caval tapes around the caval catheters or by occlusion of the pulmonary artery, and then ventilation can be stopped. Decompression of the left side of the heart is accomplished by inserting a vent directly into the left ventricle or left atrium or by passing a vent into the left side of the heart via a pulmonary vein. This venting prevents overdistention of the left ventricle, a complication that produces an immediate decrease in myocardial contractility as well as prolonged depression of cardiac function.[31] Intracardiac suckers are used to return blood from cardiac chambers to the oxygenator or reservoir after open cardiotomy has been performed, so that excessive blood loss does not occur during surgical repair. During bypass as well as before and afterward, the electrocardiogram, pulse, temperature, systemic pressure, and central venous pressure are usually monitored. Mild hypothermia to 30° C. is used by many surgeons, whereas others prefer to perform all operations at normothermia.

After closure of all cardiac incisions, the patient is rewarmed to a normothermic level and bypass is converted from complete to partial. Bypass is stopped slowly, and all catheters are clamped. If cardiac action and hemodynamics are satisfactory after a short observation period, decannulation is begun. Decannulation is accomplished in the reverse order of cannulation, with the vent and venous catheters being removed first. The arterial cannula is removed after perfusate has been slowly returned from the pump oxygenator until the right atrial pressure reaches approximately 15 mm. Hg or the left atrial pressure is 20 mm. Hg. After all catheters are removed, the effect of heparin is reversed by the administration of protamine sulfate in doses of 1.0 to 1.5 mg. for each 100 units (1 mg.) of heparin given at the initiation of perfusion.

## SELECTED REFERENCES

Galletti, P. M., and Brecher, G. A.: Heart-Lung Bypass — Principle and Techniques of Extracorporeal Circulation. New York, Grune & Stratton, 1962.
*This book represents an extensive review of the principles of extracorporeal circulation from its inception through 1961.*

Gibbon, J. H., Jr.: Application of a mechanical heart and lung apparatus to cardiac surgery. Minn. Med., 37:171, 1954.
*This is Gibbon's report of the first successful use of extracorporeal circulation in man in an operation to correct an intracardiac defect.*

Mead, R. H.: A History of Thoracic Surgery. Springfield, Ill., Charles C Thomas, 1961.
*This well written historical account of the development of thoracic surgery to 1960 provides useful background data.*

Peirce, E. C., II: The membrane lung, its excuse, present status, and promise. J. Mount Sinai Hosp. N. Y., 34:437, 1967.
*This article provides an excellent review of the problems and promise of membrane oxygenators. Prolonged perfusions await the further refinement of these oxygenators.*

Peirce, E. C., II: Extracorporeal Circulation for Open-Heart Surgery. Springfield, Ill., Charles C Thomas, 1969.
*This monograph provides much information necessary for those desiring a complete reference source in this field.*

## REFERENCES

1. Andersen, M. N., Mondelow, N., and William, O. G.: Relationship of respiratory alkalosis to metabolic acidosis during extracorporeal circulation. Surgery, 53:730, 1963.
2. Brown, I. W., Smith, W. W., and Emmon, W. O.: An efficient heat exchanger for use with extracorporeal circulation. Surgery, 44:372, 1958.
3. Clark, S. C., Gollan, F., and Gupta, V. P.: Oxygenation of blood by gas dispersion. Science, 111:85, 1950.
4. Clowes, G. H. A., Jr.: Bypass of the heart and lungs with an extracorporeal circulation. In: Gibbon, J. H., Jr., Sabiston, D. C., Jr., and Spencer, F. C., eds.: Surgery of the Chest. 2nd ed. Philadelphia, W. B. Saunders Company, 1969, pp. 610–642.
5. Clowes, G. H. A., Jr., Hopkins, A. L., and Neville, W. E.: An artificial lung dependent upon diffusion of oxygen and carbon dioxide through plastic membranes. J. Thorac. Surg., 32:630, 1956.
6. Cooley, D. A., Beall, A., and Grondin, P.: Open heart operations with disposable oxygenators, 5 per cent dextrose prime and normothermia. Surgery, 52:713, 1962.
7. DeBakey, M. E.: Simple continuous flow blood transfusion instrument. New Orleans Med. Surg. J., 87:386, 1934.
8. Dennis, C., Spreng, D. S., Nelson, G. E., Karlson, K. E., Nelson, R. S., Thomas, J. V., Eder, W. P., and Varco, R. L.: Development of a pump-oxygenator to replace the heart and lungs: An apparatus applicable to human patients and application to one case. Ann. Surg., 134:709, 1951.
9. Gadboys, H. L., Slomin, R., and Litwak, R. S.: Homologous blood syndrome. I. Preliminary observations on its relationship to clinical cardiopulmonary bypass. Ann. Surg., 156:793, 1962.
10. Galletti, P. M., and Brecher, G. A.: Heart-Lung Bypass— Principle and Techniques of Extracorporeal Circulation. New York, Grune & Stratton, 1962.
11. Gibbon, J. H., Jr.: Artificial maintenance of circulation during experimental occlusion of pulmonary artery. Arch. Surg., 34:1105, 1937.
12. Gibbon, J. H., Jr.: The maintenance of life during experimental occlusion of the pulmonary artery followed by survival. Surg. Gynec. Obstet., 69:602, 1939.
13. Gibbon, J. H., Jr.: Application of a mechanical heart and lung apparatus to cardiac surgery. Minn. Med., 37:171, 1954.
14. Gibbon, J. H., Jr., Miller, B. J., and Fineberg, C.: An im-

proved mechanical heart-lung apparatus. Med. Clin. N. Amer., *37*:1603, 1953.

15. Gordon, A. S.: Heat exchangers as hypothermia inducers in heart surgery. Ann. Rev. Med., *13*:75, 1962.

16. Howell, W. H., and Holt, E.: Two new factors in blood coagulation – heparin and proantithrombin. Amer. J. Physiol., *47*:328, 1918.

17. Kay, E. B., and Cross, F. S.: Direct vision repair of intracardiac defects utilizing a rotating disc reservoir oxygenator. Surg. Gynec. Obstet., *140*:701, 1957.

18. Kessler, J., and Patterson, R.: The production of microemboli by various blood oxygenators. Ann. Thorac. Surg., *9*:221, 1970.

19. Kirklin, J. W., and Theye, R.: Whole body perfusion from a pump oxygenator for open intracardiac surgery. In: Gibbon, J. H., Jr., ed.: Surgery of the Chest. Philadelphia, W. B. Saunders Company, 1962, pp. 694–707.

20. Lee, W. H., Krumhaar, D., Derry, G., Sachs, D., Lawrence, S. H., Clowes, G. H. A., and Maloney, J. V.: Comparison of the effect of membrane and non-membrane oxygenators on the biochemical and biophysical characteristics of blood. Surg. Forum, *12*:200, 1961.

21. Lee, W. H., Krumhaar, D., Fonkalsrud, E. W., Sehjeide, O. A., and Maloney, J. V.: Denaturation of plasma proteins as a cause of death after intracardiac operations. Ann. Surg., *50*:29, 1961.

22. Legallois, J. J. C.: Experiments on the Principle of Life. Translated by N.C. and J.C. Nancrede. Philadelphia, 1813.

23. Lesage, A., Tsuchioka, H., Young, W. G., and Sealy, W. C.: Pathogenesis of pulmonary damage during extracorporeal perfusion. Arch. Surg., *93*:1002, 1966.

24. Lillehei, C. W., Cohen, M., Warden, H. E., and Varco, R. L.: Direct vision intracardiac correction of congenital anomalies by controlled cross circulation. Surgery, *38*:11, 1955.

25. Meade, R. H.: A History of Thoracic Surgery. Springfield, Ill., Charles C Thomas, 1961.

26. Miyauchi, Y., Inoue, T., and Paton, B. C.: Comparative study of priming flows for two hour hemodilution perfusion. J. Thorac. Cardiovasc. Surg., *52*:413, 1966.

27. Neville, W. E.: Extracorporeal circulation. Curr. Probl. Surg., July, 1967.

28. Osborn, J. J., Swank, R. L., Hill, D. J., Aguilar, M. J., and Gerbode, F.: Clinical use of a Dacron wool filter during perfusion for open heart surgery. J. Thorac. Cardiovasc. Surg., *60*:575, 1970.

29. Paton, B. C., and Rosenkrantz, H.: Non-hemic priming fluids for extracorporeal circulation. Dis. Chest, *48*:311, 1965.

30. Peirce, E. C., II: The membrane lung, its excuse, present status and promise. J. Mount Sinai Hosp. N. Y., *34*:437, 1967.

31. Peirce, E. C., II: Extracorporeal Circulation for Open Heart Surgery. Springfield, Ill., Charles C Thomas, 1969.

32. Sealy, W. C., Brown, I. W., Jr., and Young, W. G., Jr.: Report on the use of both extracorporeal circulation and hypothermia for open heart surgery. Ann. Surg., *147*:603, 1958.

33. Trinkle, J. K., Helton, N. E., Bryant, L. R., and Griffin, W. O.: Pulsatile cardiopulmonary bypass: Clinical evaluation. Surgery, *68*:1074, 1970.

34. Wesolowski, S. A., and Welch, C. S.: Experimental maintenance of the circulation by mechanical pumps. Surgery, *31*:769, 1952.

# XVII

# Assisted Circulation

*John E. Connolly, M.D.*

The explosive advances in cardiovascular surgery over the past two decades have clearly indicated both the feasibility of mechanical cardiopulmonary assistance for a few hours and the need for practical methods for mechanical assistance of the failing circulation for several days. Many new diagnostic devices and methods for repair of cardiac dysfunction are now available if the patient can be kept alive long enough for these techniques to be put to use. Likewise, temporary mechanical support of some hearts that are successfully repaired may be necessary for some days until recovery from surgery is complete. Finally, in spite of the surgeon's ability to repair most varieties of cardiac disease, some patients with cardiomyopathy, advanced coronary artery disease, or irreparable congenital anomalies will be successfully treated only by a heart transplant or a totally implantable permanent artificial heart.

In the search for a simple, practical, and successful long-term method of mechanically assisting the failing circulation, three problems have been elucidated that are of minor importance during short periods of support for open heart surgery but are major limiting factors for prolonged assistance. These are (1) control of clotting in the extracorporeal circuit without causing bleeding from the patient, (2) prevention of damage to blood cells and proteins associated with the prolonged use of currently available oxygenators, and (3) regulation of a physiologic pulse contour. Availability of durable materials that resist clotting and a self-contained power source are additional unsolved problems confronted in the development of a permanent implantable artificial heart.

At present, the only practical and widely accepted method of mechanical circulatory assistance is a partial vein to artery bypass using a non-blood-primed oxygenator and pump that can be preassembled and connected to a patient in a matter of minutes through the femoral vessels (Fig. 1). The power source may be a battery; this allows the system to be portable for emergency use. Such apparatus can maintain perfusion and oxygenation in a patient with massive pulmonary embolism until the diagnosis is confirmed and

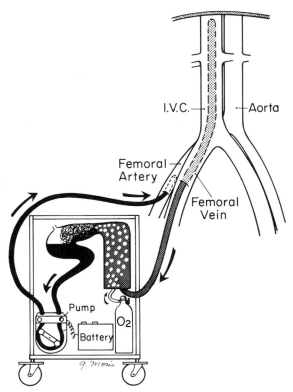

**Figure 1** Diagram of venoarterial bypass with a disposable non-blood-primed pump-oxygenator connected to the patient through the femoral vessels.

operative embolectomy performed. Patients suffering from cardiogenic shock secondary to myocardial infarction can be kept alive by such a portable pump-oxygenator until angiographic studies are performed which may delineate surgically correctable cardiac lesions and thus permit immediate operative correction. This method of mechanical circulatory assistance with a gas-interface oxygenator is dangerous when used for more than 6 hours. The use of membrane oxygenators has permitted extension of this type of assisted circulation to several days, but the problems of an implantable mechanical heart have not been solved.

Experimental approaches to the problems of circulatory support listed earlier can be classified as: (1) direct mechanical compression of the heart, (2) mechanically changing pressure and volume relationships to decrease systolic systemic resistance and improve diastolic coronary filling, (3) shunting portions of venous blood around the heart and back into the systemic circulation, (4) pumping oxygenated blood from the lungs into a systemic artery, bypassing and resting the left ventricle, and (5) pumping venous blood through an oxygenator and into an artery, bypassing and resting the heart and lungs.

## EXTERNAL CARDIAC MASSAGE

Kouwenhoven and associates[25] in 1960 demonstrated that adequate systolic pressures of 60 to 100 mm. Hg could be obtained by repeated manual compression of the sternum toward the spine in patients with cardiac arrest. This technique of external cardiac massage has been widely applied and has saved many lives by maintaining the circulation until cardiac resuscitation could be performed. Harkins and Bramson[21] in 1961 described an ingenious mechanical device for providing prolonged external cardiac massage in patients who cannot be revived rapidly. They also speculated on the possibility of use of their mechanized unit to increase cardiac output in a failing but still beating heart. The apparatus consists of a cushioned piston rod that intermittently descends upon the sternum and compresses it toward the dorsal spine in a manner similar to external manual cardiac compression.

The compression is electronically synchronized with the electrocardiogram and occurs at the beginning of ventricular systole. This apparatus has subsequently been modified and simplified and is now widely used by rescue teams, in ambulances, and in hospitals. A commercially available external heart massager is shown in Figure 2. It is strapped about the patient's chest, and an oxygen mask is used to provide concomitant ventilatory support.

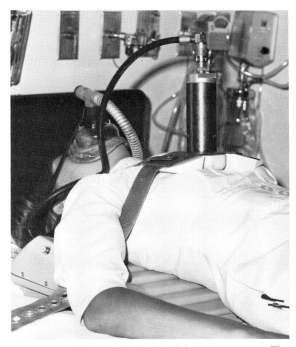

**Figure 2** External mechanical heart massager. The mechanical pressure-driven pump is strapped to the chest. Note also the oxygen mask supplying positive-pressure breathing, which is part of the portable resuscitation apparatus.

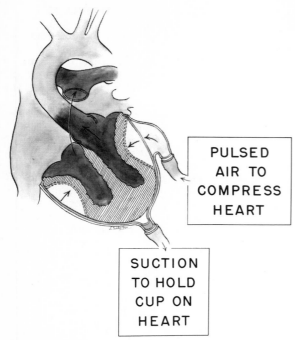

PULSED
AIR TO
COMPRESS
HEART

SUCTION
TO HOLD
CUP ON
HEART

**Figure 3** Diagram of cup ventricular assistance. Suction holds the cup on the heart, and compressed air causes the cup to intermittently squeeze the ventricles. If desired, the cup assistance can be synchronized with the electrocardiogram.

## CUP VENTRICULAR ASSISTANCE

Mechanical ventricular assistance has also been provided by the direct application of a plastic cup pump held about the ventricles by continuous negative pressure[1] (Fig. 3). A pneumatic pump applies alternating negative and positive pressure between a rigid outer shell and a flexible diaphragm to squeeze the ventricles. While such a mechanism can provide adequate circulation for a number of hours with only modest trauma to the myocardium, the technique requires direct exposure of the heart, which entails an extensive surgical procedure that is undesirable in the patient suffering from cardiogenic shock. Also, the presence of the cup may prevent adequate angiographic study of the heart if this technique is to be used as a prelude to corrective cardiac surgery. Cup ventricular assistance would appear to be useful only temporarily after cardiac surgery or for the preservation of organ perfusion during donor organ procurement.

## COUNTERPULSATION

Clauss et al.[11] in 1961 described another approach to mechanical assistance of the failing circulation called counterpulsation. This technique was based on observations of Sarnoff and Braunwald, who showed that myocardial oxygen consumption is related to ventricular pressure during systole and not to blood flow. If a quantity of blood is withdrawn from the arterial system immediately after the instant of isometric contraction, the pressure required during the phase of the maximal rate of ejection is reduced considerably. The same quantity of blood is then returned during diastole to enhance coronary artery perfusion in relation to the decreased myocardial work. Initial problems with counterpulsation or diastolic augmentation were related to inaccurate timing, with increased cardiac work resulting rather than assistance to the circulation. While more sophisticated electronic apparatus has provided more reliable counterpulsation, clinical application of the technique has shown the necessity of cannulation of both femoral arteries for adequate augmentation volume and a relatively high degree of hemolysis associated with the technique.

### Counterpulsation by Body Compression

A number of investigators (Birtwell et al.[6] and Osborn et al.[32]) have proposed and studied the effects of counterpulsation by encasing various portions of the body in alternating pressure suits to decrease peripheral resistance during systole and augment flow in diastole. The instant of compression is synchronized with the diastolic phase of the cardiac cycle. In most instances, the venous return, cardiac output, and systolic and diastolic pressures could be modified to reduce left ventricular work and at the same time increase cardiac output. From a practical standpoint, such pressure suit augmentation has lent itself most readily to the lower extremities. However, the amount of circulatory assistance provided by such devices is small and does not appear to be sufficient to answer the needs of most patients in cardiogenic shock.

An ingenious alternative to external pressure counterpulsation is the development by Arntzenius[2] of internal assistance or body acceleration synchronous with the heart (BASH). The entire patient in a BASH-bed is rapidly accelerated caudally during systole, and cranially during diastole; thus systolic resistance is reduced, and diastolic aortic root pressure is increased. Initial clinical trials in patients with cardiogenic shock have been very encouraging.

### Counterpulsation by Intra-aortic Balloon Pumping

A simplified approach to counterpulsation or diastolic augmentation has been provided by intra-aortic balloon pumping.[8, 9] A thin-walled polyurethane balloon is introduced retrograde from a femoral or subclavian artery into the descending thoracic aorta. The polyurethane helium-filled balloon is inflated during diastole and deflated at the beginning of systole, in electronic synchronization with the patient's electrocardiogram (Fig. 4). The theoretical physiologic benefits of this technique have been outlined earlier.

This technique has been used as supportive

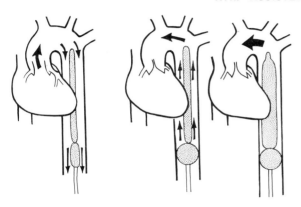

SYSTOLE                    DIASTOLE

**Figure 4**   Intra-aortic balloon pumping. The double balloon deflates at the beginning of systole to decrease the work of ventricular ejection. The distal balloon, followed by the proximal balloon, inflates during diastole to increase the aortic root pressure and, in turn, the coronary blood flow.

treatment in cardiogenic shock and as an adjunct to the preoperative and postoperative care of selected patients requiring open heart surgery or myocardial revascularization. Laboratory investigation of this technique has shown its effectiveness in increasing coronary blood flow and decreasing left ventricular work. Improved survival in induced cardiogenic shock in animals after balloon pumping has been reported by some investigators. It would appear that diastolic augmentation by phasic balloon pumping may be helpful in sustaining circulation if the amount of infarcted or impaired ventricular muscle is not too great. A number of reports of the clinical application of balloon pumping have been published, with only occasional successes. Although controls are not available, balloon pumping may be helpful if applied within the first 20 hours of cardiogenic shock, and particularly if used in conjunction with surgical correction of ventricular aneurysm or myocardial revascularization or both. There is at present some disagreement about the design and number of balloons employed, but the major problems with this technique appear to be (1) difficulty in its introduction in patients with peripheral vascular occlusive disease, (2) problems with synchronization, and (3) the possibility of balloon rupture.

## LEFT HEART BYPASS

Another approach to mechanical support of the failing circulation is left heart bypass. Open-chest left heart bypass (left atrium to femoral artery shunting) has been a well recognized adjunct to facilitate prolonged cross-clamping of the thoracic aorta since 1957.[15] However, few patients in cardiogenic shock can be expected to tolerate thoracotomy for institution of circulatory support. Closed chest left heart bypass for support of the failing circulation was first suggested by Dennis and associates in 1967.[17] Drainage of the left atrium was accomplished by passing a large metal cannula from a jugular vein through the right atrium, piercing the interatrial septum in the fashion of transseptal left heart catheterization, and entering the left atrium. This ingenious form of support has many theoretical advantages. Use of the patient's own lungs for oxygenation eliminates a major source of difficulty in prolonged bypass. The work of the left ventricle is decreased. Here, as in venoarterial bypass, unless all or nearly all of the blood flow to the left ventricle is bypassed, the value of the technique is questionable.

Experiments have been performed to measure the oxygen consumption of the heart during left heart bypass. This was accomplished by determining arteriovenous oxygen differences between the root of the aorta and the coronary sinus and by measuring coronary blood flow during left heart bypass. Coronary blood flow was measured by placing a flowmeter directly on the coronary sinus. With these determinations, the oxygen consumption of the heart was calculated by means of the Fick principle and shown to be reduced 50 per cent or more with total or near-total left heart bypass.

Four hours of closed-chest left heart bypass significantly improved the survival of animals subjected to experimental cardiogenic shock.[10] It appears that even short periods of myocardial rest may reverse otherwise fatal cardiogenic shock. However, attempts to conduct closed-chest left heart bypass in animals for more than 12 hours were rarely successful. Both pulsatile flow for better organ perfusion and the elimination of anticoagulation appeared to be necessary to permit successful left heart bypass beyond 12 hours.

### Pulsatile Versus Nonpulsatile Pumping

Several investigators have demonstrated that nonpulsatile flow for several hours provides inadequate perfusion for normal metabolism demands (Many,[29] Trinkle,[38] German[19]). In the study of German and associates,[19] the kidney was selected for assessment of the tissue effects of the two types of pumping. If renal oxygen flow (renal blood flow × oxygen content) was maintained at a constant level, oxygen uptake of the kidney was significantly higher with pulsatile than with nonpulsatile bypass; this indicated improved tissue perfusion with pulsatile pumping. Lactate production was significantly less in kidneys subjected to pulsatile as compared with nonpulsatile perfusion. One can conclude from these experiments that mechanical assistance to the circulation for prolonged periods of hours or days can be carried out with less physiologic derangement if a pulsatile pump rather than a nonpulsatile pump is employed, regardless of the variety of assistance employed.

### Pulsatile Nonthrombogenic Left Heart Bypass

Success in providing a surface coating that would prevent blood clotting in extracorporeal

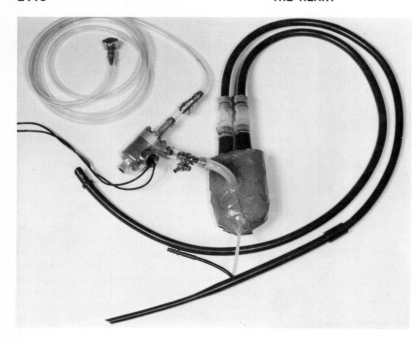

**Figure 5** Nonthrombogenic pulsatile pump and tubing used for open-chest left heart bypass in humans. Note fiberglass-encased chamber, which is yellow, with solenoid valve and compressed-air source. Directly above the pump are housings containing pig valves. Dark color of polyvinyl tubing is due to athrombogenic graphite coating.

circuits was first reported by Gott and associates,[20] using graphite, benzalkonium, and heparin. Wakabayashi[40] modified the coating technique by employing graphite impregnated in plastic. Wakabayashi combined his graphite-coated tubing with a pulsatile left ventricle pump coated with Dacron velour. He employed this type of pump and circuit to conduct prolonged left heart bypass without the use of heparin.[39] Bypass for 30 hours in dogs was successful. An endothelial-like membrane covered the velour lining and no clots were found in the pump or tubing after 30 hours of left heart bypass. These results were significantly better than those in control animal experiments in which left heart bypass was performed with uncoated tubing, heparin, and conventional nonpulsatile pumping. This athrombogenic left heart bypass circuit has been employed to provide partial bypass for up to 4 hours in 10 patients undergoing thoracic aortic aneurysm resection and graft interposition (Fig. 5). No heparin was employed, and throughout bypass the mediastinum was remarkably free of bleeding. Postoperative bleeding also was significantly decreased as compared to that found when bypass techniques requiring heparin are used. Inspection of the pump, valves, and tubing at the end of these operations did not disclose any significant thrombi.

A diagram is shown in Figure 6 of a closed-chest left heart bypass circuit employing a nonthrombogenic pulsatile pump and coated tubing to permit prolonged circulatory assistance without heparin. The left atrial catheter is inserted either by the Dennis technique mentioned earlier (Fig. 6, inset *a*) or by a transseptal technique from a femoral vein (Ross). The blood is returned to an axillary artery in preference to a femoral artery because of the abdundance of collaterals in the arm.

### Transarterial Closed-Chest Left Ventricular Bypass

In 1969, Zwart[41] proposed bypass of the left ventricle by direct removal of left ventricular blood through a catheter introduced retrograde into the left ventricular cavity. The blood was then returned to a peripheral artery. Figure 6, inset *b*, shows the left ventricular catheter entering from an axillary artery. Experience with this apparatus has demonstrated that a catheter of a size that can be introduced retrograde into the left ventricular chamber will permit total left heart bypass for several hours in sheep with a fibrillating heart. There is some question, however, whether a catheter of such a size can remove most of the left ventricular output in a beating heart. Initial clinical trials have been technically successful but have not yet produced long-term survival.

### Direct Left Ventricle–Femoral Artery Bypass

For circulatory assistance at the completion of heart surgery, a coated athrombogenic cannula can be inserted through the apex of the left ventricle to aspirate blood which is then pumped through coated tubing to a femoral or axillary artery. The chest can be closed, with a stab wound for exit of the cannula. This technique has been employed in patients for periods of 6 to 9 hours, without the use of heparin, to decrease the work of the heart. None of the patients were long-term survivors, but all appeared to benefit during the bypass. The ultimate place for this type of bypass depends upon the ability of the heart to recover during the time of assistance.

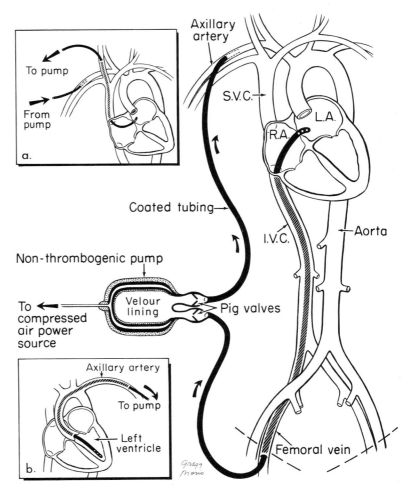

**Figure 6** Diagram of nonthrombogenic closed-chest left heart bypass for treatment of cardiogenic shock in man. Left atrial blood is removed transseptally via a femoral vein and returned by a pulsatile pump to an axillary artery. The pump employs biologic (pig) valves and a velour lining. Inset *a* demonstrates a transatrial catheter introduced into the left atrium through a jugular vein as described by Dennis. Inset *b* shows a left ventricular catheter inserted via an axillary artery after the technique of Zwart.

## VENOARTERIAL BYPASS

### Without Oxygenation

It is well known that phlebotomy can be life-saving in the treatment of cardiac failure and that intra-arterial transfusion can raise the aortic root pressure, increasing coronary perfusion, in patients with cardiogenic shock. Used separately, these techniques can be employed only briefly. However, in combination they can be maintained for hours or days. In experimental animals subjected to a fixed severe cardiac load, employment of partial venoarterial bypass has been shown to produce a remarkable restoration of myocardial strength.[13] The effectiveness of venoarterial bypass is directly related to its ability to raise the aortic root pressure and increase coronary blood flow.[14]

In 1958, emergency venoarterial bypass through the femoral vessels without oxygenation was performed at the bedside of four patients suffering from medically refractory cardiogenic shock due to myocardial infarction. The circulatory dynamics of all four patients improved during perfusions of up to 4 hours, but only one patient survived for any significant period beyond completion of the bypass.[3] Animal experiments were subsequently conducted to determine the length of time venoarterial bypass without oxygenation could be performed. With a roller nonpulsatile pump and total-body anticoagulation, 12 hours of bypass was tolerated with a high degree of success. However, significant mortality occurred with longer periods, and there were few surviving animals bypassed for 24 hours. Postmortem examination showed gross and microscopic findings similar to those seen in hemorrhagic shock. These included loss of circulating blood volume and hemorrhage into the bowel. Bleeding associated with repeated heparin dosage, the adverse effects of prolonged nonpulsatile pumping, and effects of perfusing with hypoxic blood appeared to limit the feasibility of venoarterial bypass for longer than 12 hours.

Sarnoff et al.[36] in 1958 and Salisbury et al.[34,35] in 1959 and 1960 demonstrated that myocardial oxygenation consumption was directly related to the systolic pressure in the ventricle, as mentioned earlier. Therefore, it appeared that cardiac work was not significantly reduced unless all or almost all of the blood was diverted from the ventricle. This would not be possible with venoarterial bypass unless an oxygenator were added to the circuit, thus limiting the technique to the short periods of extracorporeal oxygenation possible with conventional oxygenators. The clinical usefulness of venoarterial bypass without oxygenation might be in the treatment of acute right ventricular failure as seen with massive pulmonary embolism or secondary to tight mitral stenosis, but it appears to be of no value in left ventricular support.

### With Oxygenation

Total venoarterial bypass with oxygenation is routinely used for open heart surgery, and partial venoarterial bypass with an oxygenator in circuit is an excellent method of assisting the circulation for a few hours. Beyond that time a toxic effect is observed, which may become lethal after 6 hours of oxygenation.

**With a Membrane Oxygenator.** It has been recognized that this "toxic effect" is due to direct exposure of blood proteins to gas (Dobell[18] and Lee[28]) and can be alleviated by interposing a plastic film between gas and blood. Membrane oxygenators of this type were first described and used by Clowes in 1957.[12] However, the membrane lung was not a practical possibility until silicone polymer membranes with excellent gas-transfer properties were substituted for Teflon membranes in 1962. Bramson and colleagues[7] first demonstrated that an oxygenator employing such membranes could be successfully employed routinely for open heart surgery in 1965. Subsequently, a number of investigators (Hill,[22] Kolobow,[24] Landé,[27] and Bartlett and Drinker[4]) demonstrated that partial bypass can be carried out for periods up to 2 weeks without detrimental effects. The limiting factor is control of clotting and bleeding. Prolonged cardiopulmonary support using venoarterial bypass with a membrane oxygenator has been used clinically for 3 days with success (Hill and O'Brien[23]) and is undergoing clinical testing in many centers (Landé[27] and Peirce[33]).

## CONTROLLED VENTILATORY SUPPORT

Controlled ventilatory support of patients following cardiac surgery reduces the work of breathing and, in turn, cardiac work and is thus an ancillary method of providing assistance to the circulation. Such ventilatory support is being increasingly employed after cardiac surgery principally to maintain normal blood gases, but at the same time it provides some circulatory assistance.

## IMPLANTABLE ARTIFICIAL HEART

A considerable amount of laboratory investigation has been directed to the development of a permanent mechanical replacement for the heart. At present, a totally implantable power source capable of operating such a heart has not been developed. All such devices require external power sources with transmission lines penetrating the chest, and this leads to a high incidence of eventual infection. Likewise, all currently described artificial hearts are subject to the problems of clotting, with the resulting expected incidence of embolic phenomena similar to that seen with mechanical heart valves and requiring permanent anticoagulation.

Some progress has been made in solving some of the problems attendant upon use of artificial mechanical hearts by concentrating on implantable left heart bypass devices. In 1963 DeBakey and Liotta reported successful use of such a device in one of six patients.[16] However, this technique was subsequently discarded because of the problems previously mentioned. Bernhard and co-workers[5] have developed a pneumatically activated, double-valved pump that is interposed between the left ventricular apex and the descending thoracic aorta. The device accepts blood from the left ventricle during systole and ejects it into the descending thoracic aorta in diastole. Anticoagulant requirements are diminished by the culturing of a neo-intima of fibroblasts on the velour lining. Studies in calves have shown that this method of intermittent left heart bypass can be effective for several months.

Several groups (Akutsu,[37] Kloff,[26] Nosé[31]) have developed total artificial hearts of silicone or polyurethane and have employed them successfully for full support of the circulation in calves and sheep for longer than 100 hours. Multiple thromboses and infection continue to limit the long-term success of these experimental total replacement artificial hearts. These investigators, however, have shown that such devices can totally replace the heart and support life for short periods. They offer promise of success if the aforementioned problems can be solved.

## FUTURE OF ASSISTED CIRCULATION

Although thousands of patients die each year of cardiogenic shock who might be kept alive with mechanical circulatory assistance, only those with borderline needs of assistance might be expected to recover after hours or days of assistance. In the majority of patients, the underlying cardiac lesion will remain and result in demise after termination of the bypass. Clearly, the place of assistance in patients with cardiogenic shock is to support the patient until diagnosis and surgical treatment of the underlying disease can be accomplished. In most patients, this will consist of cardiac catheterization and angiography followed by coronary artery bypass surgery or ventricular aneurysm resection or perhaps valve replacement.

An increasing number of patients are being supported by peripheral venoarterial cannulation and temporary pump-oxygenator bypass or by aortic balloon pumping while angiography is performed. Figure 7 shows a patient being transported to an angiography room while his circulation is supported by a portable pump-oxygenator. Following such definitive radiologic examination, corrective surgery on the impaired ventricle

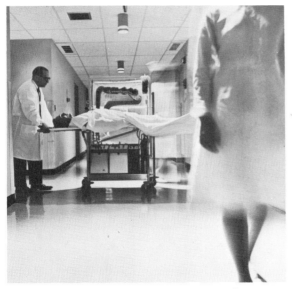

**Figure 7** Emergency pump-oxygenator. Patient is being transferred to angiography room or operating room with circulatory support supplied by a portable pump-oxygenator.

or coronary vessels resulting in adequate myocardial function has been successfully performed (Mundth[30]). If left ventricular function is not adequate postoperatively, mechanical assistance may be required for several days or weeks until heart function improves or cardiac transplantation can be arranged. Intra-aortic balloon augmentation would not appear to be applicable in such situations. Left heart bypass without heparinization (extracorporeal or implanted) or the use of partial venoarterial bypass with a membrane oxygenator appears to provide the most promise in such situations requiring prolonged assistance.

While a totally implantable mechanical heart is not yet a reality, it is the author's belief that it will be in the next decade and that experience currently being gained with mechanical circulatory assistance for hours or days will contribute to the advances needed to solve the problems of a permanent artificial heart.

## SELECTED REFERENCES

Dennis, C., Carlens, E., Senning, A., Hall, D. P., Moreno, J. R., Capelletti, R. R., and Wesolowski, S. A.: Clinical use of a cannula for left heart bypass without thoracotomy. Ann. Surg., *156*:623, 1962.
*This paper describes an ingenious method of performing left heart bypass with a closed chest. A cannula is introduced through the jugular vein into the right atrium. It then pierces the atrial septum to enter the left atrium. Blood removed from the left atrium is pumped back to a peripheral artery.*

Hill, J. D., Bramson, M. L., Osborn, J. J., and Gerbode, F.: Observations and management during clinical venovenous bypass for respiratory insufficiency. Advances Cardiol., *6*:133, 1971.
*This paper describes the use of the Bramson membrane oxygenator to support six patients with severe respiratory insufficiency by continuous venovenous perfusion for up to 6 days. The problems encountered are discussed and suggestions for improvement made. Although these six patients*

eventually died, a more recent patient with pulmonary insufficiency whose circulation was assisted for 3 days with the Bramson membrane oxygenator survived.

Mundth, E. D., Yurchak, P. M., Buckley, M. J., Leinbach, R. C., Kantrowitz, A., and Austen, W. G.: Circulatory assistance and emergency direct coronary-artery surgery for shock complicating acute myocardial infarction. New Eng. J. Med., *283*:1382, 1970.
*This paper describes the successful use of intra-aortic balloon pumping to sustain the failing circulation while coronary arteriography and subsequently emergency coronary artery bypass surgery was performed in a patient suffering from an acute myocardial infarction and cardiogenic shock.*

Salisbury, P. F., Bor, N., Lewin, R. J., and Reiben, P. A.: Effects of partial and total heart lung bypass on the heart. J. Appl. Physiol., *14*:458, 1959.
*The work described in this paper demonstrated that the oxygen requirement of the heart is determined principally by the mean left ventricular pressure. Thus, total bypass appears to be necessary to provide significant rest for the heart.*

Salisbury, P. F., Cross, C. E., Rieben, P. A., and Lewin, R. J.: Comparison of two types of mechanical assistance in experimental heart failure. Circ. Res., *8*:431, 1960.
*In this study, left heart bypass was shown to be superior to venoarterial bypass. In several types of experimental heart failure, left heart bypass consistently produced increased systemic pressure and lowered left atrial and left ventricular end-diastolic pressures. From the experiments it was concluded that left heart bypass ameliorates both left and right heart failure.*

Wakabayashi, A., Yim, D., Dietrick, W., Hirai, J., and Connolly, J. E.: Left ventricular bypass: A new nonthrombogenic device with homograft aortic valves. Amer. J. Cardiol., *25*:450, 1970.
*A new pulsatile disposable nonthrombogenic left ventricular bypass unit is described. Plastic cannulas and tubing of the unit are coated with a polyurethane-polyvinyl graphite film. The blood pump and valve housings are lined with Dacron velour. Two dog aortic valves are used as pump valves. In vivo tests in normal dogs showed that they could tolerate near-total left ventricular bypass for 30 hours with no evidence of clotting even though heparin was not used. Dogs subjected to acute heart failure and then treated with the nonthrombogenic left ventricular bypass unit for 10 hours showed a remarkable increase in survival over control animals. The elimination of heparin during bypass greatly reduced blood loss and, in turn, mortality.*

## REFERENCES

1. Anstadt, G. L., Blakemore, W., and Baue, A.: A new instrument for prolonged mechanical cardiac massage. Circulation, Supp., *32*:43, 1965.
2. Arntzenius, A. C.: Discussion of Ware, R. W., et al.: Inertial cardiac assistance. Trans. Amer. Soc. Artif. Intern. Organs, *17*:219, 1971.
3. Bacaner, M.: Human heart failure and shock treated by means of a mechanical veno-arterial bypass without oxygenation. Ann. Intern. Med., *55*:837, 1961.
4. Bartlett, R. H., Isherwood, J., Moss, R. A., Olezewski, W. L., Polet, H., and Drinker, P. A.: A toroidal flow membrane oxygenator. Four-day partial bypass in dogs. Surg. Forum, *20*:152, 1969.
5. Bernhard, W. F., LaFarge, C. G., Husain, M., Yamamura, N., and Robinson, T. C.: Physiologic observations during partial and total left heart bypass. J. Thorac. Cardiovasc. Surg., *60*:807, 1970.
6. Birtwell, W. C., Giron, F., Ruiz, U., Norton, R. L., and Soroff, H. S.: The regional hemodynamic response to synchronous external pressure assist. Trans. Amer. Soc. Artif. Intern. Organs, *16*:462, 1970.
7. Bramson, M. L., Osborn, J. J., Main, F. B., O'Brien, M. F., Wright, J. S., and Gerbode, F.: A new disposable membrane oxygenator with integral heat exchange. J. Thorac. Cardiovasc. Surg., *50*:391, 1965.
8. Bregman, D., Goetz, R. H., and State, D.: Clinical experience with a new cardiac assist device: The dual-chambered

intra-aortic balloon assist. J. Thorac. Cardiovasc. Surg., 62:577, 1971.

9. Buckley, M. J., Leinbach, R. C., Kastor, J. A., Laird, J. D., Phil, D., Kantrowitz, A. R., Madras, P. N., Sanders, C. A., and Austen, G. W.: Hemodynamic evaluation of intra-aortic balloon pumping in man. Circulation, Suppl. II, 41:130, 1970.

10. Chapple, J. C., and Connolly, J. E.: Efficacy of left heart bypass in the treatment of acute heart failure. Surg. Forum, 15:262, 1964.

11. Clauss, R. H., Birtwell, W. C., Albertal, G., Lunzer, S., Taylor, W. J., Fosberg, A. M., and Harken, D. E.: Assisted circulation: 1. The arterial counterpulsator. J. Thorac. Cardiovasc. Surg., 41:447, 1961.

12. Clowes, G. H., and Neville, W. E.: Further development of a blood oxygenator dependent upon the diffusion of gases through plastic membranes. Trans. Amer. Soc. Artif. Intern. Organs, 3:52, 1957.

13. Connolly, J. E., Bacaner, M. B., Bruns, D. L., Lowenstein, J. M., and Storli, E.: Mechanical support of the circulation in acute heart failure. Surgery, 44:255, 1958.

14. Connolly, J. E., Bacaner, M. B., Bruns, D. L., Lowenstein, J. M., and Storli, E.: The effect of venoarterial bypass on coronary blood flow. Arch. Surg., 81:58, 1960.

15. Connolly, J. E., Kountz, S. L., and Boyd, R. J.: Left heart bypass: Experimental and clinical observations on its regulation with particular reference to maintenance of maximal renal blood flow. J. Thorac. Cardiovasc. Surg., 44:577, 1962.

16. DeBakey, M. E.: Left ventricular bypass pump for cardiac assistance. Clinical experience. Amer. J. Cardiol., 27:3, 1971.

17. Dennis, C., Carlens, E., Senning, A., Hall, D. P., Moreno, J. R., Cappelletti, R. R., and Wesolowski, S. A.: Clinical use of a cannula for left heart bypass without thoracotomy. Ann. Surg., 156:623, 1962.

18. Dobell, A. R. C., Mitri, M., Galva, R., Sarkosy, M., and Murphy, D. R.: Biologic evaluation of blood after prolonged recirculation through film and membrane oxygenators. Ann. Surg., 161:617, 1965.

19. German, J. C., Chalmers, G. S., Hirai, J., Mukherjee, N. D., Wakabayashi, A., and Connolly, J. E.: Comparison of nonpulsatile and pulsatile extracorporeal circulation on renal tissue perfusion. Chest, 61:65, 1972.

20. Gott, V. L., Whiffen, J. D., Koepke, D. E., Daggett, R. L., Boake, W. C., and Young, W. P.: Techniques of applying a graphite-benzalkonium-heparin coating to various plastics and metals. Trans. Amer. Soc. Artif. Inter. Organs, 10:213, 1964.

21. Harkins, G., and Bramson, M. L.: Mechanical external cardiac massage for cardiac arrest and for support of the failing heart. A preliminary communication. Surg. Res., 1:197, 1961.

22. Hill, J. D., Bramson, M. L., Osborne, J. J., and Gerbode, F.: Observations and management during clinical venovenous bypass for respiratory insufficiency. Advances Cardiol., 6:133, 1971.

23. Hill, J. D., and O'Brien, T. G.: Personal communication.

24. Kolobow, T., and Zapol, W. M.: Partial and total extracorporeal respiratory gas exchange with the spiral membrane lung. Advances Cardiol., 6:112, 1971.

25. Kouvenhoven, W. B., Jude, J. R., and Knickerbocker, G. G.: Closed-chest cardiac massage. J.A.M.A., 173:1064, 1960.

26. Kwan-Gett, C., Backman, D. K., Donovan, F. M., Jr., Eastwood, N., Foote, J. L., Kawai, J., Kessler, T. R., Kralios,

A. C., Peters, J. L., Van Kampen, K. R., Wong, H. K., Zwart, H. H. J., and Kolff, W. J.: Artificial heart with hemispherical ventricles II and disseminated intravascular coagulation. Trans. Amer. Soc. Artif. Intern. Organs, 17:474, 1971.

27. Landé, A. J., Edwards, L., Bloch, J. H., Carlson, R. G., Subramanian, V. A., Ascheim, R. S., Scheidt, S., Fillmore, S., Killip, T., and Lillehei, C. W.: Clinical experience with emergency use of prolonged cardiopulmonary bypass with a membrane pump-oxygenator. Ann. Thorac. Surg., 10:409, 1970.

28. Lee, W. H., Jr., Krumhaar, D., Fonkalrud, E. W., Schjeide, O. A., and Maloney, J. V.: Denaturation of plasma proteins as a cause of morbidity and death after intracardiac operations. Surgery, 50:29, 1961.

29. Many, M., Giron, F., Birtwell, W. C., Deterling, R. A., and Soroff, H. S.: Effects of depulsation of renal blood flow upon renal function and renin secretion. Surgery, 66:242, 1969.

30. Mundth, E. D., Yurchak, P. M., Buckley, M. J., Leinbach, R. C., Kantrowitz, A., and Austen, W. G.: Circulatory assistance and emergency direct coronary-artery surgery for shock complicating acute myocardial infarction. New Eng. J. Med., 283:1382, 1970.

31. Nosé, Y., Tajima, K., Imai, Y., Klain, M., Mrava, G., Schriber, K., Urbanek, K., and Ogawa, H.: Artificial heart constructed with biological material. Trans. Amer. Soc. Artif. Intern. Organs, 17:482, 1971.

32. Osborn, J. J., Russi, M., Salel, A., Bramson, M. L., and Gerbode, F.: Diastolic augmentation by external pulsed pressure. Fifteenth Conference on Engineering in Medicine and Biology, Chicago, November 4, 1962.

33. Peirce, E. C., II: A comparison of the Landé-Edwards, the Peirce, and the General Electric-Peirce membrane lungs. Trans. Amer. Soc. Artif. Intern. Organs, 16:358, 1970.

34. Salisbury, P. F., Bor, N., Lewin, R. J., and Rieben, P. A.: Effects of partial and total heart-lung bypass on the heart. J. Appl. Physiol., 14:458, 1959.

35. Salisbury, P., Cross, C. E., Rieben, P. A., and Lewin, R. J.: Comparison of two types of mechanical assistance in experimental heart failure. Circ. Res., 8:431, 1960.

36. Sarnoff, S. J., Braunwald, E., Welch, G. H., Jr., Case, R. D., Stamsby, W. N., and Cruz, R.: Hemodynamic determinants of oxygen consumption of the heart with special reference to the time tension index. Amer. J. Physiol., 192:148, 1958.

37. Takano, H., Takagi, H., Turner, M. D., Henson, E. C., Crowell, J. W., and Akutsu, T.: Problems in total artificial heart. Trans. Amer. Soc. Artif. Intern. Organs, 17:449, 1971.

38. Trankle, J. K., Helton, N. E., Bryant, L. R., and Griffen, W. O.: Pulsatile cardiopulmonary bypass: Clinical evaluation. Surgery, 68:1074, 1970.

39. Wakabayashi, A., Dietrick, W., and Connolly, J. E.: Closed-chest left heart bypass without anticoagulation. J. Thorac. Cardiovasc. Surg., 58:811, 1969.

40. Wakabayashi, A., Yim, D., Dietrick, W., Hirai, J., and Connolly, J. E.: Left heart bypass: A new nonthrombogenic device with homograft aortic valves. Amer. J. Cardiol., 25:450, 1970.

41. Zwart, H. H. J., Kralios, A. C., Kwan-Gett, C. S., Backman, D. K., Foote, J. L., Andrade, J. D., and Kolff, W. J.: Transarterial closed-chest left ventricular bypass for desperate heart failure. Advances Cardiol., 6:157, 1971.

# 57

# THE SURGEON

*Loyal Davis, M.D.*

Surgery is the application of the knowledge of the basic biologic and physical sciences to the care of the patient. In that it is based on accepted and applicable principles of anatomy, physiology, chemistry, bacteriology, and related disciplines, it is a science.

Surgery is also an art. The surgeon must translate his knowledge and apply his skills by a series of mental, moral, and physical acts into their highest potential for the care of each patient under certain circumstances and at a specific time.

## EDUCATION OF THE SURGEON

In the nineteenth century and early years of the twentieth century, it was unusual for a graduate to pursue his medical education beyond commencement day, or a year of internship. It was possible to graduate, pass a state board examination, and practice without having the experience of an internship in some states. The colonial pattern of the practice of medicine prevailed generally. Physicians learned to perform surgical operations by cutting upon patients willing to mount a table and exercise the degree of patience, confidence, and courage necessary under the conditions imposed. These operators wielded their knives indiscriminately within the abdomen and pelvis and about the periphery.

The surgical courses were designed for undergraduate medical students, with the goal of preparing them to practice surgery, within the bounds of their own conscience and belief in the Golden Rule. A course in surgical anatomy might be given in the senior year, by which time it was hopefully assumed that the cadaver dissection of the freshman year, and the combined experiences of the intervening years, had prepared the student for a valuable review of the intricacies of blood vessels, nerves, and viscera. There was also the course listed as "dog surgery" or "operative surgery," the goal of which was to teach students to remove the gallbladder, kidneys, spleen, and portions of the small and large intestines, perform end-to-end and end-to-side anastomoses, and reduce fractures.

Today, only the principles of surgery, based upon the application of medical scientific facts, should be taught undergraduate medical students. No attempt should be made to teach them to be surgeons; in fact, every effort should be made to discourage them from believing they have received instruction that prepares them to operate upon patients. The principles of immediate,

emergency care of the injured patient, the goals to be reached for the best definitive care of the surgical patient, and the proper diagnostic methods to be pursued to arrive at an opinion, without wasting the finances and physical and mental capacities of the patient, should be the basic elements of the philosophy of a course in surgery.

These goals can best be arrived at by the introduction of medical students to patients and their care as early as possible in the curriculum. Taking histories, examining patients and informally discussing with the doctor responsible for the care of the patient, the procedures to be carried out, with the realization that teaching and learning are a reciprocal business, and following the patient to the operating room and participating in surgical procedures and techniques should be the basis for the teaching of surgery. One more item should be added. The chairman of the department of surgery should have personal, individual contact with every member of the class of students to whom surgery is being taught. This has been accomplished and is not impossible, even in this day of multiple committee meetings and the peripatetic leanings of many professors of surgery. He should be willing to listen to his students' suggestions about course content and their evaluations of the teaching talents of his faculty, but he alone must be responsible for the disciplined teaching and learning that is necessary in surgery.

Medical students today have a far better preliminary education for medicine, and this perhaps leads to the conclusion that a basic education in the art of the practice of medicine is not important. It may lead a medical-student clinical clerk to state confidently to an experienced attending physician during a discussion of the treatment of a patient that, in his experience, the attending physician was grossly in error.

There is the appearance in greater numbers of undergraduate medical students who wear the badges of an emancipated generation and rebellion toward the established habits, customs, and practices of the profession. It must be admitted that the wearing of a beard, long, artistically shaved sideburns, or long hair is not the heart of the problem. The history of medicine bears witness to the fact that the physician's beard, his frock coat, his ornate heavy watch chain, his starched shirt, and his detachable cuffs were accoutrements that substituted for his lack of knowledge about disease processes and their treatment. The problem for students and faculty is not with the neatly dressed, clean individual with long hair or a beard, but with his unkempt, casually dressed, barefooted, bead-adorned fellow student. A form of appearance has developed among a small group of students who mark themselves with their symbols. It probably is fair to say that these symbols represent a means of freeing them from constricting, restricting, and confining rules which, they believe, deprive them of their individuality.

These individuals who wish to become physicians and surgeons present a paradox. To become a doctor, one must be a dedicated person who is quite free of most of the hang-ups of society. He must confront the problems of another human being's body and soul daily. This requires that he be comfortable and confident within himself, as well as knowledgeable. He must know his patient as a person and not as a disease entity alone. He must present to the patient the image of secure confidence that inspires confidence in return. The patient who believes he is being treated by someone who views him as an experiment or a lump of flesh, or by one who, himself, is obviously insecure and slovenly, is more frightened and more ill than his disease process predicts.

The art and the science of the practice of medicine demand the acceptance of more and more responsibility and less freedom. By definition, it is a constricting education not like that of the philosopher, the historian, the political scientist, or the chemist, all of whom may retain, throughout their education and practice, freedom of action that the doctor must deny himself. The physician or surgeon should maintain his freedom and individuality but must be sufficiently mature that he no longer needs the external exhibition of the fact that his freedom is limited only by himself and the needs of the patients whom he, alone, has chosen to serve.

Those who will push forward the boundaries of surgical treatment must have a thorough, applicable knowledge of all the sciences involved in the mechanisms of living tissue. Surgery is no longer a mechanical art; it is the coalition of several sciences, and those who would contribute to its advancement in the future, and who would give their patients the best possible care, must be educated and trained accordingly. To become a surgeon today requires postgraduate education and training. This period of study must be one of teaching, learning, and training. Too often, the words "residency training" are interpreted as an apprenticeship in techniques.

There are programs available for those who voluntarily wish to devote years of their life and career to become a surgeon. There are no excuses today for short cuts for those unwilling to make all the sacrifices necessary, or unable intellectually and mentally to accept the disciplined education necessary to become a surgeon.

Regardless of the special field of surgery in which the postgraduate surgical student becomes interested, he should be educated and trained basically in the principles of surgery that apply to all parts of the body. The minimum should be 2 years, and it is to be hoped that eventually the pendulum may return to a 3:1 or 3:2 proportion between so-called general surgery and a special field of surgery.

A philosophy has developed that if one has an elementary education in diagnosis and examination, and an interest and experience in research, he is automatically a fully equipped surgeon. This is a completely false assumption, one that denies the art of surgery. It is as indefensible as the viewpoint of a surgeon who takes satisfaction in the number of patients he has operated upon that day, without careful thought of their preoperative and postoperative problems, without a study of the pathologic condition found, or a meticulous record which may become part of an enlightening clinical study, and who has no interest in or sympathy with contributions from the research laboratory. Neither of these attitudes is the attitude of a surgeon.

There are other reasons for a broad, basic education and training in the principles of surgery. Not every young graduate can make a fixed decision at the beginning about a special field of surgery. He may change more than once, to his own and his patients' advantage, and he should analyze his decision and keep his mind open as he becomes temporarily a surgical specialist in each field in his progress through the program.

Of more importance is the fact that if he decides to live and prosper in a smaller community without a medical school, he should have knowledge in all fields of surgery. He should be able to recognize and confidently deal with an impacted fracture of the surgical neck of the humerus or femur, for example. He must also be professionally and ethically honest, and direct his patient to the orthopedic surgeon for the introduction of a prosthetic head of the femur.

Lack of basic education and training for all surgical residents is one of the weakest areas of many postgraduate programs. Each surgical specialty seeks its own medical school department, autonomous and in many instances unwilling to cooperate in the education and training of surgeons in the true sense.

On the other hand, there are chairmen of departments of surgery who are reluctant to provide places in their programs of basic surgical training for young men who have decided to devote themselves to a particular field of surgery. This separation into compartments of surgery should be stopped, both in the medical school, where administration and teaching can be decentralized but coordinated under the department of surgery chairman, and in the hospital, so that residents may receive basic education and training in every aspect of surgery. Ideally, both medical school and hospital staffs should be so organized, not only for the best immediate interests of young men, but also for the best surgical care for the patient, the goal so often taken for granted in the struggle of men to build their own little empires.

There are at least two problems of present residency programs that are difficult to resolve.

One deals with the methodology of education and training, and the other with remuneration for the postgraduate student in surgery.

No essential difference in the opportunities for education and training of the resident exist between patients who pay the attending surgeon and teacher for his services and those who are unable to pay a professional fee but are, or are not, able to finance their hospitalization costs. That resident can become an envied surgeon who is taught step by step the proper technique of the repair of an inguinal hernia and the gentle handling of tissues; the thought that should be devoted to each patient's surgical problem before operation; the critical review of how each operation might have been performed more skillfully and expeditiously, from incision to placement of the last suture and dressing; the art of dealing with the patient's relatives for the protection of the patient; and the discussion of the proper fee based completely upon the patient's ability to pay in relation to the magnitude of the surgical procedure, though his experiences have been confined wholly to so-called "private" patients.

It must be recognized that the resident and his surgical teacher have reciprocal responsibilities to teach and to learn, and a joint responsibility to give the patient the best possible surgical treatment. One surgical chief once said that every young doctor who aspired to become a surgeon should evaluate both his inherent ability to use his hands and his brain cooperatively and the breadth and integrity of his imagination. He did not mean an imagination to conceive new procedures, new operating table attachments, or instrumental gimmicks but the ability to imagine himself, his wife, mother, father, or child as the patient.

Such an aspiring resident, as he sits in a comfortable chair in his quarters, can perform an operation upon an imaginary patient. He should be able to imagine difficulties in finding the appendix, or identifying the cystic duct, and then deal with them successfully, as would Walter Mitty. He should collect many questions for his chief, to be asked at the propitious moment, under the proper circumstances, not when the great man is having difficulty in identifying the common duct.

This is not to say that teaching beds supported by endowment, taxes, and, in part, insurance hospitalization benefits are unnecessary and superfluous. It is to say, however, that patients who occupy such beds should not be under the complete, sole authority of the senior resident and his assistant residents. The best education and training for surgery require that the professor and his associates assume responsibility for the best possible surgical care and act as the residents' first assistants. This requires energy, time, and dedication to the task of teaching, and it does interfere with the professional staff's personal interests in surgical practice, laboratory investigations, administrative committee meetings, which multiply according to Parkinson's law, and peripatetic desires supported by boxes of large and small lantern slides.

It requires that the patient admitted to the hospital under these circumstances be informed and made to understand that the resident will operate and have responsibility, assisted by the surgeon-in-chief or his associates. This, too, requires time and effort, but it prevents the criticism of ghost surgery, and ensures the best care for the patient. It may help the resident realize that, regardless of his seniority and his youthful, admirable self-confidence, there will always be something he can learn about surgery, and that if he does not have an inner stimulus to continue to learn, he will fail as a surgeon.

With understanding of the changing social and economic structure of the United States, it is reasonable to ask why students engaged in postgraduate study in surgery should be remunerated. It is difficult to accept the statement that because he is married and has children, someone else should be responsible for his economic security during the period of his continued education. It is only fair to accept the premise that biologic urges in men of the same age group were the same 50 years ago as they are now. The question is whether or not the postgraduate student is present primarily to be educated and trained as a surgeon.

In a voluntarily supported hospital, funds to support such an educational program come from the hospital's operating income; none have an endowment sufficiently large to fund residency graduate teaching programs. In state- or county-supported institutions, these funds are derived from taxes. In either case, the expense becomes an item in the increased cost of medical care. In a recent survey of 96 hospitals in 10 cities, representing all types of ownership and management, and geographically distributed, the average cash remuneration received by the house staff averaged $6900 annually for interns, and from $7500 for first-year residents to $9800 for fifth-year residents. In the analysis of fringe benefits, or perquisites, the survey found that almost 50 per cent of the institutions paid the full cost of hospitalization for their house staffs and 30 per cent of the institutions paid the full cost for coverage of dependents. It indicated that two-thirds of the hospitals provided laundry services and supplied duty uniforms for their house staffs. Other benefits included parking privileges, food, housing, attendance at professional meetings, and free tuition at nearby colleges. The majority of the hospitals relied on patient revenues for the financial support of salaries and perquisites; other sources, but far less frequent, were federal grants and state appropriations. Very few hospitals reported that medical schools were a source of funding for those programs of postgraduate educations.

In addition to being sick and used for teaching, the patient must also pay for the latter privilege. Teaching by a university and a hospital is a charitable gift, and perhaps the patient should be able to deduct all of his hospital bill, since a great share of the bill supports medical teaching. But, it is said, insurance companies pay for most of the hospital bill; but who pays the premiums, which necessarily are being increased? Every other school and every other department of a voluntarily supported university gets its funds for teaching from the university. There isn't anyone like the patient to support the chemistry department, the law school, or the school of business.

It is true that postgraduate students in surgery have been placed at a disadvantage with their college classmates in engineering and in the physical or biologic sciences. Their contemporaries earn respectable incomes immediately after graduation from college; the medical school graduate is more certain to give military service, and the postgraduate educational years have been assumed voluntarily, since they are unnecessary for the qualifications required by state licensure bodies.

There should be several criteria to judge the value received from the expense involved. Does it provide better surgeons to give the best possible care for the patient? Are young surgeons equitably distributed geographically to provide the improved care? Are there too many candidates for education and training in the multiple fields of specialization? Does specialism produce doctors who know much about one thing and nothing about the art of the practice of surgery?

The tendency toward specialization and research and away from teaching students to care for patients has been most marked in universities, the very place it should be condemned. At present, members of a medical school faculty are able to devote about 40 per cent of their time to research activities. As the faculty has engaged more and more in appropriate scholarly activities within the medical school and hospital, it has become less and less closely associated with the practice of medicine in the community in which many of its graduates participate. Sir William Osler foresaw the unfortunate impact of the "full-time" system on the teaching of medicine. He wrote: "The danger would be the evolution throughout the country of a set of clinical prigs, the boundary of whose horizon would be the laboratory and whose only human interest was research, forgetful of the wider claims of the clinical professor as a trainer of the young, a leader in the multiform activities of the profession, an interpreter of science to the generation, and a counselor in public and private of the people in whose interests after all the school exists."

## SURGICAL SOCIETIES AND COLLEGES

In medieval times, certain monks were appointed to perform the tasks of shaving, bleeding, pulling teeth, and dressing wounds. In 1163, at the Council of Tours, the activities of the monks were restricted to their religious duties, and they were forbidden to leave the monastery to attend the sick and injured. Consequently, elementary surgical practices fell into the hands of military surgeons, barbers, bath-keepers, and traveling charlatans, and it became necessary to belong to a guild to practice a craft. Guilds, like unions today, exerted great power. The members had specific religious and civic duties, wore their own livery, participated in processions, and contributed to the treasury of

the city. Soon, barbers took on more of the duties originally performed by the monks and became barber-surgeons.

The red and white striped pole represented the blood and bandages of the barber-surgeon's craft. The number of members of the guild trained in anatomy and surgery gradually increased, and the guild became a union of barbers and surgeons, which existed mainly for civic and economic reasons. Eventually, the surgeons formed companies of their own and gained authority to train apprentices, conduct examinations, license practitioners, and guard the public health. As charters were granted by kings with permission to use the royal favor, these companies became royal colleges.

The oldest royal college is that of Edinburgh, which was incorporated in 1505 by the favor of James IV, who was interested in medicine and tried his skill at surgery. The charter required that each member be acquainted with anatomy, and the company was entitled to receive each year the body of one criminal "efter he be deid" for dissection. The organization had a bath house, a laboratory, and a library. In 1695, the surgeons were separated from the barbers, and in 1778, the corporation became the Royal College, though it remained a municipal body until 1850.

The chronologic development of the Royal College of Surgeons in England was similar. From 1300 to 1540, there was an incorporated Company of Barbers, and the Guild of Surgeons was unincorporated; from 1540 to 1745, it was the Company of Barber-Surgeons; the Company of Surgeons existed from 1745 to 1800; and the Royal College of Surgeons of London existed from 1800 to 1843, when the present name was adopted. Henry VIII granted the charter to the Company of Barbers in 1540, and this is depicted in a famous painting by Holbein. Of the 10 identified members, four were barbers, four were surgeons, and two were "foreigners."

After complete separation of the surgeons and the receipt of their charters, examinations for fellowship were initiated, and today a fellowship is required for qualification to practice surgery in Great Britain. Each of the royal colleges of surgeons has devoted its efforts to postgraduate education and research to elevate the standards of care to patients.

The American College of Surgeons, founded in 1913, was patterned in many respects after the royal colleges in Great Britain. Its primary goal is to improve the care of surgical patients, and this has been contributed to by its efforts in improving postgraduate surgical education, elevating the standards of hospitals, and educating the lay public. Gradually, the qualifications for fellowship have been raised until at present they consist of an education and training that qualify the candidate for examination by the boards of surgery and its specialities, and evidence of high personal and professional moral and ethical standards.

There are hundreds of medical societies, surgical associations, and colleges in the United States. Doctors voluntarily join county medical societies, membership in which entitles them to membership in their state medical society and the American Medical Association. These basic medical organizations require graduation from an approved medical school, a state license to practice medicine, and evidence of good ethical and professional practices. Their activities include the presentation of scientific papers by their members and invited guests and discussion of problems that influence the practice of medicine. Each state has a medical society, as does each county except in those instances when two or three contiguous small counties have joined together to form one society.

The American Medical Association was founded in 1847 through the efforts of Nathan Smith Davis. It is a confederation of state societies. It has a Board of Trustees, which is the policy-making body, but, in effect, this power lies within the House of Delegates. This body consists of 244 delegates, including those chosen by each state society in a number proportionate to the number of doctors practicing in the state who are members of the state society and the American Medical Association; representatives from the scientific sections of the Association; and representatives from the government medical services.

There is a multitude of more exclusive societies representing specialty areas in the practice of medicine and surgery, and others dedicated to specific diseases or organs of the body. The specialty societies require evidence of proper education and training in the specific field, and the disease and organ societies limit their membership to those who have shown interest by their work and contributions.

The American Surgical Association is typical of associations and societies formed by doctors who have an interest in a special area of medicine and is one of the oldest. It was founded in 1881 by a group of surgeons whose leader and first president was Samuel Gross. Objections to it centered around the supposition that a new association was being organized that would usurp the functions of the American Medical Association and destroy its influence as the representative body of the medical profession. It was argued that all the objectives sought by such an association of surgeons could be accomplished through the section on surgery of the American Medical Association. There had been many discussions of the rights of surgical specialists compared with those of general practitioners; the economic, scientific, and social aspects of specialization were attracting increasing attention. Gross replied that the new organization would strengthen the American Medical Association "by rousing it from its Rip Van Winkle slumbers and infusing new life into it."

It is doubtful that any new medical or surgical society has been formed without meeting opposition from the members of an older society. Often, the members of exclusively small, special societies become so conservative that they oppose the admission of younger men. So the younger men band together and form a new society; they in turn become older and more reactionary; young, aggressive men rebel and form a society, and the cycle is repeated. Or, when certain geographic areas of the country are not represented in the membership of national societies, directions of the compass designate new associations of surgeons. The ever increasing multiplicity of medical and surgical societies is not bad; it only emphasizes the desire of doctors to meet together, discuss their problems, learn from each other, and indulge their inherent peripatetic personalities.

## ETHICS AND PRACTICES

Surgeons should always be proud of belonging to a profession that stands alone in the enforcement of adherence of its members to a high code of ethical conduct that guides the relationship between its members and their patients and dates back to the Hippocratic oath.

The Principles of Medical Ethics of the American Medical Association contain the code of ethics to which all medical organizations subscribe. However, neither the Principles nor their interpretation by the Judicial Council of the Association has always been clear and precise. Violations by the more enterprising members of the profession have been frequent. Therefore, the Board of Regents of the American College of Surgeons, in no way a subsidiary organization of the American Medical Association, has made its own interpretation and requires its Fellows to observe a more stringent course of ethical conduct than that specified in the Principles. The Regents have held that the College has the right and responsibility to do this in the interest of the welfare and best professional care of the patient and disciplines its Fellows for infractions.

The most controversial interpretation of the Board of Regents has been that of the principles governing the financial relations in the professional care of patients. A pledge against fee-splitting has been required of its Fellows since the founding of the College, and was also required of every physician practicing in a hospital approved by the College when it originated and conducted the program of hospital standardization.

It has been well established that the practice of return by the operating surgeon of a portion of the patient's fee to the referring doctor, without the patient's knowledge, has not been prevalent in every state of the Union, but where it has existed, it has been a serious threat to the advancement of the best care of the patient. The result has been that the patient has been referred for care to the surgeon who proved to be the highest bidder and not necessarily the best qualified surgeon.

Many do not understand the serious implications of fee-splitting; in fact, lawyers make a practice of returning a percentage of a client's fee to the referring firm. Lawyers deal with estates, properties, and businesses and not with human lives. Errors by inept attorneys can be judged in money lost, not lives.

When a patient is referred for care and treatment, the surgeon is morally and legally responsible for the preoperative diagnosis, the decision to operate, preoperative care, performance of the operation, and postoperative care as long as the surgical condition of the patient is of major importance. Consultation with and advice from colleagues in other fields of practice should be sought freely, and when surgical care is no longer needed, the patient should be referred back to his physician, with a complete and detailed report of the care given and the progress of the patient.

The concept of surgical care as a combined effort of several doctors is important, and the patient should be informed that he may be cared for by several individuals working under the direction of the responsible surgeon. The attending surgeon is also responsible for the acts of residents, and in order to discharge fully this responsibility to the patient, he must actively supervise operations performed by the resident and so inform the patient. The active supervisory participation provides excellent teaching for the resident, ensures the best possible surgical care, and obviates the charge of ghost surgery that exists when the patient is unaware of the identity of the operating surgeon.

Discussion between the doctor and the patient or his relatives before a statement for professional fees is submitted may prevent misunderstandings and the resentment of patients about a fee they learn about for the first time when they receive the doctor's billhead in the mail. A satisfactory agreement can be reached by a frank discussion of all the considerations involved in determination of a fee. The fee should be commensurate with the services given and the reasonable ability of the patient to pay. In the case of the physician, the value of the services performed depends upon the nature of the disease and the skill required to treat it, as well as the length of time the patient is ill. The surgeon's fee depends upon the nature and extent of the operation, and the special skill required, and should include those services given by him personally, by his employees, or by surgical associates under his direction.

Reasonable ability to pay a fee should be based upon all the expenses of the family, regardless of the existence of insurance against the cost of the medical or surgical care. Medical or surgical insurance is not designed to serve as a platform upon which to erect an additional fee not justified by the economic circumstances of the family. To abuse insurance in such a way nullifies the individual's benefits for which he has paid a premium and will quickly destroy voluntary insurance programs.

A surgical assistant who has no other professional relationship with the patient may be compensated by the surgeon. The referring physician, or consultant, should submit his individual bill directly to the patient for the services he performs. Ethically, a surgeon should not pay the referring physician for any services the latter may perform in the care of the patient; nor should he resort to any subterfuge to assist the referring physician to collect an unjustifiable fee, such as permitting

him to render unnecessary services in the operating room.

Combined statements of the fees of two or more doctors should be itemized to show clearly to the patient the services performed by each doctor and the amount each is to be paid. It is far better if separate statements are sent to the patient, or to an insurance carrier. In the submission of statements to patients, clinic groups and formal partnerships are regarded as single contractors, and it is ethical and proper to submit one bill for all the services given by individual members of the group clinic or partnership.

Some insurance companies will pay only one physician for the care given by all doctors in the treatment of the patient, stating that multiple bills complicate their accounting practices. This is not an ideal arrangement because it encourages unethical financial arrangements. If the insurance benefit specifically covers the entire medical care of the patient, and not merely the surgical operation, the surgeon may receive the single check and then pay the fees submitted individually by other physicians for their services by his own check, if it is made payable jointly to the patient and the doctor.

The sole point at issue is the interests of the patient, which should be the primary responsibility of the physician; referral of the patient for surgical care, or expert care in any special field, should be based solely upon the quality of the care expected. Acceptance of any other inducement is a violation of the trust that should exist between the patient and his doctor. The most common unethical inducements are division of the surgical fee between the surgeon and the referring physician, regardless of the source of the payment, be it an insurance carrier or the patient; permitting the referring physician to collect the total bill from the patient and pay the surgeon; alternate billing of surgical patients, whereby the surgeon and the referring physician collect and retain the entire fee from alternate patients; disproportionate reduction of the surgeon's fee to enable the referring physician to charge excessively for his services; and payment of office rent on a percentage of professional income, particularly when the owners or lessees of the space can refer patients to the surgeon.

It is also unethical to accept a rebate from a manufacturer or dealer who has supplied a patient with drugs, appliances, or any other adjunct to treatment, such as eye glasses, or to accept a rebate or reduction in cost from clinical pathology or roentgenology laboratories for work referred to them.

With the idea of voluntary health insurance in the United States came the insistence that whatever was covered must be quantifiable so that it could be priced. The cost of hospitalization was a tangible item, and Blue Cross came into existence. But the definitions of hospital costs are so complex that there were bound to be constant haggles with state insurance departments over rates.

Some Blue Cross plans cover in-hospital doctors' fees, a function reserved by other plans for Blue Shield. Whatever have been the limitations and deficiencies, commerical insurance companies have followed Blue Cross and Blue Shield plans. Though widely misrepresented as health insurance, the premium is on sickness. At present, most Blue Cross plans cover diagnostic procedures, which need not necessarily be done in a hospital.

Blue Cross insurance pays virtually all the hospital bill and, if a family has coverage by Blue Shield, the doctor's bill. However broad the coverage of Blue Cross, Blue Shield, and commercial insurance companies may become, competition with prepaid group-practice plans increases. In 1966, the Blue Cross plans paid for 876 patient-days in the hospital per 1000 subscribers, while the group-practice plans paid for 408; Blue Shield subscribers had 73 surgical procedures per 1000, while the groups' subscribers had 31.

Voluntary insurance, regardless of its organization, has encountered competition from the federal law that created Medicare. This provided every citizen 65 years of age or older, except retired federal employees, with 60 days of free hospital care, after an original $40 deductible that was designed to discourage unnecessary hospitalization. Thirty or more days of hospital care at a charge of $10 a day was provided; 20 days of free nursing-home care; 80 more days of nursing-home care at a cost of $5.00 a day; 100 home visits by nurses or other health specialists after hospitalization; and 80 per cent of the cost of hospital diagnostic tests, after a $20 deductible for each series. To finance this coverage, the taxable wage base of Social Security was raised and the tax increased for both employee and employer.

The voluntary supplement to Medicare provided payment of 80 per cent of reasonable charges for all physicians' services over $50; another 100 home visits, whether or not the patient was hospitalized and the costs of nonhospital diagnostic tests, surgical dressings, splints, and rented medical equipment. Those citizens 65 years of age and older who wished to participate voluntarily were to pay $3.00 a month, and these contributions were to be supplemented from general revenues of the Treasury. Both the taxable wage base of Social Security and the monthly contributions to cover physicians' fees have been increased to finance the plan.

To avoid abuse of the distribution of benefits of medical care insurance, and innumerable interpretations of what is and is not ethical practice, the benefits should be paid directly to the patient, thus strengthening an important part of the patient-doctor relationship, and giving to the policy holder the benefits he is entitled to by the payment of his premiums.

The benefits of medical insurance should be based upon the premium costs of the policy coverage and not upon the name of the operation or disease. Insurance companies have obtained the cooperation of county and state medical societies in setting fee schedules for various operations, and many of the designated surgical fees are ridiculously scheduled. Moreover, fee schedules thus established tend to be the fee understood as acceptable to the profession, regardless of the skill and talent required or the economic ability of the patient to pay. It makes a trades union of a profession and encourages the establishment of a level of mediocrity.

## SURGEON AND PATIENT

The reputation of a surgeon is more sensitive than that of a member of any other profession, and his good name is exquisitely reactive to patients' gossip. The most stimulating, most gratifying, and at the same time most exasperating experiences in a surgeon's life can be the relations with patients and their families. It is quite simple for a surgeon to become careless and assume that patients know as much about their illness as he does; or to become frustrated when, after a careful explanation to them in as simple language as he can use, they give evidence by their next question that they have comprehended little. It is easy to form the habit of telling them nothing, and to rationalize it by believing this is the best for their psychologic state. Many patients learn of their forthcoming surgical treatment only that their operation will be on Friday.

The indications for an operation, what it is hoped can be accomplished, and the extent of the continued follow-up care should be explained in detail to the patient and his family. The most fantastic errors can be encountered in the relay of this information from the patient to his relatives, or from one relative to another, so that sometimes multiple explanations must be given patiently.

These meetings afford another method of learning about the responsibilities of the family and their ambitions and aims, in short, an opportunity to establish a personal relationship of the type enjoyed by the old-style family doctor. The less personal the relationship, the more certain it is that the patient and his family will think bitterly in terms of percentage of the patient's recovery, based upon his condition as a healthy youth, when they are dissatisfied with the results of his surgical operation.

There is, of course, a difference between the patients of today and those of yesterday; it is too easy to place all the onus for a poor doctor-patient relationship upon changes in the doctor. With some modern patients, a major surgical operation is followed by a minor degree of gratitude. The patient's life may be saved only to have him complain that his sutures stick, the nurses have cold hands, the hospital bed is hard, the coffee abominable, and the hospital bills outrageous. The final summing up consists in the conclusion that the high cost of medical care is due solely to the surgeon's fee.

Today's patient may rush off to the law courts after surgery if he wakes up from an extensive life-saving operation and finds a safety pin sticking him, or if he incurs a backache at his work. If he coughs in front of a jury, or limps into the court-room on a cane, he gets an award, the size of which is increasing, as is, naturally, the fee of his lawyer, who encouraged him to file the suit. Citizens have become more and more security-minded and more dependent upon unions and governmental agencies. The world, they say, owes them a living. What is more natural than for a citizen to turn to his surgeon's or employer's insurance company, which appears to be a limitless source of wealth? He rationalizes this by saying that it won't take anything out of an individual's pocket.

The increasing interest of the public in medicine and a more widespread knowledge of medical facts are factors that exert a profound influence upon the practice of surgery. Articles fill magazines and newspapers, and scenes of the operating room are as familiar on television screens as scenes of frontier saloons. The general effect of public interest and knowledge of medicine has been good, but often the popular presentation of a surgical procedure has been exaggerated to make it effective to the layman. The result may be that the reader or viewer, who is not very discerning at best, may be misled to anticipate a more favorable outcome of an illness or injury than even the best surgeon, or the best operation, can deliver. Weekly picture magazines vividly portray the surgical anatomy, pathology, and operative steps in the treatment of heart disease or low back ailments, so clearly, in fact, that a patient may regard his surgeon as slightly mentally retarded if he expresses a reservation.

There is no justification for the surgeon who releases an announcement of the results of his experimental or clinical investigations, or an impending new operation, to the press prior to presentation before a scientific society of his peers. He is helpless to stop the press from reporting upon his presentation, but, with the cooperation of his colleagues in the society, he can attempt to influence a reasonably factual report upon his experiences. However, regardless of all efforts, the headlines that cover the story are under the control of neither the writer, the surgeon nor the society. They are written for the single purpose of selling newspapers and can, therefore, be entirely misleading to patients.

## SOCIAL, ECONOMIC, AND EDUCATIONAL FACTORS IN THE PRACTICE OF SURGERY

The practice of surgery is being influenced by social, economic, and educational factors far more strongly than at any other time in its history.

The United States is experiencing the trials, tribulations, and penalties of an era of the half-done job. To put it another way, this is an era in which there are constant attempts to legislate all facets of enterprise to the level of mediocrity. It is the age of plumbers who may come to fix a leaky faucet some day, maybe; of salesmen and saleswomen who at their pleasure respond to inquiries about their merchandise; of teachers who demand a single salary schedule so that achievement cannot be rewarded; of students who take cinch courses and believe that they know more about what should be taught than their professors; and of doctors who sponsor fee schedules that reward the unqualified surgeon equally with the well educated and well trained surgeon. There appears to be a stampede away from the goal of first-rateness and responsibility.

With the basic tenets of democracy that all men are born free and equal and are entitled to life, liberty, and the pursuit of happiness, no one can take issue. It is manifestly absurd, however, to maintain that a physician with no education and training in surgery, who calls himself a surgeon and has the legal right to operate upon a patient without restriction, is the equal of the surgeon who has voluntarily spent many years in formal education and training to become qualified to express an authoritative opinion, which he can implement with skill and talent. Yet a study of specific categories of the most commonly performed surgical operations in hospitals of varying bed capacities in the United States showed that 50 per cent of these operations are performed by doctors who have sought the short cut, those who have not been willing to pursue the hard path toward the goal of first-rateness in surgery.

Self-declared surgeons have attempted to establish certifying boards by edict, with standards below the accepted minimum. Failing to receive acceptance, they used the goon tactics of labor union leaders in an attempt to force their will upon men who strive to maintain the first-rate in the care of surgical patients.

To strive for the first-rate in surgery entails the willingness to listen to the suggestions of the young, and to modify and adopt them if possible in education, training, and practice. It does not mean, however, the abandonment of experience and tradition, or substitution of the mediocre for the excellent. This pursuit of the first-rate often encounters a philosophy that what is right is not as important as what is momentarily beneficial to the individual or the organization.

There is reason to have knowledge of and respect for orthodoxy in the education, training, and practice of surgeons. This means the holding of the correct views that are in the best interests of the public, and the care of the surgical patient is a matter of public interest. The difficulty is in preventing orthodoxy from passing into stagnation, or assuming prerogatives that do not permit discarding theories and practices that have ceased to be commonly accepted or have no further value.

Gradually, medical school faculties and universities have relinquished what little influence they have had in the determination of the character and maintenance of the quality of surgical education to groups that should function only as completely independent and unprejudiced examiners. These examining bodies should not be accountable for the review, approval, or disapproval of the requirements and conduct of graduate study in surgery. The surgical faculty of the medical school should state that the candidate has fulfilled its prescribed course of graduate study in a satisfactory manner, and that he has been granted an advanced degree, which indicates that it believes him to be a properly educated surgeon. The faculty should state that the candidate is prepared for an examination of his qualifications as a surgeon. The faculty should publish the contents of its course of study in postgraduate surgical education just as is done in other fields of postgraduate study.

The existing boards of surgery and the surgical specialties should examine the products of these university-directed programs of education in surgery. The method and scope of examination should be determined independently by each board of examiners. The quality of the product of graduate programs in surgical education may be judged by the results of the examinations.

In recognition of completing the course of graduate surgical study and successfully passing the board examination, fellowship in the American College of Surgeons should be granted after a satisfactory demonstration of adherence to, and support of, the principles of ethical and professional practices and conduct promulgated by the College and the American Medical Association.

There can be no question about the important influence the Committee on Graduate Training in Surgery of the American College of Surgeons, the Council on Medical Education and Hospitals, the Advisory Board for Medical Specialties, and the boards of surgery and the surgical specialties have had upon raising the standards of education for surgeons, and thus elevating the care of surgical patients. It is time, however, that universities and their medical school faculties play a more dominant and direct role in the postgraduate education of surgeons.

It is doubtful if a young man completing a surgical educational program can be examined properly by any method, or by any group of men, and graded justly or accurately. His chief and his associates are the ones who can judge most fairly and completely the breadth of his surgical knowledge, his integrity, and his search for the first-rate in his surgical performances without thought of monthly remuneration or hours off duty.

The surgeon must learn to analyze himself and establish his highest level of performance and integrity. The initiative and responsibility for becoming first-rate rest with the individual. These qualities of the resident in surgery can be recognized and encouraged by his teachers but they cannot be measured and graded. They are the elements that finally distinguish the surgeon whose greatest reward is his own satisfaction with his individual performance.

Education in surgery is a continuing process. What will result from the shortening of the education process of a doctor to permit him to begin his surgical educational and training program at an earlier age? Is there an hour of a day in a certain month of a specific year when the surgical student can say, "Now I am a surgeon," and stop his learning process? Does it matter what name is given the year following graduation from medical school? Is it not a time for study and teaching, experience, and self-analysis just as is the tenth or twentieth postcommencement year?

There is a preoccupation with the problems of teaching students how to be good surgeons and care for patients among a group who have never practiced surgery competitively, or have found it beyond their talents. Thus, these men, in their own opinions, qualify to establish dicta and introduce the schism-producing phrase, "academic surgeon." Does this mean that he is the one who does not operate upon patients, but is academically or theoretically a surgeon? Does it mean that the surgeon who operates upon and cares for patients is not a scholar, cannot teach, and cannot investigate? Does it mean that the practicing surgeon who voluntarily gives his time, thought, and energy to teaching students and residents is not a good teacher because he receives no money for his teaching duties because his medical school does not have sufficient financial support to remunerate him?

There is an obligation to understand the privileges and responsibilities inherent in becoming a surgeon. He must be dedicated to keeping his own score in the pursuit of the first-rate. This involves his own code of personal and professional ethics, a feeling of obligation to contribute to the best of his ability and talents to the improvement of the care of surgical patients, a duty to uphold the values in education and training for which he will have sacrificed so much, a feeling for taste and style, and the capacity to recognize and enjoy the first-rate.

Guy de Chauliac (1300–1370) wrote a prescription for a surgeon that needs little modification today:

Let the surgeon be bold in all sure things, and fearful in dangerous things; let him avoid all faulty treatments and practices. He ought to be gracious to the sick, considerate to his associates, cautious in his prognostications. Let him be modest, dignified, gentle, pitiful and merciful; not covetous nor an extortionist of money; but rather let his reward be according to his work, to the means of the patient, to the quality of the issue, and to his own dignity.

# NORMAL LABORATORY VALUES

*Prepared by* REX B. CONN, M.D.,

## NORMAL HEMATOLOGIC VALUES

| | | |
|---|---|---|
| Acid hemolysis test (Ham) | No hemolysis | |
| Alkaline phosphatase, leukocyte | Total score 14–100 | |
| Bleeding time | | |
| Ivy | Less than 5 min. | |
| Duke | 1–5 min. | |
| Carboxyhemoglobin | Up to 5% of total | |
| Cell counts | | |
| Erythrocytes: Males | 4.6–6.2 million/cu. mm. | |
| Females | 4.2–5.4 million/cu. mm. | |
| Children (varies with age) | 4.5–5.1 million/cu. mm. | |

| Leukocytes | | | |
|---|---|---|---|
| Total | | 5000–10,000/cu. mm. | |
| Differential | *Percentage* | *Absolute* | |
| Myelocytes | 0 | 0/cu. mm. | |
| Juvenile neutrophils | 3– 5 | 150– 400/cu. mm. | |
| Segmented neutrophils | 54–62 | 3000–5800/cu. mm. | |
| Lymphocytes | 25–33 | 1500–3000/cu. mm. | |
| Monocytes | 3– 7 | 285– 500/cu. mm. | |
| Eosinophils | 1– ʻ3 | 50– 250/cu. mm. | |
| Basophils | 0– 0.75 | 15– 50/cu. mm. | |

(Infants and children have greater relative numbers of lymphocytes and monocytes)

| | |
|---|---|
| Platelets | 150,000–350,000/cu. mm. |
| Reticulocytes | 25,000– 75,000/cu. mm. |
| | 0.5–1.5% of erythrocytes |
| Clot retraction, qualitative | Begins in 30–60 min. |
| | Complete in 24 hrs. |
| Coagulation time (Lee-White) | 5–15 min. (glass tubes) |
| | 19–60 min. (siliconized tubes) |
| Cold hemolysin test (Donath-Landsteiner) | No hemolysis |
| Corpuscular values of erythrocytes | |

(Values are for adults; in children, values vary with age)

| | |
|---|---|
| M.C.H. (mean corpuscular hemoglobin) | 27–31 picogm. |
| M.C.V. (mean corpuscular volume) | 82–92 cu. micra |
| M.C.H.C. (mean corpuscular hemoglobin concentration) | 32–36% |
| Fibrinogen | 200–400 mg./100 ml. |
| Fibrinolysins | 0 |
| Hematocrit | |
| Males | 40–54 ml./100 ml. |
| Females | 37–47 ml./100 ml. |
| Newborn | 49–54 ml./100 ml. |
| Children (varies with age) | 35–49 ml./100 ml. |

| | |
|---|---|
| Hemoglobin | |
| Males | 14.0–18.0 grams/100 ml. |
| Females | 12.0–16.0 grams/100 ml. |
| Newborn | 16.5–19.5 grams/100 ml. |
| Children (varies with age) | 11.2–16.5 grams/100 ml. |
| Hemoglobin, fetal | Less than 1% of total |
| Hemoglobin A₂ | 1.5–3.0% of total |
| Hemoglobin, plasma | 0–5.0 mg./100 ml. |
| Methemoglobin | 0.03–0.13 grams/100 ml. |
| Osmotic fragility of erythrocytes | Begins in 0.45–0.39% NaCl |
| | Complete in 0.33–0.30% NaCl |
| Partial thromboplastin time | 60–70 sec. |
| Kaolin activated | 35–45 sec. |
| Prothrombin consumption | Over 80% consumed in 1 hr. |
| Prothrombin content | 100% (calculated from prothrombin time) |
| Prothrombin time (one stage) | 12.0–14.0 sec. |
| Sedimentation rate | |
| Wintrobe: Males | 0–5 mm. in 1 hr. |
| Females | 0–15 mm. in 1 hr. |
| Westergren: Males | 0–15 mm. in 1 hr. |
| Females | 0–20 mm. in 1 hr. |

(May be slightly higher in children and during pregnancy)

| | |
|---|---|
| Thromboplastin generation test | Compared to normal control |
| Tourniquet test | Ten or fewer petechiae in a 2.5 cm. circle after 5 min. with cuff at 100 mm. Hg |

| Bone marrow, differential cell count | *Range* | *Average* |
|---|---|---|
| Myeloblasts | 0.3– 5.0% | 2.0% |
| Promyelocytes | 1.0– 8.0% | 5.0% |
| Myelocytes: Neutrophilic | 5.0–19.0% | 12.0% |
| Eosinophilic | 0.5– 3.0% | 1.5% |
| Basophilic | 0.0– 0.5% | 0.3% |
| Metamyelocytes ("juvenile" forms) | 13.0–32.0% | 22.0% |
| Polymorphonuclear neutrophils | 7.0–30.0% | 20.0% |
| Polymorphonuclear eosinophils | 0.5– 4.0% | 2.0% |
| Polymorphonuclear basophils | 0.0– 0.7% | 0.2% |
| Lymphocytes | 3.0–17.0% | 10.0% |
| Plasma cells | 0.0– 2.0% | 0.4% |
| Monocytes | 0.5– 5.0% | 2.0% |
| Reticulum cells | 0.1– 2.0% | 0.2% |
| Megakaryocytes | 0.03– 3.0% | 0.4% |
| Pronormoblasts | 1.0– 8.0% | 4.0% |
| Normoblasts | 7.0–32.0% | 18.0% |

## NORMAL BLOOD, PLASMA, AND SERUM VALUES

For some procedures the normal values may vary depending upon the methods used.

| | |
|---|---|
| Acetone, serum | |
| Qualitative | Negative |
| Quantitative | 0.3–2.0 mg./100 ml. |
| Aldolase, serum | 0.8–3.0 ml.U./ml. (30°) (Sibley-Lehninger) |
| Alpha amino nitrogen, serum | 4–6 mg./100 ml. |
| Ammonia nitrogen, blood | 75–196 mcg./100 ml. |
| plasma | 56–122 mcg./100 ml. |
| Amylase, serum | 80–160 Somogyi units/100 ml. |
| Ascorbic acid | See Vitamin C |
| Base, total, serum | 145–160 mEq./liter |
| Bilirubin, serum | |
| Direct | 0.1–0.4 mg./100 ml. |
| Indirect | 0.2–0.7 mg./100 ml. (Total minus direct) |
| Total | 0.3–1.1 mg./100 ml. |
| Calcium, serum | 4.5–5.5 mEq./liter (9.0–11.0 mg./100 ml.) (Slightly higher in children) (Varies with protein concentration) |
| Calcium, serum, ionized | 2.1–2.6 mEq./liter (4.25–5.25 mg./100 ml.) |
| Carbon dioxide content, serum | 24–30 mEq./liter Infants: 20–28 mEq./liter |
| Carbon dioxide tension (Pco₂), blood | 35–45 mm. Hg |
| Carotene, serum | 50–300 mcg./100 ml. |
| Ceruloplasmin, serum | 23–44 mg./100 ml. |
| Chloride, serum | 96–106 mEq./liter |
| Cholesterol, serum | |
| Total | 150–250 mg./100 ml. |
| Esters | 68–76% of total cholesterol |
| Cholinesterase, serum | 0.5–1.3 pH units |
| RBC | 0.5–1.0 pH units |
| Copper, serum | |
| Male | 70–140 mcg./100 ml. |
| Female | 85–155 mcg./100 ml. |
| Cortisol, plasma | 6–16 mcg./100 ml. |
| Creatine, serum | 0.2–0.8 mg./100 ml. |

| | |
|---|---|
| Creatine phosphokinase, serum | |
| Male | 0–50 mI.U./ml. (30°) (Oliver-Rosalki) |
| Female | 0–30 mI.U./ml. (30°) (Oliver-Rosalki) |
| Creatinine, serum | 0.7–1.5 mg./100 ml. |
| Cryoglobulins, serum | 0 |
| Fatty acids, total, serum | 190–420 mg./100 ml. |
| Fibrinogen, plasma | 200–400 mg./100 ml. |
| Folic acid, serum | 7–16 nanogm./ml. |
| Glucose (fasting) | |
| blood, true | 60–100 mg./100 ml. |
| Folin | 80–120 mg./100 ml. |
| plasma or serum, true | 70–115 mg./100 ml. |
| Haptoglobin, serum | 40–170 mg./100 ml. |
| Hydroxybutyric dehydrogenase, serum | 0–180 mI.U./ml. (30°) (Rosalki-Wilkinson) 114–290 units/ml. (Wroblewski) |
| 17-Hydroxycorticosteroids, plasma | 8–18 mcg./100 ml. |
| Icterus index, serum | 4–7 |
| Immunoglobulins, serum | |
| IgG | 800–1500 mg./100 ml. |
| IgA | 50–200 mg./100 ml. |
| IgM | 40–120 mg./100 ml. |
| Iodine, butanol extractable, serum | 3.2–6.4 mcg./100 ml. |
| Iodine, protein bound, serum | 3.5–8.0 mcg./100 ml. (May be slightly higher in infants) |
| Iron, serum | 75–175 mcg./100 ml. |
| Iron binding capacity, total, serum | 250–410 mcg./100 ml. |
| % saturation | 20–55% |
| 17-Ketosteroids, plasma | 25–125 mcg./100 ml. |
| Lactic acid, blood | 6–16 mg./100 ml. |
| Lactic dehydrogenase, serum | 0–300 mI.U./ml. (30°) (Wroblewski modified) 150–450 units/ml. (Wroblewski) 80–120 units/ml. (Wacker) |
| Lipase, serum | 0–1.5 units (Cherry-Crandall) |
| Lipids, total, serum | 450–850 mg./100 ml. |

# OF CLINICAL IMPORTANCE

*The Johns Hopkins School of Medicine, Baltimore*

## NORMAL BLOOD, PLASMA, AND SERUM VALUES (*Continued*)

| | |
|---|---|
| Magnesium, serum | 1.5–2.5 mEq./liter |
| | (1.8–3.0 mg./100 ml.) |
| Nitrogen, nonprotein, serum | 15–35 mg./100 ml. |
| Osmolality, serum | 285–295 mOsm./liter |
| Oxygen, blood | |
|   Capacity | 16–24 vol. % (varies with Hb) |
|   Content    Arterial | 15–23 vol. % |
|              Venous | 10–16 vol. % |
|   Saturation  Arterial | 94–100% of capacity |
|              Venous | 60–85% of capacity |
|   Tension, $P_{O_2}$ Arterial | 75–100 mm. Hg |
| pH, arterial, blood | 7.35–7.45 |
| Phenylalanine, serum | Less than 3 mg./100 ml. |
| Phosphatase, acid, serum | 1.0–5.0 units (King-Armstrong) |
| | 0.5–2.0 units (Bodansky) |
| | 0.5–2.0 units (Gutman) |
| | 0.0–1.1 units (Shinowara) |
| | 0.1–0.63 unit (Bessey-Lowry) |
| Phosphatase, alkaline, serum | 5.0–13.0 units (King-Armstrong) |
| | 2.0–4.5 units (Bodansky) |
| | 3.0–10.0 units (Gutman) |
| | 2.2–8.6 units (Shinowara) |
| | 0.8–2.3 units (Bassey-Lowry) |
| | 30–85 milliunits/ml. (I.U.) |
| | (Values are higher in children) |
| Phosphate, inorganic, serum | 3.0–4.5 mg./100 ml. |
| | (Children: 4.0–7.0 mg./100 ml.) |
| Phospholipids, serum | 6–12 mg./100 ml. as lipid phosphorus |
| Potassium, serum | 3.5–5.0 mEq./liter |
| Proteins, serum | |
|   Total | 6.0–8.0 grams/100 ml. |
|   Albumin | 3.5–5.5 grams/100 ml. |
|   Globulin | 2.5–3.5 grams/100 ml. |
|   Electrophoresis | |
|     Albumin | 3.5–5.5 grams/100 ml. |
| | 52–68% of total |
|     Globulin | |
|       Alpha₁ | 0.2–0.4 gram/100 ml. |
| | 2–5% of total |

| | |
|---|---|
|       Alpha₂ | 0.5–0.9 gram/100 ml. |
| | 7–14% of total |
|       Beta | 0.6–1.1 grams/100 ml. |
| | 9–15% of total |
|       Gamma | 0.7–1.7 grams/100 ml. |
| | 11–21% of total |
| Pyruvic acid, plasma | 1.0–2.0 mg./100 ml. |
| Serotonin, platelet suspension | 0.1–0.3 mcg./ml. blood |
|   serum | 0.10–0.32 mcg./ml. |
| Sodium, serum | 136–145 mEq./liter |
| Sulfates, inorganic, serum | 0.8–1.2 mg./100 ml. (as S) |
| Thyroxine, free, serum | 1.0–2.1 nanogm./100 ml. |
| Thyroxine binding globulin | |
|   (TBG), serum | 10–26 mcg./100 ml. |
| Thyroxine iodine (T₄), serum | 2.9–6.4 mcg./100 ml. |
| Transaminase, serum: SGOT | 0.19 mI.U./ml. (30°) |
| | (Karmen modified) |
| | 15–40 units/ml. (Karmen) |
| | 18–40 units/ml. |
| | (Reitman-Frankel) |
|                 SGPT | 0.17 mI.U./ml. (30°) |
| | (Karmen modified) |
| | 6–35 units/ml. (Karmen) |
| | 5–35 units/ml. |
| | (Reitman-Frankel) |
| Triglycerides, serum | 0–150 mg./100 ml. |
| Urea, blood | 21–43 mg./100 ml. |
|   plasma or serum | 24–49 mg./100 ml. |
| Urea nitrogen, blood (BUN) | 10–20 mg./100 ml. |
|   plasma or serum | 11–23 mg./100 ml. |
| Uric acid, serum | |
|   Male | 2.5–8.0 mg./100 ml. |
|   Female | 1.5–6.0 mg./100 ml. |
| Vitamin A, serum | 20–80 mcg./100 ml. |
| Vitamin B₁₂, serum | 200–800 picogm./ml. |
| Vitamin C, blood | 0.4–1.5 mg./100 ml. |

## NORMAL URINE VALUES

| | |
|---|---|
| Acetone and acetoacetate | 0 |
| Addis count | |
|   Erythrocytes | 0–130,000/24 hrs. |
|   Leukocytes | 0–650,000/24 hrs. |
|   Casts (hyaline) | 0–2000/24 hrs. |
| Alcapton bodies | Negative |
| Aldosterone | 3–20 mcg./24 hrs. |
| Alpha amino nitrogen | 50–200 mg./24 hrs. |
| | (Not over 1.5% of total nitrogen) |
| Ammonia nitrogen | 20–70 mEq./24 hrs. |
| Amylase | 35–260 Somogyi units/hr. |
| Bence Jones protein | Negative |
| Bilirubin (bile) | Negative |
| Calcium | |
|   Low Ca diet (Bauer-Aub) | Less than 150 mg./24 hrs. |
|   Usual diet | Less than 250 mg./24 hrs. |
| Catecholamines | |
|   Epinephrine | Less than 10 mcg./24 hrs. |
|   Norepinephrine | Less than 100 mcg./24 hrs. |
| Chloride | 110–250 mEq./24 hrs. |
| | (Varies with intake) |
| Chorionic gonadotrophin | 0 |
| Copper | 0–30 mcg./24 hrs. |
| Creatine | |
|   Male | 0–40 mg./24 hrs. |
|   Female | 0–100 mg./24 hrs. |
| | (Higher in children and during |
| | pregnancy) |
| Creatinine | 15–25 mg./kg. of body weight/24 hrs. |
| Cystine or cysteine, qualitative | Negative |
| Delta aminolevulinic acid | 1.3–7.0 mg./24 hrs. |

Estrogens

| | Male | Female |
|---|---|---|
| Estrone | 3–8 | 4–31 |
| Estradiol | 0–6 | 0–14 |
| Estriol | 1–11 | 0–72 |
| Total | 4–25 | 5–100 |

(Units above are mcg./24 hours.)
(Markedly increased during pregnancy)

| | |
|---|---|
| Glucose (reducing substances) | Less than 250 mg./24 hrs. |
| Gonadotrophins, pituitary | 5–10 rat units/24 hrs. |
| | 10–50 mouse units/24 hrs. |
| | (Increased after menopause) |
| Hemoglobin and myoglobin | Negative |
| Homogentisic acid, qualitative | Negative |

| | |
|---|---|
| 17-Hydroxycorticosteroids | |
|   Male | 3–9 mg./24 hrs. |
|   Female | 2–8 mg./24 hrs. |
| | (Varies with method used) |
| 5-Hydroxyindole-acetic acid (5-HIAA) | |
|   Qualitative | Negative |
|   Quantitative | Less than 16 mg./24 hrs. |
| 17-Ketosteroids | |
|   Male | 6–18 mg./24 hrs. |
|   Female | 4–13 mg./24 hrs. |
| Osmolality | 38–1400 mOsm./kg. water |
| pH | 4.6–8.0, average 6.0 |
| | (Depends on diet) |
| Phenylpyruvic acid, qualitative | Negative |
| Phosphorus | 0.9–1.3 gm./24 hrs. |
| | (Varies with intake) |
| Porphobilinogen | |
|   Qualitative | Negative |
|   Quantitative | 0–0.2 mg./100 ml. |
| | Less than 2.0 mg./24 hrs. |
| Porphyrins | |
|   Coproporphyrin | 50–250 mcg./24 hrs. |
|   Uroporphyrin | 10–30 mcg./24 hrs. |
| Potassium | 25–100 mEq./24 hrs. |
| | (Varies with intake) |
| Pregnanetriol | Less than 2.5 mg./24 hrs. in adults |
| Protein | |
|   Qualitative | 0 |
|   Quantitative | 10–150 mg./24 hrs. |
| Sodium | 130–260 mEq./24 hrs. |
| | (Varies with intake) |
| Solids, total | 30–70 grams/liter, average |
| | 50 grams/liter |
| | (To estimate total solids per liter, |
| | multiply last two figures of specific |
| | gravity by 2.66, Long's coefficient) |
| Specific gravity | 1.003–1.030 |
| Sugar | 0 |
| Titratable acidity | 20–40 mEq./24 hrs. |
| Urobilinogen | Up to 1.0 Ehrlich unit/2 hrs. (1–3 P.M.) |
| | 0–4.0 mg./24 hrs. |
| Vanillylmandelic acid (VMA) | 1–8 mg./24 hrs. |

# NORMAL LABORATORY VALUES

## NORMAL VALUES FOR GASTRIC ANALYSIS

Basal gastric secretion (one hour)

| | Concentration<br>Mean ± 1 S.D. | Output<br>Mean ± 1 S.D. |
|---|---|---|
| Male | 25.8 ± 1.8 mEq./liter | 2.57 ± 0.16 mEq./hr. |
| Female | 20.3 ± 3.0 mEq./liter | 1.61 ± 0.18 mEq./hr. |

After histamine stimulation
- Normal    Mean output = 11.8 mEq./hr.
- Duodenal ulcer    Mean output = 15.2 mEq./hr.

After maximal histamine stimulation
- Normal    Mean output   22.6 mEq./hr.
- Duodenal ulcer    Mean output   44.6 mEq./hr.

| Diagnex blue (Squibb): | Anacidity | 0–0.3 mg. in 2 hrs. |
|---|---|---|
| | Doubtful | 0.3–0.6 mg. in 2 hrs. |
| | Normal | Greater than 0.6 mg. in 2 hrs. |
| Volume, fasting stomach content | | 50–100 ml. |
| Emptying time | | 3–6 hrs. |
| Color | | Opalescent or colorless |
| Specific gravity | | 1.006–1.009 |
| pH (adults) | | 0.9–1.5 |

## NORMAL VALUES FOR CEREBROSPINAL FLUID

| | |
|---|---|
| Cells | Fewer than 5 cu. mm., all mononuclear |
| Chloride | 120–130 mEq./liter<br>(20 mEq./liter higher than serum) |
| Colloidal gold test | Not more than 1 in any tube |
| Glucose | 50–75 mg./100 ml.<br>(20 mg./100 ml. less than blood) |
| Pressure | 70–180 mm. water |

| | |
|---|---|
| Protein, total | 15–45 mg./100 ml. |
| Albumin | 52% |
| Alpha$_1$ globulin | 5% |
| Alpha$_2$ globulin | 14% |
| Beta globulin | 10% |
| Gamma globulin | 19% |

## NORMAL VALUES FOR SEMEN

| | | | |
|---|---|---|---|
| Volume | 2–5 ml., usually 3–4 ml. | Count | 60–150 million/ml.<br>Below 60 million/ml. is abnormal |
| Liquefaction | Complete in 15 min. | Motility | 80% or more motile |
| pH | 7.2–8.0; average 7.8 | Morphology | 80–90% normal forms |
| Leukocytes | Occasional or absent | | |

## NORMAL VALUES FOR FECES

| | | | |
|---|---|---|---|
| Bulk | 100–200 grams/24 hrs. | Nitrogen, total | Less than 2.0 grams/24 hrs. |
| Dry matter | 23–32 grams/24 hrs. | Urobilinogen | 40–280 mg./24 hrs. |
| Fat, total | Less than 6.0 grams/24 hrs. | Water | Approximately 65% |

## NORMAL VALUES FOR SEROLOGIC PROCEDURES

| | |
|---|---|
| Anti-hyaluronidase | Less than 1:200. Significant if rising titer can be demonstrated at weekly intervals. |
| Anti-streptolysin O titer | Normal up to 1:128. Single test usually has little significance. Rise in titer or persistently elevated titer is significant. |
| Bacterial agglutinins | Significant only if rise in titer is demonstrated or if antibodies are absent. |
| Complement fixation tests | Titers of 1:8 or less are usually not significant. Paired sera showing rise in titer of more than two tubes are usually considered significant. |
| C reactive protein (CRP) | Negative |

| | | |
|---|---|---|
| Proteus OX-19 agglutinins | 1:80 | Negative |
| | 1:160 | Doubtful |
| | 1:320 | Positive |
| R. A. test (latex) | 1:40 | Negative |
| | 1:80 –1:160 | Doubtful |
| | 1:320 | Positive |
| Rose test | 1:10 | Negative |
| | 1:20 –1:40 | Doubtful |
| | 1:80 | Positive |
| Tularemia agglutinins | 1:80 | Negative |
| | 1:160 | Doubtful |
| | 1:320 | Positive |

Heterophile titer

| | Unabsorbed | Absorbed<br>With<br>G.P. | Absorbed<br>With<br>Beef |
|---|---|---|---|
| Normal | 1:160 | 1:10 | 1:160 |
| Inf. mono. | 1:160 | 1:320 | 1:10 |
| Serum sickness | 1:160 | 1:5 | 1:10 |

## TOXICOLOGY

| | |
|---|---|
| Arsenic, blood | 3.5–7.2 mcg./100 ml. |
| Arsenic, urine | Less than 100 mcg./24 hrs. |
| Barbiturates, serum | 0<br>Coma level: Phenobarbital approximately 11 mg./100 ml.; most other barbiturates 1.5 mg./100 ml. |
| Bromides, serum | 0<br>Toxic levels above 17 mEq./liter |
| Carbon monoxide, blood | Up to 5% saturation<br>Symptoms occur with 20% saturation |
| Dilantin, blood or serum | Therapeutic levels 1–11 mcg./ml. |

| | |
|---|---|
| Ethanol, blood | Less than 0.005% |
| Marked intoxication | 0.3–0.4% |
| Alcoholic stupor | 0.4–0.5% |
| Coma | Above 0.5% |
| Lead, blood | 0–40 mcg./100 ml. |
| Lead, urine | Less than 100 mcg./24 hrs. |
| Lithium, serum | 0<br>Therapeutic levels 0.5–1.5 mEq./liter<br>Toxic levels above 2 mEq./liter |
| Mercury, urine | Less than 10 mcg./24 hrs. |
| Salicylate, plasma | 0 |
| Therapeutic range | 20–25 mg./100 ml. |
| Toxic range | Over 30 mg./100 ml. |
| Death | 45–75 mg./100 ml. |

## LIVER FUNCTION TESTS

| | | | |
|---|---|---|---|
| Bromsulphalein (B.S.P.) | Less than 5% remaining in serum 45 minutes after injection of 5 mg./kg. of body weight | Hippuric acid | Excretion of 3.0–3.5 grams hippuric acid in urine within 4 hours after ingestion of 6.0 grams sodium benzoate, |
| Cephalin cholesterol flocculation | 0–1 in 24 hours. | | *or* |
| Galactose tolerance | Excretion of not more than 3.0 grams galactose in the urine 5 hours after ingestion of 40 grams of galactose. | | Excretion of 0.7 gram hippuric acid in urine within 1 hour after intravenous injection of 1.77 grams sodium benzoate. |
| Glycogen storage | Increase of blood glucose 45 mg./100 ml. over fasting level 45 minutes after subcutaneous injection of 0.01 mg./kg. body weight of epinephrine. | Thymol turbidity | 0–5 units. |
| | | Zinc turbidity | 2–12 units. |

## PANCREATIC (ISLET) FUNCTION TESTS

**Glucose tolerance tests**

**Oral** — Patient should be on a diet containing 300 grams of carbohydrate per day for 3 days prior to test. After ingestion of 100 grams of glucose or 1.75 grams glucose/kg. body weight, blood glucose is not more than 160 mg./100 ml. after 60 minutes, 140 mg./100 ml. after 90 minutes, and 120 mg./100 ml. after 120 minutes. Values are for blood; serum measurements are approximately 15% higher.

**Intravenous** — Blood glucose does not exceed 200 mg./100 ml. after infusion of 0.5 gram of glucose/kg. body weight over 30 minutes. Glucose concentration falls below initial level at 2 hours and returns to preinfusion levels in 3 hours or 1 hour. Values are for blood; serum measurements are approximately 15% higher.

**Cortisone-glucose tolerance test** — The patient should be on a diet containing 300 grams of carbohydrate per day for 3 days prior to test. At 8½ and again 2 hours prior to glucose load patient is given cortisone acetate by mouth (50 mg. if patient's ideal weight is less than 160 lb., 62.5 mg. if ideal weight is greater than 160 lb.). An oral dose of glucose 1.75 grams/kg. body weight, is given and blood samples are taken at 0, 30, 60, 90, and 120 minutes. Test is considered positive if true blood glucose exceeds 160 mg./100 ml. at 60 minutes, 140 mg./100 ml. at 90 minutes, and 120 mg./100 ml. at 120 minutes. Values are for blood; serum measurements are approximately 15% higher.

## RENAL FUNCTION TESTS

Clearance tests (corrected to 1.73 sq. meters body surface area)

Glomerular filtration rate (G.F.R.)
Inulin clearance,
Mannitol clearance, or
Endogenous creatinine clearance

| | |
|---|---|
| Males | 110–150 ml./min. |
| Females | 105–132 ml./min. |

Renal plasma flow (R.P.F.)
p-Aminohippurate (P.A.H.), or
Diodrast

| | |
|---|---|
| Males | 560–830 ml./min. |
| Females | 490–700 ml./min. |

Filtration fraction (F.F.)

$$FF = \frac{G.F.R.}{R.P.F.}$$

| | |
|---|---|
| Males | 17–21% |
| Females | 17–23% |

Urea clearance ($C_u$)

| | |
|---|---|
| Standard | 40–65 ml./min. |
| Maximal | 60–100 ml./min. |

Concentration and dilution — Specific gravity > 1.025 on dry day; Specific gravity < 1.003 on water day

Maximal Diodrast excretory capacity $T_{M_D}$ — Males 43–59 mg./min.; Females 33–51 mg./min.

Maximal glucose reabsorptive capacity $T_{M_G}$ — Males 300–450 mg./min.; Females 250–350 mg./min.

Maximal PAH excretory capacity $T_{M_{PAH}}$ — 80–90 mg./min.

Phenolsulfonphthalein excretion (P.S.P.) — 25% or more in 15 min.; 40% or more in 30 min.; 55% or more in 2 hrs. After injection of 1 ml. P.S.P. intravenously

## THYROID FUNCTION TESTS

| | |
|---|---|
| Protein bound iodine, serum (P.B.I.) | 3.5–8.0 mcg./100 ml. |
| Butanol extractable iodine, serum (B.E.I.) | 3.2–6.4 mcg./100 ml. |
| Thyroxine iodine, serum ($T_4$) | 2.9–6.4 mcg./100 ml. |
| Free thyroxine, serum | 1.4–2.5 nanogram/100 ml. |
| $T_3$ (index of unsaturated T.B.G.) | 10.0–14.6% |
| Thyroxine-binding globulin, serum (T.B.G.) | 10–26 mcg. $T_4$/100 ml. |
| Thyroid-stimulating hormone, serum (T.S.H.) | 0 up to 0.2 milliunits/ml. |
| Radioactive iodine ($I^{131}$) uptake (R.A.I.) | 20–50% of administered dose in 24 hrs. |
| Radioactive iodine ($I^{131}$) excretion | 30–70% of administered dose in 24 hrs. |
| Radioactive iodine ($I^{131}$), protein bound | Less than 0.3% of administered dose per liter of plasma at 72 hrs. |
| Basal metabolic rate | Minus 10% to plus 10% of mean standard |

## GASTROINTESTINAL ABSORPTION TESTS

**d-Xylose absorption test** — After an 8 hour fast 10 ml./kg. body weight of a 5% solution of d-xylose is given by mouth. Nothing further by mouth is given until the test has been completed. All urine voided during the following 5 hours is pooled, and blood samples are taken at 0, 60, and 120 minutes. Normally 26% (range 16–33%) of ingested xylose is excreted within 5 hours, and the serum xylose reaches a level between 25 and 40 mg./100 ml. after 1 hour and is maintained at this level for another 60 minutes.

**Vitamin A absorption test** — A fasting blood specimen is obtained and 200,000 units of vitamin A in oil is given by mouth. Serum vitamin A level should rise to twice fasting level in 3 to 5 hours.

---

### REFERENCES

Castleman, B., and McNeely, B. U.: New Eng. J. Med., 283:1276, 1970.
Davidsohn, I., and Henry, J. B.: Clinical Diagnosis by Laboratory Methods. 14th ed. Philadelphia, W. B. Saunders Company, 1969.
Department of Laboratory Medicine, The Johns Hopkins Hospital: Clinical Laboratory Handbook. Baltimore, July 1, 1971.
Henry, R. J.: Clinical Chemistry – Principles and Techniques. New York, Harper & Row, 1964.
Long, C.: Biochemists' Handbook. Princeton, D. Van Nostrand Company, 1961.
Miale, J. B.: Laboratory Medicine – Hematology. 3rd ed. St. Louis, C. V. Mosby Company, 1967.
Miller, S. E., and Weller, J. M.: Textbook of Clinical Pathology. 8th ed. Baltimore, Williams and Wilkins Company, 1971.
Stewart, C. P., and Stolman, A.: Toxicology, Mechanisms and Analytic Methods. New York, Academic Press, 1960.
Sunderman, F. W., and Boerner, F.: Normal Values in Clinical Medicine. Philadelphia, W. B. Saunders Company, 1949.
Tietz, N. W.: Fundamentals of Clinical Chemistry. Philadelphia, W. B. Saunders Company, 1970.
Wintrobe, M. M.: Clinical Hematology. 6th ed. Philadelphia, Lea & Febiger, 1967.

# INDEX

# INDEX

*So essential did I consider an index to be to every book, that I proposed to bring a bill into Parliament to deprive an author who publishes a book without an index of the privilege of copyright, and, moreover to subject him for his offence to a pecuniary penalty.*

—LORD CAMPBELL, *Lives of the Chief Justices*

VOLUME I — PAGES 1–1002
VOLUME II — PAGES 1003–2135

Page numbers in *italics* indicate illustrations; page numbers followed by (t) indicate tables.